W9-CEI-327

Rockwood and Green's

Fractures in Adults

FOURTH EDITION

Rockwood and Green's

Fractures in Adults

Volume 1

EDITED BY

Charles A. Rockwood, Jr., MD
Professor and Chairman Emeritus
Department of Orthopaedics
The University of Texas
Health Science Center at San Antonio
San Antonio, Texas

Robert W. Bucholz, MD
Professor and Chairman
Department of Orthopaedic Surgery
The University of Texas Southwestern
Medical Center
Dallas, Texas

David P. Green, MD
Clinical Professor
Department of Orthopaedics
Former Chief, Hand Surgery Service
The University of Texas
Health Science Center at San Antonio
San Antonio, Texas

James D. Heckman, MD
Professor and Chairman
Department of Orthopaedics
The University of Texas
Health Science Center at San Antonio
San Antonio, Texas

With 58 Contributors

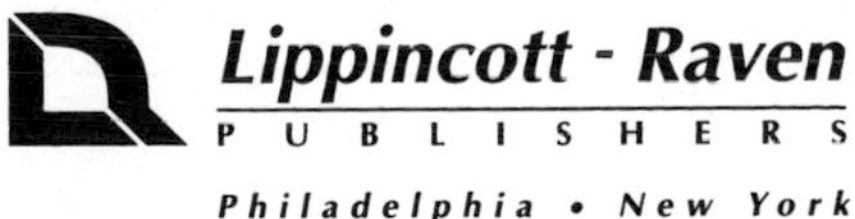

Philadelphia • New York

Acquisitions Editor: James Ryan
Associate Editor: Delois Patterson
Project Editor: Bridget Hannon Meyer
Production Manager: Caren Erlichman
Production Coordinator: David Yurkovich
Design Coordinator: Doug Smock
Indexer: Ann Cassar
Compositor: Tapsco, Incorporated
Printer/Binder: Quebecor/Kingsport

Copyright © 1996, by Lippincott-Raven Publishers.
Copyright © 1991, 1984, 1975 by J. B. Lippincott Company. All rights reserved. This book is protected by copyright. No part of it may be reproduced, stored in a retrieval system, or transmitted, in any form or by any means—electronic, mechanical, photocopy, recording, or otherwise—without the prior written permission of the publisher, except for brief quotations embodied in critical articles and reviews. Printed in the United States of America. For information write Lippincott–Raven Publishers, 227 East Washington Square, Philadelphia, PA 19106.

Library of Congress Cataloging-in-Publication Data

Rockwood and green's fractures in adults/edited by Charles A. Rockwood, Jr. . . . [et al.] with 58 contributors.—4th ed.
p. cm.
Vol. 3 published separately as: Fractures in children/edited by Charles A. Rockwood, Jr., Kaye E. Wilkins, James H. Beaty.
ISBN 0-397-51509-X (3 vol. set: alk. paper).—ISBN 0-397-51602-9 (2 vol. set: alk. paper).—ISBN 0-397-51510-3 (v. 1: alk. paper).—ISBN 0-397-51511-1 (v. 2: alk. paper).
1. Fractures. 2. Dislocations. I. Rockwood, Charles A., 1936-. II. Green, David P. III. Fractures in children.
[DNLM: 1. Fractures. 2. Dislocations. WE 175 R684 1996]
RD101.F739 1996
617.1′5—dc20
DNLM/DLC
for Library of Congress 95-38992
CIP

The material contained in this volume was submitted as previously unpublished material, except in the instances in which credit has been given to the source from which some of the illustrative material was derived.

Great care has been taken to maintain the accuracy of the information contained in the volume. However, neither Lippincott–Raven Publishers nor the editors can be held responsible for errors or for any consequences arising from the use of the information herein.

The authors and publisher have exerted every effort to ensure that drug selection and dosage set forth in this text are in accord with current recommendations and practice at the time of publication. However, in view of ongoing research, changes in government regulation, and the constant flow of information relating to drug therapy and drug reactions, the reader is urged to check the package insert for each drug for any change in indications and dosage and for added warnings and precautions. This is particularly important when the recommended agent is a new or infrequently employed drug.

Materials appearing in this book prepared by individuals as part of their official duties as U.S. Government employees are not covered by the above-mentioned copyright.

9 8 7 6 5 4 3 2 1

WE
175
R684
1996
V.1

DEDICATION

To the past, present, and future students, residents, and fellows of the wonderful specialty of orthopaedics.

3 0001 00344 0015
33206804

Contributor List

Daniel R. Benson, MD
Professor
Department of Orthopaedics
University of California, Davis;
Chief, Spine Surgery
University of California, Davis, Medical Center
Sacramento, California

Louis U. Bigliani, MD
Professor of Orthopaedic Surgery
College of Physicians and Surgeons
Columbia University;
Chief, The Shoulder Services
New York Orthopaedic Hospital
Columbia-Presbyterian Medical Center
New York, New York

Mark E. Bolander, MD
Consultant in Orthopaedic Surgery
Mayo Clinic;
Professor of Orthopaedics
Mayo Medical School
Rochester, Minnesota

Michael J. Bolesta, MD
Assistant Professor of Orthopaedic Surgery
The University of Texas Southwestern Medical Center
Dallas, Texas

Robert J. Brumback, MD
Associate Professor
Department of Surgery
Division of Orthopaedics
University of Maryland School of Medicine
Baltimore, Maryland

Robert W. Bucholz, MD
Professor and Chairman
Department of Orthopaedic Surgery
The University of Texas Southwestern Medical School
Dallas, Texas

Joseph A. Buckwalter, MD
Professor of Orthopaedics
University of Iowa Hospitals
Iowa City, Iowa

Andrew R. Burgess, MD
Assistant Professor of Surgery
Division of Orthopaedics
University of Maryland School of Medicine;
Associate Professor of Orthopaedic Surgery
Department of Surgery
The Johns Hopkins University;
Chief, Orthopaedic Traumatology
R Adams Cowley Shock Trauma Center
University of Maryland Medical Center
Baltimore, Maryland

Thomas E. Butler, Jr, MD
Hand Surgeon
Tuscon Orthopaedic Institute
Tuscon, Arizona

Kenneth P. Butters, MD
Clinical Instructor
University of Oregon Health Science University
Eugene, Oregon

Robert Chandler, MD
Associate Clinical Professor
Department of Orthopaedic Surgery
University of Southern California School of Medicine
Los Angeles, California;
Assistant Clinical Professor
University of California, Irvine
Irvine, California

Michael W. Chapman, MD
Professor and Chair
Department of Orthopaedics
University of California, Davis;
Chief, Department of Orthopaedic Surgery
University of California, Davis, Medical Center
Sacramento, California

William P. Cooney III, MD
Professor
Department of Orthopaedic Surgery
Mayo Medical School
Rochester, Minnesota

Fred G. Corley, Jr., MD
Associate Professor
Department of Orthopaedics
The University of Texas Health Science Center
San Antonio, Texas

Edward V. Craig, MD
Professor of Clinical Surgery (Orthopaedics)
Cornell University Medical College
New York, New York

Richard L. Cruess, MD
Dean, Faculty of Medicine
Professor of Surgery
McGill University
Montreal, Quebec

Jesse C. DeLee, MD
Associate Clinical Professor
The University of Texas Health Science Center
San Antonio, Texas

James H. Dobyns, MD
Professor (Emeritus) of Orthopaedic Surgery
Mayo Medical School
Rochester, Minnesota;
Consultant Associate
The Hand Center of San Antonio
San Antonio, Texas

Thomas A. Einhorn, MD
Professor of Orthopaedics
Mount Sinai School of Medicine
New York, New York

C. McCollister Evarts, MD
Senior Vice President for Health Affairs;
Dean, College of Medicine;
Professor of Orthopaedics
Pennsylvania State University,
Hershey Medical Center
Hershey, Pennsylvania

Evan L. Flatow, MD
Herbert Irving Associate Professor of Orthopaedic Surgery
Associate Chief, The Shoulder Service
New York Orthopaedic Hospital
Columbia-Presbyterian Medical Center
New York, New York

William B. Geissler, MD
Associate Professor
University of Mississippi Medical Center;
Associate Professor
Department of Orthopaedic Surgery
Hand/Upper Extremity Surgery,
Sports Medicine, Arthroscopic Surgery
Jackson, Mississippi

David P. Green, MD
Clinical Professor
Department of Orthopaedics
University of Texas Health Science Center;
President and Fellowship Director
The Hand Center of San Antonio
San Antonio, Texas

James W. Harkess, MD
Assistant Professor of Orthopaedic Surgery
University of Tennesse
Memphis, Tennessee

James W. Harkess, MD
Clinical Professor of Orthopaedic Surgery
University of Louisville School of Medicine
Louisville, Kentucky

James D. Heckman, MD
Chairman
Department of Orthopaedics
The University of Texas Health Science Center
San Antonio, Texas

Robert N. Hotchkiss, MD
Assistant Professor of Surgery (Orthopaedics)
Cornell University Medical College;
Chief of Hand Service
The Hospital for Special Surgery
New York, New York

James Langston Hughes, MD
Professor
University of Mississippi School of Medicine;
Chairman
Department of Orthopaedic Surgery
University of Mississippi Medical Center
Jackson, Mississippi

John N. Insall, MD
Director
Insall Scott Kelly Institute for Orthopaedics and Sports Medicine
New York, New York

L. Candace Jennings, MD
Instructor in Orthopaedic Surgery
Harvard Medical School
Boston, Massachusetts

Eric E. Johnson, MD
Professor of Orthopaedic Surgery;
Chief Orthopaedic Trauma Service
University of California School of Medicine
Los Angeles, California

Alan L. Jones, MD
Assistant Professor
The University of Texas Southwestern Medical Center
Dallas, Texas

Kenneth J. Koval, MD
Chief, Fracture Service
Department of Orthopaedics
Hospital for Joint Disease
New York, New York

Ronald L. Linscheid, MD
Professor of Orthopaedic Surgery
Mayo Medical School;
Consultant in Orthopaedic Surgery and Surgery of the Hand
Mayo Clinic
Rochester, Minnesota

Jay D. Mabrey, MD
Assistant Professor
Department of Orthopaedics
The University of Texas Health Science Center
San Antonio, Texas

Michael MacMillan, MD
Associate Professor
Department of Orthopaedics
University of Florida;
Associate Professor
Shands Hospital at University of Florida
Gainesville, Florida

Pasquale X. Montesano, MD
Private Practice
Orthopaedic Surgery, Spine
Carmichael, California

James V. Nepola, MD
Professor
Department of Orthopaedics
University of Iowa College of Medicine
Iowa City, Iowa

Steven A. Olsen, MD
Assistant Professor
Department of Orthopaedics;
Co-Director of Trauma
University of California, Davis
Sacramento, California

William C. Pederson, MD
Clinical Associate Professor of Surgery and Orthopaedic Surgery
The University of Texas Health Science Center
San Antonio, Texas

Vincent D. Pellegrini, Jr., MD
Michael and Myrtle Baker Professor and Chair
Department of Orthopaedics
Pennsylvania State University College of Medicine
Hershey, Pennsylvania

Roger G. Pollack, MD
Assistant Professor of Orthopaedic Surgery
Columbia University
New York, New York

William C. Ramsey, MD
Clinical Instructor
Orthopaedic Surgery
University of Louisville
Louisville, Kentucky

J. Spence Reid, MD
Assistant Professor
Department of Orthopaedics and Rehabilitation
Pennsylvania State University College of Medicine
Hershey, Pennsylvania

Robin R. Richards, MD
Associate Professor
Division of Orthopaedic Surgery
Department of Surgery
University of Toronto;
Head, Division of Orthopaedic Surgery
St. Michaels Hospital
Toronto, Ontario

Charles A. Rockwood, Jr, MD
Professor and Chairman Emeritus
Department of Orthopaedics
The University of Texas Health Science Center
San Antonio, Texas

Thomas A. Russell, MD
Associate Professor of Orthopaedic Surgery
University of Tennessee
Memphis, Tennessee

William E. Sanders, MD
Clinical Associate Professor of Orthopaedics
Department of Orthopaedics
The University of Texas Health Science Center
San Antonio, Texas

W. Norman Scott, MD
Director, Insall Scott Kelly Institute for Orthopaedics and Sports Medicine;
Chief, Division of Orthopaedics
Beth Israel Hospital North
New York, New York

Giles R. Scuderi, MD
Director
Insall Scott Kelly Institute for Orthopaedics and Sports Medicine;
Attending Orthopaedic Surgeon
Beth Israel Medical Center North Division
New York, New York

Dempsey Springfield, MD
Associate Professor in Orthopaedic Surgery
Harvard Medical School
Boston, Massachusetts

E. Shannon Stauffer, MD
Professor and Chairman
Division of Orthopaedics and Rehabilitation
Southern Illinois University School of Medicine;
Medical Director Spinal Injury Center
Memorial Medical Center
Springfield, Illinois

Marc F. Swiontkowski, MD
Professor
Department of Orthopaedics
University of Washington;
Chief of Orthopaedics
Harborview Medical Center
Seattle, Washington

Marvin Tile, MD
Professor of Surgery
University of Toronto;
Surgeon-in-Chief
Sunnybrook Health Science Center
Toronto, Ontario

Audrey K. Tsao, MD
Associate Professor
University of Mississippi Medical Center;
Associate Professor
University Hospitals and Clinics
Jackson, Mississippi

Robert G. Viere, MD
Assistant Professor of Orthopaedic Surgery
The University of Texas Southwestern Medical Center;
Chief, Spinal Cord Injury Service
Department of Veterans Affairs
VA Medical Center
Dallas, Texas

J. Tracy Watson, MD
Senior Staff
Henry Ford Hospital
Detroit, Michigan

Gerald R. Williams, Jr, MD
Assistant Professor of Orthopaedic Surgery
Director, Shoulder Study Group
Hospital of the University of Pennsylvania
Philadelphia, Pennsylvania

Michael A. Wirth, MD
Assistant Professor
Department of Orthopaedics
The University of Texas Health Science Center
San Antonio, Texas

Donald A. Wiss, MD
Southern California Orthopaedic Institute
Van Nuys, California

D. Christopher Young, MD
Orthopaedic Surgeon
West End Orthopaedic Clinic
Richmond, Virginia

Joseph D. Zuckerman, MD
Chairman
Department of Orthopaedic Surgery
Surgeon-in-Chief
Hospital for Joint Disease Orthopaedic Institute;
Associate Professor of Orthopaedic Surgery
New York University School of Medicine
New York, New York

Preface

"Old editors never die. . .they just get tired." Nearly 25 years ago we set out to compile a comprehensive reference source on musculoskeletal injuries for orthopaedic surgeons and residents. The ride has been exhilarating and not unlike a roller coaster—the highs coming from the intense gratification we've enjoyed from the widespread acceptance of this book, and the lows from those dark moments when innumerable problems plagued various stages in the preparation, delivery, and ultimate publication of this text. The changes in fracture care over that span of time have been truly phenomenal, far exceeding our ability to edit by ourselves this vast body of knowledge, with its many pockets of specialized information and techniques. For this reason, we have added new editors who have been responsible for substantial portions of this 4th edition and who will bear increasingly more of the editorial load for future editions. By helping us select new authors and by contributing their expertise and editorial skills, Drs. Bucholz, Heckman, and Beaty have raised the quality of the book to a higher level.

Aside from including a huge amount of new information, this edition has a major change in format from previous editions. When we published the first edition in 1975, we specifically intended to exclude details of operative technique, in part because these were so well covered at that time in Campbell's Operative Orthopaedics. However, operative intervention has assumed a far greater role in the management of many fractures, and we now believe that our original goal of providing a *comprehensive* fracture text cannot be achieved without including precise descriptions of each author's "procedures of choice." We have *not* changed our original focus—the emphasis is still upon providing the reader with whatever information he or she needs to make the best possible educated decision about how to treat any given injury. It is *in addition* to those basic principles and knowing more than one way to treat a fracture that we have included in this edition detailed descriptions and illustrations of operative techniques.

Charles A. Rockwood, Jr., MD
David P. Green, MD
Kaye E. Wilkins, M.D.

Preface to the First Edition

Orthopaedists agree on the need for a comprehensive, up-to-date reference book on fractures. Texts that once filled this role are now either out of date or unavailable. Since the most recent of those books was published—a short span of some 14 years—significant advances have been made in the recognition and management of bone and joint injuries. For example, improved methods of external and internal fixation have been devised, a more sophisticated appreciation of the ligamentous anatomy of the knee has led to improved operative repair of damaged structures, and innovative thinking in regard to the management of spine injuries has revolutionized the management of patients with spinal cord injuries.

One cannot properly discuss fractures and exclude dislocations and ligamentous injuries and, indeed, our intent has been to cover the entire range of bone and joint injuries in adults.

We recognize that much controversy exists in the treatment of musculoskeletal injuries and that there may be several "correct" methods of treating any given injury. Realizing this, our goals in this book are (1) to present the historical background, diagnosis and pathological anatomy of virtually every bone and joint injury the orthopaedist is called upon to treat; (2) to offer a thorough discussion of the various alternative methods of treating each injury, discussing, when pertinent, the relative advantages and disadvantages of each; (3) to allow each author, chosen for his recognized competence in the management of the injuries about which he is writing, to present the methods he has come to prefer; and (4) to provide a comprehensive list of references at the end of each chapter, in order to give the reader as complete a compilation as possible of valuable sources for further study. It is our hope that we have succeeded.

Charles A. Rockwood, Jr., M.D.
David P. Green, M.D.

Contents

VOLUME I

General Principles 1

Upper Extremity **605**

VOLUME II

Rockwood and Green's

Fractures in Adults

Volume 1

General Principles

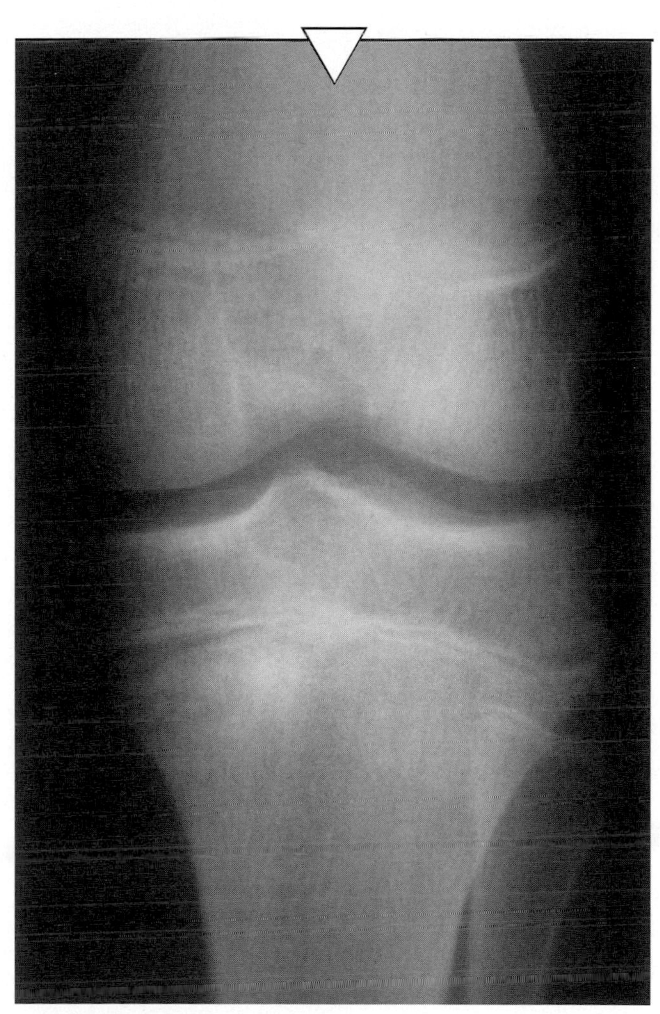

Rockwood and Green's Fractures in Adults, Fourth Edition,
edited by Charles A. Rockwood, David P. Green, Robert W. Bucholz and James D. Heckman.
Lippincott-Raven Publishers, Philadelphia © 1996.

CHAPTER 1

Principles of Fractures and Dislocations

James W. Harkess, William C. Ramsey, and James W. Harkess

DESCRIPTION OF FRACTURES

Fractures may be categorized in several ways: (1) by anatomical location (proximal, middle, or distal third of the shaft; supracondylar; subtrochanteric); (2) by the direction of the fracture line (transverse, oblique, spiral); and (3) by whether the fracture is linear or comminuted (ie, with multiple extensions, giving rise to many small fragments). Greenstick fractures, so common in children, are rarely found in adults, but occasionally an incomplete fracture or infraction may be seen. When the shaft of a long bone is driven into its cancellous extremity, it is said to be *impacted.* This is common in fractures of the upper humerus, but we believe that the so-called impacted fracture of the femoral neck is really a misnomer for an incomplete or partial fracture.

Fractures are termed *open* when the overlying soft tissues have been breached, exposing the fracture to the external environment, or *closed* when the skin is still intact. The archaic terms *compound* and *simple* have nothing to recommend them and should be dropped.

Although most fractures occur as the result of a single episode by a force powerful enough to fracture normal bone, there are two types of fractures in which this is not so: pathologic and stress fractures.

Pathologic Fractures

A *pathologic fracture* is one in which a bone is broken through an area weakened by preexisting disease, by a degree of stress that would have left a normal bone intact. Osteoporosis, from whatever cause, may be a source of pathologic fracture and is one of the important factors implicated in the high incidence of fractures in the elderly. Although fractures through any type of lesion may reasonably be called pathologic, sometimes the term is used in a more restricted sense to denote a fracture through a malignant lesion, such as an osseous metastasis or a primary tumor (eg, myeloma). Pentecost and associates[308] have suggested the term *insufficiency fracture* for those fractures occurring in bones affected with nontumorous disease.

Stress Fractures

Bone, like other materials, reacts to repeated loading. On occasion, it becomes fatigued and a crack develops, which may lead to a complete fracture—a *stress fracture.* These fractures are seen most frequently in military installations where recruits undergo rigorous training. However, they are sometimes found in ballet dancers and athletes, and no age group or occupation is immune.[126,127,160] Baker and associates[24] suggested that stress fractures occur only after muscle fatigue, and the absence of functioning muscles allows abnormal stress concentration with subsequent failure of the bone.

BIOMECHANICS OF FRACTURES

Biomechanics, for many persons, is an inherently dry subject, but an understanding of some principles is necessary to treat fractures rationally. What follows constitutes an elementary review of the subject, which we hope will serve as an introduction for the uninitiated. Whether a bone fractures under stress depends on both extrinsic and intrinsic factors.

Extrinsic Factors

The extrinsic factors important in the production of fractures are the magnitude, duration, and direction of the forces acting on the bone, as well as the rate at which the bone is loaded.[149,159]

For the purposes of subsequent discussion, it might be well to define some terms. A *force* is an action or influence, such as a push or pull, which, when applied to a free body, tends to accelerate or deform it (force = mass × acceleration). Forces having both magnitude and direction may be represented by vectors. A *load* is a force sustained by a body. If no acceleration results from the application of a load, it follows that a force of equal magnitude and opposite direction (ie, a reaction) opposes it (Newton's third law).

Stress may be defined as the internal resistance to deformation or the internal force generated within a substance as the result of the application of an external load. Stress is calculated by the formula

$$\text{Stress} = \frac{\text{Load}}{\text{Area on which the load acts}}$$

Stress cannot be measured directly. Both stress and force may be classified as tension, compression, or shear. *Tension* attempts to pull a substance or material apart; *compression* does the reverse. The stresses evoked by such forces resist the lengthening or squashing; because these stresses act at right angles to the plane under consideration, they are called *normal stresses.* A *shear stress* acts in a direction parallel to the plane being considered.

Stress is usually expressed as pounds per square inch (psi) or kilograms per square centimeter (kg/cm^2). However, purists point out that kilograms and pounds are measurements of mass and not force, so that the rather clumsy terms *pound force* and *kilogram force* have been introduced to differentiate force from mass. To further complicate matters, other units of force have

TABLE 1-1
Glossary

Dyne. That force that, if applied to 1 gram mass, gives it an acceleration of 1 cm per second per second (cm/s^2)

Poundal. That force that, if applied to 1 pound mass, gives it an acceleration of 1 foot per second per second (ft/s^2)

Newton. That force that, if applied to 1 kilogram mass, gives it an acceleration of 1 meter per second per second (m/s^2)

Kilopond (Kp). The force required to give 1 kilogram mass an acceleration of 9.80665 meters per second per second (9.8 m/s^2) or a force of 9.80665 newtons. "This force is equivalent to the weight of one kilogram mass under standard earth gravity; it represents the force with which this mass is attracted toward the center of the earth."

Hectobar. 1 Hectobar = 100 bars and 1 bar = 10^6 dynes/cm^2 or 10^5 pascals.

been created: dynes, poundals, newtons, kiloponds, and hectobars (Table 1-1).

Currently, stress is likely to be expressed in newtons (N) per square meter or in pascals (Pa) (1 pascal = 1 newton/m^2, 1 megapascal = 1 newton/mm^2, 1 gigapascal = 1 billion or 10^9 pascals).

Strain is defined as the change in linear dimensions of a body resulting from the application of a force or a load. *Tensile strain* and *compression strain* are, respectively, the increase or decrease in length per unit of the starting length and may be expressed as inches per inch, as centimeters per centimeter, or merely as a percentage of the starting length. Tensile and compressive strains are normal—that is, they act perpendicular to the cross section of the structure and are designated as ϵ (epsilon) (Fig. 1-1).

Shear strain has been defined as the relative movement of any two points perpendicular to the line joining them, expressed as a fraction of the length of that line, and it is produced when an external load is applied, producing an angular deformity (Fig. 1-2). This may be demonstrated by drawing a right angle on the surface of an object and noting the angular change after load. This angle is denoted γ (gamma), and shear strain is defined as tan γ. Because this is a small angle, it can be assumed that tan γ is equal to the angle measured in radians (360° = 2π radians or 1 radian = 57.3°).[280]

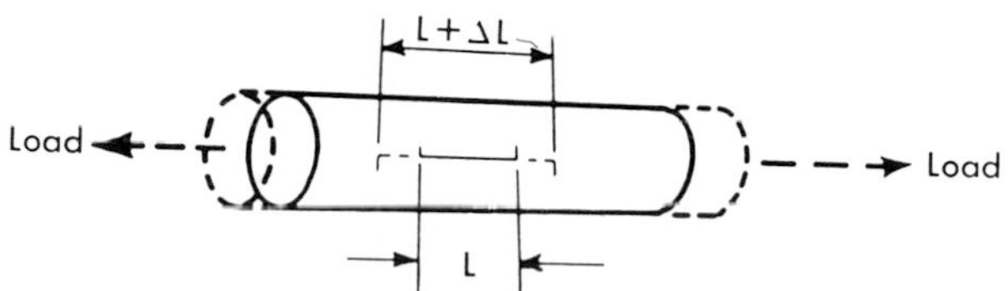

FIGURE 1-1. Normal strain. (*Murphy, E.F., and Burstein, A.H.: Physical Properties of Materials Including Solid Mechanics. In A.A.O.S. Atlas of Orthotics: Biomechanical Principles and Application, p. 7. St. Louis, C.V. Mosby, 1975.*)

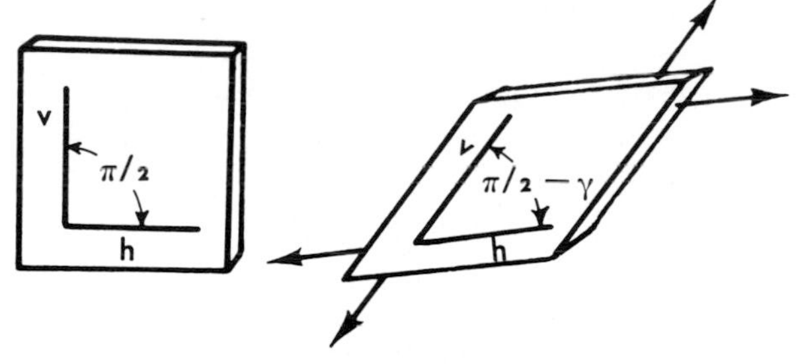

FIGURE 1-2. Shear strain. (*Murphy, E.F., and Burstein, A.H.: Physical Properties of Materials Including Solid Mechanics. In A.A.O.S. Atlas of Orthotics: Biomechanical Principles and Application, p. 7. St. Louis, C.V. Mosby, 1975.*)

Normal and shear strains are not mutually exclusive. Tension and compression strains are always associated with shear strains. If a square is drawn on the surface of an object that is then subjected to a compression load (Fig. 1-3), the consequent shortening of sides a and c has changed the angles of the diagonals, thus demonstrating shear strain. Similarly, Figure 1-4 demonstrates strain produced by an oblique load. The angles of the square have changed, indicating shear strain, but diagonal f is shortened and e is lengthened, indicating compressive and tensile strain. However, these diagonals still intersect each other at 90°, indicating that there is no shear strain in these directions.[280]

Intrinsic Factors

Gaynor Evans[149] listed the properties of bone that are important in determining its susceptibility to fracture as energy-absorbing capacity, modulus of elasticity (Young's modulus), fatigue strength, and density.

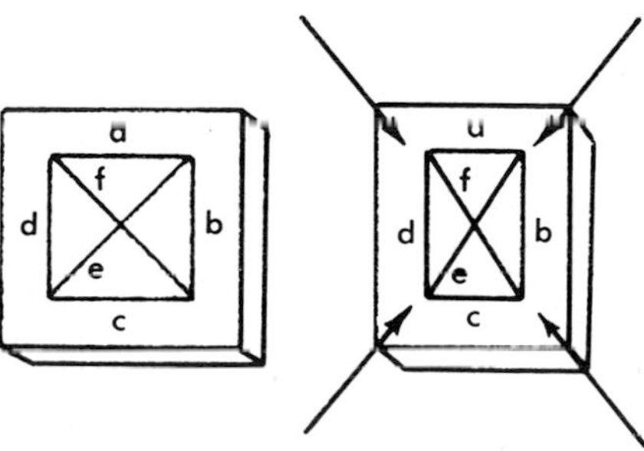

FIGURE 1-3. Compressive and shear strain. (*Murphy, E.F., and Burstein, A.H.: Physical Properties of Materials Including Solid Mechanics. In A.A.O.S. Atlas of Orthotics: Biomechanical Principles and Application, p. 7. St. Louis, C.V. Mosby, 1975.*)

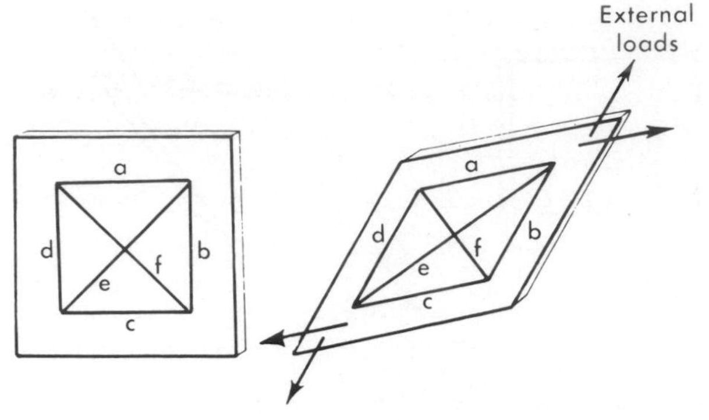

FIGURE 1-4. Shear, tensile, and compressive strains. (*Murphy, E.F., and Burstein, A.H.: Physical Properties of Materials Including Solid Mechanics. In A.A.O.S. Atlas of Orthotics: Biomechanical Principles and Application, p. 8. St. Louis, C.V. Mosby, 1975.*)

Energy-Absorbing Capacity

Energy is the capacity to do work, and work is the product of a force moving through a displacement (ie, work = force × distance). Work and energy are measured in foot pounds (ft lbs), kilogram centimeters (kg cm), or newton meters (Nm).

The unit of force in the Système International is the *newton (N),* which is the force required to give 1 kg mass an acceleration of 1 meter per second per second (m/s^2), and 1 kg force (kgf) is equal to 9.80665 N. One newton meter (Nm), which would be the unit of work or energy, has been named the *joule (J),* which is also the measure of energy represented by a current of 1 ampere at a voltage of 1 volt.

Strain energy is the energy a body is capable of absorbing by changing its shape under the application of an external load. The more rapidly a bone is loaded, the greater will be the energy absorption before failure. Thus, fractures associated with slow loading are generally linear, whereas rapid loading infuses enormous strain energy so that an explosion of the bone takes place at failure, giving rise to the severe comminution of high-energy fractures.

According to Frankel and Burstein,[159] the energy absorbed to produce failure of a femoral neck has been found experimentally to be 60 kg cm. However, in falls, kinetic energy far in excess of this level is produced. This energy—if it can be dissipated by muscle action, elastic and plastic strain of the soft tissues, and other mechanisms—will not produce a fracture. In old age, these mechanisms become progressively impaired, and this is a potent factor in the production of fractures in the elderly.

Young's Modulus and Stress-Strain Curves[52,149,159,400,414]

When a rubber band is stretched, once the deforming force is removed, the band will revert to its resting length; in other words, there has been a stretch deformation that is recoverable, and this is known as *elastic strain.* However, if greater stress is applied to the material, its power to recover may be exceeded, and it remains permanently deformed. This is known as *plastic strain.* Eventually, if the strain increases, a point will come when the material fails. This is known as the *break point.*

If a specimen of a substance is subjected to a tensile stress and the strain is measured, the stress may be compared to the strain by plotting a graph. Figure 1-5 shows such a stress–strain curve for mild steel.

It can be seen that the first portion of this curve is linear; the strain increases proportionately to the stress, until point b is reached. Point b, known as the *yield point* or *limit of proportionality,* denotes the end of the elastic region of the curve. If at any point along this gradient up to the point b the load is removed, the substance will regain its resting shape. The slope of this curve is a measure of the material's stiffness. The steeper the curve, the stiffer the material; the gradient is known as the *modulus of elasticity (E)* or *Young's modulus.*

The curve from point b to x (the break point where failure occurs) shows that strain increases much more rapidly with each increment of stress. This is the plastic region of the curve, where permanent strain or deformity has been produced in the material. If the load is removed at point c, there will be some recovery and the curve will parallel Young's modulus, but permanent deformity remains, represented by point e.

With the application of a load, a maximum stress will be achieved (point f). This is the *ultimate tensile strength* (UTS), the maximum stress the material can sustain before fracturing. Beyond this point, strain increases with diminished stress. This is because the ma-

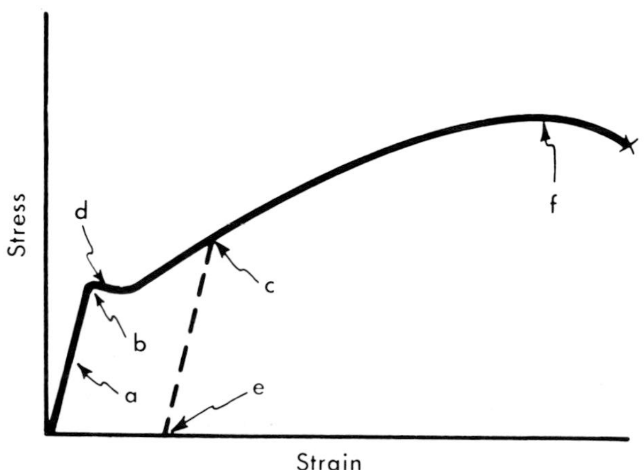

FIGURE 1-5. Effect of simple tension of mild steel. (*Murphy, E.F., and Burstein, A.H.: Physical Properties of Materials Including Solid Mechanics. In A.A.O.S. Atlas of Orthotics: Biomechanical Principles and Application, p. 11. St. Louis, C.V. Mosby, 1975.*)

terial "necks"; that is, the cross section diminishes, owing to shear strains at 45° to the long axis. A material that undergoes plastic deformity is said to be *ductile,* and those that fail soon after the yield point are *brittle.*

The amount of energy absorbed by the material is represented by the area under the curve. In a comparison between two types of steel (Fig. 1-6), one can see that the hard steel has a much higher yield point and UTS than the soft ("mild") steel, but it is much more brittle and its ability to absorb energy before failure is quite inferior; thus, the mild steel has greater "toughness." *Toughness* then is the amount of energy a material is able to absorb before failure and is measured in joules per cubic meter or foot pounds per cubic inch.

Fatigue Strength

When a material is subjected to repeated or cyclical stresses, it may fail, even though the magnitude of the individual stresses is much lower than the UTS of the material. This is known as *fatigue failure* (see Fig. 1-19**C**). In metal, the process starts as one or more cracks on the surface that gradually propagate until the cross-sectional area becomes so reduced that the metal fails by conventional overload mechanisms. The initial crack may start as a defect in the metal, a surface scratch, corrosion, or other stress riser. Once the crack has been initiated, it cannot be cured by resting. There is no self-healing mechanism in metals.

The fatigue strength of a metal may be illustrated by plotting the stress range against the number of cycles necessary to produce failure. From this curve the fatigue or endurance limit can be read. The *endurance limit* is the greatest repetitive stress for which the metal does not fail. Steel used in manufacturing orthopaedic

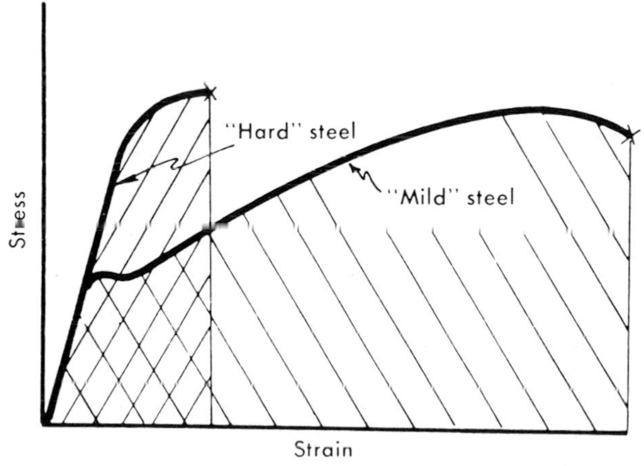

FIGURE 1-6. Stress–strain curve for steel. (*Murphy, E.F., and Burstein, A.H.: Physical Properties of Materials Including Solid Mechanics. In A.A.O.S. Atlas of Orthotics: Biomechanical Principles and Application, p. 12. St. Louis, C.V. Mosby, 1975.*)

implants may tolerate 1000 N/mm^2 for a single load but only half that amount when subjected to more than 100,000 cycles. Providing the stress level never rises above that of the endurance limit, a ferrous alloy can withstand an infinite number of cycles. This is not necessarily true of other metals, however, and aluminum alloys are particularly liable to fatigue. The endurance limit for a metal is between 30% and 50% of its yield strength, or about 0.4 times the UTS.

Biomechanical Properties of Bone

When compared with cast iron, bone is three times as light and ten times more flexible, but both materials have about the same tensile strength. Bone is a two-phase material consisting of matrix, which is mostly collagen, and bone mineral. Bone mineral (hydroxyapatite) is more rigid than bone with a modulus of 114 giganewtons/m^2 compared with 18 giganewtons/m^2 for bone (1 giganewton = 1 billion newtons) and is stronger in compression than in tension. Bone collagen, on the other hand, offers no resistance to compression but has a tensile strength five times that of bone. It would seem that this composite owes its tensile strength to its collagen and its rigidity and resistance to compression to its mineral content. Bone has a tensile strength of about 140 meganewtons/m^2 and a compression strength of 200 meganewtons/m^2.[3a]

The arrangement of apatite crystals closely packed, but in discrete units, may protect bone from crack propagation, because a crack traversing a crystal will meet an interface, thus forming a T-shaped crack that dissipates energy and prevents the crack from extending (Cook-Gordon mechanism). This is the same mechanism seen when the propagation of a crack in a wooden structure is halted when a hole is drilled at the advancing end of the crack. Furthermore, stiffness and static strength increase with the degree of mineralization of bone so that its ultimate strength is three times greater at 70% mineralization than at 60%.

A stress–strain curve for bone shows that it is ductile; but, being anisotropic (ie, having different mechanical properties when stressed in different directions), its tensile strength and Young's modulus are greater when bone is loaded in its longitudinal axis than in other directions. Bone has a "grain" or profound direction due to the longitudinal alignment of the haversian systems so that cortical bone withstands 17 gigapascals in a longitudinal direction and 12 gigapascals in a transverse direction.[415] Bone can be strained 0.75% before plastic deformity occurs, and the breaking strain is 2% to 4%. During plastic deformation it can absorb six times as much energy before fracture than during the elastic phase. As bone elongates, the cross section diminishes. This is known as the *poisson effect,* and Poisson's ratio, change in diameter over change in length $\delta d/\delta L$, varies from 0.28 to 0.45.[20]

However, bone is not a simple elastic substance as is mild steel. If one loads a spring, the deformation will be immediate, and no matter how long the load is applied for, there will be no change in the strain unless the load is altered. Bone is a viscoelastic material, and the addition of viscosity introduces a rate-dependent element to the effects of loading.

The simplest model of a viscoelastic material is the combination of a dashpot and spring in parallel (Fig. 1-7).[159] A dashpot is a device for cushioning or dampening a movement to prevent sudden shock and consists of a cylinder filled with air or fluid and a piston. When a load is applied to the piston, it will move at a rate proportional to the load as long as the force is applied or until there is no more fluid to be displaced. A hypodermic syringe has the same mechanics as a dashpot. Owing to the viscosity of the fluid, the velocity with which it flows through the needle is proportional to the pressure applied to it, and much greater force must be applied to the plunger to inject quickly than slowly. The greater the viscosity of the fluid, the longer it takes to empty. Viscoelastic materials behave differently at different load and strain rates; the elastic element determines the maximum deformity and the viscous component the time that will be taken to reach it.

The spring, because it conforms to Hooke's law, is known as a *hookean body*; the dashpot, as a *newtonian body*; and the combination, hooked up in parallel, as a *Kelvin body* (see Fig. 1-7). A hookean body and

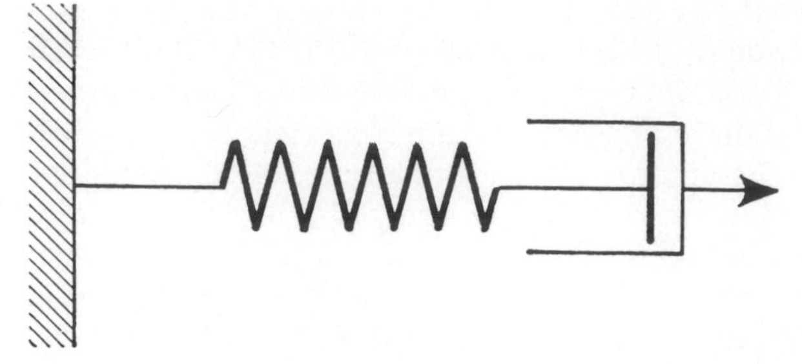

FIGURE 1-8. A series combination of a hookean body and a newtonian body is known as a Maxwell body. (*Frankel, V.H., and Burstein, A.H.: Orthopaedic Biomechanics, p. 105. Philadelphia, Lea & Febiger, 1970.*)

a newtonian body in series is called a *Maxwell body* (Fig. 1-8).

Energy is required to deform both hookean and newtonian bodies; however, whereas the energy is recoverable in the former when the load is removed (ie, when the spring regains its former length), this is not true of the dashpot. There is no tendency to restitution in the newtonian body, and the energy is lost.

Figure 1-9 shows the load-deformation curves for a Kelvin body produced by a constantly increasing load and increasing strain. The straight-line portion of both of these curves is equal to the spring constant. The first part of the curve on the left represents the immediate resistance of the newtonian element.

If the loading direction is reversed under conditions of a constant-loading rate, the load-deformation curve

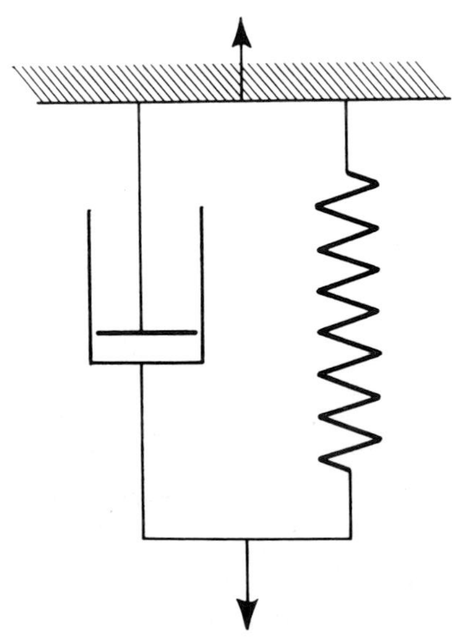

FIGURE 1-7. The Kelvin body is the parallel combination of a newtonian body and a hookean body. (*Frankel, V.H., and Burstein, A.H.: Orthopaedic Biomechanics, p. 102. Philadelphia, Lea & Febiger, 1970.*)

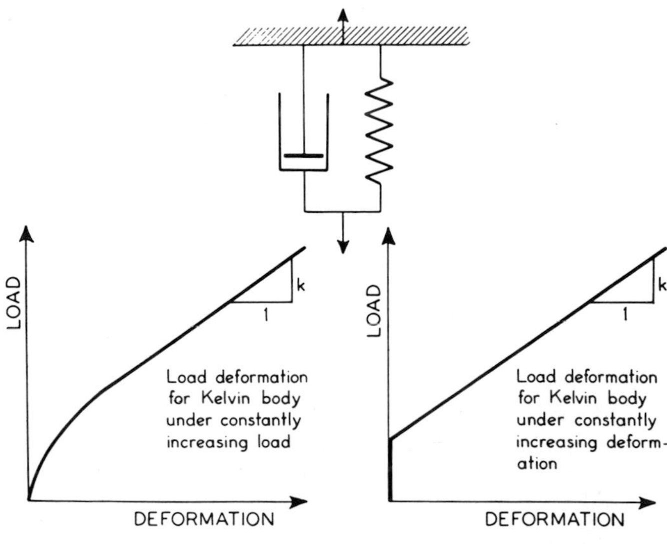

FIGURE 1-9. (*Left*) The load-deformation curve for a Kelvin body produced by a constantly increasing load. The curve is asymptotic to a line of slope k. (*Right*) Load-deformation characteristics for a Kelvin body under the application of a constant strain rate. (*Frankel, V.H., and Burstein, A.H.: Orthopaedic Biomechanics, p. 103. Philadelphia, Lea & Febiger, 1970.*)

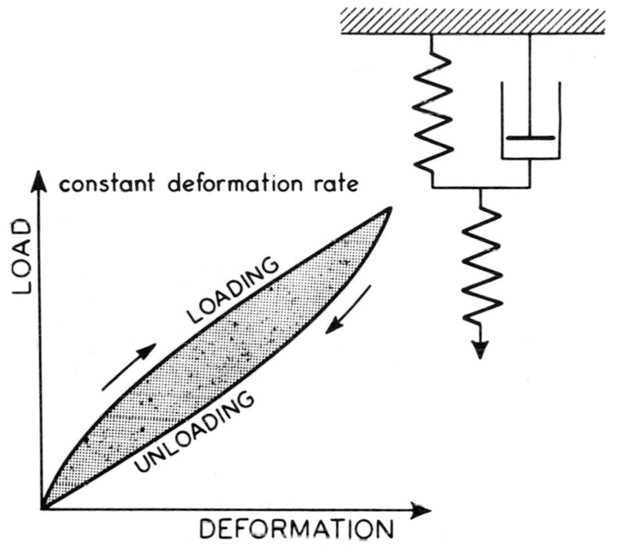

FIGURE 1-10. Loading–unloading curve for constant strain rate. The shaded area is a hysteresis loop and represents energy loss during the loading and unloading cycle. (*Frankel, V.H., and Burstein, A.H.: Orthopaedic Biomechanics, p. 104. Philadelphia, Lea & Febiger, 1970.*)

(Fig. 1-10) shows a *hysteresis loop*, the area of which corresponds to the energy loss.

Similar curves are shown for the Maxwell body in Figure 1-11. As can be seen, deflection continues to increase without increase in load after the resistance generated by the hookean body is taken up (see Fig. 1-11). It is also evident that, unless the loading procedure is reversed, the model cannot return to its original dimensions.

Various rheologic models for bone have been suggested by Sedlin, Piekarski, and Currey (Fig. 1-12).[108a,317,376]

Because bone is a viscoelastic material, the rate of application of stress is a major factor in determining the degree of damage to both bone and soft tissues when fractures occur. The higher the loading speed, the greater the bone's ability to absorb energy; however, if the loading is carried to failure, the greatly enhanced amount of energy, when dissipated, wreaks havoc with the bone. Low-energy fractures are generally linear without much displacement, but with increasing amounts of energy the comminution and displacement of the fractures will increase, as will the damage to the soft-tissue components of the extremity.

Fatigue (Stress) Fractures

Just as metal subjected to repeated stresses will fail, so will bone. Fatigue fractures are most commonly seen in military installations where recruits, unaccustomed to vigorous activity, are exercised. Such fractures are also seen in highly trained athletes, ballet dancers, and even greyhounds. Frankel and Burstein[159] believe that a key factor in stress fractures is muscle fatigue, which leads to abnormal loading of the bones. Normally, muscles allow the body to shunt stress from the bones. This stress shielding is lost when the muscle action is no longer optimal.[126,127,211,270] It is likely that this is also a factor in stress fractures in the elderly.

Carter and Hayes[77] examined specimens of cortical bone that were fractured by a single flexural loading and compared them with flexural fatigue specimens. The pattern of fracture was similar in both groups: a transverse fracture formed on the tension side and an oblique fracture formed on the compression side. However, the oblique fracture surface was much

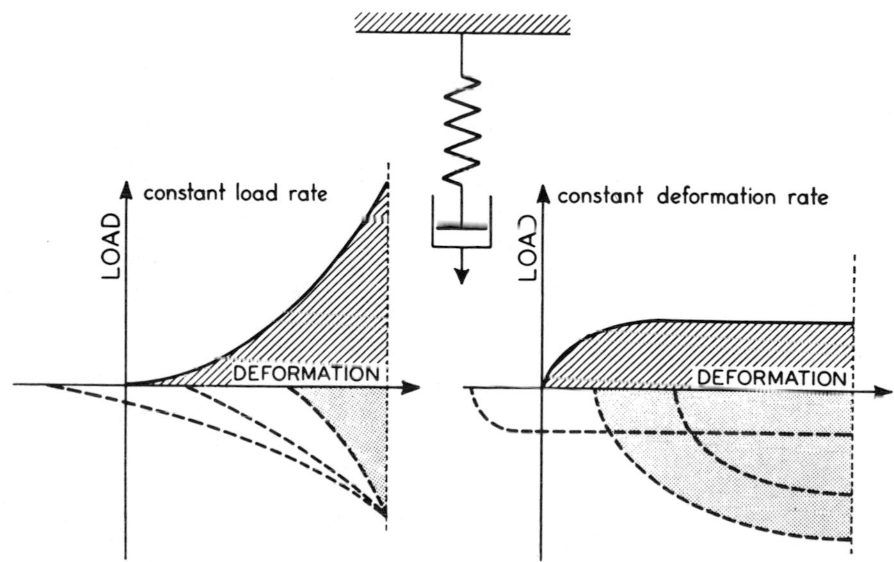

FIGURE 1-11. (*Left*) The load deformation characteristics for a Maxwell body under a constantly increasing load. (*Right*) The load-to-deformation characteristics for a Maxwell body under constantly increasing deformation. (*Frankel, V.H., and Burstein, A.H.: Orthopaedic Biomechanics, p. 106. Lea & Febiger, 1970.*)

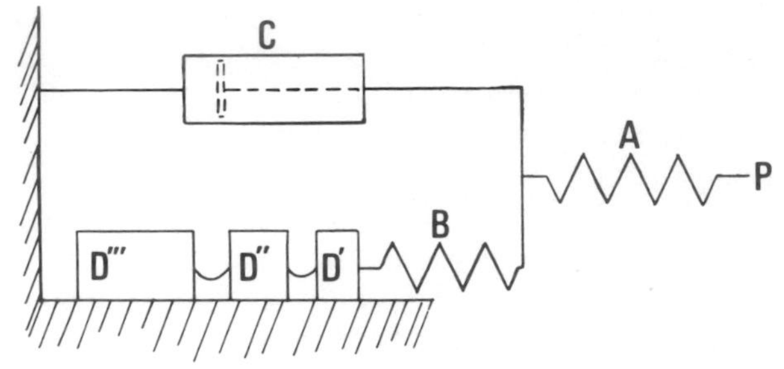

FIGURE 1-12. Curry's model for the viscoelastic behavior of bone. (*Currey, J.D.: The Mechanical Properties of Bone. Clin. Orthop., 73:222, 1970.*)

greater in the fatigue specimens. Specimens that were not fatigued to complete fracture showed diffuse microscopic damage. Repeated loading caused a progressive loss of stiffness, a decrease in yield strength, and an increase in permanent deformation and hysteresis. The damage was most marked on the compressive side, where there was oblique cracking and longitudinal splitting. The damage on the tension side was more subtle and consisted mainly of separation at cement lines and interlamellar cement bonds.

Bone, when tested in the laboratory, has no endurance limit and ultimately will fail when subjected to enough cycles. But bone in vivo, unlike other materials, has the property of self repair, so that rest and protection from stress will allow these fractures to heal. Indeed, it has been suggested that Wolff's law might be contingent on the healing of microstress fractures, thus buttressing the regions of highest stress.

The strength of bone is dependent on the density of the bone, the mineral content, and the quality and amount of collagen. It follows that any condition that diminishes these attributes (eg, osteoporosis, osteomalacia, scurvy) will increase susceptibility to fracture. An increase in density alone, however, is no guarantee of strength. Osteopetrosis and Paget's disease are both associated with increased liability to fracture.

Holes in Bone

Holes of any size significantly weaken bones,[55] but when the diameter of the hole is greater than 30% of the diameter of bone, the weakening effect becomes exponential. Worse still is the effect of an open section, as would result from the harvesting of a cortical bone graft or resection of a lesion from bone. After such procedures the affected bone must be protected from stress, and it is good practice to graft defects with cancellous bone after removing lesions. When an open section is left in the shaft of a bone and the bone is subjected to torsional stress, there is a redistribution of the shear stresses (Fig. 1-13) so that the more central stresses are in the same direction as the applied torque and, rather than resisting it, are additive.[159] Theoretically, sharp corners in a defect also act as stress risers, but this effect is negligible when compared with the effect of the open section.

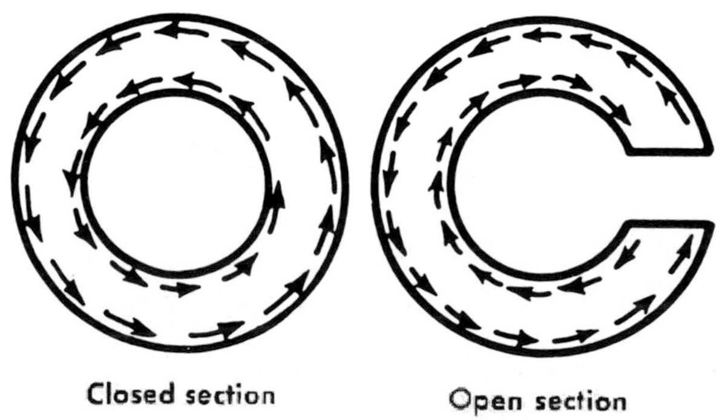

FIGURE 1-13. The effect of an open section on torsional stress patterns in the shaft of a bone. (*Murphy, E.F., and Burstein, A.H.: Physical Properties of Materials Including Solid Mechanics. In A.A.O.S. Atlas of Orthotics: Biomechanical Principles and Application, p. 222. St. Louis, C.V. Mosby, 1975.*)

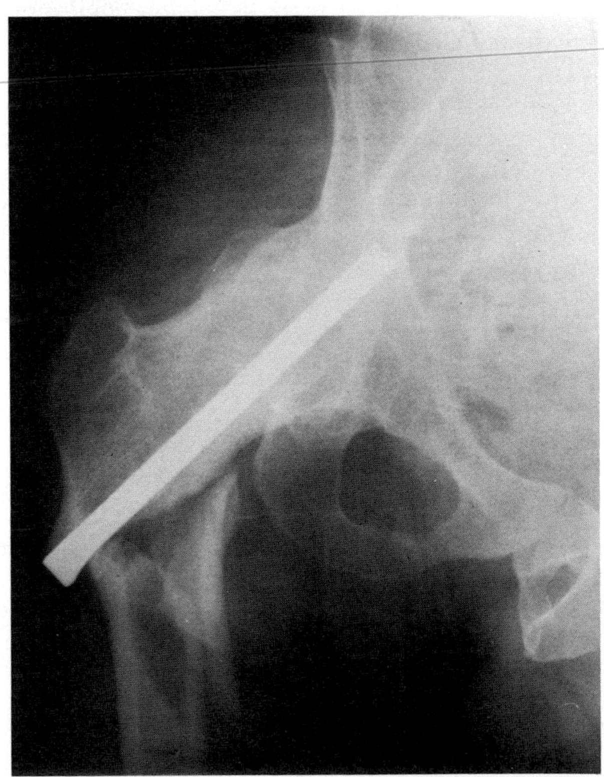

FIGURE 1-14. This radiograph shows an arthrodesed hip of a middle-aged man who stumbled and fell in a restaurant. Because of the long lever arm of his lower extremity, considerable moments were applied in the region of the Smith-Peterson nail, which acted as a stress riser, resulting in a fracture below the nail.

Effect of Metallic Implants

Orthopaedic implants weaken bone by stress shielding,[417,418] but they also predispose to fracture by increasing the stiffness of a segment of bone so that there is an abrupt transition between the degree of elasticity of the supported and unsupported segments of bone. This is a *stress riser,* and fractures at the lower end of an implant are distressingly common (Fig. 1-14).

The strength of any structure depends not only on the material from which it is made but also on how that material is distributed in relation to the forces that act on it. Thus, one can take a ruler and bend it easily in one direction but when one tries to angulate it across its broadest axis it will not deflect. The resistance to bending is related to the amount of material resisting the applied force and the distance of this material from the neutral axis. Resistance to bending can be calculated by the area moment of inertia; for a rectangular beam this resistance is calculated by the formula $BH^3/12$ where B = width and H = height.[159,281] For example, for a beam with a cross section of 2 inches by 4 inches, there will be an area moment of inertia of $(2 \times 64)/12 = 10.67$ in one axis and $(4 \times 8)/12 = 2.67$ in the other, so that in one configura-

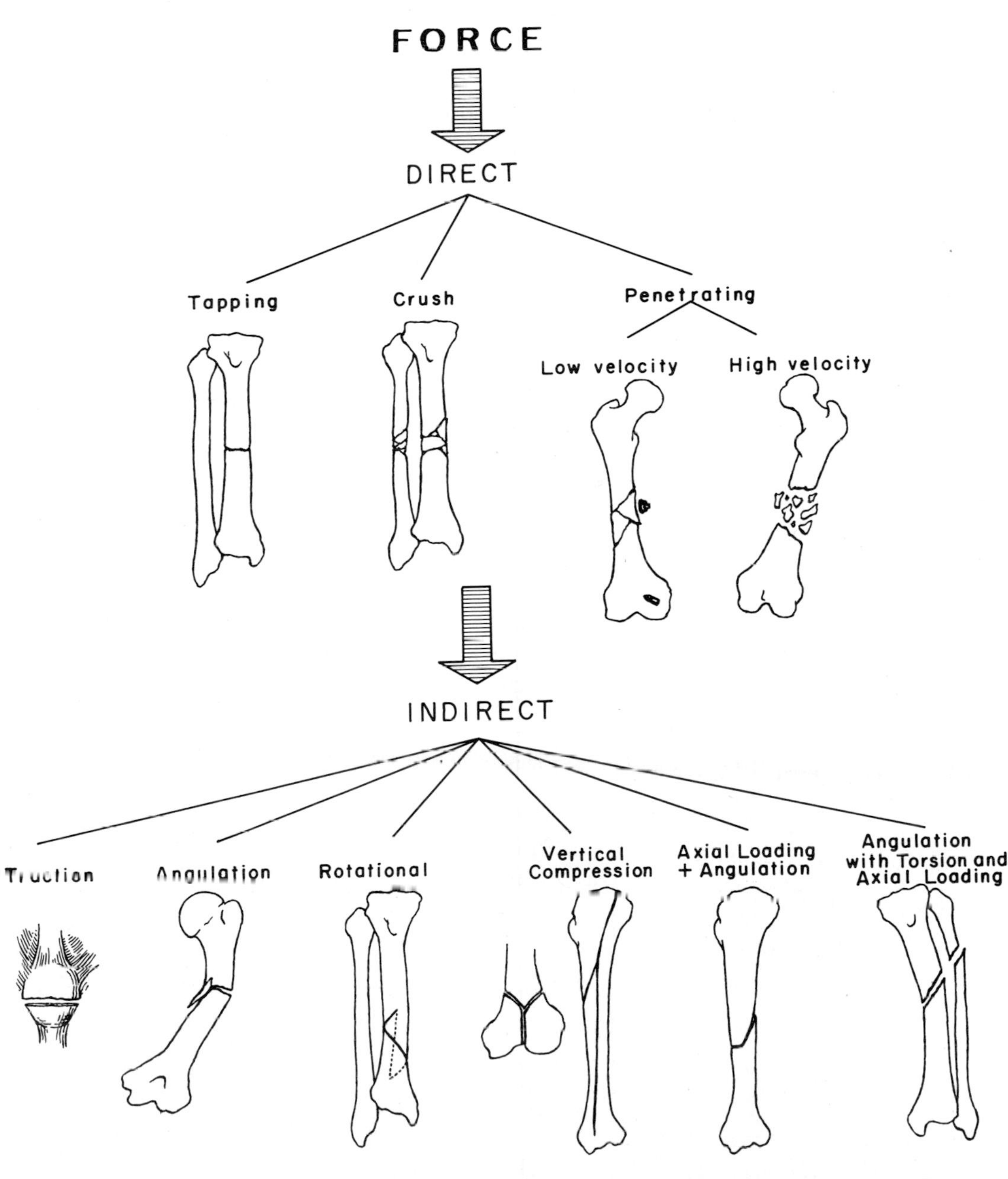

FIGURE 1-15. Classification of fractures according to the mechanism of injury.

tion the beam will be four times as resistant to bending than in the other.[159,281]

It is also evident that a solid rod will have less resistance to bending than a hollow cylinder with a larger radius, even though the amount of material in each is the same. The area moment of inertia for a cylindrical structure is $(\pi r^3)/2$.[159,281] If the cylinder is hollow, the value would be diminished by subtracting $(\pi r_2^3)/2$, where r_2 is the radius of the hollow portion.

Because bending moments are proportional to the length of the lever, it follows that persons with long, slender bones are at greater risk than those with short bones with large diameters. It follows, too, that fusion or ankylosis of the hip or knee will preclude a person from shortening the lever arm of the extremity in a fall. These factors, in addition to removing the energy-dissipating function of the mobile joint, predispose to fracture. Supracondylar fracture of the femur is a price that may be paid for arthrodesis of the knee, and subtrochanteric fracture for fusion of the hip.

Resistance to torsional stress is dependent on the distance of material from the neutral axis. It is described by the polar moment of inertia, which is calculated for a circular cross section by the formula $(\pi r^4)/2$.[159,281]

CLASSIFICATION OF FRACTURES BY THE MECHANISM OF INJURY

Deducing the probable mechanism of injury by interpreting the clinical and radiographic features of a fracture is not merely a sterile academic exercise. Knowing how a fracture was produced has therapeutic implications. Bone fractures from both direct and indirect forces, which may be classified (Fig. 1-15).

Direct Trauma

Perkins[309] divided fractures produced by direct application of the force to the fracture site into tapping fractures, crush fractures, and penetrating fractures. Essentially these are caused, respectively, by a small force

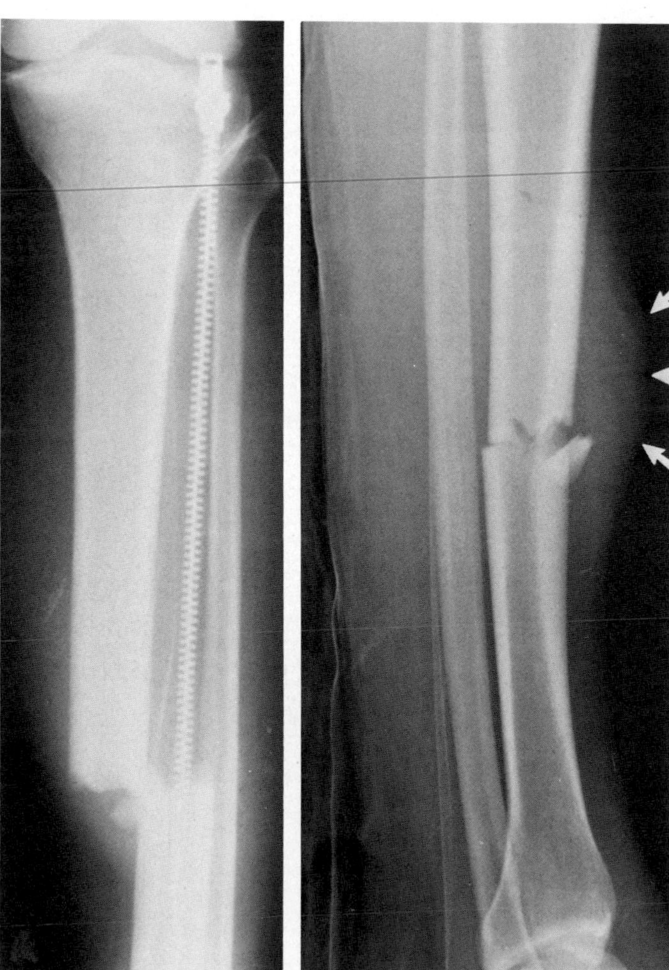

FIGURE 1-16. Anteroposterior and lateral views of the left tibia, showing a typical tapping fracture. The fracture is transverse with comminution of one cortex, and the fibula is intact. Note the fracture hematoma overlying the point of impact (*arrows*).

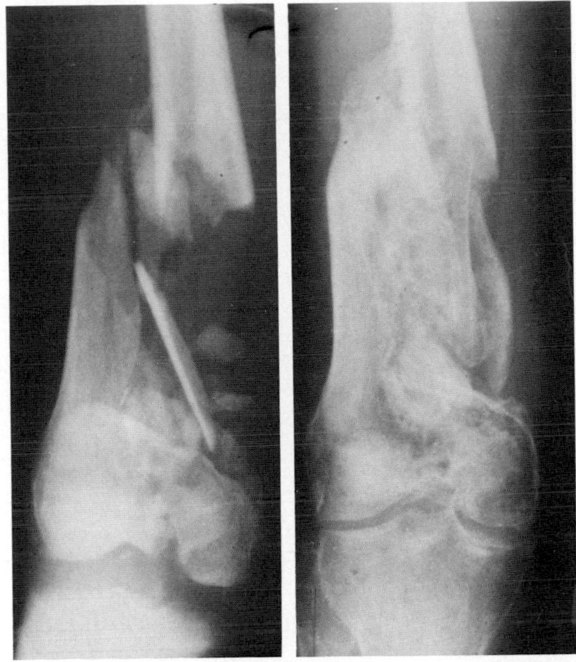

FIGURE 1-17. (*Left*) A crush fracture of the distal end of the right femur. This woman attempted suicide by jumping from an overpass on an interstate highway and was struck by a speeding truck. Note the gross comminution of the fracture. (*Right*) The end result of this fracture after treatment by traction and active motion of the knee. After 8 months the defects in the femur were healed in by periosteal new bone.

acting on a small area, a large force acting on a large area, and a large force acting on a small area.

Tapping Fractures

Tapping fractures occur when a force of dying momentum is applied over a small area. The identifying features are a transverse fracture line and the frequent finding in the forearm or leg that only one bone is fractured. Because most of the energy is absorbed by the bone, there is very little soft-tissue damage, although a small area of overlying skin may be split or bruised. Tapping fractures frequently are inflicted by kicks on the shin or blows with nightsticks or other blunt weapons (Fig. 1-16).

Crush Fractures

Crush fractures are accompanied by extensive soft-tissue damage. The bone is either extensively comminuted or broken transversely. In the forearm or leg, both bones fracture at the same level (Fig. 1-17).

Penetrating (Gunshot) Fractures

Penetrating fractures are produced by projectiles, and for all intents and purposes they can be called gunshot fractures. A distinction should be made between high-

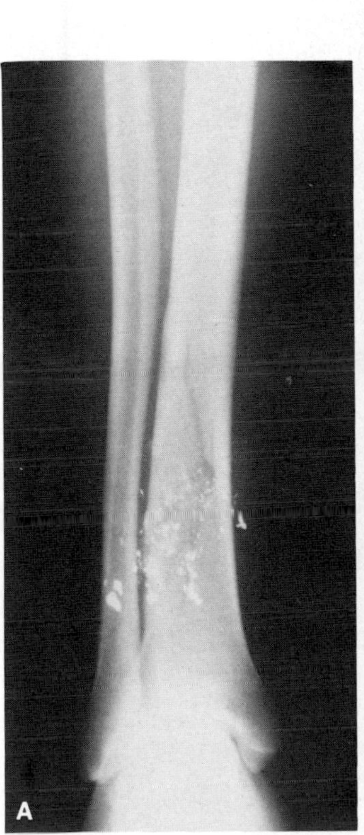

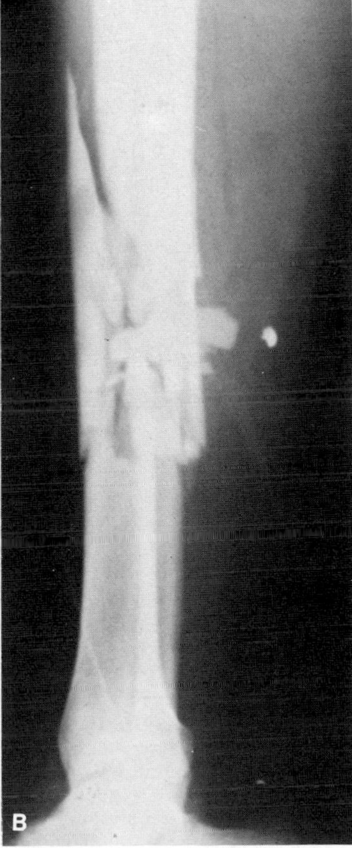

FIGURE 1-18. (**A**) Low-velocity gunshot wound of the left tibia. The fracture line is linear without displacement, and the bullet has disintegrated on contact with the bone. (**B**) High-velocity gunshot wound sustained during a robbery attempt. The patient was shot by the police with an M-16 rifle. Note in this case the extreme comminution of the fracture fragments caused by the greater energy imparted to the bone.

velocity and low-velocity missiles. There is some disagreement in the literature as to what constitutes a high-velocity weapon. Dimond and Rich,[130] quote the Wound Ballistics Manual of the Office of the Surgeon General as stating that a muzzle velocity greater than 2500 ft/s constitutes high velocity. DeMuth and Smith[124] considered anything over 1800 ft/s high velocity, and Russotti and Sim[359] use 2000 ft/s as the cut-off point. Regardless of the precise definition of a high-velocity missile, however, the distinction has important implications in the management of gunshot wounds. Because the kinetic energy of the bullet varies directly with the square of its velocity and only linearly with its mass, any increase in velocity produces an exponential increase in tissue damage. For example, the M16 rifle has a muzzle velocity of 3250 ft/s, so that in spite of using a smaller projectile than a .300 caliber rifle, it has greatly increased destructive properties. Low-velocity missiles produce little in the way of soft-tissue damage. They may splinter the shaft of a bone or embed themselves in cancellous ends (Figs. 1-18**A** and 1-19). High-velocity wounds from military rifles, on the other hand, involve extensive soft-tissue damage, and the fragments of the bone, which disintegrates on being struck, become secondary missiles (see Fig. 1-18**B**).

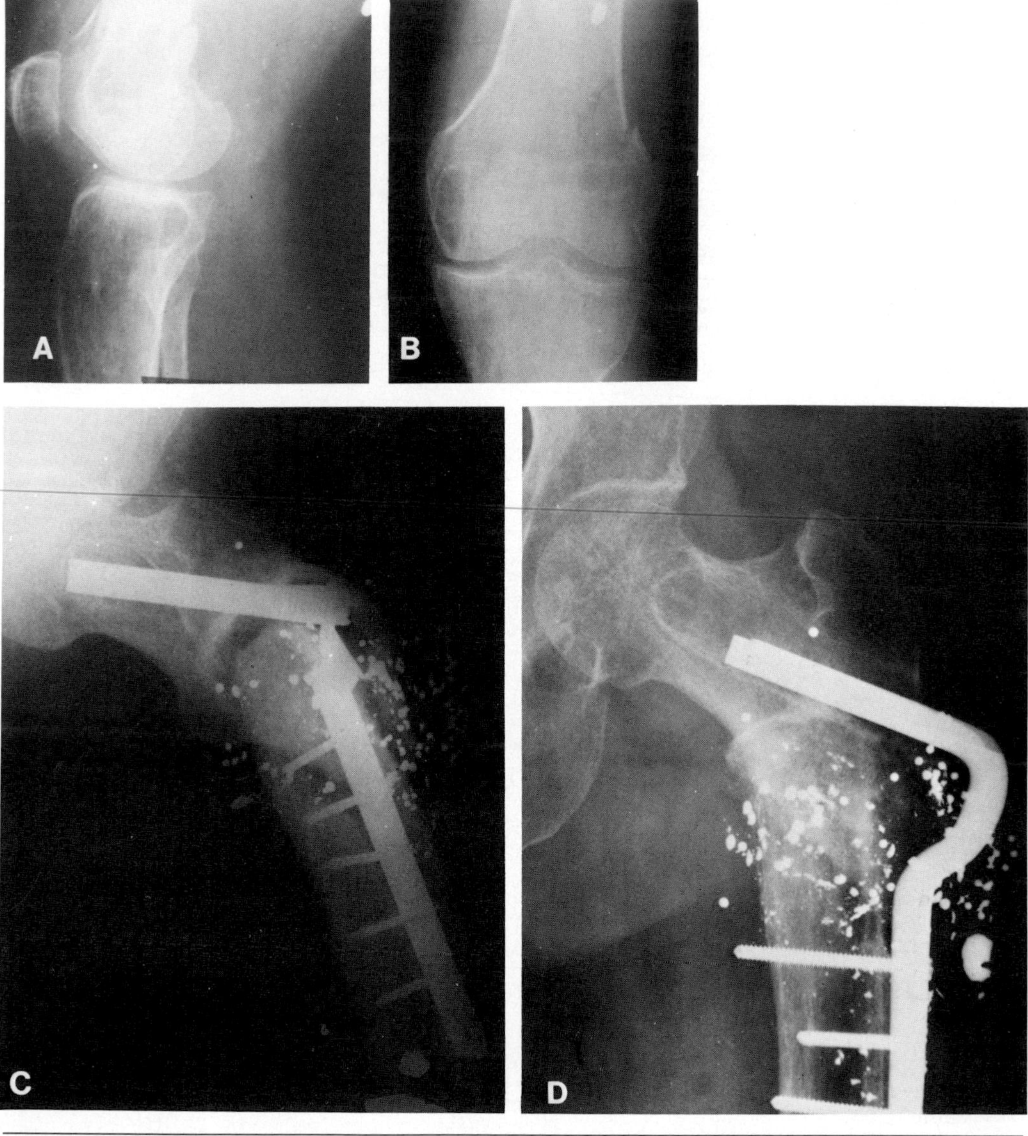

FIGURE 1-19. (**A** and **B**) Radiographs of the knee in a patient who lived an adventurous life and was admitted with a fracture produced by a .22-caliber bullet. (**C**) Radiograph of the ipsilateral hip demonstrated a nonunion of an old shotgun fracture fixed by a bladeplate assembly. Nonunion had resulted with breakage of the plate through the first screw hole. This type of fixation is inadequate for subtrochanteric fractures, which are better treated with a Zickel or similar type nail. (**D**) This fracture went on to union after the insertion of a compression plate device.

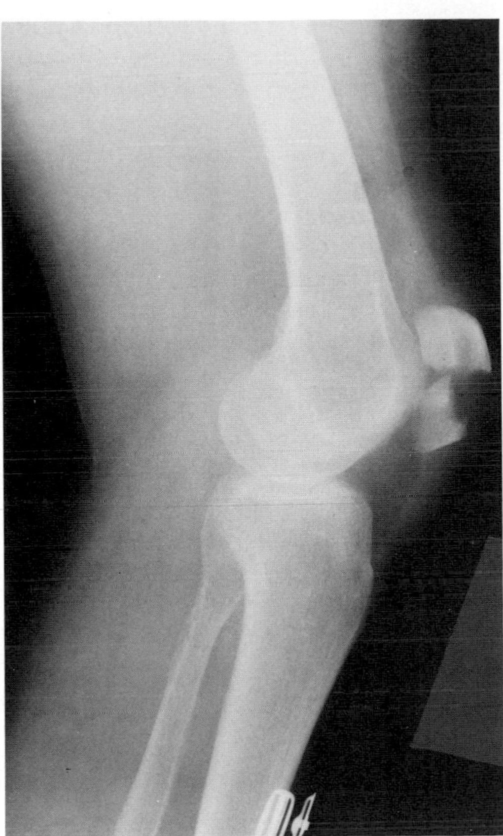

FIGURE 1-20. Fractures of the patella may occur as the result of a flexion force being applied to the knee while the quadriceps is in contraction, leading to a separated transverse fracture.

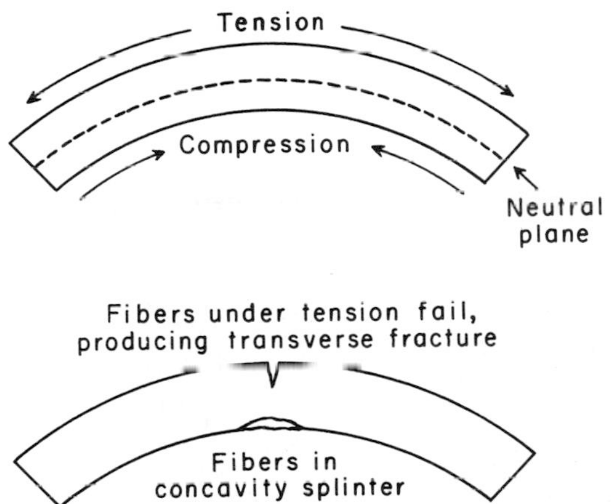

FIGURE 1-21. Mechanism of an angulation fracture. If a bone is angulated, tension stresses will be present over the convexity, while compression stresses will be present in the concavity. Because bone is most likely to fail in tension, the fibers over the convexity will rupture first, throwing the stress onto the fibers immediately adjacent until a transverse fracture is produced. Commonly, the bone in the concavity of the angulation will fail in compression, causing some splintering of the cortex.

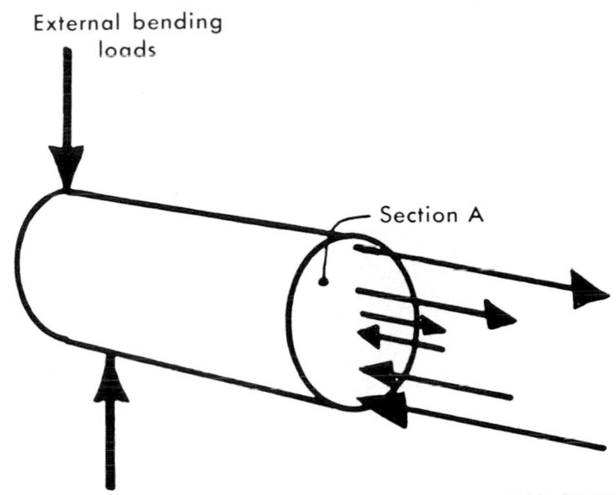

FIGURE 1-22. Effect of external bending forces on internal forces within the beam. (*Murphy, E.F., and Burstein, A.H.: Physical Properties of Materials Including Solid Mechanics. In A.A.O.S. Atlas of Orthotics: Biomechanical Principles and Application, p. 15. St. Louis, C.V. Mosby, 1975.*)

Indirect Trauma

Fractures produced by a force acting at a distance from the fracture site are said to be caused by indirect trauma.

Traction or Tension Fractures

The shaft of a long bone is most unlikely to be pulled apart by a traction or tension force, but this can happen to the patella or olecranon when the knee or elbow is forcibly flexed while the extensor muscles are contracting (Fig. 1-20). Similarly, the medial malleolus may be pulled off by the deltoid ligament in eversion and external rotation injuries of the ankle. The fracture line in tension fractures is transverse, which is what one would expect if the bone fibers fail under

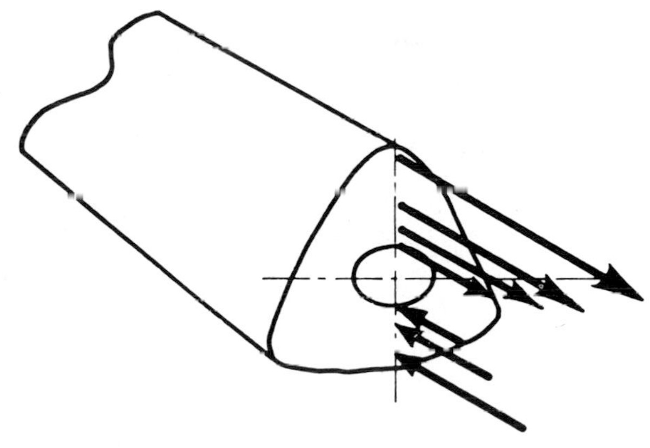

FIGURE 1-23. Unequal effect of bending loads on the tibia. (*Murphy, E.F., and Burstein, A.H.: Physical Properties of Materials Including Solid Mechanics. In A.A.O.S. Atlas of Orthotics: Biomechanical Principles and Application, p. 15. St. Louis, C.V. Mosby, 1975.*)

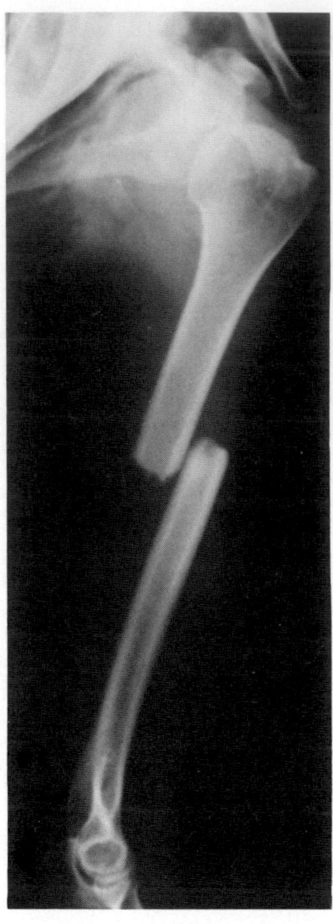

FIGURE 1-24. Transverse fracture of the humerus secondary to an angulation force.

tension at right angles to the direction of pull. It has been stated, however, that the plane of fracture may be along shear lines at 45° to the direction of pull.[3a]

Angulation Fractures

When a lever is angulated (Fig. 1-21), the convexity is under a tension stress, the concavity is under compression, and somewhere in between there is a neutral plane under neither compression nor tension. The farther from the neutral plane, the greater will be the magnitude of these stresses (Fig. 1-22), and in a bone with an asymmetric cross section these forces may be greater on one side than on the other (Fig. 1-23). Because bone is stronger in compression than in tension, the fibers over the convexity fail first, thereby throwing more stress on the adjacent fibers, which in turn fail. By this progression a transverse fracture line is propagated (Fig. 1-24). Not uncommonly, however, the bone in the concavity that is under compression will fail in shear at an angle to the main fracture line, breaking off a triangular fragment of variable size.[10]

Rotational Fractures

When a piece of chalk is twisted until it breaks, a characteristic spiral fracture line is produced that makes one complete rotation around the circumference, each end of which is joined by a vertical compo-

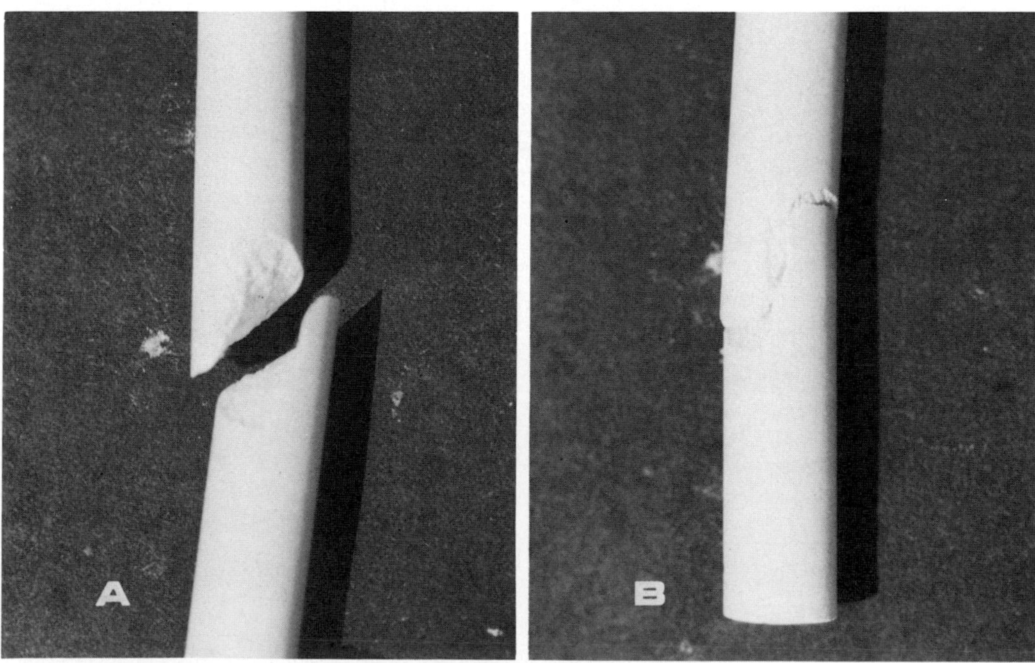

FIGURE 1-25. (**A**) A model of a spiral fracture produced by torque. (**B**) The vertical fracture line joining the upper and lower extremities of the spiral fracture.

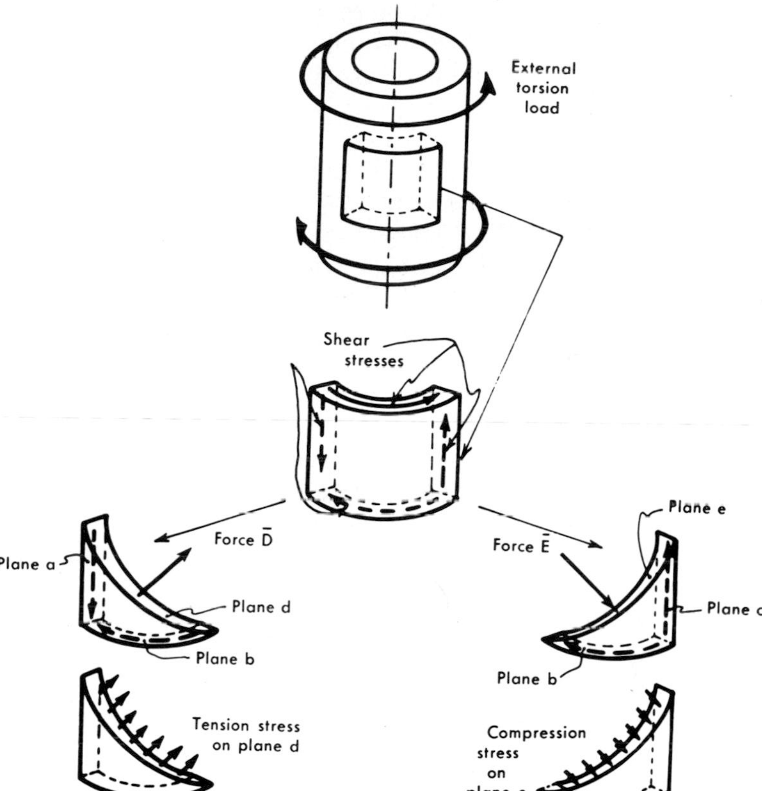

FIGURE 1-26. Effect of torsion on shear and compressive stress. (*Murphy, E.F., and Burstein, A.H.: Physical Properties of Materials Including Solid Mechanics. In A.A.O.S. Atlas of Orthotics: Biomechanical Principles and Application, p. 11. St. Louis, C.V. Mosby, 1975.*)

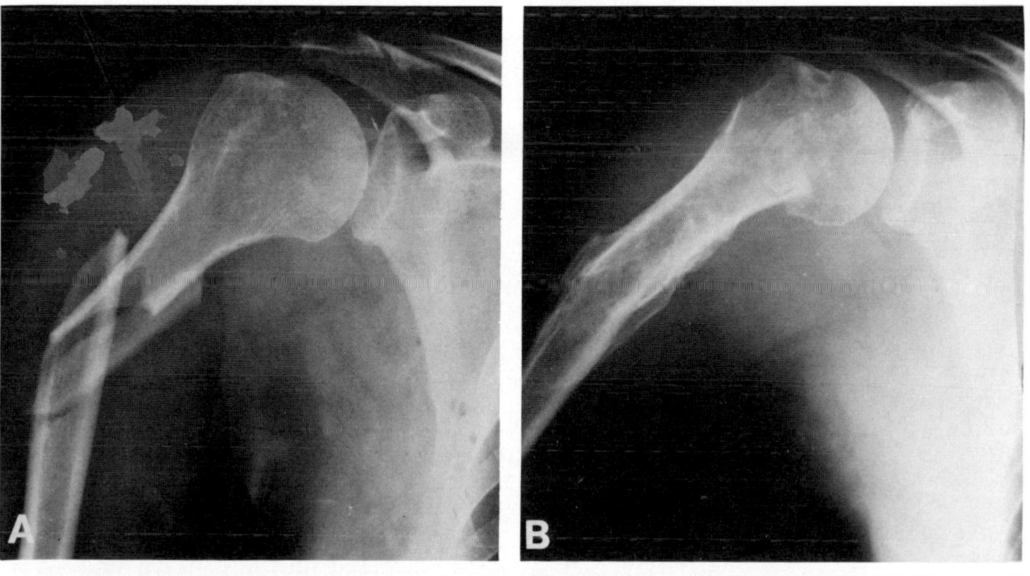

FIGURE 1-27. (**A**) Radiograph of a spiral fracture of the left humerus with a loose butterfly fragment in a 67-year-old man. (**B**) Ten years later the fracture seems to be well healed. After a subsequent fall, he sustained an impacted fracture of the humeral neck.

nent with or without some splintering (Fig. 1-25). Formerly it was contended that this spiral was caused by shear forces at 45° to the long axis, but this is not the case.[10] It is now generally agreed that the spiral is caused by failure in tension. Reilly and Burstein[334] have shown that the vertical component is a shear failure and initiates the fracture.

Netz and associates[286] described torsional fractures as occurring in two stages: in stage I, an increasing number of cracks occur in the cortex; in stage II, at maximum torque, ultimate failure is brought about by the sudden propagation of the cracks to form the spiral fracture. However, because all the fragments fit together without distortion, they believe that the nonlinear portion of the stress–strain curve does not result from viscoelasticity but rather from the stage I cracking of the cortex.

If torque or a twisting force is applied to a bone, vertical and horizontal shear stresses result (Fig. 1-26). The horizontal shear can be resolved into compression and tension forces, which are maximal at 45° to the plane of maximum shear. Because bone is more likely to fail in tension, it is along this line that the fracture runs (Fig. 1-27).

Torsional stresses are greatest the farther they are removed from the axis of rotation, but they are inversely proportional to the polar moment of inertia $(\pi r^4)/2$, which explains why such fractures are more common in the distal third of the tibia than in the proximal third, even though the cortex of the former is much thicker and denser (Fig. 1-28).

Compression Fractures

If one were to take a uniform cylinder of a homogeneous material and load it axially until it failed, it would fracture along a linear plane at an angle of almost 45° along the line of maximum shear strain (Fig. 1-29). However, long bones are not uniform cylinders or columns and are only rarely fractured by a pure compression force. When this happens, the hard shaft of the long bone is driven into the cancellous end, giving rise to the T- or Y-shaped fracture (eg, at the lower end of the humerus or femur) (Fig. 1-30).[10] Experimentally, it has been shown that a compressive load applied in the long axis of a bone will produce a fracture in a plane 30° to the direction of force.[108a] This suggests that the fracture is initiated with the production of shear lines formed by buckling of lamellae that probably first appear in areas of stress concentration such as a vessel or resorption space. With increasing strain, the bone eventually cracks along these lines by a combination of compression and shear.

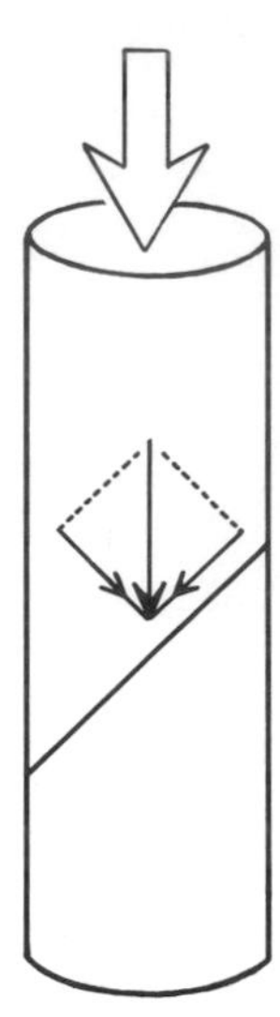

FIGURE 1-29. If a column of a uniform material is vertically loaded, it will tend to fail in shear at an angle of 45° to the long axis of the column. If the force is resolved into two components, as shown here, the maximum shear force will be at 45° to the long axis of the column.

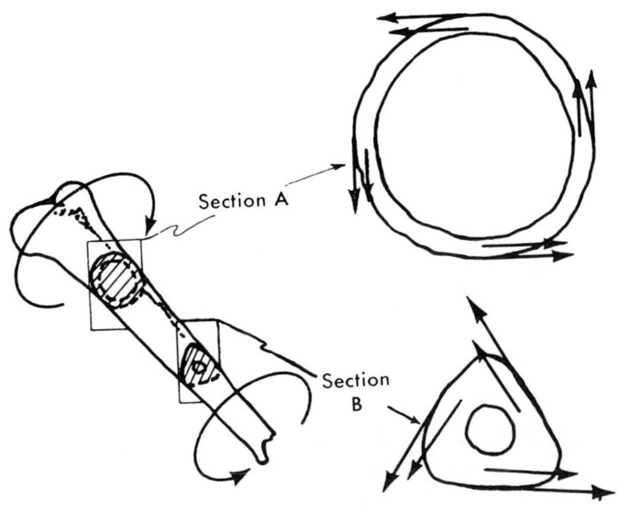

FIGURE 1-28. Effect of torsional loading of the tibia. (*Murphy, E.F., and Burstein, A.H.: Physical Properties of Materials Including Solid Mechanics. In A.A.O.S. Atlas of Orthotics: Biomechanical Principles and Application, p. 17. St. Louis, C.V. Mosby, 1975.*)

Less commonly, compression in the longitudinal axis of the tibia sometimes produces longitudinal fractures without displacement. Perkins has christened these "teacup fractures," comparing them to a cracked cup that does not break and is still usable (Fig. 1-31**A**).[310] These fractures do not become displaced, need no treatment, and always heal. A similar fracture, "cleavage intercondylar fracture of the femur," has been described by Pogrund and associates,[320] which is also caused by a longitudinal force applied through the patella. This fracture, too, does not appear to displace.

Fractures are usually produced by a combination of forces rather than by one acting alone. In his analysis of fracture mechanics, Alms[10] stated that when a beam is loaded axially with a force insufficient to cause failure, and then angulated, this will result in the compressive force being diminished on the convex side of the beam and increased on the concave side. As a result, failure might start by shearing at an angle of 45° where the bone is under compression; alternatively, the failure may start at right angles to the shaft, owing to tension stress over the convexity. In either case, the resultant fracture line is

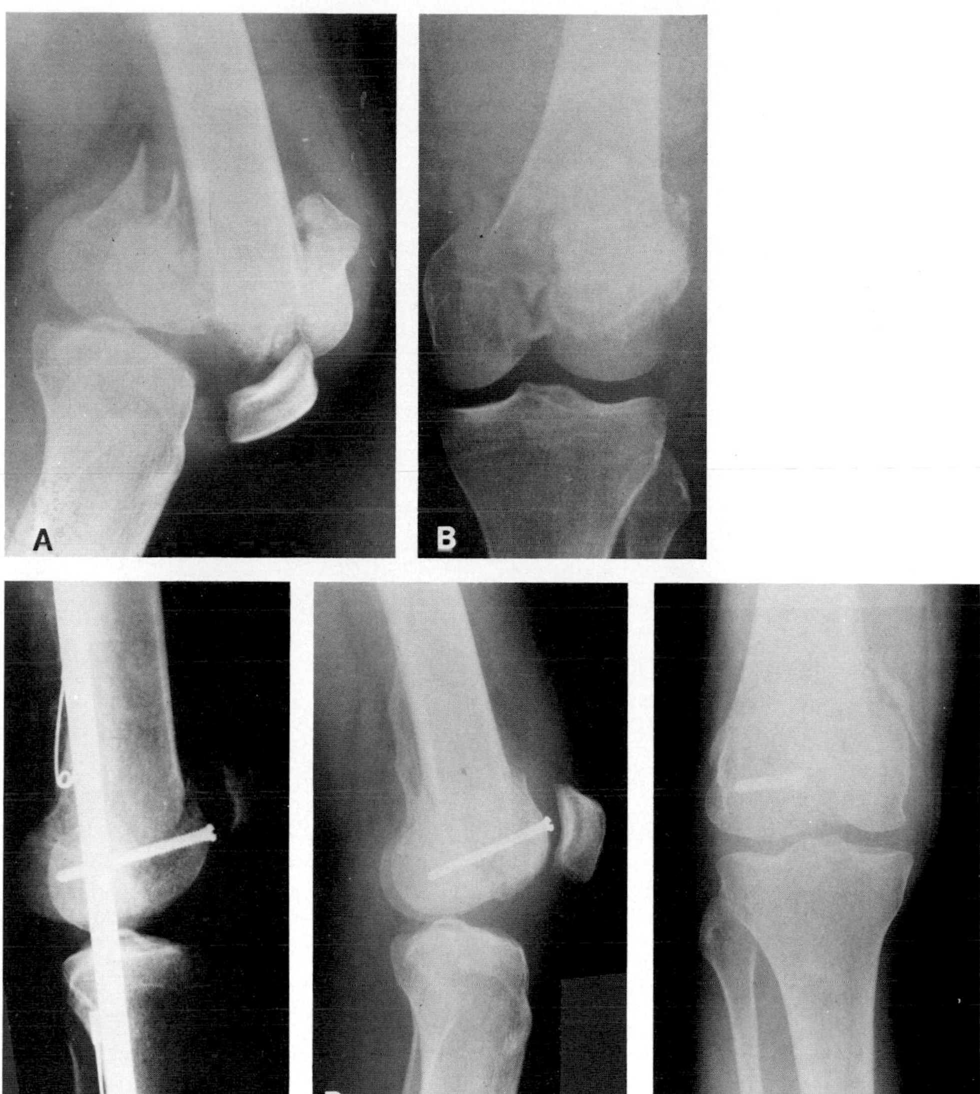

FIGURE 1-30. (**A** and **B**) Compression fracture of the lower end of the femur where the femoral shaft has been driven through the condyles, giving rise to a supracondylar T fracture plus a vertical fracture of the lateral femoral condyle. (**C**) Open reduction was carried out with internal fixation of the lateral condyle by a screw. (**D** and **E**) Long-term follow-up showing healing of the fracture. This patient has a full range of motion of the knee in spite of a defect in the lateral femoral condyle.

curved, consisting of an oblique component caused by compression and a transverse component caused by angulation (Fig. 1-31**B**). The magnitude of each component will be proportional to the respective forces. Frequently, the fragment of bone bearing the oblique surface is sheared off, forming a butterfly fragment.

Fractures Due to Angulation, Rotation, and Axial Compression

The result of combined angulation and rotation is the equivalent of an angulation about an oblique axis, which causes an oblique fracture.[8,10] If the shaft of a long bone is also loaded axially, the tendency to fracture is increased with a shear force at 45° to the long axis (Fig. 1-32). It could be argued, however, that these are merely angulation fractures around an oblique axis.

This type of fracture is sometimes confused with a spiral fracture. Perkins[310] stated that the broken ends of a spiral fracture are "long and sharp and pointed like pen nibs" (Fig. 1-33), whereas in oblique fractures they are "short, blunted and rounded like a garden trowel." Charnley[86] noted that, "if [a fracture is] truly spiral it will be impossible for a clear gap to be seen through the fracture by any orientation of the radiograph."

CLINICAL FEATURES OF FRACTURES

In the majority of fractures the diagnosis is self-evident, but the following signs and symptoms, alone or in combination, should alert the surgeon to the possibility of a fracture.

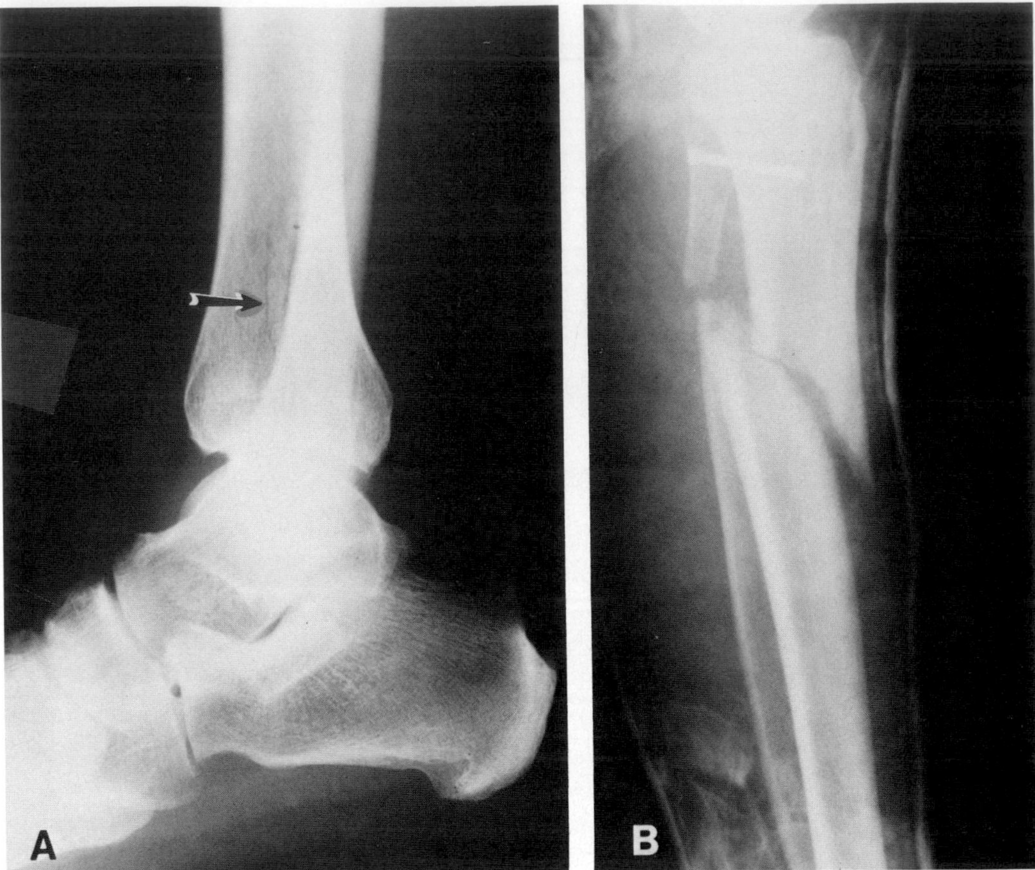

FIGURE 1-31. (**A**)Radiograph of the ankle in a 45-year-old man who fell from a chair and landed heavily on his foot. Pain developed in his distal tibia and ankle. He has vertical fracture lines traversing the articular surfaces of the joint (*arrow*), but without displacement. This is a typical "teacup fracture," as described by Perkins. (**B**) Radiograph of the lower leg in a patient who was riding a motorcycle and sustained this fracture in a collision when his foot struck the ground. The fracture has both oblique and transverse elements, caused by a combination of vertical compression and angulation. The head of the fibula was also dislocated, and resection of the fibular shaft was necessary to reduce the dislocation and relieve the tension on the common peroneal nerve. The tibial fracture became very unstable and required stabilization by a plate.

Pain and Tenderness

All fractures cause pain in neurologically intact persons, although the intensity may vary considerably. Minor compression fractures of the vertebrae, for example, often go untreated because the pain is not severe enough for the patient to seek medical advice. On the other hand, pain and tenderness may be the only evidence of fracture (eg, fractured scaphoid and fatigue fractures). A possible exception to this rule is the finding of Grosher and associates[180] that, on examining military recruits with radioactive bone scans, some fatigue fractures were asymptomatic.

The diagnosis of stress fractures is likely to be missed by the unwary. Satku and coworkers[367] have reported on 16 elderly patients who had sustained 18 such fractures around the knee. Thirteen of these fractures were misdiagnosed and attributed to other pathologic processes in the knee, but all were tender over the fracture.

Heel pain after unwonted activity in middle-aged and elderly persons is often due to stress fracture and when evaluated radiographically after 2 or 3 weeks will show a band of increased density from the fracture callus (Fig. 1-34). In cases of doubt, a radioactive bone scan will resolve the difficulty.

In an examination of the injured patient, gentle palpation generally confirms the presence of tenderness; and once this has been established, there is little point in reconfirming the observation at the expense of the patient's discomfort.

Loss of Function

Function is lost owing to pain and the loss of a lever arm in most fractures. In incomplete fractures of the femoral neck, for example, it is not uncommon for the patient to continue to walk or even ride a bicycle.

(text continues on page 23)

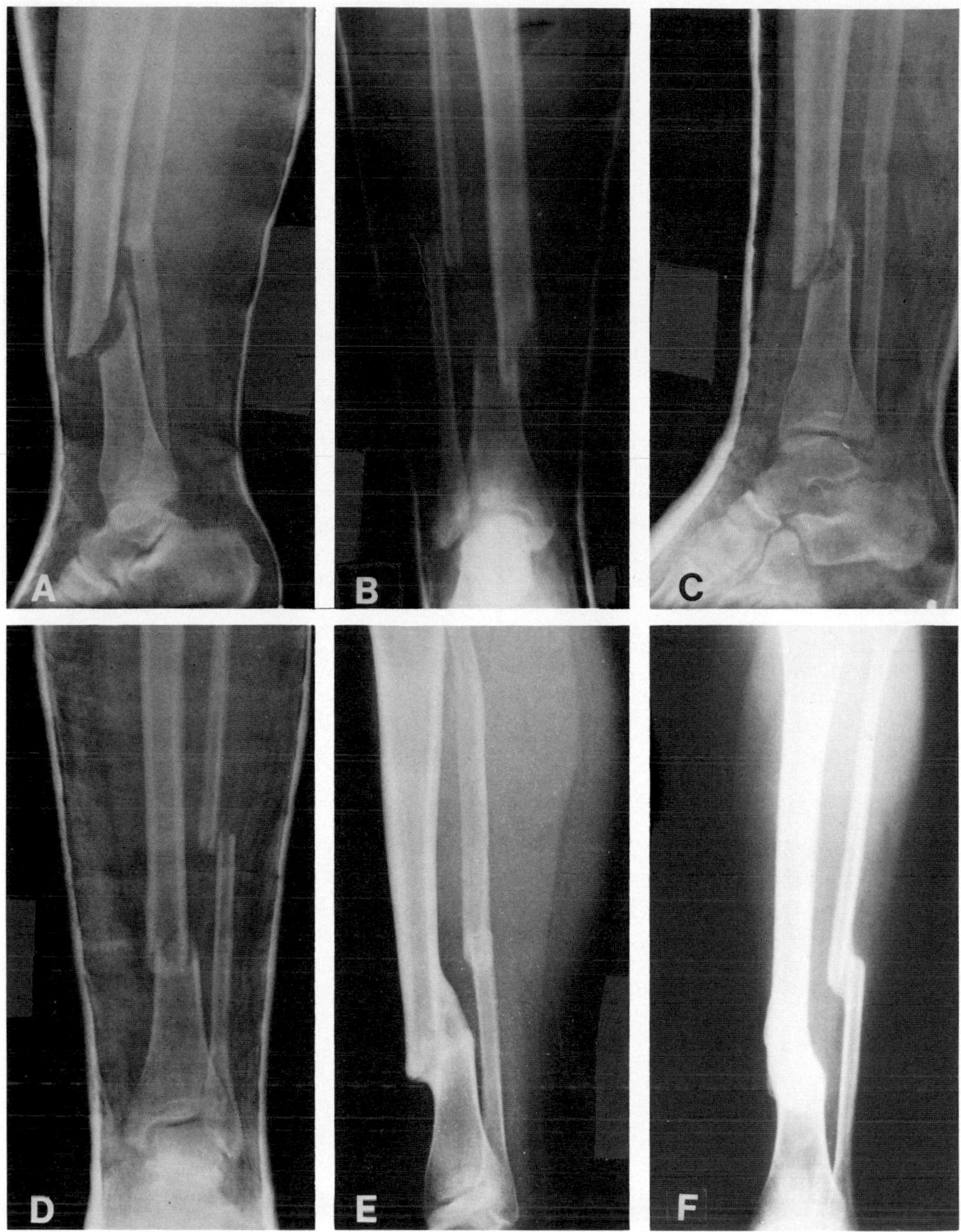

FIGURE 1-32. (**A** and **B**) Anteroposterior and lateral views of an oblique fracture. The proximal fragment is shaped like a trowel. This reduction, obtained by a tyro, is inadequate. Note the large air space at the upper end of the tibia where the cast has lost contact with the tibia. (**C** and **D**) After remanipulation and the application of three-point fixation, the proximal and distal fragments are parallel in both planes, and there is little or no shortening. (**E** and **F**) The fracture has united by periosteal callus. In spite of the offset, the cosmetic and functional results are excellent.

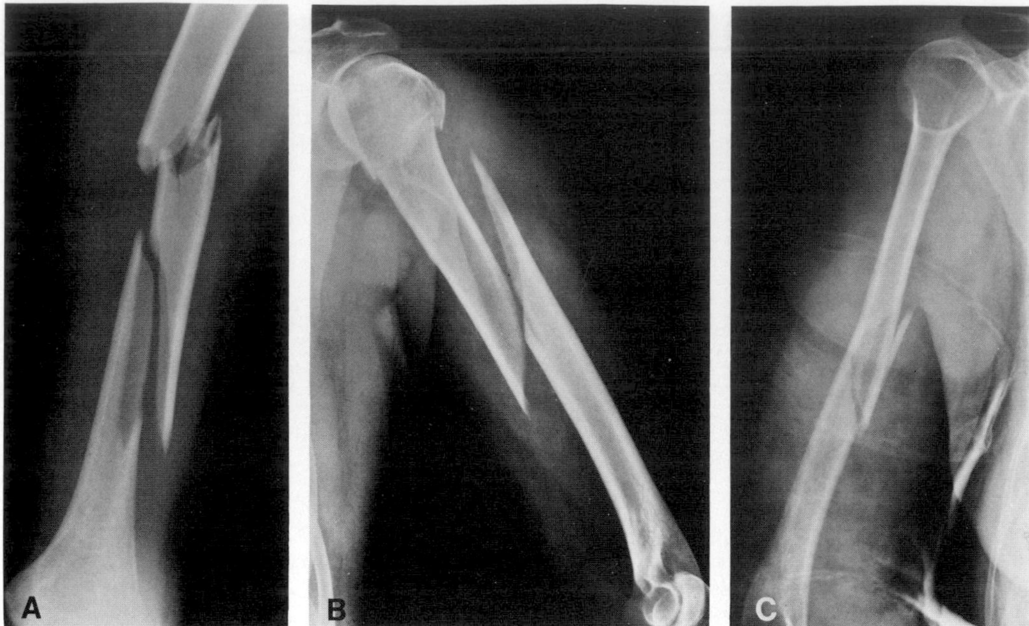

FIGURE 1-33. (**A**) Radiograph of a fractured humerus in a girl who was riding the pillion of a motorcycle that ran off the road. The segmental fracture is produced by an oblique fracture proximally and a spiral fracture distally. (**B**) A combination of an impacted humeral neck proximally and spiral fracture distally as a result of a fall and torque to the humerus. (**C**) Spiral fracture of the humerus with butterfly fragment. Note the sharp ends of the fracture fragments "like pen-nibs" that, according to Perkins, characterize spiral fractures.

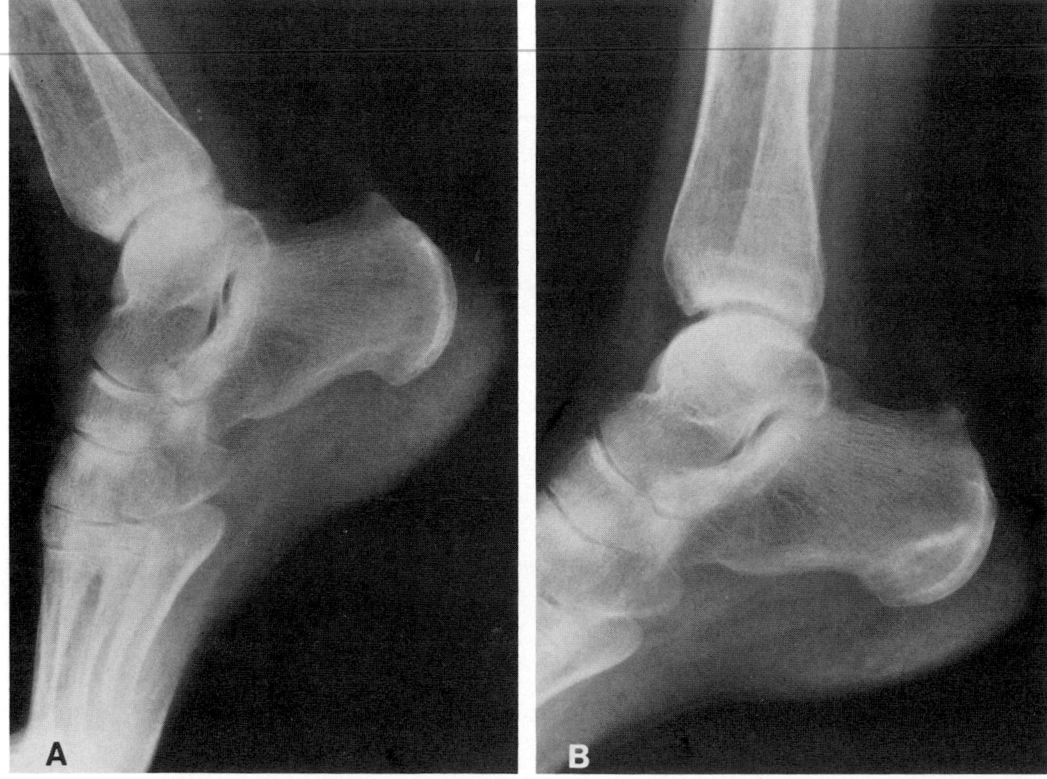

FIGURE 1-34. (**A**) Lateral view of the foot in a woman who complained of severe pain in her heel reveals no evidence of fracture. (**B**) Films taken 1 month later show a linear density of endosteal callus in the posterior of the os calcis, indicating a healing fatigue fracture.

Deformity

The hemorrhage resulting from fracture generally gives rise to perceptible swelling, and fractures commonly produce angulation or rotational deformities and, especially where there is marked muscle spasm, shortening.

Attitude

The attitude of patients is sometimes diagnostic. Patients with a fractured clavicle generally support the affected upper extremity with the opposite hand and rotate their head to the side of the fracture. When patients sit up from the supine position holding their head with their hands, a fracture of the odontoid is very probably the cause.

Abnormal Mobility and Crepitus

When motion is possible in the middle of a long bone, there can be little doubt that it is fractured. Such motion may also provoke crepitus, the transmitted grating sensation of bone fragments rubbing on each other. Because eliciting these signs is painful to patients and potentially dangerous, they should never be sought deliberately.

Neurovascular Injury

No examination for suspected fracture is complete without careful evaluation of peripheral nerve function and vascularity. One must be particularly alert in supracondylar fractures of the humerus and femur, where both nerves and vessels are at serious risk.

Radiographic Findings

Ultimately, the proof is the radiographic demonstration of a fracture. There are pitfalls to avoid in this regard.[310] Fractures will be missed if the proper views are not requested. The x-ray films should include the joints at each end of the bone. Technically poor films should not be accepted. Fractures of the carpal bones may not show immediately or if the proper view has not been taken, and stress fractures may not be evident until a considerable time after the onset of pain (see Fig. 1-34).

Fractures of the axial skeleton are the most likely to be missed, and cervical spine films should always be taken when patients have head injuries and are unconscious.

The introduction of computed tomograms (CT scans) has been of inestimable benefit in the evaluation of injuries to the spine and acetabulum, and increasingly so with three-dimensional reconstruction (Fig 1-35). Magnetic resonance imaging is not helpful in fracture diagnosis other than delineating associated injury to the central nervous system, soft-tissue disruption, or occasionally fatigue fracture.

CLINICAL FEATURES OF DISLOCATIONS

A *dislocation* is a complete disruption of a joint so that the articular surfaces are no longer in contact. *Subluxations* are minor disruptions of joints where articular contact still remains. Perkins[310] stated that most subluxations are associated with fractures of the joint, and we agree with this. It is rare to have dislocations or subluxations of the wrist or ankle without an associated fracture, and a large number of patients with posterior dislocations of the hip have fractures of the posterior lip of the acetabulum (Fig. 1-36).

Pain

Like other injuries, dislocations are associated with pain, which may be severe, and persist until the joint is relocated.

Loss of Normal Contour and Relationship of Bony Points

In anterior dislocation of the shoulder, the flattening of the deltoid and the loss of the greater tuberosity as the most lateral point of the shoulder confirms the diagnosis. When the elbow is flexed 90°, the epicondyles and olecranon form an equilateral triangle. With the joint fully extended, the epicondyles and the olecranon form a straight line. These relationships are disrupted when the joint is dislocated.

Loss of Motion

In most dislocations, active and passive motion is grossly limited or impossible.

Attitude

The position in which the limb is held is diagnostic in dislocations of the hip. The flexed, adducted, internal rotation deformity of the posterior dislocation and the abducted, externally rotated lower extremity with apparent lengthening of an anterior dislocation are both diagnostic.

Radiographic Findings

As in fractures, x-ray films are an indispensable part of the evaluation. If this step is omitted, catastrophes will occur, because associated fractures will go unrec-

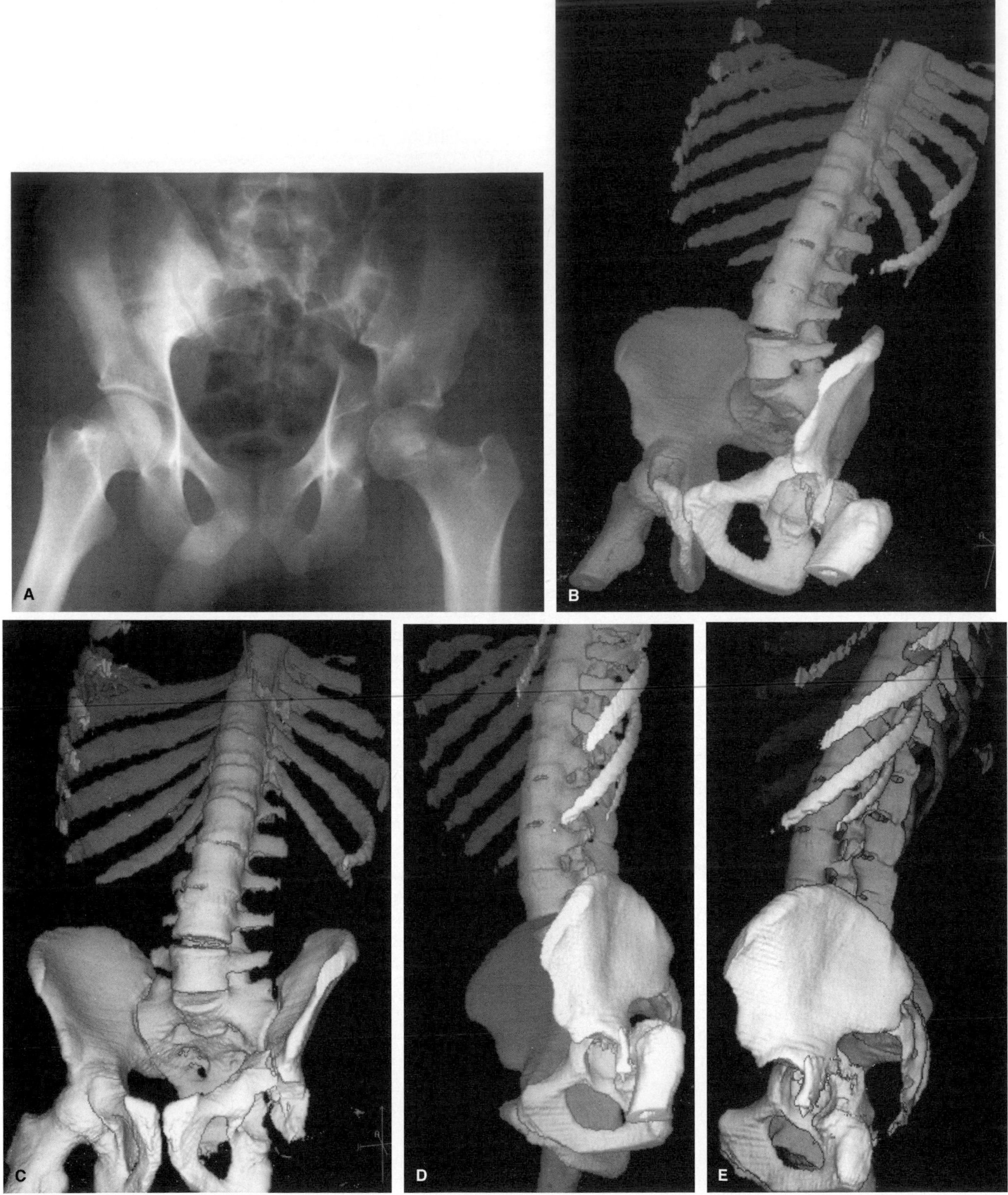

FIGURE 1-35. (**A**) Anteroposterior radiograph of pelvis showing a transverse fracture of the left acetabulum. (**B**) CT scan showing the same fracture and posterior dislocation of hip. (**C**) Same fracture with femoral head subtracted showing both ends of fracture line. (**D**) Lateral view demonstrating dislocation and distortion of acetabulum. (**E**) Head of femur subtracted showing comminution of posterior lip of acetabulum.

continues

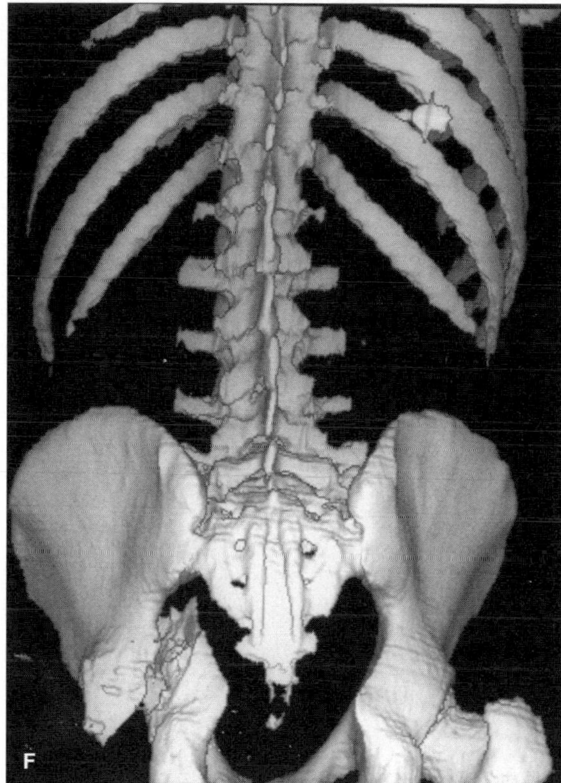

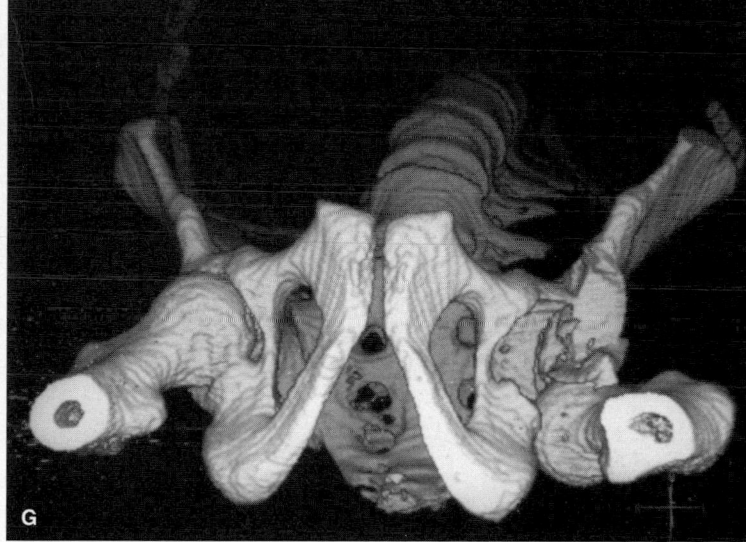

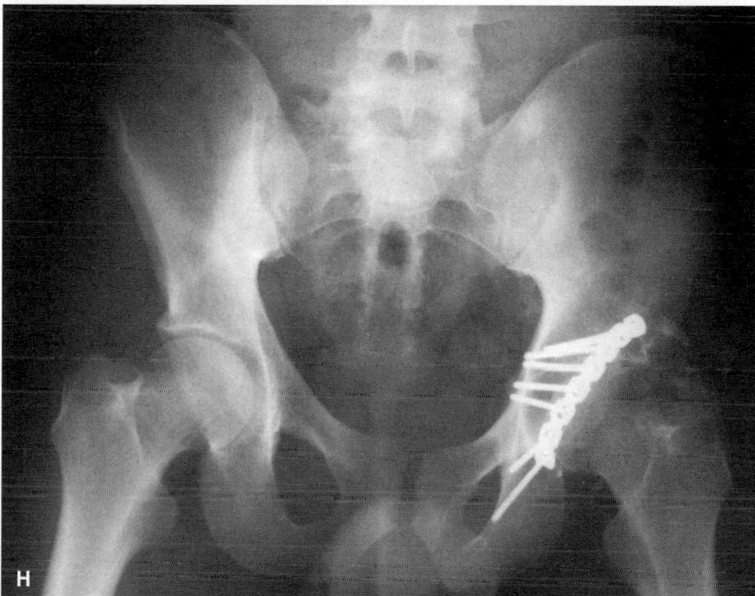

FIGURE 1-35. (continued) (**F**) Posterior view with medial displacement of distal fragment with femoral head subtracted. (**G**) Perineal view. (**H**) Anteroposterior radiograph showing reduction and stabilization by reconstruction plate. The ability to manipulate CT scans by computerized three-dimensional reconstruction and to remove obstructing structures to see clearly the geography of a fracture, allows the surgeon to plan the procedure knowing precisely what will be found at operation.

ognized. Radiographic examination without clinical examination is equally reprehensible. A distressingly high proportion of posterior dislocations of the shoulder go unrecognized because the limitation of motion is not elicited and the appropriate axillary or angle-up views are not obtained.

Neurovascular Injury

As in the case of fractures, a neurologic examination must be done. The incidence of neurologic damage is much higher with dislocations than with fractures. The sciatic nerve is often contused in posterior dislocations of the hip, with the common peroneal division taking the brunt. The common peroneal nerve is also pulled asunder by varus dislocations of the knee. Shoulder dislocations are often associated with brachial plexus or axillary nerve stretching, and radial head dislocations are associated with injury to the posterior interosseous nerve. One must always be alert to the danger of occult vascular damage, particularly in dislocations of the knee, where damage to the popliteal artery may vary from complete disruption to internal tears that

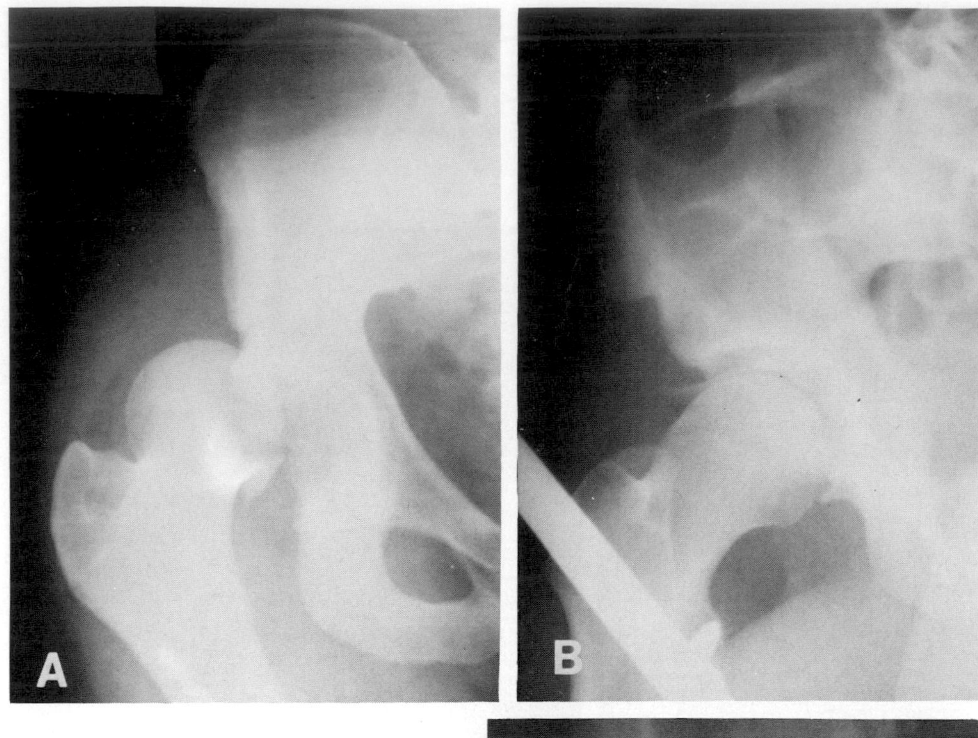

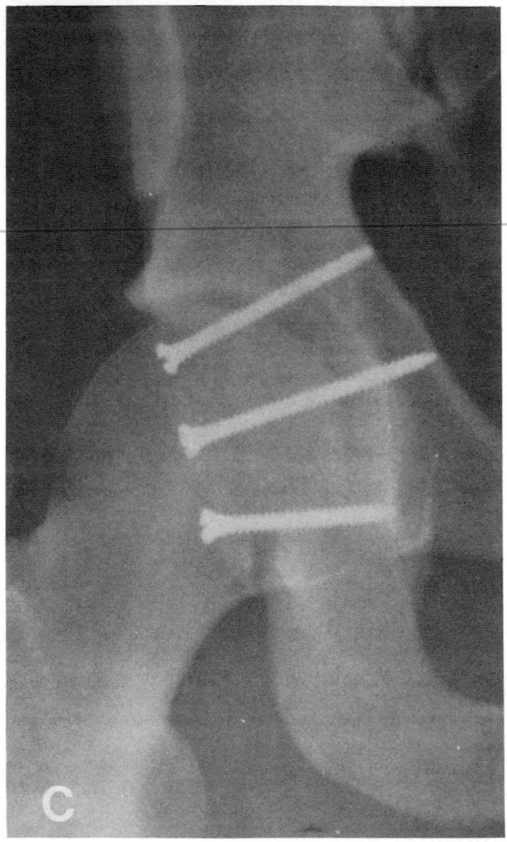

FIGURE 1-36. (**A**) A classic posterior dislocation of the hip, with the hip held in the flexed, adducted, and internally rotated position. (**B**) On closed reduction bony fragments have been reduced into the acetabulum and the hip is unstable. (**C**) The result following open reduction and internal fixation of the fragments from the posterior lip.

initiate occlusion clots. An early arteriogram is indicated when there is any suspicion of vascular damage. The presence of weak pedal pulses or Doppler flow is no guarantee that major damage to the popliteal artery has not occurred.

EMERGENCY MANAGEMENT OF FRACTURES

The treatment of fractures may be divided into three phases: emergency care, definitive treatment, and rehabilitation.

Unfortunately, physicians are rarely present to give the initial treatment at the site of the accident, and of necessity we have delegated this role to others. We cannot, however, completely abrogate our responsibility in this matter. The burden of teaching emergency medical service technicians, ambulance attendants, firemen, policemen, and others must rest with the medical profession.

Splinting

> *. . . Not only should the technical use (of splints) be appreciated by the men, but it should also be appreciated that all unnecessary handling of the injured part without splinting should be avoided. It cannot be too strongly emphasized that a wound which may be of moderate seriousness may become greatly increased in importance by careless or incompetent handling in the transport to or from the hospital.**

One of the most highly touted and least frequently obeyed maxims in emergency care is, "Splint them where they lie." London,[249] in his investigation of ambulance services in England, stated, "Little formal splintage was used; when questioned, crews often said that with a journey that was usually short they did not think that the time spent on applying splints was justifiable." In the same paper, London made the following observations: "Crews were encouraged to think in terms of comfortable support rather than splintage or immobilization. . . .What was disappointing was the infrequent use of inflatable splints."

What is true in England is, we believe, equally true in the United States. Even after being seen in emergency departments, the majority of patients are shuffled off to radiology departments without splints. Even worse, those arriving with splints not infrequently have them removed before they are sent for radiographic studies. In an informal survey of five emergency departments in Louisville, Kentucky, we found that fewer than 20% of patients with fractures had been splinted before being seen by an orthopaedist.

Adequate splinting is desirable for the following reasons:

1. Further soft-tissue injury (especially to nerves and vessels) may be averted and, most importantly, closed fractures are saved from becoming open.
2. Immobilization relieves pain.
3. Splinting may well lower the incidence of clinical fat embolism and shock.
4. Patient transportation and radiographic studies are facilitated.

Improvised Splints

The excuse should never be used that no splints were available. Almost anything rigid can be pressed into service—walking sticks, umbrellas, slats of wood—padded by almost any material that is soft. Folded newspapers or magazines make admirable splints for the arm or forearm; and when all else fails, bandaging the lower extremities together or fixing the arm to the trunk will help. For injuries of the legs and ankles, a pillow pinned or bandaged around the injured limb immobilizes by its bulk.

Conventional Splints

Basswood Splints
Basswood splints, still found in first aid kits and some hospitals, are hallowed by tradition and really fall in the category of improvised splints.

Universal Splints
Universal arm and leg splints, which are ludicrous looking, are aluminum and prefabricated to fit the leg or upper limb. These splints look like portions of discarded armor and are designed to fit everyone, and so fit no one.

Cramer Wire Splints
Cramer wire splints resemble miniature ladders with malleable metal uprights and wire rungs. They can be bent into appropriate shapes, padded, and bandaged to the extremities. They do not appreciably interfere with radiographic examinations and are most useful. This is the type of splinting advocated in *Emergency War Surgery*, the North Atlantic Treaty Organization's handbook for armed forces.[142]

Thomas Splints
Thomas splints have a long and honorable history in the emergency care of lower extremity fractures. Their introduction in World War I by Sir Robert Jones reduced the horrendous mortality from fractures of the

*Joel E. Goldthwait, Lt. Col. M.C. In Jones, Robert (ed.): Orthopaedic Surgery of Injuries. London, Oxford Medical Publications. Published by the Joint Committee of Henry Frowde, Hodder, & Stoughton, 1921.

femur from 80% to 20%. Use of the Thomas splint was continued by the British Army into World War II where, with the addition of plaster of Paris, it became the Tobruk splint.

The Thomas splint and its modifications are still in widespread use. In most emergency services, the half-ring type is used; and in fact this is required ambulance equipment by national standards. Traction is usually accomplished by a padded hitch over the shoe with a Spanish windlass, and the leg is held firmly in place with Velcro fasteners. Such special accessories for the Thomas splint are not essential. We prefer to apply the splint with triangular bandages. A narrow-fold bandage made into a clove hitch and placed over the shoe or boot without constricting the ankle provides the traction. Devices, such as the Millbank clip, are used to grasp the heel of the shoe, and spats with traction tapes are also available. Broad-fold bandages are then tied at intervals along the splint to support the limb. The whole process takes only a few minutes.

Inflatable Splints

Inflatable splints consist of a double-walled polyvinyl jacket with a zip fastener that is placed around the injured limb. A valve on the outer wall then allows the jacket to be inflated, either by mouth or by a pump.

In the past these splints were endorsed as being easy to apply, comfortable, effective, and safe. They were said to control swelling and bleeding, and are thought by some to be the splint of choice in fractured limbs that were burned.[423] We are considerably less enthusiastic about inflatable splints than these authors. Frequently, we found that they had been applied to the leg to splint fractures of the femur but barely reached the fracture site. Meanwhile, the ambulance attendant or police officer believed he or she has splinted the fracture, and the patient was certainly no better—and perhaps even worse—as a result of his or her ministrations. Although the air splints are excellent for forearm, wrist, and ankle injuries, the belief that they are the answer to all extremity injuries is unfounded.

Ashton and associates[21] have shown that these splints, when inflated to a pressure of 40 mm Hg, markedly reduced blood flow in the limbs of all 15 subjects tested and that there was complete cessation of flow in 6 of them. Inflation to 30 mm Hg caused a similar but less pronounced reduction in flow, which was further aggravated by elevation of the extremity, so that 5 of the 6 subjects tested had complete cessation of flow. It would seem that when splints are inflated to pressures that are efficient, there is danger of circulatory embarrassment, and at lower pressures they are ineffective.

The application of pneumatic splints and their effects has also been studied.[380] In one study it was found that when trained ambulance attendants inflate the splints the median pressure is 25 mm Hg (range, 15–35 mm Hg). This pressure is transmitted directly into the limb and is added to the preexisting pressure within the soft-tissue compartments. In contrast, when uneven pressure is applied to an extremity by a compressive dressing, direct transmission does not occur. It was also noted that there is a gradual loss of pressure with time with pneumatic dressings. In numerical terms, if an initial pressure of 50 to 60 mm Hg is obtained with an air splint, 75% of this pressure is transmitted to the anterior compartment of a leg. It is likely that this pressure is an additive to the preexisting compartment pressure. The same stability could be obtained easily with a firm wool and crepe dressing, without the additive pressure to the anterior compartment.

Inflatable splints should not be applied over clothing, because folds can cause high-pressure points and blistering. We have also had trouble removing splints that had adhered to an area of abrasion and other exudating surfaces such as burns.

Structural Aluminum Malleable (SAM) Splints

If one were to enumerate the properties of the ideal first-aid splint, they might be as follows: it should be efficient, light, inexpensive, easily applied to a variety of anatomical locations, easily stored or carried, and radiolucent.

Scheinberg (personal communication, 1974) invented the structural aluminum malleable (SAM) splint, which is a strip of soft aluminum 0.02-inch thick and coated with polyvinyl. Subsequently he modified the splint by coating 0.016-inch-thick aluminum foil with low-density, closed-coil polyethylene foam. Cut into 34 × $4\frac{1}{2}$-inch strips, this composite can be rolled up like a bandage or packed flat, weighs $5\frac{1}{2}$ oz, takes up very little room, and is easily carried by soldiers, ski patrols, and ambulances. When folded longitudinally (the "structural bend"), these floppy, malleable strips change as if by magic to rigid members. The structural bend gives the splint a configuration like the slat from a venetian blind. Sugar-tong splints can be made to immobilize the forearm and humerus. A two-poster splint can be made to stabilize the cervical spine, and the femur can be splinted by an aluminum Liston splint. The excess length may either be folded on itself or easily trimmed with bandage scissors. Much to our surprise, we found that SAM splints could be used many times without developing fatigue fractures. They are self-padded, are stain resistant, can be trimmed to size by scissors, and conform to any contour. Happily, they present no impediment to x-ray films, and excellent films can be obtained without removing them.

The U.S. Army is now using SAM splints, and they have also been adopted by many emergency medical services. They do not seem to be adversely affected by extremes of climate, are water and blood repellent, and have been carried by members of an expedition to climb Mt. Everest.

Splinting Open Fractures

Open fractures should be splinted exactly as closed fractures, except that the wound should be covered as early as possible. Even if sterile dressings are unavailable, a clean handkerchief over the wound is better than nothing. Gratuitous interference with wounds outside the operating room is the worst kind of meddling, and external bleeding is best managed by local pressure over the wound. We deprecate the undoing of dressing over open fractures, even in the emergency department. The only place to investigate such wounds is in the operating room under sterile conditions.

DEFINITIVE TREATMENT OF FRACTURES

Definitive treatment of fractures must be delayed until the general condition of the patient has stabilized. The establishment and maintenance of an adequate airway and the treatment of chest, abdominal, and other life-threatening injuries all take precedence over the management of fractures.

The fact that large volumes of blood may be lost even in closed fractures should not be forgotten. Fractures of the femur may be associated with a blood loss of 1 to 2.5 L and tibial fractures with a loss of 0.5 to 1.5 L. Fractures of the pelvis are notoriously treacherous in this regard and may result in exsanguination. Any patient who has sustained multiple fractures has lost a lot of blood and should have a blood sample drawn immediately for cross matching. Even if the patient appears in no great distress, it is circumspect in these cases to have a large needle or catheter in at least one vein to keep it open with saline or some other physiologic solution. Open fractures, of course, are even more dangerous from this point of view. It is good practice to estimate what the blood loss has been and to monitor the patient's physical signs, hemoglobin, and hematocrit.[90–92,154]

The objectives of the treatment of a fracture are to have the bone heal in such a position that the function and cosmesis of the extremity are unimpaired and to return patients to their vocation and avocations in the shortest possible time with the least expense. Unfortunately, these objectives are sometimes incompatible, and the goals that are to be stressed depend on the desires and needs of the patients.

It is customary to talk about the "conservative" and the "operative" treatment of fractures. Conservative does not necessarily mean nonoperative. The meaning of this word has become so corrupted by modern usage that this connotation should be dropped. We much prefer to talk of open and closed methods of treatment. Either may, on occasion, be radical or conservative, depending on one's point of view.

In North America, and I suspect in most other technically advanced countries, closed methods of fracture management are in a marked decline. The ability to produce anatomical alignment and maintain it by internal fixation, particularly by interlocking nails, is apparently making such methods passé. It has been our observation during the past 5 years that orthopaedic residents are incapable of applying casts with any degree of dexterity, although they are very expert in inserting a variety of nails. Similarly, the application of traction is an arcane, antique procedure of historical interest alone.

This state of affairs was deprecated in an editorial entitled "Fixation is Fun" in the *Journal of Bone and Joint Surgery* by Apley and Rowley,[17] who thought that open reductions were done because orthopaedists enjoyed doing them. They believed that surgeons who treat fractures should be equally adept in both methods. "Only then will every patient have the chance of being treated by the method which is best for him and also the most cost-effective for the community."[17] It is difficult to know how this should be achieved when apprentice surgeons do not see such methods employed by their preceptors.

We have struggled with this problem and have considered expunging a great deal of what follows. But we hope that this volume will be read by surgeons who might have a need for some of the information set down here. In our travels we have seen many persons very adequately treated by traditional methods, including the bone-setters of Guangzhou (Canton) from whom we can all learn something of value. There are still many parts of the world where image intensifiers, interlocking nails, and sophisticated fixators are not readily available, and the patients cannot afford them even if they were.

Closed Treatment

The closed treatment of fractures generally consists of some form of manipulation or "reduction", followed by the application of a device to maintain the reduction until healing has occurred.

Reduction

The sooner the reduction of a fracture is attempted the better, because swelling of the extremity tends to increase for 6 to 12 hours after the injury. This hemorrhage and edema in the soft tissues make them inelastic and pose a barrier to adequate reduction. Although the closed fracture is never a surgical emergency—the late Dr. John Royal Moore deferred all of his closed reductions to 1 day a week—it is easier to effect a reduction early than late.

Before embarking on the manipulative reduction, adequate x-ray films must be obtained to determine what the objectives of the manipulation are to be or if, indeed, a reduction is necessary. Perkins[310] stated that closed reduction is contraindicated when:

1. There is no significant displacement.
2. The displacement is of little concern (eg, humeral shaft).
3. No reduction is possible (eg, comminuted fracture of the head and neck of humerus).
4. The reduction, if gained, cannot be held (eg, compression fracture of the vertebral body).
5. The fracture has been produced by a traction force (eg, displaced fracture of the patella).

To achieve a reduction, the following steps usually are advised: (1) apply traction in the long axis of the limb; (2) reverse the mechanism that produced the fracture; and (3) align the fragment that can be controlled with the one that cannot.

Traction

Traction can achieve a reduction only when the fragments are connected by a soft-tissue bridge (Fig. 1-37). Indeed, no manipulative reduction can be successful without some form of soft-tissue linkage, and great care must be taken not to disrupt these soft-tissue connections by ill-advised, overstrenuous manipulation. When traction is applied to a limb, the distal fragment, guided by the soft-tissue hinge, falls into place.

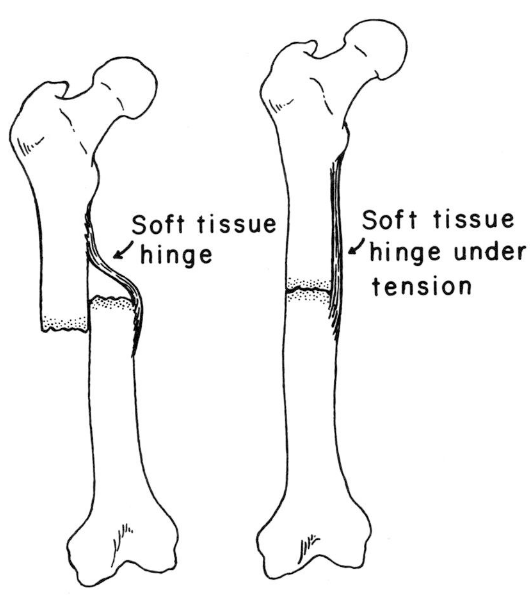

FIGURE 1-37. In most fractures a soft tissue hinge will be present between the bone ends. This hinge will lie in the concavity of the angulation in a transverse fracture, or along the vertical component of a spiral fracture. This soft tissue hinge is the linkage that allows the fracture to be reduced, and under appropriate tension it will stabilize the fracture once it has been reduced.

Unhappily, traction by itself does not always achieve this result. Where bone fragments penetrate overlying muscles, it may be impossible to disengage the fragments, so that there is a soft-tissue obstruction to reduction. One might suspect this to be so when no sensation of crepitus is present on manipulation.

A second obstruction to reduction by traction, described by Charnley,[86] is the presence of a large hematoma in the thigh with a fracture of the femur. To accommodate this blood, the thigh becomes grossly swollen and tense with an increase in its transverse diameter. As a result, the elasticity of the soft tissues is grossly reduced, and the fragments cannot be pulled out to length owing to the soft-tissue resistance.

A third mechanism, the description of which Charnley[86] ascribed to Beveridge Moore, is that of soft-tissue interlocking (Fig. 1-38). In this circumstance, the bone ends are overlapped, and the soft-tissue hinge then acts as an obstruction to the reduction. Traction, if pursued with vigor, will rupture the hinge, making the fracture completely unstable, and will lead to over-distraction. To reduce such a fracture, it must be "toggled" (ie, the angulation is increased until the bone ends disengage, after which the bone ends are latched on and the fracture is reduced by gentle traction and reversal of the angulation).

By and large, traction should be reserved for fractures that are overlapped (eg, fractures of the femur where the pull of the quadriceps shortens the bone). Unless the bone ends can be locked on and are stable, once traction is discontinued the shortening will recur.

Reversing the Mechanism of Injury

It seems axiomatic that if a fracture is produced by an external torque, it should be reduced by making the distal fragment retrace its steps—by twisting it internally. Similarly, angulation in one direction should be reduced by angulation in the opposite direction. An initial period of longitudinal traction may aid in fracture reduction by overcoming muscle pull and disimpacting the fracture, but the definitive reduction should be accomplished by reversing the mechanism of injury. For example, a Colles' fracture, which is produced by supination and dorsal angulation, should be reduced not by prolonged traction on the fingers but by pronating and flexing the distal fragment. Reduction by this method depends on the presence of a soft-tissue linkage, which, when put on the stretch, stabilizes the reduction. In oblique and transverse fractures, the soft-tissue hinge is in the concavity of the angulation, and in spiral fractures, it is in the region

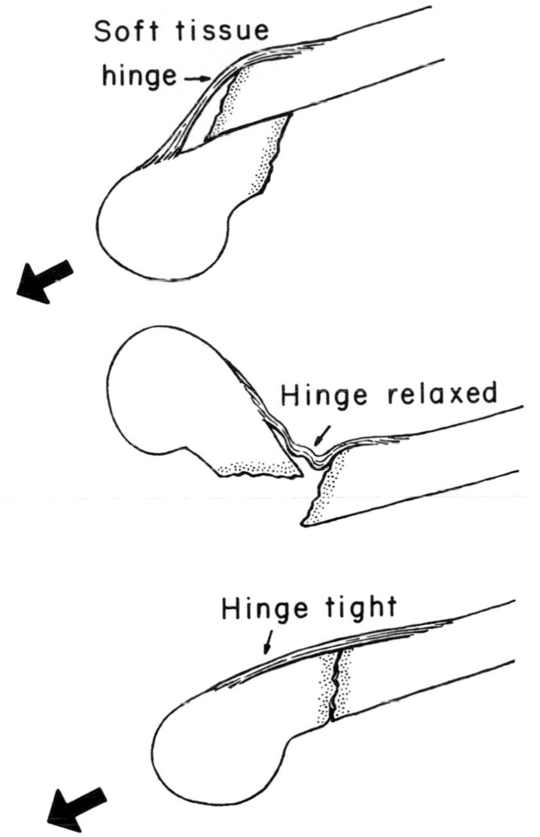

FIGURE 1-38. The soft tissue hinge may act as an obstruction to reduction by traction when the fragment ends are interlocked. Excessive traction will rupture the soft tissue hinge, making further attempts at reduction fruitless. Under these circumstances the fracture should be angulated to relax the soft tissue hinge, and then further traction and angulation in the opposite direction will reduce and stabilize the fracture.

of the vertical fracture line. Where there is no soft-tissue hinge, closed reduction is not feasible.

Aligning the Fragment That Can Be Controlled

By and large, the recommendation to align the fragment that can be controlled with the one that cannot be is somewhat simplistic. Essentially, the fragment that can be controlled is the distal fragment, and this should be lined up with the proximal fragment. The proximal fragment adopts a position dictated by the pull of the muscles attached to it. In fractures of the forearm, the key to reduction is the position of the proximal radial fragment. If the fracture is through the proximal third, the proximal fragment will be strongly supinated by the supinator and biceps, and the forearm must be manipulated accordingly. A fracture at a lower level adds the action of the pronator teres, so that the proximal fragment is in a position midway between full supination and full pronation. A slavish adherence to this dictum may lead one astray on occasion and should be tempered by what the x-ray shows. Similarly, in the closed management of transverse subtrochanteric fractures, the proximal fragment is flexed, abducted, and externally rotated, and the distal fragment must be aligned with the proximal fragment to effect a successful reduction.

Immobilization

Once a satisfactory reduction has been achieved, it must then be maintained until primary union has taken place. Immobilization may be provided by a cast, continuous traction, or some form of splint.

Plaster-of-Paris Casts†

The use of splints for the maintenance of fracture reduction has been practiced from time immemorial. Albucasis immobilized fractures by bandages made stiff with egg albumin. The genius who first impregnated a dressing with dehydrated gypsum to be used in the treatment of battlefield injuries was a Flemish military surgeon named Antonius Mathijsen.[255] This invention, which eventually developed into the modern plaster bandage, is second in importance only to x-rays in the history of fracture treatment.

The plaster-of-Paris bandage consists of a roll of muslin stiffened by dextrose or starch and impregnated with the hemihydrate of calcium sulfate. When water is added, the calcium sulfate takes up its water of crystallization ($CaSO_4 \cdot H_2O + H_2O \rightleftharpoons CaSO_4 \cdot 2H_2O$ + heat). This is an exothermic reaction, and after a few minutes the plaster-of-Paris becomes a homogeneous, rocklike mass. Accelerator substances are added to the bandages to afford a spectrum of available setting rates ranging from slow to extra fast. Setting may be accelerated by increasing the temperature of the water or by adding alum and slowed by adding common salt.

Methods of Application. Every orthopaedist has his own preferred method of applying plaster-of-Paris casts, but in essence there are three schools.

Skin-Tight Cast. The skin-tight cast was advocated by Böhler, the famous Viennese fracture surgeon. The plaster-of-Paris bandage is applied directly to the skin without any intervening padding, in an effort to gain the most efficient immobilization possible. This type of cast is rarely used now. It required a great deal of skill to apply and was fraught with the danger of pressure sores and circulatory embarrassment. It was uncomfortable to remove because the patient's hair was incorporated into the cast.

Bologna Cast. The Bologna cast, emanating from the Rizzoli Institute, was advocated by Charnley.[86] In contrast to Böhler's method, generous amounts of cotton

---

†Although the correct term is plaster-of-Paris cases, or casings, it does seem rather pedantic, and we shall use the incorrect but common appellation, cast.

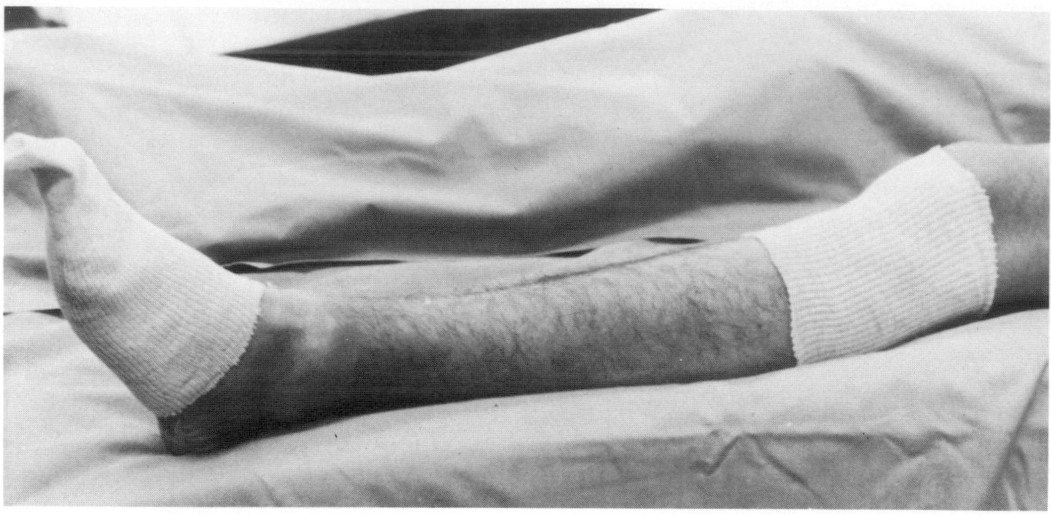

FIGURE 1-39. It is necessary to use stockinette only at the upper and lower ends of the cast. Not only is this economical, but it also prevents tension of the stockinette over bony prominences that may later give rise to burning pain and even pressure sores.

wadding are applied to the limb and compressed by the plaster bandage with "just the right amount of tension." This technique is said by Charnley to be demanding, so most surgeons (including us) split the difference and apply a padded cast without tension. We shall call this the "third way."

Third Way. In the third way, most orthopaedists use stockinette, a tubular knitted stocking that stretches freely in diameter but sparingly in length. Stockinette may be applied over the entire member to be immobilized, but our preference is to apply just two segments, to cover the upper and lower ends of the casts (Fig. 1-39). The stockinette makes the cast look tidy and pads its sharp margins. It is probably best to avoid stockinette in postoperative casts where swelling is anticipated.

Sheet wadding is applied over the stockinette from the distal to the proximal end of the limb, as smoothly as possible. Each turn should be applied transversely, tearing the border that traverses the greater diameter of the limb so that it lies smoothly (Fig. 1-40). Various types of wadding are available; our preference is for the rather soft, quilted variety that can be stretched easily. The more densely compressed forms of wadding are more likely to exert a tourniquet effect if they become wadded or displaced. The amount of wadding to be used depends on how much swelling one anticipates after the application of the cast. Too much padding reduces the efficacy of the cast, and the more padding that is used, the more plaster that is necessary. Thighs are so well padded by nature that we apply the plaster directly on the stockinette without any padding. It is circumspect to apply a little extra padding to bony prominences such as the heel and malleoli. If felt pads are to be used, they must be applied as the most superficial layer, immediately under the plaster. Since they adhere to the plaster, they cannot displace. When not fixed by this means, pads may wander and give rise to embarrassing pressure sores.

The rolled plaster bandage must be thoroughly immersed in water until air bubbles stop rising. At this point the bandage is saturated with water and should be held with one end in each hand and gently squeezed. It never should be wrung out like a washcloth, since this tends to leave the plaster of Paris in

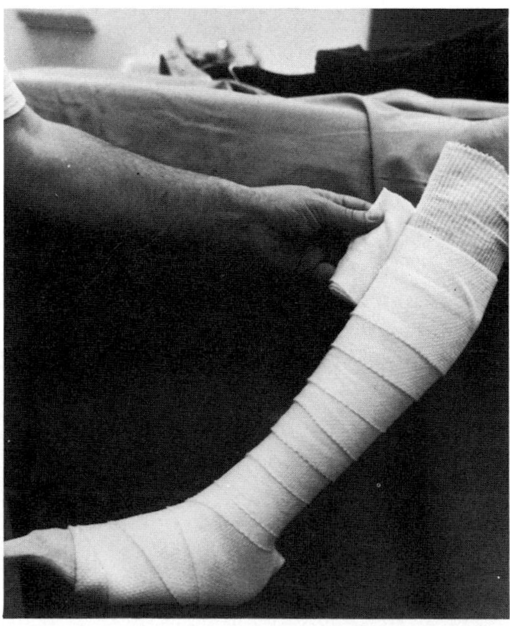

FIGURE 1-40. Padding should be applied from distal to proximal, taking care to apply the padding evenly. Each turn should be overlapped by 50% of the succeeding turn.

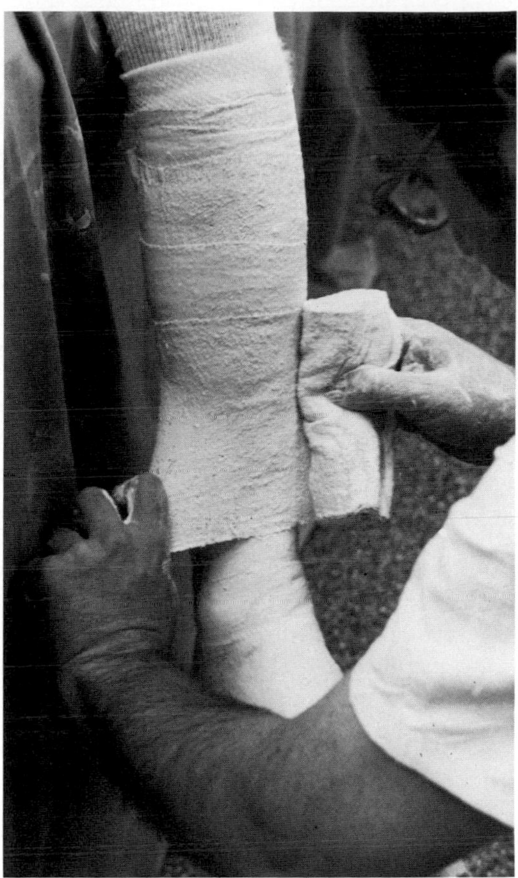

FIGURE 1-41. The plaster-of-Paris bandage should be applied in the same direction as the wadding. The roll should be applied with the fingertips and must never be removed from the extremity. To make the bandage conform to the varying circumferences of the arm or leg, tucks should be taken in it with the left hand.

the pail rather than in the bandage. It is also prudent to unwrap the first 2 or 3 inches before wetting so that the tail of the bandage can be located easily. It has been our practice to use cold water only, especially when using extra-fast-setting plaster. This allows more time to mold the cast and rub the layers of the cast together. We formerly believed that cold water also gave us the strongest cast, but Callahan and associates[74] have showed this is not true. They found that when the dip water was 35°C, the resulting cast was stronger than when the dip water was 10°C. However, in their conclusions they believed that this difference in strength was not great enough to be of major importance clinically.

The largest bandage that can be handled should be used: 8-inch for the thigh, 6-inch for the leg, 4-inch for the hand and forearm. When the plaster is applied with the bandage held vertically, the central core tends to drop out. This can be prevented by pushing it back at intervals with the opposite thumb. The plaster bandage should be rolled onto the limb in the same direction as the wadding. At all times the bandage should be in contact with the limb; if it is rolled on by the fingertips, it can never be too tight. Each turn of the bandage should overlap the preceding turn by half, and the bandage should always be moving (Fig. 1-41). It is permissible to put two turns in the same place only at the upper and lower extremities of the cast. In this way the cast is uniformly thick throughout its length. Areas of uneven thickness act as stress risers; the cast tends to break at the juncture between thick and thin.

The bandage should always be laid on transversely, and tucks are taken in the lower border by the left hand to accommodate for the changing circumference of the limb. Each turn is smoothed by the left thenar eminence as it is laid down, and the bandage is smoothed by the palms of both hands after it is applied, so that every layer is melded with the other into a homogeneous whole. Where this is not done, the cast is lamellated and much weaker than it should be. A plaster bandage should never be reversed, as may be done when applying a gauze bandage. If one does so, the bandage runs against the grain and cannot be applied easily.

A plaster-of-Paris cast should always be made too long and then trimmed to size with a sharp knife or a cast saw. We prefer a scalpel, which should be held

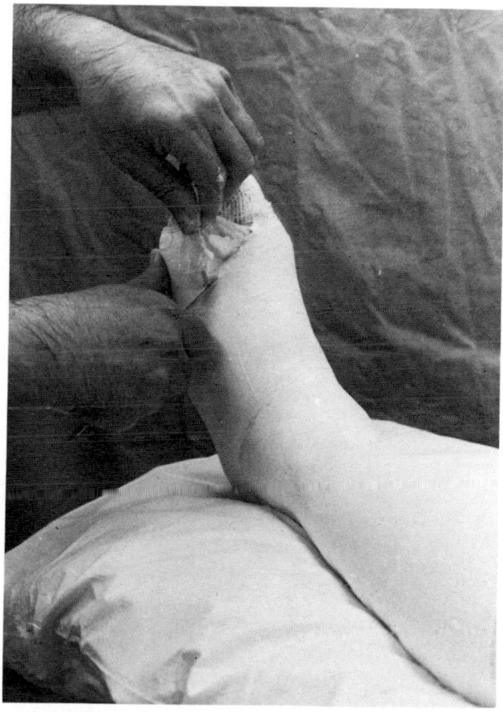

FIGURE 1-42. In trimming the extremities of plaster-of-Paris casts, a good method is to brace the thumb against the plaster and hold a sharp knife in the remaining four fingers. Tension is applied to the plaster to be removed by the other hand as the knife cuts.

with the four fingers and the palm while the thumb is braced against the cast to prevent slipping. The plaster to be removed is held in the left hand and pulled while the blade cuts (Fig. 1-42). After trimming, the stockinette is folded over the cut edge and fixed by a turn of bandage or by a plaster strip (Fig. 1-43).

In reducing fractures, it is often necessary to manipulate the fracture through the wet cast for the final adjustment. This requires the cast to be applied as quickly and as dexterously as possible. These manipulations must be done with the palms and thenar eminences (Fig. 1-44). On no account must the cast be indented by a fingertip, because this will almost certainly produce a pressure sore in the underlying skin. In molding the cast to achieve three-point fixation, one hand must exert pressure over the fracture site on the side opposite the soft-tissue bridge, while the other hand gently massages the distal fragment in the proper direction to close the gap. As Charnley advised, "It takes a curved cast to produce a straight bone" (Fig. 1-45).

Once the plaster is felt to "set," all manipulations must be halted until the cast gains functional strength. During this "green period" it is very easy to crack the cast, and this defect can be remedied only by the addition of further layers of plaster, making the cast heavier than desirable. The ultimate strength of the cast depends on its thickness, the degree to which the layers are fused together, and the smoothness of the finish. To achieve the maximum strength for a given amount of plaster, rubbing with wet hands is essential. The operator should always have the bucket nearby so that he or she may easily dip his or her hands in the water. Rubber gloves are said to help make the cast smoother,[263] but they also make the bandage slippery and less easy to control. (The parsimonious senior author of this chapter [JWH] decries the use of rubber gloves merely to apply a cast and considers it effete, but he is a minority of one.)

The removal of troublesome plaster of Paris adhering to the hairs of the surgeon's forearm can be facilitated by adding some sugar to the hands when washing.

For most purposes a cast that is $^{1}/_{4}$-inch thick will be adequate and, in general, upper extremity casts need

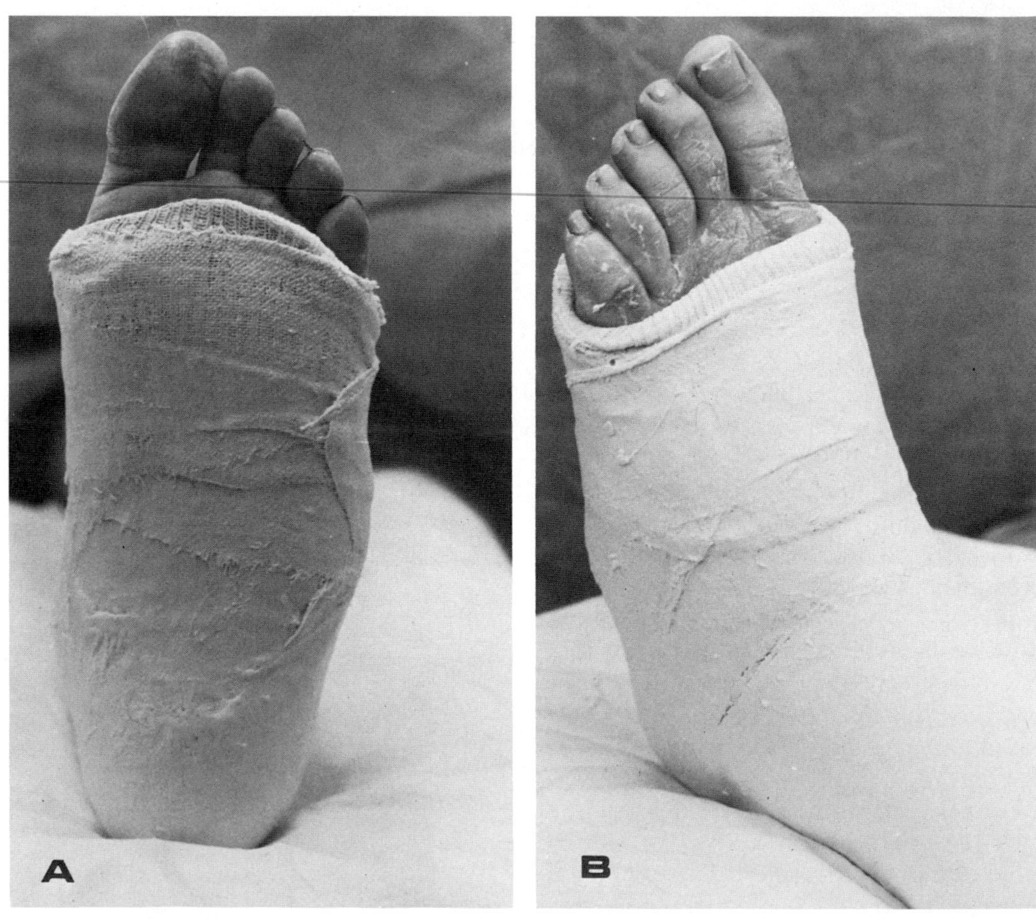

FIGURE 1-43. (**A** and **B**) Casts should be trimmed so that the fingers and toes are free to move. The stockinette is then folded over the edges of the cast and anchored with a plaster-of-Paris strip. Care should always be taken to make sure that the lateral border of the cast does not impinge on the fifth toe.

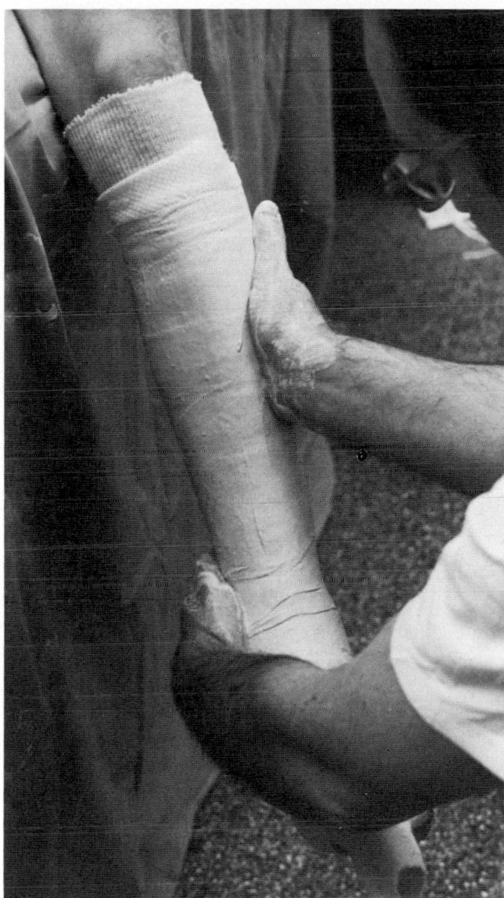

FIGURE 1-44. When manipulating through a wet cast or rubbing in the turns of the bandage, always use the palms of the hands and thenar eminences and never the fingertips.

much less plaster than do weight-bearing casts of the lower extremity. A forearm gauntlet cast can be applied with no more than one 4-inch bandage in a woman and a below-knee cast can be applied with three or four 6-inch bandages.

A cast that looks good might conceivably be wrong, but a cast that looks bad cannot be right. The expeditious, efficient application of plaster is as important a skill for the apprentice orthopaedist to acquire as the use of a scalpel, and an ill-applied cast can negate the results of an impeccable surgical procedure.

Upper-Extremity Casts. Casts on the upper extremity may extend above the elbow or be limited to the forearm and hand. In either case, the cast should be trimmed along the line of the knuckles on the dorsum and obliquely across the proximal flexion crease of the palm on the volar side to allow unrestricted motion of the fingers. A hole should be cut out around the thumb just large enough to allow unrestricted motion. The edges of this thumb hole must be carefully everted, so that the sharp edge does not cut the skin (see Fig. 1-62). Occasionally, the thumb may be included in the cast, as in treating scaphoid fractures.

Lower-Extremity Casts. Long-leg casts may be applied with the knee flexed or extended, but if weight-bearing is to be allowed, the knee should be neutral or in 5° of flexion. The cast should be trimmed in line with the metatarsal heads on the plantar aspect and at the base of the toes dorsally. The fifth toe must be entirely free; this is a common site for a plaster sore (see Fig. 1-43). Perkins[309] stated that it is most important not to immobilize the forefoot in varus, and he left the metatarsal heads free to bear weight. If a toe plate is used, the metatarsophalangeal joints must not be held in hyperextension. In fractures of the lower third of the tibia, dorsiflexion of the foot frequently causes angulation of the fracture. It is quite permissible under these circumstances to immobilize

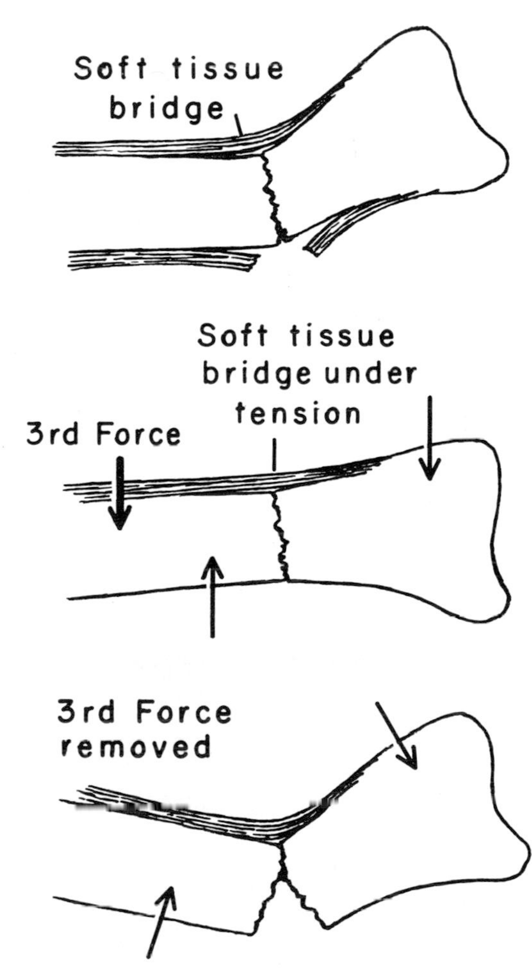

FIGURE 1-45. To maintain the reduction of the fracture, a three-point system must be used. The cast should be molded so that the soft tissue bridge is under tension. This means that the forces must be applied as in this diagram. Should one of the three forces be removed, the system becomes unstable. (*After Charnley, J.: The Closed Treatment of Common Fractures, 3rd ed. Edinburgh, E. & S. Livingstone, 1968.*)

the foot in plantarflexion, although in fractures of the ankle this would be proscribed. When the foot is immobilized in plantarflexion and a walking heel is applied, the contralateral shoe should be raised to equalize leg lengths.

Böhler walking irons and rubber walking heels have largely become supplanted by plaster boots or cast shoes. These have the advantage of being removable at bedtime, and the patient walks with a better gait. The only indication for a rubber heel in our practice is when we employ early weight bearing in a tibial fracture where the foot is in equinus.

Many orthopaedists reinforce their casts by applying splints to the posterior aspect of the cast. This adds weight without adding much strength. The same amount of plaster applied anteriorly as a fin strengthens the cast immeasurably, making fracture of the cast at the ankle virtually impossible (Fig. 1-46).

Patellar Tendon-Bearing Casts. Patellar tendon-bearing (PTB) casts were devised by Sarmiento[23,364] to immobilize fractures of the tibial shaft and at the same time allow the knee to bend. We have tended to use an above-knee cast, as recommended by Dehne,[114,115] for the first 2 or 3 weeks after reduction, and then replace it with a PTB cast. This type of cast must be applied with care over minimal padding and is applied in segments. In applying the upper portion of the cast, the knee should be flexed to a right angle and the cast molded flat over the upper calf to give a triangular cross section. The cast is molded anteriorly around the patella, and an indentation is made over the patellar tendon (Fig. 1-47). The cast is trimmed to look like a PTB prosthesis, and it is most important to trim the cast like a wing-back chair around the femoral condyles to prevent rotation of the proximal tibia on weight bearing (see Figs. 1-47 and 1-48).

Cast Braces. Cast braces enjoyed a considerable vogue during the 1970s for the management of femoral fractures and fractures of the tibial plateau. After preliminary treatment by traction, the cast brace is applied when the fracture is "stable and firm." In essence, a long-leg cast is applied over a long Spandex stocking, with the upper end molded to the shape of a quadrilateral socket, or a plastic socket is incorporated in the cast. The knee is then cut out and hinged. Although excellent results were obtained by this method of treatment especially in the distal third of the femur, it required meticulous care and a great deal of supervision of the patient. Complications were common, and the method is no longer popular in the United States (see Fig. 1-96).

Hip and Shoulder Spicas. We abhor the use of hip and shoulder spicas because they are large, heavy, and cumbersome and are highly inefficient in the immobilization of fractures in adults. In the past, patients were frequently sent home in hip spicas to make space in hospitals. In their home environment, if no one cares for them, they may lie unturned, soaking in their own urine and feces and manufacturing immense decubitus ulcers. We have seen a paraplegic woman with a fractured spine transported in a double hip spica, who on arrival had bone showing over both iliac spines, both greater trochanters, and her sacrum (Fig. 1-49). It is hazardous to place patients in spicas when they lack sensation, and it is only under the most unusual circumstances that we would now advocate the use of

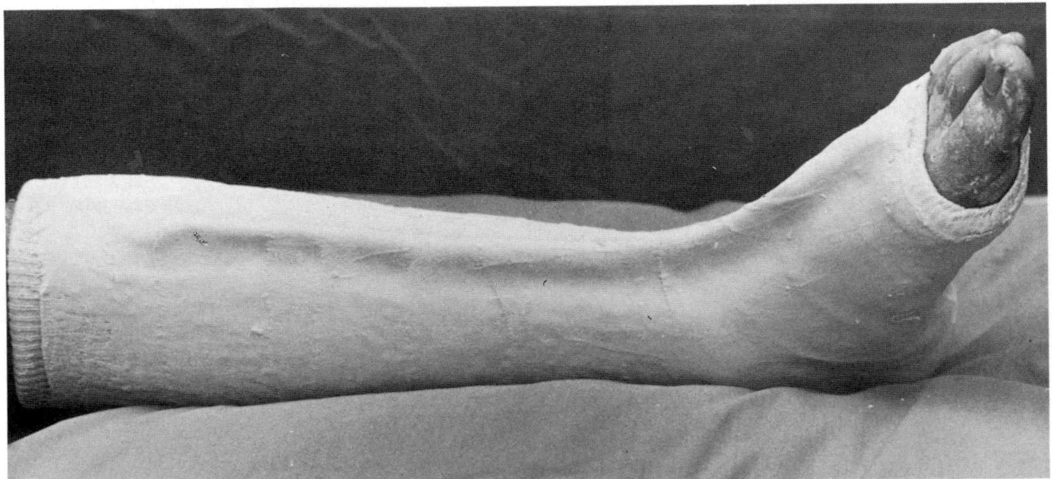

FIGURE 1-46. To reinforce the cast with a splint, it is much better to apply it in the concavity of an angulation, as an I-beam or fin, than to apply it over a convexity, such as a lamina. Such a fin substantially increases the strength of the ankle, whereas the same amount of plaster applied posteriorly would have very little effect.

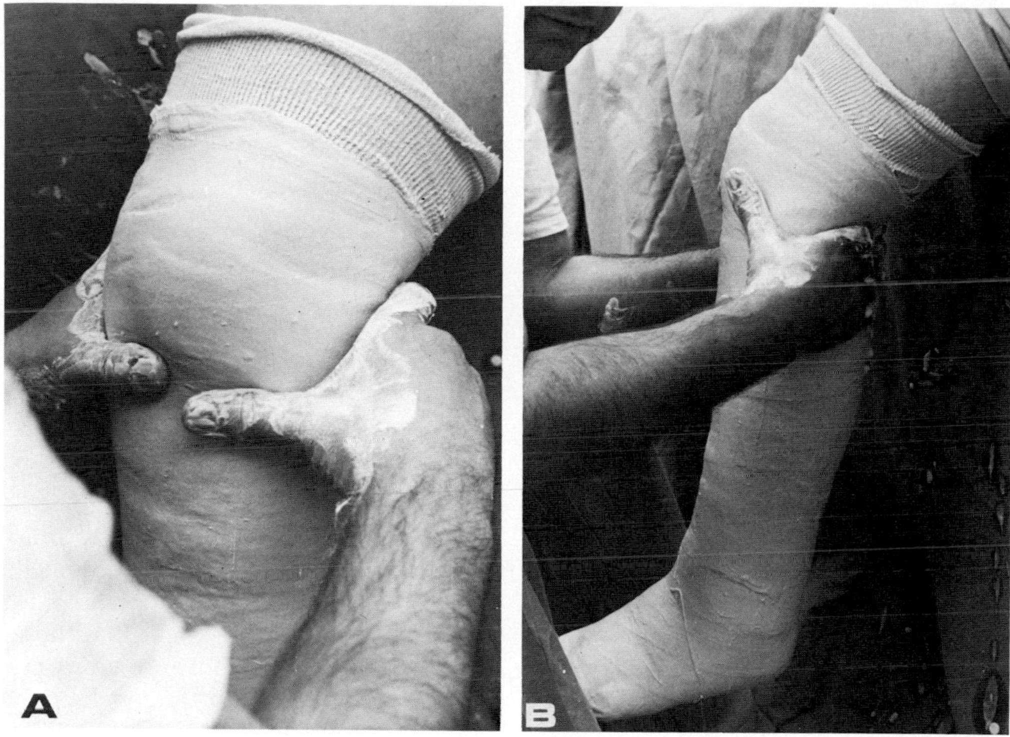

FIGURE 1-47. (**A** and **B**) In the application of a patellar tendon–bearing cast, indentation must be made over the patellar tendon, and the cast must be carefully molded around the patella. At the same time, the posterior calf must be molded to make a triangular cross section at the upper end of the leg.

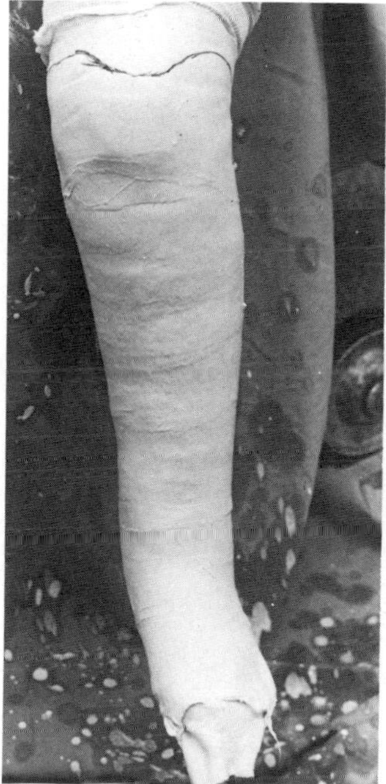

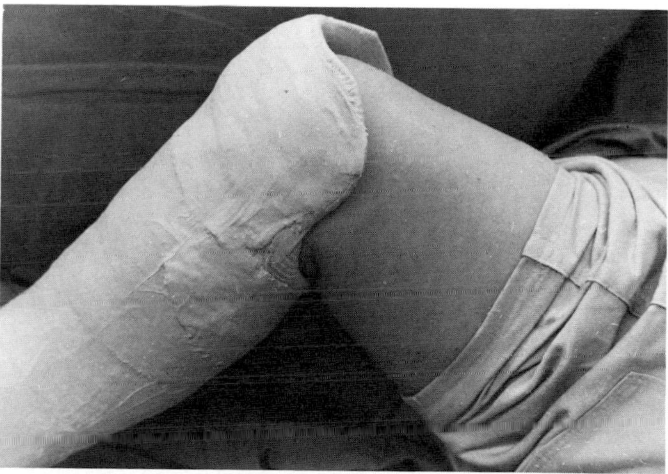

FIGURE 1-48. The patellar tendon-bearing cast should be cut out to resemble a patellar tendon-bearing prosthesis, and it is particularly important to trim the lateral portion like a wing-back chair. When the knee is flexed, pressure is taken from the patellar tendon, but in full extension, pressure is exerted on the thick skin over the tendon.

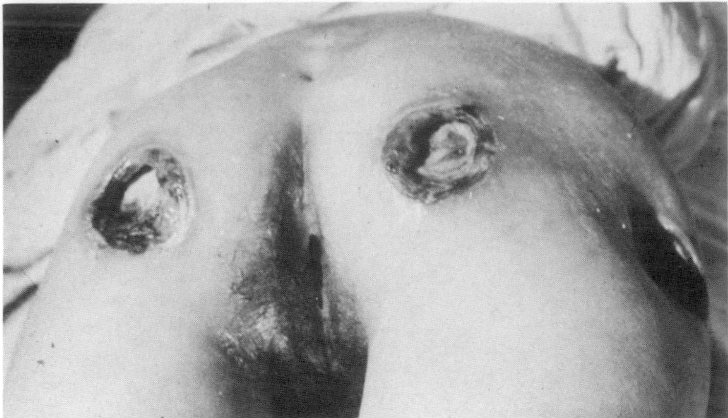

FIGURE 1-49. This paraplegic woman was transported in a double hip spica. On arrival at her new hospital she had large decubiti over both ischial tuberosities, both greater trochanters, and both anterior superior iliac spines. The application of circular casts or spicas in patients without sensation is fraught with terrible danger and should rarely be done.

the hip spica in adult fractures; however, they may still play a role in childrens' fractures.

To reduce the weight of these casts and make the patient more comfortable, a substantial window should be cut out over the belly. This portion of the cast contributes nothing to its strength, but the window should always be circular or oval and never rectangular, because corners act as stress risers. This means that it is best cut with a knife. If one waits too long, cutting the hard plaster can be tedious. The task is made easier by outlining the window with the knife and then making a cross with the plaster saw within the circle. The free corners may then be pried up and the cutting of the circumference completed with ease (Fig. 1-50).

Older orthopaedists at some time or other in their career have been embarrassed by the disconcerting habit that spicas have of breaking at the hip. This is sometimes caused when a triangular area, commonly known as the "intern's angle," at the junction of the limb and trunk does not receive its fair share of the plaster. It also results, as Strange[397] pointed out, from the juncture of the body and leg being an open section and thus very much weaker than the circular portions of the cast (Fig. 1-51). To strengthen this weak point, fin-like reinforcements are applied anteriorly, posteriorly, and laterally, much in the same way that a walking cast might be reinforced (see Fig. 1-46).

Wedging Plaster-of-Paris Casts. After an attempted closed reduction and the application of a circular cast,

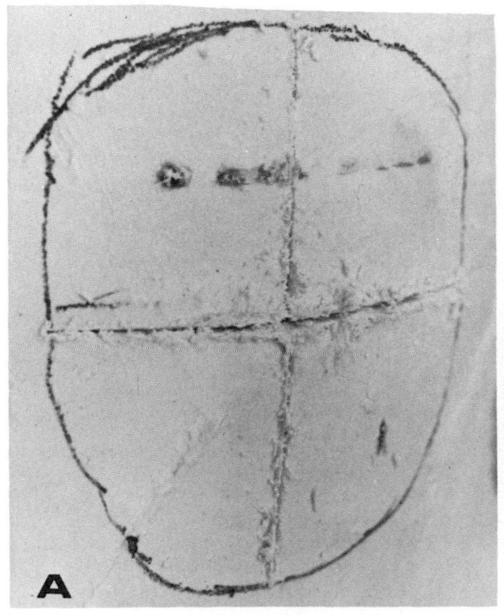

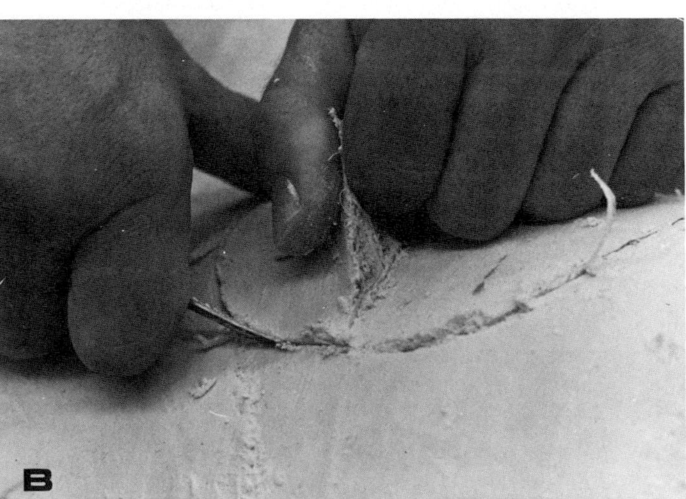

FIGURE 1-50. (**A** and **B**) Cutting a belly hole in a plaster jacket or spica can be tedious, especially when the plaster is hard. The easiest method is to outline the dimensions of the hole with a pencil and then divide the area into four quadrants with a reciprocating plaster saw. The circle is then outlined with a knife along the pencil marks, and the free edges of the quadrant can be pried upward and the periphery cut with the knife. It is always safer to brace the thumb against the cast to prevent the knife from slipping.

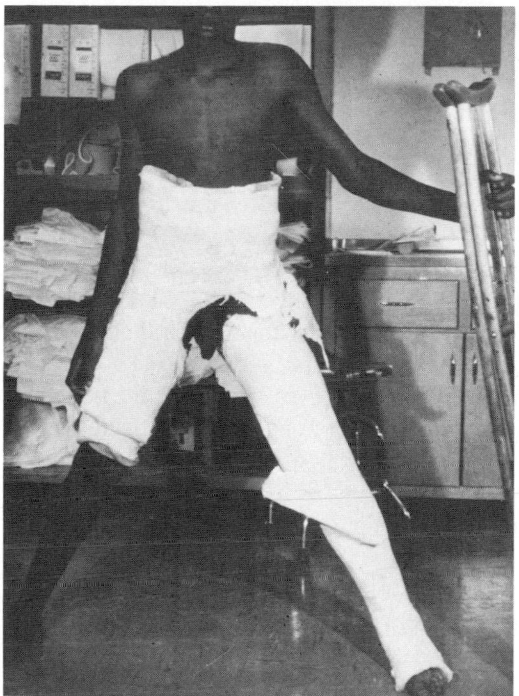

FIGURE 1-51. This sporting patient walked in his spica, which failed at its weakest point, the open section of the thigh at the "intern's angle."

there may be some residual varus or valgus angulation or posterior bow. Under these circumstances, it is quite permissible to make a transverse cut two thirds of the way around the cast (leaving a hinge opposite the convexity of the angulation) and open up the cut until the angulation is adequately corrected. The cut edges of the cast must then be everted with molders, or, if these are not available, pliers. Some surgeons place little blocks of wood or corks to hold the wedge open, but these are unnecessary and potentially dangerous because they may exert pressure on the underlying skin. We generally pack some sheet wadding in the defect and repair the cast while holding the limb in the corrected position. To gain the greatest mechanical advantage, the wedge should be made at the point where the central long axes of both fragments intersect; this point can be ascertained by drawing the appropriate lines on the x-ray film.[86] The geometry and technique of wedging has been described in some detail by Husted.[213] It must be stressed, however, that wedging will correct only angulation, never lateral shift or rotation. We find the greatest use for wedging in fractures of the tibia, where the correction tends to be comparatively small. If large corrections are to be made, a combination of an opening wedge on the concave side and closing wedge on the convex side is safer, because a large opening wedge will elongate the cast and apply undue pressure on the dorsum of the foot. However, if large corrections are necessary, we usually apply a new cast.

Windows in Casts. There are times when it is necessary to inspect wounds under casts, and making windows to do so seems reasonable. If at the time of cast application such a window is known to be necessary, it is a good plan to apply a large bolus of dressings over the wound, so that it sticks out. One may then take a sharp knife and cut around the periphery of this wad, leaving an oval hole. A rectangular hole cut with a saw makes the cast weak, because the corners act as stress risers. The cast might reasonably be reinforced by a dorsal fin to make up for the weakness of the open section.

Windows in casts are hazardous if left open, especially if there is any tendency for the limb to swell. The soft tissue may herniate through the hole, becoming grossly edematous, and the skin tends to break down from the pressure produced by the margins of the defect. To avoid this complication, we generally cut a piece of felt or sponge rubber to the size of the hole and bandage this snugly in place over the dressings with an elastic bandage to provide uniform compression.

Plaster-of-Paris Splints

Thus far we have been describing only circular casts, where the entire circumference of the anatomical part is encased. However, plaster-of-Paris may be used in the form of splints, either as first aid or, in some cases, as the definitive treatment of fractures.

The two most common types of splint used in the upper extremity are the radial slab and the sugar tong. In adult fracture work, both of these splints may be used in the treatment of a Colles' fracture.

Radial Slab. The radial slab consists of eight to ten thicknesses of 6-inch plaster with a thumb hole cut in it. No padding other than stockinette is used, and the wet plaster is applied to the radial side of the forearm, overlapping the dorsal and volar surfaces of the wrist and forearm. This splint is applied and then wrapped with a wet gauze bandage (2- or 3-inch) and allowed to set. Owing to the tendency of the fingers to swell after Colles' fractures, we sometimes apply a hand dressing of fluffs or absorbent cotton on top of the splint with only the fingertips showing and elevate the arm. Should there be any circulatory embarrassment, the splint is easily removed with a pair of scissors. Increasingly in our practice we have used the Ullson nail in Colles' fractures but supplement it initially by plaster splints.

Sugar Tong Splint. Although the radial slab has not been popular in the United States, the sugar-tong splint has. After reduction of the fracture, a splint is run from the knuckles on the dorsum over the flexed elbow and the volar aspect of the forearm to the mid-palmar crease. Padding is applied either before the plaster or as a longitudinal strip along with the plaster. It is molded while setting and wrapped with gauze or an elastic wrap. This, of course, limits the motion of the elbow and, like the radial slab, is easily removed. We have an aversion to using the sugar tong splint for Colles' fractures, probably because of our own ineptitude, but we never feel that we can adequately control the radial shift, which is the key to mastery of this troublesome fracture. We do not have the same reservations, however, about the treatment of fractures of the humeral shaft. A sugar tong splint running from the axilla medially to the shoulder laterally, combined with a collar and cuff or a stockinette Velpeau, is an admirable way to treat these fractures.

In the lower extremity, posterior splints are frequently used for the temporary splintage of fractures or for immobilization after open reduction when circular casts may be contraindicated because of the danger of postoperative swelling. When such splints are used, particularly when the knee is to be included, they must be made thick enough to support the load without breaking. Thick splints incur the danger of thermal injury so that one must take steps to prevent burns (see Thermal Effects of Plaster, p. 52).

The Efficacy of Plaster Immobilization

The object of applying a plaster-of-Paris cast is to keep the bone ends in apposition and the fracture aligned until the fracture heals. It has been said that immobilization by plaster will work only where the soft-tissue hinge is intact, where there is inherent stability of the reduced fracture, and where the cast is properly applied using a three-point system. When a bone is fractured and not widely separated, the soft-tissue hinge in the concavity of the angulation or around the vertical fracture in a spiral fracture is, as we have seen, the linkage that allows us to reduce the fracture with manipulation. If no soft-tissue bridge is present, reduction by manipulation is not feasible and a fracture will stay reduced only if the soft-tissue bridge remains under tension. This requires three-point fixation, which is achieved by molding the wet cast in a similar manner to the way the fracture was reduced initially. Two of these three points, therefore, are applied by the hands. Two forces acting alone *cannot* stabilize a fracture; a third force must be present. This third force is supplied by the portion of the cast over the proximal portion of the limb (see Fig. 1-45). With overreduction, the bridge is under the greatest tension and the reduction is even more stable—"a curved plaster is necessary in order to make a straight limb."[86]

Charnley[86] divided fractures into three categories: (1) those with inherent stability against shortening (transverse fractures), (2) those with potential stability against shortening (oblique fractures less than 45° to the long axis of the bone), and (3) those with no stability against shortening (oblique, spiral, and comminuted fractures). Only the first two categories, he believed, are suitable for immobilization by casts alone.

However, there is another factor: the hydrodynamic effect of the cast. Because the soft tissues are semifluid, the hydrostatic pressure increases when they are compressed by a cast. This increased tension tends to keep the limb from shortening as it most certainly would do were it unsupported. We believe it is this factor that makes possible the success of the Dehne method[114,115] of early ambulation in fractures of the tibia. Initially, Sarmiento[364] believed that by the application of a PTB cast, he would be able to bypass the tibial fracture and transfer weight from the foot to the proximal tibia. After making a series of biomechanical studies, he no longer believes this and attributes the success of his cast to the "hydraulic container" effect.[365] However, Sven Hansen and associates[398b] have studied above-knee, below-knee, and PTB casts by measuring the load on the heel while weight bearing. The results were identical for all three casts, and it was concluded that there was no fracture-suspending effect produced by PTB casts.

We have treated many oblique, spiral, and, indeed, comminuted fractures of the tibia with weight-bearing casts with no more than 1.25 cm of shortening after healing. We would admit, however, that some such fractures do need a little help with transfixation pins for 3 or 4 weeks to prevent undue shortening. However, this is now generally achieved by an external fixator rather than by pins and plaster. The need to resort to such measures is perhaps more related to the skill of the surgeon in applying the cast than to the inherent instability of the fracture.

It would be very naive to believe that absolute immobilization can ever be achieved by any type of external splint. Patients are often quite conscious of movement of the fracture fragments in the early days of treatment, but, with the production of callus and its progressive stiffening, this disappears.

Hicks[200] applied casts to two lower limbs with simulated tibial fractures that had been amputated through the distal third of the femur. These casts were applied "more tightly than would ever have been risked in clinical practice." When he windowed the casts over the fracture sites, he was able to produce a lateral shift of 2.5 cm in one and more than 3 cm in the other merely by pushing with his fingers. "Rotation to the extent of 20° and angulation to the extent of 6° were just as easily obtained."

Hicks[200] has also shown that plaster-of-Paris casts applied ostensibly to immobilize fracture fragments may have the reverse effect and increase the amplitude of motion at the fracture site. A slavish obedience to the rule of immobilizing the joints proximal and distal to the fracture does not necessarily ensure better fixation of the fracture. In fractures of the forearm, an above-elbow cast prevents the muscles spanning the elbow from exerting their action on the elbow joint. As a result their pull is transmitted distally to the fracture sites. The action of the brachioradialis that inserts in the distal radius is a deforming force in Colles' and Galeazzi fractures. London[250] has shown that when forearm fractures in children are treated with forearm casts, late redisplacement of the fractures does not occur. Although this method of treatment does not seem applicable to fractures of the forearm in adults, owing to their "inherent lack of stability," Sarmiento reported on the management of 42 forearm fractures by a functional brace that allows "early freedom of motion of all joints."[212a,212b,366] No one who has suffered through the travail of trying to achieve union in indolent supracondylar fractures of the humerus or femur with ankylosis of the elbow or knee can doubt that the immobilization of a joint has a deleterious effect on the healing of a contiguous fracture.

Furthermore, Hicks[200] has also demonstrated that if, in an amputated specimen with a fractured tibia, the action of the peroneal tendon is simulated, the subtalar joint is fixed by the cast and the lower fragment of the tibia is rotated externally. Similarly, simulated inverter action is accompanied by rotation of this fragment in the reverse direction. A total range of 12° rotation is produced by this means. This experimental evidence lends credence to the clinical observation of Sarmiento[364,365] that free motion of the foot and ankle is not deleterious in the treatment of tibial fractures.

It would appear, then, that for at least some fractures of the forearm and leg better immobilization is obtained by casts employing three-point fixation of the fractures and not of the joints.

Fiberglass Casts

Until recently there had been no challenge to the plaster-of-Paris bandage as the material to employ in the making of casts. Plastic materials requiring ultraviolet light to "cure" the casts gave a lightweight, durable product but were time-consuming and inconvenient to apply.[245] In recent years, however, a variety of knitted materials—cotton, rayon, and fiberglass—have been impregnated with polyurethane pre-polymer, which when soaked in water cures to form a light, durable, material that is radiolucent. The pre-polymer molecules have isocyanate end-groups that react with any molecule containing an active hydrogen,[445] and the chemical reaction is:

$$\text{Pre-polymer} + H_2O \begin{cases} CO_2 \\ \text{Polyurethane polymer} \end{cases}$$

The most popular bandage material is knitted fiberglass, and typically there is a ratio of 45% polyurethane resin to 55% fiberglass. The pre-polymer is methylene bisphenyl di-isocyanate (MDI), which converts to a nontoxic polymeric urea substance.[445] Although this is an exothermic reaction, the temperatures reached during curing pose no hazard of thermal injury.[324] Although this material is capable of burning, it is not readily set afire and the patient would be cognizant of the temperature long before the cast would ignite.[343]

The technique of applying fiberglass is somewhat different from that for plaster of Paris. One cannot easily make the generous "tucks" of the plaster bandage, so bandages of smaller width should be used and the tucks eliminated. Rather than making turns of bandage at right angles to the limb, fiberglass conforms more easily if applied spirally, squaring the upper and lower ends by horizontal turns. We generally use 4-inch bandages for the leg (and even 3-inch in small women), 2-inch bandages around the hand and forearm, and 3- or 4-inch bandages around the arm.

It is permissible to apply fiberglass with a little more tension than plaster of Paris since fiberglass is more elastic. Because fiberglass bandages cannot easily be trimmed with a knife, we try to limit the cast to what would be the trim lines of a plaster cast. This ensures a smooth edge, whereas trimming may produce an irregular, jagged border. When trimming cannot be avoided, Böhler's scissors are recommended when the cast is still "green" or a saw may be used after it has set. Either way, the edges should be everted by molders to prevent erosion of the skin. Reversing the bandage is permissible and helpful when bandaging around the hand and thumb.

Much to the dismay of penny-pinching Scotsmen, rubber gloves are mandatory for all who handle these bandages to prevent the monomer from polymerizing on the skin. Furthermore, the use of the specially designed nylon padding and stockinette is advised, so that if the cast becomes wet, it may easily be dried by the judicious use of a hair dryer. We are, however, reluctant to advise patients that it is permissible to go swimming with such casts, particularly if there is a recent wound.

Immobilization by Continuous Traction

Some fractures are so unstable that maintenance of a reduction by plaster-of-Paris casts is impossible, or casts may be, for one reason or another, impractical. In these circumstances the bone can be reduced and held to length by means of continuous traction, provided a soft-tissue linkage still exists.

Traction has been shown to be a safe and dependable way of treating fractures for more than 100 years. It does, however, require constant care and vigilance, and it is costly in terms of the length of hospital stay. All of the hazards of prolonged bed rest—thromboembolism, decubiti, pneumonia, and atelectasis—must be considered when traction is used.

It does seem extraordinary that, although traction had been used for millenia in the reduction of fractures and dislocations, and many elaborate machines and devices were invented to apply it, continuous traction was not employed until the 19th century.[306]

Continuous traction may be applied through traction tapes attached to the skin by adhesives or by a direct pull through pins transfixing the skeleton.

Skin Traction. Although Gurdon Buck did not invent skin traction (nor did he claim to have done so), isotonic skin traction has come to be known by his name. It was used extensively in the Civil War in the treatment of fractured femurs and later spread to Europe and Great Britain, where it was called "the American method."[306] Skin, however, is designed to bear compression forces and not shear. If much more than 8 pounds is applied for any length of time, the superficial layers of the skin are pulled off, leaving an irritated, exuding surface. The force exerted by skin traction is dissipated in the soft tissues, so that this form of traction in adult fracture work is used only as a temporary measure to make the patient comfortable while awaiting definitive therapy.

When skin traction is to be used, we prefer moleskin for the traction tape. Ordinary adhesive tape must never be used, because it is impervious to moisture and thus allows the underlying skin to become sodden with perspiration; the tape then creeps, pulling off the superficial layers of the skin, leaving a weeping, angry excoriation (Fig. 1-52). On no account should the limb be shaved. The superficial layers of the skin have a protective function, and tape on shaved skin causes irritation and discomfort. Some surgeons believe that tincture of benzoin applied to the skin before the application of adhesive traction protects the skin, but there is no good evidence to support this contention.

The malleoli must be protected from the traction tape by padding proximal to them. Pressure sores may result from padding applied directly to the malleoli. The moleskin tapes should be applied evenly without wrinkles, and, if necessary, oblique cuts may be made in the borders to make them conform to the limb. The traction tapes are applied to a block or a spreader and through this to a cord, which passes over a pulley to an attached weight. The moleskin is held in place by an elastic bandage carefully applied from the ankle to the knee, which must be checked regularly to ensure that it does not exert a tourniquet effect by becoming disarranged (Fig. 1-53**A**).

A variety of prepackaged skin traction devices are available that can be applied easily and quickly. Some of these are adherent, whereas others exert their action by the friction of sponge rubber against the skin so that they may be removed and reapplied as often as is desired.

We seldom use skin traction in adults, and when we do, as a temporary measure in hip fractures, we tend to use the sponge rubber boot. In the elderly in whom the skin is fragile, great care must be exercised and no more than 5 pounds applied. There is also a great danger of friction burn to the heel, so that we frequently place a water-filled rubber glove under the heel.[1]

We are all prisoners of tradition and previous ex-

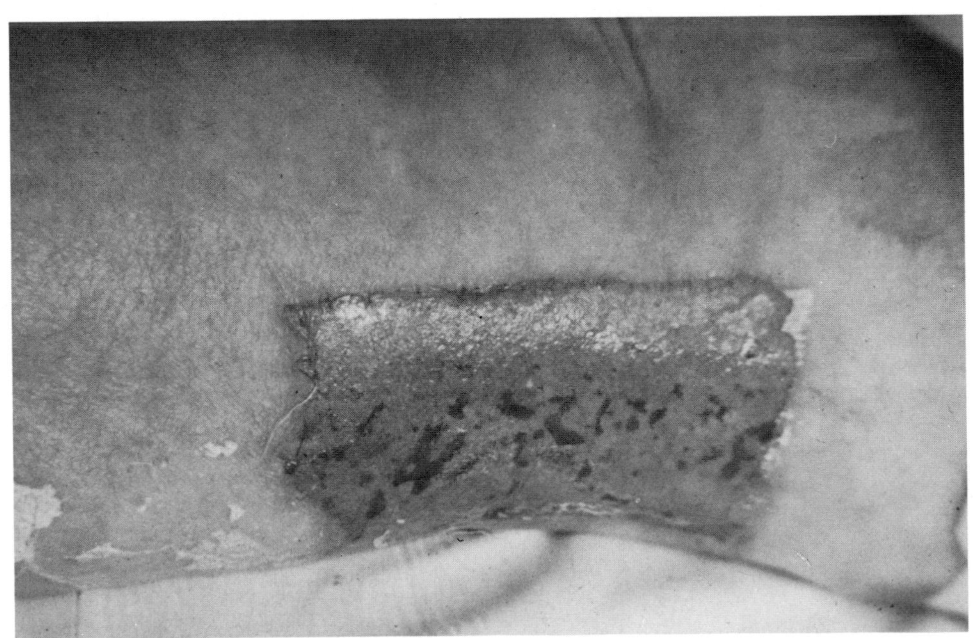

FIGURE 1-52. When skin traction is applied using regular adhesive tape, superficial layers of the skin may be avulsed. The result is a weeping, angry excoriation.

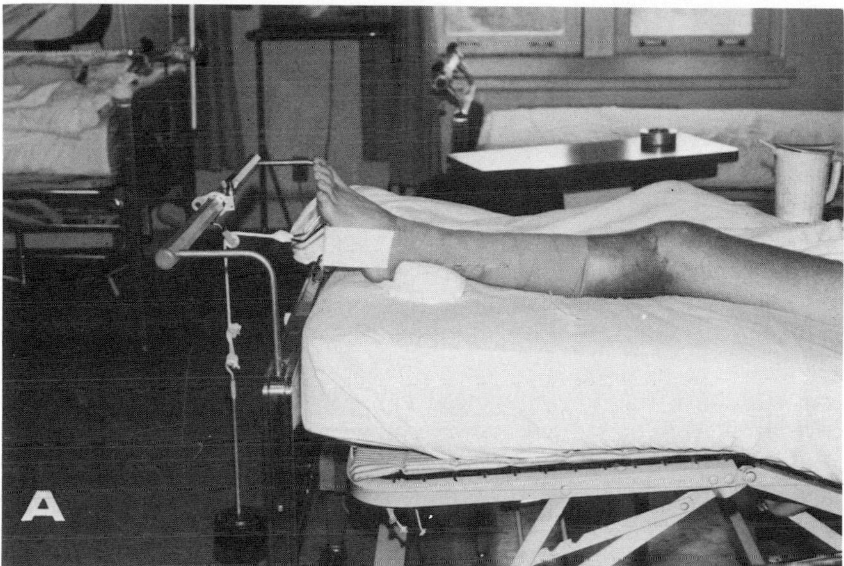

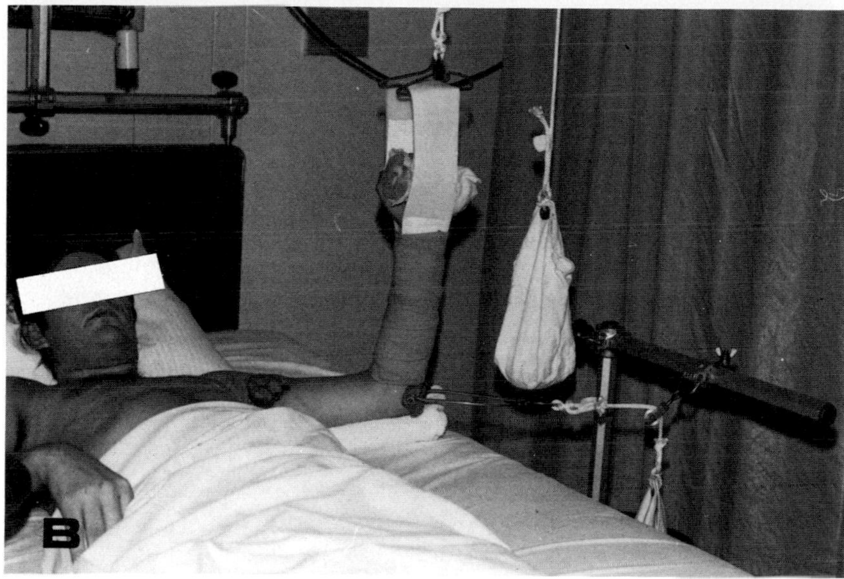

FIGURE 1-53. (**A**) Skin traction should be applied only as a temporary expedient. Padding is applied *superior* to the malleoli, and the traction tapes are bandaged by an elastic bandage from the ankle to the knee. (**B**) Olecranon traction is sometimes used in the treatment of fractures of the humerus, especially supracondylar fractures. The pin is inserted through the ulnar shaft immediately distal to the olecranon, taking care to avoid the ulnar nerve. The forearm and hand are supported by skin traction.

perience, and it has been our custom to apply skin traction to the limbs of elderly women pending the operative management of their fractured hips. But Finsen and colleagues[152] studied a number of such patients and assigned them to three groups: one group with 3-kg skin traction on a Braun splint, another group with tibial pin traction equivalent to 10% of their body weight, and the remainder, who were allowed to lie with their fractured limb on a pillow. They found that there was no difference in the amount of pain medication consumed or in patient complaint, and indeed it was easier to give nursing care to those patients whose limbs were not tied down.[152] A similar study by Anderson and associates found no advantage to preoperative traction in a randomized study and our recent experience would confirm their observations.[12]

Skeletal Traction. Skeletal traction was first achieved by the use of tongs. As we know it today, skeletal traction is applied by a pin transfixing bone, introduced by Fritz Steinmann. Kirschner also invented a similar device using a very fine wire that required a special traction bail to keep the wire under tension.[313] The idea of using a wire of small diameter that does minimal damage to the tissues is most attractive; but, unhappily, Kirschner wires, especially over the long term, have a propensity for cutting through the bone like wire through cheese.

Our own preference is Steinmann pin traction, using a threaded pin rather than one that is smooth. Smooth pins tend to loosen rapidly, so they slip in and out, frequently leading to soft-tissue infection and, on occasion, to osteomyelitis of the host bone. Recently, partially threaded Steinmann pins have been introduced.

These combine the strength of the smooth pin with the holding power of the threaded pin, and this, we believe, is the best option for skeletal traction.

To insert Steinmann pins, the skin must be prepared as for any surgical procedure. Gloves are worn, the area is isolated with towels, and sterile precautions are observed.

Frequently the patient will be under general or spinal anesthesia, but there is no reason why the pins cannot be inserted under local infiltration anesthesia, provided care is taken to infiltrate the periosteum adequately.

In drilling a Steinmann pin, particularly when a skin incision has not been used, the skin may be caught by the pin and become puckered. If left like this it will slough, and tension should be relieved by nicking it with a knife at three points equidistant from each other.[86] The pin holes should be dressed by sponges impaled on the pins and soaked with tincture of benzoin or Ace Adherent or, if desired, by sponges soaked in an antiseptic such as povidone-iodine (Betadine).

The most common indication for skeletal traction is for fractures of the femur. Posterior bowing and late varus deformities in fractures of the femur owing to the pull of the adductors will plague the unwary, but abduction of the hip and the use of posterior pads prevent these untoward deformities. Overdistraction of the fracture with consequent delayed union or nonunion is a major complication. With improvements in intramedullary fixation and the high cost of hospital care, continuous traction as primary treatment for femoral fractures is entirely passé in current practice but may be used whenever internal fixation must be deferred.

Occasionally, skeletal traction is indicated for humeral fractures in patients with multiple injuries. It is also commonly used in supracondylar fractures of the humerus and in tibial plateau fractures when these difficult fractures are to be treated with early motion (Apley's traction).[16] On occasion, it is used in the treatment of tibial fractures, particularly where there are associated burns; however, because nonunion or delayed union of the tibia has been attributed to skeletal traction, we are inclined to use an external fixator in such circumstances.

Traction for Femoral Fractures. The proximal tibia is the site of choice for traction in femoral fractures. (Although one would imagine that traction through the distal femur would be much more efficient, it has the inherent disadvantage that the pin may provoke binding down of the quadriceps, particularly when the pin tract becomes infected.)

The tibial tubercle is palpated, and the pin is drilled from the lateral to the medial side, 2 cm posterior to the tibial tubercle. In osteoporotic patients, it is prudent to go more distally into the bone of the shaft. This purchase is less likely to fail than one in the weak bone of the metaphysis.

Although femoral fractures may be treated by traction alone in the "90–90" position (ie, with both the hip and knee flexed to 90°) or merely over a pillow as Perkins[309] described, most fractures of the femur are treated with some form of additional splintage.

The most popular method is balanced suspension in a Thomas splint, or variant of it, with a Pearson attachment and isotonic traction with weights. Commonly, the reduction of these fractures is achieved by the traction and the secondary use of pads, slings, or pushers. We much prefer, whenever possible, to reduce the fracture by gentle manipulation under anesthesia and to hold the position gained by maintenance traction. This technique was also preferred by Charnley,[86] who made an excellent case for isometric traction in a straight Thomas splint.

Charnley[86] also recommended the use of a "traction unit," which is a short-leg cast incorporating a tibial Steinmann pin. Whenever a smooth Steinmann pin is used for traction, we believe that it should be anchored in plaster. Other advantages claimed for this "traction unit" are (1) it prevents equinus of the foot; (2) the popliteal nerve and calf muscles are protected from the pressure of the slings of the splint; (3) external rotation of the foot and distal femur is controlled; (4) the tendo calcaneus is protected from pressure; (5) it is comfortable; and (6) fractures of the tibia and ipsilateral femur can be treated in this way.

Hugh Owen Thomas personally made his bed splints to fit the patient, but made-to-measure splints are a luxury not obtainable in many hospitals. In most institutions it is difficult to find a splint of exactly the right size. The leather covering the rings is often hard, dry, cracked, and, frequently, soiled by the last patient to use it. For this reason, the Harris splint (which has no ring) is useful, but we have had some problems with the medial upright impinging in the patient's perineum (Fig. 1-54).

Many hospitals use a variant of the Thomas splint with a half ring (Keller-Blake) that can be swiveled so that one splint can be used for both right and left extremities. When the ring is positioned posteriorly, the ring is uncomfortable and tends to collapse. If such a splint is used, it is better to place the solid half ring anteriorly and pass the webbing strap posteriorly over an abdominal pad.

In 1924, Hamilton Russell[353] described a method of treating fractures of the femur in which a single rope is attached to a sling, which supports the thigh and also exerts a longitudinal pull through a pulley on a foot plate. The traction applied to the femur is the result of the forces acting at the thigh sling and on the foot. By the arrangement of pulleys at the distal end, a 10-pound weight exerts a 20-pound pull. We believe

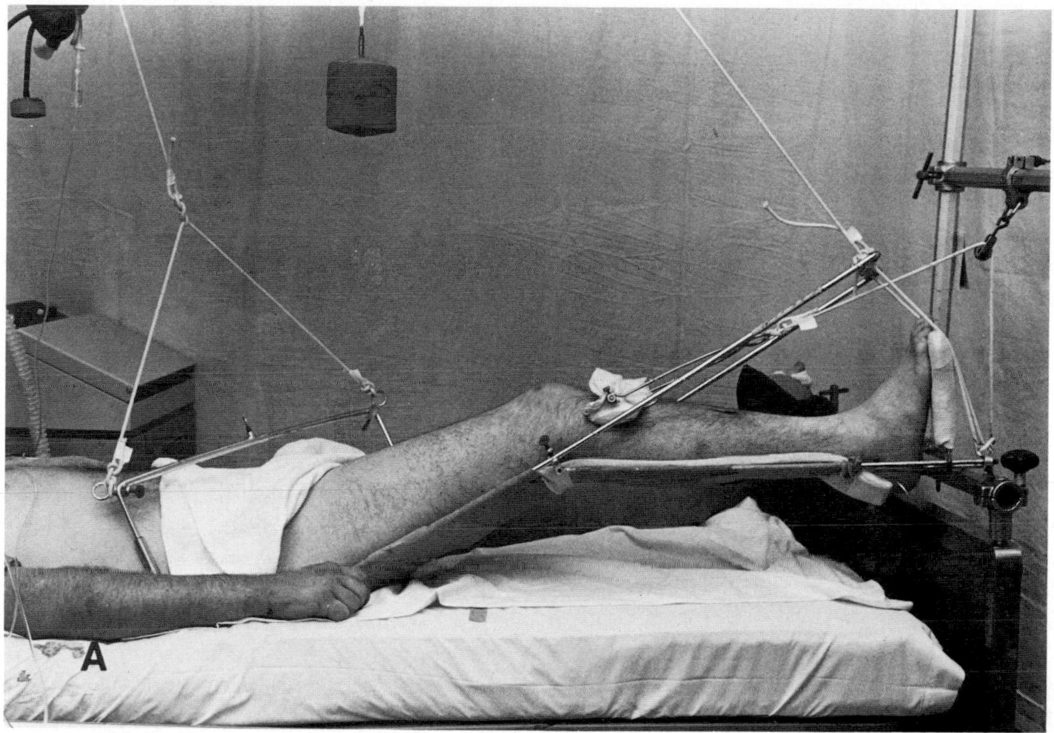

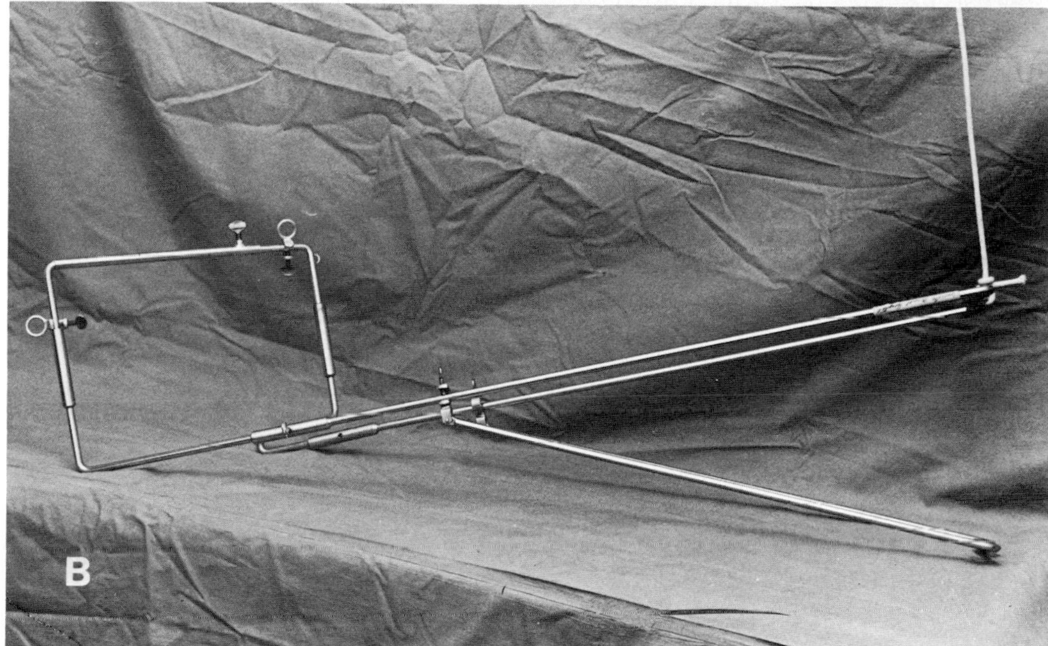

FIGURE 1-54. (**A** and **B**) Balanced traction in a Harris splint with Pearson attachment. The entire system is counterbalanced by a 10-pound weight. Longitudinal traction is applied to a pin through the tibia, and the foot is kept out of equinus position by a plantar support. Care must be taken to see that the tendocalcaneus is well padded and that pressure over bony prominences or the peroneal nerve does not occur.

the reason this method was popular was the perception of getting something for nothing—a 20-pound pull for 10. In practice, we find this traction a tedious business requiring continual readjustment and attention. However, a development of this traction is a method known as "split Russell's traction," where traction is applied through both a supracondylar pin and an os calcis pin attached to separate weights. Again, the pull on the femur is the result of these two forces.

Yet another modification (Litchman and Duffy[247]) employs two slings, one under the thigh and the other under the calf, and replaces the weights with a constant-force spring. This arrangement dispenses with the pillow under the limb as described by Russell. Although we use this arrangement for children, it can easily be modified for adults by using a pin through the os calcis.

We prefer to use another variation, invented by Kenneth G. Tomberlin and Orhan Alemdaroglu (unpublished work), in which a Pearson attachment is attached to a tibial Steinmann pin and held in place by a traction bow. A pulley is braised to the end of this splint so that longitudinal traction is applied through the Pearson attachment. As in Russell's traction, a single rope provides traction in two planes: in an upward direction from the traction bow and longitudinally through the splint; the pull on the femur is the result of the two-plane traction. The traction rope runs from the traction bow to an overhead pulley, from there to a pulley on a bar at the end of the bed, then through the pulley on the splint, and finally through a second pulley at the end of the bed and to the weights. This pulley arrangement doubles the pull of the traction weights. Finally, a supportive sling is placed under the thigh with a 5- to 10-pound pull on it (Fig. 1-55).

Pressure over the tendo Achilles or heel is a problem for patients in traction. We use a rubber glove, partially filled with water and tied, as a localized water bed for the heel. This is an invention of Dr. George Wright, and we have used it for a number of years with success. It is important that the glove remain soft and not overdistended.

A most ingenious traction system for femoral fractures was invented by the late Alonzo Neufeld,[287] which he called the "dynamic method." A Steinmann pin is inserted through the proximal tibia, which is anchored in a plaster gaiter or below-knee cast. A half-ring Thomas splint with a Pearson attachment is applied with the half ring placed anteriorly. The distal end of the Thomas splint is cut off, making the assembly very similar to a Fisk splint. The leg is affixed to the Pearson attachment by more plaster of Paris, and the leg and splint assembly is suspended by ropes attached to the splint at mid-leg and mid-thigh. These ropes are attached to the ends of a crossbar, which is suspended by a single rope at its midpoint. This single rope runs over a union traction pulley, which is free to run on an overhead bar. The weight for this traction is transmitted by the pulley over the foot of the bed and is between 10 and 20 pounds. Immediate knee motion is permitted with this apparatus, and in a short time the patient is able to stand up in bed. This traction has been used for patients aged 5 to 90 years.

Distal Femoral Traction. The main indication for distal femoral traction is where the ligaments of the knee have been injured on the ipsilateral side of a femoral fracture. In supracondylar fractures, where the posterior tilt of the distal fragment cannot be controlled by

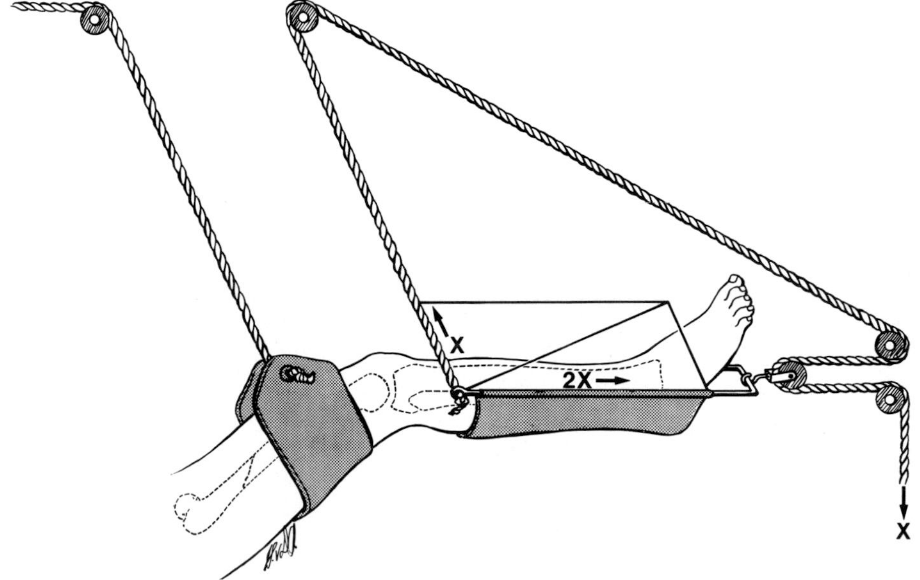

FIGURE 1-55. Tomberlin's traction. The Steinmann pin in the tibia is subjected to a longitudinal pull through the Pearson attachment and a pull in a cephalad and vertical direction through the traction bow. The arrangement of two pulleys at the end of the bed and the pulley on the Pearson attachment doubles the effect of the applied weights. By adjusting the overhead pulley, the resultant pull is in the long axis of the femur, with a magnitude of 1.5 to 1.75 times the added weights. The thigh sling is for comfort and has a weight of 5 pounds to support the limb.

other means, a pin or a Kirschner wire may be inserted at the level of the superior border of the patella and the recalcitrant fragment pulled anteriorly (Fig. 1-56). The Steinmann pin is best inserted from the medial to the lateral side (to avoid any risk to the femoral vessels) and immediately proximal to the condyles.

Calcaneal Traction. Traction through the os calcis may be used in the treatment of tibial or femoral fractures, but we tend to avoid it whenever possible, because osteomyelitis of the calcaneus is such a chronic and disabling condition. When it must be used, great care should be exercised to avoid skewering the subtalar joint. The preferred location is a point 2.5 cm posterior and 2.5 cm inferior to the lateral malleolus or, as Charnley[86] advised, "a point 1 inch superior and 1 inch anterior to the profile of the heel."

Traction Through the Olecranon. A medium or small threaded Steinmann pin is inserted from the medial side $1\frac{1}{2}$ inches distal to the tip of the olecranon. The course of the ulnar nerve must be kept in mind. The flat posteromedial surface of the ulna is palpated, and the pin is drilled through. The traction may be in the side-arm position, or the humerus may be held vertically with the forearm supported by a felt sling. In the side-arm position, skin traction with a spreader may be used to support the forearm (see Fig. 1-53*B*).

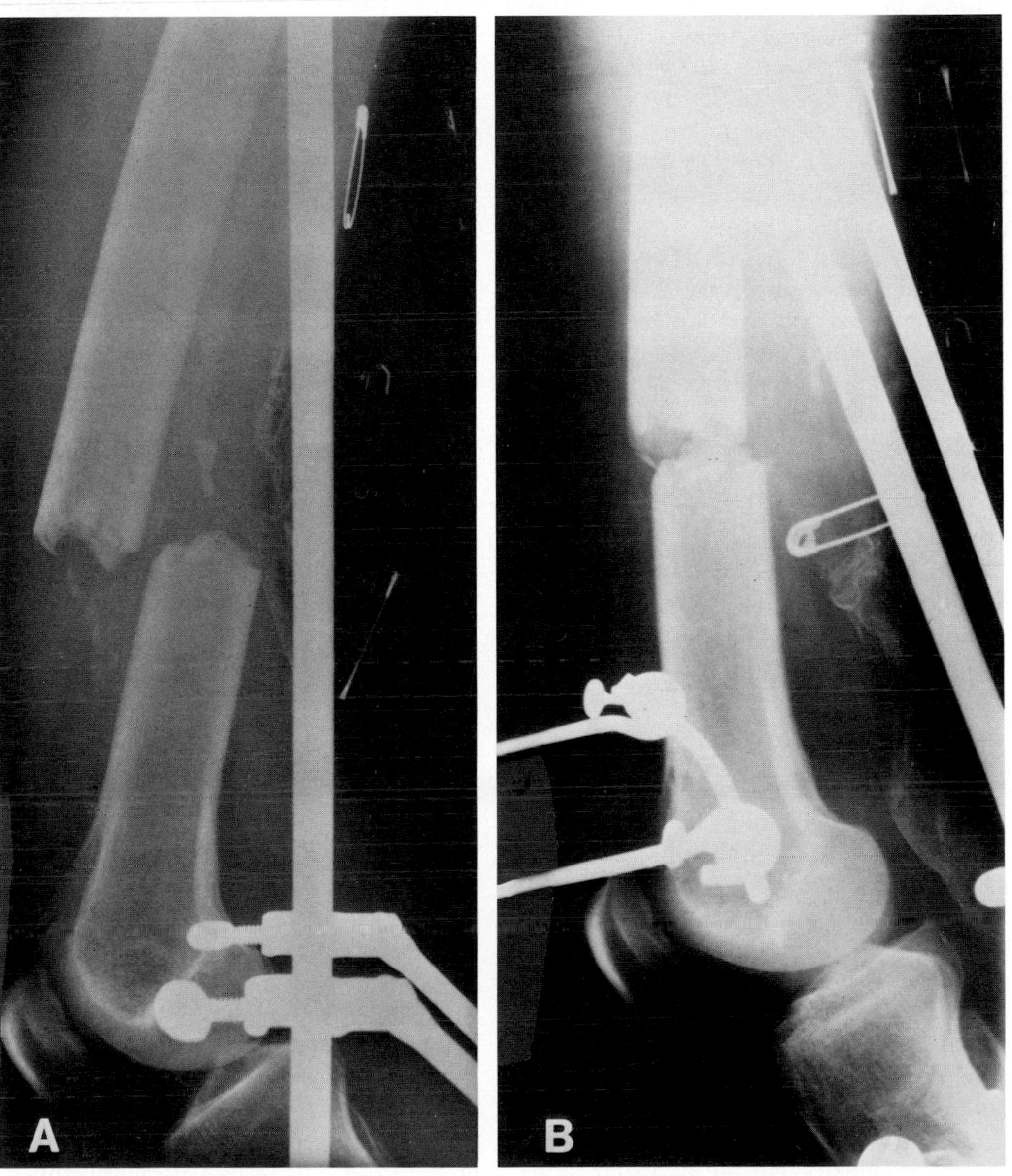

FIGURE 1-56. (**A** and **B**) This femoral fracture could not be reduced by simple longitudinal traction alone. A better position was produced with the addition of a Steinmann pin through the distal fragment at the level of the upper border of the patella and anterior traction.

To avoid problems with the ulnar nerve, traction may be applied to the head of an AO spongiosa screw or a small screw hook inserted directly into the olecranon.

Traction by Plaster. Traction may also be applied by means of plaster-of-Paris casts. In fractures of the humerus a very light "hanging" cast[73,396] is applied from the knuckles to a point no higher than 2.5 cm above the fracture site and suspended at the wrist from a string around the neck. The combined weight of the upper extremity and cast applies traction to the humeral fracture. Anteroposterior bowing may be corrected by shortening or lengthening the string; varus or valgus angulation is addressed by altering the suspension point at the wrist.

Pins and Plaster. In very unstable fractures of the leg, particularly where there has been marked comminution, it may be impossible to prevent gross shortening in a conventional cast. Under these circumstances, pins may be inserted through the proximal tibia and os calcis. The fracture is pulled out to length and a cast is applied incorporating the pins, thereby applying continuous distraction of the fracture.

Pins and plaster have been advocated for a number of fractures other than those of the tibia, including the femur[166,375] and the distal end of the radius. Although this method works, it demands meticulous care and is complicated by nonunion or delayed union, pin tract infection, and, especially in the lower extremity, pin breakage.[378] At the present time, the combination of pins and plaster has been supplanted entirely by external fixators.

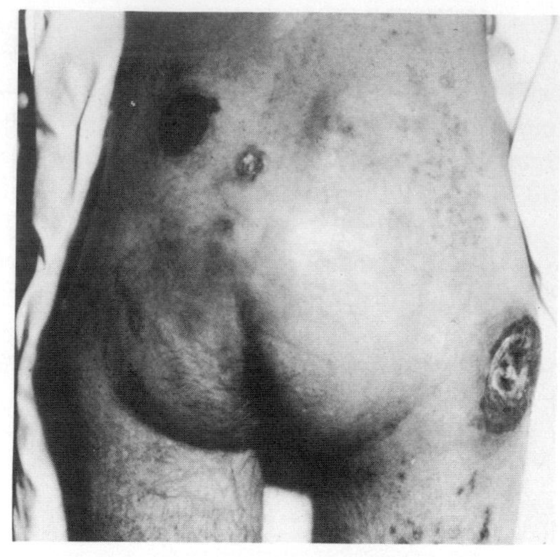

FIGURE 1-57. This young man with multiple fractures was sent to convalesce at home in a plaster-of-Paris spica. Although he did suffer some discomfort, his pain disappeared along with the skin over the trochanters, sacrum, and left posterior-superior iliac spine. All complaints of pain under plaster-of-paris casts must be taken seriously.

Complications of Plaster Casts and Traction

Many successful malpractice suits against orthopaedists and fracture surgeons are based on complications of plaster casts and traction.

Plaster Sores. The skin is not designed to be compressed without relief over extended periods of time. When such pressure occurs for as little as 2 hours, irreversible damage may occur. The skin and the underlying fat, which has a poor blood supply, may necrose, and a plaster sore—nasty-smelling and usually infected—occurs.

These unhappy events do not occur without warning unless the patient is unconscious or the skin is insensate. Circular casts should be used with circumspection and trepidation in paraplegics or those who have impaired sensation (see Fig. 1-49). The patient harboring a potential plaster sore invariably complains of burning pain or discomfort, and these complaints must always be taken seriously. If neglected, the discomfort eventually disappears, but by then so has the skin and its nerve endings (Fig. 1-57). In all cases, the site of the patient's complaints should be inspected without delay. Irritating trips to the hospital in the middle of the night and the mutilation of one's elegant plaster casts can be avoided to some extent by paying attention to minor details during cast application.

It is not good practice to have your assistant support the lower extremity by holding the stockinette while you apply the plaster (Fig. 1-58). This creates pressure over the heel and burning pain. Similarly, in finishing the cast, pulling too vigorously on the stockinette may cause pressure on bony prominences.

Finger indentations on a cast produce high-pressure points to a much greater extent than do broad indentations made by the palm of the hand. In any case, indentations rarely occur when the cast is supported by the flat of the hand, and nurses and other helpers must be instructed accordingly (Fig. 1-59). After the cast is completed, it should not be allowed to rest on a sharp edge that will indent it but should be supported by a pillow or something soft.

The upper end of a cast may be unduly sharp and cause an excoriation. This is particularly common in the fold of the buttock, especially in obese patients. It can be avoided by bending out the upper edge of the cast with the fingers so that it flares. Not infrequently the patient may compound the difficulty by inserting tissues or something soft between the cast and the skin or by cutting away the offending plaster, often leaving a jagged edge that produces another sore. Patients should be told that if the cast cuts, the border should be bent out with a pair of pliers. This also applies to the margins of a thumb hole (Fig. 1-60).

Immobilization of the metacarpophalangeal joints, especially in extension, must be avoided like the

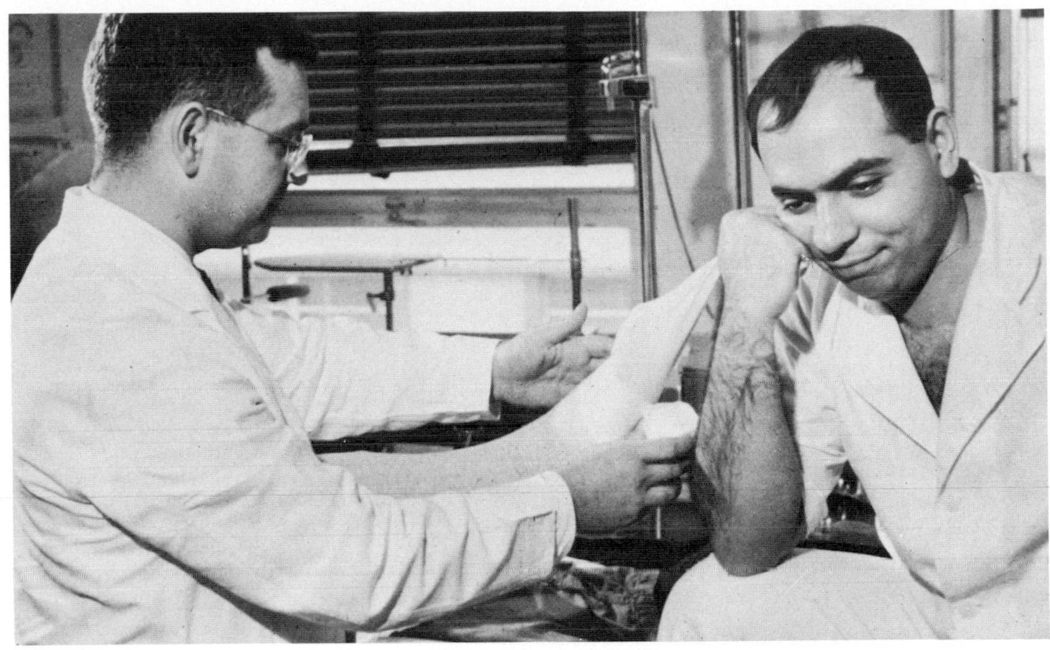

FIGURE 1-58. It is not good practice to have the lower extremity supported by an assistant holding the stockinette. This inevitably causes undue pressure of the stockinette over the heel, and it may cause burning pain or even a sore. The same effect can be produced by pulling too vigorously on the stockinette when folding it over the sharp edges of the cast.

plague, owing to the danger of permanent stiffness (Fig. 1-61) (see Chapter 11).

On occasion, patients in casts will be seized by uncontrollable itching. In their efforts to get relief, they commonly unravel a wire coat hanger and use it to scratch under the cast. Not only do they produce excoriations but, by wadding up the padding, they may produce sores too.

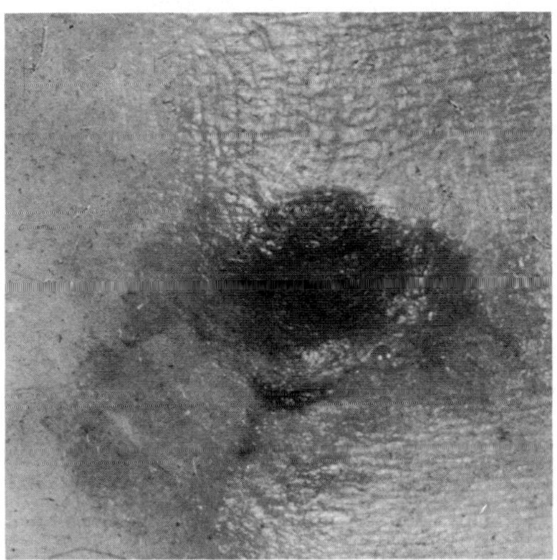

FIGURE 1-59. The surgeon in this case inadvertently made an indentation with his thumb while modeling the fractured ankle. The result was skin necrosis over the medial malleolus.

Felt pads placed over bony prominences may migrate and have the opposite effect from that intended. To prevent this, the felt should be applied as the last layer of padding so that it adheres to the plaster.

The Tight Cast. Care should always be taken not to wrap a plaster bandage too tightly. However, even when a cast is not too tight when applied, if the limb swells, it may become tight later. Pain is the first and most constant complaint of the patient with a tight cast; even if the peripheral circulation appears unimpaired, the prudent course is to split the cast (Fig. 1-62). Garfin and co-workers[165] applied padded plaster-of-Paris casts to the hind legs of dogs and monitored compartment pressures after the injection of autologous serum into the leg. When the casts were univalved (ie, a single cut made longitudinally), the intracompartmental pressures fell 30%; spreading the cut caused a 60% drop; and cutting the padding, a further 10%. Complete removal of the cast reduced the pressure by 85%.

Similar results were recorded when the padding was soaked in povidone-iodine and blood or when the Webril had been soaked and dried, but the percentage drop was less.

In comparing the rise of pressure in the anterior compartments after injection in casted and noncasted legs, it was found that 40% less fluid was required in casted legs than in noncasted legs to produce the same increase in pressure.

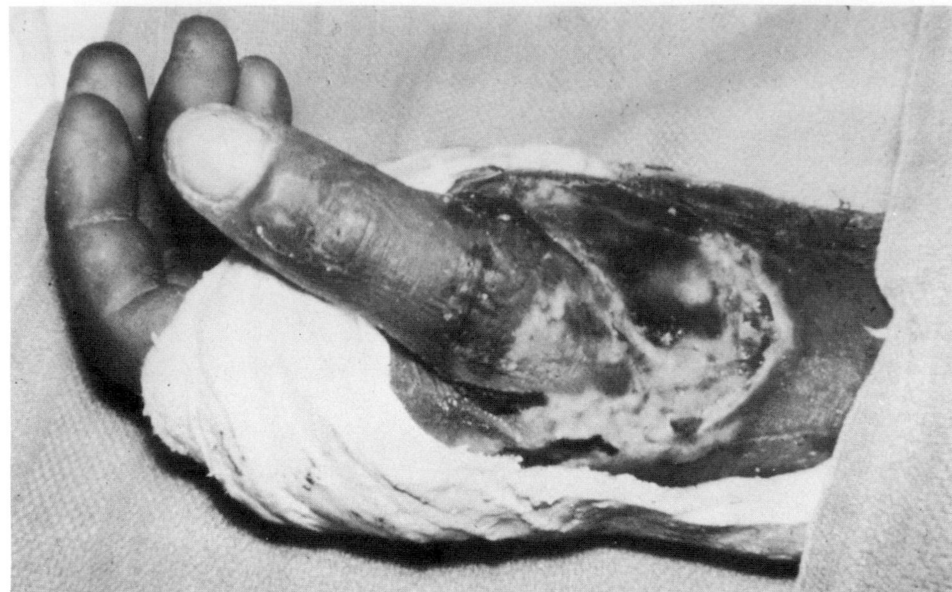

FIGURE 1-60. This is the end result of pressure exerted by an improperly applied cast over the thumb metacarpal. The patient had a large, full-thickness skin slough and lost the abductor and extensor tendons of his thumb in the bargain. The sharp edges of the thumb hole must always be everted, and undue pressure over the base of the thumb metacarpal must be avoided.

What is not immediately apparent is that the position of the foot will influence the tension in the fascial compartment in the leg. Weiner and associates[432] measured pressures in the anterior and deep posterior compartments by transducer-tipped catheters and found that pressures were lowest when the foot was immobilized in a position between 0° and 37° of flexion. They also found that when the cast was split and spread 1 cm that the pressure was reduced in the anterior compartment by 47% and by 33% in the deep compartment. Younger and associates[448] also approached this problem by comparing

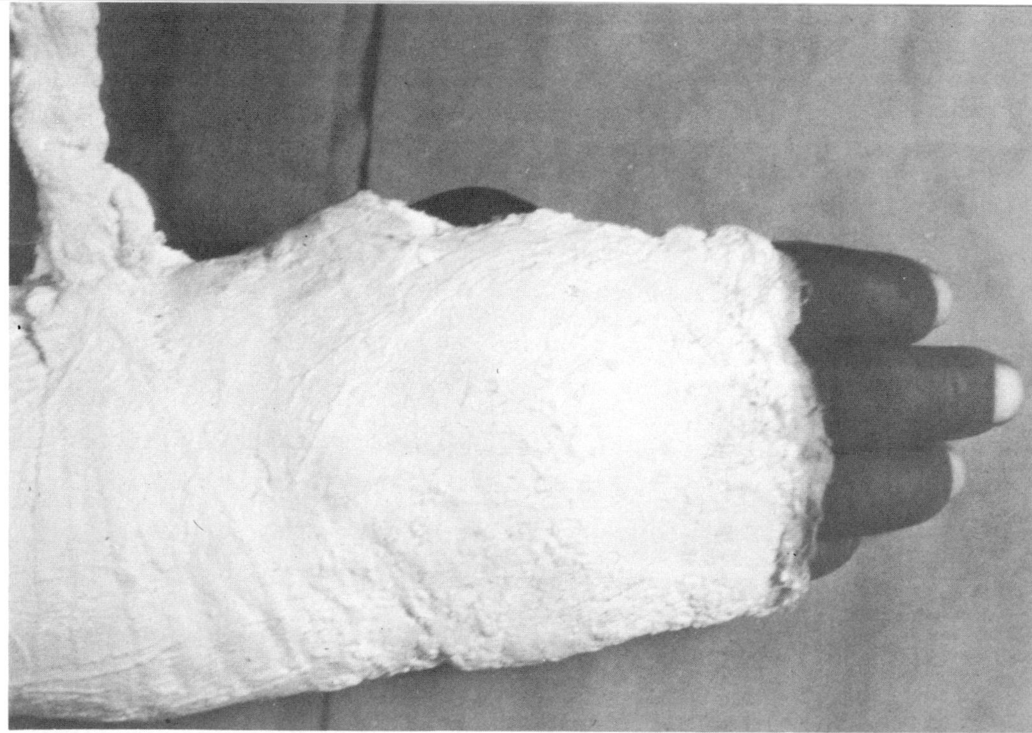

FIGURE 1-61. This is the hand portion of a poorly applied hanging cast. Not only is this plaster rough and improperly applied, but by extending over the fingers, it limits their motion and holds the metacarpophalangeal joints in extension. Such a monstrosity, applied for even a short time, can cripple a hand.

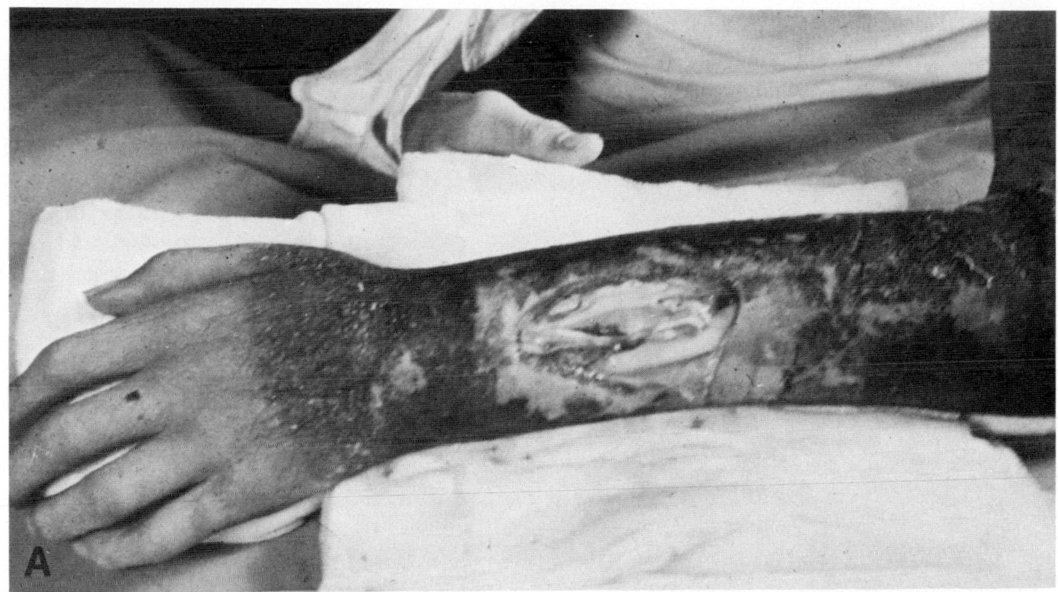

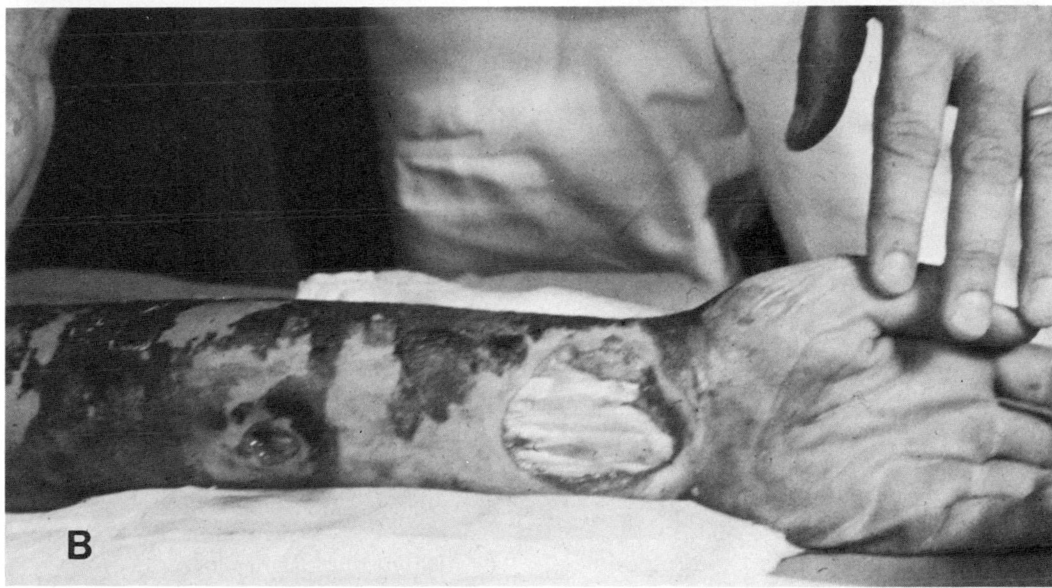

FIGURE 1-62. (**A** and **B**) This young man had an open fracture of his left forearm treated by a plaster-of-Paris cast. When, subsequently, the arm became infected and swollen, his complaints of pain were disregarded. Ultimately his entire forearm became necrotic. This is how it looked immediately before amputation.

the ability of plaster-of-Paris splints to accommodate to increasing intracompartmental pressures with that of circular casts. To do so, they made mock-ups of those devices and inflated a sphygmomanometer cuff to simulate a swelling limb. Rather surprisingly, they found that a circular cast split immediately at the time of application and spread 1 cm was superior to splint immobilization and a circular cast split after 12 hours. The former spread with an internal pressure of 150 mm Hg, and the latter remained intact at 300 mm Hg.

It has been our practice to univalve casts at the time of application and to spread them if we are at all concerned that significant swelling might occur.

It would seem logical that in a patient having symptoms from a tight cast, sequential decompression should be carried out until symptoms are relieved. However, blood-soaked padding appears to be as hard and as unyielding as the plaster of Paris itself, and one would never be wrong in bivalving the cast and cutting the padding to the skin.

Circular bandages of gauze or encircling adhesive tape should never be applied under a cast, because these, too, may have a tourniquet effect (Fig. 1-63).

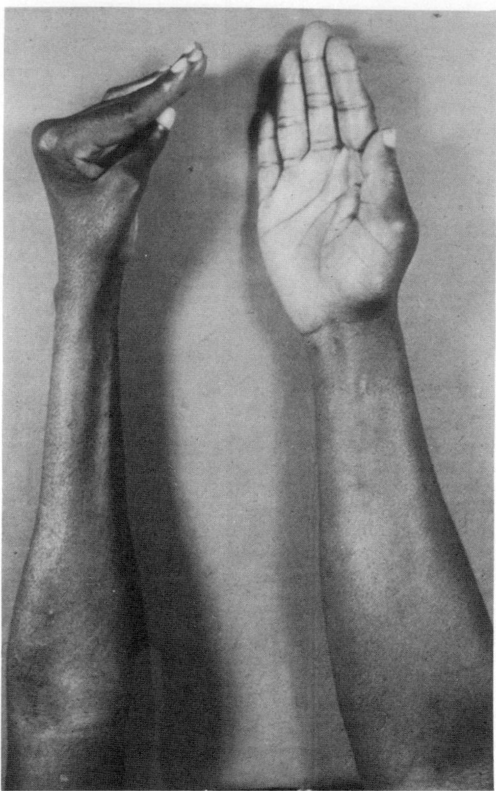

FIGURE 1-63. The end result of circular constriction may be Volkmann's ischemic contracture, which in this case involved the intrinsic muscles of the left hand. This is the "main d'accoucheur." When a patient complains of pain, all encircling dressings and casts must be split.

Patrick and Levack[302] studied the pressure over the prominence of the distal radius after the application of a forearm cast. They found that the highest pressure was recorded immediately after the application of the cast. The pressure dropped over the next 2 or 3 hours, only to rise again to a submaximal peak at an average of 13 hours. Over the next 72 hours the pressure gradually fell, but at no time after the first hour did they record a pressure of more than 30 mm Hg. Five of the nine cases studied had edema of the hand and fingers after 48 to 72 hours. On the basis of this study they recommended initial immobilization by sugar tong splints rather than by circular casts.

In the past, we have frequently employed the Jones dressing post-operatively where we anticipated significant swelling particularly in injuries around the knee. However, our innate laziness and the easy availability of "post-op" knee splints has significantly reduced our dependence of this safe and useful immobilization. The Jones dressing is a bulky dressing usually applied after knee surgery. It consists of a thick layer of absorbent cotton wrapped with domette or elastic bandages followed by two more layers of cotton and bandage. We have modified this by using Kling or Kerlex bandages and cheap cotton batting instead of absorbent cotton and finishing the last layer with an elastic bandage. Where additional stability is required, slabs of plaster are placed on the medial and lateral sides of the limb as the most superficial layer under the last bandage. A similar sort of bulky dressing may also be used in the upper limb. This should not be called a compression dressing, because persons will be encouraged to apply it too tightly. It should be applied without much tension and, if too tight, it is easily removed with scissors in seconds.

Thermal Effects of Plaster. When dehydrated gypsum takes up its water of crystallization, an exothermic reaction takes place. How high the temperature becomes depends on the amount of plaster, its surface area, and the external environment's ability to allow the plaster to lose heat. Other factors such as chemical accelerators, temperature of the water, and the water content of the bandage are also important. Although in most circumstances this exothermic reaction does nothing more than make the patient pleasantly warm, it is possible to produce thermal burns with the application of thick plaster-of-Paris splints.[222] This is particularly so in preformed splints, 16-ply thick and backed by sponge padding to obviate the need of supplementary sheet wadding.

Williamson and Scholtz[439] have shown that thermal injuries are temperature and time related and that second-degree burns will be produced by a temperature of 50°C after 12 minutes. Third-degree burns may result after a 50°C temperature has been maintained for 5 to 15 minutes.[128]

Occasionally, temperatures as high as 82°C may be produced by curing plaster.[29]

Lavalette and associates[243] found that dip water warmer than 24°C, a cast thicker than eight ply, and the insulation of a pillow were conducive to temperatures hot enough to burn skin, especially when present in combination.

The circumspect orthopaedist should wet the plaster with water from the cold faucet; limit the thickness of splints or circular casts to the thinnest strong enough for his purpose; and leave the bandage manageably sloppy, because a dry bandage sets more quickly and is without the heat sink provided by the excess water. The danger is even more acute in comatose or unconscious patients or where the skin is insensitive. It is possible that, in shock, the lack of circulation in the skin might further impair the ability to dissipate heat. Furthermore, in these patients in whom emergency splintage is being applied, it makes sense to apply cast padding, a poor conductor, to the limb and to make sure that as much surface is exposed to the circulating air as possible.

Thrombophlebitis and Equinus Position. Ochsner noted 30 years ago that thrombophlebitis or phlebothrombosis was uncommon in patients treated by lower extremity casts. He pointed out that, on a theoretical basis, one would expect to have more episodes rather than fewer when a lower limb was injured and immobilized. This comparative immunity, he believed, was related to the casted leg's being warmer than normal. Micheli,[269] however, reported six cases of patients with lower-extremity casts who developed pulmonary embolism in four instances and severe thrombophlebitis in two. Three of these patients had rupture of the tendo calcaneus, and the others had a subtalar dislocation, a fractured tibial shaft, and a tibial plateau fracture, respectively. We have had two patients, treated for heelcord rupture by immobilization in equinus, develop pulmonary embolism. We have attributed this to pooling of blood in the veins of the calf with subsequent clotting secondary to the loss of the "pumping" action of the triceps surae. In the extreme equinus position these muscles become so relaxed that they are unable to generate enough tension to strip the calf veins. Although we still treat fractures of the distal third of the tibia by a cast with the foot in equinus, we are careful not to overdo it, while at the same time not dorsiflexing the foot enough to angulate the fracture. The equinus position, contrary to popular belief, does not give rise to stiffness of the ankle in 2 or 3 weeks time—unless there is also a fracture involving the mortise.

Hooper and associates[209] have studied fractures of the shaft of the tibia in which the fibula is intact. In these fractures there is an inherent tendency for the tibial fracture to collapse to the fibular side, producing a varus malalignment. This they attribute to the tibia's being displaced by dorsiflexion of the ankle. Although this can be averted by immobilization in equinus or by internal fixation, they prefer to osteotomize the fibula. The major lesson to be learned, however, is that extreme equinus is to be avoided.

Clark and Winson[89] have raised the question of whether lower extremity casts predispose to pulmonary embolism. They reviewed 691 patients who had sustained a pulmonary embolism over a 5-year period. Of these, 22 had sustained a lower extremity injury that had been treated by a cast and 10 of those were for management of fractured ankles. They found that "the middle-aged female patient with an undisplaced fracture would seem to typify the patient at risk." It would seem to us that the mechanism is venous pooling due to lack of triceps surae function.

The Cast Syndrome. In the past, compression fractures of the spine have been treated with hyperextension body jackets. Occasionally, patients treated in this way developed pernicious vomiting and electrolyte imbalance, and some even died. This "cast syndrome" is caused by an obstruction of the third portion of the duodenum resulting from constriction by the superior mesenteric vessels.[285] Few people now believe that immobilization of stable compression fractures of the spine is necessary, and certainly the position of extreme hyperextension should be avoided.

Some nervous persons feel unduly constricted by any type of cast that encloses the body, a condition akin to claustrophobia. They, too, are likely to vomit and have a variety of psychosomatic complaints, which lead to the cast having to be removed. The vomiting in such cases is rarely as severe and life threatening as in the true cast syndrome.

Infection Secondary to Cast Application. It is rare to have wounds infected by contaminated plaster-of-Paris, sheet wadding, or dip water, but such cases have been reported. It would seem that sterilization of plaster-of-Paris or the use of distilled water for dip water is not indicated, but the circumspect surgeon will use sterile dressings and sheet wadding after surgery or where there is an open wound. It is also mandatory that plaster buckets be cleaned or replaced after use and not allowed to stand full of stagnant water as a potential culture medium.

The rather naive idea that one should be able to swim with a fiberglass cast on is potentially dangerous because this tends to promote maceration of the skin unless thorough drying by hot air is carried out and the padding is nylon. One case of ringworm has been reported under these circumstances,[253] and we have had an infection of a transcutaneous Kirschner wire in an operated foot that was dangled in a swimming pool. The absolute contraindication to this practice is the presence of a recent operative wound.

Allergic Reactions. We have never seen an allergic reaction to plaster-of-Paris, but we have one patient with a sensitivity to cotton stockinette. There have, however, been two cases in which sensitized patients have had allergic responses to the benzalkonium in the plaster bandage.[251,389]

Traction Hazards. Patients in traction develop pressure ulcers just as readily as those treated by plaster. The skin in contact with the ring of a Thomas splint, the sacrum, and other pressure areas must be inspected daily. In some high-risk patients, the sacrum should be protected by an "antigravity pad." A sheepskin, real or synthetic, or a commercially available "egg crate" foam pad is also helpful to preserve the back of a patient who will be in traction for extended periods. The heels and heel cords are particularly likely to develop decubiti and should be protected by heel cups, sponge rubber pads, or water-filled gloves.

If the foot is allowed to lie in the equinus position, a permanent dropfoot contracture may develop. This should be prevented by active exercise and the provision of some type of device to hold up the foot.

Circular bandages should be checked and reapplied as necessary to prevent constriction of the circulation

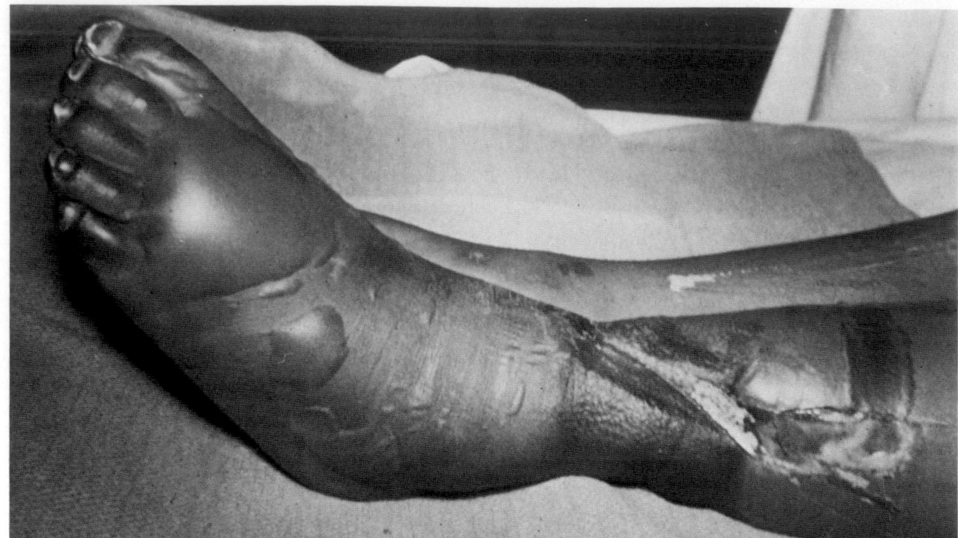

FIGURE 1-64. This child had a fractured femoral shaft treated at home in Bryant's traction. Disarranged bandages acted as a ligature around the ankle, and the foot of the uninjured extremity had to be amputated.

and to ensure that the skin tapes are not slipping. This is particularly true in children who are being treated by Bryant's or gallows traction. In general, this method is best used in very small children up to 20 pounds, and the absolute upper limit is 30 pounds. For larger children we advise Weber's method if catastrophic circulatory problems are to be avoided (Fig. 1-64).[368,431]

Under no circumstances should the lower extremity be allowed to rotate externally in a Thomas splint. This may cause pressure on the common peroneal nerve with subsequent paralysis.

In treatment of fractures of the cervical spine, traction by means of a head halter should be used only for a short time, because sores develop readily over the chin. Skull tongs should be inserted as early as possible (Fig. 1-65).

External Fixation of Fractures

It is not wise to use external fixation everywhere and for everything.

W. Taillard[402]

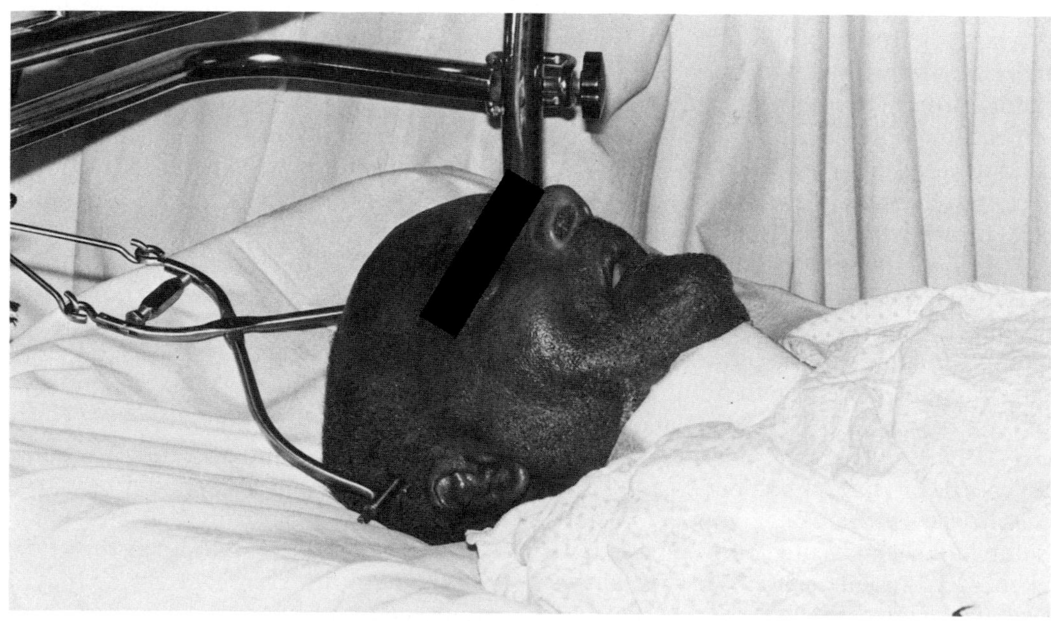

FIGURE 1-65. Traction for injuries of the cervical spine should be by means of some type of skull tongs. The use of the head halter for more than a short period of time, especially if heavy weight is to be used, will give rise to excoriation of the skin over the chin.

Although Alvin Lambotte has generally been given the credit for introducing, in 1907, the use of transfixing pins attached to an external frame to treat fractures, Seligson[379] has pointed out that Parkhill[301] was using such a device before 1897. Nevertheless, the European tradition of external fixation has been predicated on Lambotte's pioneer work.

In the United States, Roger Anderson[14] devised a frame with transfixion pins in 1934 that allowed him to line up difficult tibial fractures and then apply a cast that incorporated the pins. In cases in which there was severe soft-tissue trauma, he used the apparatus as the primary means of fixation.

Otto Stader,[388] a veterinarian, described an external fixator for use in animals in 1937, and this was adopted by surgeons treating persons. Although the use of external fixators declined in this country, probably owing to the complication of pin tract infection, its use continued in Europe.

The Hoffmann apparatus, originally described in 1939,[205] was modified and improved by Vidal and Ardrey,[427] and the excellent results achieved by surgeons in France, Switzerland, and elsewhere using this equipment sparked a revival of interest in this method worldwide. Many different types of fixators are now available, ranging from very expensive, elaborate machines to "do-it-yourself" frames of methyl methacrylate.[18,215]

External fixators allow stabilization of a fracture at a distance from the fracture site without increasing soft-tissue damage. They maintain the length and alignment of a fractured extremity without casting so that soft-tissue wounds can be easily inspected and treated, and the stability engendered may allow early mobilization and activity.[31]

External fixation is particularly helpful in open fractures of the tibia, but it may be used under certain circumstances in the femur, pelvis, humerus, and other bones.

In our practice, we have used external fixation much less frequently in recent years on account of the introduction of interlocking tibial nails that have most of the virtues of external fixators without the burden of pin care and pin tract infection.

Types of External Fixation

In recent years there has been a plethora of external fixators described and advocated, and it would not be productive to give the details of every device in this discourse. Behrens[30] has divided these devices into two groups: pin fixators and ring fixators (Fig. 1-66). Pin fixators can be further subdivided into simple and clamp devices.

In ring fixators, a frame is built consisting of rings or partial rings and connecting rods that encompass the extremity, from which transfixion pins or wires suspend the bone. In pin fixators, the rigid pins are an intrinsic component of the frame as well as the means of anchorage to bone. In simple fixators, the pins are attached by independent articulations to a longitudinal rod, but in the other type of pin fixator, the pins are held by clamps, which in turn are attached to the longitudinal rod by an articulation.

Simple Pin Fixators

Examples of simple fixators are the Roger Anderson device and the AO/ASIF types. These devices provide much more latitude in pin placement than other fixators, both in the separation or spread of the pins and the angle of approach to the bone, which, in turn, enhances the rigidity of the frame. The number of configurations possible is legion and, occasionally, even nowadays, we fall back on the Roger Anderson (Tower) apparatus, but the AO/ASIF is our fixator of choice.

The major defect of simple fixators is that they allow very little adjustment after application, without replacing pins, so that the fracture must be reduced before the application of the frame.

Clamp Fixators

Clamp fixators such as the Hoffman or Kronner devices allow for final reduction of the fracture after application of the device, but adjustments can be made by loosening the articulations. The pin spread and direction of the pins is dictated by the clamp, and the variety of frames that can be built is significantly abridged. Furthermore, gradual adjustment is not possible, and once the articulations are released, there is an inherent danger of losing the reduction.

Ring Fixators

Ring fixators such as the Ilizarov or Ace-Fischer devices allow gradual and precise correction of angulatory and rotational deformity but, unlike pin fixators,

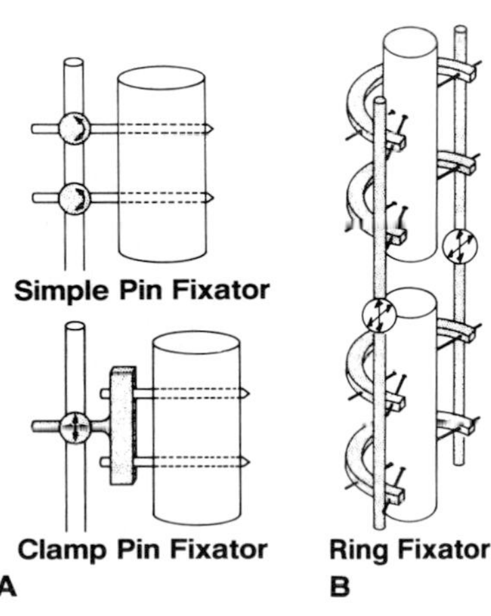

FIGURE 1-66. (**A**) Simple and clamp pin fixators. (**B**) Ring fixator. (*Behrens, F.: A Primer of External Fixation. Clin. Orthop., 241:8–9, 1989.*)

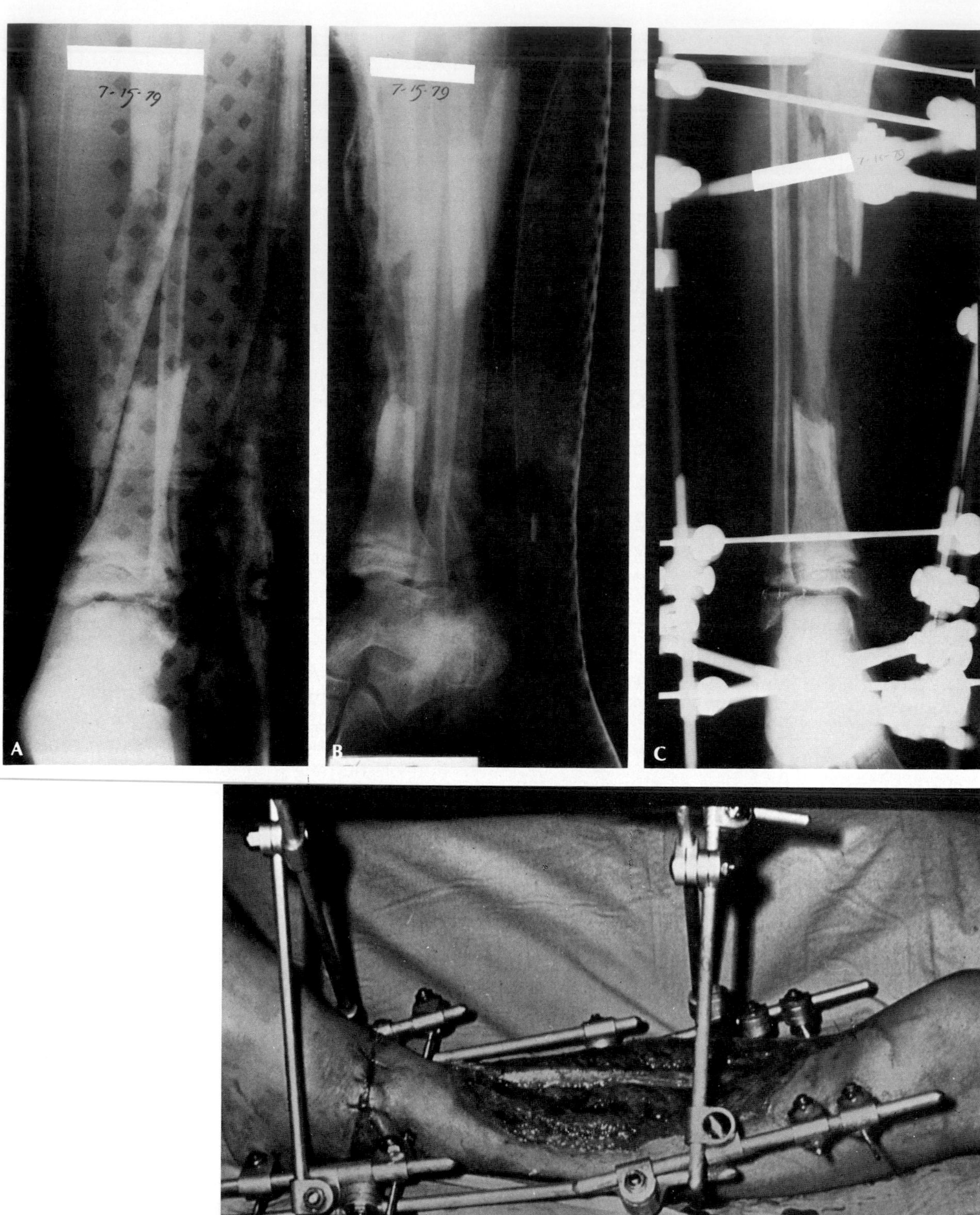

FIGURE 1-67. Radiographs and clinical photos of the lower leg in a 10-year-old boy who inadvertently fell into a feeding augur and had his left leg chewed up. (**A** and **B**) The initial films show segmental fractures of the tibia and fibula and an open disruption of the ankle joint. (**C**) The leg after debridement and the application of a Roger-Anderson fixator. Unfortunately, the loose middle fragment became a sequestrum and had to be removed. (**D**) An intraoperative photograph at the time the fragment was removed.

continues

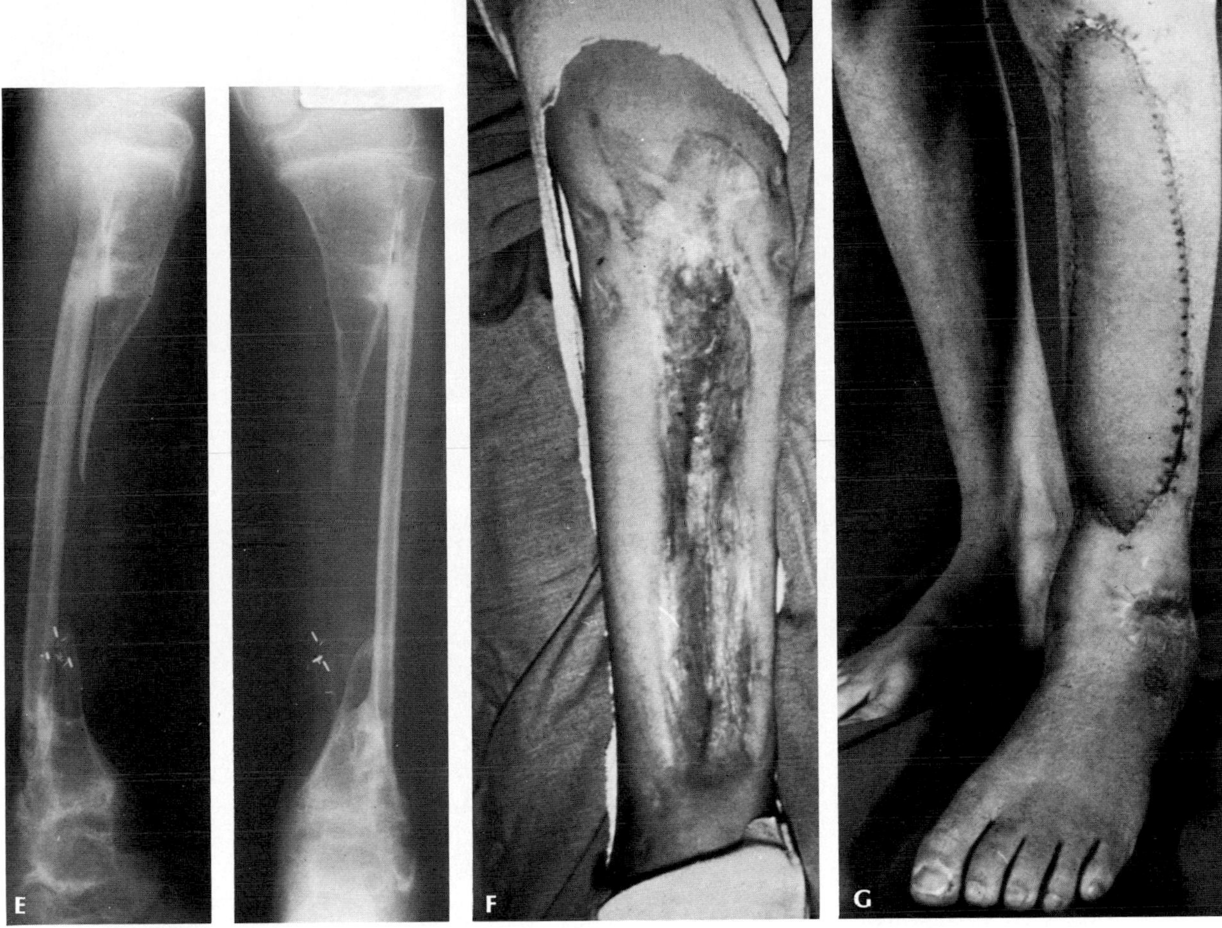

FIGURE 1-67. (continued) (**E**) The leg 2 years later, after multiple debridements and the creation of a tibiofibular synostosis proximally and distally by bone grafts. (**F**) A clinical photograph at this stage with split-thickness grafts covering the defect. These grafts were liable to break down with trauma and had to be replaced. (**G**) The leg after the application of a latissimus dorsi free flap.

tend to limit access to wounds of the extremities and make free tissue transfer difficult or impossible.

Simple Pin Fixators

The Roger Anderson System

In the Roger Anderson system, multiple pins can be inserted either as transfixion pins or as half pins. Each pin is connected to a clamp that also has a connection for an aluminum rod. There are also double connectors for the aluminum rods so that a frame can be built. Although we used this apparatus extensively in our earliest essays in external fixation it has been supplanted by better, albeit more expensive, devices (Figs. 1-67 and 1-68).

The Wagner Apparatus

The use of frames with transfixion pins for fractures of the femur is tedious and inherently dangerous. As a rule we prefer to fix femurs internally, but we have found the Wagner apparatus[212,390] helpful when internal fixation is not an option (eg, long-standing, shortened malunions and nonunions; infected, plated nonunions; fractures with large bone deficits; and neurovascular injuries) (Figs. 1-69 through 1-71).

It is probably best to line up the fracture by traction, inserting two Schanz screws proximally and distally, using a guide to keep them parallel. The screws should be inserted by hand. Alignment can be adjusted at the ends of the apparatus and the fracture distracted or compressed by turning the screw. This is particularly useful when a gradual reduction of a severe overlap is called for (Fig. 1-72).

The Orthofix Fixator (Dynamic Axial Fixator)

The Wagner apparatus, while providing excellent axial fixation and the ability to compress or distract a fracture, must be applied to a fracture already reduced and allows little or no adjustment once applied. The Orthofix fixator

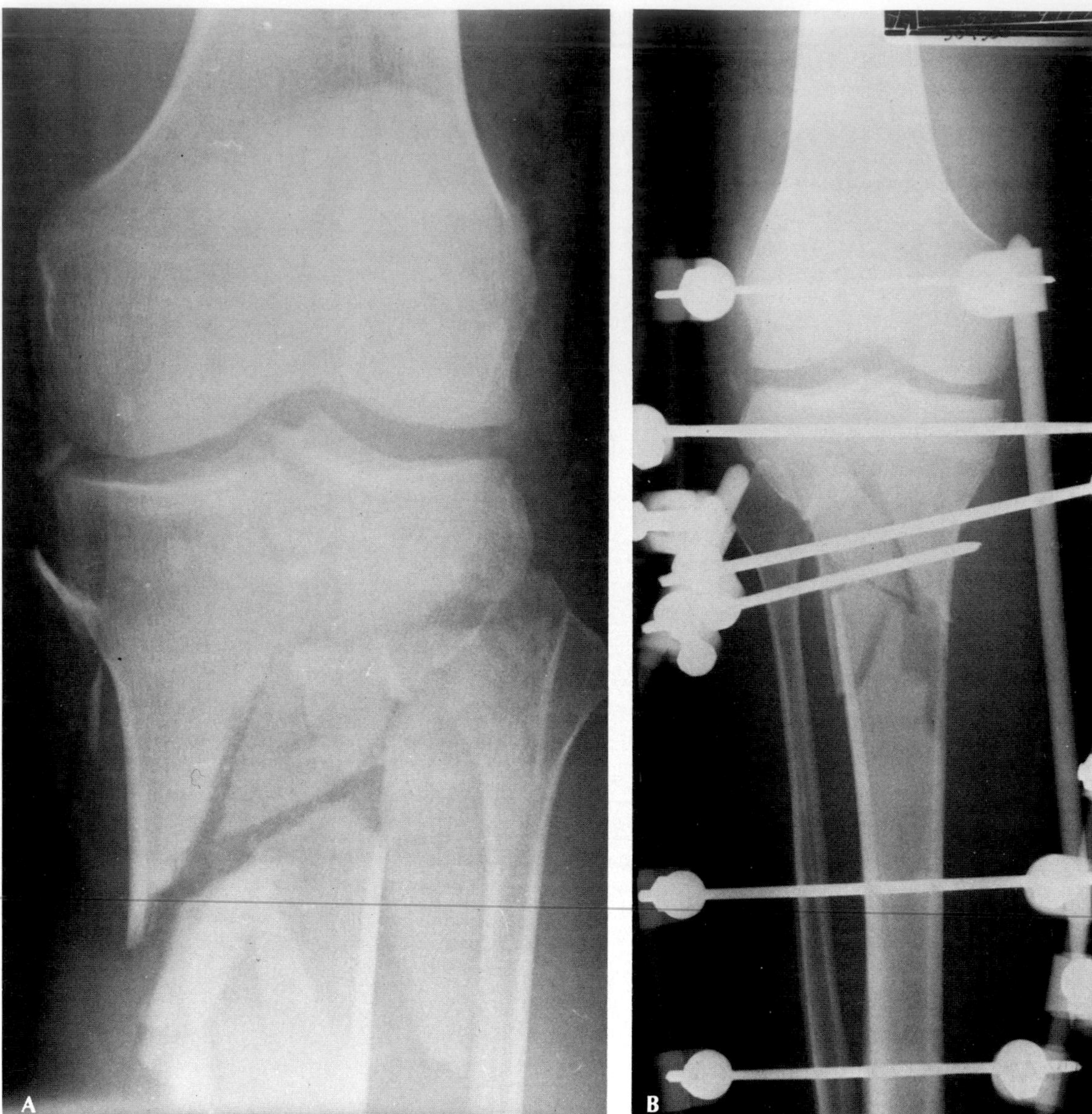

FIGURE 1-68. (**A** through **E**) Radiographs of the knee in a man who drove his motorcycle off the road and sustained a severely comminuted fracture of the proximal end of the tibia with disruption of the ligamentum patellae and the pes anserinus. (**A**) The comminuted fracture. (**B** and **C**) The tibia after application of a Roger-Anderson external fixator. Note that the patella has also been included in the assembly. This allowed immediate mobilization of the knee, even in the presence of a repaired ligamentum patellae. During movements of the knee the patella was maintained in its proper relationship to the tibia by the external fixator.

continues

provides the same advantages as the Wagner but in addition allows the surgeon to carry out the reduction of the fracture after the application of the device and to make subsequent adjustments to correct angulatory and rotational discrepancies; it also allows dynamic axial compression after the appearance of callus.

The device is a single bar with a ball-and-socket joint at each end, to which is attached a clamp with five slots to provide a choice in the number and location of the anchoring pins (Fig. 1-73). These pins are self-tapping and are tapered, 5 mm at the point and 6 mm in the shaft. The body of the fixator contains a telescoping shaft controlled by a compression/distraction device. When the requisite degree of compression or distraction is reached, the shaft is locked, and the compression/distraction device removed. When dynamic axial compression is required, the shaft is unlocked.

The device is applied by inserting a screw through both cortices of one diaphyseal fragment after predrilling with a drill guide. Three more screws are inserted in a similar

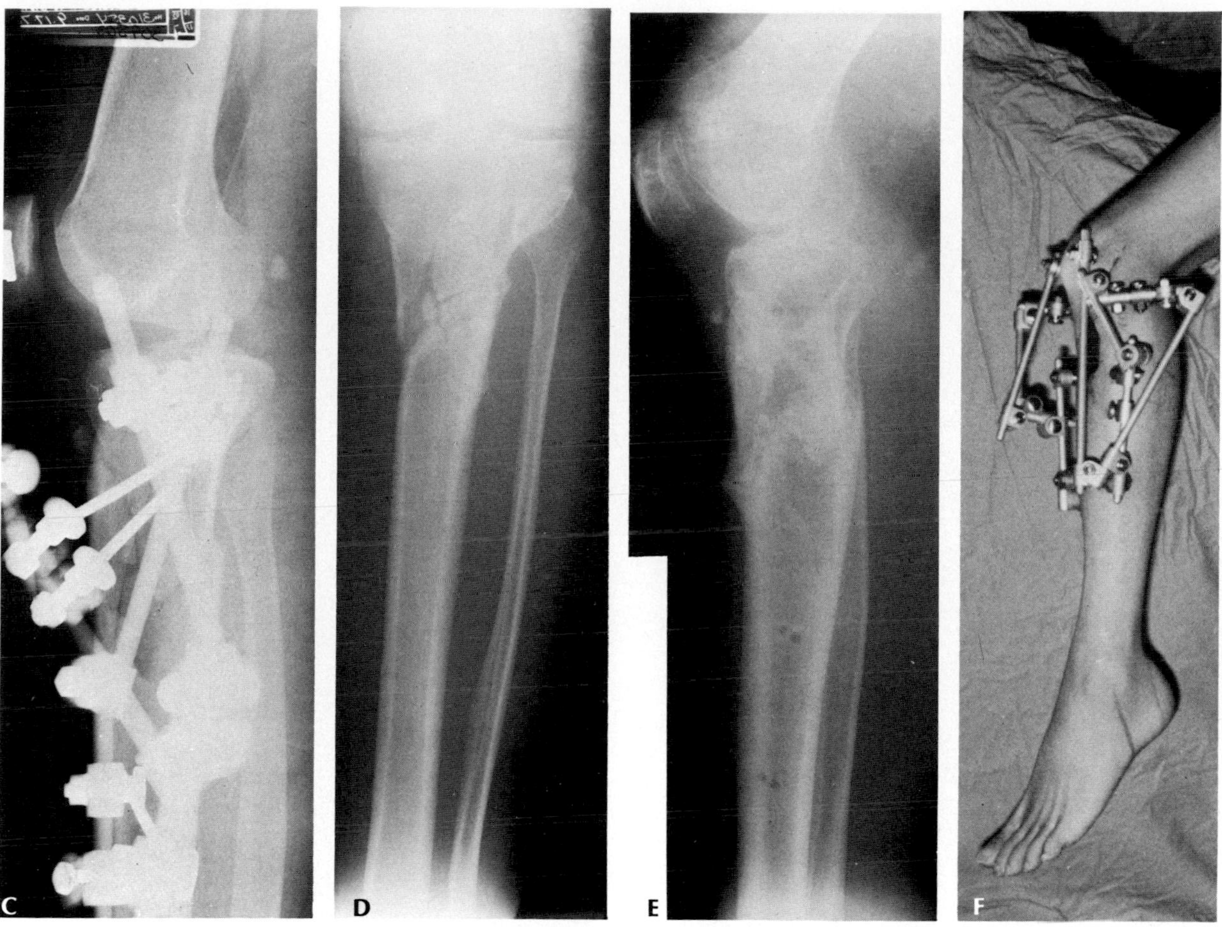

FIGURE 1-68. (continued) (**D** and **E**) The end result with complete healing of the fracture and the joint space well maintained. (**F**) Clinical photograph of a similar patient showing the external fixator with transfixion of the patella.

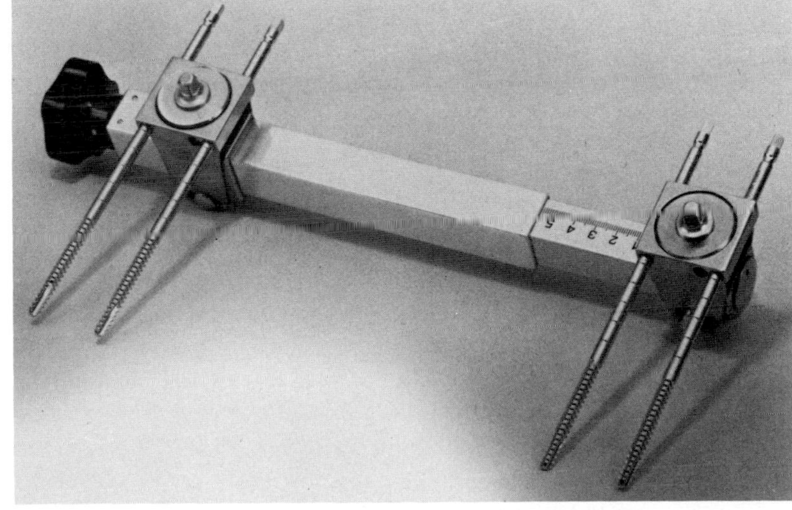

FIGURE 1-69. The Hoffmann modification of the Wagner leg-lengthening apparatus. (*Courtesy of Howmedica, Inc., 1981.*)

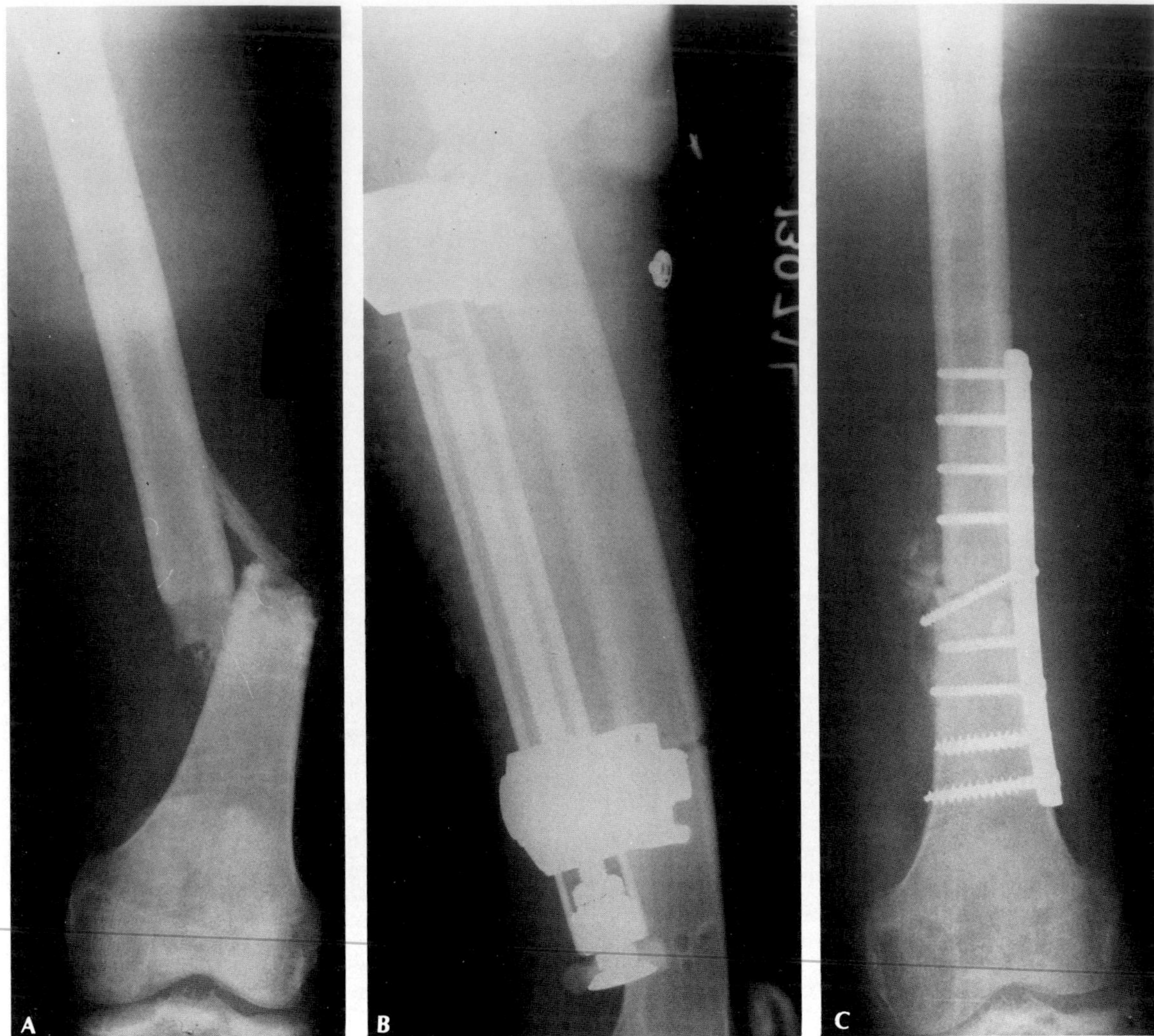

FIGURE 1-70. Radiographs of the femur in a 20-year-old blind man who was involved in an automobile accident. He sustained an open fracture of the left tibia, a closed fracture of the right tibia, a crushing injury of the right foot that necessitated a Syme's amputation, and a fracture of the right femur. The right femur was temporarily stabilized with a Wagner apparatus and then plated. The use of the Wagner apparatus enabled this patient to be mobilized and facilitated the treatment of his leg injuries until the definitive treatment of the femur was performed. (**A**) The preoperative condition of the femur. (**B**) The Wagner apparatus, rather inexpertly applied, with the lower pins too close to the fracture site. (**C**) The femur with a plate on the tension side and an oblique screw through the fracture site to achieve satisfactory interfragmental compression. These fractures now would be treated immediately with interlocking nails.

manner using a template for placement. In the tibia, the screws are inserted through the subcutaneous surface; and in the femur, a direct lateral approach is used.

After insertion of the screws, the bar is adjusted to the appropriate length and applied to the screws. When reduction of the fracture has been achieved, the pin clamps are locked by a cam arrangement at the ball joints and the telescopic central bar is locked in its sleeve. The joints allow 30° of angulation and free rotation. The positions of the locking cams are ascertained by pairs of markers on the camshaft end and the encasing collar. When these markers are aligned, the ball joint is unlocked. Locking occurs between 45° and 75° of rotation.

Chao and Hein[81] investigated the mechanical properties of this device and found it to be comparable to quadrilateral fixators with transfixing full pins and advised that multiple usage was permissible for four consecutive 6-month periods, providing that "careful inspection and routine replacement of crucial parts is performed on the used apparatus before reapplication."

De Bastiani and associates[111] (in their initial report in English), treated 288 fresh fractures, of which 239 were closed and 49 were open; 117 were in the femur, 160 in the tibia, 44 in the humerus, 1 in the radius, and 16 in the pelvis. In closed fractures their success rates were 91% in the tibia and 98% in the femur and humerus. In open fractures their success rates for the

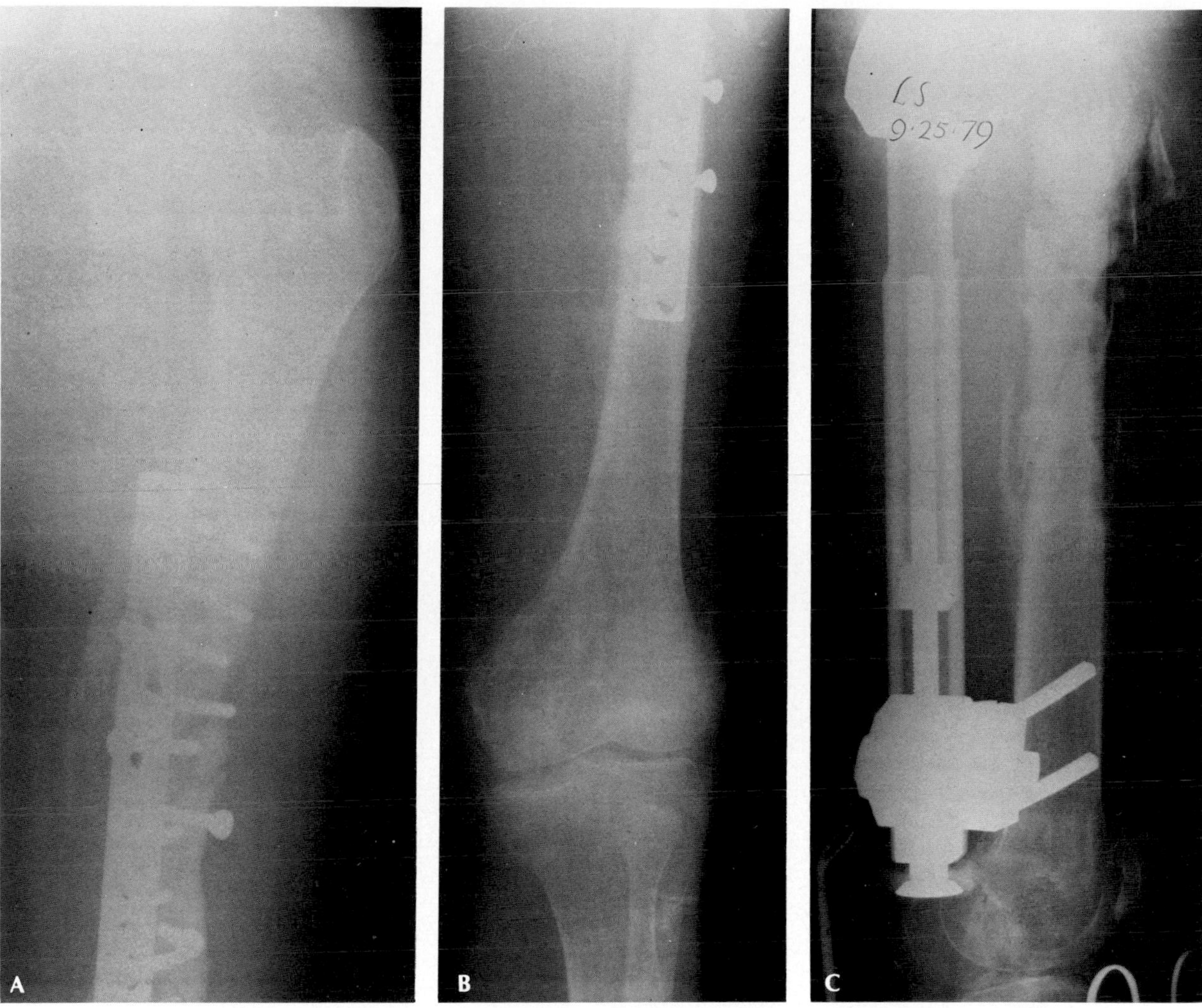

FIGURE 1-71. Radiographs of the leg in a 16-year-old boy who sustained a femoral shaft fracture that was treated by the application of a plate. (**A** and **B**) Anteroposterior and lateral films of the femur show that the plate has been applied to the anterior aspect of the femur instead of the lateral side, and the fracture at this point is infected with loose internal fixation and broken screws. (**C**) Because the internal fixation was performing no useful function, it was removed and a Wagner external fixator applied. Cancellous bone grafting was performed during the operation.

continues

tibia and femur were 88% and 89%, respectively. Their pin tract infection rate was incredibly low: only 14 (in ten patients) of 1525 pins inserted. The average time taken to apply the apparatus was a mere 15 minutes.

The AO/ASIF Fixator

The inventors of the AO/ASIF device[204] set out to provide a fixator that would be versatile, stable, and simple (Fig. 1-74).[7] It consists of four components: Steinmann pins, Schanz screws, a tube with an outer diameter of 11 mm, and an adjustable clamp to fix the pins to the tube.

The tubes come in a variety of lengths from 100 to 600 mm and are approximately two and one-half times as strong as the threaded bar of the earlier AO fixator.

The Steinmann pins are 5 mm in diameter (150–250 mm in length) and have a modified drill bit-point to eliminate thermal damage to the bone. The Schanz screws are also 5 mm in diameter and are available in lengths from 100 to 200 mm. These screws have been modified by making the threaded portion only 18 mm long so that it engages only the far cortex, while the near cortex is occupied by the smooth, unthreaded 5-mm shaft.

The adjustable clamp connects the Steinmann pins or the Schanz screws to the tubes and allows for correction in all planes. To insert the pins and screws, 3.5- and 4.5-mm drill bits are necessary, as well as a

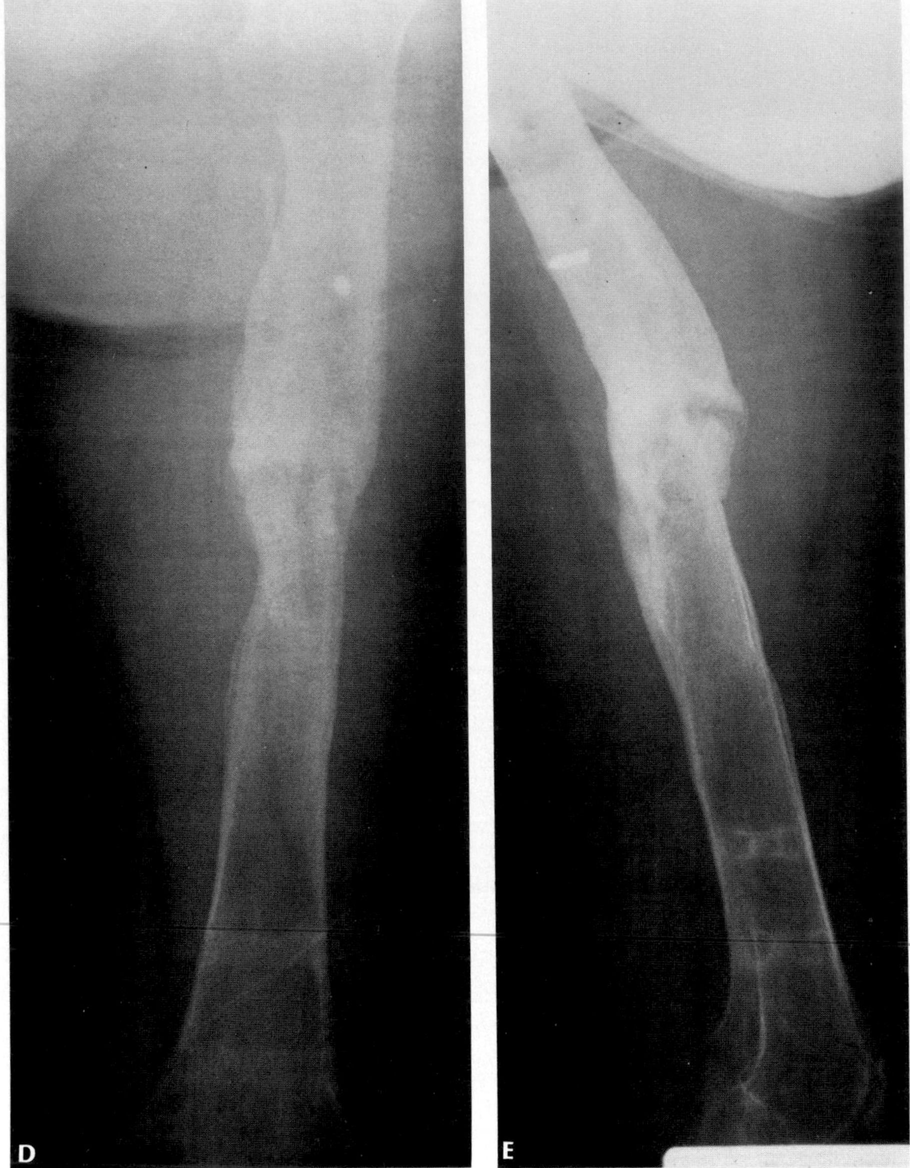

FIGURE 1-71. (continued) (**D** and **E**) The end result 16 months later, after having been maintained in the Wagner apparatus for 13 months.

3.5-mm trocar and drill sleeves with inner diameters of 3.5 and 5 mm.

To insert a Schanz screw, the drill sleeves and trocar are assembled and inserted through a stab wound until the trocar impinges on the surface of the bone. After removal of the trocar, both cortices of the bone are drilled through with a 3.5-mm drill. The 3.5-mm sleeve should then be removed and the near hole enlarged with the 4.5-mm drill. The Schanz screw is then introduced by a hand chuck and the 5-mm drill sleeve removed.

Steinmann pins are introduced in a similar fashion; the combined drill sleeves and trocar are introduced as before, but in this case, the trocar and 3.5-mm drill sleeve are both removed and both cortices drilled with the 4.5-mm bit. However, when quadrilateral or delta frames are applied, the aiming device should be used (Fig. 1-75). The aiming device ensures that the drills and subsequently the Steinmann pins pass accurately from the clamp on one tube to its companion on the other tube. In this case, the 3.5-mm sleeve of the aiming device is used to drill both cortices of the bone and then the aiming device is removed and the 4.5-mm drill is used to overdrill the 3.5-mm hole.

Although a large variety of configurations are possible using the AO components, three configurations are particularly recommended (Fig. 1-76): type I—unilateral frame; type II—bilateral frame; and type III—triangulated assembly.

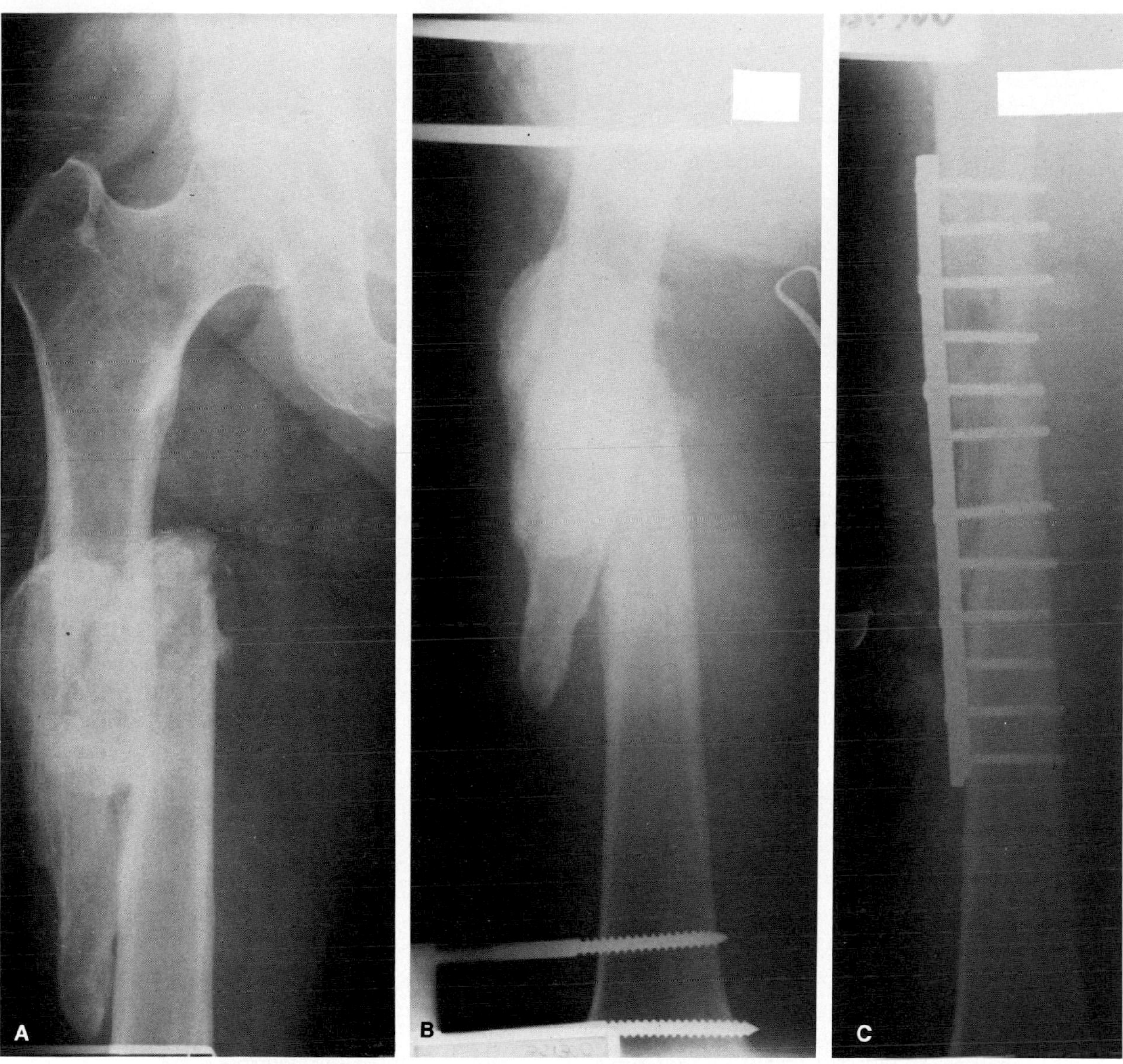

FIGURE 1-72. The use of the Wagner device for gradual lengthening. A 44-year-old man fractured his femur when he overturned a tractor. He was treated at a military installation by a cast-brace. After removal of the cast-brace he developed pain in his thigh but kept walking anyway. He was seen by four orthopaedists for disability evaluation, all of whom reported different leg-length discrepancies, which they believed to be secondary to shortening with malunion. (**A**) This radiograph shows that no union had been achieved. (**B**) The femur was pulled out to length gradually by a Wagner apparatus. (**C**) Internal fixation by a plate after the femur had been pulled out to length.

Unilateral Frame. The unilateral frame is particularly indicated where anatomical or functional conditions make the other frames inadvisable (eg, the humerus and forearm). It is also appropriate for open fractures of the femur and has been particularly advocated by Behrens and Solls for the management of tibial fractures. In the tibia, the pins are inserted in the tibial crest. A Schanz screw is placed in each fragment in the metaphysis close to the joint. Four (or six) clamps are placed on a tube of appropriate length that is fixed to the Schanz screws. A closed reduction of the fracture is then carried out, and the clamps are tightened. It is essential that rotational alignment be achieved at this juncture. Screws are then inserted through the remaining clamps and the assembly tightened. The closer the tube is placed to the tibial crest, the more rigid the fixation will be, and it may be further enhanced by adding a second tube. If a second tube is added, it must be done before the third and fourth screws are inserted, so that the screws can be inserted through each pair of clamps simultaneously. The frame may be made even stiffer by applying two unilateral frames at an angle to each other and cross linking the tubes. This is the V-frame.

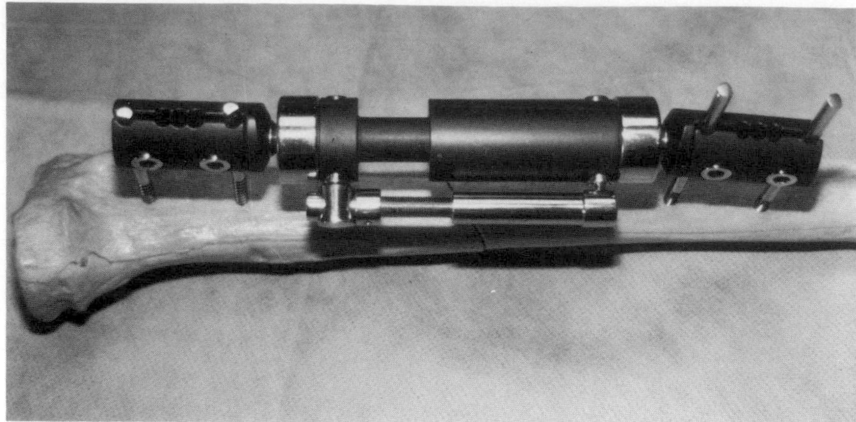

FIGURE 1-73. The Orthofix fixator. (*Courtesy of EBI Medical Systems, Inc., 1989.*)

Bilateral Frame. The bilateral AO/ASIF configuration is used primarily in fractures of the tibia. The first Steinmann pin is inserted through the distal tibia, anterior to the fibula, and parallel to the ankle joint. If the bone is hard, it should be predrilled with the 3.5-mm drill and then with the 4.5-mm drill. In osteoporotic bone, however, predrilling with the 3.5-mm drill is adequate and the 5-mm Steinmann pin is inserted. Insertion of a proximal pin is carried out from lateral to medial immediately anterior to the fibula while an assistant applies traction and corrects rotational malalignment of the leg. The pins should be parallel and be inserted by a hand chuck. Clamps corresponding to the number of pins desired are threaded on the longitudinal tubes and care is taken to place them in such a manner that their

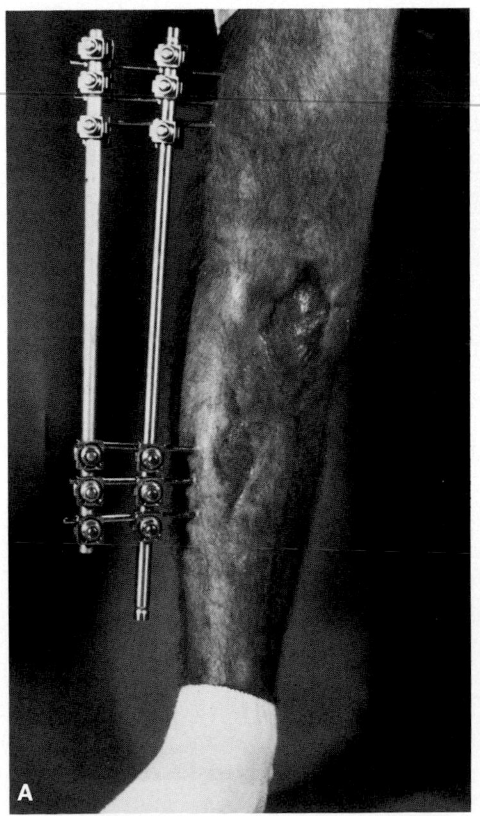

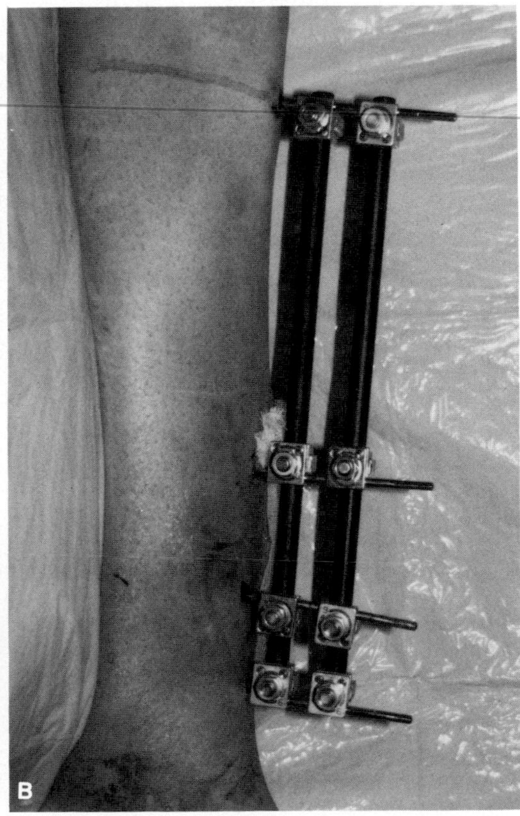

FIGURE 1-74. (**A**) The AO/ASIF external fixator, type I unilateral frame with double bar. Note that the upper pins are in the distal femur to reduce a comminuted plateau fracture by ligamentotaxis and to stabilize a comminuted fracture of the shaft. (**B**) Immobilization of a tibial fracture by an anterior unilateral frame with double bars (Trauma Fix). Note that these bars are made of a radiolucent fiber composite.

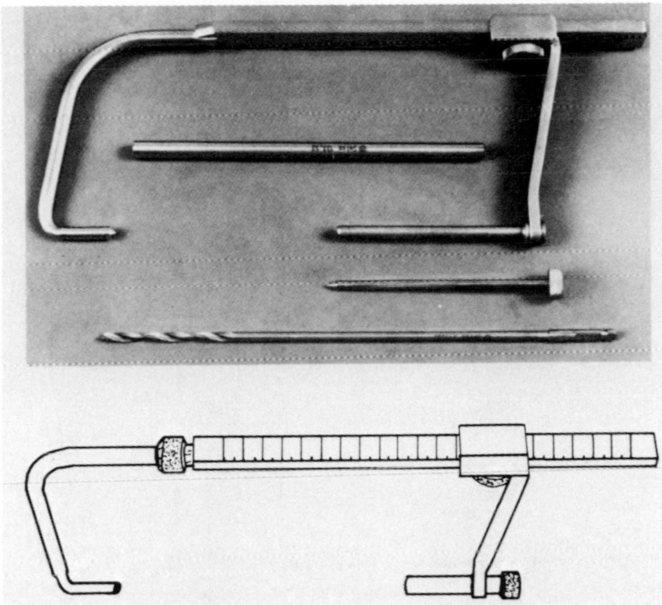

FIGURE 1-75. The AO aiming device. (*Hierholzer, G., Rüedi, T., Allgower, M., and Schatzker, J.: Manual on the AO/ASIF Tubular External Fixator, p. 27. New York, Springer-Verlag, 1985.*)

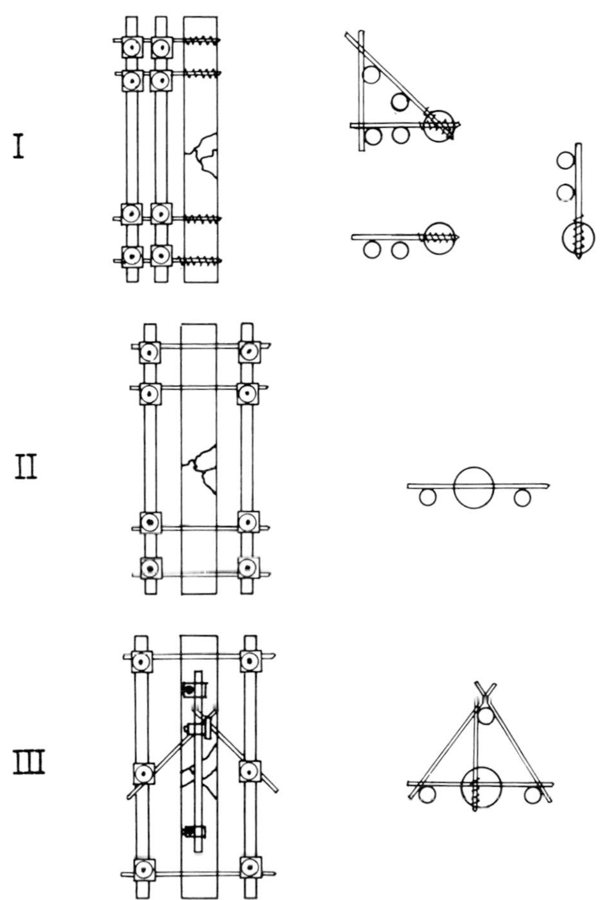

FIGURE 1-76. The AO fixator assemblies. (**I**) Unilateral frame, one-plane and two-plane (V-shaped). (**II**) Bilateral frame. (**III**) Triangulated frame. (*Hierholzer, G.; Rüedi, T, Allgöwer, M., and Schatzker, J.: Manual on the AO/ASIF Tubular External Fixator, p. 31. New York, Springer-Verlag, 1985.*)

broad part lies anterior to the Steinmann pins, and the tube posterior to them. The clamps should be tightened minimally to allow later final reduction of the fracture. The screws are then tightened and the remaining Steinmann pins inserted using the pin guide to make the drill holes.

If the definitive treatment of the fracture is to be by fixator, pins should be inserted close to the fracture site; if internal fixation is planned for later, the pins should be inserted as far as possible from the fracture.

When this frame is used and there is adequate bony contact, axial compression may be exerted on the fracture site by preloading the Steinmann pins (ie, bending them toward the fracture) (Fig. 1-77). On the other hand, if there is a bony defect or no inherent stability because of comminution, the Steinmann pins should be preloaded within each fragment by bending the pins toward each other (see Fig. 1-77).

This preloading may be produced by applying the AO compressor or a Verbrugge clamp, or by one's fingers.

Triangulated Assembly. The axial and lateral stability are about the same in type II and type III AO/ASIF configurations, but the triangulated assembly has greater torsional stability than is achieved by fewer anchoring pins in the bone. It is mostly used in the tibia, where fewer pins pierce the anterolateral compartment, but is sometimes indicated in fractures of the distal femur.

To build this frame, one Steinmann pin is inserted proximally and one distally in the same manner as when applying the type II bilateral frame. Three clamps are applied to each tube and the tubes are

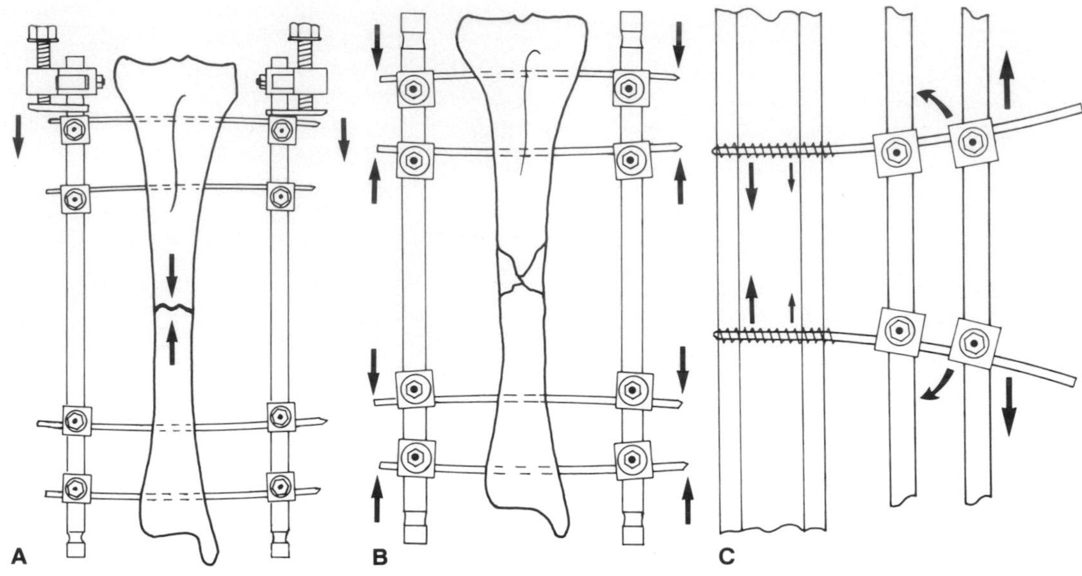

FIGURE 1-77. To prevent loosening, Steinmann pins and Schanz screws should be preloaded. (**A**) Where compression of the fracture site is indicated, the pins are bent toward the fracture. (**B**) Loading Steinmann pins within each fragment by bending them toward each other. (**C**) Preloading Schanz screws within the same fragment. (*Hierholzer, G., Rüedi, T., Allgöwer, M., and Schatzker, J.: Manual on the AO/ASIF Tubular External Fixator, p. 54, 58, and 68. New York, Springer-Verlag, 1985.*)

applied to the Steinmann pins loosely. After reducing the fracture the clamps are tightened and one Schanz screw is inserted anteroposteriorly in each fragment. A third tube with four clamps attached is fitted to the Schanz screws, and the lateral tubes are cross linked to the sagittal tube using Steinmann pins and the previously applied clamps. As in the type II frame, the Steinmann pins in the bone are preloaded (see Fig. 1-76).

Clamp Fixators

The Hoffmann System (Figs. 1-78 through 1-80) The Hoffmann system is a clamp fixator. The resurgence of interest in external fixation was sparked by Vidal and colleagues' use of the quadrilateral frame in conjunction with an improved Hoffmann system.[427]

The Hoffman quadrangular frame was attached to

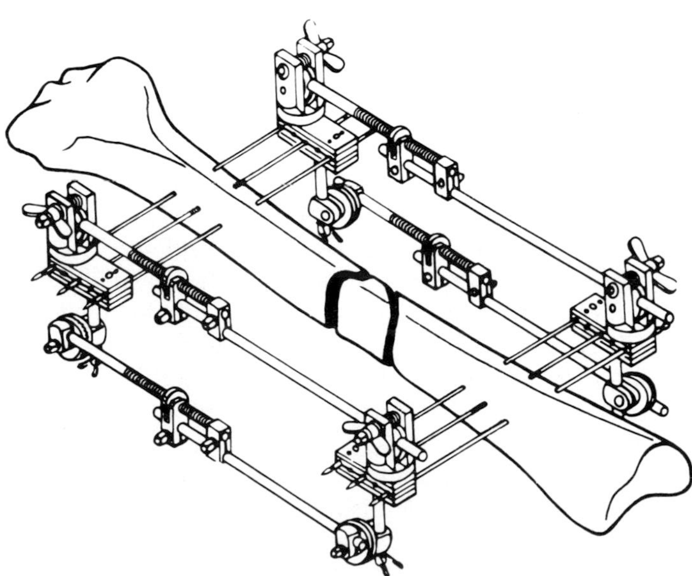

FIGURE 1-78. Complete quadrilateral tibial frame (Hoffmann). (*Connes, H.: Hoffmann's External Anchorage, Edition GEAD, Paris, 1977.*)

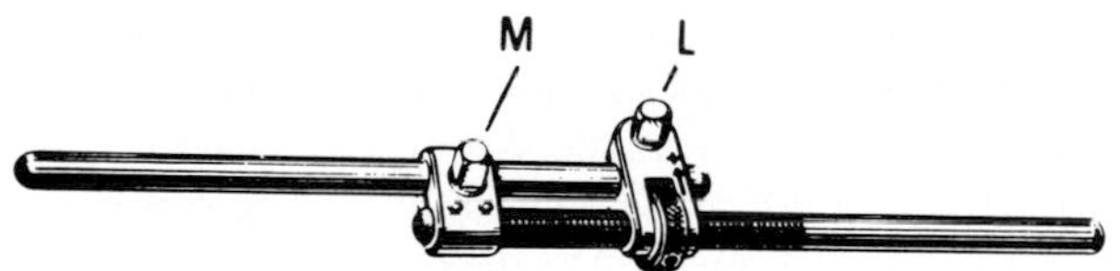

FIGURE 1-79. The adjustable connecting rod for the Hoffmann device. To lengthen or compress, the two-sided screw (*L*) is locked and the square head (*M*) is loosened. In the original version, turning the knurled nut in the direction of the arrow will produce lengthening. When the desired effect is gained, *M* is locked. (*Connes, H.: Hoffmann's External Anchorage, Edition GEAD, Paris, 1977.*)

transfixing Steinman pins by Bakelite clamps, which dictated the placement of the pins that were all inserted in the same plane. The apparatus was bulky, interfered with the patient's ambulation, and even with modifications (the triple and chalet frames [see Fig. 1-80**B** and **C**]) did not provide any great advantage over less cumbersome fixators. Any device that uses transfixion pins in the tibia is likely to interfere with ankle motion by anchoring the muscles of the anterior compartment and to endanger the neurovascular bundle. Furthermore, the insertion of pins through fleshy sites greatly increases the chance of pin tract infection.

Carbon-Fiber Fixators

One of the irritating aspects of external fixation is the difficulty in obtaining serial x-ray films of a fracture that is obscured by a metal frame. Witschger and Wegmüller[442] have addressed this problem by experimenting with a variety of materials to replace the metal longitudinal bars (plastics reinforced with fiberglass, Kevlar, nylon, and carbon-reinforced epoxy). Of these alternatives, carbon-reinforced epoxy was found to be the most suitable, and Synthes has marketed a fixator made of this material under the trade name TraumaFix (see Fig. 1-74**B**).

The carbon rod is more rigid than the metal tube and is 40% lighter. It is also more resistant to fatigue. With an applied torque of 20 N, a metal tube breaks after 32,000 cycles whereas the carbon rod withstands up to 100,000 cycles without failure. The manufacturers recommend this fixator for single use, although the rod could reasonably be used more than once, and it comes, prepackaged and sterile, complete with 5-mm Schanz screws, 3.5-mm drill with drill sleeve, depth gauge, and an 11-mm wrench. The clamps are aluminum and have captive nuts, and the entire assembly weighs 12.3 oz.

A very similar, disposable, carbon-fiber fixator is marketed by the Howmedica Company under the name of Ultrafix. In this system both single- and double-pin clamps are available as well as rod-to-rod clamps; all of these clamps allow 360° of rotation providing a great deal of versatility in pin placement and frame construction. Half pins 5 mm in diameter are used with this fixator, which is not designed to employ transfixion pins. It does allow two-plane fixation with linkage (delta frame) or double-bar unilateral fixation similar to the AO fixator.

The Hex Fix fixator now has a carbon version to facilitate radiographic examination.

Rigidity of Fixation

Although it might be argued that quadrilateral frames, especially with additions in other planes, are more rigid than unilateral frames, this disparity can be substantially reduced. In all pin fixators rigidity depends more on the pins than on any other factor.[76] Rigidity is greatly enhanced by increasing the number of pins, the size of pins, and their stiffness or modulus of elasticity.[33,76] It would be unwise, however, to increase the diameter of pins to more than 6 mm because of the weakening effects of a large hole in the bone. Greater stability is also gained by increasing the distance between pins and by having pins in different planes.[76]

Behrens,[30–35] who has studied this problem extensively, compared the Hoffmann frame with a unilateral AO frame and found the AO frame to be stiffer in all planes. To add rigidity to frames employing half pins, he advised decreasing the distance between the bone and the longitudinal rod, increasing the pin-to-pin distance, use of two-plane configurations, and use of an anterior frame with two longitudinal bars. He stated that unilateral frames are more desirable because they provide better wound access, cause less joint stiffness, and diminish the chance of neurovascular damage.

Behrens found that, overall, the two-plane or delta configuration (see Fig. 1-76) was the stiffest, but exceeded the anterior, one-plane, double-bar (at 25 mm and 80 mm from the tibia) by only a negligible degree.[35] These principles do not apply to the AO system alone but can be adapted to any pin fixation system.

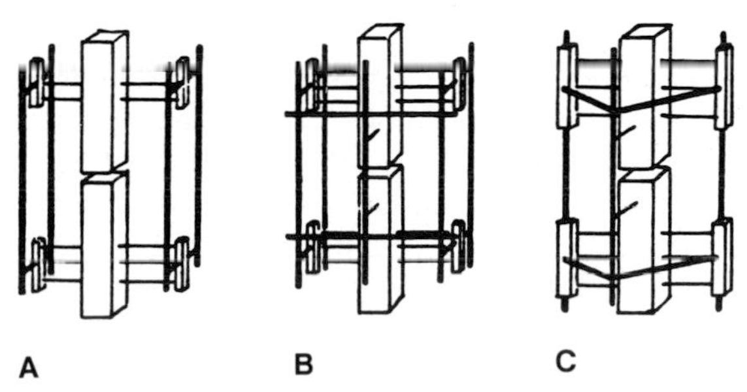

FIGURE 1-80. (**A**) Original Hoffmann-Vidal quadrilateral double frame. (**B**) Quadrangular triple frame. (**C**) Triangular triple frame. (*Vidal, J., Nakach, G., and Orst, G.: New Biomechanical Study of Hoffmann® External Fixation. Orthopedics 7:654, 1984.*)

Ring Fixators

The Ilizarov Frame

Several devices for external fixation using wires under tension suspended from metal rings have been designed. Both the Volkov-Oganesian and the Ilizarov[155,214,296,297,298] frames from Russia are examples of this method. Wires of small diameter (less than 2 mm) pass through the bone and are placed under tension of about 100 kg and secured to circumferential rings (Fig. 1-81). The stability of the apparatus has been demonstrated both clinically and in the laboratory. The smaller wires may cause less skin irritation and reduce pin tract infections. Two potential liabilities are the bulk of the frame and the resultant lack of access for soft-tissue care.

The principles and apparatus of Ilizarov have created great interest and offer a substantially different approach to skeletal reconstruction after trauma. The fixator was used for more than 40 years by its originator, the late Professor Gavriel Abramovich Ilizarov, who performed feats of legerdemain in an institute dedicated to his methods in Kurgan, Siberia. The primary focus in this country has been application of the technique in pseudarthrosis, bone defects, and deformity. However, in the republics of the former Soviet Union the device has been used for years in the management of acute trauma and soft-tissue defects.

The technical details and use of the frame are quite complex and beyond the scope of this chapter. For fractures that require stabilization or correction of deformity, the frame is applied to maintain alignment, allowing early weight bearing and longitudinal loading. End-to-end compression is applied when the fracture configuration allows. If deformity is present, the apparatus can be used to realign the fragments and maintain anatomical alignment. The use of the frame in this setting differs little from most external fixation devices.

In acute fractures with soft-tissue defects, the principles of Ilizarov differ from the more traditional approach. Rather than maintain length with external fixation and treat the soft-tissue loss with muscle flaps and bone grafting, the Russians allow shortening at the site of bone and soft-tissue loss to achieve primary healing, irrespective of acute limb shortening. A corticotomy and lengthening is then performed at a site *away* from the zone of injury to reestablish limb length. According to Ilizarov, the use of autogenous bone grafting and soft-tissue coverage procedures are virtually eliminated. The experience with these methods in acute trauma in the United States is limited and unreported at this time.

In comparing the Ilizarov fixator with a variety of the common half-pin fixators, the Ilizarov fixator is significantly less stiff in lateral bending than uniplanar fixators, comparable in anteroposterior bending and torsion, and 75% less stiff in axial loading.[155]

The frame is most stable when the Kirschner wire is inserted at a 90° angle to its mate at the same level, but anatomical constraints make this impractical. A 45°/135° placement decreases the stiffness in anteroposterior, but not lateral, bending. Increasing the wire tension from 900 to 1300 N increases bending and axial stiffness but decreases torsional stiffness.[155]

The small diameter of the transfixion pins should not lull one into a sense of false security regarding their potential to damage neurovascular structures. One must pay the same meticulous attention to the anatomical hazards as when using larger transfixion pins. Partial rings to which large diameter half pins may be clamped are available. These are particularly helpful in anchorages to the upper end of the femur where transfixion wires are hazardous (Fig. 1-82).

The Monticelli Spinelli Fixator

The Monticelli Spinelli device is a modified Ilizarov frame and has been designed primarily for limb-lengthening procedures (Fig. 1-83). There are three sizes of color-coded rings: small (blue), medium (green), and large (gray). These rings are constructed by bolting two segments together—a $^{3}/_{4}$ ring and a $^{1}/_{4}$ ring. Each of these segments may be used separately in building a frame or combined to form a complete ring. A $^{3}/_{4}$ ring may be used in the proximal tibia to prevent the limiting of knee flexion that a full ring would engender. The $^{1}/_{4}$ ring may be used with half pins in the proximal femur in fixation of femoral fractures or in lengthenings.

The Ace-Fischer Fixator

The Ace-Fischer device is a ring fixator in which the rings are connected by rods that have universal joints at each end and are capable of either compression or distraction by rotating a compression wheel (one revolution equals 1 mm). Both $^{1}/_{3}$ and $^{2}/_{3}$ rings may be used, and their fixation to bone is by transfixion pins, half pins, or Kirschner wires. The fixation pins are predrilled and are either fixed directly to the rings or through pin holders that accept up to three pins.

In fracture treatment, two distractors are attached to a proximal and a distal ring and rotational deformity is corrected with the universal joints unlocked. After the rotational deformity is corrected, the joints are relocked. Angular deformity is then corrected by unlocking the universal joints in the plane of the required reduction and by lengthening and shortening the appropriate distractors. Similarly, displacement is corrected by loosening the four universal joints in the plane of displacement and manually correcting it. After reduction, additional rods may be added and "dynamization" may be achieved by loosening the

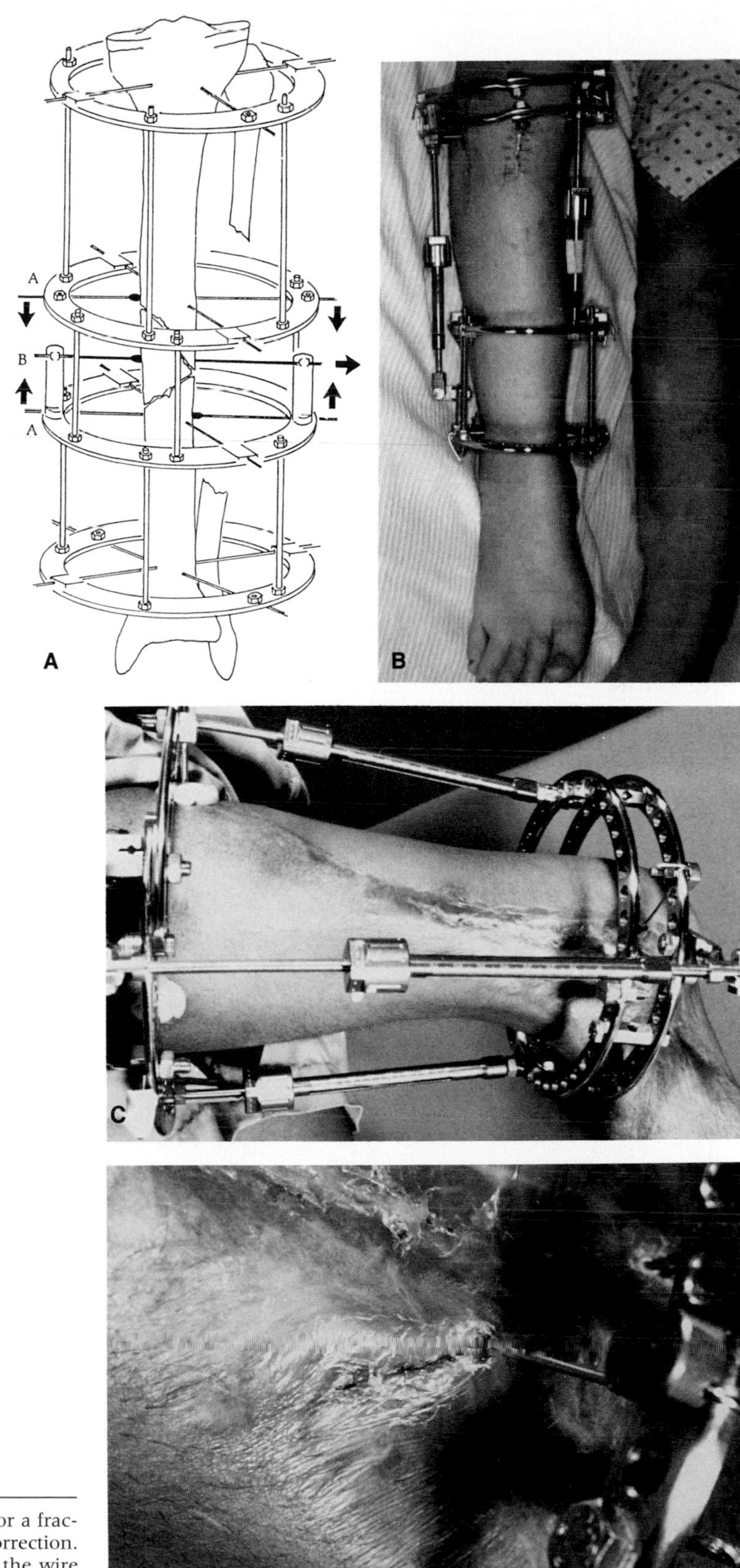

FIGURE 1-81. The Ilizarov apparatus. (**A**) The frame for a fractured tibia. (**B**) Lengthening of the tibia after angular correction. (**C**) Lengthening of the femur. (**D**) During lengthening, the wire cuts through skin with immediate healing as the wire progresses.

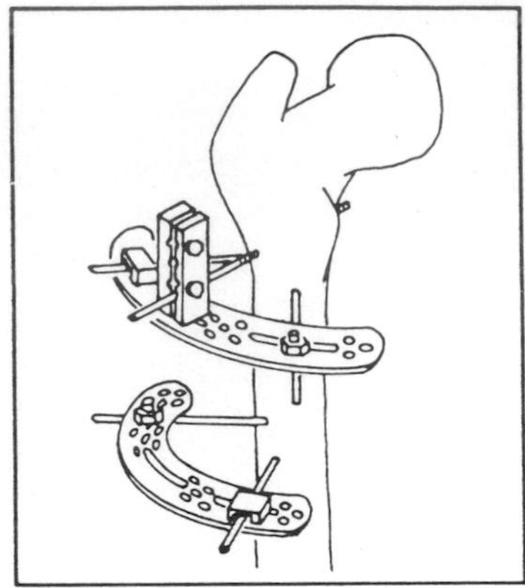

FIGURE 1-82. Half rings carrying Steinmann pins for use where wires are not applicable. (*Courtesy of Richards Medical Company.*)

"fast-adjust" mechanism on the distraction rods. This allows axial loading without loss of reduction.

The Hex Fix Fixator

The Hex Fix fixator (Smith and Nephew Richards, Inc., Memphis, TN) consists of a single hexagonal bar that is made of anodized aluminum, stainless steel, or carbon fiber. "Spools" may be threaded over these rods, which in turn carry pin clamps on which titanium or stainless steel pins are mounted that may be 4, 5, or 6 mm in diameter. The spools, which may be moved freely up and down the rod, are locked in position by a set screw and may be single or double. The double spool is able to mount two pin clamps and the single, one. The pin clamps come in four varieties: the single and double as well as the single and double swivel clamps that carry, as their name suggests, either one or two pins held in place by two set screws (Fig. 1-84).

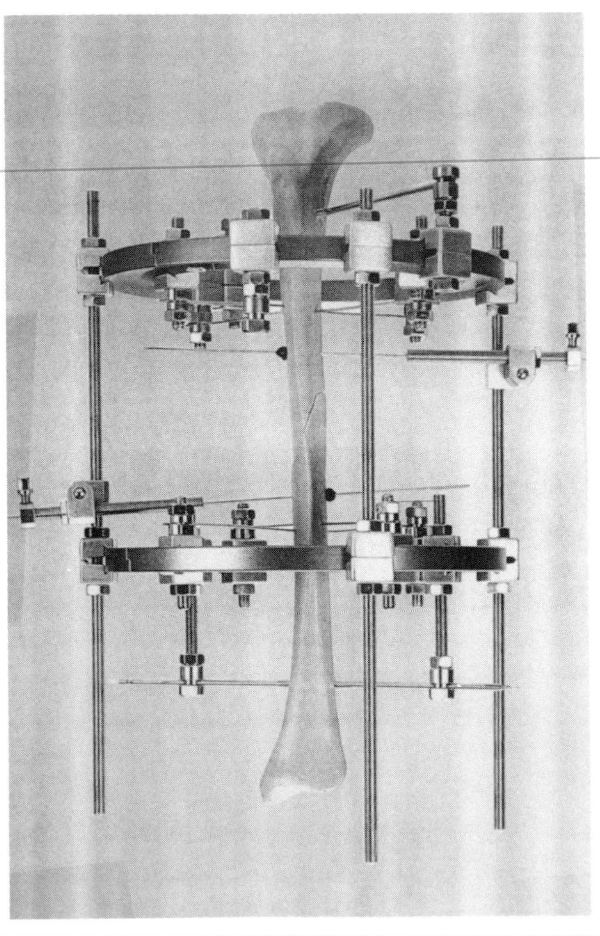

FIGURE 1-83. Monticelli Spinelli external fixator. Note the stop-wires exerting interfragmentary compression. (*Courtesy of Richards Medical Company.*)

Locking rings on the spools allow the pin clamps to be rotated in the transverse plane and be locked in the desired position. Single and double swivel clamps allow rotation in the longitudinal plane and locking is accomplished by a 10-mm nut.

The universal swivel clamp allows a major fragment to be fixed with a two-pin cluster so that it can be manipulated in any direction at any time without pin removal or revision.

To apply the frame to manage a tibial diaphyseal fracture, the bar is fitted with four single spools and four single swivel pin clamps. The first pin is inserted in the proximal diaphysis close to the knee joint, and the second pin is inserted in the distal fragment in the same plane and close to the ankle joint. The bar with the four spools and pin clamps is now attached to these pins and the fracture distracted and reduced. When the reduction has been effected the locking screws and nuts are tightened. The remaining two spools and clamps are adjusted so that the pins can be directed 2 cm above and below the fracture site.

The system is very versatile, allowing multiplanar pin fixation, and an Ilizarov ring adapter may be added for management of pilon or tibial plateau fractures. The addition of a drive unit allows the frame to be used for leg-lengthening or segment transport. Each turn of the screw distracts the fragments by 1 mm (see Fig. 1-84**C**).

It is recommended that femoral fractures be managed by a single-axis frame mounting six pins (see Fig. 1-84**A**)

The Pinless External Fixator

AO/ASIF has developed an innovative type of external fixator that is attached to the tibia by clamps that are inserted through the soft tissues.[392] These clamps are tightened by means of removable handles, which allows the surgeon to adjust the tension by feel until the fixation is stable. After removing the handles the clamps are connected to an AO/ASIF fixator.

The results in experimental animals have shown that the fixation is satisfactory and after 5 weeks there was no evidence of infection. This may be the fixation of choice when immediate intramedullary fixation is contraindicated but is going to be used at a later date.

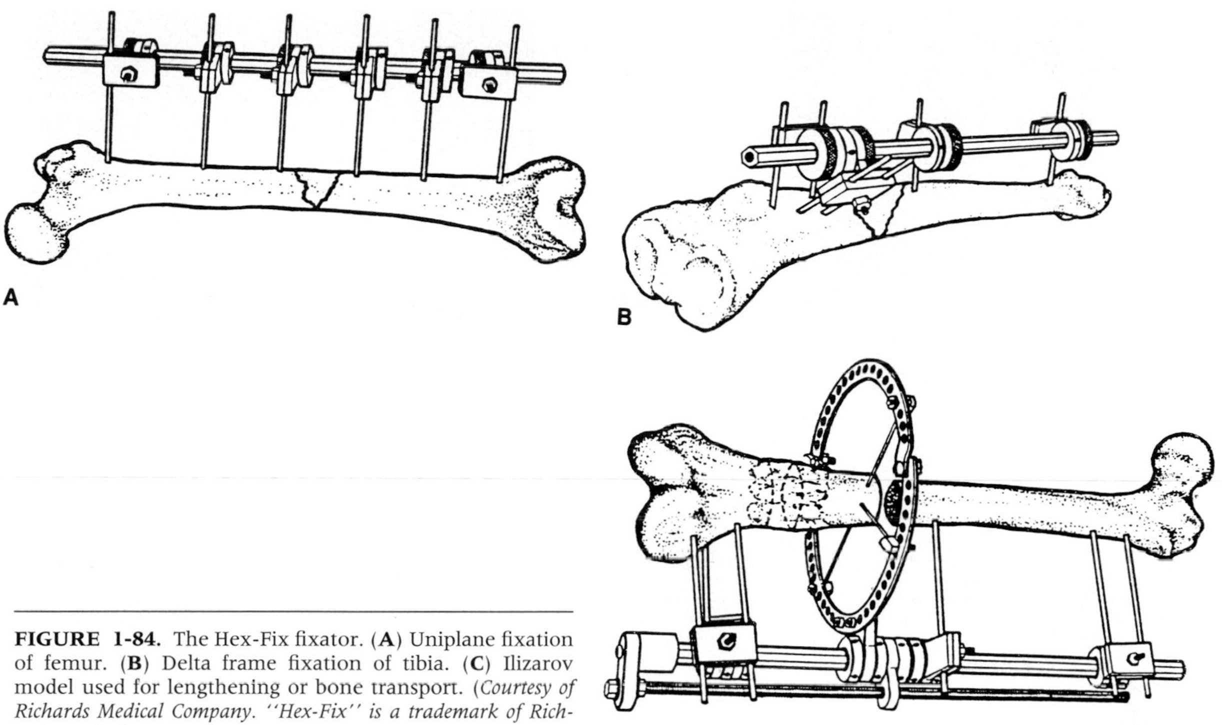

FIGURE 1-84. The Hex-Fix fixator. (**A**) Uniplane fixation of femur. (**B**) Delta frame fixation of tibia. (**C**) Ilizarov model used for lengthening or bone transport. (*Courtesy of Richards Medical Company. "Hex-Fix" is a trademark of Richards Medical Company.*)

Combined Internal and External Fixation of Fractures

The stability of the frame, as we have seen, is greatly enhanced by contact of the bone ends of an inherently stable fracture, which allows compression to be applied. This desirable condition may also be achieved by limited open reduction and minimal internal fixation with a screw or even cerclage (Fig. 1-85).[204]

A rebuttal of this principle, however, is the view of Krettek and coworkers,[237] who found no perceptible advantage in supplemental lag screw fixation in open tibial fractures managed by external fixation. In their experience they had a greater incidence of refracture and delayed union requiring bone grafting.[237]

What is not generally advocated in the literature on external fixation, but we have found most useful in unstable fractures of the tibia, is the principle of internally fixing the fibula as advocated by the late George Eggers. Even in the most catastrophic fractures of the leg, the skin over the fibula tends to be intact and one may plate the fibula with impunity. This immediately restores the length of the leg and supplements the stability of the external fixator (Fig. 1-86).

Confirmation of the usefulness of this approach has been supplied by Morrison and his associates,[278] who studied the effect of fibular plating on five cadaver limbs where a 2-cm segment was removed from the tibia and the fibula resected. Plating of the fibula increased stiffness on axial loading by a factor of 2.2.[278]

The importance of the intact fibula is also underscored by Van der Werken and colleagues.[420] They treated 11 patients with displaced tibial fractures in whom there was no fibular fracture by inserting only one 4.5-mm half-pin above and below fracture. Distraction of those pins automatically restored length and alignment. The patients were allowed to walk with crutches without weight bearing for 6 weeks, and active motion of the knee and ankle was encouraged. The pins were then removed and the patients resumed walking in a functional brace for 4 weeks. The results were uniformly excellent.

Another stratagem to increase stability where a segment of tibia has been lost was devised by Dr. Douglas Hanell (personal communication, 1984) when he was a fellow in microsurgery in Louisville. In the case illustrated in Figure 1-87, an 18-month-old child sustained a shotgun blast to her leg resulting in a segmental loss of the tibia. She was treated by the application of a fixator and a latissimus dorsi free flap. To make the construct more stable, Hanell inserted a hand-carved block of high-density polyethylene into the tibial defect. Later, when tissue homeostasis had been reached, this spacer was removed and replaced with an adult radial allograft. Unhappily, the allograft lay inert in the leg for several months before we belatedly supplemented it with cancellous autograft. The end result has been most satisfactory.

We are not purists and have no compunction about combining external fixation with a supplementary fiberglass cast that need not incorporate the pins of the fixator. This has the advantage of preventing equinus

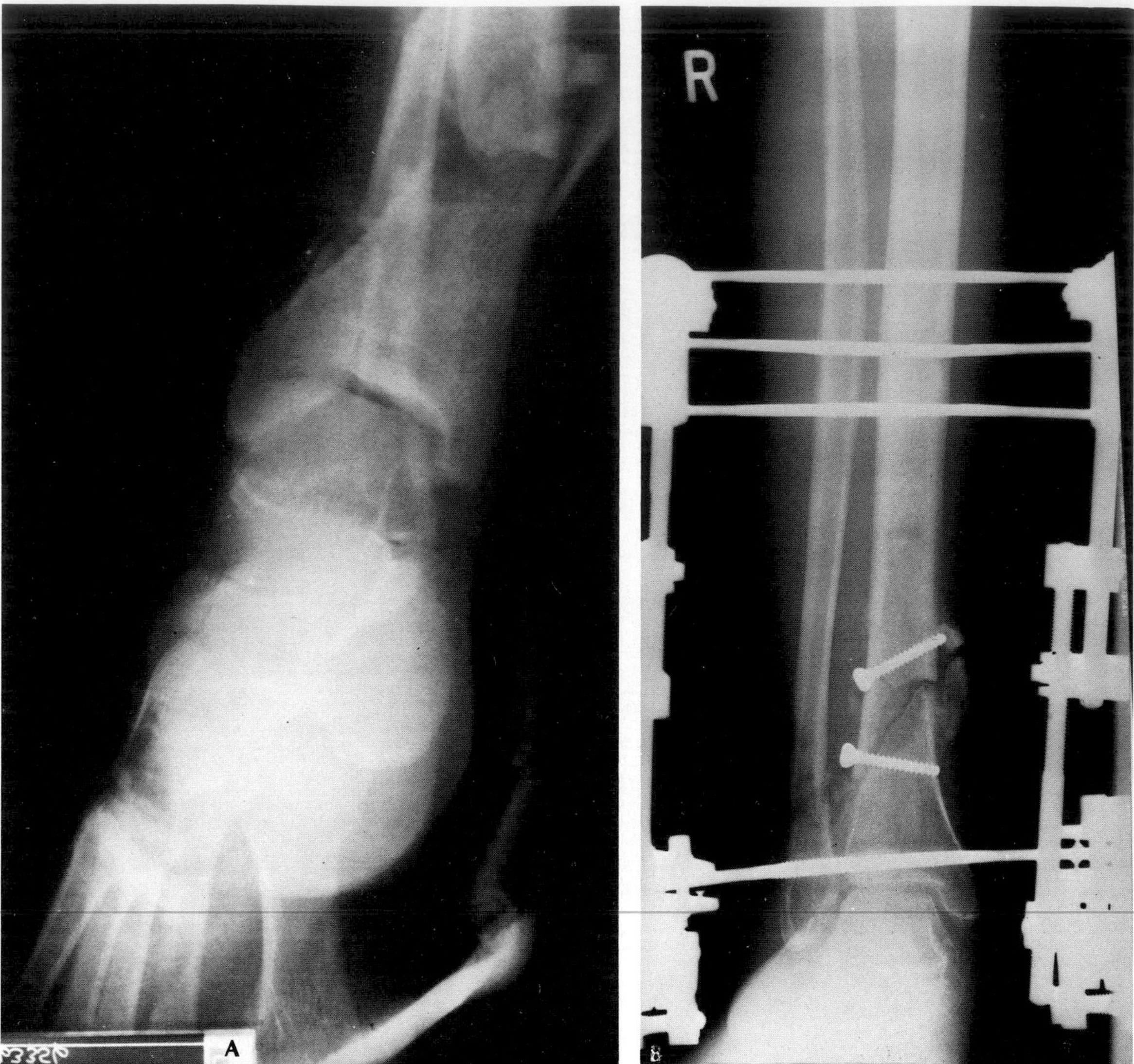

FIGURE 1-85. Combination of external and internal fixation used to treat an open tibial fracture incurred in a motorcycle accident. (**A**) Preoperative fracture. (**B**) Hoffman fixator and loose butterfly fragment fixed by two screws.

continues

deformity of the ankle and increases resistance to bending stresses (Fig. 1-88).

Complications of External Fixation

Pin Tract Infection

The history of external fixation is rife with pin tract infection, which led to discontinuation of the technique in the past. It is said that Roger Anderson, when entertaining a group of visiting orthopaedists, was asked if there was not pus draining from a pin tract of one of his patients. "No, no," he said, "that's only a little serum." This apparently is the origin of the euphemism "Seattle serum" for pus.

Burny[67] stated that percutaneous implants in general are associated with infection and tissue proliferation. Smooth-surfaced implants undergo either marsupialization or deep sinus tract formation, and skin epithelium grows along the percutaneous portion of the implant and eventually surrounds it. Rough implants allow tissue ingrowth, providing a site for bacterial sequestration. Infection, commonly from *Staphylococcus aureus,* originates on the body surface around the entry sites.

Pin tract infections may be classified, in ascending order of severity, as:

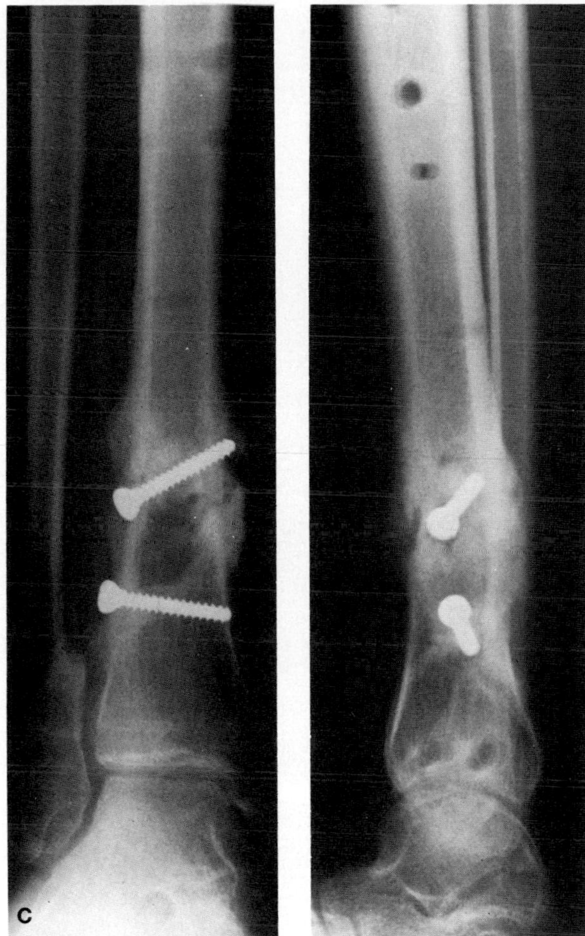

FIGURE 1-85. (continued) (**C**) Healing after removal of fixator.

Grade I—Serous drainage
Grade II—Superficial cellulitis
Grade III—Deep infection
Grade IV—Osteomyelitis.

As noted previously, placing pins through fleshy areas predisposes to infection, so pretibial placement is the site of choice in tibial fractures. Significant infection of pins is infrequent with the Ilizarov system, perhaps owing to the small diameter of the transfixion pins; those infections that do occur tend to be grade I and are easily dealt with.[297]

Rommens and colleagues[345] reported a minor infection rate of 9.4% and a major infection rate of 9.1% in a series of 95 patients treated with the Vidal-Ardrey frame for tibial fractures, and Clifford and associates[93] had a 43% overall infection rate. However, in the latter report, when broken down into rates for transfixion and half pins, the infection rates were 78% and 17%, respectively. De Bastiani and coworkers,[111] as we have seen, had a comparatively negligible infection rate; the reason for their unusual success is not obvious.

Prophylaxis consists of ensuring that pin incisions are adequate and that the threaded portion of a pin is not evident in the wound. Pin care (ie, the meticulous washing of the pin sites several times per day with soap and water and mechanical cleansing with cotton swabs) is the sheet anchor of pin management. Some surgeons use povidone-iodine, which is fine, but we deprecate the use of hydrogen peroxide, which is a tissue poison.

When infection does supervene, free drainage by enlarging the wound and therapy with appropriate antibiotics are indicated. When this is ineffective, the pin should be removed and replaced, and curettage of the pin tract may be necessary to remove a sequestrum. We have no experience in the use of locally injected antibiotic solutions in pin tract infections and are somewhat skeptical regarding their usefulness.

We have looked on pin tract infections as a squalid nuisance or at best an inconvenience since most of them respond to treatment. However, pin tract infection may compromise the result of subsequent tibial nailing. McGraw and associates[260] reported that 7 of 16 patients treated by sequential external fixation and intramedullary fixation developed severe deep infections. Maurer and colleagues[256a] had 24 patients treated sequentially, of whom 7 had previous pin tract infections. Tornquist[413] treated 18 tibial nonunions by intramedullary nailing, and 6 of those had been managed by external fixation. Two healed without incident, but the remaining 4 developed deep infections by the organisms that had previously been cultured from infected pin sites.

The length of time between removal of the fixator and the nailing was immaterial in these cases, and the pinholes were all healed. Perioperative antimicrobial therapy was used in these cases, and none appeared infected before surgery. All of these authors advised against this sequential treatment.

In contradistinction, Wheelwright and Court Brown in Edinburgh used nailing in 26 patients after treating the pin tracts and allowing them to granulate. The only infection in the series was a previously infected type IIIB fracture.[435]

Blachut and his colleagues[53] have reported a series in which 41 open tibial fractures were treated by a protocol in which the wounds were debrided and immobilized by external fixation for an average of 17 days followed by intramedullary nailing. There were only 2 infections (5%) that healed without the development of chronic osteomyelitis. With a relatively short period of external fixation, the incidence of pin tract infection is less than with chronic application. This problem, however, might well have been solved by the introduction of the AO/ASIF "pinless fixator"

(text continues on page 76)

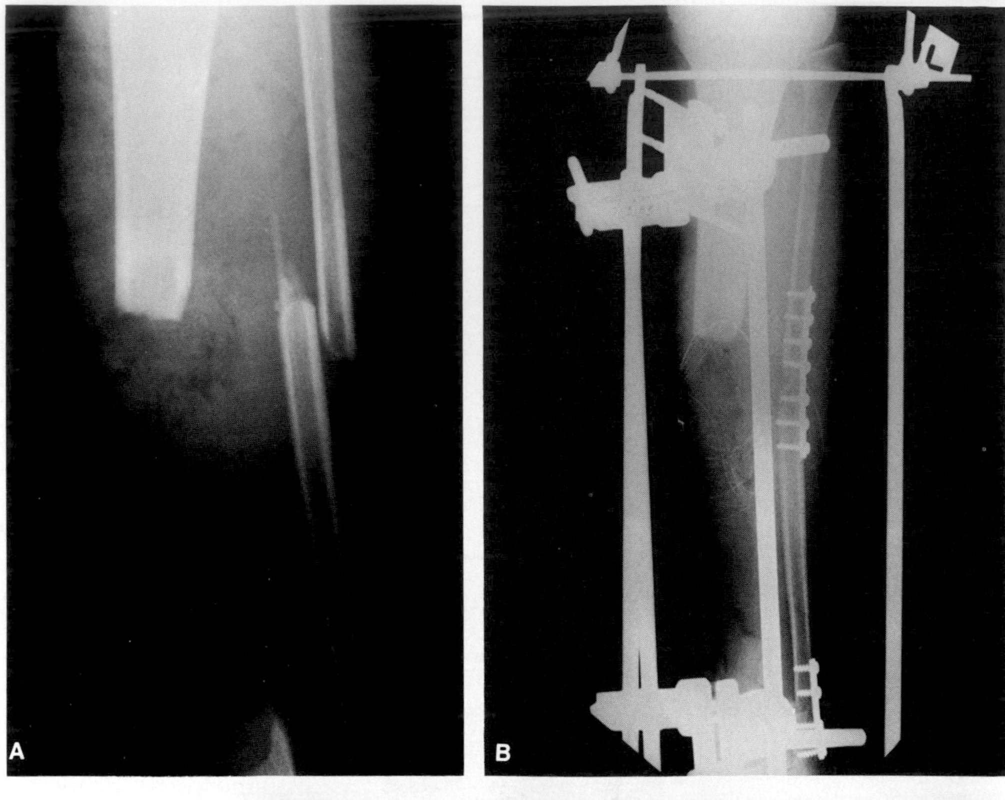

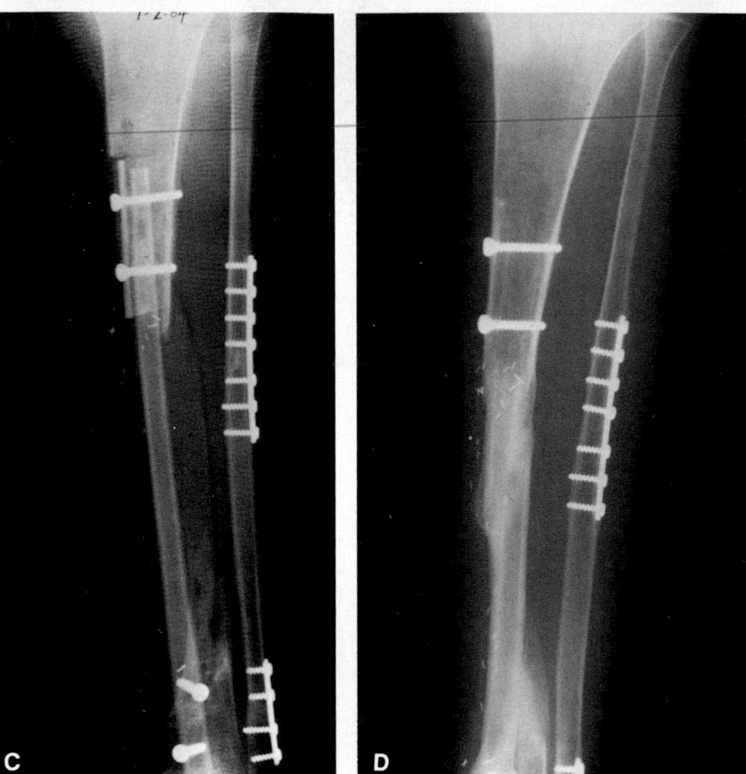

FIGURE 1-86. In unstable fractures of the tibia, fibular plating enhances the stability of external fixation. Radiographs of the leg in a 15-year-old boy who was riding on a motorcycle and sustained ipsilateral femoral and tibial fractures. (**A**) On admission to hospital, the shaft of the tibia was missing. (**B**) The fibula was plated and an external fixator and Tomberlin traction were applied. (**C**) A vascularized fibular graft was used to bridge the defect in the tibia. (**D**) The end result.

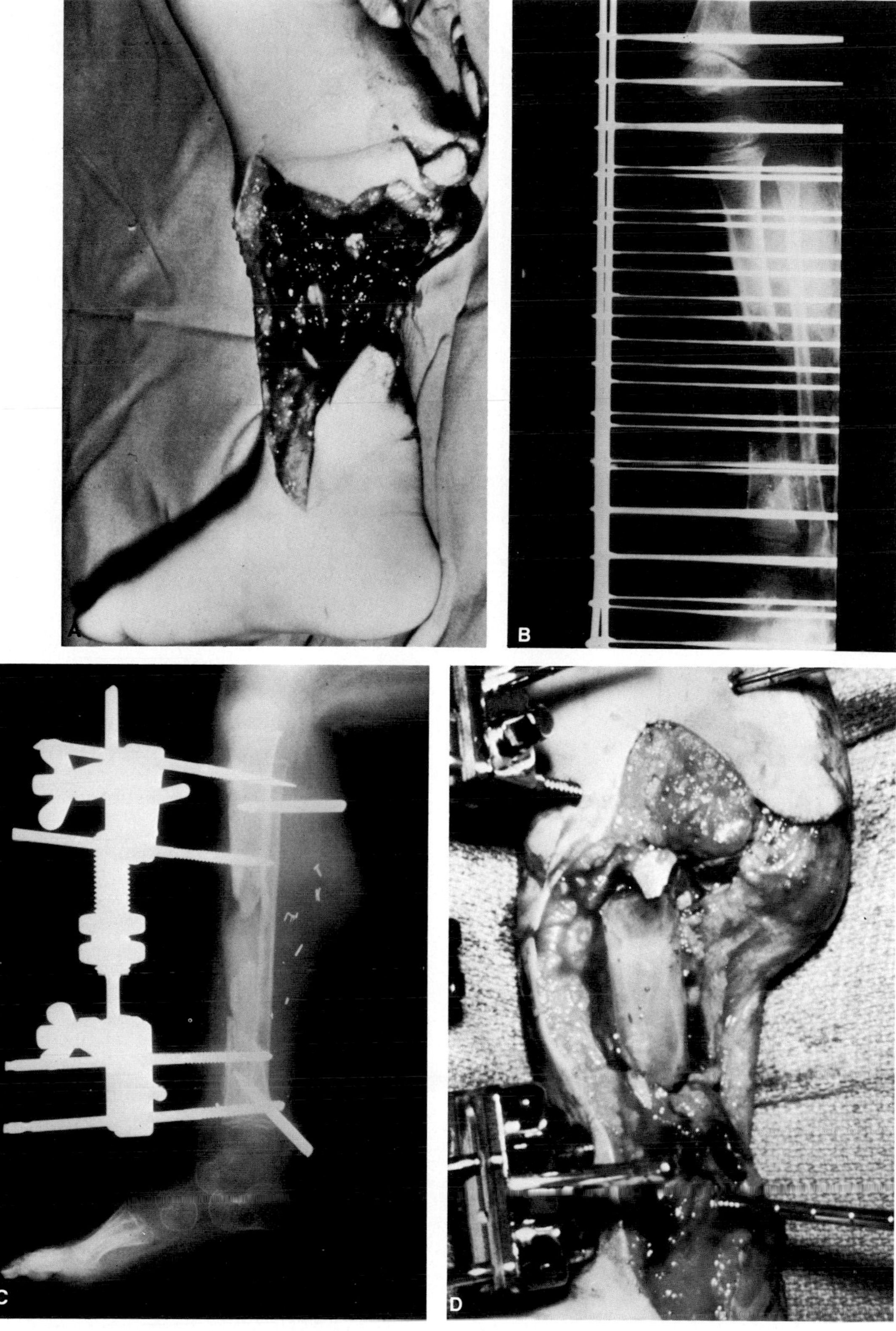

FIGURE 1-87. An 18-month-old girl sustained an accidental close-range shotgun wound resulting in a massive soft tissue wound and loss of a portion of the shaft of the right tibia. (**A**) Clinical photograph of the leg. (**B**) Radiograph on admission. (**C**) Application of an external fixator with a polyethylene spacer between the bone ends. (**D**) Intraoperative photograph showing the polyethylene spacer *in situ*.

continues

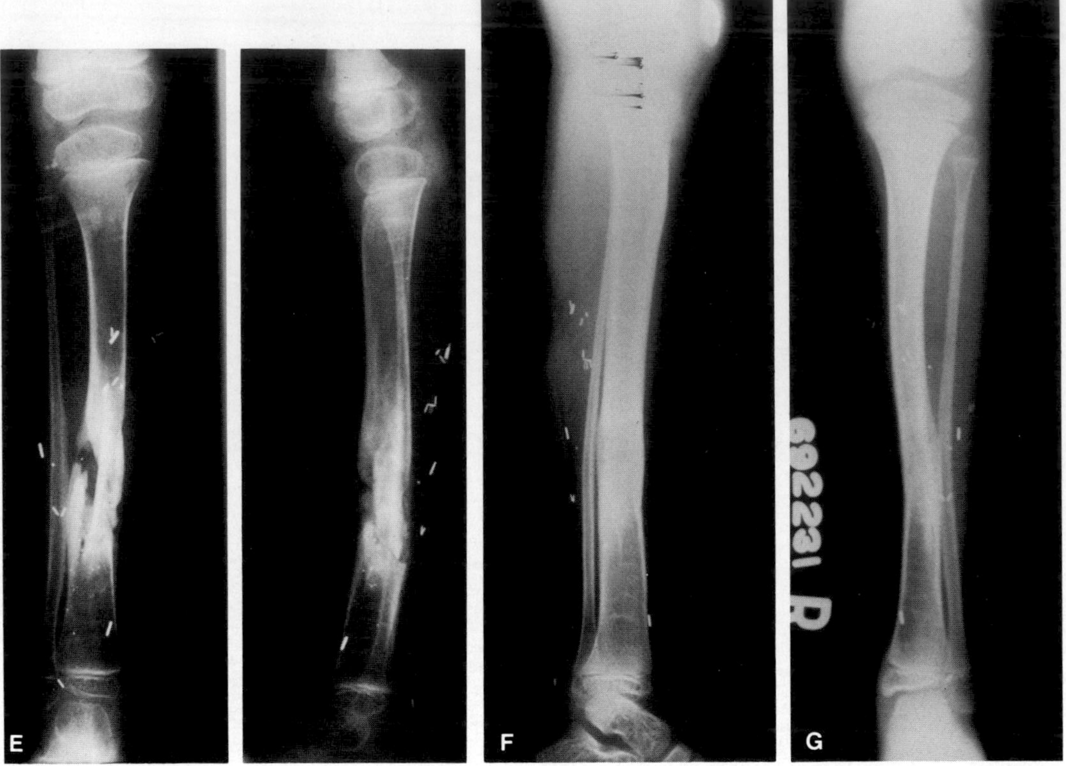

FIGURE 1-87. (continued) (**E**) The spacer was later removed and replaced with an allograft. (**F** and **G**) Radiographs of the end result.

that will allow fixation of tibial fractures without infection.[392]

It would appear that the circumspect surgeon should be very hesitant to nail a tibia in the presence of even a remote pin tract infection while it is permissible to carry out sequential nailing after short-term external fixation uncomplicated by infected pins.

Pin Loosening and Breakage

Pin loosening is inevitable if external fixators are on for long periods, and the loosening rate increases with time. Pin anchorage is of prime importance; a loose pin is nonfunctional and, furthermore, contributes to pin tract infection.[67] Obviously the anchorage is dependent on the quality of the bone; cortical bone provides a better anchor than metaphyseal bone, and young healthy bone is better than osteoporotic bone. Although we can do nothing about the quality of the bone, we can prevent the problems of improper pin insertion and select well-designed pins.

If bone is burned during pin insertion, a ring sequestrum forms, which can lead to infection and subsequent loosening.[67] Drilling bone with a Steinmann or other pin that does not allow the escape of bone chips increases the local temperature.[176a] It follows that either the holes should be predrilled or a pin with a drill tip should be used. We prefer the former option and use a trocar with a drill-guide cannula to allow predrilling of the pin.

The best half pins are those with a small threaded region that engages only the far cortex, with the near hole occupied by the smooth shaft.[31] By this arrangement the effective stiffness of the pin is doubled, the bone fit is tighter, and the stress at the bone–pin interface is reduced. The use of tapered half pins that may be advanced to regain fixation is of doubtful utility and inevitably results in further protusion of the pin through the far cortex.

The bone–pin interface is subjected to compression because of bending of the pin and to shear stress because of tension and compression loads. Failure may occur from a simple overload or by fatigue. In 1173 tibial fractures treated by external fixation with 4-mm pins, Burny[69] reported a 0.5% incidence of interface fracture and a 5.2% incidence of pin fracture.

Burny and his associates[68] investigated pin loosening by measuring the maximum torque at the time of pin removal and by the changes in the frequency of vibration of the external portion of the pin. They proposed the following clinical classification of loosening:

Stage 1—Perfect anchorage; no perceptible motion between pin and bone

Stage 2—Slight motion noticeable between pin and

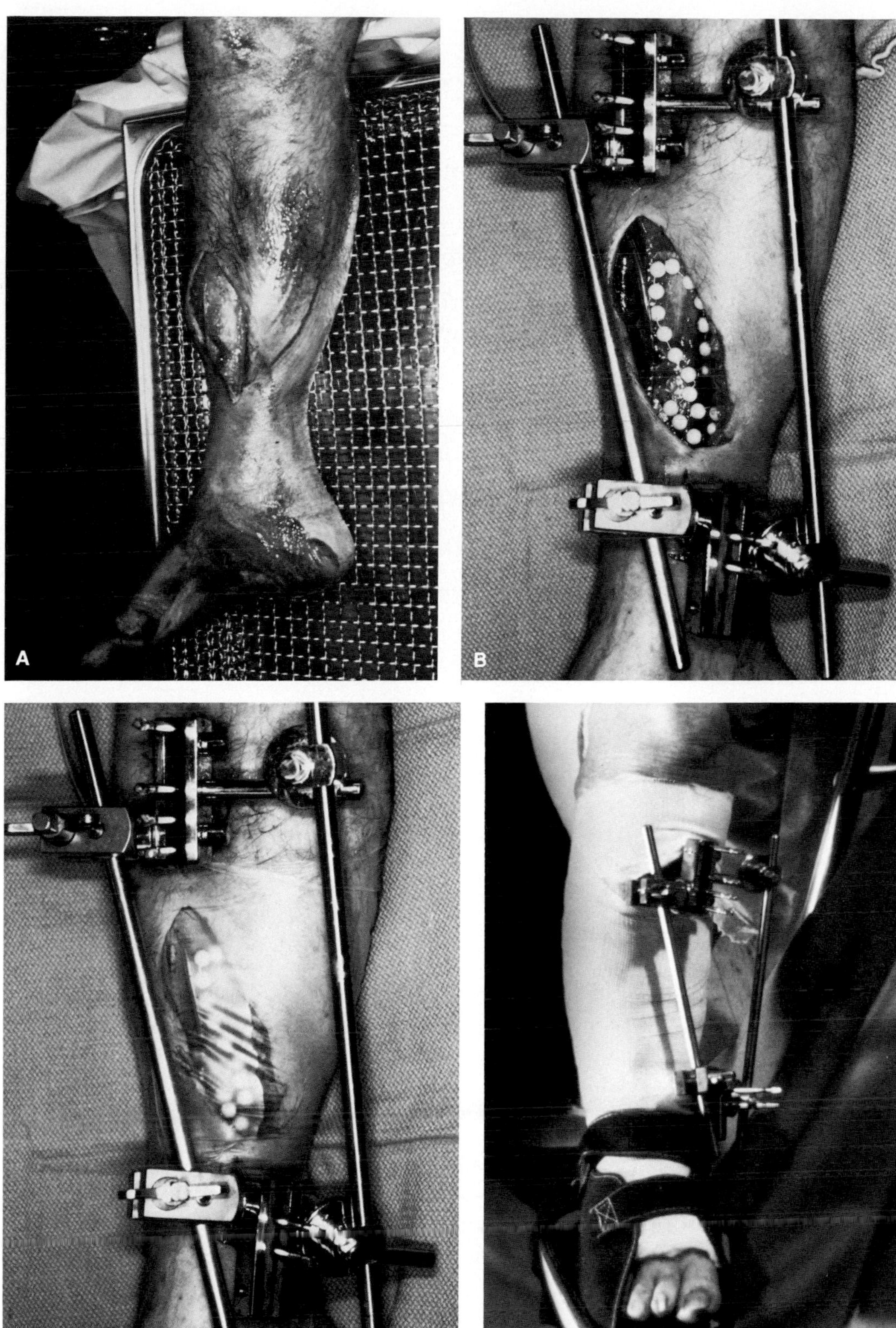

FIGURE 1-88. Clinical and radiographic views of a fractured tibia in an elderly woman who had been inebriated when injured, was unattended until the following morning, and did not remember how she was hurt. (**A**) Condition of the leg on admission. (**B**) After wound debridement and insertion of tobramycin beads and fixation by a one-plane, double-bar, Hoffmann fixator. (**C**) Bead pouch. (**D**) Cast supplementation of fixator.

continues

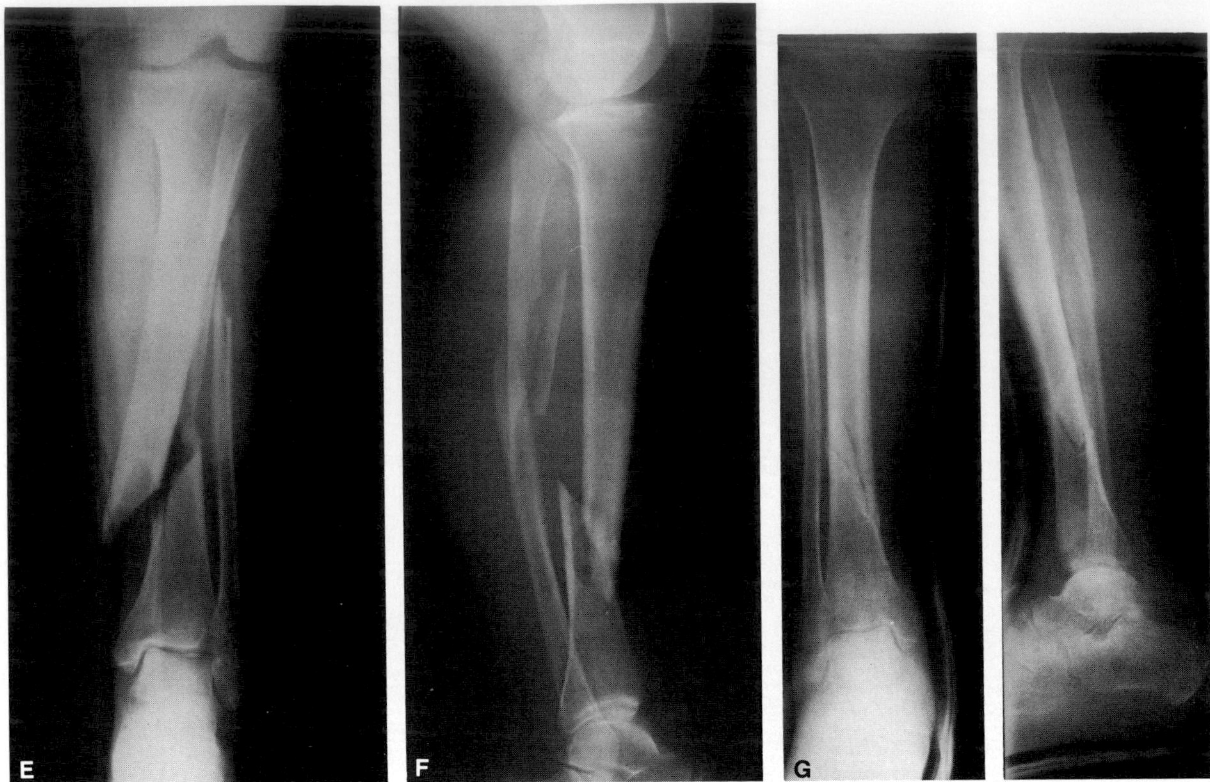

FIGURE 1-88. (continued) (**E** and **F**) Initial radiographs. (**G**) Early healing after 4 months.

bone (sensation of "contact" on fast oscillations by hand)

Stage 3—Considerable motion between pin and bone (clinical loosening)

Stage 4—Possibility of manual extraction (or spontaneous pull out) of pin.

Because one of the major causes of pin loosening is failure at the pin–bone interface, it follows that early weight bearing in unstable fractures is contraindicated, although this apparently does not apply to the Ilizarov method, in which early weight bearing is encouraged. Bone–pin stress is reduced by having the near hole occupied by the unthreaded, smooth shank of the fixation pin, and the pin breakage that occurs with early weight bearing results from both overload and fatigue.[31]

The AO/ASIF group believes that straight pins under zero load cause bone resorption and loosening owing to micromovement and that this can be eliminated by preloading the pins. Their experiments show that bending paired Steinmann pins toward each other can reduce the linear displacement of each fragment by 45%; the horizontal displacement is also reduced, but to a lesser degree. This increase in stability decreases the pin loosening and the danger of slippage.[204]

Limitation of Joint Motion

By transfixing muscles, the mobility of the contiguous joint may be limited, and this is particularly so where the muscles of the anterolateral compartment of the leg are involved. When a quadrilateral frame is applied to the tibia, the foot should be dorsiflexed to the neutral position before inserting the transfixing pins. Knee motion may also be limited by supracondylar pins or screws, and it is good practice to put the knee through a full range of motion to enlarge the puncture holes in the iliotibial tract.[204] Should a supracondylar pin become infected, there is some danger of the quadriceps scarring down to the underlying femur and permanently limiting knee flexion.

Neurovascular Damage and Compartment Syndrome

When applying an external frame, the surgeon should always have in the forefront of his or her mind the important anatomical structures at risk and the location of both safe and hazardous corridors for pin placement (Fig. 1-89). It is safer to place half pins than transfixion pins, but even half pins are not without risk, especially when the point of the pin protrudes in a hazardous area. One should always flex the patient's knee when placing an anteroposterior penetrating pin

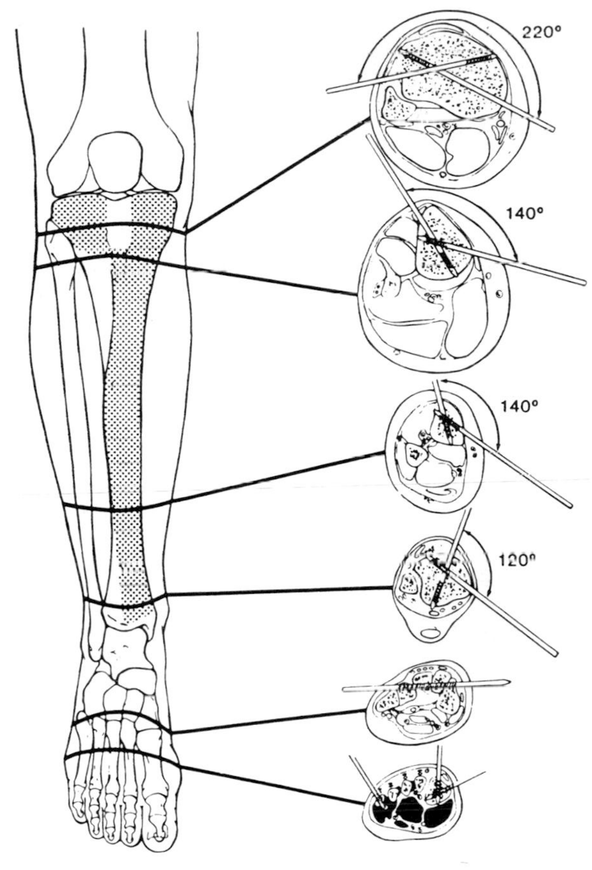

FIGURE 1-89. "Safe corridors" and arcs of insertion in the leg. (*Behrens, F., and Searls, K.: External Fixation of the Tibia: Basic Concepts and Prospective Evaluation. J. Bone Joint Surg., 68B:246–254, 1986.*)

in the proximal tibia to avoid damage to the posterior tibial neurovascular bundle.

In a retrospective study of 28 femoral and 91 tibial fractures treated by external fixation between 1985 and 1990, there were four iatrogenic vascular injuries: two arterial thromboses with distal ischemia and two false aneurysms. The vessels involved were the deep and superficial femoral and the anterior and posterior tibial arteries. The authors caution that one should pay attention to excessive bleeding from the pin holes and the signs of compartment syndrome and distal ischemia.[304]

The investing fascia converts the anterolateral compartment of the leg into a tight, unyielding box. A pin in this compartment, especially when the leg has been severely contused by a closed injury, may initiate enough bleeding to produce a compartment syndrome, so constant vigilance is necessary to prevent catastrophe.

Malalignment and Malunion

It is easy to apply a fixator to the tibia in malrotation, especially when the uninvolved leg, which might be used for comparison, is covered. Lining up the medial border of the patella with the first interdigital space is a good generalization, but there is a wide range of tibial torsion, and the safest plan is to make both legs match. Many frames allow little or no adjustment after application, and it saves a great deal of embarrassment to get it right the first time.

Even if the initial reduction has been perfect, pin loosening and weight bearing may allow angular deformities to occur, so the circumspect surgeon checks alignment clinically and radiologically throughout the healing period.

Delayed Union or Nonunion

Detractors of external fixation refer to frames as "nonunion machines," and indeed delayed union and nonunion are common with this form of treatment.

Rommens and associates[345] treated tibial fractures by a Vidal-Ardrey frame and reported that only 21% of the fractures healed within 4 months without other intervention. In 12.9% an overt pseudarthrosis developed, and 32.6% required a second procedure such as bone grafting, internal fixation, or both to achieve union.

Believing that the external fixator keeps the fracture distracted, some have advocated replacing the fixator with a cast after 6 weeks. But compression, per se, does not increase bone healing. Hart and associates[194] have shown experimentally that in the healing of osteotomies in dog tibias, compression increased the rigidity of fixation but not the rate of healing, and there was significantly more periosteal bone formation in noncompressed osteotomies.

Kenwright and Goodship[227,228] studied the effect of a short period of axial micromovement in simulated and clinical fractures of the tibia. Both in osteotomized sheep and in clinical cases treated by a Dynabrace fixator, healing was enhanced when 500 cycles of micromovement were applied over 17 minutes at 0.5 Hz daily.

It now appears to be widely accepted that micromovement in the axial plane enhances bone formation and healing in externally fixed fractures. To achieve this axial micromotion, the frame may be destabilized by removal of pins; moving longitudinal bars farther away from the bone; removing supplementary frames; or allowing the frame to telescope. In uniplanar fixation with two longitudinal bars or tubes, rigidity may be reduced by removing one of the bars or by replacing it with a shorter bar. This production of intermittent axial motion has come to be known as *dynamization,* a neologism deprecated by Allgöwer[6] (a prejudice that we share), and has also been called *build down* by Behrens,[33] although this term would seem to be an oxymoron. Nonetheless, Melendez and Colon[266] treated 45 open tibial fractures (89% type III) using an Orthofix frame and dynamized the fractures at 8 weeks.

All but one of these fractures healed in 22.6 weeks, although 58% had supplementary bone grafting and the overall complication rate was 53%. DeBastiani and associates,[111] using the same device, had a 91% success rate with tibial fractures that were dynamized when callus showed at 3 weeks. How long rigidity should be maintained or to what degree motion at the fracture site is beneficial is still to be determined. The process of destabilizing the frame and the timing of weight bearing have been discussed by Allgöwer and Sequin[7] and Behrens and Johnson,[33] but no one presently has determined if motion other than axial—angulation, rotation, or both—is helpful or deleterious.

Nishimura[290] studied the stiffness of healing fractures by adding strain gauges to a longitudinal rod of a tibial fixator. The knee was extended against 1- and 2-kg loads and the strain measured. He established that there are five healing curves: normal, slow healing, nonunion, arrest in development, and breakage of callus. The strain on the connecting rod decreased hyperbolically as the callus strength and mass increased and became constant when the strength reached a level equal to 50% of the intact bone. It would seem that this scale gives the surgeon an indication of whether a fracture is healing and provides a clue as to the appropriate time to "dynamize" the frame.

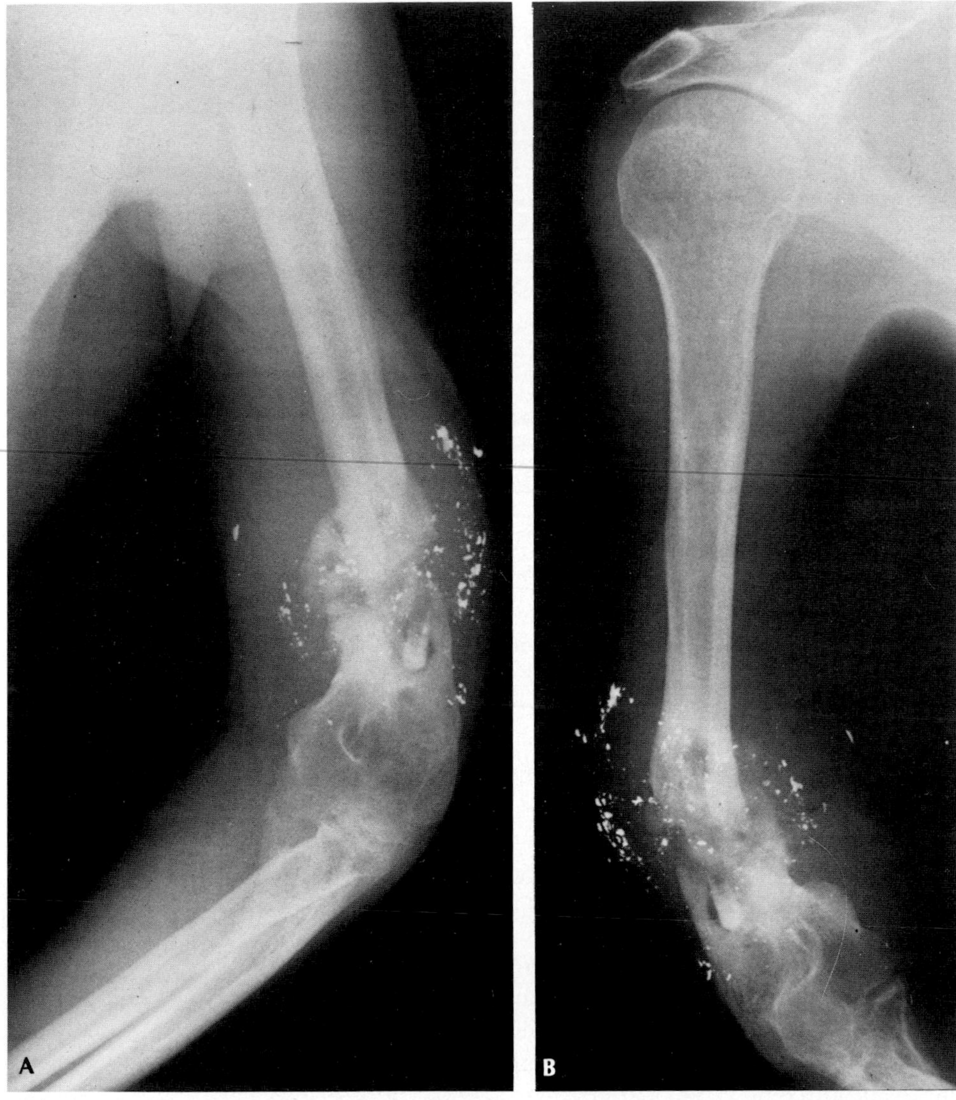

FIGURE 1-90. Radiographs in a man who had been shot in the left arm and left leg in an altercation and was seen many months later with infected nonunions of both bones as well as a radial nerve deficit in the left arm. Several sequestrectomies of the humerus were required. Neither external nor internal fixation alone gave sufficient stability for healing, but the combination of both combined with cancellous grafting eventually produced a satisfactory union and an arm that no longer drained. (**A** and **B**) Views of the left humerus with sequestra and lead fragments from the bullet.

continues

Indications for the Use of External Fixation

The prime indication for external fixation is when other means of fixation clearly are inappropriate. Fractures associated with extensive soft-tissue injuries are the most common indication in the United States, and most class III and many class II injuries are treated by this means, which allows free access to the wounds and does not preclude free tissue transfer, cancellous grafting, or hydrotherapy. External fixation certainly has a role in grossly comminuted, unstable fractures; where there is a bony deficit; in fractures associated with burns; and in the preliminary fixation of pelvic fractures. We have also found it useful in comminuted metaphyseal fractures where the principle of "ligamentotaxis"[425] can be applied, as in Colles' fracture.[112,218,333,337] In our practice we also have found external fixation very useful in the management of the fractured calcaneus and in achieving preliminary reduction in pilon fractures. An external frame is also useful to supplement an unstable osteosynthesis or in osteoporotic patients where conventional implants do not hold (Fig. 1-90).

The emergence of effective unreamed tibial nails and their use in open tibial fractures has in many centers supplanted the use of external fixation except in the severe type IIIC fractures. Tornetta and associates[412] compared the end results in 15 patients with grade IIIB open tibial fractures treated by unreamed interlocking nails with 14 similar patients treated by external fixators. All of these fractures healed, and the complication rate was about the same in each group.

Dell'Oca,[120] who is an advocate of simple pin fixators with extensive experience, lists the advantages of external fixation as being less damaging to the vascularity of the bone and being less likely to produce significant infection, although he has a 10% pin infection rate. When infections do develop, they are much more easily handled than when internal fixation has been used.

Perhaps the most clear-cut indication for the use of external fixation is in warfare or in dealing with mass

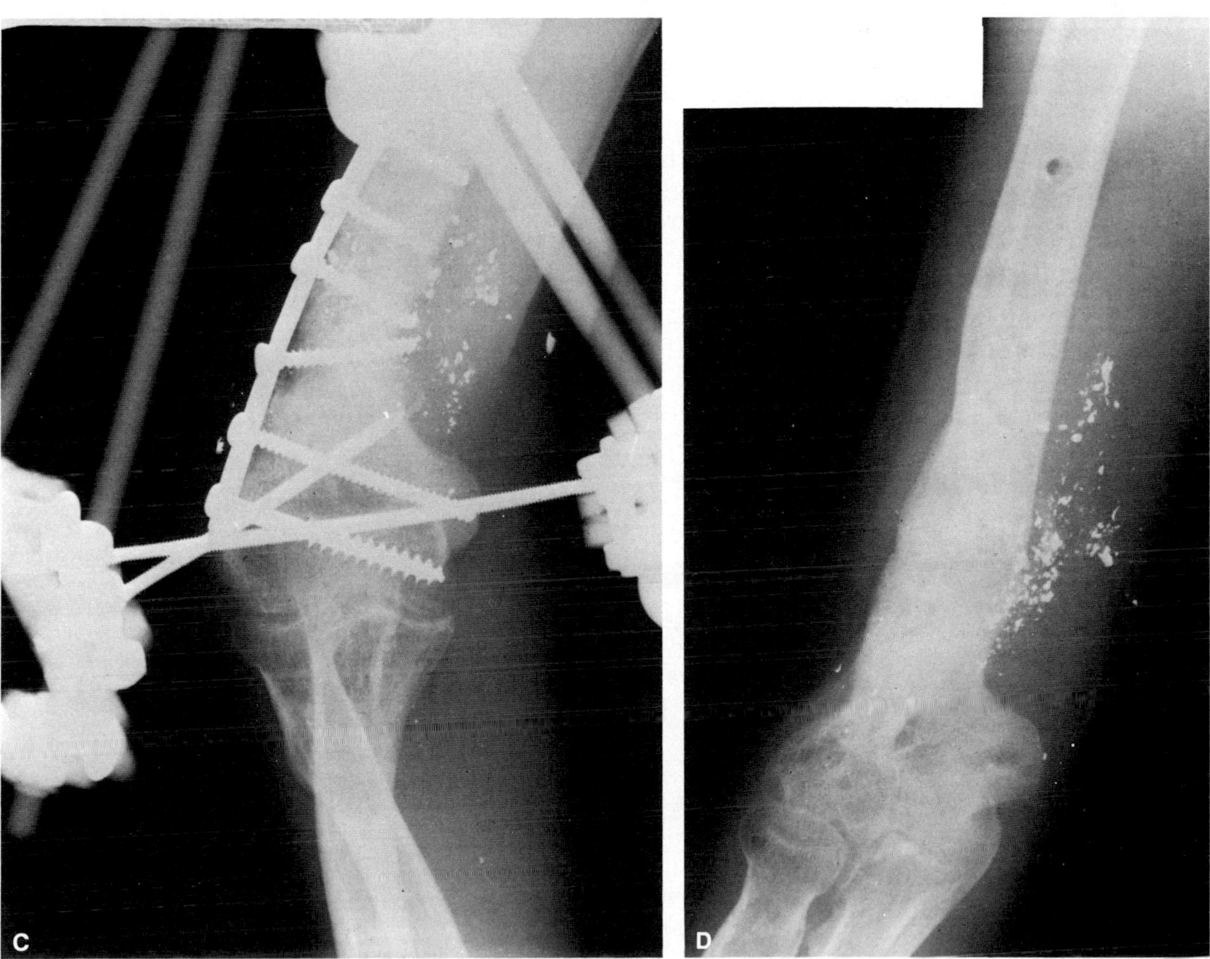

FIGURE 1-90. (continued) (**C**) A combination of plating and Roger-Anderson external fixation. (**D**) The end result. Similar techniques were employed for the nonunion of the tibia. Hyperbaric oxygen and antibiotic therapy were also used in the treatment of this man's infections.

casualties in a disaster. Fixators can be applied quickly and expeditiously even by unexperienced surgeons, and the instruments necessary and operating room requirements are minimal. In Third World countries where finances preclude intramedullary nailing, the external fixator, which can be reused many times, is an inexpensive, effective way of managing fractures where operating facilities are primitive.

The use of fixators for closed fractures of the tibia is controversial, but Burny[69] has treated these fractures successfully by uniplane fixation and early weight bearing.

In general, external fixators are a very useful means of treating a variety of complicated fractures. We see no virtue in using them in the treatment of most fractures where either plaster immobilization or internal fixation would be better. Healing is much quicker in fractures of the tibia managed by a cast and immediate weight bearing, and intramedullary fixation is a better solution for combined closed fractures of the femoral and tibial shafts. External fixators do poorly in the management of epiphyseal or intra-articular fractures, except in Colles' fractures[112,218,333,337] and some tibial plateau fractures, where again the principle of ligamentotaxis[425] can be applied. On the other hand, we believe that open fractures with massive soft-tissue damage can be handled much more expeditiously by external fixation. This allows the application of free flaps (latissimus dorsi or composite flaps with bone), so limbs that otherwise would have to be amputated are saved. Such wounds are easily inspected and redebrided and can be treated by hydrotherapy. In polytrauma this method allows instantaneous stabilization, especially where there is neurovascular injury, without subjecting a seriously ill patient to further trauma and blood loss. External fixation is also the only feasible means of fixation in infected fractures where the primary fixation is loose or broken and the bone is osteoporotic or necrotic.

We prefer to insert pins through viable skin whenever possible, but this is not mandatory and we have no compunction about placing pins through an open wound or denuded area if this is the only way. A little forethought in pin placement is necessary when soft-tissue cover is going to be required, and access to the vascular bundles should not be obstructed.

It is not our purpose to advocate any particular fixator. The reader must make up his or her own mind regarding the competing claims of the manufacturers of the various devices and, indeed, the choice may be determined by what is available in one's own hospital. In our practice we are reluctant to use the Ilizarov frame for acute trauma, especially in the multiply injured patient. The device requires a large inventory of parts, it is time consuming to apply, and it precludes free tissue transfer; however, it undoubtedly has an important role in the management of nonunion and segmental defects. Our experience with the Ilizarov frame has been largely confined to leg-lengthening and the correction of angular deformities, in which it has been enormously helpful. In general, we believe that the best fixators are those that may be applied quickly, are applicable to a variety of fractures and anatomical sites, and supply adequate fixation.

Internal Fixation of Fractures

Corrosion of Implants

When two dissimilar metals are in contact with each other in an electrolyte solution, one of these metals will be positive relative to the other, according to their positions in the electromotive series. Atoms from the anode go into solution as positively charged ions, leaving the anode negatively charged. Were there no cathode, the negative charge on the anode would tend to attract these metallic ions back. However, at the cathode another reaction is going on, which takes electrons from the cathode metal surface: $4e^- + O_2 + 2H_2O = 4OH^-$. With contact of the metal surfaces, there is a flow of electrons (ie, an electric current is produced, and the negative charge is reduced on the anode so that the attack on the anode continues). This is sometimes called a *battery effect,* because it is essentially the same process that goes on in a galvanic cell. Even in a single metal, a battery effect can be produced. If a strip of iron is immersed in a salt solution, the portion nearest the surface, where the oxygen tension is greatest, becomes the cathode; the anode is a zone at a deeper level.

Where the cathode is large and the anode small, the corrosion is greatest.[52,80,178,263] If the cathode is a plate and the anode a screw, severe corrosion takes place (Fig. 1-91**B** and **C**). For this reason, different metals should not be used in the same assembly, especially if they are far apart in the electromotive series. However, Hicks and Cater[203] have shown that mixing of plates and screws made of the more inert metals such as Vitallium and titanium does not give rise to significant corrosion.

Mears[263,264] concurred with this view and pointed out that electrochemical techniques are available to test combinations of alloys and to classify them into three types:

1. Combinations that do not appreciably alter the corrosion resistance of either component
2. Combinations in which the presence of one alloy improves the corrosion resistance of the other alloy by anodic protection, without deterioration of its own corrosion resistance
3. Combinations in which an alloy improves the corrosion resistance of another alloy but simultaneously provokes more rapid corrosion of itself.

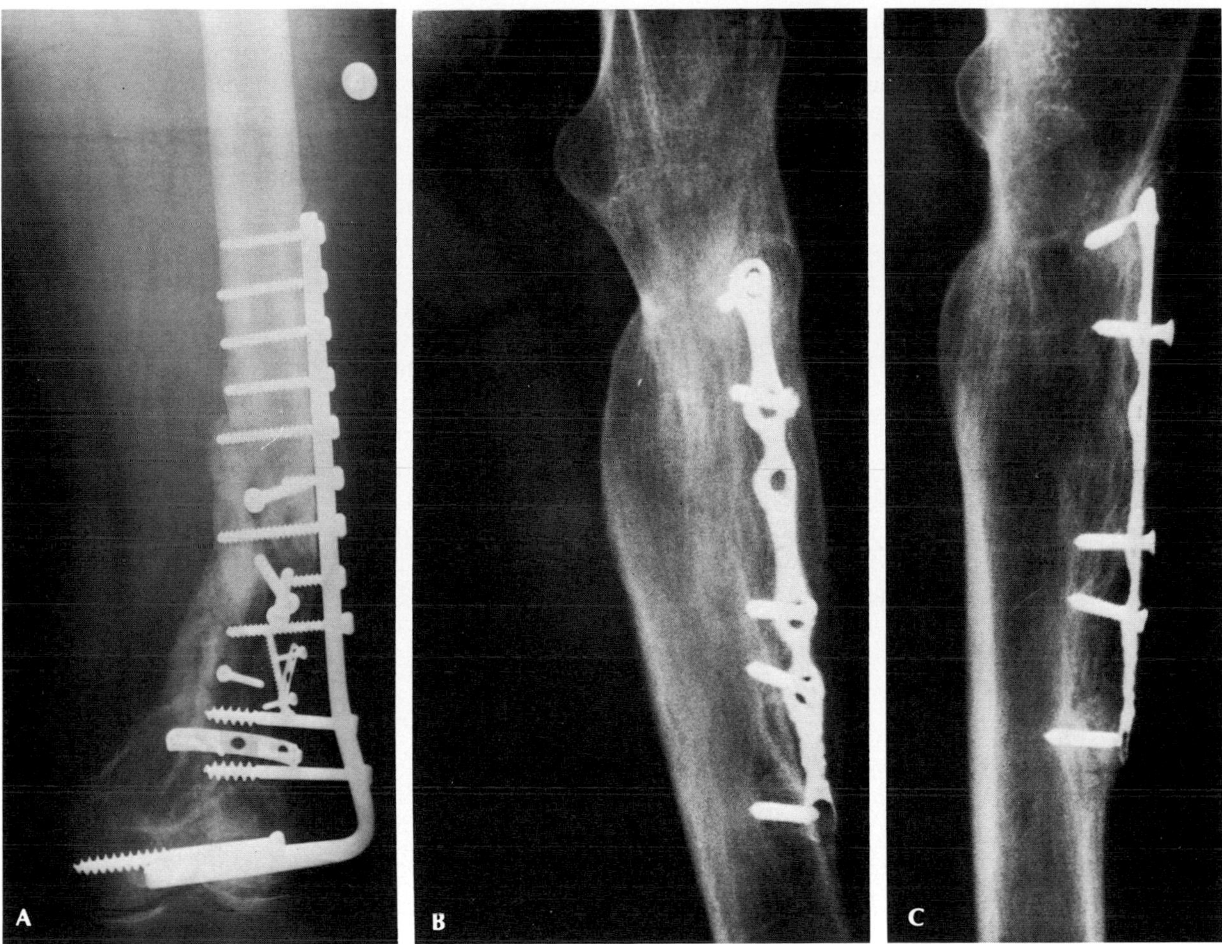

FIGURE 1-91. Examples of inappropriate internal fixation. (**A**) Multiple injuries to a woman's left lower extremity including a comminuted fracture of the supracondylar region of the femur. This is the appearance of the bone 18 months after the injury, at which time she had a draining, immobile knee. The surgeon obviously embarked on the treatment of this fracture without a good preoperative plan. The reduction is inadequate, no bone grafts were used, and the use of the many screws and plates violated the principles of sound internal fixation. (**B** and **C**) This femoral fracture healed in spite of rather inadequate plating more than 50 years ago. There is advanced corrosion of the plate and screws that apparently is causing the patient no discomfort.

This latter principle was used to protect the copper sheathing of wooden ships by the addition of zinc, but it seems unlikely that this mechanism would have a useful role in orthopaedics.

Mears did not intend for orthopaedists to "mix and match" metals for themselves, but pointed out that combinations of alloys carefully selected by metallurgical methods will be useful for certain functions. Although this may be so, we concur with the AO that it is safer to have all components of identical composition and that they should be as inert as possible.

If a layer of oxide is present on the surface of the metals, it acts as a block to the passage of ions. The presence of molybdenum in a ferrous alloy helps in the formation of a passive oxide barrier, and stainless steel used in the manufacture of implants should contain 2.5% to 3.5% molybdenum. The oxide layer can be thickened artificially by treating it with nitric acid (passivation) or electrochemically (anodization).

Chloride ions interfere with oxidation and the formation of a passivation layer in stainless steel implants. The practice of steam sterilization of implants with saline in the environment gives rise to surface corrosion in both instruments and implants and should be prohibited.[263] Furthermore, rough usage and scratches will break the oxide film on the surface of an implant and be the nidus where corrosion, especially stress corrosion, may start. Implants should be handled with delicacy, never thrown around in basins or shaken together in a basket or immersed in saline. Indeed, implants should be kept in their packages or placed in protective containers until the time of use.

In spite of the improvements in stainless steels, corrosion still occurs, and some of the mechanisms postulated to explain these cases are described below.

Transfer of Metals From Tools to Implants

Using radioactive tracer techniques, Bowden and associates[45] showed that significant amounts of metal were transferred from screwdrivers to screw heads and from drill bits to plates. This difficulty could be solved by using tools made from the same material as the implant, by making the screwdrivers harder, and by using drill guides to prevent contact between drill and plate. Hicks and Cater,[203] however, stated that this transfer of metal is not clinically significant.

Crevice Corrosion

Differences in oxygen tension or concentrations of electrolytes or changes in pH in a confined space, such as in the crevices between a screw and a plate, may result in local corrosion called *crevice corrosion* or *contact corrosion*.[151]

Fretting Corrosion

Cohen[95] subjected plate-and-screw assemblies to cyclic stress in saline solutions and found the greatest corrosion in the screw assemblies where the heads rubbed on the plate and where the nuts and washers were in contact. He believed that this was most probably secondary to abrasion of the metal surfaces removing the protective oxide coating (ie, fretting). Similar assemblies not subjected to the cyclical stresses did not show this marked effect.

Stress-Corrosion Cracking

Stress-corrosion cracking is a phenomenon in which a metal in certain environments, especially those rich in chlorides, is subjected to stress and fails at a much lower level than usual as a result of corrosion.[178]

In austenitic steels a process called *sensitization* may result when implants are subjected to heat treatments during manufacture. It is believed that some of the chromium becomes converted to chromium carbide, so that the grain boundaries of the metal lose their protective coating of chromium. This gives rise to increased corrosion because (1) the metallic grains lose the passivation effect of chromium oxide; and (2) a galvanic effect accentuates corrosion because of differences in the composition of the grain itself and its boundary region. Stress accentuates this destructive effect, leading to failure.

Choice of Metals for Surgical Implants

If one could create the ideal implant material, it would be inert, nontoxic to the body, and absolutely corrosion-proof. It would be inexpensive, easily worked, and capable of being wrought in a variety of shapes without expensive manufacturing techniques. It would have great strength and high resistance to fatigue.

Unfortunately, this material is not available at the present time. Implants are made of stainless steel; cobalt, chromium, and molybdenum alloys (eg, Vitallium); and titanium. The characteristics of these materials have been detailed by Brettle[51,52] in his excellent reviews of this subject and more recently by Disegi and Wyss.[133]

Stainless steel contains 18% chromium and 8% nickel and may be cast or forged. Of the materials available, stainless steel has the best mechanical properties. It is strong and has good fatigue resistance. It is easily worked and inexpensive to manufacture, but it has the serious drawback of corrodibility.

Vitallium has much better corrosion resistance than stainless steel, but it is in every way mechanically inferior. It has to be cast by the very complicated and expensive lost-wax process, and quality control is harder to achieve than with stainless steel. Vitallium also has a low ductility, and screws made of this material bond quite securely to bone. In removing a screw that has become securely anchored, it is easy to break the head off. Wrought Vitallium is a cobalt, chromium, nickel, and tungsten alloy with much more desirable mechanical properties than standard Vitallium and excellent corrosion resistance. It differs from cast vitallium, which has 6% molybdenum, by having no molybdenum content at all.

Titanium is the most inert of all. It is easily worked, and $^{1}/_{16}$-inch plates are radiolucent. Unfortunately, this admirable metal has an extremely low modulus of elasticity (15×10^6 psi, which is much less than the 28 to 30×10^6 psi for Vitallium and stainless steel) and has a lower tensile strength. Although titanium alloys may be used instead of titanium alone, it is Brettle's opinion that titanium's modulus of elasticity will not be appreciably altered. Titanium plates and implants, therefore, have to be bulkier than stainless steel to provide the same rigidity.

Titanium can be modified by alloying it with aluminum and vanadium (Ti-6Al-4V), and in the United States it is made into implants by the Zimmer Company, who market it under the trade name Tivanium. They have given the implants a surface treatment that makes them gold colored for easy identification. The alloy is said to have a greater tensile strength than either stainless steel or the chrome-cobalt alloys and has almost twice the fatigue strength of these materials. It is extremely hard and resistant to scratching, is corrosion proof, and has a ductility equal to that of stainless steel. The high resistance to corrosion is due to the coating of titanium dioxide that forms on the surface by contact with air and forms an inert layer, titanium is "self-passivating." It does have a low modulus of elasticity, so that if plates were to be made of it, they would have to be substantially thicker to provide the rigidity of stainless steel. On the other hand, by being less stiff, the problem of stress protection may be alleviated.

Perren and Pohler[310] are also advocates of titanium as an implant material on account of its corrosion resistance and the tolerance of tissues to it. They aver that there have been no allergic reactions to titanium but deprecate the use of titanium alloys containing vanadium, a soluble metal that they consider more toxic than nickel.

The AO/ASIF has developed a pure titanium from which to manufacture its implants.[134] Commercially pure titanium comes in four grades (1, 2, 3, and 4) depending on the oxygen content of the metal, and the strength of the metal increases as the oxygen content. By annealing and cold-working grade 4 titanium they have produced a metal with a very fine grain size that has a modulus that is 55% to 56% of stainless steel and 41% to 42% of chrome cobalt. Implants made from this titanium will therefore be much less likely to produce stress-shielding of bone than either steel or chrome cobalt. In comparison with stainless steel, pure titanium's tensile strength is similar but its minimum yield strength is superior. Its minimal yield strength is comparable to cast chrome cobalt, and its minimum elongation is less so that it is much superior in contourability.

Matter and Burch[256] have reported on the results of implantation of 271 limited contact dynamic compression plates made of this material, and of the 57 that have been retrieved none was found to be corroded and there was minimal tissue reaction to their presence.

In 1977, researchers at Sulzer Brothers of Wintertur, Switzerland, developed a new alloy: titanium with 6% aluminum and 7% niobium (TAN) that was used to make total hip prostheses and marketed by Protek as Protasul in 1986. This alloy has a modulus of elasticity that is similar to titanium 4, but its ultimate tensile strength is much higher (900 megapascals as opposed to 500 megapascals). Its strength endurance level is equivalent to Ti-6Al-4V, and it is substantially superior to cold-worked titanium so that it will be used by the AO for the next generation of implants.[135]

A number of alloys have been discovered that have "memory" (eg, gold-cadmium, copper-zinc, titanium-niobium).[27,185] If these metals are deformed at low temperatures, they will recover their original configuration when the temperature is raised to the requisite level. Another such alloy is titanium-nickel. Originally discovered in the United States, this alloy (55% nickel and 45% titanium by weight) is known as Nitinol, and implants have been made from this material, which is inert in the tissues.

Small changes in the composition of these alloys may alter their behavior significantly, but in China a very similar alloy, Nitalloy (54% nickel and 46% titanium), has been used clinically.[240] A staple made of this material and deformed at 0°C may be implanted in bone. When heated to 34°C to 40°C it will regain its original configuration, allowing the staple to exert a compression force. In a similar manner, a rod or cable may be overstretched at low temperatures and then contract at body temperatures after implantation.

In the last report on this alloy, 158 fractures were fixed by staples, and of these, 121 were intra-articular. The staples were cooled to 4°C to 7°C and deformed so that the legs of the staple made an angle of 70°. When reading a temperature of 37°C the staples regain their normal shape of 90°, thereby exerting compression. This is known as the *Marmen effect.*[109]

A significant number of implant failures result from implants being used improperly or being applied in the wrong location. Even in the best-regulated circumstances, however, implant failure will sometimes occur. As Howard Rosen has said, "Any time metal is put into the body in the treatment of fracture, it's the start of a race between bone healing and implant failure." Obviously, quality control of implants is extremely important, and most manufacturers go to great lengths to make sure that their products are not defective.

However, Cahoon and Paxton[72] selected 35 implants at random from the stock of a hospital and subjected them to a rigorous examination. They found that more than 50% of these were unacceptable from a metallurgical viewpoint owing to large grain size, inclusions, porosity, cracks, pitting, and a molybdenum content below 2% in stainless steel. Molybdenum, of course, protects against pitting, corrosion, and fatigue failure and should be above the 2% level. They also found Jewett nails that had been manufactured by welding the nail to the side plate, so that large amounts of delta ferrite were formed, thereby reducing the implant's corrosion resistance.

Such studies should prompt prudent orthopaedists to ensure that the manufacturer of the implants they use adopts the recommended metallurgical standards, fabricates the implants with care, and maintains adequate testing facilities. In the increasingly litigious environment in which we live, it would be circumspect to retain a broken implant for subsequent metallurgical examination, if necessary. These words should not be taken in any way as an indictment of the orthopaedic implant industry. Indeed, we have been most impressed by the quality control provisions in the implant factories we have visited.

The reuse of implants is not permissible in the United States. Implants become seriously attenuated after being subjected to repeated stresses in the hostile environment of the body and are much more likely to fail with a second use. It may be permissible to allow their use in a country where implants are unavailable owing to their high cost, but even that is for purely economic reasons and certainly is not a desirable situation.

Allergic Responses to Implants

It has been known for some time that in certain individuals cutaneous eruptions will arise after implant surgery secondary to sensitivity to nickel, chrome, or cobalt. Kubba and associates,[243] in a prospective study, found 19 such patients. Six of these had transient exanthematic dermatitis, which was recurrent in two cases, and 13 had a persistent reaction.

In patients who have such problems it makes sense to use titanium implants, which are unlikely to evoke an allergic response.

Although titanium is the most inert of the metals used for implants and the AO believes that there is no allergic response to titanium implants, this may not be entirely true. Lalor and associates found large amounts of particulate titanium in the soft tissues of five patients undergoing total hip arthroplasty revision. In four of these cases the titanium screws used to fix a cobalt-chrome acetabular component had undergone fretting of their necks. Macrophages in the fibrous tissue removed were loaded with titanium particles.[241]

Patch tests of titanium salts produced no allergic reactions in the patients' skin. However, when patch tests were carried out on four of these patients with Metanium ointment, two developed eczematous reactions after 48 hours. Metanium ointment is a cream used to treat diaper rash and contains titanium. The authors concluded that not only did titanium particles evoke osteolysis and component loosening, but it may also evoke sensitization.

Although the use of titanium for fracture fixation is now well established, its use in total joint components is still being questioned.[64,79,217,241,438]

Carcinogenic Effects of Metals

An article in the lay press[41,372] has been published regarding the possibility of metallic induction of malignant tumors. Such tumors have been reported in conjunction with total hip prostheses,[307,399] but only six cases have been reported in which a tumor has arisen at the site of a metallic plate.[119,136,137,258,259,407] Of these plates, four were stainless steel and two cobalt-chrome. In one of these instances, an infant had bilateral derotational osteotomies carried out for congenital dislocation of the hip, which were fixed by stainless steel plates. After removal of the plates, Ewing's sarcoma developed on one side. In all of these cases the association of malignancy and plates may well have been coincidental.

Black,[40] in his review of oncogenesis by metallic ions, summarized the experimental evidence regarding the release of cobalt, chromium, and nickel from implants and the induction of tumors. He stated that chromium may be released either in trivalent or hexavalent forms and that the latter is able to penetrate cell membranes and is probably a potent carcinogen.

Black's conclusions, which pertain more to hip prostheses than plates and screws, were as follows:

1. There is adequate evidence to conclude that there is a finite, non-zero risk of oncogenesis in humans associated with the implantation of F75 alloy (chrome-cobalt).
2. This risk increases with increasing dosage and increasing period of exposure.
3. It is prudent to act on these conclusions while awaiting a definite determination of risk.

It does seem that significant quantities of chromium, cobalt, and nickel may be liberated from metallic implants—especially when corrosion occurs.

Metallic debris from total arthroplasty does seem to provoke changes in immunologic function: the macrophages ingest the particles, lymph nodes fibrose, and bursal lymphocytes diminish. It is conceivable that tumor may result from modification of immune surveillance. However, tumor induction would appear to be much more common in veterinary practice than it is in humans.[193,382] The cases cited, even if all *are* related to metallic tumor induction, represent an infinitesimal percentage of patients subjected to implant insertion. The risk perhaps is much greater in implants with sintered or pore-coated surfaces, where presumably the loss of ions will be much greater owing to the greatly enlarged surface area. A comprehensive review of this subject has been published by Vahey and coworkers[419] describing 20 cases from the literature in which tumors have developed at the site of metallic implants as well as the increased incidence of lymphoma and hematopoietic tumors in patients with metallic arthroplasties.

The circumspect fracture surgeon will avoid the use of stainless steel or chrome-cobalt when the patient has a demonstrated sensitivity to metal. On the other hand, the magnitude of the problem scarcely dictates eschewing stainless steel and chrome-cobalt in favor of titanium on this account alone or giving up the use of metallic implants.

Removal of Metallic Implants

It is common practice to remove metallic implants after radiologic evidence of healing, and indeed patients are told that these procedures are mandatory to avoid future complications. That this advice is true is open to question, and these operations are not free of complications. Brown and associates[58] reported a 19% incidence of significant complications after removing metal from 42% of 297 healed fractures. When there was a clear cut indication for removal of a device the patients usually did well but in those operated routinely there was an 11% incidence of postoperative infection and an overall complication rate of 15%. Sanderson and his colleagues[361] removed implants from 188 patients, 34% of these for cause, and had a complication rate of 20%.

It seems that removal of forearm plates gives rise to the greatest number and most severe complications. Sanderson[361] had a 42% complication rate, and Langkamer and Ackroyd[242] had a 40% complication rate. The complications, in addition to infection, included a variety of nerve injuries and refractures after insignificant trauma. Rosson and Shearer[351] removed forearm plates from the forearms of 80 patients (115 plates). They had no refractures in removing 48 plates from children, but had four refractures after removing 73 plates from 51 adults. Significantly, all four of these refractures occurred in the 6 patients whose plates were removed in less than 12 months after the osteosynthesis. These authors recommend that only 3.5-mm screws be used in forearm fractures and that no plates be removed in less than 18 months.

Refracture may occur through empty screw holes, through the original fracture site, or through the attenuated bone that was under the plate. Single photon absorptiometry studies have shown that screw-hole healing is not complete at 18 weeks after removal of plates, and on this basis it has been advised that athletic activity should be eschewed for 4 months postoperatively.[349] Using this method, Rossen and coworkers[349] have studied the bone mass, bone density, and cortical width of forearm bones after removal of plates in 14 patients. In only one of these cases were all three of these parameters diminished in comparison to the uninjured side when the plates were removed at 16 months. The AO recommends that forearm plates be retained for 18 to 24 months so that 21 months would be in the middle of that range. Six patients had the plates removed before 21 months, and six had them removed later. Four of the former had diminished bone density, and in only one of the latter did this occur. The authors concluded that bone atrophy did not contribute to refracture as long as the plates were not removed prematurely.

Drilling a hole in a bone immediately reduces its breaking strength, especially when it is made in a tension area. The size of the hole is immaterial unless it exceeds 20% or 30%[70] of the diameter of the bone. Such defects make bones susceptible to fracture by any type of applied stress,[55] but after internal fixation is inserted the bone gradually becomes stronger by remodeling of the bone around the hole. On removing the screw, however, the hole again becomes a stress riser. Overdrilling the hole or filling the holes with plastic plugs is not helpful and the bone remains vulnerable for several months.

Rosson and his associates[350] also compared the effect of demineralization with that of a single screw hole in predisposing a rabbit tibia to fracture. By using matched pairs, one tibia was demineralized by Gooding and Stewart's demineralizing fluid to between 75% and 80% of normal. The other tibia had a drill-hole made in it. These tibiae were subjected to three-point bending to failure. The demineralized specimens had a mean diminution in maximum bending moment to 75% and in energy absorbing capacity to a mean of only 90%. The drill hole, on the other hand, produced a reduction in energy-absorbing capacity to 53% of normal and a maximum bending moment to 70% of normal. In no demineralized specimen did the energy absorbing capacity fall below 60% of normal, and none of the bones with drill holes exceeded this level. Since energy-absorbing capacity is more relevant to resistance to fracture, they concluded that the effect of screw holes was more important than cortical atrophy.

There has been an ongoing battle between the proponents of "stress-shielding," producing cortical porosity under plates,[279,280,319,418] and the AO school, which believes it to be a transitory problem due to circulatory impairment that corrects itself with time.[167,168,314,315] The reports that confirm that refracture is less common when the plates are retained for longer periods clearly support the AO view.

Even the removal of intramedullary nails is not without its problems, especially when the appropriate extractors are not available; all of us with gray hair have unhappy memories of struggling with incarcerated nails of various types. Miller and associates[271] removed 60 femoral rods, and their complications were hematomas of the thigh and five nails that were broken. The distal ends of three of these nails were left in situ.

It would seem that the consensus is to remove only implants causing symptoms and, as Lord Chesterfield advised, "to let sleeping dogs lie." The only dissenting vote would seem to be by Richards and associates,[339] who reported a 3% complication rate—one refracture, one radial nerve injury, one gluteal hematoma, and no infections. Even they, however, say that patients with implants who are asymptomatic should have the risks and benefits of surgery discussed with them and a decision reached based on informed consent.

In our own practice, we prefer to remove intramedullary nails in young persons after satisfactory healing to obviate the possibility of having to deal with a bent or broken nail after a subsequent injury.

The question before the modern surgeon is not whether operative treatment is to supersede manipulative treatment. The problem before each of us is how can we improve our skill and technique in both manipulative and operative treatment and what means we must adopt in each individual case to give to our patients the surest, safest, and most complete restoration of function.

Those who have a large and varied experience of the manipulative treatment of deformity will probably have greater confidence in their ability to deal with deformities resulting from fractures by manipulation and external splinting. They will reserve direct operation for those cases in which they have found that their manipulative skill has not proved equal to returning the limb in a correct position until union of the fragments has taken place.

The crying evil of our art in these times is the fact that much of our surgery is too mechanical, our medical practice too chemical, and there is a hankering to interfere, which thwarts the inherent tendency to recovery possessed by all persons not actually dying.—H. O. Thomas, 1833

The case that starts botched up stays botched up.—Michael Rosco, 1967

 Indications for Operative Treatment

Open Reduction and Internal Fixation of Fractures

Until comparatively recently the orthodox position was that closed management was good and that open reduction, if not actually bad, should be avoided if at all possible and be reserved for cases in which closed reduction had failed, in which joint incongruency, especially in the lower limb, was present, or in which cumulative experience had shown that closed methods were unlikely to be successful.

The advent of better implants, improved technology, and better trained surgeons, schooled in biomechanics, has changed orthopaedic philosophy so that now one would be hard-put to name a fracture for which no one has advocated operative management.

No one can deny that intramedullary fixation of the femur, especially with interlocking nails, produces vastly better results at lower cost than treatment by continuous traction. Although we have treated tibial shaft fractures by casting and early weight bearing with relatively good results for many years, contemporary papers on their management by interlocking nails, reamed and unreamed, would suggest that nailing is better. Hooper and associates have written the only paper of which we are aware that compares the results of the two methods in a prospective series.[210] Twenty-three patients were managed by manipulation of the fracture and the application of a long-leg cast that was replaced by a PTB cast at 4 weeks. Interlocking intramedullary nailing with weight bearing was used in 29 patients, and there was a higher proportion of open fractures in this group. All of the fractures healed, but there was more shortening and angulation in the non-operated group, although two of the patients who had undergone nailing had significant external rotational deformity. If one critically evaluates one's patients treated by casting, one will find significant limitation of subtalar motion in many of these patients that interferes with the patient's ability to compensate for malalignment of the fracture, which will not be present in the patients who have been operated on who are able to exercise their joints early. No one nowadays would seriously argue with the concept of early fixation of fractures in the polytraumatized patient.

There has been a curious shibboleth about operating on patients with head injuries and lower extremity fractures, but Poole and his associates in reviewing 114 patients with such injuries found that pulmonary complications depended on the severity of the head injury and were not related to fixation of their fractures. Delay in operation did not help their neurologic condition, but internal fixation of their fractures made their care easier.[322]

But Pape and associates[299,300] have reported a higher incidence of adult respiratory distress syndrome when patients with pulmonary contusion were subjected to intramedullary nailing of the femur within the first 24 hours (33% vs 7.7%) and a higher mortality (21% vs 4%). However, Charash and coworkers[85] have written a rebuttal to this paper and claim better results when patients undergo nailing within 8 hours.

Gustilo and coworkers[183] also have found that open reduction and internal fixation during the first week in polytraumatized patients reduced the incidence of adult respiratory distress syndrome and fat embolism.

Open reduction is like the girl who when she was good, she was very, very good but when she was bad, she was horrid.[17] Certainly the results of badly performed, ill-planned surgery are catastrophic (see Figs. 1-91 and 1-92). In many parts of the world the money and facilities for open surgery are not universally available and closed reduction is still a valid treatment.

Bone Substitutes in Fracture Surgery

The use of autogenous bone grafts has been helpful to enhance healing of nonunion and delayed union and to improve stability by filling voids in the injured bone. But this undoubted benefit comes with a price. The operating time is lengthened, more scars are foisted on the body, and there are a galaxy of complications: hematomas and blood loss, infection, fracture through the graft site, injury to superficial nerves with hypesthesia, neuromas, and meralgia paresthetica.

It is not surprising that there has been considerable effort expended to provide a substitute for the patient's own bone. Allograft bone is not osteogenetic and often needs to be supplemented by autogenous grafts or mixed with bone marrow.[383] Xenografts such as bovine bone have been tried and found wanting in the

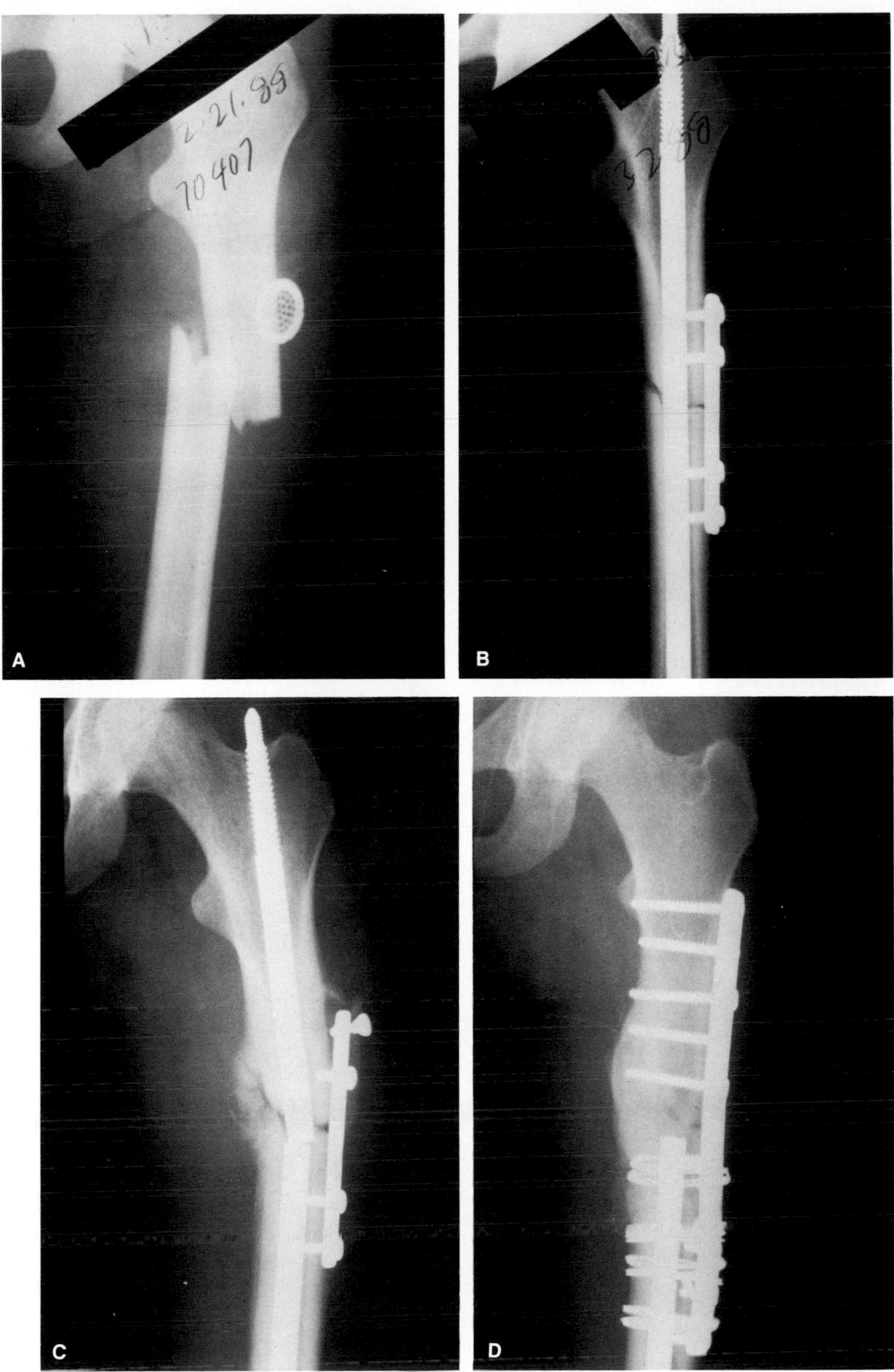

FIGURE 1-92. A 17-year-old girl sustained a fracture of the proximal third of the femur in an automobile accident. (**A**) The original radiograph. (**B**) The surgeon elected to insert a 9-mm Schneider nail, which did not fill the unreamed medullary cavity. Rotational stability could only be achieved by adding a four-hole unicortical plate. (**C**) Inevitably this small nail failed with disruption of the reduction and plate fixation. (**D**) The surgeon was unable to extract the distal fragment of the nail and elected to leave it *in situ*. This precluded the insertion of screws through the distal portion of the plate, which was then fixed with cerclage wires. This fixation was so insecure that a second surgeon applied a hip spica for 3 months, leaving the broken nail entombed in the medullary cavity of the femur.

past, but a product that is a mixture of bovine collagen and hydroxyapatite has been recommended for filling bony cavities. Another product derived from marine coral has been advised for similar purposes but neither of these products are as strong as bone.

Collagraft is a ceramic mixture of hydroxyapatite and tricalcium phosphate. The tricalcium phosphate may be resorbed, creating a space for bony ingrowth and leaving the hydroxyapatite to provide structural strength. Koclalkowski and his associates[236] have found that the pathways of bone ingrowth resulted in retardation of bone healing and remodeling. They also filled bone defects by a mixture of this material ground up into small granules and suspended in a nonimmunogenic bovine collagen gel to which was added autogenous bone marrow. They found that new bone growth was directly proportional to the amount of added bone marrow and the optimum mixture contained 60% bone marrow. The 11 cases they managed by this mixture all healed in an average of 58.7 weeks (range, 25 to 135 weeks). In experimental nonunions, cancellous bone grafting was more effective and these investigators found it difficult to keep the fluid mixture in bone defects. A multicenter investigation of Collagraft compared 128 patients treated by conventional bone grafting with 139 cases treated by a Collagraft marrow mixture. They found no adverse effects attributable to the Collagraft mixture, but the complication rate and infection rate was higher in the Collagraft group (8.1% vs 6.0%).[104]

We have a strong attachment to autogenous bone grafts and have no experience with the bone substitutes, but it does seem to us that there are two very exciting developments that are close to general release: recombinant human bone morphogenetic bone protein and the Norian SRS (Skeletal Repair System).

Bone Morphogenetic Protein

LaCroix[240a] postulated a humeral factor, osteogenin, that stimulates connective tissue cells to produce bone; and, more recently, Urist[418a] has shown that demineralized bone matrix is able to induce the formation of bone and cartilage when implanted in extraskeletal sites. Further research has resulted in the discovery of a proteinacious substance that is capable of inducing bone formation, bone morphogenetic protein. Seven bone morphogenetic proteins have been identified, numbered 1 through 7. Bone formation will be induced when there is an inducer substance, a permissive substrate, and responsive cells. Stevenson and colleagues[395] found that bone morphogenetic protein 3 (Osteogenin) applied to a cylinder (composed of hydroxyapatite [60%] and tricalcium phosphate [40%]) induced bone formation when placed in a bone defect produced in the long bones of rats. Yasko and associates[446] treated bone defects in rats by a mixture of 10 mg of inactivated rat bone matrix to which was added either 1.4 or 11 micrograms of recombinant human bone morphogenetic protein (rhBMP2). Both mixtures produced bone in proportion to the dose of bone morphogenetic protein, but the fractures healed only with the higher dose. Cook and his associates[101] were able to heal defects in rabbit tibiae in a similar manner using RhBMP1. This ability to manipulate bone healing by natural products has far-reaching possibilities in fracture management.

Norian Skeletal Repair System

Constantz,[100,321] devised a material that would set and immobilize a fracture and then be replaced by bone. The material is made by dry-mixing monocalcium phosphate monohydrate (MCPM)—$Ca(H_2PO_4)_2 \cdot H_2O$, α-tricalcium phosphate (TCP)—$Ca_3(PO_4)_2$ and calcium carbonate (CC)—$CaCo_3$. The addition of sodium phosphate solution to this mixture forms a paste that remains formable or injectable for 5 minutes. After 10 minutes it sets, and after 12 hours it reaches its maximum strength. Its tensile strength is equal to that of cancellous bone, and its compression strength is greater. This ceramic material holds the fracture firmly in place and eventually it will be replaced by ingrowth of bone. The setting of the mixture is not exothermic, and the pH is physiologic. A multicenter study is underway in which Colles' fractures are being treated by closed reduction and the percutaneous injection of this material. It is obvious that tibial plateau and other metaphyseal comminuted fractures might similarly be managed.

It seems likely that we shall see increasing use of naturally occurring humoral agents to manipulate the rate and magnitude of healing of various tissues. Our own experience in this realm has been the use of platelet growth factors to heal trophic and varicose ulcers, and our clinical assessment is that they are helpful.

FRACTURE CARE

Adequacy of Reduction

What constitutes adequate position must vary with the location of the fracture. Nothing short of anatomical restoration is adequate in the forearm, but in the humerus almost any position is compatible with good function. In general, one tries to line up the distal fragment with the proximal fragment. An overlap of 2 cm in the femur or tibia can be compensated for by pelvic tilt; but if it is greater than this, the shoe must be raised to avoid stress on the lumbar spine. It is said that valgus or varus angulation must be no more than 5° in the tibia to avoid shear stresses on the knee and ankle. However, in a follow-up study 29 years after fractures of the tibia, Merchant and Dietz[268] found that the magnitude of varus, valgus, and anteroposterior angulation made no appreciable difference to the incidence of arthritis of the knee or ankle. These surprising results are at variance with most of the opinions expressed in the literature and are of considerable medicolegal importance.

Green and Green[177] have pointed out the futility of measuring angulation on x-rays if only the standard anteroposterior and lateral views are taken. The magnitude of the angulation, they say, will always be underestimated unless the plane of deformity is parallel to the plane of the film. When an angulated bone is rotated under the image intensifier there is constant change in the magnitude of the apparent angulation. "If the maximal angulation is shown on one view the orthogonal view will show no angulation. Conversely, if angulation is shown on both views, the maximum angle will be shown in an intermediate plane."[177] It is possible to calculate the apex angle and plane trigonometrically from standard anteroposterior views and they have derived a formula to do so.

Green and Green studied 100 fractures and found that 93% of the angular deformities and 94% of the transitional deformities occurred in planes oblique to the standard views. The maximum error in diminution of deformity occurs when the plane of the x-ray plate is at 45° to the maximum angulation, which gives an error of 41.4%.

Visualization error

$$= \frac{\text{Actual magnitude} - \text{worst view on radiograph}}{\text{Worst view on radiograph}} \times 100$$

This formula calculates the percentage error in measuring angulations or translations, and the "actual magnitude" is calculated from the trigonometric formula. In Green and Green's study of 100 fractures, the anteroposterior and lateral views alone underestimated the true angulation by an average of 13.8% (a range of 0% to 40%). Similarly, translational deformities were underestimated by 14%. If four views are taken rather than two, the maximum possible error decreases from 41.4% to 8.2%, and in the study series the angulation error fell to 2% for angulation and 2.5% for translation.

The authors make a plea that instead of splitting the angulation into two components such as 10° valgus and 15° recurvatum, it makes much more sense to describe it three-dimensionally by measuring the true angle and the direction in which it points (eg, a 22° angulation, apex 25° posterolaterally).

The Greens have made an estimation chart (Table 1-2) that allows one to categorize an angulation from anteroposterior and lateral views, and the circumspect surgeon should at least check his reduction by making four views to uncover egregious error.

TABLE 1-2
Estimation Chart

AP:Lateral or Lateral:AP	Rotation of True Plane From Larger View (degrees)	True Angle or Translation (%)
1:1	45	40 greater
1:1.5 (2:3)	33	20 greater
1:2	25	10 greater
1:3	17	5 greater
1:4	12	2.5 greater

A method of quickly estimating the plane and magnitude of either translation or small angular deformities from standard anteroposterior (AP) and lateral roentgenograms. Determine the *ratio* of the deformities on the two standard views; the true apex angle (or the actual amount of transverse translation) will be larger than the worst visualized view by the percentage shown in the third column, and the deformity plane (or plane of transverse translation) will be rotated away from the plane of the worst visualized view by the angle shown in the second column. To increase the accuracy of the chart for estimating angular deformities, decrease the values in the third column by 2 percentage points for every 5 degrees that the lesser visualized deformity exceeds 10 degrees.

For those who are mathematically oriented, the trigonometrical formulae are as follows:

Translational Deformities

$$\text{Plane of translation } t = \tan^{-1} \text{Lat/AP}$$

$$\text{Magnitude of translation } d = \sqrt{\text{Lat}^2 + \text{AP}^2}$$

Angulation Deformities

$$\text{Plane of angulation } A = \tan^{-1}(\tan \text{Lat}/\tan \text{AP})$$

$$\text{True deformity angle } \psi = \tan^{-1}\sqrt{\tan^2 \text{Lat} + \tan^2 \text{AP}}$$

We believe that these papers should be required reading for every orthopaedic surgeon. The parameters of what constitutes an acceptable reduction can only be established when we can define the direction and magnitude of residual deformity.

Malalignment in the lower extremity manifestly alters stress on the hip, knee, and ankle joints and has a role in the development of degenerative arthrosis, although there are as yet few good studies confirming this contention.[139,409] Nonetheless, fracture surgeons should strive, insofar as they are able, to restore the normal alignment of the limb and the relationship of one joint to another.

Alignment may be defined as the colinearity of the three major joints and is determined by the mechanical axis of the limb, that is, a line drawn from the center of the femoral head to the center of the ankle joint. Malalignment is measured by the vertical distance from the center of the knee to this line that normally passes medial to and close to the center of the knee.[409]

The orientation of a joint is determined by measuring the angle subtended by the two bones forming it. The anatomical axis of the femur forms an angle of 1.2° varus ± 2.2°.[409]

Measurements of mechanical axis, alignment, and joint orientation are best made with the patient standing with the patella pointing forward on a "chiropractic" film that encompasses the entire lower extremity.

Angulations in the coronal plane in the proximal femur have traditionally been believed to be relatively benign, but increasing varus diminishes the lever arm of the hip abductors and valgus angulation increases pressure on the femoral head. As the angulation proceeds distally down the femoral shaft, the effect on the knee becomes increasingly pernicious. Similarly in the tibia, proximal angulation affects the knee and distal angulation affects the ankle.

Conventional wisdom has stated that anteroposterior angulations of the ankle in the axis of motion of the contiguous joint are benign since the angulation may be compensated by movement of the joint. This assertion is open to serious question. Tetsworth and Paley,[409] in cadaveric studies of the ankle, found that the contact area of the articular surfaces was drastically reduced by anterior bowing and recurvatum, and to a greater extent than by angulation in the coronal plane. They also found that restriction of motion of the subtalar joint also diminished contact area, especially when the joint was fixed in varus.

In the upper extremity, anterior or posterior angulation of the humerus is compensated by elbow motion and minor degrees are benign. Similarly, the magnitude of shoulder motion mitigates rotational malalignments and proximal angulations. But in the forearm, angulation or malrotation drastically impairs pronation and supination.

Malrotation is no less pernicious than angulation deformity and is frequently unappreciated by the surgeon.

Malrotation of the tibia leads to perceptible deformity and ruins the alignment of the knee and ankle. According to Perkins,[309] "When the joint above the fracture is a ball and socket joint, correction (of rotation) is not essential." This is just as well, because one can only correct the rotation accurately at an operation where one can see exactly how the fragments fit and can maintain the reduction with a plate.

It would appear that some degree of malrotation occurs after both traction treatment and blind nailing of the femur. Schatzker,[371] in his defense of open intramedullary nailing of the femur, notes that malrotation is avoided by being able to line up the linea aspera under vision. Although 10° of malrotation is common and asymptomatic, Sudmann[398a] had one patient with 25° of malrotation who walked with an obvious external rotation deformity and had pain, presumably on this account.

Mayfield,[257] in his review of 75 femoral shaft fractures, discovered that 31 patients had an internal malrotation deformity. Those with severe deformity manifested a Trendelenburg sign and hip abductor weakness during walking owing to the functional reduction of the lever arm of the femoral neck.

A middle-aged woman sustained an intertrochanteric fracture that was produced by an internal rotation torque. An attempt was made to reduce the fracture by internal rotation, and she underwent nailing in this position. She complained of discomfort that was not relieved by removing the nail. Derotational osteotomy and trochanteric realignment were necessary to restore her gait and relieve her discomfort (Fig. 1-93).

It would appear that rotational malunions correct spontaneously in children. Brouwer[56] examined 55 patients 27 to 32 years after a childhood fracture and could find only one patient with significant rotational malalignment, and he was asymptomatic. Hägglund and associates[186] confirm that these malalignments correct spontaneously in 1 to $4^1/_2$ years even if the deformity is as much as 20°.

Connolly[97] has stressed that depending on two-dimensional x-ray films alone in the management of three-dimensional fracture deformities is inadequate. Apparent valgus and varus deformity may be secondary to rotational malalignment and will not be cured in the tibia by wedging a cast.

A woman with a comminuted fracture of the tibia was treated by closed reduction and plaster casting. Subsequently a plate was applied to her tibia to treat her nonunion. She was distressed after removal of her cast because her foot did not point ahead as it should. She consulted another orthopaedist who told her that this was only a cosmetic deformity and of no functional importance. After several years she developed pain in her ankle that was mitigated, but not cured, by a derotational osteotomy (Fig. 1-94).

Schandelmaier and associates[370] treated 169 fractures of the tibial shaft either by external fixation or by interlocking nails. None of these cases was believed to have more than 20° of malrotation by clinical assessment, but when 90 of these patients underwent measurement by the Clementz method, 10 patients were found to have a malrotation greater than that. Furthermore, a comparison of clinical and radiologic measurement revealed that in 23 of these patients there was a discrepancy of 20°. Sixty percent of the patients had a malrotation of one standard deviation and 25% had two standard deviations.

Although none of the 10 patients with malrotation

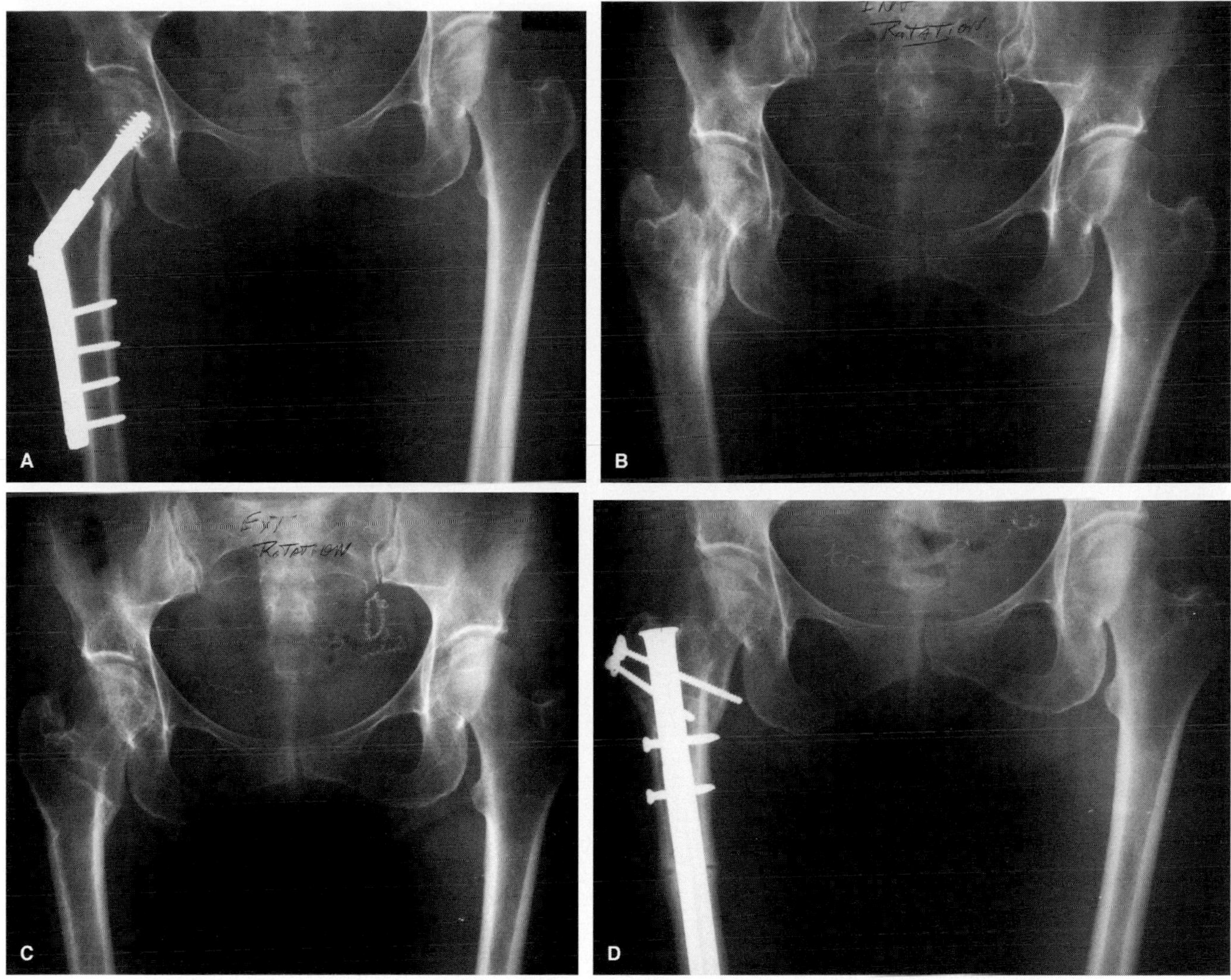

FIGURE 1-93. A 50-year-old woman sustained an intertrochanteric fracture of the right hip that was treated by open reduction and internal fixation. She complained thereafter of a limp, pain in the groin, and discomfort on lying on her right side that was not alleviated by removal of the sliding hip screw. Clinical examinations showed that she had a gluteus medius limp, a high-riding greater trochanter, inability to externally rotate beyond neutral, and 60° of internal rotation. (**A**) Initial radiograph with sliding screw *in situ.* (**B** and **C**) Comparison views in internal and external rotation. Note the shortening of the right femoral neck in both views, the high-riding greater trochanter, and the change in contour of the femoral shaft. (**D**) Postoperative radiograph after derotational osteotomy and realignment of the greater trochanter that was found to be displaced anterior to the femoral neck. We have postulated that this woman's fracture was due to an internal torque and should have been reduced by external rotation. Her malrotation was on the order of 45° and effectively shortened the lever arm of the gluteus medius. She was significantly improved by surgery but continued to have discomfort in the hip.

in excess of 20° had significant interference with function, the authors stressed that the follow-up was only 30 months.

The Clementz Method

This method is dependent on intact knee ligaments and medial malleolus and the use of an image intensifier. The knee to be examined must be fully extended, and the beam of the image intensifier shone horizontally through the distal femur. The limb is rotated until the posterior borders of the femoral condyles are superimposed and the limb is locked in this position. The C-arm is then moved distally to shoot horizontally through the ankle and the tube tilted 5° craniad. The tube is then rotated until a tangential view of the medial malleolus is obtained. The number of degrees the tube is rotated can be read on the protractor on the x-ray tube. The same procedure is then repeated on the other extremity and the results compared.

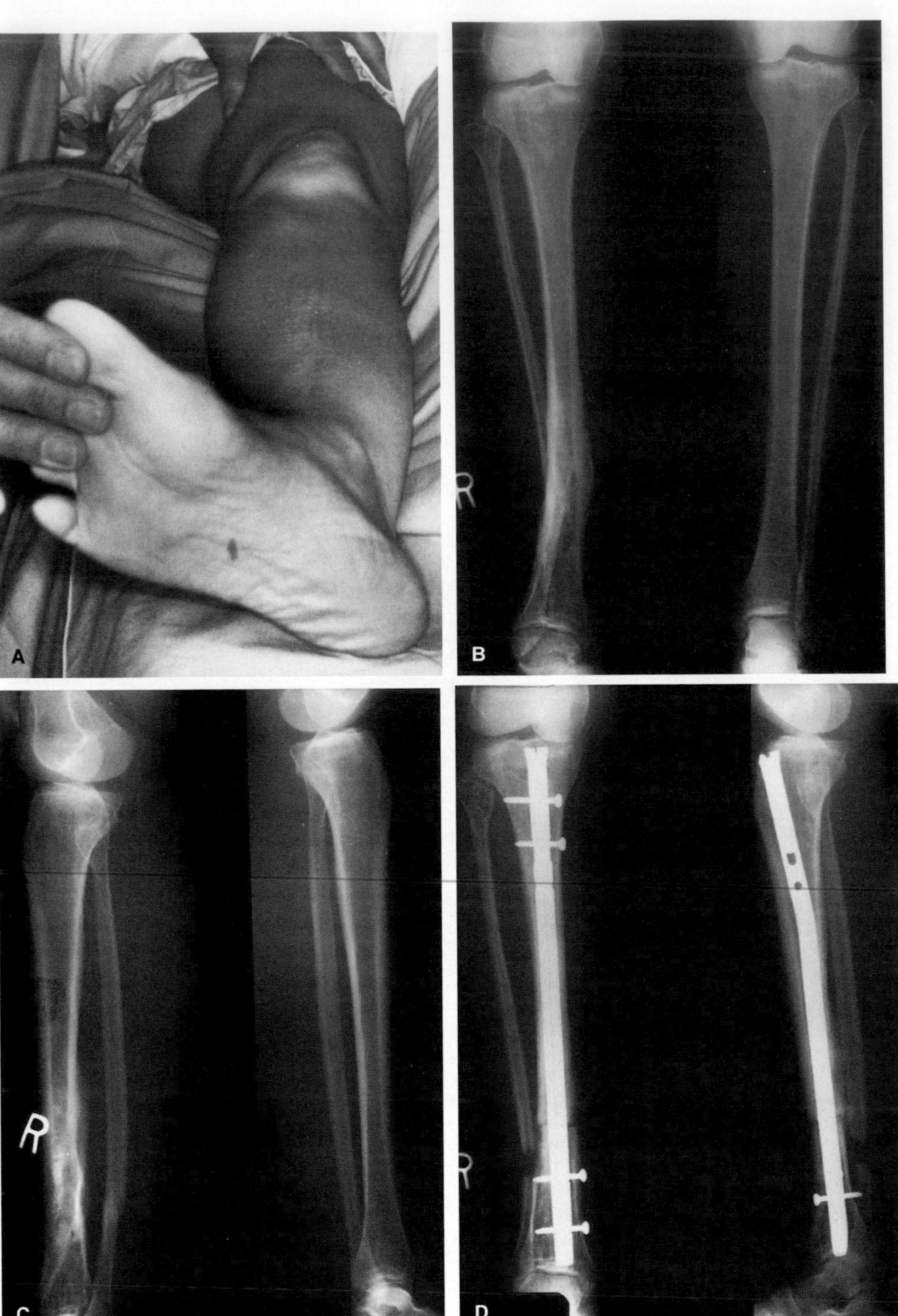

FIGURE 1-94. This woman with malunion of the right tibia following a comminuted fracture of the right tibia has residual angulation and malrotation. (**A**) Clinical photograph. (**B** and **C**) Anteroposterior and lateral radiographs of tibia. Note the valgus angulation in the anteroposterior view is no longer seen in the lateral view so that the maximum angulation is in a plane at 45° to these views. The malrotation is evident by comparing the ankle mortices of the two sides. (**D**) Postoperative films after correcting the angulation and malrotation and osteotomizing the fibula. The osteotomy was made through the apex of the angulation, the medullary canal opened up, and the 30° maltotation corrected.

Overlapping finger deformities associated with fractures of the phalanx may not be evident on radiologic examination and are best prevented by "buddy splinting" to an adjacent digit (see Chapter 11).

Merwyn Evans[148] described a method of avoiding malrotation of the radius in his classic paper on forearm fractures. Using the contour of the radial tuberosity as a marker, he compared films of the normal forearm in varying degrees of pronation and supination with those of the reduced, fractured forearm to make sure that the distal fragment was anatomically aligned.

One should always suspect malrotation when there is an abrupt change in diameter from one fragment to another at a fracture site where there is no comminution.[284]

Prevention of Infection

When an operation is undertaken, a closed fracture is converted into an open one with the potential danger of its becoming infected. This complication may be catastrophic. It can lead to the loss of a limb and, at best, it prolongs the period of morbidity, may make more operations necessary, and impairs the quality of the final result. It follows, then, that every precaution must be taken to prevent this dismal series of events.

Care of the Soft Tissues

A fracture was defined, we believe by Clay Ray Murray, as a "soft-tissue injury complicated by a break in a bone." The most important single factor in the management of fractures is the treatment of the overlying soft tissues;[60,61,144,169,170] in fractures of the tibia especially, this may determine the success or failure of treatment. Incisions made through traumatized, compromised skin may cause its demise. The management of tibial fractures has been revolutionized by intramedullary nailing,[5,48,107,221,430,443] and even open fractures may be safely managed by unreamed nails.[15,47,108,113,184,196,266,363,436] The indications for tibial plating and extensive exposures have been correspondingly reduced.

There is still a tremendous compulsion for surgeons to close wounds primarily, even though it has been shown quite conclusively that delayed primary closure or secondary closure by skin grafting is much safer.[60,61] Certainly in well-debrided wounds seen early, where the soft-tissue damage and contamination have not been severe, it is permissible to suture primarily. On the other hand, ill-advised attempts to provide skin cover for fractured tibias by suturing wounds under tension, by making "relaxing" incisions, and by the rotation of flaps is so fraught with danger that it should rarely be done.[60] If cover is mandatory, it has been suggested that Ger's technique, in which the bone is covered by a transposed muscle belly followed by skin grafting on the fifth postoperative day, is the best means of achieving it.[169,170] We believe that this adds insult to injury in a severely traumatized limb and do not advocate it as an immediate measure. In Louisville, we are most fortunate in having a number of highly skilled microsurgeons, so that tissue cover, in catastrophic soft-tissue loss, is often provided by a latissimus dorsi or other composite free flap. This has revolutionized the management of leg injuries and has salvaged limbs that would inevitably have been amputated in other times. The timing of applying such composite, free grafts is a matter that has not been satisfactorily resolved. If the graft is delayed for more than 48 hours the recipient site becomes secondarily invaded by undesirable opportunistic organisms, so that immediate application of the graft after debridement is desirable. On the other hand, one hesitates to perform a procedure requiring several hours on a patient who is severely injured and who already may have been anesthetized for a considerable time. Furthermore, one is reluctant to compromise vessels in a traumatized limb until the total insult to the extremity can be accurately assessed. The full extent of tissue damage is sometimes not ascertainable, and redebridement may be required later. Nevertheless, when conditions have been favorable, we have had excellent results from primary free tissue transfer.

Godina,[173] whose experience in covering exposed tibias was unrivaled, has shown that the results of cover in the first 48 hours are vastly superior to delayed cover. The infection rate, graft survival, and time in hospital are markedly better. Godina pointed out that edema and infection make the vascular anastomoses technically much more difficult and thus compromise the result. Furthermore, when the anterior tibial artery is transected it may be used as the donor artery only in the first 48 hours. After this time the flow in the vessel drops to 10% of normal and cannot sustain a free flap. (For a more extensive discussion of soft-tissue management and free flaps, see Chapter 7.)

A temporizing stratagem popularized by Seligson and Henry[196a] is the "bead pouch." After debriding the wound, tobramycin-impregnated or other antibiotic-impregnated beads are placed in the wound and covered by Op-Site, an adhesive plastic wound dressing that allows transpiration. The closed space is drained by a small Hemovac catheter. The wound is reexamined after 48 hours; if necessary, it is redebrided and new beads are inserted or, if the wound is clean, it is closed by whatever method is most appropriate (see Fig. 1-84)

The use of antiseptics on open wounds has nothing to recommend it, and we deprecate the use of Dakin's solution, hydrogen peroxide, povidone-iodine, or whirlpool treatment with povidone-iodine scrub. Esterhai and Queenan[146] recommend dressings that will prevent desiccation of the wound and provide a barrier to bacterial contamination. Such dressings are:

1. Semipermeable films (eg, Opsite, Tegaderm, and Bio-occlusive)
2. Hydrogels (eg, Vigilian)
3. Occlusive hydrocolloids (eg, Duoderm)
4. Artificial skin (eg, Epigard).

In the management of chronic nonhealing wounds such as trophic ulcers, we have been helped by the use of hyperbaric oxygen therapy and platelet growth factors. Hyperbaric oxygen has been shown to enhance neutrophil and macrophage function as well as to inhibit a variety of organisms, especially anaerobes and microaerophilic bacteria. We frequently employ it in type IIIB and IIIC tibial fractures.

All would agree that the most important predisposing causes of infection are the presence of dead or devitalized tissue, hematoma, dead space, and foreign bodies. It follows, therefore, that these conditions must be eliminated or controlled as far as possible. The management of open fractures and these problems is discussed in Chapter 6.

Prophylactic Antibiotics

Although formerly there was dispute regarding the value of prophylactic antibiotic therapy in fracture surgery, and even evidence that it increased the rate of infection,[156,394] the use of antimicrobial drugs to prevent infection perioperatively and to eliminate contamination of open wounds is now firmly established.[156,283,369,438]

Especially in the management of open fractures the early institution of systemic antibiotic therapy is a sine qua non, and a broad-spectrum antibiotic or a combination of antimicrobials is given to cover the spectrum of likely contaminating organisms. We still prefer to use a first-generation cephalosporin such as cephazolin or cephalothin and, in grossly contaminated wounds, add tobramycin or ciprofloxacin. The primary defense against infection, however, is adequate wound excision; and we culture the material removed to help with subsequent addition to the antibiotic regimen. We prefer to debride the obviously contaminated and damaged tissue first and then irrigate, rather than in the reverse order.

We have usually given antibiotics for 48 hours in the absence of overt infection, but Wilkins and Patzakis[437] advise 3 days administration for type I and II tibial fractures and 5 days of antibiotic therapy for type III fractures. Certainly the greater the magnitude of the soft-tissue injury, the longer the periods of antibiotic administration, especially when repeated debridements are necessary.

The use of local irrigants or aerosols containing antibiotics has also been shown to be effective in reducing the rate of postoperative infection.[157,232,429] Gingrass and associates,[171] in experimental studies, found that gentle scrubbing of contaminated wounds and irrigation with neomycin solution was superior to irrigation with saline or scrubbing with hexachlorophene (pHisoHex), either alone or in combination, in preventing infection in contaminated wounds. Parenteral neomycin, while ineffective by itself, did improve the results when used as an irrigant and was complemented by gentle scrubbing.

Dirsch and Wilson[132] advocate topical antibiotic irrigation but believe that irrigation with saline solution alone is not helpful and indeed washes out the antibiotics in the tissues that had been given systemically.

When surgery is being performed on a previously open or infected fracture, we start antibiotics intravenously with the induction of anesthesia and continue them for 24 hours.

Internal Fixation and Infection

It used to be held that an internal fixation device, being a foreign body, in some way enhanced the chances of wound infection and was absolutely proscribed in the treatment of open fractures. This contention has been supported by published series. Gustilo and associates[183] analyzed 511 open fractures and found that of the 112 fractures treated by primary fixation, 11.6% became infected, whereas in the 299 without primary internal fixation, the infection rate was only 6.68%.

When infection occurred after internal fixation, it was formerly advised that the metal should be removed to control the sepsis. The idea that metal per se is responsible for infection is open to serious doubt.

McNeur[261] has shown that both in war wounds and open fractures in civilians, adequate management of the soft-tissue wound and the use of antibiotics allow the use of primary internal fixation without incurring prohibitively high infection rates. Of 145 cases treated at the Alfred Hospital, early skin healing was obtained in 125. Twelve patients had delayed wound healing, and only 5 developed infection. In the total series, there were only six infected fractures (3.6%), and in none of these was the metal removed early. Four of the fractures went on to union in spite of infection.

There is now a plethora of reports of unreamed interlocking nailings of the tibia and femur with very low infection rates.[15,47,108,184,265,363,436] Low-velocity gunshot fractures of the femur have also been shown to be amenable to immediate intramedullary nailing without infection supervening.[444]

Experience seems to confirm that when internal fixation is secure it should not be removed in the presence of infection and that with debridement, irrigation, and antibiotic therapy, union will eventually occur.[201,231] It may be that the optimum management of an infected nonunion is to combine aggressive treatment of the infection with secure, rigid, internal fixation.

Nutrition and Infection

We all pay lip service to the notion that well-nourished patients cope better with stress and are less likely to become chronically infected than the homeless and the poor whose nutrition is poor. An elderly woman living by herself is also likely to be undernourished.

In practice it seems to us that this aspect of care is frequently neglected.

Smith[384] avers that body weight is a poor measure of adequacy of nutrition and recommends screening patients by assessing total lymphocyte count, serum albumin value, and, more importantly, serum transferrin level.

A serum albumin value below 3.5 g/dL is associated with much higher complication rates than in patients with higher levels, and when associated with a total lymphocyte count below 1500 cells/mm^3 there is an enhanced risk of infection, wound breakdown, and impaired fracture healing. Smith states that a 10% weight loss during the previous year or a weight that is less than 90% of the ideal should be a trigger to investigate the patient's nutritional state. In our hospital our dietitians have been enormously helpful in both the investigation and correction of nutritional deficits.

Immunodeficiency and Infection

With the increasing numbers of patients being immunosuppressed to protect renal, pancreatic, hepatic, cardiac, and pulmonary transplants, one must be meticulous when they sustain fractures to protect them from wound infections. But those patients are instantaneously recognized.[50] What is not so apparent are those patients who are positive for infection with human immunodeficiency virus (HIV) but do not have the overt stigmata of the acquired immunodeficiency syndrome. Paiment and associates[295] in a study of 476 asymptomatic, HIV-seropositive patients operated on for orthopaedic trauma found an overall 16.7% infection rate as opposed to a 5.4% rate in HIV-negative patients. This discrepancy was even greater in open fractures, where the comparative rates were 55.6% and 11.3%, respectively. They noted that in Gustilo type IIIA and IIIB fractures the patients were at "ominous risk" and required aggressive therapy.

It used to be that a surgeon's only concern was the prevention of infection of the patient during surgery, but now the shoe is on the other foot. That surgeons may be infected by fluids from patients is exemplified by their having an incidence of positivity to hepatitis B virus of 28.4% as compared with 3.7% for the general population. Hepatitis B, however, has a much higher infectivity than HIV. Fortunately, the hepatitis vaccine gives complete protection from this potentially lethal disease.

The Centers for Disease Control and Prevention estimates the risk of HIV seroconversion by inoculation at 0.4% per incident. But contamination of the skin may allow infection through minute breaks in the skin. As little as 0.3 mL of infected blood may carry an infecting dose. Ippolito[216] has calculated the risk of seroconversion as being 0.1% per parenteral exposure and 0.6% for each exposure of the mucous membranes. The incidence of HIV in orthopaedists is very low at this time, although it might be underestimated since few surgeons are going to advertise their infection for obvious reasons. After screening of the surgeons attending the annual meeting of the American Academy of Orthopaedic Surgeons in 1991, the yield of seropositivity was only 0.06% and both those men had exposure to risks other than from their occupation. Gruen and Gruen[181] have reported that three orthopaedic surgeons have already been infected. Nonetheless, this should not be a source of complacency, and these numbers will inevitably rise. It has been estimated that the cumulative risk of HIV infection for an orthopaedic surgeon may be as high as 20% if the surgeon is working in a high risk area where there is a 10% seroprevalence. Circumspect fracture surgeons should take every precaution to protect themselves because their clientele has a higher incidence of seropositivity than the general population, particularly if they work in a trauma center in a large city. In some trauma subsets, seropositivity may be as high as 19%.[189]

Hammond and associates[189] surveyed 81 trauma rooms and found that only 16% observed universal precautions. Sharp technique, protective eye wear, protection of the body by gowns or aprons, and ankle and foot protection were defective.

Surgeons should protect themselves with goggles, face shield, or space suit; protect the body with gowns and aprons; and wear bootees or protective footwear.[11,37] It has been suggested that gloves should be changed every 25 minutes because often at the end of a procedure there are blood stains on the fingers without the surgeon being aware of a tear in a glove.[316] Double-gloving makes sense to protect the skin; furthermore, an inadvertent needle stick of the finger will carry a reduced inoculum because the passage through the two layers of gloves wipes off the needle. Solid suture needle sticks carry a smaller inoculum than hollow needles.

When a surgeon operates, he or she must assume that the patient is HIV positive. Should the surgeon have a needle stick or other potential hazard he or she should ask the patient's permission to test for HIV. The surgeon, if the patient is seropositive, should be tested immediately, at 6 weeks, 3 months, and 6 months. Further testing is unnecessary.[37]

Prophylactic treatment by zidovudine is controversial and is probably ineffectual.

The dimensions of this problem would be significantly diminished if HIV were to be treated as a public health problem rather than a social one. The routine Wasserman test on hospital admission served a very useful purpose in yesteryear, and HIV testing would be even more valuable to protect health care workers from an incurable disease.

ANESTHESIA IN FRACTURE TREATMENT

Most fracture work is carried out under general or regional anesthesia administered by an anesthesiologist. The choice of method and agents under these circumstances must be left to the anesthesiologist and is dictated by the age and condition of the patient as well as the experience of the person administering the anesthetic. It is axiomatic that the patient should be resuscitated and stabilized before the administration of anesthesia, and whenever possible anesthesia in a patient with a full stomach should be deferred to avoid the danger of aspiration pneumonia. If anesthesia is mandatory, the patient may be intubated while awake to avoid the danger of aspirating gastric contents. Spinal anesthesia in an acutely injured patient is hazardous and is best avoided.

On occasion the surgeon is obliged to work without the services of an anesthesiologist. Fractures of the tibia seen soon after injury may often be reduced and immobilized without anesthesia or under analgesics such as morphine or meperidine. When these drugs are used, we prefer to administer them intravenously (eg, 8 to 10 mg of morphine or 75 to 100 mg of meperidine), because their action is produced rapidly and predictably. They should be given slowly and should be well diluted. In general, fractures reduced without the services of an anesthesiologist tend to be minor ones in the upper extremity—especially those involving the wrist and hand.

The methods commonly used to provide such anesthesia are local infiltration of local anesthetics, intravenous regional anesthesia (Bier's block), and regional nerve block. Hypnosis or the use of ataractic drugs may also be employed.

Local Infiltration

If a needle is introduced into a fracture hematoma, blood is easily aspirated, and analgesia may be obtained by injecting lidocaine, mepivacaine, or some similar drug into the hematoma.[131] This method is most frequently used in the treatment of Colles' fracture. The fracture is palpated, and 10 mL of 1% lidocaine or a similar agent is injected into the hematoma. Another 5 mL must be injected around the ulnar styloid, or analgesia will be incomplete. Furthermore, at least 10 to 15 minutes should be allowed before starting to manipulate the fracture. Theoretically, this method would seem to carry the risk of infecting the hematoma, but in practice this rarely occurs. Case[78] treated a series of 136 Colles' fractures; 79 were anesthetized by infiltration of the hematoma, 30 by Bier's block, and 26 by general anesthesia. He found that there was no difference in the ease of reduction or in the end result, although the simplicity of induction and the economy of time in a busy casualty department made hematoma infiltration the method of choice. Case used 5 mL of 2% lignocaine and reduced the fracture after a 10- to 15-minute wait. There were no infections in his series.

Intravenous Regional Anesthesia

Intravenous regional anesthesia, originally described by Bier in the 19th century, has been revived and is used in surgery of the forearm and hand, as well as in the leg and foot. A needle or venous catheter is inserted into a convenient superficial vein. The arm or leg is then elevated and exsanguinated by wrapping with an Esmarch or Ace bandage. A pneumatic tourniquet is inflated (250 mm Hg in the arm; 400 mm Hg in the leg), and the bandage is removed. In the arm 20 to 40 mL of 0.5% lidocaine is injected into the vein (for larger volumes, 0.25% solution can be used), and in the foot and leg 40 to 80 mL is required. Atkinson and associates[22] recommended that no more than 50 mL of 0.5% lidocaine should be used in the arm, and they used an average dose of 224 mg of lidocaine. Sorbie and Chacha[386] used no more than 200 mg in the arm and 400 mg in the leg. After this injection, anesthesia is usually produced within 5 minutes. At this point a second tourniquet is inflated distal to the first, and the original tourniquet is deflated.

This method gives excellent anesthesia for an hour or more, although some patients complain of tourniquet pain. Should the tourniquet become deflated before 20 minutes after the injection, a toxic dose of lidocaine may be released into the general circulation. Great care should be taken to ensure that this does not happen, and drugs and equipment for dealing with reactions to local anesthetics must be on hand. No type of anesthetic should be undertaken without having another person in the room or at least within easy earshot. No patient with a history of idiosyncrasy to local anesthetic agents should be treated by this means.

If this method is to be used, never use a long-acting agent such as bupivacaine (Marcaine). In one misadventure, a young man lost his life and an orthopaedist his reputation when this agent was used and the tourniquet was not inflated. Although Hollingsworth and associates[207] recommended this agent for intravenous regional anesthesia, when there is a misadventure, prolonged resuscitation is necessary and death may result.

Brachial Block

Excellent anesthesia of the upper extremity can be produced by interscalene or supraclavicular brachial block. Because there is some danger inherent in both of these techniques, and because pneumothorax has been reported in up to 20% of supraclavicular blocks, we believe that these methods are best left to those skilled in their use. Brachial block by the axillary route, on the other hand, is a simple, efficient, and relatively risk-free means of producing anesthesia of the upper extremity. This technique has been described well by Burnham, DeJong, and others.[53,116,440] Kleinert and associates[233] reported the results of 647 blocks in 1963, and since that time axillary block has become our anesthetic method of choice in the upper extremity. More than 90% of the hands operated on in Louisville are anesthetized in this manner, as well as Colles' fractures and other minor injuries of the upper extremity. A subsequent paper from the same authors reported their experience with more than 10,000 cases.[224]

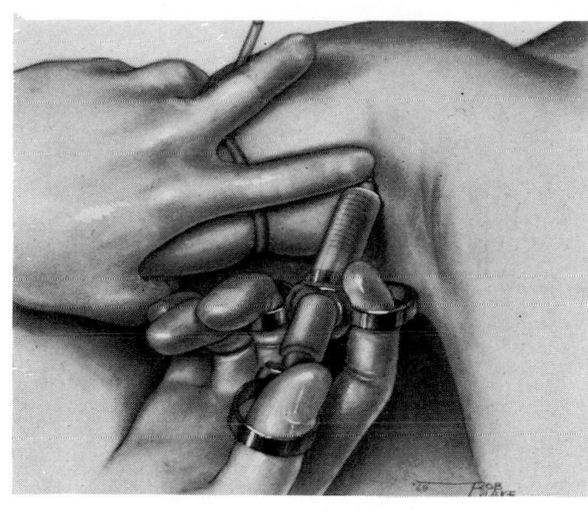

FIGURE 1-96. The artery is palpated in the axilla, and the needle is passed close to the fingertips. A tourniquet prevents peripheral leakage and diffusion of the agent and allows the block to be produced by smaller dosages of local anesthetic. (*Kasdan, M.L., Kleinert, H.E., Kasdan, A.P., and Kutz, J.E.: Axillary Block Anesthesia for Surgery of the Hand. Plast. Reconstr. Surg., 46:256, 1970.*)

Technique

The patient lies in the supine position, and the shoulder is externally rotated and abducted to 90°. The elbow is also flexed to a right angle, and the patient is placed in a comfortable position. After preparing the skin, the axillary artery is palpated where it lies under the cover of the pectoralis major. With the use of a 10-mL syringe and a $^5/_8$-inch, 25-gauge needle, a wheal is raised in the skin overlying the artery, as high in the axilla as possible, and the needle is inserted into the neurovascular sheath (Figs. 1-95 through 1-97). A distinct sensation is felt as the sheath is pierced, and after detaching the syringe, the needle can be seen to pulsate owing to the proximity of the artery. At this point the patient should be questioned regarding paresthesias in the limb, which confirms that the sheath has been entered. To avert the hazard of intravascular injection, the needle should be aspirated before the anesthetic agent is injected. The duration of the block is enhanced by the addition of epinephrine, 1:200,000, to the anesthetic agent. If lidocaine is used, 20 mL of 1% solution may be adequate to produce anesthesia of the hand and forearm; and where more extensive anesthesia of the extremity is required, the dosage may

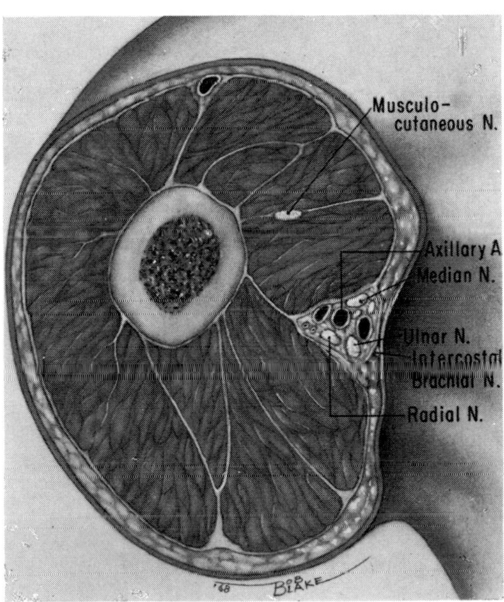

FIGURE 1-95. A cross section of the axilla demonstrating the superficial position of the neurovascular bundle. (*Kasdan, M.L., Kleinert, H.E., Kasdan, A.P., and Kutz, J.E.: Axillary Block Anesthesia for Surgery of the Hand. Plast. Reconstr. Surg., 46:256, 1970.*)

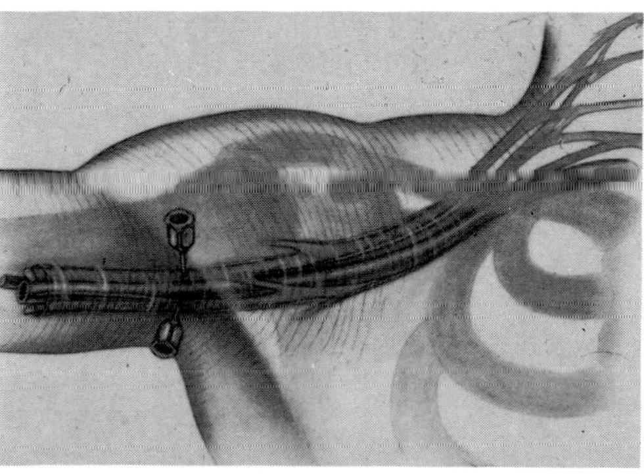

FIGURE 1-97. The injection should be high in the axilla, and a two-needle technique may be used to make sure that all three nerves are blocked. (*Kasdan, M.L., Kleinert, H.E., Kasdan, A.P., and Kutz, J.E.: Axillary Block Anesthesia for Surgery of the Hand. Plast. Reconstr. Surg., 46:256, 1970.*)

be increased to 40 mL. Smaller doses may suffice if a tourniquet is placed around the arm before the insertion of the needle (Erickson technique) (see Fig. 1-96). This tourniquet prevents peripheral leakage and diffusion of the agent. To make sure that all three cords are blocked, two needles may be inserted, one above and one below the artery, but in general one needle is sufficient (see Fig. 1-97). A $^5/_8$-inch needle is adequate for all but the most gargantuan arms, owing to the superficial location of the neurovascular bundle. If a longer needle is used, it is possible to inject the coracobrachialis muscle and produce no block at all. Although there will inevitably be a small percentage of unsuccessful blocks (Kasdan and associates[224] reported 90% success), the most common cause of failure is impatience. Although profound anesthesia may occur within 10 minutes, it may take 30 minutes. On occasion the patient awakes from general anesthesia with an excellent block because the surgeon was unwilling to wait.

In reported series of nerve blocks, the neurologic complication rate has been reported from 0% to greater than 5%. Most of the complications are minor and transitory and some, indeed, may be secondary to faulty positioning, complications of surgery or casting, tourniquet injury, or some other factor unrelated to the block per se. However, serious complications do occur, such as chronic pain, persistent loss of sensation, and paralysis.

Because modern anesthetic agents are unlikely to have direct toxic effects on nerves when used according to the manufacturer's directions, mechanical injury to the nerve by needling must be considered as a possible cause when untoward symptoms occur.

Selander and his group[377] have investigated this problem both clinically and experimentally. In the technique of axillary block, one may identify the major nerves by provoking paresthesia with the probing needle and then injecting around the nerve. An alternative technique is the Eriksson method of inserting two needles in the axillary sheath and gauging their position by the transmitted pulsations of the artery. In his clinical study, Selander divided his patients into two groups: 290 were blocked by evoking paresthesias and 243 by the Eriksson technique. Of the latter group, 40% had paresthesia inadvertently evoked during the insertion of the needles. Eight complications resulted in the paresthesia group (2.8%), and only 2 (0.8%) had complications in the other group.

Selander also investigated histologically the effects of puncturing sciatic nerves in rabbits, using needles with short (14°) and long (45°) bevels. The long-beveled needles were most likely to produce injury, but this depended on the orientation of the bevel to the long axis of the nerve. If the bevel was parallel to the nerve fascicles, comparatively little damage was done; but in other orientations, distortions or transections of nerve fibers resulted or perineural gaps were produced with herniation of fibers. Damage could be produced by short-beveled needles but was less severe and independent of orientation.

It would seem, therefore, that the safest method of axillary block would be the Eriksson method, using 4-mm needles with 45° bevels.

Scott[374] has published a superb manual of regional anesthesia with detailed and explicit instructions and anatomical diagrams; this is an excellent guide for those who must do their own anesthesia.

Intravenous Diazepam

Diazepam (Valium) is a benzodiazepine derivative that has ataractic and muscle relaxant properties. It is recommended for the treatment of anxiety and tension states. Diazepam is also used for the relief of skeletal muscle spasm such as in cerebral palsy, athetosis, and the stiff-man syndrome. This drug is contraindicated in patients with acute, narrow-angle glaucoma and should not be administered to patients in shock, coma, or acute alcohol intoxication who have depressed vital signs.

Bultitude and associates[65] reported on the intravenous use of diazepam as the sole anesthetic agent for the reduction of Colles' fractures. They advised a dose of 20 mg given intravenously, or 30 mg in heavy adults, administered over a period of seconds equal to twice the number of milligrams given (eg, 20 mg over 40 seconds). In their experience this was a useful anesthetic. They thought that the drug had little or no analgesic action but did induce transient amnesia. (One of our anesthesiologist friends has described this method as being the pharmacological equivalent of "biting the bullet.") Their patients were quick to recover, could sit up in 5 minutes, and were able to return home in 2 hours.

Of the 71 patients treated, only two 85-year olds became unrousable for 2 minutes, and one of them had a fall in blood pressure for 10 minutes after the injection. Both of these patients made a full recovery. The only other complications reported in this study were pain at the injection site and thrombophlebitis. Others have noted respiratory depression after intravenous injection of diazepam.

We have used this technique, too, but have given somewhat smaller doses (10 to 20 mg). It has been useful in reducing dislocations of the shoulder and elbow as well as in minor fractures. Care must be taken with inebriated patients, however, because alcohol and diazepam appear to have a synergistic action. Diazepam or regional block should never be used when there is no one to help or if oxygen and some means of ventilating the patient are not easily available.

In some emergency departments, fractures will be reduced without the services of an anesthesiologist in attendance using intravenous drugs.

Grant and associates[176] describe the use of midazolam (Versed) to anesthetize patients to reduce Colles' fractures. A solution of midazolam, 1 mg/mL, is injected by 1-mL increments with intervening pauses until the patient evinces slurring of speech and yawning and the fracture is reduced. The average dose required is 4.5 mg (2–7 mg), but in those older than 70 the average dose is only 2.7 mg (2–3.5 mg).

Bono and associates[43] use methohexital (Brevital), a short-acting barbiturate, to induce deep sedation or unconsciousness for a period of less than 10 minutes. Five hundred milligrams of the drug is dissolved in 50 mL of sterile water (10 mg/mL). The initial dose is 0.75 to 1.00 mg/kg and is repeated as necessary. An average of 2.5 doses was given per patient to provide anesthesia for 7.6 ± 5.0 minutes. Supplemental oxygen and bag breathing were given as necessary, and the methohexital was supplemented by diazepam, morphine, and meperidine without additive or synergistic effect on the hemodynamic or respiratory systems.

This method, however, did call for special training for the physicians, nurses, and personnel in the emergency department. In the litigious environment of the United States, orthopaedists would be ill advised to carry out anesthetic procedures that incur significant risk especially since they will not be remunerated anyway for acting as their own anesthetist.

Relief of Pain After Surgery

Most surgeons have their own pet regimen for the relief of pain, but the medical profession in general has been castigated both in the lay press and by pain experts for not being aggressive enough in this regard.

In our practice we use personally controlled analgesia (PCA) devices that deliver a solution of morphine (1 mg/mL) or meperidine (10 mg/mL) intravenously for the first 24 to 48 hours after operation. In normal adults younger than the age of 70, we set the computer to deliver on demand a maximum of 1 mL every 10 minutes. However, unless a threshold of analgesia is achieved this dose will often be inadequate, so that we start the patient off with a 3-mL bolus that may be repeated, if necessary, in 1 hour. In addition, we add a 2-mL/h continuous flow during the night. In the elderly, continuous flow may be dangerous and is best avoided and we also diminish the maximum dose by 50%. If the patient has senile dementia or is confused, then PCA is clearly contraindicated and more conventional means are employed to relieve pain.

PCA to our mind is ideal in many ways: the medication is given intravenously, which is the most effective route; there is no delay waiting for a nurse to answer the patient's call and prepare a "shot"; and it reduces the burden on the nursing staff especially at night. On occasion, when complete relief is not achieved the morphine or meperidine may be supplemented by ketorolac (Toradol) intravenously without increasing the danger of narcotic overdose. Ketorolac is a nonsteroidal anti-inflammatory drug with analgesic properties that is useful postoperatively; it should be given intravenously initially, according to the manufacturer's instructions, although it may be given later by mouth. Subsequently, we generally switch to oral analgesics and particularly to codeine derivatives. Oxycodone (Percodan, Percocet, Tylox) is an excellent analgesic comparable to morphine and is more effective when given orally.[321] Unhappily, it is equally addictive, so that we have used it sparingly and usually use hydrocodone (Vicodin, Synalgos DC) instead.

Narcotic dosage may be significantly diminished by the appropriate use of local anesthetic block. We frequently infiltrate incisions with 0.5% bupivacaine and where the patient has had a nerve block for anesthesia, it will frequently last 6 to 8 hours postoperatively. When we manipulate shoulders, we have the anesthesiologist perform an interscalene block to allay pain and, indeed, this might be done for the relief of pain after any shoulder surgery.

When epidural anesthesia is used during surgery, the catheter may be left in situ and the anesthesia continued. More frequently, opioids may be substituted for anesthetic drugs; and small doses of morphine will exert their action directly on the spinal cord, giving superb analgesia. We are somewhat jaundiced by our own experience, on account of the side effects of nausea, vomiting, urinary retention, and problems with the catheter. Ventilatory depression is the most serious complication of this treatment, so that nurses looking after these patients must be alert to recognize it. The toxic effects of morphine may be reversed by naloxone.[340]

But there is a price to pay for the relief of pain. Maletis and associates[252] had a 27% incidence of compartment syndrome in 41 patients who had reduction of tibial fractures under intravenous regional anesthesia. When general anesthesia was used, the rate dropped to 13%.

If a patient has long-acting analgesia, will it mask the pain of ischemia or compartment syndrome? There are reports in which the diagnosis of compartment syndrome has been delayed in patients having epidural analgesia.[398] Montgomery and Ready[273] rebut this contention and describe two patients who developed a compartment syndrome after being in the lithotomy position for an extended period of time. In neither case was the ischemic pain relieved by epidural morphine, and the diagnosis was made in a timely manner by intracompartmental pressure measurement.

If continuous analgesia is maintained after procedures likely to be followed by compartment ischemia, then these patients must be closely followed by a competent staff who are alive to the dangers and signs of this condition.

Choice of Agent

Most of the commonly used local anesthetic agents are effective, but bupivacaine (Marcaine) has the advantage of being extremely long-acting.[275] It lasts two to three times as long as lidocaine (Xylocaine) or mepivacaine (Carbocaine) and 20% to 25% longer than tetracaine (Pontocaine). It is relatively less toxic than other similar drugs, and in our hands 0.5% solutions have been excellent for both local infiltration and nerve blocks.

Etidocaine (Duranest)[208,248] is a long-acting agent that is comparable to bupivacaine in the duration of its action and is midway between lidocaine and bupivacaine in toxicity. An excellent axillary block may be obtained using 30 mL of 0.5% or 1.0% etidocaine with epinephrine, which will give 6 to 7 hours of surgical anesthesia. Onset of anesthesia occurs in 10 to 12 minutes, and total recovery takes up to 10 hours.

At Louisville Jewish Hospital, where nearly 7000 nerve blocks are done annually, the agent of choice is a mixture of etidocaine (30%) and bupivacaine (70%). This has been found to be more effective than either agent alone and capitalizes on the advantages of both drugs.

REHABILITATION FOLLOWING FRACTURES

The concept that rehabilitation is a process that should start after the healing of a fracture and may safely be delegated to physical therapists and physiatrists is fallacious. Rehabilitation is the business of the entire medical team, and it should start the minute the patient is admitted to the hospital.

The prime goals of rehabilitation in the fracture patient are: (1) to maintain or restore the range of motion of joints, (2) to preserve muscle strength and endurance, (3) to enhance the rate of fracture healing by activity, and (4) to return the patient to function and employment at the earliest juncture.

Maintenance of Joint Motion

The stiffness that results after immobilization of a joint is proportional to the length of time involved. The main factor in the production of this contracture is shortening of the surrounding musculature and, to a lesser degree, changes in the joint capsule. Intra-articular changes also occur (eg, proliferation of the subsynovial fatty tissue that encroaches on and may obliterate the synovial cleft). In time this soft-tissue overgrowth may cover the articular cartilage and become confluent with it. Where articular surfaces are in contact, especially under pressure, fibrillation and degeneration occur, and fibrous adhesions or even bony fusion may result. The articular cartilage must depend on synovial fluid for its nutrition. The obliteration of the joint and the lack of motion to "pump" the fluid in and out may also add to the decrease in thickness of the cartilage.[57,143]

It follows that no joint should be immobilized unnecessarily and all joints should be put through a full range of motion every day. The elderly woman with a Colles' fracture should never be left to vegetate in a sling and develop a frozen shoulder and stiff fingers. Proper exercise (including the shoulder) is as much a part of her treatment as the application of a cast or fixator.

The shoulder is particularly likely to develop stiffness in persons who are middle-aged and older, and circumduction exercises must be started as soon as they can be tolerated by patients with fractures of the humeral neck. When a frozen shoulder does develop, an active program of exercises may mobilize the shoulder. In recalcitrant cases, gentle manipulation under general anesthesia may be tried, keeping in mind the danger of fracturing an osteoporotic humerus. The manipulation is best carried out by stabilizing the scapula and abducting the shoulder by pressure on the proximal third of the humerus. No sudden stress should be applied, and on no account must the whole lever-arm of the humerus be used by grasping the elbow, nor should rotational stress be applied.

The elbow does not tolerate injury well and frequently becomes stiff. Early active motion in elbow injuries is desirable, and any attempt to force motion by passive manipulation may incite myositis ossificans.

Limitations of knee motion may follow fractures of the femur, especially when there is scarring binding the quadriceps down to the underlying femur. For this reason we have followed the admonition of the AO group to maintain the knee in flexion after fixing distal femoral fractures. When femoral fractures were treated by continuous traction, surely a rare occurrence nowadays, limited knee motion was not uncommon and manipulation of the knee sometimes resulted in a refracture of the femur or a spontaneous fracture of the osteoporotic patella. Such problems are rare now unless there has been associated soft-tissue damage complicating the fracture.

Continuous Passive Motion

Salter,[358] in his presidential address to the Canadian Orthopaedic Society, reviewed the history of the management of bone and joint injuries and showed that most authorities favored rest and immobilization on a purely empiric basis. Hugh Owen Thomas, the father of British orthopaedics, advocated that immobilization should be "complete, prolonged, uninterrupted and enforced." This tradition dominated orthopaedic thinking, and Lucas-Championniere, a late 19th-century French surgeon often castigated as a quack, promulgated the heresy of massage and motion to prevent muscle atrophy and joint stiffness in the treatment of fractures.

On the basis of experimental work on rabbits, Salter[360] has shown that continuous passive motion (CPM) enhances healing in both articular and ligamentous injuries of joints.

The practical application of this work has been the invention of passive motion devices to exercise the joints of both the upper and lower extremities after operation or injury. Some devices on the market have variable speed controls, but Salter believes that the optimum rate is one cycle per 45 seconds and has designed his apparatus accordingly. In all of these CPM machines the arc of motion may be preset to the needs of each patient and increased at will.

Although we embraced this treatment with enthusiasm initially, both for fracture patients and knee arthroplasty, we have largely given it up and start out patients on early active motion. Rosen and associates[347] compared the results of using CPM, early active motion, and a combination of both in the rehabilitation of anterior cruciate ligament reconstruction. The results were identical among the three groups.

An invariable concomitant of joint immobilization or disease is muscle atrophy. When a knee is immobilized the quadriceps atrophies disproportionately to the hamstrings and this is also true of the triceps in the elbow. It would also seem that the less tension on the muscle, the more it will atrophy (ie, the quadriceps atrophies more when the knee is immobilized in extension and the muscle atrophies most in the first 5 days).[403] Free fluid in the knee joint also invokes atrophy, but the exact mechanism is unknown.

> *. . .the urgent need to document the effectiveness of rehabilitation procedures, specifically therapeutic exercise procedures. The widespread disregard for measurement issues has allowed a vast but flawed body of literature to grow and to retard the advance of the science of therapeutic exercise.*[352]
>
> Jules M. Rothstein

Muscular Exercise

To increase muscular power and endurance the muscle must be exercised. When one reads the literature on exercise, he or she is faced by an enormous mélange of papers by a heterogeneous collection of professionals, some of whom are long on opinion and, regrettably, short on fact.

Muscular contraction or exercise may be concentric, eccentric, isometric, isotonic, isokinetic, or plyometric.[447]

Concentric exercise is when a muscle moves a load by shortening, such as flexing the elbow with a dumbbell in the hand. Eccentric contraction used to be called a *lengthening contraction* and occurs when the muscle contracts as it lengthens, such as in gently lowering a heavy box to the floor by allowing the elbow to extend while the elbow flexors "pay out the slack." Both concentric and eccentric contractions are classified as *isotonic* exercise since the load is constant. This term may be imprecise since the muscle tension changes with joint position even although the speed of motion is kept constant. It has been suggested that a better term might be *dynamic* exercise,[447] but the utility of this suggestion escapes us.

Isometric contraction is where the tension increases in the muscle without any change in its length (ie, muscle setting).

In isokinetic exercise the movement velocity is controlled by an external machine and the patient or subject controls the torque or force of contraction that is matched by the computer-controlled resistance of the apparatus.

Plyometric exercise is when a concentric contraction is preceded by a quick prestretch to enhance the force of contraction. This is more concerned with athletic training perhaps than with therapeutic exercise.

The limbs and their joints may be looked on as an integrated chain with the motion of one joint having an influence on the others. Open-chain exercises are those performed with the limb free in space (eg, quadriceps exercised by extending against weights on the foot); and in closed-chain exercise, the terminal segment is fixed (eg, strengthening the quadriceps by climbing stairs).

Muscle Strength

Muscle strength is the maximum force or tension that a muscle can generate with a single contraction. It is frequently measured by adding weight to the load the muscle has to move until the maximum load is achieved. This is known as the one repetition maximum (1 RM), but it may be inaccurate owing to the fatigue factor that occurs with repeated trials. A similar measure is the 10 repetition maximum (10 RM), which is the maximum load that can be lifted ten times and is 70% to 80% of the 1 RM.

The determinants of strength are listed below:

1. *Muscle size.* Big muscles are stronger than little muscles, and there is a direct relationship between muscle cross section and strength.[117,387]
2. *Muscle education.* The more muscle fibers that contract synchronously, the stronger will be the

muscle contraction. By exercise and training, muscles can be made "smarter." It is said that weight lifters can achieve a 20% increase in the strength of isometric contraction by doubling the synchronization ratio of their muscles.[117]

3. *Age.* With aging there is a progressive decrease in the number of functioning motor fibers and muscle bulk. Although exercising in the elderly will increase muscle strength it will not necessarily produce muscular hypertrophy. Moritani and de Vries[276] studied five young men aged 18 to 26 and five elderly men aged 67 to 72. In each group the men were subjected to an identical, 8-week training program to strengthen elbow flexors and the results were compared. Both groups had comparable increases in strength, but only the young men demonstrated muscular hypertrophy.[163]
   This contention is denied by Frontera and associates,[163] who were able to produce muscular hypertrophy in elderly men, and by Evans and Rosenberg,[150] who were able to produce dramatic results in nursing-home patients in Boston. Evans and Rosenberg documented the improvement by CT scans of the thigh that showed marked hypertrophy of the muscle mass. It is their contention that Moritani and de Vries did not sufficiently load the elderly group, and they recommend exercising at 80% of the 1 RM.
4. Fiber type profile. There are three types of muscle fiber: Type I is a "slow twitch" red fiber that is "slow oxidative" and fatigue resistant. Type IIa fibers are stronger, faster, and bigger than type I fibers and although relatively fatigue-resistant are not so much so as type I fibers. These fibers contain both aerobic and anaerobic enzymes and are sometimes referred to as fast oxidative glycolytic (FOG) fibers or fast red fibers. Type IIb fibers are the "fast twitch" fibers. They are strong but readily fatigable because they do not contain aerobic enzymes. There is some controversy whether the mix of fibers may be changed by exercise.[387] The strength endurance curve will be modified by the mix of muscle fibers.

Exercising to Increase Strength

DeLorme[121–123] is the father of progressive resistance exercise (PRE) and described his technique in 1943. By and large, we seem to spend more time rehabilitating the quadriceps femoris muscle than any other muscle. Although DeLorme wrote more about strengthening this muscle in his original paper, the technique is equally applicable to any muscle.

Strength training is predicated on the "overload principle," that is, taxing the muscle beyond ordinary, customary loads. DeLorme tested the patient for the 10 RM and for the next 5 days the patient would lift 50% of this load ten times, then 75%, and finally 100% of 10 RM ten times. At the end of this period, a new 10 RM level would be determined and the process repeated every 5 days until adequate quadriceps strength was regained.

It might be thought that it would be better to start with the 100% load and reverse the order to allay the effect of fatigue. This is the Oxford technique.[449] In point of fact it seems immaterial which technique is used. Strength may also be enhanced by having patients carry out one maximal contraction every day, although this technique is more applicable to athletes. The subject is loaded to the point where he or she can barely extend the knee and then holds it in extension for 5 seconds. The load is then increased daily by 1.25 lb thereafter for 8 weeks. It is claimed that the strength of the quadriceps can be increased 80% to 400% by this combination of isotonic and isometric exercise.[346]

For many patients, especially early in their rehabilitation, *short arc exercises* in which the knee is exercised through the last 30% of extension rather than the conventional 90° are used, particularly when the knee is painful or very weak.

It is claimed by some that eccentric exercise is more effective than concentric exercise in regaining strength.[3,161] The muscle is loaded and gradually lengthens as the weight is lowered. It is possible to use much larger weights than in concentric exercise, and thereby the chance of muscle damage is increased.[110] The muscle is able to generate more tension with less energy consumption in such exercise.

The *force velocity curve,* in which muscle tension is plotted against velocity of contraction, shows that there is an inverse relationship between these two entities—the slower the contraction, the greater the tension. It follows then that the greatest tension of all will be developed when the velocity of contraction is zero (ie, in isometric contraction).[387] Although strength may be enhanced by isometric exercise substantially, this improvement is mainly at the joint angle at which the muscle is exercised but drops off progressively as this angle is changed. Isometric exercise is most useful when a joint is immobilized and other types of exercise precluded (eg, quadriceps setting and straight-leg raising when the knee is immobilized).

Isokinetic exercise,[145] also known as constant velocity or accommodating resistant exercise, is where the movement velocity, imposed by an external dynamometer, is constant and the force of contraction or torque produced is controlled by the patient. Both concentric and eccentric exercise may be carried out in such devices and the slower the rate, the greater is the muscle tension generated.[272] The dynanometer is programmed to resist whatever torque the subject generates. It has been shown that those subjects that are exercised at slow rates (6 rpm or 36/s) made much greater gains in strength than those exercised at fast rates (18 rpm or 108/s). However, when both groups were tested at a variety of velocities, the high-velocity group showed improvement at all speeds, whereas in the slow group improvement was confined to exercising at slow velocity.

Strength may be increased by both concentric and eccentric isokinetic exercise, but muscular hypertrophy only occurs with eccentric exercise. It is recommended that both types of exercise be employed.[105]

Winter and associates[441] have pointed out that if the effect of gravity is not considered in testing with constant velocity dynamometers substantial errors will result. In a study of knee flexion and extension the error in mechanical work varied from 26% to 43% in extension and from 55% to 510% in flexion.

Almekinders and Oman,[9] in a review of isokinetic exercise, state that there has been no consistent relationship between isokinetic and athletic performance or that it is superior to traditional isometric and isotonic exercise. Furthermore, eager patients may overdo things by putting out more effort than is appropriate and cause joint pain and swelling. Perhaps the greatest virtue of isokinetic exercise is that it allows submaximal exercise within a patient's tolerance to pain.

However muscle strength is enhanced, it is not a good idea to produce asymmetry between a muscle and its antagonists. Both groups of muscles should be strengthened so that they work in balance (eg, hamstring strengthening with quadriceps exercises).[447]

Exercise for Endurance

DeLorme believed that endurance would best be improved by exercising with small loads with high repetitions. Furthermore, he was of the opinion that endurance would not be improved by strengthening exercises or strength by endurance exercises (the DeLorme axiom). This is not entirely true, and both parameters will be increased by both types of exercise to some degree.[118]

It would seem from our perusal of the pertinent literature that no particular method of reconditioning has been shown to be clearly better than the others, and traditional methods of progressive resistance exercise not requiring expensive apparatus are capable of producing the desired effect. Isotonic exercise that uses both concentric and eccentric contraction is cost effective and efficient.

Aquatic Exercises

Exercise in water has the enormous advantage of decreasing the weight of the body by the upthrust of the water displaced. Weight bearing, especially in the obese, is facilitated, and there is little danger from falling. The resistance from the water when walking helps strengthen muscle, and the rhythmic coordination of swimming helps to increase joint motion.

Walkers

It is quite unrealistic to expect elderly patients to walk with crutches because they have neither the strength nor the agility and coordination to use them. In such cases a simple walker made from tubular aluminum that they can lift up and place before them is the most stable and foolproof device. It is also unreasonable to prescribe non–weight-bearing ambulation for elderly persons with fractured hips, and, indeed, the work of Rydell and Frankel would seem to show that partial weight bearing is more benign than many maneuvers carried out in bed. For this reason, in stable, well-fixed fractures of the hip we now start weight bearing as soon as possible.

Canes

Canes are useful but less efficient than crutches for maintaining balance and relieving weight. The patient's natural tendency is to hold the cane with the hand on the side of the injury, which gives rise to a very awkward gait. The patient should be instructed to use the cane in the opposite hand and bear weight on the injured limb and cane simultaneously. The use of a solitary crutch should be discouraged, because it, too, gives rise to an awkward gait. By and large, if a patient needs one crutch, he or she needs two.

Heat

In most departments of physical medicine, there are a number of expensive machines whose main purpose is to supply some form of heat to the tissues. We are not aware of any evidence that heat per se has any beneficial effect in rehabilitation after injury. Ultrasound has been shown to be more efficient in the heating of deep tissues, but the therapeutic benefits of this are somewhat nebulous. The daily application of ultrasound to neck injuries sustained in rear-end vehicular collisions seems to us to benefit mainly the owner of the ultrasound machine.

The application of heat to painful joints and muscles does relieve pain and discomfort and is a useful preliminary measure to active exercises. In this regard, one method does not appear to be superior to another. Hot packs or immersion in warm water are as good as more sophisticated methods and have the advantage of being available at home. If short-wave diathermy is used, it must never be applied over implants, because it induces high temperatures in the metal with damage to the tissues.

Cold applications may also be used to reduce pain before exercise, and we usually ask the therapist to try both and see which is most efficacious.

Ambulation Aids

Most patients with lower-extremity fractures require some form of ambulation aid. Although most rehabilitation centers appear to prefer other than simple axillary crutches, these have the advantage of being inexpensive and readily available. Because the large majority of patients uses them for only a short time, the expense of providing more sophisticated crutches does not seem reasonable. In adjusting these crutches, there should be a handbreadth between the pad of the crutch and the axilla. The pad is designed to take pressure on the lateral side of the chest and not in the axilla, where pressure on the brachial plexus can produce a "crutch palsy." The handpiece should allow the elbow to be flexed comfortably while bearing weight. For comfort, the axillary portion and the handpiece should be padded with sponge rubber and, for safety, the largest rubber tips should be added.

It is a mistake to believe that crutch-walking diminishes physical effort and expenditure of energy. Crutch-walking is an athletic feat requiring muscular strength, increased cardiac output, respiratory effort, balance, and muscle coordination. Everyone cannot use crutches. Cardiac and respiratory disease, age, and lack of coordination preclude crutch-walking and we find that most women of middle age or older do better with walkers. It is best to give instruction in parallel bars first and to prepare patients for ambulation by crutches or walker by strengthening exercises of the upper extremities while the patient is still confined to bed.

Crutch Gaits

Swing-to and swing-through gaits are the most rapid and energy-consuming gaits. The crutches are placed in front of the body and the body pulled level with them (swing-to) or propelled through them (swing-through). Weight may be borne on both feet or, more commonly, on the foot of the uninjured extremity.

In the alternating two-point gait, the left foot is advanced with the right crutch and the right foot with the left crutch so that partial weight bearing is allowed bilaterally.

The three-point gait is perhaps the most useful of all the crutch gaits. In this gait the injured extremity and both crutches are advanced simultaneously and either partial or non–weight bearing may be prescribed. The noninjured extremity is then advanced and the cycle repeated.

Four-point crutch walking is a slow, laborious gait in which the left crutch is advanced followed by the right foot and then the right crutch and left foot in turn.

Purposeful Exercise

Exercise is dull, and most persons prefer carrying out purposeful tasks. This fact is used by devising projects for patients that use the motion desired (eg, using a screwdriver to gain supination range and power). Such therapy not only achieves a therapeutic aim but is also a diversion for the patient that breaks the tedium of a stay in the hospital.

It is also important to make the patient as self-sufficient as possible before he or she returns home. The use of the occupational therapist in supervising activities of daily living is extremely helpful, but unfortunately these functions are rarely to be found outside rehabilitation centers and almost never in general or community hospitals.

Massage

Massage is a time-honored treatment, but the laying on of hands has little place in the rehabilitation of patients with fractures, except as a means of softening up and mobilizing scars that are impeding joint motion. It is extremely unlikely that massage will dissipate edema or improve circulation to an extremity.

Orthoses

Conventional bracing has very little place in the treatment of fractures. Long-leg braces with ischial seats or quadrilateral sockets and pelvic bands are sometimes prescribed to "protect" fractures of the femur or even fractures of the hip. Mechanically, such braces are ineffective and much inferior to cast braces.

Sarmiento[364,365] has shown that tibial fractures may be handled by PTB casts with free ankle joints and later by braces of orthoplast with a similar free ankle. Now there is a variety of off-the-shelf braces designed to be used after a 4- to 6-week immobilization in a cast. Polyethylene braces have also been devised by Sarmiento that are effective in the management of humeral shaft fractures and have supplanted sugar tong splints and "hanging casts."[366]

The major application for bracing in the treatment of fractures is to compensate for associated nerve injuries such as dropfoot secondary to peroneal palsy. Dynamic bracing is also frequently used in the after-treatment of hand injuries, both to compensate for nerve deficits and to stretch out contractures gently and restore joint motion.

INJURY AND THE LAW

A surgeon treating fractures must inevitably become involved with the law. On occasion, patients sue for disabilities incurred; those injured at work are entitled to benefits under workers' compensation laws; and, unhappily, some patients, discontented with the results of the surgeon's ministrations, may sue for malpractice. In addition, surgeons will also be asked to render independent medical opinions on patients treated by other surgeons.

Most physicians do not enjoy giving testimony in court and resent the time and effort in writing legal reports or filling out the routine reports for insurance companies. These duties can only be performed by physicians; and should they be carried out in a perfunctory manner, the patient will suffer, and the physician's professional competence may be brought into question in any ensuing litigation.

The Medical Report

For a variety of legal purposes, a medical report is necessary. Some examples of these reports do not support the contention that medicine is a learned profession. R. M. Fox,[158] a personal-injury attorney who has a somewhat slanted view of these matters, made a valid criticism: "No medical school in the United States today offers a course in medicolegal report writing, in spite of its obvious socioeconomic importance and the billions of dollars type of claim. Little, if any, postgraduate medical education on this subject is available."

A few words on the preparation of such reports would seem to be in order. If the report is on a patient other than our own, we make a practice of prefacing the report by naming the party who has requested the examination and the date on which this examination was performed. When the report is on our own patient, permission to release the information must be given by the patient.

History

Although the patient may give a lengthy account of the circumstances of the accident, only that which is germane to the assessment of the injury should be included in the report, and certainly no judgment as to culpability should appear in the medical report. Although the patient's account to a physician of the circumstances of the accident is inadmissible as evidence bearing on the actionable event itself, it will be admissible to the extent it is relevant in establishing the basis on which the physician's ultimate opinion is based. If, in some way, these notes are erroneous, they may damage the credibility of the patient or in some way influence the outcome of the case.

The past history of the patient must be recorded, especially when previous injury or disease is directly concerned in the production or aggravation of the problem being assessed. If the report is on a patient whom you have treated yourself, a detailed report of the initial examination and subsequent events should be included. The patient should be questioned regarding his or her current condition, and the nature, severity, duration, and frequency of the patient's specific complaints should be listed and described.

Increasingly, the medical records of other treating physicians, physical therapists, and chiropractors are being furnished by those requesting the examination. Much of the material sent is repetitious, frequently illegible, and often not very helpful. But it must be read and commented on, especially if the findings in these records are at variance with your own examination.

Clinical Examination

The clinical examination is carried out in a meticulous manner. Notes are taken during the examination rather than depending on memory; care is taken to differentiate left from right. In most jurisdictions, the medical witness is permitted to refer to these notes to refresh his or her recollection, provided the notes were made at the time of the examination or shortly thereafter. Thorough notes can be invaluable for responding intelligently and consistently in the event of a far-reaching, extended cross examination. The sooner the formal report is dictated, the more accurate it will be. That which can be measured should be, with tape or goniometer. Scars should be noted, especially where they interfere with function or where cosmesis is important. Negative findings, where indicated, should also be noted.

Medical Assessment

After describing the medical findings in technical terms, we generally give a résumé of the findings in nontechnical, lay terms or translate the technical language as we go, depending on the complexity of the case. This is very helpful to the recipient of the report if he or she is a lawyer or other lay person. In the summation of the report the diagnoses should be listed, some opinion should be expressed about the compatibility of the patient's injuries with the patient's history of how they were incurred, and whether the complaints are consonant with the physical findings. There is no place, however, for gratuitous and unnecessarily pejorative remarks regarding the patient.

The prognosis should be discussed when it can be reasonably determined. No one can expect an absolutely accurate forecast of events, but an educated guess is much more helpful than saying that the prognosis is undetermined. The possible and probable end results and the length of time the patient is likely to be incapacitated should be estimated. If further surgery or rehabilitative treatment is necessary, this should be listed and justified.

Physical Impairment and Disability

In the event that the patient's condition is stable and no further treatment is indicated, many agencies and insurance companies will ask for an estimate of permanent disability, or permanent physical impairment expressed as a percentage. There is a distinction between these two terms. *Disability* is a measure of the loss of a person's ability to engage in his or her occupation or earn a living, and therefore is not a purely medical determination. *Physical impairment* is a measure of loss of function or assessment of anatomical defect, which is the same for all similar patients, irrespective of how they earn their living. To quote a hackneyed example: If two men each lost their left fifth fingers, their physical impairments would be identical. If one was a concert violinist and the other a manual laborer, their permanent disabilities would be vastly different. Obviously, disability has to be predicated on physical impairment, but the former is a legal determination and the latter, a medical one.

The physician is the final arbiter of physical impairment. He or she will be helped in this task by the use of various tables that have been devised by the American Medical Association, as well as other publications by authorities in the field.[26,230]

In previous editions of the American Medical Association's *Guide to the Assessment of Physical Impairment* the determination of impairment of orthopaedic defects was predicated largely on limitation of joint motion determined by a standard goniometer. In the latest (fourth) edition, this method of assessment has been retained to a large extent but another method has been added, the diagnosis-related estimate, which has supplanted the former technique for a variety of conditions. The other major change has been the introduction of the use of one or two inclinometers to measure joint motion, especially of the spine (Fig. 1-98).

This volume is used in many jurisdictions now, and especially in workers' compensation cases, so the orthopaedist should be conversant with this book, which is more comprehensive but more difficult to use.

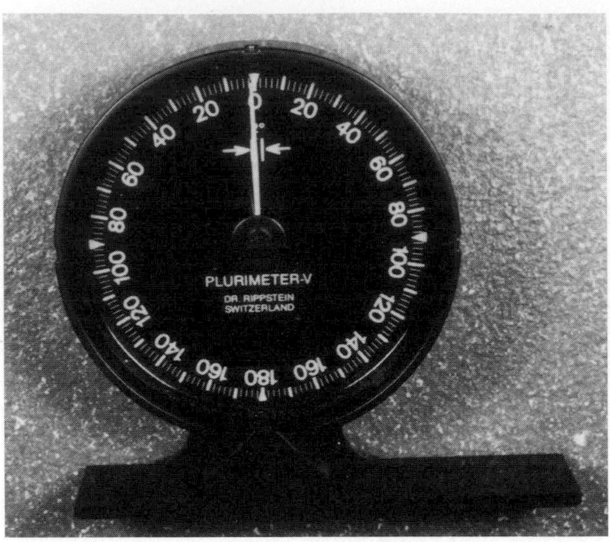

FIGURE 1-98. The American Medical Association's *Guide to the Evaluation of Permanent Impairment* recommends that inclinometers be used to measure the range of motion of the back.

Increasingly physicians are being asked to state whether a patient can push, pull, crawl, and so on, which is usually easy to answer. What is not easy to answer is how much can the patient lift and how often can he or she lift it? To answer such questions honestly requires patient testing and observation, functions that the busy physician obviously cannot perform. Such requests may be reasonably referred to evaluation centers where trained personnel can carry out such studies. Increasingly such centers carry out "objective" evaluation using apparatus such as recording isokinetic dynamometers. Perhaps such apparatus can measure improvement in a particular patient, but the results depend on which brand of machine is used.[9] We have serious doubt that such investigations unerringly identify malingerers.

One should be prepared to show how the percentage of impairment was ascertained; it is not enough to pick a figure from the air or add another 20% because the patient is a sweet person or needs money badly. There are few functions undertaken by the orthopaedist that are more difficult and taxing than the fair, impartial determination of physical impairment.

Testimony in Court

The large majority of personal-injury claims are settled out of court, and this process is facilitated in many instances by a comprehensive and lucid medical report. In those cases in which settlement cannot be reached amicably, the surgeon will usually be asked to give a deposition before the formal trial. A *deposition* is a pretrial examination of a witness by the opposing attorneys without the presence of a judge. The proceedings are recorded by a court stenographer, and the evidence is given under oath. If the case goes to trial, the surgeon will answer the same or similar questions in more formal circumstances, or, in the event that he or she is unable to attend in person, the deposition may be entered as evidence. Should the medical witness give substantially different replies in court to similar questions asked in a deposition, one or either of the attorneys will pick up the discrepancy, and this will inevitably vitiate the testimony of the witness.

The attorney and physician who are brought together in litigation should have a common goal—to assist the court or jury in arriving at the truth. Although this is a time-consuming and occasionally frustrating experience, it is absolutely necessary for the physician to educate the lawyer about the medical aspects of the case. Failure to do so may do a great disservice to the patient, because the lawyer may never ask the questions most pertinent to the case.

A common legal device is the *hypothetical question.* The lawyer, in asking the hypothetical question on which the medical opinion will be based, must include all relevant material findings, including essential negative findings. On that assumed set of facts, the medical witness is asked, "Do you have an opinion and, if so, what is that opinion?" The most frequently encountered gambit in cross examination of the physician is to rephrase the hypothetical question with some omissions or possibly new inclusions. The experienced physician generally avoids traps by being alert and, where necessary, by clarifying the question—"are you asking me if it was the injury that produced this defect?"

As a witness, one should testify to that which one believes to be true, and if one does not know the answer to the question or if it is beyond the area of one's expertise, the witness should say so. Before a deposition the prudent physician refreshes his or her memory of the pertinent literature. Although quotations from the medical texts or papers as such are not admissible as evidence, lawyers in many jurisdictions introduce such material in the process of cross examination and ask the medical witness if the authors are recognized authorities and if the witness agrees with the opinions they have expressed. The surgeon should be at least as well read as the attorney.

Not infrequently the attorney who has requested the surgeon to testify asks for a pretrial or predeposition conference in which the attorney goes over the evidence, asks for clarifications, and reviews the questions he or she will ask. There is nothing unethical in such conferences, but the surgeon should not lose his or her objectivity and become a partisan for one side or the other. The surgeon is a witness, not an advocate.

In the adversary system of justice each attorney attempts to dispose of his or her opponent's arguments, and this may extend to discrediting the medical testimony, too. A lawyer is duty-bound to try to throw doubt on all evidence inimical to a case. This should not be construed as a personal attack by the medical witness.

It is sometimes said that lawyers try to make fools of doctors on the witness stand. This they cannot do without generous help from the physician. If the physician sticks to the facts of which he or she is sure, no lawyer will be able to shake the physician's testimony. Many physicians go wrong by becoming advocates; they become emotionally involved. After losing their sang-froid on the witness stand, not only is their testimony suspect, but they also look foolish. The duty of the medical witness is to state the facts of the case as he or she knows them, to offer his or her best medical opinion when he or she has sufficient grounds to formulate one, and to confine his or her testimony to what he or she is asked. Because members of juries are lay persons, explanations should be as simple and straightforward as possible with a minimum of medical jargon. The witness's remarks should be addressed to the jury, because they, not the attorneys, are charged with the duty of determining the facts of the case and assessing the credibility of witnesses. In the rare event that a lawyer harries a medical witness, the opposing attorney or the judge will invariably intervene. To lose one's temper or argue with counsel is unprofessional and diminishes the value of one's testimony. At all times the medical witness should speak up clearly and distinctly and act like a member of a learned profession.

Workers' Compensation

Workers' compensation statutes vary from state to state, and the practicing physician should acquaint himself or herself with the laws of his or her own state. In essence, these laws have been enacted to compensate employees injured while at work for loss of earnings and permanent disability. This compensation is paid by the employer or an insurance carrier, whether or not the employer was in any way negligent or whether the employee contributed to the accident by his or her own negligence. There is no attempt to compensate the employee for pain and suffering but only for loss of earnings. Because workers' compensation claims are usually settled by a referee and the physician is normally not present at these hearings, the quality of the medical report is of major importance in the settlement of these claims. However, increasingly in our state, depositions are being held in preparation for such hearings.

Physician Liability

A physician is liable to be sued whenever a patient believes his or her treatment has been inadequate. Whether these complaints have any substance is immaterial, and even the most careful and competent surgeon may be sued. It is commonly held by physicians that the present unhappy situation is related to the pernicious system of contingency payments to attorneys, but this overlooks the fact that the suit must be brought in the first place by a disgruntled patient. It seems to us that the causes for such actions are as outlined below.

Negligence

Many suits are related to the complications of tight or improperly applied casts, and precedents are so well established in such cases that the surgeon who does not take appropriate steps when a patient complains of pain under a cast is not only negligent, he or she is stupid. It is a pity that the five *P*s of impending Volkmann's ischemia (pallor, pulselessness, pain, paresthesia, and paralysis) have been taught so well. The only one that is universally reliable is pain. Unreasonable pain in an immobilized limb must be investigated; the cast should be split to the degree that is necessary to relieve the patient's pain and, if necessary, the cast should be bivalved and the padding divided to the skin. If a compartment syndrome is likely, a decompression should be done without delay.

Another potent source of trouble is neglecting to make a radiographic examination of a painful area, so that a fracture goes undetected. The desire to spare the patient expense is a false economy, and prudent surgeons make such examinations even though they are reasonably sure that no fracture is present. They also must make sure that the examination is complete (eg, the hip and knee must be included in x-rays in fractures of the femur to rule out coexisting injuries of these joints). Furthermore, if the quality of the films is unsatisfactory, they must ensure that the examination is repeated and better films obtained. When a case is not progressing satisfactorily, a surgeon should not hesitate to call for assistance from more experienced or knowledgeable colleagues.

Undesirable Cosmetic or Functional Result

Even with the most assiduous care, it is impossible in all cases to restore an injured person to a condition comparable to that which he or she was in before the accident. The surgeon should make a realistic prognosis early on in the patient's management so that no unrealistic expectations will be entertained by the patient or the patient's relatives. All operative procedures other than those life-saving measures that require action without delay should be discussed frankly with the patient and with the appropriate family members. The scope and aim of the procedure and a frank appraisal of the inherent risks should be explained, and this should be reflected in the operative permit that the patient signs and in the surgeon's notes.

Breakdown in Physician–Patient Rapport

Many suits, perhaps the majority, are engendered when a patient becomes angry because a physician belittles or berates him or her or in some way shows a lack of concern, unapproachability, or offhandedness in the patient's treatment. This may be of no importance when the result is good; but when the result is poor, it may be the factor that precipitates a suit. The patient should be treated as you would like your spouse or child to be treated in similar circumstances. A little kindness and encouragement costs nothing and improves rapport. Remember that the patient who irritates you the most is the one who is most likely to sue you. Gratuitous, pejorative descriptions of your patient in the chart will antagonize him or her if the patient reads these descriptions and may well identify you as a curmudgeon if they are read in court. In general, for example, it is better to say that a patient "weighs 360 pounds" than to say that he or she is "grossly obese."

Remarks Critical of Treatment

The surgeon, another physician, or ancillary personnel can make remarks that can be construed as being critical of the treatment received. It goes without saying that everything that is said about treatment, especially that given by someone else, should be carefully worded, so that no pejorative inference may be picked up by the patient. Criticism of another without knowing all the circumstances is unfair and unjust, and the instigation of a lawsuit against another physician is unethical.

Medical Records

The best defense a surgeon has against groundless suits is obviously to give patients competent, assiduous, and courteous service. The only way that this can be documented for legal purposes is by the completeness of the patient's records, both those in the hospital and in the surgeon's office. Voluminous notes may not prove the treatment has been excellent, but a paucity of records suggests a lack of care. In any case, the medical record may be the only evidence to corroborate the physician's story. The sooner these notes are written or dictated after the events they describe, the greater is their value. In many hospitals the dates of dictation and transcription appear on such documents as operative reports. Obviously, an operative report dictated 3 months after the event does not carry as much weight in a court of law as one dictated immediately after the operation.

After a suit has been initiated, some misguided physicians attempt to doctor the record by additions or alterations. Almost always this is picked up by an alert attorney, and it damages the physician's case irreparably. Inevitably, errors creep into hospital records, owing to mistakes in transcription. When such errors are corrected, or when anything is added to the record, these additions should be dated and initialed. Considerable caution should be exercised when operative notes are dictated by an assistant. These should be read carefully, countersigned, and amended when necessary. It is even more prudent, however, for the surgeon to do his or her own dictation.

Good Samaritan Laws

Some states have seen fit to enact legislation that exempts physicians from legal action because they gave emergency medical treatment at the scene of an accident. Opinions vary as to whether such laws are really necessary. There is no legal compulsion for a physician to stop at any accident and give aid; but if he or she does so, the physician establishes a physician–patient relationship and his or her conduct is then governed by what a reasonably prudent physician would do under similar circumstances. Suit being brought under these circumstances is highly unlikely and is even less likely to be sustained in a court of law, unless there has been gross mismanagement. The remote threat of a possible malpractice suit, at any rate, is a rather poor excuse for not carrying out one's obvious duty, and we believe that few physicians would refuse to render aid on this account.

REFERENCES

1. Adams, J.P., Kenmore, P.I., Russell, P.H., and Haas, S.S.: Regional Anesthesia in the Upper Limb. *In* Adams, J.P. (ed.): Current Practice in Orthopaedic Surgery, vol. 4, pp. 238–261. St. Louis, C.V. Mosby, 1969.
2. Agnew, S.G., Peter, R., and Henley, B.: The Role of the Unreamed Nail. Orthop. Trans., 18:8, 1994.
3. Albert, M.: Eccentric Muscle Training in Sports and Orthopaedics. Churchill Livingstone, 1991.

3a. Albright, J. A.: Bone Physical Properties in the Scientific Basis of Orthopaedics. *In* Albright, J.A. and Brand, R.A., pp 155–183. New York, Appleton-Century-Crofts, 1979.

4. Alho, A.: Mineral and Mechanics of Bone Fragility Fractures. A Review of Fixation Methods. Acta Orthop. Scand., 64:227–232, 1993.
5. Alho, A., Ekeland, A., Strsoe, K., Folleras, G., and Thoreson, B.A.: Locked Intramedullary Nailing for Displaced Tibial Shaft Fractures. J. Bone Joint Surg., 72B:805–809, 1990.
6. Allgower, M., and Sequin, F.: Dynamization of the AO/ASIF Tubular External Fixator. AO/ASIF Dialogue, 1(3):12–13, 1987.
7. Allgöwer, M., Sequin, F., and Ruedi, T.: Simplicity is the Rule of the Game: The AO/ASIF Tubular External Fixator. AO/ASIF Dialogue, 1(1):5–6, 1985.
8. Allum, R.L., and Mowbray, M.A.S.: A Retrospective Review of the Healing of Fractures of the Shaft of the Tibia With Special Reference to the Mechanism of Injury. Injury, 11:304–308, 1980.
9. Almekinders, L.C., and Omam, J.: Isokinetic Muscle Testing: Is It Clinically Useful? J. Am. Acad. Orthop. Surg., 2:221–225, 1994.
10. Alms, M.: Fracture Mechanics. J. Bone Joint Surg., 43B:162–166, 1961.
11. American Academy of Orthopaedic Surgeons: Recommendations for the Prevention of Human Immunodeficiency Virus (HIV) Transmission in the Practice of Orthopaedic Surgery. Park Ridge, Ill., American Academy of Orthopaedic Surgeons, 1989.
12. Anderson, G.H., Harper, W.M., Connolly, C.D., Badham J., and Goodrich, N.: Preoperative Skin Traction for Fractures of the Proximal Femur. J. Bone Joint Surg., 75B:794–796, 1993.
13. Anderson, J.T., and Gustilo, R.B.: Immediate Internal Fixation in Open Fractures. Orthop. Clin. North Am., 11:569–578, 1980.
14. Anderson, R.: An Automatic Method of Treatment for Fractures of the Tibia and the Fibula. Surg. Gynecol. Obstet., 58:639–646, 1934.
15. Anglen, J., Unger, D., di Pasquale, T., et al: The Treatment of Open Tibial Shaft Fractures Using an Unreamed Interlocked Intra-Medullary Nail. Orthop. Trans., 18:7, 1994.
16. Apley, A.G.: Fractures of the Lateral Tibial Condyle Treated by Skeletal Traction and Early Mobilization. J. Bone Joint Surg., 38B:699–708, 1956.
17. Apley, A.G., and Rowley, D.: Fixation is Fun (Editorial). J. Bone Joint Surg., 74B:485–486, 1992.
18. Aron, J.D.: Methylmethacrylate External Fixation Splints. Orthop. Rev., 9:35–44, 1978.
19. Ash, A.: Medico-legal Aspects of Traumatic Neurosis. Indust. Med. Surg., 37:30–36, 1968.
20. Ashman, R.B., Cowin, S.C., VanBuskirk, W.C., and Rice, J.C.: A Continuous Wave Technique for the Measurement of the Elastic Properties of Cortical Bone. J. Biomech., 17:349–361, 1984.
21. Ashton, H.: Effect of Inflatable Plastic Splints on Blood Flow. Br. Med. J., 2:1427–30, 1966.
22. Atkinson, D.I., Modell, J., and Moya, F.: Intravenous Regional Anesthesia. Anesth. Analg., 44:313–317, 1965.
23. Austin, R.T.: The Sarmiento Tibial Plaster: A Prospective Study of 145 Fractures. Injury, 13:10–22, 1981.
24. Baker, J., Frankel, V.H., and Burstein, A.H.: Fatigue Fractures: Biomechanical Considerations (Abstract). J. Bone Joint Surg., 54A:1345–46, 1972.
25. Basmajian, J.V.: Crutch and Cane Exercises. *In* Basmajian, J. V., and Wolf, S. L. (eds.): Therapeutic Exercise, 5th ed. Baltimore, Williams & Wilkins, 1990.
26. Bateman, J.E.: An Introduction to Disability Evaluation of the Extremities. Instr. Course Lect., XVII:332–336, 1960.
27. Baumgart, F., Bensmann, G., and Haaster, J.: Memory Alloys—New Material for Implantation in Orthopaedic Surgery. *In* Uhthoff, H.K. (ed.): Current Concepts of Internal Fixation of Fractures, pp. 122–127. New York, Springer-Verlag, 1980.
28. Beckenbaugh, R.D.: Colles' Fractures: A Closer Look. Cont. Ed., 13:19, 1980.
29. Becker, D.W., Jr.: Danger of Burns from Fresh Plaster Splints Surrounded by Too Much Cotton. Plast. Reconstr. Surg., 62:436–437, 1980.
30. Behrens, F.: A Primer of Fixator Devices and Configurations. Clin. Orthop., 241:5–14, 1989.
31. Behrens, F.: General Theory and Principles of External Fixation. Clin. Orthop., 241:15–23, 1989.
32. Behrens, F.: Unilateral External Fixation for Severe Lower Extremity Lesions: Experience With the ASIF (AO) Tubular Frame. *In* Seligson, D., and Pope, M.: Concepts in External Fixation, pp. 279–291. New York, Grune & Stratton, 1982.
33. Behrens, F., and Johnson, W.: Unilateral External Fixation: Methods to Increase and Reduce Frame Stiffness. Clin. Orthop., 241:48–56, 1989.
34. Behrens, F., and Searls, K.: External Fixation of the Tibia: Basic Concepts and Prospective Evaluation. J. Bone Joint Surg., 68B:246–254, 1986.
35. Behrens, F., Johnson, W.D., Koch, T.W., and Kovacevic, N.: Bending Stiffness of Unilateral and Bilateral Fixator Frames. Clin. Orthop., 178:103–110, 1983.

36. Behrman, S.W., Fabian, T.C., Kudsk, K.A., and Taylor, J.C.: Improved Outcome With Femur Fractures: Early vs Delayed Fixation. J. Trauma, 30:792–798, 1990.
37. Benson, D.R.: Special Consideration for Surgeons. *In* DeVita V. T., Hellman, S., and Rosengery S. A. (eds.): AIDS: Etiology, Treatment and Prevention, 3rd ed. Philadelphia, J.B. Lippincott, 1992.
38. Beyer, J.C. (ed.): Wound Ballistics. Washington, D.C., Department of the Army, Office of the Surgeon General, 1962.
39. Blachut P.A., Meek R.N., and O'Brien P.J., External Fixation and Delayed Intramedullary Nailing of Open Fractures of the Tibial Shaft: A Sequential Protocol. J. Bone Joint Surg., 79A:729–735, 1990.
40. Black, J.: Metallic Ion Release and Its Relationship to Oncogenesis. *In* Fitzgerald, R.H., Jr (ed.): The Hip, pp. 199–213. St. Louis, C.V. Mosby, 1985.
41. Blakeslee, S.: New York Times, July 25, 1987, pp. 17–18.
42. Blockey, N.J.: An Observation Concerning the Flexor Muscles During Recovery of Function After Dislocation of the Elbow. J. Bone Joint Surg., 36A:833–840, 1954.
43. Bono, J.V., Rella, J.G., Zink, B.J. and Reilly, K.M.: Methohexitol for Orthopaedic Procedures in the Emergency Department. Orthop. Rev., 22:833–838, 1993.
44. Bostman, O.M.: Refracture After Removal of a Condylar Plate from the Distal Third of the Femur. J. Bone Joint Surg., 72A:1013–1018, 1990.
45. Bowden, F.P., Williamson, J.B.P., and Laing, P.G.: The Significance of Metallic Transfer in Orthopaedic Surgery. J. Bone Joint Surg., 37B:676–690, 1955.
46. Bowker, P., and Powell E.S.: A Clinical Evaluation of Plaster-of-Paris. Injury, 23:13–20, 1992.
47. Boynton, M.D., and Schmeling, G.J.: Nonreamed Intramedullary Nailing of Open Tibial Fractures. J. Am. Acad. Orthop. Surg., 2:107–114, 1994.
48. Boynton, M.D., Curcin, A., Marnio, A.R., et al.: Intramedullary Treatment of Open Tibia Fractures: A Comparative Study. Orthop. Trans., 16:662, 1992.
49. Braten, M. Terjesen, T., and Rossvoll, I.: Torsional Deformity After Intramedullary Nailing of Femoral Shaft Fractures: Measurement of Anteversion Angles in 110 Patients. J. Bone Joint Surg., 75B:799–803, 1993.
50. Brennan, P.J., and Girolamo, M.P.: Musculoskeletal Infections in Immuno-compromised Hosts. Orthop. Clin. North Am., 22:389–399, 1991.
51. Brettle, J.: A Survey of the Literature on Metallic Surgical Implants. Injury, 2:26–39, 1970.
52. Brettle, J., Hughes, A.N., and Jordan, B.A.: Metallurgical Aspects of Surgical Implant Materials. Injury, 2:225–234, 1971.
53. Bromage, P.R.: Local Anaesthetic Procedures for the Arm and Hand. Surg. Clin. North Am., 44:919–923, 1964.
54. Brooker, A.F., Jr., and Edwards, C.C.: External Fixation: The Current State of the Art. Baltimore, Williams & Wilkins, 1979.
55. Brooks, D.B., Burstein, A.H., and Frankel, V.H.: Biomechanics of Torsional Fractures: Stress Concentration Effect of a Drill Hole. J. Bone Joint Surg., 52A:507–514, 1970.
56. Brouwer, K.J.: Torsional Deformities After Fractures of the Femoral Shaft in Childhood: Retrospective Study, 27–32 Years After Trauma. Acta Orthop. Scand., 52(Suppl. 195):79–163, 1981.
57. Brower, T.D., Akahoshi, Y., and Orlic, P.: The Diffusion of Dyes Through Articular Cartilage In Vivo. J. Bone Joint Surg., 44A:456–463, 1962.
58. Brown R.M., Wheelwright E.F., and Chalmers J.: Removal of Metal Implants After Fracture Surgery: Indications and Complications. J. R. Coll. Surg. Edinb., 38:96–100, 1993.
59. Brown, P.W., and Urban, J.G.: Early Weight-Bearing Treatment of Open Fractures of the Tibia: An End Result of 63 Cases. J. Bone Joint Surg., 51A:59–75, 1969.
60. Brown, P.W.: The Fate of Exposed Bone. Am. J. Surg., 137:464–469, 1979.
61. Brown, R.F.: Compound Fractures of the Tibia—The Soft Tissue Defect. Proc. R. Soc. Med., 65:625–626, 1972.
62. Brown, S.A., and Mayor, M.B.: The Biocompatibility of Materials for Internal Fixation of Fractures. J. Biomed. Mater. Res., 12:67–82, 1978.
63. Brumback, R.J., Ellison, P.S. Jr., Poka, A., Lakatos, R., Bathon, G.H., and Burgess, A.R.: Intramedullary Nailing of Open Fractures of the Femoral Shaft. J. Bone Joint Surg., 71A:1324–1330, 1989.
64. Bullough, P.J.: Metallosis (Editorial). J. Bone Joint Surg., 76B:687–688, 1994.
65. Bultitude, M.I., Wellwood, J.M., and Hollingsworth, R.P.: Intravenous Diazepam: Its Use in the Reduction of Fractures of the Lower End of the Radius. Injury, 3:249–253, 1972.
66. Burke, J.F.: The Effective Period of Preventive Antibiotic Action in Experimental Incisions and Dermal Lesions. Surgery, 50:161–168, 1961.
67. Burny, F.: The Pin as a Percutaneous Implant: General and Related Studies. Orthopedics, 7:610–615, 1984.
68. Burny, F., Domb, M., Donkerwolcke, M., and Andrianne, Y.: Maximum Torque at the Time of Retrieval (MTR). Orthopedics, 7:627–628, 1984.
69. Burny, F.L.: Elastic External Fixation of Tibial Fractures: Study of 1421 Cases. *In* Brooker, A.F., and Edwards, C.C. (eds): External Fixation: The Current State of the Art, pp. 55–73, Baltimore, Williams & Wilkins, 1979.
70. Burstein, A.H., Currey, J., Frankel, V.H., Heiple, K.G., Lunseth, P., and Vessely, J.C.: Bone Strength: The Effect of Screw Holes. J. Bone Joint Surg., 54A:1143–1156, 1972.
71. Byrd, H.S., Cierny, G., III, and Tebbetts, J.B.: Management of Open Tibial Fractures With Associated Soft Tissue Loss: External Pin Fixation With Early Flap Coverage. Plast. Reconstr. Surg., 75:73–79, 1981.
72. Cahoon, J.R., and Paxton, H.W.: A Metallurgical Survey of Current Orthopaedic Implants. J. Biomed. Mater. Res., 4:223–244, 1970.
73. Caldwell, J.A.: Treatment of Fractures of the Shaft of the Humerus By Hanging Cast. Surg. Gynecol. Obstet., 70:421–425, 1940.
74. Callahan, D.J., Carney, D.J., Daddario, N., and Walter, N.E.: The Effect of Hydration Water Temperature on Orthopaedic Plaster Cast Strength. Orthopedics, 9:683–685, 1986.
75. Callahan, D.J., Carney, D.J., Daddario, N., and Walter, N.E.: A Comparative Study of Synthetic Cast Material Strength. Orthopedics, 9:679–681, 1986.
76. Campbell, D., and Kempson, G.E.: Which External Fixation Device? Injury, 12:291–296, 1981.
77. Carter, D.R., and Hayes, W.C.: Compact Bone Fatigue Damage: A Microscopic Examination. Clin. Orthop., 127:265–274, 1977.
78. Case, R.D.: Haematoma Block—A Safe Method of Reducing Colles' Fractures. Injury, 16:469–470, 1985.
79. Case, C.P., Langkamer, V.G., James, C., et al.: Widespread Dissemination of Metal Debris from Implants. J. Bone Joint Surg., 76B:701–712, 1994.
80. Cater, W.H., and Hicks, J.H.: The Recent History of Corrosion in Metal Used for Internal Fixation. Lancet, 2:271, 871–873, 1956.
81. Chao, E.Y.S., and Hein, T.J.: Mechanical Performance of the Standard Orthofix External Fixator. Orthopedics, 11:1057–69, 1988.
82. Chao, E.Y.S., Aro, H.T., Lewallen, D.G., and Kelly, P.J.: The Effect of Rigidity on Fracture Healing in External Fixation. Clin. Orthop., 241:24–35, 1989.
83. Chao, E.Y.S., Neluheni, E.V.D., Hsu, R.W.W., and Paley, D.: Biomechanics of Malalignment. Orthop. Clin. North Am., 25:379–386, 1994.
84. Chapman, M.W.: The Role of Intramedullary Fixation in Open Fractures. Clin. Orthop., 212:26–34, 1986.
85. Charash, W.E., Fabian, T.C., and Croce, M.A.: Delayed Surgical Fixation of Femur Fractures is a Risk Factor for Pulmonary Failure Independent of Thoracic Trauma. J. Trauma, 37:667–672, 1994.
86. Charnley, J.: The Closed Treatment of Common Fractures, 3rd ed. Edinburgh, E. & S. Livingstone, 1968.
87. Christensen, K.S., Frautner, S., Stickel, M., and Nielsen, J.F.:

Inflatable Splints: Do They Cause Tissue Ischaemia? Injury, 17:167–170, 1986.

88. Christie, J.: Surgical Heat Injury of Bone. Injury, 13:188–190, 1981.
89. Clark, A.M., and Winson, I.G.: Does Plaster Immobilization Predispose to Pulmonary Embolism. Injury, 23:533–534, 1992.
90. Clarke, R.: Assessment of Blood Loss Following Injury. Br. J. Clin. Pract., 10:746–769, 1956.
91. Clarke, R., Fisher, M.R., Topley, E., and Davies, J.W.L.: Extent and Time of Blood Loss After Civilian Injury. Lancet, 2:381–385, 1961.
92. Clarke, R., Topley, E., and Flear, C.T.G.: Assessment of Blood Loss in Civilian Trauma. Lancet, 1:629–638, 1955.
93. Clifford, R.P., Lyons, T.J., and Webb, J.K.: Complications of External Fixation of Open Fractures of the Tibia. Injury, 18:174–176, 1987.
94. Cochran, G. vanB.: Kilograms and Kilopounds: Mass Force or Weight? J. Bone Joint Surg., 53A:181–182, 1971.
95. Cohen, J.: Corrosion Testing of Orthopaedic Implants. J. Bone Joint Surg., 44A:307–316, 1962.
96. Connes, H.: The Hoffman External Fixation Techniques: Indications and Results. Paris, Editions Gead, 1977.
97. Connolly, J.F.: Torsional Fractures and the Third Dimension of Fracture Management. South Med. J., 73:884–891, 1980.
98. Connolly, J.F., Whittaker, D., and Williams, E.: Femoral and Tibial Fractures Combined With Injuries to the Femoral or Popliteal Artery: A Review of the Literature and Analysis of 14 Cases. J. Bone Joint Surg., 53A:56–68, 1971.
99. Connolly, J.: Management of Fractures Associated With Arterial Injuries. Am. J. Surg., 120:331, 1970.
100. Constantz, B.R., Ison, I.C., Fulmer, M.T., et al.: Skeletal Repair by In Situ Formation of the Mineral Phase of Bone. Science, 267:1796–1798, 1995.
101. Cook, S.D., Baffles, G.C., Wolfe, M.W., Kuber-Sampath, T., and Rueger, D.C.: Healing of Large Segmental Defects With Recombinant Human Osteogenic Protein (rh OP-1). Orthop. Trans., 8:674–675, 1992.
102. Cooney, W.P., III, Fitzgerald, R.H., Jr., Dobyns, J.H., and Washington, J.A., II: Quantitative Wound Cultures in Upper Extremity Trauma. J. Trauma, 22:112–117, 1982.
103. Cornelissen, M., Burny, F., VanderPerre, G., and Donkerwolcke, M.: Standardized Method to Measure the Fixation Quality of a Pin: Theoretical Derivation and Preliminary Results. Orthopedics, 7:623–626, 1984.
104. Cornell, C.N., Lane, J.M., Chapman, M., et al.: Multicenter Trial of Collagraft as Bone Graft Substitute. J. Orthop. Trauma, 5:1–8, 1991.
105. Cote, C., Simoneau, J.A., Lagasse, P., et al.: Isokinetic Strength Training Protocols: Do They Induce Skeletal Muscle Fiber Hypertrophy? Arch. Phys. Med. Rehabil., 69:281–285, 1988.
106. Court Brown, C.M., Keating, J.F., and McQueen, M.M.: Infection After Intramedullary Nailing of the Tibia. J. Bone Joint Surg., 74B:770–774, 1992.
107. Court-Brown, C.M., Christie, J., and McQueen, M.M.: Closed Intramedullary Nailing: Its Use in Closed and Type I Open Fractures. J. Bone Joint Surg., 72B:605–611, 1990.
108. Curcin, A., Bonyton, M.D., Marino, A., and Trafton, P.G.: Results in Open Tibial Shaft Fractures Treated With a Nonreamed Interlocking Nail. Orthop. Trans., 18:663, 1992.
108a. Currey, J.D.: The Mechanical Properties of Bone. Clin. Orthop., 73:222, 1970.
109. Dai, K.R., Hou, X.K., Sun, Y.H., Tang, R.G., Qui, S.J., and Ni, C.: Treatment of Intra-articular Fractures With Shape Memory Compression Staples. Injury, 24:651–655, 1993.
110. Davies, C.T.M., and White, M.J.: Muscle Weakness Following Eccentric Work in Man. Pflugers Arch., 392:168–171, 1981.
111. DeBastiani, G., Aldeghiri, R., and Brivio, L.R.: The Treatment of Fractures With a Dynamic Axial Fixator. J. Bone Joint Surg., 66B:538–545, 1984.
112. deBruijn, H.P.: Functional Treatment of Colles' Fracture. Acta Orthop. Scand., 58(Suppl. 223), 1987.
113. Dechan, M.A., Oppenheim, W., and Aurori, B.: Assessment of Prognostic Indicators in Tibial Fractures Treated With Unreamed Interlocking Intramedullary Nails. Orthop. Trans., 18:7, 1992.
114. Dehne, E.: Treatment of Fractures of the Tibial Shaft. Clin. Orthop., 66:159–173, 1969.
115. Dehne, E., Deffer, P.A., Hall, R.M., Brown, P.W., and Johnson, E.V.: The Natural History of the Fractured Tibia. Surg. Clin. North Am., 41:1495–1513, 1961.
116. DeJong, R.H.: Axillary Block of the Brachial Plexus. Anesthesiology, 22:215–225, 1961.
117. DeLateur, B.J.: Strength and Local Muscle Endurance. Phys. Med. Rehabil. Clin. North Am., 5:269–294, 1994.
118. DeLateur, B.J., Lehmann, J.F., and Fordyce, W.E.: A Test for the DeLorme Axiom. Arch. Phys. Med. Rehabil., 49:245–248, 1968.
119. Delgado, E.R.: Sarcoma Following a Surgically Treated Fractured Tibia: A Case Report. Clin. Orthop., 12:315–318, 1958.
120. Dell'Oca, A.A.F.: External Fixation Using Simple Pin Fixators. Injury, 23(Suppl. 4):S1–S6, 1992.
121. DeLorme, T.L., and Watkins, A.L.: Progressive Resistance Exercise. New York, Appleton-Century-Crofts, 1951.
122. DeLorme, T.L., and Watkins, A.L.: Technics of Progressive Resistance Exercise. Arch. Phys. Med. 29L:263–273, 1948.
123. DeLorme, T.L.: Restoration of Muscle Power by Heavy Resistance Exercise. J. Bone Joint Surg., 27A:645–647, 1945.
124. DeMuth, W.E., and Smith, J.M.: High-Velocity Bullet Wounds of Muscle and Bone: The Basis of Rational Early Treatment. J. Trauma, 6:744–755, 1966.
125. Devas, M. (ed.): Geriatric Orthopaedics. New York, Academic Press, 1977.
126. Devas, M.B.: Stress Fractures. Practitioner, 197:70–76, 1966.
127. Devas, M.B.: Compression Stress Fractures in Man and the Greyhound. J. Bone Joint Surg., 43B:540–551, 1961.
128. Diacke, A.W., Schultz, R.D., and Nohlgren, J.E.: Technique for Quantifying Low-Temperature Burns. J. Surg. Res., 4:270–274, 1964.
129. Dickinson, A.L., Jackson, C.G.R., Layne, D.L., and Ringet, S.P.: The Effect of Different Sequences of High and Low Intensity Resistance Exercises on Muscular Performance and Cellular Change (Abstract). Med. Sci. Sports Exer., 15:154–155, 1983.
130. Dimond, F.C., Jr., and Rich, N.M.: M-16 Rifle Wounds in Vietnam. J. Trauma, 7:619–625, 1967.
131. Dinley, R.J., and Michelinakis, E.: Local Anaesthesia in the Reduction of Colles' Fracture. Injury, 4:345–346, 1973.
132. Dirschl, D.R., and Wilson, F.C.: Topical Antibiotic Irrigation in the Prophylaxis of Operative Wound Infections in Orthopaedic Surgery. Orthop. Clin. North Am., 22:419–426, 1991.
133. Disegi, J.A., and Wyss, H.: Implant Materials for Fracture Fixation: A Clinical Perspective. Orthopedics, 12:75–79, 1989.
134. Disegi, J.: AO/ASIF Unalloyed Titanium Implant Material, 3rd ed.
135. Disegi, J.: AO/ASIF Titanium—6% Aluminum—7% Niobium Implant Material. AO/ASIF Materials Technical Commission, 1993.
136. Dodion, P., Putz, P., Amiri-Lamraski, M.H., Efira, A., deMartelaere, E., and Heimann, R.: Immunoblastic Lymphoma at the Site of an Infected Vitallium Bone Plate. Histopathology, 6:807–813, 1982.
137. Dube, V.E., and Fisher, D.E.: Hemangioendothelioma of the Leg Following Metallic Fixation of the Tibia. Cancer, 30:1260–66, 1972.
138. Dugas, R., and D'Ambrosia, R.: Civilian Gunshot Wounds. Orthopedics, 8:1121–25, 1985.
139. Eckhoff, D.G.: Effect of Limb Malrotation on Malalignment and Osteoarthritis. Orthop. Clin. North. Am. 25:405–414, 1994.
140. Edwards, C.C., Jaworski, M.F., Solana, J., and Aronson, B.S.: Management of Compound Tibial Fractures Using External Fixation. Am. Surg., 45:190–203, 1979.
141. Ekholm, R.: Nutrition of Articular Cartilage: A Radioautographic Study. Acta Anat., 24:329–338, 1955.

142. Emergency War Surgery (NATO Handbook). Washington, D.C., U.S. Dept. of Defense, 1958.
143. Enneking, W.F., and Horowitz, M.: The Intra-articular Effects of Immobilization on the Human Knee. J. Bone Joint Surg., 54A:973–985, 1972.
144. Epps, C.H., Jr., and Adams, J.P.: Wound Management in Open Fractures. Am. Surgeon, 27:766–769, 1961.
145. Esselman, P.C., and Lacerte, M.: Principles of Isokinetic Exercise. Phys. Med. Rehabil. Clin. North Am., 5:255–268 1994.
146. Esterhai, J.L. Jr., and Queenan J: Management of Soft Tissue Wounds Associated With Type III Open Fractures. Orthop. Clin North Am., 22:427–432. 1991.
147. Evans, E.B., Eggers, G.W.N., Butler, J.K., and Blumel, J.: Experimental Immobilization of Rat Knee Joint. J. Bone Joint Surg., 42A:737–758, 1960.
148. Evans, E.M.: Fractures of the Radius and Ulna. J. Bone Joint Surg., 33B:548–561, 1951.
149. Evans, F.G.: Relation of the Physical Properties of Bone to Fractures. Instr. Course Lect., XVIII:110–121, 1961.
150. Evans, W.E., and Rosenberg I.H.: Biomarkers: The 10 Determinants of Aging You Can Control. New York, Simon & Schuster, 1991.
151. Ferguson, A.B., Jr., and Laing, P.G.: Corrosion and Corrosion-Resistant Metals in Orthopaedic Surgery. Instr. Course Lect., XV:96–103, 1958.
152. Finsen, V., Borset, M., Buvik, G.E., and Hauke, I.: Preoperative Traction in Patients With Hip Fractures. Injury, 23:242–244, 1992.
153. Finsterbush, A., and Friedman, B.: Reversibility of Joint Changes Produced by Immobilization in Rabbits. Clin. Orthop., 111:290–298, 1975.
154. Fisher, M.R.: Clinical Signs Following Injury in Relation to Red Cell and Total Blood Volume. Clin. Sci., 17:181–204, 1958.
155. Fleming, B., Paley, D., Kristiansen, T., and Pope, M.: A Biomechanical Analysis of the Ilizarov External Fixator. Clin. Orthop., 241:95–105, 1989.
156. Fogelberg, E.V., Zetzmann, E.K., and Stinchfield, F.E.: Prophylactic Penicillin in Orthopaedic Surgery. J. Bone Joint Surg., 52A:95–98, 1970.
157. Forbes, G.B.: Staphylococcal Infection of Operation Wounds With Special Reference to Topical Antibiotic Prophylaxis. Lancet, 2:505–509, 1961.
158. Fox, R.M.: The Medicolegal Report Theory and Practice. Boston, Little, Brown, & Co., 1969.
159. Frankel, V.H., and Burstein, A.H.: Orthopaedic Biomechanics. Philadelphia, Lea & Febiger, 1970.
160. Freeman, M.A.R., Todd, R.C., and Pirie, C.J.: The Role of Fatigue in the Pathogenesis of Senile Femoral Neck Fractures. J. Bone Joint Surg., 56B:698–702, 1974.
161. Friden, J.: Changes in Human Skeletal Muscle Induced by Long-Term Eccentric Exercise. Cell Tissue Res., 236:365–372, 1984.
162. Frigg, R.: The Development of the Pinless External Fixator: From Idea to the Implant. Injury, 23(Suppl. 3):S3–S8, 1992.
163. Frontera, W.R., Meredith, C.N., O'Reilly, K.P., Knuttgen, H.G., and Evans, W.J.: Strength Conditioning in Older Men: Skeletal Muscle Hypertrophy and Improvement of Function. J. Appl Physiol., 64:1038–1044, 1988.
164. Gallinaro, P., and Biasibetti, A.: External Fixation—Why, Which, When? *In* Ilizarov Techniques: Manual for the Course Sponsored by the Program of Continuing Medical Education, University of Maryland School of Medicine, May 16–18, 1988.
165. Garfin, S.R., Mubarak, S.J., Evans, K.L., Hargens, A.R., and Akeson, W.H.: Quantification of Intracompartmental Pressure and Volume Under Plaster Cast. J. Bone Joint Surg., 63A:449–453, 1981.
166. Garland, D.E., Chick, R., Taylor, J., and Salisbury, R.B.: Treatment of Proximal-Third Femur Fractures With Pins and Thigh Plaster. Clin. Orthop., 160:86–93, 1981.
167. Gasser, B., Perren, S.M., and Schneider, E.: Parametric Numerical Design Optimization of Internal Fixation Plates. Transactions of the 7th Meeting. Aarhus, Denmark: European Society of Biomechanics, 1990.
168. Gautier, E., Cordey, J., Mathys, R., Rahn, B.A., and Perren, S.M.: Porosity and Remodeling of Plated Bone After Internal Fixation: Result of Stress Shielding or Vascular Damage? *In* Ducheyne P, Van der Perre, G., and Aubert, A. E., (eds.): Biomaterials and Biomechanics, pp. 196–200. Amsterdam, Elsevier Science Publishers, 1984.
169. Ger, R.: The Management of Pretibial Skin Loss. Surgery, 63:757–763, 1968.
170. Ger, R.: The Management of Open Fractures of the Tibia With Skin Loss. J. Trauma, 10:112–121, 1970.
171. Gingrass, R.P., Close, A.S., and Ellison, E.H.: The Effect of Various Topical and Parenteral Agents on the Prevention of Infection in Experimental Contaminated Wounds. J. Trauma, 4:763–783, 1964.
172. Gissane, W.: Symposium on the Treatment of Fractures of the Shafts of the Long Bones. Proc. R. Soc. Med., 52:291–295, 1959.
173. Godina, M.: The Tailored Latissimus Dorsi Free Flap. Plast. Reconstr. Surg., 80:304–306, 1987.
174. Goto, M., and Ogata, K.: Experimental Study on Thermal Burns Caused by Plaster Bandage. Nippon Seikeigeka Gakkai Zasshi, 60:671–680, 1986.
175. Grana, W.A., and Kopta, J.A.: The Roger Anderson Device in the Treatment of Fractures of the Distal End of the Radius. J. Bone Joint Surg., 61A:1234–38, 1979.
176. Grant, A., Hoddinott, C., and Evans, R.: Midazolam Sedation for the Reduction of Colles' Fractures. Injury, 24:461–463, 1993.
176a. Green, C.A., and Matthews, L.S.: The Thermal Effects of Skeletal Fixation Pin Placement in Human Bone (Abstract). Trans. Orthop. Res. Soc. 6:103, 1981.
177. Green, S.A., and Green, H.D.: The Influence of Radiographic Projection on the Appearance of Deformities. Orthop. Clin. North Am., 25:467–475, 1994.
178. Greener, E., and Lautenschlager, E.: Materials for Bioengineering Applications. *In* Brown, J.H.V., Jacobs, J.E., and Stark, L. (eds.): Biomedical Engineering. Philadelphia, F.A. Davis, 1971.
179. Griffiths, D.L.: Hazards of Closed Reduction of Fractures. Tex. Med., 642:46–50, 1968.
180. Groshar, D., Lam, M., Even-Sapir, E., Israel, O., and Front, D.: Stress Fractures and Bone Pain: Are They Closely Associated? Injury, 16:526–528, 1985.
181. Gruen, G.S., Gruen, R.G.: Human Immunodeficiency Virus: Occupational Risk for Surgeons. Orthopedics, 15:135–137, 1992.
182. Gustilo, R.B.: Use of Antimicrobials in the Management of Open Fractures. Arch. Surg., 114:805–808, 1979.
183. Gustilo, R.B., Simpson, L., Nixon, R., Ruiz, A., and Indeck, W.: Analysis of 511 Open Fractures. Clin. Orthop., 66:148–154, 1969.
184. Haas, N., Kretteck, C., Schandesmaier, P., Frigg, R., and Tscherne, H.: A New Solid Unreamed Tibial Nail for Shaft Fractures With Severe Soft Tissue Injury. Injury, 24:49–54, 1993.
185. Haasters, J., Vensmann, G., and Baumgart, F.: Memory Alloys—New Material for Implantation in Orthopaedic Surgery: II. *In* Uhthoff, H.K. (ed.): Current Concepts of Internal Fixation of Fractures, pp. 128–135. New York, Springer-Verlag, 1980.
186. Hägglund, G., Hansson, L.T., and Norman, O.: Correction by Growth of Rotational Deformity After Femoral Fracture in Children. Acta Orthop. Scand., 54:858–861, 1983.
187. Häggmark, T., Eriksson, E., and Jansson, E.: Muscle Fiber Type Changes in Human Skeletal Muscle After Injuries and Immobilization. Orthopedics, 9:181–185, 1986.
188. Häggmark, T., Liedberg, H., Ericksson, E., and Wredmark, T.: Calf Muscle Atrophy and Muscle Function After Nonoperative vs Operative Treatment of Achilles Tendon Ruptures. Orthopedics, 9:160–164, 1986.
189. Hammond, J.S., Eckes, J.M., Gomez, G.A., and Cunningham,

D.N.: HIV, Trauma, and Infection Control: Universal Precautions are Universally Ignored. J. Trauma, 30:555–561, 1990.

190. Hardaker, W.T., Jr., Ward, W.T., and Goldner, J.L.: External Fixation in the Management of Severe Musculoskeletal Trauma. Orthopaedics, 4:437–444, 1981.
191. Hardy, N., Burny, F., and Deutsch, G.A.: Pin Tract Histological Study: Preliminary Clinical Investigations. Orthopedics, 7:616–618, 1984.
192. Harris, J.D., Kenwright, J., Evans, M., Tanner, K.E., and Gwillim, J.: Control of Movement and Fracture Stiffness Monitoring With External Fixation. Orthopedics, 7:485–490, 1984.
193. Harrison, J.W., McLain, D.L., Holm, R.B., Wilson, G.P., III, Chalman, J.A., and MacGowan, K.N.: Osteosarcoma Associated With Metallic Implants: Report of Two Cases in Dogs. Clin. Orthop., 116:253–257, 1976.
194. Hart, M.B., Wu H.-J., Chao, E.Y.S., Kelly, P.J.: External Skeletal Fixation of Canine Tibial Osteotomies: Compression Compared With No Compression. J. Bone Joint Surg., 67A:598–605, 1985.
195. Hassard, H.: Medical Malpractice: Risks, Protection, Prevention. Oradell, NJ, Medical Economics, 1966.
196. Helfet, D.L., Howey, T., DiPasquale, T., Sanders, R., Zinar, D., and Brooker, A.: The Treatment of Open and/or Unstable Tibial Fractures With an Unreamed Double-Locked Tibial Nail. Orthop. Rev., 23(Suppl.):9–17, 1994.
196a. Henry, S.L.; Ostermann, P.A.W.; and Seligson, D.: Prophylactic Management of Open Fractures with the Antibiotic Bead Pouch Technique. Presented at the Orthopaedic Trauma Association Meeting, Dallas, TX, Oct. 27, 1988.
197. Hey-Groves, E.W.: Methods and Results of Transplantation of Bone in the Repair of Defects Caused by Injury or Disease. Br. J. Surg., 5:185–242, 1918.
198. Hey-Groves, E.W.: Modern Methods of Treating Fractures. New York, William Wood, 1922.
199. Hicks, J.H.: Letter to the Editor. Injury, 4:361, 1973.
200. Hicks, J.H.: External Splintage as a Cause of Movement in Fractures. Lancet, 1:667–670, 1960.
201. Hicks, J.H.: High Rigidity in Fractures of the Tibia. Injury, 3:121–134, 1971.
202. Hicks, J.H.: The Fallacy of the Fractured Clavicle. Lancet, 1:131–132, 1958.
203. Hicks, J.H., and Cater, W.H.: Minor Reactions Due to Modern Metals. J. Bone Joint Surg., 44B:122–128, 1962.
204. Hierholzer, G., Rüedi, T., Allgöwer, M., and Schatzker, J.: Manual on the AO/ASIF Tubular External Fixator. New York, Springer-Verlag, 1985.
205. Hoffmann, R.: Retules à Os Pour la Reduction Dirigée, Non Saglante, des Fractures (Osteotaxis). Helv. Med. Acta, 5:844–850, 1938.
206. Holden, C.E.A.: The Role of Blood Supply to Soft Tissue in the Healing of Diaphyseal Fractures. J. Bone Joint Surg., 54A:993–1000, 1972.
207. Hollingsworth, A., Wallace, W.A., Dabir, R., Ellis, S.J., and Smith, A.F.M.: Comparison of Bupivacaine and Prilocaine Used in Bier Block: A Double-Blind Trial. Injury, 13:331–336, 1982.
208. Hollmen, A., and Mononen, P.: Axillary Plexus Block With Prilocaine. Acta Anaesthesiol. Scand. (Suppl.), 60:25–28, 1975.
209. Hooper, G., Buxton, R.A., and Gillespie, W.J.: Isolated Fractures of the Shaft of the Tibia. Injury, 12:283–287, 1981.
210. Hooper, G.J., Keddell, R.G., and Penny, I.D.: Conservative Management or Closed Nailing for Tibial Fractures: A Randomised Prospective Trial. J. Bone Joint Surg., 73B:83–85, 1991.
211. Howse, A.J.G.: Orthopaedists Aid Ballet. Clin. Orthop., 89:52–63, 1972.
212. Hughes, L.J., and Jackson, M.S.: Use of the Wagner Apparatus in Fractures of the Femur. Presented at the 46th Annual Meeting of the American Academy of Orthopaedic Surgeons, San Francisco, February 22–24, 1979.
212a. Hughston, J.C.: Fractures of the Distal Radial Shaft: Mistakes in Management. J. Bone Joint Surg., 39A:249–264, 1957.
212b. Hughston, J.C.: Fractures of the Forearm: Anatomical considerations. J. Bone Joint Surg., 44A:1664–1667, 1962.
213. Husted, C.M.: Technique of Cast Wedging in Long Bone Fractures. Orthop. Rev., 15:373–378, 1986.
214. Ilizarov, G.A., and Frankel, V.H.: The Ilizarov External Fixator: A Physiologic Method of Orthopaedic Reconstruction and Skeletal Correction: A Conversation With Prof. G.A. Ilizarov and Victor H. Frankel, M.D., Ph.D. Orthop. Rev., 17:1142–1154, 1988.
215. Inoue, S.A., Ichida, M., Imai, R., Suzu, F., Ohashi, J., and Sakakida, K.: External Skeletal Fixation Using Methylmethacrylate-Technique and Indication With Clinical Report. Int. Orthop. (SICOT), 1:64–69, 1977.
216. Ippolito, G., Puro, V., and DeCarli, G.: The Risk of Occupational Human Immunodeficiency Virus Infection in Health Care Workers. Arch. Intern. Med., 153:1451–1458, 1993.
217. Jacobs, J.J., Rosenbaum, D., Hay, R.M., Gitelis, S., and Black, J.: Early Sarcomatous Degeneration Near a Cement-less Hip Replacement. J. Bone and Joint Surg., 74B:7400–744, 1992.
218. Jenkins, N.H., Jones, D.G., Johnson, S.R., and Mintowt-Czyz, W.J.: External Fixation of Colles' Fractures: An Anatomical Study. J. Bone Joint Surg., 69B:207–211, 1987.
219. Jensen, J.S., Hansen, F.W., and Johansen, J.: Tibial Shaft Fractures: A Comparison of Conservative Treatment and Internal Fixation With Conventional Plates or AO Compression Plates. Acta Orthop. Scand., 48:204–212, 1977.
220. Jones, R.: An Orthopaedic View of the Treatment of Fractures. Am. J. Orthop. Surg., 11:314–335, 1913.
221. Kaltenecker, G., Wins, O., and Quaicoe, S.,: Lower Infection Rate After Interlocking Nailing in Open Fractures of Femur and Tibia. J. Trauma, 30:474–479, 1990.
222. Kaplan, S.S.: Burns Following Application of Plaster Splint Dressings: Report of Two Cases. J. Bone Joint Surg., 63A:670–672, 1981.
223. Karlström, G., and Olerud, S.: Percutaneous Pin Fixation of Open Tibial Fractures. J. Bone Joint Surg., 57A:915–924, 1975.
224. Kasdan, M.L., Kleinert, H.E., Kasdan, A.P., and Kutz, J.E.: Axillary Block Anesthesia for Surgery of the Hand. Plast. Reconstr. Surg., 46:256–261, 1970.
225. Kellam, J.F.: The Role of External Fixation in Pelvic Disruption. Clin. Orthop., 241:66–82, 1989.
226. Kempson, G.E., and Campbell, D.: The Comparative Stiffness of External Fixation Frames. Injury, 12:297–304, 1981.
227. Kenwright, J., Goodship, A., and Evans, M.: The Influence of Intermittent Micromovement Upon the Healing of Experimental Fractures. Orthopedics, 7:481–484, 1984.
228. Kenwright, J., and Goodship, A.E.: Controlled Mechanical Stimulation in the Treatment of Tibial Fractures. Clin. Orthop., 241:36–47, 1989.
229. Keon-Cohen, B.T.: Fractures at the Elbow. J. Bone Joint Surg., 48A:1623–39, 1966.
230. Kessler, H.H.: Disability-Determination and Evaluation. Philadelphia, Lea & Febiger, 1970.
231. Key, J.A., and Reynolds, F.C.: The Treatment of Infection After Medullary Nailing. Surgery, 35:749–757, 1964.
232. Kia, D., and Dragstedt, L.R., II: Prevention of Likely Wound Infections: Prophylactic Closed Antibiotic-Detergent Irrigation. Arch. Surg., 100:229–231, 1970.
233. Kleinert, H.E., DeSimone, K., Gaspar, H.E., Arnold, R.E., and Kasdan, M.L.: Regional Anesthesia for Upper Extremity Surgery. J. Trauma, 3:3–12, 1963.
234. Knapp, U.: Synthetic Skin Substitute in the Treatment of Wounds Marked by Loss of Substance. Chir. Praxis, 23:173–183, 1977–78.
235. Knapp, U., and Weller, S.: Care of Soft Tissues in Open Fractures. Akt. Traumatol., 8:319–327, 1978.
236. Koclalkowski, A., Angus Wallace, W., and Prince, H.G.: Clinical Experience With a New Artificial Bone Graft: Preliminary Results of a Prospective Study. Injury, 21:142–144, 1990.
237. Krettek, C., Haas, N., and Tscheme, H.: The Role of Supplemental Lag-Screw Fixation for Open Fracture of the Tibial Shaft Treated With External Fixation. J. Bone Joint Surg., 73A:893–897, 1991.

238. Kubba, R., Taylor, J.S., and Marks, K.E.: Cutaneous Complications of Orthopaedic Implants: Two Year Prospective Study. Arch. Dermatol., 117:554–560, 1981.
239. Kumar, P., Bryan, C.E., Leech, S.H., Mathews, R., Bowler, J., and D'Ambrosia, R.D.: Metal Hypersensitivity in Total Joint Replacement: Review of the Literature and Practical Guidelines for Evaluating Prospective Recipients. Orthopaedics, 6:1455–1458, 1983.
240. Kuo, P.O., Yang, P., Zhang, Y., et al.: The Use of Nickel-Titanium Alloy in Orthopaedic Surgery in China. Orthopedics, 12:111–116, 1984.
240a. Lacroix, P.: The Organization of Bones, p. 90. London, Churchill Livingstone, 1951.
241. Lalor, P.A., Revel P.A., Gray, A.B., Wright, S., Railton, G.T., and Freeman M.A.R.: Sensitivity to Titanium: A Cause of Implant Failure? J. Bone Joint Surg., 73B:25–28, 1991.
242. Langkamer, V.G., and Ackroyd, C.E.: Removal of Forearm Plates: A Review of the Complications. J. Bone Joint Surg., 72B:601–604, 1990.
243. Lavalette, R., Pope, M.H., and Dickstein, H.: Setting Temperatures of Plaster Casts. J. Bone Joint Surg., 64A:907–911, 1982.
244. Lawyer, R.B., and Lubbers, L.M.: Use of the Hoffman Apparatus in the Treatment of Unstable Tibial Fractures. J. Bone Joint Surg., 62A:1266–1273, 1980.
245. Leach, R.E.: New Fiberglass Casting System. Clin. Orthop., 103:109–117, 1974.
246. Lesmes, G.R., Costill, D.L., Coyle, E.F., and Fink, W.J.: Muscle Strength and Power Changes During Maximal Isokinetic Training. Med. Sci. Sports, 10:266–269, 1978.
247. Litchman, H.M., and Duffy, J.: Lower Extremity Balanced Traction: A Modification of Russell Traction. Clin. Orthop., 66:144–147, 1969.
248. Loftström, B. (ed.): Clinical Experience With Long-Acting Local Anaesthetics. Acta Anaesthesiol. Scand. (Suppl.), 60:1975.
249. London, P.S.: Observations on Medical Investigation of Ambulance Services. Injury, 3:225–238, 1972.
250. London, P.S.: Observations on the Treatment of Some Fractures of the Forearm by Splintage That Does Not Include the Elbow. Injury, 2:252–270, 1971.
251. Lovell, C.R., and Staniforth, P.: Contact Allergy to Benzalkonium Chloride in Plaster of Paris. Contact Dermatitis, 7:343–344, 1981.
252. Maletis, G.B., Watson, R.C., and Scott, S: Compartment Syndrome: A Complication of Intravenous Regional Anesthesia in the Reduction of Lower Leg Shaft Fractures. Orthopaedics, 12:841–846. 1989.
253. Marks, M.T., Guruswamy, A., and Gross, R.H.: Ringworm Resulting From Swimming With a Polyurethane Cast. J. Pediatr. Orthop., 3:511–512, 1983.
254. Mathews, L.S., and Hirsch, C.: Temperatures Measured in Human Cortical Bone When Drilling. J. Bone Joint Surg., 54A:297–308, 1972.
255. Mathijsen, A.: Plaster-of-Paris in the Treatment of Fractures. Liege, Granmont-Doners, 1854.
256. Matter, P., and Burch, H.B.: Clinical Experience With Titanium Implants, Especially With the Limited Contact Dynamic Compression Plate System. Arch. Orthop. Trauma Surg., 109:311–313, 1990.
256a. Maurer, D.J., Merkow, R.L.; Gustilo, R.B.: Infection After Intermedullary Nailing of Severe Open Tibial Fractures Initially Treated With External Fixation. J. Bone Joint Surg., 71A:835–838, 1989.
257. Mayfield, G.W.: Rotational Malunion of Femoral Shaft Fractures and Its Functional Significance (Abstract). J. Bone Joint Surg., 56A:1309, 1974.
258. McDonald, I.: Malignant Lymphoma Associated With Internal Fixation of Fractured Tibia. Cancer, 48:1009–1011, 1981.
259. McDougall, A.: Malignant Tumor at the Site of Bone Plating. J. Bone Joint Surg., 38B:709–713, 1956.
260. McGraw, J.M. and Lui, E.V.A.: Treatment of Open Tibial Shaft Fractures, External Fixation and Secondary Intramedullary Nailing. J. Bone Joint Surg., 76A:900–911, 1988
261. McNeur, J.C.: Management of Open Skeletal Trauma With Particular Reference to Internal Fixation. J. Bone Joint Surg., 52B:54–60, 1970.
262. Meachim, G., Pedley, R.B., and Williams, D.F.: A Study of Sarcogenicity Associated With Co-Cr-Mo Particles Implanted in Animal Muscle. J. Biomed. Mater. Res., 16:407–416, 1982.
263. Mears, D.C.: Materials and Orthopaedic Surgery. Baltimore, Williams & Wilkins, 1979.
264. Mears, D.C.: The Use of Dissimilar Metals in Surgery. J. Biomed. Mater. Res., 9:133–148, 1975.
265. Meek, R.N., Vivoda, E.E., and Pirani, S.: Comparison of Mortality of Patients With Multiple Injuries According to Type of Fracture Treatment: A Retrospective Age- and Injury-Matched Series. Injury, 17:2–4, 1986.
266. Meleher, G.A., Ryf, C., Laubenegger, A., and Rendi, T.: Tibial Fractures Treated With the AO Unreamed Nail. Injury, 24:407, 1993.
267. Melendez, E.M., and Colón, C.: Treatment of Open Tibial Fractures With the Orthofix Fixator. Clin. Orthop., 241:224–230, 1989.
268. Merchant, T.C., and Dietz, F.R.: Long-Term Follow-Up After Fractures of the Tibial and Fibular Shafts. J. Bone Joint Surg., 71A:599–606, 1989.
269. Micheli, L.J.: Thromboembolic Complications of Cast Immobilization for Injuries of the Lower Extremities. Clin. Orthop., 108:191–195, 1975.
270. Miller, E.H., Schneider, H.J., Bronson, J.L., and McLain, D.: A New Consideration in Athletic Injuries. Clin. Orthop., 111:181–191, 1975.
271. Miller R., Renwick, S.E., DeCoster, T.A., Shonnard, P., and Jabczenski, F.: Removal of Intramedullary Rods After Femoral Shaft Fracture. J. Orthop. Trauma, 6:460–463, 1992.
272. Moffroid, M.T., and Whipple, R.H.: Specificity of Speed of Exercise. Phys. Ther., 50:1692–1700, 1970.
273. Molster, A.O.: Effects of Rotational Instability on Healing of Femoral Osteotomies in the Rat. Acta Orthop. Scand., 55:632–636, 1984.
274. Montgomery, C.J., and Ready, L.B.: Epidural Opioid Analgesia Does Not Obscure Diagnosis of Compartment Syndrome Resulting from Prolonged Lithotomy Position. Anesthesiology, 75:541–543, 1991.
275. Mooney, V., Nickel, V.L., Harcey, J.P., and Snelson, R.: Cast-Brace Treatment for Fractures of the Distal Part of the Femur: A Prospective Controlled Study of 150 Patients. J. Bone Joint Surg., 52A:1563–1578, 1970.
276. Moore, D.C., Bridenbaugh, L.D., Bridenbaugh, P.O., and Tucker, G.T.: Bupivacaine: A Review of 2,077 Cases. J.A.M.A., 214:713–718, 1970.
277. Moritani, T., de Vries, H.A.: Potential for Gross Muscle Hypertrophy in Older Men. J. Gerontol., 35:672–682, 1980.
278. Morrison, K.M., Ebraheim, N.A., Southworth, S.R., Sabin, J.J., and Jackson, W.T.: Plating of the Fibula: Its Potential Value as an Adjunct to External Fixation of the Tibia. Clin Orthop., 266:209–213, 1991.
279. Moyen, B.J.-L., Lahey, P.J., Jr., Weinberg, E.H., and Harris, W.H.: Effects on Intact Femora of Dogs of the Application and Removal of Metal Plates: A Metabolic and Structural Study Comparing Stiffer and More Flexible Plates. J. Bone Joint Surg., 60A:940–947, 1978.
280. Moyen, B., Comtet, J.J., Roy, J.C., Basset, R., and deMourgues, G.: Refracture After Removal of Internal Fixation Devices: Clinical Study of 20 Cases and Physiopathologic Hypothesis. Lyon Chir., 76:153–157, 1980.
281. Murphy, E.F., and Burstein, A.H.: Atlas of Orthotics: Biomechanical Principles and Application. Chicago, American Academy of Orthopaedic Surgeons, 1975.
282. Mustard, W.T., and Simmons, E.H.: Experimental Arterial Spasm in the Lower Extremities Produced by Traction. J. Bone Joint Surg., 35B:437–441, 1953.
283. Nach, D.C., and Keim, H.A.: Prophylactic Antibiotics in Spinal Surgery. Orthop. Rev., 2(6):27–30, 1973.
284. Naumark, A., Kossoff, and Leach, R.E.: The Disparate Diameter: Sign of Rotational Deformity in Fractures. J. Can. Assoc. Radiol., 34:8–11, 1983.

285. Nelson, J.P., Ferris, D.O., and Ivins, J.C.: The Cast Syndrome: Case Report. Postgrad. Med., 42:457–461, 1967.
286. Netz, P., Eriksson, K., and Stromberg, L.: Non-Linear Properties of Diaphyseal Bone: An Experimental Study on Dogs. Acta Orthop. Scand., 50:130–143, 1979.
287. Neufeld, A.J., Mays, J.D., and Naden, C.J.: A Dynamic Method for Treating Femoral Shaft Fractures. Orthop. Rev., 1:19–21, 1972.
288. Nichols, P.J.R.: Rehabilitation After Fractures of the Shaft of the Femur. J. Bone Joint Surg., 45B:96–102, 1963.
289. Nicoll, E.A.: Fractures of the Tibial Shaft: A Survey of 705 Cases. J. Bone Joint Surg., 46B:373–387, 1964.
290. Nishimura, N.: Serial Strain Gauge Measurement of Bone Healing in Hoffman External Fixation. Orthopedics, 7:677–684, 1984.
291. O'Brien, J.P.: The Femoral Shaft Refracture. Aust. N.Z. J. Surg., 39:194–197, 1969.
292. Olerud, S., and Danckwardt-Lilliestrom, G.: Fracture Healing in Compression Osteosynthesis. Acta Orthop. Scand. (Suppl), 137:1971.
293. Olix, M.L., Klug, T.J., Coleman, C.R., and Smith, W.S.: Prophylactic Penicillin and Streptomycin in Elective Operations of Bones, Joints, and Tendons. Surg. Forum, 10:818–819, 1959.
294. Oonshi, H., Tatsumi, M., and Hasegawa, T.: Biomechanical Studies on Framework and Insertion of Pins of External Fixation. Orthopedics, 7:658–668, 1984.
295. Paiement, G.D., Hymes, R.A., LaDouceur, M.S., Gosselin, R.A., and Green, H.D.: Postoperative Infections in Asymptomatic HIV-Seropositive Orthopaedic Trauma Patients. J. Trauma, 37:545–551, 1994.
296. Paley, D.: Ilizarov Fracture Reduction Method With Preconstruction. *In* Ilizarov Techniques: Manual for the Course Sponsored by the Program of Continuing Education, University of Maryland School of Medicine, May 16–18, 1988.
297. Paley, D.: Insertion and Fixation Tips for Ilizarov Wires. *In* Ilizarov Techniques: Manual for the Course Sponsored by the Program of Continuing Education, University of Maryland School of Medicine, May 16–18, 1988.
298. Paley, D.: The Biomechanics of the Ilizarov Fixator. *In* Ilizarov Techniques: Manual for the Course Sponsored by the Program of Continuing Education, University of Maryland School of Medicine, May 16–18, 1988.
299. Pape, H.C., Dwenger, A., Regel, G., et al.: Pulmonary Damage After Intramedullary Femoral Nailing in Traumatized Sheep—Is There an Effect From Different Nailing Methods. J. Trauma, 33:574–581, 1992.
300. Pape, H.C., Auf'm'Kolk, Paffrath, T., Regel, G., Sturm, J.A., and Tscherne, H.: Primary Intramedullary Femur Fixation in Multiple Trauma Patients With Associated Lung Contusion—A Cause of Post Traumatic ARDS? J. Trauma, 34:540–548, 1993.
301. Parkhill, C.: A New Apparatus for the Fixation of Bones After Resection and in Fractures With a Tendency to Displacement. Trans. Am. Surg. Assoc., 15:251–256, 1897.
302. Patrick, J.H., and Levack, B.: A Study of Pressures Beneath Forearm Plasters. Injury, 13:37–41, 1981.
303. Patzakis, M.J., Harvey, J.P., and Ivler, D.: The Role of Antibiotics in the Management of Open Fractures. J. Bone Joint Surg., 56A:532–541, 1974.
304. Paul, M.A., Patka, P., vanHenzen, E.P., Koomen, A.R., and Rauwerda, J.: Vascular Injury from External Fixation: Case Reports. J. Trauma, 33:917–920, 1992.
305. Pavel, A., Smith, R.L., Ballard, A., and Larson, I.J.: Prophylactic Antibiotics in Elective Orthopaedic Surgery: Prospective Study of 1591 Cases. South. Med. J., 70(Suppl. 1):50–55, 1977.
306. Peltier, L.F.: A Brief History of Traction. J. Bone Joint Surg., 50A:1603–1617, 1968.
307. Penman, H.G., and Ring, P.A.: Osteosarcoma in Association With Total Hip Replacement. J. Bone Joint Surg., 66B:632–634, 1984.
308. Pentecost, R.L., Murray, R.A., and Brindley, H.H.: Fatigue, Insufficiency, and Pathologic Fractures. 187:1001–1004, 1964.
309. Perkins, G.: Fractures and Dislocations. London, Athlone Press, 1958.
310. Perkins, G.L.: The Ruminations of an Orthopaedic Surgeon. London, Butterworth, 1970.
311. Perren, S., and Pohler, O.: News From the Lab: Titanium as Implant Material. AO/ASIF Dialogue, 1(3):11–12, 1987.
312. Perren, S.M.: Physical and Biological Aspects of Fracture Healing With Special Reference to Internal Fixation. Clin. Orthop., 138:175–196, 1979.
313. Perren, S.M.: The Biomechanics and Biology of Internal Fixation Using Plates and Nails. Orthopedics, 12:21–33, 1989.
314. Perren, S.M., Cordey, J., Rahn, B.A., Gautier, E., and Schneider, E.: Early Temporary Porosis of Bone Induced by Internal Fixation Implants: A Reaction to Necrosis, Not to Stress Protection? Clin. Orthop. Rel. Res., 232:139–151, 1988.
315. Perren, S.M., Klaue, K., Pohler, O., Predieri, M., Steinemann, S., and Gautier, E.: The Limited Contact Dynamic Compression Plate (LC-DCP). Arch. Orthop. Trauma Surg., 109:304–310, 1990.
316. Perugia, L., and Traina, G.C.: Current Concept: AIDS and Surgery. Int. Orthop., 18:397–399, 1994.
317. Piekarski, K.: Structure, Properties and Rheology of Bone. *In* Ghista, D.N., and Roaf, R. (eds.): Orthopaedic Mechanics: Procedures and Devices, pp. 1–20. New York, Academic Press, 1978.
318. Piekarski, K., Wiley, A.A., and Bartels, J.E.: The Effect of Delayed Internal Fixation on Fracture Healing: An Experimental Study. Acta Orthop. Scand., 40:543–551, 1969.
319. Pilliar, R.M., Cameron, H.U., Binnington, A.G., Szivek, J., and MacNab, I.: Bone Ingrowth and Stress Shielding With a Porous Surface Coated Fracture Fixation Plate. J. Biomed. Mater. Res., 13:799–810, 1979.
320. Pogrund, H., Husseini, N., Bloom, R., and Finsterbush, A.: The Cleavage Intercondylar Fracture of the Femur. Clin. Orthop., 160:74–77, 1981.
321. Pool, R: Coral Chemistry Leads to Human Bone Repair. Science, 267:1771, 1995.
322. Poole, G.V., Miller, J.D., Agnew, S.G., and Griswold, J.A.: Lower Extremity Fracture Fixation in Head-Injured Patients. J. Trauma, 32:654–659, 1992.
323. Poyhia, R., Vainio, A., and Kalso, E.: A Review of Oxycodone's Clinical Pharmokinetics and Pharmacodynamics. J. Pain Symptom Management, 8:63–67, 1993.
324. Pope, M.H., Callahan, G., and Lavalette, R.: Setting Temperatures of Synthetic Casts. J. Bone Joint Surg., 67A:262–264, 1985.
325. Pratt, D.J., Papagiannoupoulos, G., Rees, P.H., and Quinnell, R.: The Effects of Intramedullary Reaming on the Torsional Strength of the Femur. Injury, 18:177–179, 1987.
326. Pringle, R.G.: Missed Fractures. Injury, 4:311–316, 1973.
327. Puno, R.M., Teynor, J.T., Nagano, J., and Gustilo, R.B.: Critical Analysis of Results of Treatment of 201 Tibial Shaft Fractures. Clin. Orthop., 212:113–121, 1986.
328. Puno, R.M., Vaughan, J.J., vanFraunhofer, J.A., Stettin, M.L., and Johnson, J.R.: A Method of Determining the Angular Malalignments of the Knee and Ankle Joints Resulting from Tibial Malunion. Clin. Orthop., 223:213–219, 1987.
329. Puno, R.M., Vaughan, J.J., Stetten, M.L., and Johnson, J.R.: Long-Term Effects of Tibial Angular Malunion on the Knee and Ankle Joints. J. Orthop. Trauma, 5:247–254, 1991.
330. Rasmussen, P.S.: Tibial Condylar Fractures as a Cause of Degenerative Arthritis. Acta Orthop. Scand., 43:566–575, 1972.
331. Rattner, I.N.: Injury Ratings: How to Figure Dollar Values in the U.S.A. New York, Crescent Publishing, 1970.
332. Regan, L.J.: Doctor and Patient and the Law, 3rd ed. St. Louis, C.V. Mosby, 1956.
333. Regazzoni, P., and Brunner, R.: External Fixation of the Distal Radius. AO/ASIF Dialogue, 1(3):8–9, 1987.
334. Reilly, D.T., and Burstein, A.H.: The Elastic and Ultimate Properties of Bone Tissue. J. Biomech., 8:393–405, 1975.
335. Rhinelander, F.W.: Instruments for Use With Flexible Steel Wire in Bone Surgery. J. Bone Joint Surg., 40A:365–374, 1958.
336. Rhinelander, F.W.: The Normal Microcirculation of Diaphy-

seal Cortex and Its Response to Fracture. J. Bone Joint Surg., 50A:784–800, 1968.

337. Ricciardi, L., and Diquigiovanni, W.: The External Fixation Treatment of Distal Articular Fractures of the Radius. Orthopedics, 7:637–641, 1984.
338. Rich, N.M., Metz, C.W., Jr., Hutton, J.E., Jr., Baugh, J.H., and Hughes, C.W.: Internal Versus External Fixation of Fractures With Concomitant Vascular Injuries in Vietnam. J. Trauma, 11:463–473, 1971.
339. Richards, R.H., Palmer, J.D., and Clarke, N.M.P.: Observations on Removal of Metal Implants. Injury, 23:25–28, 1992.
340. Riegler, F.X.: Update on Perioperative Pain Management. Clin. Orthop., 305:283–292, 1994.
341. Riska, E.B., von Bondsdorff, H., Hakkinen, S., Jaroma, H., Kiviluoto, O.L., and Paavolain, T.: External Fixation of Unstable Pelvic Fractures. Int. Orthop., 3:183–188, 1979.
342. Riska, E.B., von Bonsdorff, H., Hakkinen, S., Jaroma, H., Kiviluoto, O., and Paavolain, T.: Primary Operative Fixation of Long Bone Fractures in Patients With Multiple Injuries. J. Trauma, 17:111–121, 1977.
343. Ritchie, I.K., Wytch, R., and Wardlaw, D.: Flammability of Modern Synthetic Bandages. Injury, 19:31–32, 1988.
344. Rodriquez-Merchan, E.C.: The Risks of HIV Transmission from Haemophilic Patients to Orthopaedic Surgeons (Editorial). Int. Orthop., 18:331, 1994.
345. Rommens, P.M., Broos, P.L.O., Stappaerts, K., and Gruwez, J.A.: Internal Stabilization After External Fixation of Fractures of the Shaft of the Tibia: Sense or Nonsense? Injury, 19:432–435, 1989.
346. Rose, D.L., Radzyminski, S.F., and Beatty, R.R.: Effect of Brief Maximal Exercise on the Strength of the Quadriceps Femoris. Arch. Phys. Med. Rehabil., 33:157–164, 1957.
347. Rosen, M.A., Jackson, D.W., and Atwell, E.A.: The Efficacy of Continuous Passive Motion in the Rehabilitation of Anterior Cruciate Ligament Reconstruction. Am J. Sports Med., 20:122–127, 1992.
348. Rosson, J.W., Perley, G.W., and Shearer, J.R.: Bone Structure After Removal of Internal Fixation Plates. J. Bone Joint Surg., 73B:65–67, 1991.
349. Rosson, J., Murphy, W., Tonge, C., et al.: Healing of Residual Screw Holes After Plate Removal. Injury, 22:383–384, 1991.
350. Rosson, J., Eagan, J., Shearer, J., and Monro, P.: Bone Weakness After the Removal of Plates and Screws: Cortical Atrophy or Screw Holes. J. Bone Joint Surg., 73B:283–286, 1991.
351. Rosson J.W., and Shearer J.R.: Refracture After Removal of Plates From the Forearm. J. Bone Joint Surg., 73B:415–417, 1991.
352. Rothstein, J.M.: Outcome Assessment of Therapeutic Exercise. *In* Basmajian, J. V., and Wolf, S. L. (eds.): Therapeutic Exercise, 5th ed. Baltimore, Williams & Wilkins, 1990.
353. Russell, R.H.: Fracture of the Femur: A Clinical Study. Br. J. Surg., 11A:491–502, 1924.
354. Russell, G.G.: Primary or Delayed Closure for Open Tibial Fractures. J. Bone Joint Surg., 72B:125–128, 1990.
355. Russotti, G.M., and Sim, F.H.: Missile Wounds of the Extremities: A Current Concept Review. Orthopedics, 8:1106–15, 1985.
356. Rutter, J.E., de Vries, L.S., and van der Werken, C.: Intramedullary Nailing of Open Femoral Shaft Fractures. Injury, 25:419–422, 1994.
357. Rybicki, E.F., Simonen, F.A., Mills, E.J., et al.: Mathematical and Experimental Studies on the Mechanics of Plated Transverse Fractures. J. Biomech., 7:377–384, 1974.
358. Salter, R.B.: Presidential Address to the Canadian Orthopaedic Association. J. Bone Joint Surg., 64B:251–254, 1982.
359. Salter, R.B., and Field, P.: The Effects of Continuous Compression on Living Articular Cartilage: An Experimental Investigation. J. Bone Joint Surg., 42A:31–49, 1960.
360. Salter, R.B., Clements, M.D., Ogilvie-Harris, D., et al.: The Healing of Articular Tissues Through Continuous Passive Motion: Essence of the First 10 Years of Experimental Investigation (Abstract). J. Bone Joint Surg., 64B:640, 1982.
361. Sanderson, P.L., Ryan, W., and Turner, P.G.: Complications of Metalwork Removal. Injury, 23:29–30, 1992.
362. Santavirta, S., Karaharju, E., and Korkalla, O.: The Use of Osteotaxis as a Limb Salvage Procedure in Severe Compound Injuries of the Upper Extremity. Orthopedics, 7:642–648, 1984.
363. Sargeant, I.D., Lovell, M., Casserley, H., and Green, D.A.L.: The AO Unreamed Tibial Nail: A 14 Month Follow-up of the 1992 T.T. Experience. Injury, 25:423–425, 1994.
364. Sarmiento, A.: A Functional Below-the-Knee Cast for Tibial Fractures. J. Bone Joint Surg., 49A:855–875, 1967.
365. Sarmiento, A.: Functional Bracing of Tibial and Femoral Shaft Fractures. Clin. Orthop., 82:2–13, 1972.
366. Sarmiento, A., Kinman, P.B., Galvin, E.G., Schmitt, R.H., and Phillips, J.G.: Functional Bracing of Fractures of the Shaft of the Humerus. J. Bone Joint Surg., 59A:596–601, 1977.
367. Satku, K., Kumar, V.P., and Chacha, P.B.: Stress Fractures Around the Knee in Elderly Patients. J. Bone Joint Surg., 72A:918–922, 1990.
368. Saxer, U.: Fractures of the Shaft of the Femur. *In* Weber, B.G., Brunner, C., and Freuler, F. (eds.): Treatment of Fractures in Children and Adolescents, pp. 268–293. New York, Springer-Verlag, 1980.
369. Scales, J.T., Towers, A.G., and Roantree, B.M.: The Influence of Antibiotic Therapy on Wound Inflammation and Sepsis Associated With Orthopaedic Implants: A Long-Term Clinical Survey. Acta Orthop. Scand., 43:85–100, 1972.
370. Schandelmaier, P., Krettek, C., Schmitt, A., and Tscherne H.: Comparison of Clinical and Fluoroscopic Assessment of Posttraumatic Tibial Malrotation. Presented before the Orthopaedic Trauma Association Meeting, 1992. Orthop. Trans., 18:8, 1994.
371. Schatzker, J.: Open Intramedullary Nailing of the Femur. Orthop. Clin. North Am., 11:623–631, 1988.
372. Scheer, L.: Asbestos Again? Forbes Magazine, June 12, 1989.
373. Schemitsch, E.H., and Richards, R.R.: The Effect of Malunion on Functional Outcome After Plate Fixation of Both Bones of the Forearm in Adults. J. Bone Joint Surg., 74A:1068–1077, 1992.
374. Scott, D.B.: Introduction to Regional Anaesthesia. New York, Appleton & Lang, 1989.
375. Scudese, V.A.: Femoral Shaft Fractures: Percutaneous Multiple Pin Fixation, Thigh Cylinder Plaster Cast and Early Weight Bearing. Clin. Orthop., 77:164–178, 1971.
376. Sedlin, E.D., and Hirsch, C.: Factors Affecting the Determination of the Physical Properties of Femoral Cortical Bone. Acta Orthop. Scand., 37:29–48, 1966.
377. Selander, D., Dhuner, K.-G., and Lundborg, G.: Peripheral Nerve Injury Due to Injection Needles Used for Regional Anesthesia: An Experimental Study of the Acute Effects of Needle Point Trauma. Acta Anaesthesiol. Scand., 21:182–188, 1977.
378. Seligson, D., and Harman, K.: Negative Experiences With Pins-in-Plaster for Femoral Fractures. Clin. Orthop., 138:243–245, 1979.
379. Seligson, D., and Pope, M.: Concepts in External Fixation, New York, Grune & Stratton, 1982.
380. Shakespeare, D.T., Henderson, N.J., and Sherman, K.P.: Transmission of Pressure Into the Human Limb From Pneumatic Splints. Injury, 16:38–40, 1984.
381. Simmons, E.H.: An Experimental and Clinical Study of Vascular Spasm. Arch. Surg., 73:625–634, 1956.
382. Sinibaldi, K., Rosen, H., Liu, S.K., and De Angelis, M.: Tumours Associated With Metallic Implants in Animals. Clin. Orthop., 118:257–266, 1976.
383. Skoff, H.D.: Bone Marrow/Allograft Component Therapy: A Clinical Trial. Am. J. Orthop., 24:40–47, 1995.
384. Smith, T.K.: Nutrition: Its Relationship to Orthopaedic Infections. Orthop. Clin. North Am., 22:373–377. 1991.
385. Solheim, K.: Tibial Fractures Treated According to the AO Method. Injury, 4:213–220, 1973.
386. Sorbie, C., and Chacha, P.: Regional Anaesthesia by the Intravenous Route. Br. Med. J., 1:957–960, 1965.
387. Spielholz, N.I.: Scientific Basis of Exercise Programs. *In* Basmajian, J. V., and Wolf, S. L. (eds.): Therapeutic Exercise, 5th ed. Baltimore, Williams & Wilkins, 1990.

388. Stader, O.: A Preliminary Announcement of a New Method of Treating Fractures. North Am. Vet., 18:37–38, 1937.
389. Staniforth, P.: Allergy to Benzalkonium Chloride in Plaster of Paris After Sensitisation to Cetrimide: A Case Report. J. Bone Joint Surg., 62B:500–501, 1980.
390. Stein, H., and Makin, M.: Use of the Wagner Apparatus in Fractures of Lower Limb. Orthop. Rev., 9(7):96–99, 1980.
391. Stein, H., Horer, D., and Horesh, Z.: The Use of External Fixators in the Treatment and Rehabilitation of Compound Limb Injuries. Orthopedics, 7:707–709, 1984.
392. Stene, G.M., Frigg, R., Schlegel, U., and Swiontkowski, M.: Biomechanical Evaluation of the Pinless External Fixator. Injury, 23(Suppl. 3):S9–S27, 1992.
393. Stetson, W.B., Brian, W.W., Williams, B., and Wiss, D.A.: Unstable Fractures of the Tibia Treated With a Reamed Interlocking Nail. Orthop. Trans., 16:662, 1992.
394. Stevens, D.B.: Postoperative Orthopaedic Infections: A Study of Etiological Mechanisms. J. Bone Joint Surg., 46A:96–102, 1964.
395. Stevenson, S., Cunningham, N., Toth, J., Davy, D., and Reddi, H.: The Effect of Osteogenin (A Bone Morphogenetic Protein) on the Formation of Bone in Orthotopic Segmental Defects in Rats. J. Bone Joint Surg., 76A:1676–1691, 1994.
396. Stewart, J.J.: Fractures of the Humeral Shaft. Curr. Pract. Orthop. Surg., 2:140–162, 1964.
397. Strange, F.A.St. Clair: The Hip. London, Heinemann, 1965.
398. Strecker, W.B., Wood, M.B., and Bieber, E.J.: Compartment Syndrome Masked by Epidural Anaesthesia for Post-Operative Pain. J. Bone Joint Surg., 68A:1447–1448, 1986.
398a. Sudmann, E.: Rotational Displacement After Percutaneous Intramedullary Osteosynthesis of Femur Shaft Fractures. Acta. Orthop. Scand. 44:242–248, 1973.
398b. Sven-Hansen, H.; Bremerskov, V.; and Ostri, P.: Fracture-Suspending Effect of the Patellar-Tendon-Bearing Cast. Acta. Orthop. Scand. 50:237–239, 1979.
399. Swann, M.: Malignant Soft-Tissue Tumour at the Site of a Total Hip Replacement. J. Bone Joint Surg., 66B:629–631, 1984.
400. Swanson, S.A.V.: Biomechanical Characteristics of Bone. *In* Kenedi, R.M. (ed.): Advances in Biomedical Engineering, vol. 1. New York, Academic Press, 1971.
401. Tachdjian, M.O., and Compere, E.L.: Postoperative Wound Infections in Orthopaedic Surgery: Evaluation of Prophylactic Antibiotics. J. Int. Coll. Surg., 28:797–805, 1957.
402. Taillard, W.: External Fixation: Past, Present, Future: Introduction to the Tenth International Conference on Hoffman External Fixation. Orthopedics, 7:398–400, 1984.
403. Tardieu, C., Tabary, J.C., Tabary, C., and Tardieu, G.: Adaptation of Connective Tissue Length to Immobilization in the Lengthened and Shortened Positions in Cat Solens Muscle. J Physiol 78–214, 1982.
404. Taylor, A.R.: Wrinkle Corner: External Fixation of Fractures: A Simple Method. Injury, 12:258–259, 1980.
405. Taylor, D.C., Salvian, A.J., and Shackleton, C.R.: Crush Syndrome Complicating Pneumatic Antishock Garment (PASG) Use. Injury, 19:43–44, 1988.
406. Tayton, K., and Bradley, J.: How Stiff Should Semirigid Fixation of the Human Tibia Be? A Clue to the Answer. J. Bone Joint Surg., 65B:312–315, 1983.
407. Tayton, K.J.J.: Ewing's Sarcoma at the Site of a Metal Plate. Cancer, 45:413–415, 1980.
408. Teitz, C.C., Carter, D.R., and Frankel, V.H.: Problems Associated With Tibial Fractures With Intact Fibulae. J. Bone Joint Surg., 62A:770–776, 1980.
409. Tetsworth, K., and Paley, D.: Malalignment and Degenerative Arthropathy. Orthop. Clin. North Am., 25:367–377, 1994.
410. Thunold, J.: Fractura Cruris: An Analysis of a Six-Year Material. Acta Chir. Scand., 135:611–614, 1969.
411. Thunold, J., Varhaug, J.E., and Bjerkeset, T.: Tibial Shaft Fractures Treated by Rigid Internal Fixation. Injury, 7:125–133, 1975.
412. Tornetta P, III, Bergman, M., Watnik, N., Berkowitz, G., and Sstener, J.: Grade III B Open Tibia Fractures: External Fixation vs Non-reamed Interlocked IM Nail. Orthop. Trans., 18:7, 1992.
413. Tornquist, H.: Tibia Nonunions Treated By Interlocked Nailing: Increased Risk of Infection After Previous External Fixation. J. Orthop. Trauma, 4:109–114, 1990.
414. Turen, C.H., and DiStasio, A.J.: The Treatment of Grade III B and Grade III C Open Tibial Fractures. Orthop. Clin North Am., 25:561–571, 1994.
415. Turner, C.H., and Burr, D.B.: Basic Biomechanical Measurements of Bone: A Tutorial. Bone, 14:595–608, 1993.
416. Uhthoff, H.K.: Preface. *In* Uhthoff, H.K.: Current Concepts of Internal Fixation. New York, Springer-Verlag, 1980.
417. Uhthoff, H.K., and Dubuc, F.L.: Bone Structure Changes in the Dog Under Rigid Internal Fixation. Clin. Orthop., 81:165–170, 1971.
418. Uhthoff, H.K., Boisvert D., and Finnegan M: Cortical Porosis Under Plates. J. Bone Joint Surg., 76A:1507–1512, 1994.
418a. Urist, M.R., Mikulski, A.; and Boyd, S.D.: A Chemosterilized Antigen-Extracted Autodigested Autoimplant for Bone Banks. Archives of Surgery 110:416–428, 1975.
419. Vahey, J.W., Simonian, P.T., and Conrad E.U., III: Carcinogenicity and Metallic Implants. Am. J. Orthop., 24:319–324, 1995
420. Van der Werken, C., Meeuwis, J.D., and Oosstvogel, H.J.M.: The Simple Fix: External Fixation of Displaced Isolated Tibial Fractures. Injury, 24:46–48, 1993.
421. Venable, C.S., and Stuck, W.G.: Electrolysis Controlling Factor in the Use of Metals in Treating Fractures. J.A.M.A., 111:1349–1352, 1938.
422. Venable, C.S., and Stuck, W.G.: Results of Recent Studies and Experiments Concerning Metals Used in the Internal Fixation of Fractures. J. Bone Joint Surg., 30A:247–250, 1948.
423. Vere-Nicoll, E.D.: Air Splints for the Emergency Treatment of Fractures. J. Bone Joint Surg., 46A:1761–1764, 1964.
424. Vidal, J., and Orst, G.: External and Internal Fixation as Complementary Procedures in the Treatment of Trauma. Orthopedics, 7:715–717, 1984.
425. Vidal, J., Buscayret, C., and Connes, H.: The Treatment of Articular Fractures by "Ligamentotaxis" With External Fixation. *In* Brooker, A.F., and Edwards, C.C. (eds.): External Fixation: The Current State of the Art, pp. 75–81. Baltimore, Williams & Wilkins, 1979.
426. Vidal, J., Nakach, G., and Orst, G.: New Biomechanical Study of Hoffmann External Fixation. Orthopedics, 7:653–657, 1984.
427. Vidal, J., Rabischong, P., Bonnel, F., and Ardry, J.: Étude Biomechanique du Fixateur Externe d' Hoffmann Dans les Fractures de Jambe. Montpellier Chir., 16:43–52, 1970.
428. Ward, E.F., and White, J.L.: Interlocked Intramedullary Nailing of the Humerus. Orthopedics, 12:135–141, 1989.
429. Waterman, N.G., and Pollard, N.T.: Local Antibiotic Treatment of Wounds. *In* Maibach, H.I., and Rovee, D.T., (eds.): Epidermal Wound Healing, pp. 267–280. Chicago, Year Book Medical Publishers, 1972.
430. Watson, J.T.: Current Concepts Review: Treatment of Unstable Fractures of the Shaft of the Tibia. J. Bone Joint Surg., 76A:1575–1584, 1994.
431. Weber, B.G.: Fractures of the Femoral Shaft in Childhood. Injury, 1:65–68, 1969
432. Weiner, G., Stye, N., Nakhostine, M., and Gershuni, D.H.: The Effect of Ankle Position and a Plaster Cast on Intramuscular Pressure in the Human Leg. J. Bone Joint Surg., 76A:1476–1481, 1994.
433. Weise, K., Holz, U., and Sauer, N.: Second and Third Degree Open Fractures of Long Hollow Bones: Therapeutic Management and Results of Treatment. Akt. Traumatol., 13:24–29, 1983.
434. Weissman, S.L., and Khermosh, O.: Orthopedic Aspects in Multiple Injuries. J. Trauma, 10:377–385, 1970.
435. Wheelwright, E.F., and Court-Brown, C.M.: Primary External Fixation and Secondary Intramedullary Nailing in the Treatment of Tibial Fracture. Injury, 23:373–376, 1992.
436. Whittle, A.P., Russell, T.A., Taylor, J.C., and Lavelle, D.G.: Treatment of Open Fractures of the Tibial Shaft With the Use

of Interlocking Nails Without Reaming. J. Bone Joint Surg., 74A:1162–1171, 1992.

437. Wilkins, J., and Patzakis, M.: Choice and Duration of Antibiotics in Open Fractures. Orthop. Clin. North Am., 22:433–437, 1991.

438. Williams, D.F.: Titanium: Epitome of Biocompatibility or Cause for Concern (Editorial). J. Bone Joint Surg., 76B:348–349, 1994.

439. Williamson, C., and Scholtz, J.R.: Time Temperature Relationships in Thermal Blister Formation. J. Invest. Dermatol., 12:41–47, 1949.

440. Winnie, A.P., and Collins, V.J.: The Subclavian Perivascular Technique of Brachial Plexus Anesthesia. Anesthesiology, 25:353–363, 1964.

441. Winter, D.A., Wells, R.P., and Ott, G.W.: Errors in the Use of Isokinetic Dynanometers. Eur J. Appl. Physiol., 46:397–408, 1981.

442. Witschger, P., and Wegmüller, M.: Carbon Fiber Rods for the AO/ASIF External Fixator. AO/ASIF Dialogue, 1(3):9–10, 1987.

443. Woll, T.S., and Duwelius, P.J.: The Segmental Tibial Fracture. Clin. Orthop., 281:204–207, 1992.

444. Wright, D.G., Levin, J.S., Esterhai, J.L., and Heppenstall, R.B.: Immediate Internal Fixation of Low-Velocity Gunshot Related Femoral Fractures. J. Trauma, 35:678–682, 1993.

445. Wytch, R., Mitchell, C., Ritchie, I.K., Wardlaw, D., and Ledingham, W.: New Splinting Materials: Prosthet. Orthot. Int., II:42–45, 1987.

446. Yasko, A.W., Lane, J.M., Fellinger, E.J., Rosen, V., Wozney, J.M., and Wang, E.A.: The Healing of Segmental Bone Defects, Induced by Recombinant Human Bone Morphogenetic Protein (rhBMP-2). J. Bone Joint Surg. 74A:659–670, 1992.

447. Young, J.L., and Press, J.M.: The Physiologic Basis of Sports Rehabilitation. Phys. Med. Rehabil. Clin. North Am., 5:9–36, 1994.

448. Younger, A.S.E., Curran, P., and McQueen, M.M.: Backslabs and Plaster Casts: Which Will Best Accommodate Increasing Intracompartmental Pressures? Injury, 21:179–181, 1990.

449. Zinovieff, A.N.: Heavy Resistance Exercise: The "Oxford Technique." Br. J. Phys. Med., 14:129–132, 1951.

Rockwood and Green's Fractures in Adults, Fourth Edition,
edited by Charles A. Rockwood, David P. Green, Robert W. Bucholz and James D. Heckman.
Lippincott-Raven Publishers, Philadelphia © 1996.

CHAPTER 2

The Multiply Injured Patient With Musculoskeletal Injuries

Marc F. Swiontkowski

High-velocity trauma is the number one cause of death in the 18- to 44-year age group worldwide. In the United States, loss of income due to death and disability resulting from high-velocity trauma totals 75 billion dollars annually.[53,148,171] This is an economic loss of staggering proportions.[202] The goal of all governmental agencies responsible for health care decisions must be to minimize mortality and maximize return to function in this large, economically productive segment of the population.[8] Despite the major economic productivity losses due to this public health problem, injury receives less than 2% of the total research budget in the United States. In this light, difficult decisions must be made regarding funding of research into injury prevention and trauma management, and legislation must be passed that is designed to minimize morbidity and mortality from vehicular accidents.[44,55,56] Within the local health care system, much effort has been directed toward optimizing the care of the trauma victim to quick return of these individuals to productive life.[201] These efforts must continue in the foreseeable future because of the enormous impact of this problem on the individual and society.[248]

PHILOSOPHY AND TRAUMA TEAM ORGANIZATION

The treatment of complex injuries in multiple organ systems demands a team approach. The team must be able to evaluate the patient swiftly, be willing to discuss the effect of the management of one problem on another, and be able to arrive at decisions quickly and efficiently in regard to performing life-saving procedures.

Every team must have a final decision-maker, the captain. In the case of the patient who has sustained multiple injuries, this should be the individual most experienced in performing procedures to maintain the airway, manage shock from multiple causes, manage emergent situations affecting cardiac output (ie, cardiac tamponade or injury to the great vessels), diagnose and treat intrathoracic or intra-abdominal hemorrhage, and make appropriate decisions regarding the early management of central nervous system (CNS) and extremity trauma. In most settings, this will be the general surgeon with an interest and background in the care of the multiply injured patient. This need not be the case, however, because a neurologic, urologic, or musculoskeletal trauma surgeon with the same qualifications may be the critical decision-making individual in some settings, especially in more rural areas. Effective leadership is the key to coordinating the activities of numerous consultants, who may be prone to focus on specific problems and lose sight of the overall patient. Therefore, the responsibilities of the team leader are to (1) assess the patient's status, (2) determine the need for specific diagnostic tests and delegate these to team members, (3) coordinate the activities of ancillary services (eg, respiratory technicians) and specialty consultants, and (4) make critical treatment and triage decisions, inclusive of setting limits on operating time and blood loss when multiple options from the consultant are available.[123] To perform these tasks, the team captain must have great familiarity with the team members' skills and capabilities for facilitating an optimal outcome for the injured patient.

Team members must be identified and their duties known and well rehearsed long before the arrival of the trauma victim. In the community, nonteaching setting, the team members consist of on-call surgeons, emergency physicians, primary care physicians, and nurse anesthetists. In the level I setting, these roles are assumed by general surgery and emergency residents with accompanying medical students. As described by Jurkovich,[123] preassigning duties and positions around the patient after arrival facilitates the resuscitation phase. The team leader is at the head of the patient and is responsible for airway management, protection of the cervical spine, and nasogastric tube insertion while directing the activities of the other team members (Fig. 2-1). The physician on the patient's right performs intravenous access, Foley catheter insertion, and tube thoracostomy or peritoneal tap when indicated. If a second physician is available for the patient's left side, this individual can begin the initial survey or assist with venous access. Rehearsal of these roles minimizes confusion and limits noise during the resuscitation phase. These physicians provide important feedback to the team leader and must refrain from making independent clinical decisions without direction from the captain. Trauma team nurses are critical to the resuscitation of the trauma victim. Their primary responsibility is to record vital signs and report them to the team leader. They also administer drugs and fluids, draw or assist in obtaining blood samples, and assist with tube thoracostomy or peritoneal lavage. An organized trauma care flow sheet is critical to accurate

(*text continues on page 125*)

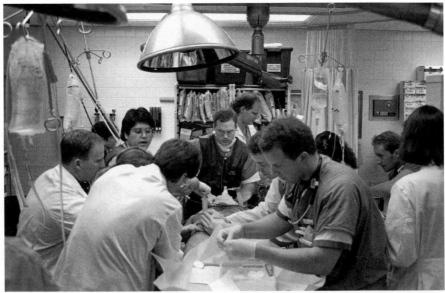

FIGURE 2-1. The trauma team functions optimally with the general surgeon as the team captain at the head of the patient, where attention can be directed toward airway management, protection of the cervical spine, and completion of the primary survey. Other team members with their own tasks can be supervised best from this location.

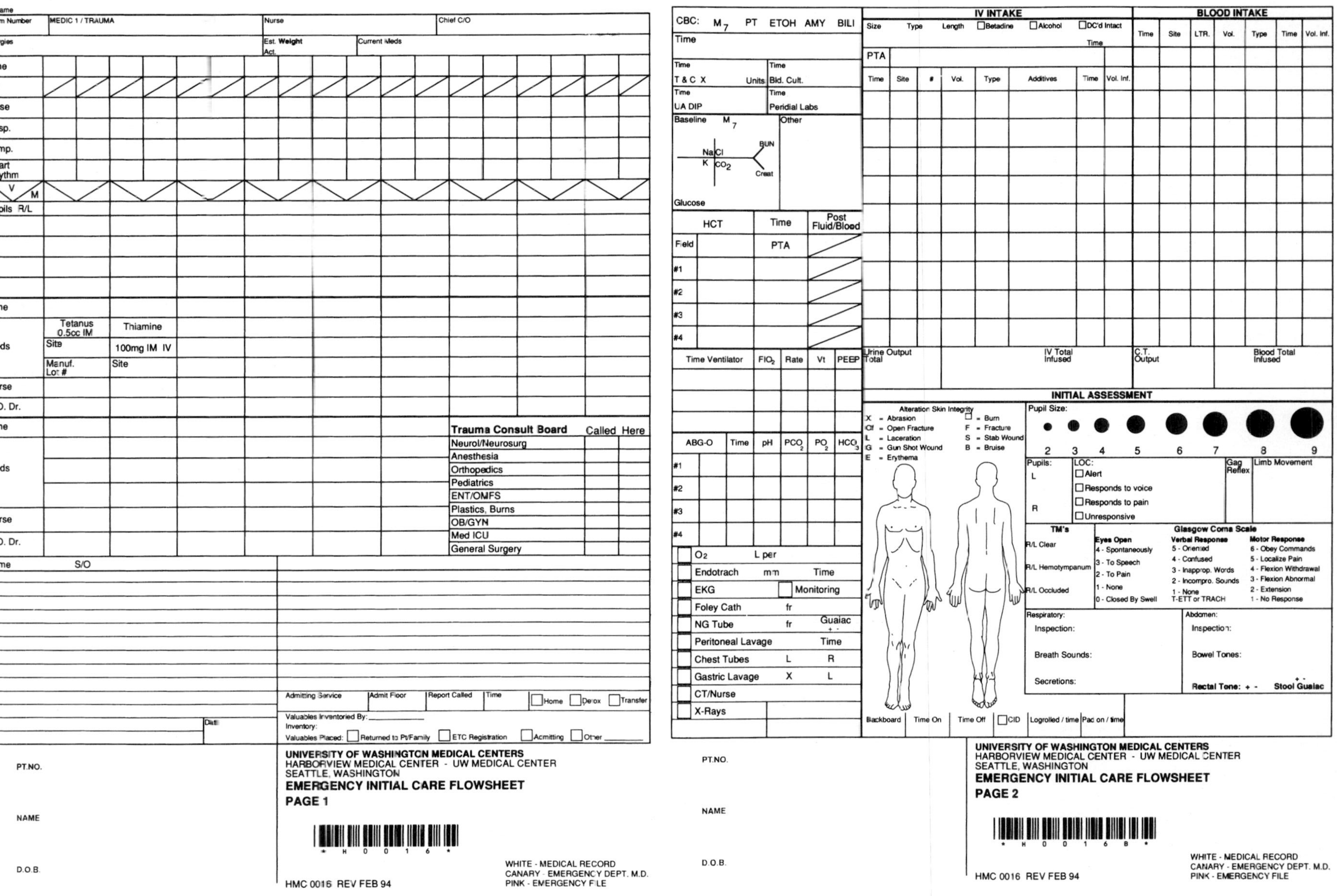

Pt. Name
Room Number | MEDIC 1 / TRAUMA | Nurse | Chief C/O
Allergies | Est. Weight Act. | Current Meds
Time
BP
Pulse
Resp.
Temp.
Heart Rhythm
E V M
Pupils R/L
Time
Meds | Tetanus 0.5cc IM | Thiamine
Site | 100mg IM IV
Manuf. Lot # | Site
Nurse
V.O. Dr.
Time
Meds
Nurse
V.O. Dr.

Trauma Consult Board	Called	Here
Neurol/Neurosurg		
Anesthesia		
Orthopedics		
Pediatrics		
ENT/OMFS		
Plastics, Burns		
OB/GYN		
Med ICU		
General Surgery		

Time S/O
Date
Admitting Service | Admit Floor | Report Called | Time | ☐ Home ☐ Detox ☐ Transfer
Valuables Inventoried By: __________
Inventory:
Valuables Placed: ☐ Returned to Pt/Family ☐ ETC Registration ☐ Admitting ☐ Other ________

PT.NO.
NAME
D.O.B.

UNIVERSITY OF WASHINGTON MEDICAL CENTERS
HARBORVIEW MEDICAL CENTER - UW MEDICAL CENTER
SEATTLE, WASHINGTON
EMERGENCY INITIAL CARE FLOWSHEET
PAGE 1

* H 0 0 1 6 *

HMC 0016 REV FEB 94

WHITE - MEDICAL RECORD
CANARY - EMERGENCY DEPT. M.D.
PINK - EMERGENCY FILE

A

CBC: M_7 PT ETOH AMY BILI
Time
Time | Time
T & C X Units | Bld. Cult.
Time | Time
UA DIP | Peridial Labs
Baseline M_7 | Other
Na Cl BUN
K CO_2 Creat
Glucose

HCT	Time	Post Fluid/Blood
Field	PTA	
#1		
#2		
#3		
#4		

Time Ventilator	FIO_2	Rate	Vt	PEEP

ABG-O	Time	pH	PCO_2	PO_2	HCO_3
#1					
#2					
#3					
#4					

☐ O_2 L per
☐ Endotrach mm Time
☐ EKG ☐ Monitoring
☐ Foley Cath fr
☐ NG Tube fr Guaiac + -
☐ Peritoneal Lavage Time
☐ Chest Tubes L R
☐ Gastric Lavage X L
☐ CT/Nurse
☐ X-Rays

IV INTAKE
Size | Type | Length | ☐ Betadine | ☐ Alcohol | ☐ DC'd Intact Time
PTA
Time | Site | # | Vol. | Type | Additives | Time | Vol. Inf.

BLOOD INTAKE
Time | Site | LTR. | Vol. | Type | Time | Vol. Inf.

Urine Output Total | IV Total Infused | C.T. Output | Blood Total Infused

INITIAL ASSESSMENT

Alteration Skin Integrity
X = Abrasion ☐ = Burn
Of = Open Fracture F = Fracture
L = Laceration S = Stab Wound
G = Gun Shot Wound B = Bruise
E = Erythema

Pupil Size: 2 3 4 5 6 7 8 9
Pupils: L R
LOC: ☐ Alert ☐ Responds to voice ☐ Responds to pain ☐ Unresponsive
Gag Reflex
Limb Movement

TM's: R/L Clear; R/L Hemotympanum; R/L Occluded

Glasgow Coma Scale
Eyes Open: 4 - Spontaneously; 3 - To Speech; 2 - To Pain; 1 - None; 0 - Closed By Swell
Verbal Response: 5 - Oriented; 4 - Confused; 3 - Inapprop. Words; 2 - Incompro. Sounds; 1 - None; T-ETT or TRACH
Motor Response: 6 - Obey Commands; 5 - Localize Pain; 4 - Flexion Withdrawal; 3 - Flexion Abnormal; 2 - Extension; 1 - No Response

Respiratory: Inspection: Breath Sounds: Secretions:
Abdomen: Inspection: Bowel Tones: Rectal Tone: + - Stool Guaiac + -

Backboard | Time On | Time Off | ☐ CID | Logrolled / time | Pac on / time

PT.NO.
NAME
D.O.B.

UNIVERSITY OF WASHINGTON MEDICAL CENTERS
HARBORVIEW MEDICAL CENTER - UW MEDICAL CENTER
SEATTLE, WASHINGTON
EMERGENCY INITIAL CARE FLOWSHEET
PAGE 2

* H 0 0 1 6 B *

HMC 0016 REV FEB 94

WHITE - MEDICAL RECORD
CANARY - EMERGENCY DEPT. M.D.
PINK - EMERGENCY FILE

INJURY TIME (EST):	ADMITTING R3 NOTE	
ER ARRIVAL TIME:	NAME / SERVICE / TEAM / ATTENDING (Print)	DATE/TIME
REFERRING M.D./ADDRESS/PHONE#		
CONSULTANTS: NAME		
☐ NEUROSURG.:		
☐ ORTHO.:		
☐ BURN / PLASTICS:		
☐ EYE:		
☐ UROLOGY:		
☐ ORAL SURG.:		
☐ OTO / HNS:		
GLASCOW COMA SCALE		
EYE OPENING RESPONSE: Spontaneous 4, To Voice 3, To Pain 2, None 1		
BEST VERBAL RESPONSE: Oriented 5, Confused 4, Inappropriate 3, Incomprehensible 2, None 1		
BEST MOTOR RESPONSE: Obeys Command 6, Localizes Pain 5, Withdraws (Pain) 4, Flexion (Pain) 3, Extension (Pain) 2, None 1		
☐ **INTUBATED** ☐ **PARALYZED** **GCS:** ______		
REVISED TRAUMA SCORE		
RESPIRATORY RATE: 10 - 29 / min. 4, > 29 / min. 3, 6 - 9 / min. 2, 1 - 5 / min. 1, 0 0		
SYSTOLIC BLOOD PRESSURE: > 89 mm Hg 4, 76 - 89 mm Hg 3, 50 - 75 mm Hg 2, 1 - 49 mm Hg 1, No BP 0		
GLASCOW CONVERSION SCORE: 13 - 15 4, 9 - 12 3, 6 - 8 2, 4 - 5 1, 3 0		
TOTAL TRAUMA SCORE: ______ (RR + BP + GCS) (0 - 12)		

PT.NO.

NAME

D.O.B.

UNIVERSITY OF WASHINGTON MEDICAL CENTERS
HARBORVIEW MEDICAL CENTER - UW MEDICAL CENTER
SEATTLE, WASHINGTON
ETC TRAUMA ADMIT NOTES PG. 1

* H 0 5 8 3 *

HMC N 0583 REV NOV 93

WHITE - MEDICAL RECORD
CANARY - DEPARTMENT
PINK - NURSING

B

Physician's Order for Spine Clearance
Check one box only
***Some patient care situations may require seperate orders**

[ ] **Full Spine Precautions - CTLS spine injury has not been cleared or an injury has been identified:**
- patient requires hard cervical collar at all times
- full log roll when moving the patient
- patient may not be placed on an air fluidized or air loss specialty bed
- mattress to remain flat at all times (reverse trendelenberg OK) - bedrest only
- additional information/orders:

[ ] **Partial Spine Precautions - Cervical spine has been cleared radiographically, but patient is unable to cooperate with a physical exam and has a low probability of ligament injury - upright films have NOT been done:**
- T,L,S spines are cleared or stabilized
- patient should wear a hard cervical collar at all times
- patient requires care when moving but log rolling with manual cervical immobilization is not necessary
- mattress to remain flat at all times (reverse trendelenberg OK) - bedrest only
- additional orders/information:

[ ] **Partial Spine Precautions - Cervical spine has been cleared radiographically, but patient is unable to cooperate with a physical exam and has a low probability of a ligament injury UPRIGHT FILMS COMPLETED**
- in addition to the above listed Partial Spine Precaution orders - patient may be up in chair with hard cervical collar in place and HOB may be elevated prn
- additional orders/information:

[ ] **Patient's CTLS spines are cleared:**
- patient may be mobilized as appropriate
- additional information/orders:

Additional Appliance / Orthotic Orders:

Physician signature__________ Date__________ Time__________

PATIENT NUMBER

PATIENT NAME

D.O.B.

UNIVERSITY OF WASHINGTON MEDICAL CENTERS
HARBORVIEW MEDICAL CENTER
UNIVERSITY OF WASHINGTON MEDICAL CENTER
SEATTLE, WASHINGTON

PHYSICIANS ORDERS

UH N 0093 DEC 89

C

FIGURE 2-2. Several trauma patient forms help with patient management while optimizing data recording. (**A**) The trauma patient flow sheet has areas where organ system injury diagnostic maneuvers are recorded, vital sign flow is tracked, and laboratory results are recorded. (**B**) A consultation sheet helps with keeping information at hand for the trauma team leader and with facilitating communication between consulting services. (**C**) This cervical spine injury order form has proven helpful for communication between nursing, managing service, and consulting spine physicians.

record keeping for the resuscitation (Fig. 2-2*A*) because the environment is not conducive to reflective long-hand note recording. The nursing team is also responsible for removal of the victim's clothing and assisting with the primary and secondary survey. The radiology technician is responsible for supplying high-quality chest, lateral cervical spine (to the superior end-plate of T1), and anteroposterior pelvic films without adding confusion or noise to the resuscitation process. Respiratory technicians should be available to assist with supplemental oxygen and suction, setting up ventilators, and monitoring pulse-oximetry, again without adding noise or confusion. Clerks to move specimens and supplies, phone for consultants, and communicate with the operating room are necessary to the smooth completion of this phase.

At a minimum, the definitive care setting must have adequate laboratory facilities to perform quick and accurate hematologic and blood chemistry determinations, arterial blood gas analysis, and alcohol and drug screens and to provide emergent blood product support services. The facilities and manpower requirements have been well laid out in the American College of Surgeons regional trauma systems guidelines.[51,52] The level I facility must have a radiologic suite to provide high-quality plain radiographs of the spine, abdomen, chest, pelvis, and extremities, as well as emergent angiography and computed tomography (CT) services. An operating room must be staffed and ready 24 hours a day to manage emergency chest, abdominal, head, pelvic, and extremity trauma. The senior trauma surgeon must be in house with consultants available within 15 to 20 minutes. Surgical house staff must be available. The radiology technician, anesthesiologist, CT technician, and operating room staff must be in the facility. A trauma registry must be in place to review trends in management and outcome. A trauma nurse coordinator acts as the main support person for the registry and functions as a discharge coordinator while acting as a liaison between consultants during the acute phase of management. Requirements for the level II facility are the same, with the exception of the need for surgical house staff. Hospital administration must be willing to support these services, expensive as they are, to deliver high-quality care to the multiply injured patient. Equally important, the team captain must have the support of surgical specialists. These individuals who make up the trauma consultation team must be familiar with the problems unique to the trauma patient, must be committed to the trauma program, and must be willing to work together to optimize the patient's recovery—that is, they must be "team players" (see Fig. 2-2*B*).

This team approach requires a forum for discussion of problems, review of poor outcomes, dissemination or development of new protocols, and improvement of rapport. This group meeting should take place on a monthly basis and can also function in the quality assurance mode for the trauma program. The trauma nurse coordinator is responsible for the collection of data to monitor the program. These data include emergency department and operating room response times, unplanned repeat trips to the operating room, and length of time to perform diagnostic tests. Other criteria to be monitored are provided by the Committee on Trauma of the American College of Surgeons.[51,52] Individual patient management is discussed in the general forum described earlier, particularly emphasizing unexpected morbidity and mortality.

The trauma registry is an integral part of this review process because it can provide a screening tool to discover victims who fall outside the established objective treatment guidelines. In most settings, the trauma nurse coordinator is responsible for accurate data collection, data entry, and routine program analysis. The level of detail included in the registry is dependent on the needs of the individual institution. Several commercially developed packages are available for trauma registry purposes, and several states have developed unique registries. The American College of Surgeons has developed a national trauma registry software package with tightly defined minimal criteria and well-defined data collection processes.[172] The Orthopaedic Trauma Association has similarly developed a registry package with greater detail for musculoskeletal injury and treatment available to all its members.[96] The goal for this tool is to allow individual institutions to determine the level of detail of data to be collected beyond minimal standards and to facilitate multicenter outcomes trials.

It has been suggested that trauma deaths follow a trimodal distribution: immediate, early, and late.[251] Immediate death by severe head injury or transected aorta can only be dealt with by prevention and public education. Patients who die early often have a correctable injury, such as an epidural or subdural hematoma, hemopneumothorax, spleen or liver wound, or blood loss from multiple extremity injury. Coordinated prehospital care and definitive care at a level I center can benefit these individuals the most.[38,175] Those who die later often succumb to sepsis or multiple organ failure, often as a consequence of their initial management. These patients also benefit from trauma center care because of the concentration of expertise and facilities available to treat these patients. The concept of concentration of patients in centers to benefit from the experience and commitment has been well documented for 12 surgical procedures and for other technical procedures, such as coronary angioplasty.[121,144] It naturally follows that trauma care, an even more complex situation because of the nearly unlimited injury variables, would demonstrate a volume/improved outcomes relationship. Definitive documentation of improved functional outcome for survivors apart from preventable death has not yet been published, however.[164,201]

Institution of graded trauma care systems has been definitively shown to have a major positive impact on preventable trauma deaths.[38,111,143,222,250,251] West's classic studies documented the fall in mortality by 50% after the institution of the trauma system in Orange County, California.[270,271] Audit of trauma care before and after the implementation of a regional trauma care system in San Diego showed significant improvement in the following: suboptimal care of the trauma victim, delay in evaluation of the victim, delay in disposition, suboptimal assessment, and trauma mortality.[225] Most critically, the preventable death rate fell from 13.6% to 2.7%. Trunkey and Lim[252] reviewed 425 fatalities in the San Francisco region. They found that preventable deaths at the trauma center were disproportionately lower than those at other area hospitals. Six deaths among the 142 patients treated at the designated trauma center were deemed preventable, compared with 13 patients treated elsewhere. More recently, a preventable death rate in trauma patients without CNS injury of 21% in Dade County, Florida, was reported.[131] The rate of preventable death at the county's level I center was 12%, compared with 26% at the other 22 hospitals in the county. The causes of death were attributed to delay in surgery or to the lack of an appropriate surgical procedure. Although it has been suggested that a minimal number of 200 trauma admissions is optimal, it has been demonstrated that the salutary benefits of trauma care systems on preventable death can be derived from systems that deal in smaller volumes of trauma admissions.[263] Similar findings are apparent in other countries using identical methods for calculating injury severity with nearly identical observed effect for the impact of the lack of an organized trauma care system (Tables 2-1 and 2-2).[7,9,10,37,55,56,89] A published survey of the state chairmen of the American College of Surgeons Committee on Trauma found 29 states were totally lacking a trauma care system, 19 were deficient in one or more components, and only 2 fulfilled all requirements.[6,53] Several highly functional regional systems serve as models (Oregon, Pennsylvania), and the step-by-step approach to system implementation has been published.[51] National norms for trauma mortality have been published.[42] Financial stability of hospitals committing to participating in a trauma care system have been a concern; these financial disincentives must be dealt with at the federal and regional level.[6,43,70,71,148,202,222] The widespread movement of managed care systems must be done in such a way as to preserve graded trauma care systems.[3,238] Although much work remains to be done, it seems clear that trauma care systems are effective in preventing loss of life. These systems have also been shown to be beneficial in regard to outcome for specific organ system involvement, such as subdural hematoma,[237] as well as to benefit all age groups inclusive of children and the elderly.[65,115,142,159,198,216,255] Although it follows empirically that these systems also result in decreasing morbidity, these data are less available.

The majority of the more severely injured patients return to economic productivity; however, a large percentage of these patients require and benefit from rehabilitation services.[164,201,223] Rehabilitation of the injured patient has not received the appropriate emphasis in the development of trauma care systems. This is emphasized in the National Research Council's report "Injury in America."[53] The efficacy of rehabili-

TABLE 2-1
Evaluation of Multiple Trauma Patient Injury Severity Score (ISS)

ABBREVIATED INJURY SCALE DEFINED BODY AREAS

1. Soft tissue
2. Head and neck
3. Chest
4. Abdomen
5. Extremity and/or pelvis

SEVERITY CODE

1. Minor
2. Moderate
3. Severe (non–life threatening)
4. Severe (life threatening)
5. Critical (survival uncertain)
6. Fatal (dead on arrival)

ISS = $A^2 + B^2 + C^2$

TABLE 2-2
Abbreviated Injury Scale for Injuries to the Extremity or Pelvis

CODE

1. Minor
2. Moderate injury
   - Minor sprains and fractures
   - Dislocation of digits
   - Compound fracture and digits
   - Undisplaced long bone or pelvic fracture
   - Major sprains of major joints
3. Serious, non–life-threatening displaced simple long-bone fracture or multiple hand and foot fracture
4. Severe, life-threatening; survival probable
   - Single open long-bone fracture
   - Pelvic fracture with displacement
   - Dislocation of major joints
   - Multiple amputation of digits
   - Laceration of major nerve or vessels of extremities
   - Multiple closed-bone fractures
   - Amputation of limbs
5. Critical; survival uncertain; multiple open limb fractures
6. Fatal (dead on arrival)

tation services is well documented for patients with spinal cord injuries. Approximately 85% of patients who are rehabilitated after spinal cord injury are able to live independently with fewer complications and resultant hospitalizations, and thereby lower costs.[53]

Legislation regarding the establishment of trauma care systems in the United States occurs at the state level. Approximately 60% of states have enacted trauma care system legislation. Legislation to support injury prevention often accompanies the establishment of trauma care systems. Measures such as mandatory use of seat belts, motorcycle helmets, and child safety restraints have been shown to be efficacious in reducing injury.[190,245,248]

TRANSPORT OF THE TRAUMA PATIENT

The multiply injured patient must reach the definitive care setting in a timely fashion. He or she must be appropriately cared for during extrication and transport to avoid a preventable death due to airway obstruction, and shock treatment should be initiated. The ambulance crews of the 1950s and 1960s who simply threw the individual into the back of the vehicle and drove to the nearest hospital have, for the most part, been replaced by skilled emergency medical technicians (EMTs). EMTs are generally affiliated with local fire departments and emergency care regional authorities, and are dispatched by local emergency operators to reported accidents. The EMT is generally well trained in the initial management of the multiply injured patient and arrives at the scene in a well-maintained vehicle that has the equipment needed for extrication, special support, airway management, vital sign monitoring, administration of intravenous solutions, cardiac arrest management, and fracture splintage (Table 2-3). Increasingly, the EMT may arrive in a similarly equipped helicopter.

In the management of the multiply injured patient with musculoskeletal injury, EMTs are trained to perform a thorough assessment of the sensory, motor, and circulatory function of the limb in the field, documenting the external appearance of the limb and dressing traumatic wounds appropriately.[109] After the limb is aligned in the field, premade padded splints or pillow splints are applied for distal extremity injuries. Air splints are popular but can be difficult to use when zippers fail or the injured limb must be pulled through the tubular splint before inflating. They are not advised for air transport because changes in cabin pressure result in deflating or inflating the splint. Pneumatic antishock garments are applied to patients with suspected pelvic fracture based on a stability examination and hypotension. The patient is log-rolled onto a backboard with the open garment in place, and the leg and abdominal sections are zippered closed and the sections inflated. The recommended inflation pressures are 50 to 100 mm Hg in each section, with no more than 30 mm Hg for long-term application. Use of these garments has a down side because they have been associated with compartmental syndrome, missing of open fractures, and decreased ventilatory capacity.[5,46,204] The efficacy of these resuscitation tools has been questioned in the literature, but they remain in widespread use.[155]

TABLE 2-3
Basic Emergency Medical Technician Skills

1. Perform technically sound cardiopulmonary resuscitation.
2. Maintain an airway (endotracheal intubation?).
3. Obtain intravenous access and start Ringer's lactate therapy.
4. Reduce and splint fractures.
5. Perform primary survey of patient and report findings to destination center.
6. Act in concert with physician in early treatment decisions (radio/telephone contact).

There exists a degree of controversy as to the function of the EMT in the United States today. On one side is the "scoop and run" philosophy, which holds that EMTs should swiftly and safely extricate the patient with spinal precautions and place the victim on a backboard.[233] The airway should be cleared; and if spontaneous respirations are occurring, the individual should be placed in the vehicle and transported to the definitive care unit designated by the dispatcher. En route, intravenous access should be obtained, vital signs checked, and fluid therapy initiated. In cases of absent spontaneous respirations, cardiopulmonary resuscitation should be initiated en route. With this theory, speed of transport is critical. Cowley and coworkers[57] reported a threefold increase in mortality for every 30 minutes of elapsed time without care.

The second philosophy, held by Copass and colleagues,[79] is that EMTs can be trained to do procedures that will begin the resuscitation efforts in the field. In cases in which spontaneous respiration is absent or when the patient has profound hypovolemic hypotension, EMTs can safely intubate the patient and start central venous lines. Flutter valve needles can be placed in the patient's thorax to manage tension pneumothoraces temporarily. These procedures are performed under physician supervision via radio contact. Copass' group has shown that significant improvements in morbidity and mortality rates can be expected with this system.[79] The benefits of this more aggressive approach have been confirmed for serious head injury.[12,197] The advantages were also recognized by Hervé and associates,[111] who demonstrated a decreased mortality from spinal, chest, abdominal, and pelvic trauma after the establishment of an emergency medical aid system that provided early high-level care at the accident site.

Regardless of the philosophy employed, all agree that EMTs should be able to perform certain basic tasks (see Table 2-3). There must be frequent open-ended dialogue among the dispatchers, EMTs, and the director of the regional EMT program to improve skills of the EMTs and thus optimize the care of critically injured individuals.

Air transport systems began in the late 1970s to deal with geographic boundaries to prompt trauma victim transport. In Seattle, helicopter transport began in response to the difficult situation of island populations with limited scheduled ferry service. Initially, this incorporated the military emergency transportation system, which then evolved into an independent entity for the transport of trauma victims with leased jet-powered helicopters and fixed-wing aircraft. These air transport programs have allowed for the transport of victims over greater distances to level I centers, where higher patient volume allows for more facile management of injured patients with very acceptable safety records.

The critical role of prehospital management requires a dedicated medical director; tested, designated lines of communication; tested and rehearsed triage criteria; effective transport in a graded fashion; and a highly trained dedicated cadre of prehospital care workers trained in the specific interventions described previously. The importance of establishing these features has been well documented by Ornato and associates.[175] This study documented the decline by 24% of the deaths due to trauma in Nebraska between 1972 and 1982 after improvement in prehospital emergency medical services.

PLAN OF TREATMENT

Musculoskeletal injury is extremely common in the multiply injured patient. One study has identified a 78% incidence of significant orthopaedic injury in a large series of patients with multiple injury, which is nearly equivalent to the incidence of head injury, twice that of major thoracic injury, and four times the incidence of significant abdominal injury.[207] Although patterns of seat belt use, air bag technology, and other preventative strategies have had an impact on this very high figure, it remains apparent that orthopaedic surgeons need to be involved in the management of these patients; their skills are frequently called on. It behooves us, then, to understand the treatment of the entire patient as well as the interrelationship between the management of these injuries and their impact on the other needs of the patient.

Wolff and coworkers[274] have identified five phases in the care of the multiply injured patient after arrival at the definitive care center. They include (1) resuscitation, (2) emergency procedures, (3) stabilization, (4) delayed operative procedures, and (5) rehabilitation.

Resuscitation

The principles of initial assessment and management described in the American College of Surgeons Advanced Trauma Life Support (ATLS) course are accepted as the guideline for resuscitation of the trauma victim. The key to this system is the ability to teach people the management of injuries based on their life-threatening potential; this is generally known as the ABC (airway, breathing, circulation) system of trauma resuscitation. The following summary is modified from an article by Jurkovich.[123]

Airway

The first priority in management of the injured patient is the establishment of a clear airway, followed by ventilation and oxygenation. Removal of oral debris and jaw-thrust maneuvers are performed in the field by the EMT team as the initial maneuver in patients with less severe trauma. If, however, the adequacy of the airway is in question because of head or facial trauma, shock, or thoracic trauma, definitive airway control must be achieved. This generally involves endotracheal intubation, which may be achieved in the field by EMT personnel. Concern for potential cervical spine injury frequently becomes an issue in these patients. As stated by Jurkovich,[123] "No patient should expire from lack of an airway because of concern over a possible cervical spine injury." Gentle maneuvers are possible to manipulate the neck into a position that will allow intubation; this generally requires an assistant to apply gentle linear traction, grasping the cranium at the occiput. Nasotracheal intubation can alternatively be performed in the patient who has not sustained a midfacial injury and who is breathing spontaneously. Only in rare circumstances is tracheotomy required; however, personnel must be trained in this technique for this eventuality.

Breathing

The most common reasons for ineffective ventilation (breathing) after successful establishment of an airway are malposition of the endotracheal tube, pneumothorax, and hemothorax. Critically hypotensive patients rarely have a chest radiograph available; therefore, when tension pneumothorax is suspected by auscultation, large-bore needle catheter decompression is indicated and, where findings indicate, this should be fol-

TABLE 2-4
Indications for Immediate Surgery

1. Hemorrhage secondary to
   a. Liver, splenic, renal parenchymal injury; laparotomy
   b. Aortic, caval, or pulmonary vessel tears; thoracotomy
   c. Depressed skull fracture or acute subdural hemorrhage; craniotomy
   d. Pelvic fracture—stabilization
2. Prevention of pulmonary failure
   a. Femoral shaft fractures
   b. Pelvic fractures

lowed rapidly by tube thoracostomy or flutter valve placement. This can then be followed by the radiograph as the resuscitation progresses. The respiratory therapist can be directed to set up mechanically assisted ventilation at the direction of the team captain when the patient has decreased ventilatory drive due to head injury, flail chest wall segment, or chemical paralysis that may have been used to assist in intubation.

Circulation

Fluid replacement and pressure control of obvious external bleeding will have been initiated in the field and should be continued in the emergency department. Additionally, a large-bore venous catheter may be placed to facilitate fluid and blood replacement, which is performed based on the patient's blood pressure, pulse, and hematocrit. At a minimum, two large-bore (16-gauge) catheters are necessary for this phase of treatment. They are generally placed in the antecubital fossae or groin; injured extremities should be avoided for line placement. Alternative sites include saphenous vein cutdowns in adults and intraosseous (tibia) infusion for children younger than 6 years of age. Many trauma surgeons agree that subclavian access is best reserved for patient monitoring of correction of fluid loss (central venous pressure or pulmonary artery catheter) unless No. 8F catheters are used. The initial fluid bolus is 1000 mL of Ringer's lactate in adults or 20 mL/kg in children. The response to the bolus is monitored by skin perfusion (color, temperature), urine output, and central venous pressure readings, if available. This may be repeated in 5 minutes if the response is inadequate. If the blood pressure is not responding and the hematocrit level is less than about 30% to 35% in adults, type-specific blood becomes a consideration. The need for continuing fluid boluses to maintain a normal blood pressure indicates ongoing blood loss. If the patient has a femoral shaft fracture, hypotension cannot be attributed to this injury, and another source will be identified on the primary or secondary survey.[176] Here, *hemodynamic stability* is defined as normal vital signs that are maintained with only maintenance fluid replacement volumes.

Other aspects of management of hemorrhage are equally important as the principles of fluid replacement. Direct pressure control is always preferable to blind clamping or using tourniquets for extremity hemorrhage. Traction with Thomas splints and distal extremity splints should be applied or maintained during this phase of patient management to help limit continued hemorrhage from unstable fractures. If there are no apparent reasons to go directly to the operating room for hemorrhage control (this assumes that the primary survey has been completed), abdominal or pelvic angiography should be considered during this phase of management (Table 2-4).

Disability/Neurologic Assessment

Continuing with the alphabet,"D" is for disability. A brief examination follows at this point to determine the level of neurologic function. The patient's level of consciousness, pupillary response sensation, and motor activity in all extremities is rapidly assessed. A rectal examination to determine sphincter tone must be performed to complete the assessment. A precise measurement of neurologic function is provided by the Glasgow Coma Scale developed by Teasdale and Jenett (Table 2-5).[243] In the authors' institution, the modifiers "T" for intubated and "P" for partially chemically paralyzed are used to indicate that the calculated score may not reflect true pathology.

TABLE 2-5
Glasgow Coma Scale

Criteria	Score
EYE OPENING (E)	
Spontaneous	4
To speech	3
To pain	2
Nil	1
BEST MOTOR RESPONSE (M)	
Obeys	6
Localizes	5
Withdraws	4
Abnormal flexion	3
Extensor response	2
Nil	1
VERBAL RESPONSE (V)	
Oriented	5
Confused conversation	4
Inappropriate words	3
Incomprehensible sounds	2
Nil	1
COMA SCORE (E + M + V) = 3 to 15	

Exposure for Complete Examination

A complete physical examination is done at this point inclusive of analysis of early laboratory results and radiographs. This requires completely undressing the patient, which is generally done by the trauma nurse as patient management progresses. The results of the pooled data may determine new treatment priorities and direct further investigations. If the patient is not adequately resuscitated by this time the ABCs are reviewed (continuing the alphabet, G = go back to the beginning). The most common causes for inadequate response to resuscitation are unrecognized cardiac tamponade, delayed tension pneumothorax, or unrecognized retroperitoneal bleeding. Continued lack of response warrants getting another opinion, preferably from an experienced trauma surgeon (H = help).

Maintenance of blood pressure is accomplished initially with crystalloid, followed by type O blood in emergent situations and type-specific blood whenever possible. Administration of crystalloid and the use of type O blood has proven efficacy.[221,249] Elevation of the hematocrit beyond 30% has no physiologic benefit for the patient.[80] Fluids, both blood and crystalloid, used in resuscitation of the patient must be warmed to prevent the negative effect on core body temperature with resultant negative effects on platelet function and cardiac contractility.[162,254] As long as adequate blood pressure can be maintained in combination with ventilatory support, diagnostic studies can be performed. In many instances, tube thoracostomy, placement of pneumatic antishock trousers, or pericardiocentesis may be required to restore normal blood pressure. One randomized study has, however, identified no salutary effect of antishock trousers on survival, cost of treatment, or length of hospital stay of hypotensive patients, given the caveat that they reach the trauma center within 30 minutes.[155] The routine trauma admission requires an anteroposterior chest radiograph, lateral view of the cervical spine down to the superior end-plate of T1, and anteroposterior pelvis radiograph. If normal blood pressure proves difficult to maintain with appropriate fluid management, abdominal peritoneal lavage may be performed to rule out intra-abdominal hemorrhage.[52,77,93,160] If the blood pressure is stable in a moderate range, abdominal CT can be extremely helpful in establishing a diagnosis of a liver or splenic injury, ruptured viscus, or renal injury.[185] CT is especially useful in patients with head or spinal cord injury, hematuria, or pelvic fracture.[68,117,189] In the comparative study of these two technologies, peritoneal lavage has been found to be a reliable method for detecting ongoing hemorrhage.[68,77,93] When used as a diagnostic maneuver in patients with pelvic fracture, diagnostic peritoneal lavage has been reported to have a positive predictive value of 98% and a negative predictive value of 97%.[160]

In the presence of a head injury, mid-face injury, or cervical spine injury, CT of the head must be conducted during this phase as well to rule out intracerebral injury. Plain radiographs of the entire spine (anteroposterior and lateral views of the entire cervical, thoracic, and lumbar spine centered over the appropriate vertebrae—C3, T6, and L3 with an open-mouth view) should be obtained at this stage if indicated (see Fig. 2-2*C*). Appropriate indications would be a spinal fracture already diagnosed, an unconscious patient who cannot be adequately examined, and a mechanism of injury consistent with high-velocity impact. If the patient's blood pressure is not maintained within a reasonable range at any point, there is no indication for further diagnostic studies and the patient must enter the second phase of treatment. One randomized study has called into question the re-establishment of a normal blood pressure in the patient with penetrating trauma, citing increases in blood loss, morbidity, and mortality when this treatment algorithm is applied before the institution of surgical management of the bleeding.[19] It is unknown if these findings could be generalized to the blunt trauma patient; most authorities advocate continuation of the principle of establishing a normal blood pressure as expediently as possible for the trauma victim.

Immediate Surgery

During this phase of treatment, the patient is generally moved to the operating theater. Here, all maximally invasive life-saving surgical procedures are performed. As noted earlier, an extremely unstable patient in whom an adequate systolic blood pressure (as indicated by capillary perfusion of the distal extremities and urinary output of 30 mL/hr) has not been restored may have to be moved to the operating room before all diagnostic procedures have been performed. In rare circumstances, major surgical procedures may be instituted in the emergency department, as typified by a thoracotomy for open cardiac massage. This maneuver, however, has generally only been successful for penetrating trauma, and its indications in blunt trauma are subject to debate.

Most patients are brought to the operating room having already been intubated and placed on a volume respirator, with two large-bore intravenous access lines (volume replacement ongoing) and a urinary catheter in place. If there has been inadequate opportunity to obtain a clear lateral cervical spine radiograph all the way to C7 and to examine a cooperative patient, the individual must be assumed to have a cervical spine fracture and a hard cervical collar should be in place[129] (see Fig. 2-2*C*). Endoscopic assisted intubation may be indicated. In many instances, trauma victims will have full stomachs or may have ingested alcohol within 8 hours, and this must be taken into consideration for all victims who arrive in the operating room unintubated. This complicates the situation, and techniques to apply cricothyroid pressure during intubation to minimize the risk of aspiration must be used. The trauma anesthesiologist will generally choose shorter-acting intravenous and inhalation agents along with paralyzing drugs for the multiply injured patient.[197]

The majority of life-saving operations in this phase will be performed for ongoing hemorrhage (see Table 2-4). This would include laparotomy for splenic, liver, or renal parenchymal injury or thoracotomy for injury to the aorta, vena cava, or pulmonary vessels. Penetrating trauma results in injuries to the same structures, but the types of lesion found vary according to the type of projectile involved. Neurosurgical procedures for ongoing mass effect of depressed skull fractures or subdural hematoma are also indicated at this stage and can be performed in concert with the abdominal or thoracic procedures. Rarely, ongoing hemorrhage due to extremity arterial trauma will require vascular repair in conjunction with stabilization of the fractures by the orthopaedist.

Stabilization of femoral and pelvic fractures prevents the pulmonary failure state in blunt trauma.[25,31,120,224] Therefore, after hemorrhage due to the these fractures has been controlled, femoral shaft fractures and unstable pelvic injuries should be stabilized under the initial anesthesia. Noncritical orthopaedic injuries to the tibia, foot and ankle, and upper extremities can await the next phase of treatment. If, however, the patient is hemodynamically stable, all open fractures and displaced fractures of the femoral or talar neck should be managed under the initial anesthesia. Attention must be directed toward maintaining body temperature because hypothermia (which may be present from exposure at the accident scene and the use of unwarmed fluids for resuscitation) has devastating effects on cardiac contractility, platelet function, and drug metabolism.[162,254]

During this phase of treatment, the overall injury severity, age, premorbid nutritional status, and general medical condition of the patient must be taken into consideration. To this end, many systems of trauma scoring have been developed to aid in prognostic decisions in the multiply injured patient and to assist in research into the problem of polytrauma.[145] These systems include the Triage Index (TI),[43] Trauma Score (TS),[163] Abbreviated Injury Scale (AIS),[10,98] and the Injury Severity Score (ISS).[9,10,54,145] The ISS grew out of the AIS and is the most widely used at this time. In this scale, a severity rating is applied to each injury within each organ system and the results are squared and summed (see Tables 2-1 and 2-2). General condition and age of the patient cannot be taken into account in this system, but it has been demonstrated that the LD_{50} for the age group of 15 to 44 is an ISS of 40; for patients aged 45 to 64 it is 29; and for those 65 and older it is 20. This information must be considered during the phase of emergent surgery. As an example, a severe crush injury to a tibia associated with an ISS of 40 in a 19-year-old motorcyclist should be managed with debridement and application of an external fixator, while the same injury in a 70-year-old with an ISS of 40 should be managed with an immediate open below-the-knee amputation.[106] This illustrates the importance of communication on the part of the orthopaedist with the general surgeon during this phase of treatment.

Stabilization

The goals for this phase of care of the multiply injured patient and the procedures subsequently performed depend to a large extent on the condition of the patient before entry into the phase of immediate surgery. If a stable blood pressure was maintained during the resuscitation and the majority of the major diagnostic work was completed, there will be far less diagnostic work to do during this phase than if the patient was rushed to the operating theater. Claudi and Meyers[48] have outlined the goals of this phase of treatment to include (1) restoration of stable hemodynamics, (2) restoration of adequate oxygenation and organ perfusion, (3) restoration of adequate kidney function, and (4) treatment of bleeding disorders.

This phase of treatment begins after the phase of immediate surgery and after the initial treatment of shock has proven effective. It may last hours to days. During this phase, all open wounds should be optimally managed and all fractures splinted in the position of function. In general, this phase of therapy is conducted in an intensive care unit under the continued direction of the trauma surgeon. In many settings, an intensive care specialist familiar with the evaluation and treatment of the trauma victim will take over the stabilization. The goal is to stabilize the patient rapidly to prevent parenchymal damage and to prepare as soon as possible for return to the operating room for other procedures.

The management of shock remains the top priority during the prior phase of treatment and continues into the stabilization phase. The clinical signs of skin color and temperature, pulse, and blood pressure are followed closely as a rough guide to the severity of shock. These can be unreliable in younger patients, who have extensive physiologic reserves; a loss of up to 20% of blood volume may not be associated with changes in these clinical monitors. The signs of severe shock, a loss of 40% of blood volume, are tachypnea, tachycardia, hypotension, and metabolic acidosis. Shock must be treated rapidly to avoid organ failure. Patients who have prolonged shock must be carefully observed for compartmental syndrome, which can occur even in uninjured limbs (Figs. 2-3 through 2-5).

In the restoration of stable hemodynamics, the usual monitoring tools are central lines, often including Swan-Ganz catheters for measuring pulmonary artery capillary wedge pressures and cardiac output, arterial lines (continuous measurement of arterial blood pressure and access for multiple arterial blood gas samples), and a urinary catheter. Appropriate crystalloid and colloid replacement therapy will be selected based on physiologic parameters as well as on frequent packed hematocrit measurement, arterial blood gas levels, urinary output, cardiac output, wedge pressures, and arterial blood pressure. Urine output may be falsely elevated when contrast agents have been administered to the patient for radiographic studies, thereby rendering this measure of organ perfusion unreliable. Mixed venous oxygen saturation is an especially useful tool because it is a measure of the average oxygen delivery to the major organs.[125] Changes in this measure do not directly reflect changes in cardiac output (measured by Swan-Ganz catheter directly as an adjunctive measure) but are a good indicator of the adequacy of resuscitation. Mixed-venous oxygen saturation at or near 70% and arterial blood gases with a base deficit of 5 mEq/L or less ensure that oxygen delivery is equal to demand and that resuscitation of the patient has been adequate.[125,215,257]

For most trauma victims, volume-controlled mechanical ventilation is selected for this phase. The early use of positive end-expiratory pressure (PEEP) is extremely valuable in preventing pulmonary failure.[21,40,58,94,218,268] Frequent arterial blood gas analysis should direct changes in the mechanical ventilator and PEEP settings. Weaning from mechanical ventilation may be systematically conducted based on the patient's responses to intermittent assisted ventilation and trials of removal from ventilator support once the patient's blood pressure, oxygenation, and ventilation function have stabilized and if, in the absence of facial or tracheal injury, extubation can safely be performed. Evaluation of the admission chest film and repeated daily chest films are helpful in managing a patient on a ventilator. The number of fractured ribs correlates closely with the incidence of hemothorax or pneumothorax.[116] Early stabilization of pelvic and femoral fractures to avoid traction is critical in this phase of patient management.[224]

Adequate renal function can be maintained by appropriate management of shock. Maintaining adequate blood pressure and urinary output during the two preceding phases is nearly 100% effective in preventing renal failure. Diuretics should be used in a limited fashion in this phase only when sufficient volume has been documented by adequate cardiac output and pulmonary capillary wedge pressure, and in general is only indicated in elderly patients. If hypovolemic acute renal failure follows high-output failure, as documented by serum and urinary electrolytes, appropriate use of renal dialysis directed by a nephrologist during this phase is indicated.

Bleeding disorders in the multiply injured patient are nearly always due to hemodilution (ie, dilution of platelets and coagulation factors) or shock-related hepatic dysfunction, with the former being far more common. Occasionally, a transfusion reaction may be encountered when O-negative (in females of childbearing age, otherwise O-positive blood) or type-specific blood has been used during the resuscitation phase. Whenever possible, crossmatched blood should be used and 6 units of platelets should be given with every 8 to 10 units of blood transfused. Fresh-frozen plasma should be used when prolonged prothrombin and partial thromboplastin times are evident in patients receiving massive transfusions. Disseminated intravascular coagulation is best treated by prevention, because it is very difficult to reverse once the process begins. Adequate initial shock treatment is critical to avoid these complications.

Deep venous thrombosis is common in trauma patients; in one publication an incidence of 58% was noted in 349 trauma patients, with an 18% incidence of proximal vein thrombosis.[87] The injuries that are most often associated with thrombosis are spinal cord injury, femur fracture, tibia fracture, and pelvic fracture. The incidence of pulmonary emboli as a result is ten times higher in multiply injured patients with pelvic fracture compared with those who do not have a pelvic fracture (2% versus 0.2%).[36] Duplex ultrasound scanning for detection of deep venous thrombosis has been found to be effective and reliable with a sensitivity of 100%, accuracy of 97%, and specificity of 97%.[82] Prophylaxis seems to be clearly indicated for trauma patients,[130] along with close follow-up surveillance. Prophylaxis with sequential compression devices alone does not appear to be as efficacious as these devices with subcutaneous heparin or low-dose warfarin.[130] Prophylaxis with subcutaneous heparin or low-dose warfarin is not recommended for patients with head injury apparent on CT. Duplex scanning is indicated for patients who will be unable to mobilize for 2 days or more or for those with pelvic, femur, spine, or tibia fractures; the two groups are nearly the same because of the amount of injury and the complexity of treatment required. Prophylaxis for the non–head-injured patient includes sequential compression stockings and subcutaneous heparin at 5000 units twice daily for those patients awaiting further operative in-

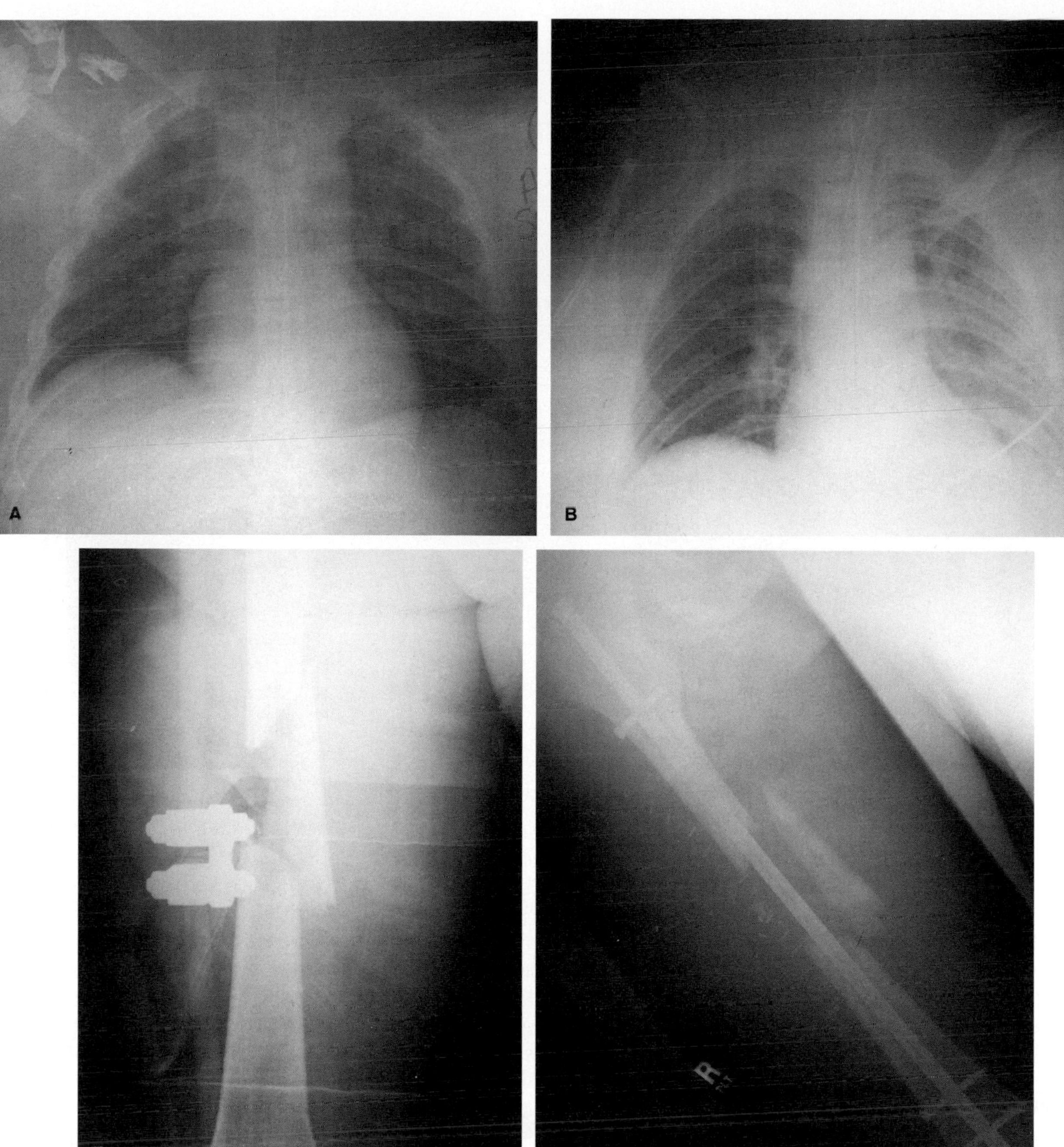

FIGURE 2-3. (**A**) Hypotension remains the most significant factor to be considered when trying to avoid tissue loss due to compartmental syndrome. In this 22-year-old man, more than 80 units of blood were required to support blood pressure during management of a severe hepatic injury, a scapulothoracic disassociation with brachial plexus and axillary artery injury, and an open femur fracture. The scapular injury was treated with prompt open forequarter amputation, and the liver injury was treated with laparotomy and packing. (**B**) However, adult respiratory distress syndrome resulted, requiring 10 days of positive end-expiratory pressure therapy to resolve. (**C** and **D**) The femur fracture was not treated with debridement for 3 days because of the severity of the patient's other injuries. Ultimately, deep infection resulted despite delaying the intramuscular nailing for 10 days by temporizing with an external fixator bridging from pelvis to tibia. (**E**) The fracture ultimately healed with multiple debridements and antibiotic bead therapy; the drainage resolved with removal of the nail at 1 year, with overreaming of the femoral canal. (**F**) The patient had a missed diagnosis of compartmental syndrome, the diagnosis being delayed by 36 to 48 hours after he became normotensive. This resulted in loss of anterior and lateral compartment function.

continues

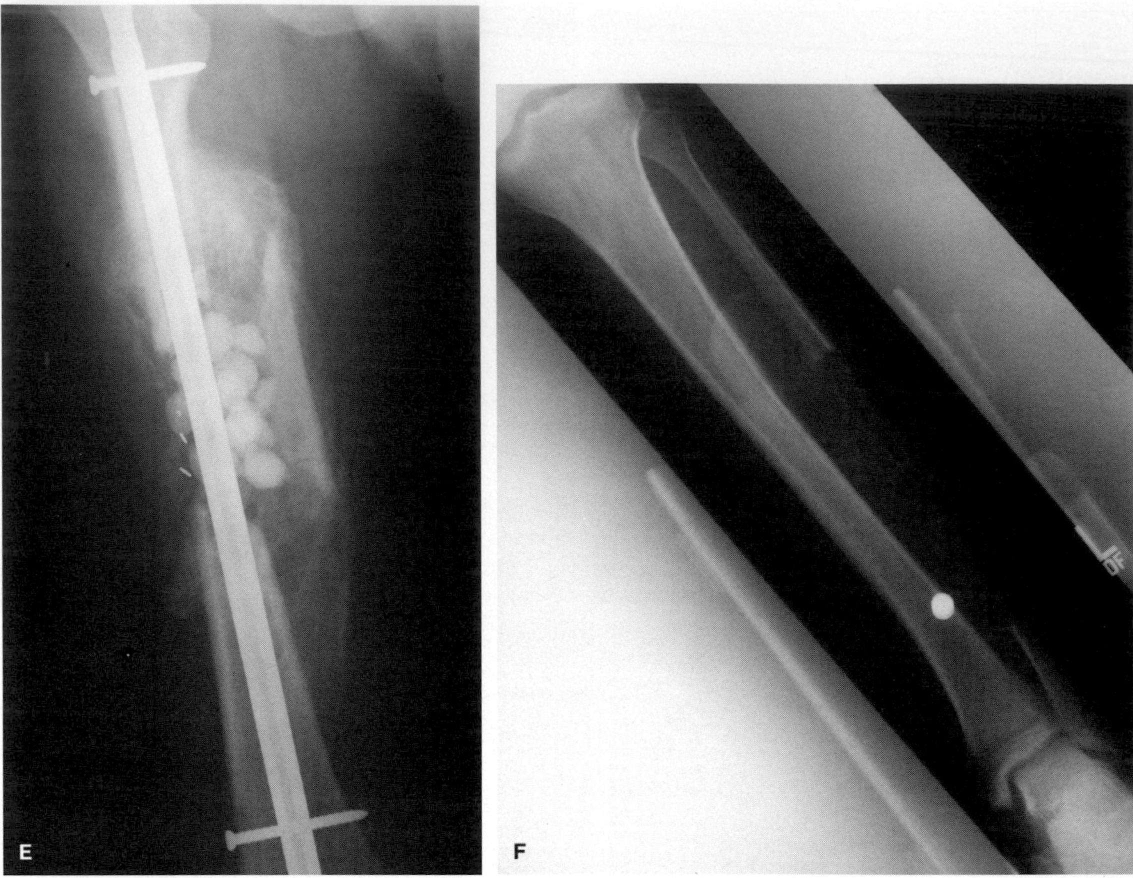

FIGURE 2-3. (continued)

tervention and compressive stockings as well as low-dose oral warfarin therapy for those who require no further invasive procedures. Most surgeons continue the anticoagulation until the patient has been mobilized and spends most of the day out of bed. In the patient who develops proximal venous thrombosis and who requires a major pelvic, acetabular, or femur reconstruction, vena cava filters have proven to be of value and should be used before the operative stabilization of the proximal injury.[97]

Delayed Operative Procedures

Because the length of the preceding phase is highly variable, all open wounds must be optimally managed and all fractures splinted in the position of function during that phase of treatment. This is done in an attempt to minimize the complications of infection and to offer the pain relief of fracture stability to decrease the use of narcotics. Narcotics act as CNS depressants as well as respiratory and gastrointestinal function depressants, and should be used as little as possible.[27,62] In most cases, however, the phase of stabilization is complete within 3 to 4 hours, and the patient can then be brought to the operating theater for care of non–life-threatening problems. If high ventilatory pressures or PEEP is required to optimize oxygenation, special arrangements must be made to bring a high-pressure ventilator with the patient to the operating room because there are limitations on pressure and flow rates for standard anesthesia machines.[153]

As mentioned in the previous section, operative management of femoral fractures and pelvic fractures prevents the pulmonary failure state, and these fractures should be managed whenever possible under the initial anesthesia. Several other musculoskeletal problems must be treated within the first 6 to 8 hours for avoidance of complications. Compartmental syndromes, most often associated with fractures of the tibia and forearm in the multiple trauma setting, must be managed with fasciotomy early to prevent permanent muscle cell death or loss of nerve function or both. Compartmental syndromes are associated with hypotension and poor peripheral perfusion, and vigilance is mandatory for patients who have required a lengthy resuscitation phase. These syndromes can occur even in limbs without fracture or open soft-tissue injury (see Figs. 2-3 and 2-4). Open fractures must

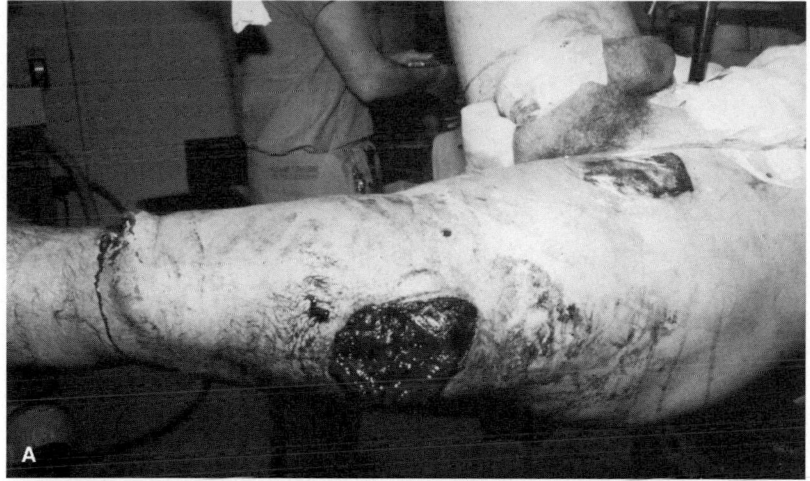

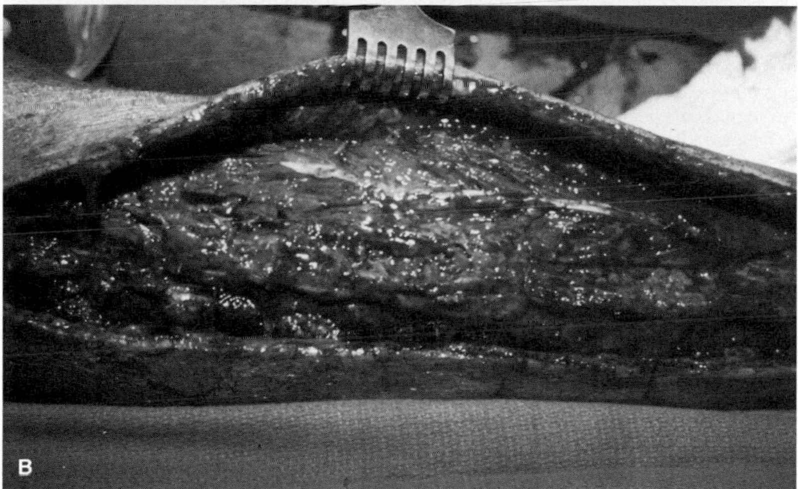

FIGURE 2-4. (**A**) This 18-year-old man required 140 units of blood and blood products to resuscitate him from a pelvic fracture with bilateral open femur fractures. External fixation was used for the pelvic injury after the pneumatic antishock trousers were removed. The femur fractures were treated with debridement and interlocking nailing. (**B**) Lower leg compartmental syndromes were diagnosed at day 2; and with delay in fasciotomy, necrotic muscle was found in all four compartments. Vigilance is the key to prevent tissue loss in profoundly hypotensive patients.

also be managed with irrigation and debridement in this time frame to avoid higher rates of infection.[102] Similarly, fractures with associated vascular injury must be reconstructed within 6 hours to avoid loss of muscle and nerve function. When revascularization times are delayed beyond this range, compartmental syndromes distal to the lesion due to prolonged ischemia time must also be considered. There is some evidence to suggest that emergent capsulotomy, open reduction, and internal fixation with compression minimizes the risk of late necrosis of the femoral head.[239] These fractures, along with displaced fractures of the talar neck, should be managed in this early acute phase to avoid the devastating complications of bone necrosis in these major weight-bearing joints.

Major fractures of the metaphyseal distal femur, proximal tibia, distal tibia, ankle and foot, and wrist and elbow should be considered in the next line of priority. Especially in the case of severe fractures around the elbow, ankle, and hind foot, if management is not completed within 8 to 10 hours of injury, major swelling and fracture blisters ensue, making it wise to delay operative procedures to 8 to 12 days. Reduction in this time frame will be much more difficult, and therefore early intervention is recommended. Delay in operative management for reasons of institutional referral has been shown to lead to higher complication rates.[39] Internal fixation of closed tibial fractures should be classed in the next, less-urgent group, especially when associated with an ipsilateral femoral fracture. Conservative treatment in this setting has been shown by Veith and associates[260] to be associated with higher rates of nonunion and a greater loss of knee motion. Operative fixation of upper extremity shaft fractures can be grouped here as well. Patients with blunt trauma, especially those who are intubated or have head injuries, can be particularly hard to examine, resulting in missed injury. Repeated, at least daily, examinations of all four extremities minimizes delay in diagnosis, which has been reported to involve nearly 10% of injuries in a mass casualty situation.[240,264] Continuous clinical monitoring for the potential of compartmental syndrome is mandatory, especially when the patient has experienced a period of

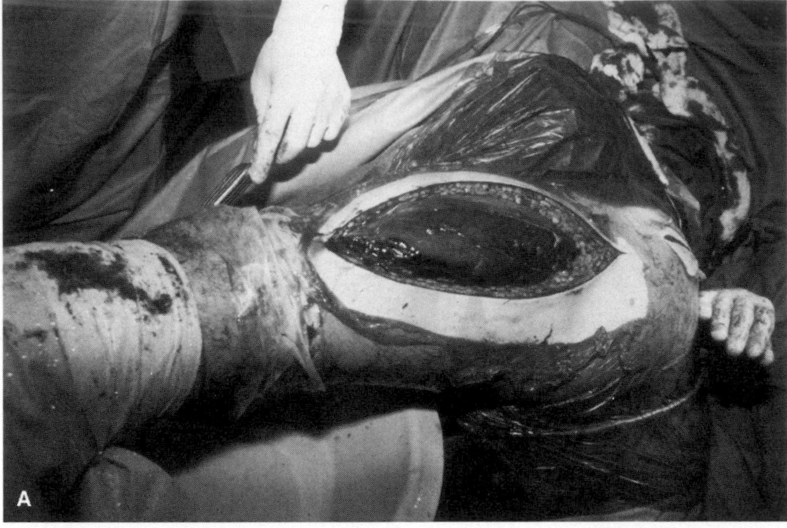

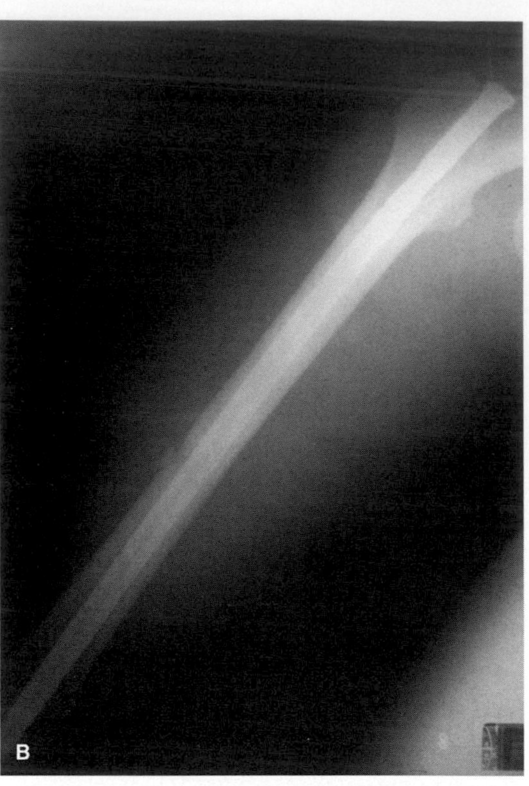

FIGURE 2-5. (**A** and **B**) Vigilance is the key to avoiding failure to diagnose compartmental syndrome. In addition to the most common regions of the lower leg and forearm, the diagnosis must be considered in the arm, hand, foot, buttock, and thigh in the patient with multiple injuries. In this 19-year-old man, who fractured his femur in a fall in a fraternity house, compartmental pressure was measured after stabilizing his femoral shaft when a tense thigh was noted and documented to be 100 mm Hg. Thigh fasciotomy was performed; no tissue loss ensued.

hypotension; both the foot and ankle must be evaluated,[152] along with the forearm.

The management of unstable cervical and thoracolumbar spine fractures varies as to whether the patient is neurologically intact or not. Patients with complete loss of neurologic function distal to the fracture who have return of cord level reflexes (ie, bulbocavernosus reflex) are best managed with early stabilization to enhance the rehabilitation phase. Recumbent, conservative treatment is not indicated in this group. Operative stabilization, which for the most part will be posterior internal fixation and fusion, is best accomplished within the first 5 to 7 days in this phase to return the patient to the upright position and improve the ventilation-perfusion efficiency of the pulmonary circulation. These patients, because of their lack of motor function, are at risk for deep venous thrombosis and need to be mobilized early.[169] Patients with cervical, thoracic, or lumbar spine fractures and no loss of neurologic function should similarly be managed in the same time frame to allow early mobilization and to prevent the complications of prolonged recumbency. Patients with spine fractures and partial loss of neurologic function represent a group of different considerations and are discussed in detail later in this chapter.

Careful attention must be paid to the nutritional status of the patient at this point because the multiply injured patient has extremely high caloric requirements at this juncture.[118] This caloric intake may be accomplished by tube feedings whenever possible. If the patient, due to head injury, loss of gut, or maxillofacial injuries, is unable to take in 2000 to 3000 calories per day, parenteral nutrition must be initiated. Nutritional consultation and a dietary plan based on calorie counts, skin tests, and lymphocyte counts can be extremely useful.

Before institution of this phase in the patient's postinjury course, sepsis may intervene with resultant multisystem organ failure. Border and colleagues[27] have clearly described the influence of nonviable tissue and bacterial translocation in this process. Injured tissue is the source of humeral factors that effect the host immune response.[137] Trauma produces nonviable tissue by the direct application of external force. Penetrating trauma generally produced a smaller volume of nonviable tissue than blunt trauma because the zone of injury is more focused. Nonviable tissue is always surrounded by an area of marginally viable tissue, which is imbedded in a region of normal tissue. Bacterial growth in the marginally viable zone can convert this area into nonviable tissue. With intravenous antibiotics, because this zone has a partially intact microcirculation, this can be avoided because delivery of the antibiotic to the area will occur. The timely and judicious use of antibiotics is thus particularly effective in preventing wound complications in injured patients.[63,64]

Shock and the resuscitation process produces systemic activation of the leukocyte system, with production of oxygen-free radicals producing further tissue damage.[2,259] Some of the sources of further tissue injury relate to the gut mucosa. Bacterial translocation occurs that allows access to the gut lymphatic system and portal venous system, thereby activating the gut and liver leukocyte system.[7,62] This activation appears to be directly related to the detrimental effect on the lung and multiple organ failure.[174] This occurs because of activation of the lung leukocyte system as well as due to embolic phenomenon composed of fat, platelets, and leukocytes and can also be related to atelectasis. Therefore, in blunt multiple system trauma, there are multiple sources for activation of the leukocyte oxygen-free radical system in the gut, liver, lung, and wounds, with subsequent septic organ failure. The lung produces the most readily apparent and early effect of adult respiratory distress syndrome (ARDS).[2,58]

Recovery and Rehabilitation

This is the phase during which musculoskeletal injuries play a critical role. The vast majority of permanent disability after multiple trauma is due to musculoskeletal or CNS trauma.[161,164] These injuries must be optimally managed in the emergent and delayed operative procedures phases. Closed-head injury and complete spinal cord injury are little affected by management, but major improvements can be made by optimum management of musculoskeletal injury. These injuries are best treated as soon as possible. Fracture reductions are much easier to perform if done before the healing process has begun. Intra-articular fractures are therefore best dealt with operatively in the first 24 hours after injury. Open fractures, fractures with vascular injury, femoral and talar neck fractures, femoral shaft fractures, unstable pelvic fractures, and fractures of emergent nature are discussed in subsequent sections. The best results with incomplete spinal cord injury and optimum return of nerve root function also seem to be obtained with urgent reduction and stabilization of the spine.[1]

The recovery and rehabilitation phase begins at the conclusion of the operative phase. In cases of head injury, maxillofacial trauma, or genitourinary injury, great care must be taken to ensure optimal patient nutrition. Therefore, the input of the nutritionist becomes critical at this juncture. Similarly, because of post-traumatic depression, the role of the consulting psychologist or psychiatrist becomes important. Physical and occupational therapists play a critical role in optimizing return of function.

In cases of severe multiple musculoskeletal injury, especially those that occur in conjunction with head injuries, transferring the patient to a rehabilitation center is appropriate at this point. In this setting, a physiatrist with specialized training in rehabilitation medicine serves as a critical team leader. This individual organizes the input of the rehabilitation nurse specialists, occupational and physical therapists, and the orthopaedists, urologists, and neurosurgeons. Those patients who do not require speech or occupational therapy, do not have a spinal cord injury, and do not have neurologic injuries that would benefit from an admission to a rehabilitation unit may be best treated at home. To obtain optimal functional results, the orthopaedist should supervise the physical therapists and visiting home nurses. Patients with severe musculoskeletal injury must be seen by the treating physician fairly frequently in the first 6 weeks after discharge and at 3- to 4-week intervals thereafter until functional results have been maximized.

CRITICAL MUSCULOSKELETAL ISSUES

The Patient is Too Sick!

That the patient is too sick is the most common argument against aggressive early management of multiple trauma. Frequently, anesthesiologists and surgeons unfamiliar with the care of this type of patient raise this objection when the orthopaedist indicates his or her desire, for example, to place intramedullary nails in the femoral and tibial fracture or to internally fix an intra-articular distal humerus fracture while the patient is under the initial anesthesia. Several authors have retrospectively reviewed the efficacy of aggressive early management in polytrauma and have concluded that mortality and morbidity are significantly decreased by early operative intervention in the management of long-bone fractures.[13,24,120,208] Meek and associates[159] retrospectively reviewed a series of 71 patients with multiple long-bone fractures who were assigned to one of two groups according to the treating physician, who performed either rigid stabilization of long-bone fractures within 24 hours or traction and cast treatment. The cases were matched according to ISS scores. Of the 22 patients treated with early stabilization, 1 died; and of the 49 treated in traction and casts, 14 died, which represents a highly significant difference. Johnson and colleagues[120] retrospectively reviewed a series of 132 consecutive cases of patients with musculoskeletal injuries (minimum of two long-bone fractures) and ISS scores greater than 18. They compared a group of patients in which all major fractures (long bones, pelvis, and spine) were stabilized in the first 24 hours (N = 83) to a group of patients who had their operative stabilization delayed (N = 49), basing their analysis of the effect of these treatment regimens on ARDS. They concluded that there is a significant increase in the incidence of ARDS associated with a delay in operative stabilization of major fractures. This was most dramatic in the group with an ISS of greater than 40. Retrospective reviews addressing similar issues by Wolff and associates,[274] Rüedi,[212] Riska and colleagues,[207] Goris and coworkers,[94] Gustilo and associates,[103] Hansen,[105] Fahkry and associates,[78] and others have confirmed the fact that early operative stabilization of major long-bone and pelvic fractures decreases the pulmonary failure state, morbidity, and mortality.[170] Retrospective data,[103] however, did not show a difference in ARDS and in mortality rates in patients treated with fracture stabilization within the first 24 hours and 24 hours to 1 week. Aggressive management of major fractures in multiply injured patients with burns has also been shown to be advisable, but controlled data are lacking.[69]

Border's group in Buffalo, New York,[224] prospectively studied 56 patients with blunt multiple trauma (ISS of 22 to 57) and evaluated the effect of three musculoskeletal injury management schemes on the pulmonary failure septic state. One group had immediate internal fixation of long-bone fractures and postoperative ventilatory support, a second group had 10 days of femur traction and postoperative ventilator support, and the third group was immediately extubated after surgery and had 30 days of femur traction. Ten days of femur traction doubled the duration of the pulmonary failure state and increased the number of positive blood cultures by a factor of 10, the use of injectable narcotics by a factor of 2, and the number of fracture complications by 3.5. Thirty days of femur traction increased the duration of the pulmonary failure state by a factor of 3 to 5 (relative to the first group), the number of positive blood cultures by a factor of 74, the use of narcotics by a factor of 2, and the number of fracture complications by 17. In one retrospective comparison study, Bone and colleagues[26] compared the mortality rates of 676 patients treated at well-established level I trauma centers in six states that practice "early total care" or immediate stabilization of long-bone fractures, with 906 from the American College of Surgeons Multiple Trauma Outcome Study (MTOS).[42] In patients younger than the age of 50 years with an ISS of 18 to 34, the mortality in the total care group was 5.1%, compared with 11.8% in the patients in the MTOS. In those with an ISS of 35 to 45, it was 11.5% in the total care group compared with 25.8% in the MTOS group. Similar data were forthcoming in patients 50 years of age and older. In a prospective randomized trial, Bone and colleagues[25] demonstrated advantages to early (within 24 hours) stabilization of femoral fractures with intramedullary nailing in patients with multiple injuries in terms of ventilator days, length of stay, and hospital charges. In 177 patients, early stabilization significantly decreased the incidence of ARDS, pulmonary dysfunction, fat embolism syndrome, pulmonary emboli, and pneumonia; there was a 2.2% incidence in the early treated group versus 38% in the group stabilized more than 48 hours after injury. However, there were fewer patients who required thoracotomy in the delayed nailing, multiply injured group (three versus none in the acute nailing, multiply injured group).[25] These advantages held for the management of patients with isolated femur shaft fractures. Delay in surgical stabilization of long-bone fractures to optimize outcome from severe head trauma does not appear to be a valid concept.[194] Early stabilization of long-bone fractures in this setting appears to have benefits for head injury outcome; however, this area deserves further study in controlled trial format.[112,258] Head injury does appear to speed fracture union through humeral factors.[61,235]

Trauma patients with long-bone fractures, even those with multiple injuries as manifested by high ISS, clearly benefit from early (within 24 hours) fixation of the fractures. Although some (very few) patients may indeed be so physiologically deranged as to warrant a delay in long-bone fracture stabilization this should be done only with clear consideration of the disadvantages of such a delay. Every effort must be made to rapidly prepare these patients for fracture stabilization.

Long-Bone Fractures

The indications for fixation of long-bone fractures are clear, and the techniques for this type of management are worthy of discussion. For fractures of the femoral shaft, there is no doubt that closed intramedullary nailing is the procedure of choice. Winquist and colleagues,[267] in a series of 520 femoral shaft fractures, demonstrated that the rate of infection is 0.9% and that of nonunion is 0.9%—rates that have not been duplicated with any other method of treatment. Fat embolism syndrome as determined by clinical signs, hemoglobin level, and PaO_2 is common in patient with isolated fractures of the femur (75%) and tibia (19%) and rarely is a cause of morbidity.[75,76,83,156,241] Previously, there was concern about increasing the risk of fat embolism in the victim of multiple trauma by reaming the femoral shaft fracture; however, there has not been any clinical increase in the incidence of ARDS after the nailing of femoral shaft fractures.[45,167,186,244,269] Manning and associates[151] have shown that both in the laboratory and clinically (including 86 open fractures) the reaming of a fractured femur does not produce an increase in fat release. The timing of fixation of isolated femur fractures has been analyzed in terms of complications, mortality, and resource utilization.[208] Patients with fixation performed between 24 hours and 72 hours had morbidity similar to those who had fixation in the first 24 hours with more efficient utilization of operating room resources.

However, controlled trials have documented a cost savings for the practice of stabilization of isolated femoral shaft fractures in the first 24 hours of hospitalization.[25]

Of all fractures of the long bones, the femur fracture is the most critical. Conservative care of femoral shaft fractures requires the use of traction with the concomitant problems of poor chest position, difficulty with moving the patient for subsequent studies, and the inability to get the patient out of bed. The femoral shaft fracture must receive the orthopaedist's highest priority in the multiply injured patient and should be stabilized with an intramedullary nail whenever possible. Immediate fixation of femoral shaft fractures does not have a negative effect on fracture healing.[74,177] In the multiply injured patient, excellent results have been obtained by plate fixation using indirect reduction techniques.[203] Plate fixation has the advantage of not requiring a change in the patient's supine position on the operating table but requires a larger wound, thereby creating a larger metabolic demand. When nailing is not advisable owing to the patient's general condition, temporary external fixation or plating is the next best choice.

Interlocking nailing has extended the use of the closed nailing technique to include very proximal and distal fractures, as well as highly comminuted fractures. In the vast majority of patients with polytrauma, the side-lying position for intramedullary nailing of the femur can be used. After the surgical management of intrathoracic or intra-abdominal hemorrhage, the patient's condition is generally stable once blood loss has been corrected. If the patient's blood pressure has been difficult to maintain, the supine position can be used. The affected limb must be abducted past the midline to allow ease of exposure of the greater trochanter to develop the starting point for the intramedullary nail.[126] Another indication for the supine position in nailing the femoral shaft fracture is an associated pelvic fracture. Placing the patient in the side-lying position places stress across the posterior elements of the pelvis and can restart bleeding from fracture surfaces or minor sacral venous plexi. Many authors prefer the supine position for the nailing of comminuted fractures using interlocking nails, because they believe that the techniques for inserting the distal locking screws are much easier to employ with the patient in this position. In either position, the C-arm must be used throughout the procedure for the closed intramedullary nailing technique. Another advantage of the supine nailing position is that surgical conditions of the abdomen, chest, and head can be more easily treated simultaneously by surgical teams working together to expedite the management of the patient.

The closed intramedullary nailing technique has been safely extended to grade I, II, and III open fractures with no significant increase in the rate of chronic bone infection.[139] To avoid the need for traction after debridement of the wound, external fixation should be employed to allow mobilization of the patient if the surgeon is unsure of the patient's hemodynamic status or is unfamiliar with unreamed nailing techniques for grade IIIa or IIIb fractures. The fixation should be applied with the patient in the supine position, using the C-arm for pin placement after a thorough debridement of the wound. In general, lateral pin placement is preferred to avoid scarring within the quadriceps muscle mass and subsequent loss of knee motion (Fig. 2-6). The frame should be removed and an interlocking nail placed once the patient's condition has stabilized, preferably in the first 2 weeks after injury to minimize the risk of deep infection from pin tract contamination of the medullary canal.

Occasionally, when a humeral shaft fracture is present, intramedullary nailing is indicated to allow axial weight bearing with crutches early on. This is generally done in the secondary phase of procedures but may be indicated when the patient is stable and tolerating the initial operative session well. Closed tibial fractures may be managed with closed interlocking nailing in the multiply injured patient. Closed fractures can be splinted to partially immobilize the fracture fragments so that stabilization procedures can be delayed to the second visit to the operating room. Reamed or unreamed tibial nailing may be used in this setting. For open fractures, unreamed interlocking nailing is the procedure of choice. This must be done after the initial debridement during the first anesthesia to allow for adequate wound care without compromising fracture stability. Half-pin fixation frames have proven to be far superior to the old through-pin Hoffman type of frames when external fixation is chosen. This is because the pins do not impale the muscle-tendon units and allow early motion of the adjacent joints. The half-pin constructs have also proven to have superior biomechanical characteristics. These frames can be used temporarily and safely converted to reamed interlocking nails in the first 2 weeks after injury.[20] External fixators have been developed that do not violate the medullary canal and can be rapidly applied and allow conversion to a reamed or unreamed interlocking nail while the frame is left in place.[200] These may be most appropriate for the unstable critically ill multiply injured patient and can be applied (since they only require a scalpel to place; no drilling is necessary) in the intensive care unit, emergency department, or angiography suite. Immediate reamed intramedullary nailing may have a limited role in open tibial shaft fractures because of a slight increase in the risk of chronic bone infection. Evidence does exist that suggests that immediate fixation of diaphyseal fractures speeds fracture union.[72–74,112]

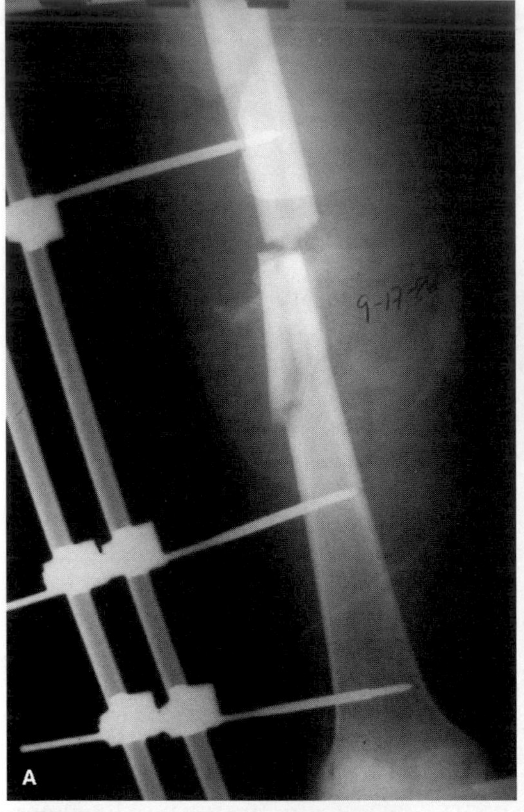

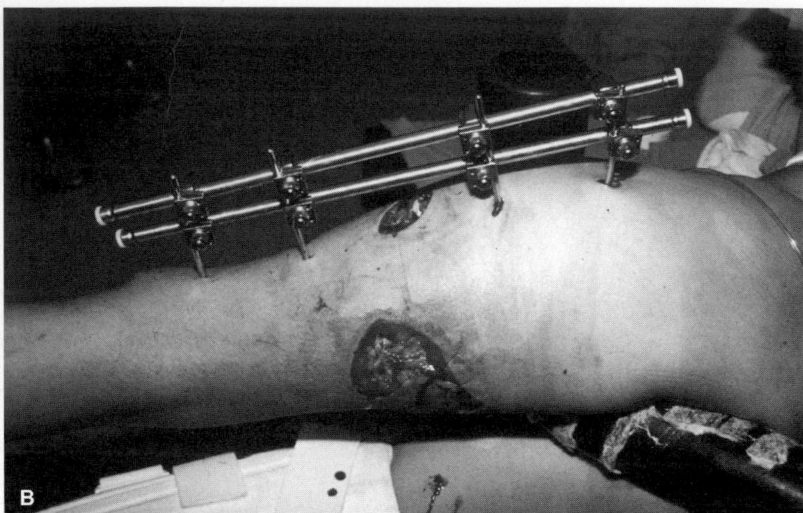

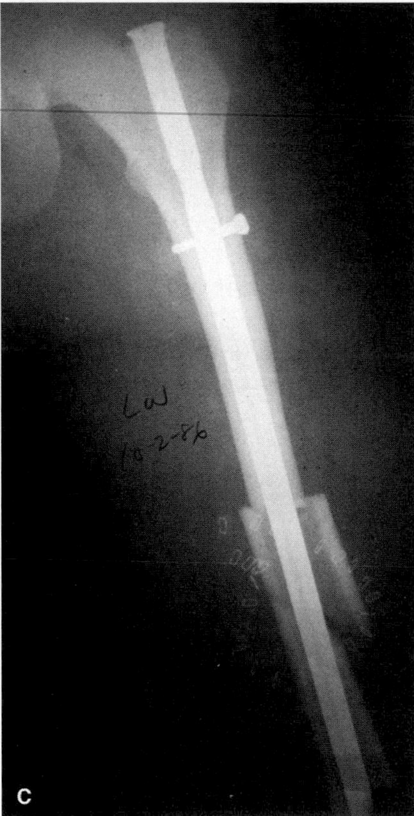

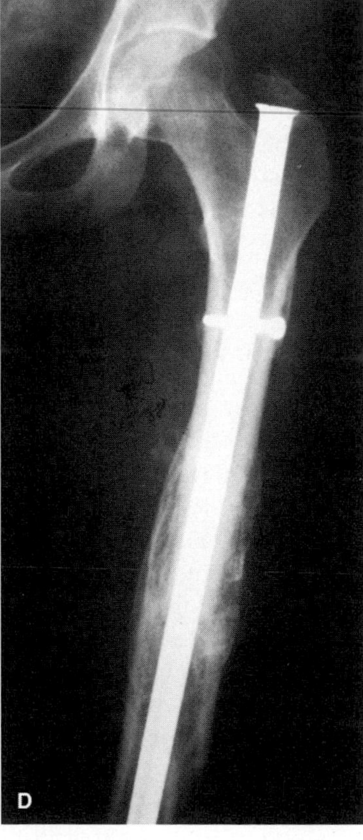

FIGURE 2-6. (**A** and **B**) External fixation is an excellent way to temporarily stabilize femoral shaft fractures while avoiding the use of traction. In this 18-year-old woman with a Glasgow Coma Score of 6 and a subdural hematoma and frontal contusion requiring craniotomy, the external fixation was rapidly placed, after debridement of the open femoral shaft fracture, under the initial anesthesia after the neurosurgical procedure. (**C** and **D**) At day 7, after her condition had stabilized, the frame was removed and the fracture treated with standard interlocking nail, resulting in rapid union. Her functional recovery was excellent given the severity of her injury.

In general, once the femoral shaft fracture has been stabilized and the open long-bone fractures debrided and stabilized, the decision to proceed with further intramedullary stabilization of other long-bone fractures can be made. The factors to be considered must include expertise of the surgical and nursing staff, availability of implants, condition of the patient, and level of fatigue of the surgical and nursing staff. In most trauma centers, a second surgical or nursing team can be brought in if it is in the patient's best interest to stabilize all the long-bone fractures in the first surgical sitting.

Reaming and Pulmonary Failure

Attention has been drawn to the association between blunt chest injury, reamed femoral nailing, and ARDS.[180–183] This phenomenon had been previously reported by Tallucci and colleagues.[241] However, the weight of the clinical evidence regarding the positive effects of femoral nailing has been substantial.[24–26] In patients with blunt trauma, pulmonary shunt is most commonly associated with chest trauma.[86,122] The clinical situation is rare in which the mortality is solely attributable to pulmonary pathology.[122] Several investigators have confirmed the presence of marrow emboli and reaming of intramedullary canals in the clinical setting and in laboratory models.[47,187,188,199,269,275] Great caution must be used in interpreting these studies because many are conducted in animals or patients (arthroplasty) with intact femora. This is a vastly different scenario than that which occurs with a broken femur in which the medullary contents from the proximal fragment are not pressurized to the same degree. This association deserves further intense clinical study when adequate statistical power can be achieved, which was a limitation of the study of Pape and coworkers.[182] The suggestion that unreamed femoral nailing offers less marrow emboli effects deserves critical scrutiny. Studies that have critically measured intramedullary pressures show the majority of the effect to be from the size of the reamer shaft[165]; equivalent pressures are generated from unreamed nails and reamers of equivalent size. Reamer sharpness also plays a role in the generation of pressure and cortical temperature.[166] Clinicians are best advised to use limited reaming or smaller unreamed nails when patients have definite significant chest trauma.[256] In addition to anticipated benefits for patient physiology, using unreamed nails has biologic advantages for fracture healing.[217] Alternatively, plate fixation can be used with anticipation of good results.[203] Delay in fixation of the fracture is to be avoided because multiple well-done clinical studies have confirmed the detrimental effect of this delay.[13,25,120,208]

The pathophysiology of lung injury associated with blunt trauma is a subject of intense clinical and laboratory research. Interstitial lung water increases as a result of hypotensive-hypovolemic shock.[181,196] Forced immobilization has been documented to produce pulmonary fat embolism in rabbits.[276] The most reliable predictive laboratory test for ARDS is the platelet count.[2] There may be a protective effect from this phenomenon delivered by ketoconazole, ibuprofen, and corticosteroids.[11,95,124,141,219,231] PEEP has been demonstrated to be an effective treatment against ARDS.[40,173] Some investigators have demonstrated a positive effect of low doses of corticosteroids for prevention of fat embolism, but the effect needs further study, preferably in the form of randomized trials because of the possibility that this therapy may be related to a higher incidence of other complications.[124,138,141,219] Management techniques inclusive of pharmacologic and mechanical ventilation apart from new techniques for stabilizing femoral shaft fractures are likely to be important for the limitation of the effects of ARDS on patient survival and long-term lung morbidity.[205,206]

Fractures and Severe Head Injury

Outcomes from the management of head injury are improving at a steady pace with improvement on mortality and functional outcomes in specialized trauma units.[150] Not infrequently the clinical situation arises in which the patient presents with multiple fractures and a severe head injury as manifested by low Glasgow Coma Scale score[178,243] (see Table 2-5). Diagnosis and initial management of the head injury generally take priority in the earliest phase of treatment. Patients who are combative after head injury can benefit by intubation with chemical paralysis to prevent neurologic injury from associated spine fracture.[197] Mortality rates in large trauma patient studies are driven by severe head injury more than any other organ system.[37,54] The patient will need to be taken to the CT scanner to define the injury after the initial neurologic examination is complete. If emergent craniotomy is not indicated, intracranial pressure monitoring is nearly always indicated. The pressure monitoring catheter is generally inserted in the emergency department or can be placed in the operating room before the onset of orthopaedic skeletal stabilization procedures. Great care must be taken to avoid hurried transfer of head-injured patients to neurologic trauma specialty centers because noncranial, life-threatening injuries can frequently be overlooked in the rush to move the patient.[110]

Head injury in itself is not a contraindication to stabilization of fractures. In the limited literature on this topic, head-injured patients have fared better with early stabilization of long-bone fractures.[112,191,194] When intracranial pressures are high or extremely labile, and there exists no neurosurgical solution to this phenomenon, communication with the orthopaedist must be well founded so that the proper line between risking raising the intracranial pressure due to fracture surgery and the morbidity of traction treatment can be chosen. A general guideline is that when the intracranial pressure is stable below 20 mm Hg, extremity surgery can be safely undertaken. This surgery must be done quickly, limiting blood loss and consequent fluid shifts. The pelvis and femur take priority in this situation. This is a clinical scenario in which temporary stabilization of femoral shaft fractures with external fixation with delayed conversion to interlocking nails is an excellent solution to the treatment dilemma for a femoral shaft fracture (see Fig. 2-6). Prognosis based on Glasgow Coma Scale score or ISS should not be used as a decision-making tool to determine not to treat the patient with optimum orthopaedic management.[178] Patients who generally would not recover meaningful function based on these criteria often make full recovery.[150]

Pelvic Fractures: Stabilization or Angiography?

Pelvic fractures are often life threatening. Several series report mortality rates of 5% to 20%.[189,195,209,210,229] In reviewing these series, it becomes evident that there is an important difference between simple and complex fractures in terms of morbidity, mortality, and treatment techniques. Simple fractures include simple avulsion fractures of the anterior superior (or inferior) iliac spines, iliac ring fractures, and minimally displaced pubic or ischial rami fractures. These are generally low-velocity fractures and rarely occur in association with multiple trauma. It is important to classify the complex fractures, because this yields important information with respect to associated injuries, risk of bleeding, and mortality.[91,189,277] Reports suggest that it is indeed rare for hemorrhage due to pelvic fracture alone to result in the death of the patient.[101,195]

Classification

Pennal and associates[189] have classified pelvic fractures according to the direction of the applied force. Anteroposterior compression fractures, lateral compression fractures, and vertical shear fractures are thereby defined. The anterior half of the pelvis includes the pubic and ischial rami, while the posterior portion includes the ilia, the sacroiliac joint, the sacrum, and the strong posterior sacroiliac ligaments. In general, injury to the anterior structures is associated with bladder rupture and urethral tears, while injury to the posterior structures is associated with a higher incidence of severe hemorrhage, as well as injury to the sacral nerve roots. Anteroposterior compression fractures include the so-called "open book" fracture (the widened symphysis pubis) as well as the "straddle fracture" (displaced fractures of all four anterior rami). Anteroposterior compression fractures are generally associated with a higher incidence of bladder and urethral injuries. The lateral compression group of fractures generally consists of an impacted sacral fracture or a fracture through the posterior ilium associated with an ipsilateral or contralateral pubic and ischial rami fracture. These fractures may be associated with injuries to the sacral nerve roots, as well as, less commonly, bladder or urethral injury. Because the critical posterior sacroiliac ligament complex is generally not violated, severe hemorrhage (more than 4 to 6 units) is generally not a problem. The vertical shear fracture includes a disruption through the sacroiliac joint, posterior ilium, or sacrum associated with a disruption of the symphysis or an ipsilateral fracture of the ischial and pubic rami. The hemipelvis will frequently migrate superiorly, and the posterior sacroiliac ligament complex is disrupted. These are the fractures most often associated with major hemorrhage as well as disruption of the sacral plexus. Tile has modified this classification scheme to fit the ABC schema developed by Müller and the AO.[246]

Burgess and associates[91,277] have studied the influence of fracture pattern on hemorrhage and death. They added an additional classification to the original Pennal and Tile groups called combined mechanism injuries. These are fractures that have radiographic features attributable to more than one of the three mechanisms or patterns. Data from this group of investigators seem to indicate that it is not the vertical sheer injuries that most frequently result in severe hemorrhage. Rather, it is the anteroposterior injuries, lateral compression injuries, and combined mechanism injuries that most frequently are associated with these severe consequences.[60,91]

Based on the initial radiographs, the orthopaedist can focus attention on the associated injuries. With the anteroposterior compression injury, a more careful search for bladder, vaginal, or urethral disruption should be conducted. With posterior ring disruptions associated with anteroposterior compression, vertical shear, or combined mechanism injury, a careful neurologic examination must be performed and repeated; attention must always be directed toward ensuring that the patient has been adequately resuscitated and that ongoing hemorrhage is not occurring.[123] Fracture patterns do not always correlate with blood loss, so vigilance is the key in dealing with the multiply injured patient with a pelvic fracture.[114]

Emergent Pelvic Fracture Care

Patients with severe pelvic fractures may frequently be transported in pneumatic antishock trousers on backboards. These trousers must be removed after the patient's blood pressure has been stabilized to allow for examination of the pelvis and limbs and for operative procedures to be performed. Their use has been associated with missed open fractures and compartmental syndrome in the lower extremity (especially at pressures greater than 30 mm Hg).[5,46] The use of antishock trousers is not a definitive treatment for pelvic fractures, and the trousers should not be left on the patient indefinitely. One negative effect of this tool is a decrease in vital capacity; therefore, early removal is generally advised.[204] One prospective randomized trial concerning the use of antishock trousers found no benefit for survival, length of hospital stay, or hospital cost provided patients reached the hospital within 30 minutes.[155]

Open pelvic fractures carry a mortality rate of up to 50%, because they are frequently the most high energy type of fracture, with the greatest displacement and a high risk of deep infection.[209,210] Generally, the ischial rami produce the open wounds in the perineum. In the female, the pubic rami can produce an open wound into the vagina and a digital pelvic examination is therefore mandatory. In open fractures, a diverting colostomy is indicated, and if the anterior rami fractures are amenable to simple internal fixation with plates and screws and the surgeon has the skills to do so, this should be performed because stability of the fracture fragments will decrease the risk of infection. If the injury is not amenable to this type of management and instability is detectable on examination, an anterior external fixator should be applied.

Determining whether intra-abdominal injury is or is not the source of ongoing blood loss in the presence of a pelvic fracture can be difficult. Peritoneal lavage is a reliable method for quickly and accurately ruling out intra-abdominal hemorrhage.[160] The technique must be modified slightly in the setting of a pelvic fracture such that the entry point for the catheter is above the umbilicus. This modification will prevent the inadvertent entry into a retroperitoneal hematoma in the reflection of the peritoneum that follows the round ligaments below the umbilicus. Gross blood or red blood cell counts greater than 300,000 cm^3 are positive and constitute indications for laparotomy.

In the case of continuing hemorrhage, aggressive management of the pelvic fracture is mandatory. If other sources of blood loss have been dealt with and the patient has lost more than 4 to 6 units of blood, stabilization of the pelvic fracture is indicated. The simplest way to accomplish this is by applying a bilateral long-leg spica cast with distal femoral pins (Fig. 2-7*G*). This prevents motion of the pelvis when the patient is transported and turned in bed. A large abdominal hole must be cut out for continued observation of the abdomen. The critical feature of this treatment is that the legs are stabilized and patient movement does not cause movement of fracture surfaces. This type of management is most appropriate for hospitals and physicians who do not frequently manage patients with hemorrhage due to pelvic fracture. The treating physician must be familiar with spica cast application, and the facility must have a table that will allow for application of such casts on adults. It is most helpful to have at least two individuals available who are experienced with cast application so that the spica can be put on relatively quickly and the patient moved to an intensive care unit.

The next simplest way to treat hemorrhage due to fracture surfaces or motion is to apply an anterior external fixator. These frames do not offer tremendous support to the posterior disruptions in the case of the vertical shear fractures and cannot hold posterior reductions. In one retrospective study, a mortality rate of 11% was reported due to associated injury (not pelvic fracture) and the need for routine application of external fixators was questioned.[195] These frames are useful, however, for stabilizing fracture surfaces to markedly decrease their motion and thereby aid in promoting clotting.[32] New posterior ring reduction clamps have been developed and are in clinical trials (see Fig. 2-7*A* through *F*).[84] They are more difficult to apply because the pins must be placed precisely on the lateral surface of the ilium overlying the sacroiliac joint; I recommend using fluoroscopy to ensure proper placement and to avoid misplacement into the sciatic notch, further injuring the patient. Ultimately, displaced posterior disruptions should be reduced and internally fixed. The fixation may be accomplished with lag screws across the ilium and into the sacrum placed posteriorly or with small plates placed in screws across the fracture or sacroiliac joint from the anterior side.[211] Although several groups are investigating the role of emergent internal fixation,[92,136] these reconstructions are generally done as delayed operative procedures when progressive hemorrhage is not apparent, because they often will decompress tamponaded bleeding surfaces and promote further bleeding. Early (within 8 hours) internal or external fixation has been shown to have a lower complication rate and less blood loss in one comparative, retrospective study.[136] As is the case with femoral shaft fractures, traction generally should not be used in the acute management of pelvic fractures in multiply injured patients because of the enforced recumbency of the patient and inadequate stabilization of the fracture.[224]

Once the pelvis has been adequately stabilized by spica cast, external fixator, or rarely, internal fixation, hemorrhage will usually cease. For the rare patient who experiences continuing blood loss, pelvic arteriography is indicated.[15,113,179] Because only 10% to 15% of the sources of blood loss is from minor arterial injury, many surgeons believe that this technique is not

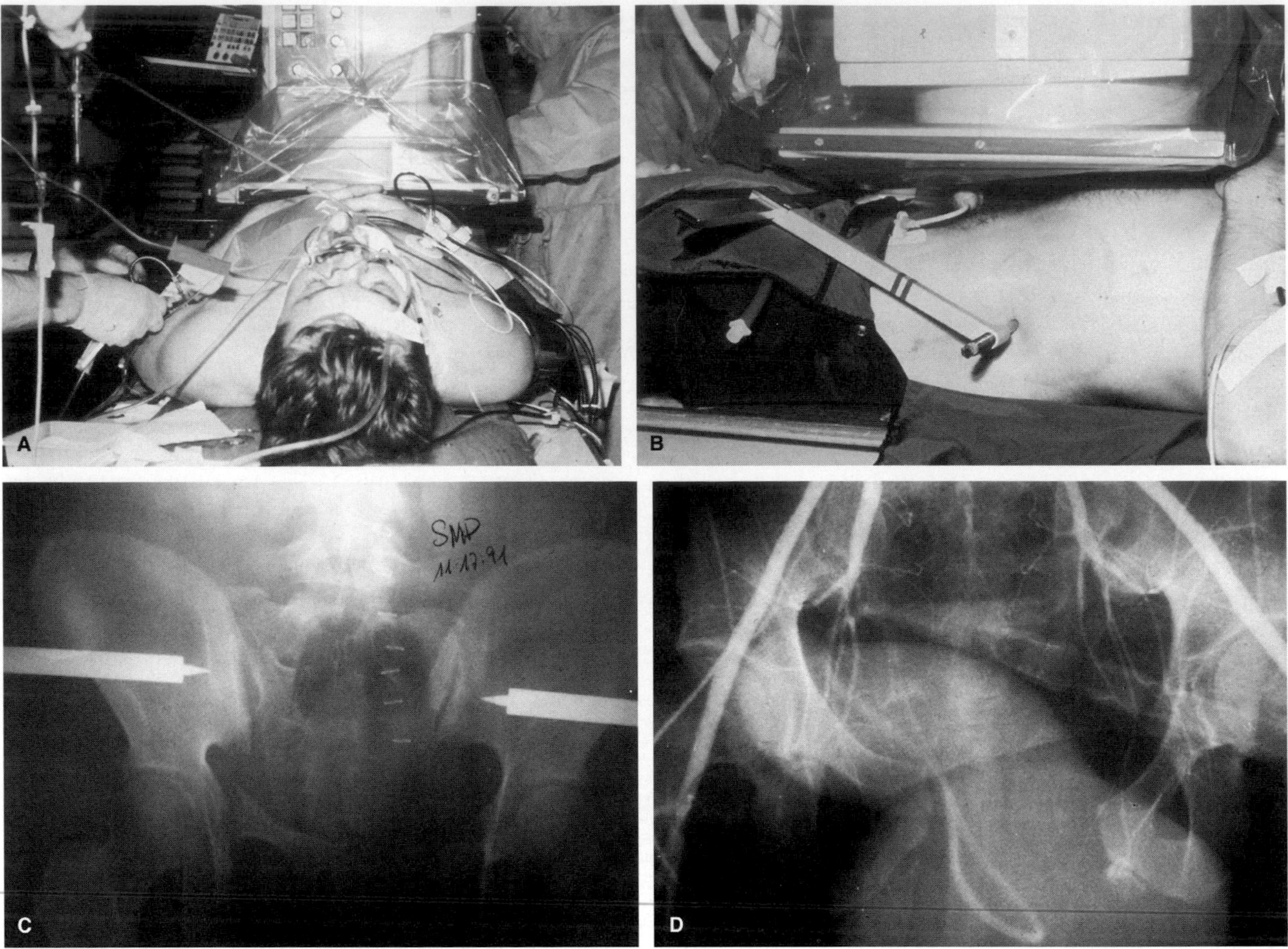

FIGURE 2-7. (**A** and **B**) In hypotensive patients with pelvic fracture, the posterior pelvic ring disruption is best addressed with a posterior pelvic clamp. When the patient's condition is unstable, it can be placed in the patient in the angiography suite, where fluoroscopy is available to optimize the placement of the pins, while the angiographer is setting up. (**C**) Good reduction of a complete sacroiliac disruption is demonstrated. (**D**) The patient must be carefully monitored in the angiography suite to prevent falling behind in fluid management and resuscitation. At a minimum, this generally requires the presence of the trauma surgeon as well as an emergency department or intensive care unit nurse. Pudendal artery bleeding is identified here just before embolization. (**E** and **F**) After the patient has become stable, the clamp can be removed and internal fixation substituted. (**G**) A simple alternative in centers where this equipment is unavailable is a bilateral spica cast.

indicated as a first-line management of hemorrhage secondary to a pelvic fracture[229]; however, this is controversial. Monitoring of the hemodynamically unstable patient in the angiography suite is critical. A skilled intensive care unit nurse and a physician responsible for managing the patient's resuscitation should accompany the patient to the angiography suite. This protects the patient and also serves as a stimulus for the angiographer to consider the patient and his or her general condition rather than getting lost in the details of the study. One current management plan allows for application of external fixation or posterior resuscitation clamp using fluoroscopy in the angiography suite while the angiography team is setting up for their procedure. Eighty-five percent of the sources of bleeding are fracture surfaces or minor pelvic or sacral veins, and angiography and embolization cannot address these. After stabilization of the pelvis has been performed, angiography and embolization is undertaken. If blood loss continues with loss of 6 to 8 more units over the next 12 to 24 hours and does not appear to be slowing, the patient should be returned to the radiology suite. Arteriography and embolization with absorbable gelatin sponge (Gelfoam) or coils can be very effective in experienced hands in controlling blood loss from gluteal or pudendal arteries.[15] Rarely, a patient who experiences continued blood loss despite management of hypothermia and correction of coagu-

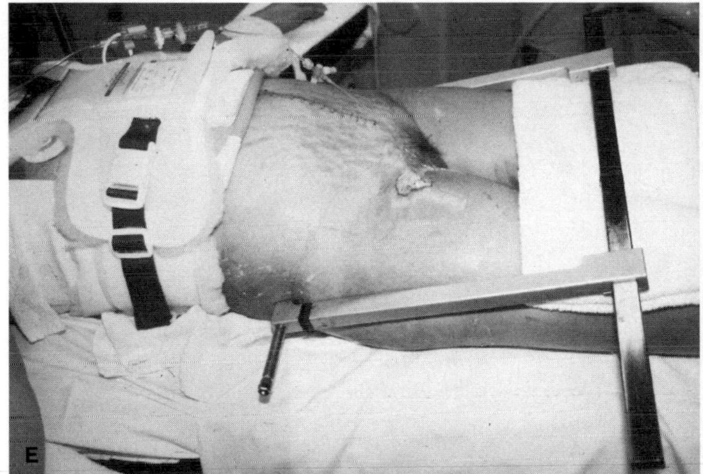

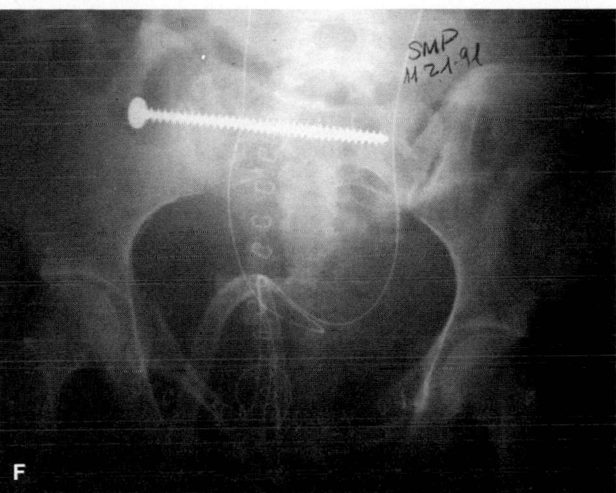

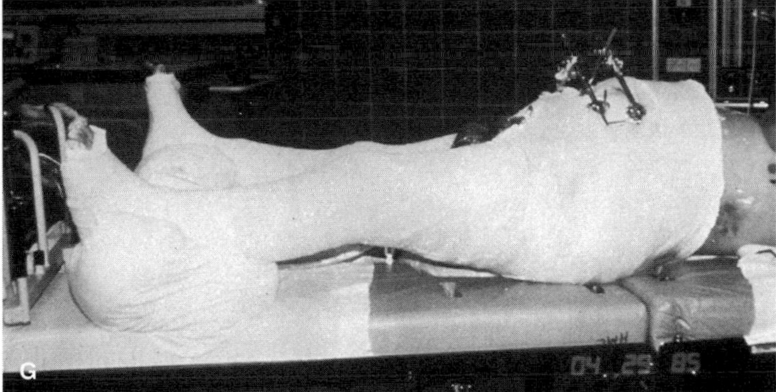

FIGURE 2-7. (continued)

lation disorder, stabilization of the pelvis by one of the methods discussed, and arteriography and embolization will require exploratory surgery. This is the procedure of last resort, and patients who reach this point have a very poor prognosis. Hemipelvectomy has been reported to save patients in this situation.[149] Throughout the early course of resuscitation and management, attention must be paid to treating hypothermia because of its negative influence on cardiac contractility, clotting processes, and drug metabolism and to appropriate replacement of platelets and clotting factors based on frequent laboratory monitoring.[2,162]

Spinal Cord Injuries

Multiply injured patients with head injuries should be assumed to have a spine fracture until it can be proven otherwise. They should be transported with hard cervical collars and on backboards. The initial screening examination of every patient with presumed spinal cord injury must include a lateral cervical spine film down to C7–T1. In the presence of a head injury, during the stabilization phase, complete thoracic and lumbar films must be obtained. Only when the spine films have been cleared should the cervical collar be removed (see Fig. 2-2*C*). Patients should be removed from the backboard early in the course and managed with log-rolling to prevent decubitus ulcers.

Patients with spinal cord injuries will have special requirements in regard to fluid replacement during resuscitation. This is due to autonomic dysreflexia and loss of vascular tone. Fluid requirements due to vasodilatation must be carefully assessed because patients in neurogenic shock with no other source for blood loss are euvolemic. Trendelenburg positioning should be used liberally to support perfusion of the CNS, and atropine may be used to counteract the resultant bradycardia.[232] Details of the management of neurogenic shock are covered in Chapter 17. Methylprednisolone therapy has been shown to be efficacious in terms of improved neurologic outcomes from spinal cord injury.[30] The initial intravenous bolus dose is 30 mg/kg, with a maintenance intravenous dose of 5.4 mg/kg/h for 24 hours. To optimize outcome, methylprednisolone therapy must be started within 8 hours of injury. A small prospective randomized study has shown GM_1 ganglioside to be efficacious in improving motor outcomes at 1 year.[89] The 21 aminosteroids are presumed to act as an antioxidant and do not have the glucocorticoid systemic effects.[81] These compounds are in being tested in clinical trials in patients with spinal cord and head injuries.

The initial survey in patients with spinal cord injury must include examination for the bulbocavernosus reflex. In the patient with quadriparesis or hemiparesis, the absence of this reflex indicates the presence of spinal shock. The final neurologic status of the patient with complete paraplegia or quadriplegia cannot be determined until these cord level reflexes return. Individuals with paraparesis or quadriparesis must be carefully examined for any sign of residual motor or sensory sparing, because this function indicates a partial cord injury and has important prognostic and treatment significance. Spinal cord injury makes complete diagnosis of all injuries difficult; one study reported missed injuries in 42% of patients with spinal cord injuries (approximately half with spinal fractures at another level).[214] Although concomitant abdominal injury is not common, it does occur and is common in vehicular accidents when only the lap belt is used.[117] Vigilance in this clinical setting must be heightened.

Cervical Spine Fractures

The initial treatment of cervical spine fractures is similar with respect to presence or absence of cord injury. Patients with C1 or C2 fractures are generally neurologically intact on presentation. They should be left in a hard cervical collar until more definitive immobilization can be performed. In general, this means application of a halo and placement in temporary traction or attachment to a vest or cast. For lower cervical fractures, the patient should remain in a hard cervical collar until a definitive diagnosis of the fracture can be made. Frequently, this will include CT to determine the status of the neural canal. For most lower cervical fractures or single or bilateral dislocated facets, the patient should be placed immediately into a halo or Gardner-Wells tongs as soon as it has been determined that the patient's other injuries do not require immediate operation. Heary and associates[108] have demonstrated that early placement of these patients into a halo or vest, even when the definitive treatment is operative stabilization, facilitates further workup of the trauma patient without compromising the outcome for the management of the cervical spine injury.

When the patient has complete quadriparesis, stabilization of the spine with fusion to the intact levels above and below (generally posterior) is indicated to allow early rehabilitation.[16,232] Recovery of one additional distal nerve root function after stabilization is common.[16] In this way, the recumbent position with the concomitant risk of pulmonary problems is avoided. With posterior wiring techniques to supplement bone graft arthrodesis, little more than a cervical collar is necessary for postoperative immobilization. In the instance of partial quadriparesis with distal sparing of function, the general course is a posterior cervical fusion for spinal realignment and indirect reduction, followed by an anterior decompression of the canal (removal of bone fragments).[1,129] This has been accompanied by an improvement of distal function in many cases.[4,22] Depending on the status of the resuscitation and the management of other injuries to the head and body cavities, urgent decompression and surgical realignment may be advisable for patients with partial lesions because there are data to suggest improved functional outcomes for patients with distal sparing, even that as little as some sacral roots.[1]

Patients who have sustained polytrauma with cervical spine fracture require special handling during the evaluation and early treatment phase. If the spine fracture requires reduction, this is best done with tong traction, and the patient should be kept in traction during laparotomy, thoracotomy, or stabilization of femur or pelvis if required during the emergency procedure phase of treatment. This requirement also influences the choice of anesthetic technique; endoscopically aided orotracheal or nasotracheal intubation that can be done without manipulating the neck is necessary. The patient's spinal column is kept aligned during these procedures, which mandates continuation of supine positioning for stabilization of the femur.[125,129]

Thoracolumbar Fractures

The three-column theory of Denis has been helpful in distinguishing stable from unstable fractures.[66] With an anterior body fracture (the anterior column) with disruption of the posterior wall of the vertebral body (the middle column) and the interspinous ligaments (the posterior column), the fracture is unstable. Disruption of two of the three columns at any single level also indicates instability. Instability implies the potential for further neurologic injury. Once these fractures are properly diagnosed with plain radiographs and CT scans, the patient must be log-rolled, maintaining spinal alignment until the fracture can be definitively treated. Stryker-framed or Roto Kinetic beds can be helpful adjuncts, especially when there are associated injuries.

The general principles of treatment for cervical spine fractures apply for fractures of the thoracolumbar spine. If the patient has complete paraplegia, posterior fusion with rod placement should be carried out to allow mobilization of the patient and a timely rehabilitation. The spine fusion is protected with a plastic thoracic lumbosacral orthosis until the fusion is solid. In the case of a partial injury, a two-stage procedure is preferred, with initial posterior rodding and fusion, followed by anterior decompression shortly thereafter. Most authors believe that early decompression and stabilization (as early as the patient's general condition allows) is also appropriate for patients with partial paraplegia. The indication for an emergent stabilization and decompression is neurologic deterioration. Great vigilance must be maintained in dealing with the patients with multiple injuries. In one series of 201 patients with femoral shaft fracture, 7 patients had thoracolumbar fracture, for an associated incidence of 3.5%, and 4 of these 7 patients had their spine fracture go undiagnosed until after the femoral fracture was internally stabilized.[213]

Distal Extremity Injury and Limb Salvage

Injuries to the distal extremity includes fractures and dislocations distal to the wrist and ankle. As a general principle, these fractures should be managed with splintage until the patient has been fully resuscitated and injuries of the head, abdomen, chest, pelvis, and long bones have been optimally managed. Certain injuries must be managed with greater care, particularly fractures around the ankle. Fracture-dislocations must be reduced and placed in well-padded splints. If it is possible to manage these injuries in the early setting in which the patient's condition remains clinically stable, this should be done. Late management of fracture-dislocations of the ankle, particularly after institutional transfer, have a much higher complication rate.[39]

Open wounds should be carefully debrided before splintage in the most critically ill patients. For open tibial fractures, the pinless external fixator can be applied in minutes and provides excellent wound access and adequate stabilization for temporary fixation.[200] Exceptions to this rule include dysvascular distal limbs in which arterial reconstructions must be performed to save limbs. This is when communication as directed by the team captain becomes critical.

Decisions for limb salvage attempts may be inappropriate in the setting of the patient with polytrauma, especially in older patients who lack vast physiologic reserves.[134,255] Prolonged attempts at limb salvage have been shown to be associated with higher risk of sepsis and death, as well as higher cost[23,41,135] and psychosocial morbidity.[90,106] Absolute indications for amputation include a limb with no potential for function or documented disruption of the posterior tibial nerve.[135] Scales to assist with decisions of salvage versus amputation have been developed to aid in decision making.[99,119] The Mangled Extremity Severity Scale (MESS) is one particularly useful scale that assigns points for soft-tissue injury (1–4), ischemia time (1–6), age of the patient (0–2), and hypotension (0–2) (Table 2-6) Retrospective application of this scale and limited prospective applications have seemed to indicate that a score of 7 points or less is nearly always compatible with salvageable limb.[119] Although the scale was developed for lower extremity applications, one publication has demonstrated, based on retrospective application, that it may also be useful for the upper extremity.[230] Other attempts at more comprehensive scaling of the individual tissue injury in the limb have not been widely accepted, probably due to complexity.[99]

These scales are particularly useful in guiding the clinician to think about all the major factors that may be relevant for a successful salvage of the limb. They are not the complete answer to the dilemma in the majority of clinical situations, however. The assignment of the critical number for the soft-tissue injury (0–4) requires great experience and judgment—it will always remain a subjective assessment based on these elements. The severity of the bone injury and what it will take to get union in terms of morbidity and the status of the tibial nerve based on a visual assessment of the injury[134,135] are just two of many components that must figure heavily into the assignment of points for soft-tissue injury. Unlisted factors that have a major influence include smoking history, nutritional status, and arteriosclerosis. Job requirements and educational level also must be considered. Therefore, it seems clear that scales will never be more than a helpful framework. Consultation with the team captain among experienced clinicians who understand what reconstructive procedures and recovery times will be necessary is the most effective way of making this deci-

TABLE 2-6
Mangled Extremity Severity Score (MESS) Variables

Factor	Points
A. Skeletal/soft tissue injury	
• Low energy (stab, simple fracture, low-velocity gunshot wound)	1
• Medium energy (open or multiple fractures, dislocation)	2
• High-energy (close-range shotgun or high-velocity gunshot wound, crush injury)	3
• Very high energy (above plus gross contamination, soft tissue avulsion)	4
B. Limb ischemia	
• Pulse reduced or absent but perfusion normal	1
• Pulseless; paresthesias, diminished capillary refill	2
• Cool, paralyzed, insensate	3
*score doubled for ischemia >6 hours	
C. Shock	
• Systolic blood pressure always >90 mm Hg	0
• Hypotension transiently	1
• Persistent hypotension	2
D. Age	
• <30 y	0
• 30–50 y	1
• >50 y	2

sion. After the conclusion is reached, the injury should be carefully photographed and detailed notes from the various clinicians involved should be placed in the medical record in case the decision-making process is later questioned.

INJURY CLASSIFICATION SYSTEMS AND DATA SYSTEMS

Müller and associates[168] have stated that a classification system is "useful only if it considers the severity of the bone lesion and serves as a basis for treatment and for evaluation of the results." In terms of communication between members of the treatment team, it is apparent that clinicians are better off using descriptors than classification schemes because of their apparent unreliability.[34,88,227,228] It remains to be seen whether fracture or soft-tissue injury severity as measured by scales in common use are important predictors of clinical or functional outcome because they have been so rarely accompanied by these types of relevant data in the published literature. Some recent data call this predicted association into question, thereby bringing forth the possibility that such factors as educational level, general health, and mental outlook play as important a role in the ultimate outcome as the particulars of the injury do.[146,147] We need, however, injury severity classification systems to study these associations and to increase the usefulness of the published literature for pooling published results.[50]

To study the effect of injury severity on clinical and functional outcomes for groups of patients, fracture and soft-tissue severity scales must be available. Fracture classification scales have been widely proliferated and generally not validated. It has been the trend for each author to publish new classification systems with each retrospective review. Colton[50] has pointed out the hazards of this prolific approach. The literature becomes increasingly difficult to use in a comparative sense, thus severely limiting the usefulness of aggregate data. The worse case identified is that of fractures of the olecranon, with 22 different scales having been published.[50] A more rationale approach would be to have a broadly accepted lexicon analogous to the International Classification of Disease, 9th revision, codes but specific for fractures and soft-tissue injury. The Orthopaedic Trauma Association has taken the lead in developing such a consensus-based document. This system has not been validated as being predictive of either injury severity or outcome. The concept for this scheme is to be used either primarily or as a supplemental classification for future publications of articles related to musculoskeletal injury. It may be wise for editors of relevant journals to consider this a requirement for publication. The goal is to enhance the usefulness of the published literature by consistently using the same system. This will help with retrospective analysis of published cases and with planning future prospective trials.

Many injury classification schemes have been systematically studied regarding intraobserver and interobserver variability. A partial list includes the Neer classification of proximal humerus fractures, the Evans classification of intertrochanteric fractures, and the Gustilo classification for open fractures.[34,88,103,104,227,228] These systems have all been found to be lacking in terms of interobserver consistency, bringing criticism from editors and authors alike. They are thought to be "bad systems," and many individuals believe they can be improved upon. On closer study, it seems they are not "bad systems." Rather, this is a problem of trying to force a continuous variable (the infinite number of possibilities for fracture pattern and soft-tissue injury in each region) into a dichotomous variable (the classification). Because of the limitless variability in injuries, judgments are required to categorize them according to any classification scheme. Increasing reliability regarding this task occurs with clinician experience; however, it rarely exceeds 70% reproducibility. This problem will not be addressed by developing new classification systems but rather by improved methods for applying the most accepted systems. The optimum method of applying these systems for publication is blinded (to clinical result and treatment group, if possible) assessment of the radiographs or clinical photographs (or videotapes) with patient identifiers removed, by three to four individuals of the highest level of experience that is practical. The results of the classification should then be statistically analyzed; and where there is lack of agreement, the consensus method should be used to develop the categorization with each member of the assessment team arguing his or her rationale for placing the injury in a particular category. This more scientific methodology allows for optimum use of any injury classification scheme.

MEASUREMENT OF OUTCOMES

Trauma Registries

As defined by the American College of Surgeons Committee on Trauma Resources for Optimal Care of the Injured Patient, the trauma registry forms the backbone for the evaluation of effectiveness and quality for each institution's trauma program.[51,265] Details regarding the data elements that should be collected are provided in this document. The critical elements used to monitor the trauma program include timing of prehospital care, mechanism of injury, vital signs in the field and on arrival, and outcome measures, such as ventilator days, days in an intensive care unit, and mortality. This concept of quality assessment or "end result measurement" stems from the seminal work of Codman in 1934, who suggested that all hospitals should have a good handle on their patient outcomes so the effectiveness of care from the physician and institutional aspects could be improved.[49] Much later in the century, cancer registries began to be developed to go about the business of systematically measuring the effectiveness of chemotherapy and radiation therapy protocols.[59] To deal with widespread difference of opinion as to what trauma registries should monitor,[28] the Centers for Disease Control (given the responsibility for studying prevention and treatment of the disease of injury) convened a lengthy workshop on trauma registries in 1988.[192,193] Participants included organizations with major interest in the field, such as the American College of Surgeons Committee on Trauma, the American College of Emergency Physicians, the American Medical Association's Committee on Emergency Medical Services, and the National Highway Traffic Safety Administration. Patient inclusion criteria and core data elements were defined by consensus methodology.[192] Further development sponsored by the American College of Surgeons has led to the development of a standardized preformatted software package available to all institutions for trauma program monitoring.[172] Before this development, many institutions had created their own registries and several states (Pennsylvania, Oregon) and Canadian provinces had successfully implemented state-wide programs.[261] By 1992, 48% of states had implemented trauma registries.[226] The ACS Tracs system in the future will save important registry development costs for institutions and regional systems.[172]

Controversy exists regarding the inclusion or exclusion of lower energy trauma cases into comprehensive regional trauma system registries. Many of patients with an ISS of less than 10 are elderly patients with limited physiologic reserve and are at risk for significant morbidity and even mortality from these lower energy injuries.[33] Because of this high potential for long-term disability and the fact that populations throughout the world are aging, it is believed to be appropriate to include cases with lower levels of injury into these surveillance registries. This will increase their usefulness as injury prevention tools in addition to serving the other key functions of quality assessment and monitoring of outcome for this population.[104,247,272,273]

In many hospital systems, discharge databases form a critical source for data elements for the trauma registry. The addition of the "E Codes" (injury mechanism codes) to the universally applied diagnosis-related groups (DRGs) and ICD-9 codes has greatly enhanced the usefulness of this data source for trauma registries.[178,234] These data combined with ISS[9,10] and length of stay, mortality, and resource utilization information make the hospital discharge database a useful tool for monitoring trauma programs.[261] It is anticipated that the use of standardized databases for the monitoring of trauma programs[172] will, because of uniformity of data collection, allow for greater ease of monitoring for regional and statewide systems. These data are important to monitor programs that have been established in response to US Public Law 101-590—the Trauma Care Systems and Planning Act of 1990.

Trauma registries and discharge databases use as their measure of injury severity the ISS, which grew out of the AIS (see Tables 2-1 and 2-2).[9,10] Although analysis of this data element has proven useful for analysis of resource utilization for hip fractures in large populations,[272] the level of detail regarding musculoskeletal injury is insufficient. Critical components of injury severity such as soft-tissue injury detail and fracture classification as well as details of treatment and, most critically, non–mortality-based clinical outcomes are totally lacking. This has led the Orthopaedic Trauma Association to develop a software package, available to its membership, that allows tracking of more detailed skeletal and soft-tissue injury information, details regarding treatment, and a patient-based outcome module inclusive of relevant clinical outcomes (eg, range of motion, fracture union) and health status.[96,236] This type of decentralized data collection tool is absolutely key toward developing information on the effectiveness of management strategies for musculoskeletal injury.

Resources are required to use such registries in a trauma center, proportional to the volume of patients seen. Data forms are most accurately completed by the most senior individuals who are available in terms of injury classification and treatment description. "Buy in" is required by the departmental chief and members of the attending staff for the registry to be comprehensive for the institution. Data entry clerks are required to enter data and obtain complete information when forms are lacking. New software programs are available from the Orthopaedic Trauma Association that allow the surgeon to directly enter data, thus bypassing the forms. In general, one clerk is required for 1500 orthopaedic injuries per year, and more are needed if radiographs are being stored with the injury data. A research coordinator is necessary to develop a program to systematically obtain functional outcome data as a routine. It is strongly suggested that specific research questions or quality assurance program issues be studied using this approach. Routinely obtaining functional outcome data on all trauma patients is expensive and impractical, resulting in the collection of huge volumes of data that will not be used for any meaningful analysis. In essence, because of the broad range of injury in terms of bone and soft-tissue severity dealt with in the field of musculoskeletal traumatology, the only way to gather sufficient cases to study outcome is with multicenter study designs. The use of the decentralized database format will become the necessary linking component allowing all centers to collect the same data in the same format, thus greatly enhancing data management.

Outcome Assessment

Orthopaedic clinical research has focused on outcomes relevant to the practitioner and not the patient. The published clinical literature regarding management of musculoskeletal injury is retrospective in design with rare exception and is focused on these "clinical outcomes."[262] These include traditional orthopaedic measures such as range of motion, alignment, stability, and radiographic assessments. This relative lack of controlled trials in the entire field of orthopaedics has made the definition of optimum management strategies impossible. Even in the most highly investigated areas of the field such as joint replacement, deficiencies are severe. Both Gartland[85] and Gross[100] have confirmed that research regarding hip arthroplasty is "process based," meaning that it is focused on elements important to the technical aspects of the procedure (eg, cement lucency, dislocation rates) and not on the effect of the procedure on patient function. This paucity of patient-oriented data is true for injured patients as well. When these data are assessed, important and interesting findings are the result.[14,114] It is the opinion of many informed researchers that it is this fundamental lack of "end-result" information, relevant to patient function, that is responsible for the variations in medical and orthopaedic practice that have become so apparent in recent years.[128,266] Improvement in the situation will mandate new emphasis on clinical trial methodology in studying musculoskeletal injury, and where this is not feasible due to low incidence conditions, standardized outcome assessment (multicenter) is used whenever possible.[220] Outcome assessment must include relevant clinical outcomes important to the process of care as well as patient-derived, health-oriented outcomes generally obtained by questionnaire.[127] Additionally, improved training for clinician researchers in the appropriate use of statistics must be undertaken.[262]

The retrospective clinical literature is replete with scales used to divide patient results into good, fair, or poor. These scales are surgeon derived, are rarely used in more than one retrospective review, and have internal weighting for scoring (eg, relative value of pain to that of range of motion, alignment, and so on) that is determined by the author and not by patient input.[67,238] This lack of the use of well-validated scales has further served to undermine the usefulness of the literature for the assessment of efficacy of injury treatment strategies. The lack of adequate numbers of randomized trials for most topics in orthopaedics makes the technique of meta-analysis to determine effectiveness issues unavailable.[132,133,253]

Several well-validated health status instruments have been developed and are available for use in assessing patient function after musculoskeletal injury. The four most widely used and evaluated scales that are appropriate for use in musculoskeletal disease or injury are the Short Form-36 (SF-36), Sickness Impact Profile (SIP), Nottingham Health Profile, and the Quality of Well-Being Scale (QWB), which forms the backbone of the Quality Adjusted Life Years (QALYs) methodology.[273] These scales share the common characteristic of assessing all "domains" of human activity inclusive of physical, psychological, social, and role functioning. Additionally, they share the characteristic of assessing the patient as a whole (from the patient's perspective) and not as an organ system, disease, or limb. They are internally consistent, are reproducible, can discriminate between clinical conditions of different severity, and are sensitive to change in health status over time.[140] There are added benefits derived from the fact that they are not physician administered, which increases their reliability. Brief descriptions of these instruments follow.

The SF-36 was developed by Ware and associates and the Rand corporation as a part of the Medical Outcomes Study.[235,242] It is perhaps the most widely applied general health status instrument and has certain features that make it the most appealing for studying musculoskeletal injury. Its 36 scaled questions relate to six different functional subscales: bodily pain, role function (physical and mental health), social function, physical function, energy/fatigue, and general health perceptions. The scales are scored separately, and there is no aggregate scale, a feature that seems to limit its usefulness somewhat. It has been validated to be a reliable and reproducible questionnaire that has been applied to numerous health conditions. Furthermore, it has been validated to be reliable as administered by the patient, by interviewer, by telephone, and by mail; it takes 5 to 7 minutes to complete. These features make its use appealing; it is the most practical for use in a busy office or clinic setting. This instrument may well have a "floor effect" for musculoskeletal conditions, however. This means that clinically important functional problems may not be adequately characterized by this scale—the disability is too minimal to be picked up by the questions in the scale. This scale is more often recommended to researchers who wish to study musculoskeletal injury than the other scales discussed here.

The SIP has 136 endorsable statements and was developed by Bergner and associates at the University of Washington. It is best administered by trained interviewers and takes 25 to 35 minutes to complete.[17,18] It has 12 different domains, which are addressed by the endorsable statements (the patient simply affirms yes or no if the statement of function applies to his or her current situation). These 12 areas are scored independently and aggregated into a physical and a psychosocial subscale as well as one aggregate score. The scale is 0 to 100 points; the higher the score, the worse the disability. Scores in excess of the mid-30s bring into question whether the patient is better off not living. The SIP, too, has been used in multiple health conditions that make comparisons of impact of disease on health possible. It has been used in musculoskeletal trauma with good success.[146,147] Because of the difficulty and length of administration it may be most useful for well-funded outcome studies or controlled trials. It is likely that it also suffers from the "floor effect" of lesser degrees of musculoskeletal function not being picked up.

The Nottingham Health Profile is interviewer administered and has been successfully used to assess functional outcomes of limb salvage versus early amputation.[90,157,158] It has been shown to be valid in trials in Great Britain and Sweden. Part I of the profile measures subjective health status through a series of 38 weighted questions that assess impairments in the categories of sleep, emotional reaction, mobility, energy level, pain, and social isolation. In each category 100 points represents maximal disability and 0 represents no limitations. Part II consists of seven statements that require yes or no responses. These assess the influence of health problems on job, home, family life, sexual function recreation, and enjoyment of the holidays. The responses to both parts of the profile can be compared to the average scores for the population as a whole with similar age and sex distributions.

The QWB is the foundation for QALYs and was designed to be a commonly used effectiveness measure for policy analysis and resource allocation. Patients are asked to respond to questions regarding their level of physical activity (three levels), mobility (three levels), and social activity (5 levels) and according to the one symptom or problem that bothers them the most on the day the questionnaire is administered (choice of 22 symptom complexes). The QWB is calculated by combining preference weights that were derived from responses to a household survey that asked respondents to rate their preferences for various health states on a 1 to 10 scale, ranging from death to perfect health. Multiple QWB scores are calculated separately for each of 6 days preceding the interview, and the final score is taken as the average of the 6 scores. The scale ranges from 0 equals death to 1 equals perfect health. The QWB is interviewer administered. By using data from large populations and multiplying times years of life expectancy and cost per intervention gives the QALY, which is the cost per year of well life expectancy. The QALY provides a methodology for making difficult decisions regarding resource allocation. When orthopaedic interventions such as hip arthroplasty and hip fracture fixation have been studied using this methodology, they have fared well.[184] The QWB physical function scale also likely suffers from the "floor effect."

The National Institutes of Health has sponsored the development of a musculoskeletal functional scale that is widely applicable to musculoskeletal injury and disease. The Musculoskeletal Functional Assessment Instrument (MFAI) is being validated, and it is anticipated that incremental improvement will be made in avoiding the floor effect these other general health status instruments suffer from.[154] It is anticipated that a long 100-item scale that can be interviewer administered or mail or telephone administered, takes 15 to 17 minutes to complete, and is most appropriate for controlled trials will be the end product. A separate short form of 30 to 40 items, validated for the same modes of administration, will be the second product. It is anticipated that the shorter instrument will have wide appeal for office-based assessments and for multicenter outcomes assessments where efficiency and cost are major issues.

ACKNOWLEDGMENTS

The author appreciates the helpful review and input from Gregory Jurkovich, MD, and the editorial assistance of Renee Schurtz.

REFERENCES

1. Aebi, M., Mohler, J., Zach, G.A., and Morscher, E.: Indication, Surgical Techniques and Results of 100 Surgically Treated Fractures and Fracture-Dislocations of the Cervical Spine. Clin. Orthop., 203:244–257, 1986.
2. Alberts, K.A., Noren, I., Rubin, M., and Torngren, S.: Respiratory Distress Following Major Trauma: Predictive Value of Blood Coagulation Tests. Acta Orthop. Scand., 57:58–262, 1986.
3. American Association of Trauma Surgery Policy Statement: Managed Care and the Trauma System, May 1994.
4. Anderson, P.A., and Bohlman, H.H.: Anterior Decompression and Arthrodesis of the Cervical Spine: Long Term Motor Improvement: I and II. J. Bone Joint Surg., 74A:671–692, 1992.
5. Apprahamian, C., Gessert, G., Bandyk, D.F., Bell, L., Stiehl, J., and Olson, D.W.: MAST-Associated Compartment Syndrome (MACS): A Review. J. Trauma, 29:549–555, 1989.
6. Apprahamian, C., Wolferth, C.C., Darin, J.C., McMahon, J., and Weitzel-DeVeas, C.: Status of Trauma Center Designation. J. Trauma, 29:566–570, 1989.
7. Baker, J., Deitch, E., Li, M., Berg, R., and Specian, R.: Hemorrhagic Shock Induced Bacterial Translocation From the Gut. J. Trauma, 28:896–906, 1988.
8. Baker, S.P.: Injuries: The Neglected Epidemic. Stone Lecture, 1985 American Trauma Society Meeting. J. Trauma, 27:343–348, 1987.
9. Baker, S.P., and O'Neill, B.: The Injury Severity Score: An Update. J. Trauma, 16:882–885, 1976.
10. Baker, S., O'Neill, B., and Haddlon, W.: The Injury Severity Score: A Method for Describing Patients With Multiple Injuries

and Evaluating Emergency Care. J. Trauma, 14:187–196, 1974.
11. Balk, R.A., Jacobs, R.F., Tryka, A.F., Townsend, J.W., Walls, R.C., and Bone, R.C.: Effects of Ibuprofen on Neutrophil Function and Acute Lung Injury in Canine Shock. Crit. Care Med., 16:1121–1127, 1988.
12. Baxt, W.G., and Moody, P.: The Impact of Advanced Pre Hospital Emergency Care on the Mortality of Severely Brain-Injured Patients. J. Trauma, 27:365–369, 1987.
13. Behrman, S.W., Fabian, T.C., Kudsk, K.A., et al.: Improved Outcome With Femur Fractures: Early Versus Delayed Fixation. J. Trauma, 30:792–798, 1990.
14. Benirschke, S.K., Melder, I., Henley, M.B., et al.: Closed Interlocking Nailing of Femoral Shaft Fractures: Assessment of Technical Complications and Functional Outcomes by Comparison of a Prospective Database With Retrospective Review. J. Orthop. Trauma, 7:118–122, 1993.
15. Ben-Menachem, Y., Coldwell, D.M., Young, J.W.R., and Burgess, A.R.: Hemorrhage Associated With Pelvic Fractures: Causes, Diagnosis and Emergent Management. Am. J. Radiol., 157:1005–1014, 1991.
16. Benzel, E.C., and Larson, S.J.: Recovery of Nerve Root Function After Complete Quadriplegia From Cervical Spine Fractures. Neurosurgery, 19:809–812, 1986.
17. Bergner, M., Bobbitt, R.A., Carter, W.B., et al.: The Sickness Impact Profile: Development and Final Revision of a Health Status Measure. Med. Care, 19:787–805, 1981.
18. Bergner, M., Bobbitt, R.A., Pollaro, W.E., et al.: The Sickness Impact Profile: Validation of a Health Status Measure. Med. Care, 14:57–67, 1976.
19. Bickell, W.H., Wall, M.J., Pepe, P.E., et al.: Immediate Versus Delayed Fluid Resuscitation for Hypotensive Patients With Penetrating Torso Injuries. N. Engl. J. Med., 331:1105–1109, 1994.
20. Blachut, P.A., Meek, R.N., and O'Brien, P.J.: External Fixation and Delayed Intramedullary Nailing of Open Fractures of the Tibial Shaft. J. Bone Joint Surg., 72A:729–735, 1990.
21. Blaisdell, F.W., and Lewis, F.R., Jr. (eds.): Respiratory Distress Syndrome of Shock and Trauma in Post-traumatic Failure. Philadelphia, WB Saunders, 1977.
22. Bohlman, H.H.: Acute Fractures and Dislocations of the Cervical Spine. J. Bone Joint Surg., 61A:1119–1142, 1979.
23. Bondurant, F., Cotler, H.B., Buckle, R., Miller-Crotchett, P., and Browner, B.D.: The Medical and Economic Impact of Severely Injured Lower Extremities. J. Trauma, 28:1270–1273, 1988.
24. Bone, L.B., and Bucholz, R.: The Management of Fractures in the Patient with Multiple Trauma. J. Bone Joint Surg., 68A:945–949, 1986.
25. Bone, L.B., Johnson, K.D., Weigelt, J., and Scheinbeng, R.: Early Versus Delayed Stabilization of Fractures: A Prospective Randomized Study. J. Bone Joint Surg., 71A:336–340, 1989.
26. Bone, L.B., McNamara, K., Shine, B., and Border, J.: Mortality in Multiple Trauma Patients with Fractures. J. Trauma, 37:262–265, 1994.
27. Border, J.R., Hansen, S.T., Jr., Reudi, T.P., and Allgower, M.: Bacterial Growth and Infections: Antibiotics and Other Effective Measures. *In* Border, J. R. (ed.): Blunt Multiple Trauma: Comprehensive Pathophysiology and Care. New York, Marcel Dekker, 1990.
28. Boyd, D.R.: Trauma Registries Revisited (Editorial). J. Trauma, 25:186–187, 1985.
29. Boyd, C.R., Tolson, M.A., and Copes, W.S.: Evaluating Trauma Care: The TRISS Method. J. Trauma, 27:370–378, 1987.
30. Bracken, M.B., Shepard, M.J., Collins, W.F., et al.: A Randomized Controlled Trial of Methylprednisolone or Naloxone in the Treatment of Spinal Cord Injury. N. Engl. J. Med., 322:1405–1411, 1990.
31. Broos, P.L.O., Stappaerts, K.A., Luiten, E.S.T., and Gruwez, J.A.: The Importance of Early Internal Fixation in Multiply Injured Patients to Prevent Late Death due to Sepsis. Injury, 18:235–237, 1987.
32. Broos, P., Vanderschot, P., Craninx, L., and Reynders, P.: Internal Hemorrhages Associated With Fractures of the Pelvic Girdle: Importance of Early Stabilization With an External Fixator. Acta Orthop. Belg., 59:130–138, 1993.
33. Brotman, S., McMinn, D.L., Copes, W.S., Rhodes, M., Leonard, D., and Konvolinka, C.W.: Should Survivors With an Injury Severity Score Less Than 10 Be Entered in a Statewide Trauma Registry? J. Trauma, 31:1233–1239, 1991.
34. Brumback, R.J., and Jones, A.L.: Interobserver Agreement in the Classification of Open Fractures of the Tibia: The Results of a Survey of Two Hundred and Forty-five Orthopaedic Surgeons. J. Bone Joint Surg., 76A:1162–1166, 1994.
35. Bucholz, R.W. (ed.): Orthopaedic Decision Making.
36. Buerger, P.M., Peoples, J.B., Lemmon, G.W., and McCarthy, M.C.: Risk of Pulmonary Emboli in Patients With Pelvic Fractures. Am. Surg., 59:505–508, 1993.
37. Bull, J.P.: The Injury Severity Score of Road Traffic Casualties in Relation to Mortality, Time of Death, Hospital Treatment Time and Disability. Accid. Anal. Prev., 7:249–255, 1975.
38. Cales, R., and Trunkey, D.: Preventable Trauma Deaths: A Review of Trauma Care Systems Development. J.A.M.A., 254:1059–1063, 1985.
39. Carragee, E.J., and Csongradi, J.J.: Increased Rates of Complications in Patients With Severe Ankle Fractures Following Institutional Transfers. J. Trauma, 35:767–771, 1993.
40. Carroll, G.C., Tuman, K.J., Braverman, B., et al.: Minimal Positive End-Expiratory Pressure (PEEP) May Be "Best PEEP." Chest, 93:1020–1025, 1988.
41. Caudle, R.J., and Stern, P.J.: Severe Open Fractures of the Tibia. J. Bone Joint Surg., 69A:801–807, 1987.
42. Champion, H.R., Copes, W.S., Sacco, W.J., et al.: The Major Trauma Outcome Study: Establishing National Norms for Trauma Care. J. Trauma, 30:1356–1365, 1990.
43. Champion, H.R., Sacco, W.J., Hannan, D.S., et al.: Assessment of Injury Severity: The Triage Index. Crit. Care Med., 8:201–208, 1980.
44. Champion, H.R., and Teter, H.: Trauma Care Systems: The Federal Role. J. Trauma, 28:877–879, 1988.
45. Chan, K.M., Tham, K.T., Chiu, H.S., Chow, Y.N., and Leung, P.C.: Post-traumatic Fat Embolism: Its Clinical and Subclinical Presentations. J. Trauma, 24:45–49, 1984.
46. Christensen, K.S.: Pneumatic Antishock Garments (PASG): Do They Precipitate Lower-Extremity Compartment Syndromes? J. Trauma, 26:1102–1105, 1986.
47. Christie, J., Burnett, R., Potts, H.R., and Pell, A.H.C.: Echocardiography of Transatrial Embolism During Cemented and Uncemented Hemiarthroplasty of the Hip. J. Bone Joint Surg., 76B:409–412, 1994.
48. Claudi, B.F., and Meyers, M.H.: Priority in the Treatment of the Multiply Injured Patient With Musculoskeletal Injuries. *In* Meyers, M.H. (ed.): The Multiply Injured Patient With Complex Fractures, pp. 3–8. Philadelphia, Lea & Febiger, 1984.
49. Codman, E.A.: The End Result Concept. *In* The Shoulder, pp. 1–29. Malaber, Fla., Kreiger, 1934.
50. Colton, C.L.: Telling the Bones (Editorial). J. Bone Joint Surg., 73B:362–364, 1991.
51. Committee on Trauma, American College of Surgeons, eds. Resources for the Optimal Care of the Injured Patient. Chicago, American College of Surgeons, 1990.
52. Committee on Trauma, American College of Surgeons, eds. Advanced Trauma Life Support Manual. Chicago, American College of Surgeons, 1993.
53. Committee on Trauma Research: Injury in America: A Continuing Public Health Problem. Washington, D.C., National Academy Press, 1985.
54. Copes, W.S., Champion, H.R., Sacco, W.J., Lawnick, M.M., Keast, S.L., and Bain, L.W.: The Injury Severity Score Revisited. J. Trauma, 28:69–77, 1988.
55. Court-Brown, C.M.: Care of Accident Victims. Br. Med. J. 298:115–116, 1989.
56. Court-Brown, C.M.: The Treatment of the Multiply Injured Patient in the United Kingdom. J. Bone Joint Surg., 72B:345–346, 1990.
57. Cowley, R.A., Hudson, F., and Scanlan E: An economical and proved helicopter program. J. Trauma, 13:1029–1038, 1973.
58. Cryer, H.G., Richardson, J.D., Longmire-Cook, S., and Brown,

C.M.: Oxygen Delivery in Patients With Adult Respiratory Distress Syndrome in Patients Who Undergo Surgery. Arch. Surg., 124:1378–1385, 1989.
59. Cutler, S.J., and Latourette, H.B.: A National Cooperative Program for the Evaluation of End Results in Cancer. J. Natl. Cancer Inst., 22:633–646, 1959.
60. Dalal, S., Burgess, A.R., Siegel, J., et al.: Pelvic Fracture in Multiple Trauma: Classification by Mechanism is the Key to Pattern of Organ Injury, Resuscitative Requirements and Outcome. J. Trauma, 29:981–1002, 1989.
61. DeBastiani, G., Mosconi, F., Spagnol, G., Nicolanto, A., Ferrari, S., and Aprili, F.: High Calcitonin Levels in Unconscious Polytrauma Patients. J. Bone Joint Surg., 74B:01–104, 1992.
62. Deitch, E.A., and Bridges, R.M.: Effect of Stress and Trauma on Bacterial Translocation From the Gut. J. Surg. Res., 42:536–542, 1987.
63. Dellinger, E.P., Caplan, E., Weaver, L., et al.: Duration of Preventative Antibiotic Administration for Open Extremity Fractures (Double Blind Prospective). Arch. Surg., 123:333–339, 1988.
64. Dellinger, E., Miller, S., Wertz, M., Grypma, M., Droppert, B., and Anderson, P.: Risk of Infection After Open Fracture of the Arm or Leg. Arch. Surg., 123:1320–1327, 1988.
65. DeMaria, E.J., Kenney, P.R., Merriam, M.A., Casanova, L.A., and Gann, D.S.: Aggressive Trauma Care Benefits the Elderly. J. Trauma, 27:1200–1206, 1987.
66. Denis, F.: The Three Column Spine and Its Significance in the Classification of Acute Thoracolumbar Spinal Injuries. Spine, 8:817–831, 1983.
67. Deyo, R.A., Inui, T.S., Leninger, J.D., and Overman, S.S.: Measuring Functional Outcomes in Chronic Disease: A Comparison of Traditional Scales and a Self-Administered Health Status Questionnaire in Patients With Rheumatoid Arthritis. Med. Care, 21:180–192, 1983.
68. Donohue, J.H., Federle, M.P., Griffiths, B.G., et al.: Computed Tomography in the Diagnosis of Blunt Intestinal and Mesenteric Injuries. J. Trauma, 27:11–17, 1987.
69. Dosett, A.B., Hunt, J.L., Purdue, G.F., and Schlegel, J.D.: Early Orthopedic Intervention in Burn Patients With Major Fractures. J. Trauma, 31:888–893, 1991.
70. Eastman, A., Lewis, F. Jr,, Champion, H., and Mattox, K.: Regional Trauma System Design: Critical Concepts. Am. J. Surg., 154:79, 1987.
71. Eastman, A.B., Rice, C.L., Bishop, G.S., and Richardson, J.D.: An Analysis of the Critical Problem of Trauma Center Reimbursement. J. Trauma, 31:920–926, 1991.
72. Elasser, J.D., Moyer, C.F., and Lesker, P.A.: Improved Healing of Rabbit Osteotomies via Delayed Fixation. J. Trauma, 15:869–876, 1975.
73. Emery, M.A., and Murakomi, H.: Fracture Healing in Cats After Immediate and Delayed Open Reduction. J. Bone Joint Surg., 49B:571–579, 1967.
74. Eriksson, E., Wallin, C.: Immediate or Delayed Kuntscher Rodding of Femoral Shaft Fractures? Orthopedics, 9:201–204, 1986.
75. Fabian, T.C.: Unraveling the Fat Embolism Syndrome. N. Engl. J. Med., 329:961–962, 1993.
76. Fabian, T.C., Hoots, A.V., Stanford, D.S., Patterson, C.R., and Mangiante, E.C.: Fat Embolism Syndrome: Prospective Evaluation in 92 Fracture Patients. Crit. Care Med., 18:42–46, 1990.
77. Fabian, T.C., Mangiante, E.C., White, T.J., Patterson, C.R., Boldreghini, S., and Britt, L.G.: A Prospective Study of 91 Patients Undergoing Both Computed Tomography and Peritoneal Lavage Following Blunt Abdominal Trauma. J. Trauma, 26:602–608, 1986.
78. Fakhry, S.M., Rutledge, R., Dahners, L.E., and Kessler, D.: Incidence, Management and Outcome of Femoral Shaft Fracture: A Statewide Population-Based Analysis of 2805 Adult Patients in a Rural State. J. Trauma, 37:255–261, 1994.
79. Fortner, G.S., Oreskovich, M.R., Copass, M.K., and Carrico, C.J.: The Effects of Prehospital Trauma Care on Survival From a 50-Meter Fall. J. Trauma, 23:976–981, 1983.
80. Fortune, J.B., Feustel, P.J., Saifi, J., Stratton, H.H., Newell, J.C., and Shah, D.M.: Influence of Hematocrit on Cardiopulmonary Function After Acute Hemorrhage. J. Trauma, 27:243–249, 1987.
81. Francel, P.C., Long, B.A., Malik, J.M., Tribble, C., Jane, J.A., and Kron, I.L.: Limiting Ischemic Spinal Cord Injury Using a Free Radical Scavenger 21-Aminosteroid and/or Cerebrospinal Fluid Drainage. J. Neurotrauma, 79:742–751, 1993.
82. Froehlich, J.A., Dorfman, G.S., Cronan, J.J., Urbanek, P.J., Herndon, J.H., and Aaron, R.K.: Compression Ultrasonography for Detection of Deep Venous Thrombosis in Patients Who Have a Fracture of the Hip: A Prospective Study. J. Bone Joint Surg., 71A:249–256, 1991.
83. Ganong, R.B.: Fat Emboli Syndrome in Isolated Fractures of the Tibia and Femur. Clin. Orthop., 291:208–214, 1993.
84. Ganz, R., Krushell, R.J., Jakob, R.P., and Kuffer, J.: The Antishock Pelvic Clamp. Clin. Orthop., 267:71–78, 1991.
85. Gartland, J.J.: Orthopaedic Clinical Research: Deficiencies in Experimental Design and Determination of Outcome. J. Bone Joint Surg., 70A:1357–1364, 1988.
86. Gbaandor, G.B.M., Dunham, C.M., Rodriguez, A., et al.: Does Pulmonary Contusion Contribute to Mortality in Multiple Injured Patients? Panam. J. Trauma, 2:26, 1990.
87. Geerts, W.H., Code, K.I., Jay, R.M., Chen, E., and Szalai, J.P.: A Prospective Study of Venous Thromboembolism After Major Trauma. N. Engl. J. Med., 331:1601–1606, 1994.
88. Gehrchen, P.M., Nielson, J.O., and Olesen, B.: Poor Reproducibility of Evans Classification of the Trochanteric Fracture: Assessment of Four Observers in Fifty-two Cases. Acta Orthop. Scand., 64:71–72, 1993.
89. Geisler, F.H., Dorsey, F.C., and Coleman, W.P.: Recovery of Motor Function After Spinal Cord Injury: A Randomized, Placebo-Controlled Trial With GM-1 Ganglioside. N. Engl. J. Med., 324:1829–1838, 1991.
90. Georgiadis, G.M., Behrens, F.F., Joyce, M.J., Earle, A.S., and Simmons, A.L.: Open Tibial Fractures With Severe Soft Tissue Loss–Limb Salvage Compared With Below Knee Amputation. J. Bone Joint Surg., 75A:1431–1441, 1993.
91. Gokcen, E.C., Burgess, A.R., Sigel, J.H., Mason-Gonzalez, S., Dischinger, P.D., and Ho, S.M.: Pelvic Fracture: Mechanism of Injury in Vehicular Trauma Patients. J. Trauma, 36:789–796, 1994.
92. Goldstein, A., Phillips, T., Sclafani, S.J., et al.: Early Open Reduction and Internal Fixation of the Disrupted Pelvic Ring. J. Trauma, 26:325–333, 1986.
93. Gomez, G.A., Alvarez, R., Plasencia, G., et al.: Diagnostic Peritoneal Lavage in the Management of Blunt Abdominal Trauma: A Reassessment. J. Trauma, 27:1–5, 1987.
94. Goris, R.J.A., Gimbere, J.S.F., Van Neikerk, J.L.M., Schoots, F.J., and Booy, L.H.: Early Osteosynthesis and Prophylactic Mechanical Ventilation in the Multitrauma Patient. J. Trauma, 22:895–903, 1982.
95. Gossling, H.R., and Pellegrini, V.D.: Fat Embolism Syndrome: A Review of the Pathophysiogy and Physiological Basis of Treatment. Clin. Orthop., 165:68–82, 1982.
96. Graef, R.: Synthes USA, 1690 Russell Road, Paoli, PA 19301, 1-800-345-1272.
97. Greenfield, L.J., Peyton, R., Crute, S., and Barnes, S.: Greenfield Vena Caval Filter Experience. Arch. Surg., 116:1451–1456, 1981.
98. Greenspan, L., McLellan, B.A., and Greig, H.: Abbreviated Injury Scale and Injury Severity Score: A Scoring Chart. J. Trauma, 22:60–64, 1985.
99. Gregory, R.T., Gould, R.J., Peclet, M., et al.: The Mangled Extremity Syndrome (MES): A Severity Grading System for Multisystem Injury of the Extremity. J. Trauma, 5:1147–1150, 1985.
100. Gross, M.: A Critique of the Methodologies Used in Clinical Studies of Hip Joint Arthroplasty Published in the English Literature. J. Bone Joint Surg., 70A:1364–1371, 1988.
101. Gruen, G.S., Leit, M.E., Gruen, R.J., and Peitzman, A.B.: The Acute Management of Hemodynamically Unstable Multiple Trauma Patients With Pelvic Ring Fractures. J. Trauma, 36:706–713, 1994.
102. Gustilo, R.B., and Anderson, J.T.: Prevention of Infection in

the Treatment of One Thousand and Twenty-five Open Fractures of Long Bones. J. Bone Joint Surg., 58A:453–458, 1976.
103. Gustilo, R.B., Corpuz, V., and Sherman, R.E.: Epidemiology, Mortality, and Morbidity in Multiple Trauma Patients. Orthopedics, 8:1523–1528, 1985.
104. Gustilo, R.B., Mendoza, R.M., and Williams, D.N.: Problems in the Management of Type III (Severe) Open Fractures: A New Classification of Type III Open Fractures. J. Trauma, 24:742–746, 1984.
105. Hansen, S.: Concomitant Fractures in Long Bones. *In* Meyers, M. (ed.): The Multiply Injured Patient With Complex Fractures, pp. 401–411. Philadelphia, Lea & Febiger, 1984.
106. Hansen, S.T., Jr.: The Type IIIC Tibial Fracture: Salvage or Amputation? (Editorial) J. Bone Joint Surg., 69A:799–800, 1987.
107. Hardin, G.T.: Timing of Fracture Fixation: A Review. Orthop. Rev. Supp., 19:861–867, 1990.
108. Heary, R.F., Hunt, C.D., Krieger, A.J., Antonio, C., and Livingston, D.H.: Acute Stabilization of the Cervical Spine by Halo/Vest Application Facilitates Evaluation and Treatment of Multiple Trauma Patients. J. Trauma, 33:445–451, 1992.
109. Heckman, J.D. (ed.): Emergency Care and Transportation of the Sick and Injured, 5th ed, pp. 260–311. Chicago, American Academy of Orthopaedic Surgeons, 1992.
110. Henderson, A., Coyne, T., Wall, D., and Miller, B.: A Survey of Interhospital Transfer of Head-Injured Patients With Inadequately Treated Life-Threatening Extracranial Injuries. Aust. N.Z. J. Surg., 62:759–762, 1992.
111. Hervé, C., Gaillard, M., and Huguenard, P.: Early Medical Care and Mortality in Polytrauma. J. Trauma, 27:1279–1285, 1987.
112. Hofman PAM, Goris RJA: Timing of Osteosynthesis of Major Fractures in Patients With Severe Brain Injury. J. Trauma, 31:261–263, 1991.
113. Holting, T., Buhr, H.J., Richter, G.M., Roeren, T., Friedl, W., and Herfarth, C.: Diagnosis and Treatment of Retroperitoneal Hematoma in Multiple Trauma Patients. Arch. Trauma Surg., 111:323–326, 1992.
114. Horne, G., Iceton, G., Twist, J., and Malony, R.: Disability Following Fractures of the Tibial Shaft. Orthopedics, 13:423–426, 1990.
115. Hurst, A.M., Obeid, F.N., Sorenson, V.J., and Bivins, B.A.: Factors Influencing Survival of Elderly Trauma Patients. Crit. Care Med., 14:681–684, 1986.
116. Inderbitizi, R., Ludi, D., Luder, P., and Stirnemann, P.: Significance of Rib Fractures in Simple and Multiple Trauma. Helv. Chir. Acta, 57:791–797, 1991.
117. Jeanneret, B., and Holdener, H.J.: Vertebral Fractures and Abdominal Trauma: A Retrospective Study Based on 415 Documented Vertebral Fractures. Unfallchirurg, 95:603–607, 1992.
118. Jensen, J.E., Jensen, T.G., Smith, T.K., Johnson, D.A., and Dudrick, S.J.: Nutrition in Orthopaedic Surgery. J. Bone Joint Surg., 64A:1263–1272, 1982.
119. Johansen, K., Daines, M., Howey, T., Helfet, D., and Hansen, S.T., Jr.: Objective Criteria Accurately Predict Amputation Following Lower Extremity Trauma. J. Trauma, 30:568–573, 1990.
120. Johnson, K.D., Cadambi, A., and Seibert, G.B.: Incidence of Adult Respiratory Distress Syndrome in Patients With Multiple Musculoskeletal Injuries: Effect of Early Operative Stabilization of Fractures. J. Trauma, 25:375–384, 1985.
121. Jollis, J.G., Peterson, E.D., DeLong, E.R., et al.: The Relation Between the Volume of Coronary Angioplasty Procedures at Hospitals Treating Medicare Beneficiaries and Short-Term Mortality. N. Engl. J. Med., 331:1625–1629, 1994.
122. Julien, M., Lemoyne, B., Denis, R., and Malo, J.: Mortality and Morbidity Related to Severe Intrapulmonary Shunting in Multiple Trauma Patients. J. Trauma 27:970–973, 1987.
123. Jurkovich, G.J.: The Role of the Trauma Surgeon in the Management of Orthopaedic Trauma. *In* Hansen, S.T., Jr., and Swiontkowski, M.F. (eds.): Trauma Protocols. New York, Raven Press, 1993.
124. Kallenbach, J., Lewis, M., Zaltzman, M., Feldman, C., Orford, A., and Zwi, S.: "Low-Dose" Corticosteroid Prophylaxis Against Fat Embolism. J. Trauma, 27:1173–1176, 1987.
125. Kandel, G., and Aberman, A.: Mixed Venous Oxygen Saturation: Its Role in the Assessment of the Critically Ill Patient. Arch. Intern. Med., 143:1400–1402, 1983.
126. Karpos, P.A.G., McFerran, M., and Johnson, K.D.: Intramedullary Nailing of Acute Femoral Shaft Fractures Using Manual Traction Without a Fracture Table. J. Orthop. Trauma, 9:57–62, 1995.
127. Keller, R.B.: Outcomes Research in Orthopaedics. J. Am. Acad. Orthop. Surg., 1:122–129, 1993.
128. Keller, R., Soule, D.N., Wennberg, J.E., and Hanley, D.F.: Dealing With Geographic Variations in the Use of Hospitals: The Experience of the Maine Medical Assessment Foundation Orthopaedic Study Group. J. Bone Joint Surg., 72:1286–1293, 1990.
129. Kohler, A., Friedl, H.P., Kach, K., Stocker, R., and Trentz, O.: Patient Management in Polytrauma With Injuries of the Cervical Spine. Helv. Chir. Acta, 60:547–550, 1994.
130. Knudson, M.M., Collins, J.A., Goodman, S.B., and McCrory, D.W.: Thromboembolism Following Multiple Trauma. J. Trauma, 32:2–11, 1992.
131. Kreis, D., Plasencia, G., Augenstein, D., et al.: Preventable Trauma Deaths: Dade County, Florida. J. Trauma, 26:649–654, 1986.
132. L'Abbé, K.A., Detsky, A.S., and O'Rourke, K.: Meta-analysis in Clinical Research. Ann. Intern. Med., 107:224–233, 1987.
133. Labelle, H., Guibert, R., Joncas, J., Newman, N., Fallaha, M., and Rivard, C.H.: Lack of Scientific Evidence for the Treatment of Lateral Epicondylitis of the Elbow: An Attempted Meta-analysis. J. Bone Joint Surg., 74:646–651, 1992.
134. Lange, R.H.: Limb Reconstruction Versus Amputation Decision Making in Massive Lower Extremity Trauma. Clin. Orthop., 243:92–99, 1989.
135. Lange, R.H., Bach, A.W., Hansen, S.T., and Johansen, K.: Open Tibial Fractures With Associated Vascular Injuries: Prognosis for Limb Salvage. J. Trauma, 25:203–207, 1985.
136. Latenser, B.A., Gentillelo, L.M., Tarver, A.A., Thalgott, J.S., and Batdorf, J.W.: Improved Outcome With Early Fixation of Skeletally Unstable Pelvic Fractures. J. Trauma, 31:28–31, 1991.
137. Lazarou, S.A., Barbul, A., Wasserkrug, H.L., and Efron, G.: The Wound Is a Possible Source of Post-traumatic Immunosuppression. Arch. Surg., 124:1429–1431, 1989.
138. Levy, D.L.: The Fat Embolism Syndrome: A Review. Clin. Orthop., 261:281–286, 1990.
139. Lhowe, D.W., and Hansen, S.T.: Immediate Nailing of Open Fractures of the Femoral Shaft. J. Bone Joint Surg., 70A:812–820, 1988.
140. Liang, M.H., Fossel, A.H., and Larson, M.G.: Comparisons of Five Health Status Instruments for Orthopaedic Evaluation. Med. Care, 28:632–642, 1990.
141. Lindeque, B.G.P., Schoeman, H.S., Dommisse, G.F., Boeyens, M.C., and Vlok, A.L.: Fat Embolism and the Fat Embolism Syndrome: A Double Blind Therapeutic Study. J. Bone Joint Surg., 69B:128–131, 1987.
142. Loder, T.T.: Pediatric Polytrauma: Orthopaedic Care and Hospital Course. J. Orthop. Trauma, 1:48–54, 1987.
143. Lowe, D.K., Gately, H.L., Gross, J.R., Frey, C.L., and Peterson, C.G.: Patterns of Death, Complications and Error in Management of Motor Vehicle Accident Victims: Implications for a Regional System of Trauma Care. J. Trauma, 23:503, 1983.
144. Luft, H., Bunker, J., and Enthoven, A.: Should Operations be Regionalized? The Empirical Relation Between Surgical Volume and Mortality. N. Engl. J. Med., 301:1364–1369, 1979.
145. MacKenzie, E.J.: Injury Severity Scales: Overview and Directions for Future Research. Am. J. Emerg. Med., 2:537–549, 1984.
146. MacKenzie, E.J., Burgess, A.R., McAndrew, M.P., et al.: Patient-Oriented Functional Outcome After Unilateral Lower Extremity Fracture. J. Orthop. Trauma, 7:393–401, 1993.
147. MacKenzie, E.J., Cushing, B.M., Jurkovich, G.J., et al.: Physical Impairment and Functional Outcomes Six Months After Severe Lower Extremity Fractures. J. Trauma, 34:528–539, 1993.
148. MacKenzie, E.J., Morris, J.A., Smith, G.S., and Fahey, M.:

Acute Hospital Costs of Trauma in the United States: Implications for Regionalized Systems of Care. J. Trauma, 30:1096–1101, 1990.
149. Malawer, M., and Zielinsky, C.: Emergency Hemipelvectomy in the Control of Life-Threatening Complications. Surgery, 93:778–785, 1983.
150. Malisano, L.P., Stevens, D., and Hunter, G.A.: The Management of Long Bone Fractures in the Head-Injured Polytrauma Patient. J. Orthop. Trauma, 8:1–15, 1994.
151. Manning, J.B., Bach, A.W., Herman, C.M., and Carrico, C.J.: Fat Release After Femur Nailing in the Dog. J. Trauma, 1983; 23:322–326.
152. Manoli, A., Fakhouri, A.J., and Weber, T.G.: Concurrent Compartmental Syndromes of the Foot and Leg. Foot Ankle, 14:339–342, 1993.
153. Marks, J.D., Shapara, A., Kraemer, R.W., and Katz, J.A.: Pressure and Flow Limitations of Anesthesia Ventilators. Anesthesiology, 71:403–408, 1989.
154. Martin, D., Engelberg, R., Carter, W., et al.: Development of the Musculoskeletal Functional Assessment Instrument. J. Orthop Res, in press.
155. Mattox, K.L., Bickell, W.H., Pepe, P.E., Mangelsdorff, A.D.: Prospective Randomized Evaluation of Antishock MAST in Post-traumatic Hypotension. J. Trauma, 26:779–786, 1986.
156. McCarthy, B., Mammen, E., LeBlanc, L.P., et al.: Subclinical Fat Embolism: A Prospective Study of 50 Patients With Extremity Fractures. J. Trauma, 13:9, 1976.
157. McDowell, I, and Newell, C. (eds.): Measuring Health: A Guide to Rating Scales and Questionnaires, pp. 125–133. New York, Oxford University Press, 1987.
158. McEwen, J.: The Nottingham Health Profile; A Measure of Perceived Health. *In* Teeling-Smith, G. (ed.): Measuring the Social Benefits of Medicine, pp. 75–84. London, Office of Health Economics, 1983.
159. Meek, R., Vivoda, E., and Pirani, S.: A Comparison of Mortality in Patients With Multiple Injuries According to the Method of Fracture Treatment: A Retrospective Age- and Injury-Matched Series. Injury, 17:2–4, 1986.
160. Mendez, C., Gubler, D., and Maier, R.V.: Diagnostic Accuracy of Peritoneal Lavage in Patients With Pelvic Fractures. Arch. Surg., 129:477–482, 1994.
161. Miller, J.D., Jones, P.A., Dearden, N.M., and Tocher, J.L.: Progress in the Management of Head Injury. Br. J. Surg., 79:60–64, 1992.
162. Miller, R.D., Robbins, T.O., Tong, M.J., and Barton, S.L.: Coagulation Defects Associated With Massive Blood Transfusion. Ann. Surg., 174:794–801, 1971.
163. Morris, J.A., Auerbach, P.S., Marshall, G.A., Bluth, R.F., Johnson, L.G., and Trunkey, D.D.: The Trauma Score as a Triage Tool in the Prehospital Setting. J.A.M.A., 256:1319–1325, 1986.
164. Morris, J.A., Sanchez, A.A., Bass, S.M., and MacKenzie, E.J.: Trauma Patients Return to Productivity. J. Trauma, 31:827–834, 1991.
165. Müller, C., Frigg, R., and Pfister, U.: Effect of Flexible Drive Diameter and Reamer Design on the Increase of Pressure in the Medullary Cavity During Reaming. Injury 3(Suppl. 24):S40–S47, 1993.
166. Müller, C., McIff, T., Rahn, B.A., Pfister, U., and Weller, S.: Intramedullary Pressure, Strain on the Diaphysis and Increase in Cortical Temperature When Reaming the Femoral Medullary Cavity—A Comparison of Blunt and Sharp Reamers. Injury, 3(Suppl.):S22–S30, 1993.
167. Müller, C., Rahn, B.A., Pfister, U., and Meinig, R.P.: The Incidence, Pathogenesis, Diagnosis and Treatment of Fat Embolism. Orthop. Rev., 107–117, 1994.
168. Müller, M.E., Nazarian, S., Koch, P., and Scatzker, J.: The Comprehensive Classification of Fractures of Long Bones. Berlin, Springer Verlag, 1990.
169. Myllynen, P., Kammonen, M., Rokkanen, P., Bostman, O., Lalla, M., and Laasonen, M.D.: Deep Venous Thrombosis and Pulmonary Embolism in Patients With Acute Spinal Cord Injury: A Comparison With Nonparalyzed Patients Immobilized due to Spinal Fractures. J. Trauma, 25:541–543, 1985.
170. Nast-Kolb, D., Waydhas, C., Jochum, M., Spannagl, M., Oswald, K.H., and Schweiberer, L.: Gunstiger Operationszeitpunkt fur die Verzorgung von Femurschaftfrakturen beim Polytrauma? Chirurg, 61:259–265, 1990.
171. National Safety Council: Accident Facts. Chicago, 1990.
172. National Tracs, 55 E. Erie St., Chicago, IL 60611, 1-800-435-3590.
173. Norwood, S.H., and Civetta, J.M.: The Adult Respiratory Syndrome. Surg. Gynecol. Obstet., 161:497–508, 1985.
174. Nuytinck, J., Goris, R., Weerts, J., Schillings, P.H., and Stekhoven, J.K.: Acute Generalized Microvascular Injury by Activated Complement and Hypoxia: The Basis of the Adult Respiratory Distress Syndrome and Multiple Organ Failure? Br. J. Exp. Pathol., 67:537–548, 1986.
175. Ornato, J., Craren, E., Nelsonk, N., Kimball, K.: Impact of Improved Emergency Medical Services and Emergency Trauma Care on Reduction in Mortality From Trauma. J. Trauma, 25:575–579, 1985.
176. Ostrum, R.F., Verghese, G.B., and Santner, T.J.: The Lack of Association Between Femoral Shaft Fractures and Hypotensive Shock. J. Orthop. Trauma, 7:338–342, 1993.
177. Pahud, B., and Vasey, H.: Delayed Internal Fixation of Femoral Shaft Fractures: Is There an Advantage? J. Bone Joint Surg., 69B:391–394, 1987.
178. Pal, J., Brown, R., and Fleiszer, D.: The Value of the Glasgow Coma Scale and ISS: Predicting Outcome in Multiple Trauma Patients With Head Injury. J. Trauma, 29:746–751, 1989.
179. Panetta, T., Scalafani, S., Goldstein, A.S., Phillips, T.F., and Shaftan, G.W.: Percutaneous Transcatheter Embolization for Massive Bleeding From Pelvic Fractures. J. Trauma 25:1021–1029, 1985.
180. Pape, H.C., Auf'm'Kolk, M., Paffrath, T., Regel, G., Sturm, J.A., and Tscherne, H.: Primary Intramedullary Fixation in Polytrauma Patients With Associated Lung Contusion—A Cause of Post-traumatic ARDS? J. Trauma, 34:540, 1993.
181. Pape, H.C., Dwenger, A., Regel, G., et al.: Pulmonary Damage After Intramedullary Femoral Nailing in Traumatized Sheep—Is There an Effect From Different Nailing Methods? J. Trauma, 33:574–581, 1992.
182. Pape, H.C., Regel, G., Dwenger, A., et al.: Influences of Different Methods of Intramedullary Femoral Nailing on Lung Function in Patients With Multiple Trauma. J. Trauma, 35:709–716, 1993.
183. Pape, H.C., Regel, G., Dwenger, A., Sturm, J.A., and Tsherne, H.: Influence of Thoracic Trauma and Primary Femoral Intramedullary Nailing on the Incidence of ARDS in Multiple Trauma Patients. Injury, 3(Suppl.):S82–S103, 1993.
184. Parker, M.J., Myles, J.W., Anand, J.K., and Drewett, R.: Cost-Benefit Analysis of Hip Fracture Treatment. J. Bone Joint Surg., 74B:261–264, 1992.
185. Peitzman, A.B., Makaroun, M.S., Slasky, B.S., and Ritter, P.: Prospective Study of Computed Tomography in Initial Management of Blunt Abdominal Trauma. J. Trauma, 26:585–592, 1986.
186. Pelias, M.E., Townsend, M.C., and Flancbaum, L.: Long Bone Fractures Predispose to Pulmonary Dysfunction in Blunt Chest Trauma Despite Early Operative Fixation. Surgery, 111:576–579, 1992.
187. Pell, A.H.C., Christie, J., Keating, J.F., and Sutherland, G.R.: The Detection of Fat Embolism by Transesophageal Echocardiography During Reamed Intramedullary Nailing: A Study of 24 Patients With Femoral and Tibial Fractures. J. Bone Joint Surg., 75B:921–925, 1993.
188. Pell, A.H.C., Hughes, D., Keating, J., et al.: Brief Report: Fulminating Fat Embolism Syndrome Caused by Paradoxical Embolism Through a Patent Foramen Ovale. N. Engl. J. Med., 329:926–929, 1993.
189. Pennal, G.F., Tile, M., Waddell, J.P., and Garside, H.: Pelvic Disruption: Assessment and Classification. Clin. Orthop., 151:12–21, 1980.
190. Petrucelli, E.: Seat Belt Laws: The New York Experience—Preliminary Data and Some Observations. J. Trauma, 27:706–710, 1987.
191. Phillips, T.F., Contreras, D.M.: Timing of Operative Treatment

Hematoma: Direct Admission to a Trauma Center Yields Improved Results. J. Trauma, 26:445–450, 1986.

238. Swiontkowski, M.F., and Chapman, J.R.: Cost and Effectiveness Issues in Care of Injured Patients. Clin. Orthop., in press.

239. Swiontkowski, M.F., Winquist, R.A., and Hansen, S.T.: Fractures of the Femoral Neck in Patients Between the Ages of Twelve and Forty-Nine Years. J. Bone Joint Surg., 66A:837–846, 1984.

240. Tait, G.R., Rowles, J.M., Kirsh, G., Martindale, J.P., and Learmonth, D.J.: Delayed Diagnosis of Injuries From the M1 Aircraft Accident. Injury, 22:475–478, 1991.

241. Talucci, R.C., Manning, J., Lampard, S., Bach, A., and Carrico, C.J.: Early Intramedullary Nailing of Femoral Shaft Fractures: A Cause of Fat Embolism Syndrome. Am. J. Surg., 146:107–111, 1983.

242. Tarlov, A.R., Ware, J.E., Greenfield, S., Nelson, E.C., Perrin, E., and Zubkoff, M.: The Medical Outcomes Study: An Application of Methods for Monitoring the Results of Medical Care. J.A.M.A., 262:925–930, 1989.

243. Teasdale, G., and Jennett, B.: Assessment of Coma and Impaired Consciousness: A Practical Scale. Lancet, 2:81–84, 1974.

244. ten Duis, H.J., Nijsten, M.W.N., Klausen, H.J., and Binnendijk, B.: Fat Embolism in Patients With an Isolated Fracture of the Femoral Shaft. J. Trauma, 28:383–390, 1987.

245. Tideiksaar, R.: Geriatric Falls: Assessing the Cause, Preventing Recurrence. Geriatrics, 44:57–61, 1989.

246. Tile, M.: Pelvic Ring Fractures: Should They Be Fixed? J. Bone Joint Surg., 70B:1–12, 1988.

247. Tinetti, M.E., Speechley, M., and Ginter, S.F.: Risk Factors for Falls Among Elderly Persons Living in the Community. N. Engl. J. Med., 319:1701–1707, 1988.

248. Trauma Care Systems: Position Paper, Third National Injury Control Conference: Setting the National Agenda for Injury Control in the 1990's. Atlanta, US Department of Health and Human Services, Centers for Disease Control, 1991.

249. Traverso, L.W., Lee, W.P., and Langford, M.J.: Fluid Resuscitation After an Otherwise Fatal Hemorrhage: Crystalloid Solutions. J. Trauma, 26:168–175, 1986.

250. Trunkey, D.D.: Trauma Care Systems. Emerg. Med. Clin. North Am., 2:913, 1990.

251. Trunkey, D.D.: Trauma. Sci. Am., 249:28–35, 1983.

252. Trunkey, D.D., and Lim, R.: Analysis of 425 Consecutive Trauma Fatalities: An Autopsy Study. J. Am. Coll. Emerg. Phys., 3:1364–1369, 1974.

253. Turner, J.A., Ersek, M., Herron, L., and Deyo, R.: Surgery for Lumbar Spinal Stenosis: Attempted Meta-analysis of the Literature. Spine, 17:1–8, 1992.

254. Valeri, C.R., Feingold, H., Cassidy, G., Ragno, G., Khuri, S., and Altschule, M.D.: Hypothermia-Induced Reversible Platelet Dysfunction. Ann. Surg., 205:175–181, 1987.

255. vanAllst, J.A., Morris, J.A., Yeats, H.K., Miller, R.S., and Bass, S.M.: Severely Injured Geriatric Patients Return to Independent Living: A Study of Factors Influencing Function and Independence. J. Trauma, 31:1096–1102, 1991.

256. van Os, J.P., Roumen, R.M.H., Schoots, F.J., Heystraten, F.M.J., and Goris, R.J.A.: Is Early Osteosynthesis Safe in Multiple Trauma Patients With Severe Thoracic Trauma and Pulmonary Contusion? J. Trauma, 36:495–498, 1994.

257. Vaughn, S., and Puri, V.K.: Cardiac Output Changes and Continuous Mixed Venous Oxygen Saturation Measurement in the Critically Ill. Crit. Care Med., 16:495–498, 1988.

258. Ve'csei, V., Trojan, J., Euler, F., et al.: Der Zeitpunkt der Osteosynthese von Extremitatenfrakturen bei Scwerem Schadelhirn-trauma. Hefte Unfallheilk., 132:263–267, 1978.

259. Vedder, N., Fouty, B., Winn, R., Harlan, J., and Rice, J.: Role of Neutrophils in Generalized Reperfusion Injury Associated With Resuscitation From Shock. Surgery, 106:509–516, 1989.

260. Veith, R.G., Winquist, R.A., and Hansen, S.T.: Ipsilateral Fractures of the Femur and Tibia: A Report of Fifty-Seven Consecutive Cases. J. Bone Joint Surg., 66A:991–1002, 1984.

261. Vestrup, J.A., Phang, T., Vertresi, L., Wing, P.C., and Hamilton, N.E.: The Utility of a Multicenter Regional Trauma Registry. J. Trauma, 37:375–378, 1994.

262. Vrbos, L.A., Lorenz, M.A., Peabody, E.H., and McGregor, M.: Clinical Methodologies and Incidence of Appropriate Statistical Testing in Orthopaedic Spine Literature: Are Statistics Misleading? Spine, 18:1021–1029, 1993.

263. Waddell, T.K., Kalman, P.G., Goodman, S.J.L., and Girotti, M.J.: Is Outcome Worse in a Small Volume Canadian Trauma Center? J. Trauma, 31:858–961, 1991.

264. Ward, W.G., and Nunley, J.A.: Occult Orthopaedic Trauma in the Multiply Injured Patient. J. Orthop. Trauma, 5:308–312, 1991.

265. Weddel, J.M.: Registers and Registries: A Review. Int. J. Epidemiol., 2:221–228, 1973.

266. Wennberg, J., and Gittelsohn, A.: Small Area Variations in Health Care Delivery. Science, 182:1102–1108, 1973.

267. Winquist, R.A., Hansen, S.T., and Clawson, D.K.: Closed Intramedullary Nailing of Femoral Fractures: A Report of Five Hundred and Twenty Cases. J. Bone Joint Surg., 166A:529–539, 1984.

268. Weigelt, J., Mitchell, R., and Snyder, W.: Early Positive End-Expiratory Pressure in the Adult Respiratory Distress Syndrome. Arch. Surg., 114:497–501, 1979.

269. Wenda, K., Ritter, G., Degrief, J., et al.: Zur Genese Pulmonaler Komplikationen nach Marknagelosteosynthesen. Unfallchirurg, 91:432, 1988.

270. West, J.G., Cales, R.H., and Gazzinga, A.B.: Impact of Regionalization: the Orange County Experience. Arch. Surg., 118:740, 1983.

271. West, J.G., Trunkey, D.D., and Lim, R.C.: Systems of Trauma Care: A Study of Two Counties. Arch. Surg., 114:455, 1979.

272. White, B.L., Fisher, W.D., and Laurin, C.A.: Rate of Mortality for Elderly Patients After Fracture of the Hip in the 1980's. J. Bone Joint Surg., 69A:1335–1340, 1987.

273. Williams, A.: Setting Priorities in Health Care: An Economist's View. J. Bone Joint Surg., 73B:365–367, 1991.

274. Wolff, G., Dittman, M., Ruedi, T., et al.: Koordination von Chirurge und Intensivmedizin zur Vermeidung der Posttraumatischen Respiratorischen Insuffizienz. Unfallheilkunde, 81:425–442, 1978.

275. Wozasek, G.E., Simon, P., Redl, H., and Schlag, G.: Intramedullary Pressure Changes and Fat Intravasation During Intramedullary Nailing: An Experimental Study in Sheep. J. Trauma, 36:202–207, 1994.

276. Xue, H., Zhang, Y.-F.: Pulmonary Fat Embolism in Rabbits Induced by Forced Immobilization. J. Trauma, 32:415–419, 1992.

277. Young, J.W.R., Burgess, A.R., Brumbach, R.J., and Poka, A.: Pelvic Fractures: Value of Plain Radiography in Early Assessment and Management. Radiology, 160:445–451, 1986.

Rockwood and Green's Fractures in Adults, Fourth Edition,
edited by Charles A. Rockwood, David P. Green, Robert W. Bucholz and James D. Heckman.
Lippincott-Raven Publishers, Philadelphia © 1996.

CHAPTER 3

Principles of Internal Fixation

Robert W. Chandler

FUNDAMENTAL BIOMECHANICAL AND SURGICAL PRINCIPLES

Historical Perspective

The history of internal fixation of fractures is long and its beginning somewhat hazy (Table 3-1). The first recorded medical history until the mid 1800s can be considered to be the time of nonoperative fracture management because of the lack of safe and effective surgical technology.[113,115,331,473] Operative intervention during this phase of history consisted of caring for open fractures, and the result was often a severe infection.[331] Painful pseudarthrosis was one of the few indications for open surgery of fractures.[473]

TABLE 3-1
Chronology of Internal Fixation

Date	Contribution (Author-Originator)
1861	Silver wire ORIF patella (Cooper)
1870	Advocate of internal fixation (Féraud)
1877	Silver wire ORIF of Closed Patella Fracture (Lister)
1886	Plate and screw fixation removable percutaneously (Hansmann)
1889	CRIF hip fractures fixation with bone peg (Senn)
1892	ORIF with screws and wires (Lane)
1893	Promoted internal fixation: Intermedullary pegs, Ferrule (Senn)
1893	Ivory pegs and clamps for internal fixation (Bircher)
1897	Promoted ORIF for Irreducible fractures (Ransohoff)
1900	ORIF tibial fractures: silver plates, galvanized steel screws (Steinbach)
1901	Used barbed staples for fractures (Jacoel)
1904	Temporary fixation with small nails (Niehans)
1904	Abduction and casting of femoral neck fractures (Whitman)
1906	Discussed technical problems of internal fixation (Martin)
1907	Closed reduction internal fixation using AP Xrays and bone peg +/− screw (Delbet)
1907	Lane Plate (Lane)
1907	Developed and promoted internal fixation methods (Lambotte)
1912	106 patients treated with wires, nails, screws, dowels, pins, and plates (Blake)
1912	Plate fixation of diaphyseal fractures (Beckman)
1912	Intramedullary pegs (Hey-Groves)
1912	Vanadium steel bone plates and self tapping screws. (Sherman)
1912	ORIF of femoral neck fractures through two incisions using bone peg (Albee)
1913	Silver pins foreclosed I. M. fixation of forearm fractures under fluoroscopy (Schone)
1913	I. M. nailing (Nicholaysen)
1913	Forearm Nailing (Schone)
1913	Flexible threaded pins and nuts used as cerclage (Milne)
1914	Oval hole modified Lane plate for compression after resorption at the fracture (MacLean)
1914	Nail plate combination for hip fractures (Preston)
1914	Narrow bands used as cerclage (Putti)
1916	Cerclage with bands (Parham)
1916	IM fixation, interfragmentary fixation, double onlay plates, curved plates (Hey-Groves)
1918	Intramedullary nailing (Hey-Groves)
1923	Closed reduction, percutaneous fixation with two wood screws (Martin)
1924	Treatment of femoral neck fractures 306 cases with union in 67% (Lofberg)
1925	Trans articular pinning of metacarpal fractures (Lambotte)
1929	Manchon or muff, a collar to surround bone ends (Contremoulins)
1930	ORIF femoral neck fractures with ivory, beef bone, or autogenous graft (Hey-Groves)
1931	Triflanged nail for ORIF of femoral neck fractures (Smith-Petersen)
1932	Orthopaedic table, Xrays, for femoral neck fractures care (Hawley)
1932	Cannulated nail and percutaneous nailing (Johansson)
1932	Use of external compression device for arthrodesis of knee (Key)
1933	I. M. Fixation (Müller & Meernach)
1934	Screw bolt device for hip fixation (Henry)
1934	Closed reduction and percutaneous fixation under image control (Wescott)
1934	Connected Smith-Petersen nail to a side plate (Thornton)
1935	Multiple small pin fixation of hip fractures (Gaenslen)
1935	Multiple small pins for hip fractures (Telson & Ransohoff)
1935	Concepts of tension band fixation applied to bone (Pauwels)
1936	Small screws with nuts for hip fractures (Knowles)
1936	Intramedullary Steinmann pins (Rush)
1937	I. M. Fixation of diaphysis (Chigot)
1937	Specialized small screws for femoral neck fractures, adjustable (Moore)
1938	Studied pressure as related to bone mechanics (Glucksmann)
1940	Extensive research and development of intramedullary surgery (Kuntscher)
1940	Intramedullary Kirschner wires (Lambrinudi)
1941	Smith-Petersen nail joined to a Hawley side plate (Jewett)
1943	Extendable bone plate, oval hole to allow manual impaction (Townsend & Gilfian)
1944	Single piece nail plate device for proximal femoral fractures (Neufeld)
1944	Three nails for femoral neck fractures (Nystrom)
1945	Depth Gauge (Flanagan)
1948	Slotted Plate. Believed compression aided bone healing. Internal splint idea (Eggers)
1948	Positive pressure for arthrodesis (Charnley)
1949	Improvement in compression hip screw (Danis)
1949	Axial compression with coapteurs, compression and rigid fixation (Danis)
1949	Corkscrew bolt for hip fractures (Lippmann)
1950	Precise technique of screw application (Petersen)
1950	Sliding nail plate (Pohl)
1950	Solid femoral nail (Street)
1951	Inboard compression device (Venable)

continues

TABLE 3-1
***Chronology of Internal Fixation** (continued)*

Date	Contribution (Author-Originator)	Date	Contribution (Author-Originator)
1952	Optimum pressure across an osteotomy 12–18 lbs., >30 lbs. caused necrosis (Friedenberg)	1958	Telescoping nail plate device (Massie)
1952	Triflanged tibial nail (Lottes)	1958	Injected medullary polyurethane polymer with reinforcing rods (Mandarino & Salvatore)
1952	Dual plates for compression osteosynthesis (Boreau & Hermann)	1958	Formation of AO/ASIF Group in 1958 to develop internal fixation (Müller)
1953	Perforated cruciate, locking nail (Modney)	1959	Multiple small nails through plate with impaction for femoral neck fractures (Deyerle)
1955	Self adjusting nail plate for hip fractures (Pugh)	1964	Wide clinical application of tension band methods (Weber)
1955	Sliding hip nail plate (Schumpelick & Jantzen)	1972	Locking reamed I. M. Nailing (Klemm & Schellmann)
1956	Self compression plate (Bagby)	1972	Use of Methacrylate and metal for fracture fixation (Harrington)
1957	I. M. nailing of forearm fractures (Sage)		
1957	Self compressing hip screw and plate (Charnley)		

From Peltier, L.: Fractures: A History and Iconography of their Treatment. San Francisco: Norman Publishing. 273, 1990.

By the time of the Civil War, amputation was recommended for fractures caused by gunshot.[185] Immobilization of the injured extremity was by means of wood splints, braces of leather, and gypsum-impregnated gauze. The doctrine of immobilization of a joint above and a joint below the fracture became gospel. Long bone fractures of the lower extremity such as the femur were treated in extension as a position of rest and with traction as a means of realignment. Kirschner wires and Steinmann pins were developed for techniques of traction rather than for internal fixation.[394]

Not until the mid-19th century did innovation in internal fixation methods begin to appear with some regularity.[394] From about 1860 until the mid-20th century, virtually all contemporary internal fixation methods were developed in some form, and basic scientific aspects of fracture healing were studied (see Table 3-1). Intensive efforts to improve operative technique and implant materials occurred in the second half of the 20th century, with an emphasis on perfecting methods that were created earlier. Improved outcome in terms of reliability and function with the least complication is the goal of internal fixation. In most areas throughout the world, not only risk-benefit analysis is considered but increasingly, cost-benefit analysis.

Biology of Bone and Fracture Relative to Internal Fixation

Fundamental understanding of biologic and mechanical aspects of fracture repair is key to selection of fracture management techniques. Fracture management is guided by results of laboratory research that is related to cellular biology, vascular physiology, and biomechanics.* Microcirculation of bone and soft tissues has been studied in intact and in fractured bone. Much of the basic research on internal fixation and fracture healing is focused on the effects of fixation on the vascular supply of bone and the study of the interplay between mechanics and healing.

One major area of interest has been the association of fracture healing and motion at the fracture site. The perceived association of motion and healing for a long time created a dichotomy of treatment, in which one school of thought believed that fracture motion produced union, whereas the other believed that motion impeded union. A basic unifying theory was proposed by Perren based on a complex relation between fracture gap size, strain across the gap, and the ability of diverse cells types to proliferate and differentiate according to level of strain.[399,403] Strain refers to the mechanical force that produces elongation and is represented as a change in length divided by original length. Only with low strain across a fracture gap (less than 2%) does bone form. The orderly progression from blood clot to mature remodeled bone in a fracture crevice is governed by strain, such that primitive mesenchymal cells differentiate into fibroblasts, which lay down a collagen matrix, reducing strain and allowing further differentiation of cell types, culminating in bone-producing elements. Low strain and no gap creates direct formation of bone or primary healing, whereas large gaps and low strain promotes callus or secondary bone formation.

Mechanical testing of bone formed under such differing mechanical environments revealed qualitative

---

* References 28, 251, 270, 282, 372, 374, 397, 399–403, 422, 424, 425, 483, 495–498, 522–524.

and quantitative differences. Compacting of fragments having no gap combined with a rigid implant (typically a plate) results in low gap-strain and represents compression fixation. At the other extreme, larger gaps in combination with a comparatively flexible implant lowers strain equally. Primary healing occurs with rigid compression fixation (plate) and callus formation or secondary healing occurs in the gap-flexible fixation model.

Fracture stabilization through external support, such as casts, braces, and external fixators, and internal fixation are all forms of splintage. Rigidity of the bone-fixation construct is a complex continuum, ranging from freely moving bone ends having essentially zero stiffness to rigidly fixed fracture fragments having tight bone contact, small gaps, and compression loading. Internal fixation in this chapter is approached as though there were two discrete regions on the continuum: rigid compression fixation and noncompression fixation. Attempts to prove superiority of one method over another have been overshadowed and dominated by the clinical success and reliability of both—a testament to the vitality of bone.

Classification

Fracture classification systems are beneficial in planning treatment and comparing results. Many classification systems have arisen is the past few years, which helps the clinician to understand the fracture, communicate with others, select treatment, and if surgery is to be performed, select the operative incision and plan reconstruction. Müller has presented a complete and systemic classification that is based largely on morphology, which lends itself readily to computerization because of its complete symbolic representation.[359] The Orthopaedic Trauma Association also has developed a useful classification system based on ICD-9 codes and Hennepin County Medical Center trauma registry codes.[190]

Approach to Internal Fixation

Hans Willenegger, one of the founders of the Association for the Study of Internal Fixation (ASIF), recognized the importance of judgment regarding operative indication because he promoted excellence of treatment, whether operative or nonoperative. When the basic tenets of internal fixation are observed correctly, reliable and predictable outcome is attainable. Weber, defining the foundation for successful application of internal fixation wrote that "Crucial to the success of these techniques (internal fixation) are: (a) an appropriate indication, (b) observance of correct biomechanical principles, and (c) strict aseptic technique."[71] These critical elements form the basis of this chapter.

Indications for Operative Treatment

Superior Outcome

Closed intramedullary nailing of the femoral shaft fracture is not only cost-effective but also produces a superior result in terms of patient comfort and functional outcome.[263,286] Similarly, few disagree that fractures of both bones of the forearm in adults or Monteggia's and Galeazzi's fractures are unlikely to be handled adequately by closed methods, so that open reduction and internal fixation is the method of choice.[269,272,328,349] Fractures of the femoral neck would be poorly treated by traction or plaster immobilization. The list of such fractures having superior outcome with internal fixation has grown substantially during the past three decades and is discussed in greater detail in the chapters that follow.

Failure of Closed Methods

Closed management techniques fail in the hands of even the most skilled clinician in a certain percentage of cases. If the bone fragments are impaled in soft tissues, if a secondary displacement occurs, or if bony apposition and adequate alignment cannot be achieved, an operation is indicated. Commonly, fractures of the distal radius are prone to secondary displacement and need realignment and fixation. Stubborn committment to an unsuccessful initial nonoperative plan despite failure to restore adequate position of the fracture is not in the patient's best interest. Factors other than the fracture alone must be considered when constructing a treatment plan.

Articular Fractures

Even minor incongruities in the articular surfaces of joints result in loss of function and the eventual appearance of degenerative arthritis. Anatomic reduction, rigid stabilization, and rapid mobilization is recommended for many joint fractures.† Criteria of acceptable reduction are converging on a 1-mm standard.

Pathologic Fractures

Pathologic fractures include the following: primary and secondary tumors, osteopenia, and failed replacement arthroplasty.‡ Internal fixation of pathologic

† References 45, 136, 164, 197, 217, 259–261, 271, 273, 278, 312, 325, 337, 339, 340, 416, 433, 441, 470, 489, 491, 506, 534.

‡ References 10, 13, 31, 56, 89, 95, 131, 144, 180, 194, 195, 198, 204, 206, 250, 344, 418.

fractures from tumor relieves pain, improves nursing care, and often allows the patient to return home and spend precious time with his or her family in relative comfort. Special internal fixation techniques are generally required to overcome deficiencies in bone quality and quantity. Use of allograft combined with acrylics and metal (composite fixation) is necessary for some of these problems. In many such cases, fixation may act as a prosthesis if the local biologic situation is not compatible with bone union. The goal of such surgery in some situations is to provide stability and pain relief for a certain period. In other cases, union is expected.

Associated Vascular Injury

The difficulty in recommending treatment for fractures having associated vascular lesions lies in the variability of the numerous components of the injury, all of which need to be assessed and treated in a timely manner. Of major concern in this assessment are extent of soft-tissue destruction, amount of contamination, degree of vascular damage, degree of ischemia, ischemia tolerance of the patient, associated pressure-mediated ischemia, associated multiple organ injuries and time to successful revascularization, and the nature and extent of bone injury. It is no surprise that a single recommendation is impossible. External fixation is usually the treatment of choice in fractures having associated vascular injuries, with an external fixator being preferable to casting or traction.[17,449]

Rich and associates reviewed fractures with associated arterial injuries sustained in Vietnam.[427] Of 29 patients who had simultaneous arterial repair and internal fixation of the associated fracture, ten later came to amputation. Five of these amputations were directly related to infection of the fracture and the anastomosis and half the patients had complications from the intramedullary nail, necessitating its removal. Although a series of 29 patients is comparatively small, the amputation rate in these patients was 36%, compared with an overall rate of 13.5% in similar injuries treated without internal fixation. Zehntner noted fewer complications with external fixation than with internal fixation.[535]

After a study of 17 patients having fractures complicated by vascular injuries, Karavias and colleagues recommended external fixation for open injuries and internal fixation for closed ones.[276] In a more focused review of 13 patients having femur fractures and associated vascular lesions, Dichristina and coworkers advocated posterolateral plating when ischemia time was less than 6 hours, as long as it could be accomplished at least provisionally within 30 minutes.[118] Thus, when time permits, when associated soft-tissue lesions are not severe, and when ischemia of tissues is reversed expediently, internal fixation of fractures having associated vascular lesions may be indicated.[450,477,518]

Multiple Injuries

The association of several fractures or fractures with other organ system injuries makes internal fixation of fractures desirable for comfort of the patient, ease of nursing, transportation, or to prevent joints from becoming stiff. Even survival is enhanced with aggressive internal fixation.[100,214,253,429,525] Meek and colleagues compared two groups of patients having multiple injuries; one group was treated early and aggressively by internal fixation and the other group was treated "conservatively."[343] The former group had a mortality rate of 4.5% and the latter 28.5% in the 30 days after the injury. Gustilo and coworkers found that the incidence of adult respiratory distress syndrome and fat embolism syndrome was least in the polytraumatized patients who were operated on within the first week after injury; the most severely injured patients underwent surgery on the day of admission, of necessity.[191]

Stabilization of fractures protects soft tissues from further injury from unstable bone ends and thereby decreases bleeding and reduces pain and the need for narcotic analgesia. The more fractures that a patient has sustained, the more potential benefit is available with operative stabilization. Rehabilitation begins immediately after the operation, allowing the patient to achieve independence earlier. Transfer out of an acute-care setting is possible at an earlier date, making such care cost-effective. Furthermore, mobilization reduces atrophy, bone demineralization, and venous stasis, thereby lessening ultimate disability.

Mobilization

Intertrochanteric fractures of the femur may be treated by traction, with excellent healing of the fracture. This regimen requires skilled nursing, however, if bed sores are to be avoided. Many older patients have pulmonary emphysema, heart disease, hiatal hernia, and other ailments that make it mandatory for them to sit up. Satisfactory internal fixation under these circumstances appears to be the treatment of choice, especially when it allows them to be transferred to an extended-care facility.

Devas, in his excellent book *Geriatric Orthopaedics*, underscores the desirability of restoring older people to function and walking at the earliest juncture and keeping them in the hospital as short a time as possible or preferably not at all.[116] He advocates open reduction and internal fixation only if it will provide an early return to function. "Under no circumstances should any procedure be done for a fracture which does not allow the patient to be up and walking by the next day."[116] The very old cannot walk with crutches or without weight bearing. Intertrochanteric fractures must be firmly fixed; in femoral neck fractures, prostheses may be better than internal fixation.

Reconstruction

Stable reliable internal fixation is indicated in reconstruction of skeletal deformities due to traumatic injury and in those of nontraumatic origin. Such indications include arthritis, pseudarthrosis, and malunion, in addition to congenital and developmental angular, rotatory, and length deformities.[507] Principles developed for management of acute fracture problems are well suited to application of procedures such as osteotomy and arthrodesis bacause they involve stabilizing a surgically created instability.[158,226,258,361,379]

Host Factors

After proper diagnosis and evaluation of the patient and before selecting internal fixation as the desired treatment, full consideration of the host's healing potential is advisable. Appropriate attention needs to be given to the acute physiologic state of the patient and his or her underlying medical problems. Cardiac, pulmonary, neurologic, vascular, urologic, and alimentary injury should be diagnosed and treated in concert with the musculoskeletal injury.

Chronic medical problems may have an adverse effect on the outcome of fracture management and should be defined. Impaired wound healing and increased susceptibility to infection have been associated with protein deficiency, diabetes mellitus, essential fatty acid depletion, vitamin C deficiency, vitamin A deficiency, zinc deficiency, over- or underproduction of glucocorticoids, after parathryroidectomy, immunodeficiency, and impaired vascularity.[314] Decreased tissue oxygen content is a detriment to wound healing and may be produced by a variety of conditions, including arteriosclerosis, frostbite, burns, cigarette smoking, and diabetic small vessel disease.[176] Lawrence summarized these data as being intrinsic or extrinsic factors (Table 3-2).[308]

Clearly, the presence of any of the correctable disorders noted above should be addressed with care of the primary problem but open fracture surgery may have to wait until the condition or deficiency no longer adversely affects the patient.

TABLE 3-2
Factors Associated With Compromised Host Response to Injury and Wounding

Intrinsic Factors	Extrinsic Factors
Infection	Hereditary healing disorders
Foreign bodies	Nutritional deficiencies
Ischemia	Distant malignancies
Cigarette smoking	Old age
Radiation	Diabetes
Mechanical trauma	Jaundice
Local toxins	Alcoholism
Cancer	Uremia
	Glucocorticoids steroids
	Chemotherapeutic agents
	Other medications

From Lawrence, W.T.: Clinical Management of Nonhealing Wounds. *In* Cohen, R.F. and Linblad, W.J. (eds): Wound Healing Biochemical and Clinical Aspects, p. 541. Philadelphia; W.B. Saunders, 1992.

Operative Plan

Surgeons working at the Insalsspital in Bern, Switzerland, under Müller were required to prepare a detailed drawing of the plan of surgery for all operations involving implants, whether fractures, total joint replacements, or osteotomies. The mentor's final evaluation considered how closely the postoperative radiographs matched the preoperative drawings. Such operative plans help to improve the flow of surgery by improving preparation and have proven their value sufficiently over time to become standard practice. The drawing must show not only the final product but must detail the steps and equipment used during the procedure. Operating-room personnel also appreciate having a copy of the operative plan in advance. Texts detail the preparation and use of these orthopaedic drawings.[336,361] The degree of preparation before surgery should be tailored to the difficulty of the operation. Common routine procedures need implant and equipment checks only, whereas those having higher levels of difficulty should trigger preparation of preoperative plans.

Timing of Surgery

Optimal timing of surgery is a matter of opinion for which there is no simple summary. Immediate surgery has the potential advantage of reducing the overall time of disability and the complications associated with immobility. In cases of an emergent nature, such as ischemia or open wounds, the need for early operation is imperative. Certain fractures, including femoral neck fractures in young patients, fracture dislocations, and displaced fractures having associated neurologic deficit (otherwise requiring surgery), should be addressed expediently to avoid late sequelae of avascular necrosis, skin necrosis, and permanent neurologic loss, respectively. Polytrauma also warrants an aggressive approach to timing of fixation. Less urgent situations must be weighed when staffing, equipment, and expertise considerations may favor a delay. A rapidly performed but poorly done osteosynthesis has a less favorable outcome than a delayed but properly performed one.

Prophylactic Antibiotics

Prophylactic antibiotic use is prevalent but has questionable efficacy in closed fracture operations.[62,384] Fogelberg and associates, in their literature review, found that most prophylactic antibiotics either were of no value or enhanced the likelihood of postoperative infection.[146] Stevens, reviewing postoperative infections in Lexington, Kentucky, found that the infection rate increased significantly after procedures lasting more than 90 minutes and that prophylactic antibiotics in clean cases increased the prevalence of sepsis.[472]

Scales and associates reviewed 1816 patients operated on at the Royal National Orthopaedic Hospital and the Queen Elizabeth II Hospital.[443] There was no correlation between the infection rate and such factors as age, sex, vacuum drainage, site of implant, weight bearing, corrosion of metal, or chemical composition of the implant. Those patients given pre- and postoperative antibiotics for a total of 5 to 7 days had the lowest prevalence of wound infection, whereas those given antibiotics only after surgery had the highest rate of infection for the group.

Fogelberg and associates used pre- and postoperative penicillin for patients undergoing spinal surgery and mold arthroplasty of the hip and were able to reduce the prevalence of infection from 8.9% in the control group to 1.7% in the treated group.[146] Similarly, Nach and Keim found that prophylactic oxacillin, penicillin, or lincomycin given before, during, and after surgery was effective in reducing both major and minor infections.[367] The treated group had a prevalence of 1.6% major infection, whereas the control group had an 11.4% prevalence of major infections and 3.8% of minor infections.

Gerber reported an infection rate of 1.5% in hip fracture patients undergoing surgery without prophylactic antibiotics and in 0.7% of patients given antibiotics but the series had only 54 patients.[168] Hughes, on the basis of absent statistical significance, concluded that low-energy closed fractures did not require prophylactic antibiotics, although five patients of the untreated group had superficial wound infection, compared with none in the treated group.[242] Rubinstein and colleagues did a prospective, randomized study of patients undergoing clean spinal surgeries. Nine of 71 placebo patients had wound infections, compared with 3 of 71 who received a single dose of 1 g of cephazolin ($p < 0.07$).[434] Oishi, after reviewing literature on the subject, concluded that the preponderance of evidence favored prophylactic use of cephazolin administered on induction of anesthesia and 10 minutes before inflation of the tourniquet.[375]

The use of local irrigants or aerosols containing antibiotics has also been shown to be effective in reducing the rate of postoperative infection. Gingrass and associates, in experimental studies, found that gentle scrubbing of contaminated wounds and irrigation with neomycin solution was superior to irrigation with saline or scrubbing with pHisoHex (either alone or in combination) in preventing infection in contaminated wounds.[172] Parenteral neomycin, although ineffective by itself, improved the results when used as an irrigant and complemented by gentle scrubbing. In agreement, Rosenstein and coworkers found reduced infection with *Staphylococcus*-inoculated bone surgery in dogs after bacitracin wound irrigation, compared with no treatment or irrigation with saline alone.[432]

Incisions

An operation that begins with a poorly selected incision often is plagued by continuing difficulties that extend beyond the operating room. Part of the preop-

TABLE 3-3
Indications for Use of Cerclage

Provisional fixation[361]
Combined with intramedullary devices for control of rotational instability
Long bone fractures[196,263,377,493]
Stemmed prostheses
Combined with Steinmann pins or Kirschner wires to produce tension band
Olecranon*
Patella†
Malleolus[380]
Repair of tendon–bone or ligament–bone avulsion††
Greater tuberosity
Lesser tuberosity
Greater trochanteric
Calcaneus
Symphysis
AC dislocations
Primary fracture fixation combined with or without external support
Allograft fixation and compression[87,182,212,385]
Compression arthrodesis
Spinal surgery: sublaminar wire, posterior spinous processes[137,162,413,437,460,512]
To neutralize tension forces and compress a graft under the wire

* References 37, 94, 134, 150, 232, 257, 265, 306, 322, 348, 364, 365, 368, 388, 433, 510, 521.
† References 34, 41, 49, 78, 90, 193, 246–248, 313, 326, 341, 404, 428, 442.
†† References 105, 106, 110, 140, 208, 243, 244, 254, 255, 277.

erative plan must be consideration of the options available in terms of operative exposure. Inadequate visualization of a fracture makes reduction and fixation almost impossible. It is suggested that the operating surgeon consider first the possibilities of percutaneous fixation after indirect reduction. Such methods are common with diaphyseal long bone fractures of the lower extremities. Second in order of preference is an adequate but limited open procedure, perhaps arthroscopically assisted. Arthroscopic assistance for fracture surgery has not yet developed sufficiently to be considered a standard of care but progress continues in this area.[11,38,97,112,149,188,234,288,370,500] Traditional open surgery should be performed through a carefully selected incision that is long enough to avoid traction on soft tissue and adequate to gain exposure of the fracture.

Care of Soft Tissues

Murray defined a fracture as a ''soft-tissue injury complicated by a break in a bone.''[366] The most important single factor in the operative management of fractures is the treatment of the overlying soft tissues.[63,64,130,165,166] Incisions made through traumatized compromised skin may be complicated by wound necrosis and infection, with spread of the infection to the fracture site. The condition of the soft tissues may dictate operative approach and timing or simply closed management. The best barrier to infection is viable tissue.[492] Soft-tissue preservation is necessary so that a satisfactory internal fixation is not compromised by tissue necrosis.

Gerber has defined three stages of soft-tissue damage in an effort to reduce soft-tissue complications of surgery:[167]

- Stage I: compromised soft tissues; standard techniques of internal fixation are possible if further devitalization by surgery is avoided
- Stage II: partial, noncircumferential destruction of soft tissues; alternative techniques of fixation are necessary to prevent complications
- Stage III: soft tissues about the fracture site are destroyed; soft-tissue reconstruction is needed.

Careful handling of the soft tissues, with correct operative exposure, efficient and short time of operation, and use of indirect reduction techniques, contributes to the safety margin and improved outcome after internal fixation.[25,42,167,216,218,291,451]

Reduction Techniques

Methods to achieve fracture reduction are either direct or indirect. Direct methods are used after the fracture has been exposed, the edges cleared of debris and obstruction, and the fracture manipulated with bone-holding forceps or levers of various types. The ideal manipulation instrument has limited contact with the bone, little need for dissection of soft tissues for application to the bone surface, and fits the size and curvature of the bone. Specially designed periosteal elevators (eg, Cobb elevators) are useful to lever an impacted fracture apart, using their long handles and thin tips. Once the fracture has been mobilized and can be displaced slightly, bone spreaders modeled on lamina spreaders may be placed in the fracture crevice to further displace the fragment, allowing cleaning and reduction. Finally, fracture reduction clamps may be applied to hold the reduced fracture or fracture implants, such as a plate. Bone pushers further round out the direct fracture-reduction inventory.

Direct reduction methods are essential for fracture surgery but add an additional measure to the negative biologic impact of the injury. Methods that accomplish fracture reduction without additional injury are preferable. These methods are called indirect fracture-reduction techniques.[71,336,361] Small areas of the bone, sometimes remote to the fracture, are used as fixation points to apply a distraction force to disengage the fracture and accomplish realignment without disturbing additional soft tissues. The oldest indirect reduction technique is traction. Delayed intramedullary nailing of the femur and tibia is considerably easier if the original length of the bone has been restored and slightly increased by skeletal traction before surgery. The same is true for other fractures, such as complex fractures of the articular portions of the tibia (plateau and plafond) and pelvis.

Traction in the operating room is provided by fracture tables, which are available in various designs. Femoral, tibial, and humeral fractures are often reduced and stabilized by longitudinal fracture-table traction during operations, whereas fixation is performed percutaneously, without opening of the fracture site. Fresh long bone fractures may be manipulated by hand and held manually while the fracture is nailed. A portable traction device called the femoral distractor was created by the ASIF to accomplish the same objectives as the fracture table, without the bulk (Fig. 3-1).[361] This device is useful for a wide assortment of fracture problems, including most comminuted fractures of the lower extremities, particularly intra-articular fractures such as supracondylar femur, tibial plateau, and plafond, talus, and calcaneus. Variations consisting of downsized distractors are also available. A monoframe external fixator may be used to help disengage and then hold the fracture while permanent fixation is applied.

The hook on the ASIF articulated-tensioning device may be reversed to generate a distraction force rather than a compression force, adding to the array of indirect reduction techniques. Provisional fixation of a

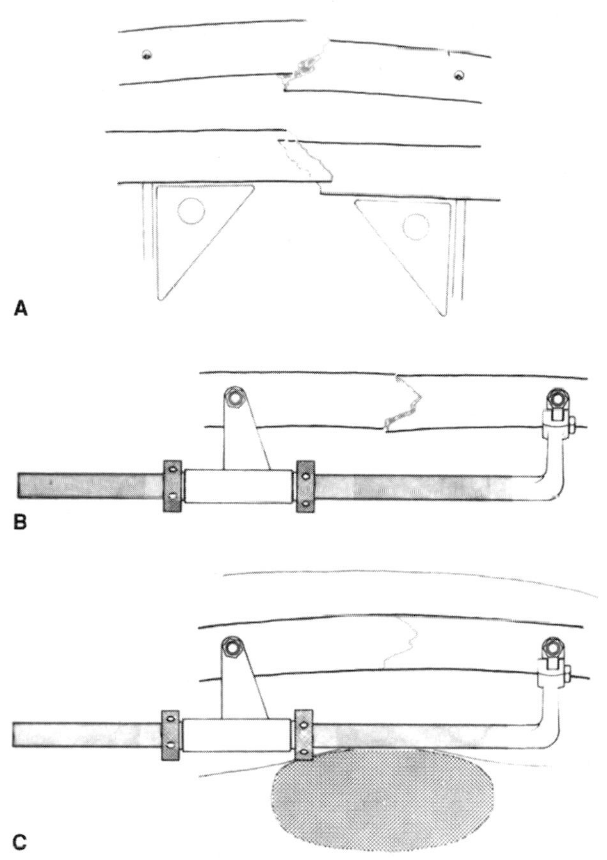

FIGURE 3-1. Femoral-distractor device insertion technique. (**A**) The fracture is aligned by manipulation. Schanz screws are placed perpendicular to the long axis of the bone. (**B**) The distractor is assembled and connected to the screws. (**C**) The fracture is reduced with use of a bump, correcting sagittal plane angulation. (Müller, M.E., Allgower, M., Schneider, R., and Willenegger, H.: Manual of Internal Fixation, 3rd Ed, p. 171. Berlin, Springer-Verlag, 1992.)

plate to one side of a still shortened fracture is followed by gentle distraction with the articulated tensioner in distraction mode, with final fracture reduction. The tensioner is then converted to compression mode and the fracture is compressed. A lamina spreader placed between the end of the plate and a screw outside of the plate has the same effect as the tensioner in distraction mode. Proper rotation must be restored before the implementation of either of these methods.

Permanent fixation may also serve as an indirect reduction aid. A slightly angulated pseudarthrosis of the tibia is reduced with an intramedullary nail. A plate applied to the convex side of an angulated pseudarthrosis also aligns the bone, while at the same time creating a dynamic tension band. Fresh fractures can also be manipulated by judicious use of internal fixation. Care in the planning and use of such methods is advisable because the mechanical effects of the fixation device must be well understood to avoid an adverse shift of the bone. It should be remembered that bone moves to metal. Undesirable shifts of the fracture during final fixation are due to imperfect contouring of the metal, in most cases.

INTERNAL FIXATION: COMPRESSION FIXATION

Internal fixation creates a drastic alteration in the mechanical environment of the injured extremity. The design and material composition of the implant are both relevant and important but a key element is in the technique of implantation. A specific piece of metal such as a screw may be applied in differing ways, creating diverse mechanical effects. A screw may be inserted, creating a compression force across a fracture plane, thereby decreasing shear force and providing stability. Conversely, it may applied in such a manner as to push the fracture apart, thereby impeding union. Biologic and mechanical failure soon follow. Similarly, a plate may act as either a distraction or compression device, depending on fracture configuration and technique of application. Compression should be understood as being a method of stabilization, not a way of accelerating union.[207] Compression fixation methods create bony stability and thereby protect metal from fatigue.[71] Exact interdigitation of jagged bone edges increases friction at the fracture site, substantially reducing load on the fixation device and neutralizing harmful shear forces across bone interfaces. A stable reduction combined with mechanically sound fixation and biologically viable bone are the essential ingredients for osseous union with internal fixation.

Lag Effect

One of the most powerful and useful compression methods is that of the lag screw. Lag literally means "to follow." Lag screws are one of the most common forms of internal fixation. Any screw type may be used to produce a lag effect (squeeze) as long as three criteria are met:

1. The screw in the near side fragment, threaded or nonthreaded, must glide freely in the near side screw hole without engaging the bone.
2. Threads in the far side fragment screw hole must continue to progress through the bone as the screw turns and must firmly grip the bone without stripping.
3. The advancement of the head of the screw must be solidly arrested on the surface of the near side.

A screw may be inserted to produce a lag effect, whether it is fully threaded or not. A screw with a smooth shank can be used as a lag screw with one

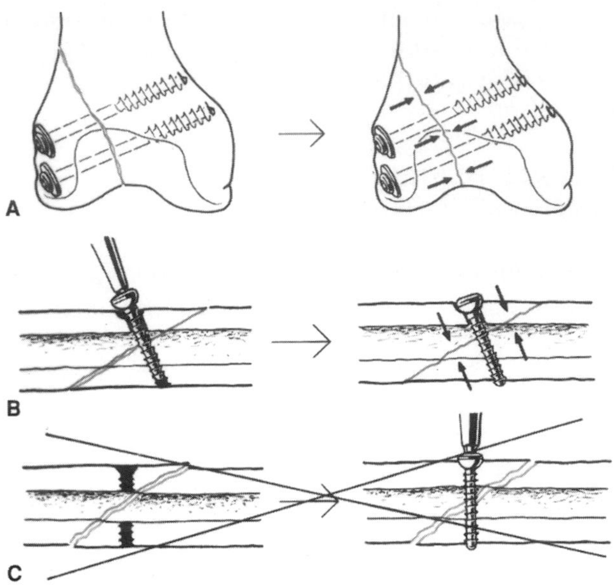

FIGURE 3-2. Lag screws. (**A**) Smooth shank screws used as lag screws, with a single drill-bit technique. (**B**) Fully threaded screws, requiring preparation of a glide hole on the near side. (**C**) When a fully threaded screw is placed without a glide hole, the fracture is held apart. (Müller, M.E., Allgower, M., Schneider, R., and Willenegger, H.: Manual of Internal Fixation, 3rd Ed, p. 189. Berlin, Springer-Verlag, 1992.)

drill bit, whereas a fully threaded screw requires two drill bits to produce the same effect mechanically. A smooth-shank lag screw must be inserted such that all threads cross the fracture site (Fig. 3-2). Because the number of threads on such screws are fixed and available in only a few lengths, there are applications in which—in proportional terms—only a few threads reside in the thread hole. The advantage of the two drill bit method and the fully threaded screw lies in maximizing the number of threads actually used for fixation because the glide hole replaces the smooth shank mechanically and all of the screw in the thread hole is threaded, regardless how long the length of the far side fragment.

Lag effect using screws is adequate as the only fixation for some metaphyseal or epiphyseal fractures (eg, tibial plateau fractures and medial malleolar fractures). Otherwise, particularly in cortical bone, lag screws must be protected with a plate or plate equivalent, such as an external fixator. The protective device is referred to as a neutralization device because it controls bending, translational, and torsional forces. Use of lag screws only without a neutralization plate for long bone diaphyseal fixation invites mechanical failure. Proper insertion of lag screws produces compression between fracture elements and is referred to as interfragmentary compression. Optimal compression is achieved with the axis of the screw perpendicular to the axis of the plane of the fracture. Interfragmentary compression is achievable with other fixation devices in addition to lag screws but less efficiently.

Buttress and Antiglide

A simple definition of ''buttress'' is a support or prop. An unstable hillside can be supported with a wooden fence, which acts as a buttress. A more active buttress in the same situation would be the shovel of a bulldozer, which literally braces the hillside by pushing the dirt back up the hill. The ideal application of a buttress device in fracture fixation mimics the latter example and literally acts to push bone fragments together, thereby producing interfragmentary compression with a pushing action. Appropriate plate contouring facilitates the compression effect of a buttress plate as, during screw application, elastic deformation of the plate is converted into antishear and compres-

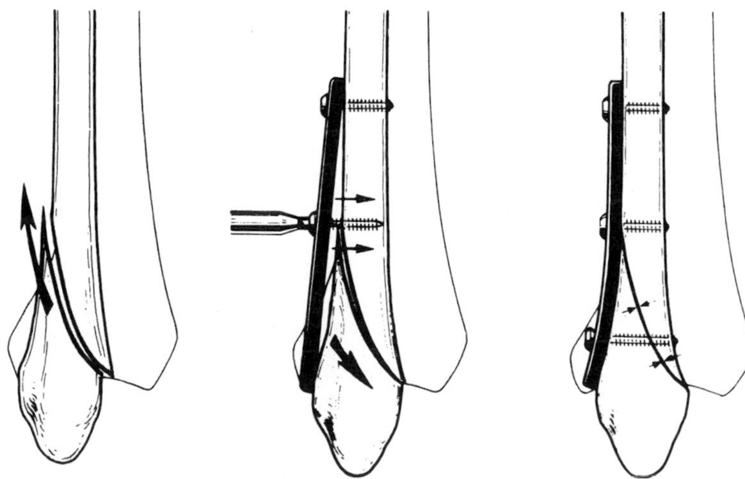

FIGURE 3-3. An antiglide buttress plate with a lag screw through the plate is indicated for an oblique distal fibula fracture (*left*). The plate creates fracture compression with a pushing action from the flat plate as the second screw is tightened (*middle*). Interfragmentary compression is further enhanced with the lag screw (*right*). (Brunner, C.F., and Weber, B.G.: Special Techniques in Internal Fixation, p. 125. Berlin, Springer-Verlag, 1982.)

sion forces. A buttress plate, however, does not necessarily produce a compression effect. It can be applied without compression; it then functions as a rigid splint rather than a compression device.

Plates are most effective in producing interfragmentary compression using buttress action and may take advantage of lag screws applied through the plate. A special case of buttress action called "antiglide" counteracts the tendency of inclined planes of cortical bone to slide as compressive loading is applied. An antiglide buttress plate may include a lag screw placed through the plate, further enhancing stability (Fig. 3-3).

Axial Compression

Another useful technique for producing fracture compression takes advantage of a fixation device that is applied to one side of the fracture but crosses to the other side. A pulling or tensioning force delivered to the unfixed side forces the fragments into each other as tension is applied. Successful application of this technique requires stability of the loaded construct. Direction of pull may be critical. If the fracture consists of two oblique components, load may be applied inappropriately, shifting the fragments over each other and offsetting the fracture (Fig. 3-4). Comminution may make compression problematic.

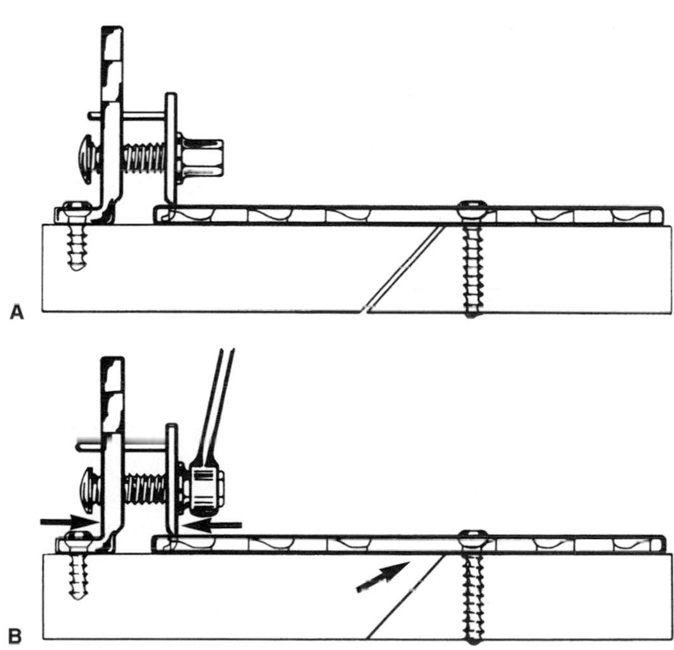

FIGURE 3-4. Compression of a plate with an external tensioning device. (**A**) A holding screw is placed close to the acute angle of an oblique fracture. (**B**) Tension is applied from the obtuse angle side, resulting in compression of the fracture. (Schauwecker, F.: Practice of Osteosynthesis, 2nd Revised Ed, p. 31. Stuttgart, Thieme Stratton, 1982.)

Axial compression is achievable with self-compressing plates, plates compressed with removable tensioning devices, compression nails, and external fixators (Fig. 3-5), which illustrates the use of a nail to produce static axial compression. Ideal plate fixation uses axial compression followed by interfragmentary compression, with a lag screw preferably applied through the plate. To avoid stress on the lag screw, axial compression is applied before interfragmentary compression.

Static and Dynamic Tension Band

Frederick Pauwels developed early concepts of load transfer within bone (Fig. 3-6).[393] Long bones, being curved tubular structures, have a tension side and a

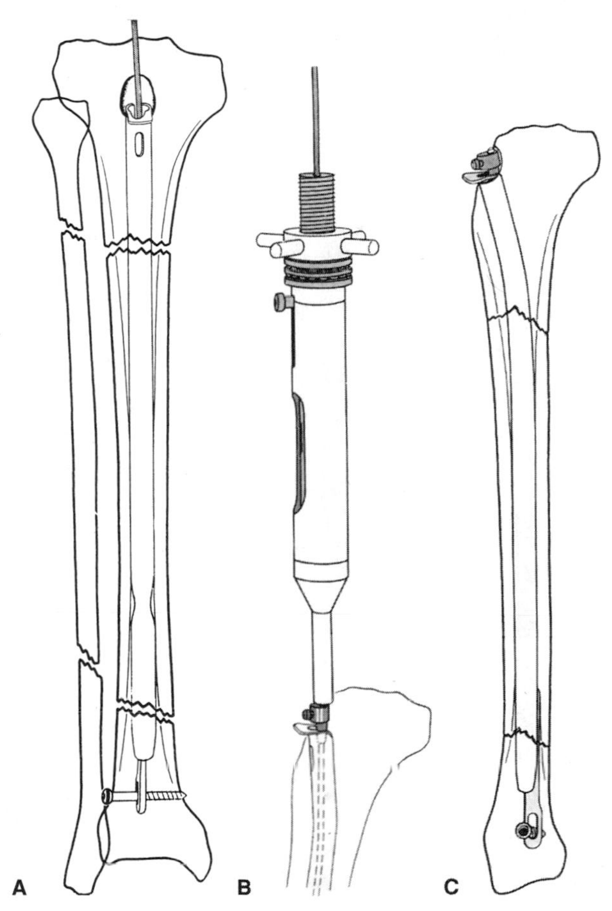

FIGURE 3-5. The technique of compression-nailing of a transverse segmental fracture is illustrated using the Kaesmann nail. (**A**) The nail is composed of two implanted elements, one of which is anchored in the distal tibia with a locking bolt. The other encompasses the first and rests on the insertion portal. (**B**) A tensioning device is applied to the nail at the entry portal and pulls the bolt component upward, compressing the fractures. (**C**) The final construct. (Hempel, D., Fischer, S.: Intramedullary Nailing, p. 120. Stuttgart, Georg Thieme Verlag, 1982.)

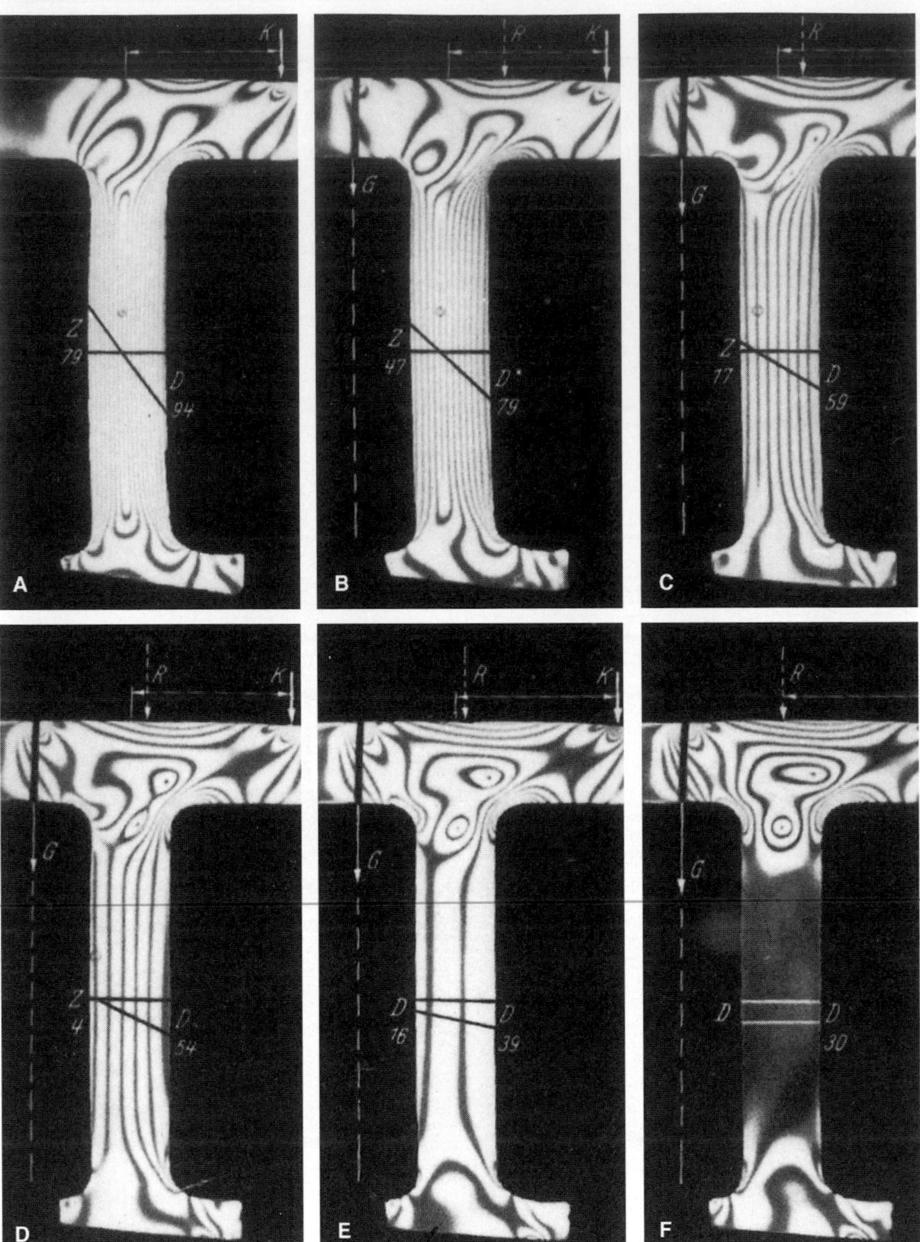

FIGURE 3-6. Pauwels used photoelastic models to illustrate the effectiveness of tension-band mechanics. Eccentric loading produces a stress–strain differential within the material, which can be made uniform by a tension band and has the same function as a counterweight. (**A**) Eccentric force *K* is applied at a distance from the neutral axis *o*, creating a tensile force of 79 kp/cm^2 (*Z*) and compression force of 94 kp/cm^2 (*D*). (**B**) A weak tension band *G* is applied to the left of the column, creating a resultant force *R* more closely aligned with the neutral axis. The tensile force *Z* is reduced to 47 kp/cm^2 and compression force *D* becomes 79 kp/cm^2. (**C–F**) A progressively stronger tension band *G* further shifts the resultant force *R* toward neutral force *o* until they become collinear in **F**. There is now a uniform compressive force of 30 kp/cm^2. (Pauwels, F.: Biomechanics of the Locomotor Apparatus, p. 157. Berlin, Springer-Verlag, 1980.)

compression side. His famous load–strain diagrams displayed schematic representations of bone under load conditions and led to a technique of fixation applied to the tension side of bone called a "tension band." A tension band is a structure that converts tension forces into compression forces. Bone as a material fails easily under tension, compared with compression. Similarly, bone forms under compression and resorbs under tension. Finally, a fracture fixed with a tension band bears load and thereby reduces the load applied to the fixation device, thereby protecting the device from failure under cyclic loading conditions.

A tension band is mechanically efficient, meaning that a small amount of material can be used for maximum stabilization (Fig. 3-7). No specific implant is implied by the term tension band because a tension-band effect can be produced by an array of implants, including a wire loop (Fig. 3-8*A*), a wire and screw (see Fig. 3-8*B*), a staple, and plate.[71,114,361,393,507] Diaphyseal plating methods may take advantage of plate tension-band methods, whereas metaphyseal avulsions are ideal for wire loop, screw and wire, or staple methods.[§] Critical to all tension-band techniques is knowledge of

[§] References 34, 41, 78, 94, 99, 103, 105, 110, 122, 150, 208, 219, 232, 236, 246, 247, 265, 313, 322, 352, 365, 380, 386, 521.

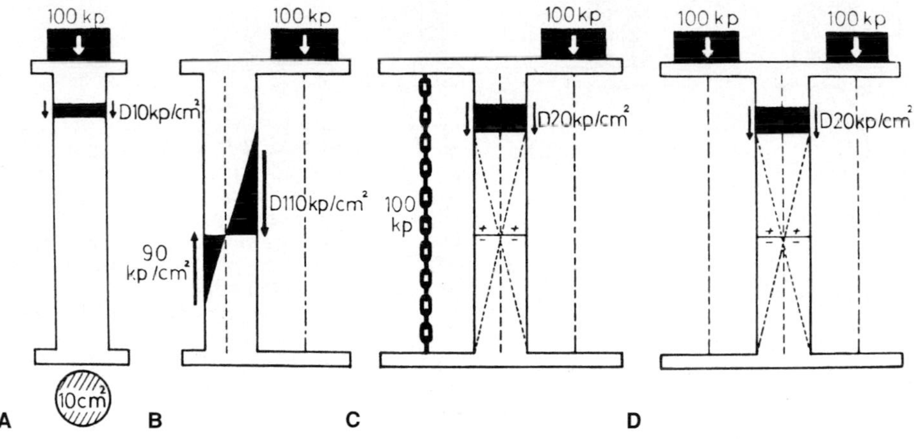

FIGURE 3-7. Schematic of a tension band illustrates the equivalency of the tension band to a counterbalancing weight. (**A**) One hundred kp are applied to the top of the column, resulting in uniform compression loading within each unit-volume of column material. (**B**) Eccentric applied load of the same magnitude as in **A.** results in compression forces in the side of the column closest to the applied load and tensile forces on the other side. (**C**) Uniform compression forces within each unit-volume may be restored with a tension band applied to the tensile side. (**D**) The net effect is to double the unit-volume compressive load, compared with **A.** (Müller, M.E., Allgower, M., Schneider, R., and Willenegger, H.: Manual of Internal Fixation, 3rd Ed, p. 227. Berlin, Springer-Verlag, 1992.)

prestressing effects, bone geometry, and correct fixation technique.

If a tension band creates the desired compression effect only at the time of application, it is referred to as a static tension band. If, in addition to this static compression effect, the fixation produces an additional tension-band effect during physiologic loading, it becomes a dynamic tension band. Dynamic tension-band effects are possible when the static tension-band device is placed on the convex side of a curved tubular bone (Fig. 3-9). Cyclic compression loading then occurs with activity of the patient.

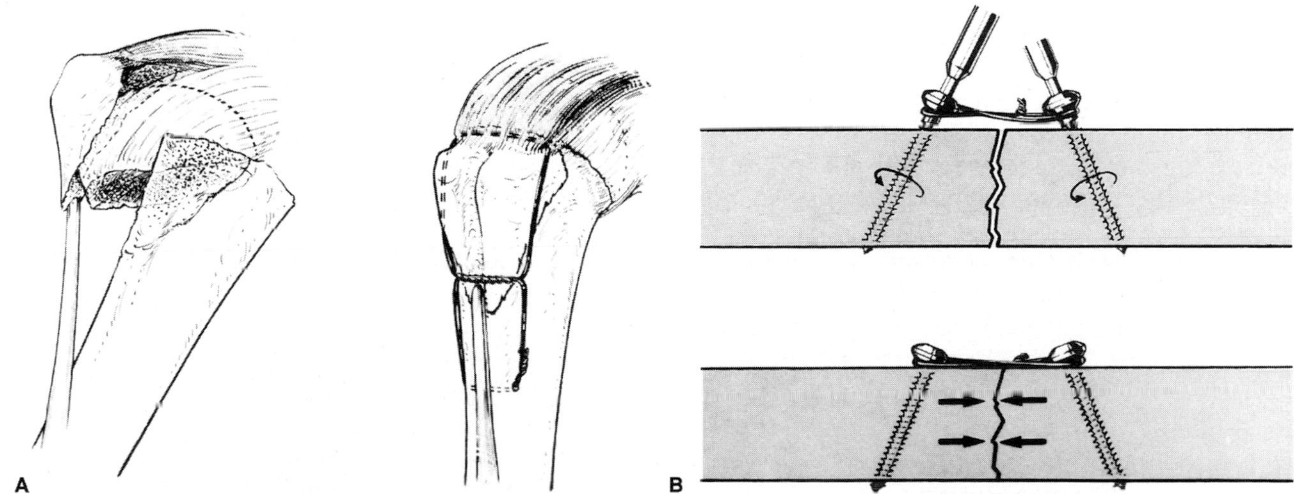

FIGURE 3-8. (**A**) Only wire may be used to created both a static and dynamic tension-band effect for a fracture of the greater tuberosity of the humerus. This construct requires stable reduction of the head and shaft, most effectively with the head impacted in slight valgus. (Brunner, C.F., and Weber, B.G.: Special Techniques in Internal Fixation, p. 41. Berlin, Springer-Verlag, 1982.) (**B**) Screws are inserted at an angle. A loop of wire is tightened before final tightening of the screws. The screws are then tightened and the fracture is compressed. A corticocancellous bone graft strut may be placed under the tension band to enhance healing in pseudarthrosis cases. (Brunner, C.F., and Weber, B.G.: Special Techniques in Internal Fixation, p. 80. Berlin: Springer-Verlag, 1982.)

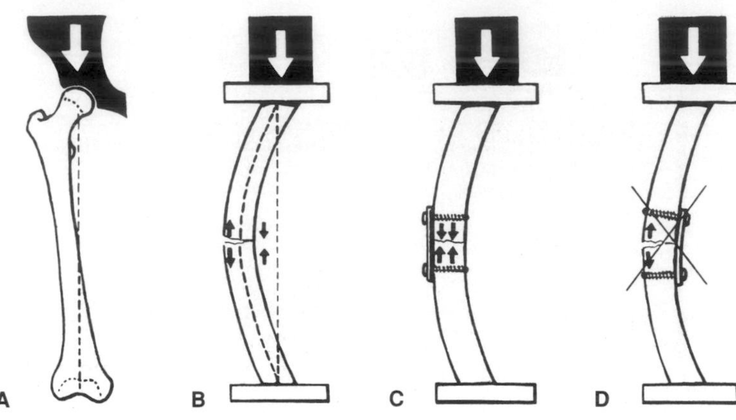

FIGURE 3-9. Dynamic tension-band effect depends on application of the fixation to the tension side of the bone. (**A**) The femur is curved, creating medial compression force and a lateral tension force. (**B**) Tension and compression forces are generated as load is applied. (**C**) A lateral tension-band plate creates uniform compression forces within the unit-volume affected by the fracture. (**D**) A medial tension band does not counteract lateral tension forces. (Müller, M.E., Allgower, M., Schneider, R., and Willenegger, H.: Manual of Internal Fixation, 3rd Ed, p. 227. Berlin, Springer-Verlag, 1992.)

Prestressing

Robert Soeur, an early advocate of diverse fixation methods, including Küntscher's methods, discussed the desirable effects of prestressing when discussing internal fixation.

> *In 1928 the French engineer Freyssinet devised a means of avoiding the disadvantages of the truss,girder: this was the method of making prestressed concrete. When a specimen is compressed from both ends it becomes considerably more resistant to bending, because its material is in some way consolidated. If this longitudinal prestressing is operating along the central axis its effects are distributed throughout.*
>
> *This comes back to saying that under a bending stress the tensile stresses that had been the cause of cracking are nullified. Some books are lined up on a library shelf. To move then en bloc, we press the row together between our hands. No volume falls or separates from its neighbors. Our compression is the prestressing.*[465]

Soeur attempted to apply the ideas of material prestressing to bone in the form of wire loops passed through the medullary canal and anchored in the cortex above and below the fracture site (Fig. 3-10). Before twisting the free ends of the loop, the wire was tensioned. These early attempts at prestressing were of limited success, and the method of extramedullary longitudinal rods affixed with multiple wire loops never caught on. Prestressing, however, has become an invaluable aspect of plate fixation technique, which is discussed more fully in the section on plates.

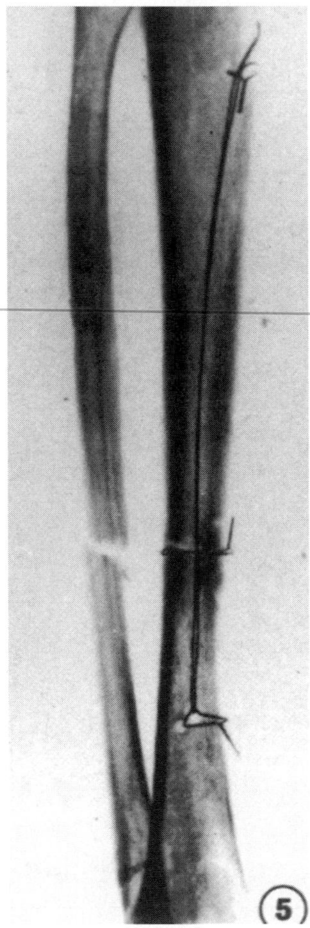

FIGURE 3-10. Pretensioned wires were used to stabilize a tibia fracture. Special conditions of stable fracture configuration and correctly positioned wires are necessary and rarely present in cases needing surgery but the mechanical principle is demonstrated. (Soeur, R.: Fractures of the Limbs. Brussels, La Clinique Orthopedique, 1981.)

INTERNAL FIXATION: NONCOMPRESSION TECHNIQUES

Splints

Techniques that do not create a compression effect at the immediate time of application are noncompression fixation techniques. The classic noncompression technique is a device occupying the center of the medullary canal, such as an intramedullary nail or rod. As are plates, noncompression devices are forms of splints. A gliding splint allows compression from physiologic loading conditions, whereas a nongliding splint incorporates design features that prevent fragment compaction.[361] Intramedullary devices may be nongliding or gliding, whereas plates are intended to be strictly nongliding splints. Early attempts to create gliding splints with slotted plates (eg, Eggers' plate) were abandoned when dynamic gliding effects proved unreliable.[127]

The terms "rod and nail" are used interchangeably at times, although they are fundamentally different. A rod is loosely applied, so that contact with the endosteal bone is limited and almost inadvertent (Fig. 3-11). In distinction, a nail is tightly applied to the endosteal bone to the point of firm wedging. Examples from the home are a carpenter's nail driven into a board, displacing wood and becoming firmly wedged. A rod suspends a roll of paper towels, allowing free motion between the paper towel tube and the rod.

Küntscher is given deserved credit for the origination and development of intramedullary fixation by means of nailing.[297–299] Rigid, stable fixation was the goal of such surgery:

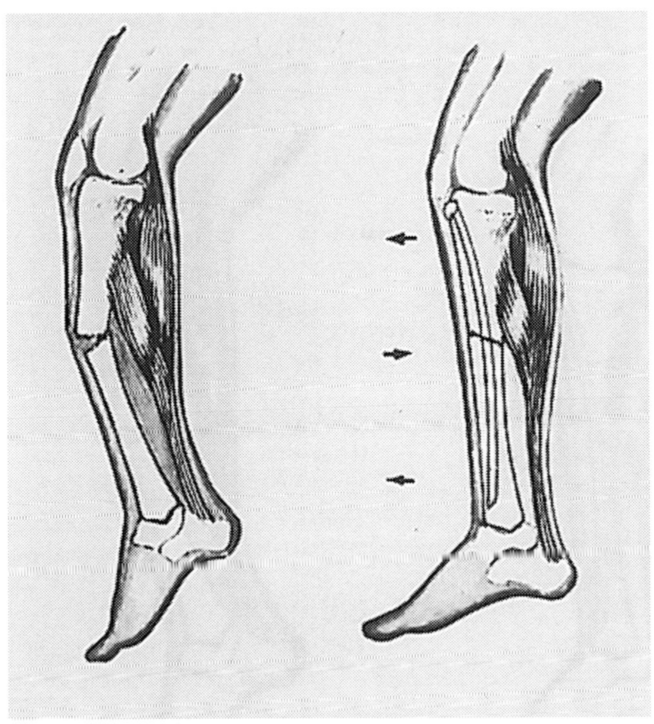

FIGURE 3-11. A Rush rod combined with an intact soft-tissue hinge posteriorly functions dynamically to maintain fracture position and provide stability. This intramedullary device works as a spring, storing and releasing energy. (Rush, L.V.: Atlas of Rush Pin Techniques, p. 32. Meridian, Miss: Berivon, 1976.)

> *The basic idea of intramedullary nailing is the achievement of stable osteosynthesis. Union of fragments by means of a suitable internal splint is so solid that all additional external splinting is unnecessary. If an extremity is to be used immediately, it is understandable that the internal splint has to have about the same stability as the bone which it is replacing mechanically.*[299]

Reaming was developed as a method to improve stability by better fit of the nail in the reamed bone, use of a larger diameter nail, and to extend the indications for the method. A hollow slotted nail was developed to allow what Küntscher called "elastic adherence," which simply put meant collapse of the nail with elastic deformation and recoil. Actually, such collapse does not occur and the nail simply jams in the bone. Compression at the fracture site is a byproduct of functional activity rather than design. With increasing comminution, the prospects of stable compression diminish. Furthermore, compression, whether or not present, was thought to not be essential for union to occur.

From inadvertent dynamic compression to deliberate distraction or detensioning was a simple step that took almost 30 years to develop.[96] Cross-locking of the nail to the bone above and below the fracture to control instability had occurred to others before Küntscher but was perfected by Klemm and others.[96,283–287] The novelty of this innovation was revolutionary in its impact on fracture care and was the key necessary to realize the full potential of intramedullary splintage.[‖] Compression is seldom achieved with interlocking methods and fragments often are grossly displaced. Union reliably occurs anyway.

Biologic Fixation

Undergoing close scrutiny are newer plate methods, sometimes referred to as "biologic" fixation.[24,25,71,167,291,336,400,507] Biologic fixation can be rephrased as follows: fixation in which the utmost respect is given to soft tissues and vascularity of bone. Fixation rigidly maintains fracture alignment without compression (nongliding splint). The term may be applied to nail methods but was created in the context of plating. Within that context, biologic fixation principles may be summarized as:

Repositioning and realigning by manipulation at a distance to the fracture site, preserving soft-tissue attachments

Leaving comminution fragments out of the mechanical construct while preserving their blood supply;

‖ References 27, 33, 36, 44, 46, 69, 70, 104, 123, 124, 128, 145, 222, 240, 263, 279, 286, 392, 410, 439, 464, 467, 486, 529, 530, 536.

if a fragment is incorporated, it is manipulated on its vascular pedicle
Using low-elastic modulus, biocompatible materials
Decreasing contact between the bone and the implant (endosteal and periosteal)
Limiting operative exposure when possible

When a plate is applied "biologically" to maintain a defect due to comminution, it is called a bridge or gap plate. Vascularized comminution acts as a graft, and no added grafting is needed. If bone loss has occurred, graft is harvested and placed in the defect. Such a construct is a special example of splintage.

Baumgaertel and coworkers studied standardized segmentally comminuted subtrochanteric femur fractures in sheep treated with lag screw and condylar plate reconstruction, indirect reduction and gap plating, or indirect reduction and gap plating with a special point contact condylar plate.[24] All fractures healed in both groups using indirect methods and bone mass was increased, compared with conventional methods. Time and further clinical research will ultimately help to refine indications for these methods.

EXTRAMEDULLARY FIXATION TECHNIQUES

Cerclage

Cerclage may have been the first or one of the first internal fixation techniques. Documentation of early cases is sketchy and Evans dispelled notions of a case reputed to have been the first documentation of metallic cerclage in a 1775 French manuscript.[133] Malgaigne credits Flaubert of Rouen with fixing an open humerus fracture with thread suture in 1839.[331] Cerclage fixation has been an important part of the orthopaedic armamentarium since.[#]

Despite concern expressed by Charnley,[87a] wires and narrow cables contact bone over a small region and do not interfere substantially with cortical blood flow, according to the microangiographic studies of Rhinelander.[422,424,425] Blood does not flow through the cortex longitudinally, so there is no obstruction to flow as long as the surface area of contact is small—a millimeter or less.

This time-honored technique has been strongly condemned on the ground that a circumferential wire loop strangles bone. The periosteal blood supply, however, enters the cortex through innumerable small vessels. No periosteal arteries of the long bones run longitudinally to be pinched off with encircling wires. Callus grows abundantly over the wires, which are tight and hold the fracture reduced. It is only when the immobilization is insufficient that troubles arise (Fig. 3-12).[422]

Parham bands cover a larger surface area than do cables or wires and therefore interfere with cortical blood flow, leading to necrosis.[424] In later animal studies, Rhinelander found that Partridge bands, which were meant to improve on Parham bands by minimizing circulatory disturbance of bone with flow channels under the band, did not impede circulation because they loosened after application and cortical blood flow was restored.[426] Jones, however, reported three clinical cases of cortical necrosis with Partridge-band use (Fig. 3-13).[268]

Cerclage may consist of a wide variety of types of implants, from various diameters of stainless steel or titanium wire measured in gauge or millimeters to cables with filaments of steel or titanium to bands of steel or nylon. Monofilament wires are primarily used for tension-band fixation or primary fracture fixation,

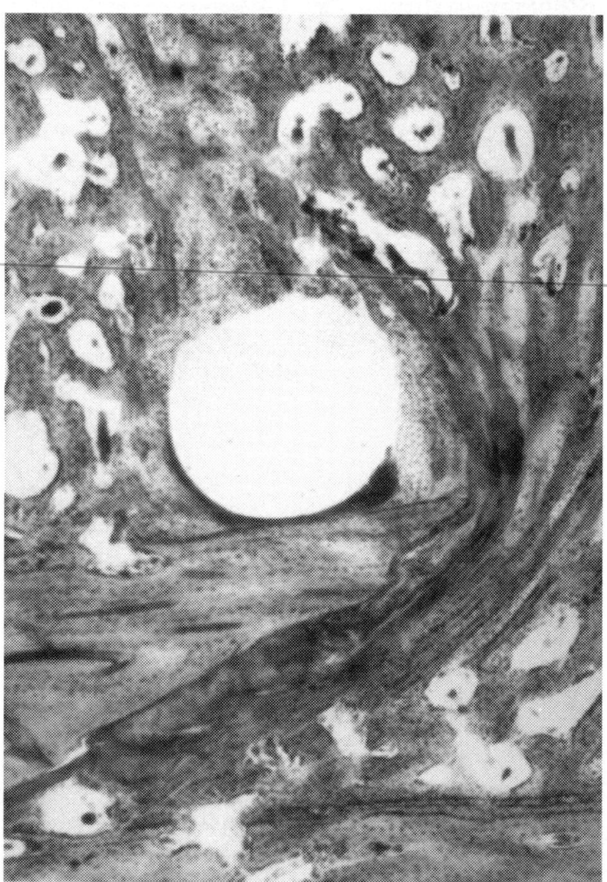

FIGURE 3-12. A single small-diameter wire has little effect on vascularity of bone. This photomicrograph of a fracture fixed with wire cerclage shows that abundant new bone has formed around the implant (*large circle* at center). (Rhinelander, F.W.: The Normal Microcirculation of Diaphyseal Cortex and Its Response to Fracture. J. Bone Joint Surg. 50(4):798, 1968.)

[#] References 75, 78, 125, 143, 181, 189, 193, 223, 231, 281, 318, 326, 451, 459, 461, 490, 493, 520.

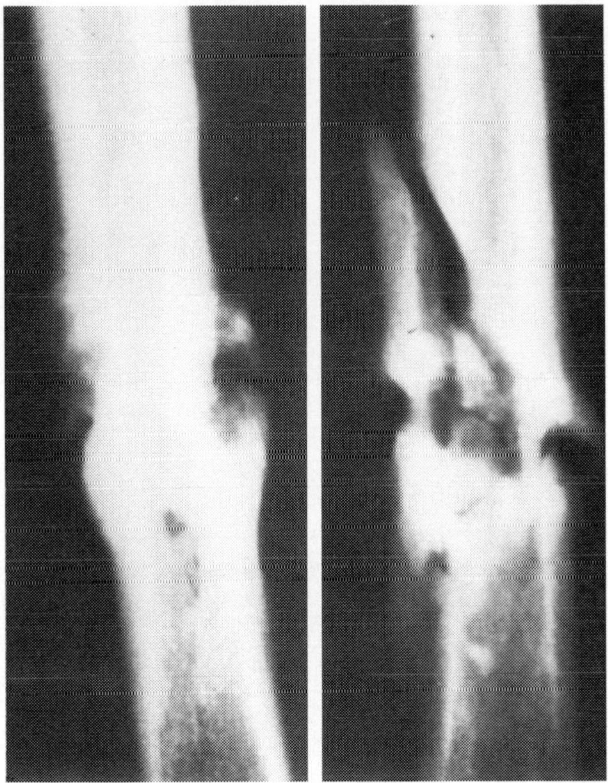

FIGURE 3-13. Cortical necrosis associated with Partridge bands on the human femur. On the *left,* a paucity of new bone formation is seen, whereas on the *right,* a nonunion has developed. The damage may have occurred during placement rather than as a result of continued presence of the implant. (Jones, D.G.: Bone Erosion Beneath Partridge Bands. J. Bone Joint Surg. 68(3):476, 1986.)

whereas cables have been developed for trochanteric or allograft fixation.

Indications

Cerclage is simply a means of producing interfragmentary compression when applied to fracture fragments, acting in a manner similar to interfragmentary screws. Kanakis and Corday found that cerclage for interfragmentary compression, combined with a neutralization plate for a three-fragment long bone shaft fracture in plastic bone, was mechanically more stable than lag screws in torque and equal in axial load.[275]

Wires may be used when a compressive force is necessary and space is limited. Additionally, cerclage is a satisfactory method of neutralizing tension forces, either as a single implant or combined with other fixation (eg, Kirschner wires, Steinmann pins, or screws).

Indications for use of cerclage are listed in Table 3-3.

Mechanical Features

A variety of cerclage designs and materials are available, from monofilament wires and braided cables to straps and bands made of metals and synthetics having differing mechanical properties. Figure 3-14 illustrates a selection of such devices.

Wang and coworkers tested 18-gauge (1-mm) Vitallium, 16-gauge 316L stainless steel, and three braided strands of 24-gauge stainless steel for yield strength and elongation.[504] The Vitallium had the greatest strength and the braided wire the least, whereas the elongation percentages were just the opposite, with that for Vitallium almost double that for the braided steel. A full knot or a half-knot with twists was stronger than a twist.

Guadagni and Drummond studied strengths of various wire-fastening techniques and concluded that the wire-wrap and ASIF methods were inadequate (Fig. 3-15).[187] Their conclusion was based on comparison of the yield strength of 18-gauge (1-mm) wire of 400 to 450 N with the yield strength of the knot, reasoning that elongation would produce failure just as untying would. Consistent with the findings of Wang,[504] Guadagni found that the square knot and the knot twist had superior strength to the twist. They argued that twisting was strong enough, simple, and produced tension during the twist.

Data from the work of Schultz and coworkers agree with these conclusions; the knot exceeded the twist, which exceeded the bend (ASIF).[453] Again, the twist was thought to be adequate and preferred for clinical use. Commercial wire tighteners produced greater strength due to more consistent twists and were recommended. Doubling the wire diameter from 0.45 to

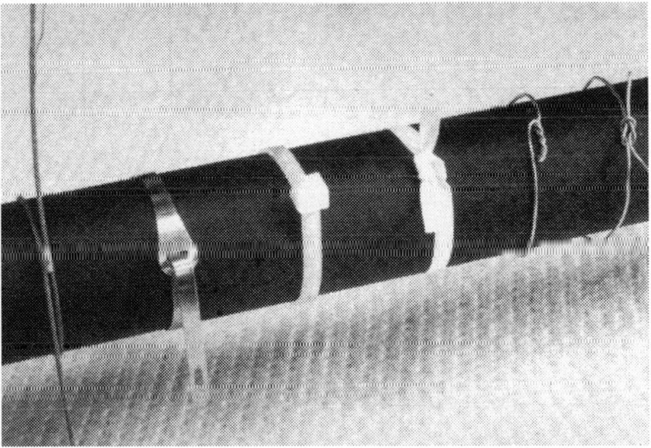

FIGURE 3-14. Cerclage systems, including (*left* to *right*) titanium cable, Parham band, cable tie, Mersilene tape, and stainless steel wire. (Shaw, J.A., and Daubert, H.B.: Compression Capability of Cerclage Fixation Systems. Orthopedics 11:1170, 1988.)

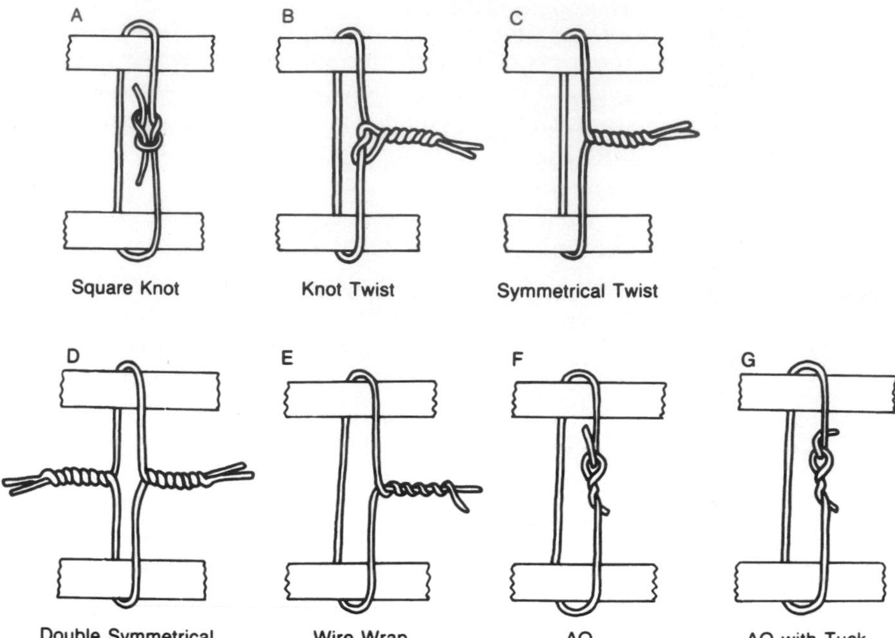

FIGURE 3-15. Techniques of fastening wire cerclage in clinical use. (Guadagni, J.R., and Drummond, Denis S.: Strength of Surgical Wire Fixation. Clin Orthop 209:177, 1984.)

0.98 mm increased the load-to-failure more than 300%. More than two twists added no additional strength. A tensioning twist opposite the fastening twist decreased strength 10% to 15%.

Shaw extended the mechanical analysis from wire only to include Parham bands, swage-lock titanium cables, and Mersilene tape.(Table 3-4).[458] It is interesting to note that although the knot produced higher ultimate strengths, the twist produced superior compressive force. The titanium cable overall performed best, given its high compressive strength combined with high ultimate strength. Mersilene was more limited in terms of both ultimate yield strength and compressive strength but was thought to be advantageous for improved fatigue resistance.

Finally, Cheng and coworkers proposed a further modification of fastening technique called the hairpin knot, which produced superior compressive force and load versus strain performance, compared with knotting and twisting (Figs. 3-16 and 3-17).[88] This technique is essentially a double loop made with a single continuous length of wire fastened with a single throw of knot and then a twist, thereby improving strength with double wire and compression with the twisted knot. The vascular implications of this method have not been evaluated. The double loop may occupy a relatively large surface area of bone, similar to a Parham band, and may have a similar impact on cortical blood flow.

Clinical Aspects

Cerclage may be used as a tension-resisting device and in such applications, technique is straightforward. Twisting wire of adequate diameter has proved successful in clinical practice for the many indications listed. Clinical application of cerclage techniques demands preservation of compressive forces and reliability of the fastening method. It does little good to struggle to make a knot if in the process all the compressive load becomes dissipated. A simple fastening method, such as the twist or double twist, in which compressive load is applied symmetrically across the plane of the fracture is more important in fracture fixation than a stronger fastening method because the twist method is easy to apply, even when space is limited. Stable fracture reduction combined with clever exploitation of tension-band principles reduces the strength requirements of the implant. Wire techniques should be replaced with cables for allograft strut fixation. Finally, the metal must lie directly on the bone. If soft tissue is interposed between wire and the bone, the system may loosen as the soft tissues creep or necrose.

Cerclage and Strut

Cerclage has proved useful in combination with struts made of various materials. Soeur developed a system of fracture fixation consisting of Steinmann pins placed parallel to the long axis of the bone at 90° or 180° angles to each other and fastened with loops passed around the rod across the canal.[465] Not a true cerclage by definition, this technique was nevertheless the predecessor of contemporary methods of cerclage (Fig. 3-18).

Fractures in close proximity to arthroplasties pose difficult fixation problems. Conservative care, long-

TABLE 3-4
Cerclage Fixation Data

Cerclage System	Maximum Compression Force-kg (x̄ ± SEM)	Ultimate Strength-kg (x̄ ± SEM)
18 Gauge Wire		
Square knot	1.74 ± 0.18	98.48 ± 0.68
Moderate square knot	13.64 ± 0.91	80.53 ± 2.70
Knot twist	11.73 ± 2.10	81.36 ± 1.28
Twist knot	9.22 ± 1.08	55.06 ± 2.45
Twist knot (clinical)	4.18 ± 0.88	50.40 ± 0.67
20 Gauge Wire		
Square knot	1.97 ± 0.22	69.55 ± 0.61
Moderate square knot	8.94 ± 0.99	55.33 ± 2.81
Knot twist	4.66 ± 0.73	54.77 ± 1.32
Twist knot	5.72 ± 0.44	35.05 ± 0.73
Twist knot (clinical)	0.98 ± 0.32	35.08 ± 1.47
Parham Bands		
0.64 mm thick	28.98 ± 1.82	128.52 ± 3.39
0.44 mm thick	13.79 ± 3.47	73.26 ± 3.89
Titanium Cable	26.36 ± 3.19	104.70 ± 1.52
Mersilene Tape	3.56 ± 0.46	38.33 ± 1.0
Nylon Cable Ties		
Dry	7.73 ± 0.88	60.00 ± 0.51
Autoclaved	7.78 ± 0.68	26.97 ± 0.85
Soaked	6.23 ± 0.42	22.45 ± 0.59
Polypropylene Cable Ties		
Dry	8.05 ± 0.44	46.23 ± 1.26
Autoclaved	9.86 ± 0.32	24.77 ± 1.31
Soaked	7.09 ± 0.24	17.77 ± 0.84

A comparison of different materials and fastening techniques with respect to compression achieved by the method and the ultimate strength. Not surprisingly, cables and bands outperformed wires and synthetics.
Reprinted with permission from Shaw, J.A., and Daubert, H.B.: Compression Capability of Cerclage Fixation Systems. Orthopedics, 11:1172, 1988.

stemmed arthroplasties, cerclage alone, and plates alone have all been used in such cases with variable success.[138,223,456,471,509] Additional methods have combined cerclage with a plate of metal or cortical allograft.** A metallic plate is available having the option of screw fixation or cable cerclage. The cables are threaded through a block, which is fitted into a groove in the plate and then crushed over the cables with a special tool (Fig. 3-19).

Periprosthetic fractures are special examples of pathologic fracture, and techniques of fixation using allograft struts and cerclage may find wider application in other types pathologic fracture. As the population ages and osteoporosis takes its toll, fragility fractures should become more prevalent. Cerclage of allograft may be of value in augmentation of a plate–bone construct in such cases.

Transfixion

In 1875, Volkmann described an operation in which a pseudarthrosis was stabilized by placing ivory pegs across the fracture site, thereby transfixing the bone (Fig. 3-20).[473] Transfixion is fixation by means of piercing or penetrating. It is the simplest of all internal fixation methods and is applicable as a percutaneous technique and by open operation. Such fixation is not likely to be intrinsically secure, even in fractures of the hand, and usually must be supplemented by some form of external splintage or reinforcement. If Kirschner wires are used alone, movement of the fracture fragments tends to occur, with possible backing out or failure of the wires.

** References 129, 182–184, 210–212, 334, 347, 373, 385, 502, 514.

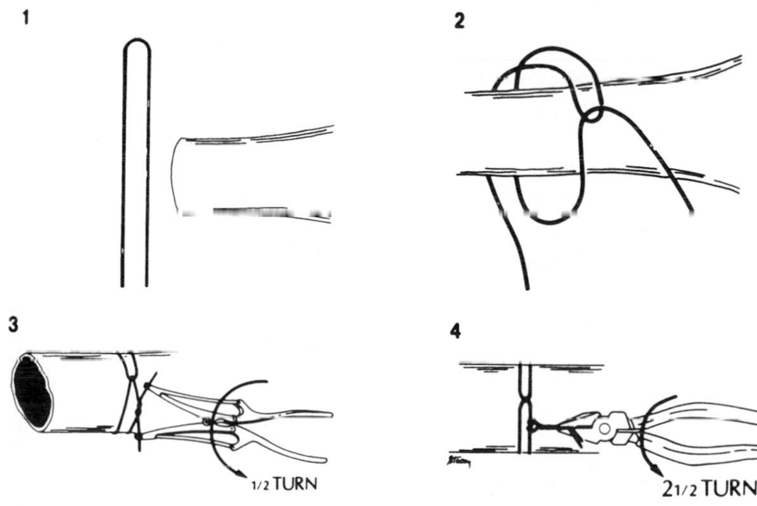

FIGURE 3-16. The technique of the hairpin knot makes a double loop around the bone and fastens with a knot twist. (Cheng, S.L., Smith, T.J., and Davey, J.R.: A Comparison of the Strength and Stability of Six Techniques of Cerclage Wire Fixation for Fractures. J. Orthop. Trauma 7(3):222, 1993.)

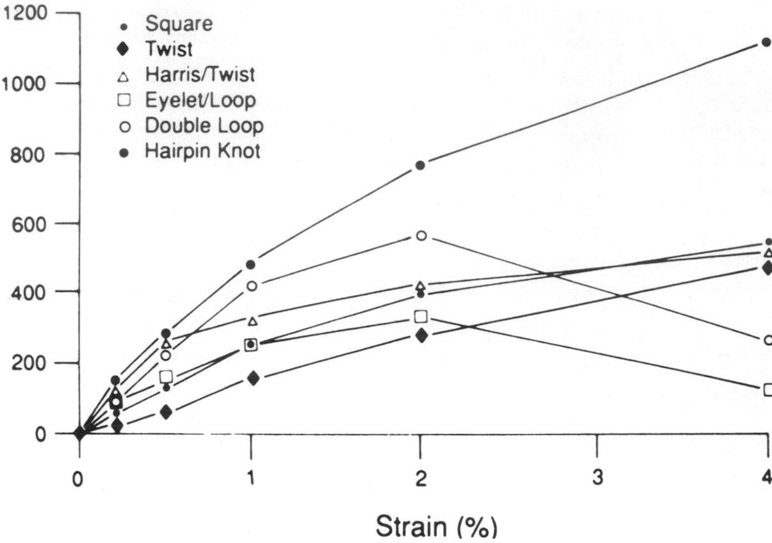

FIGURE 3-17. Applied load and strain of various fastening techniques. The hairpin knot outperformed the others in this test. (Cheng, S.L., Smith, T.J., and Davey, J.R.: A Comparison of the Strength and Stability of Six Techniques of Cerclage Wire Fixation for Fractures. J. Orthop. Trauma 7(3):223, 1993.)

Although Kirschner wires were originally designed to provide skeletal traction with minimal bone damage, they are virtually never used in this manner. Instead, they are used to provide fixation for fractures in the hand, wrist, foot, proximal humerus, and in pediatric fractures.[††] A common use of transfixion pins or wires is as provisional fixation to hold a fracture before placement of final fixation.

A tension-band system can be created by joining together a transfixion device with wire cerclage.[‡‡] Technically demanding, this combination is useful in fractures of the olecranon (Fig. 3-21), patella, phalanges, and occasionally the medial malleolus. Transfixion

[††] References 1–3, 23, 61, 76, 98, 110, 119, 132, 142, 154, 161, 170, 171, 173, 177, 192, 197, 252, 289, 305, 353, 369, 383, 396, 405, 406, 417, 419, 421, 431, 452, 474, 479.

[‡‡] References 34, 41, 49, 50, 78, 90, 193, 246, 247, 313, 335, 380, 428, 442.

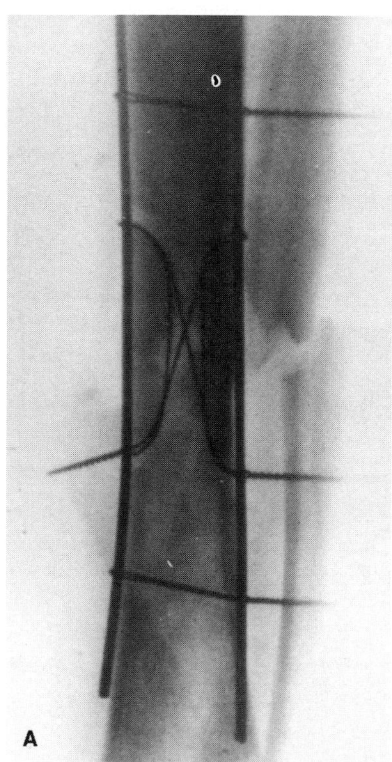

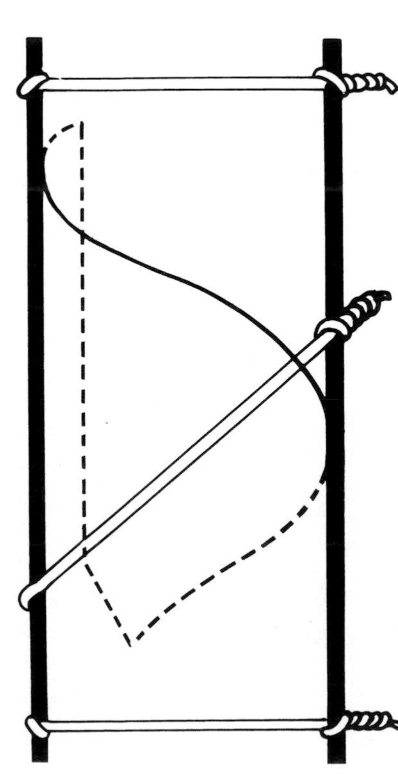

FIGURE 3-18. (**A**) Wire loops were used to generate interfragmentary compression and stability while angular forces were controlled with longitudinal rods wired to each other in this tibial shaft fracture. (**B**) Wire loops anchor rods to the cortex to control bending forces while interfragmentary compressive loading is produced by interfragmentary wires. (Soeur, R.: Fractures of the Limbs. Brussels, La Clinique Orthopedique, 1981.)

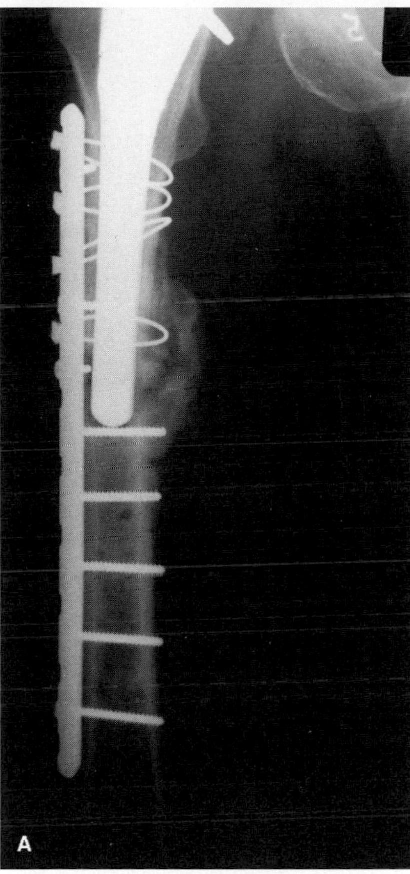

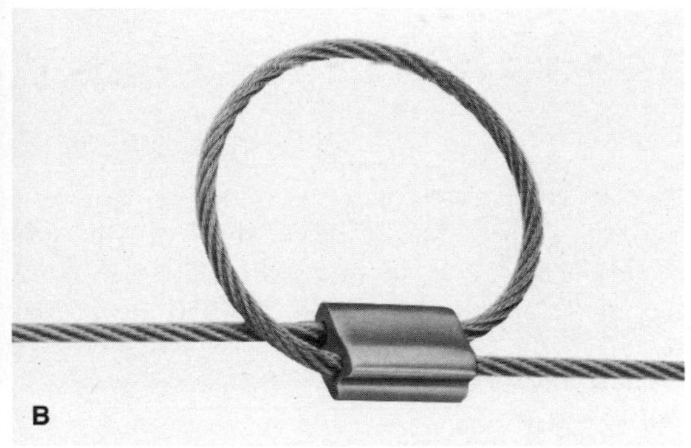

FIGURE 3-19. (**A**) A femoral shaft fracture occurred distal to a total hip prosthesis, which fills the canal. Repair was successful, with a plate fixed with a few unicortical screws, cables and blocks proximally, and bicortical screws distally. Limited control of axial shear force is provided by cerclage. (**B**) Close-up photograph of the Dall Miles cable implant. (*Courtesy of Howmedica, Rutherford, NJ.*)

pins must have firm hold on the far side fragment. The wire loop is tightened, compressing the fracture. It is essential for the wire loop to be seated at the junction of the transfixion device and bone. Soft-tissue interposition at this interface leads to tissue necrosis and loosening of the construct.

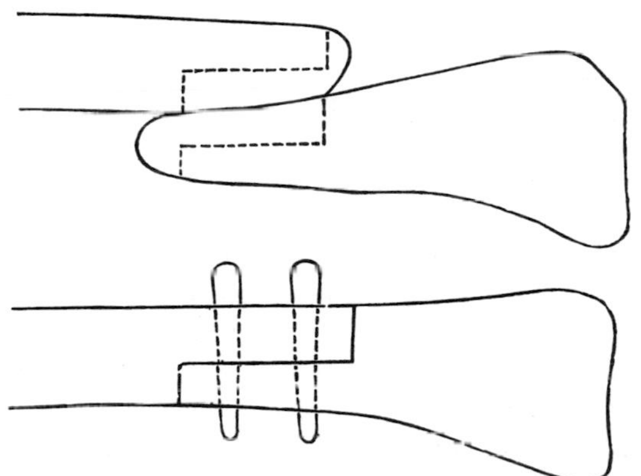

FIGURE 3-20. Volkmann's technique of resection of pseudarthrosis and fixation with two ivory pegs in 1875. (Stimson, L.A.: A Treatise on Fractures, p. 216. 1883, Philadelphia, Henry C. Lea's Son & Co, 1883.)

A final indication for transfixion is as temporary stabilization of an unstable joint. Dislocations of the distal radioulnar joint, the proximal radiocapitellar joint, the distal tibia fibular joint, and the metatarsal cuneiform joint are some examples of problems requiring temporary transfixion. Three to 6 weeks of fixation is typically long enough for soft-tissue healing.

Screws

Screw Design and Properties

Screws used for internal fixation are based on machine screws, threaded from head to tip and having a blunt end. To insert these screws in bone, a preliminary drill hole is made. After this, threads may be cut by a tap before the insertion of the screw, or the screw may be designed to cut its own path with a fluted tip. The screw commonly has a hexagonal head for ease of insertion or removal.

The pitch of a screw (Fig. 3-22) is the distance between the threads, and the lead is the distance through which a screw advances with one turn. If the screw has only one thread, the pitch and lead are identical. If there is more than one thread, however, the lead of

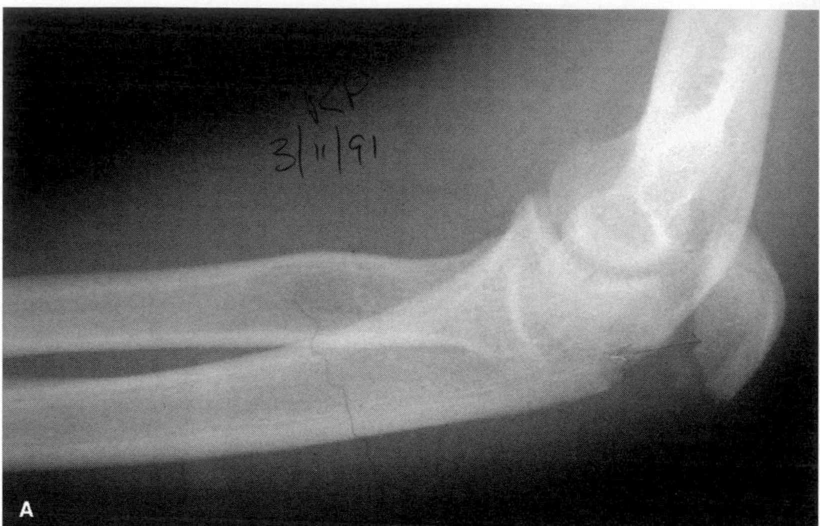

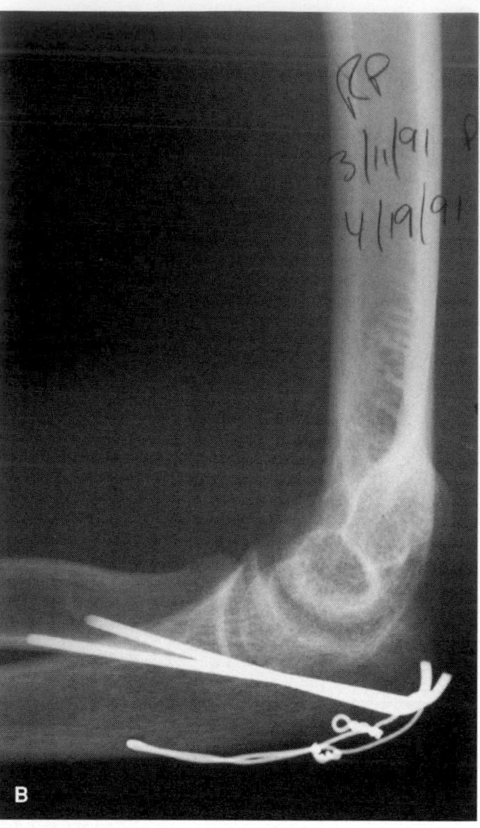

FIGURE 3-21. Displaced olecranon fracture, treated with transfixion wires and tensioned wire loop. (**A**) Preoperative lateral radiograph. (**B**) Union at 5 weeks.

the screw is increased proportionally to the number of threads. A double-threaded screw has a lead double the pitch, and this allows the screw to be tightened more rapidly.[151] Screws are named according to their major diameters. They are either fully or partially threaded.

The tensile strength of a screw, or its resistance to breaking, depends on its root diameter (ie, the diameter of the screw between the threads), whereas the pull-out strength depends on the outside diameter of the threads. Shear strength is proportional to the cube of the root diameter, and tensile strength is proportional to its square. The number of threads per inch has no effect on the pull-out strength of the screw if five or six threads are in the cortex.

Bechtol and Lepper[30] advised that the diameter of the drill be midway between that of the root of the screw and that of the thread. They also believed that the screws should be inserted by a torque equal to 75% of that required to strip the screw. The ASIF group advises 80% of stripping torque. Although Bechtol and Lepper[30] believed that thread configuration is of little importance, Frankel and Burstein[151] disagreed, contending that the ability to resist stripping depends on the total cross-sectional area of material presented to the root of the thread.

Koranyi and associates[290] found no difference in the holding power of the V-threads of coarse and fine Sherman screws and the buttress threads of the ASIF screws but in comparing the holding power of fluted ends of the fine and coarse Sherman screws with the shanks of the screws, they found a reduction of 17% and 24%, respectively.

When a screw is inserted into bone, torque is applied through the screw head, so that the screw advances through its pretapped path or cuts its way if it is self-tapping. With impingement of the screw head on the cortex or on the countersink of a plate, tension is generated in the screw. Torque stress is also induced in the screw to a varying degree and is enhanced by drilling too small a hole and by the increased friction engendered by a self-tapping screw. A screw's resistance to tensile stress is reduced by super-added torque shear and vice versa. The strength of the screw is further impaired by bending moments induced by improper insertion. Screws should be inserted at 80% of the torque that would cause them to strip. Hughes and Jordan[241] have shown that stainless steel and titanium

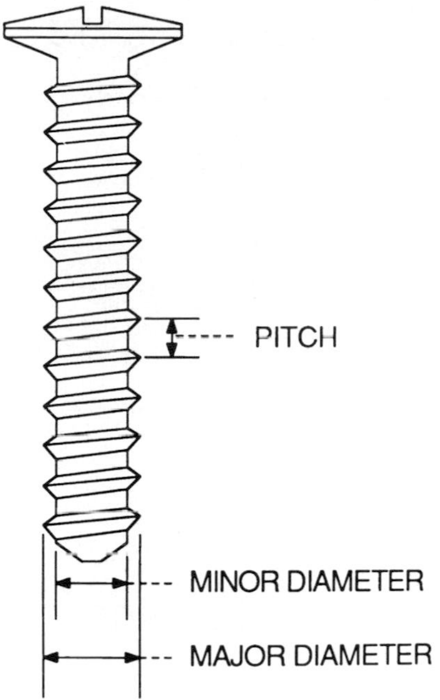

FIGURE 3-22. Schematic of a fully threaded screw. The sharpness of the thread tip, angle, and symmetry of the thread help to define holding power. (DeCoster, T.A., Heetderks, D.B., Downey, D.J., Ferries, J.S., and Jones, W.: Optimizing Bone Screw Pullout Force. J. Orthop. Trauma 4(2):172, 1990.)

alloy (Ti-6A1-4V) screws have greater shear strength than those of pure titanium or Vitallium.

Schatzker and associates[241,446–448] made a series of studies on the holding power of screws in the living bone of dogs. Most other studies have been in bovine or cadaver bone or nonliving material. They compared the "push-out" rather than "pull-out" strength of 3.5- and 4.5-mm ASIF screws with that of Vitallium screws (a pretapped 4-mm buttress-thread screw and a 3.5-mm self-tapping screw). They showed that the predominant factor in the holding power of a screw immediately after insertion is the diameter of the screw thread. Other determinants such as thread profile, mode of insertion, and ratio of the drill hole to the external diameter of the screw were of minor importance.

The contention that a self-tapping screw, if removed and reinserted into the same hole, loses holding power by stripping its threads was also discredited by these studies. Self tapping screws inserted at 80% of their torque-out value were removed and reinserted 12 times without significant loss of holding power. Histologic studies showed no difference in the extent of bone death, splintering, or bone remodeling produced by tapped and self-tapped screws or between Vitallium and stainless steel. The mean values of holding power for all the screws tested increased between 150% and 190% at the end of 6 weeks but declined to between 125% and 160% at the end of 12 weeks.

Movement of screws in bone provoked bone resorption and marked fibrous tissue proliferation. In contrast, a screw at rest, even when placed in a hole drilled too large, became enveloped in bone. Bone resorption is caused by motion of the screw rather than screw loosening being secondary to resorption of bone. Furthermore, if a screw is stripped, it may be beneficial to leave it in situ if no motion occurs between it and the bone. When a screw was inserted with overdrilling of the near cortex, new bone formed around the screw in the oversized hole. Granulation tissue did not form at the screw–bone interface in the far cortex but the dead bone around the screw threads remodeled so that compression at the interface ultimately fell to zero.

ASIF Screws

The ASIF has developed bone screws for a wide variety of internal fixation situations. In comparing ASIF screws with other types of screws, it is difficult to demonstrate marked superiority of the ASIF screw in any single parameter. Nevertheless, as Mears[342] has noted, where a measurable difference exists, it is always in the favor of the ASIF screw and furthermore, it is part of a well-engineered complete system of internal fixation.

Cortex Screws

Cortical screws are available in diameters from 1.5 to 4.5 mm. The insertion characteristics for all are similar, so that once the pattern is learned, it may be applied to the entire screw family. The drill for the pilot hole is slightly larger than the core or minor diameter of the screw. For the glide hole, the drill matches the major diameter of the screw. The tap is the same diameter and pitch as the screw (Fig. 3-23).[339]

Holding Screw or Neutral Screw

The large-fragment ASIF cortical screw[342,361–363] has a thread diameter of 4.5 mm and a core diameter of 3 mm. The head, which has a diameter of 8 mm, has a deep hexagonal recess that mates accurately with the screwdriver, providing a large contact surface between the screw head and screwdriver for the efficient transfer of torque. The assembly of screw and instrument is stable and there is no mechanism to lock and unlock, so that no time is wasted in loading the screwdriver (Fig. 3-24).

The pilot hole is drilled (with the aid of a centering guide when a plate is used) with a 3.2-mm drill bit. The length of the screw to be used is measured by a

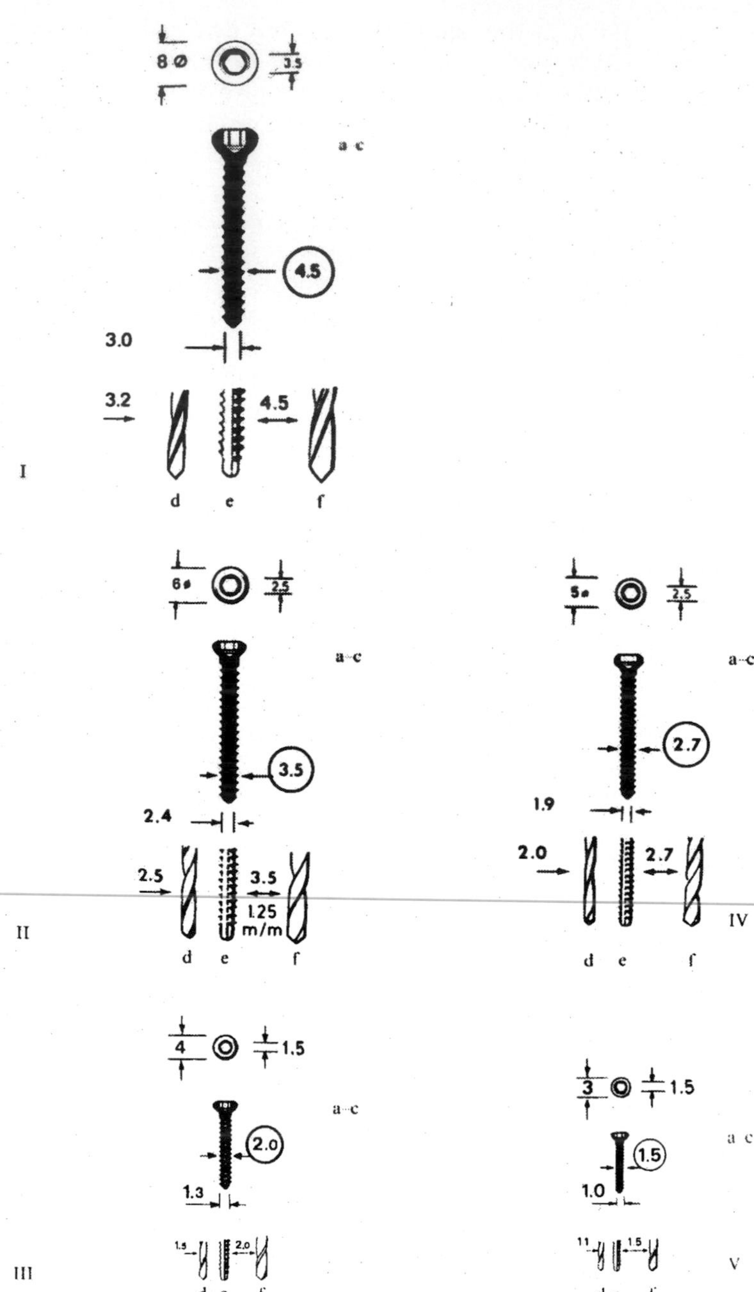

FIGURE 3-23. Available ASIF cortical screws and their drill bits, taps, and washers. (**I**) 4.5-mm cortex screw: *a.* 8-mm screw head and 3.5-mm hexagonal recess; *b.* fully threaded, with 1.75-mm pitch; *c.* core diameter of 3 mm and outer diameter of 4.5-mm; *d.* 3.2-mm thread-hole drill bit; *e.* 4.5-mm glide-hole drill bit; *f.* 4.5-mm tap. (**II**) 3.5-mm cortex screw: *a.* 6-mm screw head, with 2.5-mm hexagonal recess; *b.* fully threaded, with 1.75-mm pitch; *c.* 2.4-mm core; *d.* 2.5-mm thread-hole drill bit; *e.* 2.7-mm glide-hole drill bit; *f.* 3.5-mm tap. (**III**) 2.7-mm cortex screw: *a.* 5-mm head, with 2.5-mm hexagonal recess; *b.* fully threaded, with 1-mm pitch; *c.* core diameter of 1.9-mm and outer diameter of 2.7-mm; *d.* 2-mm thread-hole drill bit; *e.* 2.7-mm glide-hole drill bit; *f.* 2.7-mm tap. (**IV**) 2-mm cortex screw: *a.* 4-mm head, with 1.5-mm hexagonal recess; *b.* fully threaded, with 0.8-mm pitch; *c.* core diameter of 1.3-mm and outer diameter of 2 mm; *d.* 1.5-mm thread-hole drill bit; *e.* 2-mm glide-hole drill bit; *f.* 2-mm tap. (**V**) 1.5-mm cortex screw: *a.* 3-mm head, with 1.5-mm hexagonal recess; *b.* fully threaded, with 0.6-mm pitch; *c.* core diameter of 1-mm and outer diameter of 1.5-mm; *d.* 1.1-mm thread-hole drill bit; *e.* 1.5-mm glide-hole drill bit; *f.* 1.5-mm tap. (Müller, M.E., Allgower, M., Schneider, R., Willenegger, H.: Manual of Internal Fixation, 3rd Ed, p. 183. Berlin, Springer-Verlag, 1992.)

depth gauge and the thread cut with a 4.5-mm tap inside a tap sleeve to protect the soft tissues. The screw is inserted. The process occurs during Ringer's lactate irrigation to cool the metal and clear debris. The tap and screwdriver may be operated by hand but there are quick-change couplings for the small air drill for power insertion. The sequence of screw insertion is the same as for other screws, substituting the appropriate size taps and drills. Figure 3-23 gives the sizes of the cortical screws and their appropriate drills and taps.

Cortex Screw as a Lag Screw

Lag effect is created when the near hole (gliding hole) is drilled with a 4.5-mm drill bit. A drill sleeve with an outer diameter of 4.5 mm is inserted into this hole until it abuts on the far cortex. A 3.2-mm drill bit is inserted through the drill sleeve and the far or thread hole is bored (Fig. 3-25). The far hole is then threaded with a 4.5-mm tap. Alternatively, the far hole may be drilled first, even before the reduction of the fracture. The fracture is then reduced, the far hole guide

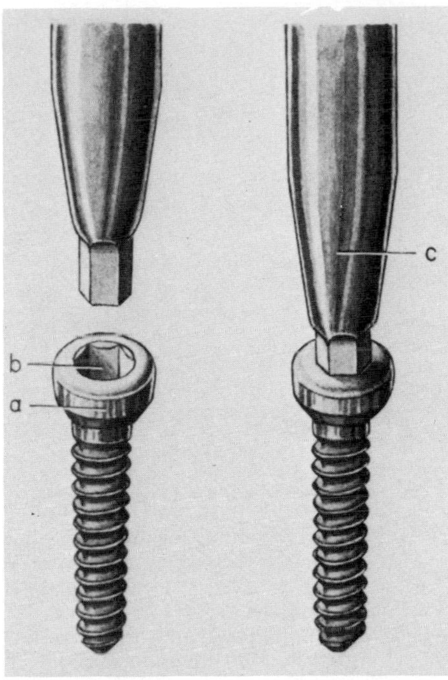

FIGURE 3-24. The ASIF screw and driver. The screw head has a shallow cylindrical flank that gives better contact with the hole in the plate, and the hexagonal screwdriver, with matching recess in the screw, gives a much larger surface area for transmission of the torque from the screwdriver to the screw. (Müller, M.E., Allgower, M., Schneider, R., and Willenegger, H.: Manual of Internal Fixation. New York, Springer-Verlag, 1970.)

is inserted in the hole, and the near hole is drilled (Fig. 3-26).

A countersink is inserted into the gliding hole to provide a recess for the spherical head of the screw in areas of hard cortical bone when the screw resides outside of the plate. The depth gauge should be used after preparation of the countersink hole because the screw will penetrate deeper into the bone. Countersinking a screw gives more even load transfer from screw to bone and irritates the skin less. Care must be taken to not penetrate the cortex with the countersink and lose purchase, however.

Shaft Screw

A special titanium cortical screw (shaft or shank screw) has been developed for the titanium limited-contact dynamic compression plate (LC-DCP) system for use as a lag screw or to anchor a plate being loaded with the external tensioning device. The smooth shank of the screw has an outer diameter of 4.5 mm for improved stiffness and strength.[282,361] A 40% loss of compression was noted with a 4.5-mm cortical screw of conventional design when placed as a lag screw through the plate due to indentation of the screw within the glide hole.[398]

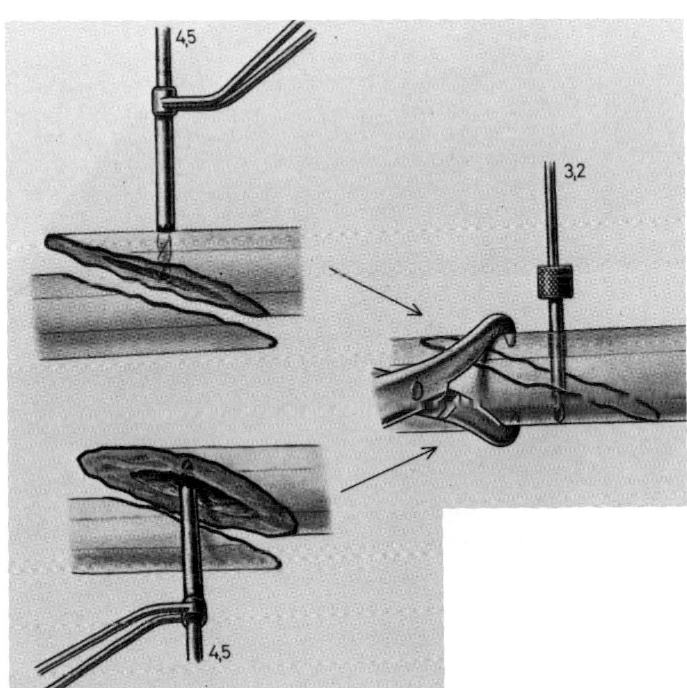

FIGURE 3-25. Technique of lag-screw fixation. Predrilling the gliding hole (*top left, bottom left*). A 4.5-mm hole is drilled in one cortex from inside or outside. After reduction, the opposite cortex is drilled, using the drill guide that has a 4.5-mm outer diameter and a 3.2-mm inner diameter. (Müller, M.E., Allgower, M., Schneider, R., and Willenegger, H.: Manual of Internal Fixation. Techniques Recommended by the AO Group, 2nd Ed, p. 39. New York, Springer-Verlag, 1979.)

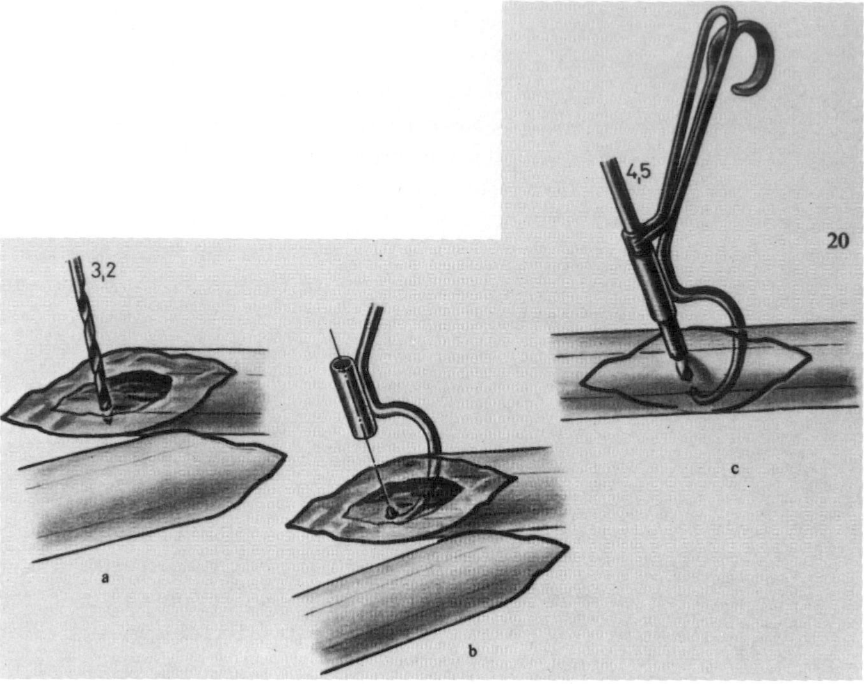

FIGURE 3-26. Alternative technique of lag screw fixation. The thread hole may be drilled first and the gliding hole aligned with the far hole guide. (Müller, M.E., Allgower, M., Schneider, R., and Willenegger, H.: Manual of Internal Fixation. Techniques Recommended by the AO Group, 2nd Ed, p. 39. New York, Springer-Verlag, 1979.)

Self-Tapping Screw

Advantages of self-tapping screws are reduced operative time and decreased instrumentation (Fig. 3-27).[26] The potential disadvantages of a self-tapping screw are damage to the bone by bone tissue deformation and destruction caused by displacement pressure and heat. The ideal self-cutting screw will cut a sharp path and clear the debris from the cuttings. Cutting flutes positioned in cortical bone lead to decreased pull-out strength. The ASIF self-tapping screw has three flutes: a positive rake angle, a short and large cutting flute, and a tapered tip (Fig. 3-28).[26]

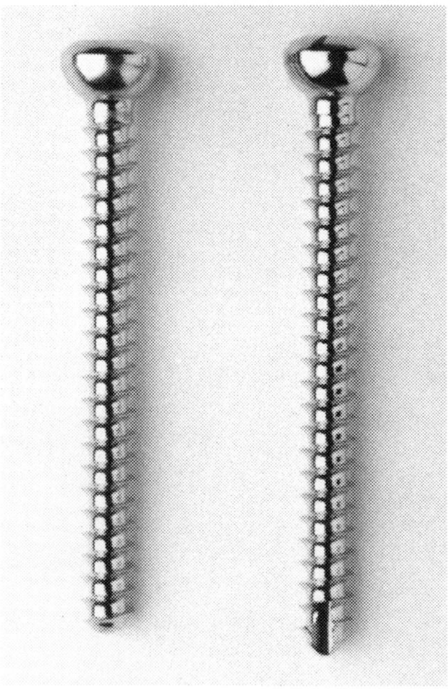

FIGURE 3-27. The ASIF self-tapping screw (*right*) has a cutting tip to save a step in the insertion procedure. (*Courtesy of Synthes, Paoli, PA.*)

The cutting efficiency of the flute is determined by the sharpness of the cutting edge, which in turn is related to the manufacturing process. Additionally, the volume of the flute must be adequate to accommodate debris from the cutting process, which is related to the thickness of the bone in which the screw is placed. Baumgart and coworkers have estimated that a 4.5-mm cortex screw in a 3.2-mm pilot hole gathers about 1 mm^3 of bone per revolution.[26] Furthermore, with a pitch of 1.75 mm, three revolutions are required to advance one point on the outer surface of the screw through the cortex, producing 3 mm^3 of bone debris. Information concerning the influence of the cutting angle on insertion torque is available on a theoretic basis but little is known about optimization of cutting angle for biologic materials.[26]

Studies of insertion torque and pull-out force of tapped, self-tapping, and untapped 4.5-mm cortex screws found insertion torque similar for pretapped and self-tapping screws, compared with two to three times higher values for untapped insertion.[26] Pull-out strength was comparable between the pretapped and self-tapping screws but considerably lower for untapped screw. If the cutting tip does not protrude through the cortex, the pull-out strength is reduced by 10%.[26]

Cancellous Screws

In contrast to cortical screws, cancellous screws have a greater difference between major and minor diameters. Cancellous screws are intended for metaphyseal and epiphyseal fixation, wherein bone has greater porosity. Cancellous screws gather a greater volume and surface area between the threads.

Cancellous screws are available in diameters from 4 to 7.3 mm, with a 4.5-mm self-tapping screw in between (malleolar). Figure 3-28 lists the screws, with their appropriate drill and tap. Cancellous tap use is optional in most applications. The 4.5-mm screw has a cortical thread design (for dense cancellous bone), a sharper point than cancellous screws, a core diameter of 3 mm, and a thread diameter of 4.5 mm.

Cancellous Screws as Lag Screws. To use cancellous screws as lag screws, a single drill bit is used for the pilot hole, a 2.5-mm bit for the 4.0-mm screw, a 3.2-mm bit for the 6.5-mm screw, and a 4.5-mm bit for the 7.0-mm screw. A tap is available but is used for only the first few turns (if any) because these screws

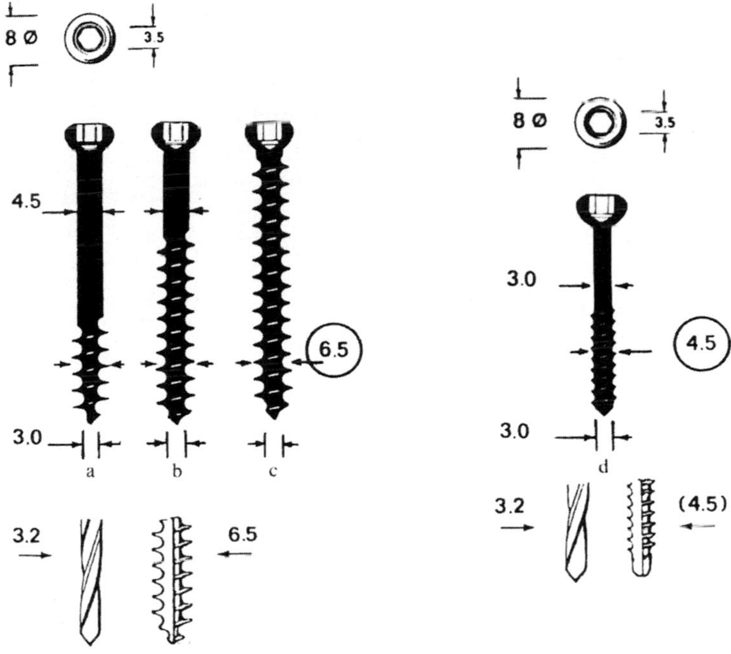

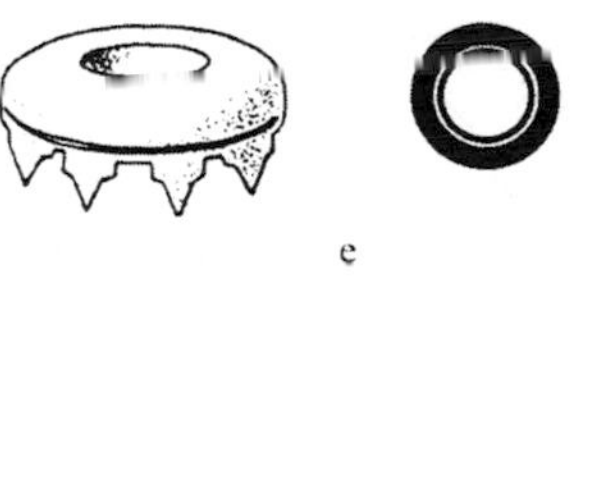

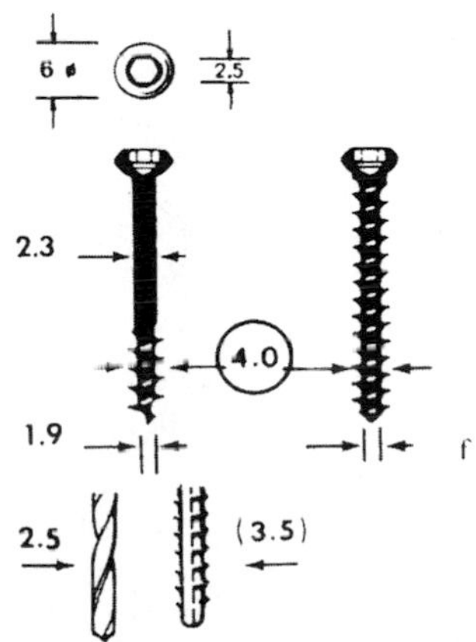

FIGURE 3-28. ASIF cancellous screws and their drill bits, taps and washers: *a,b,c.* 6.5-mm screw with 8-mm head having a 3.5-mm hexagonal recess, shaft core of 4.5-mm, and thread core of 3-mm; 3.2-mm drill bit and 6.5-mm tap; *a.* 16-mm thread length; *b.* 32-mm thread length; *c.* fully threaded; *d.* 4.5-mm screw, with 3-mm core, 4.5-mm thread diameter, 3.2-mm drill, and optional 4.5-mm tap (has cutting tip on screw); *e.* Plastic and metal washers; *f.* 4-mm screws with 6-mm head having 3.5-mm hexagonal recess; core diameter is 1.9-mm, pitch 1.75-mm, and requires a 2.5-mm drill and 4-mm tap. (Müller, M.E., Allgower, M., Schneider, R., Willenegger, H.: Manual of Internal Fixation, 3rd Ed, p. 185. Berlin, Springer-Verlag, 1992.)

gain better purchase when they cut their own way into cancellous bone. Lag effect depends on glide of the smooth screw shank in the near side screw hole. Thread length must be chosen such that all threads are in the far side hole and do not cross the fracture site.

Cannulated Screws

Hollow screws modeled on the cortical and cancellous screws discussed above have been developed to allow provisional fixation to become part of the final construct (Fig. 3-29). Operative trauma and the number of steps necessary to place final fixation are thus reduced. A guide pin is placed where desired, the position is verified, the depth is read with an external depth gauge, and a cannulated drill makes the pilot hole over the guide pin. The pin is removed and the hole tapped. The screw is then placed. Screws are available in a wide range of sizes. Hearn and coworkers studied pull-out strength of cannulated large-diameter (7-mm) cancellous screws and found no difference, compared with noncannulated screws (6.5 mm).[213] Similarly Leggon and coworkers reported similar results after testing pull-out strength of both cannulated and noncannulated cortical and cancellous screws (3.5-mm cortical cannulated and noncannulated, 6.5-mm cancellous noncannulated, and 7-mm cannulated cancellous).[309]

Interference Screws

Bone-ligament-bone graft reconstruction of torn cruciate ligaments has become a standard procedure for the cruciate-deficient knee.[§§] Significant improvement in the results of these procedures occurred with development of fixation methods sufficient to allow immediate mobilization of the patient and motion of the knee.[303] The bone side of the graft is pulled into a bone tunnel and wedged firmly into the substance of the tunnel with a 7- or 9-mm diameter headless screw (Fig. 3-30). Kurosaka and colleagues[300] compared six different types of bone pedicle fixation, including staples, sutures tied over buttons, and screws. The headless 9-mm screw outperformed other methods in terms of highest linear load and stiffness. The bone-ligament-bone unit failed at 1600 N, the 9-mm headless screw at 600 N, and the AO/ASIF 6.5-mm screw failed at 200 N. Stapling and suturing over buttons were less effect than the 6.5-mm AO/ASIF screw method.

[§§] 18, 60, 135, 155, 169, 174, 178, 201, 245, 267, 300, 311, 323, 371, 469, 532

Effects on Bone of Drilling

The drilling of a hole in a bone immediately reduces its breaking strength. Bechtol and Lepper[30] stated that when holes are placed in an area of tension, the weakening effect is greatest. The size of the hole has little effect on the breaking strength, so long as it is less than 20% of the diameter of the bone. When this size is exceeded, the degree of weakening is proportional to the size of the hole. The presence of a screw also weakens the bone to the same extent as an unfilled hole but the effect diminishes with the production of new bone.

Laurence[307] found that the bending moment required to fracture an intact tibia varied from 59 Nm to 226 Nm (mean, 137 Nm). When a 3-mm drill hole was made in the tibia, however, the moment required

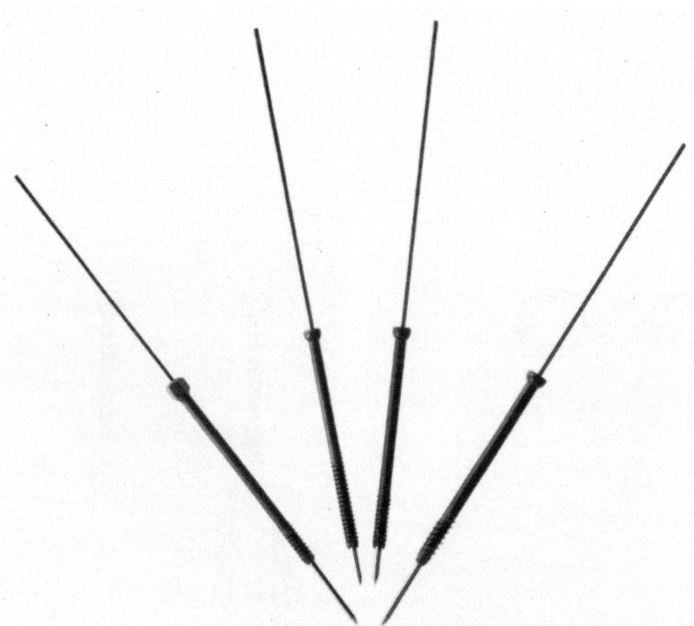

FIGURE 3-29. Self-tapping cannulated cancellous titanium screws. (*Courtesy of Ace Orthopaedic Company, El Sequando, CA.*)

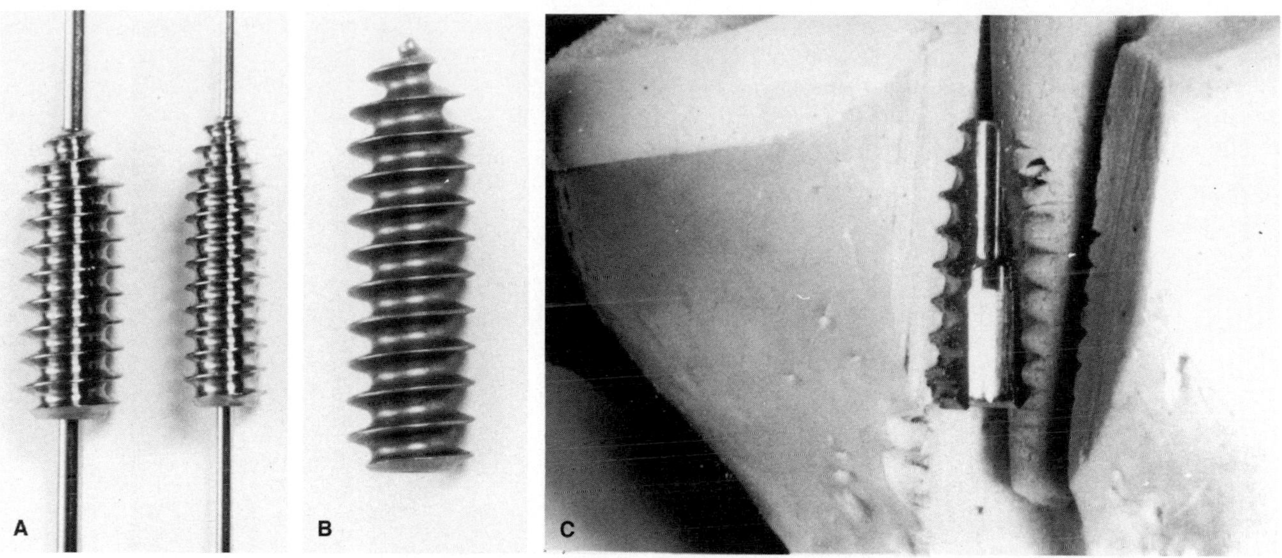

FIGURE 3-30. (**A**) Cannulated headless 7- and 9-mm titanium interference screw. (**B**) Noncannulated 9-mm Kurosaka interference screw with hexagonal recess. (**C**) The interference screw threads into the bone of both the graft and bone tunnel, displacing the graft into the substance of the tunnel producing secure fixation. (*Courtesy of the DePuy Corporation, Warsaw, IN.*)

was reduced from 229 to 147 Nm (mean, 98 Nm). Brooks and associates[58] studied the influence of drill holes on torsional fractures in paired canine femurs. With a 2.8-mm hole and a load applied for 0.1 second, the mean reduction in energy absorption was 58.5% and for 3.6-mm holes, 51.9%. Because the energy absorbed by these bones with holes is reduced, these fractures have less comminution (Fig. 3-31).

Burstein and associates,[77] at Case Western Reserve University, also found that a fresh screw hole weakened bone in bending and torsional loading. Whereas Bechtol found 20% to be the critical level, Burstein[77] determined that the size of the screw hole had no effect on breaking strength until it exceeded 30% of the diameter of the bone. When torque was applied to the drilled bone, the stresses around the hole were 1.6 times greater than those over the remainder of the bone; when failure occurred, the fracture line passed through the drill hole in more than 90% of the bones tested. With time, however, the strength of the bone increased, even with the screw in situ, but after removal of the screw, the bone is again unduly susceptible to fracture. Surprisingly, in these latter cases, the experimental fracture line passed through the screw hole in only 6 of 38 fractures.

Although the effects of having a screw in bone are mitigated by remodeling, once the screw is removed, the hole again becomes a stress riser. It follows that the bone must be protected after the removal of screws, at least until the defect heals. After removal of a screw, the hole remains evident on radiographs for an extended period. Just because there is an obvious sclerotic margin does not mean that the hole has not healed. Histologic examination shows that the defect is filled with woven bone in 6 to 8 weeks. Remedies for screw-hole weakness, such as overdrilling or filling the holes with plastic plugs, are not helpful.

Screw-Fixation Technique

The angle of screw insertion is of great importance (Fig. 3-32). At the time of insertion, the greatest compressive loading along the fracture interface is with the screw perpendicular to the plane of the fracture. Placed perpendicular to the long axis of the bone, the screw may create a shear plane and offset the fracture (Fig. 3-33). Arzimanoglou and Skiadaressis[12] compared the results of fixing a standard fracture by screws inserted at right angles to the shaft, at right angles to the fracture line, and by a combination of the two. The greatest stability under conditions of compression loading was obtained by screws inserted at right angles to the shaft and the least by those inserted perpendicular to the fracture line (dynamic loading conditions; Fig. 3-34). Conversely, optimal compression of the fracture is produced with a lag screw inserted perpendicular to the plane of the fracture and is the preferred orientation for most lag screw applications.[361]

Müller and associates[361] have endorsed this principle; however, for treating spiral fractures with a loose butterfly fragment, they recommend fixing the two major fragments with a transverse screw and inserting the remaining screws at an angle midway between the perpendiculars to the shaft and the fracture line (Fig.

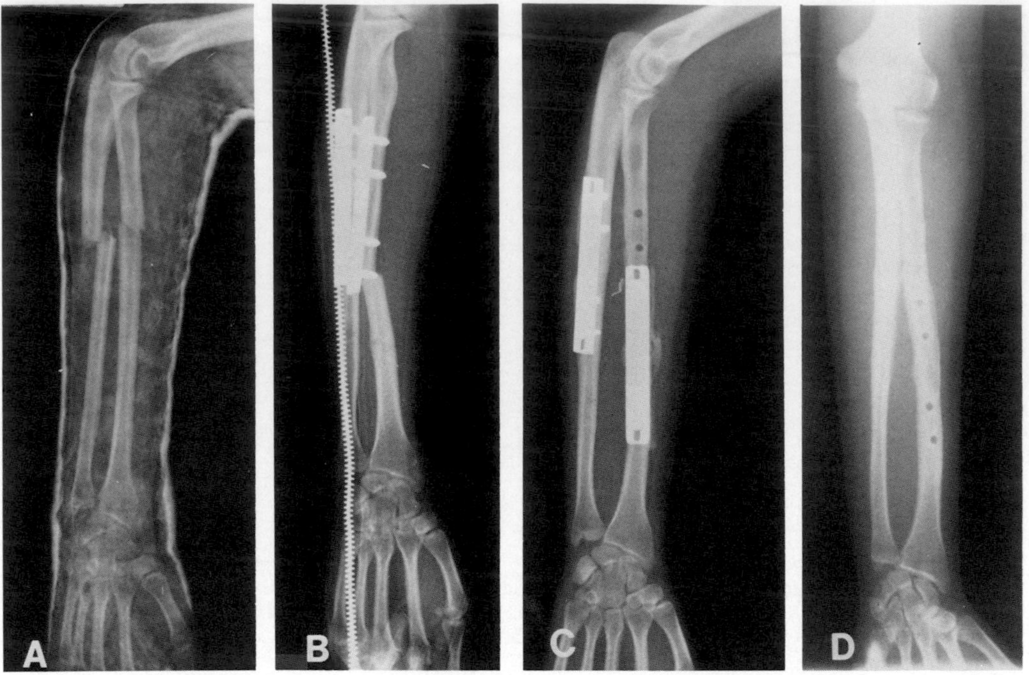

FIGURE 3-31. (**A**) Radiograph showing fractures of both bones of the forearm in a 14-year-old girl. (**B**) Eight months after compression plating, she sustained a refracture through the lower screw in the radius. (**C**) This fracture also was treated with a compression plate and the addition of an osteoperiosteal graft from her rib. (**D**) Four months later, after removal of both plates. The holes persisted for a considerable time radiographically but histologically the holes healed by woven bone despite the radiographic appearance (see also Fig. 1-111).

3-35). Although transverse screws give the greatest stability against displacement with compression loading, the midway position gives more protection against bending in an axis perpendicular to the screws. Lag screw fixation only for diaphyseal fractures is not advisable. Protection with a plate or external fixator is recommended.

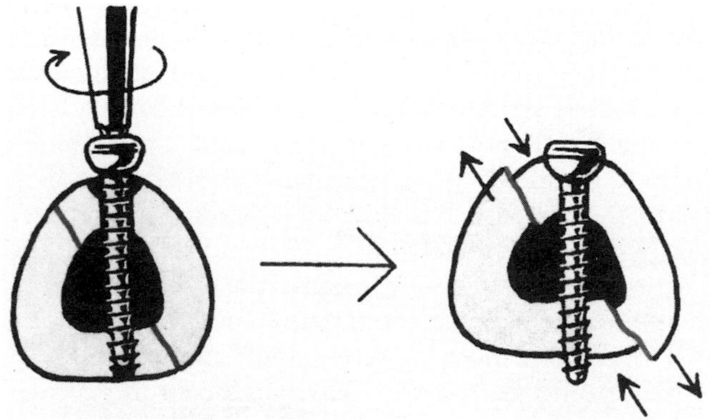

FIGURE 3-32. Poor assessment of the fracture plane leads to fracture displacement as bone aligns itself with the resultant force vector created by lag effect of the screw. (Müller, M.E., Allgower, M., Schneider, R., and Willenegger, H.: Manual of Internal Fixation, 3rd ed, p. 189. Berlin: Springer-Verlag, 1992.)

Plates

History

According to Mears, plating of fractures is traceable into the last century, when Hansmann[342] described a percutaneously removable plate in 1886. Later, Lane, Lambotte, and Sherman developed implants and techniques of plate osteosynthesis.[394] Pauwels defined tension-band techniques in 1935. Danis pioneered techniques of compression osteosynthesis and defined primary union biologically.[394] In 1950, Peterson[407] defined basic principles of bone plating:

Careful handling of implants
Proper orientation of the screw head in the plate
Measurement of screw holes with a depth gauge
Final tightening of all screws
Drill diameter slightly smaller than screw diameter
Correct plate contouring before application

Compression plating is meant to achieve rigid fixation of the fracture. Rigid fixation promotes primary bone healing, in which contact healing occurs across the apposed bone ends by cutting cones of revascularization that cross the fracture site. In such healing, periosteal callus is scant or absent. The appearance of ex-

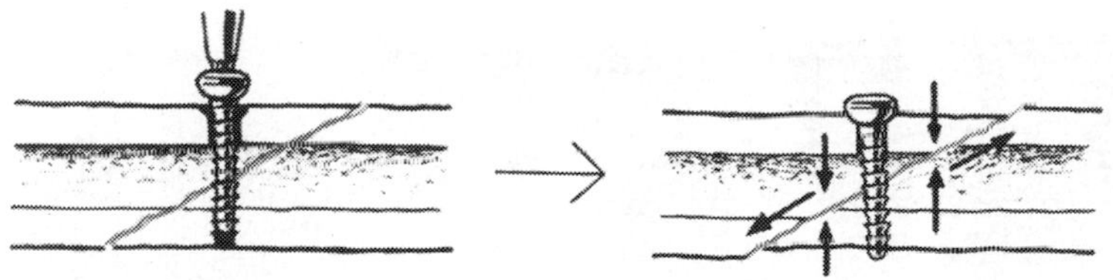

FIGURE 3-33. A cortical lag screw placed perpendicular to the long axis of the bone may displace the fracture as the two inclined planes act to transform the applied load into a horizontal shear producing force. Such a screw is best positioned to resist displacement with compression loading. (Müller, M.E., Allgower, M., Schneider, R., and Willenegger, H.: Manual of Internal Fixation, 3rd ed, p. 189. Berlin: Springer-Verlag, 1992.)

ternal callus, sometimes referred to as irritation callus, may be evidence of motion or infection.

Methods of plate compression have undergone transformation from the coaptor attachment on the plate of Danis to the external and removable external tensioning devices of the AO/ASIF system to the auto compression plate developed first by Eggers[126,127] and later Bagby and coworkers.[15,16] Both autocompression and external-tensioning methods are important in plate fixation techniques.

Biology

Plate fixation techniques, as mainly practiced, necessitate exposure of the fracture site, evacuation of the hematoma, and violation of the periosteal circulation of the bone in proportion to the degree of soft-tissue release performed by the surgeon. Whether the fracture hematoma is a source of cellular elements contributing to fracture healing is still unknown[44a] but preservation of the hematoma may be of value. Rhinelander has shown that after fracture, the periosteal circulation becomes dominant, primarily through dense connective-tissue attachments.[422,423] Careless soft-tissue technique adversely affects bone healing through circulatory impairment. In a study of the effect of osteotomy on blood flow in the canine tibia, Smith and coworkers observed a decrease in blood flow of 50% at 10 minutes and 66% at 4 hours, compared with controls.[463] Internal fixation also decreased blood flow substantially, with the most enduring and profound decreased flow occurring with intramedullary nails when compared with plates. The least alteration in flow was seen with external fixation.

Superb studies of bone healing under rigid compression have been made by Schenk in collaboration with Willenegger.[361–363] They have shown that where bone is under compression such that no fracture gap is present, dead bone is resorbed; resorption cavities, produced by cutting cones of osteoclasts, traverse the fracture plane. Blood vessels accompanied by mesenchymal cells and osteoblast precursors soon follow to reconstitute the haversian systems.

If the axial compression opens up a gap in the cortex opposite the plate, usually about 200 μm, the healing process is a little different. Primary bone formation takes place but the orientation of this bone is not longitudinal but parallel to the fracture surface (gap healing). In the second stage of gap healing, the longitudinal haversian systems are reconstituted by cutting cones from each fragment, and the bone is united primarily without the need for ensheathing callus.

Olerud and Danckwardt-Lilliestrom[376] studied healing in dog tibias in which a double osteotomy had

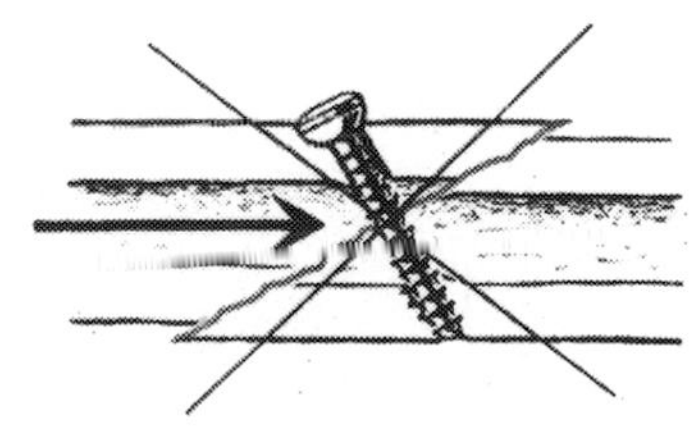

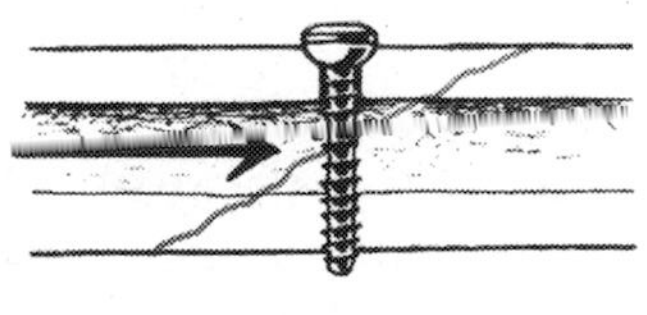

FIGURE 3-34. Optimal compression force across the fracture is produced by a lag screw placed perpendicular to the plane of the fracture but under physiologic loads has a greater tendency for displacement than a screw placed perpendicular to the long axis of the bone. Most lag screw applications require the lag screw to be perpendicular to the plane of the fracture, with shear being controlled with a plate or external fixator. (Müller, M.E., Allgower, M., Schneider, R., and Willenegger, H.: Manual of Internal Fixation, 3rd Ed, p. 191. Berlin, Springer-Verlag, 1992.)

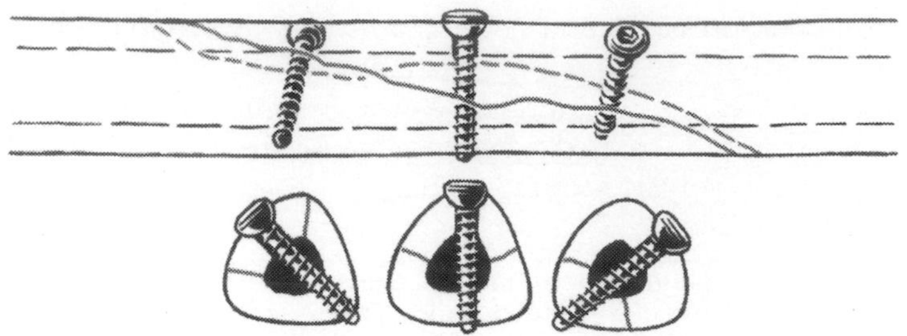

FIGURE 3-35. A spiral fracture is best stabilized with lag screws that follow the variable perpendiculars of the spiral. Additional fixation in the form of a plate or external fixator completes the construct by controlling bending and torsion. (Müller, M.E., Allgower, M., Schneider, R., and Willenegger, H.: Manual of Internal Fixation, 3rd ed, p. 191. Berlin, Springer-Verlag, 1992.)

been performed, with removal of the loose segment to ensure its complete avascularity. When this loose fragment was replaced and fixed by a compression plate, they found that within 2 weeks, 80% of the intermediate fragments had vessels in the haversian canals that were derived from the endosteal circulation. Both the intermediate fragment and the bone ends were being remodeled by simultaneous bone resorption and new bone formation in the haversian systems.

The provision of rigid internal fixation to facilitate primary healing exacts a price. The large, strong plates that eliminate micromotion at the fracture site also "stress-protect" the bone (ie, they absorb stress that normally would be borne by the bone). If is not adequately stressed, bone atrophies and where plates have been in situ for some time, the bone breaks down and is vulnerable to refracture after removal of the metal.[354,355] This further aggravates the problem of the empty screw holes.

Uhthoff and associates[494] studied dog femurs having transverse fractures treated by four-hole compression plates and found osteopenia, which was most pronounced in the cortex underlying the plate. There was subperiosteal resorption, with a reduction in the caliber of the shaft. Histologically, there was a persistence of woven bone but these changes reversed after removal of the plates.

Paavolainen and associates[381,382] also studied the healing of experimental fractures in rabbit tibiofibular bones that were fixed by six-hole stainless steel Dynamic Compression Plates (DCPs, Synthes, Paoli, PA). These fractures were tested for torsional strength at intervals from 3 to 24 weeks postoperatively. During the first 9 weeks, there was progressive improvement in maximum torque capacity, energy absorption, and torsional rigidity, reflecting the advancement of the union. From 9 to 24 weeks, the torque capacity and energy absorption decreased, whereas torsional rigidity reached a steady state. They concluded that after healing, the continued presence of the implant has an adverse effect on the cortical bone, which loses strength. The rabbit normally obtains bony union at 6 to 8 weeks. In histologic studies, they found that after 9 weeks there was rapid excavation and breakdown of the cortical wall, and porosity increased from 9% to 37.5%. The osteoporosis was accompanied by new subperiosteal bone, increasing the overall diameter of the bone and the medullary cavity.

If the fixation is made even better, the cortical porosity is enhanced. Pilliar and associates[409] applied a porous coating of cobalt-based alloy on the surface of 316L stainless steel plates. The powder was sintered to the plates in hydrogen at 1270°C. The control was a steel plate annealed at 1270°C for 3 hours. Six months after applying the plates in dogs, there was no difficulty in prying the control plates off but the coated plates were removed only with great difficulty. There was greater intracortical porosity and bone resorption on the side of the coated plate.

When a plate is applied to bone, the modulus of the plated section is higher than the rest of the bone and there is an abrupt transition at the juncture of plated and unplated bone. This acts as a stress riser, and attempts have been made to mitigate this action by tapered plates and the use of a unicortical screw in the last hole to smooth out the difference. Both problems conceivably may be solved by using plates that are less stiff. Uthoff and coworkers[499] have compared stainless steel and titanium plates in the healing of osteotomies in beagles and found that radiologic bone loss was 19% for stainless steel and only 3% for the titanium plates.

Coutts and associates[101] compared stainless steel plates with plates made of a composite of carbon fibers laminated in polymethylmethacrylate. This was a short-term study on six mongrel dogs. The bending stiffness of the steel plates was 5.5×10^4 kg/cm^2 and of the composite, 6×10^3 kg/cm^2. There appeared to be no qualitative difference between the two plates in radiologic healing of the fractures nor was there a difference in torque, deformation, or energy absorption at refracture. The computed maximal shear strengths were identical. Intracortical porosity, however, was 14% with steel plates and only 6.8% for the composite.

Tayton and his associates[482] have used semirigid carbon fiber–reinforced plates both experimentally and in clinical practice. In sheep with both simple transverse and segmental osteotomies fixation with these plates was uniformly successful in achieving union. The carbon fiber–reinforced implants used clinically were of two varieties. In the first seven cases, a copy of the ASIF DCP was used but the large slotted holes weakened the plate to such an extent that the design was changed to an eight-hole, broad plate in which the holes were round. This latter plate was used in 13 patients.

All the patients selected for the study had sustained transverse or short oblique fractures of the mid-shaft of the tibia, some of which included butterfly fragments. After surgery, the patients were encouraged to walk with a cane as soon as they were comfortable (3 to 10 days). Of the seven patients in the initial ASIF DCP group, six went on to union, whereas the seventh developed a hypertrophic pseudarthrosis after failure of the plate. Three of the patients with healed fractures complained of pain on weight bearing. All of the patients whose fractures were treated by the noncompressing round-hole plates healed. Only two of these complained of pain and both were found to be harboring deep infections.

When the implants were removed from these 20 patients, they were tested by four-point bending to destruction. The round-hole plates were half as rigid as stainless steel and the DCPs were one third as stiff but both of the carbon fiber designs had greater fatigue strengths than metal. Most interesting was the correlation between stiffness and the patients' complaints of pain. Most of those complaining had plates with a stiffness varying from 1 to 1.7 Nm per degree. Tayton[481] concluded that the stiffness of tibial plates should therefore be greater than 1.75 Nm per degree and subsequently has used plates having stiffness of 2 Nm per degree.

All of the fractures in this series healed with bridging callus. As Uhthoff[496] has observed, it is difficult to tell when a fracture has healed when held under rigid compression, and the implant must be removed after an arbitrary period. With flexible implants, healing can be ascertained more easily, the area moment of inertia can be increased, and presumably the stress-shielded osteoporosis should be less.

Realizing that not all agree, the understanding of the ASIF is that porosis under a plate is not entirely secondary to "stress protection" but perhaps largely due to disturbance of the blood supply. The amount of bone contact of the plate has undesirable effects on the previously normal bone under the plate. Perren and coworkers have observed that:

> *Damage to blood perfusion is produced by the close plate-to-bone contact (periosteal damage) and drilling through the bone for bicortical screw anchorage (endosteal and intramedullary damage). Due to the resulting local bone necrosis, fracture healing may be delayed by the slow bone substitution through the process of remodeling or even complicated by sequester formation.*[420]

Allgower[8] writes that osteoporosis secondary to vascular damage is rapidly reversible but enough time should be allowed for cortical remodeling and restoration of structure. He recommends that the minimal times for the removal of a plate should be 1 year for the tibia, 18 months for the forearm and humerus, and 2 years for the femur.

Design

Dynamic Compression Plates. Dynamic Compression Plates are available in 4.5-mm narrow, 4.5-mm broad, and 3.5-mm sizes to be used for long bone diaphyseal fractures, osteotomies, and arthrodeses. Plate size should be matched to bone size but the 4.5-mm broad plates generally are used for the humerus and the femur, the 4.5-mm narrow plates are used for the

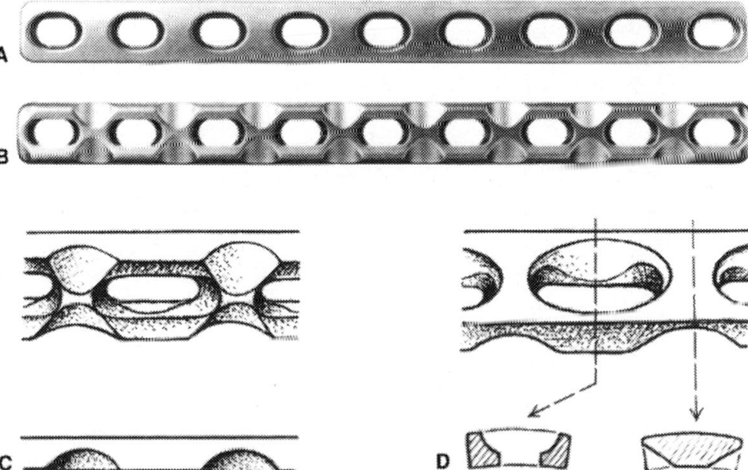

FIGURE 3-36. Titanium LC-DCP illustrated: (**A**) Top view. (**B**) Notching on the undersurface. (**C**) Revascularization channels (illustration). (**D**) Double-ramp configuration of the holes (*top*). The two bottom views contrast the geometry of the hole area of the plates with the solid areas. (Müller, M.E., Allgower, M., Schneider, R., and Willenegger, H.: Manual of Internal Fixation, 3rd ed, p. 243. Berlin, Springer-Verlag, 1992.)

tibia, and the 3.5-mm plates [398] for the forearm; 2.7-mm plates also are available.

Limited Contact-Dynamic Compression Plates. In an effort to decrease possible stress-shielding and dysvascularity under the plate, titanium LC-DCPs have been designed (Fig. 3-36).[282,402] Titanium plates are available in a wide array of sizes and designs (Fig. 3-37). Conventional DCPs have almost 100% contact with bone under the plate, whereas the LCPs have only 50% bone contact. Cortical porosity after plating is reduced with the LC plate. Additional advantages of the LC-DC plate are listed in Table 3-5.[398]

Less favorable is the ultimate tensile strength of 680 MPa for ASIF titanium, compared with 980 MPa for ASIF steel. To have mechanical strength comparable with steel, titanium plates must be larger, have a different configuration, be alloyed with other metals, or be hardened in the manufacturing process.[121] Table 3-6 presents results of four-point bending tests of 3.5- and 4.5-mm narrow and broad DCPs and LC-DCPs. Largely through trial and error and long clinical experience, various plate sizes and configurations have been developed. Little is known about optimization of strength and stiffness variables of plates relative to the wide range of clinical situations. A family of plates has been created for diverse fracture problems; within guidelines, treatment outcome depends more on appropriate indications and good technique rather than plate configuration or material.

Internal Fixator

Ramotowski and Granowski[414] published results of long bone fracture treatment in 850 fractures and 445 pseudarthroses using a plate system comprised of a plate elevated from the cortex (Fig. 3-38). The plate is mounted on platform screws, which in turn are affixed to the plate with nuts. The plate may be located internally or externally, depending on the specific application. Additional implant modifications to decrease bone contact by offsetting the implant from the bone are being developed. Plates may be mounted on nuts, through which screws are passed, locking neutralization screws to the plate and offsetting the plate from the bone. The nut may be changed such that contact with the bone occurs over a smaller area yet the screw is still locked to the plate and the plate offset from the bone (Fig. 3-39). The screw head does not toggle in the plate, further enhancing fixation.

TABLE 3-5
Advantages of the Limited-Contact Dynamic Compression Plate

Uniform material stiffness due to even placement of screw holes from one end of the plate to the other
Wider angle of screw orientation relative to screw hole (40° compared with 20° for the DCP in the line of the long axis)
Auto compression from either side of the hole allowing sequential compression between holes
Improved tissue compatibility
Grooves in the undersurface of the plate to allow circulation under the plate and formation of callus bridges
Improved fatigue life of LC-DCP titanium
Decreased stiffness: Young's modulus for steel is twice that of titanium

From Perren, S.: The Concept of Biological Plating Using the Limited Contact-Dynamic Compression Plate (LC-DCP). Injury: AO/ASIF Scientific Supplement, 22(4): S1–S41, 1991.

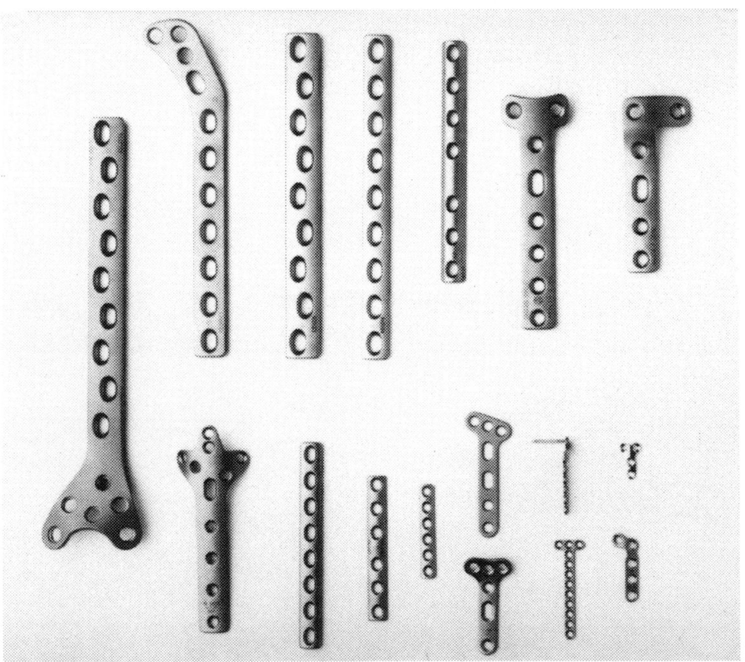

FIGURE 3-37. Titanium ASIF plates include (from left) femoral buttress plate; (*top*) tibial buttress plate, 4.5-mm broad LC-DCP, 4.5-mm narrow LC-DCP, semitubular T and L buttress; and (*bottom*) cloverleaf, 3.5-mm LC-DCP, one-third tubular, one-fourth tubular, oblique and straight T buttress, and assorted minifragment plates. (*Courtesy of Synthes.*)

TABLE 3-6

Mechanical Properties of Chemically Pure Grade IV Titanium Plates Compared With Steel

Material	Design	Mean Bending Strength	Mean Bending Stiffness
		(NM)	(NM2)
Ti	3.5 LC-DCP	14.5 ± 0.5	1.6 ± 0.1
Ti	4.5 Narrow LC-DCP	25.1 ± 1.1	3.9 ± 0.1
Ti	4.5 Broad LC-DCP	51.1 ± 0.4	9.1 ± 0.1
316 L	3.5 DCP	17.3 ± 0.3	3.1 ± 0.1
316 L	4.5 Narrow DCP	23.3 ± 0.4	5.2 ± 0.3
316 L	4.5 Broad DCP	55.2 ± 2.6	12.1 ± 1.5

Disegi, J.A., and Cesarone, D.M.: Metallurgical Properties of Unalloyed Titanium Limited Contact Dynamic Compression Plates. *In:* Harvey, G. Jr. (ed): Clinical and Laboratory Performance of Bone Plates, p. 36, Philadelphia, American Society for Testing and Materials, 1994.

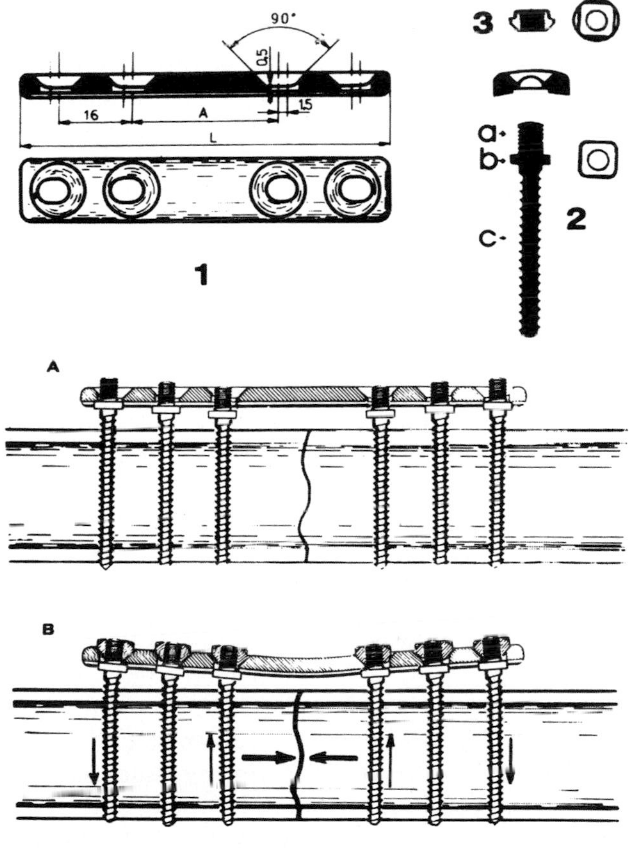

FIGURE 3-38. Zespol plate fixator: (**1**) plate; (**2**) platform screw (*a*, tapped pin; *b*, screw platform; *c*, screw); (**3**) nut. (**A**) Screw platforms may be placed variable distances from the bone to create compressive loading (**B**) with tightening of the nuts. (Ramotowski, W., and Granowski, R.: Zespol. An original method of stable osteosynthesis. Clin. Orthop. 272:68, 1991.)

Perren[398] has advanced the concept of the internal fixator as a device placed internally without touching the bone other than by pins or screws. Reporting on experiments in sheep having a plate designed to make contact only at a few points (point contact plate [PCP]), Remiger and coworkers[420] found that none of the PCP-treated bones failed at the original fracture site at 12 weeks (65% normal strength). In contrast, two of six specimens fixed with the DCP failed at 24 and 48 weeks. They concluded that the plate-protective function of the PCP lasted fewer than 12 weeks, compared with 24 weeks with the DCP (plate protection is the time needed for the bone at the fracture site to become mature).

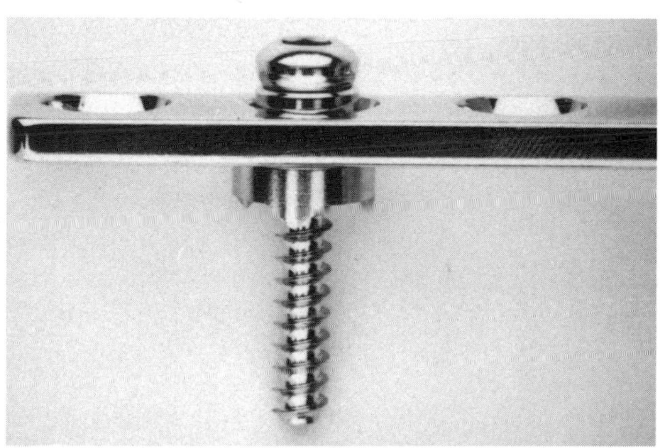

FIGURE 3-39. A modified nut (Schüli) locks the screw to the plate and offsets the plate from the bone. (*Courtesy of Synthes, Paoli, PA.*)

Further efforts to decrease adverse effects of plates on bone consist of percutaneous insertion technique combined with noncontact between bone and plate. Van der Werken[163] of the Netherlands, Ganz of Switzerland,[163] and Mast[336] of the United States are developing percutaneous plate insertion methods with little or no bone–plate contact. Small skin incisions are made for plate insertion and screw placement. Fracture reduction is indirect and plating is applied subfascially, with little disturbance of soft tissues. Plates are locked to the screws with 4.5-mm nuts applied under the plate. Long bone fractures stabilized with plates applied in this manner resemble interlocking nails (Fig. 3-40). Such methods are under investigation and have yet to become routine in clinical practice.

Curved Plate

Semitubular plates were introduced in 1960 as self-compressing plates and were originally designed to be used on the anterior crest and medial edge of the tibia. These plates are delicate (only 1 mm thick) and easily deformed but their semitubular conformation gives them greater rigidity than a flat plate of similar dimensions. The semitubular plates have oval holes, so that by placing screws at the far end of the hole from the fracture line, the plate is self-compressing. The semitubular plate has indications as a buttress plate in combination with solid lag screws or as a blade plate device.[71,274] Plates with smaller curvatures are also available. One-third and one-fourth tubular plates have been introduced, which are fastened by 3.5- and 2.7-mm screws, respectively. These plates have their greatest usefulness in fibula, metatarsal, and metacarpal fractures.

Angled Plates

Also called blade plates, angle plates are useful in repair of metaphyseal fractures primarily of the femur and may be used as compression plates with the external tensioning devices. Angled plates are compatible with 7.3-, 7-, 6.5-, and 4.5-mm steel screws. The popularity of the angled plates has declined with the development of sliding screw plate implants.

Buttress Plates

Flat buttress plates with specialized indications consist of the cloverleaf or "C" plate, the "H," "L," and "T" plates, and finally the "S" or spoon plate. These implants are intended for buttressing fractures of the epiphyseal-metaphyseal zones of the long bones. Femoral and tibial buttress plates are available with a DCP extension for fractures extending from metaphyseal into diaphyseal bone. Efforts to improve the user-friendliness of these plates has resulted in a host of precontoured small profile plates for special regions, such as the tibial plateau (Fig. 3-41).

Reconstruction Plates

Plates with intermediate thickness between the DCP and buttress plates have been created that have scallop-like notches in the side of the plate between the holes (Fig. 3-42). These implants may be contoured in three planes to fit complex surfaces such as the pelvis, the distal humerus, and the calcaneus. Because of the diminished mass of material, these plates are not as strong as comparable DCPs.

Wave Plate

A plate may be contoured such that the lateral cortex is not in immediate contact with the plate (Fig. 3-43). The space between the plate and the bone is filled with bone graft. Such a construct was devised by Weber to reduce the prevalence of refracture after plate removal.[43] The result of the construct is a greatly enhanced tension-reducing lateral bone mass.

Mechanics of Plating

Prestress of the plate facilitates axial compression of a transverse fracture. The plate should be contoured such that it sits off the bone 1 to 2 mm adjacent to the fracture site. As the plate is tensioned, a more even compression effect across the fracture site is delivered than if the plate had been tensioned without prestress. Haas and Tscherne[492] have measured the magnitude of prestressing with transverse fractures. Data from their work are presented in Figure 3-44. Prestressing of a compression plate applied to the tension side of a bone produces an enhanced dynamic tension-band effect.

Perren[397] has shown that bone can tolerate up to 300 Kpa/cm^2 without undergoing pressure necrosis and that this compression enhances the rigidity of fixation. The level of the compression does not remain

FIGURE 3-40. (**A**) Comminuted (grade IV) middle third femur fracture in a 32-year-old man after a traffic accident. (**B**) Flexibility of a long ASIF plate. (**C**) Radiographs after subfascial plating, with restoration of length and alignment. (**D**) Callus is visible at 6 weeks after operation. (**E**) Full weight bearing was started at 12 weeks. (**F**) Mature bridging callus is present at 18 weeks. (*Courtesy of Y.E.A. van Riet, M.D., and Professor Chr. van der Werken, Utrecht, Holland.*) ►

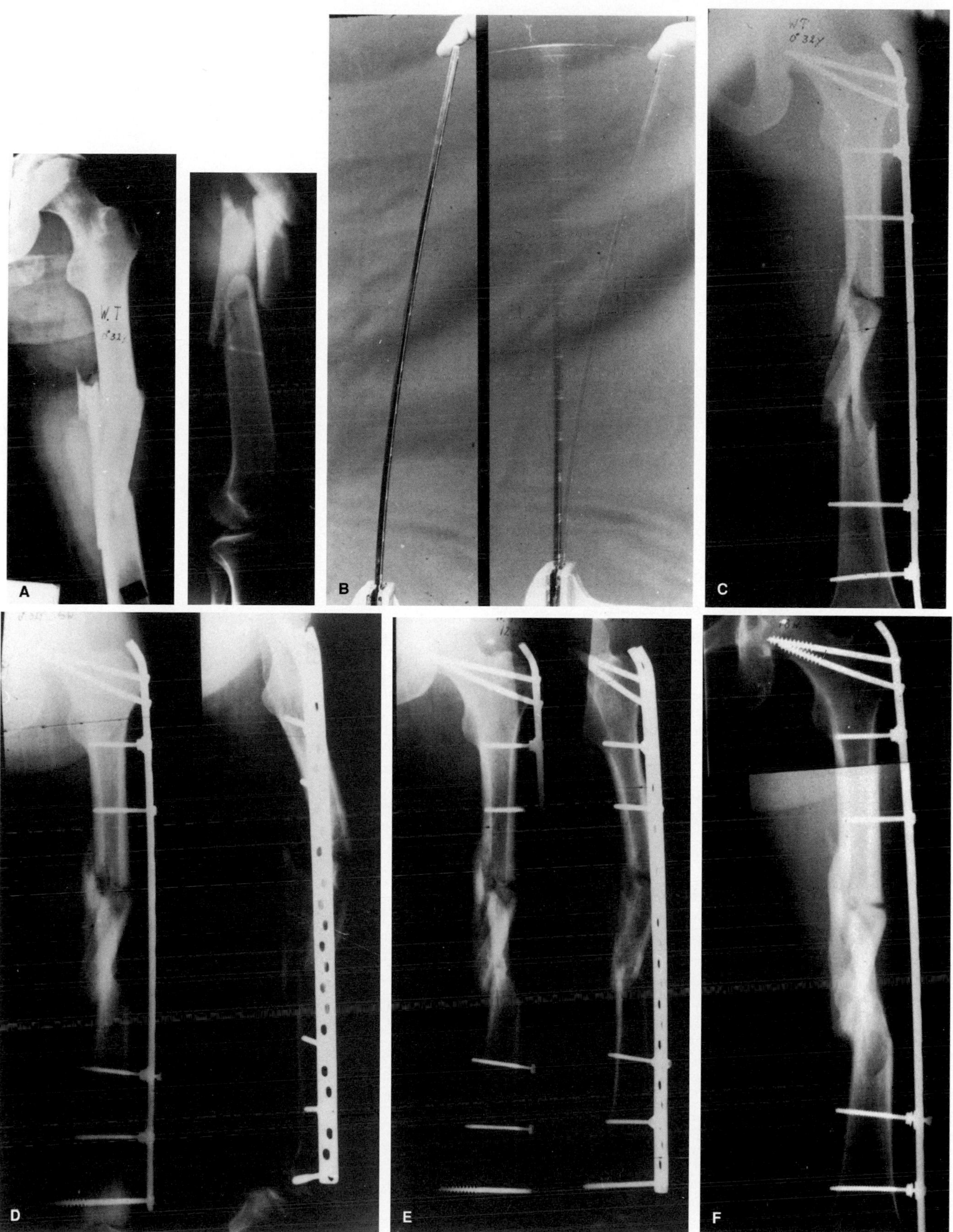

FIGURE 3-40.

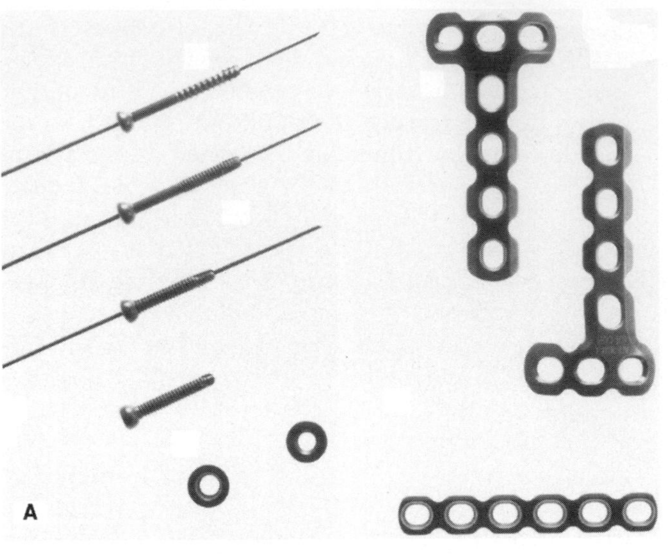

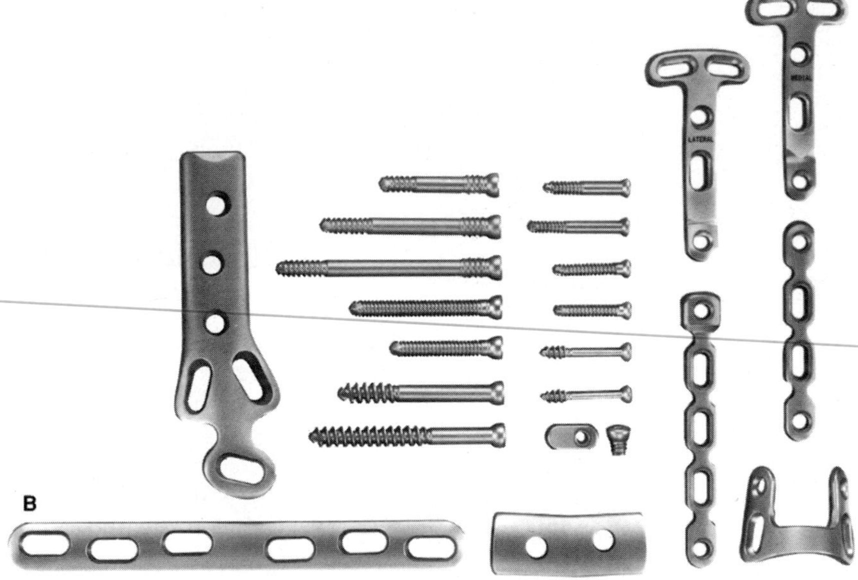

FIGURE 3-41. (**A**) Specially designed low-profile 4.5/5-mm titanium buttress plates and cannulated cortical screws. (*Courtesy of Ace Orthopaedic Company, El Sequindo, CA.*) (**B**) The titanium Alta system of plate osteosynthesis includes extensile long bone shaft plates and low-profile buttress plates. (*Courtesy of Howmedica, Inc, Rutherford, NJ.*)

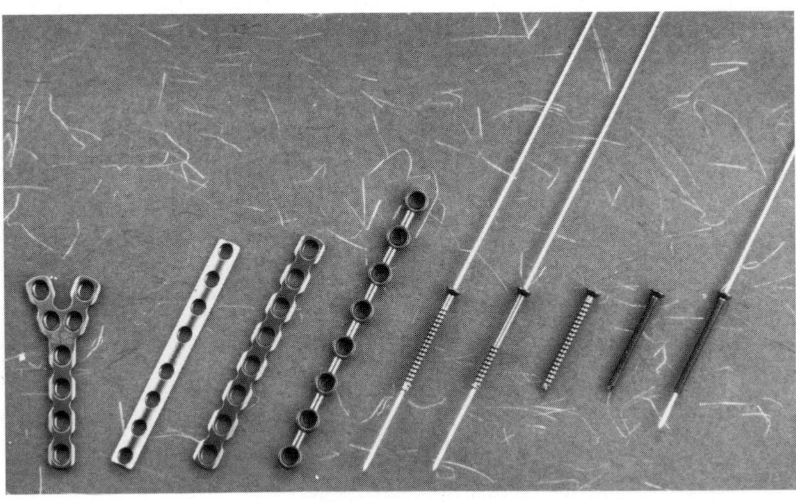

FIGURE 3-42. Reconstruction plates made of titanium are useful for fractures of the distal humerus, pelvis, and calcaneus. Cannulated and noncannulated titanium screws are available for plate fixation and lag-screw application. (*Courtesy of Ace Orthopaedic Company, El Sequando, CA.*)

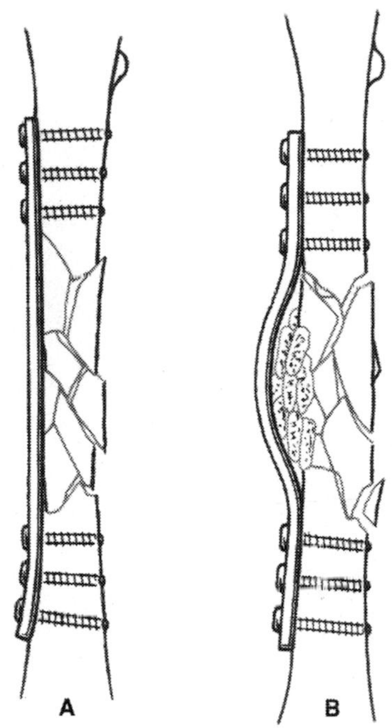

FIGURE 3-43. The Wave plate of Weber for strain protection of the lateral cortex. (**A**) Biologic plating of a femur shaft fracture. (**B**) The 4.5-mm broad dynamic compression plates or LC-DCP is modified to allow bone graft under the plate laterally. (Müller, M.E., Allgower, M., Schneider, R., and Willenegger, H.: Manual of Internal Fixation, 3rd Ed, p. 231. Berlin, Springer-Verlag, 1992.)

this high, however, but gradually diminishes as the bone remodels and the fracture heals. After 2 months, the compression falls well below 50% of the initial level (Fig. 3-45).

When a plated bone is subjected to flexural loading, the weakest configuration is obtained when the plate is under compression, the strongest when the bone is loaded from the side opposite to the plate. In the first example, the fracture tends to open up and the whole load is borne by the plate. Conversely, loads that tend to close the fracture place the plate under tension, and a significant portion of the load is supported by bone, thereby diminishing the bending moment on the plate. In this latter configuration, Bynum and associates[80] found that no benefit accrued from increasing either the breadth of the plate or the size of the screws but when the plate was increased in length from 3 to 6 inches, the strength of the assembly was doubled.

Laurence and associates[307] studied the stress on the screws of a four-hole plate subjected to a load that tended to open up the fracture. Almost the entire load was carried by the two central screws on either side of the fracture. The stress on these two screws was unaffected by changing either the length of the plate or the distance between the screws. Even when an eight-hole plate was substituted for the four-hole, only the central two screws were significantly stressed. The remaining screws were under compression stress rather than tension. In this study, the load on the screws never exceeded their pull-out strength, so the plate became the vulnerable component of the assembly. They concluded that a four-hole plate is adequate to resist stresses that open up the fracture, even if the screws engage only one cortex. Clinically, we know that four-hole plates have little place in the management of long bone fractures, and it appears that plates should have sufficient length to withstand bending and torsional moments and screws should be strong enough to resist the tensile, shear, and angulatory stresses placed on them.

The strength of a bone–plate assembly is influenced by the character of the fracture. Transverse fractures are stronger under compression than oblique fractures; however, when tested in rotation, the reverse is true. Comminution, inadequate reduction, and missing fragments contribute to weakness of the assembly. In plating metacarpal fractures in horses, Bynum[80] found that the maximum strength that could be achieved was 60% of that of the intact contralateral metacarpal. Because horses are obliged to stand up and are unable to run on three legs as dogs do, in his clinical series, Bynum had only one successful outcome in 15 cases. Similarly, quiet walking in humans imposes a bending moment of 80 nm on the tibia, and a tibia fixed with a Stamm plate fails at 24 nm.[81] Early, unrestricted weight bearing is not feasible in plated fractures.

Rybicki and associates[440] have shown that in compression loading, the bone bears 80% of the load and the plate 20%. The stress is not evenly distributed across the bone, however, so that the cortex on the plated side is protected from 75% of the applied stress, whereas on the opposite side, the stress was 150% the applied value.

Hayes and Perren[209] determined the coefficient of friction for both titanium and stainless steel dynamic compression plates and found that there was no significant difference between these plates when the design was the same. They calculated that a normal force of 200 kp would generate a frictional force of up to 75 kg at the plate–bone interface; this maximal friction force is commensurate with the total interfragmentary compressive forces (75 to 135 Kpa) measured in vivo with instrumented compression plates. They concluded that frictional forces may transmit a significant proportion of the longitudinal, interfragmentary compressive force to a healing bone.

Compression Plating

External Tensioning Device. After reduction of the fracture, the plate is applied to the bone and secured to one fragment. A drill guide for the external com-

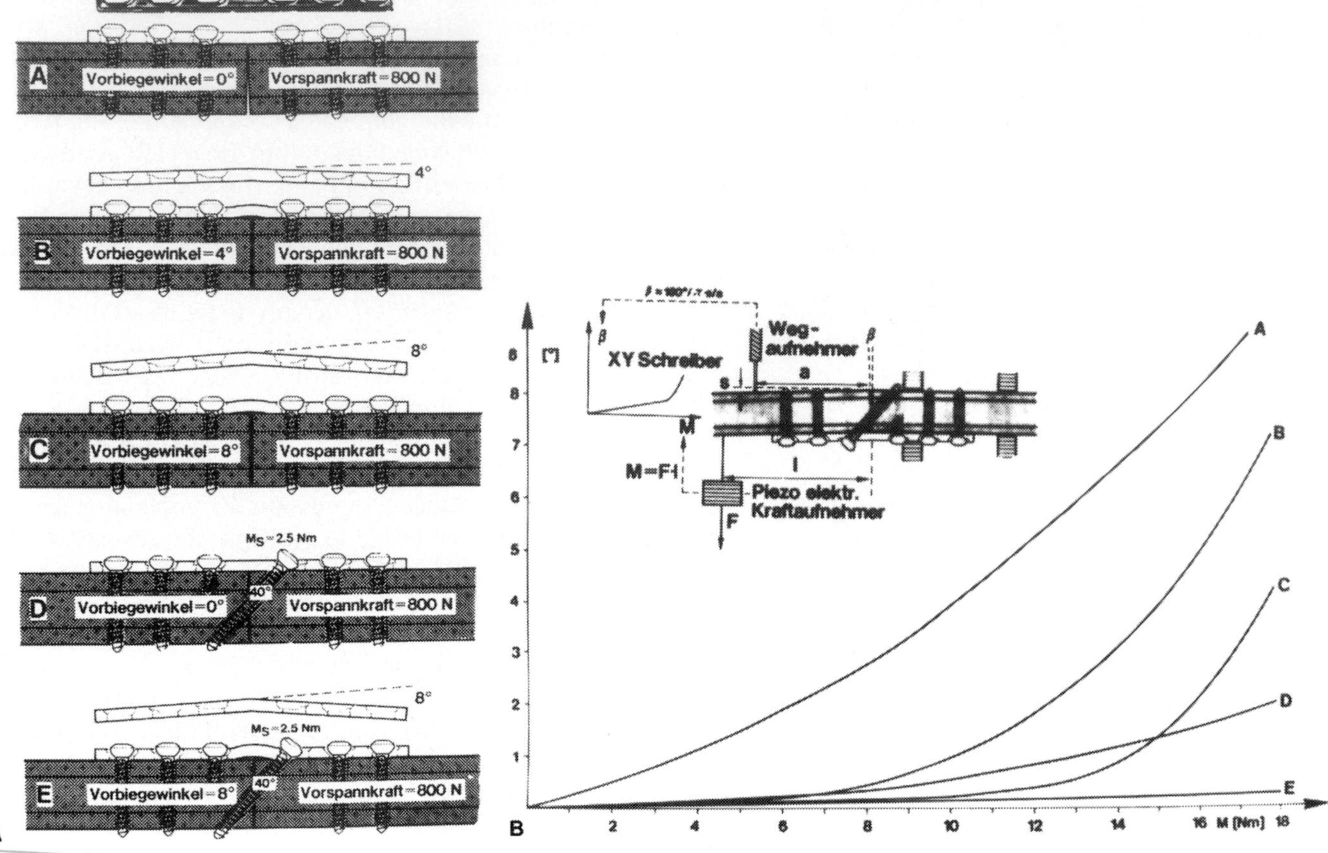

FIGURE 3-44. (**A**) Plate techniques tested in **B:** *A,* No preload compression only; *B,* preload (4°) and compression; *C,* preload (8°) and compression; *D,* compression and lag screw but no preload; *E,* Preload (8°), compression, and lag screw. (**B**) Load deflection curve, showing progressive increase in stability with preload, greater preload, and lag effect. The greatest rigidity was achieved with axial load, 8° of preload, and interfragmentary compression with a lag screw through the plate. (Tscherne, H., and Gotzen, L.: Fraktur und Weichteilschaden. In: J. Rehn Schweiberer, L. (ed.): Hefte zur Unfallheilkunde, vol. 28, p. 60. Berlin, Springer-Verlag, 1983.)

pression device is inserted into the last hole of the opposite end of the plate, a hole is drilled external to the plate and tapped, and the compression device is screwed to the bone, with the free end hooked into the plate. Turning a worm screw pulls the plate toward the device, compressing the fracture site.

Two versions of tensioner are available. The latest model, having an excursion of 20 mm contrasted with the 8 mm of the original, has a direct-reading strain gauge with red, green, and yellow zones, indicating excessive (red), inadequate (yellow), and optimal pressurization of the fracture site. The original device has no such quantitative feature. These tensioners are made for use with 4.5-mm plates. The new version has one additional improvement: the hook is reversible so that it may be used in a distraction mode for reducing an overlapped fracture. A smaller version of the original tensioner is available for 3.5-mm plate tensioning.

Either side of a transverse fracture may be affixed first without affecting the mechanics at the fracture site. Such is not true of an oblique fracture, which creates a definite directionality to compression plating (Fig. 3-46). The first screw should be located next to the acute angle of the fracture. The plate is then tensioned from the acute angle side, either with an autocompression screw or with the external tensioner. If the external tensioner is used, a neutral or holding screw is next placed in the hole second closest to the fracture site on the obtuse angle side. The first hole on the obtuse side is used for a lag screw. Interfragmentary compression follows application of axial compression, so that the lag screw is not deformed or destroyed by axial loading. If the optimal plate orientation is not adjacent to the obtuse and acute angles of the fracture, the fracture is fixed first with a lag screw and secondly with a neutralization plate, not a compression plate.

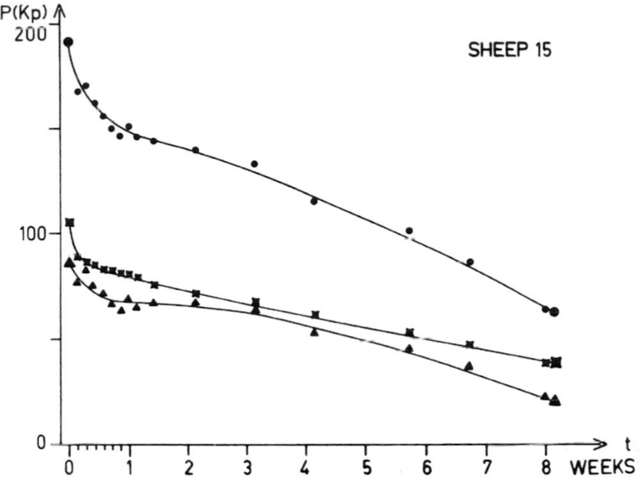

FIGURE 3-45. Compressive force (pressure) at an osteotomy site in a sheep (measured with an instrumented plate as a function of time) follows a decay curve, with 50% loss of plate-induced compression within 5 weeks. (Rittmann, W.W., and Perren, S.M.: Cortical Bone Healing After Internal Fixation and Infection, p. 33. Berlin, Springer-Verlag, 1974.)

Self-Compression. The DCP derives its name from its ability to provide axial compression without the use of the tensioning device, although this may be used when necessary. The DCP operates on the same basic principle as the Bagby plate,[15,16] which exerts its compression by the eccentric insertion of screws (Fig. 3-47). The slot for the screw has a sloping surface at one end. When the spherical head of the screw impinges on this surface, the plate moves away from the fracture, thereby compressing the fracture plane. The magnitude of this movement and consequently of the compression is determined by the drill guide that sites the screw hole (Fig. 3-48).

The load guide (see Fig. 3-48*B*), which is color-coded yellow, has an eccentrically placed hole. When this guide is used, the screw meets the inclined load plane 1 mm from its end. When the fracture is accurately reduced, the horizontal displacement produces 60 to 80 kp or axial interfragmentary compression. When using the drill guide, it is important to have the arrow engraved on the device pointing to the fracture site, so that the screw is appropriately placed (see Fig. 3-48*B*). The LC-DCP differs only in the use of a shaft screw in the compression hole and as a lag screw (Fig. 3-49).

If more compression is necessary, subsequent screws may be inserted in the compression mode. When additional compression is added, the tension on the initially inserted screws must be released by backing off one or two turns. Each screw is then tightened in turn when all the screws have been inserted. Use of one of the external tensioning devices is preferable to repeating this sequence, however. Non–load-holding screws are placed using the green neutral drill guide (see Fig. 3-48*A*). It is not quite neutral because it is inserted eccentrically 0.1 mm along the load plane and thus exerts additional compression. Any plate having an oval screw hole may be used as a self-compressing plate (Fig. 3-50).

Drill jigs are available to place the first two screw holes in exactly the same positions as they would be if they had been inserted in the plate with the load

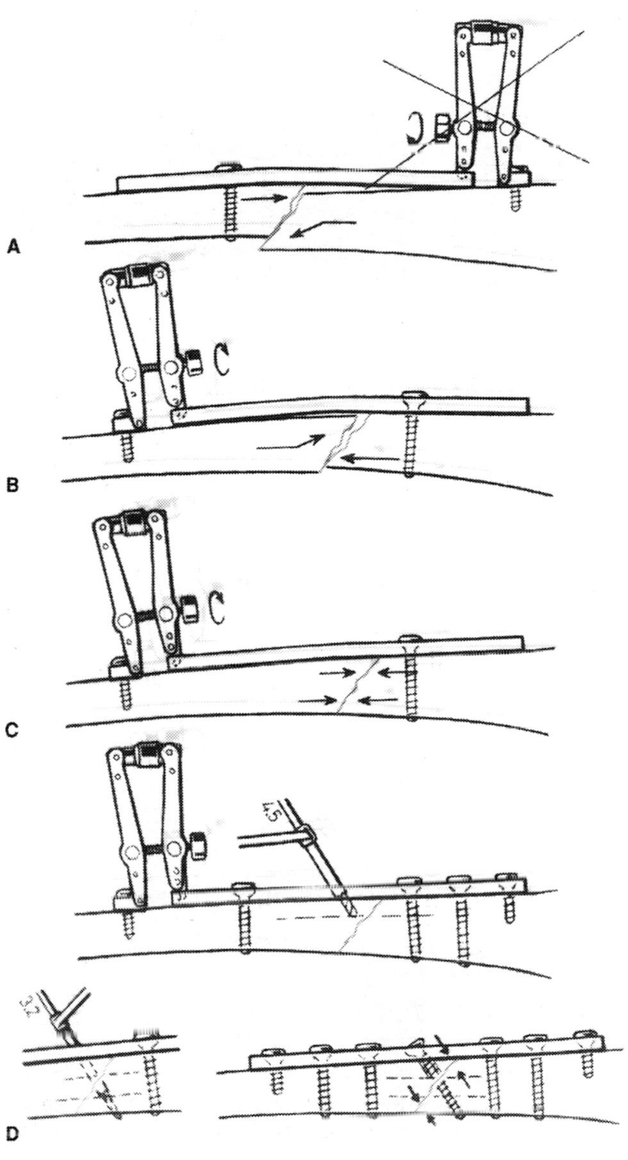

FIGURE 3-46. (**A**) Incorrect sequence of axial load leads to fracture, loss of reduction, and an unstable osteosynthesis. (**B**) The correct sequence of screw insertion consists of placement of an initial screw near the obtuse angle of the fracture. (**C**) Load is applied from the acute angle side. (**D**) The lag screw is placed after axial tensioning is completed. Holding screws fix the plate on both sides of the fracture. (Müller, M.E., Allgower, M., Schneider, R., and Willenegger, H.: Manual of Internal Fixation, 3rd Ed., p. 225. Berlin: Springer-Verlag, 1992.)

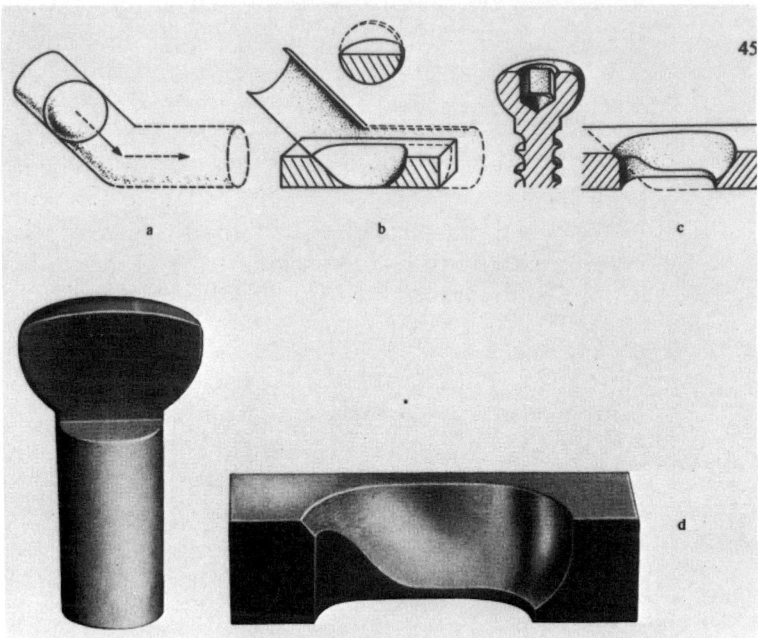

FIGURE 3-47. The spherical gliding principle of the dynamic compression plate. As the screw head is tightened, it impinges on the inclined plane. The combination of downward and horizontal movement of the screw induces horizontal movement of the underlying bone relative to a stationary plate. Compression is thus produced at the fracture. (Müller, M.E., Allgöwer, M., Schneider, R., and Willenegger, H.: Manual of Internal Fixation. Techniques Recommended by the AO Group, 2nd Ed., p. 71. New York, Springer-Verlag, 1979.)

guide (Fig. 3-51). If a plate obscures the fracture line, the reduction cannot be checked but with the drill jig, the fracture line can be observed and the drill holes made. When the screws are inserted through the plate into the predrilled holes, the accurate reduction is preserved.

There is a third drill guide in the jig (see Fig. 3-51) to allow the second screw hole from the fracture to be drilled in the compression mode, leaving the first hole in the plate to be used for a lag screw that passes obliquely through the fracture site. This should always be done in transverse and short oblique fractures of the femur and tibia but is also advisable in the humerus and even in the forearm, although care must be taken to not devascularize the tip of a spike in the radius or the ulna. This oblique screw ensures that the far cortex is under compression.

The round holes in the original ASIF plates made

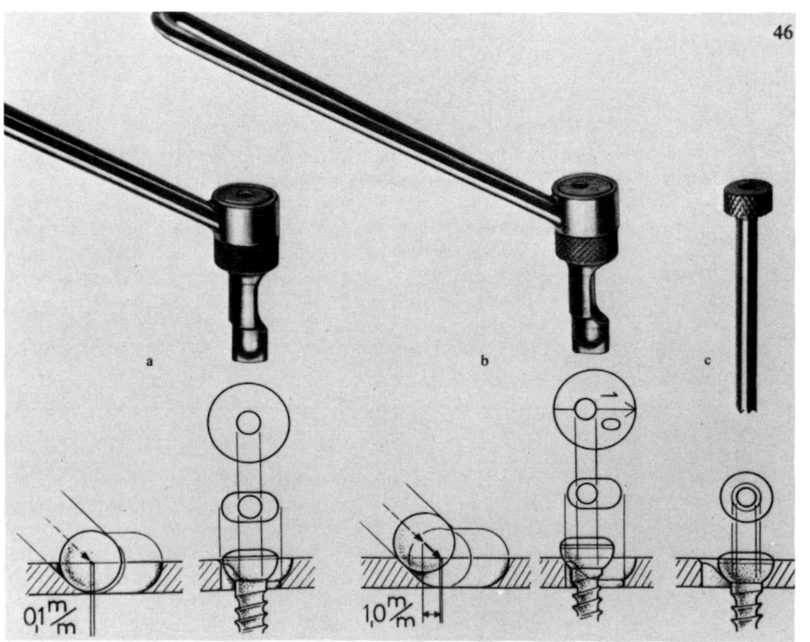

FIGURE 3-48. Drill guides for dynamic compression plates (DCP). (**A**) Neutral guide, identified with a green ring. (**B**) Load guide, identified with a yellow ring. (**C**) The 58-mm drill sleeve, called the coaxial drill sleeve, or overdrill sleeve. Drill sleeves for the LC-DCP system are similar but may be separated from the DCP guides by the presence of notching on their under surfaces. Note that the neutral guide applies a small displacement force due to the 0.1-mm offset. (Müller, M.E., Allgöwer, M., Schneider, R., and Willenegger, H.: Manual of Internal Fixation. Techniques Recommended by the AO Group, 2nd Ed., p. 73. New York, Springer-Verlag, 1979.)

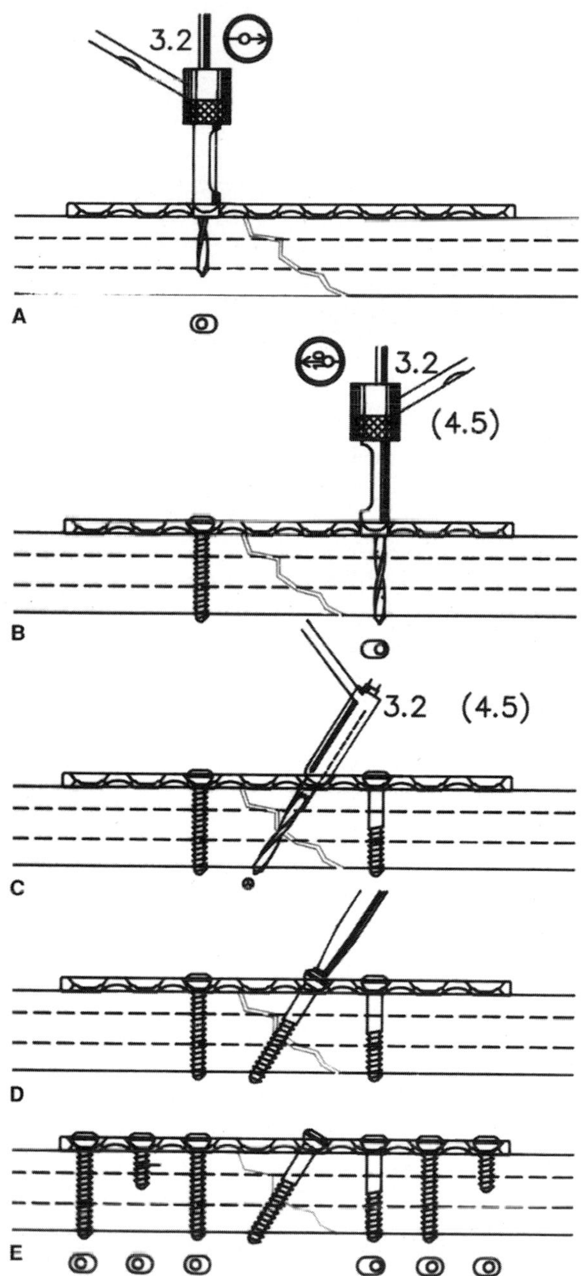

FIGURE 3-49. Technique of self-compression with the LC-DCP. (**A**) The plate is fixed with a fully threaded holding screw after anatomic reduction of the fracture and prebending of the plate. (**B**) The load drill guide is used to place a drill hole for axial compression. (**C**) Axial load is applied with a cortical shaft screw, and the gliding and fixation holes are drilled. (**D**) Interfragmentary compression is applied with a second shaft screw. (**E**) Remaining cortical holding screws are placed. (Müller, M.E., Allgower, M., Schneider, R., and Willenegger, H.: Manual of Internal Fixation, 3rd Ed, p. 249. Berlin, Springer-Verlag, 1992.)

perpendicular insertion of screws mandatory, and deviations mitigated the compression at the fracture site and stressed the screws. The design of the countersink of the DCPs and LC-DCPs allows cortical screws and spongiosa lag screws to be inserted at an angle without any deleterious effect because the spherical head of the screw mates with no angulation stress. By this means, better interfragmentary compression may be achieved.

Careful contouring of the plate is essential and requires practice and skill. Not only are bends necessary (made with a bending press) but twists in the long axis must also be contrived with bending irons. This longitudinal twisting should be left until after all the other bends are made. This modeling of the plate is facilitated by the use of a malleable aluminum template, which can be molded to the surface of the bone and then duplicated in the plate itself. Such "mutilation" of plates would formerly have been discouraged because it would have initiated cracks and thus significantly decreased the plate's fatigue life. The DCP, however, is annealed; that is, the grain size has been made larger by heating. This process makes the plate more malleable and the subsequent "cold working" of the plate increases its strength and rigidity.

Staples

Blount popularized the use of staples to accomplish physeal arrest.[5] Expansion of indications led to use in foot reconstruction and eventually to metaphyseal fractures such as the medial and lateral malleoli of the ankle.[5,84,85] Staple osteosynthesis has slowly increased to include the following indications:

Arthrodesis: subtalar, triple, wrist[‖‖]
Fractures: malleolar, trochanteric, patellar[5,20,119,125,329,378,468]
Epiphysiodesis[79,266]
Valgus osteotomy of the proximal tibia[14,102,515]

If the fracture line is transverse and the tines of the staple are elastically deformed divergently before insertion, compression occurs at the near cortex but progressively decreases away from the fixation point. Dai and coworkers[103] have reported a staple having thermally controlled compression properties (Fig. 3-52). A nickel titanium staple is deformed at 4°C, then placed across a transverse fracture. Once placed, the staple is heated with a water bath and compression occurs.

Firoozbakhsh and coworkers[139] studied pull-out strength of power- and hand-driven staples, using synthetic bone to control for uneven mechanical properties of bone. Pull-out strength was higher with higher material densities, the length of the leg of the staple, square cross section as opposed to round, and power-driven versus hand-driven staples of similar designs

‖‖ References 9, 93, 119, 141, 157, 218, 224, 261, 337, 339, 435, 468, 508, 516, 527.

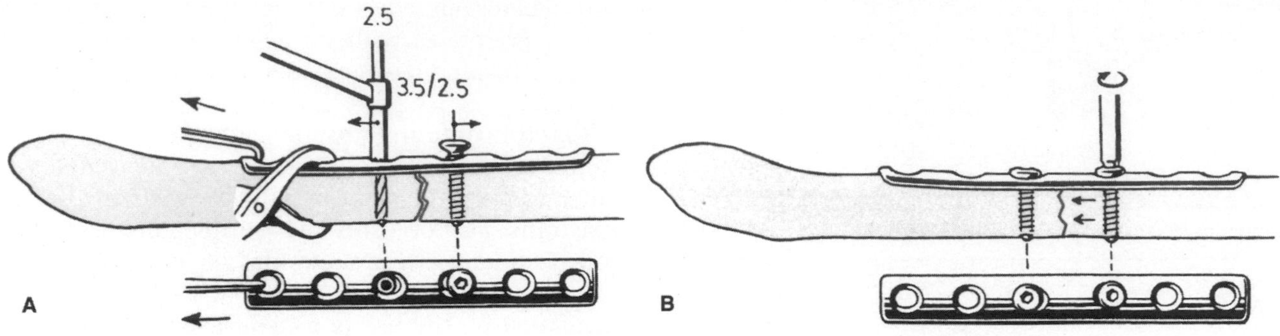

FIGURE 3-50. Eccentric screw placement in the oval holes of a one-third tubular plate applied to a transverse fibular fracture leads to compression when the screws are seated. (A) An initial 3.5-mm cortical screw is placed on one side of the fracture. The plate is pulled in a direction away from the initial screw, shifting the screw to the edge of the hole away from the fracture. A 2.5-mm drill bit is used to make a second screw hole, abutting the plate on the side away from the fracture. (B) The second screw is placed and both screws are tightened, compressing the fracture. (Müller, M.E., Allgower, M., Schneider, R., and Willenegger, H.: Manual of Internal Fixation, 3rd Ed, p. 233. Berlin, Springer-Verlag, 1992.)

(Fig. 3-53). A narrow, long, square cross-sectioned staple inserted with a power driver was recommended by the authors, based on their study. Freeland and coworkers[153] found similar results.

Suture Anchors

Before the invention of suture anchors, the surgeon had to make drill holes in the bone to reattach ligaments or tendons to their insertion points. Suture anchors simplify this procedure by affixing a sturdy suture to the bone with a screw (Fig. 3-54) or a spring-like device. Carpenter and colleagues[82] compared five commercially available suture anchor systems in terms of pull-out strength. Testing was conducted in cadaveric proximal tibias using the Mitek GII, Mitek GI, Accufex Rod TAG, Accufex Wedge TAG, and Statak. Magnitude and direction of applied load were both important in determining the pull-out strength of the different systems. Under the conditions in this set of trials, the Mitek GII pulled-out in 19% of specimens, compared with 40% for the

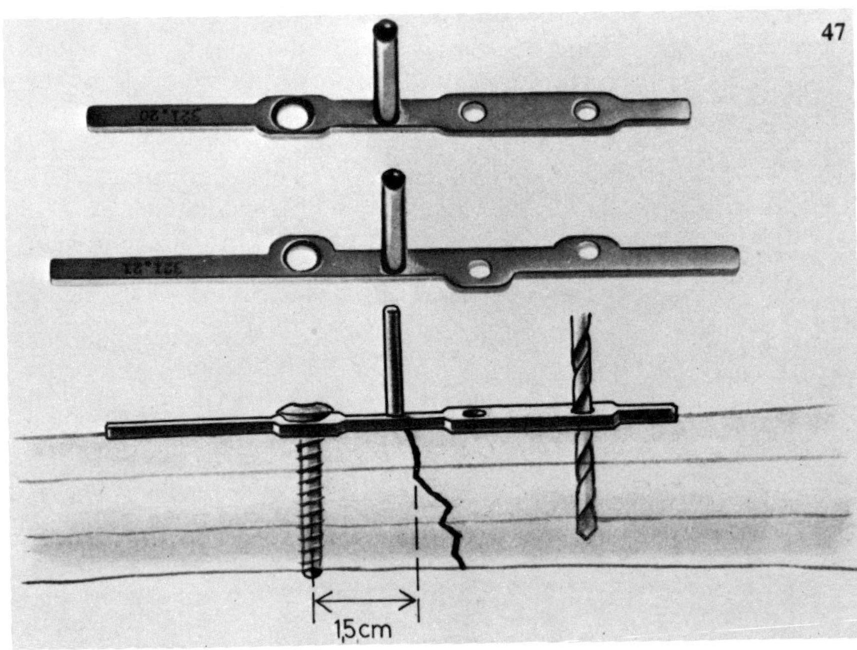

FIGURE 3-51. Drill jigs are available to place the first two screw holes in exactly the same positions they would be in if they had been inserted in the plate with the load guide. (Müller, M.E., Allgower, M., Schneider, R., and Willenegger, H.: Manual of Internal Fixation. Techniques Recommended by the AO Group, 2nd Ed., p. 73. New York, Springer-Verlag, 1979.)

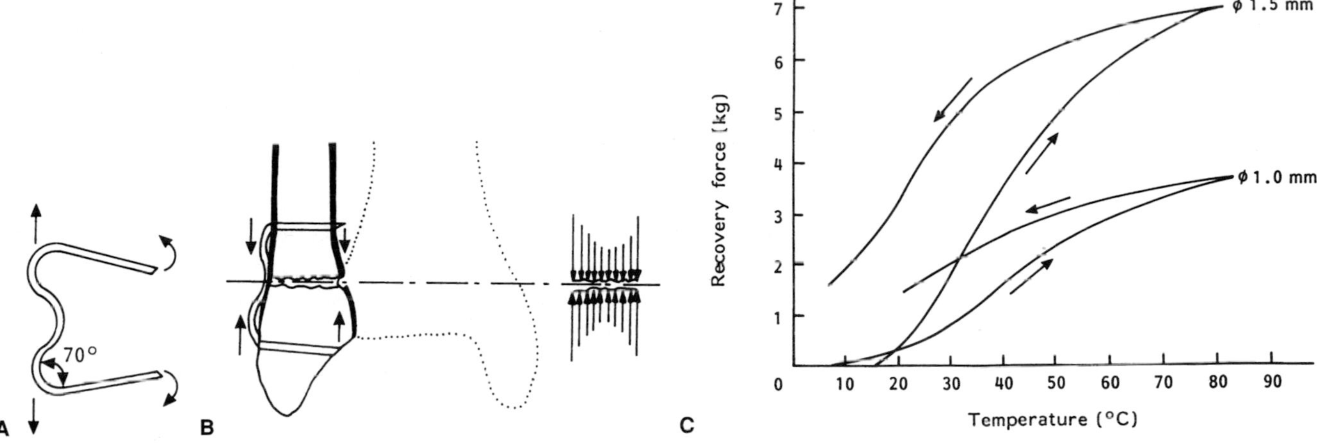

FIGURE 3-52. The thermoplastic staple may be used as a self-compressing device for transverse fractures. (**A**) The staple is manufactured with a tine-to-base angle of 70°. The staple is deformed in an ice bath to have an angle of 90° and then implanted. (**B**) Recovery of its original shape compresses the fracture as the staple is warmed. (**C**) Cold temperature plastic deformation of the staple is reversed by warming with production of a recovery force (*y axis*). (Dai, K.R., Hou, X.K., Sun, Y.H., Tang, R.G., Qiu, S.J., and Ni, C.: Treatment of Intra-Articular Fractures With Shape Memory Compression Staples. Injury 24(10):652, 1993.)

Statak, 44% for the Wedge TAG, 47% for the Mitek GI, and 60% for the Rod TAG. Such techniques were developed for rotator cuff repair and shoulder stabilization operations but may prove useful for other soft-tissue repairs.

INTRAMEDULLARY FIXATION TECHNIQUES

History

Stimson[473] references techniques of intramedullary fixation in which ivory pegs were jammed in the medullary canal in his 1883 textbook on fracture care. Hey-

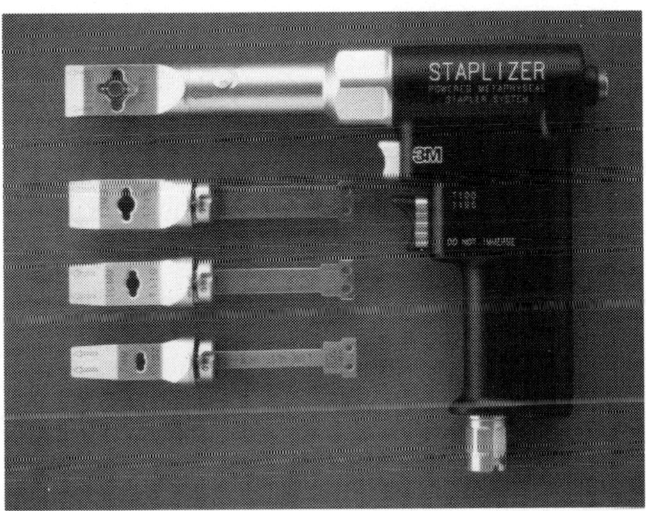

FIGURE 3-53. Staplizer® Power Staple–insertion device comes with various sizes of sterilized staples preloaded in a cartridge. (*Courtesy of the 3M Company.*)

Groves probably inserted the first metallic intramedullary device in a gunshot fracture of the femur during World War I. Writing in 1921 on ununited fractures, he stated:

> *It occurred to me, therefore, to use a long internal peg or strut, such as would render unnecessary any further fixation and would afford absolute rigidity. I have used pegs of various shapes, cylindrical, cross-sectional, and solid rods; and I am inclined to think that the last named are the best, because they give maximum strength and there is an avoidance of hollows and crevices which form dead spaces.*[225]

Smith-Petersen[394] applied a percutaneous medullary fixation technique to solve immobility problems associated with hip fractures in older patients. Küntscher,[297–299] impressed by the work of Smith-Petersen, conducted basic and clinical research on medullary surgery and fixation, ushering in the modern era of medullary fixation.[394] Knowledge of Küntscher's methods spread to Germany's neighbors during World War II as prisoners of war returned home ambulatory after medullary nailing of their femoral fractures.[465] Techniques developed for use in the femur were applied to other long bones and several systems of fixation evolved.

Development and Expansion

Since Küntscher's first report in 1939, a plethora of intramedullary implants, indications, and techniques have been developed.[##] Maatz,[327] one of the pioneers

[##] References 33, 57, 59, 91, 104, 124, 145, 160, 199, 203, 280, 283, 292, 324, 358, 392, 410, 444, 467, 486, 501, 511, 517, 528–530, 536.

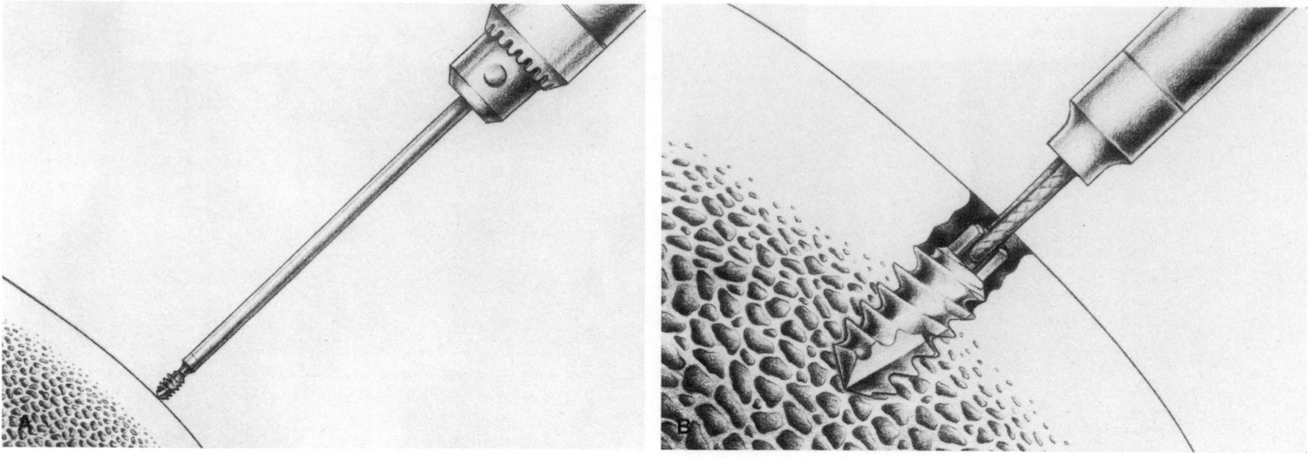

FIGURE 3-54. (**A**) The Statak® suture anchor is a screw mounted on a drill for ease of placement. Various sizes are available. (**B**) Once the screw is seated, it is disengaged from the drill stem, freeing the suture. (*Courtesy of Zimmer, Warsaw, IN.*)

of intramedullary surgery and a contemporary of Küntscher, wrote a fine monograph on the subject, identifying the wide range of nail designs in existence (Fig. 3-55). The emphasis has been on complete nail systems for reamed and unreamed applications in the femur, tibia, and humerus (Fig. 3-56). Low risk of pseudarthrosis and infection, shortened hospital stay, and rapid return to function have lent further impetus to the extension and application of these techniques to other long bones.

Device Designs

Intramedullary devices may be defined by physical characteristics:

- Length
- Width
- Curvature
- Cross-sectional geometry.
- Locking capacity and configuration
- Material

Length, Width, and Curvature

Length, width, and curvature are design features typically matched to the bone in question. Rush rods and Ender pins have small diameters relative to the medullary canal and have uniform curvature but variable lengths. Stability is achieved with stacking of multiple devices within the canal or by using the elastic properties of the rod to create a spring-like mechanism (Fig. 3-57).[250,316,358,377,412,436,513] Hacketal developed a method sometimes referred to as bundle nailing, in which as many small rods as possible are placed in the medullary space, eventually creating stability by incremental jamming.[86,148,406]

More complicated devices have curves to aid insertion, removal, and stability or to duplicate the natural curvature of the bone. Femoral nails are often curved in a sagittal plane to simulate the sagittal bow of the femur. Küntscher[299] appreciated the double sagittal curve of the femur and experimented with a nail having first a posterior curve then an anterior curve that he referred to as the "dopple nagel" or double nail. Passing a nail with a double curve through a bone having a double curve proved difficult, and the design was abandoned early. Larger and more rigid tibial and humeral nails have been designed that have curvatures to accommodate insertion portals offset from the center of the medullary canal.

Too much curvature built into the nail makes nail removal difficult and hazardous, as was discovered with the Zickel subtrochanteric device. This device has an anterversion, valgus, and anterior curvature to fit the curves of the femur. Once the fracture has healed, the bone remodels to the nail and attempted removal has led to refracture.[531]

Cross-Sectional Geometry

Intramedullary devices can be solid or hollow; open-sectioned (slotted) or closed-sectioned; cylindrical, rectangular, diamond, square, cloverleaf, triflanged, or otherwise configured. Solid nails[***] are suitable for placement without canal preparation by reaming but

*** References 66–68, 89, 179, 202, 237, 304, 319–321, 333, 338, 345, 346, 412, 438, 454, 503.

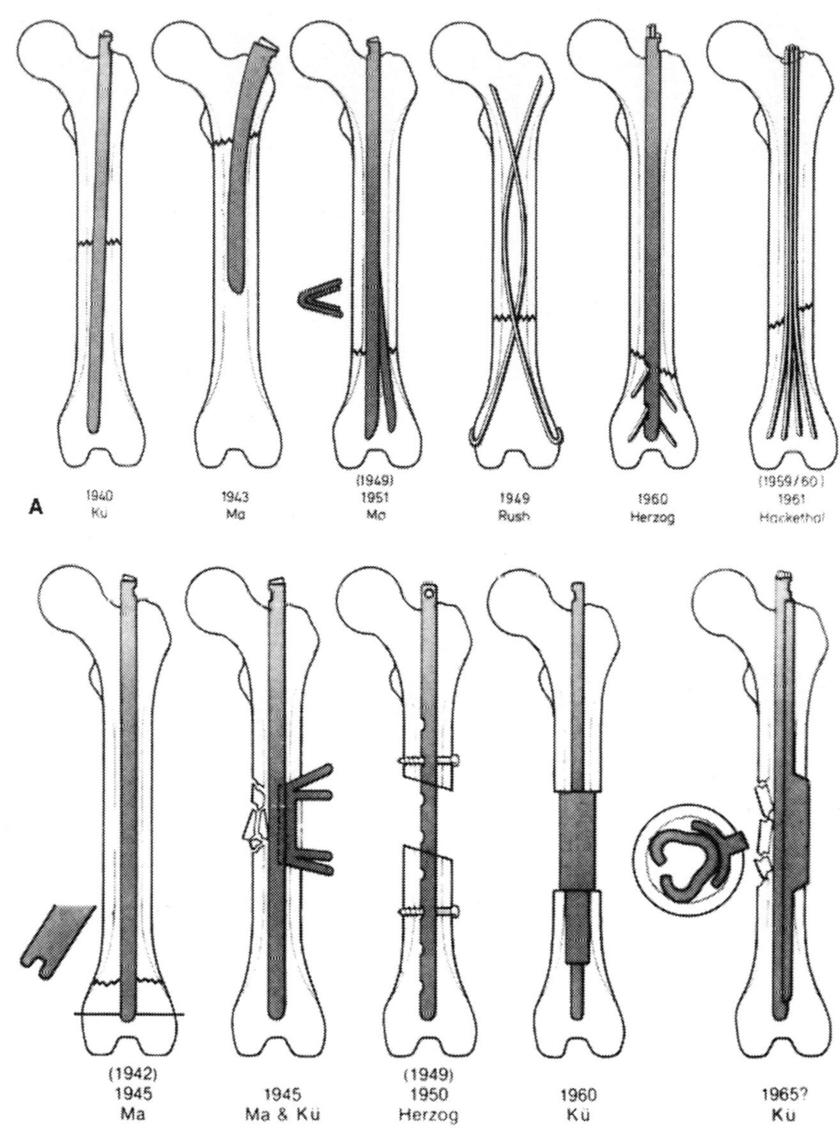

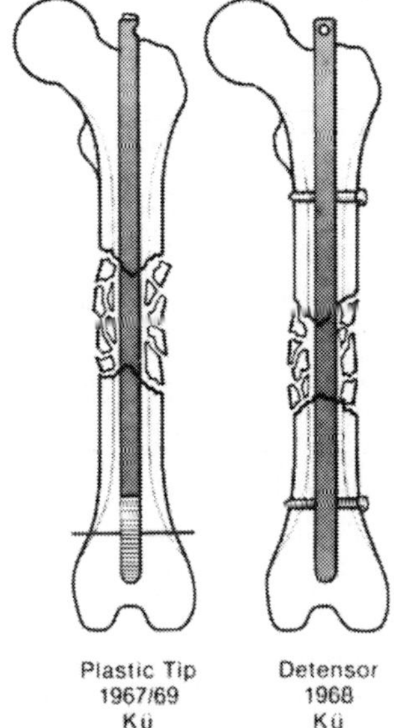

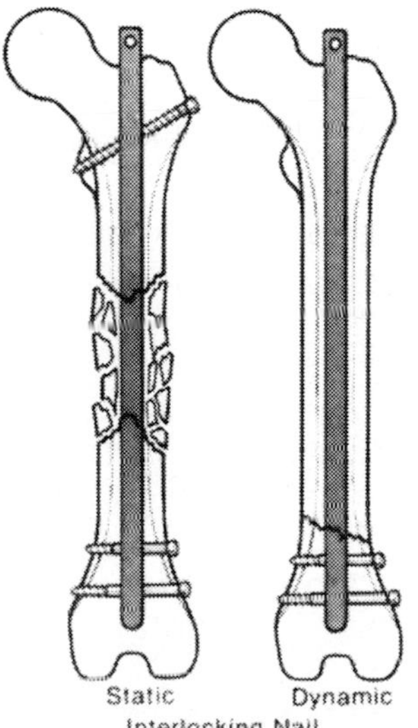

B

FIGURE 3-55. Medullary fixation has stimulated the creative instincts of orthopaedists and traumatologists. (**A**) Tactics to control rotational instability only. (**B**) Tactics to control length or rotational stability by means of blocking. (*Kü*–Küntscher; *Ma*–Maatz) (Maatz, R., Lentz, W., Arens, W., and Beck, H., (eds.): Intramedullary Nailing and Other Intramedullary Osteosynthesis, pp. 253, 254. Philadelphia, W.B. Saunders, 1986.)

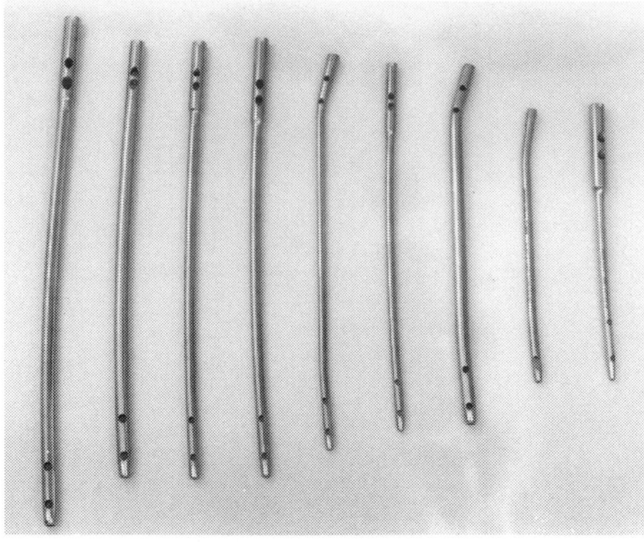

FIGURE 3-56. The Russell Taylor complete nail system. From left to right, femoral reconstruction nail, femoral nail (after reaming), delta femoral nail (without reaming), delta reconstruction nail (small diameters), delta tibial nail, delta II femoral, tibial, humeral, and delta II reconstruction nails. *(Courtesy of Smith & Nephew Richards, Inc., Memphis, TN.)*

are hard to remove if broken. Hollow nails make insertion over a guide rod possible and are ideal after canal preparation by reaming. The wall thickness of hollow nails may be variable to alter the strength and stiffness of the device. Similarly, a slot may be placed in the device to increase torsional flexibility. Cross-sectional shape influences the mechanical properties of the nail and also has an effect on the return of circulation after nailing. Channels in the nail allow better revascularization than a nail that completely fills the medullary cavity out to the endosteal cortex.[422] Flutes and corners on nails have given way to locking with screws for torsional stability.

Locking Capacity and Configuration

Most contemporary internal fixation devices are designed to allow cross-locking at both ends, so that screws can be placed through the bone and the nail above and below the fracture for additional stabilization. The number, location, and angle of screws may be varied for specific advantages. The closer to the ends of the nail that the screws are located, the more fractures that may be treated with the device.

Oblique screw orientation, common in femoral and humeral nails (Russell Taylor,[27,439] Grosse Kemf,[128, 280, 486, 536], ZMS, Klemm[96, 283]), reduces the rotational moment about the screw, eliminating the need for a second screw. Two parallel screws perpendicular to the long axis of the nail are used for distal locking in tibial and femoral nails. The ASIF tibial nail has the possibility of one its three distal screws being oriented 90° to the other two, extending the indications to include more distal fractures.[361]

The Huckstep intramedullary compression nail[238–240] differs from other nails in its quadrilateral cross section and titanium alloy composition. Holes along the length of the nail accept interlocking screws at multiple levels, and oblique proximal holes allow the insertion of lag screws up the femoral neck. Intraoperative radiographs are not routinely required and because the design is not amenable to closed nailing techniques, open reduction is mandatory.

Proximal locking in the upper femur has been extensively modified to make nailing applicable to proximal femoral fractures from the subtrochanteric region proximally. Initial fixation systems consisted of an implant driven into the head and neck, with a Küntscher nail inserted through the head–neck piece.[220,327] Even though the fixation principle has proved over time to be sound, the "Y" nail of Küntscher had limited popularity, perhaps due to technical difficulties in the insertion technique. Subsequent designs have modified proximal locking, with use of a triflanged nail (Zickel)[111,357] placed thorough the shaft nail, a "U" nail with shaft nail inside (Williams),[233] and one or two screws placed through the nail (Russell-Taylor and others[48,462]; Fig. 3-58).

Materials

Alloys that are used for nails include 316L steel, 22:13:5 steel, titanium, titanium aluminum vanadium (Ti-6Al-4V), and titanium aluminum niobium (Ti-6Al-7Nb). Except for small diameter nails used without reaming, differences in material properties are probably less significant in terms of fracture healing than nail diameter and wall thickness or biologic viability of bone at the fracture site. The smaller diameter nails, however, should be made of alloys having superior fatigue strength.

Mechanics of Intramedullary Implants

During the period of fracture healing, internal fixation aids in transmission of forces from one end of the fractured bone to the other, thereby producing stresses in the implant. The mechanical behavior of the implant is determined by both material and geometry. The rigidity or stiffness of a cylindrical structure in bending and torsion is proportional to the fourth power of the radius (ie, the polar moment of inertia). The farther that material is distributed from the bending or torsional axis, the stiffer the structure becomes. A 1-mm

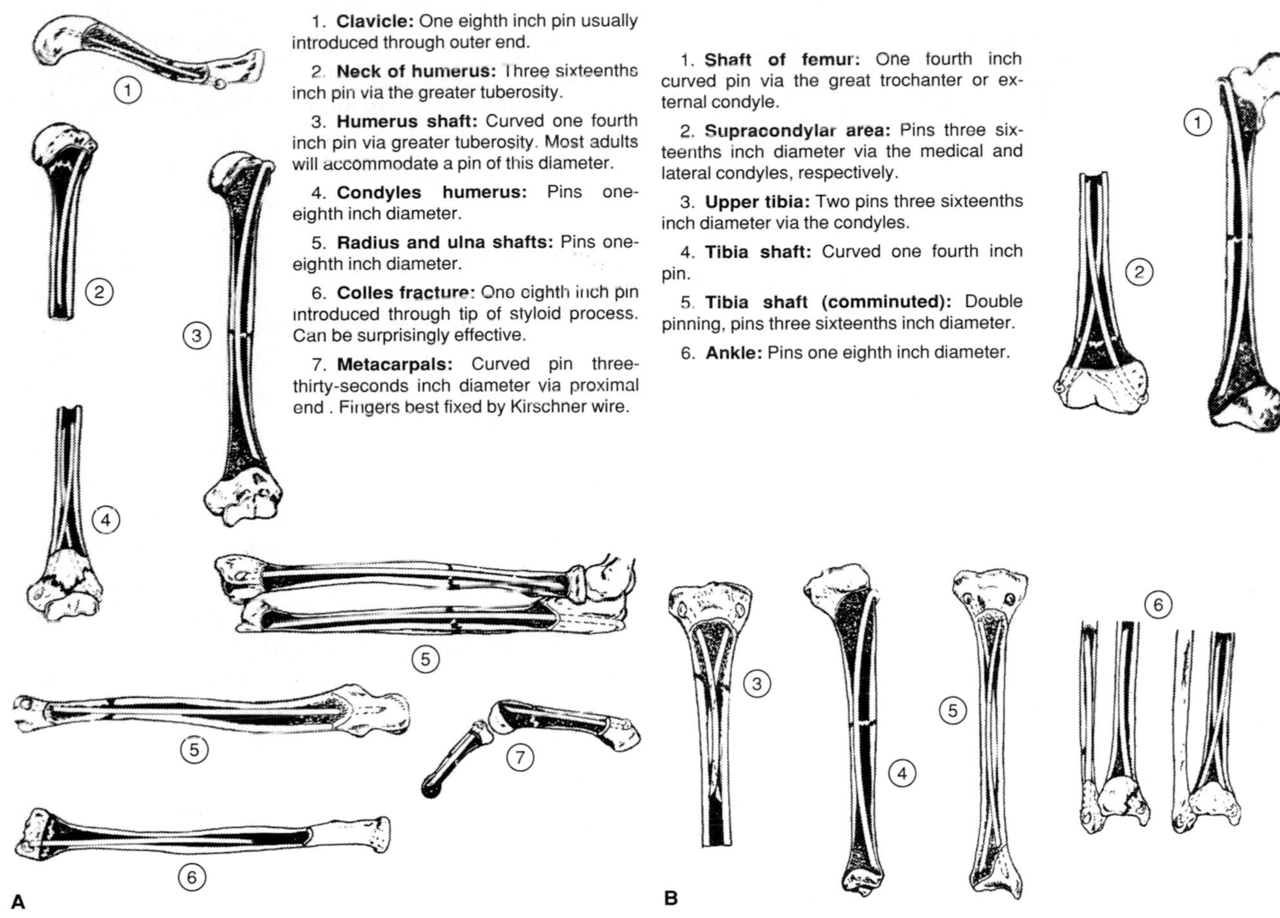

1. **Clavicle:** One eighth inch pin usually introduced through outer end.
2. **Neck of humerus:** Three sixteenths inch pin via the greater tuberosity.
3. **Humerus shaft:** Curved one fourth inch pin via greater tuberosity. Most adults will accommodate a pin of this diameter.
4. **Condyles humerus:** Pins one-eighth inch diameter.
5. **Radius and ulna shafts:** Pins one-eighth inch diameter.
6. **Colles fracture:** One eighth inch pin introduced through tip of styloid process. Can be surprisingly effective.
7. **Metacarpals:** Curved pin three-thirty-seconds inch diameter via proximal end . Fingers best fixed by Kirschner wire.
1. **Shaft of femur:** One fourth inch curved pin via the great trochanter or external condyle.
2. **Supracondylar area:** Pins three sixteenths inch diameter via the medical and lateral condyles, respectively.
3. **Upper tibia:** Two pins three sixteenths inch diameter via the condyles.
4. **Tibia shaft:** Curved one fourth inch pin.
5. **Tibia shaft (comminuted):** Double pinning, pins three sixteenths inch diameter.
6. **Ankle:** Pins one eighth inch diameter.
A
B

FIGURE 3-57. (**A**) Upper and (**B**) lower extremity long bone fractures, fixed using Rush techniques and implants. (Rush, L.V.: Atlas of Rush Pin Technics, Vol. 243, Meridian, Berivon Company, 1976.)

increase in the diameter of an intramedullary nail enhances its stiffness by 30% to 45%,[6] and a 25% increase in nail diameter doubles its bending strength.[301]

The Küntscher nail had a cloverleaf cross section with a longitudinal slot. Küntscher believed that the open section would allow compression of the nail by the isthmus of the medullary canal, thereby providing greater rotational control. Placing the slot anteriorly on the tension side of the fracture provides the strongest configuration. When the slot is placed on the compression side, local buckling occurs with high bending loads.[7] An open section has little effect on the bending stiffness of a nail but markedly reduces its stiffness in torsion. In a thin-walled cylinder, the addition of a narrow longitudinal slot reduces the torsional moment of inertia to 15% of its initial value.[7,301,480]

The working length of a nail is that portion of the nail that spans the fracture site between areas of fixation in the proximal and distal fragments (ie, the unsupported segment of the nail). This may vary from 1 to 2 mm in a transverse fracture at the isthmus to several centimeters in a comminuted diaphyseal fracture. In a comminuted fracture fixed by a static-locked nail, the working length is the distance between the proximal and distal locking screws. The working length influences nail rigidity in both bending and torsion. In bending, the stiffness is inversely proportional to the square of the working length. A nail having a working length of 0.25 inches is 16 times more rigid in bending than a nail with a working length of 1 inch. In torsion, the stiffness is inversely proportional to the working length, so that doubling the working length halves the torsional rigidity.[7] A short working length, therefore, improves nail rigidity both in bending and in torsion.

With torsional loading, a nail both twists and slips within the medullary canal. Slipping allows residual angular displacement after the load is released. Gripping strength is the resistance to slipping at the implant–bone interface and is essential for the transmission of torque between fracture fragments. Grip can be increased by cortical reaming to increase the length of

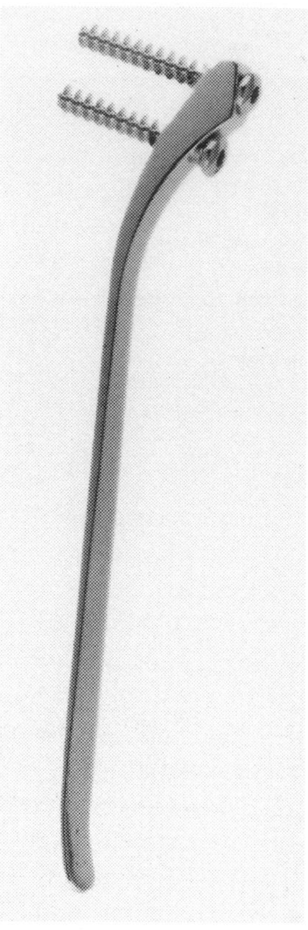

FIGURE 3-58. The Mouradian intramedullary device is used for complex proximal humeral fractures in which the head is unstable relative to the shaft. The lag screws fix the head to the nail while the nail jams in the shaft. Tuberosity fragments are then repaired to the stable head shaft construct with sutures. *(Courtesy of Howmedica, Inc., Rutherford, NJ.)*

cortical contact or by the addition of flutes.[6] Interlocking nails optimize grip by rigidly affixing the nail to the bone with screws. Kyle and associates have quantified gripping strength as the spring-back angle after in vitro torsional testing of various nail systems.[301,302] Spring-back angle is calculated by twisting a bone–nail construct through an arc of 10° and then releasing the deforming force. The final angle measured using the initial starting point as the reference plane subtracted from 10° yields the spring-back angle. The spring-back angle depends on the working length of the implant, the mode of locking (if any), and the torsional rigidity of the implant. Screw fixation proved more effective than fins. As working length is increased, torsional stiffness decreases with a small increase in spring-back angle, creating a spring-like action.[302]

Johnson and Tencer[264,483–485] have conducted extensive in vitro biomechanical evaluation of simulated comminuted subtrochanteric and femoral shaft fractures fixed by a variety of intramedullary nails. In three-point bending, fracture models having segmental subtrochanteric defects fixed with interlocking nails were 55% to 70% as stiff as intact femurs, and fractures fixed with Ender nails had less than 25% of the bending stiffness of an intact femur. Femurs with segmental defects of the shaft were significantly less rigid in bending for all intramedullary devices tested.

Models tested in axial loading showed wide variations. Ender nails failed by slippage of the nails back through their insertion sites at loads less than body weight. Nails with deployable distal fins failed by the fins cutting out distally through metaphyseal bone at 1.5 times body weight, and nails with proximal and distal interlocking screws failed only at loads of nearly four times body weight. Failure in these cases occurred by fracture at the base of the femoral neck, cutting out of the proximal screw, or bending of the nail within the fracture site. No failure of the distal locking screws was reported.

All of the systems tested demonstrated low rigidity in torsion. Ender nails and open-section interlocking nails reestablished only 3% of the torsional stiffness of the intact femur but with a closed-section nail, the torsional rigidity of the construct increased to about 50% of the intact femur.[487] Although torsional stiffness values for open-section nails are significantly lower than for closed-section nails, the bone–implant combination shows little residual angular displacement after testing. The nail deforms elastically and then springs back, with only a minor slip in the bone. Deployable fins control rotation as well as distal interlocking screws, even in those cases in which deployment of both fins is incomplete. Conversely, Ender nails show a greater degree of slip, thus allowing residual rotational deformity after release of the load.

Biologic Consequences of Intramedullary Surgery

Fracture healing proceeds mainly by the formation of periosteal callus.[400,415,422] Cortical reaming and nail insertion injure the medullary vascular system, resulting in avascularity of significant portions of the diaphyseal cortex.[107–109] The implications in open fractures are obvious, and the risk of infection must be carefully weighed against the necessity of reaming. An implant that immobilizes the fracture, however, facilitates revascularization of the fracture site.[422]

In studies of the canine tibia, fractures fixed with an intramedullary rod showed higher rates of whole bone and fracture-site blood flow than comparable fractures fixed with a plate, and they remained elevated for a longer period.[415] A delay in the maturation of callus was noted with intramedullary nails but once union was achieved, the biomechanical quality of union was similar in the two groups.

Medullary cortical reaming weakens a bone. Clawson[91] recommended removal of no more than 4 mm and cautioned that the cortex should not be reamed to less than half of its original thickness. Pratt[411] studied the effect of reaming on the torsional strength of cadaver femurs; reaming to 12 mm decreased the maximum torque to failure to 63% of that of matched controls, and further reaming to 16 mm decreased this value to 36%, with the largest increment occurring between 14 and 15 mm. He recommended reaming to less than half the bone's diameter at the mid-shaft.

Molster[351] studied the effect of medullary reaming and nail insertion on intact rat femurs and found that reaming immediately reduced the strength of the femur by 15%, although the degree of cortical reaming was not specified. Femurs, after the introduction of rigid nails, remained weaker than matched controls without nails, indicating some degree of biologic impairment from the intervention. Refracture after removal of intramedullary nails has been infrequent and this is partly related to the absence of multiple screw holes, which are stress risers.

The mechanism of osseous necrosis has been studied and appears to be pressure-mediated. Stürmer made the following observations after extensive laboratory and clinical investigation:

Pressure elevation associated with awl, guide rod, and reamers occurred in excess of 1000 mm Hg, measured both in sheep and humans (Fig. 3-59)

High intramedullary pressures caused significantly larger zones of necrosis than a special irrigation-suction reamer, which lowered pressures

High intramedullary pressure was necessary for venous drainage through the periosteal veins; "pulsating intramedullary pressure may be necessary for nourishment of the osteocytes-medullary reaming and nailing can cause a considerable disturbance of the intracortical transport mechanism"

Irrigation suction system pressure was kept at physiologic levels and thermal effects were reduced, 38.5% of the cortex remained vital, compared with 27.5% in the conventionally reamed group ($p < 0.05$)

Distal venting hole use was ineffective because of the high viscosity of the medullary contents

Unreamed rod raised pressures to 200 mm Hg and embolization occurred.[475]

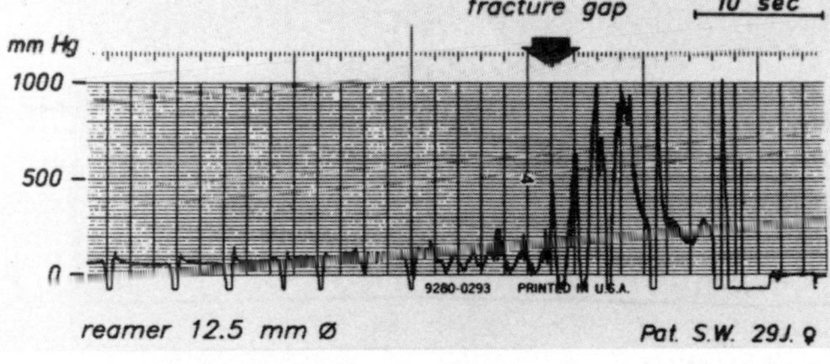

FIGURE 3-59. Intramedullary pressure measured during closed intramedullary nailing of a human tibia. Pressure approaches 1000 mm Hg in the distal fragment. (Stürmer, K.: Measurement of Intramedullary Pressure in an Animal Experiment and Propositions to Reduce the Pressure Increase. Injury: AO/ASIF Scientific Supplement 24(3):s7–s21, 1993.)

Concern over the harmful effects of reaming has led to a shift of interest back to interlocking nailing systems that do not require reaming.[104,200,215,221,228,293,296] Rhinelander[422] and others have shown more rapid revascularization with nails placed without preparatory reaming, compared with nails placed after reaming.[372,400,415,422] In a rat study, Grundnes and coworkers[186] compared reaming and fixation of 1.8-mm canals with 1.6-mm nails and 2-mm nails. Blood flow differences correlating to amount of reaming were noted but were found to be short-lived.

In animal models, variations in the rigidity of intramedullary fixation has been shown to affect fracture healing. Wang[505] studied the quality and strength of fracture callus in rabbit femurs fixed with rods of varying bending rigidity. Insufficient rigidity produced abundant callus but unreliable and widely variable bone healing. Excessive bending rigidity produced scant callus that demonstrated low energy absorption when stressed to failure. Callus formation and energy absorption to failure were optimal when the fracture was fixed by a rod of intermediate bending rigidity.

Torsional rigidity also influences fracture healing. Molster[350] studied healing of osteotomized rat femurs fixed with intramedullary rods with varying degrees of instability. Union was delayed in the femurs in which rotational instability was the greatest. Woodard[526] reported differences in fracture healing of canine femoral fractures treated with rods of differing torsional rigidity. Closed-section rods were paired with open-section rods of equal bending but differing torsional rigidity, restoring 42% and 12%, respectively, of the torsional rigidity of the femur. Pseudarthrosis occurred in 50% of these femurs treated with the more flexible slotted rods. All femurs treated by closed-section rods were united at 6 months. Grundnes[186] also found torsional flexibility was inhibitory to fracture union.

Technique of Intramedullary Surgery

The introduction of interlocking nails has expanded the variety of long-bone fractures amenable to intramedullary fixation. Closed-nailing techniques have reduced blood loss, infection rates, and length of time in hospital. The added complexity of insertion, however, has introduced new pitfalls and complications. Careful preoperative planning and operative technique, familiarity with instrumentation, and skilled radiographic monitoring are of the utmost importance.

Preoperative injury films must be carefully inspected for the fracture pattern, degree of comminution, canal size, deformity, and presence of associated injuries. Nondisplaced fractures of the femoral neck, butterfly fragments, and extensions into adjacent joints may not be appreciated intraoperatively with image intensification, and the discovery of such injuries on recovery room films is an unhappy event.

Location of the proper starting point for nail insertion is a critical step in closed nailing. An improper portal of entry allows angular deformity at the fracture site or even worse, causes comminution during reaming or nail insertion (Fig. 3-60). In femoral nailings, an excessively medial starting point may compromise the vascularity of the femoral head or produce a stress riser in the femoral neck. A lateral portal directs the nail toward the medial cortex, causing varus angulation or medial comminution that may compromise the fixation of the proximal interlocking screw. Deformity and variations in anatomy make fixed anatomic reference points unreliable. The proper starting point is that which allows access to the center of the medullary canal (Fig. 3-61).

Fracture reduction is easier when nailing is performed within a few hours of injury, before the onset of soft-tissue shortening and edema. If femoral nailing is delayed, skeletal traction is necessary, preferably with the fracture slightly distracted. Excessive intraoperative traction to achieve length compromises skin and may produce stretch injury of the sciatic or peroneal nerves or pressure on the pudendal nerve. Alternatives to use of a fracture table such as the ASIF distractor are available. Operative reduction is facilitated by placement of an internal manipulator to lever the proximal fragment into position. Intramedullary reduction devices are available, although a smaller size nail works well.

Fracture reduction is maintained by the use of a guide wire, over which cannulated flexible reamers are used. A curved ball-tip guide wire is the type most easily passed across the fracture site. A guide wire should be advanced only a few millimeters at a time. Radiographic confirmation of intramedullary passage of the wire across the fracture site is essential. Unrecognized advancement of the guide wire through soft

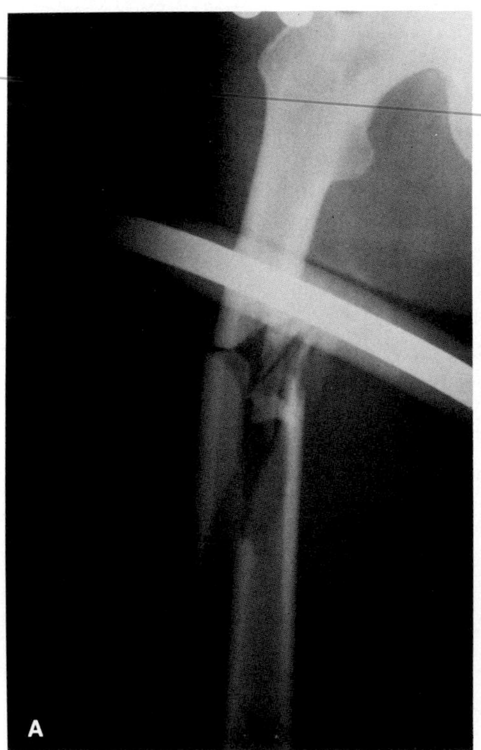

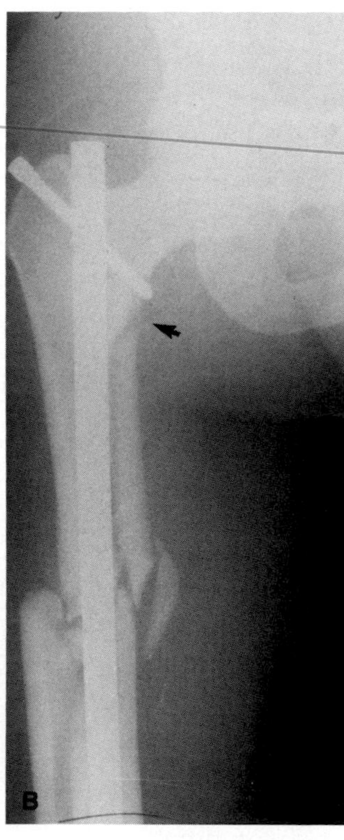

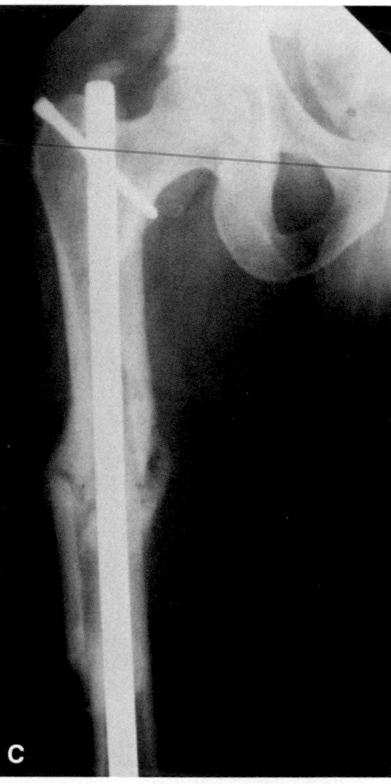

FIGURE 3-60. (**A**) A 36-year-old man sustained a comminuted mid-shaft femur fracture in a motor vehicle accident. (**B**) An aberrant entry portal directed the nail toward the anteromedial cortex, causing comminution up to the level of the lesser trochanter (*arrow*). This new fracture was not detected intraoperatively with image intensification. (**C**) Uneventful union occurred, using a statically locked nail.

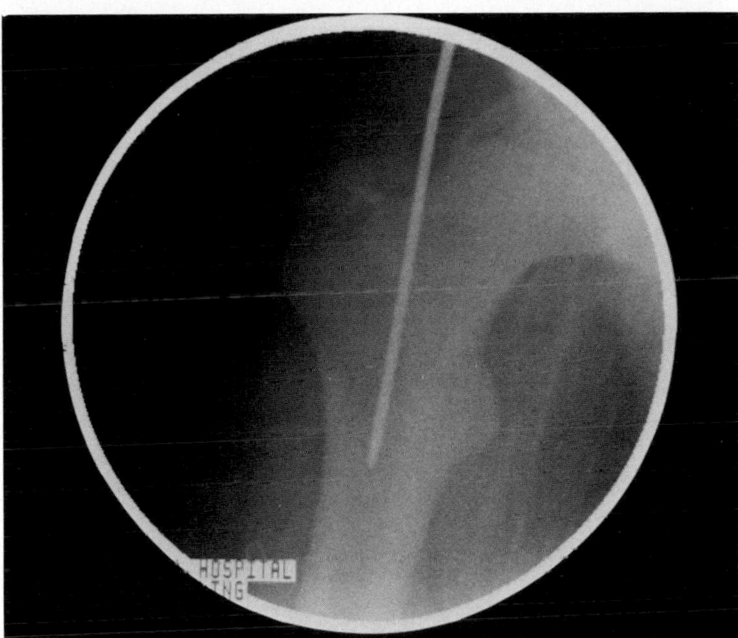

FIGURE 3-61. The safest starting point allows direct access to the center of the medullary canal in both planes. The entry portal of the tibia is the proximal most aspect of the anterior cortex, which moves the insertion point as posterior as safely possible.

tissues may produce neurologic or vascular injury, and the guide wire should be seated against subchondral bone in the distal fragment. With distal fractures, the guide wire can easily be inadvertently drawn back across the fracture site during reaming. When this occurs, replacement of the wire in the intramedullary location must always be confirmed before reaming is resumed. The first assistant should clamp and stabilize the guide wire during reaming to prevent migration.

Cannulated flexible reamers are required to prepare a curved medullary canal. Reaming should progress in 1-mm increments until the cortex is reached and in 0.5-mm increments thereafter. Sharp reamers and gentle pressure help to avoid entrapment of the reamer. An incarcerated reamer can be extricated by withdrawing the ball tip of the guide wire against the reamer and gently disimpacting the guide wire with a vise grip and mallet. Conventional spring-type flexible reamers cannot be reversed or they will unwind within the medullary canal, a most disconcerting experience.

Proper nail diameter and length is crucial. Insertion of a nail larger than the largest reamer used should never be attempted. Interlocking nails rely on transfixing screws for stabilization rather than tight endosteal contact, and slight overreaming allows greater ease of nail insertion, with less implant deformation. Interlocking nails are reamed 0.5 to 1.5 mm greater than the diameter of the nail to be used, depending on the device being used.

A nail that is too long causes soft-tissue irritation and discomfort at the insertion site or worse, penetrates the distal joint. The appropriate nail length is determined

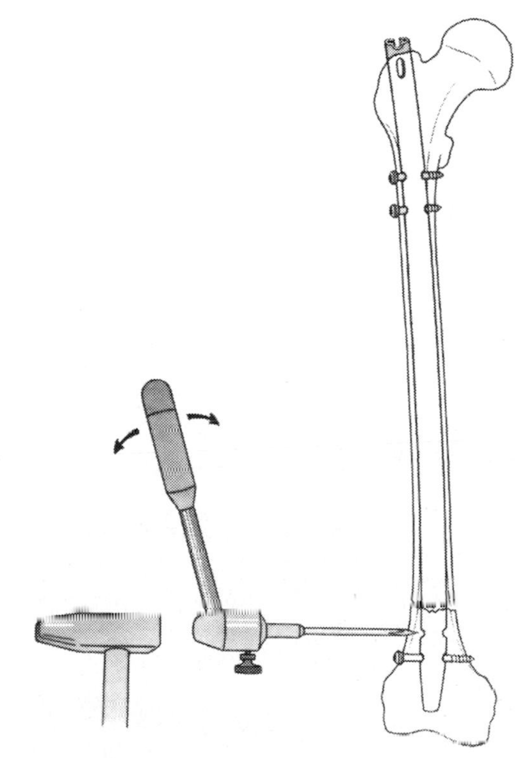

FIGURE 3-62. Klemm freehand technique of distal locking employs an awl for making the lateral bone portal after sighting in the tip with the image intensifier. Such techniques have proved to be more popular and reliable than elaborate nail- or image-mounted jigs. (Hempel, D., and Fischer, S.: Intramedullary Nailing. Stuttgart, Georg Thieme Verlag, 1982.)

intraoperatively by direct measurement of the depth of guide-wire insertion but when the fracture is comminuted, the appropriate length may be difficult to determine. Preoperative scanograms may be beneficial but are exceedingly difficult to make when a patient is in skeletal traction. It is easier to measure the uninjured side against nails of known length under the image intensifier and then adjust the traction on the injured side to ''fit'' this predetermined nail length. If both sides are fractured, the least comminuted side is nailed first. An identical nail is then used on the more comminuted side.

During insertion, the nail should advance a few millimeters with each blow of the mallet. If progress is not being made, the nail size, adequacy of reaming, starting point, and reduction should be reevaluated. The use of excessive force may result in comminution of the bone or incarceration of the nail. As the nail crosses the fracture site, its tip may impinge on the cortex of the distal fragment. If this occurs, the nail must be backed up slightly and the reduction improved before the nail is advanced.

Care must be taken to seat the nail fully before proximal screw placement, so that the screw may be correctly positioned. The nail-mounted proximal targeting jigs must be checked before nail placement to make sure that they have not become deformed by previous rough handling. The targeting device should be tightened after the nail is seated because it may loosen during driving of the nail and allow enough play to misdirect the drill bit from its proper alignment relative to the nail.

Freehand distal locking has become the most used technique as a multitude of image or nail-mounted devices have failed reliability tests over time (Fig. 3-62). Although the need for both distal screws has

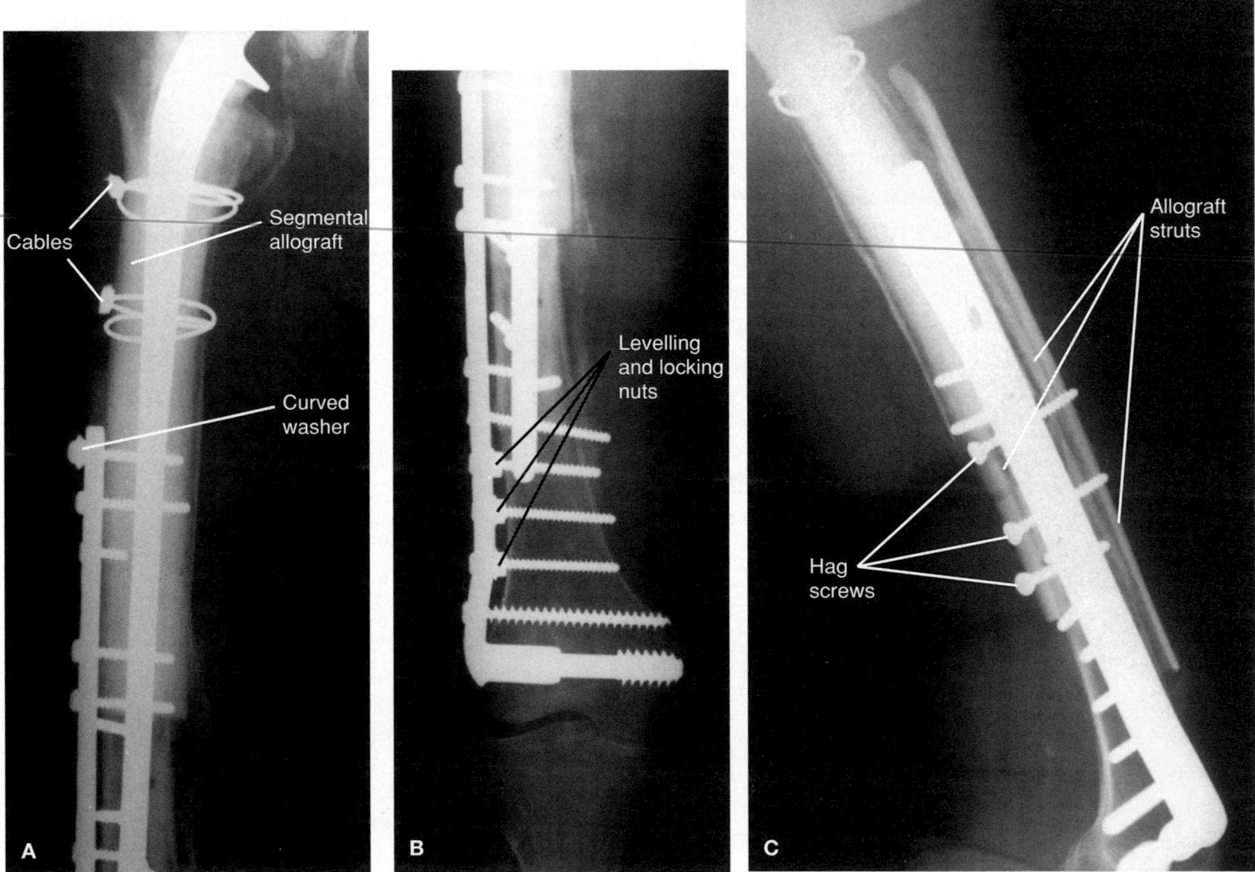

FIGURE 3-63. Proximal (**A**) and distal (**B**) anteroposterior and lateral radiographs (**C**) of composite fixation, consisting of metal and allograft struts. A fracture occurred distal to the total hip, where there was a junction between segmental prosthetic allograft, stem, and porotic native distal femur. Complete fracture occurred and was repaired with condylar plate, lag screws, and allograft struts, joining the segmental allograft and native femur. The plate was leveled relative to the allograft, using nuts under the plate (**B**).

been questioned, two screws are recommended to lessen axial and sagittal plane rotational forces.[74]

Levin[315] has measured the irradiation exposure to the surgeon's dominant hand during intramedullary nailings with freehand distal targeting. The average dose to the hand was 12 mrem. The exposure during nail insertion and proximal interlocking was 13 mrem. These figures are within the government guidelines for irradiation exposure during a 3-month period but many surgeons perform such procedures daily, and the long-term deleterious effects may be considerable. The surgeon must remain cognizant of his proximity to the radiation beam during all phases of the procedure, and the image intensifier should be used by necessity rather than by convenience. The use of a screen that has memory is mandatory.

Breakage of intramedullary nails is uncommon. In an extensive review of a series of intramedullary nails, Franklin[152] reported an aggregate incidence of breakage of 3.3% for the femur and 1% for the tibia. As would be expected, in a comminuted unstable fracture pattern, more stress is placed on the nail and breakage is more common. Before the use of interlocking nails, failure occurred at the original fracture site and often was attributed to an undersized nail. In contrast, interlocking nails often fail in proximity to the proximal and distal interlocking mechanisms.

Partially slotted nails fail most frequently at the junction of the cylindrical and cloverleaf portions of the nail.[29,152,280,486] Initially this junction was welded but such nails are produced in one piece[65] or have been redesigned with a full-length slot.[478] Distal screw holes may act as stress risers, and fatigue fracture through the more proximal of the holes may occur.[74,92] The close proximity of the fracture to this hole appears to increase the risk of breakage. Exacting technique during the distal screw insertion is required to prevent inadvertent scoring of the nail, which produces an additional stress riser.

Bending occurs more readily in solid nails, whereas cloverleaf nails tend to break. Angulation of the nail predisposes to delayed union,[249] and it is wishful thinking to anticipate union before a bent nail finally breaks. A bent nail should always be replaced by one that is new. The extremity may be manipulated immediately before exchange to facilitate removal, and specialized hooks have been devised for the removal of the distal portion of a broken nail.[152]

COMPOSITE FIXATION

Müller has been credited with the idea of using polymethylmethacrylate to supplement metallic internal fixation, known also as composite fixation.[356,360] Composite fixation consists of a mechanical linkage of at least two differing fixation materials: metal, acrylic, and allograft (Fig. 3-63). Bone loss through tumor lysis, pathologic granuloma after arthroplasty, senile osteoporosis, defect pseudarthrosis, and comminution are the typical indications for composite fixation.[†††] The most basic use of polymethylmethacrylate is as an anchor for screws in soft bone (Fig. 3-64). The drill hole is made, the depth measured, the hole tapped, and the screw placed in the hole and removed. Cement is mixed and placed in the hole; during the curing process, the screw is reinserted. Final tightening is done after the cement has hardened. In other examples, such as some fractures surrounding cemented athroplasties, the cement column predates the fracture

††† References 10, 13, 22, 89, 129, 131, 180, 194, 195, 205, 206, 230, 233, 256, 262, 295, 310, 317, 356, 360, 385, 418, 445, 502, 512.

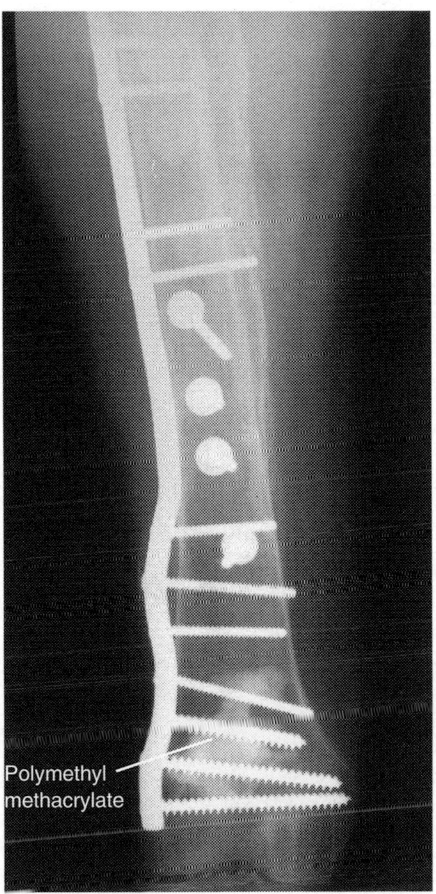

FIGURE 3-64. A femur fractured below the stem of a total hip and was fixed successfully with a plate and screws. Distal purchase was poor, requiring augmentation with methylmethacrylate. This radiograph was taken 10 years after the fixation, when the patient fell again, fracturing her the tibia just below the knee joint.

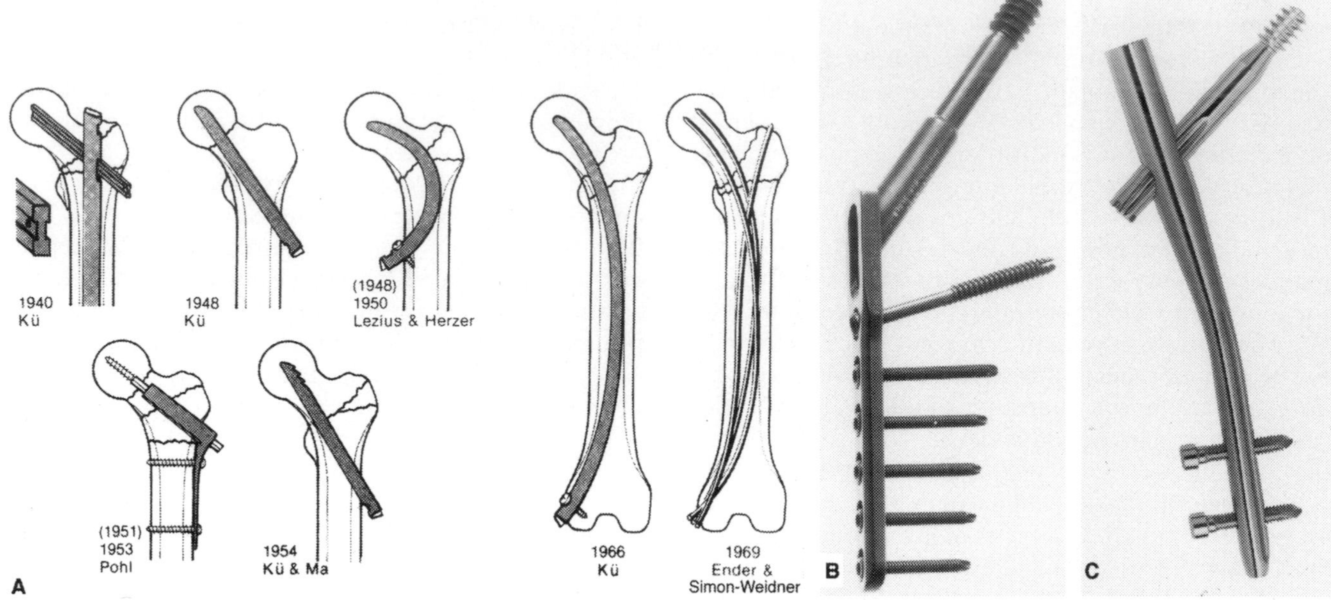

FIGURE 3-65. (**A**) Sliding hip-compression hip screw history, beginning with the Y nail of Küntscher, demonstrates its origin with intramedullary nailing advocates. (Maatz, R., Lentz, W., Arens, W., and Beck, H., (eds.): Intramedullary Nailing and Other Intramedullary Osteosynthesis. Philadelphia, W.B. Saunders, 1986.) (**B**) Titanium captured sliding hip-compression screw is a contemporary variation on the earlier hybrid theme. (*Courtesy of Ace Orthopaedic Company, El Sequando, CA.*) (**C**) The Gamma nail is intended for intertrochanteric fractures for surgeons preferring a pure intramedullary device. (*Courtesy of Howmedica, Inc.*)

and is used for screw fixation.[456] Similar techniques are occasionally useful in osteoporosis due to senility or after failed prior internal fixation surgery.[22,205,356,445,507]

Cement may be used to fill defects caused by tumor, crushing, or traumatic bone loss.[10,13,22,131,194,206,356,445] Union occurs, even with bone mass replaced by polymethylmethacrylate. When possible, techniques that reconstitute bone mass using allograft strut or cancellous bone grafts are preferable in patients in whom life expectancy is greater than a few years. A combination of limited cement filling of a defect combined with a plate or nail and allograft strut or struts may solve mechanical problems otherwise insoluble.

HYBRID FIXATION

Hybrid fixation is distinct from composite fixation: a composite consists of two or more different materials used in concert for fixation, whereas hybrid fixation may use only one material but with two or more fixation genre. An intramedullary device combined with an extramedullary device is an example of hybrid fixation. Similarly, external fixation with limited internal fixation is a form of hybrid fixation. Metallic hybrid fixation may be combined with another material such as polymethylmethacrylate to form a hybrid-composite construct. The goal of hybridization is to exploit advantages of the two types of fixation.

In 1934, Thornton[394] connected a Smith-Petersen nail (1931) to a plate and used the device for hip fractures. Jewett,[394] building on this idea, joined the intramedullary triflange with a Hawley side plate. Pohl in 1950,[394] Pugh and Schumpelick[394] and Jantzen[394] in 1955 converted the nongliding hybrid hip fixation device into a gliding one by allowing the intramedullary portion of the device to telescope inside the plate. The most commonly used hybrid device is the compression hip screw, which combines an intramedullary device (the lag screw) with an extramedullary device (the side plate; Fig. 3-65).[21,117,147,175,255,332,455,466,488,533] Interestingly, innovations joining a femoral neck–head lag screw with an intramedullary device (eg, the Gamma Nail) are both intramedullary devices and do not qualify as a hybrid implant.[128]

True to its mixed heritage, the contemporary form of the sliding hip screw blurs the lines between fixation principles. In one application, this device may be applied with static compression during surgery and with dynamic compression and gliding after resumption of physiologic loading. This combination of effects is particularly desirable in unstable intertrochanteric fractures in porotic bone and stands as an ideal indication for hybrid fixation, taking full advantage of the design properties of the implant. In another application such

TABLE 3-7
Changes in the Fractional Occurrence of Implant Polymer and Tissue Components Within the Implant Cavity During Degradation of the Polyglycolide Screws*

		Percentage of the Cross-Sectional Area				
Sample	Fields	*At 3 Wks. (N = 6)*	*At 6 Wks. (N = 5)*	*At 12 Wks. (N = 6)*	*At 36 Wks.*** (N = 5)*	*Intact Control Side*
Implant polymer	Central	100.0 +/− 0.0	100.0 +/− 0.0	72.0 +/− 21.8	0	—
	Peripheral	100.0 +/− 0.0	83.2 +/− 12.0	26.3 +/− 16.6	0	—
Loose connective tissue	Central	0	0	24.7 +/− 19.9	63.8 +/− 21.0	9.6 +/− 4.3
	Peripheral	0	15.2 +/− 10.8	69.7 +/− 16.9	49.0 +/− 8.9	5.1 +/− 2.2
Aligned connective tissue	Central	0	0	3.3 +/− 2.3	8.4 +/− 4.4	2.2 +/− 0.9
	Peripheral	0	1.6 +/− 1.1	4.0 +/− 2.5	7.0 +/− 2.0	4.3 +/− 1.7
Bone-marrow elements	Central	0	0	0	1.4 +/− 8.8	53.4 +/− 11.8
	Peripheral	0	0	0	42.7 +/− 10.5	77.5 +/− 13.6
Trabecular bone	Central	0	0	0	11.4 +/− 9.9	34.8 +/− 9.1
	Peripheral	0	0	0	1.3 +/− 0.8	13.1 +/− 4.9

* Mean and standard deviation.
** The differences were significant for all tissue components in both the central and peripheral sample fields.
Tissue type as a function of time in the screw hole of a resorbable screw with the control data in the far right column. Histologic normalization did not occur during the study period of 36 weeks.
Reprinted with permission from Bostman, O.M.: Osteolytic changes accompanying degradation of absorbable fracture fixation implants. J. Bone Joint Surg. [Br], 73(4): 679–82, 1991.

as a high subtrochanteric osteotomy, the same device can be placed to function as a compression plate having dynamic tension-band properties.

BIOABSORBABLE FIXATION

Metallic internal fixation devices often must be removed at a second operation, with considerable additional inconvenience, expense, and at some risk of operative complication. An implant that would disappear after fracture union certainly would be useful if sufficiently biocompatible and possessed of adequate mechanical properties. For almost three decades, polylactic acid and polyglycolic acid have been investigated as resorbable fixation material.[53] Initial efforts to produce resorbable fracture fixation devices were thwarted by poor material properties. Self-reinforced polyglycolic and polylactic acid rods and screws are available for limited used in fixation of fractures.[‡‡‡]

Degradation of polyglycolic acid is the result of hydrolysis and enzymatic breakdown. Polyglycolide is converted into glycine, which enters the citric acid cycle and leaves the cycle as carbon dioxide. Bostman[54] studied the sequence of cellular and tissue replacement in the wake of the degrading polymer. Table 3-7 presents a summary of his data, showing that even at the end of the study, fibrous tissue is the main component of the screw hole.[54]

Resorbable rods work as transfixion devices.[40] A pilot channel is made with a drill bit having the same diameter as the polyglycolic acid rod. The rod is then driven into the pilot hole. Additional rods are placed at angles, which are determined by the specific situation. The rods may be combined with a stout loop of nonmetallic suture to create a tension-band system for small-fragment avulsion fractures such as the olecranon or distal fibula. Cast immobilization is recommended until union. Fully threaded screws of polyglycolic acid are also available for malleolar fixation. They may be placed simply as a holding screw without compression or with overdrilling to function as a lag screw. Clinical work has largely involved resorbable fixation of ankle fractures but has

‡‡‡ References 4, 32, 35, 39, 47, 51–53, 55, 73, 83, 120, 159, 227, 229, 235, 294, 330, 387, 389–391, 395, 408, 476, 519.

TABLE 3-8
Compilation of Reports of Clinical Use of Bioabsorbable Fixation Reveals Heavy Concentration of Use in Epiphyseal Areas, Notably the Ankle

Indication	Author	#	Material
Adult radial head fractures	Pelto[395]	43	Polyglycolic acid rods
Adult capitellum fractures	Hirvensalo[227]	8	Polyglycolic acid rods
Ankle fractures	Partio[389]	71	Polylactide/polyglycolide screws
	Bostman[55]	56	Polyglycolic acid rods
	Partio[390]	152	Polyglycolide screws
	Bostman[51]	600	Polyglycolide rods or screws
	Frokjaer[159]	25	Polyglycolic acid rods
	Bucholz[73]	83	Polylactide screws
	Ahl[4]	15	Polyglycolic acid rods
Displaced elbow fractures in children	Hope[235]	13	Polyglycolic acid rods
	Makela[330]	19	Polyglycolic acid rods
Distal radius	Hoffmann[229]	40	Polyglycolic acid rods
Olecranon fractures	Partio[391]	41	Polyglycolide rods or screws
Pediatric fractures	Bostman[54]	71	Polyglycolic acid rods
Small fractures or osteotomies	Pihlajamaki[408]	27	Polylactide rods

also included osteochondral fractures, radial head fractures, olecranon fractures, and pediatric fractures of various types, in addition to an arthroscopic soft-tissue repair device (Table 3-8; Fig. 3-66).

Severe synovial reaction has been reported with polyglycolide rods used in the knee joint; use in this area should await further studies.[19,156] Significant soft-tissue problems with use in fractures of the distal radius have also been reported by Casteleyn.[83] Early reports of sinus track formation created concern over tissue compatibility[54,390] but one study showed no significant tissue reaction.[73] Sinus track formation occurs with polyglycolic acid (PGA) implants because of rapid hydrolysis. Pure polylactic acid (PLA) implants and copolymers resorb at slower rates and are not associated with such inflammatory reactions.[72]

Fixation achieved with these types of implants is often neither rigid nor stable enough to hold the frac-

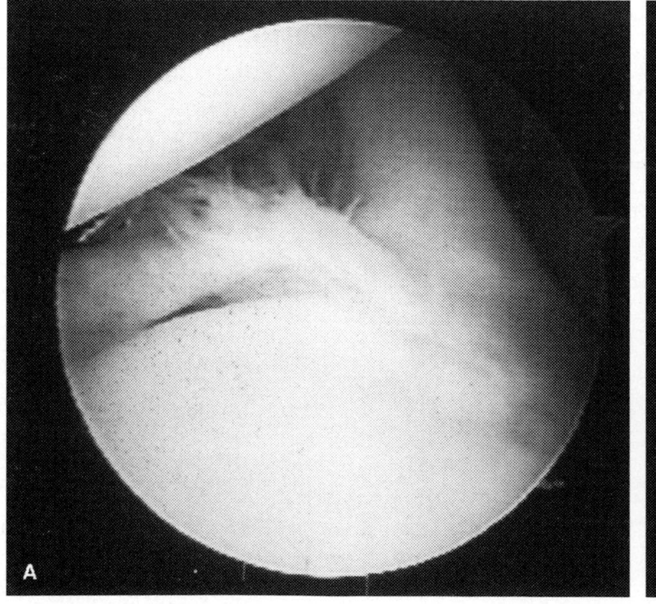

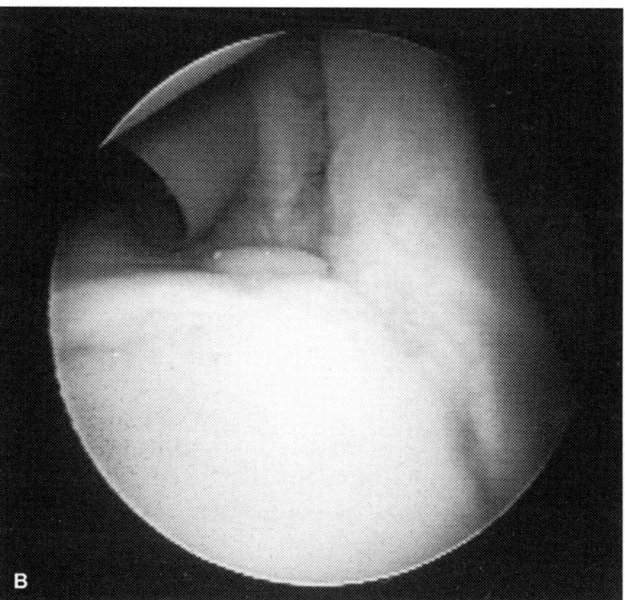

FIGURE 3-66. Bioabsorbable tacking used to stabilize torn glenoid labrum in the shoulder. (**A**) Arthroscopic view of a superior glenoid labral tear. (**B**) Percutaneous repair of the tear has been achieved with the tack. (*Courtesy of Dr. Neil ElAttrache.*)

ture stable with motion or weight bearing before union. Cast support and use of crutches for lower extremity fractures has been recommended, which limits their use further. In addition to poor mechanical properties, bioabsorbable implants have excessively low moduli resulting in backing out of screws, manufacturing problems related to polymer batch variations, and poor handling characteristics compared with metal.[72]

REFERENCES

1. Abemayor, E., Zemplenyi, J., Mannai, C., Webb, D.J., and Canalis, R.F.: The Fixation of Malar Fractures With the Transnasal Kirschner Wire. J. Otolaryngol. 17(4):179–182, 1988.
2. Adkison, J.W., and Chapman, M.W.: Treatment of Acute Lunate and Perilunate Dislocations. Clin. Orthop. 164:199–207, 1982.
3. Agee, J.M., Unstable fracture dislocations of the proximal interphalangeal joint. Treatment with the force couple splint. Clin. Orthop. 214:101–112, 1987.
4. Ahl, T., Dalen, N., Lundberg, A., and Wykman, A.: Biodegradable Fixation of Ankle Fractures. A Roentgen Stereophotogrammetric Study of 32 Cases. Acta. Orthop. Scand. 65(2):166–170, 1994.
5. Alldredge, R.H., Riordan, D.C.: The Use of Staples and Bone-Chip Grafts for Internal Fixation in Foot Stabilization Operations. J. Bone Joint Surg. 35A(4):951–957, 1953.
6. Allen, W.C.,.H., K.G., and Burstein, A.H.: A Fluted Femoral Intramedullary Rod. J. Bone Joint Surg. 60A:506–515, 1978.
7. Allen, W.C.;.P., G.; Burstein, A.H., and Frankel, V.H.: Biomechanical Principles of Intramedullary Fixation. Clin. Orthop. 60:13–20, 1968.
8. Allgöwer, M.: Modern Concepts of Fracture Treatment. AO/ASIF Dialogue 1(1):1–3, 1985.
9. Alonso, J.E., Davila R., and Bradley, E.: Extended Iliofemoral versus Triradiate Approaches in Management of Associated Acetabular Fractures. Clin. Orthop. 305:81–7, 1994.
10. Anderson, J.T., Erickson, J.M., Thompson R. Jr., and Chao, E.Y.: Pathologic Femoral Shaft Fractures Comparing Fixation Techniques Using Cement. Clin. Orthop. 131:273–278, 1978.
11. Appel, M.H., and Seigel, H.: Treatment of Transverse Fractures of the Patella by Arthroscopic Percutaneous Pinning. Arthroscopy 9(1):119–121, 1993.
12. Arzimanoglou, A., and Skiadaressis, G.: Study of Internal Fixation by Screws of Oblique Fractures in Long Bones. J. Bone Joint Surg. 34A:219–223, 1952.
13. Asnis, S.E., Lesniewski P., and Dowling T. Jr.: Anterior Decompression and Stabilization With Methylmethacrylate and a Bone Bolt for Treatment of Pathologic Fractures of the Cervical Spine. A Report of Two Cases. Clin. Orthop. 187:139–143, 1984.
14. Austin, R.T.: Compression Staples in High Tibial Osteotomy. J. R. Coll. Surg. Edinb. 18(3):177–179, 1973.
15. Bagby, G.W., and Janes, J.M.: The Effect of Compression on the Rate of Fracture Healing Using a Special Plate. Am. J. Surg. 95:761–771, 1958.
16. Bagby, G.W.: Compression Bone Plating Historical Considerations. J. Bone Joint Surg. 59A:761–771, 1977.
17. Bailey, D.E., Brinker, M.R.: Outcome Predictors in Tibial Fractures with a Vascular Injury, Are All Grade IIIC Injuries Created Equal? *In* Orthopaedic Trauma Association. 1994. Los Angeles, California: Orthopaedic Trauma Association.
18. Baker, C. Jr., and Graham, J.: Intraarticular ACL Reconstruction Using the Patellar Tendon: Arthroscopic Technique. Orthopedics 16(4):437–441, 1993.
19. Barfod, G., and Svendsen R.N.: Synovitis of the Knee After Intraarticular Fracture Fixation With Biofix. Report of Two Cases. Acta. Orthop. Scand. 63(6):680–681, 1992.
20. Bargar, W.L., Sharkey, N.A, Paul, H.A.M and Manske, D.J.: Efficacy of Bone Staples for Fixation. J. Orthop. Trauma 1(4):326–330, 1987.
21. Barrios, C., Brostrom, L.A., Stark, A., and Walheim, G.: Healing Complications After Internal Fixation of Trochanteric Hip Fractures: The Prognostic Value of Osteoporosis. J. Orthop. Trauma 7(5):438–442, 1993.
22. Bartucci, E., Gonzalez, M., Cooperman, D., Freedberg, H., and Laros, G.: The Effect of Adjunctive Methylmethacrylate on Failures of Fixation and Function in Patients with Intertrochanteric Fractures and Osteoporosis. J. Bone Joint Surg. 67A(7):1094–1107, 1985.
23. Bassett, R.L.: Displaced intraarticular fractures of the distal radius. Clin. Orthop. 214:148–152, 1987.
24. Baumgaertel, F., Perren, S.M., Rahn, B., and Gotzen, L.: Operative Treatment of Experimental Comminuted Subtrochanteric Femur Fractures in Sheep-Clinical Relevance. J. of Trauma 7(2):160–162, 1993.
25. Baumgaertel, F., and Gotzen, L.: [The biological plate osteosynthesis in multi-fragment fractures of the para-articular femur. A prospective study]. Unfallchirurg 97(2):78–84, 1994.
26. Baumgart, F.W., Cordey, J., Morikawa, K., et l.: AO/ASIF Self-tapping screws. Injury: AO/ASIF Scientific Supplement 24(1):S1–S17, 1993
27. Beals, N., Durham, G.; and Lynch, G.: Mechanical Characterizations of Interlocking Intramedullary Nails. Material Research Report ML 88-38. Memphis, Richards Medical Company, 1988.
28. Beaupre, G.S., Schneider, E., and Perren, S.M.: Stress Analysis of a Partially Slotted Intramedullary Nail. J. Orthop. Res. 2(4):369–376, 1984.
29. Beaupre, G.S., Schneider, E.; and Perren, S.M.: Stress Analysis of a Partially Slotted Intramedullary Nail. J. Orthop. Res. 2:369–376, 1984.
30. Bechtol, C.O., and Lepper, H. Jr.: Fundamental Studies in the Design of Metal Screws for Internal Fixation of Bone (Abstract). J. Bone Joint Surg. 38A:1385, 1956.
31. Behr, J.T., Dobozi, W.R., and Badrinath, K.: The Treatment of Pathologic and Impending Pathologic Fractures of the Proximal Femur in the Elderly. Clin. Orthop. 98:173–178, 1985.
32. Beiser, I.H., and Kanat, I.O.: Biodegradable Internal Fixation. A Literature Review. J. Am. Podiatr. Med. Assoc. 80(2):72–75, 1990.
33. Benirschke, S.K., Melder, I., Henley, M.G., Routt, M.L., Smith, D.G., Chapman, J.R., and Swiontkowski, M.F.: Closed Interlocking Nailing of Femoral Shaft Fractures: Assessment of Technical Complications and Functional Outcomes by Comparison of a Prospective Database With Retrospective Review. J. Orthop. Trauma 7(2):118–122, 1993.
34. Benjamin, J., Bried, J., Dohm, M., and McMurtry, M.: Biomechanical Evaluation of Various Forms of Fixation of Transverse Patellar Fractures. J. Orthop. Trauma 1(3):219–222, 1987.
35. Benz, G., Kallicris, D., Seebock, T., McIntosh, A., and Daum, R.: Bioresorbable Pins and Screws in Paediatric Traumatology. Eur. J. Pediatr. Surg. 4(2):103–107, 1994.
36. Berentey, G., and Szloboda, J.: Closed Interlocking Nailing in the Lower Extremity. Indications and Positioning. AORN J. 47(5):1203–1205, 1988
37. Berg, E.E.: Olecranon Fracture. Orthop. Nurs. 11(5):19–21, 1992.
38. Berg, E.E.: Comminuted Tibial Eminence Anterior Cruciate Ligament Avulsion Fractures: Failure of Arthroscopic Treatment. Arthroscopy 9(4):446–450, 1993.
39. Bergsma, E.J., Rozema, F.R., Bos, R.R., and de Bruijn, W.C.: Foreign Body Reactions to Resorbable Poly(L-lactide) Bone Plates and Screws Used for the Fixation of Unstable Zygomatic Fractures. J. Oral Maxillofac, Surg. 51(6):666–670, 1993.
40. Bioscience, The Treatment of Selected Indications With Totally Absorbable Osteosynthesis Implants. Tampere, Finland, Bioscience Limited, 1992.
41. Biyani, A., Mathur, N.C., and Sharma, J.C.: Percutaneous

Tension Band Wiring for Minimally Displaced Fractures of the Patella. Int. Orthop. 14(3):281–283, 1990.

42. Blatter, G., and Janssen, M.: Treatment of Subtrochanteric Fractures of the Femur: Reduction on the Traction Table and Fixation With Dynamic Condylar Screw. Arch. Orthop. Trauma Surg. 113(3):138–141, 1994.
43. Blatter, G., and Weber, B.G.: Wave Plate Osteosynthesis as a Salvage Procedure. Acta. Chir. Orthop. Traumatol. Cech. 60(5):273–277, 1993.
44. Bo, O.: New Tibial Interlocking Nail System. J. Orthop. Trauma 1(3):257–259, 1987.

44a. Bolander, M.E.: Regulation of Fracture Repair and Synthesis of Matrix Molecules. *In* Brighton, C.T., Friedlander, G., and Love, J.M. (eds): Bone Formation and Repair, pp. 186–187. Rosemont, American Academy of Orthopaedic Surgeons, 1994.

45. Bonar, S.K., and Marsh, J.L.: Unilateral External Fixation for Severe Pilon Fractures. Foot Ankle 14(2):57–64, 1993.
46. Born, C.T., DeLong W. Jr., Shaikh, K.A., Moskwa, C.A., and Schwab, C.W.: Early use of the Brooker-Wills Interlocking Intramedullary Nail (BWIIN) for Femoral Shaft Fractures in Acute Trauma Patients. J. Trauma 28(11):1515–1522, 1988.
47. Bos, R.R., Rozema, F.R., Boering, G., Nijenhuis, A.J. Pennings, A.J., and Verwey, A.B.: Bio-absorbable Plates and Screws for Internal Fixation of Mandibular Fractures. A Study in Six Dogs. Int. J. Oral Maxillofac. Surg. 18(6):365–369, 1989.
48. Bose, W.J., Corces, A., and Anderson, L.D.: A Preliminary Experience With the Russell-Taylor Reconstruction Nail for Complex Femoral Fractures. J. Trauma 32(1):71–76, 1992.
49. Bostman, O., Kiviluoto, O., and Nirhamo, J.: Comminuted Displaced Fractures of the Patella. Injury 13(3):196–202, 1981.
50. Bostman, O., Kiviluoto, O., Santavirta, S., Nirhamo, J., and Wilppula, E.: Fractures of the Patella Treated by Operation. Arch. Orthop. Trauma Surg. 102(2):78–81, 1983.
51. Bostman, O., Makela, E.A., Sodergard, J., Hirvensalo, E., Tormala, P., and Rokkanen, P.: Absorbable Polyglycolide Pins in Internal Fixation of Fractures in Children. J. Pediatr. Orthop. 13(2):242–245, 1993.
52. Bostman, O., Vainionpaa, S., Hirvensalo, E., Makela, A., Vihtonen, K., Tormala, P., and Rokkanen, P.: Biodegradable Internal Fixation for Malleolar Fractures. A Prospective Randomised Trial. J. Bone Joint Surg. 69B(4):615–619, 1987.
53. Bostman, O.M.: Absorbable Implants for the Fixation of Fractures. J. Bone Joint Surg. 73A(1):148–53, 1991.
54. Bostman, O.M.: Osteolytic Changes Accompanying Degradation of Absorbable Fracture Fixation Implants. J. Bone Joint Surg. 73B(4):679–682, 1991.
55. Bostman, O.M.: Distal Tibiofibular Synostosis After Malleolar Fractures Treated Using Absorbable Implants. Foot Ankle 14(1):38–43, 1993.
56. Bouma, W.H., and Cech, M.: The Surgical Treatment of Pathologic and Impending Pathologic Fractures of the Long Bones. J. Trauma 20(12):1043–1045, 1980.
57. Brooker, A.F., Jr.: Brooker-Wills Nailing of Femoral Shaft Fractures. Technique Orthop. 3:41–46, 1988.
58. Brooks, D.B.; Burstein, A.H.; and Frankel, V.H.: Biomechanics of Torsional Fractures: Stress Concentration Effect of a Drill Hole. J. Bone Joint Surg. 52A:507–514, 1970.
59. Broos, P., Reynders, P., van den Bogert, W., and Vanderschot, P.: Surgical Treatment of Metastatic Fracture of the Femur Improvement of Quality of Life. Acta. Orthop. Belg. 1:52–56, 1983.
60. Brown, C. Jr., Hecker, A.T., Hipp, J.A., Myers, E.R., and Hayes, W.C.: The Biomechanics of Interference Screw Fixation of Patellar Tendon Anterior Cruciate Ligament Grafts. Am. J. Sports Med. 21(6):880–886, 1993.
61. Brown, J., and Barnard, D.: The Trans-nasal Kirschner Wire as a Method of Fixation of the Unstable Fracture of the Zygomatic Complex. Br. J. Oral Surg. 21(3):208–213, 1983.
62. Brown, J.N.: An Audit of Prophylactic Antibiotic Prescribing Patterns in Orthopaedic Practice. J. R. Coll. Surg. Edinb. 39(1):55–59, 1994.
63. Brown, R.F.: Compound Fractures of the Tibia—The Soft Tissue Defect. Proc. R. Soc. Med. 65:625–626, 1972
64. Brown, S.A., and Mayor, M.B.: The Biocompatibility of Materials for Internal Fixation of Fractures. J. Biomed. Mater. Res. 12:67–82, 1978.
65. Browner, B.: Pitfalls, Errors, and Complications in the Use of Locking Kuntscher Nails. Clin. Orthop. 212:192–208, 1986.
66. Browner, B.D.; Burgess, A.R.; Robertson, R.J., Baugher, W.H., Freedman, M.T., and Edwards, C.C.: Immediate Closed Antegrade Ender Nailing of Femoral Fractures in Polytrauma Patients. J. Trauma 24:921–927, 1984.
67. Brumback, R.J., Bosse, M.J., Poka, A., and Burgess, A.R.: Intramedullary Stabilization of Humeral Shaft Fractures in Patients With Multiple Trauma. J. Bone Joint Surg. 68A(7):960–970, 1986.
69. Brumback, R.J., Reilly, J.P., Poka, A., Lakatos, R.P., Bathon, G.H., and Burgess, A.R.: Intramedullary Nailing of Femoral Shaft Fractures: Part I. Decision-making Errors With Interlocking Fixation. J. Bone Joint Surg. 70A:1441–1452, 1988.
70. Brumback, R.J., Uwagie-Ero, S., Lakatos, R.P., Poka, A., Bathon, G.H., and Burgess, A.R.: Intramedullary Nailing of Femoral Shaft Fractures: Part II. Fracture-Healing With Static Interlocking Fixation. J. Bone Joint Surg. 70A:1453–1462, 1988.
71. Brunner, C.F., and Weber, B.G.: Special Techniques in Internal Fixation. Berlin: Springer-Verlag. 1982.
72. Bucholz, R.W.: personal communication, 1994.
73. Bucholz, R.W., Henry, S., and Henley, M.B.: Fixation With Bioabsorbable Screws for the Treatment of Fractures of the Ankle. J. Bone Joint Surg. 76A(3):319–324, 1994.
74. Bucholz, R.W., Ross, S.E., and Lawrence, K.L.: Fatigue Fracture of the Interlocking Nail in the Treatment of Fractures of the Distal Part of the Femoral Shaft. J. Bone Joint Surg. 69A:1391–1399, 1987.
75. Buhler, J.: Percutaneous Cerclage of Tibial Fractures. Clin. Orthop. 105(0):276–282, 1974.
76. Burgos-Flores, J., Gonzalez-Herranz, P., Lopez-Mondejar, J.A., Ocete-Guzman, J.G., and AmayaAlarcon, S.: Fractures of the Proximal Humeral Epiphysis. Int. Orthop. 17(1):16–19, 1993.
77. Burstein, A., Currey, J., Frankel, V.H., Heiple, K.G., Lunseth, P., and Vessely, J.C.: Bone Strength: The Effect of Screw Holes. J. Bone Joint Surg. 54A: 1143–56, 1972.
78. Burvant, J.G., Thomas, K.A., Alexander, R., and Harris, M.B.: Evaluation of Methods of Internal Fixation of Transverse Patella Fractures: A Biomechanical Study. J. Orthop. Trauma 8(2):147–153, 1994.
79. Bylander, B., Hagglund, G., and Selvik, G.: Dynamics of Growth Retardation After Epiphysiodesis: A Roentgen Stereophotogrammetric Analysis. Orthopedics 16(6):710–712, 1993.
80. Bynum, D. Jr., Ray, D.R., Boyd, C.L., and Ledbetter, W.B.: Capacity of Installed Commercial Bone Fixation Plates. Am. J. Vet. Res. 32:783–791, 1971.
81. Bynum, D. Jr., Allen, G.F., Ray, D.R., and Ledbetter, W.G.: In vitro Performance of Installed Internal Fixation Plates in Compression. J. Biomed. Mater. Res. 5(4):389–405, 1971.
82. Carpenter, J., Fish, D., Huston, L., and Goldstein, S.: Pull-out Strength of Five Suture Anchors. Arthroscopy 9(1):109–113, 1993.
83. Casteleyn, P.P., Handelberg, F., and Haentjens, P.: Biodegradable Rods versus Kirschner Wire Fixation of Wrist Fractures. A Randomised Trial. J. Bone Joint Surg. 74B(6):858–861, 1992.
84. Cedell, C.A., and Wiberg, G.: Treatment of Eversion-Supination Fractures of the Ankle (2nd Degree). Acta. Chir. Scand. 124:41–44, 1962.
85. Cedell, C.A.: Supination-Outward Rotation Injuries of the Ankle. Acta. Orthop. Scand. (Suppl) 110:3, 1967.
86. Champetier, J., Brabant, A., Charignon, G., Durand, A., Letoublon, C., and Mignot, P.: [Treatment of Fractures of the

Humerus by Intramedullary Fixation]. J. Chir. 109(1):75–82, 1975.

87. Chandler, H., Clark, J., Murphy, S., McCarthy, J., Penenberg, B., Danylchuk, K., and Roehr, B.: Reconstruction of Major Segmental Loss of the Proximal Femur in Revision Total Hip Arthroplasty. Clin. Orthop. 298:67–74, 1994.

87a. Charnley, J.: The Closed Treatment of Common Fractures, 3 ed. Edinburg: E&S Livingston, 1968.

88. Cheng, S.L., Smith, T.J., and Davey, J.R.: A Comparison of the Strength and Stability of Six Techniques of Cerclage Wire Fixation for Fractures. J. Orthop. Trauma 7(3):221–225, 1993.

89. Chin, H.C., Frassica, F.J., Hein, T.J., Shives, T.C., Pritchard, D.J., Sim, F.H., and Chao, E.Y.: Metastatic Diaphyseal Fractures of the Shaft of the Humerus. The Structural Strength Evaluation of a New Method of Treatment With a Segmental Defect Prosthesis. Clin. Orthop. 248:231–239, 1989.

90. Chiroff, R.T.: A New Technique for the Treatment of Comminuted, Transverse Fractures of the Patella. Surg. Gynecol. Obstet. 145(6):909–912, 1977.

91. Clawson, D.K., Smith, R.F., and Hansen, S.T.: Closed Intramedullary Nailing of the Femur. J. Bone Joint Surg. 53A:681–692, 1971.

92. Cohn, B.T., and Bilfield, L.: Fatigue Fracture of a Tibial Interlocking Nail. Orthopedics 9(9):1355–1358, 1986.

93. Cole, J.D., and Bolhofner, B.R.: Acetabular Fracture Fixation via a Modified Stoppa Lmited Intrapelvic Approach. Description of Operative Technique and Preliminary Treatment Results. Clin. Orthop. 305:112–123, 1994.

94. Coleman, N.P., and Warren, P.J.: Tension-band Fixation of Olecranon Fractures. A Cadaver Study of Elbow Extension. Acta. Orthop. Scand. 62(1):58–59, 1991.

95. Colyer, R.A.: Surgical Stabilization of Pathological Neoplastic Fractures. Curr. Probl. Cancer, 10(3):117–68, 1986.

96. Contzen, H.: [Development of Intramedullary Nailing and the Interlocking Nail]. Aktuelle Traumatol. 17(6):250–252, 1987.

97. Cooney, W.P., and Berger, R.A.: Treatment of Complex Fractures of the Distal Radius. Combined use of Internal and External Fixation and Arthroscopic Reduction. Hand Clin. 9(4):603–612, 1993.

98. Cooper, W.E., Galorenzo, R., and Mattingly, E.H.: Delayed Open Reduction of Lisfranc's Joint Dislocation. J. Foot Surg. 22(1):45–49, 1983.

99. Cornell, C.N., Levine, D., and Pagnani, M.J.: Internal Fixation of Proximal Humerus Fractures Using the Screw-tension Band Technique. J. Orthop. Trauma 8(1):23–27, 1994.

100. Costa, P., Giancecchi, F., Tartaglia, I., and Fontanesi, G.: Immediate Multiple Osteosynthesis in Polytrauma. Ital. J. Orthop. Traumatol. 17(2):187–198, 1991.

101. Coutts, R.D., Akeson, W.H., Woo, S.L.-Y., Matthews, J.V., Gonsalves, M., and Amiel, D.: Comparison of Stainless Steel and Composite Plates in the Healing of Diaphyseal Osteotomies of the Dog Radius. Orthop. Clin. North Am. 7:223–229, 1976.

102. Coventry, M.B.: Stepped Staple for Upper Tibial Osteotomy. J. Bone Joint Surg. 51A(5):1011, 1969.

103. Dai, K.R., Hou, X.K., Sun, Y.H., Tang, R.G., Qiu, S.J., and Ni, C.: Treatment of Intra-articular Fractures With Shape Memory Compression Staples. Injury 24(10):651–655, 1993.

104. Dalton, J.E., Salkeld, S.L., Satterwhite, Y.E., and Cook, S.D.: A Biomechanical Comparison of Intramedullary Nailing Systems for the Humerus. J. Orthop. Trauma 7(4):367–74, 1993.

105. Damron, T.A., and Engber, W.E.: Surgical Treatment of Mallet Finger Fractures by Tension Band Technique. Clin. Orthop. 300:133–140, 1994.

106. Damron, T.A., Engber, W.D., Lange, R.H., McCabe, R., Damron, L.A., Ulm, M., and Vanderby, R.: Biomechanical Analysis of Mallet Finger Fracture Fixation Techniques. J. Hand Surg. 18A(4):600–607, 1993.

107. Danckwardt, L.G., Lorenzi, G.L., and Olerud, S.: Intramedullary Nailing After Reaming. An Investigation on the Healing Process in Osteotomized Rabbit Tibias. Acta. Orthop. Scand. Suppl. 134(Suppl):1, 1970.

108. Danckwardt-Lilliestrom, G.: Reaming of the Medullary Cavity and Its Effect on Diaphyseal Bone. Acta. Orthop. Scand. Suppl. 128:1–153, 1969.

109. Danckwardt-Lilliestrom, G., Lorenzi, L., and Olerud, S.: Intracortical Circulation After Intramedullary Reaming With Reduction of Pressure in the Medullary Cavity: A Microangiograhic Study on the Rabbit Tibia. J. Bone Joint Surg. 52A:1390–1394, 1970.

110. Darder, A., Darder A. Jr., Sanchis, V., Gastaldi, E., and Gomar, F.: Four-part Displaced Proximal Humeral Fractures: Operative Treatment Using Kirschner Wires and a Tension Band. J. Orthop. Trauma 7(6):497–505, 1993.

111. Davis, A.D., Meyer, R.D., Miller, M.E., and Killian, J.T., Closed Zickel Nailing. Clin. Orthop. 201:138–146, 1985.

112. De Campos, J., Vangsness C. Jr., Merritt, P.O., and Sher, J.: Ipsilateral Knee Injury With Femoral Fracture. Examination Under Anesthesia and Arthroscopic Evaluation. Clin. Orthop. 300:178–182, 1994.

113. de Chauliac, G.: On Wounds and Fractures, p. 154. Chicago, W.A. Brennan, 1923.

114. Deliyannis, S.N.: Comminuted Fractures of the Olecranon Treated by the Weber-Vasey Technique. Injury 5(1):19–24, 1973.

115. Desault, P.J.: A Treatise on Fractures, Luxations and Other Affection of the Bones, P 415. Philadelphia, Fry & Kammerer, 1805.

116. Devas, M.: Geriatric Orthopaedics. New York, Academic Press, 1977.

117. Di Fiore, M., Giacomello, A., Vigano, E., and Zanoni, A. Jr.: The Gamma Nail and the Compression-Sliding Plate in the Treatment of Pertrochanteric Fractures: Anesthesiologic Aspects. Chir. Organi Mov. 78(1):59–62, 1993.

118. Dichristina, D.G., Riemer, B.L., Butterfield, S.L., Burke, C.J., Herron, M.K., and Phillips, D.J.: Femur Fractures With Femoral or Popliteal Artery Injuries in Blunt Trauma. J. Orthop. Trauma 8(6):494–503, 1994.

119. DiGiovanni, J.E., and Martin, R.A.: Pins, Wires, and Staples in Foot Surgery. Clin. Podiatr. 1(1):211–223, 1984.

120. Dijkema, A.R., van der Elst, M., Breederveld, R.S., Verspui, G., Patka, P., and Haarman, H.J.: Surgical Treatment of Fracture-Dislocations of the Ankle Joint With Biodegradable Implants: A Prospective Randomized Study. J. Trauma 34(1):82–84, 1993.

121. Disegi, J.A., Cesarone, D.M., (eds.): Metallurgical Properties of Unalloyed Titanium Limited Contact Dynamic Compression Plates. *In*: Harvey G. Jr., J.P.; Gaines, R.F. (ed.): Clinical and Laboratory Performance of Bone Plates. Philadelphia, American Society for Testing and Materials, 1994:34–41.

122. Donecker, J.M., Bramlage, L.R., and Gabel, A.A.: Retrospective Analysis of 29 Fractures of the Olecranon Process of the Equine Ulna. J. Am. Vet. Med. Assoc. 185(2):183–189, 1984.

123. Dugas, R., and D'Ambrosia, R.: The Grosse-Kempf Interlocking Nail: Technique of Femoral and Tibial Fractures. Orthopaedics 8:1363–1370, 1985.

124. Eberle, C., Keller, H., Guyer, P., and Metzger, U.: [Stable Interlocking Intramedullary Nailing of Humeral Fractures With the Seidel Nail]. Helv. Chir. Acta. 59(4):673–677 1993.

125. Eckerwall, G., and Persson, B.M.: Fracture of the Lateral Malleolus. Comparison of 2 Fixation Methods in Cadavers. Acta. Orthop. Scand. 64(5):595–597, 1993.

126. Eggers, G.: The Contact Splint. Rep. Biol. Med. 4:42, 1946.

127. Eggers, G.W.N.: Internal Contact Splint. J. Bone Joint Surg. 30A:40–52, 1948.

128. Ekeland, A., Thoresen, B.O., Alho, A., Stromsoe, K., Folleras, G., and Haukebo, A.: Interlocking Intramedullary Nailing in the Treatment of Tibial Fractures: A Report of 45 cases. Clin. Orthop. 231:205–215, 1988.

129. Emerson, R. Jr., Malinin, T.I., Cuellar, A.D., Head, W.C., and Peters, P.C.: Cortical Strut Allografts in the Reconstruction of the Femur in Revision Total Hip Arthroplasty. A Basic Science and Clinical Study. Clin. Orthop. 285:35–44, 1992.

130. Epps, C.H. Jr., and Adams, J.P.: Wound Management in Open Fractures. Am. Surg. 27:766–769, 1961.
131. Erickson, J.M., Anderson, J.T., Thompson, R. Jr., and Chao, E.Y.: Pathologic Fractures of Femoral Shaft: Study of Internal Fixation Techniques Incorporating Methylmethacrylate. Surg. Forum 27(62):514–516, 1976.
132. Eskola, A., Vainionpaa, S., Korkala, S., Santavirta, S., Gronblad, M., and Rokkanen, P.: Four-year Outcome of Operative Treatment of Acute Acromioclavicular Dislocation. J. Orthop. Trauma 5(1):9–13, 1991.
133. Evans, P.E.: Cerclage Fixation of a Fractured Humerus in 1775. Fact or Fiction? Clin. Orthop. 174:138–142, 1983.
134. Fan, G.F., Wu, C.C., and Shin, C.H.: Olecranon Fractures Treated With Tension Band Wiring Techniques—Comparisons Among Three Different Configurations. Chang Keng I Hsueh 16(4):231–238, 1993.
135. Felli, L., and Fioravanti, P.: Reconstruction of the Anterior Cruciate Ligament With Free Grafting of the Patellar Tendon: Surgical Technique. Chir. Organi Mov. 76(4):365–367, 1991.
136. Fernandez, D.L., and Koella, C.: Combined Percutaneous and Minimal Internal Fixation for Displaced Articular Fractures of the Calcaneus. Clin. Orthop. 290:108–116, 1993.
137. Fidler, M.W.: Posterior Instrumentation of the Spine. An Experimental Comparison of Various Possible Techniques. Spine 11(4):367–372, 1986.
138. Figgie, M.P., Goldberg, V.M., Figgie, H, 3rd, and Sobel, M.: The Results of Treatment of Supracondylar Fracture Above Total Knee Arthroplasty. J. Arthroplasty 5(3):267–276, 1990.
139. Firoozbakhsh, K.K., Moneim, M.S., and DeCoster, T.A.: Pull-out Strength of Power- and Hand-driven Staples in Synthetic Bone: Effect of Design Parameters. J. Orthop. Trauma 6(1):43–49, 1992.
140. Firoozbakhsh, K.K., Moneim, M.S., Howey, T., Castaneda, E., and Pirela-Cruz, M.A.: Comparative fatigue strengths and stabilities of maetacarpal internal fixation techniques. J. Hand Surg. [Am] 18(6):1059–1068, 1993.
141. Fishmann, A.J.; Greeno, R.A.; Brooks, L.R.; and Matta, J.M.: Prevention of Deep Vein Thrombosis and Pulmonary Embolism in Acetabular and Pelvic Fracture Surgery. Clin. Orthop., 305:133–137, 1994.
142. Fitzgerald, B.E., and Zallen, R.D.: Use of Kirschner Wires for Securing Acrylic Splints to the Maxilla. J. Oral Surg., 34B(6):557–558, 1976.
143. Fitzgerald, J.A., and Southgate, G.W.: Cerclage Wiring in the Management of Comminuted Fractures of the Femoral Shaft. Injury, 18(2):111–116, 1987.
144. Flemming, J.E., and Beals, R.K.: Pathologic Fracture of the Humerus. Clin. Orthop., 203:258–260, 1986.
145. Fogarty, A.B., and Yeates, H.A.: Intramedullary Locking Femoral Nails. Experience with the AO Nail. Ulster Med. J., 60(2):129–136, 1991.
146. Fogelberg, E.V., Zetzmann, E.K., and Stinchfield, F.E.: Prophylactic Penicillin in Orthopaedic Surgery. J. Bone Joint Surg., 52A:95–98, 1970.
147. Fontanesi, G.; Costa, P.; Giancecchi, F.; and Tartaglia, I.: Intertrochanteric Valgus Osteotomy and Sliding Compression Hip Screw in Fractures of the Femoral Neck. Ital. J. Orthop. Traumatol., 17(3):293–304, 1991.
148. Foster, R.J.; Dixon, G., Jr.; Bach, A.W.; Appleyard, R.W.; and Green, T.M.: Internal Fixation of Fractures and Non-Unions of the Humeral Shaft. Indications and Results in a Multi-Center Study. J. Bone Joint Surg., 67A(6):857–864, 1985.
149. Fowble, C.D.; Zimmer, J.W.; and Schepsis, A.A.: The Role of Arthroscopy in the Assessment and Treatment of Tibial Plateau Fractures. Arthroscopy, 9(5):584–590, 1993.
150. France, M.P.: Tips of the Trade #13. Tension Band Wiring of Olecranon Fractures. Orthop. Rev., 18(6):713–715, 1989.
151. Frankel, V.H., and Burstein, A.H.: Orthopaedic Biomechanics. Philadelphia, Lea & Febiger, 1970.
152. Franklin, J.L.; Winquist, R.A.; Benirschke, S.K.; and Hansen, S.R., Jr.: Broken Intramedullary Nails. J. Bone Joint Surg., 70A:1463–1471, 1988.
153. Freeland, A.E.; Zardiackas, L.D.; Terral, G.T.; and Blickentaff, K.R.: Mechanical Properties of 3M Staples in Bone Block Models. Orthopedics, 15(6):727–731, 1992.
154. Freidline, C.W.; Gongloff, R.K.; and Porter, C., Jr.: Use of Friction Grip Contrangle for Placement of Kirschner Wire. J. Oral Surg., 39(10):785, 1981.
155. Friden, T.L.; Ryd, L.; and Lindstrand, A.: Laxity and Graft Fixation After Reconstruction of the Anterior Cruciate Ligament. A Roentgen Stereophotogrammetric Analysis of 11 Patients. Acta. Orthop. Scand., 63(1):80–84, 1992.
156. Friden, T., and Rydholm, U.: Severe Aseptic Synovitis of the Knee After Biodegradable Internal Fixation. A Case Report. Acta. Orthop. Scand., 63(1):94–97, 1992.
157. Fried, A.: Fusion of the Knee Joint with Internal Fixation by Staples. A Preliminary Report. Acta. Orthop. Scand., 41(4): 488–494, 1970.
158. Friedl, W.: Relevance of Osteotomy and Implant Characteristics in Inter- and Subtrochanteric Osteotomies. Experimental Examination Under Alternating and Static Load After Stabilisation With Different Devices Including Gamma Nail Osteosynthesis. Arch. Orthop. Trauma Surg., 113(1):5–11, 1993.
159. Frokjaer, J., and Moller, B.N.: Biodegradable Fixation of Ankle Fractures. Complications in a Prospective Study of 25 Cases. Acta. Orthop. Scand., 63(4):434–436, 1992.
160. Furrer, M.; Honegger, C.; Barandun, J.; Bereiter, H.; Leutenegger, A.; and Ruedi, T.: Interlocking Intramedullary Nailing of the Femur: Is the Advantage of Early Mobilization Gained by Risking a Malposition? Helv. Chir. Acta., 57(5):825–828, 1991.
161. Fuster, S.; Palliso, F.; Combalia, A.; Sanjuan, A.; and Garcia, S.: Intrathoracic Migration of a Kirschner Wire. Injury, 21(2):124–126, 1990.
162. Gaines, R., Jr.; Carson, W.L.; Satterlee, C.C.; and Groh, G.I.: Experimental Evaluation of Seven Different Spinal Fracture Internal Fixation Devices Using Nonfailure Stability Testing. The Load-Sharing and Unstable-Mechanism Concepts. Spine, 16(8):902–909, 1991.
163. Ganz, R.; and van Werken, C.: New Concepts of Plate Osteosynthesis. In AO/ASIF Alumni Symposium. Davos, Switzerland, 1993.
164. Georgiadis, G.M.: Combined Anterior and Posterior Approaches for Complex Tibial Plateau Fractures. J. Bone Joint Surg. 76B(2):285–289, 1994.
165. Ger, R.: The Management of Pretibial Skin Loss. Surgery, 63:757–763, 1968.
166. Ger, R.: The Management of Open Fractures of the Tibia With Skin Loss. J. Trauma, 10:112–121, 1970.
167. Gerber, C.; Mast, J.W.; and Ganz, R.: Biological Internal Fixation of Fractures [published erratum appears in Arch. Orthop. Trauma Surg. 110(4):226, 1991]. Arch. Orthop. Trauma Surg., 109(6):295–303, 1991.
168. Gerber, C.; Strehle, J.; and Ganz, R.: The Treatment of Fractures of the Femoral Neck. Clin. Orthop., 292:77–86, 1993.
169. Gertel, T.H.; Lew, W.D.; Lewis, J.L.; Stewart, N.J.; and Hunter, R.E.: Effect of Anterior Cruciate Ligament Graft Tensioning Direction, Magnitude, and Flexion Angle on Knee Biomechanics. Am. J. Sports Med., 21(4):572–581, 1993.
170. Giannini, S.; Maffei, G.; Girolami, M; and Ceccarelli, F.: The Treatment of Supracondylar Fractures of the Humerus in Children by Closed Reduction and Fixation With Percutaneous Kirschner Wires. Ital. J. Orthop. Traumatol., 9(2):181–188, 1993.
171. Gibbons, C.L.; Woods, D.A.; Pailthorpe, C.; Carr, A.J.; and Worlock, P.: The Management of Isolated Distal Radius Fractures in Children. J. Pediatr. Orthop., 14(2):207–210, 1994.
172. Gingrass, R.P., Close, A.S., and Ellison, E.H.: The Effect of Various Topical and Parenteral Agents on the Prevention of Infection in Experimental Contaminated Wounds. J. Trauma, 4:763–783, 1964.
173. Gjerloff, C., and Sojbjerg, J.O.: Percutaneous Pinning of Supracondylar Fractures of the Humerus. Acta. Orthop. Scand., 49(6):597–599, 1978.
174. Good, L., and Gillquist, J.: The Value of Intraoperative Isometry Measurements in Anterior Cruciate Ligament Reconstruc-

tion: An In Vivo Correlation Between Substitute Tension and Length Change. Arthroscopy, 9(5):525–532, 1993.

175. Goodman, S.B.; Davidson, J.A.; Locke, L.; Novotny, S.; Jones, H.; and Csongradi, J.J.: A Biomechanical Study of Two Methods of Internal Fixation of Unstable Fractures of the Femoral Neck. A Preliminary Study. J. Orthop. Trauma, 6(1):66–72, 1992.
176. Goodson, W.H.: Traumatic Injury. *In* Cohen, R.F., and Linblad, W.J. (eds.): Wound Healing Biochemical and Clinical Aspects, pp. 316–325. Philadelphia, W.B. Saunders, 1992.
177. Goossens, M., and De Stoop, N.: Lisfranc's Fracture-Dislocations: Etiology, Radiology, and Results of Treatment. A Review of 20 Cases. Clin. Orthop., 176:154–162, 1983.
178. Grana, W.A.; Egle, D.M.; Mahnken, R.; and Goodhart, C.W.: An Analysis of Autograft Fixation After Anterior Cruciate Ligament Reconstruction in a Rabbit Model. Am. J. Sports Med., 22(3):344–51, 1994.
179. Grimberg, B.; Soudry, M.; Chezar, J.; Alkalay, I.; and Daniel, M.: The Use of the Hansen-Street Intramedullary Nail in Midshaft Fractures of the Femur. Bull. Hosp. Jt. Dis., 53(1):45–50, 1993.
180. Gristina, A.G.; Adair, D.M.; and Spurr, C.L.: Intraosseous Metastatic Breast Cancer Treatment With Internal Fixation and Study of Survival. Ann. Surg., 197(2):128–134, 1983.
181. Gropper, P.T., and Bowen, V.: Cerclage Wiring of Metacarpal Fractures. Clin. Orthop., 188:203–207, 1984.
182. Gross, A.E.; Allan, D.G.; Lavoie, G.J.; and Oakeshott, R.D.: Revision Arthroplasty of the Proximal Femur Using Allograft Bone. Orthop. Clin. North Am., 24(4):705–715, 1993.
183. Gross, A.E.; Lavoie, M.V.; McDermott, P.; and Marks, P.: The Use of Allograft Bone in Revision of Total Hip Arthroplasty. Clin. Orthop., 197:115–122, 1985.
184. Gross, A.E.; McDermott, A.G.; Lavoie, M.V.; Marks, P.; and Brooks, P.J.: The Use of Allograft Bone in Revision Hip Arthroplasty. Hip, 47–58, 1987.
185. Gross, S.D.: A Manual of Military Surgery. The American Civil War Series, vol. 1. San Francisco, Norman, 1988.
186. Grundnes, O.; Utvag, E.; and Reikeras, O.: Effects of Graded Reaming on Fracture Healing. Acta. Orthop. Scand., 65(1)32–36, 1994.
187. Guadagni, J.R.; Drummond, D.S.: Strength of Surgical Wire Fixation. Clin. Orthop., 209:176–181, 1984.
188. Guanche, C.A. and Markman, A.W.: Arthroscopic Management of Tibial Plateau Fractures. Arthroscopy, 9(4):467–71, 1993.
189. Gustafsson, A.: Operative Adaptation With Cerclage in Traumatic Rupture of the Symphysis. Acta. Orthop. Scand., 41(4):446–53, 1970.
190. Gustilo, R.: The Fracture Classification Manual, 1st ed., p. 175. St. Louis, Mosby-Year Book, 1991.
191. Gustilo, R.B.; Simpson, L.; Nixon, R.; Ruiz, A.; and Indeck, W.: Analysis of 511 Open Fractures. Clin. Orthop., 66:148–154, 1969.
192. Gyrtrup, H.J., and Fosse, L.: The Use of Kirschner Wires in Diaphyseal Fractures of the Forearm. Acta. Orthop. Belg., 55(1):86–87, 1989.
193. Haajanen, J., and Karaharju, E.: Fractures of the Patella. One Hundred Consecutive Cases. Ann. Chir. Gynaecol., 70(1):32–35, 1981.
194. Habermann, E.T., and Lopez, R.A.: Metastatic Disease of Bone and Treatment of Pathological Fractures. Orthop. Clin. North Am., 20(3):469–486, 1989.
195. Habermann, E.T., Sachs, R.; Stern, R.E.; Hirsh, D.M.; and Anderson, W., Jr.: The Pathology and Treatment of Metastatic Disease of the Femur. Clin. Orthop., 169:70–82, 1982.
196. Habernek, H.: Percutaneous Cerclage Wiring and Interlocking Nailing for Treatment of Torsional Fractures of the Tibia. Clin. Orthop., 267:164–168, 1991.
197. Habernek, H.; Weinstabl, R.; Fialka, C.; and Schmid, L.: Unstable Distal Radius Fractures Treated by Modified Kirschner Wire Pinning: Anatomic Considerations, Technique, and Results. J. Trauma, 36(1):83–88, 1994.
198. Haentjens, P.; Casteleyn, P.P.; and Opdecam, P.: Evaluation of Impending Fractures and Indications for Prophylactic Fixation of Metastases in Long Bones. Review of the Literature. Acta. Orthop. Belg., 1:6–11, 1993.
199. Hajek, P.D.; Bicknell, H., Jr.; Bronson, W.E.; Albright, J.A.; and Saha, S.: The Use of One Compared With Two Distal Screws in the Treatment of Femoral Shaft Fractures With Interlocking Intramedullary Nailing. A Clinical and Biomechanical Analysis. J. Bone Joint Surg. Am., 75(4):519–525, 1993.
200. Hak, D.J., and Johnson, E.E.: The Use of the Unreamed Nail in Tibial Fractures With Concomitant Preoperative or Intraoperative Elevated Compartment Pressure or Compartment Syndrome. J. Orthop. Trauma, 8(3):203–211, 1994.
201. Halbrecht, J., and Levy, I.M.: Fluoroscopic Assist in Anterior Cruciate Ligament Reconstruction. Arthroscopy, 9(5): 533–53, 1993.
202. Hall, R.F., and Pankovich, A.M.: Ender Nailing of Acute Fracture of the Humerus. J. Bone Joint Surg., 69A:558–567, 1987.
203. Hanks, G.A., Foster, W.C., and Cardea, J.A.: Treatment of Femoral Shaft Fractures With the Brooker-Wills Interlocking Intramedullary Nail. Clin. Orthop., 226:206–218, 1988.
204. Hardman, P.D.; Robb, J.E.; Kerr, G.R.; Rodger, A.; and MacFarlane, A.: The Value of Internal Fixation and Radiotherapy in the Management of Upper and Lower Limb Bone Metastases. Clin. Oncol., 4(4):244–248, 1992.
205. Harrington, K.D.: The Use of Methylmethacrylate as an Adjunct in the Internal Fixation of Unstable Comminuted Intertrochanteric Fractures of Osteoporotic Patients. J. Bone Joint Surg., 57-A(6):744–750, 1975.
206. Harrington, K.D.: Impending Pathologic Fractures From Metastatic Malignancy: Evaluation and Management. Instr. Course Lect., 35:357–381, 1986.
207. Hart, M.B.; Wu, J.-J.; Chao, E.Y.S.; Kelly, P.J.: External Skeletal Fixation of Canine Tibial Osteotomies. Compression Compared With no Compression. J. Bone Joint Surg., 67A(4):598–605, 1985.
208. Hawkins, R.J., and Kiefer, G.N.: Internal Fixation Techniques for Proximal Humeral Fractures. Clin. Orthop., 223:77–85, 1987.
209. Hayes, W.C., and Perren, S.M.: Plate-Bone Friction in the Compression Fixation of Fractures. Clin. Orthop., 89:236–240, 1972.
210. Head, W.C.; Berklacich, F.M.; Malinin, T.I.; and Emerson, R., Jr.: Proximal Femoral Allografts in Revision Total Hip Arthroplasty. Clin. Orthop., 225:22–36, 1987.
211. Head, W.C.; Malinin, T.I.; and Berklacich, F.: Freeze-Dried Proximal Femur Allografts in Revision Total Hip Arthroplasty. A Preliminary Report. Clin. Orthop., 215:109–121, 1987.
212. Head, W.C.; Wagner, R.A.; Emerson, R., Jr.; and Malinin, T.I.: Revision Total Hip Arthroplasty in the Deficient Femur With a Proximal Load-Bearing Prosthesis. Clin. Orthop., 298:119–126, 1994.
213. Hearn, T.C.; Schatzker, J.; and Wolfson, N.: Extraction Strength of Cannulated Cancellous Bone Screws. J. Ortho. Trauma, 7(2):138–141, 1993.
214. Hegelmaier, C., and von Aprath, B.: Plate Osteosynthesis of the Diaphyseal Humerus Shaft. Indications—Risks—Results. Aktuel Traumatol, 23(1):36–42, 1993.
215. Helfet, D.L.; Howey, T.; Dipasquale, T.; Sanders, R.; Zinar, D.; and Brooker, A.: The Treatment of Open and/or Unstable Tibial Fractures With an Unreamed Double-Locked Tibial Nail. Orthop. Rev., Suppl:9–17, 1994.
216. Helfet, D.L.; Koval, K.; Pappas, J.; Sanders, R.W.; and DiPasquale, T.: Intraarticular Pilon Fracture of the Tibia. Clin. Orthop., 298:221–228, 1994.
217. Helfet, D.L.; and Schmeling, G.J.: Bicondylar Intraarticular Fractures of the Distal Humerus in Adults. Clin. Orthop., 292:26–36, 1993.
218. Helfet, D.L., and Schmeling, G.J.: Management of Complex Acetabular Fractures Through Single Nonextensile Exposures. Clin. Orthop., 305:58–68, 1994.
219. Helm, R.H.; Hornby, R.; and Miller, S.W.: The Complications

of Surgical Treatment of Displaced Fractures of the Olecranon. Injury, 18(1):48–50, 1987.
220. Hempel, D., and Fischer, S.: Intramedullary Nailing, p. 224. Stuttgart, Georg Thieme Verlag, 1982.
221. Henley, M.B.; Meier, M.; and Tencer, A.F.: Influences of Some Design Parameters on the Biomechanics of the Unreamed Tibial Intramedullary Nail. J. Orthop. Trauma, 7(4):311–319, 1993.
222. Henry, S.L.; Werner, J.; and Seligson, D.: Intramedullary Fixation of Subtrochanteric Fractures With the Williams Y-Nail: Report of Three Cases. J. Orthop. Trauma, 2(2):139–45, 1988.
223. Herzwurm, P.J., Walsh, J.; Pettine, K.A.; and Ebert, F.R.: Prophylactic Cerclage: A Method of Preventing Femur Fracture in Uncemented Total Hip Arthroplasty. Orthopedics, 15(2):143–146, 1992.
224. Hessmann, M.; Mattens, M.; and Rumbaut, J.: The Unilateral External Fixator (Monofixator) in Acute Fracture Treatment: Experience in 50 Fractures. Acta. Chir. Belg., 94(4):229–235, 1994.
225. Hey-Groves, E.W.: Methods and Results of Transplantation of Bone in the Repair of Defects Caused by Injury or Disease. Br. J. Surg, 5:185–242, 1918.
226. Hierholzer, G., and Müller, K. (eds): Corrective Osteotomies of the Lower Extremity After Trauma, p.407. Berlin, Springer-Verlag, 1985.
227. Hirvensalo, E.; Bostman, O,; Partio, E.; Tormala, P.; and Rokkanen, P.: Fracture of the Humeral Capitellum Fixed With Absorbable Polyglycolide Pins. 1-year Follow-Up of 8 Adults. Acta. Orthop. Scand., 64(1):85–86, 1993.
228. Hofer, H.P.; Seibert, F.J.; Schweighofer, F.; and Paszicsnyek, T.: The Unreamed Tibial Intramedullary Nail in Treatment of Tibial Fractures—Initial Experiences. Langenbecks Arch. Chir., 379(1):32–37, 1994.
229. Hoffmann, R.; Krettek, C.; Hetkamper, A.; Haas, N.; and Tscherne, H.: Osteosynthesis of Distal Radius Fractures With Biodegradable Fracture Rods. Results of Two Years Follow-Up. Unfallchirurg, 95(2):99–105, 1992.
230. Hofmann, D.: Technical Recommendation for Connecting Osteosynthesis. Unfallchirurgie, 18(5):291–294, 1992.
231. Hogh, J., and Jensen, P.O.: Compression-Arthrodesis of Finger Joints Using Kirschner Wires and Cerclage. Hand, 14(2):149–52, 1982.
232. Holdsworth, B.J., and Mossad, M.M.: Elbow Function Following Tension Band Fixation of Displaced Fractures of the Olecranon. Injury, 16(3):182–187, 1984.
233. Holz, U.: General Principles and Technics of Osteosynthesis in Pathological Fractures. Zentralbl Chir, 115(11):657–664, 1990.
234. Holzach, P., and Matter, P.: Arthroscopically Guided Osteosynthesis of Lateral Tibial Plateau Fractures. Z. Unfallchir. Versicherungsmed, 1:157–164, 1993.
235. Hope, P.G.; Williamson, D.M.; Coates, C.J.; and Cole, W.G.: Biodegradable Pin Fixation of Elbow Fractures in Children. A Randomised Trial. J. Bone Joint Surg., 73B(6):965–968, 1991.
236. Houben, P.F.; Bongers, K.J.; and von de Wildenberg, F.A.: Double Tension Band Osteosynthesis in Supra- and Transcondylar Humeral Fractures. Injury, 25(5):305–309, 1994.
237. Howard, M.W.; Zinar, D.M.; and Stryker, W.S.: The Use of the Lottes Nail in the Treatment of Closed and Open Tibial Shaft Fractures. Clin. Orthop., 279:246–53, 1992.
238. Huckstep, R.L.: The Huckstep Intramedullary Compression Nail. Indications, Technique, and Results. Clin. Orthop., 212:48–61, 1986.
239. Huckstep, R.L.: Stabilization and Prosthetic Replacement in Difficult Fractures and Bone Tumors. Clin. Orthop., 224:12–25, 1987.
240. Huckstep, R.L.: The Huckstep Interlocking Nail for Difficult Humeral, Forearm, and Tibial Fractures and for Arthrodesis. Techniques Orthop., 3:77–87, 1988.
241. Hughes, A.N., and Jordon, B.A.: The Mechanical Properties of Surgical Bone Screws and Some Aspects of Insertion Practice. Injury, 4:25–38, 1972.
242. Hughes, S.P.; Miles, R.S.; Littlejohn, M.; and Brown, E.: Is Antibiotic Prophylaxis Necessary for Internal Fixation of Low-Energy Fractures? Injury, 22(2):111–113, 1991.
243. Hulkko, A.; Orava, S.; and Nikula, P.: Stress Fracture of the Fifth Metatarsal in Athletes. Ann. Chir. Gynaecol., 74(5):233–238, 1985.
244. Hulkko, A.; Orava, S.; and Nikula, P.: Stress Fractures of the Olecranon in Javelin Throwers. Int. J. Sports Med., 7(4):210–213, 1986.
245. Hulstyn, M.; Fadale, P.D.; Abate, J.; and Walsh, W.R.: Biomechanical Evaluation of Interference Screw Fixation in a Bovine Patellar Bone-Tendon-Bone Autograft Complex for Anterior Cruciate Ligament Reconstruction. Arthroscopy, 9(4):417–424, 1993.
246. Hung, L.K.; Chan, K.M.; Chow, Y.N.; and Leung, P.C.: Fractured Patella: Operative Treatment Using the Tension Band Principle. Injury, 16(5):343–347, 1985.
247. Hung, L.K.; Lee, S.Y.; Leung, K.S.; Chan, K.M.; and Nicholl, L.A.: Partial Patellectomy for Patellar Fracture: Tension Band Wiring and Early Mobilization. J. Orthop. Trauma, 7(3):252–260, 1993.
248. Hunt, R.J.; Baxter, G.M.; and Zamos, D.T.: Tension-Band Wiring and Lag Screw Fixation of a Transverse, Comminuted Fracture of a Patella in a Horse. J. Am. Vet. Med. Assoc., 200(6):819–820, 1992.
249. Hunter, S.G.: Deformation of Femoral Intramedullary Nails: A Clinical Study. Clin. Orthop., 171:83–86, 1982.
250. Hyder, N., and Wray, C.C.: Treatment of Pathological Fractures of the Humerus With Ender Nails. J. R. Coll. Surg. Edinb., 38(6):370–372, 1993.
251. Inhofe, P.D.: Biomechanical Considerations in Intramedullary Fixation of Lower-Extremity Fracture. Orthop. Rev., 21(8):945–952, 1992.
252. Inoue, G.: Closed Reduction of Mallet Fractures Using Extension-Block Kirschner Wire. J. Orthop. Trauma, 6(4):413–415, 1992.
253. Ivanov, N.A.: Treatment of a Patient With Multiple Fractures of Long Bones. Orthop. Travmatol. Protez., 12:46–47, 1991.
254. Jabaley, M.E., and Freeland, A.E.: Rigid Internal Fixation in the Hand: 104 Cases. Plast. Reconstr. Surg., 77(2)288–298, 1986.
255. Jacobs, R.R.; McClain, O.; and Armstrong, H.J.: Internal Fixation of Intertrochanteric Hip Fractures: A Clinical and Biomechanical Study. Clin. Orthop., 146:62–70, 1980.
256. Jaffe, K.A.; Morris, S.G.; Sorrell, R.G.; Gebhardt, M.C.; and Mankin, H.J.: Massive Bone Allografts for Traumatic Skeletal Defects. South Med. J., 84(8):975–982, 1991.
257. Jensen, C.M., and Olsen, B.B.: Drawbacks of Traction-Absorbing Wiring (TAW) in Displaced Fractures of the Olecranon. Injury, 17(3):174–175, 1986.
258. Johnson, E.E.: Acute Lengthening of Shortened Lower Extremities After Malunion or Non-Union of a Fracture. J. Bone Joint Surg. Am., 76(3):379–389, 1994.
259. Johnson, E.E., and Davlin, L.B.: Open Ankle Fractures. The Indications for Immediate Open Reduction and Internal Fixation. Clin. Orthop., 292:118–127, 1993.
260. Johnson, E.E., and Gebhardt, J.S.: Surgical Management of Calcaneal Fractures Using Bilateral Incisions and Minimal Internal Fixation. Clin. Orthop., 290:117–124, 1993.
261. Johnson, E.E.; Matta, J.M.; Mast, J.W.; and Letournel, E.: Delayed Reconstruction of Acetabular Fractures 21–120 Days Following Injury. Clin. Orthop., 305:20–30, 1994.
262. Johnson, E.E.; Urist, M.R.; and Finerman, G.A.: Resistant Nonunions and Partial or Complete Segmental Defects of Long Bones. Treatment With Implants of a Composite of Human Bone Morphogenetic Protein (BMP) and Autolyzed, Antigen-Extracted, Allogeneic (AAA) Bone. Clin. Orthop., 277:229–237, 1992.
263. Johnson, K.D.; Johnston, D.W.; and Parker, B.: Comminuted Femoral-Shaft Fractures: Treatment by Roller Traction, Cerclage Wires and An Intramedullary Nail, or an Interlocking

Intramedullary Nail. J. Bone Joint Surg. 66A(8):1222–1235, 1984.
264. Johnson, K.D.; Tencer, A.F.; Blumenthal, S.; August, A.; and Johnston, D.W.C.: Biomechanical Performance of Locked Intramedullary Nail Systems in Comminuted Femoral Shaft Fractures. Clin. Orthop., 206:151–161, 1986.
265. Johnson, R.P.; Roetker, A.; and Schwab, J.P.: Olecranon Fractures Treated With AO Screw and Tension Bands. Orthopedics, 9(1):66–68, 1986.
266. Johnston, C.; Bueche, M.J.; Williamson, B.; and Birch, J.G.: Epiphysiodesis for Management of Lower Limb Deformities. Instr. Course Lect., 41:437–444, 1992.
267. Jomha, N.M.; Raso, V.J.; and Leung, P.: Effect of Varying Angles on the Pullout Strength of Interference Screw Fixation. Arthroscopy, 9(5):580–583, 1993.
268. Jones, D.G.: Bone Erosion Beneath Partridge Bands. J.Bone Joint Surg., 68B(3):476–477, 1986.
269. Jones, J.A.: Immediate Internal Fixation of High-Energy Open Forearm Fractures. J. Orthop. Trauma, 5(3):272–279, 1991.
270. Jones, J.K., and Van Sickels, J.E.: Rigid Fixation: A Review of Concepts and Treatment of Fractures. Oral Surg. Oral Med. Oral Pathol., 65(1):13, 1988.
271. Jupiter, J.B.; Barnes, K.A.; Goodman, L.J.; and Saldana, A.E.: Multiplane Fracture of the Distal Humerus. J. Orthop. Trauma, 7(3):216–220, 1993.
272. Jupiter, J.B.; Leibovic, S.J.; Ribbans, W.; and Wilk, R.M.: The Posterior Monteggia Lesion. J. Orthop. Trauma, 5(4):395–402, 1991.
273. Jupiter, J.B., and Lipton, H.: The Operative Treatment of Intraarticular Fractures of the Distal Radius. Clin. Orthop., 292:48–61, 1993.
274. Jupiter, J.B., and Mullaji, A.B.: Blade Plate Fixation of Proximal Humeral Non-Unions. Injury, 25(5):301–303, 1994.
275. Kanakis, T.E., and Cordey, J.: Is There A Mechanical Difference Between Lag Screws and Double Cerclage? Injury, 22(3):185–189, 1991.
276. Karavias, D.; Korovessis, P.; Filos, K.; Siamplis, D.; Petrocheilos, J.; and Androulakis, J.: Major Vascular Lesions Associated With Orthopaedic Injuries. J. Ortho. Trauma, 6(2):180–185, 1992.
277. Katznelson, A.; Volpin, G.; and Lin, E.: Tension Band Wiring for Fixation of Comminuted Fractures of the Distal Radius. Injury, 12(3):239–242, 1980.
278. Keating, J.F.; Court-Brown, C.M.; and McQueen, M.M.: Internal Fixation of Volar-Displaced Distal Radial Fractures. J. Bone Joint Surg. Br., 76(3):401–405, 1994.
279. Kempf, I.; Grosse, A.; Taglang, G.; Bernhard, L.; and Moui, Y.: Interlocking Central Medullary Nailing of Recent Femoral and Tibial Fractures. Statistical Study Apropos of 835 Cases. Chirurgie, 117(5–6):478–487, 1991.
280. Kempf, I.; Grosse, A.; and Beck, G.: Closed Locked Intramedullary Nailing: Its Application to Comminuted Fractures of the Femur. J. Bone Joint Surg., 67A:709–720, 1985.
281. Kiviluoto, O., and Santavirta, S.: Fractures of the Olecranon. Analysis of 37 Consecutive Cases. Acta. Orthop. Scand., 49(1):28–31, 1978.
282. Klaue, K.; Perren, S.M.; and Kowalski, M.: Internal Fixation With a Self-Compressing Plate and Lag Screw: Improvements of the Plate Hole and Screw Design. 1. Mechanical Investigation. J. Orthop. Trauma, 5(3):280–288, 1991.
283. Klemm, K., and Schellman, W.D.: Dynamische and Statische Verriegkling des margnagels. Unfallheikunde, 75:568–575, 1972.
284. Klemm, K.: Interlocking Nailing in Infected Pseudoarthrosis. Hefte Unfallheilkd, 161(180):180–186, 1983.
285. Klemm, K.; Schellmann, W.D.; and Vittali, H.P.: Intramedullary Nail Bolted to the Femur and Tibia. Bull. Soc. Int. Chir., 34(2):93–96, 1975.
286. Klemm, K.W., and Borner, M.: Interlocking Nailing of Complex Fractures of the Femur and Tibia. Clin. Orthop., 212:89–100, 1986.
287. Klemm, K.W.: Treatment of Infected Pseudarthrosis of the Femur and Tibia with an Interlocking Nail. Clin. Orthop., 212:174–181, 1986.
288. Kobayashi, S., and Terayama, K.: Arthroscopic Reduction and Fixation of a Completely Displaced Fracture of the Intercondylar Eminence of the Tibia. Arthroscopy, 10(2):231–235, 1994.
289. Kocialkowski, A., and Wallace, W.A.: Closed Percutaneous K-Wire Stabilization for Displaced Fractures of the Surgical Neck of the Humerus. Injury, 21(4):209–212, 1990.
290. Koranyi, E.; Bowman, C.E.; Knechi, C.D.; and Janssen, M.: Holding Power of Orthopaedic Screws in Bone. Clin. Orthop., 72:283–286, 1970.
291. Koval, K.J.; Sanders, R.; Borrelli, J.; Helfet, D.; DiPasquale, T.; and Mast, J.W.: Indirect Reduction and Percutaneous Screw Fixation of Displaced Tibial Plateau Fractures. J. Orthop. Trauma, 6(3):340–346, 1992.
292. Krettek, C.; Haas, N.; Mathys, R., Sr.; and Tscherne, H.: Initial Clinical Experience With Osteosynthesis of Femoral Shaft Fractures With a Newly Developed Intramedullary Implant (Claw Interlocking Nail). Unfallchirurg, 94(1):1–8, 1991.
293. Krettek, C.; Haas, N.; Schandelmaier, P.; Frigg, R.; and Tscherne, H.: Unreamed Tibial Nail in Tibial Shaft Fractures With Severe Soft Tissue Damage. Initial Clinical Experiences. Unfallchirurg, 94(11):579–587, 1991.
294. Kumta, S.M.; Spinner, R.; and Leung, P.C.: Absorbable Intramedullary Implants for Hand Fractures. Animal Experiments and Clinical Trial (see comments). J. Bone Joint Surg. 74B(4):563–566, 1992.
295. Kunec, J.R., and Lewis, R.J.; Closed Intramedullary Rodding of Pathologic Fractures With Supplemental Cement. Clin. Orthop., 188: 183–186, 1984.
296. Kuner, E.H.; Serif el-Nasr, M.S.; Munst, P.; and Staiger, M.: Tibial Intramedullary Nailing Without Open Drilling. Unfallchirurgie, 19(5):278–283, 1993.
297. Küntscher, G.: Die Marknagelung von Knochenbruchen. Tierexpinentaller Teil. Klin. Schr., 19:6–10, 1940.
298. Küntscher, G.: The Kuntscher Method of Intramedullary Fixation. J. Bone Joint Surg., 40A:17–26, 1958.
299. Küntscher, G.: Practice of Intramedullary Nailing, 1st ed. Springfield, Ill., Charles C. Thomas, 1967.
300. Kurosaka, M.; Yoshiya, S.; and Andrish, J.: A Biomechanical Comparison of Different Surgical Techniques of Graft Fixation in Anterior Cruciate Ligament Reconstruction. Am. J. Sports Medicine, 15(3):225–229, 1987.
301. Kyle, R.F.: Biomechanics of Intramedullary Fracture Fixation. Orthopedics, 8:1356–1359, 1985.
302. Kyle, R.F.; Schauffhausen, J.M.; and Bechtold, J.E.: Biomechanical Characteristics of Interlocking Femoral Nails in the Treatment of Complex Femoral Fractures. Clin. Orthop., 267:169–173, 1991.
303. Lambert, K.: Vascularized Patellar Tendon Graft With Rigid Internal Fixation for Anterior Cruciate Ligament Insufficiency. Clin. Orthop., 172:85–89, 1983.
304. Lancaster, J.M.; Koman, L.A.; Gristina, A.G.; Rovere, G.D.; Poehling, G.G.; Nicastro, J.F.; and Adair, D.M.: Pathologic Fractures of the Humerus. South Med. J., 81(1):52–55, 1988.
305. Larrabee, W., Jr.; Irwin, T., Jr.; Travis, L.W.; and Tabb, H.G.: Use of Transverse Kirschner Wires in Comminuted Facial Fractures. South Med. J., 72(10):1265–1267, 1979.
306. Larsen, E., and Jensen, C.M.: Tension-Band Wiring of Olecranon Fractures With Nonsliding Pins. Report of 20 Cases. Acta. Orthop. Scand., 62(4):360–362, 1991.
307. Laurence, M., Freeman, M.A.R., and Swanson, S.A.V.: Engineering Considerations in the Internal Fixation of Fractures of the Tibial Shaft. J. Bone Joint Surg., 51B:754–768, 1969.
308. Lawrence, W.T.: Clinical Management of Nonhealing Wounds. *In* Cohen, R.F., Diegelmann, R.F., and Linblad, W.J. (eds.): Wound Healing Biochemical and Clinical Aspects, pp. 541–561. Philadelphia, W.B. Saunders, 1992.
309. Leggon, R.; Lindsey, R.W.; Doherty, B.J.; Alexander, J.; Noble, P.: The Holding Strength of Cannulated Screws Compared with Solid Core Screws in Cortical and Cancellous Bone. J. Ortho. Trauma, 7(5):450–457, 1993.

310. Leggon, R.E.; Lindsey, R.W.; and Panjabi, M.M.: Strength Reduction and the Effects of Treatment of Long Bones With Diaphyseal Defects Involving 50% of the Cortex. J. Orthop. Res., 6(4):540–546, 1988.
311. Lemos, M.J.; Albert, J.; Simon, T.; and Jackson, D.W.: Radiographic Analysis of Femoral Interference Screw Placement During ACL Reconstruction: Endoscopic Versus Open Technique. Arthroscopy, 9(2):154–158, 1993.
312. Leung, K.S.; Lam, T.P.; and Poon, K.M.: Operative Treatment of Displaced Intra-Articular Glenoid Fractures. Injury, 24(5):324–328, 1993.
313. Leung, P.C.; Mak, K.H.; and Lee, S.Y.: Percutaneous Tension Band Wiring: A New Method of Internal Fixation for Mildly Displaced Patella Fracture. J. Trauma, 23(1):62–64, 1983.
314. Levanson, S.M., and Demetrou, A.A.: Metabolic Factors. *In* Cohen, R.F., Diegelmann, R.F., and Linblad, W.J. (eds.): Wound Healing Biochemical and Clinical Aspects, p.248–273. Phialdelphia, W.B. Saunders, 1992.
315. Levin, P.E., Schoen, R.W., Jr., and Browner, B.D.: Radiation Exposure to the Surgeon During Closed Interlocking Intramedullary Nailing. J. Bone Joint Surg., 69A:761–766, 1987.
316. Liang, S.C.; Liang, C.L.; and Liang, C.S.: Intramedullary Ender's Nail Fixation of Tibial Fractures. Taiwan I Hsueh Hui Tsa Chih, 81(4):470–477, 1982.
317. Linclau, L., and Dokter, G.: Osteosynthesis of Pathologic Fractures and Prophylactic Internal Fixation of Metastases in Long Bones. Acta. Orthop. Belg., 58(3):330–335, 1992.
318. Lotke, P.A., and Ecker, M.L.: Transverse Fractures of the Patella. Clin. Orthop., 158:180–184, 1981.
319. Lottes, J.O.: Intramedullary Nail of the Tibia. Instr. Course Lect., XV:65–77, 1958.
320. Lottes, J.O.: Medullary Nailing of Infected Fractures of the Femur. Clin. Orthop., 60:99–101, 1968.
321. Lottes, J.O.: Medullary Nailing of the Tibia With the Triflange Nail. Clin. Orthop., 105:53–66, 1974.
322. Low, C.K., and Low, B.Y.: Olecranon Fracture and Tension Band Wiring. Singapore Med. J., 29(5):480–484, 1988.
323. Lubowitz, J.H., and Grauer, J.D.: Arthroscopic Treatment of Anterior Cruciate Ligament Avulsion. Clin. Orthop., 294:242–246, 1993.
324. Lucas, S.E.; Seligson, D.; and Henry, S.L.: Intramedullary Supracondylar Nailing of Femoral Fractures. A Preliminary Report of the GSH Supracondylar Nail. Clin. Orthop., 296:200–206, 1993.
325. Ly, P.N., and Fallat, L.M.: Trans-Chondral Fractures of the Talus: A Review of 64 Surgical Cases. J. Foot Ankle Surg., 32(4):352–374, 1993.
326. Ma, Y.Z.; Zhang, Y.F.; Qu, K.F.; and Yeh, Y.C.: Treatment of Fractures of the Patella with Percutaneous Suture. Clin. Orthop., 191:235–241, 1984.
327. Maatz, R.; Lentz, W.; Arens, W.; and Beck, H. (eds): Intramedullary Nailing and Other Intramedullary Osteosynthesis, p. 283. Philadelphia, W.B. Saunders Company, 1986.
328. Macule Beneyto, F.; Arandes Renu, J.M.; Ferreres Claramunt, A.; and Ramon Soler, R: Treatment of Galeazzi Fracture-Dislocations. J. Trauma, 36(3):352–355, 1994.
329. Majeed, S.A., and Leithy, M.: Internal Fixation of Ipsilateral Trochanteric and Femoral Shaft Fractures by Staples and Kuntscher Nail. J. Orthop. Trauma, 2(1):33–35, 1988.
330. Makela, E.A.; Bostman, O.; Kekomaki, M.; Sodergard, J.; Vainio, J.; Tormala, P.; and Rokkanen, P.: Biodegradable Fixation of Distal Humeral Physeal Fractures. Clin. Orthop., 283:237–243, 1992.
331. Malgaigne, J.F.: A Treatise on Fractures, 1st ed., p. 683. Philadelphia, J.B. Lippincott, 1859.
332. Malkani, A.L., and Rand, J.A.: Subcapital Femoral Neck Fracture Following Open Reduction and Internal Fixation of an Intertrochanteric Hip Fracture Using a Sliding Screw and Side Plate. Orthop. Rev., 22(4):469–472, 1993.
333. Margo, M.K., and Waller, J.A.: Intramedullary Fixation of the Fractured Tibia With Lottes Nail. Clin. Orthop., 100:216–218, 1974.
334. Martin, W.R., and Sutherland, C.J.: Complications of Proximal Femoral Allografts in Revision Total Hip Arthroplasty. Clin. Orthop., 295:161–167, 1993.
335. Marya, S.K.; Bhan, S.; and Dave, P.K.: Comparative Study of Knee Function After Patellectomy and Osteosynthesis With a Tension Band Wire Following Patellar Fractures. Int. Surg., 72(4):211–213, 1987.
336. Mast, J.; Jakob, R.; and Ganz, R.: Planning and Reduction Technique in Fracture Surgery, p. 254. Berlin, Springer-Verlag, 1989.
337. Matta, J.M.: Operative Treatment of Acetabular Fractures Through the Ilioinguinal Approach. A 10-year Perspective. Clin. Orthop., 305:10, 1994.
338. Mayer, L.; Werbie, T.; Schwab, J.P.; and Johnson, R.P.: The Use of Ender Nails in Fractures of the Tibial Shaft. J. Bone Joint Surg., 67A:446–455, 1985.
339. Mayo, K.A.: Open Reduction and Internal Fixation of Fractures of the Acetabulum. Results in 163 Fractures. Clin. Orthop., 305:31–37, 1994.
340. Mayo, K.A.; Letournel, E.; Matta, J.M.; Mast, J.W.; Johnson, E.E.; and Martimbeau, C.L.: Surgical Revision of Malreduced Acetabular Fractures. Clin. Orthop., 305:47–52, 1994.
341. McCurnin, D.M., and Slusher, R.: Tension-Band Wiring of a Fractured Patella (A Photographic Essay). Vet. Med. Small Anim. Clin., 70(11):1321–1323, 1975.
342. Mears, D.C.: Materials and Orthopaedic Surgery. Baltimore, Williams & Wilkins, 1979.
343. Meek, R.N., Vivoda, E.E., and Pirani, S.: Comparison of Mortality of Patients with Multiple Injuries According to Type of Fracture Treatment: A Retrospective Age- and Injury-Matched Series. Injury, 17:2–4, 1986.
344. Menck, H.; Schulze, S.; and Larsen, E.: Metastasis Size in Pathologic Femoral Fractures. Acta. Orthop. Scand., 59(2): 151–154, 1988.
345. Merianos, P.; Cambouridis, P.; and Smyrnis, P.: The Treatment of 143 Tibial Shaft Fractures by Ender's Nailing and Early Weight-Bearing. J. Bone Joint Surg. 67B(4):686–693, 1985.
346. Merianos, P.; Pazanidis, S.; Serenes, P.; Orfanidis, S.; and Smyrnis, P.: The Use of Ender Nails in Tibial Shaft Fractures. Acta. Orthop. Scand., 53:301–307, 1982.
347. Mihalko, W.M.; Beaudoin, A.J.; Cardea, J.A.; and Krause, W.R.: Finite-Element Modelling of Femoral Shaft Fracture Fixation Techniques Post Total Hip Arthroplasty. J. Biomech., 25(5):469–476, 1992.
348. Miyagi, S.; Goto, T.; Kanazawa, C.; *et al.*: Experimental and Clinical Study of the Figure-of-Eight Wiring for Fracture of the Olecranon, Patella and Other Bones—Crossed Double Figure-of-Eight Wiring. Kurume Med. J., 32(1):37–57, 1985.
349. Mohan, K.; Gupta, A.K.; Sharma, J.; Singh, A.K.; and Jain, A.K.: Internal Fixation in 50 Cases of Galeazzi Fracture. Acta. Orthop. Scand., 59(3):318–320, 1988.
350. Molster, A.O.: Effects of Rotational Instability on Healing of Femoral Osteotomies in the Rat. Acta. Orthop. Scand., 55:632–636, 1984.
351. Molster, A.O.: Biomechanical Effects of Intramedullary Reaming and Nailing on Intact Femora in Rats. Clin. Orthop., 202:278–285, 1986.
352. Montgomery, R.J.: A Secure Method of Olecranon Fixation: A Modification of Tension Band Wiring Technique. J. R. Coll. Surg. Edinb., 31(3):179–182, 1986.
353. Moutet, F., and Frere, G.: Metacarpal Fractures. Ann. Chir. Main, 6(1):5–14, 1987.
354. Moyen, B.; Comtet, J.J.; Roy, J.C.; Basset, R.; and de-Mourgues, G.:, Refracture After Removal of Internal Fixation Devices: Clinical Study of 20 Cases and Physiopathologic Hypothesis. Lyon Chir., 76:153–157, 1980.
355. Moyen, B.J.; Lahey, P.J., Jr.; Weinberg, E.H.; and Harris, W.H.: Effects on Intact Femora of Dogs of the Application and Removal of Metal Plates: A Metabolic and Structural Study Comparing Stiffer and More Flexible Plates. J. Bone Joint Surg., 60A:940–947, 1978.
356. Muhr, G.; Tscherne, H.; and Thomas, R.: Comminuted Trochanteric Femoral Fractures in Geriatric Patients: The Results

of 213 Cases Treated with Internal Fixation and Acrylic Cement. Clin. Othop, 138:41–44, 1979.
357. Mullen, J.O., and Tranovich, M.: A Simplied Technique for Zickel Nail Insertion. Clin. Orthop., 208:195–198, 1986.
358. Muller, B.; Bonnaire, F.; Heckel, T.; Jaeger, J,H,; Kempf, I.; and Kuner, E.H.: Ender Nail With Interlocking Mechanism or Dynamic Hip Screw in Pertrochanteric Fractures? A Prospective Study Extending Its Limits. Unfallchirurgie, 20(1):18–29, 1994.
359. Müller, M.; Nararian, S.; Koch, P.; and Schatzker, J.: The Comprehensive Classification of Fractures, p. 201. Berlin, Springer-Verlag, 1990.
360. Müller, M.E.: Die Verwendung von Kunstharzen in der Knochenchirurgie. Arch. Orthop. Unfall-Chir, 54:513–522, 1964.
361. Müller, M.E.; Allgower, M.; Schneider, R.; and Willenegger, H.: Manual of Internal Fixation, 3rd ed. Berlin, Springer-Verlag, 1992.
362. Müller, M.E., Allgöwer, M., and Willenegger, H.: Manual of Internal Fixation. New York, Springer-Verlag, 1970.
363. Müller, M.E.; Allgöwer, M., Schneider, R.; and Willenegger, H.: Manual of Internal Fixation Techniques Recommended by the AO Group. New York: Springer-Verlag, 1979.
364. Murphy, D.F., Greene, W.B.; and Dameron, T., Jr.: Displaced Olecranon Fractures in Adults. Clinical Evaluation. Clin. Orthop., 224:215–23, 1987.
365. Murphy, D.F.; Greene, W.B.; Gilbert, J.A.; and Dameron, T., Jr.: Displaced Olecranon Fractures in Adults. Biomechanical Analysis of Fixation Methods. Clin. Orthop., 224:210–214, 1987.
366. Murray, W.R., Lucas, D.B., and Inman, V.T.: Treatment of Non-Union of Fractures of the Long Bones by the Two-Plate Method. J. Bone Joint Surg., 46A:1027–1048, 1964.
367. Nach, D.C., and Keim, H.A.: Prophylactic Antibiotics in Spinal Surgery. Orthop. Rev., 2(6):27–30, 1973.
368. Nap, R.C.: The Olecranon Process; Fractures and Osteotomy. Tijdschr Diergeneeskd, 113(1):55S–58S, 1988.
369. Nordback, I., and Markkula, H.: Migration of Kirschner Pinfrom Clavicle Into Ascending Aorta. Acta. Chir. Scand., 151(2):177–179, 1985.
370. O'Dwyer, K.J., and Bobic, V.R.: Arthroscopic Management of Tibial Plateau Fractures. Injury, 23(4):261–264, 1992.
371. O'Meara, P.M.; O'Brien, W.R.; and Henning, C.E.: Anterior Cruciate Ligament Reconstruction Stability with Continuous Passive Motion. The Role of Isometric Graft Placement. Clin. Orthop., 277:201–209, 1992.
372. O'Sullivan, M.E.; Chao, E.Y.; and Kelly, P.J.: The Effects of Fixation on Fracture-Healing. J. Bone Joint Surg. 71A(2):306–310, 1989.
373. Oakeshott, R.D.; Morgan, D.A.; Zukor, D.J.; Rudan, J.F.; Brooks, P.J.; and Gross, A.E.: Revision Total Hip Arthroplasty With Osseous Allograft Reconstruction. A Clinical and Roentgenographic Analysis. Clin. Orthop., 225:37–61, 1987.
374. Obara, T.: A Biomechanical Study on the Fracture Treatment—Intravital Measurement of the Strain on an Intramedullary Nail in the Healing Process of the Femoral Fracture in Goats (author's transl). Nippon Seikeigeka Gakkai Zasshi, 53(2):199–212, 1979.
375. Oishi, C.; Carrion, W.; and Hoaglund, F.: Use of Parenteral Prophylactic Antibiotics In Clean Orthopaedic Surgery: A Review of the Literature. Clin. Orthop., 296:249–255, 1993.
376. Olerud, S., and Danckwardt-Lilliestrom, G.: Fracture Healing in Compression Osteosynthesis. Acta. Orthop. Scand., (suppl), 137, 1971.
377. Olmi, R.; Graci, A.; and Moroni, A.: Osteosynthesis With the Rush Nail and Cerclage in Comminuted Fractures of the Humeral Diaphysis. Chir. Organi. Mov., 66(6):765–768, 1980.
378. Ostgaard, H.C.; Ebel, P.; and Irstam, L.: Fixation of Ankle Fractures: Power-Driven Staples Compared With a Routine Method, a 3-year Follow-Up Study. J. Orthop. Trauma, 4(4):415–419, 1990.
379. Ostrum, R.F.: Customized Plating Techniques for Juxta-Articular Fractures and Osteotomies. Orthop. Rev., 21(5):629–635, 1992.
380. Ostrum, R.F., and Litsky, A.S.: Tension Band Fixation of Medial Malleolus Fractures. J. Orthop. Trauma, 6(4):464–468, 1992.
381. Paavolainen, P.; Penttinen, R.; Slatis, P.; and Karaharju, E.: The Healing of Experimental Fractures by Compression Osteosynthesis: II. Morphometric and Chemical Analysis. Acta. Orthop. Scand., 50:375–383, 1979.
382. Paavolainen, P.; Slatis, P.; Karaharju, E.; and Holmstrom, T.: The Healing of Experimental Fractures by Compression Osteosynthesis: I. Torsional Strength. Acta. Orthop. Scand., 50:369–374, 1979.
383. Paffen, P.J., and Jansen, E.W.: Surgical Treatment of Clavicular Fractures With Kirschner Wires: A Comparative Study. Arch. Chir. Neerl., 30(1):43–53, 1978.
384. Paiement, G.D.; Renaud, E.; Dagenais, G.; and Gosselin, R.A.: Double-Blind Randomized Prospective Study of the Efficacy of Antibiotic Prophylaxis for Open Reduction and Internal Fixation of Closed Ankle Fractures. J. Orthop. Trauma, 8(1):64–66, 1994.
385. Pak, J.H.; Paprosky, W.G.; Jablonsky, W.S.; and Lawrence, J.M. Femoral Strut Allografts in Cementless Revision Total Hip Arthroplasty. Clin. Orthop., 295:172–178, 1993.
386. Palmer, R.H.; Aron, D.N.; and Chambers, J.N.: A Combined Tension Band and Lag Screw Technique for Fixation of Olecranon Osteotomies. Vet. Surg., 17(6):328–332, 1988.
387. Papagelopoulos, P.J.; Giannarakos, D.G.; and Lyritis, G.P.: Suitability of Biodegradable Polydioxanone Materials for the Internal Fixation of Fractures. Orthop. Rev., 22(5):585–593, 1993.
388. Papagelopoulos, P.J., and Morrey, B.F.: Treatment of Nonunion of Olecranon Fractures. J. Bone Joint Surg. Br., 76(4):627–635, 1994.
389. Partio, E.K.: Immobilization and Early Mobilization of Malleolar Fractures After Osteosynthesis With Resorbable Bone Screws. Unfallchirurgie, 18(5):304–310, 1992.
390. Partio, E.K.; Bostman, O.; Hirvensalo, E.; *et al.*: Self-Reinforced Absorbable Screws in the Fixation of Displaced Ankle Fractures: A Prospective Clinical Study of 152 Patients. J. Orthop. Trauma, 6(2):209–215, 1992.
391. Partio, E.K.; Hirvensalo, E.; Bostman, O.; *et al.*: Absorbable Rods and Screws: A New Method of Fixation for Fractures of the Olecranon. Int. Orthop., 16(3):250–254, 1992.
392. Pasqualini, M., and Murena, P.F.: The Grosse-Kempf Nail in Femoral and Tibial Shaft Fractures. Ital. J. Orthop. Traumatol., 17(3):321–326, 1991.
393. Pauwels, F.: Biomechanics of the Locomotor Apparatus, p. 518. Berlin, Springer-Verlag, 1980.
394. Peltier, L.: Fractures: A History and Iconography of Their Treatment, p. 273. San Francisco, Norman Publishing, 1990.
395. Pelto, K.; Hirvensalo, E.; Bostman, O.; and Rokkanen, P.: Treatment of Radial Head Fractures with Absorbable Polyglycolide Pins: A Study on the Security of the Fixation in 38 Cases. J. Orthop. Trauma, 8(2):94–98, 1994.
396. Perez Blanco, R.; Rodriguez Merchan, C.; Canosa Sevillano, R.; and Munuera Martinez, L.: Tarsometatarsal Fractures and Dislocations. J. Orthop. Trauma, 2(3):188–194, 1988.
397. Perren, S., and Pohler, O.: News From the Lab: Titanium as Implant Material. AO/ASIF Dialogue, 1(3):11–12, 1987.
398. Perren, S.: The Concept of Biological Plating Using the Limited Contact-Dynamic Compression Plate (LC-DCP). Injury: AO/ASIF Scientific Supplement, 22(1):S1–S41, 1991.
399. Perren, S.M.: Physical and Biological Aspects of Fracture Healing With Special Reference to Internal Fixation. Clin. Orthop., 138:175–196, 1979.
400. Perren, S.M.: The Biomechanics and Biology of Internal Fixation Using Plates and Nails. Orthopedics, 12:21–33, 1989.
401. Perren, S.M.; Allgower, M.; Cordey, J.; and Russenberger, M.: Developments of Compression Plate Techniques for Internal Fixation of Fractures. Prog. Surg., 12:152–79, 1973.
402. Perren, S.M.; Cordey, J.; Rahn, B.A.; Gautier, E.; and Schneider, E.: Early Temporary Porosis of Bone Induced by Internal

Fixation Implants. A Reaction to Necrosis, not to Stress Protection? Clin. Orthop., 232:139–151, 1988.
403. Perren, S.M.; Matter, P.; Ruedi, R.; and Allgower, M.: Biomechanics of Fracture Healing After Internal Fixation. Surg. Annu., 7:361–390, 1975.
404. Perry, C.R.; McCarthy, J.A.; Kain, C.C.; and Pearson, R.L.: Patellar Fixation Protected With a Load-Sharing Cable: A Mechanical and Clinical Study. J. Orthop. Trauma, 2(3):234–240, 1988.
405. Pesudo, J.V.; Aracil, J.; and Barcelo, M.: Leverage Method in Displaced Fractures of the Radial Neck in Children. Clin. Orthop., 169:215–218, 1982.
406. Peter, R.E.; Hoffmeyer, P.; and Henley, M.B.: Treatment of Humeral Diaphyseal Fractures With Hackethal Stacked Nailing: A Report of 33 Cases. J. Orthop. Trauma, 6(1):14–17, 1992.
407. Peterson, L.T.: Principles of Internal Fixation with Plates and Screws. Arch. Surg., 64:345–354, 1952.
408. Pihlajamaki, H.; Bostman, O.; Hirvensalo, E.; Tormala, P.; and Rokkanen, P.: Absorbable Pins of Self-Reinforced Poly-L-Lactic Acid for Fixation of Fractures and Osteotomies. J. Bone Joint Surg. Br., 74(6):853–857, 1992.
409. Pilliar, R.M.; Cameron, H.A.; Binnington, A.G.; Szivek, J.; and MacNab, I.: Bone Ingrowth and Stress Shielding With a Porous Surface Coated Fracture Fixation Plate. J. Biomed. Mater. Res., 13:799–810, 1979.
410. Pintore, E.; Maffulli, N.; and Petricciuolo, F.: Interlocking Nailing for Fractures of the Femur and Tibia. Injury, 23(6):381–386, 1992.
411. Pratt, D.J.; Papagiannoupoulos, G.; Rees, P.H.; and Quinnell, R.: The Effects of Intramedullary Reaming on the Torsional Strength of the Femur. Injury, 18:177–179, 1987.
412. Pritchett, J.W.: Rush Rods Versus Plate Osteosyntheses for Unstable Ankle Fractures in the Elderly. Orthop. Rev., 22(6):691–696, 1993.
413. Raco, A.; Di Lorenzo, N.; Delfini, R.; Ciappetta, P.; and Cantore, G.: The Acrylic-Wire Option in Cervical spine fixation. A retrospective study. Acta. Neurochir., 120(1–2):53–58, 1993.
414. Ramotowski, W., and Granowski, R.: Zespol. An Original Method of Stable Osteosynthesis. Clin. Orthop., 272:67–75, 1991.
415. Rand, J.A.; Chao, E.Y.S.; and Kelly, P.J.: A Comparison of the Effect of Open Intramedullary Nailing and Compression-Plate Fixation on Fracture-Site Blood Flow and Fracture Union. J. Bone Joint Surg., 63A:427–442, 1981.
416. Rao, J.P., and Femino, F.P.: Repair of a Glenoid Fracture Using a Powered Stapler. Orthop. Rev., 21(12):1449–1452, 1992.
417. Raskin, K.B., and Melone, C., Jr.: Unstable Articular Fractures of the Distal Radius. Comparative Techniques of Ligamentotaxis. Orthop. Clin. North. Am., 24(2):275–286, 1993.
418. Ray, A.K.; Romine, J.S.; and Pankovich, A.M.: Stabilization of Pathologic Fractures With Acrylic Cement. Clin. Orthop., 101(01): 182–185, 1974.
419. Reichert, K., and Caneva, R.G.: The Use of Kirschner Wire Fixation in Forefoot Surgery. J. Foot Surg., 22(3):218–221, 1983.
420. Remiger, A.R.; Predieri, M.; Tepic, S.; and Perren, S.N.: Internal Fixation Using the Point Contact Plate: An In-Vivo Study in Sheep. Journal of Orthopaedic Trauma, 7(2):176–177, 1993.
421. Reyes, G.A., Jr.: Intraoral Use of Kirschner Pins. J. Oral Surg., 33(4):304–306, 1975.
422. Rhinelander, F.W.: The Normal Microcirculation of Diaphyseal Cortex and Its Response to Fracture. J. Bone Joint Surg., 50A(4):784–800, 1968.
423. Rhinelander, F.W.: The Normal Circulation of Bone and its Response to Surgical Intervention. J. Biomed. Mater. Res., 8(1):87–90, 1974.
424. Rhinelander, F.W.: Minimal Internal Fixation of Tibial Fractures. Clin Ortho, 107:188–220, 1975.
425. Rhinelander, F.W.: Vascular Proliferation and Blood Supply During Fracture Healing. *In* Uhthoff, H.K. (ed.): Current Concepts of Internal Fixation of Fractures. New York, Springer-Verlag, 1980.
426. Rhinelander, F.W.: Experimental Fixation of Femoral Osteotomies by Cerclage with Nylon Straps. Clin Orthop, 179:298–307, 1983.
427. Rich, N.M.; Metz, C.W., Jr.; Hutton, J.E., Jr.; Baugh, J.H.; and Hughes, C.W.: Internal Versus External Fixation of Fractures with Concomitant Vascular Injuries in Vietnam. J. Trauma, 11:463–473, 1971.
428. Rink, P.C. and Scott, F.: The Operative Repair of Displaced Patellar Fractures. Orthop. Rev., 20(2):157–165, 1991.
429. Riska, E.; vonBonsdorff, H.; Hakkinen, S.; Jaroma, H.H.; Kiviluoto, O.; and Paavilainen, T.: Primary Operative Fixation of Long Bone Fractures in Patients With multiple injuries. J. Trauma, 17:111–121, 1977.
430. Rittmann, W.W., and Perren, S.M.: Cortical Bone Healing After Internal Fixation and Infection, p. 76. Berlin, Springer-Verlag, 1974.
431. Romm, S.: The Person Behind the Name: Martin Kirschner. Plast. Reconstr. Surg., 72(1):104–107, 1983.
432. Rosenstein, B.D.; Wilson, F.C.; and Funderburk, C.H.: The Use of Bacitracin Irrigation to Prevent Infection in Postoperative Skeletal Wounds. An Experimental Study. J. Bone Joint Surg. 71A(3):427–430, 1989.
433. Rowland, S.A., and Burkhart, S.S.: Tension Band Wiring of Olecranon Fractures. A Modification of the AO Technique. Clin. Orthop., 277:238–242, 1992.
434. Rubinstein, E.; Findler, G.; Amit, P.; and Shaked, I.: Perioperative Prophylactic Cephazolin in Spinal Surgery. A Double-Blind Placebo-Controlled Trial. J. Bone Joint Surg. Br., 76(1):99–102, 1994.
435. Ruesch, P.D.; Holdener, H.; Ciaramitaro, M.; and Mast, J.W.: A Prospective Study of Surgically Treated Acetabular Fractures. Clin. Orthop., 305:38–46, 1994.
436. Rush, J.: Closed Nailing of the Humerus—From Down Under. Aust. N. Z. J. Surg., 57(10):723–725, 1987.
437. Rush, L.V.: Atlas of Rush Pin Technics, vol. 243. Meridian, Berivon Company, 1976.
438. Russell, R.H.: Fracture of the Femur: A Clinical Study. Br. J. Surg., 11A:491–502, 1924.
439. Russell, T.A., and Taylor, J.C.: Interlocking Intramedullary Nailing of the Femur: Current Concepts. Semin. Orthop., 1:217–231, 1986.
440. Rybicki, E.F.; Simonen, F.A.; Mills, E.J.; Hassler, C.R.; Scoles, P.; Milne, D.; and Weis, E.B.: Mathematical and Experimental Studies on the Mechanics of Plated Transverse Fractures. J. Biomech, 7:377–384, 1974.
441. Saleh, M.; Shanahan, M.D.; and Fern, E.D.: Intra-Articular Fractures of the Distal Tibia: Surgical Management by Limited Internal Fixation and Articulated Distraction. Injury, 24(1): 37–40, 1993.
442. Satku, K., and Kumar, V.P.: Surgical Management of Non-Union of Neglected Fractures of the Patella. Injury, 22(2):108–110, 1991.
443. Scales, J.T., Towers, A.G., and Roantree, B.M.: The Influence of Antibiotic Therapy on Wound Inflammation and Sepsis Associated with Orthopaedic Implants: A Long-Term Clinical Survey. Acta. Orthop. Scand., 43:85–100, 1972.
444. Schafer, D.; Rosso, R.; Babst, R.; Marx, A.; Renner, R.; Heberer, M.; and Regazzoni, P.: Experience With the AO Universal Femoral Intramedullary Nail for Management of Femur Shaft Fractures. Helv. Chir. Acta., 60(1–2):231–234, 1993.
445. Schatzker, J., and Ha'Eri, G.B.: Methylmethacrylate as an Adjunct in the Internal Fixation of Pathologic Fractures. Can. J. Surg., 22(2):179–82, 1979.
446. Schatzker, J., Horne, J.G., and Summer-Smith, G.: The Effect of Movement on the Holding Power of Screws in Bone. Clin. Orthop., 111:257–262, 1975.
447. Schatzker, J., Horne, J.G., and Sumner-Smith, G.: The Reaction of Cortical Bone to Compression by Screw Threads. Clin. Orthop., 111:263–265, 1975.
448. Schatzker, J., Sanderson, R., and Murnaghan, J.P.: The Hold-

ing Power of Orthopaedic Screws. In Vivo. Clin. Orthop., 108:115–116, 1975.

449. Schlickewei, W., Kuner, E.H.; Mullaji, A.B.; and Gotze, B.: Upper and Lower Limb Fractures with Concomitant Arterial Injury. J. Bone Joint Surg., 74B(2):181–188, 1992.

451. Schopfer, A.; Willett, K.; Powell, J.; and Tile, M.: Cerclage Wiring in Internal Fixation of Acetabular Fractures. J. Orthop. Trauma, 7(3):236–241, 1993.

452. Schranz, P.J., and Fagg, P.S.: Trans-Radial Styloid, Trans-Scaphoid, Trans-Triquetral Perilunate Dislocation. J. R. Army Med. Corps., 137(3):146–148, 1991.

453. Schultz, R.S.; Boger, J.W.; and Dunn, H.K.: Strength of Stainless Steel Surgical Wire in Various Fixation Modes. Clin. Orthop., 198:304–307, 1985.

454. Sedlin, E.D., and Zitner, D.T.: The Lottes Nail in the Closed Treatment of Tibia Fractures. Clin. Orthop., 192:185–192, 1985.

455. Sernbo, I.; Johnell, O.; and Gardsell, A.: Locking and Compression of the Lag Screw in Trochanteric Fractures is not Beneficial. A Prospective, Randomized Study of 153 Cases. Acta. Orthop. Scand., 65(1):24–26, 1994.

456. Serocki, J.H.; Chandler, R.W.; and Dorr, L.D.: Treatment of Fractures About Hip Prostheses With Compression Plating. J. Arthroplasty, 7(2):129–35, 1992.

457. Shapiro, S.A.; Management of Unilateral Locked Facet of the Cervical Spine. Neurosurgery, 33(5):832–837, 1993.

458. Shaw, J.A., and Daubert, H.B.: Compression Capability of Cerclage Fixation Systems. Orthopedics, 11:1169–1174, 1988.

459. Simeone, L.: Dynamic Cerclage in Traumatology. Ital. J. Orthop. Traumatol., 13(1):73–80, 1987.

460. Slone, R.M.; MacMillan, M.; and Montgomery, W.J.: Spinal Fixation. Part 1. Principles, Basic Hardware, and Fixation Techniques for the Cervical Spine. Radiographics, 13(2):341–356, 1993.

461. Smith, G.H. and Green, A.L.: Cerclage Wiring of Metatarsal Fractures. A Case Report. J. Am. Podiatry Assoc., 73(1):25–26, 1983.

462. Smith, J.T.; Goodman, S.B.; and Tischenko, G.: Treatment of Comminuted Femoral Subtrochanteric Fractures Using the Russell-Taylor Reconstruction Intramedullary Nail. Orthopedics, 14(2):125–129, 1991.

463. Smith, S.R.; Bronk, J.T.; and Kelly, P.J.: Effect of Fracture Fixation on Cortical Bone Blood Flow. J. Orthop. Res., 8:471–478, 1990.

464. Soccetti, A.; Raffaelli, P.; Giovannetti, R.; Vitali, T.; and Fabrizzi, G.: Interlocking Intramedullary Nailing for the Treatment of Tibial Fractures. Ir. J. Med. Sci., 161(1):5–8, 1992.

465. Soeur, R.: Fractures of the Limbs, p. 839. Brussels, La Clinique Orthopedique, 1981.

466. Spivak, J.M.; Zuckerman, J.D.; Kummer, F.J.; and Frankel, V.H.: Fatigue Failure of the Sliding Screw in Hip Fracture Fixation: A Report of Three Cases. J. Orthop. Trauma, 5(3):325–331, 1991.

467. Stambough, J.L.; Hopson, C.N.; and Cheeks, M.L.: Stable and Unstable Fractures of the Femoral Shaft. Orthop. Rev., 20(10):855–861, 1991.

468. Stefanich, R.J., and Putnam, M.D.: The Use of Staples in Hand Surgery. Orthop. Rev., 22(3):390, 1993.

469. Steiner, M.E.; Hecker, A.T.; Brown, C., Jr.; and Hayes, W.C.: Anterior Cruciate Ligament Graft Fixation. Comparison of Hamstring and Patellar Tendon Grafts. Am. J. Sports Med., 22(2):240–246, 1994.

470. Stephenson, J.R.: Surgical Treatment of Displaced Intraarticular Fractures of the Calcaneus. A Combined Lateral and Medial Approach. Clin. Orthop., 290:68–75, 1993.

471. Stern, R.E.; Harwin, S.F.; and Kulick, R.G.: Management of Ipsilateral Femoral Shaft Fractures Following Hip Arthroplasty. Orthop. Rev., 20(9):779–784, 1991.

472. Stevens, D.B.: Postoperative Orthopaedic Infections: A Study of Etiological Mechanisms. J. Bone Joint Surg., 46A:96–102, 1964.

473. Stimson, L.A.: A Treatise on Fractures, 1st ed., p. 593. Philadelphia, Henry C. Lea's Son & Co., 1883.

474. Stromberg, L.: Compression Fixation of Bennett's Fracture. Acta. Orthop. Scand., 48(6):586–591, 1977.

475. Stürmer, K.: Measurement of Intramedullary Pressure in an Animal Experiment and Propositions to Reduce the Pressure Increase. Injury: AO/ASIF Scientific Supplement, 24(3):s7–s21, 1993.

476. Suuronen, R.: Biodegradable Fracture-Fixation Devices in Maxillofacial Surgery. Int. J. Oral Maxillofac. Surg., 22(1):50–57, 1993.

477. Swetnam, J.A.; Hardin, W., Jr.; and Kerstein, M.D.: Successful Management of Trifurcation Injuries. Am. Surg., 52(11):585–587, 1986.

478. Swiontkowski, M.F., and Seiler, J.G., III: The AO/ASIF Universal Intrameduallary Nail. Techniques Orthop., 3:33–40, 1988.

479. Szyszkowitz, R.; Seggl, W.; Schleifer. P.; and Cundy, P.J.: Proximal Humeral Fractures. Management Techniques and Expected Results. Clin. Orthop., 292:13–25, 1993.

480. Tarr, R.S., and Wiss, D.A.: The Mechanics and Biology of Intramedullary Fracture Fixation. Clin. Orthop., 212:10–17, 1986.

481. Tayton, K., and Bradley, J.: How Stiff Should Semirigid Fixation of the Human Tibia Be? J. Bone Joint Surg., 65B:312–315, 1983.

482. Tayton, K.; Johnson-Hase, C; McKibben, B.; Bradley, J.; and Hastings, G.: Use of Semi-Rigid Carbon Fiber-Reinforced Plastic Plates for Fixation of Human Fractures: Results of Preliminary Trials. J. Bone Joint Surg., 64B:105–111, 1982.

483. Tencer, A.F.; Johnson, K.D.; Kyle, R.F.; and Fu, F.H.: Biomechanics of Fractures and Fracture Fixation. Instr. Course Lect., 42:19–55, 1993.

484. Tencer, A.F.; Johnson, K.D.; Johnson, D.W.C.; and Gill, K.: A Biomechanical Comparison of Various Methods of Stabilization of Subtrochanteric Fractures of the Femur. J. Orthop. Res., 2:297–305, 1984.

485. Tencer, A.F., Johnson, K.D., and Sherman, M.C.: Biomechanical Considerations in Intramedullary Nailing of Femoral Shaft Fractures. Techniques Orthop., 3:1–5, 1988.

486. Thoresen, B.O.; Alho, A.; Edeland, A.; Stromsoe, K.; Folleras, G.; and Haukebo, A.: Interlocking Intramedullary Nailing in Femoral Shaft Fractures: A Report of 48 Cases. J. Bone Joint Surg., 67A:1313–1320, 1985.

487. Thunold, J., Verhaug, J.E., and Bjerkeset, T.: Tibial Shaft Fractures Treated by Rigid Internal Fixation. Injury, 7:125–133, 1975.

488. Tigani, D.; Laus, M.; Bettelli, G.; Boriani, S.; and Giunti, A.: The Gamma Nail, Sliding-Compression Plate. A Comparison Between the Long-Term Results Obtained in Two Similar Series. Chir. Organi. Mov., 77(2):151–158, 1992.

489. Tornetta, P., III.; Weiner, L.; Bergman, M.; Watnik, N.; Steuer, J.; Kelley, M.; and Yang, E.: Pilon Fractures: Treatment With Combined Internal and External Fixation. J. Orthop. Trauma, 7(6):489–496, 1993.

490. Tountas, A.A.; Kwok, J.M.; and Kugler, M.: The Partridge Nylon Cerclage: Its Use as a Supplementary Fixation of Difficult Femoral Fractures in the Elderly. J. Orthop. Trauma, 4(3):299–302, 1990.

491. Trumble, T.E.; Schmitt, S.R.; and Vedder, N.B.: Factors Affecting Functional Outcome of Displaced Intra-Articular Distal Radius Fractures. J. Hand Surg., 19(2):325–340, 1994.

492. Tscherne, H., and Gotzen, L.: Fraktur und Weichteilschaden. *In* Rehn, J., and Schweiberer, L. (eds): Hefte zur Unfallheilkunde, vol. 28., p. 157. Berlin, Springer-Verlag, 1983.

493. Tscherne, H.; Haas, N.; and Krettek, C.: Intramedullary Nailing Combined With Cerclage Wiring in the Treatment of Fractures of the Femoral Shaft. Clin. Orthop., 212:62–67, 1986.

494. Uhthoff, H.K.: Bone Structure Changes in the Dog Under Rigid Internal Fixation. Clin. Orthop., 81:165–170, 1971.

495. Uhthoff, H.K.: Mechanical Factors Influencing the Holding Power of Screws in Compact Bone. J. Bone Joint Surg., 55B:633–639, 1973.

496. Uhthoff, H.K. (ed): Current Concepts of Internal Fixation. New York, Springer-Verlag, 1980.
497. Uhthoff, H.K.: Current Concepts of Internal Fixation of Fractures. Can. J. Surg., 23(3):213–214, 1980.
498. Uhthoff, H.K.: Internal Fixation of Long Bone Fractures: Concepts, Controversies, Debates (Interview by Elvira Stahl). Can. Med. Assoc. J., 149(6):837–841, 1993.
499. Uhthoff, H.K.; Bardos, D.I.; and Liskova-Kiar, M.: The Advantages of Titanium Alloy Over Stainless Steel Plates for the Internal Fixation of Fractures. An Experimental Study in Dogs. J. Bone Joint Surg. 63B:427–84, 1981.
500. van Loon, T., and Marti, R.K.: A Fracture of the Intercondylar Eminence of the Tibia Treated by Arthroscopic Fixation (Published Erratum Appears in Arthroscopy 8(2):278, 1992). Arthroscopy, 7(4):385–388, 1991.
501. van Niekerk, J.L., and Schoots, F.J.: Femoral Shaft Fractures Treated With Plate Fixation and Interlocked Nailing: A Comparative Retrospective Study. Injury, 23(4):219–222, 1992.
502. Vander Griend, R.A.: The Effect of Internal Fixation on the Healing of Large Allografts. J. Bone Joint Surg. Am., 76(5):657–663, 1994.
503. Velazco, A., Whitesides, T.A., Jr., and Fleming, L.L.: Open Fractures of the Tibia Treated With the Lottes Nail. J. Bone Joint Surg., 65A:879–885, 1983.
504. Wang, G.J.; Reger, S.I., Jennings, R.L.; Mclaurin, C.A.; and Stamp, W.G.: Variable Strengths of the Wire Fixation. Orthopedics, 5(4):435–436, 1981.
505. Wang, G.J.; Reger, S.I., Mabie, K.N.; Richman, J.A.; and Stamp, W.G.: Semirigid Rod Fixation for Long-Bone Fracture. Clin. Orthop., 192:291–298, 1985.
506. Watson, J.A., and Hollingdale, J.P.: Early Management of Displaced Ankle Fractures. Injury, 23(2):87–88. 1992.
507. Weber, B.G., and Cech, O.: Pseudarthrosis, p. 323. Bern, Hans Huber, 1976.
508. Weber, T.G., and Mast, J.W.: The Extended Ilioinguinal Approach for Specific Both Column Fractures. Clin. Orthop., 305:106–111, 1994.
509. Webster, D.A., and Murray, D.G.: Complications of Variable Axis Total Knee Arthroplasty. Clin. Orthop., 193:160–167, 1985.
510. Weisband, I.D.: Tension-Band Wiring Technique for Treatment of Olecranon Fractures. J. Am. Osteopath. Assoc., 77(5):390–392, 1978.
511. Weise, K.; Grosse, B.; Hoffmann, J.; and Sauer, N.: Results of Treatment of 475 Second- and Third-Degree Open Fractures of Long Tubular Bones (1974–1988). Aktuel Traumatol, 1:2–20, 1993.
512. Whitehill, R.; Stowers, S.F.; Fechner, R.E.; *et al.*: Posterior Cervical Fusions Using Cerclage Wires, Methylmethacrylate Cement and Autogenous Bone Graft. An Experimental Study of a Canine Model. Spine, 12(1):12–22, 1987.
513. Whitelaw, G.P.; Cimino, W.G.; and Segal, D.: The Treatment of Open Tibial Fractures Using Nonreamed Flexible Intramedullary Fixation. Orthop Rev, 19(3):244–256, 1990.
514. Wilde, A.H.; Schickendantz, M.S.; Stulberg, B.N.; and Go, R.T.: The Incorporation of Tibial Allografts in Total Knee Arthroplasty. J. Bone Joint Surg. 72A(6):815–24, 1990.
515. Wildner, M.; Peters, A.; Hellich, J.; and Reichelt, A.: Complications of High Tibial Osteotomy and Internal Fixation With Staples. Arch. Orthop. Trauma Surg., 111(4):210–212, 1992.
516. Winkelmann, H.P.; Muhlich, S.; and Schmidt, M.: Normal Variants of Tibial Arteries—Anastomotic Problems in Microvascular Tissue Transfer. Aktuelle Traumatol, 24(3):99–100, 1994.
517. Winquist, R.A., and Hansen, S.T., Jr.: Comminuted Fractures of the Femoral Shaft Treated by Intramedullary Nailing. Orthop. Clin. North Am., 11:633–648, 1980.
518. Wiss, D.A.; Brien, W.W.; and Becker, V., Jr.: Interlocking Nailing for the Treatment of Femoral Fractures Due to Gunshot Wounds. J. Bone Joint Surg. 73A(4):598–606, 1991.
519. Wissing, J.C., and van der Werken, C: Tension Band Osteosynthesis of Resorbable Material. Unfallchirurg, 94(1):45–46, 1991.
520. Withrow, S.J.: Use and Misuse of Full Cerclage Wires in Fracture Repair. Vet. Clin. North Am., 8(2):201–212, 1978.
521. Wolfgang, G.; Burke, F.; Bush, D.; Parenti, J.; Perry, J.; LaFollette, B.; and Lillmars, S.: Surgical Treatment of Displaced Olecranon Fractures by Tension Band Wiring Technique. Clin. Orthop., 224:192–204, 1987.
522. Woo, S.L.; Lothringer, K.S.; Akeson, W.H.; Coutts, R.D.; Woo, Y.K.; Simon, B.R.; and Gomez, M.A.: Less Rigid Internal Fixation Plates: Historical Perspectives and New Concepts. J. Orthop. Res., 1(4):431–449, 1984.
523. Woo, S.L.; Simon, B.R.; Akeson, W.H.; Gomez, M.A.; and Seguchi, Y.: A New Approach to the Design of Internal Fixation Plates. J. Biomed. Mater. Res., 17(3):427–439, 1983.
524. Woo, S.L.; Simon, B.R.; Akeson, W.H.; and McCarty, M.P.: An Interdisciplinary Approach to Evaluate the Effect of Internal Fixation Plate on Long Bone Remodeling. J. Biomech., 10(2):87–95, 1977.
525. Wood, E.G.; Savoie, F.H.; and vander Griend, R.A.: Treatment of Ipsilateral Fractures of the Distal Femur and Femoral Shaft. J. Orthop. Trauma, 5(2):177–183, 1991.
526. Woodard, P.L.; Self, J.; Calhoun, J.; Tencer, A.F.; and Evans, E.B.: The Effect of Implant Axial and Torsional Stiffness on Fracture Healing. J. Orthop. Trauma, 1:331–340, 1987.
527. Wozasek, G.E., and Moser, K.D.: Percutaneous Screw Fixation for Fractures of the Scaphoid (Published Erratum Appears in J. Bone Joint Surg. May;73B(3):524, 1991). J. Bone Joint Surg. Br., 73(1): p. 138–142, 1991.
528. Wu, C.C., and Shih, C.H.: Biomechanical Analysis of the Mechanism of Interlocking Nail Failure. Arch. Orthop. Trauma. Surg., 111(5):268–272, 1992.
529. Wu, C.C., and Shih, C.H.: Treatment for Nonunion of the Shaft of the Humerus: Comparison of Plates and Seidel Interlocking Nails (see comments). Can. J. Surg., 35(6):661–665, 1992.
530. Wu, C.C.; Shih, C.H.; Ueng, W.N.; and Chen, Y.J.: Treatment of Segmental Femoral Shaft Fractures. Clin. Orthop., 287:224–230, 1993.
531. Yelton, C., and Low, W.: Latrogenic Subtrochanteric Fracture: A Complication of Zickel Nails. J. Bone Joint Surg., 68A: 1237–1240, 1986.
532. Yerys, P.: Arthroscopic Posterior Cruciate Ligament Repair. Arthroscopy, 7(1):111–114, 1991.
533. Yoshimine, F.; Latta, L.L.; and Milne, E.L.: Sliding Characteristics of Compression Hip Screws in the Intertrochanteric Fracture: A Clinical Study. J. Orthop. Trauma, 7(4):348–353, 1993.
534. Young, M.J., and Barrack, R.L.: Complications of Internal Fixation of Tibial Plateau Fractures. Orthop. Rev., 23(2):149–154, 1994.
535. Zehntner, M.K.; Petropoulos, P. and Burch, H.: Factors Determining Outcome in Fractures of the Extremities Associated With Arterial Injuries. J. Orthop. Trauma, 5(1):29–33, 1991.
536. Zuckerman, J.D.; Veith, R.G.; Johnson, K.D.; Bach, A.W.; Hansen, S.T.; and Solvik, S.: Treatment of Unstable Femoral Shaft Fractures With Closed Interlocking Intramedullary Nailing. J. Orthop. Trauma, 1:209–218, 1987.

Rockwood and Green's Fractures in Adults, Fourth Edition,
edited by Charles A. Rockwood, David P. Green, Robert W. Bucholz and James D. Heckman.
Lippincott-Raven Publishers, Philadelphia © 1996.

CHAPTER 4

External Fixation

James V. Nepola

'' 'Wish' the fragments into place and hold them there by 'moral suasion' and send the patient on about his business while the fracture heals.''

—Clay Ray Murray, MD.[86]

External fixation is the process of manipulating, aligning, and stabilizing bony structures with pins, wires, screws, or other bone fasteners that affix the bone to an external scaffold or frame.

HISTORY

Although other authors have begun treatises about external fixation with reference to the works of Malgaigne or Hippocrates, the first modern version of an external fixator was developed by Clayton Parkhill of Denver. Dr. Parkhill began his medical education at Jefferson Medical College in Philadelphia and ultimately became Professor of Surgery and Dean of the Medical School at the University of Colorado. In 1897, he presented the American College of Surgery with findings based on his initial experience with an early fixator he had designed.[96] Before he could popularize his device, however, Parkhill died of appendicitis at age 42, while serving as a Medical Officer during the Spanish American War. After the unfortunate and untimely death of this surgical innovator, further development of external fixation was concentrated in Europe.

Albin Lambotte is most often credited with designing the first true external fixator, even though his report on this device in 1906 came roughly a decade after Parkhill's presentation.[69] Parkhill and Lambotte never met, nor did they ever see each other's devices. Nevertheless, their versions of the external fixator look quite similar. Both are unilateral and allow for two sets of screws to be fixed to each bone fragment. Also, the screw clusters in both devices are connected by a simple adjustable frame (Figs. 4-1 and 4-2).

Various forms of external fixation that were later developed followed these early pioneers' inventions. In 1934, Roger Anderson, a surgeon from Seattle, devised a frame with transfixion pins. This device was initially designed for use with a cast that incorporated the pins for added limb support. Later, the device was refined to act as a primary means of fixation without splinting.[1] In 1937, Otto Stader, a veterinarian, further improved upon Anderson's concept by introducing a threaded adjustment bar that allowed for distraction or compression across the fracture site.[108]

External fixation devices quickly became popular with young military surgeons at the outset of World War II. The armed forces accordingly bought substantial quantities of external fixation equipment. However, it quickly became evident that when it was used by civilian surgeons with only brief training in external fixation, complications were prevalent. In November 1943, the use of this technique was restricted to ". . . carefully selected cases, only in special indications and only by surgeons trained and experienced in its application."[33] Difficulties with pinhole osteomyelitis and delayed union resulting from distraction of fractures continued. In 1944, this led the United States Surgeon General Maj. Gen. Norman T. Kirk, an orthopaedic surgeon himself, to ban the use of the technique in most war-zone medical facilities, much as he had previously banned the use of acute internal fixation.[32]

In Europe, however, such devices continued to be popular. Raoul Hoffmann, whom Vidal[118] described as "a surgeon, doctor of theology, and a master carpenter," designed a versatile device that is still used today. Vidal and Adrey refined the Hoffman system further by using multiplanar frames to increase rigidity.[117,119] The resulting Hoffman-Vidal system firmly established external fixation in the armamentarium of modern orthopaedic surgeons (Fig. 4-3).

In the 1970s, prompted by a surge of interest in external fixation, Giovanni De Bastiani of Verona, Italy, introduced an improved design he called a "dynamic axial fixator." Having extensively studied the work of Hoffman and Vidal, De Bastiani was well aware of the principal drawback in their design: the tendency for the Hoffman-Vidal system's rigid, static frame to distract and thwart union (hence, its nickname—the "nonunion machine"). De Bastiani's new design, based on a unilateral, robust frame, combined the simplicity and strength of Wagner's unilateral leg lengthening device with a telescopic, "dynamizable" fixator body. To facilitate union, the telescopic portion of De Bastiani's frame can be unlocked to provide "dynamic compression" by allowing the bone fragments to slide together. Since the introduction of the dynamic axial fixator in 1979, a number of unilateral

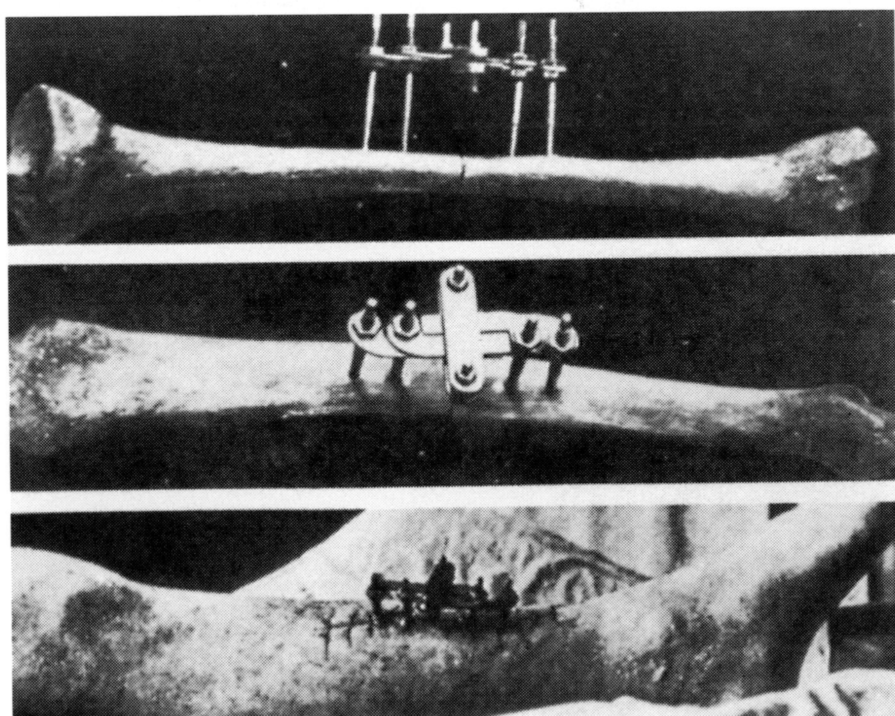

FIGURE 4-1. Views of the external skeletal fixation device of Parkhill. (Parkhill, C. A New Apparatus for the Fixation of Bones after Resection and in Fractures with a Tendency to Displacement. Trans. Am. Surg. Assoc., 15:251—256, 1897.)

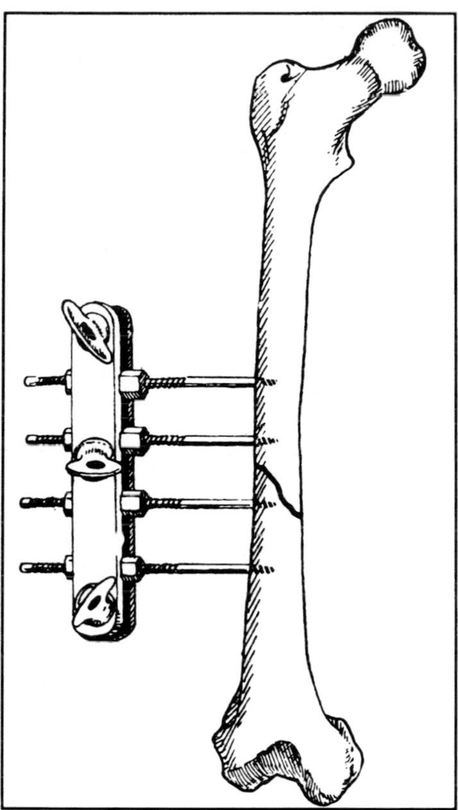

FIGURE 4-2. Lambotte's initial device. (Lambotte, A. L'Intervention Operatoire dans les Fractures Recentes et Anciennes, p. 60. Brussels, Henri Lamertin, 1907.)

dynamizable fixators have been developed, each designed to permit a degree of micromotion at the fracture or osteotomy site (Fig. 4-4).[40]

In 1951, Gavrijl Abramovich Ilizarov began his work with distraction osteogenesis techniques at what became the Pan-Soviet Scientific Center for Traumatology and Rehabilitation Orthopaedics in Kurgan, Siberia. For years, his work remained hidden behind the Soviet Union's iron curtain. But in 1980, Professor Ilizarov treated a visiting Italian explorer Carlo Mauri for an infected nonunion of the tibia. On Mauri's return to Italy, accounts of his treatment in Russia quickly circulated in the medical community, prompting Italian surgeons to invite Ilizarov to the XXII Italian AO Meeting in 1981.[72] This meeting eventually led to the collaboration of a group of Italian orthopaedic surgeons with Professor Ilizarov's clinic and the dissemination of knowledge about the technique known as distraction osteogenesis or the "Ilizarov Method." This method has become a significant part of the orthopaedic surgeon's armamentarium. It allows orthopaedic surgeons to reconstruct large defects in bone and to salvage limbs previously treated with extensive and sometimes multiple bone grafting procedures, fibular transfer techniques, or ultimately amputation. Although it was previously thought loathsome to extensively and aggressively debride open fracture wounds, surgeons with the ability to reconstruct large bony defects now have a renewed conviction to aggressively debride in cases of open injury.

Interestingly, the earliest record of distraction osteogenesis techniques may be attributed to Professor Alessandro Codivilla (1861–1912) of Bologna, Italy who used skeletal traction techniques after osteotomy to produce femoral lengthening.[34]

Currently, the variety of systems designed for external fixation is increasing. Each system incorporates more modern engineering principles and is fabricated to address specific problems of stabilizing and maintaining the pin/bone interface. For example, hybrid

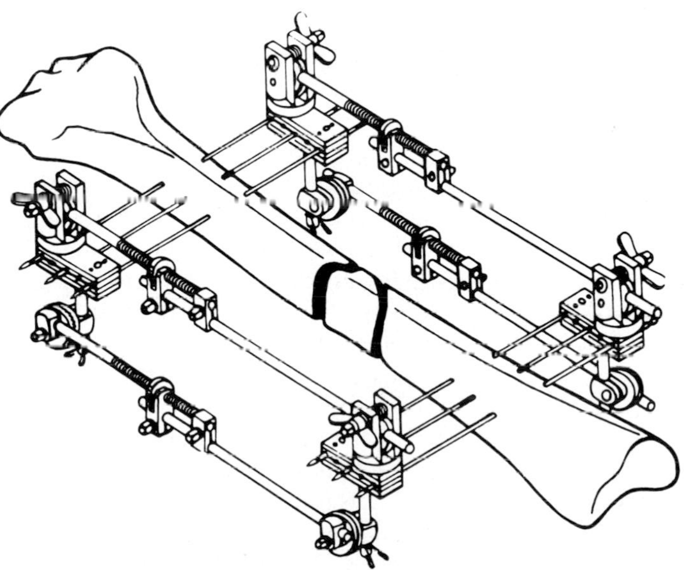

FIGURE 4-3. Complete quadrilateral tibial frame (Hoffmann). *(Connes, H.: Hoffmann's External Anchorage, Edition GEAD, Paris, 1977.)*

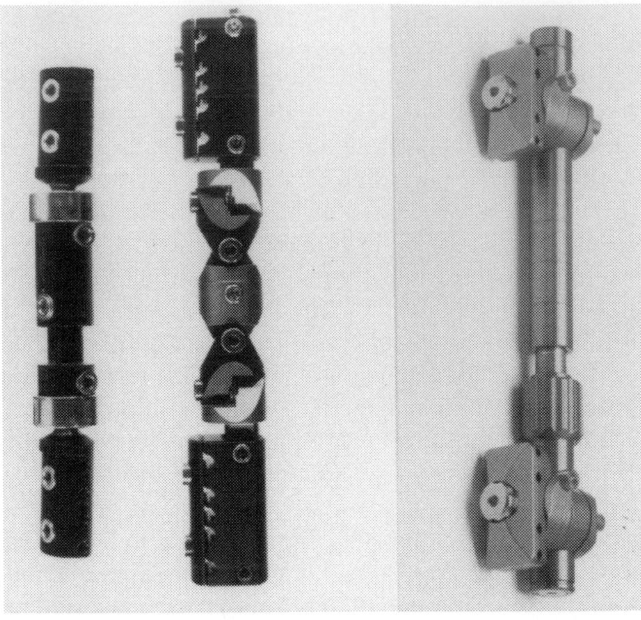

FIGURE 4-4. Stable unilateral "Maxifixators" have recently become popular. Shown are the Orthofix, Dynafix and Monotube (courtesy of Orthofix, EBI Inc., and Howmedica.)

devices that can be used to fixate complex, comminuted fractures with small metaphyseal fragments have been produced by welding unilateral half-pin frames to circular-ring tensioned-wire components (Fig. 4-5).[72] At the same time, developments in composite technology are leading to the use of radiolucent frames to enable easier radiographic evaluation of externally fixated limbs. Most recently, advances in the understanding of bone healing have led researchers to pursue the development of fixators that allow for prescribed amounts of micromotion to encourage bone healing.

FRACTURE HEALING FOLLOWING EXTERNAL FIXATION

While the early history of external fixation was characterized by clinical experiences involving numerous empirically designed hardware systems, the modern era is marked by a growing effort to generate scientifically tested hypotheses that strengthen the clinical foundations for using this technique.

The successful use of external fixation systems, like all stabilization techniques, requires an understanding of the fundamental principles of both fracture healing and the biomechanics of bone fixation. Current knowledge in these areas has underscored the uniqueness of every fracture and the need to customize the stabilization techniques for each individual injury. The one-size-fits-all mentality that frequently pervades the marketing of a technique or device is no longer acceptable.

There are basically two types of fracture healing—union through *external periosteal callus* and *primary bone healing* also known as in situ fracture remodeling. Fracture callus forms in reaction to the disruption of the periosteum and endosteum combined with the interfragmentary strain or motion associated with a bone injury. Callus bridges the fracture fragments and acts as both a stabilizing structural framework and the biological substrate that provides the cellular material for union and remodeling. In 1949, Danis recognized the phenomenon of primary healing in which fractures that are rigidly stabilized to prevent significant interfragmentary motion achieve a callusless union.[39] Such injuries primarily remodel across contact points and minute fracture gaps. Remodeling, however, takes time. In fact, the rigid plates may not be safely removed from diaphyses until 12 to 18 months after fixation. Even then, refractures after removal of rigid implants are not uncommon.[109] Thus, rigid fixation will not only preclude the development of callus; it will also typically result in a protracted, biomechanical depen-

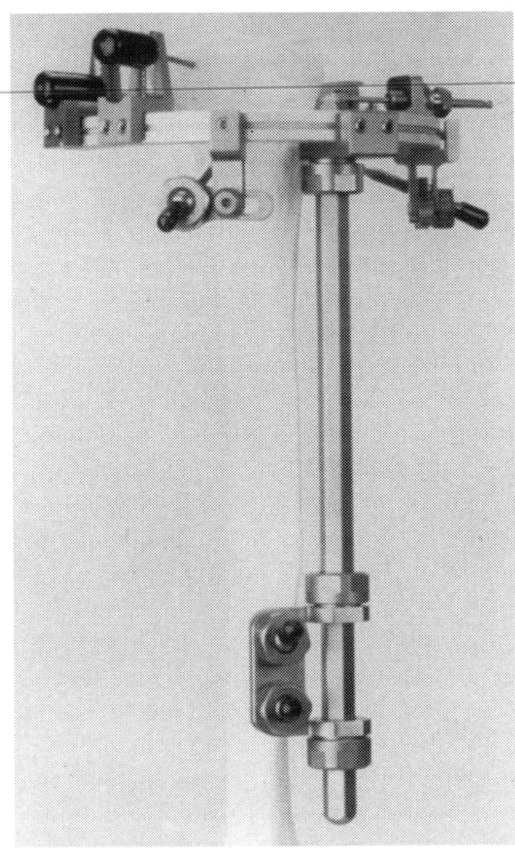

FIGURE 4-5. "Hybrid" frame with metaphyseal tensioned-wire circular-ring fixation coupled to a unilateral $^1/_2$ pin/screw fixator. (Courtesy of Zimmer Corp.)

dency of the bone-hardware construct on the fixation system itself before adequate remodeling of the bone allows for safe removal of the implant. This principle has an important bearing on the external fixation technique.

In an attempt to reproduce plate-like stability, early external fixation systems stressed the need for increasingly rigid frames in multiplanar configurations. Adjunctive interfragmentary screws were often used to increase construct stability. (Fig. 4-6) Although these rigid constructs did occasionally yield an anatomic restoration, it is now known that these techniques may have actually delayed or prevented union. While early treatment algorithms taught that external fixators were to be removed 6 weeks after application to avoid the complication of pin-track infection, the early shift from a rigid fixator construct (promoting primary healing) to a cast or brace presupposed that the fracture would have the intrinsic stability to sustain functional load bearing of the limb.

Because of the absence of callus formation, primary bone healing, whether promoted through rigid plating or rigid external fixation, requires the fracture to be supported and protected until the bone achieves sufficient strength to prevent refracture or angulation when it is once again subjected to functional stresses. Before adequate fracture remodeling, refracture may occur with a loss of reduction. A rigid external fixator that eliminates micromotion must be kept in place longer and necessarily requires prolonged maintenance of the fixator pin/bone interface.

At the time any external fixator is applied, a "race" begins between fracture healing and fixator pin failure (due to infection, loosening, etc.). External fixation depends, of course, on proper fixation of the screws, pins, or wires to the bone. Techniques that rely on frame constructs that are too rigid, and therefore require prolonged pin fixation and frame maintenance, will often fail because the fracture cannot adequately remodel by the time the pins loosen and the fixator must be removed.

In light of contemporary interfragmentary strain theories about fracture healing, current external fixation systems have been designed to allow micromotion at the fracture site to promote callus formation. Stable yet less rigid systems of external fixation maintain alignment and length while allowing and actually encouraging beneficial micromotion. By incorporating the concept of dynamization to gradually increase loading and micromotion at the fracture site without sacrificing reduction, new external fixation techniques have met with encouraging clinical results.[41]

Dynamization

The term *dynamization* describes the conversion of an external fixator or any fracture implant from a statically locked device to a more load-sharing one to promote micromotion at the fracture site. Richardson and co-workers identified two types of dynamization.[99] The first is characterized by *progressive closure* of the fracture gap by using telescopic components to promote bone contact at the fracture site (Fig. 4-7). The second type of dynamization refers to a *cyclic* movement at the fracture site. This cyclic strain can be imparted through the actual elastic deformation of the frame or through fixation wires or special components incorporated within the frame to promote spring-like

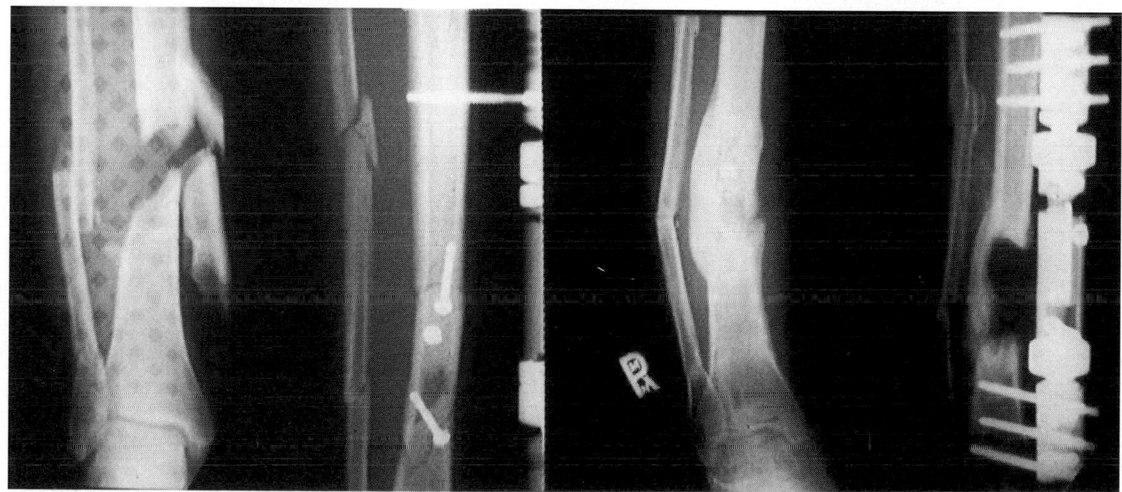

FIGURE 4-6. Although appealing, the use of combined internal "lag screws" and external fixation for diaphyseal fractures has a high incidence of refracture and infection. A 21-year-old motorcyclist sustained an open tibial injury and subsequently had this fixation. At 3 months postinjury, the fragment has been excised because of infection.

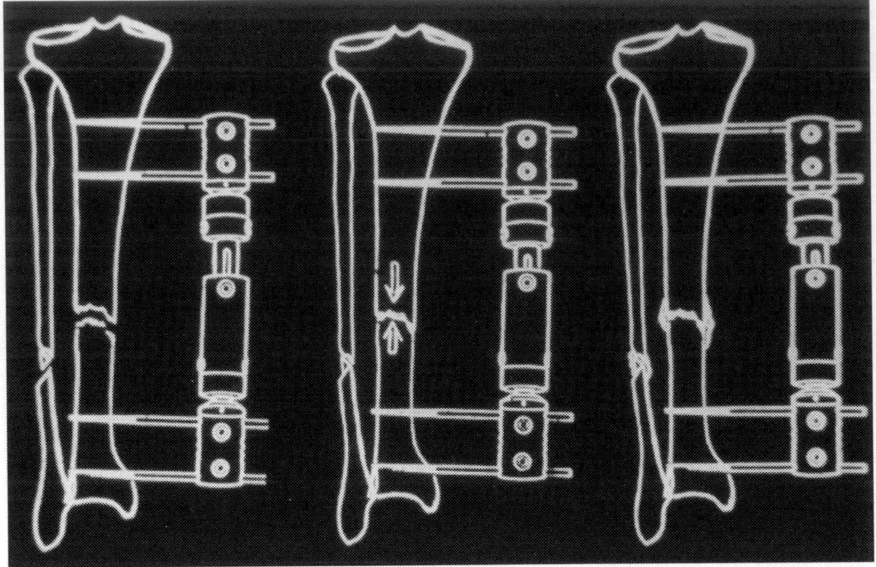

FIGURE 4-7. Progressive closure-type dynamization is achieved by sliding a telescopic component of the fixator body, approximating bone ends and avoiding the distraction associated with nonunion.

movement with weight bearing. In current practice, dynamization is usually recommended after the initial stages of fracture healing. In theory, it might be better to prescribe controlled cyclic dynamization during early phases of fracture healing to promote callus. This would be followed by *closure-type* dynamization to provide dynamic compression with weight bearing. Closure-type dynamization allows the approximation of fractured bone ends, eliminating gaps that can be created by initial overdistraction and resorption at the fracture site. Closure avoids the chronic overdistraction which has given rise to the misnomer "nonunion machine." This controlled load sharing helps to "work harden" the fracture callus and accelerate remodeling. As with a hypertrophic nonunion, once the early callus has been established, compression and stability at the fracture site promote maturation of the union.

Micromotion

Many researchers have studied the salutary effects of microstrain or micromotion on fracture healing.[42,71] In 1979, Burny advocated the concept of *flexible external fixation* to promote callus formation and enhance fracture healing.[24] This fixation method relied on elastic fixator frames to permit loading of the fracture fragments. Kenwright and Goodship have extensively studied imposed micromotion.[50] They performed experiments using an externally fixed sheep tibial osteotomy model. The fixator was adapted to permit daily controlled reciprocal micromovement of approximately 0.5 mm at relatively physiological loads for 1 hour a day. The resulting enhanced callus formation and accelerated healing clearly support the association between imposed microstrain and improved fracture healing (Fig. 4-8). Kenwright and colleagues applied a similar technique in a clinical trial at the Nuffield Orthopaedic Center and the Bristol Royal Infirmary in England. Tibial fracture patients treated with external fixation were randomized to either a cyclic dynamization or static fixed mode of treatment. Fractures treated with early controlled micromotion of 1-mm axial displacement at 0.5 Hz for 20 minutes daily healed much more quickly than those that were rigidly stabilized.[64]

Aro and coworkers studied functional closure-type dynamization using a telescoping frame external fixator on a canine osteotomy model. These experiments demonstrated more uniform callus distribution around the fracture site, but minimal acceleration of fracture healing time with dynamization.[2] Notably however, this study showed that passive dynamization resulted in a significant decrease in fixator screw loosening. Clinical studies on the external fixation treatment support this contention.[11] It appears that dynamization of the external fixation frame allows load transfer to the bone and off the pin, screw, or wire/bone interface. This off-loading of fixator pins decreases loosening and allows longer fixator treatment periods. This theory might explain the decreased rates of pin-track loosening and infection reported by De Bastiani and other proponents of the closure dynamization method.[76,83] The prevention of loosening by off-loading the fixator pins/screws/wires may thereby minimize problems, such as malunion and nonunion, associated with premature fixator removal.

Circular-ring and tensioned-wire (Ilizarov) fixation systems allow a degree of axial micromotion through

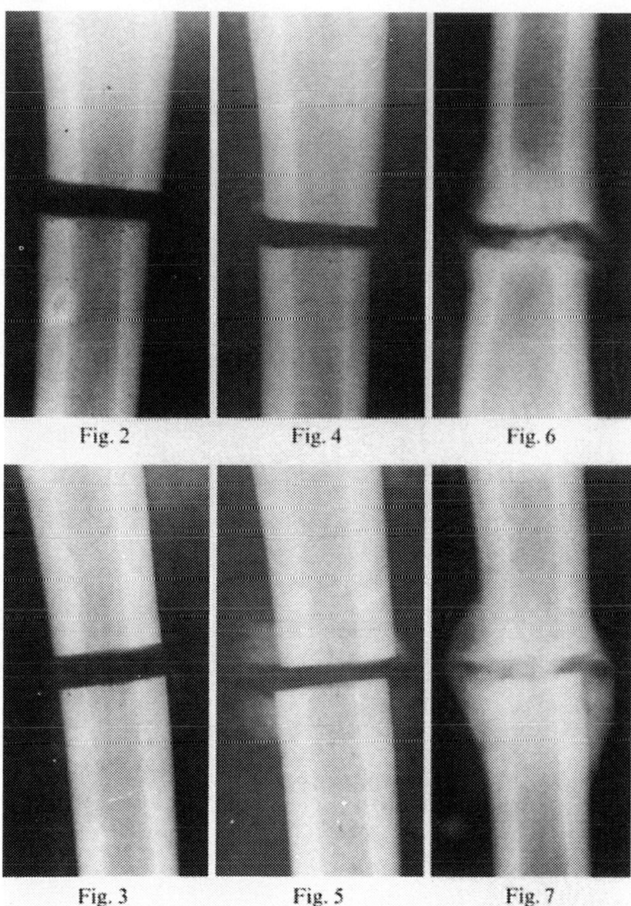

FIGURE 4-8. These radiographs show the osteotomy of two sheep at various stages of healing. Those on the top depict the rigidly fixed case and those on the bottom depict the applied micromovement case. Two weeks after operation 4 and 5 show external callus in the stimulated group and its inhibition in the rigidly fixed group. In 6 and 7, 10 weeks after operation, the difference in healing patterns is visible, with immature radiological bridging in the rigidly fixed group.[50]

the spring-like elastic deformation of the Kirschner wires. The repetitive loading associated with weight bearing imparts a form of cyclic loading to the bone fragments that are stabilized with the tensioned wires. The degree of micromotion is effected accordingly by the wire diameter, number, and tension.

The Ilizarov-type frames have mechanical stability characteristics that are similar to other external fixators in terms of medial-lateral bending, antero-posterior bending, and torsion. However, they are distinguished from other unilateral screw/pin bar constructs by this wire flexibility that allows axial cyclic dynamization.[26,68]

Unfortunately, although much is understood about the relative stability of different fixator systems and configurations, the ideal prescription for mechanical conditions that enhance fracture healing is not known. Research is ongoing to determine the proper magnitude, frequency, and timing of strain on fracture fragments to optimize healing.

EXTERNAL FIXATION COMPONENT MECHANICS

Fasteners

External fixation frames are fastened to bone using pins, screws, tension wires, or in some cases, tongs that are then affixed to frames. These fasteners may be considered transfixion or unilateral half-pin devices. Half-pins do not pass entirely through the limb, but simply cross both cortices of the bone through the soft tissue on one side. This avoids the problems associated with transfixion pins or wires which increase the risks of neurovascular compromise and myotendonous tethering (Fig. 4-9).

In principle, the most significant parameter that affects the stability of an external fixation system is the radius of the pin or screw. The bending stiffness of the pin increases as a function of the fourth power of the radius of that implant. Manufacturers have used this knowledge to create larger-diameter half-pin fixators that offer greater stability and eliminate the need for transfixion hardware.

Care must be taken to limit the diameter of any screw hole to no greater than 30% of the diameter of the diaphysis (Fig. 4-10). To exceed this significantly weakens the bone, effectively creating an open section. It has been shown that a hole greater than 30% of the diameter markedly increases the risk of fracture.[81] Burstein and colleagues demonstrated that a screw hole equal to 30% of the diameter weakened the torsional strength of that bone by 45%.[25] Over 6 to 8 weeks, the bone will remodel about the implant, restoring its strength. However, upon removal of the screw, the weakening recurs until the bone has remod-

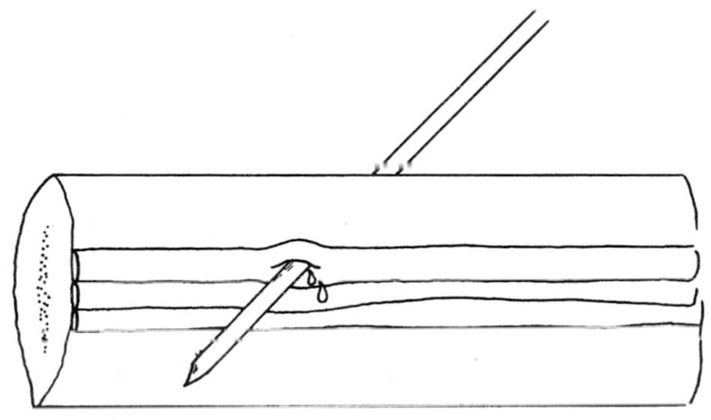

FIGURE 4-9. Transfixion pins can injure juxtaposed neurovascular structures. Care must be taken to consider the cross-sectional anatomy of any area coursed by these implants.

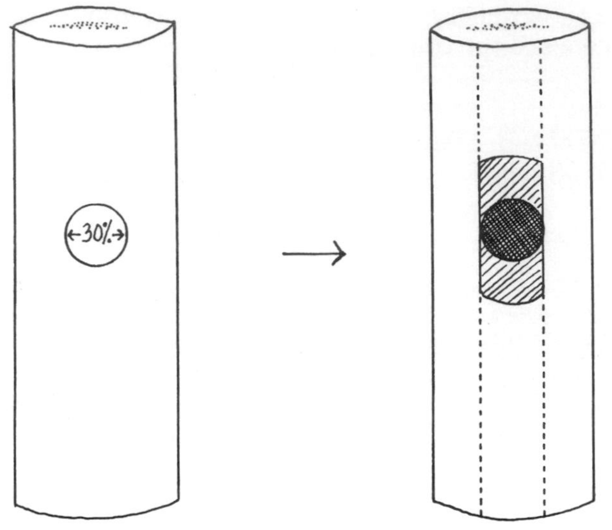

FIGURE 4-10. Holes greater than 30% of the diameter of the diaphysis markedly weaken the bone, rendering it essentially equivalent to an "open section."

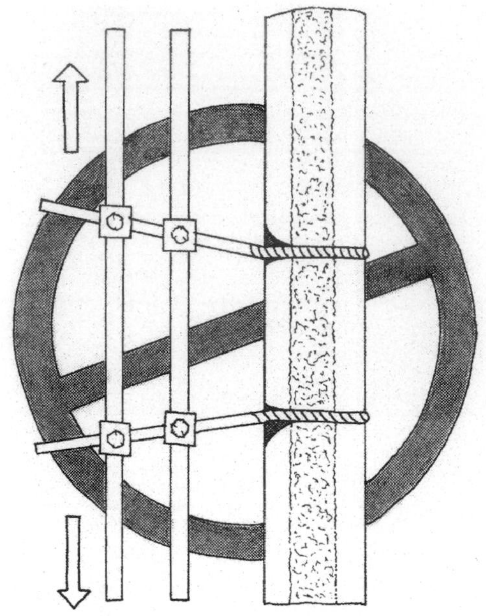

FIGURE 4-11. Bending preload is associated with accelerated implant loosening and is not recommended.

eled once more. This consideration is particularly important when treating pediatric populations with gracile bones and older patients with more brittle bone.

Screw design has concentrated on the development of implants with a greater core or root diameter to increase rigidity. In the past, some screw designs offered only a short threaded portion, based on the recommendation that the threads should only be engaged in the far cortex, leaving the thicker more rigid shank in the entry-side cortex. Because this technique was associated clinically with an increased rate of implant loosening, current recommendations favor stiffer, larger root-diameter screws with bicortical threads for better purchase and decreased loosening characteristics.

Early fixator users recommended a technique called *bending preload* (Fig. 4-11).[120] This would theoretically reduce pin loosening by allowing the elastically loaded implant to maintain three-point bending contact. Animal studies, however, have suggested that the bending preload technique actually accelerates loosening because of rapid pressure necrosis on the compression side of the preloaded pin.[59] Therefore, bending preload is discouraged.

Current theory recommends *radial preload* to improve screw fixation and prevent loosening. This can be achieved either by first drilling a pilot hole slightly smaller than the root diameter of the screw or by using a tapered root-diameter screw design to produce a radial preload as the screw is introduced (Fig. 4-12). Hydahl and coworkers demonstrated in animal studies that radial preload is preferable to bending preload techniques.[59]

Enlarging the shank diameter of screws or pins has been shown to increase the overall rigidity of the implant which, in turn, results in lower bending stresses at the entry site cortex and in a diminished rate of osteolysis and loosening.[29]

Reduction

The composite stability of the bone-fixator construct is the most important factor in treating fractures with external fixation. Fracture configuration and reduction profoundly affect stresses at the pin/bone interface. End-on-end transverse or other stably reduced fracture constructs maintained with external fixation have been shown in both in vitro and in vivo testing

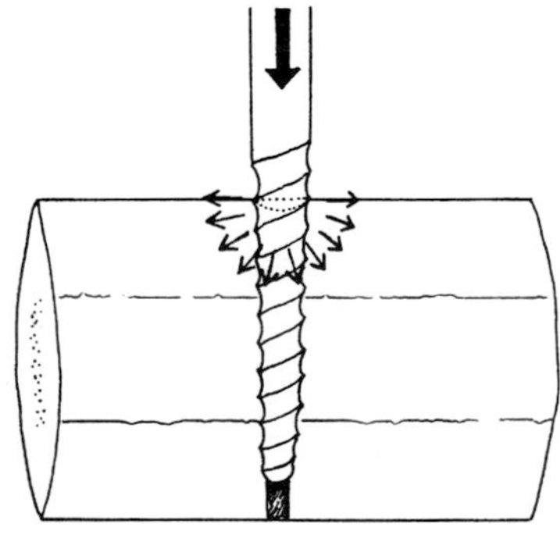

FIGURE 4-12. Radial preload of fixator screws may be imparted by using conical tapered-root implants as seen here or by predrilling with drill bits slightly smaller than the core diameter of the screw thread.

to reduce stresses at the pin/bone interface. This results in decreased rates of pin loosening. As demonstrated by Chao and Aro, bone-fixator constructs without bone-end contact, and those with very oblique (unstable) fracture patterns, tend to have increased rates of pin loosening and a longer healing time when compared with stably reduced transverse fractures with good bone-end contact.[3] This underscores the benefits of creating a stable, yet not necessarily rigid, fracture construct whenever possible when using external fixation.

Insertion Technique

The insertion technique may have mechanical effects on the initial screw/pin purchase as well as a profound biological influence on the maintenance of the implant-bone interface. The insertion of self-drilling screws has been associated with microfracture and high temperatures at the bone implant interface.[78] Thermal necrosis often results. The tensioned Kirschner wires used with circular-ring external fixation techniques are prone to thermal necrosis when inserted in harder diaphyseal bone. To reduce the potential for both thermal necrosis and the premature loosening associated with it (Fig. 4-13), an alternative technique that involves predrilling pilot holes for all screw or pin sites is now recommended to minimize microfracture and avoid excessive bone temperatures.

Unfortunately, predrilling Kirschner wires used in circular-ring tensioned-wire systems is not feasible. These wires are designed for self-drilling. Although the tips of such implants are engineered with special cutting ends to decrease thermal necrosis, they still generate significant heat upon insertion and should be cooled with saline as they are drilled into the bone. This is particularly important when drilling cortical bone. In cancellous bone, this is not as important, and wires can often be malleted into place to avoid the heat associated with drilling. Many surgeons have converted to threaded half-screws for diaphyseal fixation when using Ilizarov frames. Special coupling clamps have been designed to allow fixation of such half-screws to the circular-ring frames.[54]

Screw/Pin Materials

Chao and Aro advocate the use of high modulus materials in screw or pin design to minimize bending and thereby decrease loosening.[29] Others, however, believe that using more isoelastic materials, such as titanium alloy, improves loosening rates. This issue remains controversial.

Precious metals, such as gold and silver, have long been known to inhibit bacterial growth. It has been suggested that coating fixator pins with gold or silver might pin-track infection. Limited laboratory and clinical studies have indicated decreased pin-track infection rates when coated pins are used.[35] However, such implants are not clinically available.

Tensioned-Wire/Circular-Ring Fasteners

The Ilizarov tensioned-wire/ring method of fastening bone to the frame uses narrow-gauge 1.5- to 1.8-mm Kirschner wires under tension across circular and hemicircular rings to provide fixation. The thin wires produce minimal soft-tissue reaction. They also lend themselves to affixing smaller metaphyseal fragments with multiple wires as opposed to more rigid larger half-pins, which tend to loosen in cancellous bone and may fracture smaller fragments. Additionally, the trampoline effect of the more elastic wires achieves the cyclic-loading type of dynamization mentioned earlier.

However, tensioned wires have all the disadvantages of any transfixion implant. Soft-tissue impalement and tethering is a significant problem. The self-drilling Kirschner wires tend to produce elevated insertion temperatures in diaphyseal bone. As a result, many surgeons use thin wires only in metaphyseal areas about the knee and ankle where percutaneous placement in subcutaneous bone need not involve the more vulnerable myotendonous or neurovascular structures

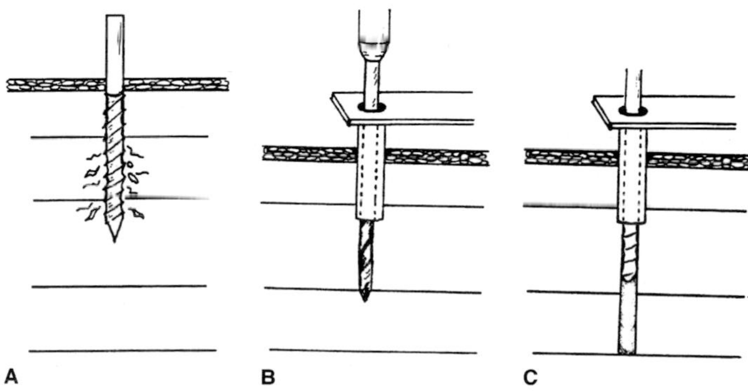

FIGURE 4-13. (**A**) Self-drilling screws tend to generate heat and microfracture during insertion. (**B**) Predrilling screw holes with a sharp drill helps minimize heat generation and bone damage. (**C**) Self-tapping screws may then be introduced without thermal necrosis and microfracture.

in the mid-leg and thigh. The Ilizarov frames have been made compatible with half-pin fixator screws through hybrid components such as the Green's Rancho cube. This allows the circular-ring fixator and its unique advantages in complex deformities and injuries to be coupled with diaphyseal half-pin implants, solving the problems associated with standard transfixion hardware. Similarly, some unilateral half-pin fixators now have attachments that permit fixation with ring components.

The stability of thin-wire fixation may depend on several variables. Increasing wire tension or wire diameter and decreasing the diameter of the ring all enhance fixation stability. In a biomechanical analysis, Gasser and associates determined that increasing wire diameter from 1.6 mm to 2.0 mm and increasing wire tension from 600 to 1200 units improved axial stiffness of a basic Ilizarov frame by 10% and bending stiffness by almost 3%.[48]

Tensile wire strength increases as a function of the square of the diameter. A biomechanically important parameter for tensioned wires is the *yield point*. This is the point at which the wire plastically deforms or permanently stretches in tension. Because it reduces the overall strength of the wire, plastic deformation can seriously compromise the stability of the construct. The yield point for typical Kirschner wires has been measured at 120 kg/mm^2, which equals 210 kg for 1.5-mm wires and 305 kg for 1.8-mm wires.[91]

Paley has characterized the optimal wire tension as no greater than 50% of the yield strength of the wire, which equals 105 kg for 1.5-mm wire and 150 kg for 1.8-mm wire.[91] Ilizarov has recommended 80 to 90 kg of tension for most trauma applications. Others prefer higher tensions: 90 kg for half-rings and 130 kg for full-ring applications.

Paley has estimated that in cases of limb lengthening, wire tension can be increased by up to 50 kg during distraction.[91] This extra load must be added to the load of initial wire pretensioning. Therefore, at application for limb lengthening, it would be prudent to pretension the wires at lower levels (80–90 kg) to allow for the possibility of increased stress associated with the lengthening procedure. This has been suggested by Paley and other proponents of the Ilizarov technique.

Optimal tensioning levels are yet to be determined in clinical trials. One can assume that different clinical situations require different wire tensions. For example, a situation requiring a more rigid compressive fixation, such as the stabilization of a hypertrophic nonunion, may require greater wire tensioning than the treatment of an acute fracture. The acute fracture, on the other hand, might call for a lower level of stiffness in the initial construct to promote callus formation.

Circular-ring tensioned-Kirschner-wire systems provide graduated wire tensioning devices (Dynamometers) to more accurately pretension the implants.

The ring diameter also directly affects the stability of the fixator construct. Decreasing the span that the wire traverses increases the overall stiffness of the construct. This, however, is limited by the space needed to accommodate the limb. Because of swelling associated with trauma and surgery, a minimum initial clearance of 2 cm around the entire ring is recommended to avoid its impingement on the limb. In situations where more severe postoperative swelling might be expected, and in the case of a crush injury, the clinician should allow even more room for potential swelling.

As noted previously, fracture reduction has a direct effect on construct stability. With thin-wire fixation techniques, beaded Olive wires may be used to apply translational forces at the fracture site and thereby maintain a reduction, particularly in cases of oblique fracture (Fig. 4-14).

Threaded Versus Smooth Fasteners

Weber and Magerl recognized that smooth implants may allow bone to translate on fixator pins.[120] Fixation with a smooth implant is therefore less stable than fixation with a threaded implant of the same core diameter. Circular-ring tensioned-wire systems depend on opposing angle wires to minimize sliding and rotation of the fragment and to increase overall stability (Fig. 4-15). Fleming and colleagues demonstrated that wires angled at 90° to one another accomplish these goals better than wires applied at smaller angles.[45] However, anatomic considerations often preclude this ideal wire position.

Number of Screws/Pins/Wires

In any system of external fixation, stability is improved by increasing the number of fixation devices to bone. Ideally, to achieve maximal effect, these additional screws, pins, or wires should be evenly distributed across the greatest possible area of the major fragments to be stabilized (Fig. 4-16).[13] Many larger body/frame external fixation systems can achieve more than adequate stability for most applications by using two closely set screw/pin clusters that are remote from the fracture to be stabilized (see Fig. 4-4).

Frame Geometry

Traditional early bar and clamp fixators, such as the ASIF or Hoffman-Vidal-Adrey systems, offer considerable versatility in exchange for stability. For simple fracture patterns with good fracture reduction, the simple uniplanar frame geometry of these systems provides adequate stability. Any unilateral application can

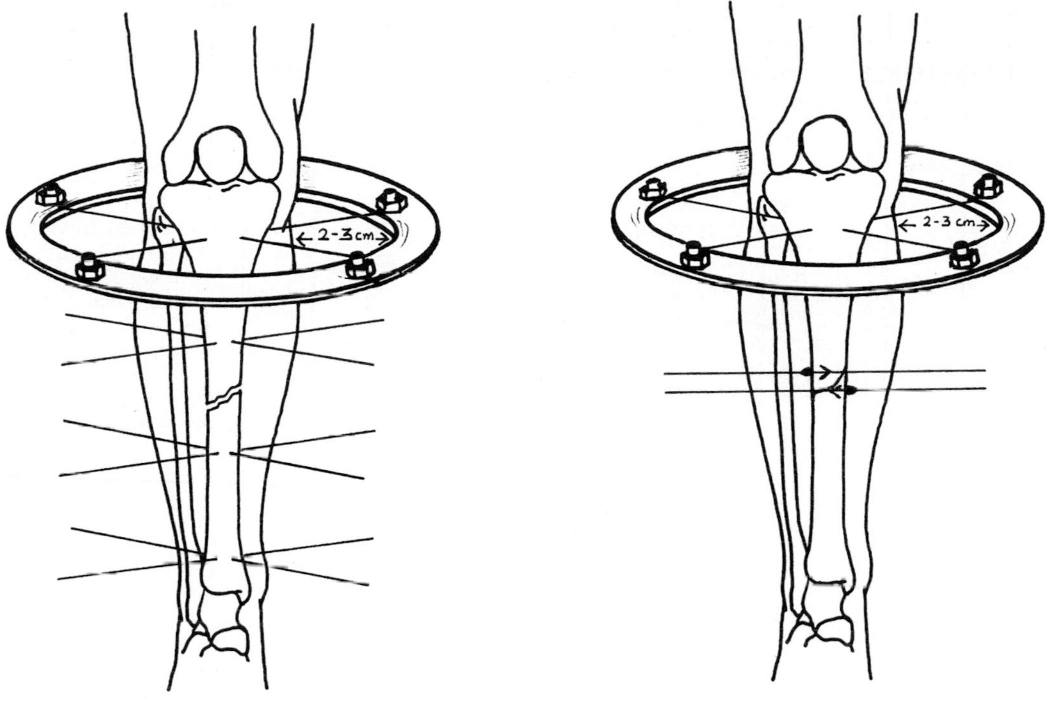

FIGURE 4-14. Beaded olive wires used in tensioned-wire fixation can effect reduction of oblique fracture lines. Small washers can be used in cancellous bone to improve fixation.

be made more resilient to the forces experienced in any one direction or plane by applying a like frame that opposes that plane of instability. When the frames are connected, they may constitute a so-called "delta configuration" (Fig. 4-17) or triangular frame (Fig. 4-18). These multiplanar configurations are rarely indicated now that stronger unilateral systems have been designed to minimize the need for such complex obstructive frames. Comparative stability studies have shown that larger unilateral systems offer a degree of

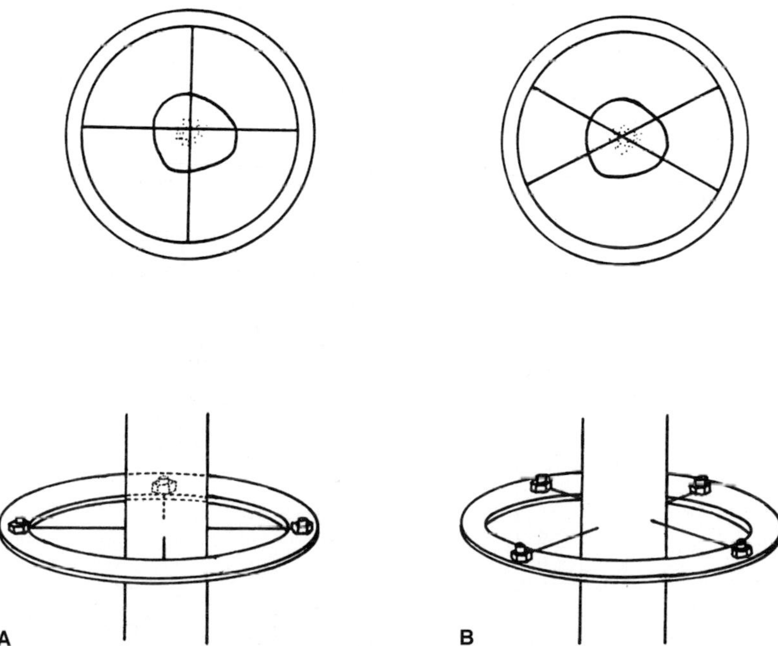

FIGURE 4-15. (**A**) Wires placed at 90° to one another ideally resist deformation of the bony fragments in both the anteroposterior and medial-lateral planes. (**B**) Wires placed at more acute angles as shown in this drawing offer less resistance to forces in the unopposed anteroposterior plane.

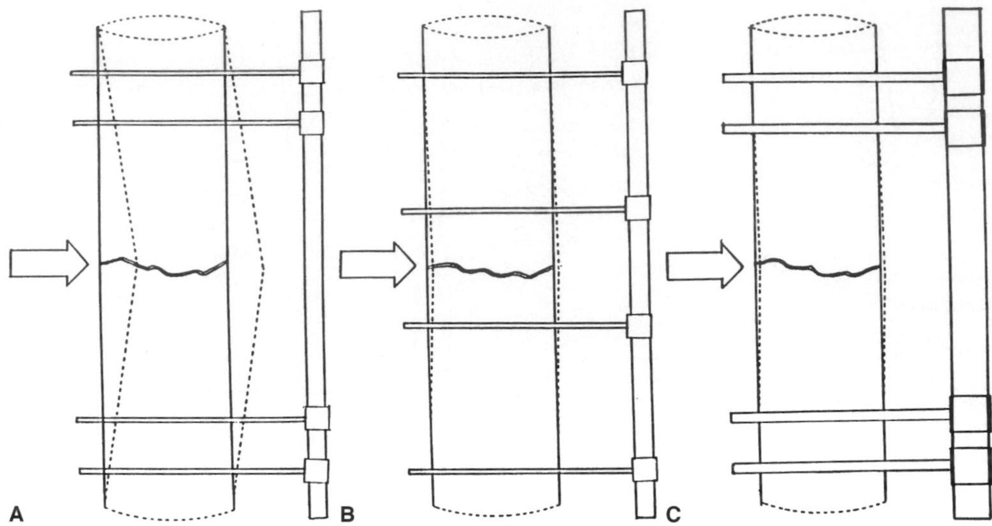

FIGURE 4-16. (**A**) External fixation with two screw clusters situated far from the fracture site offers normal stability. (**B**) External fixator systems with similar bars and clamps but screws spread evenly over the bone increases stability. (**C**) Large-framed fixators with thicker-diameter screws, on the other hand, can offer similar stability to smaller-gauged hardware despite remote placement of screws.

stability comparable to the more complex multiplanar configurations of more traditional systems.[13,19,30,45]

Mechanical tests of the ASIF tubular external fixation system, performed by Behrens' and colleagues, provides a basis for understanding how stability can be relatively increased in any system through changes in its frame geometry.[12] These analyses do not necessarily imply that complex configurations are required to provide adequate stability for most clinical situations. They merely point out the relative increases in construct stability that can be achieved by varying configurations.

Ever-increasing system rigidity is not always an asset, however, and caution is advised. As previously described, excessive rigidity can have a negative influence on healing. Inherently stronger large-body unilateral systems should almost never be applied in multiplanar configurations for routine fractures because they may inhibit callus formation. Still each situation must be individualized. Whereas a simple distal radius, humerus, or tibia fracture may not require provisions for adjunctive stabilization, added stability may be indicated in a case of femoral fixation or fixation of a knee fusion.

Bone Frame Distance

Another technique used to significantly increase the stability of any given construct involves placing the frame component as close to the bone as clinically

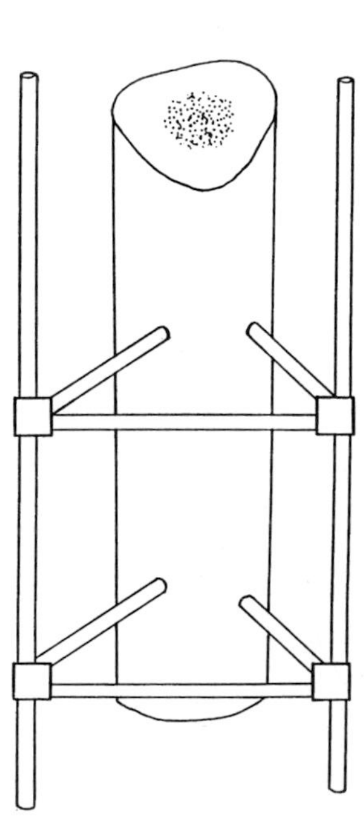

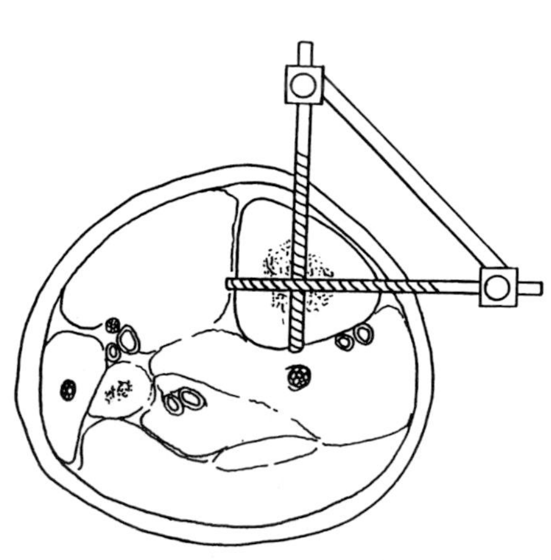

FIGURE 4-17. The "delta" configuration of external fixation offers increased resistance to deformation in two planes without transfixion implants, avoiding the attendant risk of neurovascular injury.

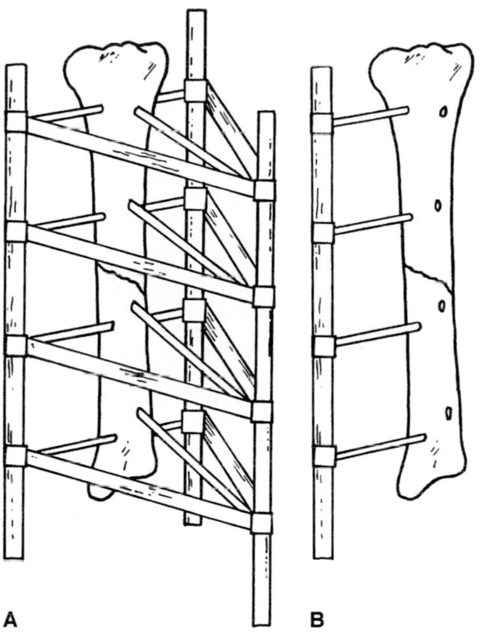

FIGURE 4-18. (**A**) A triangular frame is quite stable yet requires transfixion hardware with associated risks. (**B**) The increased rigidity of this construct requires a dynamization technique of "build down" or partial disassembly, leaving a simple unilateral frame to avoid creating a "nonunion machine."

possible. The closer the frame is to the bone, the more stable the construct will be (Fig. 4-19). This principle can also be used by clinicians who choose to produce cyclic dynamization in a frame by moving the fixator bars or body further out on the fixation pins or screws. This creates a more flexible construct. This method of decreasing frame rigidity while maintaining reduction was one of the earliest techniques of dynamization.

Implant-Clamp Fixation

In half-pin or screw fixator systems, implants are held by individual or grouped coupling clamps that affix pins or screws to the frame. To improve fixation of the half-pins to the frame, pin coupling clamps can be made wider to achieve broader, more stable fixation to the shaft of the half-pin.[4] Fixators with smaller single-coupling clamps can be used to achieve similar stability by "double stacking" them. This is another way to broaden the fixation of the pin to the frame and improve construct stability.

Articulated Fixation

In the late 1980s and early 1990s, the desire for early joint motion to theoretically improve cartilage healing and articular motion spawned the development of several articulated external fixators for stabilizing the wrist, elbow, and ankle.[15,16,31,85,103] Although each device has had some initial clinical popularity, biomechanical testing has failed to identify clinically reproducible applications of these devices, which can center the hinge of the fixator over the proper axis of a specific joint. Several authors have assessed the kinematics of articulating fixators, each citing the limited motion allowed by the uni-dimensional hinges.[31,44,112] As tested, these devices seem to allow for significant joint range of motion only with a certain degree of concomitant motion at the fracture site. These periarticular fixators remain popular, but many clinicians use them primarily in the static or locked mode (Fig. 4-20).

Biomechanics: Summary

In summary, an "ideal" degree of osseous stability for managing each clinical situation treated with external fixation is ill defined. Any fixation technique should

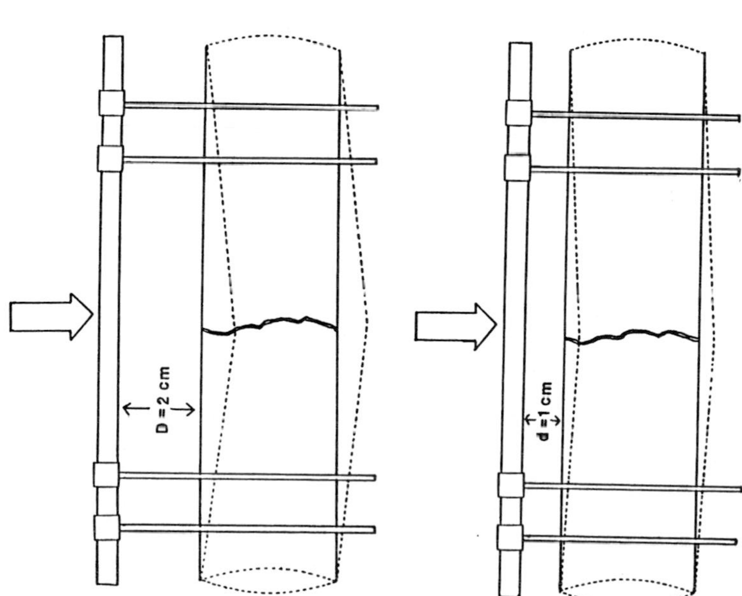

FIGURE 4-19. When fixator bars are affixed closer to bone, the overall construct is more stable as depicted by the decreased deflection (dotted lines) in reaction to an equivalent force (arrow).

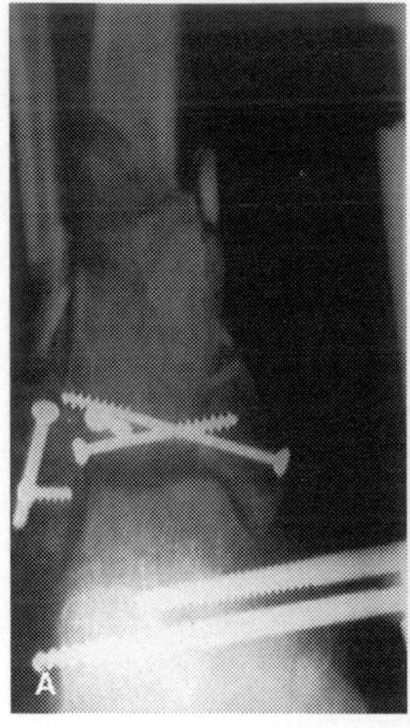

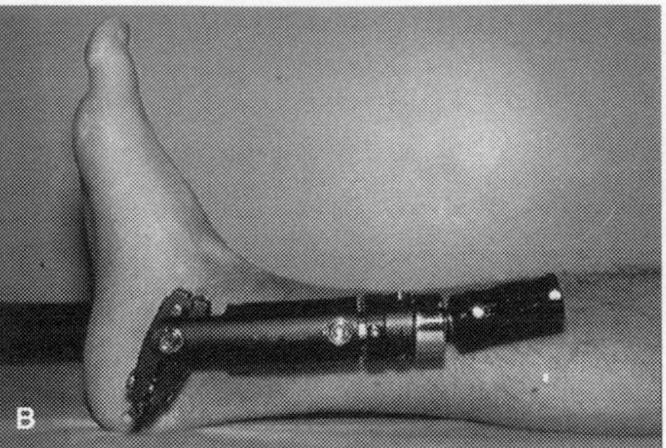

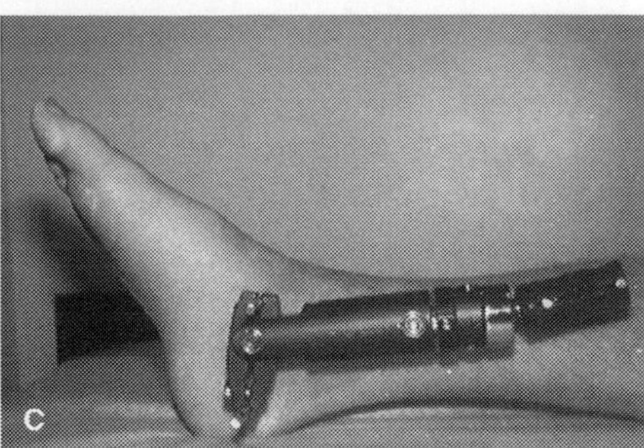

FIGURE 4-20. (**A**) A high-energy tibial plafond fracture treated with articulated external fixation allows limited (**B**) and (**C**) dorsiflexion plantar flexion of the ankle while maintaining reduction.

attempt to match the biomechanical requirement of the clinical situation with the stability of the overall construct.

Within any system of implants (pins, wires, screws, tongs), couplers (screw clamps), and frames or bodies, greater stability can be achieved by the following steps:

1. Increasing the diameter of the implant (screw, wire, pin).
2. Increasing the number of implants.
3. Increasing implant spread.
4. Using multiplanar fixation.
5. Reducing the distance between fixator frame and bone.
6. Predrilling all half-pin screw sites whenever possible, and irrigating drills and implants on insertion with a cool saline solution to avoid thermal necrosis and associated premature loosening.
7. Applying radial preload techniques to half-pin or screw fixation.
8. Improving fastener-frame fixation with improved clamp technology or double stacking.
9. Reducing fractures with fragment contact improving stability and permitting "off loading" of implants (without use of adjunctive lag screws).
10. Using circular-ring and tensioned-wire devices;
    a. Tensioning wires properly (90–130 kg).
    b. Minimizing—as much as clinically possible—circular-ring diameter placing Kirschner wires at angles that are as close to 90° to each other as clinically possible while taking care to respect neurovascular structures.
11. Dynamizing frames when possible to allow for bone-end contact, a reduction in frame/pin, screw, wire, stress, and a decrease in the tendency to loosen.

CLINICAL PRINCIPLES OF EXTERNAL FIXATION

Indications

"It is not wise to use external fixation everywhere for everything."[110]

This advice was given by W. Taillard at the Tenth International Congress on Hoffman External Fixation in 1984, and it clearly reflects the current conventional wisdom about external fixation. Still, the versatility and apparent simplicity of the technique tend to lure inexperienced clinicians who hope for an uncomplicated solution to complex problems. Because most simple closed fractures are treated with casting or internal fixation, external fixation is usually relegated to the stabilization of more severe complex injuries, especially those with associated soft-tissue wounds that are not amenable to other techniques. In many cases, internal fixation would be imprudent for fractures with soft-tissue injuries. For bone injuries, traditional fixation techniques may prove problematic. In instances of severe intra-articular fractures, external fixation may be used as a portable traction device, offering a means of reduction and stabilization through ligamentotaxis. Finally, external fixation can be an alternative method for temporary stabilization of long bone and pelvic injuries in multiply traumatized patients when the blood loss and operative time associated with definitive internal fixation are considered undesirable. The following are clinical indications and application principles that apply to each anatomic area to be addressed with external fixation.

Open Fractures

External fixation is often used to treat open fractures. Gristina and Costerton demonstrated that the presence of metallic implants increased the incidence of infection in contaminated wounds.[55] Animal models simulating severely contaminated open fractures have also demonstrated a higher rate of wound infection and osteomyelitis with internal fixation as opposed to external fixation.[6,7] For infection-prone open injuries with severe soft-tissue contamination, the desire to avoid internal fixation has led to the popularity of stabilization by external fixation remote from the zone of injury.

Severe open fractures of the tibial diaphysis are the most common injuries stabilized with external fixation. Early teaching prescribed only temporary stabilization with fixators, and prompt removal of the device was recommended to avoid pin-track problems.[53,105] Typically, fixators were removed soon after wound healing. The patient was further treated with a plaster cast, because it was difficult to judge when a fracture was adequately healed enough to have a fixator removed. This technique created an unacceptable rate of malunion, nonunion, and wound complication.

More recent authors have stressed the need to maintain the fixation until the fracture has healed sufficiently to allow for removal of the device without loss of reduction.[11,41,76] When external fixation is maintained until healing, the union rate is high (>90%) and malunion rate low (<5%). Pin-track infection rates range from 5% to 15% of pins.

Adjunctive hardware, such as lag screws, is not indicated for the treatment of diaphyseal open fractures because it is associated with an increased incidence of infection and refracture.[43,67]

Fixators should be placed through subcutaneous tissue on the anteromedial border of the tibia. The fixator body or frame position should not interfere with the wound area. This facilitates later coverage or bone grafting procedures. When pin placement is adequately remote from the fracture site, future surgical fields can be isolated and draped free of pin site involvement. This minimizes the chance of infection due to seeding from colonized pin sites (Fig. 4-21).

If initial reduction is adequate to establish a length stable construct, partial weight bearing should be initiated as soon as soft-tissue consideration permits limb dependency. If the fracture is transverse or otherwise inherently stable, the fixator can be dynamized (with progressive closure) immediately. With less stable fracture configurations, dynamization is delayed until early signs of fracture healing (callus) are evident. This usually occurs at around 6 weeks. In cases of comminuted high-energy open tibia fractures or in the event of bone loss, plans for local or posterolateral bone grafting should be made and typically performed 6 to 12 weeks postinjury to speed healing and minimize fixation time. The external fixation should be maintained whenever possible until the fracture has healed (Fig. 4-22).

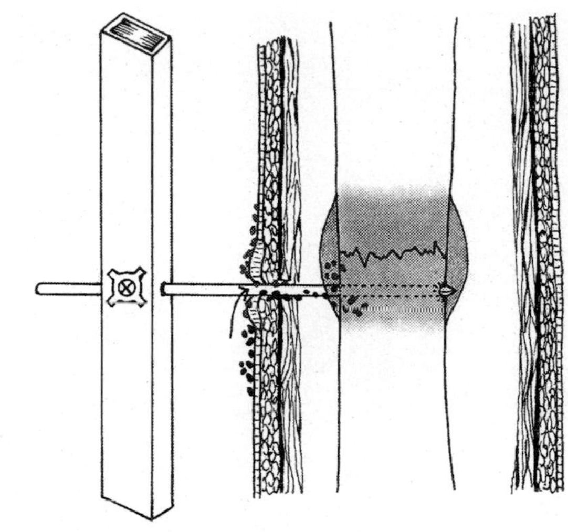

FIGURE 4-21. Fixator screws or pins should be placed remote from the zone of fracture to avoid pin-track contamination of the fracture site.

Routine conversion from external fixation to intramedullary (IM) nailing is not advisable. If IM nailing is contemplated, it is best performed acutely and without reaming as primary definitive fixation. Many authors have demonstrated that conversion to IM nailing in the tibia is complicated by higher rates of infection, particularly if there has been any evidence of pin-track infection. McGraw and Lim as well as Maurer and colleagues have demonstrated a 25% rate of infection when IM rodding procedures are undertaken after external fixation pin-site infection.[79,82] Riemer and Butterfield retrospectively studied 32 patients and found a marked increase in infection rate when reamed cannulated IM nails ($^{7}/_{16}$ pts) were used compared to solid-core nonreamed nails ($^{1}/_{16}$ pts) to stabilize tibiae previously treated with external fixation.[101]

Unilateral half-pin/screw frames are the most common devices for external fixation of open tibial shaft fractures. The advantage of nontransfixing implants has been previously discussed. The anatomically safe zones of application have been described by Green and others.[53] Proper insertion of fixation pins, screws, or wires with careful consideration of the tibial cross-sectional anatomy (Fig. 4-23) permit stabilization with minimal jeopardy to muscle, tendon, or neurovascular structures.

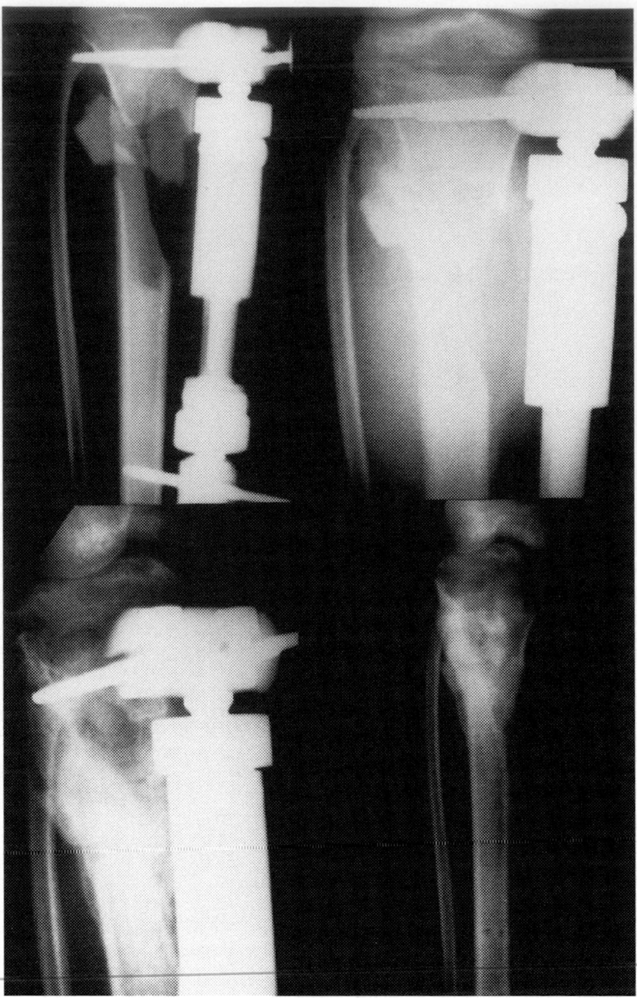

FIGURE 4-22. This comminuted high-energy open tibia fracture with bone loss was stabilized with external fixation until union. After healing of a gastrocnemius flap, bone grafting was performed. The fixator is in place at 6 months postinjury with apparent incorporation of the graft and fracture union. The fixator was removed at this point.

Multi-Trauma

The severely injured patient with multiple trauma is often best treated with early stabilization of long bone fractures.[17,51,61] Occasionally, however, such patients are physiologically unstable. They can be hypotensive and/or coagulopathic and may have suffered serious head injury. In such cases, extensive lengthy procedures associated with considerable blood loss and undesirable fluid shifts might subject the patient to unnecessary risks. However, many clinicians argue that these patients require some form of stabilization of their long bone injuries to obviate traction and permit the more upright chest position that decreases the likelihood of pulmonary complications. Many feel these patients are not too sick to be operated on, but rather, are too sick not to be.

When IM nailing is deemed an undesirable procedure because of potential blood loss and extensive operative time, external fixation can be quite helpful as a temporary means of long bone (femur) stabilization. This allows for patient mobilization with minimal operative time and little or no blood loss. Later, when the patient recovers from the critical stages of the injury, femoral fixators can be removed and more definitive stabilization techniques performed, provided there has been no intercurrent episode of pin-track infection. Indeed, if proper precautions are taken, the incidence of pin-track infections is extremely low in the first 2 weeks after application. In our institution, the policy of temporarily stabilizing femoral fractures with external fixation in the most extremely injured patients has helped to avoid traction for a number of multi-trauma victims, especially those with severe head injury. This technique has no doubt contributed to reducing morbidity and mortality.

Recent work on IM nailing has suggested that there may be some relationship between adult respiratory distress syndrome (ARDS) and instrumentation or ma-

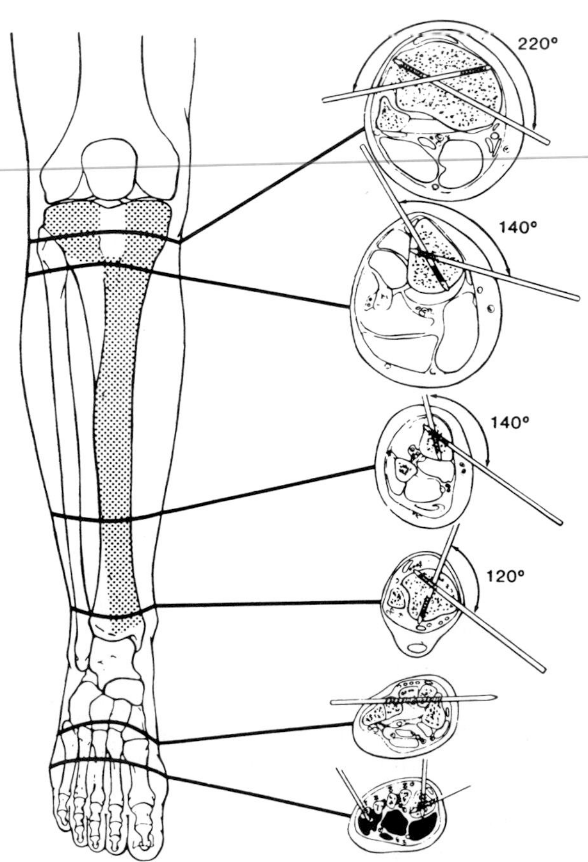

FIGURE 4-23. "Safe corridors" and arcs of insertion in the leg. (From Behrens, F., and Searls, K.: External Fixation of the Tibia. Basic Concepts and Prospective Evaluation. J. Bone Joint Surg., 68B:246—254, 1986.)

nipulation of the IM cavity with reamers or even unreamed implants.[93] This relationship is particularly noted in patients with severe chest injury.[94] The use of temporary external fixation may provide an expedient safe alternative for long-bone stabilization in these patients. Clinical experience with conversion to IM nailing in the femur has not demonstrated the same problems associated with using this technique in open fractures of the tibia. In a series of ten patients with femur fractures initially treated with external fixation, Broos and coworkers found no infections and prompt union with secondary reamed IM nailing an average of 21 days postinjury.[20] Alternatively, if the patient's condition does not permit conversion to an IM device in the femur, fractures can be treated definitively with external fixation.[9,20,52] The problems associated with pin-track infection in the bulky soft tissue of the thigh musculature as well as malunion and delayed union make this option less desirable than the more convenient nailing conversion.

In cases of femur fractures in pediatric multiple trauma patients under 13 years of age, external fixation seems to be the standard against which other methods of stabilization must be measured. The obvious convenience of IM nailing makes such techniques appealing for treatment of these injuries. However, problems with nailing, such as physeal closure and, more recently, reported incidents of aseptic necrosis of the femoral head associated with routine cephalocaudid-reamed IM nailing, requires careful consideration in these younger patients. The use of external fixation is preferable as a means of primary stabilization in this age group.[10,46,80]

There are problems associated with pin-track infection and refracture after premature fixator removal in children.[5,65] Pin-site infections are usually treatable with oral antibiotics. Chronic pin-track osteomyelitis in children is extremely rare.[5] Refractures may be related to placement of large rigid external fixator frames on children whose fractures are anatomically reduced. In 11 years of experience with this technique, I have seen a refracture of an apparently healed femoral fracture in a child only once (Fig. 4-24). The 8-year-old boy's fracture had been anatomically reduced, and little or no callus had accompanied the apparent healing at 10 weeks postinjury. Five days after fixator removal,

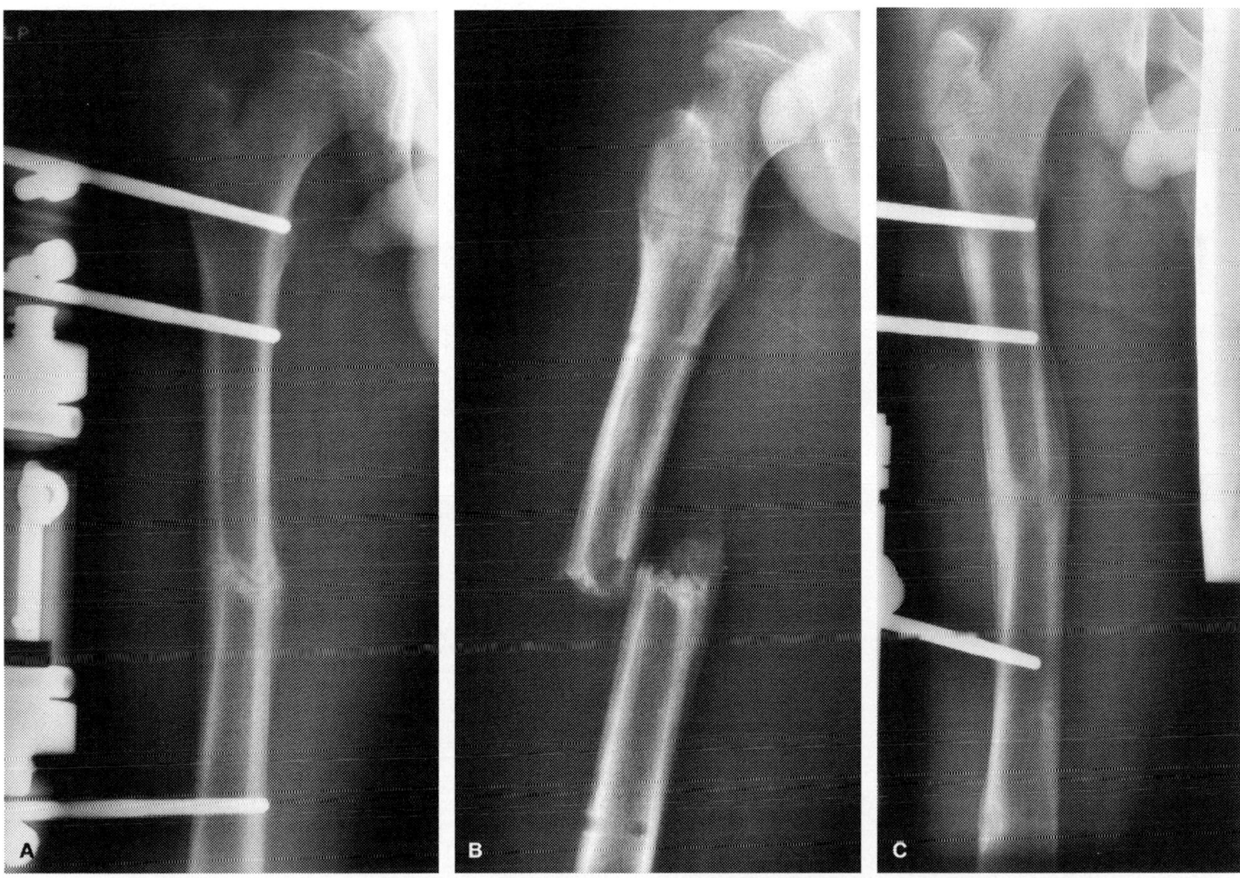

FIGURE 4-24. (**A**) Femur fracture at 10 weeks postfixation in an 8-year-old boy. The fixator was removed at this time, perhaps a bit early. (**B**) Five days after fixator removal, the femur refractured with minor trauma. (**C**) A fixator was reapplied, and healing is shown 12 weeks later.

he refractured at the same site while running. The overly rigid frame construct in this lightweight child may have contributed to his healing with minimal callus. The bone did not sufficiently remodel to tolerate early unsupported weight bearing. With reapplication of the fixator, his prompt healing was accompanied by abundant callus formation.

Pelvic Fracture

Stabilizing unstable pelvic injuries in hemodynamically unstable patients is part of the trauma surgeon's resuscitative armamentarium.[63,100,106] Biomechanical testing of cadavers devoid of any anterior or posterior ligamentous integrity has clearly implied that anterior pelvic external fixation alone is insufficient to definitively stabilize pelvic injuries with complete posterior disruptions. These limitations have been defined in numerous studies on a variety of external fixation systems that were applied in a multitude of configurations.[14,21,38] An anterior external fixator frame is biomechanically inadequate to provide sufficient stability that allows a patient with a severe anterior and posterior pelvic disruption to ambulate.[14,38,106] Attempts to achieve increased stability by changing pin placement from the traditional pelvic brim to the anterior supra acetabulum have not demonstrated significantly improved stability in bench testing.[87] Often, however, anterior frames offer sufficient stability to mobilize patients short of weight bearing. The added stability helps to control pain and improves nursing care by making it easier to transport patients and mobilize them from bed to chair. Clinical studies that show the efficacy of anterior external fixation, even in severe injuries, allude to the presence of underlying residual intact ligamentous structures that contribute to the overall bone-fixator construct stability in most situations. It is difficult to accurately assess the contributions of these residual structures. The best biomechanical analyses to date have been able to test only the worst-case scenarios with pelvises devoid of any ligamentous integrity. Tile stated that although external fixation alone is inadequate to mobilize most patients with an unstable pelvic injury, the addition of skeletal traction to the fixator may offer an acceptable option when internal fixation is not possible.[113] However, anterior external fixation with pins placed into the iliac wings offers a relatively simple way to achieve sufficient stability to assist in controlling hemorrhage.

As Ghanayem and associates clearly showed, the volume of the pelvis is well controlled by placing an anterior frame.[49] This theoretically allows for tamponade of bleeding retroperitoneal vessels. Ideally, pelvic frames should be placed low on the abdomen to enable surgical exposure for laparotomy with as little obstruction as possible. Hinged fixators for this purpose have been designed. Whenever possible, the fixator should be placed prior to incision of the abdominal fascia as laparotomy has been shown by Ghanayem and associates to contribute to pelvic instability.[49]

Huge resuscitation clamps have also been introduced (Fig. 4-25). These clamps are designed to be applied in the emergency room with large single pins that are affixed to the posterolateral aspects of each iliac wing to compress the pelvis and help control hemorrhage. Initial reports on the efficacy of these devices are encouraging.[47]

In cases of anterior pelvic injury in which the posterior ligamentous structures are left intact, such as the rotationally unstable "open-book" disruption, anterior frames provide adequate stability to rapidly mobilize the patient to ambulate. Patients with anterior pelvic external fixation generally experience reasonable pain control and tolerate bed-to-chair mobilization.

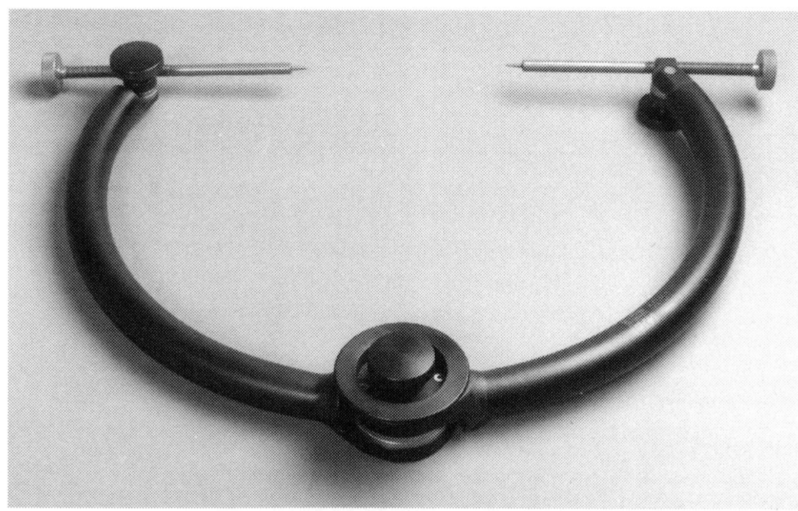

FIGURE 4-25. A large pelvic clamp for emergent temporary fixation in hemodynamically unstable patients with pelvic fractures is shown here.

However, in cases of true posterior instability, use of an anterior frame alone has been associated with loss of reduction. As a result, posterior adjunctive fixation or traction have been advised.[113]

Riemer and others, including this author, contend that despite the inaccuracy of reduction and residual displacement, treating pelvic disruption with external fixation alone results in successful functional outcomes with most pelvic fracture patterns.[77,84] In severely displaced fractures that lose reduction soon after fixation with anterior frames alone, secondary reduction and posterior instrumentation or traction can be implemented to improve and maintain reduction. In long-term studies of pelvic injuries, poor outcomes have been more clearly related to associated neurologic and urogenital problems than to reduction.[56,77] Residual pelvic displacement at neither the sacroiliac (SI) joint nor the symphysis pubis have correlated with poor functional outcome.[77,84] Nonunion of sacral fractures and persistent instability of the SI joint have often been cited as potential common sequelae of pelvic injuries treated with external fixation.[123] However, these complications have not been reported in studies by Slätis, Martin, or Miranda and their colleagues.[77,84,106] Chronic severe SI joint pain has not been a serious problem either. Malunion is quite common, however.[77,84] Pin-track infection, as with all external fixation techniques, is a problem to be reckoned with and requires vigilance and early treatment. Small-bowel obstruction has also been a complication reported in association with closed reduction and pelvic external fixation. This rare problem may arise when a loop of small bowel is trapped in a sacral fracture, presumptively at the time of reduction.[114]

External fixation remains a viable clinical option for treating displaced anterior and posterior pelvic injuries. The biomechanical limitations of anterior fixation alone must be appreciated and accounted for in posteriorly unstable injuries. Reduction and residual displacement may be problematic, yet overall functional outcome in long-term patient studies appears to be reasonable.

Complex Intra-Articular Periarticular Fracture

In general, the recommended fixation for severe displaced intra-articular fractures involves reducing and restoring the articular surface with bone grafting as needed and neutralizing fragments until healing. These are usually high-energy fractures with attendant soft-tissue injuries and may be associated with multiple trauma.

Often, complex intra-articular fractures and fracture dislocations, particularly about the knee and ankle, do not lend themselves to emergent lengthy operative procedures. This is particularly true of open injuries. These complicated reconstructive procedures should be carefully planned and are usually performed in a more elective setting. The acutely injured patient may need resuscitation and hemodynamic stabilization, during which more sophisticated imaging studies can be acquired. In such early phases of treatment, external fixation frames can be successfully used as temporary fixation devices or portable traction. Fixator pins should be placed as far as possible from any area which may be incised in the future for internal fixation. Once the patient is stable and the soft tissue about the area is safe for further intervention, definitive fixation can be done. The fixator itself can be used as an indirect reduction tool at the time of fixation.

External fixation has also been described as a definitive treatment for intra-articular fracture.[15,16,31,36,72,75,103,121] Here, the technique involves the use of both joint-spanning fixators, which rely on ligamentotaxis for reduction, and joint-sparing applications, which directly fix intra-articular fragments with fixator screws or wires. There are two main methods of stabilizing severe intra-articular fractures with external fixation. *Joint spanning* fixation completely avoids the fracture site in a portable-traction mode. *Joint sparing* interfragmentary fixation allows joint motion with fixator pins placed in the diaphysis of the bone and the metaphysis, which may or may not be comminuted with intra-articular extension. With joint-sparing fixation, placing percutaneous hardware into the fracture site raises the possibility of pin-track sepsis extending into the site and becoming an intra-articular infection. This has rarely been reported. Marsh and coworkers reported on 21 tibial plateau fractures treated with joint-sparing interfragmentary external fixation noting a 10% joint sepsis rate.[75] Anatomic studies on the proximal tibia and knee joint demonstrate that fixator pins or screws placed within 1.4 cm of the articular surface pass intra-articularly, proximal to the insertion of the collateral ligaments and synovial reflection. These implants can be problematic because pin-track infections can quickly become intra-articular. Caution should be exercised when applying percutaneous hardware near the fracture site.

The use of Ilizarov-type circular-ring and tension thin-wire fixators with opposed "dueling" Olive wires has also been advocated to reduce and stabilize severe injuries in a minimally invasive manner.[72,121] Reports of infectious complications have been few with tensioned thin-wire fixation. The possibility of infection remains of concern when using any technique that depends on the long-term maintenance of percutaneous implants around the fracture site. Patients treated with this method should be carefully monitored, and antibiotic treatment should be initiated early for any sign of pin-track infection or inflammation, particularly when hardware transgresses the fracture site.

Distal Radius

Severe injuries of the distal radius are not often amenable to internal fixation either because of the severity of comminution or the lack of sufficient bone stock in which to fix hardware. This has led many to use joint-spanning external fixators with ligamentotaxis occasionally coupled with limited open procedures to elevate depressed articular surfaces with bone graft (with or without minimal internal fixation).[70,98,104] External-fixation methods permit neutralization and reduction maintenance in these often difficult comminuted fractures that, with cast immobilization tend to deform into volar and radial angulation. Recent prospective studies that compared external fixation of distal radius fractures to closed reduction and casting demonstrated a better reduction maintenance and overall outcome with external fixation.[58,60] Because long periods of distraction may be associated with joint stiffness, care should be taken to avoid overdistraction with excessive ligamentotaxis across the wrist.[70,104] The position of immobilization should likewise avoid both hyperflexion and marked ulnar deviation and instead should tend toward the preferred neutral position as far as reduction permits. Immediate active assistive finger-joint range of motion is critical.

Care must be exercised in placing fixator pins in the radius and metacarpals. This should be managed through open incision techniques to ensure that:

1. No injury is incurred to any neurotendonous structures, particularly the superficial branch of the radial nerve on the radial dorsal forearm.
2. The screws are centrally placed in the metacarpals to minimize the possibility of stress-related metacarpal fracture.

Skin wounds can be closed around half-pins without problem.

The desire for early range of motion of the distal radius while still in the fixator prompted the development of articulated modules that reportedly allow daily intermittent supervised range of motion. However, kinematic studies of the radiocarpal joint suggest that although some motion is possible, it is meager at best.[112] The clinical benefits of articulated fixators are questionable. Sommerkamp and associates compared the treatment of unstable distal radius fractures using "dynamic" articulated fixators with treatment using static frames and concluded that the articulated fixators offered no benefit and probably increased complications.[107]

Tibial Plafond Fracture

Despite initial reports of unfettered success with open reduction and internal fixation of fractures involving the distal tibial articular surface,[102] subsequent authors caution about the potential devastating soft-tissue complications associated with acute internal fixation.[111] In severe closed and open fractures of the tibial plafond, Bonar and Marsh, Karas and Weiner, and others now recommend less invasive techniques of external fixation as a definitive way to treat more complex injuries.[15,16,62] Because of decreased incidence of wound complication and infection associated with acute internal fixation, external fixation techniques have gained in popularity.

Other authors recommend the occasional use of temporary external fixation in tibial plafond fractures. Used as portable traction, the fixator allows patient mobility while awaiting the decrease in the usual massive soft-tissue swelling associated with these injuries.[18]

In higher energy, more displaced fractures, articulated external fixation is advised for "molding" shattered, unfixable articular fragments using ligamentotaxis across the tibiotalor joint in combination with an ankle hinge to provide limited dorsi-plantar flexion (see Fig. 4-20).[15,103] However, as with the radiocarpal joint, kinematic studies of the ankle have again raised questions about the ability of hinged fixators to provide substantive range of motion without compromising fracture fixation.[44] Still, wound infection rates with external fixation of tibial plafond fractures are markedly lower than with acute internal fixation. This raises questions about the use of emergent open reduction internal fixation for serious injuries of the tibial plafond when soft-tissue damage and swelling are severe.

Bone Transport

The principle of bone transport is elegant in its simplicity. To fill an area of bone loss, one need only osteotomize a segment of that bone above or below the gap, then slowly transport the fragment across the void to "dock" against the remaining segment. This technique has proven safe and effective for treating bone loss caused by acute open fracture as well as for reconstructing limbs with loss of bone secondary to debridement in infected nonunion.[8,27,37,74,88,115] However, in practice, the technique of distraction osteogenesis is not easy for the patient or the surgeon. It is laborious, time consuming, and often frustrating. It requires perseverance and a good understanding of the treatment concepts by both the surgeon and the patient. Bone transport is based on the fact that a bone fragment transected without destruction of the periosteum may be slowly distracted or "transported" toward another fragment to fill an area of bone loss (Fig. 4-26*B* and *C*). During the osteotomy, care must be taken to preserve the periosteum and soft tissue surrounding the transected area to support osteogenesis of the regenerate bone. Previous suggestions that a corticotomy must be done without damage to the endosteal vasculature have

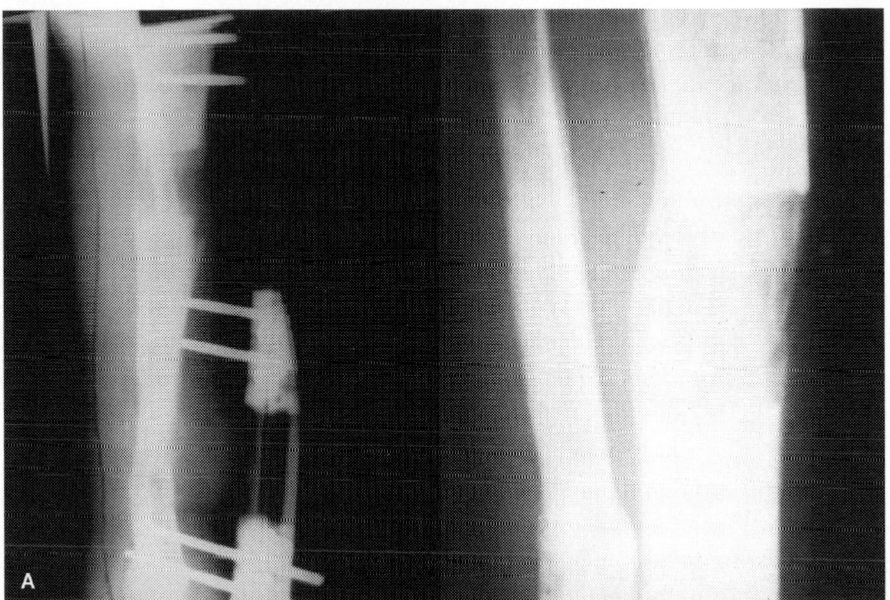

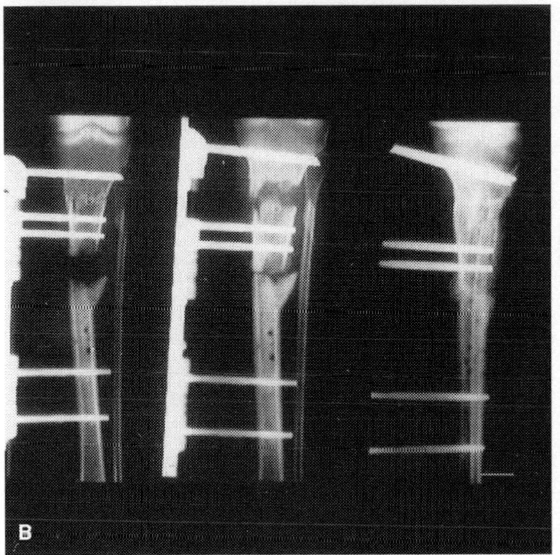

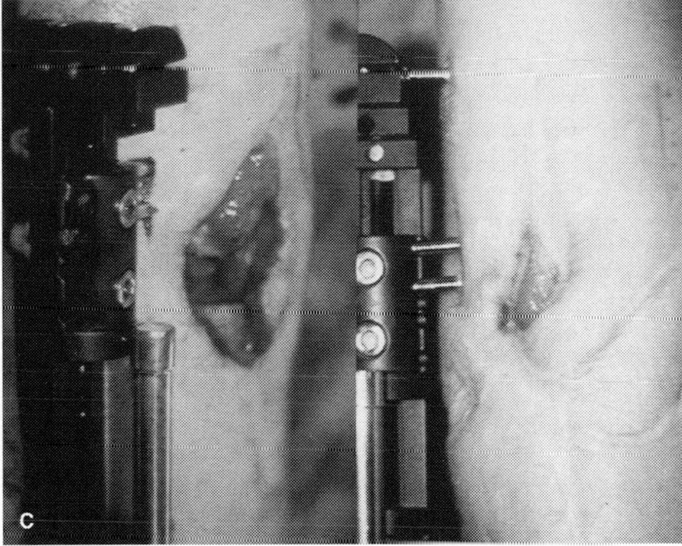

FIGURE 4-26. (**A**) Regenerate bone that forms in response to the distraction osteogenesis techniques of bone transport is quite predictable in young healthy individuals such as this 22-year-old female. (**B**) Soft-tissue defect closes as soft tissue is approximated during bone transport. (**C**) A moderate sized soft tissue defect associated with debridement of osteomyelitis.

proven less important than preserving the periosteum, as Kojimoto and coworkers showed using an animal model.[66] Brutcher and associates subsequently confirmed the efficacy of the osteotomy, but emphasized that the paucity of periosteal tissue in the adult may occasionally indicate patients for the more tedious corticotomy.[22] Stabilization for this procedure can be achieved with many different external fixation systems.

The proximal and distal ends of the bone on which the transport procedure is performed must be well aligned and should be stably fixed to ensure that the normal mechanical and anatomical axes of the limb are maintained. The transported segment must be properly aligned with the frame to ensure accurate docking with the distal fragment.

In the young healthy patient with no underlying illnesses or impediments to bone growth, such as diabetes mellitus, osteoporosis, or tobacco dependency, the usual rate of transport or lengthening is 1 mm per day divided into four increments (0.25 mm, four times daily). In healthy candidates, the formation of regenerate bone in the wake of transport is predictable (Fig. 4-26*A*). Children who are still growing may even require accelerated rates of transport to avoid premature consolidation of the regenerative bone and the need for repeat osteotomy. Older, less healthy patients will form bone less readily and are relatively poorer candidates for these techniques.

Originally, it was taught that upon docking, mere compression or sequential compression and distraction of the docking site would result in a predictable union. However, experience has suggested that, in most cases, bone grafting or so-called "freshening" of the bone ends is indicated soon after docking. When transport distances exceed 2 or 3 cm, after a time, the ends of the transported bone become covered by fibrous tissue that behaves like an atrophic nonunion after docking if they are left to heal without intervention. Early bone grafting and "rose petaling" (Fig. 4-27) of the docking site effectively promotes union.

Modest soft-tissue defects may also close with this technique (Fig. 4-25). As a segment of bone is transported, the associated soft tissue will transport as well, often achieving complete coverage of the soft-tissue defect with no need for flap or skin graft. Extremely large defects may still require coverage.

Some centers advocate facilitating difficult wound closures by acutely shortening limbs with bone and soft-tissue loss, and later regaining length by distraction at the site of a remote osteotomy.[74] This technique, often referred to as *contact lengthening,* works well with some defects up to 3 cm. In the tibia, however, attempts to shorten more than 3 cm have been associated with circulatory embarrassment that may ultimately result in amputation. Caution should be exercised, and any substantial shortening must be done gradually to minimize the tendency for already injured and indurated tissue with limited compliance to compromise the venous or arterial circulation.

Another method that can be used to expedite treatment in cases of substantial defects is bipolar transport. With this technique, two fragments of bone are osteotomized on either side of an area of bone loss. Both bone fragments are then transported toward each other, halving the time needed to span a given distance.[72]

Remember that healing times are protracted with all bone transport techniques. Paley described a "healing index" that indicates the expected duration for consolidation of each centimeter of bone lengthened.[90] This concept can be applied to bone transport as well. For the bone to completely unite, it is considered standard to require two to three times the amount of time necessary for transport. Therefore, a transport of 5 cm, a modest distance, would require 50 days for consolidation of the regenerate bone. Such a procedure would require, on average, 150–200 days or 5–7 months for a complete union. If all goes well. Infection or thrombosis that requires anticoagulation, for example, can have a profound effect on the time to union. Strict patient compliance is an absolute necessity. Patients should be apprised in advance that this technique involves at least two procedures (and possibly more) for freshening and bone grafting, for replacing screws or wires, and for correcting residual deformity at the later healing stages. Although this technique is powerful, patient selection, preoperative counseling and planning, and careful close monitoring are keys to success.

COMPLICATIONS IN EXTERNAL FIXATION

Pin-Track Infection

Pin-track infection is one problem that has clearly limited the popularity of external fixation. In the past, the frequency of pin-site problems and a lack of understanding about the etiology and proper treatment prompted many to discontinue the technique, including the US military during World War II. Indeed, there

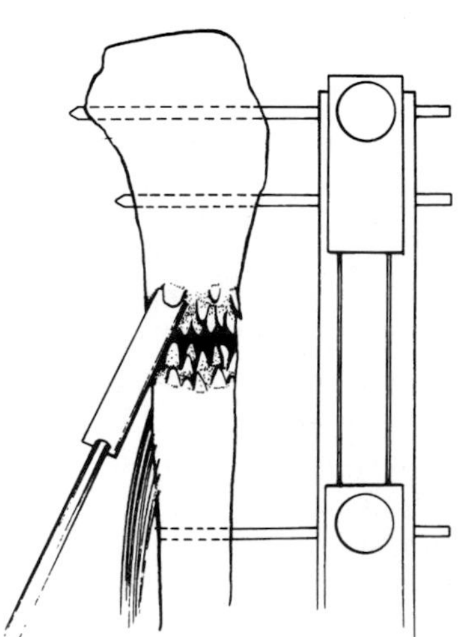

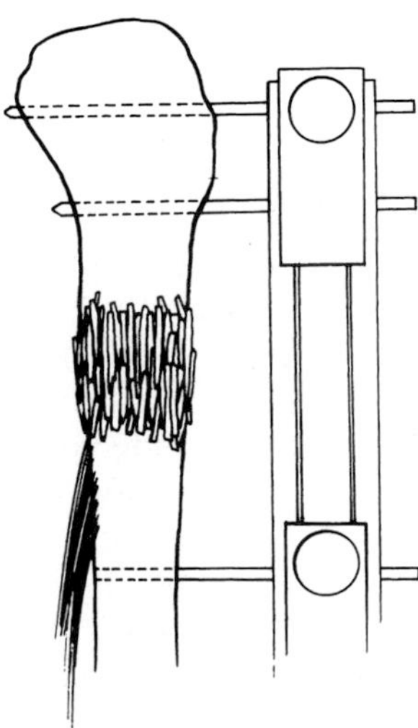

FIGURE 4-27. The "docking site" is commonly "rose petaled" and bone grafted to expedite union in bone transport cases.

are still those who would use any other fixation technique to avoid dealing with this problem.

This reluctance is humorously underscored in an anecdote involving Roger Anderson. While entertaining a group of visiting orthopaedic surgeons. Anderson was asked if it was "pus" emanating from the pin sites on one of his patients. Anderson reportedly replied, "No, no, that is only a little serum." This gave rise to the practice of euphemistically referring to purulence as "Seattle Serum". Still, those with more extensive experience with external fixation prefer to view pin-track infections merely as "obstacles" in the treatment method (to use Paley's terminology).[92] Advocates of external fixation argue that such problems are minor, treatable complications when adequate vigilance and proactive treatment protocols are followed.

To others, any pin-track difficulty is a reminder of the inherent fallibility of this technique. In their skepticism, these detractors will often remove external fixators at the first signs of trouble. This in turn starts the inevitable cascade towards nonunion, malunion, and failure of the technique so often alluded to in critiques of external fixation. Given such pessimism about the outcome of external fixation, it is no wonder that these clinicians adamantly resist its use.

The truth lies somewhere between the viewpoints of the zealot and the skeptic. To begin to accurately appreciate the magnitude of the problem, pin-track infections should be graded or staged.

Each stage characterizes a point in the continuum of the pathophysiological "natural history" of colonization, bacterial overgrowth, early soft-tissue infection, later established deep infection, and osteomyelitis.

Stage I: Inordinate Serous or Seropurulent Drainage

All pins will drain, but normal drainage should be as minimal as might be noted on the underside of a bandage about the pins. Free-flowing drainage is pathologic, as is any degree of purulence. These problems require treatment with aggressive pin-site hygiene and oral broad-spectrum antibiotics, usually involving a first generation cephalosporin. Patients who report suspicions of pin-track infection after being educated about the signs and symptoms of these problems can be prescribed broad-spectrum antibiotics over the telephone. This provides treatment as early as possible.

Stage II: Superficial Cellulitis

A halo of cutaneous erythema that extends from the pin site usually indicates a soft-tissue infection. At this stage, the problem requires oral antibiotics and increased pin-site hygiene. If this treatment meets with a discouraging response, parenteral antibiotics treatment may be indicated. European authors have advocated local injection of antibiotic (gentamycin) into infected pin sites as a means of treatment. Though described by some,[92] this technique is not yet been broadly accepted in the United States.

Stage III: Deep Infection

Fortunately, this stage is uncommon. It is characterized by deep-seated infection along the entire pin track. It can be differentiated from superficial pin-site cellulitis by purulent drainage, swelling, and severe cellulitis encompassing more than one of the pins in a cluster. Antibiotic treatment is required, often via the parenteral route. Such infections raise the suspicion of bone infection and implant loosening. Loose implants must be removed. Pins or screws may need to be replaced as stability considerations require. Reinsertion should only be done after treatment with a course of antibiotics to "sterilize" the soft-tissue sites chosen for new pin implantation. To introduce another implant through or near acutely cellulitic tissue is to invite another infection by inoculating the soft tissue and bone of the new site with the infecting organism.

It should be noted that the pin loosening most often referred to is *clinical loosening.* Frequently, very slight radiolucencies can be noted in the entry side cortex of the half-pin fixation. This radiolucency alone, in the absence of clinical loosening with sepsis, should not be mistaken for osteomyelitis. Many patients will have benign-appearing pin sites with radiographic evidence of entry-side radiolucency. This does not necessarily indicate infectious osteomyelitis and may simply represent mechanically induced resorption.[124]

Stage IV: Osteomyelitis

Clinical loosening of implants accompanied by infection and radiographic evidence of bone involvement must be interpreted as infection of bone. Acute infection can usually be treated by hardware removal and 10 to 14 days of parenteral antibiotics. If radiographic evidence of a ring sequestrum exists with persistent or recurrent drainage despite antibiotic treatment, surgical debridement is required. The author has found it useful in such cases to overdrill infected pin sites with a drill bit larger than the screw diameter on a hand brace while providing copious pulsed suction/lavage and curettage of the defect as needed to adequately debride the infected bone. Bone specimens, not swabs of drainage, should be sent for culture. Postoperative oral antibiotic treatment for 14 days is usually sufficient once the pin track has been adequately debrided. Radiographic evidence that confirms the removal of previously visualized sequestrum should be obtained intraoperatively. Care should be taken to protect the limb postoperatively for 4 to 6 weeks to avoid undue defect-related fractures.

In theory, early diagnosis and therapeutic intervention should be able to reverse the progression toward pin-track osteomyelitis and loosening and thereby help preserve the integrity of pin sites and avoid failure of the method. However, this requires both patient education about the earliest signs of problems and vigilance on the part of the clinical team to ensure prompt and effective treatment of pin-track problems.

Culturing all pin-site drainage is unnecessary and may be misleading because most pin sites will culture positive for bacterial contamination. Only documented clinical infections with purulence, pain, erythema, and swelling should be cultured for bacterial identification and antibiotic sensitivity.

Patients with external fixators should be followed closely. Regular evaluation by an experienced health-care professional on a weekly or biweekly basis can help to avoid serious complication.

Varied rates of pin-track infection are shown in Table 4-1. It is notable that with early recognition and aggressive treatment protocol, both a decrease in the incidence and severity of infections and an increase in the overall success of external fixation techniques have been seen. Both Marsh and Behrens, using different half-pin systems to treat a variety of severe open tibia fractures, have noted an acceptably low rate of pin-site infection and high rates of union with minimal deformity.[11,76]

Proponents of circular-ring and tensioned thin-wire (Ilizarov) techniques have likewise achieved successful outcomes in open-fracture treatment with a relatively low rate of serious pin-site infection.[27,37] Diaphyseal pin-track infections, though infrequent with thin-wire fixation, can sometimes be difficult to treat. When debridement is necessary, intraoperative localizing small (1–2 mm) foci of infection can be difficult. This has made many clinicians reticent to use the self-drilling thin wires in diaphyseal bone.

The best defense against pin-track infection is proper insertion technique and postoperative care. As previously noted, whenever possible, all pins should be placed through subcutaneous bone borders to avoid neurovascular and myotendonous units and the attendant risks of increased drainage and tethering. Tissue should be adequately incised during insertion, and cannulae should be used to avoid introducing skin flora into the wound and bone during drilling and insertion through contaminated soft tissues. All threaded half-pins should be predrilled with a sharp drill to avoid thermal necrosis.

A daily cycle of soft-tissue dependent swelling followed by later shrinkage with elevation causes a continuous tidal motion of the soft tissue across the exposed pin or screw surface. This allows bacteria to colonize the pin track.

Therefore, the exposed portion of the pins should be wrapped with a bulky gauze to firmly hold down the skin, prevent excessive motion, and decrease the risk that bacterial colonization levels reach infectious thresholds.

It was once assumed that exposed screw threads increased the rate of pin-track sepsis. This notion has not been substantiated, however, and most clinicians now discount the contribution of thread exposure to infection.

Daily pin care should strive to maintain a clean implant/skin interface with as little irritation as possible. In dealing with pin hygiene, it is best to keep in mind the adage "the simpler the better" or the acronym KISS (Keep It Simple with Saline). All forms of vigorous mechanical cleansing as well as the use of noxious chemical treatments have been associated with worsened rates of pin-site problems. Iodine, alcohol, or peroxide-based cleaning solutions seem to offer no benefit and have, in some studies, proved less effective than simple soap and water cleaning. In fact, many pediatric orthopaedic surgeons who have allowed their leg-length patients to swim in chlorinated pools with

TABLE 4-1
Open Tibia Fractures

	External Fixation			
	Union	*Fx Site Infection*	*Pin Site Infection*	*Malunion*
Mendes 1981	100%	4%	0	NA
Velazco 1983	92%	NA	12.5%	5%
Behrens 1986	100%	4%	6.9%	1.3%
Caudle 1987	66%	22%	NA	
Steinfeld 1988	97%	7.1%	0.5%	23%
Marsh 1991	95%	5%	10%	5%
Melendez 1989	98%	22%	14.2%	2%

their fixators report anecdotally reduced rates of pin-site sepsis over very long courses of fixation. It seems logical that keeping the limb and the external fixator device as clean as possible retards infection. Bathing in a household bath or a natural body of water is not recommended, however, as bacterial counts in most municipal water systems, lakes, rivers, and oceans may be unacceptably high. However, once other wounds are healed, patients with external fixators can shower daily as part of their overall hygiene without increased rates of infection.

Pin Loosening

As previously discussed, gradual mechanical pin loosening is to some extent a natural process in external fixation because pins or screws must withstand chronic stress. Loosening can be minimized with proper insertion techniques that stress predrilling of screw holes, radial preload (avoiding bending preload), euthermic pin insertion, and adequate soft-tissue release around the implant sites. All implants eventually loosen if subjected to continued stress. The "race" between union and implant loosening can only be won if the fracture in question heals promptly. Anything that ensures speedy union should be done. Open fractures that obviously need bone grafting should be grafted as soon as prudently possible. Off-loading implants through closure-type dynamization techniques will help to increase the longevity of pins and screws and secondarily assist healing by approximating the fracture ends.

A previously touted advantage of tapered thread-design screws was that these screws could be advanced and tightened in loosening situations. This claim has not been substantiated. Indeed, the technique of delayed tightening of loosened screws probably contributes to infection by introducing exposed and contaminated areas of the implant into the soft-tissue wound and bone.

Implant breakage poses another fortunately rare problem. A 5.2% incidence of pin fracture has been reported with the use of 4-mm diameter half-pins.[23] However, with current screws and pins of 5-mm and 6-mm diameters, this complication is now rare.

Fixator Body/Frame Failure

Frame failure represented either as breakage or bending is rare. However, many clinicians have anecdotal experience with patients who fall or trip and inadvertently overload external fixator couplers or universal joints resulting in fracture displacement. These displacements can usually be corrected by rereducing and retightening the external fixator frame. Such procedures usually require patient sedation.

Recent and growing economic pressures in the healthcare field have influenced many clinicians to reuse hardware after inspecting and replacing any obviously worn frame components. Manufacturers, though, are reluctant to warranty the use of hardware after the initial application. Without a process for formal inspection, overhaul, and recertification, the potential for fixator defects incurred during previous uses raises significant liability questions.

Apart from such legal considerations, the fact remains that most external fixator devices are inherently durable. Many medical centers reapply frames after inspection and replace only the implants (screws, pins, wires). Reuse is commonplace in Europe. Chao and colleagues have fatigue tested both Orthofix and Hoffman system hardware.[19,30] Their conclusions, based on the assumption of full-load weightbearing (600 N) of 2.5 million cycles per each use, suggest that if the fixators are appropriately monitored for screw strippage and frame cracking and if hardware is periodically tightened, each of these systems would survive four to five experimental applications. There is no clinical data to support or refute the concept of reuse. However, it remains to be seen if the present emphasis on cost cutting will render the single-use external fixator a casualty of healthcare reform. If single-use external fixator systems became more cost competitive, this discussion would be moot.

Malunion

As with any fixation technique, it is easy to apply an external fixator in a malaligned position. Angular discrepancies can easily be minimized by using fluoroscopy during application. Malrotation, however, can be easily missed and difficult to correct without repositioning pins or screws. When an external fixator is applied, care need be exercised to align the leg in proper rotation so that it is symmetrical to the normal opposite side. This may require access to the other limb during surgery. It is always best to think of any fixation method as the definitive means of stabilization at the time of application. Therefore, as with internal fixation, prefixation alignment should be acceptable to ensure that postoperative alignment is satisfactory as well. Fine tuning of reductions is possible with most external fixator systems excluding the more rudimentary bar and clamp designs. However, presupposing an unlimited degree of freedom to rereduce the fracture after inserting pins and aligning frames only invites frustration and embarrassment. It is best to get it right the first time!

Despite good initial alignment, external fixator hardware, like all hardware, may fail in some cases. Although frame and pin bending are rare, weightbearing stresses may cause implant loosening. Proper follow-up treatment requires radiographic checks during the weightbearing phase of fixation. Certainly, any comment by a patient alluding to a perception of a change in alignment or of motion should be taken seriously. Radiographs should be checked, and external fixators should be tightened as necessary. Always remember, the patient is living with the device and is the most sensitive resource for monitoring the hardware. Complaints should be investigated to avoid the risk of later complications.

Nonunion

In the past, detractors of external fixation have referred to them as nonunion machines. Indeed, delayed union and nonunion were once commonly cited as likely outcomes associated with these techniques. However, by better understanding the biology of fracture healing and the potential causes of nonunion, clinicians have achieved union rates with external fixation[96] comparable to other internal fixation techniques for injuries of like severity.[11,23,57,76,83,125]

To prevent the external fixator from keeping the fracture distracted, progressive closure dynamization techniques have evolved to eliminate gaps at the fracture site through telescopic components and other means. Compression in and of itself does not promote healing. Strain or micromovement sufficient to facilitate callus formation can be imparted through external fixation.

Park and coworkers demonstrated in an animal model that axial strain alone is not the only salutary form of stimulation to fracture healing. In their experiment on New Zealand white rabbits using an oblique tibial osteotomy model fixed with external fixators, it was clearly demonstrated that small amounts of shear strain can promote callus formation and accelerate healing just as well as axial strain.[95]

As already noted, the exact prescriptions for stress and strain magnitude have yet to be determined. But as principle precedes prescription, one can readily envision future external fixation devices that are designed to impart measured amounts of microstrain at a given phase of healing to promote union. External fixation actually lends itself to direct fracture site manipulation. The appropriate prescription for the timing and magnitude of such stimulation remains to be determined.

Soft-Tissue Impalement

Tethering

Percutaneous transfixion of soft tissue is always a concern when inserting external fixation implants. Whenever muscle or tendon structures are *tethered* by an implant, a tenodesis or myodesis-like effect restricts the motion of the joint crossed by that motor unit. After extended periods in such an external fixator, scarring may occur, requiring prolonged rehabilitation to regain joint motion. The result may be a permanent loss in motion, albeit usually a slight one, particularly if the injury is intra- or periarticular. This problem occurs much less often in children than in adults.

As a rule, after placement of an external fixator, any potentially restricted joint should be put through a full range of motion while the patient is still anesthetized. This technique can minimize the tethering effect. Whenever pins are placed in the femur, care should be taken to split the iliotibial band bluntly to make certain it is not fixed to the bone by the implant.

A rare and unique tethering complication may arise when performing bone transport techniques. Because muscle, tendon, and fascial structures may insert on transported bone segments, gradual deformity may occur with the procedure. This problem arises most often with proximal transport of a distal portion of the tibia. When there is no foot fixation, as the fragment of distal tibia is dragged proximally, the foot may be forced into an equinovarus position (Fig. 4-28). If left unaddressed, permanent deformity can occur. Vigorous daily stretching or fixation to the foot across the ankle is required to counteract this problem. In the absence of foot fixation, an ankle-foot orthosis should be used to maintain the foot in the neutral position. Knee flexion contracture has been reported but is a less common problem associated with proximal-distal transport.[92]

All joints about the foot and ankle should be in

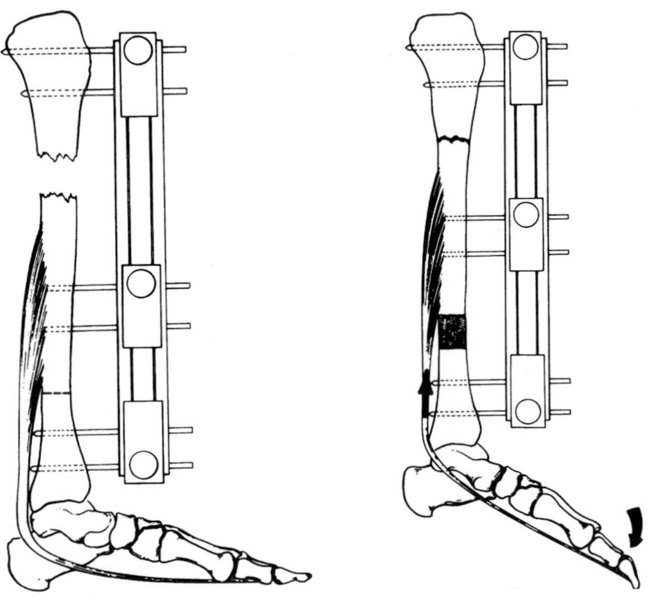

FIGURE 4-28. Distal-to-proximal transport in the tibia may be associated with tethering of muscle groups and attendant equinus deformity.

the neutral position when external fixator pins and/ or wires are placed to ensure proper plantigrade foot position at the end of treatment. Half-pins should be placed through the anteromedial safe zone over the tibial diaphysis to avoid transfixion of soft tissues. Yet it should be recognized that in half-pin techniques, bicortical purchase of the screw requires penetration of the far cortex of the tibia. Most half-screws are now blunt tipped, and this may help to minimize any unwanted soft-tissue injury. Still, the anatomy of deep compartment structures should be appreciated and fluoroscopic control used whenever possible to avoid overpenetration and compromise of the deep posterior compartment.

The knee should be relatively flexed to minimize the potential for compromise of the popliteal neurovascular structures when drilling pilot holes for placement of anteroposterior pins about the knee.[96] Likewise, care must be taken not to over insert implants. The use of lateral image intensification is quite helpful here as well.

Whenever applying an external fixator, the surgeon should have a clear understanding of the cross-sectional anatomy at the point of insertion. Large-diameter transfixion pins are no longer recommended, but the use of thinner tensioned wires with circular-ring fixation techniques demand even greater familiarity with anatomy. Cross-sectional drawings can be brought to the operating suite for those less familiar with these techniques and are helpful for instruction.

In the upper extremity, pins should always be placed with an open technique through incisions by directly visualizing the insertion site to minimize the possibility of iatrogenic neurovascular injury.

Compartment Syndrome

Compartment syndrome has been reported in association with external fixation.[87,99,116] It is a rare complication and whether induced by the presence of a pin causing compartment bleeding or by the inherent underlying preexisting injury is impossible to discern. With respect to this potentially serious complication, vigilance is the rule in any extremity injury. However, routine prophylactic fasciotomies are not advised simply because of external fixator placement in the absence of vascular compromise or crush injuries that would otherwise indicate them.

AUTHOR'S PREFERRED METHOD OF TREATMENT

External fixation should be as simple as possible. Unilateral systems now available provide adequate stability for most applications and facilitate care by using half-pins. Half-pins reduce the chance of soft-tissue impalement and often permit placement of implants through subcutaneous borders of bone. This, in turn, decreases the threat of neurovascular injury. Unilateral systems also allow better radiographic evaluation because orthogonal images are more easily acquired without fixator hardware obscuring the view. Radiolucent frames can also be used to minimize this problem. Additionally, less cumbersome frames with uniplanar pin fixation facilitate debridement, soft-tissue coverage, and/or bone grafting procedures by providing less obstructed access to soft-tissue wounds.

The use of complex multiplanar frames is rarely required in the acute setting. However, when added stability is required or when more complex injuries dictate a need, multiplanar fixation can be achieved by using delta-type fixator configurations or circular-ring and tensioned-wire components.

Incisions should be made prior to inserting wires or drills to minimize the introduction of skin flora into the wound and to protect soft tissue and skin from mechanical burns. Predrilling and screw insertion should be done through cannulae. This minimizes associated soft-tissue injury. Wherever possible, tensioned Kirschner wires should be advanced by malleting to avoid soft-tissue injury which can occur when the wire winds up tissue as it is drilled through the bone. When self-drilling of Kirschner wires is necessary, the wire should be cooled with a continuous saline irrigant during insertion. Any wire that exits the bone notably hot should be removed to avoid thermal necrosis and possible associated pin-track infection. Drills used for predrilling screw holes should be sharp. No screw should be placed into a pilot hole that has obviously been burned on predrilling. In a case of bone burning, the pin site should be changed.

Inserting half-pin/screw-threaded implants through predrilled pilot holes reduces the incidence of thermal necrosis, premature loosening, and pin-track infection. It is now considered standard.

Transfixion implants are occasionally necessary for circular-ring tensioned-wire devices. Even so, the use of transfixing wire implants through diaphyseal bone fragments is rarely needed. Half-pins may be affixed to circular ring frames to stabilize diaphyses.

Radial preload with tapered screws or down-sized pilot holes is recommended to improve implant longevity. Bending preload is to be discouraged.

Tension on soft tissue, though not initially noted at insertion, may occur during fracture manipulation and fixator realignment. Pin tracks* under tension should be carefully "released" with a scalpel after final reduc-

* Note the use of "pin track" as opposed to the more common term "tract" which, strictly speaking, is a term referring to a geographical area of land.

tion of fractures to avoid soft-tissue necrosis and pin-track infection.

All fractures should be relatively well aligned before fixator pin placement. This particularly applies to rotation. The need to markedly change fracture fragment alignment after placement of the fixator may leave the frame in an undesirable position, perhaps obscuring a wound. Ideal placement of the fixator body should be planned preoperatively. Modest adjustments in fracture alignment can be easily achieved with most systems. However, major changes may require replacing half-pins or transfixion wires for optimal fixator body alignment. It is relatively easy to provisionally align the fractured limb to get an accurate perception of the final fixator frame position and to allow for proper placement of fixator pins, screws, or wires. Whenever possible, fractures should be stably reduced to maximize contact of bone ends and minimize so-called fixator "bypass."

At the time of application, the fixator should be considered the definitive means of fixation, as it often will be. The device should be as meticulously applied as any internal fixation implant. Inaccurate or inadequate fracture reductions will ultimately result in similarly inadequate healing patterns and poor outcome.

The surgeon should be very careful to consider the appropriate level cross-sectional anatomy of any limb to be transfixed with such hardware. Figure 4-23 offers cross-sectional representations of the most common areas for application of external fixation transfixion implants. The problem of nerve compromise has been significant enough to lead some individuals to raise the possibility of using intraoperative somatosensory-evoked potentials.[73] This, however, is certainly not considered the standard of care.

Though pin tracks may not necessarily be infected, all carry a degree of bacterial contamination that can be eliminated from any prospective operative field with proper forethought. If secondary procedures, such as bone grafting, ORIF, or soft-tissue coverage involving the fracture site, are anticipated, the surgeon should apply the frame by placing pin sites well remote from the fracture site. This will allow the surgeon to prepare the operative site without involving the pin sites.

Adequate room (2–3 cm) for soft-tissue swelling should be allowed between the fixator frame and skin surface. This is particularly important in open fractures with wounds that may extend beneath the frame.

Fixator pin sites should be treated by simple daily cleansing with nonirritating solutions, such as normal saline. Chemical irritation caused by strong bactericidal agents often results in more pin-track complications than more simple treatments cause. Chronic use of oxidative solutions, such as hydrogen peroxide, may cause corrosive interactions with implant metals. Leaching of implant metals has been clinically associated with contact dermatitis-like reactions.

Patients with external fixation frames in place should be carefully monitored for problems. When detected early, common pin-track infections can usually be treated successfully with more fastidious pin-site cleansing and oral antibiotics. When appropriately treated, a purely soft-tissue pin-track infection only rarely develops into chronic osteomyelitis. The penalty for allowing a pin-site soft-tissue infection to go untreated is pin-track osteomyelitis and loosening. Truly infected implants with attendant osteolysis must be removed and replaced.

Patients with stable reductions should be encouraged to bear partial weight to enhance healing and minimize the time to union. Weightbearing helps the patient deter implant (wire, pin, screw) loosening.

When frame removal is considered, the adage "better a month late than a day too early" applies aptly to the use of external fixation. When used as a definitive means of stabilization, external fixation frames should be maintained until adequate healing allows painless, near normal full weightbearing with the frame removed from the pins. Premature removal most often results in refracture or malunion, even when postfixation bracing or casting is used. Many clinical studies have inferred less than desirable malunion and nonunion rates with the use of external fixation.[28,122] However, when carefully analyzed, such problems are usually attributable to premature frame removal either dictated by physician's treatment algorithm design or because of pin loosening and infection. Careful treatment of fixator pin sites can allow maintenance of the frame for 1 year or longer when necessary.[76]

The principles of dynamization should be used to distribute load to the fracture site, thereby promoting callus formation and accelerating remodeling, while gradually minimizing pin/bone stresses. Dynamization can be achieved with sequential disassembly techniques ("build down") or with a variety of intrinsic dynamization characteristics found in newer fixator frames and bodies.

Supplementing fixation by placing diaphyseal intrafragmentary lag screws should be avoided whenever possible as it is associated with increased infection and refracture rates in open-fracture treatment.[43,67]

Fixator pins/wires should avoid sites contiguous with the fracture hematoma. Because pin sites are frequently colonized with skin flora, placing implants through the fracture hematoma may allow seeding of the fracture site. Hematoma offers a favorable environment for bacterial growth. Implants placed through soft tissue that is stripped from the underlying bone at the injury site, as in open fractures, are likely predisposed toward infection as well. Though these mechanisms have not been proven, they are intuitively obvious, and it is imprudent to involve the pins with the fracture site. Pins are best placed well clear of the injury zone.

The aforementioned basic scientific and general clinical principles, irrespective of the specific anatomic site, form the basis for effective safe use of this clinical technique.

REFERENCES

1. Anderson, R.: Castless Ambulatory Method of Treating Fractures. J. Inter. Coll. Surg, 5:45, 1942.
2. Aro, H., Kelly, P.J., Lewallen, D.G., and Chao, E.Y.S.: The Effects of Physiologic Dynamic Compression on Bone Healing under External Fixation. Clin. Orthop Rel. Res., 256:260, 1990.
3. Aro, H.T., and Chao, E.Y.S.: Bone-Healing Patterns Affected by Loading, Fracture Fragment Stability, Fracture Type, and Fracture Site Compression. Clin. Orthop. Rel. Res., 293:8, 1993.
4. Aro, H.T., Hein, T.J., Chao, E.Y.: Mechanical Properties of Pin Clamps in External Fixators. Clin. Orthop. Rel. Res., 248:256, 1989.
5. Aronson, J., and Tursky, E.: External Fixator of Femur Fractures in Children. J. Ped. Orthop., 12:157, 1992.
6. Bach, A.W., and Hansen, S.T., Jr: Plates Versus External Fixation in Severe Open Tibial Shaft Fractures. A Randomized Trial. Clin. Orthop. Rel. Res., 241:89, 1989.
7. Baker, J., Nepola, J.V., Marsh, J.L., and Rodkey, W.: Comparison of Stabilization, External Fixation vs Nonreamed IM Nail in a Contaminated Tibial Fracture Model of the Rabbit: Effect on Infection Rate and Bacterial Distribution. Presented at Meeting of the Orthopaedic Trauma Association; November 2, 1991; Seattle, Wash.
8. Barquet, A., Svero, C., Massaferro, J., Dubra, A.: Bone Transport with the ASIF-BM Fixator for the Treatment of a 7 cm Segmental Defect of the Tibia with Run Off Only in the Posterior Tibial Artery. J. Orthop. Trauma, 7:248, 1993.
9. Barquet, A., Massaferro, J., Dubra, A., and Nin, F.: Ipsilateral Open Fracture of the Femur and Tibia Treated Using the Dynamic ASIF-BM Tubular External Fixator: Case Reports. J. Trauma, 31:1312, 1991.
10. Beaty, J.H., Austin, S.M., Warner, W.C., Canale, S.T., and Nicols, L.: Interlocking Intramedullary Nailing of Femoral-Shaft Fractures in Adolescents: Preliminary Results and Complications. J. Ped. Orthop., 14:178, 1994.
11. Behrens, F., and Searls, K.: External Fixtion of the Tibia. Basic Concepts and Prospective Evaluation. J. Bone Joint Surg., 68B(2):246, 1986.
12. Behrens, F., Johnson, W.D., Koch, T.W., and Kovacevic N.: Bending Stiffness of Unilateral and Bilateral Fixator Frames. Clin. Orth. Rel. Res., 178:103, 1983.
13. Behrens, F.: A Primer of Fixator Devices and Configurations. Clin. Ortho. Rel. Res., 245:5, 1989.
14. Bell, A.L., Smith, R.A., Brown, T.D., Nepola, J.V.: Comparative Study of the Orthofix and Pittsburgh Frames for External Fixation of Unstable Pelvic Ring Fractures. J. Orthop. Trauma, 2:130, 1988.
15. Bonar, S.K., and Marsh, J.L.: Unilateral External Fixation for Severe Pilon Fractures Foot Ankle. 14:57, 1993.
16. Bonar, S.K., and Marsh, J.L.: Tibial Plafond Fractures Changing Principles of Treatment. J. Am. Acad. Orthop. Surg., 2:297, 1994.
17. Bone, L., Johnson, J., Weigelt, J., and Scheinberg, R.: Early Versus Delayed Stabilization of Femoral Fractures. A Prospective Randomized Study. J. Bone Joint Surg. (Am), 71:336, 1989.
18. Bone, L., Stegeman, P., McNamara, K., Seibel, R.: External Fixation of Severely Comminuted Open Tibial Pilon Fractures. Clin. Orthop. Rel. Res., 292:101, 1993.
19. Brigg, B.T., and Chao, E.Y.S.: The Mechanical Performance of the Standard Hoffman-Vidal External Fixation Apparatus. J. Bone Joint Surg., 64A:566, 1982.
20. Broos, P.L., Miserez, M.J., and Rommens, P.M.: The Monofixator in the Primary Stabilization of Femoral Shaft Fractures in Multiply-Injured Patients. Injury, 23:525, 1992.
21. Brown, T.D., Stone, J.P., Schuster, J.H., and Mears, D.C.: External Fixation of Unstable Pelvic Ring Fractures: Comparative Rigidity of Some Current Frame Configurations. Med. Biol. Eng. Comp., 20:727, 1982.
22. Brutscher R., Rahn B.A., Ruter, A., and Perren, S.M.: The Role of Corticotomy and Osteotomy in the Treatment of Bone Defects Using the Ilizarov Technique. J. Orthopaedic Trauma., 7(3):261—269, 1993.
23. Burny, F.: Elastic External Fixation of Tibial Fractures: A Study of 1421 Cases: *In* Brooker, A.F., Jr., and Edwards, C.C. (eds.): External Fixation: The Current State of the Art. Baltimore, Williams and Wilkins, 1979.
24. Burny, F.: Elastic Fixation: A Biomechanical Study of the Half-Frame. In Seligson, D., and Pope, M.H. (eds): Concepts in External Fixation, p. 67. Orlando, Grune & Stratton, 1982.
25. Burstein, A.H., Currey, J., Franel, V.H., Heiple, K.G., Lunseth, P., and Vessely, J.V.: Bone Strength. The Effects of Screw Holes. J. Bone Joint Surg., 54A:1143, 1972.
26. Calhoun, J.H., Li, F., Ledbetter, B.R., and Gill, C.A.: Biomechanics of the Ilizarov Fixator for Fracture Fixation. Clinical Orthopaedics & Related Research, 290:15—22, 1992.
27. Cattaneo, R., Catagni, M., and Johnson, E.E.: The Treatment of Infected Nonunions and Segmental Defects of the Tibia by the Methods of Ilizarov. Clinical Orthopaedics & Related Research., 280:143—152, 1992.
28. Caudle, R.J., and Stern, P.J.: Severe Open Fractures of the Tibia. J. Bone Joint Surg (Am), 69:801, 1987.
29. Chao, E.Y.S., and Aro, H.T.: Chapter in Basic Orthopaedic Biomechanics, p. 293. New York Raven Press, 1991.
30. Chao, E.Y., and Hein T.J.: Mechanical Performances of the Standard Orthofix External Fixation. Orthopaedics, 7:1057, 1988.
31. Clyburn, T.A.: Dynamic External Fixation for Comminuted Intra-Articular Fractures of Distal End of the Radius. J. Bone Joint Surg. (Am), 69:248, 1987.
32. Coates, Col. John B. (ed): Orthopaedic Surgery in the European Theater of Operations, p. 116. Washington, D.C., Office of the Surgeon General, Department of the Army, 1957.
33. Coates, Col. John B. (ed): Orthopaedic Surgery in the Mediterranean Theater of Operations, p. 203. Washington, D.C., Office of the Surgeon General, Department of the Army, 1957.
34. Codivilla, A.: On the Means of Lengthening in the Lower Limbs, the Muscles and Tissues Which are Shortened Through Deformity. Clin. Orthop. Rel. Res., 301:4, 1994.
35. Collinge, C.A., Goll, G., Seligson, D., and Easley, K.J.: Pin Tract Infections: Silver vs Uncoated Pins. Orthopedics, 17(5):445—448, 1994.
36. Cooney, W.P., Linscheid, R.L., and Dobyns, J.H.: External Pin Fixation for Unstable Colles Fractures. J. Bone Joint Surg., 61A:840, 1979.
37. Dagher, F., and Roukoz, S., Compound Tibial Fractures with Bone Loss Treated by the Ilizarov Technique. J. Bone Joint Surg.-British Volume., 73(2):316—321, 1991.
38. Dahners, L.E., Jacobs, R.R., Jayaraman, G., Cepulo A.J.: A Study of External Fixation Systems for Unstable Pelvic Fractures. J. Trauma, 10:876, 1984.
39. Danis, R: Theorie et Pratique de L'Ostéosynthese, Libraries De L'Academie De Medicine. Paris, 1949.
40. De Bastiani, G., Aldegheri, R., Renzi Brivio, L.R., and Trivella, G.P.: Dynamic Axial External Fixation. Auto Medica, 10:235, 1989.
41. De Bastiani, G., Algegheri, R., and Renzi Brivio, L.R.: The Treatment of Fractures with a Dynamic Axial Fixator. J. Bone Joint Surg. (Br), 66-B:538, 1984.
42. Egger, L., Cottsavner-Wolf, F., Palmer, J., Aro, H.T., and Chao, E.Y.S.: Effects of Axial Dynamization on Bone Healing. J. Trauma, 34:185, 1993.
43. Etter, C., Burri, C., Claes, L., Kinzl, L., Raible, M.: Treatment of Open Fractures Associated with Severe Soft Tissue Damage

of the Leg. Biomechanical Principles and Clinical Experience. Clin. Orth. Rel. Res., 178:80, 1983.
44. Fitzpatrick, D.C., Marsh, J.L., and Brown, T.D.: Articulated External Fixation of Pilon Fractures: The Effects on Ankle Joint Kinematics. J. Orth. Trauma, 9:76, 1995.
45. Fleming, B., Paley, D., Kristiansen, T., and Pope, M.: A Biomechanical Analysis of the Ilizarov External Fixator. Clin. Ortho. Rel. Res., 241:95, 1989.
46. Galpin, R.D., Baxter, W.R., and Sabano, N.: Intramedullary Nailing of Pediatric Femur Fractures. J. Ped. Orthop., 14:184, 1994.
47. Ganz, R., Krushell, R., Jacob, R., Küffer, J.: Anti-Shock Pelvic Clamp. Clin. Orth. Rel. Res., 267:71, 1991.
48. Gasser, B., Boman, B., Wyder, D., and Schneider, E.: The Stiffness Characteristics of the Circular Ilizarov Device as Opposed to Conventional External Fixators. J. Biomechanics Eng., 112:15, 1990.
49. Ghanayem, A.J., Wilber, J.H., Lieberman, J.M., and Motta, A.O.: The Effect of Laparotomy and External Fixator Stabilization on Pelvic Volume in an Unstable Pelvic Injury. J. Trauma, 38:396, 1995.
50. Goodship, A.E., and Kenwright, J.: The Influence of Induced Micromovement Upon the Healing of Experimental Tibial Fractures. J. Bone Joint Surg. (Br), 67B:650, 1985.
51. Goris, R.J., Giambrere, J.S., Von Niekerk, J.L., Schotts, F.J., Booy, L.H.: Early Osteosynthesis and Prophylactic Mechanical Ventilation in the Multi-Trauma Patient. J. Trauma, 22:895, 1982.
52. Gottschalk, F.A., Graham, A.J., and Morein, G.: The Management of Severely Comminuted Fractures of the Femoral Shaft, Using the External Fixator Injury: 16:377, 1985.
53. Green, S.A.: Complications of External Skeletal Fixation, p. 93. Springfield, Charles C. Thomas 1981.
54. Green, S.A.: The Ilizarov Method: Rancho Technique. Orthopaedics Clinics of North America, 22(4):677—688, 1991.
55. Gristina, A.G., and Costerton, J.W.: Bacterial Adherence to Biomaterials and Tissue: The Significance of its Role in Clinical Sepsis. J. Bone Joint Surg. (Am), 67:264, 1985.
56. Henderson, R.C.: The Long-Term Results of Nonoperatively Treated Major Pelvic Disruptions. J. Orthop. Trauma, 3:41, 1989.
57. Hessmann, M., Mattens, M., and Rumbaut, J.: The Unilateral External Fixator (Monofixator) in Acute Fracture Treatment: Experience in 50 Fractures. Acta Chirurgica Belgica, 94(4):229—235, 1994.
58. Howard, P.W., Stewart, H.D., Hind, R.E., and Burke, F.D.: External Fixation or Plaster for Severely Displaced Comminuted Colles' Fractures? A Prospective Study of Anatomical and Functional Results. J. Bone Joint Surg., 71B:68, 1989.
59. Hydahl C., Pearson, S., Tepic, Perren, S.M.: Induction and Prevention of Pin Loosening in External Fixation: An In Vivo Study on Sheep Tibiae. J. Ortho Trauma, 5(4):485, 1991.
60. Jenkins, N.H., Jones, D.G., Johnson, S.R., and Mintowt-Czyz, W.T.: External Fixation of Colles' Fractures: An Anatoical Study. J. Bone Joint Surg., 69-B(2):207—211, 1987.
61. Johnson, K.D., Cadambi, A., and Seibert, G.B.: Incidence of Adult Respiratory Distress Syndrome in Patients with Multiple Musculoskeletal Injuries: The Effect of Early Operative Stabilization of Fractures. J. Trauma, 25:375, 1985.
62. Karas, E.H., and Weiner, L.S.: Displaced Pilon Fractures-An Update. Ortho. Cl. N.A., 25:651, 1994.
63. Kellam, J.F.: The Role of External Fixation in Pelvic Disruptions. Clin. Orthop. Rel. Res., 241:66, 1989.
64. Kenwright, J., Richardson, J.B., and Cunningham, J.L., et al.: Axial Micromovement and Tibial Fractures: A Controlled Randomised Trial of Treatment. J. Bone Joint Surg. (Br.), 73B:654, 1991.
65. Kirschenbaum, D., Albert, M.C., Robertson, W.W., Jr., and Davidson, R.S.: Complex Femur Fractures in Children: Treatment with External Fixation. J. Ped. Orthop., 10:588, 1990.
66. Kojimoto, H., Yasui, N., Goto, T., et al.: Bone Lengthening in Rabbits by Callus Distraction; The Role of the Periosteum and Endosteum. J. Bone Joint Surg. (Br), 70:543, 1988.
67. Krettek, C., Haas, N., and Tscherne, H.: The Role of Supplemental Lag-Screw Fixation for Open Fractures of the Tibial Shaft Treated with External Fixation. J. Bone Joint Surg. (Am), 73:893, 1991.
68. Kummer, F.J.: Biomechanics of the Ilizarov External Fixator. Clinical Orthopaedics & Related Research, 280:11—14, 1992.
69. Lambotte, A.: L'Intervention Opératoire dans Les Fractures Récentes et Anciennes. In Relter, L.F., Fractures, p. 59. Brussels, Henri Lamertin, 1907.
70. Leug, K.S., Shene, W.Y., Tsang, H.K., Chiu, K.H., Leung, P.C., and Hung, L.K.: An Effective Treatment of Comminuted Fractures of the Distal Radius. J. Hand Surg., 15A:11—17, 1990.
71. Lindholm, R.V., Lindholm, T.S., Torkkanen S., and Leino, R.: Effect of Forced Inter-Fragmental Movements on the Healing of Tibial Fractures in Rats. Acta Orthop. Scand., 40:721, 1970.
72. Maiocchi, A.B.: The Historical Review. *In* Maiocchi, A.B., and Aronson, J. (eds.): Operative Principles of Ilizarov Med Surgical Video Milan 1991, p. 3.
73. Makarov, M.R., Delgado, M.R., Samchukov, M.L., Welch, R.D., and Birch, J.G.: Somatosensory Evoked Potential Evaluation of Acute Nerve Injury Associated with External Fixation Procedures. Clinical Orthopaedics & Related Research, (308):254—263, 1994.
74. Marsh, J.L., Prokuski, L., and Biermann, J.S.: Chronic Infected Tibial Nonunions with Bone Loss. Conventional Techniques Versus Bone Transport. Clinical Orthopaedics & Related Research, 301:139—146, 1994.
75. Marsh, J.L., Smith, S.T., D.O., T.T.: External Fixation and Limited Internal Fixation for Complex Fractures of the Tibial Plateau. J. Bone Joint Surg. (Am.), 77:661, 1995.
76. Marsh, J.L., Nepola, J.V., Wuest, T.K., Osteen, D., Cox, K., Oppenheim, W.: Unilateral External Fixation until Healing with the Dynamic Axial Fixator for Severe Open Tibial Fractures. J. Orthop Trauma, 5 (3):341, 1991.
77. Martin, J.G., Nepola, J.V., and Marsh, J.L.: The Treatment of Unstable Pelvic Injuries with External Fixation: Orth. Trans, 18:1053, 1994—1995.
78. Matthews, L.S., Green, C.A., and Goldstein, S.A.: The Thermal Effects of Skeletal Fixation-Pin Insertion in Bone. J. Bone Joint Surg. (Am), 66A:1077, 1984.
79. Maurer, D.J., Merkow, R.L., and Gustilo, R.B.: Infection after Intramedullary Nailing of Severe Open Tibial Fractures Initially Treated with External Fixation. J. Bone Joint Surg. (Am), 71:835, 1989.
80. O'Malley, D.E., Mazur, J.M., Cummings, R.J.: Femoral Head Avascular Necrosis Associated with Intramedullary Nailing in an Adolescent. J. Ped. Ortho. 15(1):21, 1995.
81. McBroom, R.J., Cheal, E.J., and Hayes, W.C.: Strength Reductions from Metastatic Cortical Defects in Long Bones. J. Orthop. Res., 6:369, 1988.
82. McGraw, J.M., and Lim, E.V.: Treatment of Open Tibial-Shaft Fractures. External Fixation and Secondary Intramedullary Nailing. J. Bone Joint Surg. (Am), 70:900, 1988.
83. Melendez, E.M., and Colon, C.: Treatment of Open Tibial Fractures with the Orthofix Fixator. Clinic. Orthop. Rel. Res., 241:224, 1989.
84. Miranda, M.A., Riemer, B.L., Hudak, M.D., Butterfield, S.L., and Burke, C.J. III: Functional Outcome of Pelvic Ring Disruptions. Presented at Meeting of the American Association of Orthopaedic Surgeons; 1995; Orlando, Fla.
85. Morrey, B.F.: Post Traumatic Contracture of the Elbow. Operative Treatment Including Distraction Arthroplasty. J. Bone Joint Surg. (Am), 72:601, 1990.
86. McLaughlin, H.: Trauma. Philadelphia, W.B. Saunders, 1959.
87. Naden, J.: External Fixation in the Treatment of Fractures of the Tibia. J Bone Joint Surg. (Am), 31:586, 1949.
88. Nagar, L., Cheralley, F., Blanc, C.H., Livio, J.J.: Treatment of Large Bone Defects with the Ilizarov Technique. J. Trauma, 34:390, 1993.
89. Nordeen, M.H., Taylor, B.A., Briggs, T.W., and Lary, C.B.: Pin Placement in Pelvic External Fixation. Injury, 24:581, 1993.
90. Paley, D.: Current Techniques of Limb Lengthening. J Ped Orthopaedics, 8:73, 1988.
91. Paley, D.: Biomechanics of the Ilizarov External Fixation. *In*

Manocchi, A.B., Aronson, J.: Operative Principles of Ilizarov, p. 39. Med. Surgical Video, Milan, 1991.

92. Paley, D.: Problems, Obstacles, and Complications of Limb Lengthening by the Ilizarov Technique. Clin Orth Rel Res., 250:81, 1990.
93. Pape, H.C., Dwenger, A., Ragel, G., et al.: Pulmonary Damage After Intramedullary Femoral Nailing in Traumatized Sheep-Is There an Effect from Different Nailing Techniques? J. Trauma, 33:574, 1992.
94. Pape, H.C., Regel, G., Dwenger, A., Sturm, J.A., and Tscherne, H.: Influence of Thoracic Trauma and Primary Femoral Intramedullary Nailing on the Incidence of ARDS in Multiple Trauma Patients. Injury, 24(suppl. 3):582, 1993.
95. Park, S., McKellop, H., Sarmiento, A.: Shear Motion Resulted in Increased Strength and Stiffness When Compared to Axial Motion of Rigid Immobilization. Presented at the Meeting of the American Association of Orthopaedic Surgeons; 1995; Orlando, Fla.
96. Parkhill, C.: A New Apparatus for the Fixation of Bones after Resection and in Fractures with a Tendency to Displacement. Trans Am Surg. Assoc., 15:251, 1897. Abstract.
97. Raimbeau, G., Chevalier, J., and Raguin, J.: Les Risques Vasculaires du Fixateur en Cadre a la Jambe. Rev. Chir Orthop., 65supp. 11:77, 1979.
98. Raskin, K.B., Melone, C.P., Jr.: Unstable Articular Fractures of the Distal Radius. Comparative Techniques of Ligamentotaxis. Orthopaedic Clinics of North America, 24(2):275—286, 1993.
99. Richardson, J.B., Gardner, T.N., Hardy, J.R.W., Evans, M., Kuiper, J.H., and Kenwright, J.: Dynamisation of Tibial Fractures. J. Bone Joint Surg., 77B:412, 1995.
100. Riemer, B.I., Butterfield, S.L., Diamond, D.L.: Acute Mortality Associated with Injuries to the Pelvic Ring: The Role of Early Patient Mobilization and External Fixation. J. Trauma, 35:671, 1993.
101. Riemer, B.L., and Butterfield, S.L.: Comparison of Reamed and Nonreamed Solid Core Nailing of the Tibial Diaphysis after External Fixation: A Preliminary Report. Journal of Orthopaedic Trauma, 7(3):279—285, 1993.
102. Rüedi, T.P., and Allgöwer, M.: The Operative Treatment of Intra-120 Cular Fractures of the Lower End of the Tibia. Clin. Orthop., 138:105—110, 1979.
103. Saleh, M., Shannhan, M.D., and Fern, E.D.: Intra-Articular Fractures of the Distal Tibia: Surgical Management by Limited Internal fixation and Articulated Distraction. Injury, 24(1):37—40, 1993.
104. Seitz, W.H., Jr., Putnam, M.D., and Dick, H.M.: Limited Open Surgical Approach for External Fixation of Distal Radius Fractures. J. Hand Surg., 15A:288—293, 1990.
105. Siris, I.: External Pin Transfixion of Fractures: An Analysis of Eighty Cases. Ann. Surg., 120:911, 1944.
106. Slätis, P., and Karaharju, E.O.: External Fixation of Unstable Pelvic Fractures: Experiences in 22 Patients Treated with a Trapezoid Compression. Clin. Orthop. Rel. Res., 151:73, 1980.
107. Sommerkamp, T.G., Seeman, M., Silliman, J., et al.: Dynamic External Fixation of Unstable Fractures of the Distal Part of the Radius. A Prospective, Randomized Comparison with Static External Fixation. J. Bone Joint Surg. (Am)., 76(8):1149—1161, 1994.
108. Stader, O.: A Preliminary Announcement of a New Method of Treating Fractures. N. Am Vet., 18:37, 1937.
109. Stern, P.J., and Drury, W.J.: Complications of Plate Fixation of Forearm Fractures. Clin Orthop. Rel. Res., 175:25, 1983.
110. Taillard, W.: External Fixation: Past, Present and Future: Introduction to the Tenth Internal Congress on Hoffman External Fixation. Orthopaedics, 7:398, 1984.
111. Teeny, S.M., and Wiss, D.A.: Open Reduction and Internal Fixation of Tibial Plafond Fractures: Variables Contributing to Poor Results and Complications. Clin. Orthop, 392:108—117, 1993.
112. Tiedeman, J., Steyers, C., Blair, W., Skaro, E., and Brown, T.D.: Wrist Kinematics During Distraction Mobilization in the Agee External Fixation (in press).
113. Tile, M.: Pelvic Ring Fractures: Should They Be Fixed? J. Bone Joint Surg. (Br), 70:1, 1988.
114. Tillman, R.M., and Kenny, N.W.: Small Bowel Obstruction as a Complication of the Use of an External Fixator in a Pelvic Fracture. Injury, 22(1):71—72, 1991.
115. Tuikanen, E., and Asko-Seljavaara, S.: The Use of the Ilizarov Technique After a Free Micro Vascular Muscle Flap Transplantation in Massive Trauma of the Lower Leg. Clin. Orthop. Rel. Res., 297:129, 1993.
116. Van de Bossche, M.R.P., Rommens, P.M.: Open Fractures of the Femoral Shaft Treated with Osteosynthesis or Temporary External Fixation. Injury 26:323, 1995.
117. Vidal, J., Buscayref, C., Connes, H., et al.: Guidelines for Treatment of Open Fractures and Infected Pseudoarthroses by External Fixation. Clin. Orthop. Rel. Res., 180:183, 1983.
118. Vidal, J.: External Fixation, Yesterday, Today and Tomorrow. Clin. Orthop, Rel. Res., 180:7, 1983.
119. Vidal, J.: Notre experiénce du fixateur externe diHoffmann, Montpellier chir 14:451, 1968.
120. Weber, B.S., and Magerl, F.: The External Fixator. New York, Springer-Verlag, 1985.
121. Weiner, L.S., Kelly, M., Yang, E., et al.: The Use of Combination Internal Fixation and Hybrid External Fixation in Severe Proximal Tibia Fractures. J. Orth. Trauma, 9:244, 1995.
122. Whitelaw, G.P., Wetzler, M., Nelson, A., et al.: Ender Rods Versus External Fixation in the Treatment of Open Tibial Fractures. Clin Orth Rel. Res., 253:258, 1990.
123. Wild, J.J., Hanson, G.W., and Tullos, H.S.: Unstable Fractures of the Pelvis Treated by External Fixation. J. Bone Joint Surg. (Am), 64:1010, 1982.
124. Yves, A., Burny, F., Donkerwolcke, M., and Wagenknecht, M.: In Vivo Evaluation of Pin Reaction in External Fixation and Functional Bracing. *In* Coombs, R., Green, S. and Sarmiento, A. Orthotext, London, 1989.
125. Zachee, B., Roosen, P., and Mc Aechern, A.G.: The Dynamic Axial Fixator in Fractures of the Tibia and Femur. A Retrospective Study in 98 Patients. Acta Orthopaedica Belgica, 57(3):266—271, 1991.

Rockwood and Green's Fractures in Adults, Fourth Edition,
edited by Charles A. Rockwood, David P. Green, Robert W. Bucholz and James D. Heckman.
Lippincott-Raven Publishers, Philadelphia © 1996.

CHAPTER 5

Healing of the Musculoskeletal Tissues

Joseph A. Buckwalter, Thomas A. Einhorn,
Mark E. Bolander, and Richard L. Cruess

The surgeon's goal in caring for patients with acute musculoskeletal injuries is to restore their function rapidly by promoting healing of the injured tissues. Surgeons can treat injuries without extensive knowledge of tissue healing, but they are better able to select the optimal treatment if they have this knowledge. Furthermore, they can treat, and in some instances prevent, complications of musculoskeletal injuries or problems of failed or inadequate healing more effectively when they are as skilled in applying knowledge of tissue healing as they are in the use of surgical techniques. The first principles of treating musculoskeletal injuries are to prevent further tissue damage, avoid compromising the natural healing process, and create the optimal biological and mechanical conditions for healing. Following these principles requires knowledge of the capacity of tissues to heal and the variables that affect those capacities in each patient, including characteristics of the injury, the patient, and the tissue, as well as knowledge and skill in the selection and application of treatments. Recent basic and clinical studies have dramatically advanced understanding of healing and made it increasingly important that orthopaedists be experts in applied musculoskeletal biology and biomechanics as well as skilled surgeons.

Discussions of acute musculoskeletal trauma often focus on fractures and therefore on the restoration of bone structure and function. However, injuries to the other primary musculoskeletal tissues (the dense fibrous tissues [tedon, ligament, joint capsule, and meniscus][6,43,45,113]; articular cartilage[42,44,47,48]; and muscle[60,61]) frequently occur in association with fractures and can affect the result of fracture treatment. In addition, an injury that fractures bone and disrupts other primary musculoskeletal tissues often damages the supporting soft tissues (peripheral nerve, blood vessels, and lymphatic vessels). Injuries to these tissues may be more difficult to treat and leave patients with more significant permanent disability than fractures.[183,223]

In this chapter the general principles of musculoskeletal tissue healing and the variables that influence healing are described first. In subsequent sections, bone, dense fibrous tissue (tendon, ligament and joint capsule and meniscus), cartilage, and skeletal muscle healing is reviewed and how specific injury, patient, tissue, and treatment variables influence healing of these tissues is examined. The purpose is to provide a framework for understanding the healing of human musculoskeletal tissues after acute injuries, the influence of current treatments, and the potential for new treatments to improve the results of musculoskeletal tissue healing.

HEALING

Healing, the tissue response that restores tissue structure and function after injury, results from a complex interrelated series of cellular, humoral, and in most tissues, vascular events. Tissue damage combined with the hemorrhage caused by acute traumatic injury initiates a response that in vascularized tissues (eg, bone, most dense fibrous tissues, and muscle) includes inflammation, repair, and remodeling (Fig. 5-1). Inflammation, repair, and remodeling do not occur as discrete events. Instead, they form a continuous sequence of cellular, humoral, and vascular events initiated by injury. The sequence begins with the release of inflammatory mediators and ends when remodeling of the repair tissue reaches a homeostatic state. Nonvascularized tissues (e.g., cartilage and the inner regions of the menisci) cannot generate a recognizable inflammatory response, but injuries to these tissues cause a cellular response.[44–48] Unfortunately, this response cannot heal a significant injury.

INFLAMMATION, REPAIR, AND REMODELING

Inflammation

Inflammation, the cellular and vascular response to injury, includes release of inflammatory mediators, vasodilatation, exudation of plasma, and migration of inflammatory cells to the injury site. These tissue events can cause swelling, erythema, increased tissue temperature, pain, and impaired tissue function, although these clinical symptoms and signs of inflammation do not accompany every injury.

In vascularized tissues, inflammation begins immediately after injury. Release of vasoactive mediators from injured tissue promotes dilation and increased permeability of blood vessels near the injury. Blood escaping from damaged vessels forms a hematoma that temporarily fills the injury site. Within the hematoma

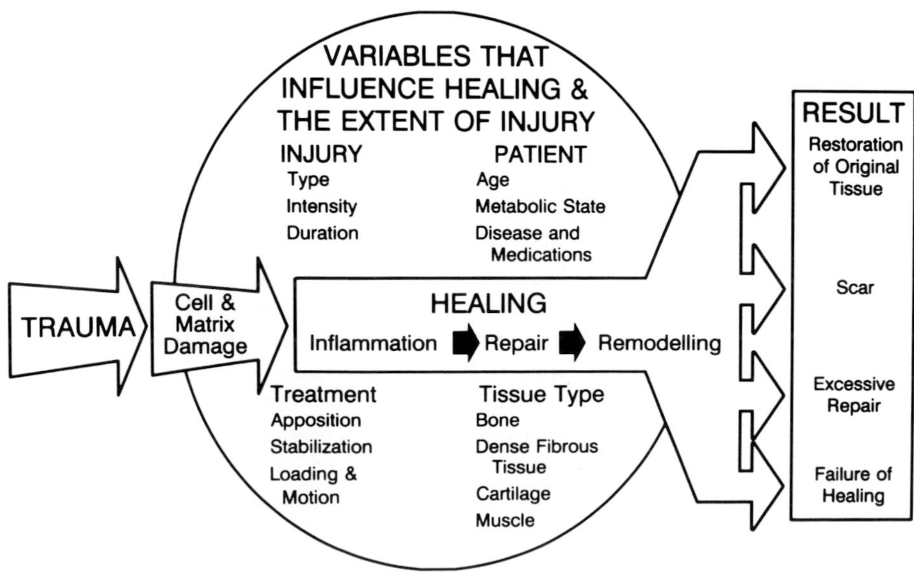

FIGURE 5-1. Schematic diagram of the response of vascularized musculoskeletal tissues to acute traumatic injury. Cell and matrix damage initiates the sequence of inflammation, repair, and remodeling. The tissue response may result in restoration of the original tissue, scar, excessive repair (scarring), or failure of repair depending on injury, tissue, patient, and treatment variables.

fibrin forms and platelets bind to fibrillar collagen, thereby achieving hemostasis. With activation of the coagulation system and platelet adherence and aggregation, the platelets release potent vasoactive mediators, including serotonin, histamine, and thromboxane A_2. They also release growth factors or cytokines. *Growth factors or cytokines,* including transforming growth factor beta (TGF-β), fibroblast growth factor, and platelet-derived growth factor as well as a large number of others, are small proteins that influence cell migration, proliferation, and differentiation, as well as matrix synthesis.[21,35,58,59,154,180,181,207,218,280,281,294] These molecules appear to have important roles in growth and development as well as healing.

Polymorphonuclear leukocytes are the first inflammatory cells to appear at the site of injury, followed by monocytes and T lymphocytes. Enzymes released from inflammatory cells may help remove necrotic tissue, and release of cytokines from monocytes and other inflammatory cells[211,271,280] may help stimulate vascular invasion of the injured tissue and the migration and proliferation of the mesenchymal cells that start the repair process. Blood vessel endothelial cells near the injury proliferate and form new capillaries that extend into the injury site. It appears that phagocytic, mesenchymal, and endothelial cells release growth factors that influence the other cells as well as the cells that produce these factors. In particular, blood vessel endothelial cells release platelet-derived growth factor, nerve tissue releases fibroblast growth factor, macrophages release interleukin-1, platelets release platelet-derived growth factor and TGF-β, and fibroblasts may also release platelet-derived growth factor and TGF-β. These observations can help explain the sequential appearance of the different cell types after injury. According to this concept, each population of cells produces factors that attract and influence the function of the next population of cells.[211] When the fibroblasts appear, they continue to produce factors that influence fibroblast function throughout repair.

Although inflammation can contribute to healing by facilitating removal of necrotic tissue and by initiating repair, especially vascular invasion and cell migration, it is not necessarily beneficial. For example, an intense prolonged inflammatory response may increase the extent of tissue damage, delay repair, or cause excessive scarring, and it is not clear that successful healing requires inflammation. Study of soft-tissue wounds in young animals shows that in fetuses and neonates healing occurs with minimal or no apparent inflammatory response.[86,89,192–194] Mesenchymal cells from the surrounding tissues migrate through a matrix with a high hyaluronic acid (hyaluronan) content and low collagen content to the injury site and heal the wound without a scar. During the early stages of growth and development, undifferentiated mesenchymal cells normally proliferate rapidly and form bone, cartilage, fibrous tissue, muscle, fat, blood vessels, and probably other tissues (Fig. 5-2). Throughout life, undifferentiated mesenchymal cells exist in the bone marrow, periosteum, and probably the peripheral blood and other tissues and retain the capacity to differentiate into specialized connective tissue cells. The observation that fetal tissues with a matrix that allows rapid cell migration and proliferation heal without inflammation and vascular invasion shows that initiating repair does not necessarily require inflammation. This work also suggests that it may be possible to heal injuries in poorly vascularized or avascular tissues and that selectively suppressing some components of inflammation and supplying appropriate cells and matrix may improve healing of other tissues.

Repair

Repair, the replacement of necrotic or damaged tissue by new cells and matrix, results from the activities of undifferentiated mesenchymal cells that migrate to the injury site during inflammation along with new blood vessels. These cells have the capacity to form bone, cartilage, fibrous tissue, blood vessels, and possibly other tissues (see Fig. 5-2).[40] Although undifferentiated mesenchymal cells probably exist in most connective tissues as well as bone marrow, and they may arise from cells that accompany the invading capillaries, their origin during the repair process remains uncertain. Soon after entering the site of clot formation and tissue damage they proliferate and synthesize a new matrix with a high concentration of collagen. Later, depending on the biological and mechanical conditions, they may differentiate into chondrocytes, osteoblasts, fibroblasts, or other cell types (see Fig. 5-2). Signals within the injured tissue—including the types of concentrations of growth factors, hormones, and nutrients, as well as pH, oxygen tension, and the electrical and mechanical environment—control proliferation, matrix synthesis, and differentiation.

Remodeling

Remodeling, the reshaping and reorganizing of tissue by removing, replacing, and reorganizing cells and matrix, completes successful healing. Repair of many acute injuries produces an excessive amount of cellular and vascular tissue with a poorly organized matrix. Remodeling reshapes and reorganizes the repair tissue so that it more closely resembles the original tissue. As remodeling progresses, cell density and vascularity decrease, the cells remove excessive repair matrix, and frequently the repair tissue matrix collagen fibrils become more highly oriented along the lines of stress. Although most appar-

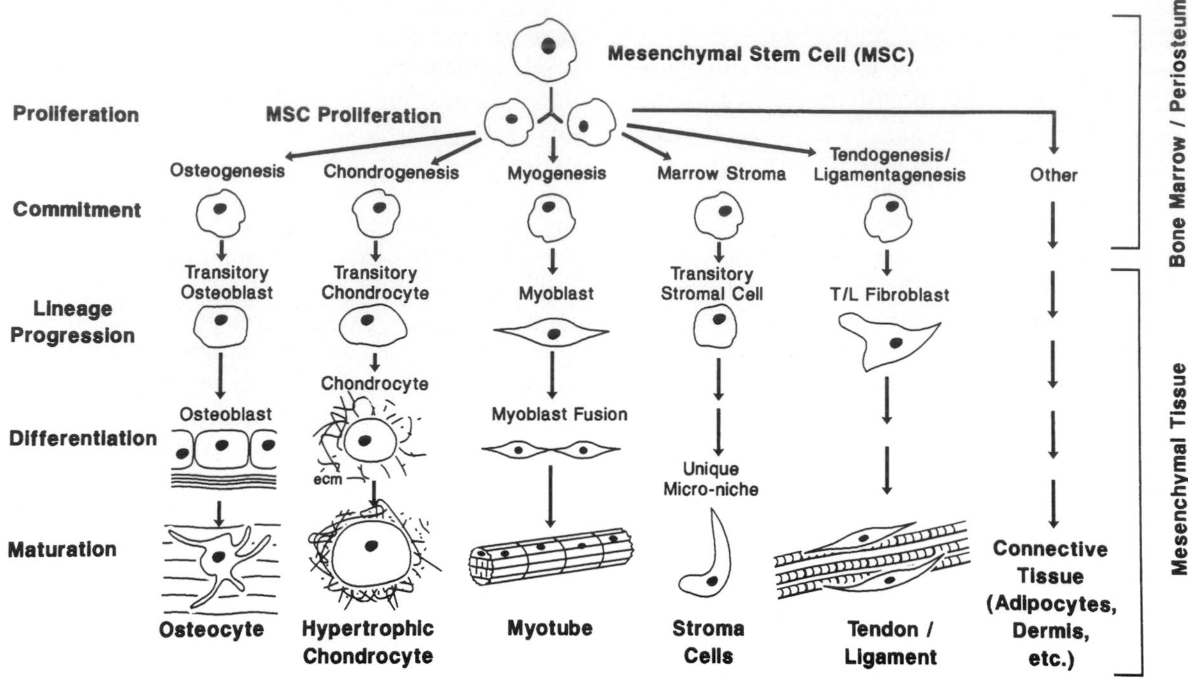

FIGURE 5-2. A diagrammatic representation of the potential of mesenchymal cells to differentiate into specialized connective tissue cells. Under appropriate conditions mesenchymal stem cells migrate to the site of injury, proliferate, and differentiate into specialized cells, including osteocytes, chondrocytes, myoblasts, fibroblasts, and others. Throughout life these cells exist in the bone marrow and periosteum. They also may be present in other tissues and in the peripheral blood. (*Courtesy of Arnold Caplan, PhD, Case Western Reserve University, Cleveland, OH.*)

ent remodeling of repair tissue ceases within months of injury, tissue removal, replacement, and reorganization continues throughout life.

RESULTS OF TISSUE INJURY

Healing, as most patients and surgeons use the term, refers not to the sequence of cell and matrix events described earlier but to a visible, palpable result of these events—that is, restoration of structural integrity to an injured tissue either with tissue identical to the original tissue or in some instances with scar tissue. Measured by this standard, the results of the tissue response to injury can be grouped into four overlapping categories (Table 5-1): (1) restoration of the original tissue; (2) scar that restores at least some structural integrity and often function; (3) excessive repair or scarring that interferes with function; and (4) failure of repair.

To add to the complexity of understanding musculoskeletal injuries, the results of treatment as measured by the degree of restoration of tissue structure, composition, and function does not necessarily determine the functional outcome for the patient. Patients with nearly identical healing of open tibia fractures may have different functional results as measured by return to work, ability to perform necessary activities of daily living, or ability to participate in recreational activities. These differences presumably are more closely related to social, economic, educational, and psychological factors than to the result of tissue healing.

VARIABLES THAT INFLUENCE HEALING

The result of a tissue injury (see Table 5-1) depends on the intrinsic tissue capacity for healing and the variables that influence healing. Animal experiments and clinical studies show that the variables that influence healing fall into four general categories: injury, tissue, patient, and treatment (see Fig. 5-1). Some of the specific injury, patient, and treatment variables have been well defined, some are presumed to influence healing based on clinical observations but have not been clearly defined, and others remain unknown.

Type of Injury

Type of Injury. In general, acute soft-tissue injuries can be identified as blunt, tearing, or penetrating injuries or combinations of these types of injury. *Blunt injuries* compress and crush tissue and range from mild contusion

TABLE 5-1
Results of Musculoskeletal Tissue Response to Injury

Result	Examples	Tissue Composition
Restoration of normal tissue (restoration of normal structural integrity, composition and function)	Most fractures Some skeletal muscle injuries Some dense fibrous tissue injuries	Bone Skeletal muscle Organized dense fibrous tissue
Scar (restoration of at least some tissue structural integrity and function)	Fibrous union of bone Most dense fibrous tissue injuries (tendon, ligament, outer meniscus regions)	Scar consisting of fibroblasts, a matrix containing primarily type I collagen, capillaries, and occasionally small myxoid regions
	Some skeletal muscle injuries Chondral portions of some osteochondral injuries	Scar with some muscle cells Scar without capillaries mixed with fibrocartilage and hyaline-like cartilage, including chondrocyte-like cells and a matrix containing type II collagen
Excessive repair or scarring (adhesions between the site of injury and the surrounding tissues restrict or prevent function)	Some tendon, ligament, joint capsule and skeletal muscle injuries (loss of muscle tendon unit or joint motion) and some osteochondral injuries (joint contractures or ankylosis)	Scar adherent to surrounding tissues
Failure of repair (persistent tissue defect or presence of tissue that does not restore structural integrity)	Fracture nonunion Many chondral and osteochondral injuries Some dense fibrous tissue injuries (eg, inner meniscus regions, tendons, ligaments) Some skeletal muscle injuries	Granulation tissue, vascular or myxoid scar, myxoid tissue, fluid, or a persistent defect

to severe crushing. *Tearing injuries* range from minimal elongation or stretching to rupture, avulsion, or tearing away of tissue. *Penetrating injuries* vary in depth and the extent to which they cleanly lacerate tissue or cause combinations of blunt and tearing injuries. Generally, the extent of tissue damage from penetrating injuries can be relatively easily determined. It is more difficult to define the extent of cell and matrix injury from blunt or tearing trauma. Surgeons usually refer to any disruptions of bone tissue as *fractures,* although disruption of bone matrix necessarily involves rupturing or tearing of the organic matrix as well as cracking or fracturing of the inorganic matrix. Visible disruptions of articular cartilage also generally are referred to as fractures when they involve both the articular cartilage and subchondral bone, that is, *osteochondral or transarticular fractures,* and when they involve only the cartilage, that is, *chondral fractures.*

Intensity and Duration of Force

If other factors are equal, including the type of injury and the condition and type of tissue, the intensity and duration of force applied to the tissue determines the severity of injury, that is, the extent of cell and matrix damage. For some injuries, it is possible to estimate the energy transferred to the tissue. For example, the kinetic energy transferred to a tissue from a bullet can be calculated from knowledge of the mass of the bullet, its tumble, and the velocity at the time it struck the tissue. This information combined with knowledge of the tissue may make it possible to estimate the extent of cell and matrix damage. In other injuries, such as complex fractures with extensive soft-tissue damage resulting from a high-speed automobile accident, determining the intensity and duration of force may not be possible.

Tissue Variables

The musculoskeletal tissues differ in their potential for healing (see Table 5-1). Fracture healing produces tissue that cannot be distinguished from uninjured bone. In contrast, the chondral portion of severe osteochondral fractures or transverse complete muscle lacerations usually heal by scar,[48,60,61] that is, tissue consisting primarily of a dense collagen matrix with a high concentration of type I collagen and fibroblasts. Not all scar tissue has the same composition, and it often contains some components of the original tissue that have re-formed within the scar (see Table 5-1). Examples of this phenomenon include the tissue that forms after some muscle, articular cartilage, and meniscal injuries. Scar may restore the structural integrity of the tissue, but in cartilage and muscle it cannot restore the original structure, composition, and function, and there is some question if it restores the original structure, composition, and function of dense fibrous tissues. After some acute injuries, excessive repair tissue may compromise function (eg, scarring of tendons to surrounding tissue or joint contractures). Occasionally, the repair phase of healing may fail to replace necrotic or lost tissue, leaving a structural defect containing granulation tissue, myxoid tissue, loose connective tissue, or fluid. Nonunions demonstrate this type of failed healing most clearly, but similar results can occur after dense fibrous tissue, cartilage, and muscle injuries.

Even though bone and the primary musculoskeletal soft tissues differ in appearance, function, and material properties, they share common features that affect healing. They all have significant mechanical functions, respond to changes in loading with alterations of cell function, and have important cell matrix interactions that influence restoration of structure and function after injury.[38,40,50] Given these common characteristics, it is not surprising that the mechanical environment or mechanical loading of these tissues after injury can significantly influence healing.[50]

In all the musculoskeletal tissues, the condition of the tissue at the time of injury and the presence or absence of other injuries influence healing. Ischemic tissues or the tissues of poorly nourished or aged patients usually suffer more severe damage from mechanical trauma than the normal tissues of well-nourished young patients. Although most acute musculoskeletal injuries are caused by mechanical damage, other types of acute injuries (eg, thermal, toxic, electrical, and radiation injuries) may occur in association with mechanical injuries. The extent of tissue damage from associated nonmechanical injuries can be deceptive in that cell death or injury may extend beyond the apparent mechanical damage.

Patient Variables

Age

In general, skeletally immature persons have the greatest healing potential and heal most rapidly.[49] Healing of injuries in adults and the elderly follows the same sequence of inflammation, repair, and remodeling, but in the elderly healing, may be slower and less effective. For some injuries the age-related differences in healing are great enough to alter the selection of treatment. For example, a minimally displaced closed femoral fracture in a 3-year-old child can heal within a month with restoration of near-normal tissue structure and function. A similar fracture in a 70-year-old patient often requires 5 months or more to heal, and the restoration of normal structure and function is less predictable. For this reason, treatment of many musculoskeletal injuries in older patients is likely to be more complex and the results often will be less satisfactory.

Nutrition

Cell migration, proliferation, and matrix synthesis require substantial energy. Furthermore, to synthesize large volumes of collagens, proteoglycans, and other matrix macromolecules, the cells need a steady supply of the components of these molecules: proteins and carbohydrates. As a result, the metabolic state of the patient can alter the outcome of injury, and in severely malnourished patients, injuries that would heal rapidly in well-nourished individuals may fail to heal. Although few surgeons in economically developed countries see many severely malnourished patients, they may see relatively large numbers of patients with milder forms of protein–calorie malnutrition and other dietary deficiencies. Jensen and associates[150] found a 42.4% incidence of clinical or subclinical malnutrition in patients undergoing orthopaedic surgical procedures. Even the less obvious forms of malnutrition may adversely affect healing.[150]

Because trauma and major surgery can cause malnutrition and thereby decrease immunocompetence,[150] surgeons must pay careful attention to nutrition and metabolic balance in patients with multiple injuries.[199] Even in well-nourished patients, the nutritional demands of healing multiple injuries can exceed intake.[79,150] Leung and colleagues[174] reported that the adenosine triphosphate (ATP) content of a 2-week rabbit fracture callus was 1000 times greater than the ATP content of normal bone. Others have suggested that a single long-bone fracture can temporarily increase metabolic requirements 20% to 25%, and that multiple injuries and infection can increase metabolic requirements by 55%.[79,150] Failure to meet these increased nutritional needs may increase mortality and surgical complications, including infection, wound dehiscence, impaired healing, and slower rehabilitation. An experimental study of fracture healing demonstrated that fracture callus does not achieve normal strength in states of dietary deficiency and that a dietary deficiency of protein reduces fracture callus strength and energy storage capacity.[91] For these reasons, optimal treatment of injured patients requires assessment of their nutritional status and treatment, which may include nutritional support.[26,79,150,199,278]

Systemic and Local Disease

Systemic diseases including diabetes, hypothyroidism, and renal failure and their associated medical treatments may adversely affect healing and increase the vulnerability of tissues to injury and the risk of complications of treatment.[2,131,145,184,273] Localized diseases including neoplasms, infections, and developmental disorders or previous injuries may also weaken musculoskeletal tissues and compromise their capacity for healing.

Medications

Experimental work shows that a variety of medications including corticosteroids, some nonsteroidal anti-inflammatory drugs, anticoagulants, diphosphonates, cancer chemotherapy agents, and possibly others may adversely affect musculoskeletal tissue healing, especially bone healing (Table 5-2).[78,130,136,255,272,283] Confirmation of the effects of medications on healing of musculoskeletal injuries in human studies is difficult because of the large number of patient and treatment variables involved, especially since patients using medications may have systemic or local diseases or metabolic abnormalities that also may affect healing.

Genetic Differences

Some genetically determined diseases, including Ehlers-Danlos syndrome, osteogenesis imperfecta, Marfan's disease, and osteopetrosis, increase the vulnerability of the musculoskeletal tissues to injury and may adversely alter the healing response. More subtle genetically determined differences may also affect healing, but these differences have not been well defined.

Treatment

The surgeon must select and apply treatment that creates the optimal biological and mechanical environment for healing. For some injuries, this consists of allowing healing to occur without intervention while providing relief of symptoms and protecting the injured tissue. Other injuries require nonsurgical or surgical intervention to create the optimal environment for healing. Currently accepted treatments include limiting progressive tissue damage from the injury; minimizing tissue damage caused by treatment; removing necrotic tissue; preventing infection; restoring and maintaining tissue alignment, apposition, and mechanical stability; restoring and maintaining the supporting nerves and blood vessels; and applying controlled loading and motion. Methods that are less well established or experimental include the use of electrical fields, ultrasound, growth factors, artificial matrices, and transplanted cells.

BONE

Structure and Composition

Like the other primary musculoskeletal tissues, bone[38,39,54,116] consists of mesenchymal cells embedded within an abundant extracellular matrix. Unlike the matrices of the other tissues, bone matrix contains

TABLE 5-2
Factors Reported to Influence Bone Healing

Factors Reported to Promote Bone Healing	Factors Reported to Impair Bone Healing
Growth hormone[12,130,138,164–166,200,217]	Growth hormone deficiency[138,215]
Thyroid hormones[98,164]	Diabetes[131,184,325]
Calcitonin[156,330]	Corticosteroids[78,130,272]
Insulin[184,274]	Anemia[257]
Vitamin A[76,298]	Malnutrition[91]
Vitamin D[76,282]	Delayed manipulation[229]
Anabolic steroids[167,168,315]	Denervation[249]
Chondroitin sulfate[53,132]	Anticoagulants[255,283]
Hyaluronidase[23]	Indomethacin[136]
Electrical fields[11,16,28,32,107,172,267,270]	Loss of fracture hematoma[122–124]
Hyperbaric oxygen[77,328]	Radiation[117,316]
Exercise[127]	Bone necrosis
Loading and micromotion[118,158–160,162,225,262]	Distraction of the fracture site
Ultrasound[125,163,327]	Infection
Cytokines[21,73,74,99,180,175,181,206,211,216,218,254]	Interposition of soft tissues
Demineralized bone matrix[20,94,208]	Decreased soft tissue vascular supply
Bone marrow cells[57,71]	Increasing age until skeletal maturity

mineral that gives the tissue great strength and stiffness in compression and bending.[54] The organic component of the bone matrix, primarily type I collagen, contributes to bone strength but also gives bone the plasticity that allows substantial deformation without fracture. Bone has an elaborate blood supply and contains nerves and lymphatics as well. The periosteum, consisting of two layers—an outer fibrous layer and an inner more cellular and vascular cambium layer—covers the external bone surfaces and participates in healing of many types of fractures.[38] The thicker, more cellular periosteum of infants and children has a more elaborate vascular supply than that of adults.[38,39,293] Perhaps because of these differences, the periosteum of children is more active in healing many fractures.

Human bones consist of two forms of bone tissue: *cortical* or *compact bone* and *cancellous* or *trabecular bone.* Long-bone diaphyses consist almost entirely of cortical bone. The metaphyses of long bones and most short and flat bones consist of relatively thin shells of cortical bone with large volumes of cancellous bone. These differences in the distribution of cortical and cancellous bone cause differences in the healing of fractures.[101,263,303]

Two types of bone can be distinguished by mechanical and biological properties: *woven* or *immature bone* and *lamellar* or *mature bone.* Woven bone forms the embryonic skeleton and is replaced by lamellar bone during development and growth. Woven bone also forms the initial fracture repair tissue and is replaced by lamellar bone as the fracture remodels. Compared with lamellar bone, woven bone has a more rapid rate of deposition and resorption, an irregular woven pattern of matrix collagen fibrils consistent with its name, approximately four times the number of osteocytes per unit volume, and an irregular pattern of matrix mineralization.[39] The frequent patchwork formation of woven bone and the spotty pattern of mineralization creates an irregular radiographic appearance that distinguishes the woven bone found in fracture callus from lamellar bone. Because of its lack of collagen fibril orientation, irregular mineralization, and relatively high cell and water concentration, woven bone is less stiff and more easily deformed than lamellar bone.[39]

Fracture Healing

A fracture initiates a sequence of inflammation, repair, and remodeling that can restore the injured bone to its original state (see Figs. 5-1 and 5-3).[139,196,261,271,306] Inflammation begins immediately after injury and is followed rapidly by repair (see Fig. 5-3). After repair has replaced the lost and damaged cells and matrix, a prolonged remodeling phase begins. The energy requirements of fracture healing increase rapidly during inflammation and reach a peak during repair, when the cells in the fracture callus are proliferating and synthesizing large volumes of new matrix. The energy requirements of fracture healing remain high until cell density and cell activity begin to decline as remodeling starts.[174]

Inflammation

An injury that fractures bone damages not only the cells, blood vessels, and bone matrix (Fig. 5-4) but also the surrounding soft tissues, including the periosteum and muscle. A hematoma accumulates within the medullary canal, between the fracture ends and beneath elevated periosteum.[123,124,245] The damage to the bone blood vessels deprives osteocytes of their nutrition, and they die as far back as the junction of collateral channels, leaving the immediate ends of the fracture without living cells (see Fig. 5-4). Severely damaged periosteum and marrow, as well as other surrounding soft tissues, may also contribute necrotic material to the fracture site.

Inflammatory mediators released from platelets and from dead and injured cells cause blood vessels to dilate and exude plasma, leading to the acute edema seen in the region of a fresh fracture.[21,59,139,211,271,280,281,294] Inflammatory cells migrate to the region, including polymorphonuclear leukocytes followed by macrophages and lymphocytes. These cells also release cytokines that can stimulate angiogenesis. As the inflammatory response subsides, necrotic tissue and exu-

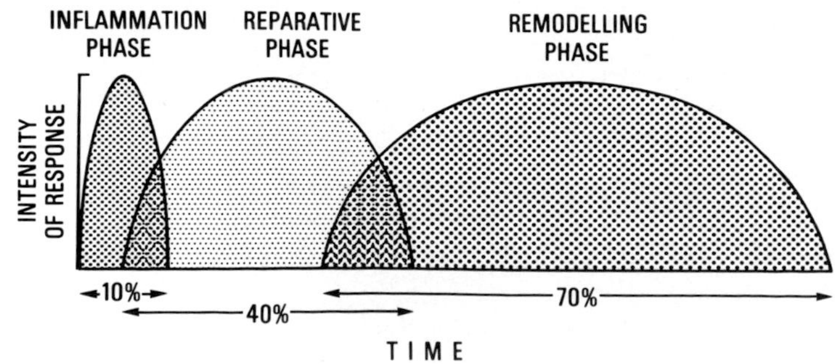

FIGURE 5-3. An approximation of the relative intensities and duration of inflammation, repair, and remodeling in fracture healing. Note that repair begins as inflammation starts to subside and that remodeling begins before repair is complete. The energy requirements of fracture healing reach the maximum during repair, corresponding with the most intense period of cell proliferation and matrix synthesis, and then gradually decrease during remodeling.

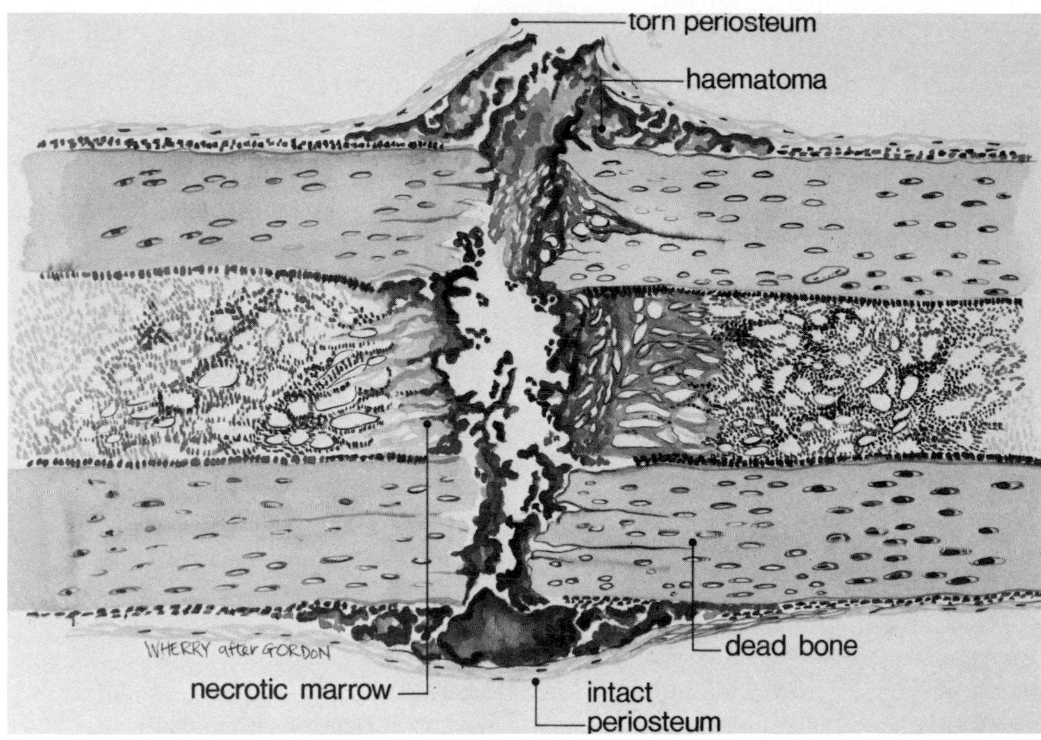

FIGURE 5-4. Diagram of the initial events after fracture of a long-bone diaphysis. The periosteum is torn opposite the point of impact and may remain intact on the other side. A hematoma accumulates beneath the periosteum and between the fracture ends. There is necrotic marrow and cortical bone close to the fracture line.

date are resorbed, and fibroblasts appear and start producing a new matrix (see Fig. 5-3).

Repair

The factors that stimulate fracture repair probably include the chemotactic factors released during inflammation at the fracture site and bone matrix proteins, including cytokines exposed by disruption of the bone tissue. Electrical stimuli may also have a role. Electronegativity is found in the region of a fresh fracture and may stimulate osteogenesis.[28,105,172] This electronegativity depends on cell viability and, unlike the currents measured in intact bones, is not generated by stress. The degree of electronegativity slowly diminishes until the fracture is united.

Although the inflammation caused by a fracture follows the same sequence for almost every fracture, the amount and composition of repair tissue and the rate of repair may differ, depending on whether the fracture occurs through primarily cancellous bone in the epiphyses, metaphyses, or vertebral bodies or through primarily cortical bone in tubular bone diaphyses. The extent of soft-tissue disruption surrounding the fracture and a variety of other factors are discussed in the section on variables that influence fracture healing. The mechanical stability of the fracture site also influences the repair process. The summaries of fracture repair and remodeling that follow immediately describe healing of closed unstable fractures, that is, fractures in which repair proceeds in the presence of motion at the fracture site. The second summary of fracture repair and remodeling describes healing of stable fractures, that is, fractures in which repair proceeds at a rigidly stable fracture site with the fracture surfaces held in contact.

Repair of Unstable Fractures

Disruption of blood vessels in the bone, marrow, periosteum, and surrounding tissue at the time of injury results in the extravasation of blood at the fracture site and the formation of a hematoma. Organization of this hematoma is usually recognized as the first step in fracture repair (Fig. 5-5). Experimental work indicates that loss of the hematoma impairs or slows fracture healing,[122–124] suggesting that the hematoma and an intact surrounding periosteal soft-tissue envelope that contains the hematoma may facilitate the initial stages of repair. Open fractures or treatment of fractures by open reduction disrupts organization of the hematoma and thereby may slow the repair process. The reasons why a hematoma may affect fracture healing remain uncertain. Presumably, the fracture hematoma pro-

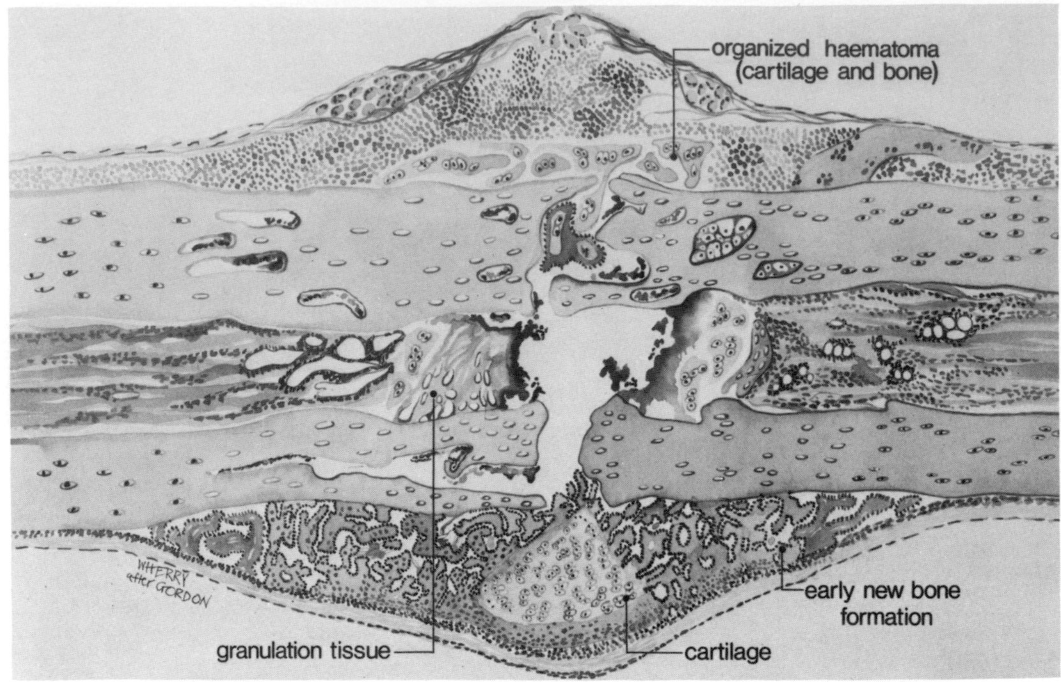

FIGURE 5-5. Diagram of early repair of a diaphyseal fracture of a long bone. There is organization of the hematoma, early woven bone formation in the subperiosteal regions, and cartilage formation in other areas. Periosteal cells contribute to healing of this type of injury. If the fracture is rigidly immobilized or if it occurs primarily through cancellous bone and the cancellous surfaces lie in close apposition, there will be little evidence of fracture callus.

vides a fibrin scaffold that facilitates migration of repair cells. In addition, growth factors and other proteins released by platelets and cells in the fracture hematoma mediate the critical initial events in fracture repair, including cell migration, proliferation, and synthesis of a repair tissue matrix.[21,139,196,211,271]

While the hematoma is organizing, the microenvironment about the fracture is acidic,[284] which may affect cell behavior during the early phases of repair. As repair progresses, the pH gradually returns to neutral, and then to a slightly alkaline level. When an alkaline pH is attained, the activity of the alkaline phosphatase enzyme is optimal and promotes mineralization of the fracture callus.

Although the volume of the vascular bed of an extremity increases shortly after fracture, presumably because of vasodilation, vascular proliferation also occurs in the region of the fracture.[250,251,324] It appears that, under ordinary circumstances, the periosteal vessels contribute the majority of capillary buds early in normal bone healing, with the nutrient medullary artery becoming more important later in the process.[250,251] Fibroblastic growth factors may be important mediators of the angiogenesis in fracture healing,[271,294] but the exact stimuli responsible for vascular invasion and endothelial cell proliferation have not been defined. When the surgeon interferes with the blood supply to the fracture site, either by stripping the periosteum excessively or by destroying the medullary system through the use of intramedullary nails, repair must proceed with vessels derived from the surviving system.[120,250,251]

The bone ends at the fracture site, deprived of their blood supply, become necrotic and are resorbed. In some fractures this may create a radiographically apparent gap at the fracture site several weeks or more after the fracture. The cells responsible for this function, the osteoclasts, come from a different cell line than the cells responsible for bone formation.[38,39,119] They are derived from circulating monocytes in the blood and monocytic precursor cells from the bone marrow,[38,39,266] whereas the osteoblasts develop from the undifferentiated mesenchymal cells that migrate into the fracture site (see Fig. 5-2). The stimulus for bone resorption remains unclear, but prostaglandins have been identified in significant amounts in the region of fresh fractures in experimental animals,[83] and these substances can increase osteoclast activity and cause recruitment of new osteoclasts.[87,253]

Pluripotential mesenchymal cells (see Fig. 5-2), probably of common origin, form the fibrous tissue, cartilage, and eventually bone at the fracture site. Some of these cells originate in the injured tissues, while others migrate to the injury site with the blood vessels. Cells from the cambium layer of the periosteum form the earliest bone.[293] Periosteal cells have an especially prominent role in healing children's fractures because the periosteum is thicker and more cellular in younger individuals.[38,39] With increasing age, the periosteum becomes thinner and its contribution to fracture healing becomes less apparent. Osteoblasts from the endosteal surface also participate in bone formation, but surviving osteocytes do not appear to form repair tissue.[292] The majority of cells responsible for osteogenesis during fracture healing appear in the fracture site with the granulation tissue that replaces the hematoma.[295] Although the appearance of these cells follows the invasion of fibroblasts and capillary loops, their precise source remains unknown.

The mesenchymal cells at the fracture site proliferate, differentiate, and produce the *fracture callus*, which consists of fibrous tissue, cartilage, and woven bone (Fig. 5-6). The fracture callus fills and surrounds the fracture site (Fig. 5-7), and in the early stages of healing can be divided into the hard or bony callus and the softer fibrous and cartilaginous callus. The bone formed initially at the periphery of the callus by intramembranous bone formation is the *hard callus*. The *soft callus* forms in the central regions with low oxygen tension and consists primarily of cartilage. Bone gradually replaces the cartilage through the process of endochondral ossification, enlarging the hard callus and increasing the stability of the fracture fragments (see Figs. 5-6 and 5-7). This process continues until new bone bridges the fracture site, reestablishing continuity between the cortical bone ends.

The biochemical composition of the fracture callus matrix changes as repair progresses (Fig. 5-8).[299] The cells replace the fibrin clot with a loose fibrous matrix containing glycosaminoglycans, proteoglycans, and types I and III collagen. In many regions they convert this tissue to more dense fibrocartilage or hyaline-like cartilage. With formation of hyaline-like cartilage, type II collagen, cartilage-specific proteoglycan, and link protein content increase. During endochondral ossification and intramembranous bone formation, the concentration of type I collagen, alkaline phosphatase, and bone-specific proteins[212] increases until the matrix mineralizes (see Fig. 5-8). Newly formed woven bone remodels to lamellar bone, and with remodeling the content of collagen and other proteins returns to normal levels.

Analysis of fracture repair demonstrates a close correlation between the activation of genes for blood vessel, cartilage, and bone-specific proteins in the cells and the development of granulation tissue, cartilage, and bone (Fig. 5-9),[152,212,260] demonstrating that fracture repair depends on regulation of gene expression in the repair cells. The simultaneous occurrence of chondrogenesis, endochondral ossification, and intramembranous bone formation in different regions of the fracture callus suggests that local mediators and

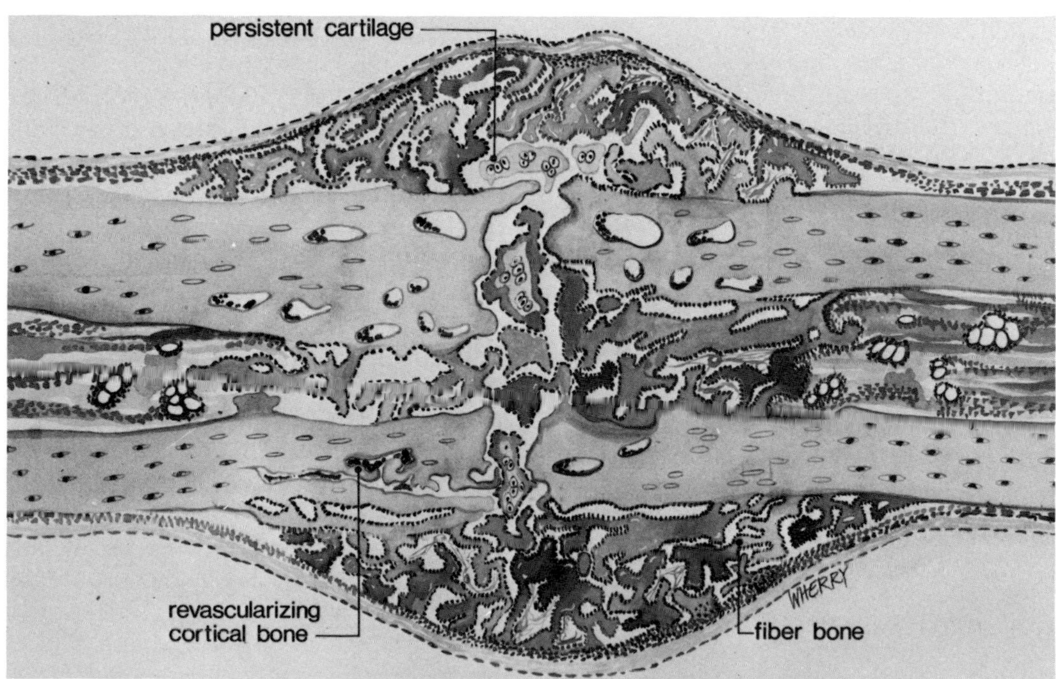

FIGURE 5-6. Diagram of a later stage in healing. Woven or fiber bone bridges the fracture gap. Cartilage remains in the regions most distant from ingrowing capillary buds. In many instances, the capillaries are surrounded by new bone. Vessels revascularize the cortical bone at the fracture site.

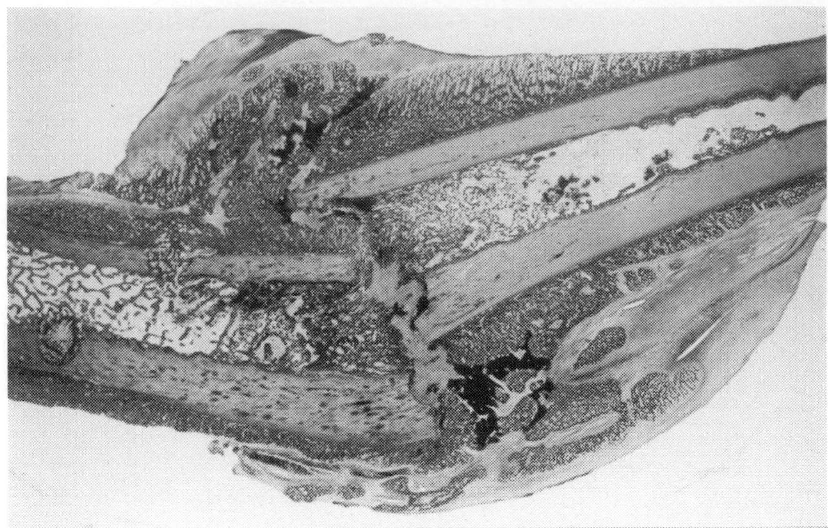

FIGURE 5-7. Light micrograph showing healing of a diaphyseal fracture. The fracture callus consisting primarily of woven bone surrounds and unites the two fracture fragments. As the callus matures it progressively stabilizes the fracture. Note that the fracture callus contains areas of mineralized and unmineralized cartilage.

small variations in the microenvironment, including mechanical stresses, determine what genes will be expressed and therefore the type of tissue the repair cells form. Compression discourages the formation of fibrous tissue. Intermittent shear forces promote normal calcification of newly formed fibrocartilage, whereas intermittent hydrostatic stress inhibits calcification.[19] Local mediators that may influence repair cell function include growth factors released from cells and platelets and oxygen tension. Acidic fibroblast growth factor (FGF), basic FGF, and TGF-β stimulate chondrocyte proliferation and cartilage formation, osteoblast proliferation, and bone synthesis.[151,208,211,218,280,281] TGF-β released from platelets immediately after injury may initiate formation of fracture callus. TGF-β synthesis is also associated with cartilage hypertrophy and calcification at the endochondral ossification front. Tissue

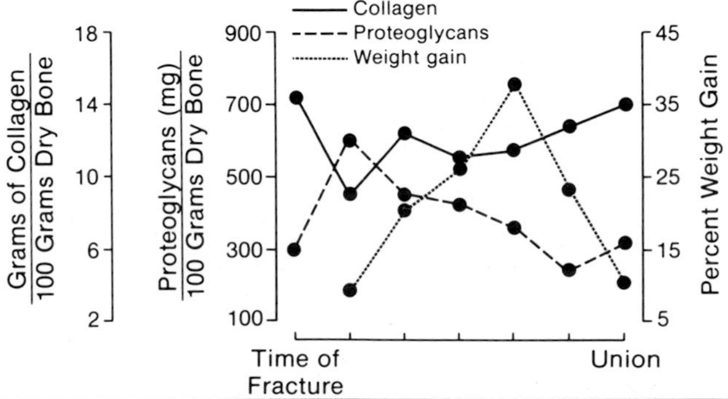

FIGURE 5-8. A schematic representation of the changing composition and mass of fracture callus. Collagen formation precedes significant accumulation of mineral. After an initial rise, proteoglycan concentration falls gradually as fracture healing progresses. The total mass of the fracture callus increases during repair and then decreases during remodeling.

oxygen tension may help determine if bone or cartilage forms. In regions with low oxygen tension, possibly because of their distance from blood vessels,[250,251] cartilage forms.[13] Cells that receive enough oxygen and are subject to the necessary mechanical or electrical stimuli form bone.[13,15,19]

Mineralization of fracture callus results from an ordered sequence of cell activities. The cells synthesize a matrix with a high concentration of type I collagen fibrils[40,116,135] that have regular spaces called "hole zones"[116,135] (Fig. 5-10) and then create conditions that promote deposition of clusters of calcium hydroxyapatite crystals within the collagen fibrils. Mineralization requires two cell functions. First, the cells must remove local conditions in the fibrocartilaginous callus matrix that inhibit mineralization, including high glycosaminoglycan concentrations. Fracture callus chondrocytes may accomplish this by secreting neutral proteoglycanases that degrade these molecules at the time of mineralization.[93] Second, after the cells prepare the matrix for mineralization, the chondrocytes, and later the osteoblasts, release "prepackaged" calcium phosphate complexes into the matrix by the budding of "matrix vesicles" from cell membranes (Fig. 5-11).[29] These membrane-derived vesicles carry neutral proteases and alkaline phosphatase enzymes that degrade the proteoglycan-rich matrix and hydrolyze ATP and other high-energy phosphate-esters to provide phosphate ions for precipitation with calcium. Figure 5-12 shows the distribution of matrix vesicle enzyme activities over time. As callus begins to mineralize (14 to 17 days after fracture in the rat), neutral proteases and alkaline phosphatase show parallel increases and peaks in activity.[93]

As mineralization proceeds, the bone ends gradually become enveloped in a fusiform mass of callus con-

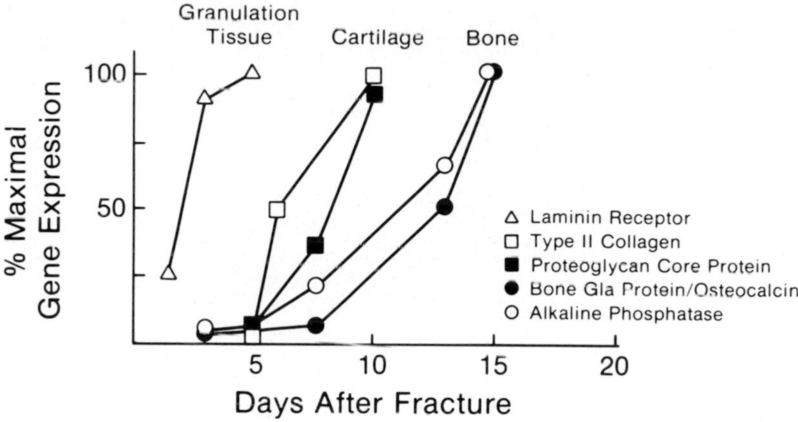

FIGURE 5-9. Relative levels of protein gene expression during fracture repair in a rat. Expression of laminin receptor, a protein found in blood vessels, is increased during granulation tissue formation. Expression of genes for cartilage (type II collagen and proteoglycan core protein) and bone-associated proteins (bone Gla protein, osteocalcin, alkaline phosphatase) is increased when these tissues are forming in the callus. (*Courtesy of Mark Bolander, Mayo Clinic, Rochester, MN.*)

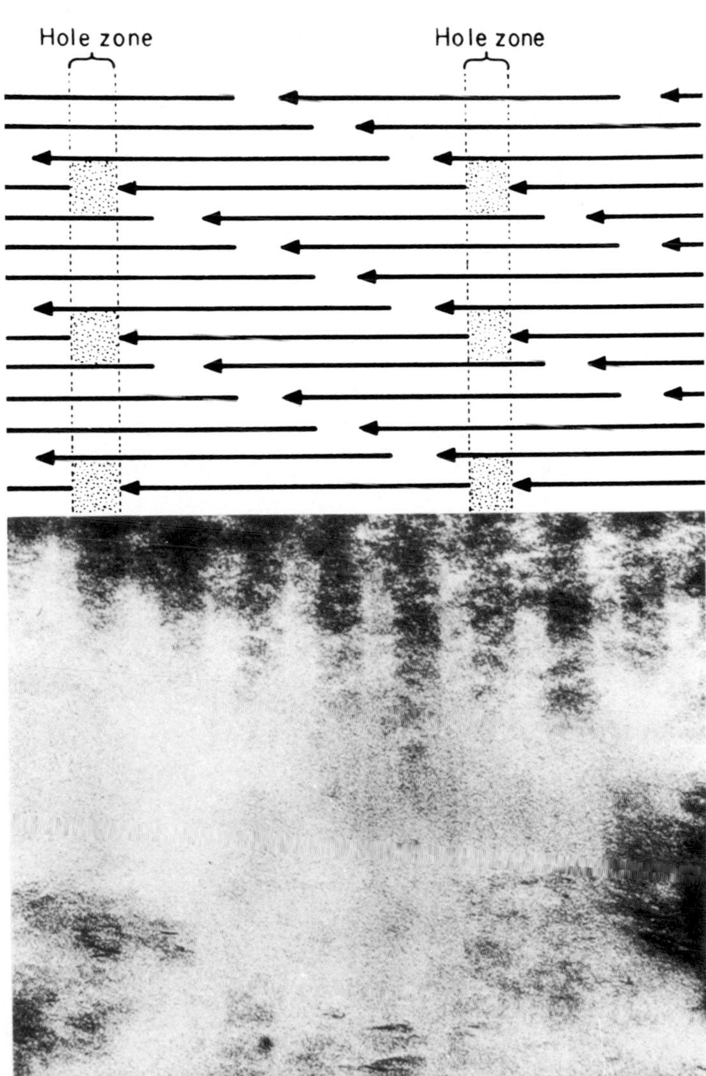

FIGURE 5-10. The initial mineralization of the collagenous matrix appears to occur in the hole zone of collagen fibrils. (*Gilmcher, M. J.: A Basic Architectural Principle in the Organization of Mineralized Tissues. Clin. Orthop., 61:16–36, 1968.*)

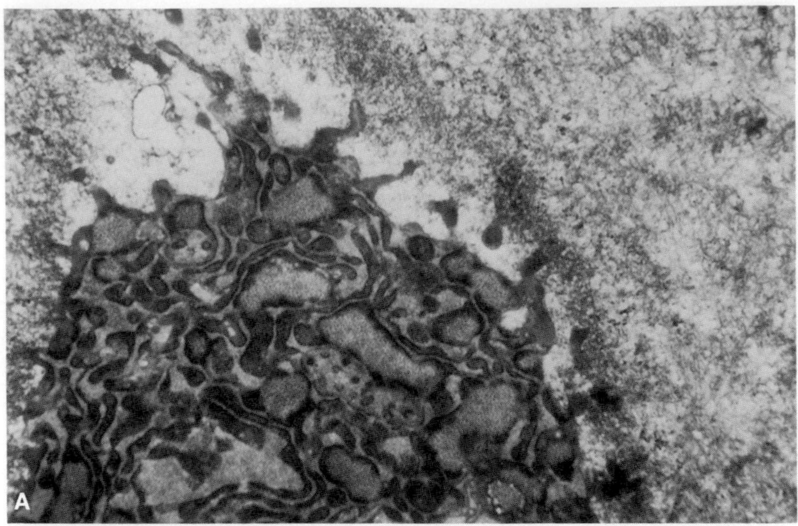

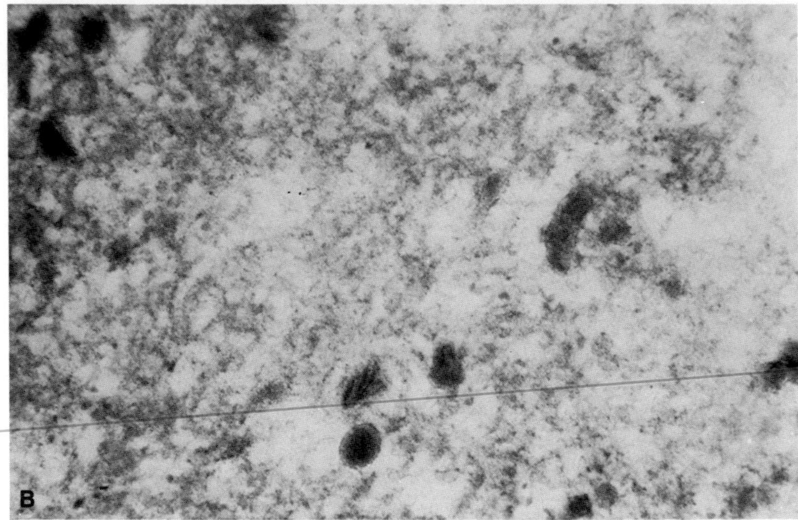

FIGURE 5-11. The release of matrix vesicles from 14-day-old fracture callus chondrocytes. (**A**) Electron micrograph of half of a fracture callus chondrocyte showing portions of the membrane budding off and forming vesicular bodies. (**B**) In the matrix, these vesicles may mediate the deposition of calcium phosphate salts and their conversion to hydroxyapatite crystals. Note the presence of dark material (amorphous mineral) within certain vesicles and needle-like structures (apatite crystals) in others. The background matrix is composed of collagen and glycosaminoglycans. (*Courtesy of Thomas Einhorn, M.D., Mount Sinai School of Medicine, New York, N.Y.*)

taining increasing amounts of woven bone. The increasing mineral content is closely associated with increasing stiffness of the fracture callus.[9] Stability of the fracture fragments progressively increases because of the internal and external callus formation, and eventually *clinical union* occurs; that is, the fracture site becomes stable and pain-free. *Radiographic union,* occurs when plain radiographs show bone trabeculae or cortical bone crossing the fracture site and often occurs later than clinical union. However, even at this stage healing is not complete. The immature fracture callus is weaker than normal bone, and it only gains full strength during remodeling.

Remodeling of Unstable Fractures

During the final stages of repair (see Fig. 5-3), remodeling of the repair tissue begins with replacement of woven bone by lamellar bone and resorption of unneeded callus. Radioisotope studies have shown increased activity in fracture sites long after the patient has full restoration of function, and plain radiographs show bone union,[313] demonstrating that fracture remodeling continues for years after clinical and radiographic union. Remodeling of fracture repair tissue after all woven bone has been replaced presumably consists of osteoclastic resorption of superfluous or poorly placed trabeculae and formation of new struts of bone along lines of stress.[108]

Electrical fields may influence fracture remodeling. When a bone is subjected to stress, electropositivity occurs on the convex surface and electronegativity on the concave surface.[15] Circumstantial evidence indicates that regions of electropositivity are associated with osteoclastic activity and regions of electronegativity with osteoblastic activity.[14] Thus the observation that changes in bone architecture are associated with changes in loading, often called *Wolff's law,*[319] may be explainable in terms of alterations in the electrical fields that affect cellular behavior. The end result of fracture callus remodeling is bone that, even if it has not returned to its original form, has been altered to perform the function demanded of it.

Although fracture callus remodeling results from an

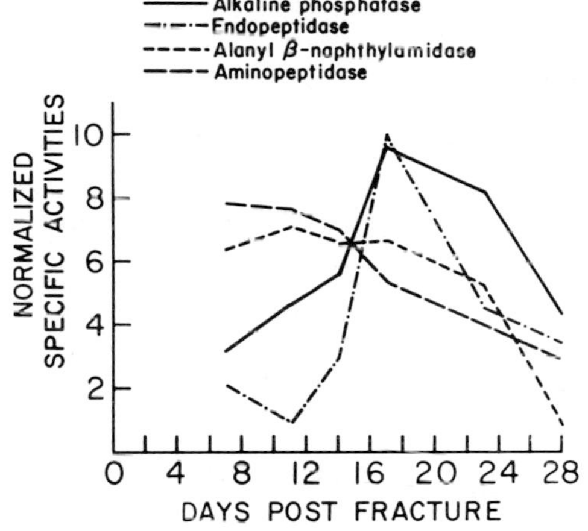

FIGURE 5-12. Distribution of the activities of alkaline phosphatase and three different neutral proteases in matrix vesicles during fracture healing. Note that the enzyme responsible for degrading glycosaminoglycans (endopeptidase) and the enzyme responsible for calcifying the callus (alkaline phosphatase) are expressed in parallel and peak between 14 and 17 days. This is when fracture callus begins to mineralize. (*Reprinted with permission from Einhorn, T. A., Hirschman, A., Kaplan, C., Nashed, R., Devlin, V. J., and Warman, J.: Neutral Protein-Degrading Enzymes in Experimental Fracture Callus. J. Orthop. Res., 7:792–805, 1989.*)

elaborate sequence of cell and matrix changes, the important functional result for the patient is an increase in mechanical stability.[314] The progressive increase in fracture stability can be described as consisting of four stages. During stage I, a healing bone subjected to torsional testing fails through the original fracture site with a low-stiffness pattern. In stage II, the bone still fails through the fracture site, but the characteristics of failure indicate a high-stiffness, hard-tissue pattern. In stage III, the bone fails partly through the original fracture site and partly through the previously intact bone with a high-stiffness, hard-tissue pattern. Finally, in stage IV, failure does not occur through the fracture site, indicating that new tissue at the fracture site duplicates the mechanical properties of the uninjured tissue.

Despite successful fracture healing, the bone density of the involved limb may be decreased for years.[157,317] In one study, patients with healed tibial fractures had decreased bone density in the involved limb decades after the injury.[157] The clinical significance of these observations remain unclear, but they suggest that fractures and possibly the decreased loading of a limb after a fracture may cause long-lasting changes in the tissues.

Repair and Remodeling of Stable Fractures

When motion occurs within certain limits at a fracture site, fracture callus progressively stabilizes the bone fragments and remodeling of the fracture callus eventually produces lamellar bone (see Fig. 5-7). However, fracture healing can occur without callus formation in either cancellous or cortical bone when the fracture surfaces are rigidly held in contact.[5,205,224,234–238,263–265] Some surgeons and investigators refer to this type of fracture healing as *primary bone healing,* indicating that it occurs without the intermediary formation and replacement of fracture callus. Many impacted epiphyseal, metaphyseal, and vertebral body fractures where cancellous and in some regions cortical bone surfaces interlock have sufficient stability to permit primary bone healing at sites where bone surfaces make direct contact. The same type of cancellous bone healing can occur at osteotomies through metaphyseal bone and at surgical arthrodesis treated with rigid stabilization. Diaphyseal osteotomies and acute diaphyseal fractures usually require use of devices that compress the fracture site as well as stabilize the fragments to allow primary healing.

Robert Danis, a Belgian surgeon, first described primary bone union and elucidated the principles of rigid internal fixation.[80] In 1958, a Swiss group, led by Maurice E. Müller, formed the AO (Arbeitsgemeinschaft für Osteosynthesfragen) and put forward four "working hypotheses" that became the principles of internal fixation: (1) anatomical reduction; (2) rigid internal fixation; (3) atraumatic surgical technique; and (4) early, pain-free, active mobilization during the first 10 postoperative days.[5]

Schenk and Willenegger[264,265] described two types of primary bone healing: gap healing and haversian remodeling. To some extent these types correspond to the repair and remodeling phases of fractures that are not rigidly stabilized. Their examinations of fractures after compression plating showed that not all cortical bone ends are in close contact, leaving gaps of varying size at the fracture site, and that the mechanism, structure, and rate of new bone formation at the fracture site depends on the size of the gaps.[264,265] When there is direct contact between cortical bone ends, lamellar bone forms directly across the fracture line, parallel to the long axis of the bone, by direct extension of osteons.[234,237,264,265] A cluster of osteoclasts cuts across the fracture line, osteoblasts following the osteoclasts deposit new bone, and blood vessels follow the osteoblasts. The new bone matrix, enclosed osteocytes, and blood vessels form new haversian systems, or "primary osteons." This process has been given the name "contact healing." In small gaps, 150 to 200 μm, or approximately the outer diameter of the osteon, the cells form lamellar bone at right angles to the axis of the bone. In larger gaps, 200 μm to 1 mm, cells fill the defect with woven bone. After gap healing, haversian remodeling begins, reestablishing normal cortical bone structure. Cutting cones consisting of osteoclasts followed by blood vessels and osteoblasts traverse the new bone in the fracture gap, depositing lamellar bone and reestablishing the cortical bone blood supply across the fracture site. Haversian remodeling presumably follows the paths of necrotic vessels and also cuts new vessel channels. If a large segment of cortical bone is necrotic, gap healing by direct extension of osteons still occurs, but at a slower rate, and areas of necrotic cortical bone remain unremodeled for a prolonged period.[224]

Perren and colleagues[234–238] reported that compression of a fracture eliminates the resorption of the cortical bone ends seen in spontaneous bone repair. They correlated the resorptive process with micromotion and resulting strain at the fracture site, and they demonstrated the importance of stability for primary bone healing. Their work indicates that rigid compression plating eliminates micromotion and strain by a combination of friction and preloading.

Failure of Fracture Healing

Despite optimal treatment, some fractures heal slowly or fail to heal.[189,275] It is difficult to set the time when a given fracture should be united, but when healing progresses more slowly than average, the slow progress is referred to as *delayed union.*[189] Watson-Jones[309] described a condition he called *slow union,* in which the fracture line remains clearly visible radiographically but there is no undue separation of the fragments, no cavitation of the surfaces, no calcification, and no sclerosis. This indolent fracture healing may be related to the severity of the injury, poor blood supply, the age and nutritional status of the patient, or other factors. It is not an ununited fracture but rather a variation of normal healing. Failure of bone healing, or *nonunion,* results from an arrest of the healing process.[189] A nonunion that occurs despite the formation of a large volume of callus around the fracture site is commonly referred to as a *hypertrophic nonunion,* in contrast to an *atrophic nonunion* where little or no callus forms and bone resorption occurs at the fracture site. In some nonunions, cartilaginous tissue forms over the fracture surfaces and the cavity between the surfaces fills with a clear fluid resembling normal joint or bursal fluid creating a *pseudarthrosis,* or false joint.[189] Pseudarthroses may or may not be painful, but they almost uniformly remain unstable indefinitely. In other nonunions, the gap between the bone ends fills with fibrous or fibrocartilaginous tissue. Occasionally, dense fibrous and cartilaginous tissue firmly stabilizes a fracture, creating a *fibrous union.* Although fibrous unions may be painless and unite the fracture fragments, they fail to restore the normal strength of the bone.

Variables That Influence Fracture Healing

Occasionally, delayed unions or nonunions occur without apparent cause, but in many instances, injury, patient, and treatment variables that adversely influenced fracture healing can be identified (see Table 5-2). These variables include severe soft-tissue damage associated with open and high-energy closed fractures, infection, segmental fractures, pathologic fractures, fractures with soft-tissue interposition, poor local blood supply, systemic diseases, malnutrition, corticosteroids, and iatrogenic interference with healing. Many other variables have been reported to retard bone healing (see Table 5-2). Some of them exert an adverse influence that can be measured in experimental studies but may not cause clinically significant impairment of fracture healing. Others, like distraction of a fracture site or interposition of soft tissues in a fracture site, have not been examined systematically in experimental studies, but clinical experience shows that they can impair fracture healing. Some investigators have identified a variety of treatments that may promote fracture healing, including electrical fields, ultrasound, controlled loading and micromotion, and cytokines (see Table 5-2).

Injury Variables. *Severity.* Severe fractures may be associated with large soft-tissue wounds, loss of soft tissue, displacement and comminution of bone fragments, loss of bone, and decreased blood supply to the fracture site. Displacement of the fracture fragments and severe trauma to the soft tissues retard fracture healing, probably because the extensive tissue damage increases the volume of necrotic tissue, impedes the migration of mesenchymal cells and vascular invasion, decreases the number of viable mesenchymal cells, and disrupts the local blood supply.[250,251] Less severe injuries leave an intact soft-tissue envelope that contains the fracture hematoma and provides a ready source of mesenchymal cells, a tube that directs the repair efforts of these cells, and an internal splint that contributes to immobilization of the fragments.

Open Fractures. Severe open fractures cause soft-tissue disruption, fracture displacement, and, in some instances, significant bone loss. Extensive tearing or crushing of the soft tissue disrupts the blood supply to the fracture site, leaving necrotic bone and soft tissue, impeding or preventing formation of a fracture hematoma, and delaying formation of repair tissue. Exposed bone and soft tissue become desiccated, increasing the volume of necrotic tissue and the risk of infection. Early use of vascularized soft-tissue flaps to cover bone exposed by severe open fractures can prevent desiccation and facilitate healing of these injuries (see Chapter 6). In addition to the problems created by the soft-tissue damage, open fractures may become infected. Management of this complication usually requires debriding infected bone and soft tissue along with antibiotic treatment. Infected fractures can unite if they are stabilized and the infection can be controlled.

Transarticular Fractures. Extension of a fracture across an articular surface can adversely influence healing and complicates treatment. Synovial fluid contains enzymes that can degrade the matrix of the initial fracture callus[169] and thereby retard the first stage in fracture healing. In addition, joint motion or loading may cause movement of the fracture fragments. Despite these problems most transarticular fractures heal, but in some instances, especially if the fracture is not rigidly stabilized, healing may be delayed or nonunion may occur (Fig. 5-13). However, rigid immobilization of a joint with a transarticular fracture frequently causes joint stiffness.[50] For these reasons, surgeons usually attempt to reduce and securely fix unstable fractures that extend across an articular surface. This approach ideally restores joint congruity and allows at least some joint motion while the fracture heals. Unfortunately, even after reduction and adequate initial stabilization, intra-articular fractures may displace due to high transarticular forces, failure of the stabilization, or collapse of the subchondral cancellous bone. This late loss of reduction occurs most frequently after comminuted fractures of the proximal and distal tibia and distal radius.

Segmental Fractures. A segmental fracture of a long bone impairs or disrupts intramedullary blood supply to the middle fragment. If there is severe soft-tissue trauma, the periosteal blood supply to the middle fragment may also be compromised. Possibly because of this, the probability of delayed union or nonunion, proximally or distally, may be increased. These problems occur most frequently in segmental fractures of the tibia, especially at the distal fracture site.[256,320] Segmental fractures of the femur less commonly develop nonunions, presumably because of the better soft-tissue coverage and resulting better blood supply. When internal fixation of a segmental fracture is performed, the soft-tissue attachments of the middle fragment should be preserved whenever possible.

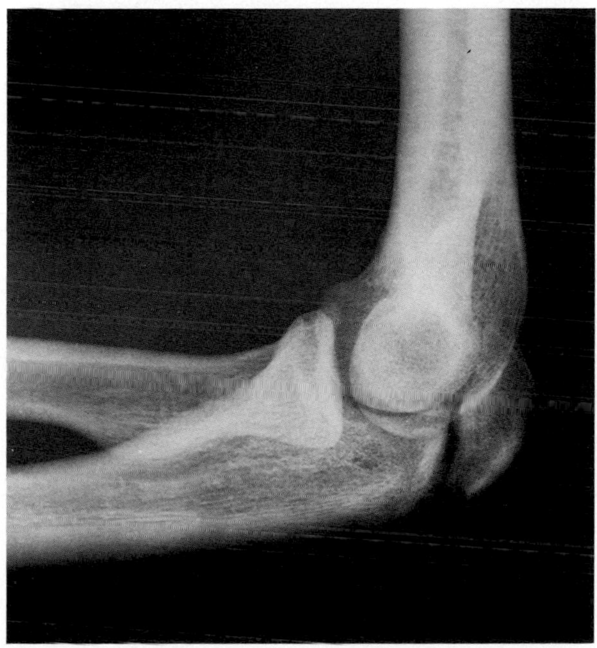

FIGURE 5-13. Radiograph of a nonunion of an intra-articular fracture of the olecranon. This 18-year-old man injured his elbow in a wrestling match. After the elbow was taped, he continued wrestling. Two years later he sought evaluation for persistent elbow pain and weakness of elbow extension.

Soft-Tissue Interposition. Interposition of soft tissue, including muscle, fascia, tendon, and occasionally, nerves and vessels, between fracture fragments will compromise fracture healing. The presence of soft-tissue interposition should be suspected when the bone fragments cannot be brought into apposition or alignment during attempted closed reduction. If this occurs, an open reduction may be necessary to extricate the interposed tissue and achieve an acceptable position of the fracture.

Inadequate Blood Supply. Lack of an adequate vascular supply can significantly delay or prevent fracture healing. Insufficient blood supply for fracture healing may result from a severe soft-tissue and bone injury or from the normally limited blood supply to some bones or bone regions. For example, the vulnerable blood supplies of the femoral head, the proximal pole of the scaphoid, distal tibia, and talar body may predispose these bones to delayed union or nonunion, even in the absence of severe soft-tissue damage or fracture displacement. Extensive surgical dissection may also compromise the vascular supply to a fracture site, especially in regions of the skeleton with a vulnerable blood supply or in fractures with associated severe soft-tissue injuries.

Patient Variables. *Age.* Patient age significantly influences the rate of fracture healing. Infants have the most rapid rate of fracture healing. The rate of healing declines with increasing age up to skeletal maturity, but after completion of skeletal growth, the rate of fracture healing does not appear to decline significantly with increasing age, nor does the risk of nonunions significantly increase. One possible reason for the greater healing potential of children may be increased availability of cells that produce repair tissue: younger cells may differentiate more rapidly from the mesenchymal pool,[illegible] and the pool of undifferentiated mesenchymal cells may be larger in children.[49] In addition, the rapid bone remodeling that accompanies growth allows correction of a greater degree of deformity in children.

Effects of Systemic Hormones. A variety of hormones can influence fracture healing (see Table 5-2). Corticosteroids compromise fracture healing,[78,130,272] possibly by inhibiting differentiation of osteoblasts from mesenchymal cells[272] and by decreasing synthesis of bone organic matrix components necessary for repair.[78] Prolonged corticosteroid administration may also decrease bone density and increase the probability of hip, distal radius, rib, and vertebral fractures.[2] The role of growth hormone in fracture healing remains uncertain. Some experimental work suggests that growth hormone deficiency adversely affects fracture healing and that growth hormone replacement can improve healing.[11,12,138,164,200,215,217] Other investigations indicate that excess growth hormone may have little or no effect[62,220] and that normal alterations in the level of circulating growth hormone probably have little effect on fracture healing. Thyroid hormone, calcitonin, insulin, and anabolic steroids have been reported in experimental situations to enhance the rate of fracture healing (see Table 5-2). Diabetes, hypervitaminosis D, and rickets have been shown to retard fracture healing in experimental situations (see Table 5-2). However, clinical experience shows that fractures will heal in patients with hormonal disturbances, although union may be slower than normal.

Bone Necrosis. Normally, healing proceeds from both sides of a fracture, but if one fracture fragment has lost its blood supply, healing depends entirely on ingrowth of capillaries from the living side or surrounding soft tissues. If a fracture fragment is avascular the fracture can heal, but the rate is slower and the incidence of healing is lower[24,189] than if both fragments have a normal blood supply. If both fragments are avascular, the chances for union decrease further. Traumatic or surgical disruption of blood vessels, infection, prolonged use of corticosteroids, and radiation treatment can cause bone necrosis. Irradiated bone, even when it is not obviously necrotic, often heals at a slower rate than normal bone.[316] Nonunion may result,[117] probably because of radiation-induced cell death in the local region, thrombosis of vessels, and fibrosis of the marrow. These changes may reduce the population of cells that can participate in repair, increase the volume of necrotic tissue, and interfere with the ingrowth of capillaries and migration of fibroblasts into the fracture site. Figure 5-14 shows an example of impaired bone healing in a femur treated with radiation.

Infection. Infection can slow or prevent healing. For fracture healing to proceed at the maximum rate, the local cells must be devoted primarily to healing the

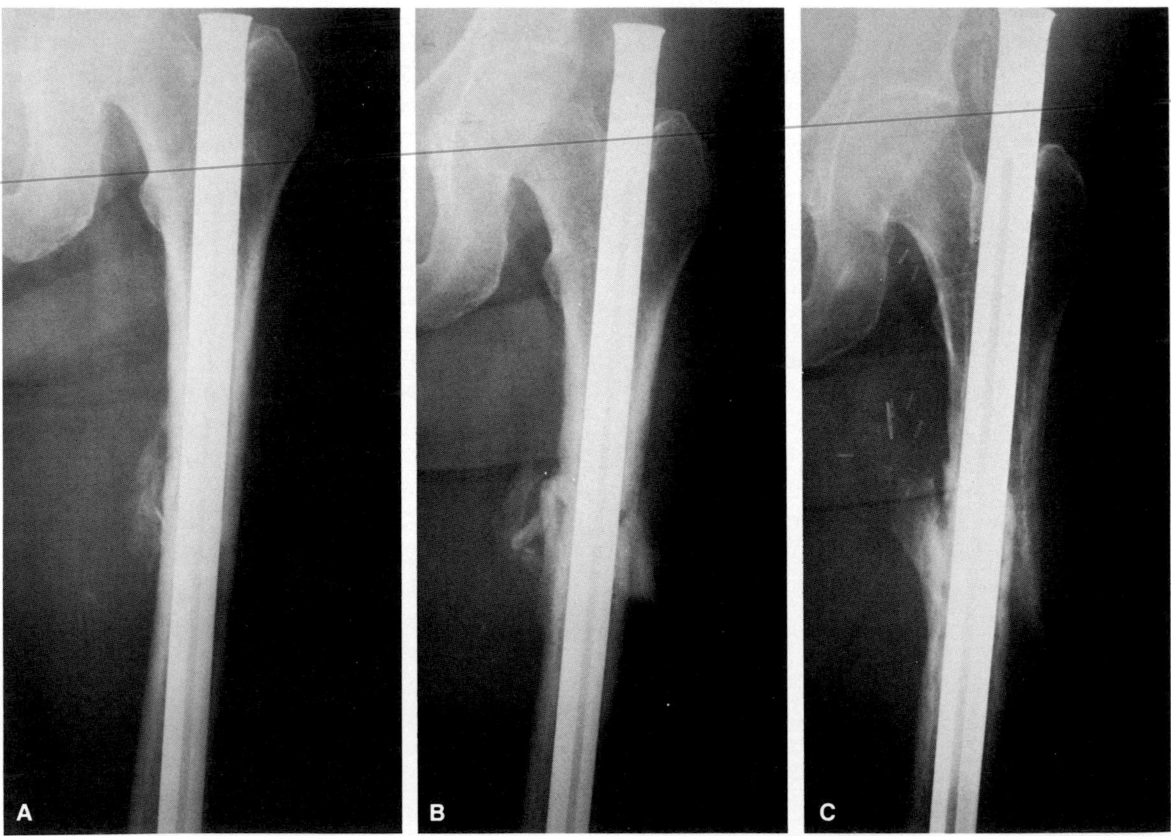

FIGURE 5-14. Radiographs showing a nonunion of a femoral fracture associated with radiation therapy. This elderly patient had a sarcoma of her thigh treated by surgical resection, followed by high-dose radiation therapy. (**A**) Five years after radiation treatment, she slipped on her laundry room floor and suffered a transverse femoral fracture that was treated by intramedullary fixation. (**B**) Three months later the bone had fragmented at the fracture site. (**C**) Four years later, the patient had been treated with bone grafts and a vascularized graft, but the bone continued to collapse and the nonunion persisted.

fracture. If infection occurs after fracture or if the fracture occurs as a result of the infection, many cells must be diverted to attempt to wall off and eliminate the infection, and energy consumption increases. Furthermore, infection may cause necrosis of normal tissue, edema, and thrombosis of blood vessels, thereby retarding or preventing healing.[7]

Tissue Variables. *Form of Bone (Cancellous or Cortical).* Healing of cancellous and cortical fractures differs,[101,263,303] probably because of the differences in surface area, cellularity, and vascularity.[39] Opposed cancellous bone surfaces usually unite rapidly, possibly because the large surface area of cancellous bone per unit volume creates many points of bone contact rich in cells and blood supply and because osteoblasts will form new bone directly on existing trabeculae. Because woven bone forms across points of cancellous bone contact, stable fractures located primarily in cancellous regions, especially impacted fractures where the trabeculae of the fracture fragments have been forced together so that they interdigitate, form little or no visible external callus[263] and rarely fail to heal. Where fractured cancellous bone surfaces are not impacted, new bone spreads from the points of contact to fill gaps.[66,263] When a gap is excessively large, two bone-forming fronts grow from the fracture fragments and eventually meet, but if excessive motion occurs, external callus (including cartilage) may develop. In contrast, cortical bone has a much smaller surface area per unit volume and generally a less extensive internal blood supply, and regions of necrotic cortical bone must be removed before new bone can form.

Bone Disease. Pathologic fractures occur through diseased bone and therefore require less force than that necessary to break normal bone. Commonly recognized causes of pathologic fractures include osteoporosis, osteomalacia, primary malignant bone tumors, metastatic bone tumors, benign bone tumors, bone cysts, osteogenesis imperfecta, fibrous dysplasia, Paget's disease, hyperparathyroidism, and infections. Fractures through bone involved with primary or secondary malignancies usually will not heal if the neoplasm is not treated. Subperiosteal new bone and fracture callus may form, but the mass of malignant cells impairs or prevents fracture healing, particularly if the malignant cells continue to destroy bone. Fractures through infected bone present a similar problem. Thus, healing fractures through malignancies or infections usually requires effective treatment of the underlying local disease or removal of the involved bone. Depending on the extent of bone involvement and the aggressiveness of the lesion, fractures through bones with nonmalignant conditions such as simple bone cysts[209] (Fig. 5-15) and Paget's disease can heal.[214] The most prevalent bone disease, osteoporosis, does not impair fracture healing, but where there is diminished surface contact of apposing cortical or cancellous bone surfaces due to decreased bone mass the time required to restore normal bone mechanical strength may be increased. Furthermore, decreased bone mass reduces the strength and stability of the interface between the bone and screws used for internal fixation. This may lead to failure of internal fixation and subsequent delayed healing or nonunion.

Treatment Variables. *Apposition of Fracture Fragments.* Decreasing the fracture gap decreases the volume of repair tissue needed to heal a fracture. Restoring fracture fragment apposition is especially important if the surrounding soft tissues have been disrupted or when soft tissues lie between the fracture fragments. When a significant portion of the periosteum and other soft-tissue components remain intact or can be rapidly restored, lack of bone fragment apposition may not impair healing.

Loading and Micromotion. The optimal conditions for fracture healing include at least some loading of the repair tissue. Based on the available evidence, it appears that loading a fracture site stimulates bone formation,[50] while decreased loading slows fracture healing.[225] Limb denervation also can retard fracture healing, possibly by diminishing loading of the fracture[249] or by inhibiting the effect of growth factors that require activation by neurotransmitters. In contrast, exercise can increase the rate of repair,[127] possibly through loading of the fracture. In addition, experimental work and clinical experience shows that early or even almost immediate controlled loading and limb movement, including induced micromotion at long-bone fracture sites, may promote fracture healing.[50,82,118,158–160,162,203,225,262]

Fracture Stabilization. Fracture stabilization by traction, cast immobilization, external fixation, and internal fixation[65,236,275] can facilitate fracture healing by preventing repeated disruption of repair tissue. Some fractures (eg, displaced femoral neck and scaphoid fractures) rarely heal if they are not rigidly stabilized. Fracture stability appears to be particularly important for healing when there is extensive associated soft-tissue injury, when the blood supply to the fracture site is marginal, and when the fracture occurs within a synovial joint. Excessive motion secondary to ineffective stabilization, repeated manipulation, or excessive loading and motion retards fracture healing and may cause nonunion.[189,229] In these injuries it is probable that the repeated excessive motion disrupts the initial fracture hematoma or granulation tissue, delaying or preventing formation of fracture callus. If excessive motion continues, a cleft forms between the fracture ends, and a pseudarthrosis develops.

Despite the importance of stability for healing some fractures, instability may not impair healing of other fractures. During the early part of repair, motion oc-

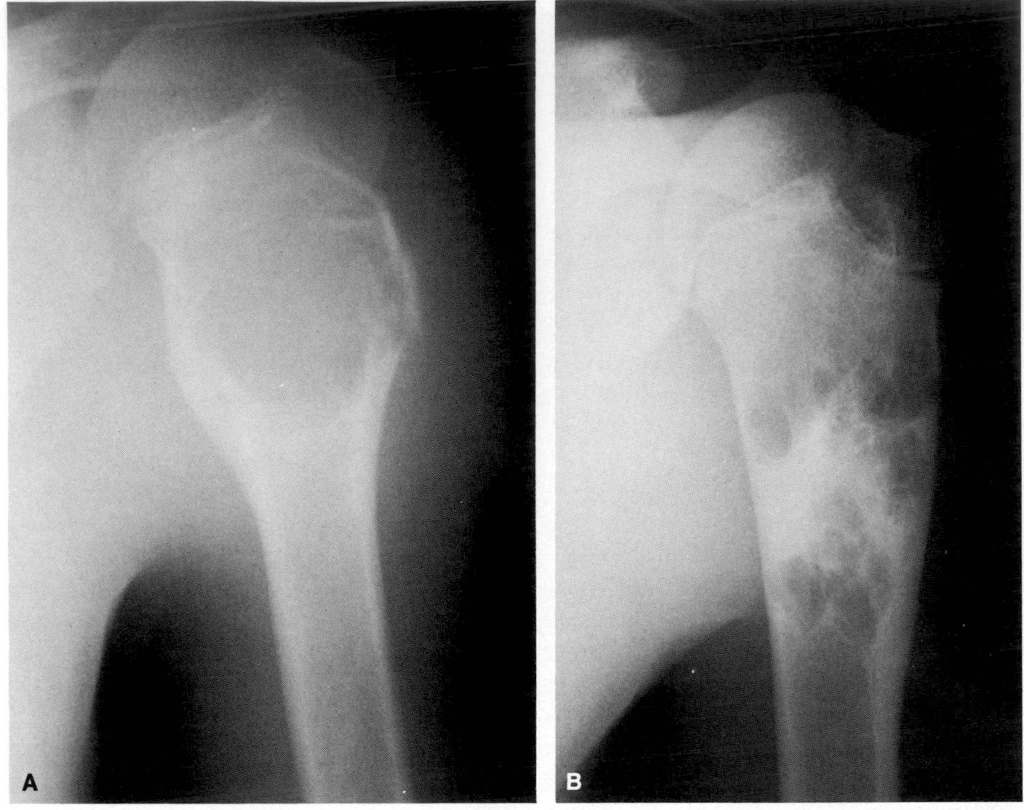

FIGURE 5-15. Radiographs showing a fracture through a simple bone cyst. (**A**) A 12-year-old boy sustained a pathologic fracture through a simple bone cyst. The fracture healed within 6 weeks. (**B**) Eighteen months after injury, the cyst has progressed toward healing.

curs at most fractures except for those treated by rigid internal fixation. Fractures with intact surrounding soft tissues that provide some stability in a well-vascularized region of bone may heal rapidly even though palpable motion of the fracture site persists for weeks after injury. For example, closed rib, clavicle, and many humeral diaphyseal and metacarpal and metatarsal fractures heal even though the fracture fragments remain mobile until fracture callus stabilizes them. As discussed previously, controlled induced micromotion can facilitate healing of some fractures.[118,158–160,262]

Unlike traction, cast immobilization, and at least some forms of external fixation, internal fixation of fractures with metallic implants can produce rigid stabilization of fractures. Although rigid stabilization of a fracture makes possible primary bone repair without cartilage or connective tissue intermediates, it does not accelerate fracture healing.[234–238] Stable fixation of fractures and the resulting primary fracture repair have the advantages of allowing early limb motion and rapid return to activity, thereby avoiding "fracture disease" (stiffness, loss of joint motion, and muscle weakness related to immobilization) and making it possible to restore anatomical apposition of fracture fragments.[5,235,236,275] This approach has proven especially beneficial in treatment of intra-articular fractures, diaphyseal fractures of the radius and ulna, unstable spine fractures, hip fractures, and some types of femoral and tibial fractures.

The surgical procedure of stabilizing a fracture with a metallic implant causes acute and later chronic inflammation.[170] Repair follows with the production of scar that remodels to form mature fibrous tissue. For totally inert implants, this would be the end of the reaction. However, no metal is completely inert, because metals release ions that may cause a tissue response after the initial inflammatory reaction. In some patients, the fibrous tissue covering the implant thickens and becomes more vascular, and microscopic examination may demonstrate the presence of giant cells; however, these tissue reactions to implants have not been shown to alter fracture healing.

Although rigid internal stabilization of fractures with metallic implants has multiple advantages, it also has potential disadvantages. Rigid fixation can alter fracture remodeling and decrease bone density because the stiffness of most implants differs from that of bone.[3,224,301,321,326] For example, steel is more than ten times as stiff as bone. When a fractured bone, rigidly fixed with a stiff implant, is loaded, the bone is shielded from normal stresses by the more rigid implant.[291,302,301] Regional loss of bone mass may occur (Fig. 5-16), which increases the probability of refracture after removal of the plate,[133,252,302] although refractures after removal of plates may also be due to screw holes, which act as stress risers. The problem of decreased bone density associated with rigid plate fixation might be avoided by use of less rigid plates (ie, plates that more closely approximate the modulus of elasticity of bone).[319,321] Attempts have been made to accomplish this by reducing the stiffness of the plate, either by decreasing its cross-sectional area or by choosing materials with a lower modulus of elasticity.[3,300,321,322]

In addition to stress shielding of bone, attempted rigid internal stabilization of fractures has other potential disadvantages. Anatomical reduction and rigid stabilization of some fractures may require extensive surgical exposure that increases the risks of infection and of compromising the blood supply to injured tissues.

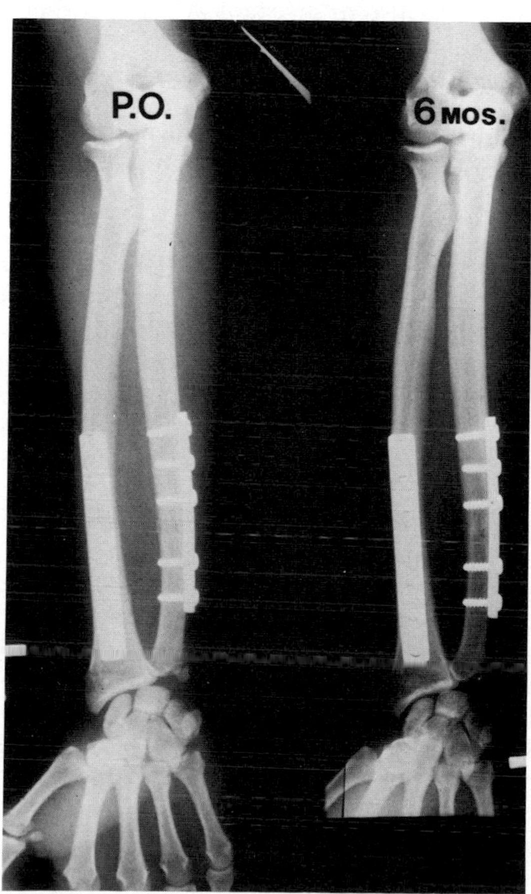

FIGURE 5-16. Radiographs showing that rigid internal fixation can decrease bone density immediately beneath the compression plate. Immediately postoperatively (*P.O.*) the bone density appears normal, but 6 months later the bone density under the plate has decreased.

Furthermore, attempted rigid stabilization of fractures may adversely affect fracture healing when anatomical reduction and rigid fixation cannot be achieved. Formation of bone in the fracture gap depends on the width of the gap and the stability of fixation. When the gap is greater than 1 mm or there is motion at the fracture site, secondary osteons do not fill the gap with bone. Complex fracture patterns and multiple bone fragments caused by high-energy trauma or the weakness of osteopenic bone may prevent the surgeon from obtaining anatomical alignment, fracture fragment compression, and rigid stabilization. If fixation devices hold a fracture site distracted or if rigid stability is not achieved after internal fixation, motion at the fracture site can result in resorption of bone in the fracture gap and the appearance of small amounts of external callus. Typically, this external callus is not adequate to stabilize the fracture site, and delayed union or nonunion may occur. Motion at the fracture site and protracted stress on the fixation device may cause failure of the device. For these reasons attempting rigid internal stabilization is not appropriate for all fractures, and when indicated it requires careful planning and attention to surgical techniques.

Bone Grafting. Surgeons frequently use grafts of cancellous, cortical, or corticocancellous bone to stimulate fracture healing and replace lost bone.[52] In addition, vascularized bone grafts bring a new blood supply to the graft site. The genetic relationship between the donor and the recipient defines the four types of bone grafts[259]:

- *Autografts* are grafts transferred from a donor site to another site in the same person.
- *Isografts* are grafts transferred between people who have identical histocompatibility antigens (ie, identical twins).
- *Allografts* are grafts transferred between genetically dissimilar members of the same species.
- *Xenografts* are grafts transferred from a member of one species to a member of another species.

Surgeons most frequently use fresh nonvascularized autografts to stimulate fracture healing. Vascularized autografts have proven useful in the treatment of selected complex fractures. Autografts can be harvested, preserved, and then implanted later, but there are relatively few situations in which this approach is used.

Fresh nonvascularized autografts contain cells that potentially can form new bone directly. In most grafts, only cells close to the surface survive and retain the potential ability to form new bone.[1,55–57,67] For this to occur, the cells must be kept viable before implantation. The grafts should not be dried, exposed to solutions that kill cells, or maintained out of the body for prolonged periods. After implantation, the graft cells must have a ready route of nutrition by diffusion. Diffusion of nutrients into the central regions of bone graft occurs if the particle size is not too large (5 mm is the maximum thickness that can be nourished in this fashion).[246,247] For this reason small cancellous autografts are assumed to be the best source of cells that can form bone after transplantation. Because cortical bone has a much smaller surface area per unit volume than cancellous bone, many cortical bone osteocytes lie far from the surface of the tissue and cannot survive by diffusion. Replacement of these necrotic cells occurs when osteoclasts resorb the graft, bringing blood vessels and osteoblasts that form new bone using the graft material as a scaffold. This process may take years and never completely restores the viability of some large cortical autografts,[318] but the recipient site cells form new bone on the surface of the autograft.

Vascularized autografts, most commonly fibular and iliac crest grafts, have the advantage of maintaining the viability of bone cells and some of the surrounding soft-tissue cells, including periosteal cells.[84,268,311] Large vascularized cortical autografts do not undergo the extensive resorption and remodeling seen in large nonvascularized cortical autografts, and they bring a new blood supply to the recipient site. These features of vascularized autografts may make them especially useful in promoting bone healing when the blood supply to the fracture site is limited or in healing large segmental defects.[84] The primary disadvantages of vascularized autografts are the technical difficulty of the surgical procedure and increased potential for surgical complications.

Fresh allografts have the potential to provide viable cells. Experimental studies indicate that viable cells from fresh allografts may participate in the repair process for about 2 weeks, but after this time they may invoke an inflammatory response that can obliterate the repair, a sequence similar to the graft rejection process described in other tissues.[22,95] For this reason, allografts usually are treated to decrease their antigenicity. Although many methods may be effective, in clinical practice freezing and freeze-drying are among the most common. The grafts may be taken and maintained under sterile conditions or sterilized with high-energy radiation.[56,67,128,296,297] The frozen, irradiated, or preserved allografts do not provide cells that form new bone and may stimulate an immunologic response despite treatment of the graft. Nevertheless, their organic matrix may possess the ability to induce local bone formation,[56,57,305] and they can provide structural support.

Selection of a bone graft to promote fracture healing should be guided by evaluation of the problems presented by the fracture. Because there is no immunologic response on the part of the host, and because it may have the capacity to form new bone, an autograft containing cancellous bone represents the best choice to stimulate new bone formation. Cancellous bone has a large surface area per unit volume, and thus it need not be resorbed before new bone formation can begin and appositional new bone can form on the surface of necrotic cancellous bone.[161] Surgeons commonly use cancellous autografts to stimulate healing of fresh fractures, delayed unions, and nonunions with minimal fracture gaps. Massive cancellous autografts can heal fractures with large gaps, including large diaphyseal segmental defects, but during the prolonged healing period the cancellous grafts do not provide mechanical stability.[68] In contrast, cortical bone autografts can provide immediate mechanical stability when they are used to replace lost diaphyseal bone segments. However, resorption and vascular invasion makes the graft porous and decreases its strength for months and possibly years after implantation.[84,96] Vascularized autografts avoid this problem, provided the vascular anastomoses remain patent until new blood vessels grow into the graft from the recipient site.[84,285,286,311] Free vascularized fibular or iliac crest grafts have been useful in treating fractures with extensive loss of bone.[84,285,286] They incorporate rapidly and can hypertrophy in response to mechanical stress in their new anatomical location.

Cancellous and cortical allografts have not been widely used to treat fractures. Host bone will unite or bond with allograft bone,[97] and allografts can replace traumatic segmental bone defects,[146,195] but their efficacy in promoting fracture healing has not been clearly demonstrated.

Bone Transport. Bone transport offers an alternative to bone graft treatment of a segmental bone loss.[227] To replace a lost portion of a long-bone diaphysis the surgeon performs a corticotomy through normal bone, creating a mobile bone segment, and then uses an external fixation device to transport the segment across the defect. As the segment moves, a column of bone forms behind it. With time, the bone that forms behind the advancing segment remodels to have a normal radiographic appearance, including a medullary cavity (Fig. 5-17). Most surgeons wait 7 to 14 days after the corticotomy to begin transporting the segment. The fixation device must stabilize the bone fragments and guide the movement of the segment being transported. The rate of transport is usually 1 mm/d (0.25 mm q.i.d.). When the leading end of the transported segment reaches the end of the defect, the external fixation device can compress the fracture site. If the fracture fails to heal, it can be treated as a nonunion without a segmental bone defect. A similar approach can be used to treat infected nonunions. The surgeon excises the infected nonunion site and transports a normal segment of bone across the defect. Although this procedure requires prolonged patient cooperation, it can be an effective method of treating

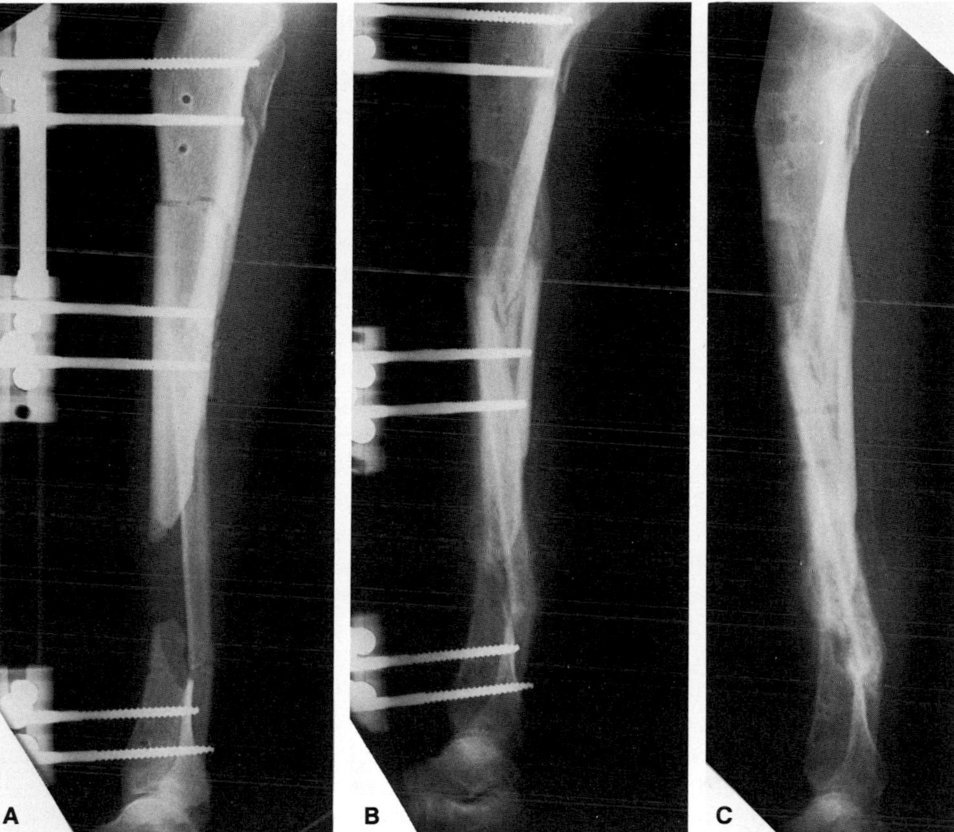

FIGURE 5-17. Radiographs showing the use of bone transport to heal a tibial nonunion secondary to segmental bone loss. (**A**) This radiograph shows a bone defect of the distal tibia occurring after an open fracture. A corticotomy has been performed in the proximal tibia and an external fixation device applied. (**B**) The external fixation device transports the proximal tibial bone across the defect. Note the column of bone that formed behind the moving segment. (**C**) After the fracture healed, the external fixation device was removed and the bone continued to remodel. (*Courtesy of J. Nepola and L. Marsh, University of Iowa Orthopaedics Department, Iowa City, Iowa.*

nonunions secondary to bone loss and infection. The clinical results of bone transport treatment of nonunions have not been extensively documented in the English medical literature, but Ilizarov, who developed the procedure, described the principles of this technique,[142,143] and other authors have reported a high success rate in healing long-bone nonunions with bone loss or infection.[10,63,121,227]

Electrical Fields. Electrical fields can alter cell proliferation and synthetic function and promote bone formation.[14,15,28,30,31,33,171,197,213,239] In addition, several reports indicate that the application of electrical fields may stimulate healing of delayed unions and nonunions,[27,28,32,106,172,267,270] including fractures that failed to respond to other treatment.[32,106,107] Although these reports describe encouraging results, defining the optimal clinical use of electrical fields to treat delayed unions and nonunions requires further study.

Ultrasound. Recent experimental and clinical reports describe acceleration of fracture healing by low-intensity pulsed ultrasound.[125,163,237] A prospective, randomized, double-blind evaluation of tibia fractures showed clinical and radiographic healing of fractures treated with ultrasound at an average of 96 days after injury, compared with 154 days for fractures treated by conventional methods alone.[125] Although the mechanism of the effect of ultrasound on fracture repair remains uncertain, this prospective clinical study indicates that it can provide a safe noninvasive method of facilitating fracture healing in humans.[125]

Demineralized Bone Matrix, Growth Factors, and Autologous Bone Marrow. New developments in cell and molecular biology have significantly increased understanding of healing and the potential for facilitating healing. In particular, demineralized bone matrix, growth factors that stimulate bone formation, and autologous bone marrow cells have the potential to improve treatment of delayed unions and nonunions.[20,21,59,71,94,151,180,181,208,211,280,281,294]

Experimental implantation of demineralized bone matrix stimulates migration of undifferentiated mesenchymal cells to the implanted matrix and differentiation of these cells into chondrocytes that synthesize a cartilaginous matrix. The cartilage then undergoes enchondral ossification, leaving bone that subsequently remodels. This sequence of events duplicates the process of fracture healing, making the use of demineralized bone matrix a potentially attractive method of stimulating fracture healing by host cells.[20,94,208]

A variety of cytokines affect all stages of bone repair. Current investigations of these factors are directed toward identifying specific molecules that might be used to stimulate fracture healing and developing methods of delivering these factors to fracture sites.[21,180,181,208,280,281,294] Experimental work shows that this approach can stimulate fracture healing and regeneration of bone that can heal segmental bone defects,[73,74,154,175,216,254] but its value in humans requires further study.

Transplantation of autologous bone marrow provides another approach to stimulating fracture healing. Bone marrow contains mesenchymal cells that can differentiate into osteoblasts and form bone[57] (see Fig. 5-2), and these cells along with other marrow elements can be harvested by bone marrow aspiration. Experimental studies show that treatment of osteotomies and delayed unions in rabbits using bone marrow preparations improved bone healing.[71,269] Based on these observations, investigators have used autologous bone marrow injections in an attempt to stimulate healing of human nonunions.[110] The results appear encouraging, but this method of promoting fracture healing needs further investigation.

Treatment That Interferes With Healing. Most fractures will heal when treated by a variety of methods. Furthermore, the healing potential of many fractures, especially those in children, can overcome less than optimal treatment, but some surgical and nonsurgical interventions interfere with healing and may cause delayed union or nonunion.[189] In particular, inadequate immobilization of some fractures (eg, scaphoid and femoral neck fractures), distraction of fracture fragments by fixation devices or traction, repeated manipulations or excessive early motion of a fracture, or excessive periosteal stripping and damage to other soft tissues during surgical exposure of a fracture may interfere with healing. Infection following surgery, or failure to achieve acceptable apposition of fracture fragments or stable fixation, may also cause delayed union or nonunion.

DENSE FIBROUS TISSUES

Structure and Composition

The musculoskeletal dense fibrous tissues form tough yet pliable sheets, bands, and cords with great tensile strength.[38,43,51,103,113] They consist of a matrix formed primarily from densely packed, highly oriented type I collagen fibrils and a sparse population of fibroblasts. Networks of blood vessels weave between dense bundles of collagen fibrils. Perivascular nerves accompany many blood vessels, and in some regions other nerve fibers have receptors sensitive to mechanical loading. The specialized forms of dense fibrous tissue include fascia, tendon, ligament, joint capsule, and meniscus. These tissues differ in shape, location, form, composition, and function but share the ability to resist large tensile loads.

Dense Fibrous Tissue Healing

Like bone, the response of vascularized dense fibrous tissue to acute injury includes inflammation, repair, and remodeling stages (see Figs. 5-1 and 5-18), and the repair tissue matrix consists primarily of type I collagen. The primary differences are that the repair tissue formed after injury to dense fibrous tissue rarely duplicates the structure and properties of the uninjured tissue, and it does not mineralize. Although the specialized forms of dense fibrous tissue follow the same general pattern of healing, because of the differences in their structure and function, tendon, ligament and joint capsule, and meniscus healing present different clinical problems.[51,103,113]

Tendon

Tendons consist of three components: the substance of the tendon,[38,113] the bone insertion,[75,323] and the muscle–tendon junction.[112,219,289] The substance of the tendon consists primarily of densely packed, longitudinally aligned bundles of collagen fibrils. Tendons contain relatively few cells, their level of metabolic activity is relatively low, and the cells in some tendon regions receive a significant proportion of their nutrition by diffusion.[137] Nonetheless, tendons deprived of their blood supply become necrotic.[241–244,276] In most regions the blood vessels that supply the tendon cells pass from the surrounding tissues through a mesotendon[70] to form a vascular network within the tendon substance.[25,34,43,70,113,230] The mesotendon consists of loose connective tissue and blood vessels so that as the tendon moves, the mesotendon extends and recoils, thereby maintaining the blood supply to the substance of the tendon. At their insertion sites, tendon collagen fibrils pass through regions of fibrocartilage and calcified cartilage before entering the bone.[75,323] The muscle–tendon junction consists of a complex interdigitation formed by muscle cells, a specialized region of extracellular matrix, and the collagen fibers of the tendon substance.[112,219,289]

All three tendon components may suffer acute traumatic injuries. Lacerations of tendon substance are the most common injuries. Avulsions or fractures through tendon insertions and tears of the muscle–tendon junction or complete avulsions of the tendon from the muscle–tendon junction occur less frequently. Complete disruption of any part of the muscle–tendon unit allows the muscle to retract, increasing the gap at the injury site. If the injury is left untreated, scar tissue may eventually fill the gap between the tendon ends, but it will leave the muscle–tendon unit longer than

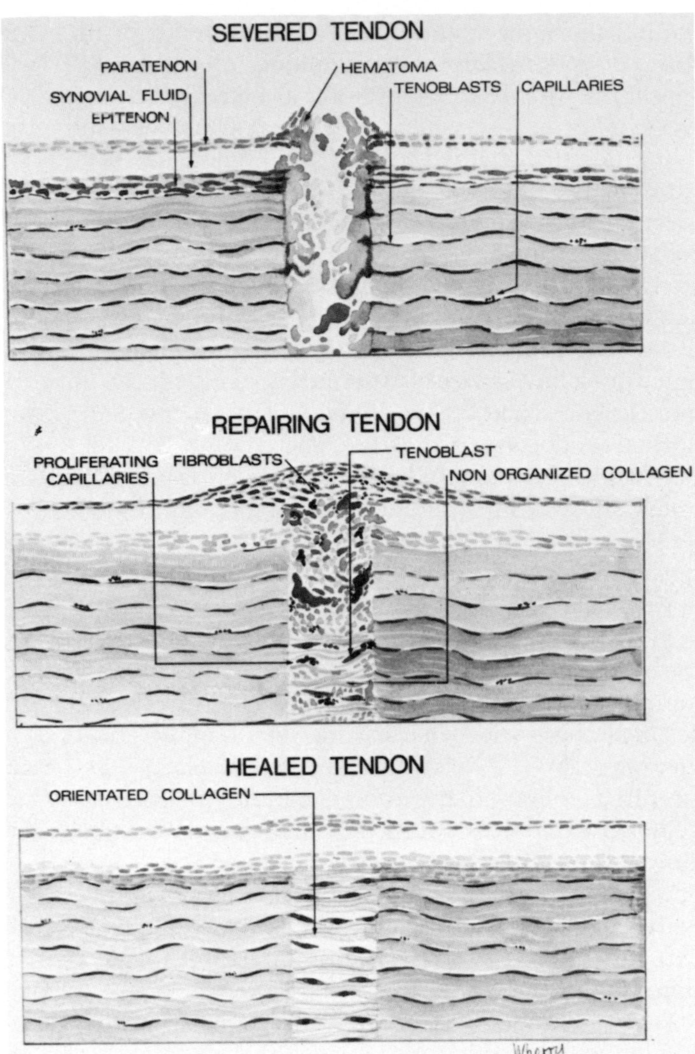

FIGURE 5-18. Sequence of events after tendon laceration: a hematoma forms between the tendon ends. Stimulated by chemotactic factors, inflammatory cells migrate into the hematoma, followed by blood vessels and fibroblasts. The fibroblasts synthesize a new matrix. They then remodel the repair tissue to restore the structure and function of the tendon. Healing of the other dense fibrous tissues follows the same pattern.

before injury and may bind the tendon to the surrounding tissues. Without restoration of normal tendon length and gliding, the function of the muscle–tendon unit will be poor. For this reason, restoration of muscle–tendon unit function after a complete disruption usually requires a surgical repair that reestablishes normal tendon length and has sufficient strength to allow immediate motion of the tendon relative to the surrounding tissues.

The specialized structure of tendons—and in some areas the structures surrounding tendons—makes it possible to transmit the force of muscle contraction to bone, thereby producing joint motion. Some tendons pass through well-defined synovial-lined sheaths and dense fibrous tissue pulleys. Achieving healing of lacerated digital flexor tendons within these tendon sheaths while preserving the pulleys and the tendon motion presents a unique problem in the treatment of musculoskeletal injuries.[113] The cut tendon ends can be sutured and will heal, but if the repair tissue scars the tendon to the sheath or the pulleys, tendon motion will be restricted and may cause joint contracture. Tendons without sheaths do not usually present this problem because scarring of their repair tissue to surrounding loose areolar tissue often will not severely restrict motion.

Because lacerated sheathed flexor tendons present the most challenging clinical tendon healing problem, many studies have concentrated on this problem. Peacock[230,231] introduced the "one wound—one scar" concept; that is, a tendon laceration creates one wound including the skin, subcutaneous tissue, tendon, and tendon sheath and these tissues form a continuous mass of repair tissue. Potenza's studies[241,242] supported this view and led to the concept that tendon healing depends on migration of mesenchymal cells into the tendon laceration from the surrounding tissues. His work showed that tendon healing begins with inflammatory cell and fibroblast migration into the site of injury (see Fig. 5-18). Granulation tissue proliferates around the injury site and between the ends of the sutured tendons, depositing randomly oriented collagen fibrils. The density of fibroblasts increases up to 3 weeks after injury, when granulation tissue fills and surrounds the repaired area. If the tendon has been sutured, the suture material holds the tendon ends together until the fibroblasts have produced sufficient collagen to form a "tendon callus."[18] The tensile strength of the repaired tendon depends on the collagen concentration and the orientation of the collagen fibrils. The collagen fibrils become longitudinally oriented by about 4 weeks, and during the next 2 to 3 months the repair tissue remodels until it resembles normal tendon (see Fig. 5-18). The amount and density of the scar tissue adhesions between the tendon injury site and surrounding tissues depend on the intensity, extent, and duration of the inflammatory and repair phases of healing and the mobility of the tendon during repair.

More recent work has emphasized the potential of intrinsic tendon cells to heal sheathed flexor tendon injuries. These cells produce collagen after injury, suggesting that they participate in tendon healing.[113,114,176–179,182,183,188] However, it is not clear that a lacerated tendon can be restored to its original strength by healing that does not include inflammation, vascular invasion, and migration of mesenchymal cells from outside the injury site. It is clear that tendons can heal within their sheaths without a mass of repair tissue extending directly from the injury into the surrounding tissues.

Early controlled mobilization of a repaired tendon can reduce scar adhesions between the tendon injury site and the surrounding tissue and facilitate healing,[113,114,190,191] but excessive loading may disrupt the repair tissue. Thus, optimal tendon healing depends on surgical apposition and mechanical stabilization of the tendon ends without excessive soft-tissue damage and on creating the optimal mechanical environment for healing. This mechanical environment includes sufficient tendon mobility to prevent adhesions and sufficient loading to stimulate remodeling of the repair tissue matrix along the lines of stress, but the loads applied to the tendon must not exceed the strength of the surgical repair.

Disruption of tendon insertions into bone often involves a fracture or avulsion of a bone fragment at the site of injury. These injuries usually can be treated by surgically reducing and stabilizing the fracture or reinserting the tendon into the bone and stabilizing the insertion. Healing occurs either by bony union or by union of the bone to the tendon substance.

Partial muscle–tendon junction injuries usually heal successfully if further injury can be prevented, but complete or nearly complete avulsions or tears can present difficult problems because attempts to suture muscle tissue consisting primarily of muscle cells to tendon are unlikely to produce a predictable result. Optimal healing of these injuries depends on approximation of the avulsed tendon and any remnants of the tendon remaining attached to the muscle or, when available, muscle fascia. Although it may appear that muscles attach to tendons over a small area, in many muscles thin extensions of their tendons penetrate long distances within the muscle bellies. Identification of these thin bands of tendon within muscle may make it possible to suture them to an avulsed or partially avulsed tendon in the proximal and distal thirds of many muscles and as far as the middle third of some muscles.[64] If this can be accomplished, the tendon–muscle injury site must then be stabilized for a sufficient time to allow repair of the muscle–tendon junction with scar tissue.

Ligament and Joint Capsule

Ligaments and joint capsules join adjacent bones with dense fibrous tissue to provide joint stability while allowing joint motion.[51,103] Like tendons, ligaments and joint capsules consist primarily of highly oriented collagen fibrils, and they have well-developed bone insertions.[75,323] Unlike tendons, they do not have elaborate synovial-lined sheaths or pulleys and usually they move less relative to surrounding tissues. Furthermore, when ligaments and joint capsules rupture or tear, the gap at the injury site is not increased by muscle pull.

Ligament and joint capsule substance healing follows the sequence described for healing of tendon substance by extrinsic cells (see Fig. 5-18). Also as in tendon healing, early motion and loading of injured ligaments can stimulate healing.[6,50,51] Because controlled normal motion of a joint does not necessarily cause large forces in the ligaments and joint capsule, limited motion will not necessarily disrupt the repair of the tissue.

If ligament or capsular tears heal with a significant gap or fail to heal, the resultant joint instability may increase the probability of subsequent joint injury and degenerative joint disease (Fig. 5-19). For this reason, restoration or maintenance of near-normal ligament and capsule length and maintenance of normal joint motion should be the objectives of treatment. The most favorable condition for healing divided ligaments and joint capsules is direct apposition of the divided surfaces. Apposition and stabilization of the injury site decreases the volume of repair tissue required to heal the injury, minimizes scarring, and may help provide near-normal tissue length. A sutured ligament can heal with a minimal gap.[221,222] When tested under tension, sutured ligaments are stronger than those that heal with a significant length of scar tissue, and liga-

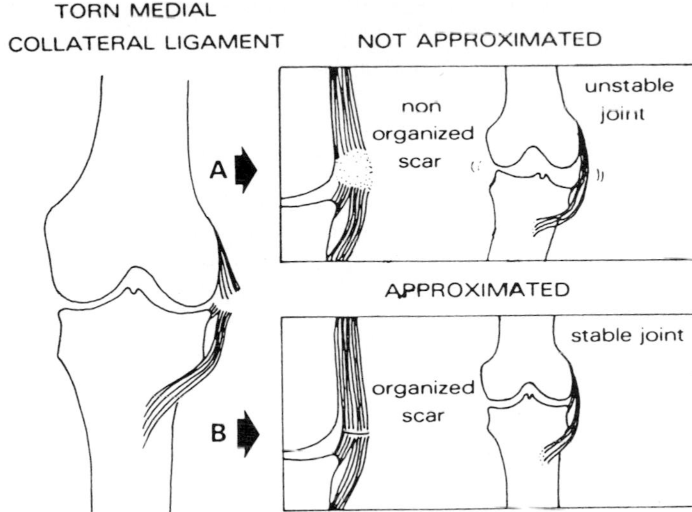

FIGURE 5-19. Approximation of a torn ligament decreases the volume of the tissue defect. When a ligament heals with a significant gap, it may fail to provide joint stability.

ments that heal with a gap between the cut ends may have a decreased ability to stabilize the adjacent joint.[6,69,290] However, many ligament and joint capsule tears will heal without surgical repair and function as well or better than surgically repaired ligaments and capsules if the torn ends do not retract and the tear occurs through tissue with an adequate blood supply.

Meniscus

Meniscal tissue has a structure, composition, and mechanical properties similar to both the dense fibrous tissues and articular cartilage.[8,45] Like the other dense fibrous tissues, it consists primarily of type I collagen and it has great tensile strength; but like articular cartilage, its matrix contains large proteoglycans and chondrocyte-like cells and it performs important mechanical functions in the knee joint, including load bearing and shock absorption, and participates in joint lubrication. Unlike articular cartilage, some regions of meniscus have a blood supply (the peripheral 25% of the lateral meniscus and the peripheral 30% of the medial meniscus) and a nerve supply (the peripheral regions of the meniscus and especially the meniscal horns).[8,45]

Within the meniscus, collagen fibril diameter and orientation and cell morphology vary from the surfaces to the deep central region.[45] The thin surface layers consist of a mesh of fine fibrils. Immediately deep to these fine fibrils, small-diameter collagen fibrils with a radial orientation relative to the body of the meniscus form a thicker subsurface layer. The flattened ellipsoid cells of this layer orient their maximum diameter roughly parallel to the articular surface. In the deeper central or middle region, making up the bulk of the meniscus, the cells assume a more spheroidal shape, similar to that of chondrocytes, and large-diameter collagen fibrils form circumferential bundles. Smaller radially oriented fibril bundles weave among the dense bundles of circumferential running collagen bundles. The circumferential collagen bundles give the meniscus great tensile strength parallel to their orientation. The radial fibers within the central region of the meniscus may help increase the strength of the tissue by resisting longitudinal splitting of the collagen framework.

The response of meniscal tissue to tears depends on whether the tear occurs through a vascular or an avascular portion of the meniscus. The vascular regions respond to injury like other vascularized dense fibrous tissues. This response can heal a meniscal injury and restore the tissue structure and function if the torn edges remain apposed and if the repair tissue is not disrupted in the early stages of healing. Providing these conditions frequently requires surgical repair of meniscal tears or tears of meniscal attachments. The avascular regions of meniscal tissue, like articular cartilage, do not repair significant tissue defects. Cells in the region of the injury, like chondrocytes in the region of the injury limited to articular cartilage, may proliferate and synthesize new matrix, but there is no evidence that the cells migrate into the defect site or produce new matrix that can fill the defect site.

Because of the ineffective repair response of meniscal cells in the avascular region of the meniscus, investigators have developed several methods to stimulate repair. These approaches include attempts to create vascular access to the injury site and to stimulate cell migration to the avascular region using implantation of a fibrin clot, an artificial matrix, or growth factors.[8] Experimental studies show that creating full-thickness channels from the periphery of the meniscus to experimentally created longitudinal lesions in the avascular portion allows blood vessels and mesenchymal cells from the peripheral meniscal tissue to migrate through the channels and heal the meniscal lesions. However, large channels may compromise the function of the meniscus by destroying the integrity of the peripheral rim. To avoid this problem, investigators have also used trephines to create vascular tunnels that connect the peripheral portion of the meniscus with lesion in the avascular region. Synovium also can provide a source of vessels and cells for meniscal healing. Abrasion of synovium to stimulate proliferation of the synovial fringe into the meniscus or suturing a flap of vascular synovial tissue into a longitudinal lesion in the avascular portion of the meniscus brings a blood supply and new cells to the injury site.[8] Although the results of these attempts to increase the blood supply appear promising, the quality of the repair tissue, its material properties, and the long-term results of these methods have not been thoroughly evaluated.

Investigators have also attempted to stimulate meniscal repair without the participation of blood vessels. This approach assumes that either the meniscal cells can repair defects in the avascular meniscal regions if appropriately stimulated or that mesenchymal cells from the vascular region can migrate into the avascular region. Several experimental studies support these assumptions. They have shown that cultured meniscal cells can proliferate and synthesize matrix when exposed to chemotactic and mitogenic factors found in hematomas.[310] Methods that might stimulate meniscal repair without participation of blood vessels include implanting a fibrin clot, presumably containing platelet-derived growth factor and possibly other growth factors that stimulate mesenchymal cell migration, proliferation, and matrix synthesis. A fibrin clot would also act as a scaffolding for migration of cells and could serve as a vehicle for implantation of specific growth factors. An experimental study showed that implanting exogenous fibrin clots in defects in the avascular regions of dog menisci stimulated proliferation of fibrous connective tissue that eventually assumed the appearance of fibrocartilaginous tissue, although it differed from normal meniscus tissue histologically and grossly.[8] The source of the repair cells was not identified, but they may have arisen from adjacent synovium and from meniscal tissue. Clinical experience with injection of fibrin clots into meniscal defects also suggests that the clots stimulate repair. In one study, 92% of isolated meniscal tears treated with fibrin clots healed compared with 59% of isolated meniscal tears treated without fibrin clots.[129] Implantation of a fibrin clot or a synthetic matrix containing growth factors or transplanted mesenchymal cells might also stimulate meniscal repair in the avascular regions.

Failure of Dense Fibrous Tissue Healing

Injuries to tendons, ligaments, joint capsules, and menisci may fail to heal despite treatment. Instead of firm scar aligned along the lines of stress, the injury site contains filmy loose connective tissue, myxoid tissue, or granulation tissue. The reasons for failure of healing are unclear in some instances, but identifiable causes include a large gap at the injury site, extensive damage to the surrounding tissue (including loss of vascular supply), excessive early loading and motion of the repair tissue, and injury-related necrosis of the tissue. Surgical treatment may also contribute to poor healing. Extensive dissection can devascularize traumatized tissue, and inappropriate suture technique may also damage the blood supply to the injury site or place excessive tension on a sutured tissue.

Excessive Repair of Dense Fibrous Tissues

Ligament, joint capsule, and tendon injuries may heal with excessive scar that restricts motion between the injury site and the surrounding tissue. When this occurs after a ligament or joint capsule injury, it causes contracture of the adjacent synovial joint. When it occurs after tendon injury, it limits tendon excursion and can lead to weakness and joint contracture. Identifiable causes of excessive repair after dense fibrous tissue injuries include severe injuries, infection, and extensive surgery that increases the volume of injured tissue. Prolonged immobilization of injured fibrous tissues does not necessarily increase the extent of scar formation, but it can allow scar adhesions to form and mature. Therefore, the best methods of preventing excessive scar and scar adhesions appear to be removing necrotic tissue and excessive hematoma when possible, minimizing surgical dissection, and using early controlled loading and motion.[6,43,50,113]

Variables That Influence Dense Fibrous Tissue Healing

Injury Variables. Segmental loss of tissue, tendon injuries that disrupt tendon sheaths and pulleys, crushing injuries that compromise the vascular supply or damage surrounding tissues, and wide separation of the disrupted ends of tendon, ligament, joint capsule, or meniscus make restoration of normal function difficult or impossible. Dense fibrous tissue injuries that produce relatively little loss of tissue and little damage to surrounding tissues and retain adequate vascular supply to the repair site have the potential for restoration of tissue function and near-normal tissue structure and composition.

Patient Variables

The influence of patient variables on repair of the dense fibrous tissues has not been extensively studied. The variables that influence bone healing—including hormonal effects, nutritional status, and systemic disease—may be important (see Table 5-2). Age does affect the composition and mechanical properties of many of the dense fibrous tissues and may also affect their vascular supply and rate of healing,[49] but the clinical importance of these possibilities has not been demonstrated.

Treatment Variables

Surgical Repair. Optimal healing of dense fibrous tissue injuries occurs when there is a minimal volume of necrotic tissue that must be resorbed; viable ends of the damaged tissue lie in close apposition, minimizing the volume of tissue that must be replaced; and the injury site is stable enough to prevent disruption of the repair tissue while allowing sufficient loading to stimulate repair and remodeling. For tendon injuries, surgeons accomplish this by irrigation and debridement, followed by repair using a technique that provides apposition of viable tissue and adequate mechanical stability, but the surgical procedure should not significantly compromise the blood supply to the injury site or leave excessive suture material in the wound.[113,114] Obtaining the best results of many complete ligament and joint capsule disruptions also requires surgical repair; but for others, healing will restore normal tissue function without operative repair. In general, surgical repair of acute meniscal tears or ruptures in vascularized regions including the meniscal attachments produces the best results.

Loading and Motion. Mechanical loading of dense fibrous tissues alters their normal organization and composition and in, general tends, to strengthen the tissues and increase their degree of matrix organization.[43,50] Investigations show that early loading and motion of the repair tissue promotes repair and matrix remodeling.[6,43,50,113] Use of early motion to promote repair and remodeling, decrease adhesions, and accelerate rehabilitation has become an accepted clinical practice for treatment of repaired tendons[113,114] and for some ligament and joint capsule injuries. However, excessive motion and loading can rupture or deform the repair tissue at a critical stage. For this reason, loading and motion treatment of dense fibrous tissue injuries must be carefully controlled.

It is likely that the optimal motion and loading treatment differs among the types of dense fibrous tissues, among the types of injuries, and among patients. For example, the optimal timing and intensity of loading and motion treatment of a clean laceration of a digital extensor tendon in a child may differ from the optimal loading and motion treatment of a crushing muscle–tendon avulsion of the Achilles tendon in an adult. Defining the appropriate loading and motion treatment for different dense fibrous tissues, different injuries, and different forms of surgical or nonsurgical treatment should improve the predictability and quality of the results of healing of these tissues.

ARTICULAR CARTILAGE

Structure and Composition

Articular cartilage consists of sparsely distributed chondrocytes surrounded by an elaborate, highly organized macromolecular framework filled with water.[41,48] Three classes of molecules (collagens, proteoglycans, and noncollagenous proteins) form the macromolecular framework. Type II collagen fibrils give the cartilage its form and tensile strength, and a variety of quantitatively minor collagens help organize and maintain the meshwork of type II collagen fibrils. The interaction of proteoglycans with water gives the tissue its stiffness to compression and its resiliency and contributes to its durability.[204] The noncollagenous proteins are less well understood than the proteoglycans and collagens, but they appear to help organize and stabilize the matrix, attach chondrocytes to the matrix macromolecules, and possibly help stabilize the chondrocyte phenotype. Unlike the other primary musculoskeletal tissues, cartilage lacks a blood supply, a nerve supply, and a lymphatic supply.

Cartilage Healing

Because cartilage lacks blood vessels, it cannot respond to cell damage with inflammation. However, injuries that disrupt subchondral bone as well as cartilage initiate the fracture healing process, and the repair tissue from bone will fill an articular cartilage defect. Cartilage healing[37,44,46–48,185–188] then follows the sequence of inflammation, repair, and remodeling like that seen in bone or dense fibrous tissue. Unlike these tissues, the repair tissue that fills cartilage defects from subchondral bone initially differentiates toward articular cartilage rather than toward dense fibrous tissue or bone.[48]

In addition to direct mechanical injury, articular cartilage can sustain damage by disruption of the synovial membrane and exposure of articular cartilage. Because of these special features, acute traumatic injuries to synovial joints can be separated into the following categories: disruption of the soft tissues of the synovial joint without direct mechanical cartilage injury and mechanical injury of articular cartilage (Table 5-3).

TABLE 5-3
Acute Articular Cartilage Injuries

Injury Type	Description	Tissue Response	Potential for Healing
I	Blunt trauma without disruption of the articular surface (damage to cartilage matrix macromolecular structure and chondrocytes, may include subchondral bone damage and cause degradation of matrix macromolecules)[37,48,88,248]	Synthesis of new matrix macromolecules Cell proliferation?	If the basic matrix structure remains intact and a sufficient number of viable cells remain, they can restore the normal tissue composition. If the matrix or cell population sustains significant damage or if the tissue sustains further damage, the cartilage may deteriorate.
II	Chondral fractures or lacerations (tissue disruption limited to articular cartilage)[37,48,115,185–187,198,201,248,287]	No fibrin clot formation or inflammation Synthesis of new matrix macromolecules and cell proliferation, but new tissue does not fill the cartilage defect.	Depending on the location and size of the lesion and the structural integrity, stability, and alignment of the joint, the lesion may remain unchanged or the remaining articular cartilage will deteriorate.
III	Osteochondral fractures (tissue disruption extends from articular cartilage into bone)[37,48,72,85,109,185–187]	Formation of a fibrin clot, inflammation, invasion of new cells, and production of new tissue Repair tissue rarely fills large articular surface defects or restores the contour of the articular surface Cartilage repair tissue usually becomes fibrocartilage, not articular cartilage or bone Bone repair tissue usually becomes normal bone	Depending on the location and size of the lesion and the structural integrity, stability, and alignment of the joint, the repair tissue may remodel and form a fibrocartilagenous articular surface, or it may deteriorate along with surrounding cartilage, leaving exposed bone.

Disruption of the Synovial Joint Soft Tissues

Exposure of cartilage to air by traumatic or surgical disruption of the joint capsule and synovial membrane can alter cartilage matrix composition by stimulating degradation of proteoglycans or suppressing synthesis of proteoglycans.[48,134,202,279] A decrease in matrix proteoglycan concentration decreases cartilage stiffness and may make the tissue more vulnerable to damage from impact loading. Prompt restoration of the synovial environment by closure of the synovial membrane will allow chondrocytes to repair the damage to the macromolecular framework of the matrix, and the tissue may regain its normal composition and function. However, prolonged exposure of the articular surface can desiccate the tissue and kill chondrocytes.

It is not clear what duration of exposure causes irreversible damage. The available evidence, based on animal experiments, suggests that damage to the matrix macromolecular framework occurs with any disruption of the synovial membrane,[134] but clinical experience suggests that permanent or progressive damage in human joints rarely occurs after temporary disruption of the synovial cavity. Furthermore, cartilage can be restored to its normal condition if the loss of matrix proteoglycans does not exceed the amount the cells can replenish, if a sufficient number chondrocytes remain viable, and if the collagenous meshwork of the matrix remains intact.[48,279]

Exposure injury to cartilage can be minimized by decreasing the period of time that the cartilage is unprotected by synovium or other soft tissues. If cartilage must remain unprotected, keeping the surface moist with a physiologic solution may be helpful. Because cartilage that has sustained exposure injury may be temporarily more vulnerable to mechanical injury, it seems advisable to minimize immediate impact loading of cartilage that has suffered this type of injury.[37,48]

Mechanical Injury to Articular Cartilage

Acute traumatic injury to articular cartilage may occur through several mechanisms.[37] Osteochondral fractures mechanically disrupt cartilage and bone tissue at the fracture site, but, in addition, osteochondral fractures may be associated with blunt trauma limited to cartilage, abrasions of the articular surface, or intracartilaginous, that is, chondral fractures.[37,287] Alternatively, blunt trauma to a synovial joint may occur without an associated bone or cartilage fracture.[37] Therefore, acute articular cartilage injuries can be separated into those caused by blunt trauma that does not disrupt or fracture tissue and those caused by blunt trauma or other mechanisms that mechanically disrupt or fracture the tissue. Injuries that fracture or disrupt cartilage can be further divided into those limited to articular cartilage and those affecting both cartilage and subchondral bone (see Table 5-3).

Blunt Trauma Without Tissue Disruption. Although the effects of acute blunt trauma on articular cartilage have not been extensively studied clinically or experimentally,[37,88,248] blunt trauma to joints occurs frequently as an isolated injury or in association with a fracture or dislocation. Among the reasons for the limited number of studies are the lack of clearly defined, clinically significant consequences of blunt trauma to cartilage, the ability of cartilage to withstand large acute loads without apparent immediate damage, the lack of a clinically detectable injury and repair response in cartilage after blunt trauma, and difficulty in defining the relationship between the intensity of blunt trauma and the extent of cartilage injury.[37] Despite these limitations, current information suggests that acute blunt trauma to articular cartilage may damage the tissue even when there is no grossly apparent tissue disruption and that these injuries may lead to later degeneration of the articular surface.

Physiologic levels of impact loading have not been demonstrated to produce cartilage injury, and clinical experience suggests that acute impact loading considerably greater than physiologic loading but less than that necessary to produce detectable fractures rarely causes significant articular cartilage injury. However, acute impact loading less than that necessary to produce visible tissue disruption may cause cartilage swelling and increased cartilage collagen fibril diameter and alter the relationships between collagen fibrils and proteoglycans.[88] This observation suggests that blunt trauma, under at least some conditions, may disrupt the macromolecular framework of the cartilage matrix and possibly injure cells without producing detectable fracture of the cartilage or bone. Presumably, this tissue damage would make cartilage more vulnerable to subsequent injury and progressive deterioration if the cells could not rapidly restore the matrix. This type of injury may help explain the development of articular cartilage degeneration after joint dislocations or other types of acute joint trauma that do not cause visible damage to the articular surface.

Trauma That Disrupts Cartilage. *Injuries Limited to Articular Cartilage.* Lacerations, traumatically induced splits of articular cartilage perpendicular to the surface, or chondral fractures kill chondrocytes at the site of the injury and disrupt the matrix. Viable chondrocytes near the injury may proliferate, form clusters of new cells, and synthesize new matrix.[37,48,185–187,198] They do not migrate to the site of the injury, and the matrix they synthesize does not fill the defect. A hematoma does not form, and inflammatory cells and fibroblasts do not migrate to the site of injury. This minimal response may be due to the inability of chondrocytes to respond effectively to injury, the inability of undifferentiated mesenchymal cells to invade the tissue defect, and the lack of a clot that attracts cells and gives them a temporary matrix to adhere to and replace with more permanent tissue. Although the response of chondrocytes to injury will not heal a clinically significant cartilage defect, most traumatic defects limited to small areas of articular cartilage do not progress.

Lacerations, fractures, or abrasions of the articular surface tangential or parallel to the surface presumably follow a similar course.[37,48,115,201] Cells directly adjacent to the injury site may die and others may show signs of increased proliferative or synthetic activity. A thin acellular layer of nonfibrillar material may form over an injured surface, but there is no evidence that the cell activity stimulated by the injury restores the articular cartilage to its original state.

Osteochondral Injury. An articular cartilage injury that also damages subchondral bone stimulates fracture healing, including inflammation, repair, and remodeling.[37,48,72,85,109,185–187] Blood from ruptured bone blood vessels fills the injury site with a hematoma that extends from the bony injury into the chondral defects. The clot may fill a small chondral defect, generally those less than several millimeters wide, but it usually does not completely fill larger defects. Inflammatory cells migrate through the clot, followed by fibroblasts that begin to synthesize a collagenous matrix. In the bone defect and the chondral defect, some of the mesenchymal cells assume a rounded shape and begin to synthesize a matrix that closely resembles the matrix of articular cartilage.[48]

Within weeks of injury the repair tissue forming in the chondral portion of the defect and the tissue forming in the bony portion of the defect begin to differ.[48] Tissue in the chondral defect has a higher proportion of repair cells and matrix that resembles hyaline cartilage, while the repair tissue in the bone defect has started to form new bone. Within 6 weeks of injury, repair tissue in the two locations is distinguished by the new bone formed in the bone defect, the absence of bone in the chondral defect, and the higher proportion of hyaline cartilage repair tissue in the chondral defect.[48]

Although the initial repair of an osteochondral injury usually follows a predictable course, subsequent changes in the cartilage repair tissue vary considerably among similar defects. In some chondral defects the production of a cartilaginous matrix continues and the cells may retain the appearance and some of the functions of chondrocytes, including production of type II collagen and proteoglycans. They rarely restore the matrix to the original state, but they may succeed in producing a form of fibrocartilaginous scar that maintains the integrity of the articular surface and provides clinically satisfactory joint function for years. Unfortunately, in many other injuries the cartilage repair tissue deteriorates rather than remodeling.[48] It becomes progressively more fibrillar, and the cells lose the appearance of chondrocytes and appear to become more fibroblastic. The fibrous matrix may begin to fibrillate and fragment, eventually leaving exposed bone. The reasons why healing of some osteochondral injuries results in formation of fibrocartilage that may provide at least temporary joint function, while others fail to repair, have not been well defined.

Variables that Influence Cartilage Healing

Injury Variables. The intensity of blunt trauma and the involvement of subchondral bone have a significant influence on the result of cartilage healing. In addition, the volume and surface area of cartilage injury and the degree of disruption of joint congruity and stability can influence healing.[37,48,72] For example, small defects, those that are unlikely to alter joint function, tend to heal more successfully than larger, clinically significant defects.

Patient Variables. As in other tissues, patient age may influence the healing potential of cartilage injuries.[49] That is, infants or young children have greater potential to heal and remodel chondral and osteochondral injuries than older individuals, although this has not been thoroughly investigated. Other patient variables such as weight, activity level, and systemic disease may be clinically important, but their influence has not been demonstrated.

Treatment Variables. *Apposition.* Because experimental work indicates that smaller defects in articular cartilage tend to heal more successfully,[48,72] it seems reasonable to expect that treatments that decrease the volume and surface area of a chondral defect, such as open reduction and internal fixation of osteochondral fractures, will increase the probability of successful cartilage repair. Experimental work indicates that 1-mm or smaller defects tend to heal more successfully than larger defects,[48,72] and eliminating the gap between fragments of an osteochondral fracture results in better anatomical restoration of an articular surface. Therefore, decreasing the width of an osteochondral fracture gap should increase the probability of a clinically acceptable result. However, depending on the location of the chondral injury within the joint and the presence or absence of other injuries to the joint, some separations of osteochondral fractures or loss of segments of the articular surface may not produce clinically significant disturbances of synovial joint function or rapid cartilage deterioration.

The clinical results of transarticular fractures show that articular surfaces can sustain limited traumatic loss of cartilage without immediate disturbance of joint function and possibly without long-term consequences. An experimental study of osteochondral defects supports these observations. Nelson and associates[210] made 6-mm diameter osteochondral defects in the weight-bearing regions of dog femoral condyles, destroying a significant portion of the width of the condylar surface. They found that the defects did not increase the cartilage stresses around the defects, and 11 months after injury there was no evidence of cartilage deterioration. Furthermore, the repair cartilage did not contribute to load bearing, suggesting that for some osteochondral injuries the success or failure of cartilage repair may not significantly influence joint function. They concluded that articular cartilage can tolerate moderate incongruities without significant increases in cartilage pressure or obvious degeneration. However, the extent of tolerable loss of articular surface has not been defined and may vary among joints.

Loading and Motion. Prolonged immobilization of a joint following osteochondral fractures can lead to significant adhesions as well as deterioration of uninjured cartilage, resulting in poor synovial joint function.[50,155,228,288] Early motion during the repair and remodeling phases of healing can decrease or prevent adhesions and immobilization-induced deterioration of uninjured cartilage. However, loading and motion must be used carefully after injury, because these measures alone will not predictably restore normal articular cartilage structure and composition in clinically significant defects, and excessive loading and motion may damage chondral repair tissue and displace fracture fragments.

Restoration of Joint Congruity. Significant traumatically induced joint incongruity causes mechanical joint dysfunction, including instability, locking, catching, and restricted range of motion, and may be associated with progressive deterioration of articular cartilage. It is not clear how much of the long-term cartilage deterioration after injuries that cause joint incongruity is secondary to the traumatic cartilage damage at the time of injury and how much is related to the long-term effects of incongruity. However, in most injuries, restoration of acceptable joint congruity avoids immediate problems with mechanical joint dysfunction and may delay or decrease the severity and rate of cartilage deterioration.

Unfortunately, the degree of joint incongruity that can be tolerated without causing long-term joint deterioration has not been well defined. A study by Brown and associates[36] of contact stress aberrations after imprecise reduction of experimental human cadaver tibial plateau fractures showed that generally peak local cartilage pressure increased with increasing joint incongruity (fracture fragment step-off), but the results varied among joints. In most specimens, cartilage pressure did not increase significantly until the fragment step-off exceeded 1.5 mm. When the step-off was increased to 3 mm, the peak cartilage pressure averaged 75% greater than normal. Brown and associates estimated that the long-term pressure "tolerance level" of cartilage may be much higher, probably about twice the normal level, indicating that simple incongruities of several millimeters should not cause immediate or long-term problems. However, they also found that in some specimens even minor incongruities, as little as 0.25 mm, caused apparently deleterious peak local pressure elevations, suggesting that results may vary even among individuals with the same degree of articular incongruity. The long-term results of traumatically induced articular incongruity may also depend on the age of the patient. Skeletally immature individuals may have a greater capacity to remodel incongruities, and age-related alterations in articular cartilage may decrease its capacity to repair injuries or withstand alterations in loading caused by joint incongruity.

Stabilization. Mechanical stabilization of an osteochondral injury in an acceptable position increases the likelihood of satisfactory healing by preventing disruption of the repair tissue and restoring articular cartilage congruity. An equally important benefit of stabilizing osteochondral fractures is that it allows early controlled loading and motion.

Experimental Treatments. Because of the limited capacity for articular cartilage healing and the severe disability that can result from joint degeneration due to loss of a significant segment of an articular surface, surgeons and investigators have been seeking methods of restoring articular surfaces.[42,44] It may be possible to significantly improve the results of treating chondral and osteochondral injuries. Digestion of small proteoglycans that interfere with clot formation and cell adhesion to the cartilage matrix followed by application of TGF-β in a fibrin matrix has led to restoration of cartilaginous tissue in animals.[140] The results of this study show that cartilage can heal without inflammation or vascular invasion; however, this method has not yet been applied to human cartilage injuries. Osteochondral allografts can effectively replace limited regions of lost or damaged articular cartilage, and other work has shown that use of artificial matrices, chondrocyte, and mesenchymal stem cell transplants can stimulate formation of a cartilaginous surface.[42]

SKELETAL MUSCLE

Structure and Composition

Unlike bone, dense fibrous tissue, and cartilage, muscle consists primarily of cells contained within a small volume of elaborate, highly organized matrix consisting of collagens, elastin, and muscle-specific molecules.[38,60,61,102,153] An elaborate system of blood vessels supports the high level of metabolic activity of muscle cells, and a complex network of nerves extends through the matrix to innervate every muscle cell. Normal function of skeletal muscle depends not only on the integrity of the cells, matrix, and blood vessels but also on the innervation of the tissue.

The muscle cells (myofibers or muscle fibers) cluster into bundles called *fascicles.* Aggregates of fascicles form muscles. Each myofiber contains multiple nuclei, a unique form of endoplasmic reticulum termed the *sarcoplasmic reticulum,* and contractile proteins organized into cylindrical organelles termed *myofibrils.* Each myofibril consists of multiple sarcomeres, the contractile units of the organelle. Membranes of the sarcoplasmic reticulum encircle the myofibrils. The interfibrillar sarcoplasm contains the organelles found in other cells, including mitochondria, lysosomes, and ribosomes.

Although the extracellular matrix makes up only a small fraction of the volume of muscle, it is critical for normal muscle function, maintenance of muscle structure, and healing. A basement membrane containing collagens, noncollagenous proteins, and muscle-specific proteoglycans surrounds each myofiber. The basement membranes, together with surrounding irregularly arranged fine collagen fibrils, form the *endomysium.* A thicker matrix sheath composed primarily of collagen fibrils and elastic fibers, the *paramysium,* covers muscle fasciculi. The *epimysium,* a more dense peripheral sheath of connective tissue, covers the entire muscle and is frequently continuous with the fascia overlying muscle. At the ends of the muscles, their extracellular matrix forms part of the muscle–tendon junctions.[112,219,289]

The blood vessels and nerves supplying the myofibers lie within the extracellular matrix between muscle fasciculi. The vessels form rich capillary networks around individual myofibers, and the nerves penetrate the matrix surrounding the myofibers to form neuromuscular junctions with the cell membranes of the myofibers. The basement membrane serves as a specialized interface for attachment of the nerves. It also binds myofiber membranes to the collagen fibrils of tendon and thereby transmits the contractile force generated by the myofibrils to the tendon.[112]

Muscle Healing

The same mechanisms of acute trauma that damage the other musculoskeletal soft tissues (ie, blunt trauma, lacerations, and tearing injuries) also injure muscle.[60,61,111,126] Muscle tendon junction tears occur frequently and clinically are often identified as muscle injuries, partially because in many muscles the muscle–tendon junction extends a great distance into the substance of the muscle and because these injuries do include damage to muscle substance. Muscle tendon junction tears were previously discussed with tendon injuries; therefore, this section will focus on injuries limited to muscle substance.

Because of its high level of metabolic activity, even temporary compromise of muscle vascular supply can cause permanent damage. Furthermore, unlike the other tissues, restoration of muscle function requires not only restoration of the original state of the tissue and its blood supply but also restoration of its nerve supply and neuromuscular junctions. For these reasons, the classification of muscle tissue injuries differs from the classification of injuries to bone, dense fibrous tissue, and cartilage. Although the healing of human skeletal muscle that occurs after acute trauma has not been extensively studied, the available evidence shows that muscle healing, like healing of the other vascularized tissues, proceeds through inflammation, repair, and remodeling (see Fig. 5-1).

Inflammation

Damage to myofibers initiates inflammation, which includes migration of inflammatory cells into the injured muscle and, in most injuries, hemorrhage and formation of a hematoma.[141] In addition to hematoma formation, and the other events seen after injury to vascularized tissues, an important part of the inflammatory process in skeletal muscle is the removal of damaged muscle fibers by phagocytic inflammatory cells that penetrate and fragment necrotic myofibers. After they enter damaged muscle fibers these cells phagocytize bundles of contractile filaments and other cytoplasmic debris. This macrophage activity not only removes damaged cell organelles but also may have an important role in stimulating regeneration of myofibers.[60]

Repair

As macrophages remove damaged or necrotic myofibers, spindle-shaped myogenic cells appear and begin to proliferate and fuse with one another to form long syncytial myotubes with chains of central nuclei.[60,141,307] Frequently, several of these early regenerating myotubes form within the basement membrane tube of a single necrotic muscle fiber. As they enlarge, the myotubes construct their sarcoplasmic reticulum and begin to assemble organized bundles of contractile filaments. The central chains of nuclei break up and migrate to the periphery of the myotube, completing the transition of the myotube into a muscle fiber. Contractile proteins continue to accumulate and form myofibrils. To become functional, a regenerating muscle fiber must be innervated, including formation of a neuromuscular junction.

At the same time myotubes are regenerating, fibroblasts are producing granulation tissue that is necessary to repair the matrix of the muscle. However, this granulation tissue can interfere with the orderly regeneration of the myofibers, producing a disorganized mass of scar and partially regenerated myofibers. This type of tissue may restore the continuity of the muscle but not its contractile function. Therefore, the optimal results of muscle healing require a balance between myofiber regeneration and synthesis of new matrix and appropriate organization and orientation of these two components of the healing muscle.

Remodeling

Once muscle fibers have appeared, the extracellular matrix continues to remodel. If excessive scar formation can be avoided and the muscle cells are innervated, controlled muscle contraction and loading increases the strength of the injured muscle.

Variables That Influence Muscle Healing

Injury Variables. Muscle injuries can be classified by the type or severity of injury and by the clinical mechanism of injury.[60]

Type of Muscle Tissue Injury. Clinically significant acute muscle injuries can be grouped into three types that differ in their potential for healing based on the components of the muscle left intact (Table 5-4).

A *type I muscle injury* damages muscle fibers but leaves the extracellular matrix, blood vessels, and nerve supply intact. Blunt trauma, including surgical trauma, mild stretching injuries, and temporary ischemia can cause a type I injury. The muscle fibers will be damaged, but the basal lamina and other components of the extracellular matrix, the blood supply, and the nerve supply remain intact. These injuries occur frequently and can heal through spontaneous muscle fiber regeneration that restores the original structure, composition, and function of the muscle.

A *type II muscle injury* damages the nerve supply and may include damage to the myofibers but leaves the extracellular matrix and blood supply intact. Type II injuries may result from isolated peripheral nerve damage, blunt trauma, or stretching of nerve and muscle. Because the matrix maintains the muscle structure, if regenerating nerve fibers reach intact neuromuscular junctions, the potential for restoration of function exists.

A *type III muscle injury* causes loss or necrosis of all muscle tissue components, including myofibers and extracellular matrix or prolonged loss of blood and nerve supply. Type III injuries result from severe blunt trauma, tearing, or penetrating trauma. If the vascular supply remains intact, the inflammatory response can remove the necrotic tissue, but some type III injuries compromise the blood supply, and the necrotic muscle is not removed and must be surgically debrided. If

TABLE 5-4
Acute Skeletal Muscle Injuries

Injury Type	Description	Tissue Response	Potential for Healing
I	Damage to muscle fibers without significant disruption of their extracellular matrix, blood vessels, and nerves. (These injuries result from blunt trauma, including surgical trauma, mild stretching injuries, and temporary ischemia.)	Organized muscle fiber regeneration Formation of fibrous tissue following an inflammatory response	A significant inflammatory response may lead to some scar formation, but most of these injuries result in normal structure and function.
II	Damage to nerves that leaves the muscle extracellular matrix and blood supply intact but may include damage to the myofibers. (These injuries may result from isolated peripheral nerve damage, blunt trauma, or stretching of nerve and muscle.)	Organized nerve fiber and muscle fiber regeneration Formation of fibrous tissue following an inflammatory response	If regenerating nerve fibers reach intact neuromuscular junctions, the potential for restoration of function exists.
III	Loss or necrosis of all muscle tissue components, including myofibers and extracellular matrix. (These injuries result from prolonged ischemia and loss of innervation and from severe blunt trauma, tearing, or penetrating trauma.)	Disorganized muscle fiber regeneration Formation of fibrous tissue	Scar formation with scattered myoblasts result in loss of function in the injured region. The scar may allow function of adjacent intact or less severely injured muscle.

Data from references 60 and 61.

the necrotic tissue is removed, repair can begin. Cells capable of differentiating into myoblasts survive even severe injuries or migrate into the injury site. However, the lack of an extracellular matrix to guide regeneration of myofibers usually prevents formation of organized muscle tissue. Even if such tissue forms, lack of guidance for reinnervation prevents regenerated myofibers from regaining function. For these reasons, the usual result of a type III muscle injury is healing by scar formation, with scattered myoblasts attempting to form myofibers.

Clinical Mechanisms of Muscle Injury. Mechanisms of acute mechanical muscle injury caused by application of an external load include blunt trauma, penetrating trauma, and tearing or stretching trauma. Muscles can also be injured by muscle contraction against resistance.[60,61,104] Because this latter mechanism of muscle injury is not a form of direct mechanical trauma, it is not included in this chapter.

Blunt trauma to skeletal muscle occurs frequently as an isolated injury or in association with fractures. The results vary from type I to type III muscle injuries. Mild blunt trauma to skeletal muscle damages myofibers without disruption of extracellular matrix, nerves, or vessels—a type I muscle tissue injury. A slightly more severe injury ruptures blood vessels as well as myofibers, causing hemorrhage and inflammation. Healing of these injuries generally results in restoration of normal function. At the other extreme, blunt trauma can crush all components of skeletal muscle, resulting in a type III muscle tissue injury that heals with scar tissue or that may not heal. If the area of the crushing injury is relatively small, muscle function may not be noticeably altered. However, after an extensive crushing injury, the cells replace large areas of the muscle with noncontractile regenerating myofibers and scar, permanently decreasing muscle strength.

Blunt trauma to muscle may also stimulate bone formation (ie, myositis ossificans).[100,144,258,308,329] A prospective study showed that 20% of patients with a quadriceps hematoma developed myositis ossificans,[258] suggesting that this type of muscle response to blunt trauma may occur frequently. The new bone can be contiguous with periosteum or lie entirely within muscle, free of any connection with underlying bone.[329] Although the clinical sequence of ossification within muscle following blunt trauma has been well described, the mechanism of this repair response has not been explained.

Most penetrating injuries of muscle result from lacerations or combinations of blunt trauma and lacerations. Because lacerations necessarily damage myofibrils, extracellular matrix, nerves, and blood vessels, they are type III tissue injuries. Given the highly organized structure of muscle with the parallel arrays of myofibrils, it would be expected that lacerations that parallel the long axes of the myofibrils would generally cause less damage than lacerations perpendicular to these axes. Muscles vary in the arrangement of their myofibrils from a simple longitudinal orientation in strap or fusiform muscles to the complex arrangement found in radial and multipennate muscles; thus, the result of a laceration transverse to the long axis of the muscle will vary among muscles depending on the arrangement of their myofibrils. Experimental studies of complete and partial transverse muscle lacerations show that after complete laceration and suture repair, the separated muscle fragments heal primarily by scar, with a small number of regenerated myotubes within the scar.[111] True regeneration of functional muscle tissue and nerves across complete lacerations has not been demonstrated, and muscle fragments separated from their nerve supply show the changes of denervation. Transected myofibers may form buds, but these buds fail to restore normal tissue across the laceration.

Tearing or stretching injuries range from mild muscle tissue damage, a type I injury, to avulsion of a segment of the muscle, a type III injury. These injuries may be deceptive in that the overlying soft tissue may remain intact over a severe internal disruption of the muscle.

Patient Variables. Patient variables including nutrition, use of corticosteroids, and systemic diseases (eg, diabetes) may influence muscle healing, but they have not been well studied. Although muscle mass and strength decline with age, it is clear that older persons can heal muscle injuries and that they benefit from treatments that increase muscle strength after injury.[49]

Treatment Variables. Preventing or relieving ischemia gives muscle tissue an opportunity for healing and should be the first consideration. Restoring innervation as soon as possible and removing necrotic tissue are also important. Other treatments that may promote muscle healing include removal of muscle hematoma,[126] temporary immobilization, and controlled loading and motion. For example, experimental studies show that immediate mobilization of injured muscles may increase scar formation and interfere with orderly regeneration of myofibers.[149] However, mobilization after a short period of immobilization produces more rapid disappearance of the hematoma and inflammatory cells; more extensive, rapid, and organized myofiber regeneration; and more rapid increase in tensile strength and stiffness.[147–149,173] In contrast, prolonged immobilization produces muscle atrophy and poor organization of the regenerating myofibers.[149,173] These results show that after a brief period of rest, controlled mobilization of an injured muscle will produce the optimal healing, and they suggest that selective suppression of inflammation after muscle injury may be beneficial. Possible future treatments for type III muscle tissue injuries include creation of artificial matrices that prevent the defect from filling with scar, allow myoblasts to form myofibers, provide a temporary framework for transmitting mechanical force, and stimulate directed growth of vessels and nerves.[60]

SUMMARY

Surgeons achieve the best results in treating acute musculoskeletal injuries when they create the optimal biological and mechanical conditions for healing. This requires understanding of tissue composition, structure, and function; the healing process; and the variables that affect healing, including tissue, injury, patient, and treatment variables.

Each of the primary musculoskeletal tissues (bone, dense fibrous tissue, cartilage, and skeletal muscle) respond to acute traumatic injury with a sequence of cellular actions that attempt to heal the injury, that is, to restore the structural integrity of the tissue. Damage to the cells of vascularized tissues initiates a response that begins with inflammation (the cellular and vascular response to injury), proceeds through repair (the replacement of damaged or lost cells and matrices with new cells and matrices), and ends with remodeling (removal, replacement, and reorganization of the repair tissue, usually along the lines of mechanical stress). Injury to nonvascularized tissues, articular cartilage, and the inner regions of the menisci does not trigger an inflammatory response, but the cells respond to injury with an effort at cell proliferation and synthesis of new matrix.

The results of musculoskeletal tissue injury can be grouped into four overlapping categories: excessive repair, failure of repair, scar, and restoration of the original state of the tissue (see Table 5-1). Excessive repair occurs when the healing response produces exuberant scar that compromises musculoskeletal function, as in the fibrous ankylosis of synovial joints that occurs after intra-articular fractures or the scarring of tendon repair tissue to the tendon sheath. Occasionally, the response to injury may fail to restore the integrity of the tissue, leaving only thin, filmy connective tissue, a poorly vascularized myxoid matrix, an organized hematoma, or other forms of structurally and functionally inadequate tissue. Examples of failure of healing include nonunions of bone or lack of functional repair after a complete ligamentous disruption. More often, musculoskeletal tissues heal by formation of scar consisting of a dense collagenous matrix containing primarily type I collagen and fibroblasts along with some elements of the original tissue. For example, scar in skeletal muscle usually contains at least some myofibrils and the tissue that fills in the chondral portions of many osteochondral defects consists of fibrocartilage with features of both dense fibrous tissue and hyaline cartilage. Scar tissue may restore clinically acceptable function of injured tissue, especially in some tendon and ligament injuries and partial lacerations of skeletal muscle. The ideal result of the healing process—restoration of the original structure, function, and composition of the tissue—occurs frequently after bone fractures and may occur after certain dense fibrous tissue injuries and even some skeletal muscle injuries.

The principles of treating acute musculoskeletal tissue injuries include preventing further tissue damage, avoiding treatments that compromise the natural healing process, and creating the optimal mechanical and biological conditions for healing. This may include removing necrotic tissue, preventing infection, rapidly restoring blood and nerve supply when necessary, and in some circumstances, providing apposition, alignment, and stabilization of injured tissue. One of the most important recent advances in the treatment of injuries of the musculoskeletal tissues has been the recognition that early controlled loading and motion of the repair and remodeling tissues improves healing of many injuries. However, as with all treatments, this intervention must be used with care, since uncontrolled or excessive loading can adversely affect or even prevent healing. At the tissue level, the effect of the mechanical environment on repair and the function of the repair tissue cells is not well understood, and at the clinical level, the optimal protocols of loading and motion of musculoskeletal tissue injuries have not been well defined. Other potentially important currently available treatments include electrical fields and ultrasound.

Although future improvements in treatment of musculoskeletal tissue injuries, including controlled motion and loading of repair and remodeling tissue, use of ultrasound and electrical fields, and surgical restoration of apposition and mechanical stability of injured tissue, undoubtedly will advance the practice of orthopaedics, it is not likely that they will restore the original state of the tissue in many of the most severe musculoskeletal tissue injuries. In particular, large segmental losses or necrosis of bone and soft tissue and most clinically significant cartilage and muscle injuries present especially difficult treatment problems. Future developments that may help promote healing of these injuries include creation and implantation of synthetic matrices and use of growth factors and implanted mesenchymal cells to guide and promote regeneration of musculoskeletal tissue.

REFERENCES

1. Abbott, L.C., Schottstaedt, E.R., Saunders, J.B., and Bost, F.C.: The Evaluation of Cortical and Cancellous Bone as Grafting Material: A Clinical and Experimental Study. J. Bone Joint Surg., 29:381–414, 1947.
2. Adinoff, A.D., and Hollister, J.R.: Steroid Induced Fractures and Bone Loss in Patients With Asthma. N. Engl. J. Med., 309:265–268, 1983.
3. Akeson, W.H., Woo, S.L.-Y., Coutts, R.D., Matthews, J.V., Gonsalves, M., and Amiel, D.: Quantitative Histological Evaluation of Early Fracture Healing of Cortical Bones Immobilized by Stainless Steel and Composite Plates. Calcif. Tissue Res., 19:27–37, 1975.
4. Allbrook, D., Baker, W., and Kirkaldy-Willis, W.H.: Muscle Regeneration in Experimental Animals and in Man: The Cycle of Tissue Change That Follows Trauma in the Injured Limb Syndrome. J. Bone Joint Surg., 48B:153–169, 1966.
5. Allgöwer, M., and Spiegel, P.G.: Internal Fixation of Fractures: Evolution of Concepts. Clin. Orthop., 138:26–29, 1979.
6. Andriacchi, T., Sabiston, P., DeHaven, K., et al.: Ligament Injury and Repair. *In* Woo, S.L.-Y., and Buckwalter J.A. (eds.): Injury and Repair of the Musculoskeletal Soft Tissues, pp. 103–127. Park Ridge, Ill., American Academy of Orthopaedic Surgeons, 1988.
7. Andriole, V.T., Nagel, D.A., and Southwick, W.O.: A Paradigm for Human Chronic Osteomyelitis. J. Bone Joint Surg., 55A:1511–1515, 1973.
8. Arnoczky, S.M., Adams, M., DeHaven, K., Eyre, E., and Mow, V.: Meniscus. *In* Woo, S.L.-Y., and Buckwalter, J.A. (eds.): Injury and Repair of the Musculoskeletal Soft Tissues. Park Ridge, Ill., American Academy of Orthopaedic Surgeons, 1988.
9. Aro, H.T., Wippermann, B.W., Hodgson, S.F., Wahner, H.W., Le Wallen, D.G., and Chao, E.Y.S.: Prediction of Properties of Fracture Callus by Measurement of Mineral Density Using Micro-Bone Densitometry. J. Bone Joint Surg., 71A:1020–1030, 1989.
10. Aronson, J., Johnson, E., and Harp, J.H.: Local Bone Transportation for Treatment of Intercalary Defects by the Ilizarov Technique: Biomechanical and Clinical Considerations. Clin. Orthop., 243:71–79, 1989.
11. Ashton, I.K., and Dekel, S.: Fracture Repair in the Snell Dwarf Mouse. Br. J. Exp. Pathol., 64:479–486, 1983.
12. Bak, B., Jorgensen, P.H., and Andreassen, T.T.: The Stimulating Effect of Growth Hormone on Fracture Healing is Dependent on Onset and Duration of Administration. Clin. Orthop., 264:295–301, 1991
13. Bassett, C.A.L.: Current Concepts of Bone Formation. J. Bone Joint Surg., 44A:1217–1244, 1962.
14. Bassett, C.A.L.: Biophysical Principles Affecting Bone Structure. *In* Bourne, G.H. (ed.): The Biochemistry and Physiology of Bone, 2nd ed., vol. 3, pp. 1–76. New York, Academic Press, 1971.
15. Bassett, C.A.L., and Becker, R.O.: Generation of Electric Potentials by Bone in Response to Mechanical Stress. Science, 137:1063–1064, 1962.
16. Becker, R.O.: Electrical Osteogenesis—Pro and Con. Calcif. Tissue Res., 26:93–97, 1978.
17. Becker, R.O., and Murray, D.G.: The Electrical Control System Regulating Fracture Healing in Amphibians. Clin. Orthop., 73:169–198, 1970.
18. Birdsell, D.C., Tustanoff, E.R., and Lindsay, W.K.: Collagen Production in Regenerating Tendon. Plast. Reconstr. Surg., 37:504–511, 1966.
19. Blenman, P.R., Carter, D.R., and Beaupré, G.S.: Role of Mechanical Loading in the Progressive Ossification of a Fracture Callus. J. Orthop. Res., 7:398–407, 1989.
20. Bolander, M.E., and Balian, G.: The Use of Demineralized Bone Matrix in the Repair of Segmental Defects. J. Bone Joint Surg., 68A:1264–1274, 1986.
21. Bolander, M.E., Joyce, M.E., Terek, R.M., and Jinguish, S.: Role of Transforming Growth Factor Beta in Fracture Healing. *In* Peiz, K.A., and Sporn, M.B. (eds.): Transforming Growth Factor Betas: Chemistry, Biology and Therapeutics. New York, New York Academy of Sciences, in press.
22. Bonfiglio, M., Jeter, W.S., and Smith, C.L.: The Immune Concept: Its Relation to Bone Transplantation. Ann. N.Y. Acad. Sci., 59:417–433, 1955.
23. Boni, M., Lenzi, L., Silva, E., and Bolognani, L.: Action of Testicular Hyaluronidase Administered In Vivo on the Miner-

alization of Fracture Callus in Rats. Calcif. Tissue Res., 2(Suppl.):30–30A, 1968.
24. Boyd, H.B., and Salvatore, J.E.: Acute Fracture of the Femoral Neck: Internal Fixation or Prosthesis? J. Bone Joint Surg., 46A:1066–1068, 1964.
25. Braithwaite, F., and Brockis, J.G.: The Vascularisation of a Tendon Graft. Br. J. Plast. Surg., 4:130–135, 1951.
26. Braun, R.M., and Schorr, R.: Surgical Nutrition in Patients With Multiple Injuries: Report of a Case. J. Bone Joint Surg., 65A:123–127, 1983.
27. Brighton, C.T.: The Semi-invasive Method of Treating Nonunion With Direct Current. Orthop. Clin. North Am., 15:33–45, 1984.
28. Brighton, C.T., Hozach, W.J., Brager, M.D., Windsor, R.E., et al.: Fracture Healing in the Rabbit Fibula—When Subjected to Various Capacitively Coupled Electrical Fields. J. Orthop. Res., 3:331–340, 1985.
29. Brighton, C.T., and Hunt, R.M.: Histochemical Localization of Calcium in Fracture Callus With Potassium Pyroantimonate. J. Bone Joint Surg., 68A:703–715, 1986.
30. Brighton, C.T., and McCluskey, W.P.: Response of Cultured Bone Cells to a Capacitively Coupled Electrical Field: Inhibition of cAMP Response to Parathyroid Hormone. J. Orthop. Res., 6:567–571, 1988.
31. Brighton, C.T., Okereke, E., Pollock, S.R., and Clark, C.C.: In Vitro Bone-Cell Response to a Capacitively Coupled Electrical Field: The Role of Field Strength, Pulse Pattern and Duty Cycle. Clin. Orthop., 285:255–262, 1992.
32. Brighton, C.T., and Pollack, S.R.: Treatment of Recalcitrant Non-union With a Capacitively Coupled Electrical Field: A Preliminary Report. J. Bone Joint Surg., 67A:577–585, 1985.
33. Brighton, C.T., Strafford, C., Gross, S.B., Leatherwood, D.R., Williams, J.G., and Pollock, S.R.: The Proliferative and Synthetic Response of Isolated Calvarial Bone Cells of Rats to Cyclic Biaxial Mechanical Strain. J. Bone Joint Surg., 73A:320–331, 1991.
34. Brockis, J.G.: The Blood Supply of the Flexor and Extensor Tendons of the Fingers in Man. J. Bone Joint Surg., 35B:131–138, 1953.
35. Brown, G.L., Curtsinger, L.J., White, M., et al.: Acceleration of Tensile Strength of Incisions Treated With EGF and TGF-beta. Ann. Surg., 208:788–794, 1988.
36. Brown, T.D., Anderson, D.D., Nepola, J.V., Singerman, R.J., Pedersen, D.R., and Brand, R.A.: Contact Stress Aberrations Following Imprecise Reduction of Simple Tibial Plateau Fractures. J. Orthop. Res., 6:851–862, 1988.
37. Buckwalter, J.A.: Mechanical Injuries of Articular Cartilage. *In* Finerman, G. (ed.): Biology and Biomechanics of the Traumatized Synovial Joint, pp. 83–96. Park Ridge, Ill., American Academy of Orthopaedic Surgeons, 1992.
38. Buckwalter, J.A.: Musculoskeletal Tissues and the Musculoskeletal System. *In* Weinstein, S.L., and Buckwalter, J.A. (eds.): Turek's Orthopaedics: Principles and Their Application, pp. 13–67. Philadelphia, J.B. Lippincott, 1994.
39. Buckwalter, J.A., and Cooper, R.R.: Bone Structure and Function. Instr. Course Lect. 36:27–48, 1987.
40. Buckwalter, J.A., and Cooper, R.R.: The Cells and Matrices of Skeletal Connective Tissue. *In* Albright, J.A., and Brand, R.A. (eds.): The Scientific Basis of Orthopaedics, pp. 1–25. Norwalk, Conn., Appleton Lange, 1987.
41. Buckwalter, J.A., Hunziker, E., Rosenberg, L., Coutts, R., Adams, M., and Eyre, D.: Articular Cartilage: Composition and Structure. *In* Woo, S.L.-Y., and Buckwalter, J.A. (eds.): Injury and Repair of the Musculoskeletal Soft Tissues, pp. 405–425. Park Ridge, Ill., American Academy of Orthopaedic Surgeons, 1988.
42. Buckwalter, J.A., and Lohmander, S.: Operative Treatment of Osteoarthritis: Current Practice and Future Potential. J. Bone Joint Surg. 76A:1405–1418, 1994.
43. Buckwalter, J.A., Maynard, J.A., and Vailas, A.C.: Skeletal Fibrous Tissues: Tendon, Joint Capsule and Ligament. *In* Albright, J.A., and Brand, R.A. (eds.): The Scientific Basis of Orthopaedics, pp. 387–405. Norwalk, Conn., Appleton Lange, 1987.
44. Buckwalter, J.A., and Mow, V.C.: Cartilage Repair as Treatment of Osteoarthritis. *In* Goldberg, V.M., and Mankin, H.J. (eds.): Osteoarthritis: Diagnosis and Management, 2nd ed. Philadelphia, W.B. Saunders, 1994.
45. Buckwalter, J.A., and Mow, V.C.: Injuries to Meniscus.*In* DeLee, J.C., and Drez, D. (eds.): Orthopaedic Sports Medicine: Principles and Practice, pp. 108–121. Philadelphia, W.B. Saunders, 1994.
46. Buckwalter, J.A., Mow, V.C., and Ratcliff, A.: Restoration of Injured or Degenerated Articular Cartilage. J. Am. Acad. Orthop. Surg. 2:192–201, 1994.
47. Buckwalter, J.A., Rosenberg, L., Coutts, R., Hunziker, E., Reddi, A.H., and Moco, V.: Articular Cartilage Injury and Repair. *In* Woo, S.L.-Y., and Buckwalter, R.A. (eds.): Injury and Repair of the Musculoskeletal Soft Tissues, pp. 465–482. Park Ridge, Ill., American Academy of Orthopaedic Surgeons, 1988.
48. Buckwalter J.A., Rosenberg, L.C., and Hunziker, E.: Articular Cartilage: Composition, Structure, Response to Injury and Methods of Facilitating Repair. *In* Ewing, J.W. (ed.): The Science of Arthroscopy, pp. 19–56. New York, Raven Press, 1990.
49. Buckwalter, J.A., Woo, S.L.-Y., Goldberg, V.M., et al.: Soft Tissue Aging and Musculoskeletal Function. J. Bone Joint Surg., 75A:1533–1548, 1993
50. Buckwalter, J.A., and Woo, S.L.-Y.: Effects of Repetitive Loading and Motion on the Musculoskeletal Tissues. *In* DeLee, J.C., and Drez, D. (eds.): Orthopaedic Sports Medicine: Principles and Practice, pp. 60–72. Philadelphia, W.B. Saunders, 1994.
51. Buckwalter, J.A., and Woo, S.L.-Y.: Ligaments. *In* DeLee, J.C., and Drez, D (eds.): Orthopaedic Sports Medicine: Principles and Practice, pp. 46–59. Philadelphia, W.B. Saunders, 1994.
52. Burchardt, H.: The Biology of Bone Graft Repair. Clin. Orthop., 174:28–42, 1983.
53. Burger, M., Sherman, B.S., and Sobel, A.E.: Observations on the Influence of Chondroitin Sulphate on the Rate of Bone Repair. J. Bone Joint Surg., 44B:675–687, 1962.
54. Burstein, A.H., Zika, J.M., Heiple, K.G., and Klein, L.: Contribution of Collagen and Mineral to the Elastic-Plastic Properties of Bone. J. Bone Joint Surg., 57A:956–961, 1975.
55. Burwell, R.G.: Studies in the Transplantation of Bone: VII. The Fresh Composite Homograft-Autograft of Cancellous Bone. J. Bone Joint Surg., 46B:110–140, 1964.
56. Burwell, R.G.: Studies in the Transplantation of Bone: VIII. Treated Composite Homograft-Autografts of Cancellous Bone: An Analysis of Inductive Mechanisms in Bone Transplantation. J. Bone Joint Surg., 48B:532–566, 1966.
57. Burwell, R.G.: The Function of Bone Marrow in the Incorporation of a Bone Graft. Clin. Orthop., 200:125–141, 1985.
58. Canalis, E.: Effect of Growth Factors on Bone Cell Replication. Clin. Orthop., 193:246–263, 1985.
59. Canalis, E., McCarthy, T., and Centrella, M.: Growth Factors and the Regulation of Bone Remodeling. J. Clin. Invest., 81:277–281, 1988.
60. Caplan, A., Carlson, B., Faulkner, J., Fischman, D., and Garrett, W.: Skeletal Muscle. *In* Woo, S.L.-Y., and Buckwalter, J.A. (eds): Injury and Repair of the Musculoskeletal Soft Tissues, pp. 213–291. Park Ridge, Ill., American Academy of Orthopaedic Surgeons, 1988.
61. Carlson, B.M., and Faulkner, J.A.: The Regeneration of Skeletal Muscle Fibers Following Injury: A Review. Med. Sci. Sports Excer. 15:187–198, 1983.
62. Carpenter, J.E., Hipp, J.A., Gerhart, T.N., Rudman, C.G., Hayes, W.C., and Trippel, S.B.: Failure of Growth Hormone to Alter the Biomechanics of Fracture-Healing in a Rabbit Model. J. Bone Joint Surg., 74A:359–367, 1992.
63. Cattaneo, R., Catagni, M., and Johnson, E.E.: The Treatment of Infected Nonunions and Segmental Defects of the Tibia by the Methods of Ilizarov. Clin. Orthop., 280:143–152, 1992.
64. Chammout, M.O., and Skinner, H.B.: The Clinical Anatomy of Commonly Injured Muscle Bellies. J. Trauma, 26:549–552, 1986.
65. Chao, E. Y-S.: Biomechanics of External Fixation. *In* Lang, J.M. (ed): Fracture Healing, pp. 105–122. New York, Churchill-Livingstone, 1987.
66. Charnley, J., and Baker, S.L.: Compression Arthrodesis of the

Knee. A Clinical and Historical Study. J. Bone Joint Surg., 34B:187–199, 1952.
67. Chase, S.W., and Herndon, C.H.: The Fate of Autogenous and Homogenous Bone Grafts: An Historical Review. J. Bone Joint Surg., 37A:809–841, 1955.
68. Christian, E.P., Bosse, M.J., and Robb, G.: Reconstruction of Large Diaphyseal Defects Without Free Fibular Transfer: In Grade IIIB Tibial Fractures. J. Bone Joint Surg., 71A:994–1004, 1989.
69. Clayton, M.L., and Weir, G.J., Jr.: Experimental Investigations of Ligamentous Healing. Am. J. Surg., 98:373–378, 1959.
70. Colville, J., Callison, J.R., and White, W.L.: Role of the Mesotenon in Tendon Blood Supply. Plast. Reconstr. Surg., 43:53–60, 1969.
71. Connolly, J., Guise, R., Lippiello, L., and Dehne, R.: Development of an Osteogenic Bone Marrow Preparation. J. Bone Joint Surg., 71A:684–691, 1989.
72. Convery, F.R., Akeson, W.H., and Keown, G.H.: The Repair of Large Osteochondral Defects: An Experimental Study in Horses. Clin. Orthop. 82:253–262, 1972.
73. Cook, S.D., Baffes, G.C., Wolfe, M.W., Sampath, T.K., and Rueger, D.C.: Recombinant Human Bone Morphogenetic Protein-7 Induces Healing in a Canine Long-Bone Segmental Defect Model. Clin. Orthop. 301:302–312, 1994.
74. Cook, S.D., Baffes, G.C., Wolfe, M.W., Sampath, T.K., Rueger, D.C., and Whitecloud, T.S.: The Effect of Recombinant Human Osteogenic Protein-1 on Healing of Large Segmental Bone Defects. J. Bone Joint Surg., 76A:827–838, 1994
75. Cooper, R.R., and Misol, S.: Tendon and Ligament Insertion: A Light and Electron Microscope Study. J. Bone Joint Surg., 52A:1–20, 1970.
76. Copp, D.H., and Greenberg, D.M.: Studies on Bone Fracture Healing: I. Effect of Vitamins A and D. J. Nutr., 29:261–267, 1945.
77. Coulson, D.B., Ferguson, A.B., Jr., and Diehl, R.C., Jr.: Effect of Hyperbaric Oxygen on the Healing Femur of the Rat. Surg. Forum, 17:449–450, 1966.
78. Cruess, R.L., and Sakai, T.: Effect of Cortisone Upon Synthesis Rates of Some Components of Rat Bone Matrix. Clin. Orthop., 86:253–259, 1972.
79. Cuthbertson, D.P.: Further Observations of the Disturbance of Metabolism Caused by Injury, With Particular Reference to the Dietary Requirements of Fracture Cases. Br. J. Surg., 23:505–520, 1936.
80. Danis, R.: Theorie et Pratique de L'Osteosyntheses. Paris, Libraries de L'Academie de Medicine, 1949.
81. Danis, R.: Étude de l'Ossification Dans les Greffes de Moelle Osseuse. Acta Chir. Belg., 3(Suppl.):1–120, 1957.
82. Dehne, E., Metz, C.W., Deffer, P.A., and Hall, R.M.: Nonoperative Treatment of the Fractured Tibia by Immediate Weight Bearing. J. Trauma, 1:514–535, 1961.
83. Dekel, S., Lenthall, G., and Francis, M.J.O.: Release of Prostaglandins from Bone and Muscle after Tibial Fracture: An Experimental Study in Rabbits. J. Bone Joint Surg., 63B:185–189, 1981.
84. Dell, P.C., Burchardt, H., and Glowczewskie, F.P. Jr.: A Roentgenographic, Biomechanical, and Histological Evaluation of Vascularized and Non-vascularized Segmental Fibular Canine Autografts. J. Bone Joint Surg., 67A:105–112, 1985
85. DePalma, A.F., McKeever, C.O., and Subin, D.L.: Process of Repair of Articular Cartilage Demonstrated by Histology and Autoradiography With Tritiated Thymidine. Clin. Orthop., 48:229–242, 1966.
86. DePalma, R.L., Krummel, T.M., Durham, L.A., et al.: Characterization and Quantitation of Wound Matrix in the Fetal Rabbit. Matrix, 9:224–231, 1989.
87. Dominguez, J., and Mundy, G.R.: Monocytes Mediate Osteoclastic Bone Resorption by Prostaglandin Production. Calcif. Tissue Res., 31:29–33, 1980.
88. Donohue, J.M., Buss, D., Oegema, T.R., and Thompson, R.C., Jr.: The Effects of Indirect Blunt Trauma on Adult Canine Articular Cartilage. J. Bone Joint Surg., 65A:948–957, 1983.
89. Dostal, G.H., and Gamelli, R.L.: Fetal Wound Healing. Surg. Gynecol Obstet., 176:299–306, 1993.
90. Duthie, R.B., and Barker, A.N.: The Histochemistry of the Preosseous Stage of Bone Repair Studied by Auto Radiography. J. Bone Joint Surg., 37B:691–710, 1955.
91. Einhorn, T.A., Bonnarens, F., and Burstein, A.H.: The Contributions of Dietary Protein and Mineral to the Healing of Experimental Fractures: A Biomechanical Study. J. Bone Joint Surg., 68A:1389–1395, 1986.
92. Einhorn, T.A., Gundberg, C.M., Devlin, V.J., and Warman, J.: Fracture Healing: Osteocalcin Metabolism in Vitamin K Deficiency. Clin. Orthop., 237:219–225, 1988.
93. Einhorn, T.A., Hirschman, A., Kaplan, C., Nashed, R., Devlin, V.J., and Warman, J.: Neutral Protein-Degrading Enzymes in Experimental Fracture Callus: A Preliminary Report. J. Orthop. Res., 7:792–805, 1989.
94. Einhorn, T.A., Lane, J.M., Burstein, A.H., Kopman, C.R., and Vigorita, V.J.: The Healing of Segmental Bone Defects Induced by Demineralized Bone Matrix. J. Bone Joint Surg., 66A:274–279, 1984.
95. Enneking, W.F.: Histological Investigation of Bone Transplants in Immunologically Prepared Animals. J. Bone Joint Surg., 39A:597–615, 1957.
96. Enneking, W.F., Burchardt, H., Puhl, J.J., and Piotrowski, G.: Physical and Biological Aspects of Repair in Dog Cortical-Bone Transplants. J. Bone Joint Surg., 57A:237–252, 1975.
97. Enneking, W.F., and Mindell, E.R.: Observations on Massive Retrieved Allografts. J. Bone Joint Surg., 73A:1123–1142, 1991.
98. Ewald, F., and Tachdjian, M.O.: The Effect of Thyrocalcitonin on Fractured Humeri. Surg. Gynecol. Obstet., 125:1075–1080, 1967.
99. Finerman, G.A.M., Gerth, N., and Urist, M.R.: Effect of Growth Factors on Chondro-osseous Induction. Trans. Orthop. Res. Soc., 14:87, 1989.
100. Finerman, G.A.M., and Shapiro, M.S.: Sports-Induced Soft Tissue Calcification. *In* Leadbetter, W.B., Buckwalter, J. A., and Gordon, S.L. (eds.): Sports-Induced Inflammation, pp. 257–275. Park Ridge, Ill., American Academy of Orthopaedic Surgeons, 1990.
101. Finnegan, M.A., and Uhtoff, H.K.: Healing of Trabecular Bone. *In* Lang, J.M. (ed.): Fracture Healing, pp. 33–38. New York, Churchill Livingstone, 1987.
102. Fishman, D.A.: Myofibrillogenesis and the Morphogenesis of Skeletal Muscle. *In* Engel, A.E., and Banker, B.Q. (eds.): Myology, vol. 1, pp. 5–37. New York, McGraw-Hill, 1986.
103. Frank, C., Woo, S.L.-Y., Andriacchi, T., et al.: Normal Ligament: Structure, Function and Composition. *In* Woo, S.L.-Y., and Buckwalter, J.A. (eds.): Injury and Repair of the Musculoskeletal Soft Tissues, pp. 45–101. Park Ridge, Ill., American Academy of Orthopaedic Surgeons, 1988.
104. Friden, J., Sjostrom, M., and Ekbolm, B.: Myofibrillar Damage Following Intense Eccentric Exercise in Man. Int. J. Sports Med., 4:170–176, 1983.
105. Friedenberg, Z.B., and Brighton, C.T.: Bioelectric Potentials in Bone. J. Bone Joint Surg., 48A:915–923, 1966.
106. Friedenberg, Z.B., and Brighton, C.T.: Biophysical Induction of Fracture Repair. *In* Lang, J.M. (ed.): Fracture Healing, pp. 75–80. New York, Churchill Livingstone, 1987.
107. Friedenberg, Z.B., Harlow, M.C., and Brighton, C.T.: Healing of Nonunion of the Medial Malleolus by Means of a Direct Current: A Case Report. J. Trauma, 11:883–885, 1971.
108. Frost, H.M.: Skeletal Physiology and Bone Remodeling. *In* Urist, M.R. (ed.): Fundamental and Clinical Bone Physiology, pp. 208–241. Philadelphia, J.B. Lippincott, 1980.
109. Furukawa, T., Eyre, D.R., Koide, S., and Glimcher, M.J.: Biochemical Studies on Repair Cartilage Resurfacing Experimental Defects in the Rabbit Knee. J. Bone Joint Surg., 62A:79–89, 1980.
110. Garg, N.K., Gaur, S., and Sharma, S.: Percutaneous Autogenous Bone Marrow Grafting in 20 Cases of Ununited Fracture. Acta Orthop. Scand., 64:671–672, 1993.
111. Garrett, W.E., Jr., Seaber, A.V., Boswich, J., Urbaniak, J.R., and Goldner, J.L.: Recovery of Skeletal Muscle After Laceration and Repair. J. Hand Surg. 9A:683–692, 1984.
112. Garrett, W., and Tidball, J.: Myotendinous Junction: Structure,

Function and Failure. *In* Woo, S.L.-Y., and Buckwalter, J.A. (eds.): Injury and Repair of the Musculoskeletal Soft Tissues, pp. 171–207. Park Ridge, Ill., American Academy of Orthopaedic Surgeons, 1988.

113. Gelberman, R., Goldberg, V., An, K.-N., and Banes, A.: Tendon. *In* Woo, S.L.-Y., and Buckwalter, J.A. (eds.): Injury and Repair of the Musculoskeletal Soft Tissues, pp. 5–40. Park Ridge, Ill., American Academy of Orthopaedic Surgeons, 1988.
114. Gelberman R.H., Vande Berg, J.S., Lundborg, G.N., and Akeson, W.H.: Flexor Tendon Healing and Rotation of the Gliding Surface: An Ultrastructural Study in Dogs. J. Bone Joint Surg., 65A:70–80, 1983.
115. Ghadially, F.N., Thomas, I., Oryschak, A.F., and Lalonde, I.M.: Long-term Results of Superficial Defects in Articular Cartilage: A Scanning Electron Microscope Study. J. Pathol., 121:213–217, 1977.
116. Glimcher, M.J.: Composition, Structure, and Organization of Bone and Other Mineralized Tissue and the Mechanism of Calcification. *In* Greep, R.O., and Astwood, E.B. (eds.): Handbook of Physiology, Section 7—Endocrinology. Washington, D.C., American Physiological Society, 7:25–116, 1976.
117. Goodman, A.H., and Sherman, M.S.: Postirradiation Fractures of the Femoral Neck. J. Bone Joint Surg., 45A:723–730, 1963.
118. Goodship, A.E., and Kenwright, J.: The Influence of Induced Micromovement Upon the Healing of Experimental Tibial Fractures. J. Bone Joint Surg., 67B:650–655, 1985.
119. Göthlin, G., and Ericsson, J.L.E.: The Osteoclast: Review of Ultrastructure, Origin, and Structure–Function Relationship. Clin. Orthop., 120:201–231, 1976.
120. Göthman, L.: Vascular Reactions in Experimental Fractures: Microangiographic and Radioisotope Studies. Acta Chir. Scand., 248(Suppl.):1–34, 1961.
121. Green, S.A., Jackson, J.M., Wall, D.M., Marinow, H., and Ishkanian, J.: Management of Segmental Defects by the Ilizarov Intercalary Bone Transport Method. Clin. Orthop., 280:136–142, 1992
122. Grundnes, O., and Reikeras, O.: Closed Versus Open Medullary Nailing of Femoral Fractures: Blood Flow and Healing Studied in Rats. Acta Orthop. Scand., 63:492–496, 1992
123. Grundnes, O., and Reikeras, O.: The Importance of the Hematoma for Fracture Healing in Rats. Acta Orthop. Scand., 64:340–342, 1993
124. Grundnes, O., and Reikeras, O.: The Role of the Hematoma and Periosteal Sealing for Fracture Healing in Rats. Acta Orthop. Scand., 64:47–49, 1993
125. Heckman, J.D., Ryaby, J.P., McCabe, J., Frey, J.J., and Kilcoyne, R.F.: Acceleration of Tibial Fracture-Healing by Noninvasive, Low-Intensity Pulsed Ultrasound. J. Bone Joint Surg., 76A:26–34, 1994.
126. Heckman, J.D., and Levine, M.I.: Traumatic Closed Transection of the Biceps Brachia in the Military Parachutist. J. Bone Joint Surg., 60A:369–372, 1978.
127. Heikkinen, E., Vihersaari, T., and Penttinen, R.: Effect of Previous Exercise on Fracture Healing: A Biochemical Study With Mice. Acta Orthop. Scand., 45:481–489, 1974.
128. Heiple, K.G., Chase, S.W., and Herndon, C.H.: A Comparative Study of the Healing Process Following Different Types of Bone Transplantation. J. Bone Joint Surg., 45A:1593–1616, 1963.
129. Henning, C.E., Lynch, M.A., Yearout, K.M., Vequist, S.W., Stallbaumer, R.J., and Decker, K.A.: Arthroscopic Meniscal Repair Using an Exogenous Fibrin Clot. Clin. Orthop., 252:64–72, 1990.
130. Herbsman, H., Kwon, K., Shaftan, G.W., Gordon, B., Fox, L.M., and Enquist, I.F.: The Influence of Systemic Factors on Fracture Healing. J. Trauma, 6:75–85, 1966.
131. Herbsman, H., Powers, J.C., Hirschman, A., and Shaftan, G.W.: Retardation of Fracture Healing in Experimental Diabetes. J. Surg. Res., 8:424–431, 1968.
132. Herold, H.Z., and Tadmor, A.: Chondroitin Sulphate in Treatment of Experimental Bone Defects. Isr. J. Med. Sci., 5:425–427, 1969.
133. Hidaka, S., and Gustilo, R.B.: Refracture of Bones of the Forearm After Plate Removal. J. Bone Joint Surg., 66A:1241–1243, 1984.
134. Hoch, D.H., Grodzinsky, A.J., Kobb, T.J., Albert, M.L., and Eyre, E.R.: Early Changes in Material Properties of Rabbit Articular Cartilage after Meniscectomy. J. Orthop. Res., 1:4–12, 1983.
135. Hodge, D.E., and Peturska, J.A.: Collagen. *In* Ramachandran, G.N. (ed.): Aspects of Protein Structure. New York, Academic Press, 1963.
136. Hogevold HE, Grogaard B, Reikeras O: Effects of Short-Term Treatment With Corticosteroids and Indomethacin on Bone Healing: A Mechanical Study of Osteotomies in Rats. Acta Orthop. Scand., 63:607–611, 1992.
137. Hooper, G., Davies, R., and Tothill, P.: Blood Flow and Clearance in Dogs. J. Bone Joint Surg., 66B:441–448, 1984.
138. Hsu, J.D., and Robinson, R.A.: Studies on the Healing of Long Bone Fractures in Hereditary Pituitary Insufficient Mice. J. Surg. Res., 9:535–536, 1969.
139. Hulth, A.: Current Concepts of Fracture Healing. Clin. Orthop., 249:265–284, 1989.
140. Hunziker, E.B., and Rosenberg, R.: Induction of Repair of Partial Thickness Articular Cartilage Lesions by Timed Release of TGF-beta. Trans. Orthop. Res. Soc., 19:236, 1994.
141. Hurme, T., Kalimo, H., Lehto, M., and Jarvinen, M.: Healing of Skeletal Muscle Injury: An Ultrastructural and Immunohistochemical Study. Med. Sci. Sports Exerc., 23(7):801–810, 1991
142. Ilizarov, G.A.: The Tension-Stress Effect of the Genesis and Growth of Tissues: I. The Influence of Stability of Fixation and Soft-Tissue Preservation. Clin. Orthop., 238:249–281, 1989.
143. Ilizarov, G.A.: The Tension-Stress Effect on the Genesis and Growth of Tissues: II. The Influence of Rate and Frequency of Distraction. Clin. Orthop., 239:263–285, 1989.
144. Jackson, D.W., and Feagin, J.A.: Quadriceps Contusions in Young Athletes: Relation of Severity of Injury to Treatment and Prognosis. J. Bone Joint Surg., 55A:95–105, 1973.
145. Jacobs, S.J., Gilbert, M.S., and Einhorn, T.A.: The Treatment of Fractures in Uremic Bone Disease: Causes of Failure and Optimization of Healing. Contemp. Orthop., 18:23–25, 1989.
146. Jaffe, K.A., Morris, S.G., Sorrell, R.G., Gebhardt, M.C., and Mankin, H.J.: Massive Bone Allografts for Traumatic Skeletal Defects. South. Med. J., 84:975–982, 1991.
147. Järvinen, M.: Healing of a Crush Injury in Rat Striated Muscle: II. A Histological Study of the Effect of Early Mobilization and Immobilization on the Repair Processes. Acta Pathol. Microbiol. Immunol. Scand., 83:269–282, 1975.
148. Järvinen, M.: Healing of a Crush Injury in Rat Striated Muscle: IV. Effect of Early Mobilization and Immobilization on the Tensile Properties of Gastrocnemius Muscle. Acta Chir. Scand., 142:47–56, 1976.
149. Järvinen, M.J., and Lehto, M.U.: The Effects of Early Mobilization and Immobilization on the Healing Process Following Muscle Injuries. Sports Med., 15:78–89, 1993
150. Jensen, J.E., Jensen, T.G., Smith, T.K., Johnston, D.A., and Dudrick, S.J.: Nutrition in Orthopaedic Surgery. J. Bone Joint Surg., 64A:1263–1272, 1982.
151. Jingushi, S., Heydemann, A., and Bolander, M.E.: Acidic FGF Injection Stimulates Cartilage Enlargement and Inhibits Cartilage Gene Expression in Rat Fracture Healing. J. Orthop. Res., 8:364–371, 1990.
152. Jingushi, S., Heydemann, A., Joyce, M.E., and Bolander, M.E.: mRNA Expression for Type I Procollagen, Alkaline Phosphatase, Osteonectin, and Bone GLA Protein in Soft Callus During Rat Femur Fracture Healing. *In* Proceedings of Conference on Bone Grafts and Bone Substitutes. Tampa, Fla., January 1989.
153. Jokl, P.: Muscle. *In* Albright, J.A., and Brand, R.A. (eds.): The Scientific Basis of Orthopaedics, pp. 407–422. Norwalk, Conn., Appleton Lange, 1987.
154. Joyce, M.E., Jingushi, S., Scully, S.P., and Bolander, M.E.: Role of Growth Factors in Fracture Healing. Prog. Clin. Biol. Res., 365:391–416, 1991.
155. Jurvelin, J., Kiviranta, I., Tammi, M., and Helminen, H.J.: Softening of Canine Articular Cartilage after Immobilization of the Knee Joint. Clin. Orthop., 207:246–252, 1986.
156. Karachalios, T., Lyritis, G.P., Giannarakos, D.G., Papanicolaou, G., and Sotopoulos, K.: Calcitonin Effects on Rabbit Bone:

Bending Tests on Ulnar Osteotomies. Acta Orthop. Scand., 63:615–618, 1992.

157. Karlsson, M.K., Nilsson, B.E., and Obrant, K.J.: Bone Mineral Loss After Lower Extremity Trauma: 62 Cases Followed for 15–38 Years. Acta Orthop. Scand., 64:362–364, 1993.
158. Kenwright, J., and Goodship, A.E.: Controlled Mechanical Stimulation in the Treatment of Tibial Fractures. Clin. Orthop., 241:36–47, 1989.
159. Kenwright, J., Richardson, J.B., Cunningham, J.L., et al.: Axial Movement and Tibial Fractures: A Controlled Randomized Trial of Treatment. J. Bone Joint Surg., 73B:654–659, 1991.
160. Kenwright, J., Richardson, J.B., Goodship, A.E., et al.: Effect of Controlled Axial Micromovement on Healing of Tibial Fractures. Lancet, 2:1185–1187, 1986.
161. Kenzora, J.E., Steele, R.E., Yosipovitch, Z.H., and Glimcher, M.J.: Experimental Osteonecrosis of the Femoral Head in Adult Rabbits. Clin. Orthop., 130:8–46, 1978.
162. Kershaw, C.J., Cunningham, J.L., and Kenwright, J.: Tibial External Fixation, Weight Bearing, and Fracture Movement. Clin. Orthop., 293:28–36, 1993.
163. Klug, W., Franke, W.G., and Knoch, H.G.: Scintigraphic Control of Bone-Fracture Healing Under Ultrasonic Stimulation: An Animal Experimental Study. Eur. J. Nucl. Med., 11:494–497, 1986.
164. Koskinen, E.V.S.: The Repair of Experimental Fractures Under the Action of Growth Hormone, Thyrotropin and Cortisone: A Tissue Analytic, Roentgenologic and Autoradiographic Study. Ann. Chir. Gynaccol. Fenn., 48(Suppl. 90):1–48, 1959.
165. Koskinen, E.V.S.: Effect of Endocrine Factors on Callus Development in Experimental Fractures. Symp. Biol. Hung., 7:315–322, 1967.
166. Koskinen, E.V.S., Ryoppy, S.A., and Lindholm, T.S.: Bone Formation by Induction Under the Influence of Growth Hormone and Cortisone. Isr. J. Med. Sci., 7:378–380, 1971.
167. Kowalewski, K., Couves, C.M., and Lang, A.: Protective Action of 17-Ethyl-19-Nortestosterone Against the Inhibition of Bone Repair in the Lathyrus-Fed Rat. Acta Endocrinol., 30:268–272, 1959.
168. Kowalewski, K., and Gort, J.: An Anabolic Androgen as a Stimulant of Bone Healing in Rats Treated With Cortisone. Acta Endocrinol., 30:273–276, 1959.
169. Lack, C.H.: Proteolytic Activity and Connective Tissue. Br. Med. Bull., 20:217–222, 1964.
170. Laing, P.G., Ferguson, A.B., Jr., and Hodge, E.S.: Tissue Reaction in Rabbit Muscle to Metallic Implants. J. Biomed. Mater. Res., 1:135–149, 1967.
171. Lavine, L.S., and Grodzinsky, A.J.: Current Concepts Review: Electrical Stimulation of Repair of Bone. J. Bone Joint Surg., 69A:626–630, 1987.
172. Lavine, L.S., and Shamos, M.H.: Electric Enhancement of Bone Healing. Science, 175:118–121, 1972.
173. Lehto, M., Duance, V.C., and Restall, D.: Collagen and Fibronectin in a Healing Skeletal Muscle Injury: An Immunohistochemical Study of the Effects of Physical Activity on the Repair of Injured Gastrocnemius Muscle in the Rat. J. Bone Joint Surg., 67:820–828, 1985.
174. Leung, K.S., Sher, A.H., Lam, T.S.W., and Leung, P.C.: Energy Metabolism in Fracture Healing. J. Bone Joint Surg., 71B:567–660, 1989.
175. Lind, M., Schumacker, B., Soballe, K., Keller, J., Melsen, F., and Bunger, C.: Transforming Growth Factor Beta Enhances Fracture Healing in Rabbit Tibiae. Acta Orthop. Scand., 64:553–556, 1993.
176. Lindsay, W.K., and Birch, J.R.: The Fibroblast in Flexor Tendon Healing. Plast. Reconstr. Surg., 34:223–232, 1964.
177. Lindsay, W.K., and McDougall, E.P.: Digital Flexor Tendons: An Experimental Study: III. The Fate of Autogenous Digital Flexor Tendon Grafts. Br. J. Plast. Surg., 13:293–304, 1961.
178. Lindsay, W.K., and Thomson, H.G.: Digital Flexor Tendons: An Experimental Study: I. The Significance of Each Component of the Flexor Mechanism in Tendon Healing. Br. J. Plast. Surg., 12:289–316, 1960.
179. Lindsay, W.K., Thomson, H.G., and Walker, F.G.: Digital Flexor Tendons: An Experimental Study: II. The Significance of a Gap Occurring at the Line of Suture. Br. J. Plast. Surg., 13:1–9, 1960.
180. Lucas, P.A.: Chemotactic Response of Osteoblast-like Cells to TGF-Beta (Abstract). Trans. Orthop. Res. Soc., 14:86, 1989.
181. Lucas, P.A., Syftestad, G.T., and Caplan, A.I.: In Vivo Ectopic Induction of Cartilage and Bone by Water-Soluble Proteins from Bone Matrix (Abstract). Trans. Orthop. Res. Soc., 13:321, 1988.
182. Lundborg, G., and Rank, F.: Experimental Intrinsic Healing of Flexor Tendons Based Upon Synovial Fluid Nutrition. J. Hand Surg., 3:21–31, 1978.
183. Lundborg, G., Rydevik, B., Manthrope, M., Varon, S., and Lewis, J.: Peripheral Nerve: The Physiology of Injury and Repair. *In* Woo, S.L.-Y., and Buckwalter, J.A. (eds.): Injury and Repair of the Musculoskeletal Soft Tissue, pp. 297–352. Park Ridge, Ill., American Academy of Orthopaedic Surgeons, 1988.
184. Macy, L.D., Kana, S.M., Jingushi, S., Terek, R.M., Borretos, J., and Bolander, M.D.: Defects of Early Fracture-Healing in Experimental Diabetes. J. Bone Joint Surg., 71A:722–733, 1989.
185. Mankin, H.J.: The Reaction of Articular Cartilage to Injury and Osteoarthritis: I. N. Engl. J. Med., 291:1285–1292, 1974.
186. Mankin, H.J.: The Reaction of Articular Cartilage to Injury and Osteoarthritis: II. N. Engl. J. Med., 291:1335–1340, 1974.
187. Mankin, H.J.: The Response of Articular Cartilage to Mechanical Injury. J. Bone Joint Surg., 64A:460–466, 1982.
188. Manske, P.R., Gelberman, R.H., Vande Berg, J.S., and Lester, P.A.: Intrinsic Flexor Tendon Repair: A Morphologic Study In Vitro. J. Bone Joint Surg., 66A:385–396, 1984.
189. Marsh, J.L., Buckwalter, J.A., and Evarts, C.M.: Nonunion, Delayed Union, Malunion and Avascular Necrosis. *In* Epps, C.H. (ed.): Complications in Orthopaedic Surgery, pp. 183—211. Philadelphia, J.B. Lippincott, 1994.
190. Mason, M.L., and Allen, H.S.: The Rate of Healing of Tendons: An Experimental Study of Tensile Strength. Ann. Surg., 113:424–459, 1941.
191. Mason, M.L., and Shearon, C.G.: The Process of Tendon Repair: An Experimental Study of Tendon Suture and Tendon Graft. Arch. Surg., 25:615–692, 1932.
192. Mast, B.A., Diegelmann, R.F., Krummel, T.M., and Cohen, I.K.: Hyaluronic Acid Modulates Proliferation, Collagen and Protein Synthesis of Cultured Fetal Fibroblasts. Matrix, 13:441–446, 1993.
193. Mast, B.A., Diegelmann, R.F., Krummel, T.M., and Cohen, I.K.: Scarless Wound Healing in the Mammalian Fetus. Surg. Gynecol. Obstet., 174:441–451, 1992.
194. Mast, B.A., Flood, L.C., Haynes, J.H., et al: Hyaluronic Acid is a Major Component of the Matrix of Fetal Rabbit Skin and Wounds: Implications for Healing by Regeneration. Matrix, 11:63–68, 1991.
195. McAndrew, M.P., and Nelson, R.L.: Allografting for Traumatic Intercalary Femoral Defects: A Report of Three Cases. J. Orthop. Trauma, 3:250–256, 1989.
196. McKibbin, B.: The Biology of Fracture Healing in Long Bones. J. Bone Joint Surg., 60B:150–162, 1978.
197. McLeod, K.J., and Rubin, C.T.: The Effect of Low-Frequency Electrical Fields on Osteogenesis. J. Bone Joint Surg., 74A:920–929, 1992.
198. Meachim, G.: The Effects of Scarification of an Articular Cartilage in the Rabbit. J. Bone Joint Surg., 45B:150–161, 1983.
199. Michelsen, C.G., and Askanazi, J: Current Concepts Review: The Metabolic Response to Injury: Mechanism and Clinical Implantations. J. Bone Joint Surg., 68A:782–787, 1986.
200. Misol, S., Samaan, N., and Ponseti, I.V.: Growth Hormone in Delayed Fracture Union. Clin. Orthop., 74:206–208, 1971.
201. Mitchell, N., and Shephard, N.: Effect of Patellar Shaving in the Rabbit. J. Orthop. Res., 5:388–392, 1987.
202. Mitchell, N., and Shephard, N.: The Deleterious Effects of Drying on Articular Cartilage. J. Bone Joint Surg., 71A:89–95, 1989.
203. Mooney, V., Nickel, V., Harvey, J.P., Jr., and Snelson, R.: Cast Brace Treatment for Fractures of the Distal Part of the Femur. J. Bone Joint Surg., 52A:1563–1578, 1970.
204. Mow, V., and Rosenwasser, M.: Articular Cartilage: Biomecha-

nics. *In* Woo, S.L.-Y., and Buckwalter, J.A. (eds): Injury and Repair of the Musculoskeletal Soft Tissues, pp. 427–463. Park Ridge, Ill., American Academy of Orthopaedic Surgeons, 1988.

205. Müller, M.E., Allgöwer, M., and Willenegger, H.: Technique of Internal Fixation of Fractures. New York, Springer-Verlag, 1965.
206. Mulliken, J.B., Kaban, L.B., and Glowacki, J.: Induced Osteogenesis—the Biological Principle and Clinical Applications. J. Surg. Res., 37:487–496, 1984.
207. Mustoe TA, Landes A, Cromack DT, et al.: Differential Acceleration of Healing of Surgical Incisions in the Rabbit Gastrointestinal Tract by Platelet-Derived Growth Factor and Transforming Growth Factor, Type Beta. Surgery, 108:324–329, 1990.
208. Muthukumaran, N., and Reddi, A.H.: Bone Matrix-Induced Local Bone Induction. Clin. Orthop., 220:159–164, 1984.
209. Neer, C.S., Francis, K.C., Marcove, R.C., Terz, J., and Carbonara, P.N.: Treatment of Unicameral Bone Cyst. J. Bone Joint Surg., 48A:731–745, 1966.
210. Nelson, B.H., Anderson, D.D., Brand, R.A., and Brown, T.D.: Effect of Osteochondral Defects on Articular Cartilage: Contact Pressures Studied in Dog Knees. Acta Orthop. Scand., 59:574–579, 1988.
211. Nemeth, G.G., Bolander, M.E., and Martin, O.R.: Growth Factors and Their Role in Wound and Fracture Healing. *In* Barbul, A., Pines, E., Caldwell, M., and Hunt, T.K. (eds.): Growth Factors and Other Aspects of Wound Healing: Biological and Clinical Implications, pp. 1–17. New York, Allen R. Liss, 1988.
212. Nemeth, G.G., Heydemann, A., Jingushi, S., Terek, R., and Bolander, M.E.: Temporal Activation and Abnormal Regulation of Cartilage and Bone Genes in Fracture Healing. *In* Proceedings of the Second International Conference on Molecular Biology and Pathology of Matrix, Philadelphia, June 1988.
213. Nerubay, J., Marganit, B., Bubis, J.J., Tadmor, A., and Katznelson, A.: Stimulation of Bone Formation by Electrical Current on Spine Fusion. Spine, 11:167–169, 1986.
214. Nicholas, J.A., and Killoran, P.: Fracture of the Femur in Patients With Paget's Disease. J. Bone Joint Surg., 47A:450–461, 1965.
215. Nichols, J.T., Toto, P.D., and Choukas, N.C.: The Proliferative Capacity and DNA Synthesis of Osteoblasts during Fracture Repair in Normal and Hypophysectomized Rats. Oral Surg., 25:418–426, 1968.
216. Nielson, H.M., Andreassen, T.T., Ledet, T., and Oxlund, H.: Local Injection of TGF-Beta Increases the Strength of Tibial Fractures in the Rat. Acta Orthop. Scand., 65:37–41, 1994.
217. Nielson, H.M., Bak, B., Jorgensen, P.H., and Andreassen, T.T.: Growth Hormone Promotes Healing of Tibial Fractures in the Rat. Acta Orthop. Scand., 62:244–247, 1991.
218. Noda, M., and Camillier, J.J.: In Vivo Stimulation of Bone Formation by Transforming Growth Factor-β. Endocrinology, 124:2991–2994, 1989.
219. Noonan, T.J., and Garrett, W.E.: Injuries at the Myotendinous Junction. Clin. Sports Med., 11:783–806, 1992.
220. Northmore-Ball, M.D., Wood, M.R., and Meggitt, B.F.: A Biomechanical Study of the Effects of Growth Hormone in Experimental Fracture Healing. J. Bone Joint Surg., 62B:391–396, 1980.
221. O'Donoghue, D.H.: Surgical Treatment of Fresh Injuries to the Major Ligaments of the Knee. J. Bone Joint Surg., 32A:721–738, 1950.
222. O'Donoghue, D.H.: An Analysis of End Results of Surgical Treatment of Major Injuries to the Ligaments of the Knee. J. Bone Joint Surg., 37A:1–13, 1955.
223. Oegema, T., An, K.N., Weiland, A., Furcht, L.: Peripheral Blood Vessel. *In* Woo, S.L.-Y., and Buckwalter, J.A. (eds.): Injury and Repair of the Musculoskeletal Soft Tissues, pp. 357–400. Park Ridge, Ill., American Academy of Orthopaedic Surgeons, 1988.
224. Olerud, S., and Danckwardt-Lillioeström, G.: Fracture Healing in Compression Osteosynthesis: An Experimental Study in Dogs With an Avascular, Diaphyseal, Intermedial Fragment. Acta Orthop. Scand. Suppl., 137:1971.
225. O'Sullivan, M.E., Bronk, J.T., Chao, E.Y.S., and Kelly, P.J.: Experimental Study of the Effect of Weight Bearing on Fracture Healing in the Canine Tibia. Clin. Orthop., 302:273–283, 1994.
226. O'Sullivan, M.E., Chao, E.V.S., and Kelly, P.J.: The Effects of Fixation on Fracture Healing. J. Bone Joint Surg., 71A:306–310, 1989.
227. Paley, D., Catagni, M.D., Argnani, F., Villa, A., Benedetti, G.B., and Cattaneo, R: Ilizarov Treatment of Nonunions With Bone Loss. Clin. Orthop., 241:146–165, 1989.
228. Palmoski, M.J., Perricone, D., and Brandt, K.D.: Development and Reversal of a Proteoglycan Aggregation Defect in Normal Canine Knee Cartilage after Immobilization. Arthritis Rheum., 22:508–517, 1979.
229. Pappas, A.M., and Radin, E.: The Effect of Delayed Manipulation Upon the Rate of Fracture Healing. Surg. Gynecol. Obstet., 126:1287–1297, 1968.
230. Peacock, E.E., Jr.: A Study of the Circulation in Normal Tendons and Healing Grafts. Ann. Surg., 149:415–428, 1959.
231. Peacock, E.E., Jr.: Biological Principles in the Healing of Long Tendons. Surg. Clin. North Am., 45:461–476, 1965.
232. Peacock, E.E., Jr., and Van Winkle, W., Jr.: Surgery and Biology of Wound Repair. Philadelphia, W.B. Saunders, 1970.
233. Penttinen, R.: Biochemical Studies on Fracture Healing in the Rat. Acta Chir. Scand., (Suppl.):432, 1972.
234. Perren, S.M.: Physical and Biological Aspects of Fracture Healing With Special Reference to Internal Fixation. Clin Orthop., 138:175–196, 1979.
235. Perren, S.M.: The Biomechanics and Biology of Internal Fixation Using Plates and Nails. Orthopedics, 12:21–34, 1989.
236. Perren, S.M., Cordey, J., and Gautier, E.: Rigid Internal Fixation Using Plates: Terminology, Principle and Early Problems. *In* Lang, J.M. (ed): Fracture Healing, pp. 139–151. New York, Churchill Livingstone, 1987.
237. Perren, S.M., Huggler, A., and Russenberger, S.: Cortical Bone Healing. Acta Orthop. Scand. Suppl., 125: 1969.
238. Perren, S.M., Russenberger, M., Steinmann, S., Müller, M.E., and Allgöwer, M.: A Dynamic Compression Plate. Acta Orthop. Scand., Suppl., 125:29–41, 1969.
239. Pienkowski, D., Pollock, S.R., Brighton, C.T., and Griffith, N.J.: Low-Power Electromagnetic Stimulation of Osteotomized Rabbit Fibulae. J. Bone Joint Surg., 76A:489–501, 1994.
240. Pilla, A.A., Mount, M.A., Nasser, P.R., et al.: Non-invasive Low-Intensity Pulsed Ultrasound Accelerates Bone Healing in the Rabbit. J. Orthop. Trauma, 4:246–253, 1990.
241. Potenza, A.D.: Tendon Healing Within the Flexor Digital Sheath in the Dog. J. Bone Joint Surg., 44A:49–64, 1962.
242. Potenza, A.D.: Critical Evaluation of Flexor Tendon Healing and Adhesion Formation Within Artificial Digital Sheaths. J. Bone Joint Surg., 45A:1217–1233, 1963.
243. Potenza, A.D.: The Healing of Autogenous Tendon Grafts Within the Flexor Digital Sheath in Dogs. J. Bone Joint Surg., 46A:1462–1484, 1964.
244. Potenza, A.D.: Flexor Tendon Injuries. Orthop. Clin. North Am., 1:355–373, 1970.
245. Potts, W.J.: The Role of the Hematoma in Fracture Healing. Surg. Gynecol. Obstet., 57:318–324, 1933.
246. Ray, R.D.: Bone Grafting: Transplants and Implants. Instr. Course Lect., 13:177–186, 1956.
247. Ray, R.D., and Sabet, T.: Bone Grafts, Cellular Survival Versus Induction: An Experimental Study in Mice. J. Bone Joint Surg., 45A:337–344, 1963.
248. Repo, R.U., and Finlay, J.B.: Survival of Articular Cartilage After Controlled Impact. J. Bone Joint Surg., 59A:1068–1076, 1977.
249. Retief, D.H., and Dreyer, C.J.: Effects of Neural Damage on the Repair of Bony Defects in the Rat. Arch. Oral Biol., 12:1035–1039, 1967.
250. Rhinelander, F.W., and Baragry, R.A.: Microangiography in Bone Healing: I. Undisplaced Closed Fractures. J. Bone Joint Surg., 44A:1273–1298, 1962.
251. Rhinelander, F.W., Phillips, R.S., Steel, W.M., and Beer, J.C.: Microangiography and Bone Healing: II. Displaced Closed Fractures. J. Bone Joint Surg., 50A:643–662, 1986.
252. Richon, A., Livio, J.J., and Saegesser, F.: Les Refractures Aprés

Osteosynthèse par Plaque á Compression. Helv. Chir. Acta., 34:49–62, 1967.

253. Rifkin, B.R., Baker, R.L., and Coleman, S.J.: Effects of Prostaglandin E_2 on Macrophages and Osteoclasts in Cultured Fetal Long Bones. Cell Tissue Res., 207:341–346, 1980.
254. Ripamonti, U., Ma, S., Cunningham, N.S., Yeates, L., and Reddi, A.H.: Initiation of Bone Regeneration in Adult Baboons by Osteogenin, a Bone Morphogenetic Protein. Matrix, 12:369–380, 1992.
255. Rokkanen, P., and Slatis, P.: The Repair of Experimental Fractures During Long-Term Anticoagulant Treatment: An Experimental Study on Rats. Acta Orthop. Scand., 35:21–38, 1964.
256. Rommens, P.M., Coosemans, W., and Broos, P.L.: The Difficult Healing of Segmental Fractures of the Tibial Shaft. Arch. Orthop. Trauma Surg., 108:238–242, 1989.
257. Rothman, R.H.: Effect of Anemia on Fracture Healing. Surg. Forum, 19:452–453, 1968.
258. Rothwell, A.G.: Quadriceps Hematoma: A Prospective Study. Clin. Orthop., 171:97–103, 1982.
259. Russell, P.S., and Monaco, A.P.: The Biology of Tissue Transplantation. Boston, Little, Brown & Co, 1965.
260. Sandberg, M., Aro, H., Multimaki, P., Aho, H., and Vuorio, E.: In Situ Localization of Collagen Production by Chondrocytes and Osteoblasts in Fracture Callus. J. Bone Joint Surg., 71A:69–77, 1989.
261. Sandberg, M.J., Aro, H.T., and Vuorio, E.I.: Gene expression During Bone Repair. Clin. Orthop., 289:292–312, 1993.
262. Sarmiento, A.: A Functional Below-the-Knee Cast for Tibial Fractures. J. Bone Joint Surg., 49A:855–875, 1967.
263. Schatzker, J., Waddell, J., and Stoll, J.E.: The Effects of Motion on the Healing of Cancellous Bone. Clin. Orthop., 245:282–287, 1989.
264. Schenk, R.K.: Cytodynamics and Histodynamics of Primary Bone Repair. *In* Lang, J.M. (ed.): Fracture Healing, pp. 23–32. New York, Churchill Livingstone, 1987.
265. Schenk, R., and Willenegger, H.: Morphological Findings in Primary Fracture Healing: Callus Formation. Simp. Biol. Hungarica, 7:75–80, 1967.
266. Scheven, B.A.A., Visser, J.W.M., and Nijweide, P.J.: In Vitro Osteoclast Generation from Different Bone Marrow Fractions, Including a Highly Enriched Haematopoietic Stem Cell Population. Nature, 321:79–81, 1986.
267. Scott, G., and King, J.B.: A Prospective Double-Blind Trial of Electrical Capacitive Coupling in the Treatment of Non-union of Long Bones. J. Bone Joint Surg., 76A:820–826, 1994.
268. Shaffer, J.W., Field, G.A., Goldberg, V.M., and Davy, D.T.: Fate of Vascularized and Non-vascularized Autografts. Clin. Orthop., 197:32–43, 1985.
269. Sharma, S., Garg, N.K., Veliath, A.J., Subramanian, S., and Srivastava, K.K.: Percutaneous Bone-Marrow Grafting of Osteotomies and Bony Defects in Rabbits. Acta Orthop. Scand., 63:166–169, 1992.
270. Sharrard, W.J.W.: A Double Blind Trial of Pulsed Electromagnetic Fields for Delayed Union of Tibial Fractures. J. Bone Joint Surg., 72B:347–355, 1990.
271. Simmons, D.J.: Fracture Healing Perspectives. Clin. Orthop., 200:101–113, 1985.
272. Simmons, D.J., and Kunvin, A.S.: Autoradiographic and Biochemical Investigations of the Effect of Cortisone on the Bones of the Rat. Clin. Orthop., 55:201–215, 1967.
273. Simpson, J.M., Silveri, C.P., Balderston, R.A., Simeone, F.A., and An, H.S.: The Results of Operations on the Lumbar Spine in Patients Who Have Diabetes Mellitus. J. Bone Joint Surg., 75A:1823–1829, 1993.
274. Singh, R.H., and Udupa, K.N.: Some Investigations on the Effect of Insulin in Healing of Fractures. Indian J. Med. Res., 54:1071–1082, 1966.
275. Sisk, T.D.: General Principles of Fracture Treatment. *In* Crenshaw, A.H. (ed.): Campbell's Operative Orthopaedics, 7th ed., pp. 1557–2013. St. Louis, C.V. Mosby, 1987.
276. Skoog, T., and Persson, B.H.: An Experimental Study of the Early Healing of Tendons. Plast. Reconstr. Surg., 13:384–399, 1954.
277. Smith, J.W.: Blood Supply of Tendons. Am. J. Surg., 109:272–276, 1965.
278. Smith, T.K.: Prevention of Complications in Orthopaedic Surgery Secondary to Nutritional Depletion. Clin. Orthop., 222:91–97, 1987.
279. Speer, K.P., Callaghan, J.J., Seaber, A.V., and Tucker, J.A.: The Effects of Exposure of Articular Cartilage to Air: A Histochemical and Ultrastructural Investigation. J. Bone Joint Surg., 72A:1442–1450, 1990.
280. Sporn, M.B., and Roberts, A.B.: Peptide Growth Factors are Multifunctional. Nature 332:217–219, March 1988.
281. Sporn, M.B., and Roberts, A.B.: Transforming Growth Factor-β: Multiple Actions and Potential Clinical Applications. J.A.M.A., 262:938–941, 1989.
282. Steier, A., Gedalia, I., Schwarz, A., and Rodan, A.: Effect of Vitamin D_2 and Fluoride on Experimental Bone Fracture Healing in Rats. J. Dent. Res., 46:675–680, 1967.
283. Stinchfield, F.E., Sankaran, B., and Samilson, R.: The Effect of Anticoagulant Therapy on Bone Repair. J. Bone Joint Surg., 38A:270–282, 1956.
284. Stirling, R.I.: Healing of Fractured Bones: Report of Investigation into Process of Healing of Fractured Bones, With Some Clinical Applications. Trans. R. Med. Chir. Soc. Edinb., 46:203–228, 1932.
285. Taylor, G.I., Miller, G.D.H., and Ham, F.J.: The Free Vascularized Bone Graft: A Clinical Extension of Microvascular Techniques. Plast. Reconstr. Surg., 55:533–544, 1975.
286. Taylor, G.I., and Watson, N.: One-Stage Repair of Compound Leg Defects With Free, Revascularized Flaps of Groin Skin and Iliac Bone. Plast. Reconstr. Surg., 61:494–506, 1978.
287. Terry, G.G., Flandry, F., Vanmangu, J.W., and Norwood, L.A.: Isolated Chondral Fractures of the Knee. Clin. Orthop., 234:170–177, 1988.
288. Thaxter, T.H., Mann, R.A., and Anderson, C.E.: Degeneration of Immobilized Knee Joints in Rats: Histological and Autoradiographic Study. J. Bone Joint Surg., 47A:567–585, 1965.
289. Tidball, J.G., and Chan, M.: Adhesive Strength of Single Muscle Cells to Basement Membrane at Myotendinous Junctions. J. Appl. Physiol., 67:1063–1069, 1989.
290. Tipton, C.M., Schild, R.J., and Flatt, A.E.: Measurement of Ligamentous Strength in Rat Knees. J. Bone Joint Surg., 49A:63–72, 1967.
291. Tonino, A.J., Davidson, C.L., Klopper, P.J., and Linclau, L.A.: Protection from Stress in Bone and its Effects: Experiments With Stainless Steel and Plastic Plates in Dogs. J. Bone Joint Surg., 58B:107–113, 1976.
292. Tonna, E.A.: An Electron Microscopic Study of Osteocyte Release During Osteoclasis in Mice of Different Ages. Clin. Orthop., 87:311–317, 1972.
293. Tonna, E.A., and Cronkite, E.P.: The Periosteum: Autoradiographic Studies on Cellular Proliferation and Transformation Utilizing Tritiated Thymidine. Clin. Orthop., 30:218–233, 1963.
294. Triffett, J.T.: Initiation and Enhancement of Bone Formation: A Review. Acta Orthop. Scand., 58:673–684, 1987.
295. Trueta, J.: The Role of the Vessels in Osteogenesis. J. Bone Joint Surg., 45B:402–418, 1963.
296. Turner, T.C., Bassett, C.A.L., Pate, J.W., and Sawyer, P.N.: An Experimental Comparison of Freeze Dried and Frozen Cortical Bone Graft Healing. J. Bone Joint Surg., 37A:1197–1205, 1955.
297. Turner, T.C., Bassett, C.A.L., Pate, J.W., Sawyer, P.N., Trump, J.G., and Wright, K.: Sterilization of Preserved Bone Grafts by High Voltage Cathode Irradiation. J. Bone Joint Surg., 38A:862–884, 1956.
298. Udupa, K.N., and Gupta, L.P.: Role of Vitamin A in the Repair of Fracture. Indian J. Med. Res., 54:1122–1130, 1966.
299. Udupa, K.N., and Prasad, G.C.: Chemical and Histochemical Studies on the Organic Constituents in Fracture Repair in Rats. J. Bone Joint Surg., 45B:770–779, 1963.
300. Uhthoff, H.K., Bardos, D.I., and Liskova-Kiar, M.: The Advantages of Titanium Alloy Over Stainless Steel Plates for the Internal Fixation of Fractures: An Experimental Study in Dogs. J. Bone Joint Surg., 63B:427–434, 1981.

301. Uhtoff, H.K., Boisvert, D., and Finnegan, M.: Cortical Porosis Under Plates: Reaction to Unloading or Necrosis. J. Bone Joint Surg., 76A:1507–1512, 1994.
302. Uhthoff, H.K., and Dubuc, F.L.: Bone Structure Changes in the Dog Under Rigid Internal Fixation. Clin. Orthop., 81:165–170, 1971.
303. Uhthoff, H.K., and Rahn, B.A.: Healing Patterns of Metaphyseal Fractures. Clin. Orthop., 760:295–303, 1981.
304. Urbaniak, J.R., Cahill, J.D., and Mortenson, R.A.: Tendon Suturing Methods: Analysis of Tensile Strengths. *In* American Academy of Orthopaedic Surgeons: Symposium on Tendon Surgery in the Hand, pp. 70–80. St. Louis, C.V. Mosby, 1975.
305. Urist, M.R., Iwata, H., and Strates, B.S.: Bone Morphogenetic Protein and Proteinase. Clin. Orthop., 85:275–290, 1972.
306. Urist, M.R., and Johnson, R.W., Jr.: Calcification and Ossification: IV. The Healing of Fractures in Man Under Clinical Conditions. J. Bone Joint Surg., 25:375–426, 1943.
307. Vracko, R., and Benditt, E.P.: Basal Lamina: The Scaffold for Orderly Cell Replacement: Observations on Regeneration of Injured Skeletal Muscle Fibers and Capillaries. J. Cell. Biol., 115:129–139, 1986.
308. Walton, M., and Rothwell, A.G.: Reactions of Thigh Tissues of Sheep to Blunt Trauma. Clin. Orthop., 176:273–281, 1983.
309. Watson-Jones, R.: Fractures and Joint Injuries, 4th ed., vol. 2. Edinburgh, Livingstone, 1955.
310. Webber, R.J.M.: In Vitro Culture of Meniscal Tissue. Clin. Orthop., 252:114–120, 1990.
311. Weiland, A.J., and Daniel, R.K.: Microvascular Anastomoses for Bone Grafts in the Treatment of Massive Defects in Bone. J. Bone Joint Surg., 61A:98–104, 1979.
312. Welsh, R.P., MacNab, I., and Riley, V.: Biomechanical Studies of Rabbit Tendon. Clin. Orthop., 81:171–177, 1971.
313. Wendeberg, B.: Mineral Metabolism of Fractures of the Tibia in Man Studied With External Counting of Strontium 85. Acta Orthop. Scand. Suppl., 52:1–79, 1961.
314. White, A.A., III., Panjabi, M.M., and Southwick, W.O.: The Four Biomechanical Stages of Fracture Repair. J. Bone Joint Surg., 59A:188–192, 1977.
315. Wiancko, K.B., and Kowalewski, K.: Strength and Callus in Fractured Humerus of Rat Treated With Anti-anabolic and Anabolic Compounds. Acta Endocrinol., 36:310–318, 1961.
316. Widmann, R.F., Pelker, R.R., Friedlander, G.E., Panjabi, M.M., and Peschel, R.E.: Effects of Prefracture Irradiation on the Biomechanical Parameters of Fracture Healing. J. Orthop. Res., 11:422–428, 1993.
317. Wiel, H.E.V., Lips, P., Nauta, J., Patka, P., Haarman, H.J., and Teule, G.J.J.: Loss of Bone in the Proximal Part of the Femur Following Unstable Fractures of the Leg. J. Bone Joint Surg., 76A:230–236, 1994.
318. Wilson, P.D., Jr.: A Clinical Study of the Biomechanical Behavior of Massive Bone Transplants Used to Reconstruct Large Bone Defects. Clin. Orthop., 87:81–109, 1972.
319. Wolff, J.: Das Gaetz der Transformation: Transformation der Knocken. Berlin, Hirschwald, 1892.
320. Woll, T.S., and Duwelius, P.J.: The Segmental Tibia Fracture. Clin. Orthop., 281:204–207, 1992.
321. Woo, S.L.-Y., and Akeson, W.H.: Appropriate Design Criteria for Less Rigid Plates. *In* Lang, J.M. (ed.): Fracture Healing, pp. 159–172. New York, Churchill Livingstone, 1987.
322. Woo, S.L.-Y., Akeson, W.H., Levenetz, B., Coutts, R.D., Matthews, J.V., and Amiel, D.: Potential Application of Graphite Fiber and Methyl Methacrylate Resin Composites as Internal Fixation Plates. J. Biomed. Mater. Res., 8:321–338, 1974.
323. Woo, S.L.-Y., Maynard, J., Butler, D., et al.: Ligament, Tendon, and Joint Capsule Insetions Into Bone. *In* Woo, S.L.-Y., and Buckwalter, J.A. (eds.): Injury and Repair of the Musculoskeletal Soft Tissues, pp. 133–166. Park Ridge, Ill., American Academy of Orthopedic Surgeons, 1988.
324. Wray, J.B.: Vascular Regeneration in the Healing Fracture: An Experimental Study. Angiology, 14:134–138, 1963.
325. Wray, J.B.: The Influence of Various Hormones on the Fracture-Healing Process. Clin. Orthop. Rel. Res., 50:324, 1967.
326. Wright, T.M.: Biomaterials for Plate Fixation. *In* Lang, J.M. (ed.): Fracture Healing, pp. 173–179. New York, Churchill Livingstone, 1987.
327. Xavier, C.A.M., and Duarte, L.R.: Estimulca Ultra-sonica de Calo Osseo: Applicaca Clinica. Rev. Bras. Ortop., 18:73–80, 1983.
328. Yablon, I.G., and Cruess, R.L.: The Effect of Hyperbaric Oxygen of Fracture Healing in Rats. J. Trauma, 8:186–202, 1968.
329. Zaccalini, P.S., and Urist, M.R.: Traumatic Periosteal Proliferations in Rabbits: The Enigma of Experimental Myositis Ossificans Traumatica. J. Trauma, 4:344–357, 1964.
330. Ziegler, R., and Delling, G.: Effect of Calcitonin on the Regeneration of a Circumscribed Bone Defect (Bored Hole in the Rat Tibia). Acta Endocrinol., 69:497–506, 1972.

Rockwood and Green's Fractures in Adults, Fourth Edition,
edited by Charles A. Rockwood, David P. Green, Robert W. Bucholz and James D. Heckman.
Lippincott-Raven Publishers, Philadelphia © 1996.

CHAPTER 6

*Open Fractures**

Michael W. Chapman and Steven A. Olson

DEFINITION

An *open fracture* is one in which a break in the skin and underlying soft tissues leads directly into or communicates with the fracture and its hematoma. The term *compound fracture* refers to the same injury, but because it is archaic and nonspecific it will not be used in this chapter. Diagnosis of an open fracture can be difficult because the wound may be a considerable distance from the fracture site. When a wound occurs in the same limb segment as a fracture, the fracture must be considered open until proven otherwise.

Depending on the extent to which the soft tissues are injured, three specific consequences may result:

* Dr. Charles F. Gregory died in 1976, less than 1 year after the publication of the first edition of this book. His chapter on open fractures in the first edition was a classic example of his clear, incisive, and articulate style, and it serves to remind us that he was indeed one of the truly great teachers and educators in American orthopaedics.

In the second edition, Gregory's chapter was retained as written in the first edition, with a second part added by Michael W. Chapman and Sigvard T. Hansen, Jr. to provide current concepts. In this edition, Drs. Chapman and Olson have combined the two parts into one unified chapter. However, the important contributions of Dr. Gregory are retained in many parts of the chapter, in particular the sections on historical perspective, etiology, and initial management (including wound treatment).

(1) The most significant is the contamination of the area of injury by bacteria from the external environment. (2) Crushing, stripping, and devascularization of soft tissues render both those tissues and the bone they cover more susceptible to infection by the contaminating bacteria. (3) The destruction or loss of soft tissues that normally ensheathe bone may affect the methods by which the fracture can effectively be immobilized and may deny the fracture site the usual contribution from overlying soft tissues in the bone healing process (generation of osteoprogenitor cells for union and consolidation); and there may be direct loss of function owing to damaged muscles, tendons, nerves, vessels, and skin.

The first of these consequences is nearly universal. The other two vary with the extent of soft-tissue damage: a minor injury managed properly arouses no great concern; a major problem may dictate immediate or early amputation.

The prognosis in open fractures is determined primarily by the amount of devitalized soft tissue caused by the injury and by the level and type of bacterial contamination. These two factors working in combination, rather than the configuration of the fracture itself, are the primary determinants of the outcome. The extent of soft-tissue devitalization is determined by the energy absorbed by the limb at the time of injury (see Etiology). The most important and ultimate goal in the treatment of open fractures is to restore limb and patient function as early and as fully as possible. To achieve this goal, the surgeon must prevent infection, restore soft tissues, achieve bone union, avoid malunion, and institute early joint motion and muscle rehabilitation. Of these goals, the most important is to avoid infection, because infection is the most common event leading to malunion, nonunion, and loss of function.

HISTORICAL PERSPECTIVE

Hippocrates, it is said, considered war the most appropriate training ground for surgeons. His greatest contribution in this regard lay in his recognition that surgeons can only facilitate healing, they cannot impose it. He recognized the need to accept certain consequences of injury, like swelling, as essential and admonished against occlusive dressings before such swelling had occurred. He opposed frequent meddling with wounds, except to extrude purulent material, so long as the wound demonstrated progress in repairing itself. He further advocated "steel" or "iron" (actually the knife) in treating wounds that did not progress. His principal misconception is generally regarded as his aphorism, which held that diseases not curable by steel (knife) are curable by fire (cautery).

Galen and his followers also recognized purulence and admired it, considering it essential to the repair process. Frequent manipulations of a wound and a continuous search for medicaments that might be applied to enhance purulence were viewed as desirable in driving the wound to heal. Subsequently, most other schools represented one or the other of these viewpoints as a base for their particular methods of treatment.

Brunschwig and Botello, in the 15th and 16th centuries, advocated the removal of nonvital tissue from wounds that did not progress properly. The practice of applying hot oil to cauterize wounds changed in 1538 when Ambroise Paré (1510–1590), a French army surgeon, ran out of hot oil during the siege of Turin. He had only "a digestive made of yolk of egg, oyle of Roses, and Turpentine" and was surprised to find that his patients "dressed with a digestive only" were alive and nearly pain free the next morning. Paré also advised that "the wound must forthwith be enlarged . . . so that there may be free passage for both the puss or matter . . . obtained therein." The significance of Paré's discoveries were largely unrecognized during his day.[172] It remained for Desault, in the 18th century, to establish the making of a deep incision to explore a wound, remove dead tissue, and provide drainage. It was he who adopted the term *debridement.* His pupil, Larrey, extended the principle and included the issue of timing. The sooner debridement is done after wounding, he contended, the better the result.

After Mathysen's development of plaster-of-Paris bandages, the principle of occlusive dressings was reintroduced, only to lapse again because of untoward effects from misapplication.

Lister's introduction of carbolic acid dressings seemed the ultimate item in the galenic search for a magic medication that would persuade wounds to heal. Seized with alacrity, it too proved disappointing, likely because the principles of debridement were too soon forgotten or abandoned—an episode destined to be repeated so many times thereafter.

The imperative of debridement of missile wounds was reestablished more firmly during World War I, first by the German army and subsequently by the Allies. Thereafter, Trueta brought together the combination of debridement and an occlusive dressing that also served as a splint (the plaster cast) in the treatment of wounded extremities during the Spanish Civil War. By contrast with prior experience, his vast number of examples demonstrated the virtues of this method when properly applied.

World War II began just after the start of the sulfa era. Sulfa agents supplanted antiseptic solutions, but like them, they were applied directly to injured tissues. Antibiotics were available during the Korean War. Yet in each of these military endeavors, the primacy of debridement and the hippocratic precept of leaving the wound open had to be relearned and then reestablished by directive. The galenic hope that medicines might circumvent the need to leave wounds open for them to heal uneventfully was dashed again. To be sure, failure was often the result of technically inadequate debridement. Yet the open wound may heal despite that, but an inappropriately closed wound seldom can, even aided by antibiotics.

It seems now that the two major schools of thought can finally be brought together because the wound that is adequately debrided and is left open (hippocratic) may benefit additionally from an appropriate antibiotic (galenic) introduced at the proper time. Such wounds probably have the best prospect for healing uneventfully, whatever their subsequent management.

ETIOLOGY

The post–World War II era saw a gradual but distinct rise in the incidence of trauma in general until the mid 1960s, when it could be said to have reached a quasi-epidemic level. Open fractures have continued to constitute a significant proportion of recorded injuries. Even as there was an absolute increase in the number of open fractures, so there has been an apparent increase in the magnitude of the injuries incurred.

Fractures occurring in two, three, or even all four limbs are no longer unusual. Moreover, one or more of the fractures is likely to be an open one.

Analyses of the patterns of injury that result from certain kinds of violence, plus some limited experimentation on the direct effects of controlled, violent forces have produced some useful information. Such knowledge of the mechanism of injury may alert the physician to seek evidence of obscure injury known to be associated with such mechanisms.

The essential equation underlying what is usually an unexpected application of a violent force to the human body is expressed as $K = MV^2/2$ where M represents mass and V the velocity of the wounding force. The contest thus arranged is a measure of how much kinetic energy (K) can be absorbed by the body's tissues before they are injured, or how much injury occurs when the kinetic energy exceeds the ability of body tissues to resist or to absorb and disperse it. Moreover, the kinds of tissue injuries that occur vary in relation to the source of the kinetic energy. The converse holds equally true when the body itself is in motion and the offending or wounding agent is essentially stationary. There are numerous examples of combinations of both.

Some of the common circumstances of injury can be measured fairly accurately; others cannot. Although the variety of conditions of injury are almost numberless, they fall in large measure into one of the following categories:

1. The body is stationary and struck by a moving object.
2. The body is in motion and strikes a stationary object.
3. The body is in motion and strikes another moving object or body.

In reviewing some examples of these three arrangements, certain other factors must be appreciated; among them is the actual kinetic energy of moving objects—be it the object striking the body or the body itself—the size of the area of impact, and the capacity of the impacted tissue to absorb and disperse energy. Analyzing a few examples may be useful.

Open fracture of the tibia is a common injury often produced when a car strikes a pedestrian. Frequently, the initial contact is made over the posterior leg in the calf area. It is to be remembered that the force that remained great enough to fracture the tibia was transmitted first across the muscle bellies in the calf, even though the integument at that point had often remained intact. The muscles must have been damaged to some extent, and indeed we have found them on some occasions to be completely transected. The fractured bone ends are deflected anteriorly, against the rather thin, overlying soft tissue and skin, which then ruptures, creating the open fracture. In the course of debridement the surgeon who recognizes the potential damage to the posterior muscles may discover a communication between the fracture hematoma and the posterior compartment containing the damaged muscle. He or she must assume that contamination may have reached all parts of the wound, including the posterior compartment. The surgeon then faces a difficult decision. Should attention be confined to the anteriorly placed tissues, which are easily accessible, or should the posterior compartment be entered to deal with the injured tissue within?

In sharp contrast to the massive, relatively slow-moving car, which usually produces a broad area of impact when it strikes a body, a missile is a dense body of comparatively small mass. Yet, in accordance with the formula $K = MV^2/2$, the missile achieves a state in which it is highly freighted with kinetic energy. Moreover, it has a small impact area at contact, so that ordinarily its point of entry is small—approximately equal to its diameter. A number of factors enter into the pattern of subsequent effects, and they are worth a brief comment.

First, we must recall that gases are compressible and liquids are not. Should such a missile penetrate the chest wall and enter living tissue, it may pass through it, producing destruction only along its direct and immediate pathway (unless it should strike a bronchus or a large vessel). The air in the lung can be compressed momentarily as air in the flight path is pushed aside. On the contrary, when a rapidly moving missile strikes tissue with a high water content, such as the liver, it produces considerable displacement of the noncompressible liquid, creating in fact a significant momentary cavity.

An excellent illustration of this behavior can be easily contrived as follows: make two targets, one a sealed can empty except for atmosphere and the other a sealed can of the same size containing sauerkraut, which has a water content approximately equal to that of muscle or liver. Using a rifle with reasonably high-velocity bullets, hit each target from the same distance. If your marksmanship is equal to it, you will see the empty can jump from its resting place, and when it is examined it will demonstrate small holes of entry and exit with little other distortion. Next hit the target can of sauerkraut, and you will note that it virtually explodes. Often its ends will be blown loose and its seam split, the whole greatly distorted. The sauerkraut will be widely spread about the area.

Muscle behaves in a similar fashion when struck by a high-velocity missile, except that the cavity that permanently disrupted the rigid can tends to be only a momentary cavity in an animal or human limb. The surrounding elastic tissues recollapse the cavity walls, leaving only the small pathway of destruction made by actual contact of the missile with tissue as the residual identifiable wound. Two corollary events may also occur, events that will not be noted unless one is aware of the foregoing mechanism. First, the fluid wave that displaces tissue as the momentary cavity comes into existence may stretch or contuse adjacent nerves and blood vessels in the vicinity of the wave effect. Second, atmospheric air tends to rush into the momentary wound cavity in response to the rapidly produced vacuum and to sweep in with it whatever material lies adjacent to the entry wound. The material thus introduced may well contain bacteria. We shall consider the clinical significance of these observations later, and their importance will become evident.

Yet another example of the usefulness of knowledge regarding the etiology of an injury is the matter of close-range shotgun wounds.[123] The shotgun shell usually contains a large number of small pellets. Although they are intended to scatter at target distance, initially they move from the gun barrel in a rather dense group called a shot cloud. If, while still quite closely packed, they strike a target, their collective impact may be somewhat like that of a bullet. However, each pellet has so much less kinetic energy than a bullet that they are soon expended. Thus, many such injuries are only penetrating ones. Occasionally, some of the shot cloud emerges from the opposite side of the limb, producing a perforating wound. There is also a danger from shell wadding, a material that used to be made of jute and hair compressed with a binding agent. Wadding is impervious to gases and literally pushes the shot down the gun barrel ahead of it when the powder is ignited. The wadding is less dense but has greater mass and tends eventually to fall behind the shot cloud in flight, although remaining fairly close to the cloud and having the same trajectory for several feet. Thus, frequently the wadding enters the wound with the shot cloud, particularly in close-range shotgun injuries. Old-style wadding, which is still being used, is extremely irritating to tissues and incites a severe inflammatory response. Thus it must be removed. Often it is difficult to locate even when its presence is suspected, and, indeed, all too frequently it has been overlooked—to the ultimate detriment of the wound and the patient. Modern shotgun shells use a plastic plug in place of wadding and are therefore less damaging. However, in close-range wounds you must look for the plug.

Two other examples of somewhat special circumstances beset with hazards to the patient and surgeon are worth consideration. Not infrequently, a limb is caught in a violent compressive force, as often occurs when a motorcycle rider catches a leg between the machine and a car in a sideswipe collision. Sometimes the visible wound of the soft tissues is only modest, and the limb is not grossly deformed. X-rays may confirm the diagnosis of fracture, but there is considerable increase in the separation between the tibia and fibula. This is a sign of severe soft-tissue injury, which usually includes stripping of the extremely tough interosseous membrane. Intense swelling often follows, which, if it does not directly injure vessels, often produces compartment syndromes. Such swelling and its consequences can be anticipated by noting this tipoff in the x-rays, and measures may be taken to prevent trouble.

Wounds incurred in a tornado are virtually always contaminated by finely dispersed soil, which literally fills the air in this awesome phenomenon. Importantly, such soil often carries a variety of usual and unusual pathogens, many anaerobic. Recorded experience has indicated clearly that closing such wounds is likely to lead to serious infections, including those produced by clostridia.

Finally, injuries involving the rotary lawn mower are unique to our time. Persons are sometimes struck by such unlikely a pseudomissile as a bit of wire or other metal set in flight by contact with a mower blade. The wounds produced are usually small, yet the pseudomissile may bury itself within a body cavity or even bone, which is some indication of the kinetic energy transferred to it by the mower blade. More importantly, it is an indication of the energy contained in the whirling tip of the mower blade itself, which in high-speed machines develops a significant, sustained blade-tip velocity. Coupled with its mass, it is capable of producing a great deal of kinetic energy.

As noted, unusual pathogenic bacteria are found in the wounds incurred by tornado victims. And in a very real sense, a wound produced by a mower blade is created in a minor tornado. The normally earthbound bacteria afloat with the detritus in the vacuum created in a mower casing may result in a wound inoculated by bacteria similar to those in a tornado. For the same reasons cited, we believe it wise never to close such wounds but to debride them and leave them open.

These few major examples of the multiple factors related to different kinds of injury illustrate the usefulness of knowing something about the "history" of how an injury was incurred. Although there are many others, of course, those mentioned should make the point. Moreover, they underscore the need for further investigation about wounding mechanisms and their immediate and late effects on tissues.

CLASSIFICATION

Classification of open fractures is important because it allows comparison of results in scientific publications, but more importantly because it gives the surgeon guidelines for prognosis and permits us to make some statements about methods of treatment. In North America and throughout most of the world, the wound classification system of Gustilo and Anderson[64] and the subsequent modification by Gustilo, Gruninger, and Davis[62,65,67] is the most widely accepted and quoted. This classification is used throughout this chapter.

We find that there is wide variation in the interpretation and use of the Gustilo-Anderson classification, and generally there is too much emphasis on wound size. The critical factors in their classification system are (1) the degree of soft-tissue injury and (2) the degree of contamination. A devastating crush injury of the leg necessitating amputation may be associated with only a small skin wound. The size of the skin wound is therefore a poor guide to the classification of the fracture. A very large wound caused by a sharp object such as a knife may have minimal associated soft-tissue crush and therefore may carry a very good prognosis. The configuration of the fracture, particularly from the standpoint of the amount of displacement and comminution evident, often points to the amount of energy absorbed by the limb at the time of injury and is helpful in the classification but is secondary to soft-tissue considerations. For these reasons, we have chosen to clarify (rather than modify) the Gustilo-Anderson classification as we use it, in the hope that the reader will find it easier to use and more accurate than descriptions presented elsewhere. Table 6-1 provides a quick reference to these guidelines.

A *type I wound* is caused by a low-energy injury that is usually less than 1 cm long (Fig. 6-1). It is generally caused by the bone piercing from the inside outward rather than by a penetrating injury. Unless the wounding occurs in a highly contaminated environment, the level of bacterial contamination is usually fairly low. A type I classification implies minimal or no muscle damage. As mentioned, a type I wound should not be judged by its size alone, because small wounds can be associated with dangerously contaminated wounds (eg, those occurring in a farmyard), and with high-energy trauma (eg, crush wounds of the tibia in pedestrians hit by automobiles). The surgeon

TABLE 6-1
Classification of Open Fractures

Type	Wound	Level of Contamination	Soft-Tissue Injury	Bone Injury
I	<1 cm long	Clean	Minimal	Simple, minimal comminution
II	>1 cm long	Moderate	Moderate, some muscle damage	Moderate comminution
III*				
A	Usually >10 cm long	High	Severe with crushing	Usually comminuted; soft-tissue coverage of bone possible
B	Usually >10 cm long	High	Very severe loss of coverage	Bone coverage poor; usually requires soft-tissue reconstructive surgery
C	Usually >10 cm long	High	Very severe loss of coverage plus vascular injury requiring repair	Bone coverage poor; usually requires soft-tissue reconstructive surgery

* Segmental fractures, farmyard injuries, fractures occurring in a highly contaminated environment, shotgun wounds, or high-velocity gunshot wounds automatically result in classification as a type III open fracture.

(Chapman, M.W.: The Role of Intramedullary Fixation in Open Fractures, Clin. Orthop., 212:27, 1986.)

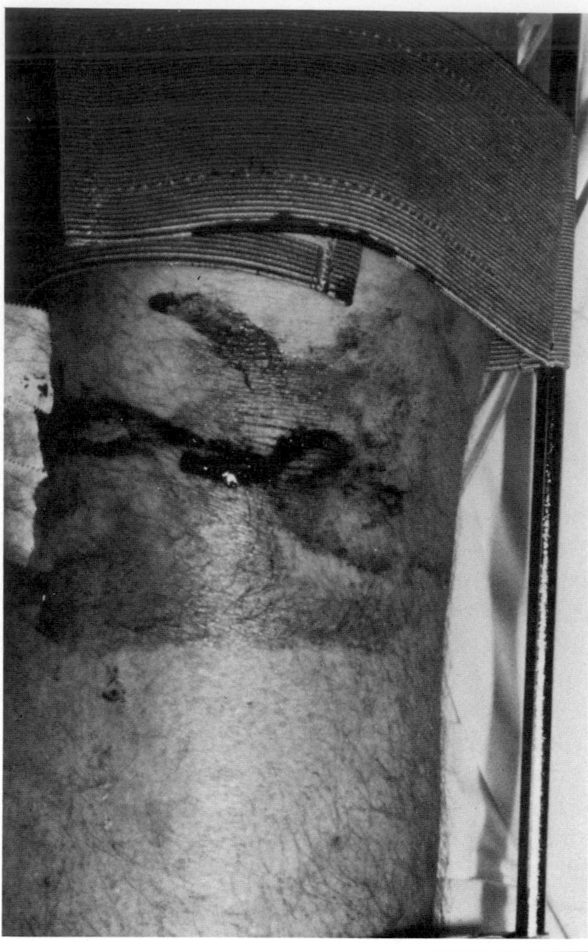

FIGURE 6-1. Type I open fracture.

must take all factors into account when classifying open fractures.

A *type II wound* is greater than 1 cm in length and has a moderate amount of soft-tissue damage, owing to a higher-energy injury (Fig. 6-2). These are generally outside-to-inside injuries. (This is a somewhat broad classification falling between type I and type III wounds.) Some necrotic muscle is usually present, but the amount of debridement required is minimal to moderate and is usually confined to one compartment. The soft tissue stripped from bone is none to minimal, and wound closure without skin grafts or local flaps should be possible.

A *type III wound* results from a high-energy, outside-to-inside injury and is generally longer than 10 cm with extensive muscle devitalization. Generally, the fracture is widely displaced or comminuted, although this is not an essential component (Fig. 6-3). The following factors always make an open fracture a type III wound: a shotgun wound, a high-velocity gunshot wound, a segmental fracture with displacement, a fracture with diaphyseal segmental loss, a fracture with an associated major vascular injury requiring repair, a wound occurring in a farmyard or other highly contaminated environment, or a fracture caused by the crushing force from a fast-moving vehicle. The energy of the injury and the degree of soft-tissue devitalization *must* be taken into account when applying this wound classification. Type III wounds can be further classified as follows:

A *type IIIA open fracture* is one in which there is limited stripping of the periosteum and soft tissues from bone, and bone coverage does not present any major problems. The overall soft-tissue envelope about the fracture is usually fairly well preserved.

A *type IIIB open fracture* is one in which there has been extensive stripping of soft tissues and periosteum from bone, and where devitalization or loss of soft tissues usually requires a local flap or free tissue transfer for closure.

A *type IIIC open fracture* is one in which there is a major vascular injury requiring repair for salvage of the extremity.

The classification of open fractures, according to the Gustillo-Anderson system requires both objective and subjective evaluation of the injured limb. The classifi-

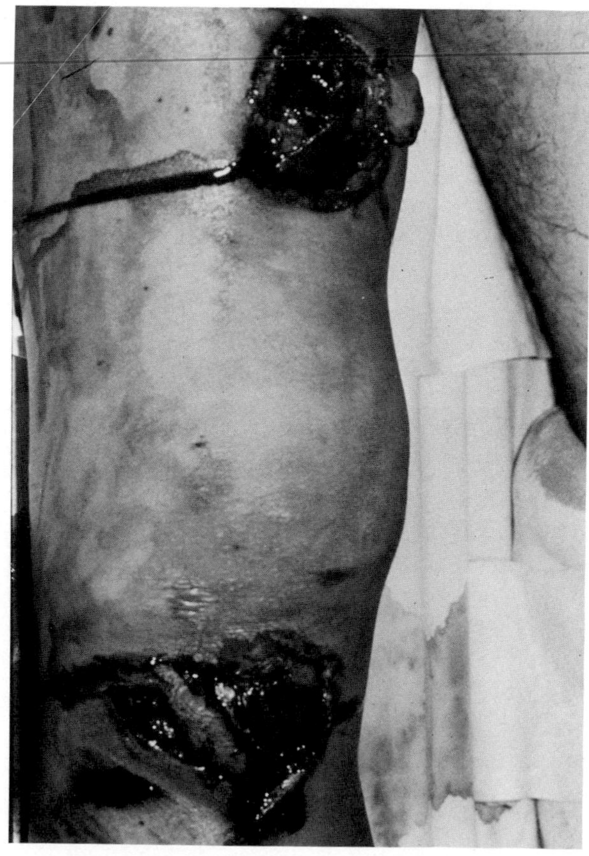

FIGURE 6-2. Type II open fracture.

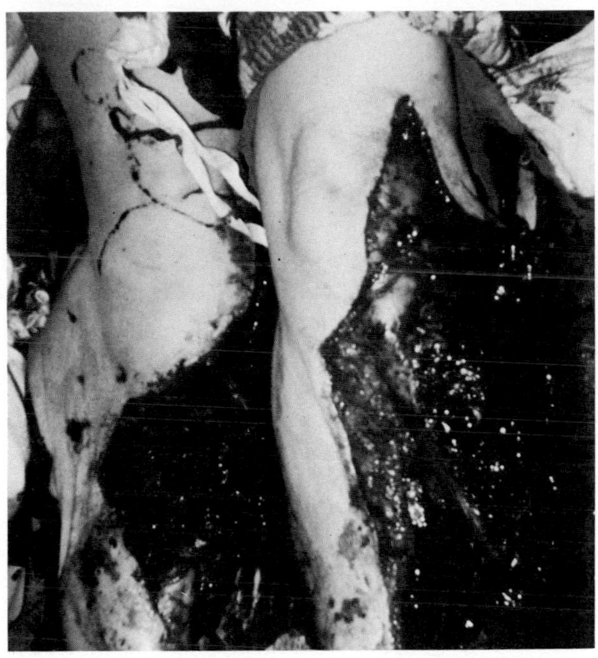

FIGURE 6-3. Type III open fracture.

cation of an open fracture should be established at the time of operative debridement of the wound. Attempts to classify an open fracture, and therefore determine treatment, before thorough debridement and assessment of the wound and soft-tissue injury, can be misleading. Brumback and associates[23] have reported on the interobserver agreement in the classification of open fractures of the tibia using the Gustillo-Anderson system. The number of respondents who agreed on the grade for each of a group of 125 randomized open fractures averaged 60%. Of the respondents who had trauma fellowship training, the agreement rose to 66% (range 40%–100%).

Attempts to modify the Gustillo-Anderson system or develop alternative open-fracture classification systems have been made. Trafton[163] proposed a classification for open tibia fractures, which combined elements of the Gustillo-Anderson and Tscherne classifications into minor, moderate, or major injuries. The AO/ASIF group has proposed an open fracture classification to grade soft-tissue injury to be used in conjunction with the AO/ASIF alpha-numeric fracture classification system. The soft-tissue grade incorporates the degree of injury to the integument (IO for open injuries), muscle tendon injury (MT), and neurovascular injury (NV).[136] Trafton's modified classification offers potential simplicity in classification, while the AO/ASIF system offers a detailed and potentially cumbersome system for grading open fractures that may be best suited for research. Neither of these systems has been validated in prospective clinical studies.

Tscherne and the Trauma Department at Hannover, Germany, have developed an open fracture score that considers the AO/ASIF fracture classification; bone loss; loss of soft tissue, skin, and muscle; neurovascular injury and the presence of compartment syndrome; foreign body contamination; final bacteriologic analysis; and time from injury to onset of treatment. This score provides four categories, types I through IV, based on points allocated for each category. This open fracture classification has been reported in a prospective series of 651 open fractures treated in Hannover, Germany, from 1984 to 1989.[136]

EXAMINATION OF THE WOUND AND INITIAL EMERGENCY MANAGEMENT

Although an obvious open fracture may attract initial attention, you must first direct your efforts at identifying life-threatening conditions and be as complete in the initial evaluation as the condition of the patient permits.[150] The "ABCs" of initial management (A—airway, B—bleeding, and C—circulation) are addressed first. The patient must have an adequate airway and ventilation, and pulmonary function must be adequate to sustain life. Compression dressings are applied to control extremity hemorrhage. Evidence of inadequate circulation (shock) requires immediate fluid resuscitation; and in severe shock, administration of blood and an immediate search for hidden, life-threatening sources of hemorrhage in the abdomen or chest should be done. When any immediate threat to the patient's life has been eliminated, a thorough, systematic examination of the patient is performed, assessing consciousness and central nervous system function, evaluating the cervical spine, and, in the multiply injured patient, applying a cervical collar until a lateral cervical spine film can be taken. The thorax, abdomen, and genitourinary systems are evaluated. The spine and pelvis are examined carefully for evidence of fractures or dislocations or both. Careful, meticulous examination of the apparently uninjured extremities is essential. Most patients require an immediate anteroposterior x-ray of the chest and pelvis. Initial sterile compression dressings and splints may be necessary before adequate evaluation of an open fracture wound, to stabilize the patient for life-salvaging procedures. As soon as possible, careful examination of the wound is performed.

In major trauma centers, surgeons from several surgical disciplines are often available for the initial resuscitation and care of the patient. This allows the orthopaedic surgeon to focus on the injuries of the musculoskeletal system. In smaller hospitals, however, the orthopaedic surgeon may be responsible for the complete care of the patient, including resuscitation and maintenance of life until a general surgeon or neurosurgeon can be summoned. In such cases, the measures outlined earlier are critical, so the surgeon can proceed with examination of the obviously injured extremity in a methodical and deliberate fashion, feeling comfortable that no other unrecognized or unassessed injury is likely to emerge suddenly or that the patient will be further compromised by neglect or oversight. This plea for a deliberate and orderly assessment underscores the fundamental principle that in dealing with the injured, one should take nothing for granted. To look offers the prospect to know—not to look is to guess. As an additional example (given by Gregory), even now one of the well-known triads of injury associated with fracture of the femoral shaft is still overlooked with distressing frequency: ipsilateral dislocation of the hip, fracture of the femoral neck, or ligamentous injury of the knee.

Initially, the circulation to the extremity and its neurologic function are assessed. If the limb is in a displaced or distorted position, we prefer to assess it before it is restored to its anatomical position to ensure that no neurovascular injury is caused by the manipulation. In most cases the limb will be in a reasonably normal position in a splint applied by emergency personnel in the field. One should note the state of circulation to the limb as indicated by capillary blush, the filling of veins, and the status of peripheral pulses. The limb should be examined meticulously for the function of the peripheral nerves. Initial sensory examination by pressure and light touch gives a gross evaluation of the sensation in the limb, but examination for two-point discrimination is often necessary to detect more subtle losses, particularly in the upper extremity. Examination for motor function is difficult in the injured limb owing to pain and splinting secondary to muscle spasm. Often, the only valid motor evaluation is that done by the initial examiner. Once the patient learns how uncomfortable the examination may be, further cooperation may be blunted and the evaluation made inadequate. For this reason, the initial examiner must do a complete examination and record all findings. The normal side must be compared with the abnormal side and results recorded using the guidelines to motor strength illustrated in Table 6-2. This is vital because a partial peroneal nerve palsy caused by the injury is often overlooked with an inadequate examination or inexact recording of the findings. Pain interfering with the examination can be minimized by good splinting of the fracture and stabilization of the joints not involved in the test for motor function. After the examination, if the limb is not in reasonably normal alignment, it should be returned to normal alignment with gentle traction, appropriately splinted, then reexamined.

Next, the skin around the wounds is examined. Is it burned? Is it contaminated with usual or unusual agents—dirt, dust, petroleum products, fertilizer? Contaminants on the skin around the wound may also have invaded it. What are the dimensions and shape of the wound? Is the surrounding tissue badly abraded, contused, or flayed from its fascial bed? The entire circumference of the wound is examined, including the patient's back and buttocks. It is surprising how often significant wounds on the posterior side of the body are overlooked initially. The danger lies, of course, in not making provisions for dealing with them when formal treatment of the limb is undertaken. Polaroid photographs of the wound and limb that can be inserted directly into the medical record at the time they are taken are invaluable, both before and after formal wound debridement. Serial photographs throughout the treatment of the limb prove to be useful in educating the patient and family and are often vital in legal proceedings. If photography is not available, then a sketch of the limb and the wound often serves better than paragraphs of written description.

Because all open fractures will be formally debrided, there is little justification for exploration of the wounds in the emergency department. Digital exploration provides little useful information, risks further contamination, and may precipitate profuse bleeding.

TABLE 6-2
Motor Strength Testing

Numerical Grade	Adjective Grade	Testing Parameters
0	Zero	No palpable muscle action
1	Trace	Muscle contraction palpable, produces no limb motion
2	Poor	Moves limb, but less than full range of motion against gravity
3	Fair	Moves limb segment through full range of motion against gravity
4	Good	Muscle strength better than fair but less than normal
5	Normal	Comparable to contralateral normal limb or expected normal strength in given individual

Local or regional anesthetics administered in the emergency department to alleviate pain or enhance wound exploration are unnecessary and can hamper subsequent care because they may preclude an accurate neurologic examination on a serial basis or by subsequent examiners. Obvious foreign bodies are removed with sterile forceps or a sterily gloved hand. If the patient will undergo formal debridement of the wound within an hour or so, then a sterile compression dressing is applied. If a delay of more than 1 hour is expected, the wound is flushed gently with 1 to 2 L of sterile saline poured from a container and then a sterile dressing is applied. Some clinicians advocate application of povidone-soaked dressings, but it has been suggested that povidone interferes with osteoblast function so we do not use it. Patzakis[125,126] advocates a predebridement culture from the wound in the emergency department before administration of antibiotics or any antiseptics; again, we are not certain that this is helpful. The validity of these cultures is discussed in more detail in the section on antibiotic management later in this chapter. Bactericidal intravenous antibiotics should be started as soon as possible.

Prehospital treatment of open fractures has improved greatly with the advent of organized emergency medical systems. Patients who arrive in the emergency department with an appropriately splinted extremity with a sterile dressing over the wound of an open fracture should be assessed for adequacy of arterial profusion and neurologic function. Under these circumstances, if there is no indication that the splint or dressing is compromising vascular perfusion, the sterile dressing applied in the field should be left in place until the patient is taken to the operating room for surgical debridement of the wound. Tscherne and associates[165] have reported that the infection rate in patients with open fractures is increased if the wound is subject to repeated inspections or careless handling before operative debridement. However, when the patient arrives with an inadequate or no splint or dressing, then examination of the wound, as described earlier, and application of a sterile dressing and splint in a timely manner is appropriate.

When a small wound in the skin overlies or is in the vicinity of a fracture, immediately the question arises as to whether the wound communicates with the fracture site, thus making it an open fracture. The safest way to answer this question is formal debridement of the wound, tracing it until its deepest extent is established. However, if the wound is treatable in the emergency department and the fracture or joint injury is treatable by closed means, formal debridement, particularly of a very minor wound, in the operating room may not be necessary. In the case of joints, particularly the knee, this question can often be answered by injecting the joint with saline or methylene blue solution and looking for egress of the solution from the wound. Although this method is not 100% dependable in revealing whether there is communication, it has been used in our facility for the past 10 years with no apparent adverse outcomes. That is, we have not failed to formally debride a wound that has subsequently proven to have penetrated a joint. The same method can be used in the case of fractures by injecting saline or methylene blue through a sterile prepared area of intact skin into the underlying fracture hematoma. If this escapes through the wound, an open fracture is present. However, there is the hazard of contaminating a closed fracture hematoma, and as with joints, a ball-valve effect of the soft tissue may prevent leakage of the fluid when, in fact, a communication does exist. If there is any suspicion at all that a wound may communicate with a joint or adjacent fracture, formal debridement should be performed.

Having resuscitated the patient, saved his or her life, and carried out initial assessment, bandaging, and splinting of the fracture, the clinician must then complete the patient's history and obtain as many details as possible about the injury.

Patient History

In severely injured patients it may not be possible to obtain more than the rudiments of an adequate history, owing to a patient's altered mental status or need to be taken immediately to the operating room. Obviously, as complete a history as possible must be obtained from the patient and from relatives, witnesses, ambulance attendants, or anyone who may have useful information.

The patient's immunity to tetanus should be determined if at all possible. If the patient has been immunized against tetanus in the past 10 years, only toxoid may be needed as a booster. If the patient has not had a recent immunization, or if the history is uncertain, 250 to 500 units of tetanus human immune globulin are administered and tetanus toxoid is given as well.

The clinician should try to elicit all points in the medical history, but particularly those that may influence management of the open fracture wound, such as a history of diabetes mellitus, chronic steroid use, or the presence of other debilitating disease. A compromised immune system (particularly a history of active acquired immunodeficiency syndrome), may push one toward early amputation in a patient with a severe type IIIB or IIIC open fracture rather than risking a severe infection that could be life threatening.

The complete history and physical examination and all information gathered to this point must be carefully and accurately recorded, including all measures taken in the treatment of the patient, the time they were carried out, and the patient's response to them.

Radiographic Examination

A discussion of x-ray examination of the open fracture has been delayed for the same reason that the taking of x-rays is usually delayed until the steps already discussed have been carried out. Several initial films are often critical to the care of the severely injured patient, including a lateral view of the cervical spine and anteroposterior views of the chest and pelvis. In well-equipped emergency departments, these are taken by overhead-mounted machines in the resuscitation room. In less well-equipped emergency departments, use of portable x-ray equipment in the resuscitation room may be necessary. Ideally, x-rays should be taken in a regular x-ray examination room rather than using portable equipment in the operating room because the quality of films that can be obtained and the various views possible are much better.

Extremity x-rays can usually be deferred until the patient's general condition has been stabilized, life-threatening emergencies have been eliminated, and the wound has been inspected and dressed and the fracture splinted as already outlined. Nothing annoys us more than to find a patient lying on an x-ray table with an open wound and an unsplinted, deformed limb. Radiographic examination is simply an adjunct to the initial evaluation of the patient, and obtaining x-rays under such conditions simply contributes to the patient's hemorrhage, contamination of the wound, and further soft-tissue injury—to say nothing of the discomfort to the patient. Although well-padded plaster splints are the quickest and most effective way of immobilizing an open fracture, the plaster will interfere with the radiographic examination, particularly in injuries about joints. We encourage the use of radiolucent splints, if at all possible. Patients with multiple injuries may require a considerable number of x-rays, including cystograms, urethrograms, intravenous pyelograms, and multiple skeletal x-rays. Computed tomographic (CT) scans of the head, abdomen, or pelvis may also be necessary. Careful planning to minimize the number of times the patient needs to be moved is not only more humane but also more efficient.

Good-quality anteroposterior and lateral x-rays of the fracture, including full visualization of the joints above and below, is the minimum examination necessary in any open fracture. Special views may be required to elucidate the full extent of the injury. In some dislocations and fracture–dislocations, adequate films can be obtained only after reduction. In such cases, a "scout" film may suffice for initial reduction, and then a more complete examination can be performed. A good example is a dislocation of the knee with compromised neurovascular function, when immediate reduction is essential. A complete radiographic evaluation is performed only after the dislocation or fracture has been reduced and the neurovascular status has been reevaluated. In most cases of this type, immediate arteriography to rule out vascular injury is indicated. Also, in the ankle and subtalar joints persistent dislocation may threaten neurovascular structures or skin, and adequate x-ray evaluation is rarely possible. After an initial scout film, closed reduction in the emergency department followed by splinting and complete radiographic examination is usually indicated. Reduction should be delayed *only* when closed reduction is not possible without a general or regional anesthetic.

Other useful findings, particularly in the soft tissues, may emerge on radiographic evaluation. Radiopaque foreign material may be seen, alerting the surgeon to seek it during debridement. Not uncommonly, air trapped in soft-tissue planes may reveal a much more extensive injury than originally suspected. In addition, this finding may help interpret similar gas shadows found in a wound a few hours later, when gas-forming bacteria may be the only other logical explanation.

Finally, preoperative planning is essential for adequate care of the fracture and complete radiographic examination is essential to this planning. It allows selection of the appropriate method for dealing with the fracture and may indicate the need to have more than one fracture stabilization system available.

PREPARATION FOR SURGICAL DEBRIDEMENT

The reader is referred to the excellent text of Mast and coauthors[102] on preoperative planning. In preoperative planning, the order in which multiple fractures will be treated, the teams necessary to treat them, and the soft-tissue and bone instruments needed are identified and made available. Open fractures often present unexpected surprises; therefore, a full set of soft-tissue and bone instruments must be immediately available. One must plan for all contingencies. The full assortment of fixation devices that might be necessary to stabilize the fracture must be available. The optimal position of the patient on the operating table and the need for an orthopaedic fracture table or fluoroscopy must be determined. Occasionally, in a clean type I open fracture where primary internal fixation is carried out (eg, a displaced fracture of the radial shaft in an adult) immediate cancellous bone grafting may be advisable. If so, a possible bone graft donor site should be selected.

Even the most grossly contaminated open fracture is not yet infected. In addition to eliminating the contaminating bacteria from the wound, it is critical to avoid further contamination by hospital-based organisms, which may prove to be far more virulent than those already in the wound. For this reason, irrigation and debridement must be carried out in a surgical suite and not in an emergency department. The approach to the fracture must be the same as for all clean elective orthopaedic surgery from the standpoint of preparation and execution. An irrigation pan (Fig. 6-4) is very useful to collect the large volumes of fluid necessary for adequate irrigation while keeping the operative field dry.

The emergency department splint and dressing are removed, and while maintaining gentle traction to prevent further injury to soft tissues, the limb is elevated for the surgical preparation. If possible, a tourniquet is applied to the upper thigh or arm. A sterile tourniquet should be available in the event that the proximal extent of the wound precludes the use of a nonsterile tourniquet. A two-phase surgical preparation of the limb helps minimize further contamination of the wound and makes the surgical preparation most effective. With one preparation set, the entire limb is washed from the fingertips or toes to the tourniquet to eliminate gross contamination. A liter of sterile saline is poured over the wound and any obvious debris is removed. The second preparation kit is opened and formal surgical preparation of the entire extremity is performed. If profuse hemorrhage is encountered during the surgical preparation, inflation of the tourniquet will limit blood loss. The limb is draped free, and the nonsterile table top is covered with a plastic or other moisture-proof drape.

IRRIGATION AND DEBRIDEMENT

Gregory noted that in discussions of debridement it is generally held that irrigation is the single most essential maneuver of the entire procedure. This is not quite true, of course, in that the critical aspect is the removal of all nonviable and contaminated tissue, and therefore the debridement itself is the essential maneuver. However, there are two adages that apply to open fracture irrigation: "If a little does some good, a lot will do a great deal more," and, "The solution to pollution is dilution." The importance of copious irrigation was emphasized by Gustilo and associates,[70] who showed that in a series in which less than 10 L of normal saline was used for irrigation there was a higher incidence of infection than in a series in which more than 10 L was used. Whether 10 L should be run through every wound is less important than the fact that irrigation must be thorough and copious. We prefer to use irrigation and debridement simultaneously. Some of the advantages of irrigation are as follows:

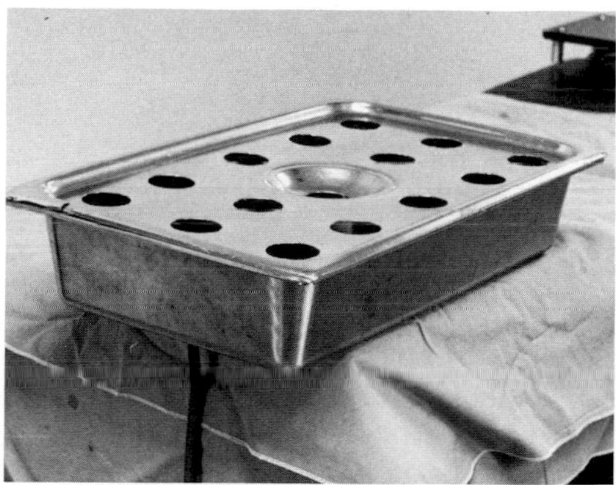

FIGURE 6-4. When a limb is to be prepped or debridement is to be performed, placing the limb on the perforated surface of a pan facilitates the necessary rinsing and sluicing with considerable quantities of fluid; because a drainage tube vents the effluent into a pail on the floor, the operative field can be kept dry.

1. Initial lavage by flushing away blood and other debris clears the wound for inspection, thus facilitating the removal of foreign material and debridement.
2. Irrigation fluid floats otherwise undetected and often necrotic fronds of fascia, fat, or muscle into the field where they can be seen and excised.
3. Lavage floats contaminated blood clots and loose pieces of tissue and debris from unseen recesses and tissue planes.
4. Lavage of the tissue restores its normal color and facilitates determination of viability.
5. Irrigation reduces the bacterial population.

Equally as important as the volume of irrigant used is the method of irrigation. Forceful streams such as those provided by a "Water Pik" may actually drive foreign material and bacteria into the tissue planes, which is obviously undesirable. Several mechanical irrigators are now widely available that pump aseptic irrigation fluids through shower heads in a pulsatile manner. These irrigators provide an ideal stream of irrigation solution over a broad area. They are far more effective than bulb syringes, and we recommend their routine use.

A number of authors have added to our knowledge of wound irrigation.[1,60,135,165] Anglen and associates[1] showed that pulse lavage with saline solution as compared with bulb syringe irrigation resulted in a 100-fold decrease in the bacterial count of a glycocalyx producing *Staphylococcus.* Similar results were encountered when either bacitracin or neomycin were added to the irrigation solution. Notable, however, was that the addition of a soap detergent (castile soap) to the pulse lavage solution decreased the bacterial count 100-fold. On the basis of their study it would appear that the addition of antibiotics to the saline used in pulse-lavage provides no added benefit.

Kellam and associates[89] reported that irrigation of fractures with solutions of povidone-iodine (Betadine) or hydrogen peroxide resulted in marked decrease in osteoblast function. No adverse effects were observed with local application of bacitracin.

Unfortunately, a prospective randomized study of actual open fractures to evaluate the clinical efficacy of these various regimens has not yet been published.

Debridement (literal translation—"unbridling") was once employed only in the treatment of infected wounds, as an incision to release the purulent contents of the wounds. Gradually it was realized that removal of necrotic tissue at the time of debridement was beneficial; and finally it was recognized that removal of wound debris and necrotic tissue is best carried out as early as possible after injury.

The objectives of debridement (and irrigation) are as follows:

1. Detection and removal of foreign material, especially organic foreign material
2. Detection and removal of nonviable tissues
3. Reduction of bacterial contamination
4. Creation of a wound that can tolerate the residual bacterial contamination and heal without infection.

Proper use of a tourniquet in the debridement of open fractures is essential. One should always have a noninflated tourniquet on the limb because it may be necessary to control severe hemorrhage encountered when a blood clot is removed from an unexpected major arterial injury. However, the tourniquet should not be inflated unless necessary to control bleeding, either for visualization or to limit blood loss, because the anoxia produced by the tourniquet interferes with evaluation of the viability of muscle. One major advantage of the tourniquet is that inflation for 10 minutes or so, followed by release, results in capillary flush of the skin distal to the tourniquet, which gives a good indication of the skin's viability. Thus, appropriate use of the tourniquet includes intermittent inflation during irrigation and debridement as indicated but *not* constant inflation throughout the procedure.

Skin and Subcutaneous Fat

An extensile incision is used that will provide effective debridement and appropriate visualization of neurovascular structures, as needed, and of the contaminated bone ends. Appropriate incisions require good judgment and a willingness to be innovative to avoid trapping oneself with a surgical approach that is not useful or produces further damage, such as distally based flaps that may become necrotic. Small puncture wounds or holes are excised as well as small, ragged flaps that are not essential to closure (Fig. 6-5). The elliptical wound thus produced is usually easily closed with sutures and can even be left open for spontaneous closure, leaving a simple linear scar. Coring wounds should be avoided because this leaves a round hole that can only close by granulation and scar formation. The cicatrix thus produced often retracts and leaves an ugly, puckered wound. Many wounds are transverse or oblique to the longitudinal axis of the limb. These can be extended by four means, illustrated in Figure 6-6. In general, we find the flaps created are smaller than the other methods, thus minimizing the risk of flap necrosis while producing the best exposure. The following points must be considered before proceeding with debridement of skin and making elective incisions:

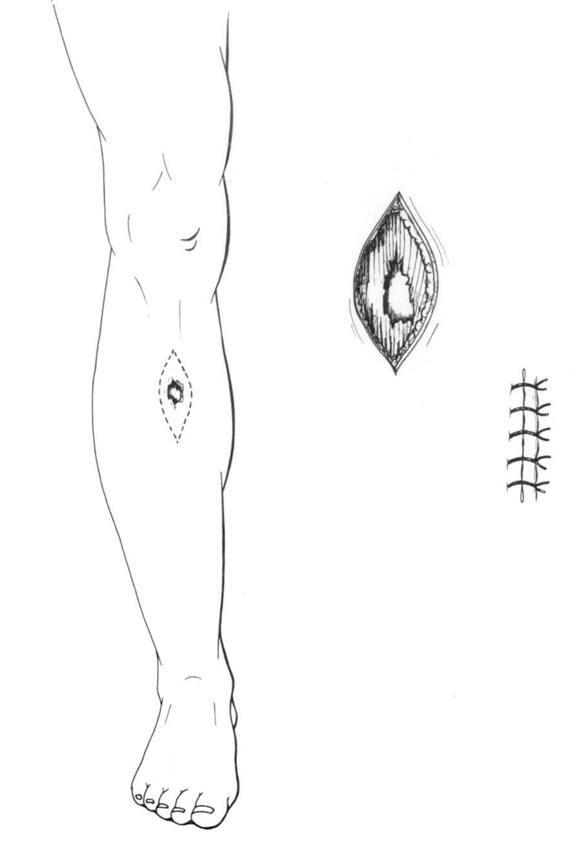

FIGURE 6-5. An elliptical excision of the fracture wound permits proper inspection of the area of injury as well as better closure if the wound is sutured.

1. The amount of gross loss of skin and subcutaneous fat
2. The extent of degloving that has occurred, which may influence the apparently viable skin remaining
3. The need to extend existing wounds for adequate exposure and the best directions for such extensions
4. The usefulness or dangers of connecting adjacent yet separate wounds

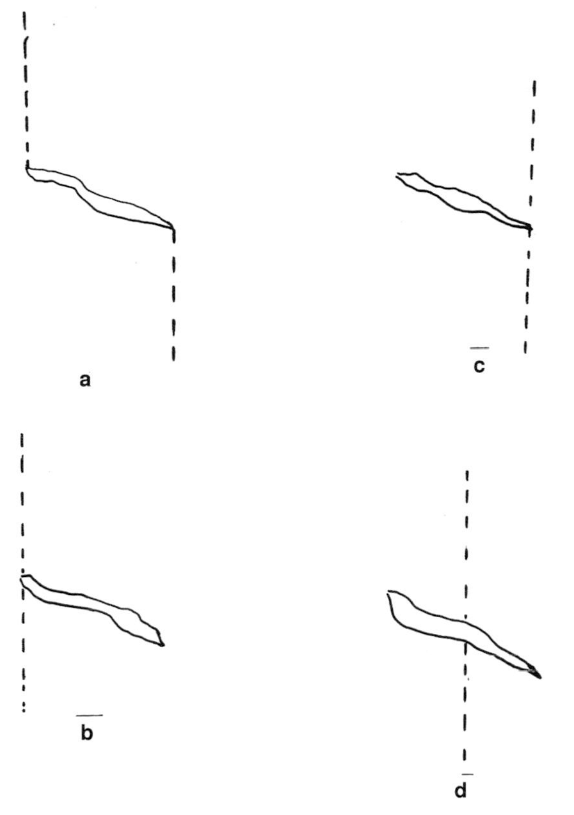

FIGURE 6-6. Methods of extension of a traumatic transverse or oblique wound. **(A)** This "2-plasty" technique produces two large flaps and risks necrosis of the tips of the flaps. **(B)** Both of these methods also produce **(C)** large flaps risking necrosis of the tips. **(D)** Crossing the wound results in the smallest flaps. This minimizes the risk of flap necrosis and is the incision of choice.

5. The prospect of survival for flaps created by the injury or by planned incisions
6. The amount of skin that can be sacrificed, if any, and its effect on subsequent closure
7. The usefulness of counterincisions to facilitate adequate debridement, arrange bone coverage, or provide for wound drainage
8. The likelihood that a planned incision may transect a major superficial vein
9. The age of the patient and the state of skin and subcutaneous tissues
10. The need to develop a sufficiently wide wound that will allow thorough inspection of its deepest recesses.

Beginning with the skin and subcutaneous fat, one should initiate a methodical, layer-by-layer debridement of the traumatic wound. One must be conservative in the excision of skin, particularly where it is at a premium (eg, over the tibia and in the foot and hand). In the hand, for example, particularly in stellate-type lacerations of the digits, excision of skin edges may be contraindicated. Where adequate skin is available, sharp excision of the contaminated and contused skin edge—1 to 2 mm into good-quality skin with a sharp blade placed at right angles to the skin—removes contaminated and nonviable skin and provides a good wound edge for subsequent closure. This gives the best cosmetic result. The forceps used on skin should always be toothed and should be used with care to avoid further contusion. Frequent changing of the knife blade is necessary to ensure a sharp, well-performed debridement.

The question of how much of an additional elective incision is required for deep exposure always arises. In wounds caused by high-energy injuries, a useful axiom is that the wound should be equal in length to the diameter of the limb at that level. A better guide is to expose the fracture site and then continue exposure until healthy tissues are encountered and all areas of periosteal stripping have been identified. Although adequate debridement is obviously necessary, one should not unnecessarily open uninvolved, clean, intact soft-tissue planes. In particular, detaching skin from its underlying fascial attachment should be avoided because the vertical vessels to the skin necessary for survival of the skin will be damaged. Meticulous hemostasis is done as debridement progresses, because considerable blood can be lost during debridement of even moderate-sized wounds.

A traumatic skin flap that has a base-to-length ratio of more than 1:2, particularly if distally based, will frequently have a nonviable tip. This can be ascertained by looking for capillary flush after deflation of a tourniquet, as described earlier. Some clinicians advocate the injection of an ampule of fluorescein and visualization of the flap with Wood's lamp. Obviously, nonviable portions should be excised, but any skin that is marginal should be left; this can always be debrided later, and skin is not the major pabulum for infection but rather, necrotic muscle. If very large wounds are produced by loss of skin and subsequent coverage is expected to be difficult, it may be possible to harvest skin from the excised flap. A Padgett dermatome works well, set at a 0.010- to 0.012-inch thickness. The graft is run through a 1-to-1 $^1/_2$ or 1-to-3 skin mesher and then widely spread. Often the graft can be applied immediately to viable muscle and fascia, because it does not actually result in closure of the wound and will rapidly epithelialize for coverage. Before an elective incision is made, the wound is irrigated with 2 L or more of saline (depending on the size of the wound) until foreign debris and blood clot are no longer visible in the wound and the tissues appear clean and fresh. It is important to do this before making the elective incisions to minimize contamination of the elective portion of the wound. At each layer of the debridement, the wound should be methodically debrided. At the level of muscle and bone, in type II or higher open fractures, at least 6 L of saline is used. When combined with the initial 2 L and the final 2 L containing antibiotic solution, this results in a minimum irrigation of 10 L for any type II or larger wound.

Fascia

Any nonviable, damaged, or contaminated fascia should be excised. No marginal fascia should be left. We believe limited fasciotomy is indicated in all open fractures secondary to high-energy injuries, and complete fasciotomy of all compartments is often indicated. This is discussed in more detail in the section on fasciotomy.

Muscle

Whereas skin tends to tear or be punctured, and fascia to split or shred, muscle, because of its high water content, is subject to hydraulic damage by fluid waves when an injuring object impacts the limb. This is particularly true of high-velocity gunshot wounds. Of equal importance is that a high-energy fracture secondary to indirect rapid loading (eg, a high-velocity skiing injury) may result in comminution of the tibia or femur, in which the bone literally explodes into many fragments. These fragments travel rapidly outward into the muscle and can cause significant muscle damage even when the outer envelope is seemingly undamaged. A small bone fragment may pierce the skin, producing what appears to be a very minor type I open fracture, when in fact there may be considerable deep muscle damage. This occurs because the more rapidly bone is loaded before fracture, the more energy is required to fracture it, and the more explosive the fracture is when it occurs. Because of this absence of direct physical trauma, it is easy to overlook nonvital muscle because it may not immediately be evident that it has been disturbed or damaged.

Necrotic muscle is the major pabulum for bacterial growth and poses a great danger in anaerobic infections. Every effort should be made to remove all nonvital muscle tissue, although often this will require careful judgment. In muscle debridement the approach of Brav[19] is the safest: "When in doubt, take it out." In type I, II, and IIIA open fractures this may be taken literally, but in types IIIB and IIIC, debridement of an entire muscle or compartment may be necessary to meet this axiom. If the major arterial supply to a severely damaged muscle has been destroyed, the only recourse is total excision. It has been our experience, however, that if even 10% of a muscle belly and its attached tendon can be preserved, significant function is retained. For that reason, there may be an indication for leaving some marginal muscle at the time of initial debridement in severe open fractures, then returning within 24 to 48 hours for redebridement, at which time the muscle will have better declared its viability. The exception to this approach is in wartime or mass casualties, where preservation of life takes precedence over the desire to preserve function.

Judgment of the viability of muscle is challenging, and the alliterative quartet provided by Gregory in his original chapter must be addressed by the surgeon: *color, consistency, contractility,* and *capacity to bleed.* Scully and associates,[147] in an attempt to correlate four features with histologic evidence of viability, concluded that consistency and capacity to bleed were the most significant. In my experience, contractility and consistency have been the most reliable, because color and capacity to bleed are easily misinterpreted. Remember that the hypoxemia associated with the use of a tourniquet, or in the presence of shock or injury to a major vessel of the involved limb, may make evaluation of these parameters difficult. The following qualifications should be observed in the applications of these indications of viability.

Color

Color can be misleading and is generally a poor guide to viability. Muscle that is dark or even black on its surface may only represent a thin layer of blood lying beneath the myonesium, or hemorrhage within the muscle substance that does not threaten viability. When freed of this thin layer, the underlying muscle may be found to be of normal color. In our experience, nonviable muscle generally is salmon, yellow, or gray and is distinctly different from the robust pink or red seen in normal muscle.

Consistency

Muscle consistency is a subjective evaluation and ranges from normal firm tissue to the stringy, friable, and even mushy state of severely damaged or disintegrating tissue. The firmer the muscle, the more certain it is viable. It is often useful to extend the wound to obviously uninjured viable muscle and compare its consistency to that in the injured area. Normal muscle, when pinched gently with a toothed forceps, immediately rebounds to its normal shape, leaving no marks from the sharp tips of the forceps. This is a delicate test, and crushing of the tissue must be avoided. When a gentle squeeze of the forceps leaves its mark in the muscle, viability is in question.

Contractility

Contractility clearly establishes muscle viability. Muscle tissue that vigorously retreats from the incising edge of a scalpel is obviously alive. Good-quality muscle will normally respond with a localized contraction to the gentle pinch of a toothed forceps or to the stimulation from a nerve stimulator unit or Bovie, set on a number 1 or 2 setting. Normally, debridement should be carried out until all muscle remaining in the wound is contractile.

Capacity to Bleed

Vigorous bleeding may produce spurious evidence of viability. The muscle may be crushed, and there may be no substantial flow through the capillary beds of the muscle, yet the arterioles may continue to bleed vigorously when transected. On the contrary, gentle, persistent oozing from capillaries tends to demonstrate adequate local perfusion, indicating that the muscle is probably viable. This distinction is subtle and demands the surgeon's attention. Muscle and other tissues injured in a point blank shotgun blast may appear "cherry red" from carbon monoxide staining. Debridement of this muscle should continue until the muscle bleeds easily and stops with routine hemostasis techniques.[171]

Tendons

Tendons, unless obviously severely damaged and contaminated, are not a major pabulum for infection; and if essential to function, they should be preserved. Where coverage of tendons by some type of soft tissue is not possible, preservation of the peritenon is essential for tendon survival. For that reason, we tend to not debride peritenon but rather copiously irrigate it. If tendon without peritenon must be left exposed in an open wound, a moist dressing must be applied and kept moist until coverage of the tendon can be obtained (see Wound Closure). If at all possible, one should try to swing some muscle, subcutaneous fat, or skin over tendon without peritenon.

Bone

Whereas muscle tissue may mount a defense against invading bacteria, bone tissue is essentially defenseless, owing to its relatively poor blood supply. If judgments about muscle viability seem troublesome, judgments about what is to be done with bone fragments are perplexing. In general, small bits of cortical bone that are free of any soft-tissue attachments should be removed. In areas of cancellous bone, a fracture may produce significant free, small fragments of cancellous bone. If these are not obviously contaminated, and if they contribute to the reconstruction of the fracture, they can be retained as bone graft. However, if a large cortical fragment constituting a significant segment of the injured bone is removed, the resulting gap will require bone grafting; this can pose treatment problems. If such a fragment has obvious soft-tissue connections, and especially if its small vessels bleed on the exposed surface, it should be retained, even if the surfaces must be trimmed to eliminate minor contamination. Unless it is grossly contaminated, the fragment probably should be preserved. The major judgment problem lies with a bone fragment that has only a tenuous soft-tissue attachment or is completely free. Its value as a bone graft, perfectly fitting the defect, is obvious. However, is it sufficiently free of contamination that it will be tolerated, or will it act as a foreign body, aggravating any infection that might occur? There are no absolute criteria, and judgment is based on experience. The inexperienced surgeon is wisest to debride the fragment. Although this risks delayed union or nonunion, it minimizes the risk of infection. There is no question that a delayed union or nonunion is a far less challenging complication than an infected nonunion.

In low-energy fractures in which a major cortical bone fragment is essential to an internal fixation construct, when the surgeon is confident that the level of contamination is low and adequate irrigation and debridement has been carried out, the fragment can be retained in the construct.[169] This allows for early redebridement if infection intervenes. In addition, retention of a large, segmental fragment of bone may lead to nonunion at one or both ends of the free fragment, and bridging of the nonviable fragment with onlay cancellous bone graft may be advisable at some time during treatment (see section on bone grafting). In the case of free butterfly fragments or segmental pieces in fractures where external fixation will provide the primary stabilization, interfragmentary screw fixation of the free fragment to the adjacent viable bone is usually indicated, followed by bone grafting across the junction site later.

As a general rule, bone debridement initially can be conservative; however, if infection intervenes, early aggressive redebridement of all nonviable bone is important. It is better to deal with the reconstruction of a large segmental defect than to allow chronic infection to result in chronic osteomyelitis, which may lead to even more bone loss. Our most common judgment error in the management of infected open fractures has been the delayed excision of nonviable bone.

Determination of the viability of bone is difficult. Although we have personally not found them to be useful, (1) injection of fluorescein and observation of bone with a Wood's lamp at the time of surgery and (2) injection with a tetracycline label before redebridement and observation with Wood's lamp have been described as useful methods in determining bone viability. The best method may prove to be laser-Doppler flowmetry to evaluate blood flow, but its efficacy in the debridement of open fractures has not yet been established.[158,159]

As described with tendons, bone without periosteum and not covered by soft tissue quickly desiccates and dies. It is critical, therefore, to preserve any periosteum attached to the bone where bone will not be immediately covered by muscle or subcutaneous fat and skin. It is usually better to thoroughly irrigate periosteum that is attached, rather than debride it, if coverage cannot be obtained (see Wound Closure).

Joints

Any wound that enters a joint mandates exploration. The wound is debrided as described earlier down to the level of the joint. The traumatic wound itself may permit adequate exploration, or an extensile incision may be necessary. In many joints, however, adequate exploration through the arthrotomy will not be possible unless the incision is very large; this is particularly true in the knee and shoulder. Under these circumstances, it may be better to combine debridement of the wound with arthroscopic examination of the joint. If fluid leakage through the wound is a problem, the synovium should be closed and arthroscopic inspection carried out in the usual fashion. It is critical that the entire joint be adequately explored, because unexpected foreign bodies or osteochondral fractures are frequently found.

Nerves and Vessels

Brisk, small vessel or arterial bleeders encountered during debridement require immediate ligation or coagulation. Methodical, layer-by-layer hemostasis is important to limit blood loss. General oozing from capillary-sized vessels generally abates with time and compression. Major vessel injuries requiring repair are usually identified before surgery and appropriately planned for but may be encountered unexpectedly during debridement. Because it is often difficult to know exactly how much time has lapsed from injury and loss of blood supply to the limb to the initiation of vascular repair, reinstitution of circulation is of primary importance. In our experience, loss of total blood supply to the limb for more than 8 hours nearly always results in amputation. If there has been a significant delay, we prefer to do a very quick irrigation and debridement of the wound to remove the grossest contamination and then proceed with vascular repair. This is particularly important if the repair must be done through the open fracture wound. There are exceptions, however; for example, if the open fracture wound is anterior to the knee and repair of a popliteal artery requires an independent elective posteromedial exposure, appropriate initial surgical preparation of the limb should be performed using the two-phase method described previously; the traumatic wound is occluded with a barrier drape and exposure is proceeded with immediately for vascular repair. In the presence of arterial injury necessitating repair, as much venous outflow as possible during the debridement is preserved.

In larger vessels, rather than carrying out immediate end-to-end anastomosis or vein grafting, it may be better to insert a temporary shunt. This permits irrigation and debridement and stabilization of the bone before final vascular repair. This may be important to establish proper limb length and avoid injury to the vessel during the bone repair.

When vascular repair is necessary, repeat debridement is frequently required, and easy visualization of the entire limb to assess circulation is important. For this reason, some clinicians advocate routine internal or external fixation in such situations. Others, notably Rich and associates[130] and Connolly,[36] have shown that nonoperative immobilization works well—especially in a mass casualty situation. (The issue of internal fixation in open fractures is dealt with later.)

Fasciotomy

After arterial repair, massive swelling distal to the site of repair is very common, particularly in the forearm or leg. Because fasciotomy so often becomes necessary in such cases, I urge you to do it prophylactically in essentially every case. If there is any doubt about its indication, it probably should be done. Moreover, it is better done too early than too late.

In the forearm, both the volar and dorsal compartments must be relieved by two incisions placed at 180° to each other over the appropriate compartment. On the volar surface, the lacertus fibrosis (proximally) and carpal tunnel (distally) must be released.

In the leg, all four compartments (anterior, lateral, superficial posterior, and deep posterior) must be released. In our opinion this is best done through one long incision over the lateral compartment. Exposure of the deep fascia for a short distance anterior and posterior to this incision, followed by a transverse incision through the fascia at the midpoint of the leg, allows easy identification of the vertical fascial planes, separating the anterior, lateral, and posterior compartments. Each compartment is released independently with a longitudinal incision extending the full length of the compartment. After release of the superficial posterior compartment, blunt dissection is done posterior to the lateral compartment and the fascia of the deep posterior compartment is released.[103]

Patman and Thompson[124] suggested four-compartment fasciotomy by resecting the fibular shaft through a single incision. We believe this is unnecessarily aggressive. Loss of the fibular shaft increases instability of the leg and removes an essential structure for reconstruction. We believe this method of compartment release is contraindicated.

In nearly all open fractures of type II or higher, or those with a crushing component, we advocate routine limited fasciotomy. This is easily accomplished by directing a pair of scissors subcutaneously to split the fascia longitudinally. Often this step will prevent a compartment syndrome, and it adds only minimal morbidity. However, it is important to continue to observe for compartment syndrome because a more complete fasciotomy may still be necessary. Medial and lateral incisions for fasciotomy of the tibia may be preferable when open reduction and internal fixation of articular injuries (eg, tibial plateau fractures) are indicated.

After formal fasciotomy, the skin should not be closed because it may be as constricting as the fascia if severe swelling occurs. Frequently, skin grafts are required to provide coverage of such wounds because swelling recedes too slowly to permit suturing. However, this added morbidity pales in contrast to that visited on the patient who needs a compartment decompression but does not receive it.

Foreign Bodies and Gunshot Wounds

Foreign bodies, especially organic ones, must be sought and removed because they often lead to significant morbidity if left in the wound. Fragments of wood are especially troublesome, because they are easily buried in tissue and, after becoming blood-soaked, resemble adjacent muscle. Cloth and leather, on the other hand, are usually found in the planes between tissues, but may find recesses remote from the site of injury. The intrinsic recesses, pits, or crevices of the foreign material may harbor pathogenic organisms or their spores. The foreign body itself, especially if organic, is likely to incite an inflammatory response.

Bullets, and especially pellets, are usually buried. Unless they are easily detected, surgical exploration to find them may entail more hazard by injury to the tissue disturbed than if they are left in situ. Shotgun pellets are removed only as they are encountered during the debridement or if they have damaged a major blood vessel or nerve. Bullets in veins have been reported on rare occasions to become emboli. An exception to the matter of removing lead bullets or particles occurs if they lie, in whole or in part, within a joint or in the subarachnoid space. Joint or subarachnoid fluid acting on lead tends to break it down and, as Leonard[96] has reported, can induce serious synovitis as well as low-grade lead poisoning. Bullet fragments and pellets thought to be in joints are generally best sought with the arthroscope, where possible; otherwise, open arthrotomy is indicated.

Shotgun wounds are less treacherous today than in the past in that horsehair wadding has been replaced by a plastic plug. However, both wadding and plugs should be sought and removed; this is most important if old shotgun shells have been used and horse hair wadding is present. Close-range shotgun wounds that perforate, and thereby create wounds of entrance and of exit, make access available to both wounds and thus facilitate thorough inspection and debridement. When the wound is simply penetrating (ie, no exit wound), thorough inspection is often difficult. Frequently, the shot cloud comes to lie against the fascia on the far side of the limb (Fig. 6-7). In this situation, a counterincision is usually justified to remove the wadding or plastic plug.

Fractures that are the result of a low-velocity gunshot wound to the extremity are an increasingly common injury in the United States. Management of these fractures requires an initial patient assessment and evaluation of the neurovascular status of the extremities as previously described. Fractures that have normal vascular perfusion can be managed with local debridement of the skin edges, without formal irrigation and debridement of the deeper soft-tissue injury.[51] Some centers continue to prefer open debridement. We recommend the routine use of intravenous antibiotics (1 g cefazolin) at the time of debridement. Antibiotic therapy is continued postoperatively if internal fixation of the fracture is performed. Dickey and coworkers,[39] in a prospective trial of no antibiotics versus 1 g of cefazolin given every 8 hours for 72 hours in a

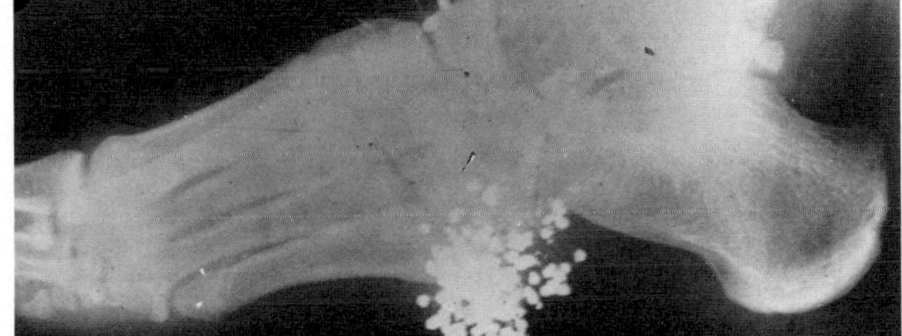

FIGURE 6-7. The shot cloud has traversed this foot from its dorsal aspect but has come to lie on the deep aspect of the plantar fascia. It serves as a clue to the location of any associated shell wadding that may also have entered the wound.

series of 67 low-velocity gunshot fractures that did not require operative stabilization, reported no difference in infection rates. Both acute and delayed intramedullary stabilization of femoral shaft fractures resulting from low-velocity gunshot wounds has been reported.[78] The incidence of infection and delayed union or nonunion is similar with these different treatment methods. Early stabilization of femoral shaft fractures did result in a decrease in hospital stay and hospital costs as well.

Gunshot wounds that pass through the abdomen and exit through the soft tissues or buttock with bowel contamination require special attention. These injuries require debridement of both the intra-abdominal and the extra-abdominal soft-tissue bullet track. In this situation, fecal contamination can spread to the soft tissues of the buttock or abdominal wall musculature, resulting in a soft-tissue abscess developing on a delayed basis if not addressed at the time of debridement.

IMMEDIATE OR EARLY AMPUTATION VERSUS LIMB SALVAGE

Immediate or early amputation through the fracture site may be indicated under the following circumstances:

1. When the limb is nonviable; that is, when there is a vascular injury that is nonrepairable or is accompanied by warm ischemia time over 8 hours; or the limb is so severely crushed that there is minimal viable tissue remaining for revascularization
2. When, even after revascularization, the limb is so severely damaged in whole or in part that function is less satisfactory than that afforded by a prosthesis
3. In severely injured limbs in the presence of severe, debilitating, chronic disease where preservation of the limb is a threat to the patient's life (eg, a severe type IIIC open fracture of the distal tibia in an elderly patient with severe diabetes with vascular disease and severe peripheral neuropathy)
4. In a limb in which the severity of the injury will demand several operative procedures and a prolonged reconstruction time that is incompatible with the personal, sociologic, and economic consequences the patient is willing to withstand (eg, a heavy equipment operator with multiple open fractures of the foot, in which reconstruction, particularly of the soft tissues, may demand a year or more, and when the outcome is uncertain; a Syme amputation could return this patient to work within a few months).

   Georgiadis and colleagues[52] compared the results of long-term functional assessment and quality of life assessments for patients who have undergone limb salvage versus immediate or early below-knee amputation. They found that patients who had limb salvage were more likely to consider themselves severely disabled and were more likely to have problems with the performance of occupational and recreational activities. However, there was no difference in their "quality of life" as measured by the Nottingham Health Profile. The economic impact of severely injured lower extremities can be substantial.[14]
5. In a military or mass casualty situation in which salvage of life or transport of the injured victim, plus the need to direct attention to more severely injured patients, would justify amputation rather than the prolonged surgical effort necessary to salvage a severely injured extremity
6. In a patient with severe, multisystem injuries with an injury severity score† of approximately 20 or more, in whom salvage of a marginal extremity may result in a systemic load of necrotic tissue and inflammatory byproducts so high that it could induce pulmonary or multiple organ failure and lead to death
7. In cases of replantation, where the function expected does not justify salvage (eg, amputation of a single finger through zone 2—the area of the proximal phalanx).

Lange and associates[94] have published absolute and relative indications for immediate amputation that are good guidelines. In fractures of the tibia their absolute indications for amputation are a type IIIC fracture in which vascular repair is required for salvage of the extremity, the injury is accompanied by complete transection of the posterior tibial nerve, and the limb is nonviable. Relative indications are items 2 through 5 in the preceding list. Attempts to develop predictive criteria for limb salvage versus amputation have included the Mangled Extremity Syndrome Index (MESI),[57] the Predictive Salvage Index (PSI),[137] the Limb Salvage Index (LSI), and the Mangled Extremity Severity Score (MESS; Table 6-3).[13,74,59,106,153] The MESS score was developed as a retrospective analysis of 26 patients with severe lower extremity injuries, all requiring arterial revascularization for potential salvage. A point score was given for each of four categories, including skeletal and soft-tissue injury, limb ischemia time, shock, and age of the patient. A total MESS score of 7 or greater is predictive of amputation. The MESS criteria have been evaluated in a prospective

† The Abbreviated Injury Scale, rev. ed. Arlington Heights, Il., American Association for Automotive Medicine, 1985.

TABLE 6-3
Mangled Extremity Severity Score (MESS)

Category	Points
A. Skeletal/soft-tissue injury	
Low energy (stab, simple fracture, low velocity gunshot wound)	1
Medium energy (open or multiple fractures, dislocation)	2
High energy (close range shotgun, high velocity gunshot, crush)	3
Very high energy (above + gross contamination, soft-tissue avulsion)	4
B Limb ischemia	
Pulse reduced or absent but perfusion normal	1*
Pulseless, paresthesias, diminished capillary refill	2*
Cool, paralyzed, insensate, numb	3*
C. Shock	
Systolic blood pressure always >90 mm Hg	0
Hypotensive transiently	1
Persistent hypotension	2
D. Age (Years)	
<30	0
30–50	1
>50	2
Mangled Extremity Severity Score (Total Points)	

* Score doubles for ischemia >6 hours.

manner with good predictive ability for limb salvage with a MESS score of 6 or below. Retrospective studies applying the MESS criteria to patients with severe soft-tissue injuries with and without vascular injury requiring revascularization have reported varying results in predictability of the MESS score.[13,57,74,86,106] The use of the MESS criteria in extremities with severe soft-tissue and bony injuries but no arterial disruption should be tempered with clinical judgment. A retrospective review of the MESS score applied to severe upper extremity long bone fractures found good correlation of a MESS score greater than 7 with amputation in 37 patients. Prospective evaluation of upper extremity injuries with the MESS has not yet been published. Attempts to modify the MESS score to provide greater emphasis on the soft-tissue injury has resulted in the NISSSA score.[106] Prospective evaluation of this modification of the MESS score is not available.

Limb salvage can also effect the patient's survival. Sudkamp and the Hannover group have emphasized the need for early amputation in the severely polytraumatized patient. They recommend early amputation for type III and type IV open fractures and type III closed fractures (Hannover classification system) when the overall survival rate is 50% or less, based on the Hannover Polytrauma Score. Roessler and associates reported three patients with isolated IIIC lower extremity injuries who died of multiple organ failure after a limb salvage attempt was made. They recommend careful monitoring of hemodynamic status after limb salvage attempts and believe early amputation is indicated if the patient is more than 3 L of fluid positive at 24 hours after reperfusion of the limb. These recommendations have not been validated in a prospective series.

Often, the full extent of injury is not known before going to the operating room. If amputation is a serious consideration, it must be discussed with the patient before the initial debridement, if possible, and consent obtained for immediate amputation if it is determined to be indicated. In unconscious patients or when appropriate informed consent is not obtainable, the limb should be amputated only if it is nonsalvageable or it is a threat to the patient's life. In such circumstances, documentation by at least two other surgeons—preferably one from another specialty—accompanied by photographs placed in the medical record, is appropriate. If the limb appears to be salvageable, it may be best to complete the initial debridement, assess the extent of the injury, and then sit down with the patient under less harried and emotional circumstances to discuss rationally the pros and cons of reconstruction versus amputation of the limb. We believe it is critical, however, to make this decision early. It is a great disservice to the patient and very costly to the patient and to society to perform multiple surgical procedures over a 1- to 2-year period to salvage a badly mutilated limb, only to finally perform an amputation because the patient grows weary of the prolonged treatment or the limb is simply not functional or is too painful.

STABILIZATION OF THE BONE

Once vascular repair has been completed and the limb salvaged, or irrigation and debridement have been done, stabilization of the bone is the next concern.

The Importance of Skeletal Stability

Achievement of stability means restoration of the fracture to as close to anatomical position as possible, with sufficient stability that multiple wound procedures will be possible and early function can be instituted. At the outset, reestablishment of good alignment realigns neurovascular structures, which provides optimal circulation to the injured extremity and minimizes the risk of compromising peripheral nerves. Restoration of normal length reduces the dead space in which blood can accumulate. Hematoma is avascular and is a pabulum for infection. Restoration of normal anatomy improves venous and lymphatic return, thereby reducing soft-tissue swelling. At the microscopic level, bone stability helps stabilize soft-tissue planes. This facilitates capillary proliferation and ingrowth to revascularize devitalized bone and soft tissues. Early revascularization of devitalized structures improves local tissue resistance to infection. Stabilization and approximation of soft-tissue planes also facilitates diffusion of nutrients and antibodies and facilitates white blood cell migration. All of these factors contribute to "local wound defense" against infection.

From the standpoint of the whole patient, fracture stability permits muscle rehabilitation and joint motion, which facilitates early return to function. The studies of Salter and associates[139] and Mitchell and Shepard[109] have shown that rigid internal fixation of osteochondral fractures and early restoration of joint motion are essential to achieve good cartilage healing and to prevent joint stiffness and intra-articular adhesions. In multiply injured patients, stabilization of major long-bone and axial skeletal fractures permits early mobilization, which facilitates cardiopulmonary care, may prevent thromboembolic phenomena, and has been shown to reduce morbidity and mortality.[15,88,104,148]

Stability can be achieved by traditional plaster-cast or traction immobilization, more functionally oriented cast bracing, cast-brace traction, pins and plaster, external fixation, internal fixation with devices including intramedullary rods, plates, and screws, or combinations of these methods.

Virtually all methods presently employed in the management of closed fractures can also be applied, within certain limits, to open fractures. However, in the open fracture, management of the bone fragments cannot logically be considered apart from the soft-tissue wound. If the wound is minor, it is usually not much of a problem; but when the soft-tissue injury is extensive, often including significant loss of skin and ensheathing muscle, it may make management of the fracture most formidable. Thus, what might be done with the fractured bone per se must often yield to what serves the best interest of the soft tissues—at least at the time of initial treatment. Whichever method of fracture treatment is chosen, it should meet certain criteria:

1. It should not compromise further the injured soft tissues.
2. It should maintain length of the bone, especially in the lower extremity and forearm.
3. It should produce good alignment of bone fragments, especially the joint surfaces in intra-articular fractures.

As in the treatment of closed fractures, it is difficult to be dogmatic about any one open fracture, and no one technique seems clearly superior to any other in *all* cases. For the surgeon who deals with open fractures only occasionally or on a temporary basis, the simpler the method, the better. Such a policy creates fewer problems for the first surgeon and provides greater latitude for definitive treatment by the last surgeon. However, the surgeon who treats open fractures on a regular basis must be aware of and consider the full range of available techniques, and even combine them or, when indicated, improvise.

Some open fractures seem to be open only "technically." A small, almost unnoticeable, wound may be associated with a minor fracture line in the underlying bone, whose fragments show no displacement on x-rays; this is indeed an open fracture. Such injuries are seductive in their appearance and treacherous. The danger of serious, even fatal infection proceeding from this circumstance has already been mentioned. The wound should receive the same consideration as any open fracture. The fracture as such may simply be splinted by a plaster slab or a cast. When the wound has healed, a definitive cast may be applied until the fracture is sufficiently united.

Larger wounds or those extended in the course of debridement and associated with displaced bone fragments frequently permit reduction under direct visualization. Yet the visualization is not always all that might be desired, because wounds, unlike incisions made for the purpose of exposure, are often neither appropriately located nor sufficiently extensive. At other times, of course, wounds are so large that the surgeon is distressed by how much of the fractured bone is so readily visible.

Immobilization in Plaster

Plaster-of-Paris casts have limitations in the treatment of open fractures because they may make access to the wound difficult and because they involve a circumferential hard dressing on a limb with the potential for swelling, which can cause compartment syndrome. In addition, a plaster cast may not provide the degree of fracture stability desired. On the other hand, in type I and low-grade type II open fractures in which the wounds are moderate and manipulative reduction of the fracture fragments produces a stable, acceptable position, plaster-of-Paris cast immobilization may be quite appropriate, particularly in children. The same type of cast used for closed management is applied, incorporating the joints above and below the fracture.

A full-length longitudinal cut is always made in the cast with a cast saw after the plaster has dried to produce a univalved cast. Any underlying webril and stocking net are cut as well. A univalved cast is superior to a bivalved cast in that it can be spread to accommodate the limb without losing adequate fracture immobilization, and it provides more uniform decompression of the limb. A bivalved cast, when spread, provides decompression in only one axis of the limb, results in increased instability, and allows swelling of the skin between the bivalved portions of the cast, which may produce blisters.

There should be a way to easily expose the wound in the cast to inspect it or to carry out delayed primary closure. Simply windowing the cast may be unsatisfactory because the window may not be accurately located over the wound. Removal of the plaster and dressing may be difficult, resulting in wound contamination, and the edges of the window (which are flush with the limb) may make application of dressings difficult. To avoid this, a bubble is made in the cast directly over the wound; the bubble should be 1 to 2 inches in diameter larger than the widest part of the wound. This is accomplished by placing a bulky pad of loosely packed cast padding directly over the wound after the dressing and circumferential cast padding have been applied. The height of the bubble depends on the size of the wound. For a wound 2 inches long, a bubble 4 inches in diameter and approximately 2 inches high works well. This bubble has several advantages. First, it indicates precisely where the wound is located. Second, when the bubble is cut off by running the cast saw around the circumference of the bubble, it leaves a smooth lip on the cast which makes removal of the underlying dressings easy and avoids getting plaster debris in the wound. The cap of the bubble is easily removed without having to use cast spreaders and other instruments that might cause discomfort to the patient. When the cast padding in the bubble is removed, a cavity is produced that provides a nice elevated rim to protect the wound and a space in which dressing changes are easy to perform. Because the bubble produces no sharp edge against the skin, cast window edema and subsequent blistering are generally avoided. The cap can be replaced over the hole to provide a nice, protective hard shell over the dressing (Fig. 6-8).

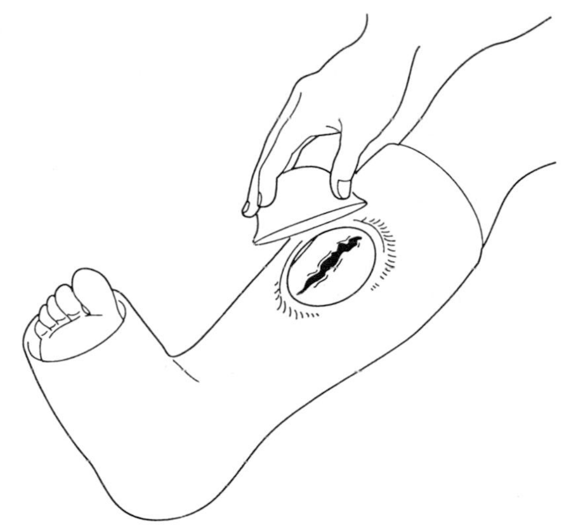

FIGURE 6-8. Bubble in plaster-of-Paris cast can be easily removed for wound care.

Another clever aid suggested by Gregory is to outline the bubble on the cast with an indelible pencil. This ensures that a surgeon unfamiliar with the patient's injury will cut in the proper site. In addition, a drawing of the fracture and a brief description of the wound can be placed on the cast, thus providing an immediately available, accurate history for subsequent persons treating the patient. When the cap is replaced, if swelling is expected, it may be important to refill the void with loosely packed cast padding to produce uniform compression over the wound site.

Pins and Plaster

When one of us (MWC) entered orthopaedic training in 1963, transverse through-and-through Steinmann pins or Kirschner wires incorporated in a plaster cast were standard methods of stabilizing unstable open fractures. Although the Roger-Anderson external fixator was available, for some reason it was used very little in open fractures. With the evolution of the external fixation frame to the currently popular single- and double-plane half-pin frames, pins and plaster have virtually disappeared as a method for immobilizing open fractures; in most cases, an external fixator can be applied more quickly. The external fixator offers the advantages of half-pin fixation, whereas pins and plaster nearly always require at least some through-and-through pins. In addition, the circumferential plaster presents problems in the swelling limb, limits wound care, and makes subsequent adjustments for fracture position difficult and certainly much more cumbersome than with most external fixation frames.

In spite of these disadvantages, pins and plaster have occasional indications. They are used frequently in underdeveloped countries as a simple, inexpensive method for fracture immobilization where the cost of external fixators precludes their use. Another excellent and inexpensive fixator that we have seen used frequently in underdeveloped countries involves simple Steinmann pins placed in a half-pin configuration and then incorporated into a bar of polymethylmethacrylate. Thus, a few comments about the technique of pins in plaster are merited.

Pins and plaster are most commonly indicated for the tibia. The most easily applied method uses Steinmann pins of sufficiently large dimension that in vivo bending of the pins will not occur. We find it best to use fully or partially threaded pins rather than smooth pins. Because the pin is incorporated in the cast and the cast tends to shift on the limb with changes in position, movement will be introduced in a smooth pin, making loosening and infection more likely. The disadvantage of a fully threaded pin is that it is more difficult to remove from the plaster cast. We find it easiest to place one through-and-through pin at approximately the level of the tibial tubercle in adults and distal to the tibial tubercle in children to avoid injury to the physeal line. A second through-and-through pin is placed approximately 1 inch proximal to the ankle joint. To avoid movement of the proximal fragment by the thigh musculature, a third half-pin is placed extending just into, but not through, the posterior cortex (Fig. 6-9). With the knee flexed to 90°, hanging off the side of the operating table with the thigh supported, traction can then be applied to the distal pin and reduction of the fracture obtained. An appropriate short-leg cast is applied, incorporating all three pins. For a secure hold, the plaster is applied directly to the pin, leaving the pins extending beyond the leg for a distance on either side equal to the width of the leg at that level. If Kirschner wires are used, the Kirschner wire bow must be left in place to maintain tension on the wire. When the cast is removed, it is easiest to cut around the base of the pin where it enters the cast to free the plaster on the pin from the remaining cast. After the cast is removed, the plaster cap on the wire can be screwed off or removed by cutting with the cast saw blade immediately against the pin.

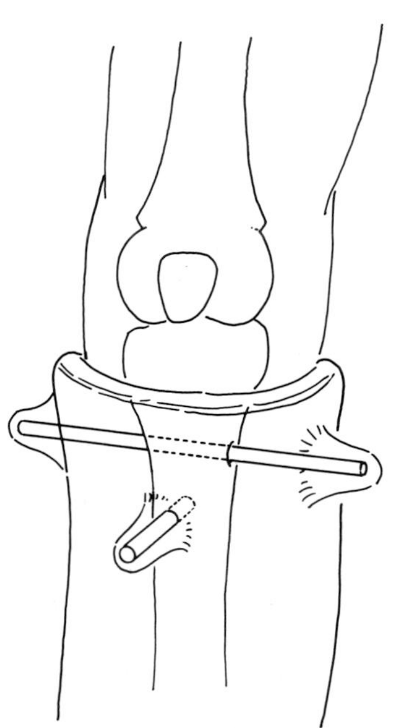

FIGURE 6-9. Two Steinmann pins incorporated in plaster give good control against rotation of the proximal fragment. The anteroposterior pin should just engage the posterior cortex, not penetrate it, to avoid neurovascular injury. (*Chapman, M.W.: Fractures of the Tibia and Fibula. In Chapman, M.W. [ed.]: Operative Orthopaedics, vol. 1, p. 441. Philadelphia, J.B. Lippincott, 1988.*)

This cuts the plaster envelope in half, which will then drop off the pin.

Pins in plaster tend to produce relative distraction of the fracture site and therefore should be used only long enough to obtain sufficient healing at the fracture site so that shortening and malrotation will not occur once the pins are removed. Generally this is possible at 6 to 8 weeks after the fracture. At this time removal of the pins and conversion to a non–weight-bearing cast or weight-bearing plaster is appropriate. This technique is useful in the upper extremity as well for fractures of the distal radius and, on occasion, for the forearm. Through-and-through pins can be placed through the bases of the second and third metacarpals and the olecranon. Half-pins can be used in the base of the metacarpals and into the shaft of the radius. Pins inserted into the radius must be inserted under direct vision to avoid injury to neurovascular structures and tendons.

Gregory described two other techniques for achieving temporary stability for cast application. In the tibia with a short, oblique fracture, the spike of one fragment can be inserted into the medullary canal of the other and placed into compression. This offers good stability; and if the obliquity is short, excessive shortening will not occur. An alternative is to reduce the fracture and percutaneously transfix it with a smooth Kirschner wire or Steinmann pin. The pin is placed through only one surface of the leg, not penetrating much beyond the cortex of the opposite side. After the cast is fully applied and dried, this smooth pin is removed. Reduction will generally thereafter be maintained. A threaded pin should not be used for this method because it may become ensnared in the padding of the cast when removal is attempted (Fig. 6-10).

Weight-Bearing Casts

Dehne,[37] Brown and Urban,[21] and Sarmiento[143,144] have demonstrated the advantages and beneficial effects of early weight bearing on the healing of fractures in the lower extremity. These advantages are equally true in the treatment of open fractures, but some practical considerations make immediate application of weight-bearing casts difficult. The wound care and potential for swelling encountered in most open fractures precludes immediate initial application of a weight-bearing cast. Once the wound has been closed, or is in a stable state where healing by secondary intention is acceptable, healing in the weight-bearing plaster may be quite appropriate. The threat of significant swelling must be passed before the application of one of these close-fitting casts. In stable, minor type I open fractures the cast may be applied within a few days after the threat of swelling has passed. In more severe

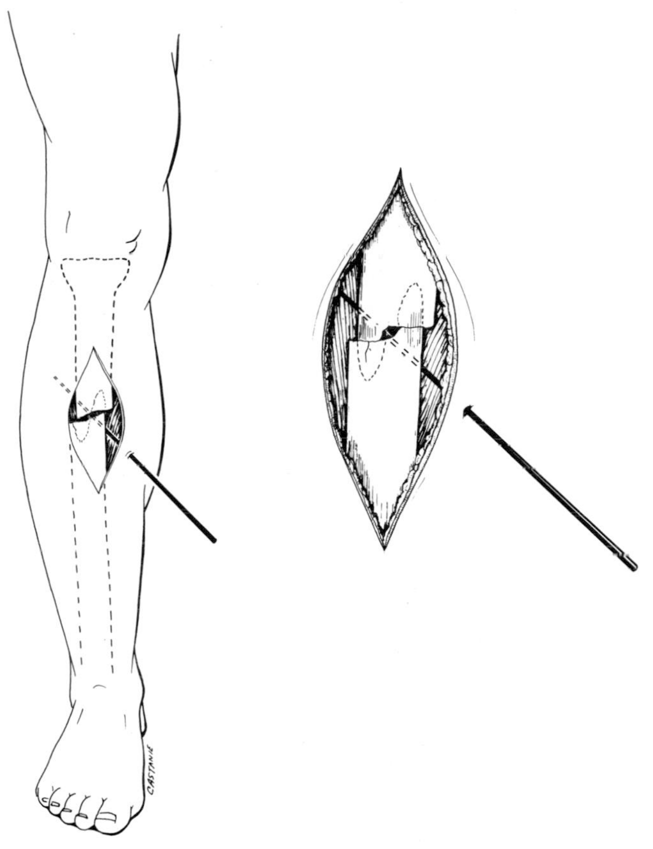

FIGURE 6-10. (*Left*) General alignment can be achieved by a temporary transfixing pin. (*Right*) Note the resulting reciprocal cortical invagination. When the plaster has set, the pin may be removed by the technique outlined in the text.

type II open fractures in which external fixation has not been used, application of a total-contact cast may have to be delayed for up to 3 to 4 weeks. The risk of late wound complications and loss of reduction of the fracture can be minimized by seeing the patient weekly after initial application of the cast for repeat x-ray films and windowing of the cast or removal to check the wound as indicated by clinical findings.

It is not necessary to have a closed wound before application of a weight-bearing plaster cast. For many years it has been noted that wounds debrided properly may heal if left undisturbed under plaster. Henry's[77] pungent observation—"Wounds may stink their way to health in plaster"—is clearly underscored by the vast experience of Orr[118] and his contemporaries in the treatment of chronic bone infection. This was further emphasized by the extensive experience of Trueta,[166] who used Orr's method to manage fresh injuries in the Spanish Civil War, and of Brown and Urban,[21] in the more recent Vietnam conflict. For success the principles of initial wound care must be meticulously followed.

Another consideration in the application of weight-bearing casts for the treatment of open fractures is the problem of split-thickness skin grafts. No matter how skillfully a cast has been applied, some telescoping occurs when the nonunited fracture is subjected to weight-bearing. The telescoping produces friction between the skin and cast surfaces. Because split-thickness skin grafts are insensitive and have poor mobility, breakdown is common. This is particularly a problem where the split-thickness graft is applied over bone, such as the anterior subcutaneous border of the tibia, where there is virtually no mobility. Breakdown of the graft can occur very rapidly, necessitating at a minimum repeat grafting to attain coverage, and at worst exposure of bone that could lead to more serious, deep-seated infection. In patients with extensive split-thickness skin grafts it may be necessary to defer treatment in a weight-bearing plaster cast until sufficient early intrinsic stability is achieved, to minimize the risk of injury to the overlying skin. In some cases circumferential casts never become practical and some other means of treatment must be adopted. The evolution from weight-bearing casts to cast-braces and prefabricated braces has been well described by Sarmiento.[143,144]

Skeletal Traction and Suspension

It is unusual for skeletal traction to be used as definitive treatment of open fractures in North America today because of the disadvantages of prolonged recumbency and because of the markedly increased costs of hospitalization compared with methods that allow earlier discharge from the hospital. However, traction is frequently used as a temporary means of fracture stabilization until more invasive methods are indicated and as definitive treatment in underdeveloped countries where internal or external fixation techniques are not readily available.

The most common indication for skeletal traction is an open fracture of the femur. In isolated open fractures of the femoral shaft, in which early mobilization is not of concern, our former practice has been to debride the fracture, leave the wound open, and place the leg in tibial pin traction with balanced suspension. After successful delayed primary closure of the wound, usually 10 to 14 days after injury, closed intramedullary nailing is done. Brumback and coworkers[22] have shown that the infection rate after primary intramedullary nailing of type I open fractures of the femur is the same as for delayed nailing; therefore, we now perform immediate fixation of these fractures (see Internal Fixation). In very unstable fractures we use a Thomas splint and Pearson attachment for suspension, but in more stable patterns when access to the wound may be important, we prefer modified skeletal Russell's traction (Fig. 6-11). The independent thigh sling

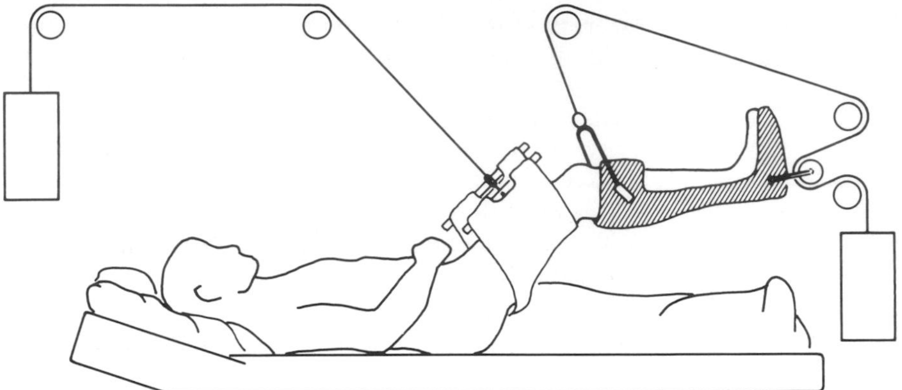

FIGURE 6-11. The "Western boot" consists of modified Russell's traction using an independent thigh sling and a proximal tibial pin incorporated into a short-leg cast with an anterior section removed. The pulley on the foot is attached by a cord to the Steinmann pin. (*Chapman, M.W., and Zickel, R.E.: Subtrochanteric Fractures of the Femur. In Chapman, M.W. [ed.]: Operative Orthopaedics, vol. 1, p. 364. Philadelphia, J.B. Lippincott, 1988.*)

permits easy access to wounds and is also more comfortable for the patient, making it much easier for nursing care and use of a bedpan. Because a large, threaded Steinmann pin is necessary to mount the patient on the fracture table used for closed intramedullary nailing, we prefer proximal tibial skeletal traction with a $^{3}/_{16}$- or $^{1}/_{4}$-inch fully threaded Steinmann pin with a bow. If intramedullary nailing is not contemplated, we prefer a Kirschner wire in the same location. We rarely use distal femoral traction unless there is a need to avoid pulling through injuries of the knee or a need for heavy traction for an acetabular or pelvic fracture. On occasion, 90°/90° traction does require a distal femoral pin (Fig. 6-12). Other than in children, our only indication for definitive treatment of a femoral fracture in traction is a decision by the patient not to proceed with internal or external fixation.

Gregory, in the first edition of this book, mentioned traction as a useful technique for the management of troublesome wounds, particularly on the proximal and posterior aspect of the thigh or buttocks. We have found external fixation, even fixation from the pelvis to the femur, to be superior to traction. In most circumstances it offers better stability, easier nursing care, and far better access to the wounds.

In injuries distal to the knee—in particular, pilon fractures of the ankle—soft-tissue swelling and injury of the skin may preclude early internal fixation. If one plans to perform internal fixation eventually, application of an external fixator may compromise later procedures, particularly if pin track complications occur. For this reason, traction through a pin in the calcaneus with suspension of the leg in slings or support on a Böhler-Braun frame may be indicated. This also permits good visualization of the extremity where impending compartment syndrome requires full exposure and careful observation of the limb. Over the past 5 years we cannot recall a fracture of the diaphysis of

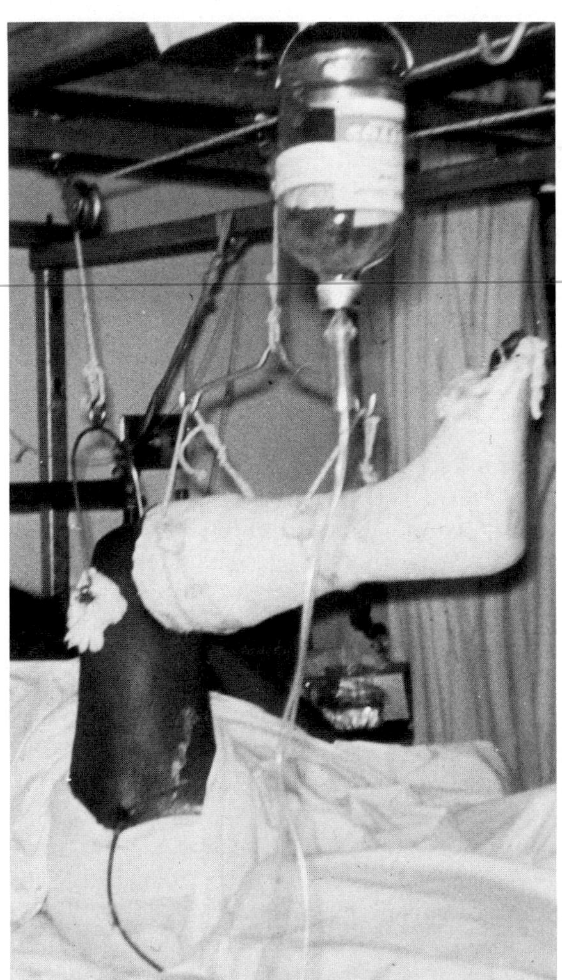

FIGURE 6-12. Simple vertical traction on the femur (90°/90°, hip and knee) makes wounds located high on the posterior thigh or the buttock easier to manage. This traction must not be used longer than necessary in the adult because of its effect on the patellofemoral joint.

the tibia that we managed definitively with traction. However, occasionally there is an indication for definitive management of a pilon fracture of the tibia in traction.

In patients who can withstand prolonged recumbency, and in whom internal fixation of a displaced open pilon fracture is contraindicated by the quality of the skin or soft tissues, poor bone stock, or severe systemic disease, treatment in traction may be of great advantage. Closed reduction of the fracture or limited internal fixation of the articular surfaces is carried out, a transverse traction pin through the calcaneus is placed in alignment with the longitudinal axis of the tibia, and sufficient traction is applied to produce slight distraction of the ankle joint. Early motion can then be instituted, which will help mold the fracture joint surfaces and preserve motion. After the threat of swelling has passed, it is sometimes useful to apply a set of mediolateral splints or occasionally a gaiter-type cast to help stabilize metaphyseal area fragments. Unfortunately, treatment in traction often requires continuous traction for 6 to 12 weeks to obtain sufficient stability that subsequent treatment in plaster or a cast brace is possible.

Open fractures of the pelvis or acetabulum, particularly if definitive treatment has been delayed, may preclude internal fixation; external fixation may be inadequate, particularly in fractures of the pelvic ring with vertical instability and in fractures of the acetabulum. In these circumstances, definitive treatment in skeletal traction becomes necessary. Again, we prefer a proximal tibial pin, if possible, because this usually permits earlier motion at the hip and knee than does a distal femoral pin. Although some of these fractures may heal quickly enough to allow traction to be discontinued by 6 weeks, very unstable injuries may require traction for as long as 12 to 16 weeks.

Traction is now rarely indicated for open fractures of the upper extremity, except in the humerus. The instability found in open fractures of the humerus is so difficult to control with overhead traction that we treat all of these injuries with either primary internal fixation or external fixation.

External Skeletal Fixation

The popularity of external skeletal fixation for the treatment of open fractures has waxed and waned throughout the middle and latter parts of the 20th century. Stader popularized its use for the treatment of fractures in domestic animals. During World War II external fixation gained considerable popularity in the military and emerged for a time as a popular method in civilian practice. The Roger-Anderson frame was used commonly throughout the 1950s and early 1960s. For the most part, early external skeletal fixation frames used through-and-through pins, and their external structure did not provide much versatility. Little was known about the biomechanics of these frames in relation to fracture healing. Because of difficulties with external fixation and the emerging popularity of internal fixation, the external methods again waned until Vidal modified the Hoffmann fixator, which quickly gained wide popularity in the 1970s.[42] Although much more versatile than previous designs, the early Hoffmann fixators also used through-and-through pins.

External fixation finally became the fracture stabilization method of choice for the treatment of most open fractures of long bones with the emergence of half-pin frames, which were popularized by Fisher[44] and the AO group.[8] Many different external fixation devices are now available, each offering unique advantages and features. (See Chapter 1 for a more complete discussion of external fixation methods.) Today external fixation is most often indicated for type IIIB and IIIC open fractures of the tibia and fibula and in open fractures of the pelvis.[41] More recently, the introduction of ring fixators using highly tensioned Kirschner wires by Ilizarov[82] and others[5,55] and half-pin or hybrid ring fixators by Green and others[48] have expanded the usefulness of external fixators.

Multiple tensioned wires on a ring are useful to stabilize juxta-articular fractures and can be combined with percutaneous cannulated screws for fixation of intra-articular fractures (Fig. 6-13**A**).[175] By using the principles of distraction osteogenesis or segment transport, bone defects can be replaced and leg length equalized without needing bone graft (see Fig. 6-13**B**).

External fixation devices offer the following advantages: for the most part, they are relatively easily and rapidly applied; excellent stability is obtained; and reasonably anatomical reduction of major fragments is possible. Minimal additional soft-tissue trauma is required for placement, so the risk of infection is minimized. In most cases, sufficient stability is achieved to allow early joint motion and muscle rehabilitation. The patient is sufficiently mobile that cardiopulmonary care is facilitated in patients with multiple injuries.

The main disadvantage of external fixators is that in complex fractures with large wounds, application can be complex and time consuming. Also, the pins may tie down musculotendon units and may interfere with soft-tissue reconstructive surgery by preventing the mobilization of flaps. These problems are worse in the femur and humerus, which are covered by thick muscle envelopes, but can be minimized with the use of half-pin fixators. Although the risk of infection at the fracture site is minimized, inappropriate technique causing bone necrosis or early

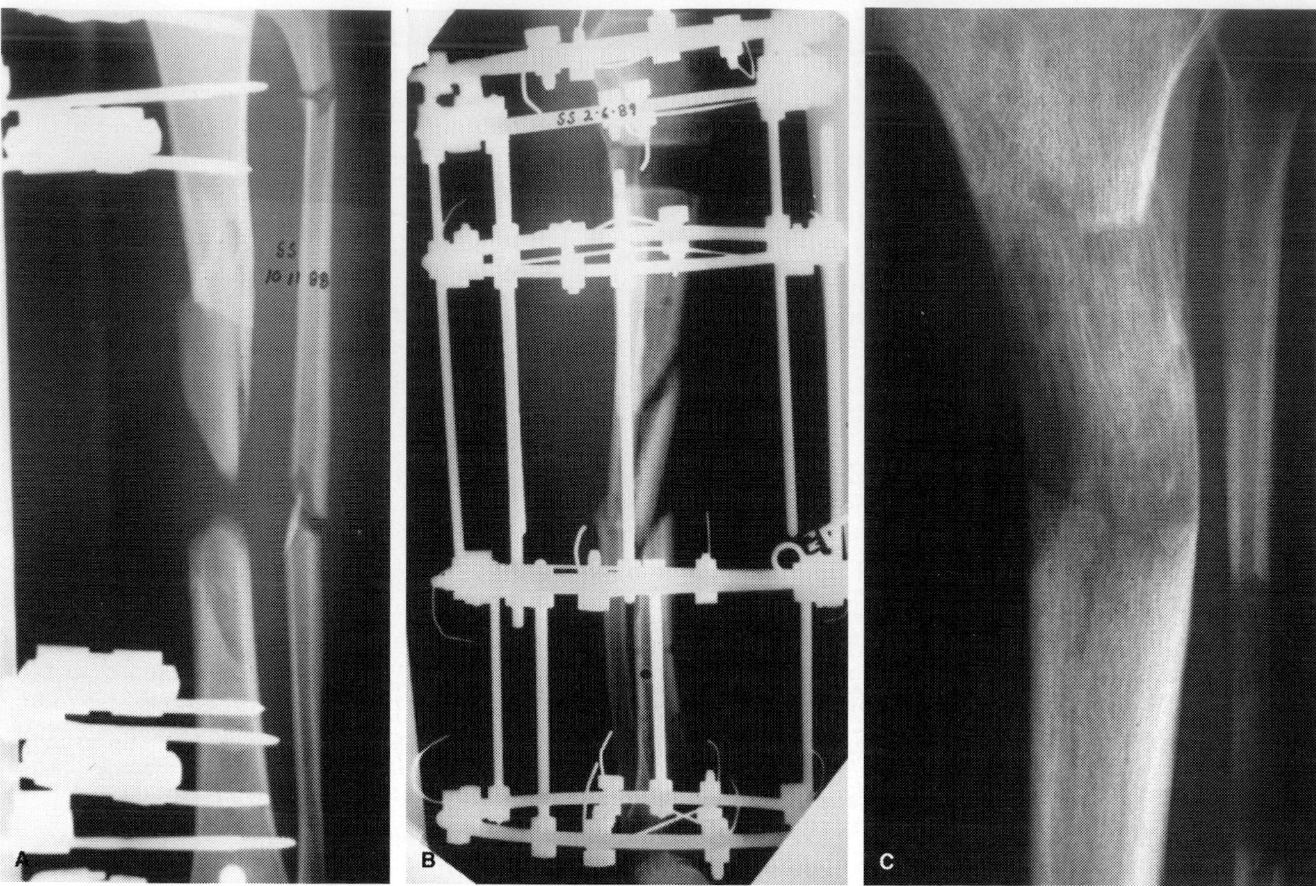

FIGURE 6-13. (**A**) Open fracture of the tibia with major segmental bone loss stabilized initially in a uniplanar external fixation. (**B**) Appearance after application of a ring fixator and proximal corticectomy for segment transport to close the defect. (**C**) Regenerate bone forming in the distraction zone.

loosening of pins, can lead to pin track infection. Loosening is more of a problem in osteopenic bone and cancellous bone. Prolonged use of external fixation devices, particularly non–weight-bearing ones, can lead to delayed union and nonunion of fractures. Many of these complications can be avoided by good surgical technique, which is discussed in other chapters in this text.

Regardless of the type of external fixation used, the following points about application apply:

1. A thorough irrigation and debridement of the fracture is essential.
2. The presence of the external fixator does not change the principles of wound management.
3. The frame must be applied to obtain as anatomical a reduction as possible and maximum contact between bone fragments.
4. Bone necrosis should be avoided by predrilling for the fixation pins using a water-cooled, sharp, drill point of the appropriate size. The fixation pins are inserted by hand following the directions of the manufacturer.
5. Injury to neurovascular structures and tying down musculotendon units should be avoided.
6. The stability of the fracture-external fixation frame construct is enhanced by the following:
   a. Use of larger pins where the threaded portion is in the far cortex and the smooth shank of the pin is within the near cortex
   b. In a standard four-pin frame, placement of two of the pins close to the fracture site and two remote to the fracture site, trying to locate all pins where sufficient cortical bone is present to provide good purchase for the pins
   c. Placement of the bar connecting the pins as close to the limb as practical; further stability can be obtained by adding more bars to the single-plane, half-pin frame, by adding additional frames as close to 90° from the original frame as possible, and by cross-connecting these two frames.

Figure 6-14 illustrates a double half-pin frame used for an unstable open fracture of the tibia employing these principles.

Indications

In fractures in which some type of internal or external fixation is required for stability, internal fixation generally is safest where the risk of infection is the lowest and external fixation is indicated where the risk of infection is the highest.[58] Thus, internal fixation is safer in type I and low-grade type II open fractures, and external fixation is most strongly indicated in type III open fractures. In the upper extremity, the violence of trauma is likely to be less than in the lower extremity and the wounds are generally of a lower grade. For this reason, internal fixation is used more commonly in the upper extremity than the lower extremity.

In the humerus, internal fixation is well tolerated because of the large muscle envelope and external fixation is less desirable. The neurovascular structures close to the humerus make insertion of external fixation pins by percutaneous or blind technique dangerous. It is necessary in most cases to expose the bone and insert the pins under direct vision to be safe, particularly around the radial nerve. In the humerus, we reserve external fixation for severe type IIIB and IIIC open fractures and in those in which comminution or poor bone quality makes internal fixation impractical or more hazardous. A single-plane, half-pin frame applied laterally works well.

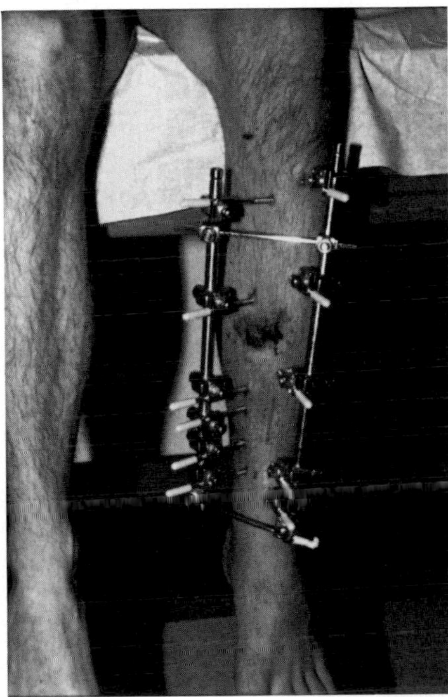

FIGURE 6-14. AO half-pin frames placed in double configuration and cross-connected. (*Chapman, M.W.: Fractures of the Tibia and Fibula. In Chapman, M.W. [ed.]: Operative Orthopaedics, vol. 1, p. 444. Philadelphia, J.B. Lippincott, 1988.*)

One of the best indications for external fixation in the upper extremity is in the management of severe "side-swipe" type III open fractures of the elbow joint that result in major soft-tissue injury, bone loss, and gross instability. A half-pin frame bridging the humerus and the ulna works quite well. If early motion is desired, a compass-hinge external fixator (Fig. 6-15**A**) is useful. The vast majority of open fractures of the radius and ulna can be safely managed by primary internal fixation, with a very low complication rate.[27,29,31] As with the elbow, external fixation is most often indicated for unstable, open, comminuted, intra-articular fractures of the distal radius; external fixation from the dorsolateral radius to the second or third metacarpals works well.

External fixation also has been advocated for spine fractures; however, this has not gained wide acceptance. We have little experience with this method. Open fractures of the spine are rare and are nearly always secondary to penetrating trauma. Most authorities advocate internal fixation when immediate stabilization is needed for these injuries.

One of the strongest indications for external fixation is open fractures of the pelvis, where stability is essential to control hemorrhage, manage the soft tissues, and allow for early mobilization. Perineal wounds and ruptured viscus increase the risk of infection in open fractures of the pelvis sufficiently that external fixation is generally the acute management of choice. Fixators work well for controlling the open-book pelvic injury but are inadequate for the stabilization of pelvic ring fractures with vertical instability. Exotic and complicated frames have not proven to be adequate for pelvic ring fractures with vertical instability; therefore, simple frames using two pins in each iliac crest are sufficient for most injuries of the pelvic ring (Fig. 6-16). Those with vertical instability require supplemental skeletal traction or delayed posterior internal fixation. Complex open, unstable fractures of the acetabulum, knee, and ankle are well managed by external fixators bridging these joints.

In the femur, we now rarely use external fixation in fresh, open fractures. Internal fixation, particularly intramedullary nailing by closed or modified open technique, is possible immediately or on a delayed basis in most cases.[27] Type III open hip fractures are exceedingly rare. Most hip fractures are inside-to-outside injuries with pinpoint wounds, where primary internal fixation is usually reasonable. The vast majority of midshaft fractures can be nailed immediately or early (see Internal Fixation). We use external fixation for diaphyseal fractures of the femur when intramedullary fixation is not possible or when there is an exceedingly

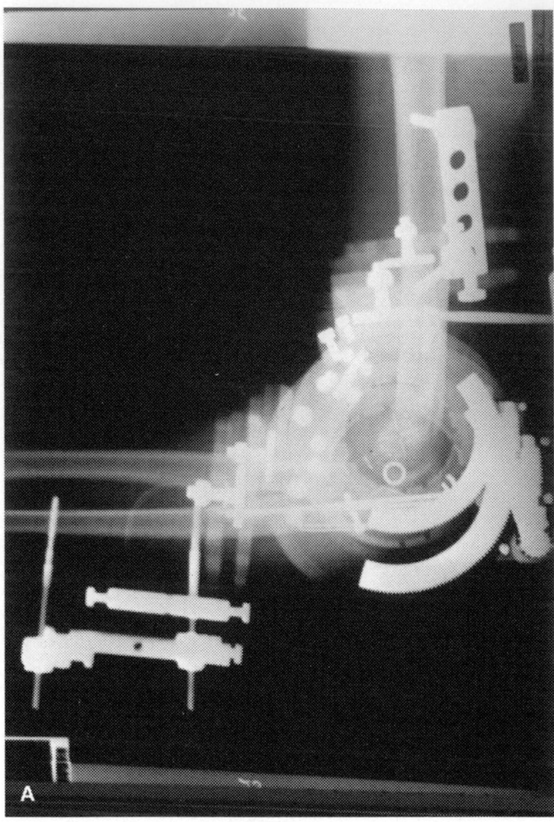

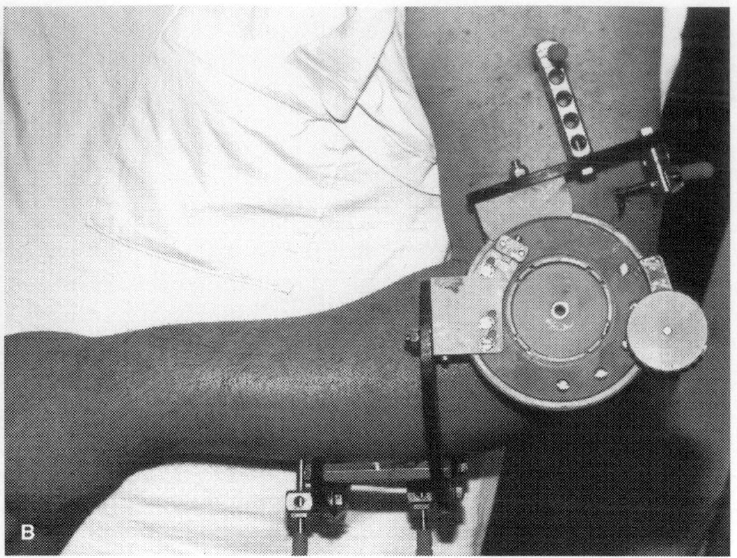

FIGURE 6-15. (**A** and **B**) This compass-hinge fixator for the elbow maintains stability and congruity of the joint with controlled motion possible.

dirty type III open fracture in which the risk of infection is simply too high. Open fractures of the supracondylar region of the femur are usually secondary to high-velocity trauma and carry a very high rate of infection, particularly after internal fixation when the rate of infection, in our experience, is 15% to 20%. In these fractures, limited internal fixation of the articular component with external fixation of the metaphyseal component is often wise. Subsequent conversion to internal fixation with a bone graft may be possible when the condition of the soft tissues permits. In open fractures of the tibia, external fixation remains one of the preferred methods of stabilization,[8] although reports suggest that nonreamed medullary nails are as effective and have some advantages[31,75,164] (see Internal Fixation). The same rationale discussed for open supracondylar fractures of the femur applies to tibial plateau fractures and pilon fractures. In pilon fractures, a triangular-type frame with fixation to the calcaneus and the forefoot is advisable to avoid an equinus deformity and to ensure adequate stabilization (Fig. 6-17).

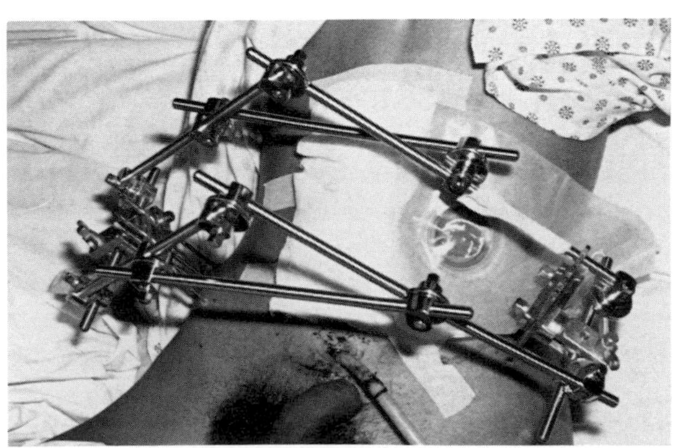

FIGURE 6-16. External fixation of an open pelvic fracture. Note colostomy and suprapubic catheter. Internal fixation was not used because of risk of infection in this open fracture.

Postoperative Management

There are nearly as many formulas for care of external fixation pin sites after insertion as there are orthopaedists in this country. We have found that the primary cause of pin infection is loosening of the pin. The other causes are movement of the skin and soft tissues about the pin, causing soft-tissue necrosis; the introduction of skin bacteria into the interface between the pin and deep soft tissues; and pressure necrosis of soft tissues owing to skin tension from improper insertion. These problems can be avoided by taking the following steps: (1) insert the pins into bone using the technique described above and (2) be absolutely certain that there is no skin tension on the pin during or after insertion.

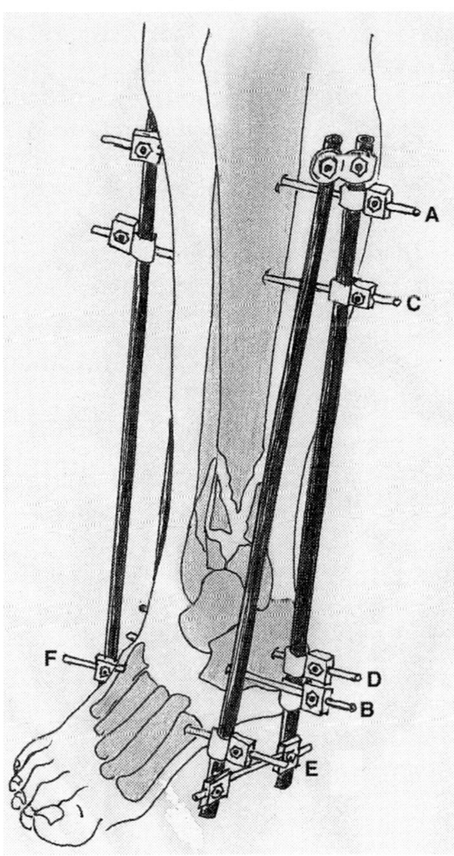

FIGURE 6-17. Double delta external fixator for open comminuted pilon fractures of the distal tibia and fibula. These are through-and-through centrally threaded pins. The fracture is aligned and then pins A and B are inserted. Half pins E and F can be used in the base of the metatarsals to support the forefoot when required. The medial or lateral half of the fixator can be removed for surgical procedures while maintaining stability of the limb.

To avoid motion of the skin about the pin, we advocate using a No. 11 blade to make a puncture wound slightly smaller than the diameter of the pin. After insertion of the pin the skin grips the pin snugly, thereby preventing differential motion. One major disadvantage of this technique is that if great care is not taken, tension of the skin against the pin can easily occur. After insertion, if the skin is gathered on one side of the pin or another, it can be released by incising the tight side to ensure that no tension is present. A couple of sutures are used to close this incision to again produce snug application of the skin to the pin. Where longitudinal incisions have been used to insert the pin, differential motion of the skin about the pin can be limited by applying a compression dressing around the pin. This is nicely done by placing a couple of 2 × 2-inch gauze pads about the pin and then putting a rubber stopcock that has been incised or a plastic clip on the pin, which is then slid down to hold the 2 × 2-inch gauze pads against the skin.

The most effective method of skin care we have found is simple cleansing of the entire external fixation frame, pin tracks, and skin daily with any standard commercial bathing soap to which the patient is not allergic. When the wounds are closed and any incisions around the pin sites have healed, this is easily accomplished during a daily shower by brushing down the frame with a surgical scrub brush and the pins and skin around the pins with a soft toothbrush. An effort must be made to remove all crusts and necrotic debris around the pin tracks. The frame and skin around the pins are then dried with a freshly laundered towel. We have found topical antiseptics to be unnecessary, and other ointments and antibiotic solutions are rarely indicated. The minute any persistent drainage is noted from a pin, or persistent discomfort is present, loosening of the pin and infection must be suspected. In such cases, the clamp holding the particular pin is loosened and the pin carefully examined. Frequently, loosening of the pin in the near cortex will be found; this can be confirmed by x-ray. Loose pins must never be left in place. These pins are removed and, if necessary, a new pin is placed in a new location. In some cases this may necessitate removal of the entire frame.

The timing of frame removal and type of subsequent fixation or mobilization are very complex issues and are beyond the scope of this chapter. Assuming that the external fixator allows good physiologic function of the extremity, we try to plan the treatment so that fracture union occurs in the fixator. This minimizes the risk of late deformity in a cast or brace and eliminates the need for secondary internal fixation. In most cases, this involves altering the frame to allow progressive loading of the fracture site for enhanced fracture union. In the case of the tibia, for example, this requires altering the frame to ensure fracture stability while permitting weight bearing. Some frames allow for "dynamization," where alignment can be maintained while weight bearing across the fracture site is permitted. When the fracture shows radiographic evidence of progression to union, the frame can be removed from the pins and the fracture checked for clinical stability. If the fracture is healed, the pins can be removed; if it is not healed, the frame can simply be replaced. In the tibia, conversion to a cast-brace or other type of removable brace is usually practical when the fracture is stable against shortening and cannot be translated, and its stiffness in bending is such that only 10° of motion in any given plane is possible.

Some surgeons advocate conversion of external fixation to internal fixation. The presence of infection in a pin track, whether previous or current, dramatically increases the risk of infection in secondary internal fixation. Pin track infection is a contraindication to conversion to internal fixation. In the absence of pin track infection, the safest measure is to first remove the fixator, temporarily immobilize the limb in a cast or in traction to allow for pin track healing (generally 10 to 14 days), and then proceed to internal fixation. The safest methods, of course, are those such as closed intramedullary nailing, where the pin tracks can be avoided.

External fixation followed by delayed intramedullary nailing some time after removal of the fixator has resulted in infection rates of 5% to 7%.[81,183,184]

The role of the pinless external fixator to provide provisional stabilization of the open tibia without intramedullary "contamination" followed with intramedullary nailing is unclear.[128] Biopsy of the intramedullary canal has not been effective in predicting infection when nonunions of the tibia are treated with intramedullary nailing.[127]

Internal Fixation

The fear of infection has led to the traditionally accepted opinion that immediate internal fixation, or for that matter any internal fixation, of open fractures is contraindicated. However, this attitude has changed markedly in the past 10 years. The prognosis in open fractures has improved dramatically since the two world wars. Military surgeons—particularly from the Korean and Vietnam wars—have effected a remarkable improvement in the infection rate by using early, meticulous, and aggressive wound debridement and irrigation; immobilizing with plaster casts or traction; and leaving wounds open, combined with parenteral bactericidal antibiotics. These advances have improved the overall prognosis and given surgeons more latitude in the treatment of open fractures.

Since 1970, reported infection rates in all types of open fractures have ranged from 2.1% to 9.4%.[62–67] Of more importance are the infection rates in each of the fracture types. In 1972, Gustilo and Anderson[64] reported no infections in type I open fractures, an incidence of 3.8% in type II, and 9% in type III. These were fractures treated without internal fixation. Their overall infection rate was 3.2%. In their later series,[62] the infection rate in type I open fractures was unchanged, in type II it was 1.8%, and in type III it was 18.4%, for an overall infection rate of 8.9%. They attributed this increase in infection rate to an increase in the percentage of severe type III open fractures in their practices. Of note is the 28% infection rate they encountered when type III fractures were internally fixed. Reports of primary internal fixation for open fractures have noted infection rates varying from 6% to 13% with the use of intramedullary fixation.[63,72,79,164,177] The infection rate in type I open fractures approximates that of clean, elective orthopaedic surgery if a formal, meticulous debridement is carried out and the traumatic wound is left open. The indications for immediate internal fixation of open fractures have changed, owing to the recent advances in wound care in open fractures, improved antibiotic therapy (and resultant improvement in infection rates), and the technical advances in internal fixation. Gristina and Rovere[59] have shown that the presence of metal per se does not promote bacterial growth in vitro. Internal fixation that results in stabilization of the fracture has been shown to have a lower susceptibility to infection than a fracture with gross instability of the fracture site.[182] Few prospective, paired, randomized studies comparing internal fixation with external fixation for stabilizing open fractures have been reported. The older literature has three such studies (Table 6-4).[32,50,170] These studies showed that external fixation had a lower infection rate and higher rate of union compared with internal fixation. On this basis, one would conclude that internal fixation is contraindicated in open fractures. During the same period, however, Lottes and colleagues[100] and D'Aubigne and coworkers[36] showed excellent results using closed tibial nailing in the treatment of open fractures of the tibia. Lottes and colleagues had a 7% infection rate and no nonunions.

Studies of internal fixation of open fractures published in the 1980s and more recently, however, have shown remarkably good results. In the four series listed in Table 6-5, the average acute infection rate

TABLE 6-4
Internal Fixation Versus External Immobilization

	Internal Fixation			External Immobilization		
Authors	*No. Cases*	*% Nonunion*	*% Infection*	*No. Cases*	*% Nonunion*	*% Infection*
Wade and Campbell[170]	51	27	14	58	9	0
Claffey[32]	48	17	35	70	0	0
Gallinaro and associates[50]	31	11	17	33	9	3
Totals	130			161		
Average Incidence		18%	33%		9%	3%

TABLE 6-5
Immediate Internal Fixation

Authors	No. Cases	Late Nonunions	Acute Infections*	Late Osteomyelitis	Secondary Amputation
Clancey and Hansen[33]	35	0	8	0	0
Rittmann and associates[133]	214	0	15	2	4†
Chapman and Mahoney[31]	101	0	10	1	1†
La Duca and associates[93]	42	0	2	0	
Totals	392	0	35	3	5
Average Incidence		0%	8.9%	0.8%	1.3%

* Up to a 40% infection rate in type III open fractures.[31]
† All in severe type III open fractures of the tibia.

was 8.9% with only three cases going on to chronic osteomyelitis—a long-term infection rate of 0.8%. Although bone grafts were required to achieve union in a number of type III open fractures of the tibia, no nonunions occurred. All of the amputations reported occurred early in severe open fractures of the tibia in which an attempt at limb salvage was made—all cases that in the previous decade would have been amputated immediately. It is evident, however, that severe type III open fractures of the tibia remain a problem.

Of significance are the excellent functional results reported by Clancy and Hanson,[33] Rittmann and associates,[133] and LaDuca and associates.[93] More recently, Bach and Henson[3] randomized 59 open tibial shaft fractures (Gustilo type II and type III open fractures) to treatment by application of a plate or external fixator. They found that the prevalence of infection after plate fixation was 35% compared with 13% after external fixation. Most reports show that reamed interlocking intramedullary nailing is associated with an increased incidence of infection as high as 33%. However, O'Brien and colleagues[91] have reported a prospective randomized trial of reamed versus nonreamed interlocked intramedullary nailing of tibial shaft fractures, and they reported a 4% incidence of infection in reamed tibial nails, and 0% incidence infection in nonreamed tibial nails. Schemitisch and colleagues[151] reported the effect of reamed versus nonreamed locked tibial nailing on callus blood flow using laser-Doppler flowmetry in a sheep model. They reported that the decrease in perfusion after reaming as compared with the nonreamed group was an immediate effect of reaming. At 2-, 6-, and 12-week follow-up there is no difference in callus formation between either group.

Prospective randomized studies comparing nonreamed interlocking tibial nails with external fixation for the treatment of type I, type II, type IIIA, and type IIIB open tibial shaft fractures have reported similar or decreased rates of infection with the use of the nonreamed locked intramedullary nail as compared with external fixation.[72,164,177] The results of these series are listed in Table 6-6.

Other than limb salvage, the most gratifying aspect of immediate internal fixation is the excellent functional results reported. The results in these series are comparable with, if not better than, studies using external fixation and nonoperative treatment. To achieve these results, however, the surgeon must be discriminating and use precise indications. The irrigation and debridement must be impeccable, and the technical execution of the internal fixation must be excellent. Meticulous postoperative care with good patient cooperation is essential. There is little room for misjudgment or error, because the consequences are usually more severe than the complications of external immobilization. There is little question that a role has been established for internal fixation in the treatment of open fractures. Because of the inherent and unavoidable risks of more extensive surgery, however, the gains to be made by internal fixation must justify its use.

Indications for Immediate Internal Fixation

When considering immediate internal fixation of an open fracture, one must take into account the "personality" of the fracture, one's capabilities as a surgeon, the abilities of the operating room team, the adequacy of surgical equipment and implants available, and the particular situation within which the fracture must be treated. For example, will the operating room team be up to the task at 2 a.m., and will the patient's general condition permit extensive surgery? Bone quality must be sufficient to hold screws, and the fracture must not be so comminuted that internal fixation is impossible. The surgeon must be skilled with rigid internal fixation methods and perform them on a sufficiently frequent basis that the problem at hand will be adequately managed. Gentleness in the management of the soft tissues is as important as technical ability in fixing the fracture.

Internal fixation of open fractures may be indicated in intra-articular fractures, in certain diaphyseal fractures where internal fixation has proven to be equal to, or more effective than, external fixation, in fractures associated with vascular injuries, in major long-bone fractures in selected victims of multiple-system trauma, and in the elderly. In type I open fractures where internal fixation would be indicated if the fracture were closed, internal fixation can be performed with minimal risk, but only after adequate irrigation and debridement. There are also social, psychiatric, and economic considerations in this decision-making process that may make internal fixation worth the additional risk.

Intra-Articular Fractures

Mitchell and Shepard[109] have shown that interfragmentary compression may play a major role in the healing of cartilage in intra-articular fractures. Studies from Llinas and colleagues[98] have demonstrated that articular step-offs heal with a different mechanism than full-thickness articular defects. In particular, they found that cartilage and subchondral bone adapt to surface incongruity by modifying their structure. This was most successful when the articular step-off was less than the thickness of the articular cartilage width. They did not find a significant benefit from continuous passive motion. Salter and colleagues[139] have shown that early institution of motion is probably necessary to achieve an optimal result. This requires rigid internal fixation of intra-articular fractures. This is especially true in weight-bearing joints, and clinical experience suggests that intra-articular fractures do best when anatomically reduced and treated with early motion for rehabilitation. These principles are applicable to open fractures as well as closed. The incidence of extensive soft-tissue injuries associated with open fractures makes this more imperative for open fractures. Intra-articular fractures not requiring internal fixation are those that are anatomically reduced and stable, those in patients with limited life expectancies, or those in selected patients with neurologic diseases or paralysis. Severe comminution or underlying bone disease, which makes adequate fixation impossible, is also a contraindication to fixation.

The majority of open intra-articular fractures have type I wounds. The low infection rate in type I injuries makes it possible to immediately internally fix these fractures with a risk of infection roughly comparable with that of closed fractures *if* meticulous irrigation and debridement have been done. Because of the increased risk of infection in type II and type III open fractures, careful judgment is required. Simple, noncomminuted fractures, such as displaced medial and lateral malleolus fractures, are easily internally fixed with minimum fixation through the open fracture wound. Such a simple procedure adds little to soft-tissue devitalization and accomplishes anatomical reduction and stability that greatly facilitates soft-tissue management. Stabilization may even lower the infection rate rather than contribute to it.[132]

Reports on primary open reduction and internal fixation in type III open articular fractures of the ankle and tibial plateau have shown good results.[9,85] Early reports of primary open reduction and internal fixation of open distal intra-articular femur fractures have shown good success with type I and type II open fractures, and infection rates in type III fractures ranging from 10% to 45%.[73,152] In severe type III open intra-articular fractures, staged surgery or limited internal fixation should be considered. Initially, irrigation and debridement are carried out and the wound is left open. The articular cartilage should be covered by soft tissue. At 5 days after injury the patient is returned to the operating room, and if there is no evidence of infection, definitive internal fixation of the fracture can be carried out. After internal fixation, for ultimate safety, the wound can be left open initially and closed 5 days later. If bone grafting is required, it can be carried out at that time. Another approach at the time of initial debridement is to anatomically reduce the articular fragments and internally fix these alone, managing the metaphyseal portion of the fracture with external fixation. After successful primary closure, usually 21 or 50 days after injury, acute effects of soft-tissue trauma have resolved and rigid internal fixation of the remainder of the fracture can be undertaken with less risk. This permits early joint mobilization. If the degree of soft-tissue devitalization and contamination causes internal fixation to be delayed longer than 3 weeks after injury, or if the fracture is too comminuted to achieve rigid fixation, it is best to proceed with early joint mobilization in traction or a functional cast-brace.

An optimal end result in intra-articular fractures requires early joint mobilization and muscle rehabilitation. The worst management is to combine the risks of internal fixation with the complications of nonfunctional, external immobilization.

Massively Traumatized Limbs

The recent increase in infection rates reported for open fractures is caused by surgeons' attempts to salvage limbs that a few years ago would never have been considered salvageable and would have been amputated. The advent of limb replantation with specialized microvascular repair techniques has been partly responsible for this change. The type III open fracture with extensive skin loss, severe muscle damage, and neurovascular injury, in which frequent operative intervention for soft-tissue care is necessary, requires stabilization to achieve limb salvage and an acceptable, functional end result. Fractures of this type are often segmental, and loss of bone substance is common. This complicates the fixation problem and makes more challenging the reconstructive surgery necessary to achieve union. This situation is most frequently encountered in car-bumper crush injuries of the tibia and in high-velocity gunshot wounds. The high infection rate in these injuries is such that rigid stabilization with an external fixation device is generally preferred.[42] In many situations, however, external fixation devices are impractical, and internal fixation is necessary. External fixators may interfere with soft-tissue management by preventing the use of muscle pedicle and skin flaps and by tying down musculotendon units. External fixators also may not offer adequate fixation for intermediate fragments.

Limited interfragmentary fixation with screws at the fracture site is often possible without additional soft-tissue dissection; this adds to stability and may prevent delayed union.

Interfragmentary fixation in the metaphyseal areas of the bone, in our experience, has not impaired bony union. Krettek and colleagues have reported an increase in delayed unions and nonunions with the use of interfragmentary fixation in the diaphyseal portion of tibial fractures when associated with external fixation. They advise that if this technique is used, early bone grafting should be incorporated as a part of the staged reconstruction protocol for the injury. Interfragmentary fixation should not be used if the fracture site is not accessible without further soft-tissue devitalization to place the screw.

In massive injuries of the humerus where external fixation is impractical, our treatment of choice has been plate fixation. This usually works well because of the large soft-tissue envelope around the humerus. Recently we have used nonreamed intramedullary nails with cross-locking. In the forearm, plate fixation is almost always the method of choice. In massive injuries, bone grafting early in treatment is nearly always necessary to avoid a nonunion.[29]

In severe open fractures of the femur, intramedullary fixation has become the standard of care.[101] This fixation works well because of the excellent muscle envelope covering the femur. Brumback and colleagues[22] have reported a retrospective review of delayed versus immediate nailing of open femoral shaft fractures in 89 patients. They reported three deep infections, all occurring in type IIIB open fractures. Two infections occurred in the group who had delayed nailing and one in the group who had immediate nailing. In Gustilo type I, II, and IIIB open fractures immediate nailing is acceptable. Type IIIB open fractures of the femur are severe injuries that usually combine contamination with massive soft-tissue injury. Careful judgment needs to be exercised in the management of these fractures. Initial stabilization should be performed either with external fixation or intramedullary fixation, depending on the characteristics of the fracture and the wound.[27] Nonreamed nails have been shown to have a lower infection rate in open femur fractures than reamed nails.[27] The newer locking nonreamed nails deserve study. Plate fixation of the open femoral shaft has also been advocated.[131] Plate fixation has potential advantages in type IIIA injuries where soft-tissue stripping has occurred at the time of injury, such that plate application can be performed easily at the time of irrigation and debridement without further soft-tissue stripping.

In the tibia, nonreamed locking intramedullary fixation is the preferred method of fracture stabilization for fractures in the middle three fifths of the bone for open type I, type II, and type IIIA fractures.[30,36,72,100,164,177,178]

Some have advocated the use of plates in selected circumstances, but these should be limited to juxta-articular fractures.[4,33,34,117] The use of plate fixation in the tibial shaft has been shown to have an increased incidence of infection in open fractures.[3] The treatment of type IIIB open fractures of the tibia remains controversial. External fixation continues to be the preferred technique, but intramedullary fixation has shown promising results. One prospective randomized study comparing external fixation and intramedullary fixation on open IIIB tibia fractures showed similar infection rates and a decreased incidence of nonunion and malunion with intramedullary fixation.[164] Experience and good clinical judgment are required to determine the appropriate treatment for these severe injuries.

In the very elderly, or in nutritionally or immunologically compromised patients with multiple, severe injuries in which the metabolic load of a massive injury is life threatening, immediate amputation may be indicated.[70] This can be a lifesaving measure.

Vascular Injuries

In the presence of vascular injuries requiring repair, we usually stabilize the fracture with internal or external fixation. This is particularly true when impingement of bone caused the vascular injury or residual instability threatens the repair. Because restoration of circulation to the limb is of primary concern, it is important that either vascular repair or temporary restoration of circulation be carried out before bone fixation. The presence of the fracture, in many instances, permits a repair through the open fracture wound that would otherwise not be possible. This is an additional reason for carrying out internal fixation after vascular repair. The surgeon must be sufficiently skilled and gentle in his or her technique that the vascular repair is not disrupted during internal fixation. Connolly,[35] through Vietnam War experience, has shown that internal fixation of fractures is not essential to protect vascular repairs; however, in open fractures with vascular injury accompanied by extensive soft-tissue injury, the advantages of internal fixation are the same as those described for massively traumatized limbs.[130]

Multiply Injured Patients

The contribution of multiple long-bone fractures to the death of the patient with multiple injuries has only recently been appreciated.[15] Because the primary cause of death in victims of multiple trauma after successful resuscitation is respiratory failure, we have attributed these deaths to chest and abdominal trauma. Trunkey and associates[167] have shown that the most important factors predisposing to the adult respiratory distress syndrome are multiple long-bone fractures, shock on admission to the emergency department, voluminous blood replacement, and comminuted fractures of the pelvis. Long-bone fractures contribute to this problem through hemorrhage, by adding to the initial quantity of injured muscle, and by preventing early mobilization because the patient is supine in bed with skeletal traction. Early stabilization of open fractures reduces hemorrhage, particularly in the pelvis. Irrigation and debridement of open fractures plus stabilization of long-bone fractures may reduce the ultimate metabolic load imposed on the patient. Pulmonary physiotherapy and achievement of a vertical chest by getting the patient out of bed are essential to avoid atelectasis and secondary infection in persistently dependent pulmonary segments.[93] Immediate stabilization of major long-bone fractures—particularly in the femur and in unstable fractures of the pelvis and spine—may be lifesaving.[7,15,17,43,88,101,104,131,148]

Any additional initial surgery in the extremities contributes to the total soft-tissue trauma; therefore, the advantages of early internal fixation must be substantial, and thoughtful consultation among the orthopaedic surgeon, general surgeon, and anesthesiologist is essential.

Whenever possible, we perform immediate open reduction and internal fixation of all extremity injuries in the polytraumatized patient. Our contraindications for proceeding with open reduction are uncontrolled hemodynamic instability, persistent disseminated, intravascular coagulopathy, persistent hypothermia with temperature below 95°F (35°C), persistent hypoxemia, and uncontrolled elevated intracranial pressure greater than 20 cm H_2O. The patient is resuscitated in the intensive care unit until stabilized and taken to the operating room for fracture fixation as soon as possible. The femur most frequently requires fixation.

Pape and colleagues,[121] from Hannover, have reported an increased incidence in pulmonary morbidity in polytraumatized patients with chest injury and femoral fractures who have been treated with a reamed intramedullary nail. They have advocated the use of nonreamed intramedullary nailing for the stabilization of femur fractures in this patient population.

The evidence for immediate fixation of the femur remains strong. Which method of fixation will prove to be the best remains controversial, but reamed or nonreamed intramedullary nail are used by most.

Fractures of the upper extremity can usually be managed with plaster immobilization, with the exception of some unstable fractures of the humerus. Injuries below the knee also can be managed initially with external fixation immobilization by plaster casts.

Although immediate internal fixation facilitates care in the intensive care unit, low tissue oxygen tensions during the immediate postinjury period may predispose to a higher wound complication rate. These advantages and disadvantages must be kept in mind when considering immediate internal fixation versus external fixation for open long-bone fractures in multiply injured patients.

Elderly Patients

The same principles apply to open fractures in elderly patients as in the young, with some exceptions. The complications of enforced bed rest, particularly with pneumonia and thromboembolic disease, are far greater in the elderly, and therefore early internal fixation to permit mobilization is even more important. As in multiply traumatized patients, the metabolic load of severe multiple injuries may necessitate early amputation to save a life.

Surgical Technique of Internal Fixation in Open Fractures

In the operating room, attention is first directed to meticulous irrigation and debridement of the open fracture. Plans for subsequent internal fixation should not divert the surgeon's attention from this essential task. Extensive surgical incisions should be planned that permit adequate exposure, do not further compromise skin flaps, and permit soft-tissue coverage of any implants that are to be placed. Internal fixation requires careful planning. The bone quality and fracture configuration must permit fixation, and the operating room team should institute rapid, facile, and adequate application of the internal fixation appliances.

The fixation must provide absolute stability and as anatomical a reduction as possible. Internal fixation without good fracture-surface contact and excellent rigidity is worse than no fixation. The fixation should require minimal additional soft-tissue dissection. The internal fixation is best applied through the open fracture wound and is placed so that soft-tissue coverage is possible even if, biomechanically, the implant is not in the most advantageous position. Indirect reduction techniques as popularized by Mast[102] and percutaneous screw fixation methods help to limit soft-tissue dissection and preserve bone blood supply. This requires flexibility on the part of the surgeon. In general, primary wound closure should *not* be performed when immediate internal fixation of an open fracture is done. Partial muscle closure in the absence of tension to achieve coverage of the fracture site or implant is important, but the skin and deep fascia should always be left open. Plastic reconstructive procedures to obtain closure or coverage of an implant are rarely indicated at the time of the initial fixation.

The difficulties in determining viability, and the additional trauma from such surgery, often lead to necrosis of flaps. Flap or pedicle coverage is best achieved at the time of delayed primary closure, which is carried out at least 5 days after injury. Some authorities believe that flap coverage as early as 48 hours gives a higher success rate. This is discussed in much greater detail in Chapter 7. If the implant and bone cannot be covered immediately, meticulous wound care, keeping the bone and surroundings moist with physiologic saline or mild antiseptic solutions (eg, Dakin's solution), is important to prevent necrosis of exposed bone. Early full-thickness tissue coverage is important to enhance revascularization and limit the risk of infection. Although coverage can usually be achieved by local muscle pedicle flaps, microvascularized flaps are sometimes required. One should try to achieve complete closure of the wound within 10 days, if possible.

Early vigorous muscle and joint rehabilitation is important to achieve the maximum benefits from internal fixation. Immediate continuous passive motion is helpful, particularly in intra-articular fractures. In most cases the postinjury pain will subside in several days, and supervised range-of-motion and strengthening exercises can be undertaken. When the fixation permits, as with intramedullary nails in stable fractures, immediate weight-bearing is important.

Bone Grafting

Autogenous, *cancellous* bone grafts are used frequently in internal fixation of open fractures.[11] Because of the risk of infection, these bone grafts are rarely applied at the time of initial internal fixation. An exception is in type I and mild type II intra-articular fractures, where cancellous bone is necessary to fill defects for obtaining anatomical reduction and stable fixation. Bone defects, particularly in diaphyseal fractures, usually heal faster if filled. There is a high incidence of delayed union in plate fixation of high-grade open diaphyseal fractures, so bone grafting should routinely be done to avoid premature plate failure from delayed union. Bone graft is best applied at the time of delayed primary closure in type I and II open fractures. In high-risk cases, in particular, type III open fractures, it may be done electively after successful delayed primary closure when infection is absent, usually 6 to 9 weeks after injury. Fischer and associates[45] demonstrated a decreased incidence of infection when bone grafting of type III open fractures was done on a delayed basis.

Good-quality, abundant, cancellous bone graft is necessary; we usually take this from the posterior ilium in the region of the posterior-superior iliac spine. In rare cases in which soft-tissue coverage of the fracture site is impossible or infection has occurred, we use the open cancellous bone grafting technique described by Papineau.[122]

Special Considerations

Foot and Hand Fractures

The foot and hand in healthy young adults have excellent blood supply; therefore, infection is not usually a major problem. Immediate internal fixation can be carried out according to the same indications used for closed fractures.[26,31] Most fixation is achieved with Kirschner wires, and the amount of additional soft-tissue dissection required is minimal. In the massively traumatized hand, internal fixation that permits immediate motion is essential for restoration of hand function.

The indications for limited internal fixation of the calcaneus with pins and screws are the same as those in closed fractures. Displaced fractures of the body and neck of the talus should be reduced anatomically and immediately internally fixed.[71] In our experience, this has resulted in an almost uniform rate of union and a much lower incidence of avascular necrosis than previously reported.[71] A similar philosophy is applied to displaced fractures of the midfoot joints.

Ankle Fracture–Dislocations

Routine fractures of one malleolus and bimalleolar and trimalleolar fractures are usually best treated by primary internal fixation.[20] In type I and low-grade type II open fractures this can be achieved with no greater risk of infection than in closed fractures.[31,133] Immediate open reduction and internal fixation of type III open ankle fractures has shown good results when soft-tissue loss is not present.[47,84] In severe type III open fractures of the ankle, extensive reconstruction that might require extensive plating at the time of initial debridement is best deferred. The articular surface can be reconstructed with wires and screws, and the remainder of the fracture may best be initially managed by external fixation or supportive hard dressing.

Internal fixation of routine ankle fractures presents few problems; however, pilon fractures are difficult to treat. Restoration of the articular surface with wires and screws to achieve anatomical position and then temporary use of external fixation for the shaft portion of the fracture is a safe approach. After 5 to 10 days, and in the absence of infection, application of a buttress plate or other implants to achieve complete stability can be done more safely. It is also possible at this time to insert cancellous bone grafts. Regardless of the approach used, early motion to restore ankle function is essential.

In those fracture–dislocations in which stability cannot be achieved with internal fixation and external fixation is not desired, early motion can be instituted while the patient is in calcaneal pin traction. Stability can be augmented with a Delbet cast.

Fractures of the ankle and talus with significant soft-tissue loss have resulted in significant disability and prolonged hospitalization and reconstructive procedures for patients. This may be an indication for early amputation.[142]

Tibial Shaft Fractures

Immobilization in a functional weight-bearing cast can produce good results in the majority of type I and mild type II open fractures of the tibia with stable fracture patterns.[21,143,144]

However, in unstable open fractures of the middle three fifths of the tibial shaft with type I, type II, and type IIIA wounds, locked nonreamed intramedullary nailing is the current fixation of choice (Table 6-6).[16,75,140,145,161]‡ More fracture patterns can be adequately stabilized by a dynamically locked nail, but more comminuted patterns require static locking. In-

‡ Excellent results have been reported with the Lottes and Ender nails as well.[24,50,60,86,43,76,54]

TABLE 6-6

Open Tibia Fractures Treated With Nonreamed Interlocking Intramedullary Nails

Author	No. Fractures	Type I	Type II	Type IIIA	Type IIIB	Type IIIC
Bonatus et al[113a]	72	27	22	11	12	0
Helfet et al[72]	37	8	14	11	2	2
Henley et al[75]	103	0	52	40	12	0
Sanders et al[140]	64	10	16	17	21	0
Tornetta et al[164]	15	0	0	0	15	0
Whittle et al[177]	50	3	13	22	13	0
		Malunion	**Delayed Union**	**Nonunion**	**Persistent Nonunion**	
Bonatus et al[113a]	72	7 (10%)	13 (18%)	12 (17%)	0	
Helfet et al[72]	37	0	2 (5%)	2 (5%)	2 (5%)	
Henley et al[75]	103	5 (5%)	14 (14%)	36 (35%)	10 (10%)	
Sanders et al[140]	64	0	17 (38%)	1 (2%)	1 (2%)	
Tornetta et al[164]	15	0	2 (13%)	0	0	
Whittle et al[177]	50	0	25 (50%)	2 (4%)	2 (4%)	

		Deep Infection Rates					
		Type I	*Type II*	*Type III3A*	*Type III3B*	*Type IIIC*	*Overall*
Bonatus et al[113a]	72	0/13	1/22 (4%)	1/12 (9%)	1/8 (8%)	0/0	4%
Helfet et al[72]	37	0/8	0/14	2/11 (18%)	0/2	0/2	5%
Henley et al[75]	103	0/0	2/52 (4%)	4/40 (10%)	1/12 (8%)	0/0	7%
Sanders et al[140]	64	0/10	0/16	1/17 (6%)	5/21 (24%)	0/0	9%
Tornetta et al[164]	15	0/0	0/0	0/0	1/15 (7%)	0/0	7%
Whittle et al[177]	50	0/3	0/13	1/22 (4%)	3/13 (23%)	0/0	8%

fection rates with nonreamed locked intramedullary nails have been comparable to treatment with external fixation, and the use of intramedullary fixation has resulted in a decreased incidence of malunion and shortening.[75,140,145] Bone and colleagues[16] have recommended early dynamization of statically locked tibial nails at 8 weeks after injury to stimulate union. We prefer to initially lock fractures with adequate bone contact into compression; then dynamization is not necessary. Templeman and colleagues[161] have advocated tomography at 3 months after injury to assess the need for further intervention to stimulate union. Moed and colleagues[111] have reported on the use of ultrasonography to predict fracture healing.

The choice of skeletal stabilization in type IIIB open tibial shaft fractures continues to be controversial. Traditionally, external fixation has been the method of choice.[25,42,87] Tornetta and associates[164] reported a prospective randomized series of type IIIB open tibial shaft fractures treated with nonreamed locked intramedullary nailing compared with external fixation. They noted a similar incidence of infection and a lower incidence of malunion in the intramedullary nailed fixation group. Schandelmair and colleagues[145] reported a retrospective review of nonreamed tibial nails compared with external fixation of open tibial fractures. They reported a 49% incidence of infection with external fixation (including pin track infection) and a 2% incidence of infection with nonreamed tibial nailing. These reports are similar to our experience at the University of California, Davis, Medical Center. A recent review of our experience reported an 8% incidence of infection in type IIIA open tibias and a 12% incidence of infection in type IIIB open tibia fractures treated with immediate nonreamed locked intramedullary nailing. Henley and colleagues,[75] in a prospective randomized study, compared nonreamed locked intramedullary nails to external fixation. They reported a higher incidence of wound problems in the external fixation group (21% vs 11%), as well as an increased incidence of malunion of 24% with external fixation versus 5% with intramedullary nailing.

Reamed intramedullary nailing of open tibial fractures has historically been reported to have an increased incidence of infection.[91] One prospective randomized comparison of nonreamed versus reamed tibial nailing has shown no difference in infection rates.

There may be an indication later for reamed nailing of some fractures treated initially with nonreamed nails to increase stability and enhance the rate of union.[162]

In much of the world, external fixation remains the treatment of choice for open fractures of the tibia. In North America and Europe, many surgeons believe that external fixators are the fixation of choice for type IIIB and IIIC fractures.

The use of external fixation and stabilization of type IIIB open tibial fractures is still practiced widely today. Stable fracture patterns can be adequately stabilized by a single plane half-pin frame; but more comminuted patterns, particularly those with segmental bone loss, may require biplane half-pin frames (delta frame) to enhance stability.

The role of circular fixators using tensional small wire fixation (Ilizarov and others) for the treatment of acute open fractures continues to evolve. Circular fixation for fractures of the periarticular regions of the tibia, either proximal or distal, when combined with half-pins in the tibial shaft, so-called hybrid external fixation, used independently or in combination with limited screw fixation of the articular fragments, is proving useful to provide good stability when comminution in the metaphysis or soft-tissue injuries precludes internal fixation.[146,174,175]

In comminuted fractures the tibia should not be shortened more than $^1/_2$ inch to achieve good bone apposition, because the muscles below the knee do not accommodate well to shortening. Larger segmental defects can be bridged with bone grafts; segment transportation and restoration of full length provides optimal muscle function.

Because external fixation is one of the most commonly used methods of fixation in the tibia, a few comments about management are merited. Unless the fracture pattern is stable and the frame is in compression, early weight bearing, other than touch-down, is usually not possible. A dorsiflexion foot support to avoid an equinus deformity is important. If the fracture is not stable when the external fixation frame is removed, maintenance of position in a cast can be exceedingly difficult. For that reason we try to keep the majority of tibial fractures in an external fixator until union occurs. We plan to adjust the frame to allow progressive weight bearing through the fracture site as the fracture consolidates. We usually do not begin weight bearing until some callus can be seen and the fracture has some early stability.

Early bone grafting is often indicated in open fractures of the tibia. In fractures with bone loss or extensive soft-tissue stripping, bone grafting should usually be performed early (6 to 8 weeks after injury). In fractures with significant bone loss being treated with conventional external fixation, early bone grafting can help facilitate earlier external fixator removal after union of the fracture has occurred at 4 to 6 months after injury. In less severe cases, if the fracture is an unstable pattern and shows no evidence of callus formation by 12 weeks, then bone grafting is indicated.

Another alternative would be the early institution of electrical stimulation, but the role of this method has not been established in fresh fractures or in delayed unions.

We remove the frame and convert the patient to either a weight-bearing cast or cast-brace when the fracture is clinically stable. There is no problem testing this in the later stages of union by removing the fixation frame and leaving the pins in place in the outpatient department. If the fracture is found to not yet be ready for conversion to a cast or brace, the frame is easily reapplied. Earlier conversion to a weight-bearing cast or brace may be necessary if pin complications mandate removal of the frame. Conversion to internal fixation is rarely necessary. In some cases in which the fracture remains quite unstable but pin complications make early removal of the external fixator necessary, insertion of a nonreamed nail may be appropriate. To minimize the risk of infection, the fixator is removed and the pin tracks are allowed to heal before nailing (this usually requires 10 to 20 days), and closed technique is used. In our experience, conversion to a plate or reamed nail is too hazardous because of the high risk of infection.[105] This is particularly true if any of the pins of the external fixator have become infected.

Because of the high rate of infection (up to 35% in the series by Bach), acute plate fixation is rarely indicated.[4,62,64] Reasonably good results have been reported in some series using compression plates combined with interfragmentary screws.[113,133] The incidence of nonunion and late osteomyelitis is quite low in these series (see Table 6-5).

When treating severe type III fractures of the tibia, particularly if complicated by infection or neurovascular injury, the indications for early amputation should be remembered (see Immediate or Early Amputation Versus Limb Salvage, p. 6-18).

Fractures of the Femur

Type I open fractures of the shaft can be immediately internally fixed with intramedullary nails with an infection rate approaching that of closed fractures.[22,24,25,28] In type II and type IIIA open fractures, the risk of infection with immediate intramedullary nailing is not increased as compared with treatment with delayed intramedullary nailing.[61,97,116] In type IIIB, very severe, highly contaminated open fractures, external fixation may have a role to play. External fixation is also useful in children and when open surgery is not feasible in patients with multiple injuries. We do not routinely use external fixation because the large soft-tissue envelope around the femur makes internal fixation safer and external fixation more troublesome. We have not found the Wagner external fixator to be very useful because the fixation pins are too distant from the fracture site: adequate stability cannot be obtained with this method unless the fracture pattern is very stable.[114] We prefer the versatility of a single-plane half-pin fixator. Long-term management usually requires a biplanar fixator. Immediate placement of external fixation followed by early removal of the fixator and intramedullary nailing has been reported for use in type IIIC open fractures.[83,183,184] In victims of multiple injuries, particularly if the patient has been placed on a regular operating table in the supine position, immediate antegrade intramedullary nailing may be difficult. In this circumstance, retrograde intramedullary nailing of open femoral shaft fractures with a through-the-knee portal or medial epicondyle portal has been advocated, although long-term results of this technique are not available.[112,141] Immediate plate fixation through the open fracture wound may be indicated in this setting. This can usually be accomplished rapidly and may be life saving.[131]

Although some type of skeletal fixation is used for the vast majority of open fractures of the femur in most trauma centers in the Western world, management by cast-braces also can work well, although the wound management is more difficult and the incidence of malunion is higher. Where fixation devices are not available, as in some Third World countries, and in mass casualty situations in which application of fixation may not be practical, immediate immobilization in a cast-brace or 1 ½ hip spica cast certainly serves a useful role. We can apply an external fixator much more rapidly than a good cast, however, and the advantages of the fixator over a cast are without question.

Open fractures of the femur often occur in conjunction with severe ipsilateral knee injuries and fractures of the hip. In these situations, internal fixation is usually indicated.[24] Intra-articular fractures involving the knee are treated with the same principles used for fractures of the ankle. Rehabilitation of severe soft-tissue injuries of the knee is usually enhanced by internal fixation of the femoral shaft fracture. Therefore, in type I, type II, and type IIIA open fractures, internal fixation is usually indicated primarily. Type IIIB open fractures of the supracondylar femur with intra-articular extension should be managed by primary limited fixation of the articular surface and bridging external fixation. This can be converted later to internal fixation when the soft tissues have been controlled. On occasion, primary plate fixation using "by-pass" indirect reduction techniques may be indicated.[102]

Upper Extremity Long-Bone Fractures

The long bones of the upper extremity have good soft-tissue coverage. This, combined with the fact that upper-extremity wounds usually involve less energy than lower-extremity wounds, makes the incidence of complications much lower.[29,31,133] In type I open fractures, internal fixation can be carried out with the same indications as in closed fractures. Care of the soft tissues in type II and type III open fractures of the humerus is facilitated with skeletal stabilization of the humeral shaft. We prefer plate fixation: however, Enders nails and newer interlocking nails have proven very useful.[66,68] Additionally, humeral shaft fractures associated with brachial plexus palsies are best treated with primary open reduction and internal fixation. Open humeral shaft fractures with radial nerve palsy are associated with a high incidence of nerve transection.[44,109] Exploration of the radial nerve at the time of debridement should be routine. Early evidence suggests intramedullary nails may have a higher incidence of nonunion in humeral shaft fractures compared with plate fixation. More prospective data are needed to clarify this issue.[12] Intra-articular fractures in the upper extremity suitable for internal fixation are best fixed immediately. Fractures of the radius and ulna can be plated immediately, particularly when combined with a bone graft, with a high rate of union and low rate of infection.[29]

DEFINITIVE WOUND MANAGEMENT

The initial decision required in the treatment of open fractures is whether the limb should be salvaged or amputated. Once a decision to attempt salvage has been made, irrigation and debridement are required and then fracture stability must be obtained. Assuming that internal or external fixation has been employed, the final decision is how to manage the open fracture wound. The options available to the surgeon are outlined below:[56]

I. Primary Options for Definitive Wound Management
   A. Primary closure by suture
   B. Primary closure with autogenous skin graft or local or microvascularized full-thickness graft
   C. Wound left open
      1. Gauze dressings
      2. Biological dressings—homografts, heterografts, or synthetic materials.[6]

When the wound is left open, a series of secondary options must be considered:

II. Secondary Options for Definitive Wound Management
   A. Delayed primary closure by suture
   B. Delayed autogenous skin graft or local or microvascularized flap
   C. Secondary closure by suture or graft
   D. Healing by secondary intention
   E. Split-thickness skin graft with the intent of subsequent excision and closure by suture or flap.

Although the preceding lists include most options, they may at times be modified and are frequently combined for unusual situations.

Primary Closure

Primary closure is rarely indicated. If it is to be done, the following criteria must be met:

1. The original wound must have been fairly clean and not have occurred in a highly contaminated environment.
2. All necrotic tissue and foreign material have been removed.
3. Circulation to the limb is essentially normal.
4. Nerve supply to the limb is intact.
5. The patient's general condition is satisfactory.
6. The wound can be closed without tension.
7. Closure will not create a dead space.
8. The patient does not have multiple-system injuries.

Type I open fracture wounds often meet these criteria; however, the type I wound is usually so small that closure by secondary intention is quite satisfactory. Type III wounds should never be closed primarily. Type II wounds require careful judgment and in general should be left open. The biggest risk of primary closure is gas gangrene, and this seems to occur in very benign-seeming wounds. If the surgeon is inexperienced or in doubt, it seems wise to invoke the axiom, "When in doubt, leave it open," or even better, "Leave all open fractures open."

On the other hand, there seems little question that fractured bones heal most rapidly when they are enclosed by infection-free, pliable, vascularized soft tissues. Thus, as Brav[19] has pointed out, one of the early objectives of treating an open fracture is to convert it to a closed one. This is probably best accomplished by delayed primary closure (see below). In most cases, the elective portion of the wound made by the surgeon can be closed, leaving the traumatic wound open. It is particularly important to cover primarily tendon without peritenon and bone not covered by periosteum, because desiccation will result in the death of these structures. Usually some local muscle or fat can be drawn across these structures, leaving the skin open. The same rationale applies to open joints, where we usually close the capsule over a suction drain and leave the remainder of the wound open.

Delayed Primary Closure

In the healthy adult, the wound healing process proceeds for the first 5 days or so whether or not the wound is closed. As long as closure is achieved before the fifth day, wound strengths at 14 days are comparable to those in wounds closed on the first day. This is why closure before the fifth day is termed *delayed primary closure*. There are several advantages to this approach: leaving the wound open minimizes the risk of anaerobic infection. Also, the delay allows the host to mount local wound defensive mechanisms, which will permit closure more safely than is possible on the first day.

Leaving Wounds Open

There is a strong tendency for surgeons to put drains into wounds that have been left open. For draining an established abscess or tissue spaces that tend naturally to reseal themselves (eg, palmar space, subgluteal space), the reasons for and usefulness of such drains are acknowledged. However, standard mechanical drains (eg, the Penrose) may irritate the tissues they contact and incite an innocent exudate. The trouble lies in the uncertainty that such an exudate is, in fact, innocent. For major soft-tissue wounds that are to be left open after debridement, gauze dressings inserted to a point just beneath the fascia are sufficient, because the fascia and skin usually create the most resistant barrier to the escape of accumulated purulent material. The dressing should just keep the fascial and skin edges separated. The wounds should not be packed because this often produces an obturator effect and thus prevents exudate and serum from draining. Loosely placed dressings conduct the exudate or transudate by capillary action to the surface. When there is no drainage, apart from the initial wound bleeding, the blood soaks into the dressing, coagulates, and may dry to a remarkable degree, leaving the dressing as a firm, rust-colored "blood shingle." Where tendon and bone lack soft-tissue coverage, it may be useful to keep the wound moist by inserting a catheter through which sterile fluid can be dripped.

Ordinarily, the wound is not exposed on the ward for inspection until the time of delayed primary closure—4 to 6 days after injury. Dressing changes in the patient's bed before that time are usually unnecessary and simply increase the risk of nosocomial infection. Of course, more severe types of fractures will have been debrided on an internal basis in the operating room before closure.

Should local symptoms of pain, odor, or obviously excessive drainage appear early on, or should more general signs of fever, leukocytosis, or other problems be noted, early return to the operating room for inspection and repeat irrigation and debridement are warranted. In type III open fractures and those that occurred in a highly contaminated environment, early return to the operating room within 36 to 48 hours may be indicated for wound inspection and repeat irrigation and debridement, particularly if the original irrigation and debridement were thought to be marginal.

When wound closure is not possible by about the fifth day, particularly when there is residual necrotic tissue in the wound that would benefit from dressing changes, then serial dressing changes in the patient's bed may be necessary. This is particularly true if infection intervenes. We prefer wet to dry dressing changes performed every 12 hours, using either normal saline or half-strength Dakin's solution. Fine mesh gauze is placed directly on the wound and overlaid with moist 4×4-inch gauze pads. The wound is covered lightly so the gauze can dry. When the dressing is changed the overlying gauze is removed dry, thus debriding the wound, and a new moist dressing is applied. When performed over several days, this technique is remarkably effective in removing superficial necrotic debris from wounds and in encouraging granulation tissue.

Wound Closure

Closure by direct suturing is possible in most cases. Only the minimum amount of suture material is placed deep in the wound. We prefer the Matthews technique advocated by Müller and colleagues.[113]

Tension in the closure is avoided because this may produce necrosis of skin edges and deeper soft tissues. If primary closure of the wound without tension is not possible, alternatives are "relaxing" incisions and split-thickness skin grafts.

Relaxing Incisions

A linear wound with minimal soft-tissue loss may be difficult to close because of underlying swelling. When it is important to obtain full-thickness coverage over bone or other structures, closure can often be effected with a relaxing incision (Fig. 6-18). It is important to understand that relaxing incisions produce different types of local flaps, the most characteristic being a bipedicle flap. Care must be exercised to place these flaps sufficiently distant from the original wound that the blood supply to the intervening skin is not threatened. This is particularly a problem if the skin between the two wounds has been injured. The relaxing incision must be long enough to allow closure of the primary wound without tension. Relaxing incisions are best suited to those areas in which there is some natural mobility of the skin and underlying tissue, such as the thigh and proximal leg, but less so where mobility is limited, as in the lower leg, ankle region, and about the wrist. Multiple, small, alternating relaxing incisions provide another technique of obtaining closure, but they must be used cautiously, particularly when the surrounding skin has been damaged (Fig. 6-19).

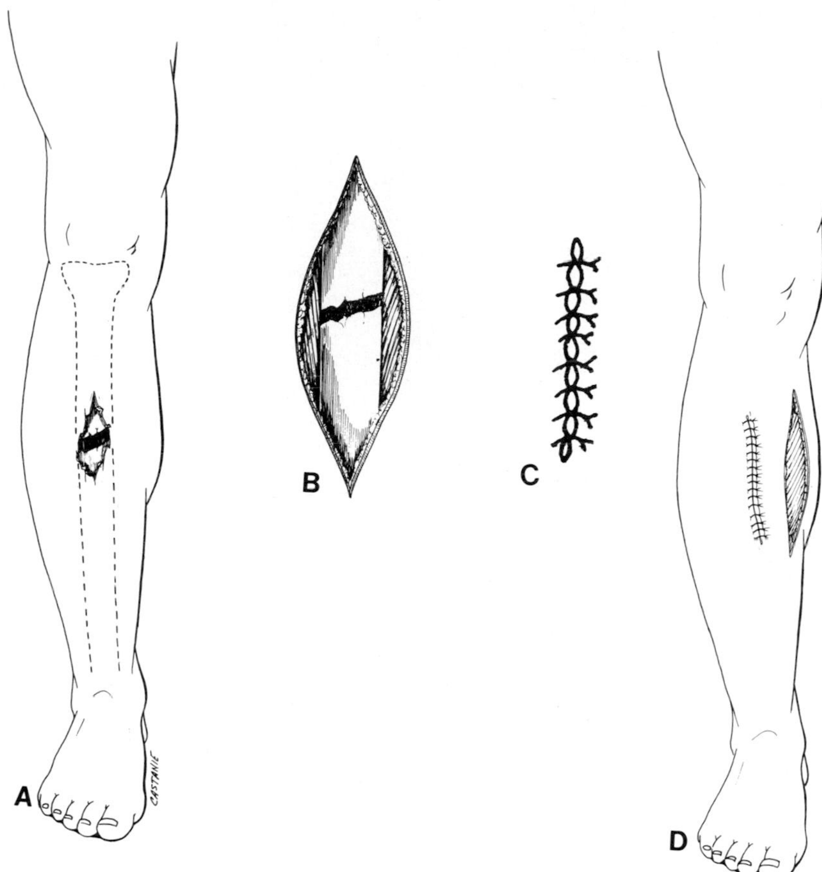

FIGURE 6-18. (**A**) A rather significant loss of tissue directly over the crest of the tibia. (**B**) The degree of tissue loss after debridement. (**C**) The excessive tension at the wound margins that results when direct suture closure is attempted. (**D**) The principle of the relaxing incision. Care must be exercised to avoid making the interval bridge of skin (essentially a bipedicled flap graft) too narrow. The primary wound can now be closed for cover without tension at the suture line. The relaxing incision can communicate with the fracture to facilitate drainage.

We mention this latter technique only for the sake of completeness because we have not used it in the last few years. Mechanical devices to aid closure (eg, Sure-Close) may be useful, but we do not have enough experience with them to advocate their use at this time.

Split-Thickness Skin Grafts

In most cases where the wound bed is composed of viable vascularized soft tissues, a split-thickness skin graft provides the best method of closure. This avoids the risk of a bipedicle flap and is better cosmetically because it leaves only one wound rather than two, as the opened relaxing incision requires split-thickness skin graft as well. In addition, when edema subsides, the skin graft will contract, and often the resulting wound will be much smaller and more cosmetically acceptable. If it is not, late excision and primary closure to produce a cosmetically acceptable wound may be possible.

Split-thickness skin grafts require support from host tissues on which they are deposited and do best when placed directly on viable muscle or well-formed granulation tissue. (Granulation tissue is not necessary as long as the underlying tissues are well vascularized.) Split grafts will not take on bare tendons or on bone not covered by periosteum. Their prospect for survival is somewhat less certain on tissues with a limited blood supply such as periosteum, fascia, and joint capsule.

Generally, relatively thin split-thickness skin grafts (0.010–0.012 inch) have demonstrated greater survival. The skin grafts mold to the wound site and drain much better if run through a 1 to $1\,^1/_2$ mesher. The less the mesh is spread, the better the cosmetic result. If the wound is marginal, spreading the mesh widely enhances drainage.[160]

Flaps

When soft-tissue loss is extensive and closure by primary suture or split-thickness skin graft is not possible, flaps become necessary. The types of flaps available are local fascial-cutaneous flaps, local muscle pedicle flaps, remote muscle pedicle flaps, and free microvascularized muscle flaps.[46,49,99,154] This is a very extensive topic in itself and is described in detail in Chapter 7. Suffice it to say that surgeons treating open fractures must be skilled in using all of these flaps or have available a colleague with such skills. Generally, flaps are

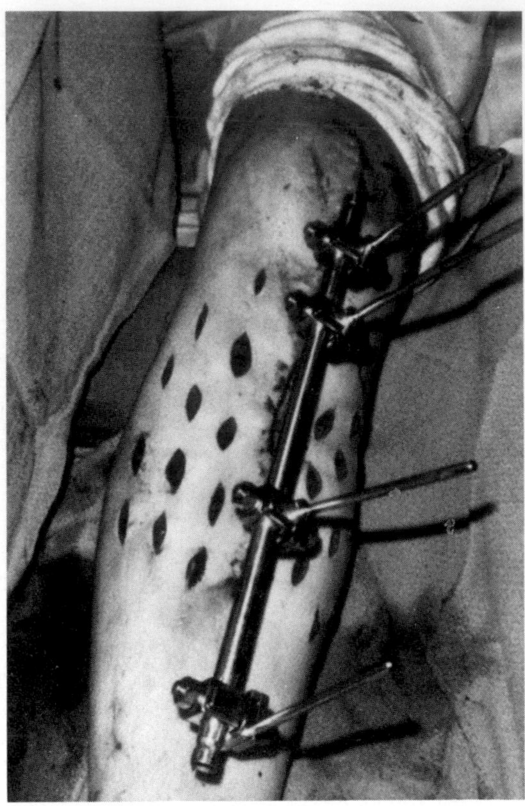

FIGURE 6-19. Multiple 1-cm stab wounds allow closure of a longitudinal wound over the exposed anterior surface of the tibia. Note the spread and alternating pattern, which is necessary to avoid skin necrosis. Do not use this technique on contused or detached skin. (*Chapman, M.W.: Fractures of the Tibia and Fibula. In Chapman, M.W. [ed.]: Operative Orthopaedics, vol. 1, p. 456. Philadelphia, J.B. Lippincott, 1988.*)

not done at the time of initial irrigation and debridement because it often is very difficult to predict the amount of progressive local tissue necrosis that may occur; a flap placed at this time may, in effect, result in primary closure of the wound. Where bone, tendon, and other structures require immediate coverage, we swing a local muscle flap without actually closing the entire wound. Otherwise, we believe most flaps are best done at about 5 days after injury.

Most coverage problems occur in the tibia (Fig. 6-20), and the fracture surgeon should be familiar with the gastrocnemius, soleus, anterior tibial, and flexor hallucis and flexor digitorum local muscle flaps (see Chapter 7).[53]

Biological Dressings

When closure is not appropriate or cannot be carried out, and arrangements cannot be made for the covering of vulnerable tissues by the transposition of local tissues, biological dressings of skin or synthetic material may be of value. Homologous human skin, heterologous porcine skin (prepared commercially), and synthetic dressings may suffice. Our personal experience with these dressings is very limited, and they have not been used on our service on a routine basis; therefore, it is difficult for us to put their role into perspective. Baxter[6] has shown that these skin dressings have several advantages in the treatment of burn patients. Changing them is considerably less painful. They seem to be a deterrent to infection, and there is some evidence that existing infection may be suppressed or controlled. Because host granulation tissue invades such grafts, allowing them to take for varying periods, the biological dressings can give evidence of the readiness of a wound bed for definitive autogenous grafting. Thus, such grafts need to be changed frequently. Salisbury[138] has shown that when granulation tissue from an autogenous graft donor site grows into a heterologous dressing, even if it is pulled away before any significant clinical take occurs, small bits of collagen from the heterologous dressing tissue remain in the host granulation tissue. This collagen apparently tends to incite a rather chronic inflammatory response, leading to some delay in epithelialization and an increase in inflammation. Because these dressings are not used commonly in the treatment of open fractures

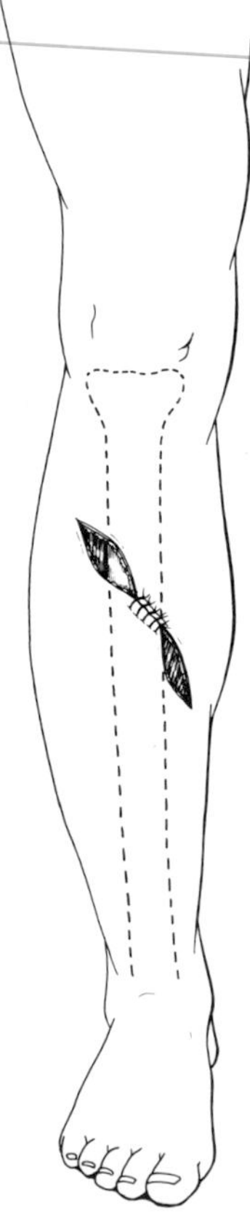

FIGURE 6-20. A method of providing "cover" for an exposed medial surface of the tibial shaft while providing for drainage at either end of the wound. This is not suitable if very much skin has been lost because tension may induce marginal necrosis of the distal edge at the sutured area.

in North America, the reader is referred to the literature on this field.

Elevation

Perhaps there is no more critical point in the control of postdebridement swelling than the simple matter of elevation. Persistent, or increased, swelling may keep tissues turgid and wound surfaces moist, thereby preventing delayed primary closure. Edematous tissues increase tension in the suture line and may lead to marginal wound necrosis. Other disadvantages of swelling include a possible increase in the prospect of infection, a loss of reduction of fracture should swelling require a cast be split and spread, and probably an increased risk of thrombophlebitis.

Limbs must be elevated in a manner that is comfortable for the patient and guarantees continuous elevation at a level above the heart; however, elevation more than 10 cm above the heart does not enhance lymphatic or venous return but does decrease the arterial input to the limb, which can be hazardous in impending compartment syndrome and in patients with peripheral vascular disease. Under most circumstances, broad slings suspended from the overhead frame serve best.

Antibiotics

Antibiotics for open fracture wounds should not be considered prophylactic, but therapeutic, because these wounds are contaminated by bacteria. (Purists would argue that in the acute wound, infection is not present and therefore antibiotics *are* prophylactic, but we argue that many organisms are present in spite of adequate irrigation and debridement.) The role of antibiotics is to kill residual organisms and at least inhibit their growth to the point where host protective mechanisms will eradicate them.[181] Irrigation and debridement are by far the most important measures in preventing infection in open fractures, and antibiotics certainly cannot be relied on to prevent infection in an inadequately debrided wound.

Patzakis and associates[126] established the basis of our current practice. In their controlled, randomized, prospective study, they compared three groups: one received immediate administration of cephalothin, one immediate administration of penicillin and streptomycin, and the third group received no antibiotics. The infection rate in the cephalothin group was 2.3%, compared with 9.7% in the penicillin/streptomycin group, and 13.9% in the final group. It is on the basis of this study and subsequent clinical experience that cephalosporins remain the antibiotics of choice for the treatment of open fractures. Early administration of antibiotics during the initial phases of resuscitation decreases the incidence of infection in open fractures. In addition, the data of Patzakis and associates support that a culture taken from the wound before any treatment is likely to yield the organisms that will subsequently cause infection. The most common organism producing infection in their series was *Staphylococcus aureus;* most of these infections were resistant to penicillin. However, recent studies have shown that predebridement cultures have no reliable correlation with the eventual infecting organism. The correlation of postdebridement cultures with the eventual infecting organism is poor at best.

Over the past decade, however, clinical experience has changed. As reflected in Gustilo's figures,[62,65] the overall infection rate in open fractures rose somewhat in the late 1970s and early 1980s, probably because the overall severity of open fractures had increased and we were salvaging limbs that previously were amputated. In the late 1980s and in the 1990s infection rates have improved owing to improved techniques and antibiotics.[176] Second, the spectrum of infecting organisms has changed. Although *S. aureus* remains a major player, gram-negative organisms have become very prevalent and mixed infections are common, particularly in type III open fractures. The precise cause for this change is not known. We hypothesize that three factors are playing a role: (1) the ubiquitous use of cephalosporins in open fractures probably is selecting out resistant gram-negative organisms; (2) gram-negative organisms such as *Pseudomonas, Enterobacter,* and enterococcus have become very prevalent nosocomial infective organisms; and (3) the severely traumatized limbs we try to salvage today may present to the population of bacteria a unique environment that was not readily available in the past.

Thus, use of antibiotics has changed. In open fractures occurring in a reasonably clean environment, and for type I or II fractures, most surgeons still use a cephalosporin—most commonly, cefazolin. In those fractures occurring in a highly contaminated environment, most surgeons add penicillin to prevent clostridial infection. In type III open fractures, aminoglycosides are frequently administered as well.[2,18,38]

The most important step a surgeon can take is to constantly monitor by cultures the organisms most frequently occurring in open fracture wounds in his or her institution and those most commonly causing infection. Constant monitoring of the antibiotic sensitivities of these organisms should provide a good guide as to the appropriate antibiotics, doses, and routes of administration.

The use of topical antibiotics remains controversial. There is enough evidence to point to their effectiveness[54,173] that we routinely place topical antibiotics in the last 2-L bag used for irrigation. In addition, the dressings can be soaked in these topical antibiotics. It seems to us that these agents remain in the wound long enough that some killing of remaining organisms will occur, thereby dropping the bacterial count in the wound. Many different antibiotics can be used for topical application; our advice regarding the selection of parenteral antibiotics applies to local antibiotics.

Kellam and colleagues have demonstrated that iodine, iodophor compounds, and hydrogen peroxide used topically are toxic to osteoblasts while bacitracin is not.[89] Anglen and associates[1] showed that topical detergents used with a mechanical pulsatile irrigator were superior in removing glycocalyx-forming bacteria than plain saline or topical antibiotics.

General principles to be followed in the use of antibiotics are (1) to administer parenteral antibiotics as soon as possible and (2) to choose antibiotics that are bactericidal and an antibiotic (or antibiotics) active against both gram-positive and gram-negative organisms. The drugs should produce bactericidal concentrations in blood, extracellular fluids, and joint fluids. They must be as hypoallergenic as possible and compatible with other antibiotics. Current recommendations for type I and type II open fracture wounds are 3 days of intravenous antimicrobial therapy, generally cefazolin, 1 g every 8 hours. For type III open fracture wounds 5 days of treatment is recommended with cefazolin and gentamicin given at 2 mg/kg initially and subsequently adjusted to serum levels. Careful monitoring of renal function is required with the use of aminoglycosides. When significant contamination is present, or the history of injury suggests significant contamination from barnyard injury, lake, or stream, the addition of penicillin, 4 million units intravenously every 6 hours to cover anaerobic organisms, specifically *Clostridium perfringens*, is advised. If cultures are positive or clinical signs of infection are present, then therapy needs to be tailored to the specific situation.

Antibiotic-Impregnated Beads

Numerous antibiotics can be incorporated in polymethylmethacrylate while maintaining their bactericidal activity. They leach out at sufficient rates that bactericidal levels are produced in the surrounding fluids and tissues.[30] Chains of methacrylate beads strung on stainless steel wire and impregnated with antibiotics have been used to treat infection and more recently have been advocated for open fractures. Seligson[149] has produced what he calls a "bead pouch" by placing over the fracture site and beads an oxygen-permeable membrane (Opsite). Local wound levels of antibiotics produced are higher than those possible by the parenteral route.[40]

Seligson has reported the use of the bead pouch technique as a supplement to parenteral intravenous antibiotics. He compared his results to 157 open fractures with systemic antibiotics only. He reported a statistically significant decrease in the infection rate in the group treated with the bead pouch, particularly in type IIIB open fractures. The control fractures had an infection rate of 39%, as compared with an infection rate of 7.3% when treated with a bead pouch.

Local wound levels of antibiotics produced are higher than those possible by the parenteral route alone. Local tissue levels of tobramycin of greater than 400 μg/mL, however, have been shown to be toxic to osteoblast cells in tissue culture.[108] The incidence of delayed union or nonunion associated with the use of the bead pouch technique has not been well studied. Bead pouch treatment for open fractures is investigational at this time but is promising.[90,119]

REFERENCES

1. Anglen, J., Apostoles, S., Christensen, G., and Gainer, B.: The Efficacy of Various Irrigation Solutions in Removing Slime-Producing *Staphylococcus*. J. Orthop. Trauma, 8:390–396, 1994.
2. Antrum, R.M., and Solomkin, J.S.: A Review of Antibiotic Prophylaxis for Open Fractures. Orthop. Rev., 16:246–254, 1987.
3. Bach, A.W., and Hanson, S.T.: Plates vs. External Fixation in Severe Open Tibial Shaft Fractures: A Randomized Trial. Clin. Orthop. Rel. Res., 241:89–94, 1989.
4. Bach, A.W., and Solomkin, J.S.: Plates Versus External Fixation in Severe Open Tibial Shaft Fractures: A Randomized Trial. Clin. Orthop., 241:89–94, 1989.
5. Bagnoli, G., and Paley, D., The Ilizarov Method. Philadelphia, B.C. Decker, 1986.
6. Baxter, C.R.: Homografts and Heterografts as a Biological Dressing in the Treatment of Thermal Injury. Presented at the First Annual Congress of the Society of German Plastic Surgeons, September 28, 1970.
7. Beckman, S., Scholten, D., Bonnell, B., and Bukrey, C.: Long Bone Fractures in the Polytrauma Patient: The Role of Early Operative Fixation. Am. Surg., 55:356–358, 1989.
8. Behrens, F., and Searls, K.: External Fixation of the Tibia: Basic Concepts and Prospective Evaluation. J. Bone Joint Surg., 68B:246–254, 1986.
9. Benirschke, S.K., Agnew, S.F., Mayo, K.A., Santoro, V.M., and Henley, M.B.: Immediate Internal Fixation Of Open, Complex Tibial Plateau Fractures. J. Orthop. Trauma, 6:78–86, 1992.
10. Blachet, P.A., Meek, R.N., and O'Brien, P.J.: External Fixation and Delayed Intramedullary Nailing of Open Fractures of the Tibial Shaft: A Sequential Protocol. J. Bone Joint Surg., 72A:729–735, 1990.
11. Blick, S.S., Brumback, R.J., Lakatos, R., Poka, A., and Burgess, A.R.: Early Prophylactic Bone Grafting of High-Energy Tibial Fractures. Clin. Orthop., 240:21–41, 1989.
12. Bolano, L.E., Iaquinto, J.A., and Vasiceck, V.: Operative Treatment of Humerus Shaft Fractures: A Prospective Randomized Study Comparing Intramedullary Nailing With Dynamic Compression Plating. Presented before the American Academy of Orthopedic Surgeons, Orlando, FL, 1995, paper No. 112.
13. Bonanni, F., Rhodes, M., and Lucke, J.F.: The Futility of Predictive Scoring of Mangled Lower Extremities. J. Trauma, 34:99–104, 1993.

13a. Bonatus, T.; Olson, S.A.; Lee, S.; Chapman, M.W.: Non-Reamed Interlocking Intramedullary Nailing for the Treatment of Open Tibial Shaft Fractures. Clinical Orthopaedics and Related Research, in press.

14. Bondurant, F., Colter, H.B., Buckle, R., Miller-Crotchett, P.,

and Browner, B.D.: The Medical and Economic Impact of Severely Injured Lower Extremities. J. Trauma, 28:1270–1273, 1988.

15. Bone, L.B., Johnson, K.D., Weigelt, J., and Scheinberg, R.: Early Versus Delayed Stabilization of Femoral Fractures: A Prospective Randomized Study. J. Bone Joint Surg., 71A:336–340, 1989.
16. Bone, L.B., Kassman, S., Stegemann, P., and France, J.: Prospective Study of Union Rate of Open Tibial Fractures Treated With Locked Un-reamed Intramedullary Nails. J. Orthop. Trauma, 8:45–49, 1994.
17. Bone, L., McNamira, K., Shine, B., and Border, J.: Mortality in Multiple Trauma Patients With Fractures. J. Trauma, 37:262–265, 1994.
18. Braun, R., Enzler, M.A., and Rittmann, W.W.: A Double-Blind Clinical Trial of Prophylactic Cloxacillin in Open Fractures. J. Orthop. Trauma, 1:12–17, 1987.
19. Brav, E.A.: Open Fractures: Fundamentals of Management. Postgrad. Med., 39:11–16, 1966.
20. Bray, T.J., Endicott, M., and Capra, S.E.: Treatment of Open Ankle Fractures: Immediate Internal Fixation Versus Closed Immobilization and Delayed Fixation. Clin. Orthop., 240:47–52, 1989.
21. Brown, P.W., and Urban, J.G.: Early Weight-Bearing Treatment of Open Fractures of the Tibia: An End-Result Study of 63 Cases. J. Bone Joint Surg., 51:59–75, 1969.
22. Brumback, R.J., Ellison, P.S., Jr., Poka, A., Lakatos, R., Bathon, G.H., and Burgess, A.R.: Intramedullary Nailing of Open Fractures of the Femoral Shaft. J. Bone Joint Surg., 71A:1324–1331, 1989.
23. Brumback, R.J., and Jones, A.L.: Intra Observer Agreement: Classification of Open Fractures of the Tibia: The Results of a Survey of 245 Orthopaedic Surgeons. J. Bone Joint Surg., 76A:1162–1166, 1994.
24. Casey, M.J., and Chapman, M.W.: Ipsilateral Concomitant Fractures of the Hip and Femoral Shaft. J. Bone Joint Surg., 61A:503–509, 1979.
25. Caudle, R.J., and Stern, P.J.: Severe Open Fractures of the Tibia. J. Bone Joint Surg., 69A:801–807, 1987.
26. Chapman, M.W.: The Use of Immediate Internal Fixation in Open Fractures. Orthop. Clin. North Am., 11(3):579–591, 1980.
27. Chapman, M.W.: The Role of Intramedullary Fixation in Open Fractures. Clin. Orthop., 212:26–34, 1986.
28. Chapman, M.W., and Blackman, R.C.: Closed Intramedullary Nailing of Femoral-Shaft Fractures: A Comparison of Two Techniques (Proceedings) (abstract). J. Bone Joint Surg., 58A:732, 1976.
29. Chapman, M.W., Gordon, J.E., and Zissimos, A.G.: Compression-Plate Fixation of Acute Fractures of the Diaphyses of the Radius and Ulna. J. Bone Joint Surg., 71A:159–169, 1989.
30. Chapman, M.W., and Hadley, W.K.: The Effect of Polymethylmethacrylate and Antibiotic Combinations on Bacterial Viability: An in Vitro and Preliminary in Vivo Study. J. Bone Joint Surg., 58A:76–81, 1976.
31. Chapman, M.W., and Mahoney, M.: The Role of Internal Fixation in the Management of Open Fractures. Clin. Orthop., 138:120–131, 1979.
32. Claffey, T.: Open Fractures of the Tibia (Proceedings) (abstract). J. Bone Joint Surg., 42B:407, 1960.
33. Clancey, G.J., and Hansen, S.T., Jr.: Open Fractures of the Tibia: A Review of One Hundred and Two Cases. J. Bone Joint Surg., 60A:118–122, 1978.
34. Clifford, R.P., Beauchamp, C.G., Kellam, J.F., Webb, J.K., and Tile, M.: Plate Fixation of Open Fractures of the Tibia. J. Bone Joint Surg., 70:644–648, 1988.
35. Connolly, J.: Management of Fractures Associated With Arterial Injuries. Am. J. Surg., 120:331, 1970.
36. D'Aubigne, R.M., Maurer, P., Zucman, J., and Masse, Y.: Blind Intramedullary Nailing for Tibial Fractures. Clin. Orthop., 105:267–275, 1974.
37. Dehne, E.: Treatment of Fractures of the Tibial Shaft. Clin. Orthop., 66:159–173, 1969.
38. Dellinger, E.P., Caplan, E.S., Weaver, L.D., et al.: Duration of Preventive Antibiotic Administration for Open Extremity Fractures. Arch. Surg., 123:333–339, 1988.
39. Dickey, R.L., Barnes, B.C., Kearns, R.J., and Tullos, H.S.: Efficacy of Antibiotics in Low Velocity Gunshot Fractures. J. Orthop. Trauma, 3:6–10, 1989.
40. Eckman, J.B., Jr., Henry, S.L., Mangino, P.D., and Seligson, D.: Wound and Serum Levels of Tobramycin With the Prophylactic Use of Tobramycin-Impregnated Polymethylmethacrylate Beads in Compound Fractures. Clin. Orthop., 237:213–215, 1988.
41. Edwards, C.C., Simmons, S.C., Browner, B.D., and Wiegel, M.C.: Severe Open Tibial Fractures: Results Treating 202 Injuries With External Fixation. Clin. Orthop., 230:98–115, 1988.
42. Edwards, C.C., Jaworski, M.F., Solana, J., and Aronson, B.S.: Management of Compound Tibial Fractures Using External Fixation. Am. Surgeon, 45:190–203, 1979.
43. Fellrath, R.F., Bohren, B., and Hanley, E.N.: Spinal Injury In Polytrauma: Influence of Surgical Timing. Presented before the Orthopaedic Trauma Association, Los Angeles, 1994.
44. Fischer, D.A.: Skeletal Stabilization With a Multiplane External Fixation Device: Design Rationale and Preliminary Clinical Experience. Clin. Orthop., 180:50–62, 1983.
45. Fischer, M.D., Gustilo, R.B., and Vareka, T.F.: The Timing of Flap Coverage, Bone Grafting, and Intramedullary Nailing in Patients Who Have a Fracture of the Tibial Shaft With Extensive Soft Tissue Injury. J. Bone Joint Surg., 73A:1316–1322, 1991.
46. Foster, R.J., Swiontkowski, M.F., Bach, A.W., and Sack, J.T.: Radial Nerve Palsy Caused by Open Humeral Shaft Fractures. J. Hand Surg., 18A:121–124, 1993
47. Franklin, J.L., Johnson, K.D., and Hansen, S.T.: Immediate Internal Fixation of Open Ankle Fractures. J. Bone Joint Surg., 66A:1349–1356, 1994.
48. Frankel, V.H.: Symposium: Current Applications of the Ilizarov Technique. Contemp. Orthop., 28:51, 1994.
49. Francel, T.J., Vander Kolk, C.A., Hoopes, J.E., Manson, P.N., and Yaremshuk, M.J.: Microvascular Soft Tissue Transplantation for Reconstruction of Acute Tibial Fractures: Timing of Coverage and Long-Term Functional Results. Plast. Reconstr. Surg., 89:478–487, 1992.
50. Gallinaro, P., Crova, M., and Denicolai, F.: Complications in 64 Open Fractures of the Tibia. Injury, 5:157–160, 1974.
51. Geisslar, W.B., Teasedall, R.D., Thomasin, J.D., and Hughes, J.L: Management of Low Velocity Gunshot Induced Fractures. J. Orthop. Trauma, 4:39–41, 1990.
52. Georgiadis, G.M., Berhrens, F.F., Joyce, M.J., Earle, A.S., and Simmons, A.L.: Open Tibial Fractures With Severe Soft Tissue Loss: Limb Salvage Compared With Below-the-Knee Amputation. J. Bone Joint Surg., 75A:1431–1441, 1993.
53. Ger, R.: The Management of Open Fracture of the Tibia With Skin Loss. J. Trauma, 10:112–121, 1970.
54. Glotzer, D.J., Goodman, W.S., and Geronimus, L.H.: Topical Antibiotic Prophylaxis in Contaminated Wounds: Experimental Evaluation. Arch. Surg., 100:589–593, 1970.
55. Golyakhovsky, V., and Frankel, V.: Operative Manual of Ilizarov Techniques. Philadelphia, CV Mosby, 1992.
56. Greene, T.L., and Beatty, M.E.: Soft Tissue Coverage for Lower-Extremity Trauma: Current Practice and Techniques. A Review. J. Orthop. Trauma, 2:158–173, 1988.
57. Gregory, R.T., Gould, R.J., Peclet, M., et al.: The Mangled Extremities Syndrome (MES): A Severity Grading System for Multisystem Injury of the Extremity. J. Trauma, 25:1147–1150, 1985.
58. Grewe, S.R., Stephens, B.O., Perlino, C., and Riggins, R.S.: Influence of Internal Fixation on Wound Infections. J. Trauma, 27:1051–1054, 1987.
59. Gristina, A.G., and Rovere, G.D.: An In Vitro Study of the Effects of Metals Used in Internal Fixation on Bacterial Growth and Dissemination. J. Bone Joint Surg. (Proceedings), 45A:1104, 1963.
60. Gross, A., Cutright, D.E., and Bhaskar, S.N.: Effectiveness of Pulsating Water Jet Lavage in Treatment of Contaminated, Crushed Wounds. Am. J. Surg., 124:373–377, 1972.

61. Grosse, A., Christie, J., Taglang, G., Court-Brown, C., and McQueen, M.: Open Adult Femoral Shaft Fractures Treated By Early Intramedullary Nailing. J. Bone Joint Surg., 75B:562–565, 1993.
62. Gustilo, R.B.: Current Concepts in the Management of Open Fractures. Instr. Course Lect., 36:359–366, 1987.
63. Gustilo, R.B.: Open Fractures. *In* Fractures and Dislocation. St. Louis, C.V. Mosby, 1993.
64. Gustilo, R.B., and Anderson, J.T.: Prevention of Infection in the Treatment of One Thousand and Twenty-Five Open Fractures of Long Bones: Retrospective and Prospective Analyses. J. Bone Joint Surg., 58A:453–458, 1976.
65. Gustilo, R.B., Gruninger, R.P., and Davis, T.: Classification of Type III (Severe) Open Fractures Relative to Treatment and Results. Orthopedics, 10:1781–1788, 1987.
66. Gustilo, R.B., Merkow, R.L., and Templeman, D.: Current Concepts Review: The Management of Open Fractures. J. Bone Joint Surg., 72A:299–304, 1990.
67. Gustilo, R.B., Simpson, L., Nixon, R., Ruiz, A., and Indeck, W.: Analysis of 511 Open Fractures. Clin. Orthop., 66:148–154, 1969.
68. Hall, R.F., and Pankovich, A.M.: Endernailing of Acute Fractures of the Humerus. J. Bone Joint Surg., 69A:558–567, 1987.
69. Hak, D.J., and Johnson, E.E.: The Use of the Un-reamed Nail in Tibial Fractures With Concomitant Preoperative or Intraoperative Elevated Compartment Pressure Or Compartment Syndrome. J. Orthop. Trauma, 8:203–211, 1994.
70. Hansen, S.T., Jr.: The Type IIIC Tibial Fracture: Salvage or Amputation (editorial). J. Bone Joint Surg., 69A:799–800, 1987.
71. Hawkins, L. G.: Fractures of the Neck of the Talus. J. Bone Joint Surg., 52A:991–1002, 1970.
72. Helfet, D.L., Howey, T., Dipasquale, T., Sanders, R., Zinar, D., and Brooker, A.: The Treatment of Open and/or Unstable Tibia Fractures With an Un-reamed Double Locked Tibial Nail. J. Orthop. Rev., February Suppl., pp. 9–17, 1994.
73. Heppenstell, T., and Hanson, S.: The Treatment of Open Distal Femur Fractures With Immediate Open Reduction and Internal Fixation. Orthop. Trans., 14:707, 1990.
74. Helfet, D.K., Howey, T., Sanders, R., and Johansen, K.: Limb Salvage vs. Amputation: Preliminary Results of the Mangled Extremity Severity Score. Clin. Orthop. Rel. Res., 256:80–86, 1990.
75. Henley, M.B., Chapman, J.R., Agel, J., Swiontkowski, M.F., Benirshke, S.K., and Mayo, K.A.: Comparison of Un-reamed Tibial Nails and External Fixators in the Treatment of Grade 2 & 3 Open Tibial Shaft Fractures. Presented before the Orthopaedic Trauma Association, Los Angeles, 1994.
76. Henley, M. B.: Intramedullary Devices for Tibial Fracture Stabilization. Clin. Orthop., 240:87–96, 1989.
77. Henry, A.K.: Extensive Exposure. Edinburgh, E. & S. Livingstone, 1952.
78. Hollmann, M.W., and Horowitz, M.: Femoral Fractures Secondary to Low Velocity Missiles: Treatment With Delayed Intramedullary Fixation. J. Orthop. Trauma, 4:64–69, 1990.
79. Howard, M.W., Zinar, D.M., and Stryker, W.S.: The Use of the Lottes Nail in the Treatment of Closed and Open Tibial Shaft Fractures. Clin. Orthop. Rel. Res., 279:246–253, 1992.
80. Howe, H.R., Poole, G.V., Hansen, K.J., et al.: Salvage of Lower Extremities Following Combined Orthopaedic and Vascular Trauma: A Predictive Salvage Index. Am. Surgeon, 53:205–208, 1987.
81. Ilizarov, G.A.: Clinical Application of the Tension-Stress Effect for Limb Lengthening. Clin. Orthop., 250:8–26, 1990.
82. Ilizarov, G.A.: Transosseous Osteosynthesis. Berlin, Springer-Verlag, 1992.
83. Iannacone, W.M., Taffet, R., DeLong, W.G., Born, C.T., Dalsey, R.M., and Deutsch, L.S.: Early Exchange Intramedullary Nailing of Distal Femoral Fractures With Vascular Injury Initially Stabilized With External Fixation. J. Trauma, 37:446–451, 1994.
84. Johnson, E.E., and Davlyn, L.B.: Open Ankle Fractures: The Indications for Immediate Open Reduction and Internal Fixation. Clin. Orthop. Rel. Res., 292:118–127, 1993.
85. Johnson, E.E., and Davlin, L.B.: Open Ankle Fractures: The Indications For Immediate Open Reduction and Internal Fixation. Clin. Orthop. Rel. Res., 292:118–127, 1993.
86. Johansen, K., Daines, M., Howey, T., Helfet, D., Hansen, S.T.: Objective Criteria Accurately Predict Amputation Following Lower Extremity Trauma. J. Trauma, 30:568–573, 1990.
87. Johnson, K.D., Bone, L.B., and Scheinberg, R.: Severe Open Tibial Fractures: A Study Protocol. J. Orthop. Trauma, 2:175–180, 1988.
88. Johnson, K.D., Cadambi, A., and Seibert, G.B.: Incidence of Adult Respiratory Stress Syndrome in Patients With Multiple Musculoskeletal Injuries: The Effect of Early Operative Stabilization of Fractures. J. Trauma, 25:375–384, 1985.
89. Kellam, J., Ramp, W., Nicholason, N., and Kaysinger, K.: Effects of Wound Irrigation Solutions on Osteoblast Function. Presented before the Orthopaedic Trauma Association, New Orleans, 1993.
90. Keating, J.F., Blachut, P.A., O'Brien, P.J., and Broekhuyse, H.M.: Reamed Nailing of Open Tibial Fractures: Does the Antibiotic Bead Pouch Reduce the Infection Rate? Presented at the 62nd annual meeting of the American Association of Orthopedic Surgeons, Orlando, FL, February 1995.
91. Keating, J.F., O'Brien, P.J., Meek, R. N., Blachut, P.A., and Broekhuyse, H. N.: Interlocking Intramedullary Nailing of Open Fractures of the Tibia: A Prospective Randomized Comparison of Reamed and Unreamed Nails. Presented at the 62nd annual meeting of the American Association of Orthopedic Surgeons, Orlando, FL, February, 1995.
92. Krettek, C., Haas, N., and Tscherne, H.: The Role of Supplemental Leg Screw Fixation for Open Fractures of the Tibial Shaft Treated With External Fixation. J. Bone Joint Surg., 73A:893–897, 1991.
93. La Duca, J.N., Bone, L.L., Seibel, R.W., and Border, J.R.: Primary Open Reduction and Internal Fixation of Open Fractures. J. Trauma, 20:580–586, 1980.
94. Lange, R.H., Bach, A. W., Hansen, S.T., Jr., and Johansen, K.H.: Open Tibial Fractures With Associated Vascular Injuries: Prognosis for Limb Salvage. J. Trauma, 25:203–208, 1985.
95. Lee, J., Goldstein, J., Madison, M., and Chapman, M.W.: The Value of Pre and Post Debridement Cultures in the Management of Open Fractures. Orthop. Trans. J. Bone Joint Surg., 15(3):776, 1991.
96. Leonard, M.H.: The Solution of Lead by Synovial Fluid. Clin. Orthop., 64:255–261, 1969.
97. Lhowe, G.W., and Hansen, S.T.: Immediate Nailing of Open Fractures of the Femoral Shaft. J. Bone Joint Surg., 70A:812–820, 1988.
98. Llinas, A., McKellop, H.A., Marshall, G.J., et al.: Healing and Remodeling of Articular Incongruities in a Rabbit Fracture Model. J. Bone Joint Surg., 75A:1508–1523, 1993.
99. Lo, L.J., Chen, Y.R., Weng, C.J., and Noordhoff, M.S.: Use of Split Anterior Tibial Muscle Flap in Treating Avulsion Injury of the Leg Associated With Tibia Exposure. Ann. Plast. Surg., 31:112–116, 1993.
100. Lottes, J.O., Hill, L.J., and Key, J.A.: Closed Reduction, Plate Fixation and Medullary Nailing of Fractures of Both Bones of the Leg: A Comparative End-Result Study. J. Bone Joint Surg., 34A:861–877, 1952.
101. Lhowe, G.W., and Hansen, S.T.: Immediate Nailing of Open Fractures of the Femoral Shaft. J. Bone Joint Surg., 70A:812–820, 1988.
102. Mast, J., Jakob, R., and Ganz, R.: Planning and Reduction Technique in Fracture Surgery. New York, Springer-Verlag, 1989.
103. Matsen, F.A., III, Mayo, K.A., Sheridan, G.W., and Krugmire, R.B., Jr.: Monitoring of Intramuscular Pressure. Surgery, 79:702–709, 1976.
104. McBroom, R.J., Tucker, W.S., and Waddell, J.P.: Early vs. Delayed Fixation of the Thoraco-Lumbar Spine in Polytrauma Patients. Presented before the Orthopaedic Trauma Association, Los Angeles, 1994.

105. McGraw, J.M., and Lim, E.V.: Treatment of Open Tibial-Shaft Fractures: External Fixation and Secondary Intramedullary Nailing. J. Bone Joint Surg., 70A:900–911, 1988.
106. McNamara, M.G., Heckman, J.D., and Corley, F.G.: Severe Open Fractures of the Lower Extremity: A Retrospective Evaluation of the Mangled Extremity Severity Score. J. Orthop. Trauma, 8:81–87, 1994.
107. Meléndez, E.M., and Colón, C.: Treatment of Open Tibial Fractures with the Orthofix Fixator. Clin. Orthop., 241:224–230, 1989.
108. Miclau, T., Edin, M.L., Lester, G.E., Lindsey, R.W., Dahners, L.E.: Bone Toxicity of Locally Applied Aminoglycosides. Presented before the Orthopaedic Trauma Association, Los Angeles, 1994.
109. Mitchell, N., and Shepard, N.: Healing of Articular Cartilage in Intra-Articular Fractures in Rabbits. J. Bone Joint Surg., 62A:628–634, 1980.
110. Moed, B.R., Kellam, J.F., Foster, R.J., Tile, M., and Hasen, S.T.: Immediate Internal Fixation of Open Fractures of the Diaphysis of the Forearm. J. Bone Joint Surg., 68A:1008–1017, 1986.
111. Moed B.R., Watson, J., Goldschmidt, P., and vanHolsbeek, M.: Ultrasound for the Early Diagnosis of Fracture Healing Following Intramedullary Nailing of the Tibia Without Reaming. Clin. Orthop. Rel. Res., 310:137–144, 1995.
112. Moed, B., and Watson, J.: Retrograde Intramedullary Nailing of Fractures of the Femoral Shaft in the Multiply Injured Patient. Presented before the Orthopaedic Trauma Association, Los Angeles, 1994.
113. Müller, M.E., Allgöwer, M., Schneider, R., and Willeneger, H.: Manual of Internal Fixation: Technique Recommended by the AO Group, 2nd ed. New York, Springer-Verlag, 1979.
114. Murphy, C.P., D'Ambrosia, R.D., Dabezies, E.J., Acker, J.H., Shoji, H., and Chuinard, R.G.: Complex Femur Fractures: Treatment with the Wagner External Fixation Device or the Grosse-Kempf Interlocking Nail. J. Trauma, 28:1553–1561, 1988.
115. Nowotarski, P., and Brumback, R.W.: Immediate Interlocking Nailing of Fractures of the Femur Caused By Low-Velocity to Mid-Velocity Gun Shots. J. Orthop. Trauma, 8:134–141, 1994.
116. O'Brien, P.J., Meek, R.N., Powell, J.N., and Blachut, P.A.: Primary Intramedullary Nailing of Open Femoral Shaft Fractures. J. Trauma, 31:113–116, 1991.
117. Olerud, S., and Karlstrom, G.: Tibial Fractures Treated by AO Compression Osteosynthesis. Acta Orthop. Scand. [Suppl.], 140:3–104, 1972.
118. Orr, H.W.: The Treatment of Osteomyelitis by Drainage and Rest. J. Bone Joint Surg., 9:730–740, 1927.
119. Osternann, P.A., Henry, S.L., and Seligson, D.: The Role Of Local Antibiotic Therapy in the Management of Compound Fractures. Clin. Orthop. Rel. Res., 295:102–111, 1993.
120. Pankovich, A.M., and Tarabishy, I.: Closed Ender Nailing of Tibial Shaft Fractures. Presented at 47th Annual Meeting of the American Academy of Orthopaedic Surgeons, Atlanta, February, 1980.
121. Pape, H.C., Regel, G., Dwenger, A., et al.: Influence of Different Methods of Intramedullary Femoral Nailing on Lung Function in Patients With Multiple Trauma. J. Trauma, 35:709–710, 1993.
122. Papineau, L. J., Alfageme, A., Dalcourt, J.P., and Pilon, L.: Chronic Osteomyelitis: Open Excision and Grafting After Saucerization [in French]. Int. Orthop. (SICOT), 3:165–176, 1979.
123. Paradies, L.H., and Gregory, C.F.: The Early Treatment of Close-Range Shotgun Wounds to the Extremities. J. Bone Joint Surg., 48A:425–435, 1966.
124. Patman, R.D., and Thompson, J.E.: Fasciotomy in Peripheral Vascular Surgery: Report of 164 Patients. Arch. Surg., 101:663–672, 1970.
125. Patzakis, M.J.: Management of Open Fracture Wounds. Instr. Course Lect., 36:367–369, 1987.
126. Patzakis, M.J., Harvey, J.P., Jr., and Ivler, D.: The Role of Antibiotics in the Management of Open Fractures. J. Bone Joint Surg., 56A:532–541, 1974.
127. Perry, C.R., Pearson R.L., and Miller, G.A.: Accuracy of Cultures of Material From Swabbing of the Superficial Aspect of the Wound and Needle Bopsy in the Preoperative Assessment of Osteomyelitis. J. Bone Joint Surg., 73A:745–749, 1991.
128. Perren S.M.: Pinless Fixation: I. Injury, 23(suppl. 3):S1–S50, 1992.
129. Prokuski, L.J., and Marsh, J.L.: Segmental Bone Deficiency After Acute Trauma. Orthop. Clin. North Am., 25:753–763, 1994.
130. Rich, N.M., Baugh, J.H., and Hughes, C.W.: Acute Arterial Injuries in Vietnam: 1,000 Cases. J. Trauma, 10:359–369, 1970.
131. Riemer, B.L., Foglesong, M.E., and Miranda, M.A.: Femoral Plating. Orthop. Clin. North Am., 25:625–633, 1994.
132. Rittmann, W.W., and Perren, S.M.: Cortical Bone Healing After Internal Fixation and Healing. New York, Springer-Verlag, 1974.
133. Ritmann, W.W., Schibli, M., Matter, P., and Allgöwer, M.: Open Fractures: Long-Term Results in 200 Consecutive Cases. Clin. Orthop., 138:132–140, 1979.
134. Roessler, M.S., Wisner, D.H., and Holcroft, J.W.: The Mangled Extremity: When to Amputate. Arch. Surg. 126:1243–1249, 1991.
135. Rosenstein, B.D., Wilson, F.C., and Thunderburk, C.H.: The Use of Bacitracin Irrigation to Prevent Infection in Post-Operative Skeletal Wounds. J. Bone Joint Surg., 71A:427–430, 1989.
136. Rüedi, T., Border, J.R., and Allgoewor, M.: Appendix B: Classification of Soft Tissue Injuries. *In* Manual of Internal Fixation. New York, Springer-Verlag, 1991.
137. Russell, W.L., Sailors, D.M., Whittle, T.B., Fisher, D.F., and Burns, R.P.: Limb Salvage vs. Traumatic Amputation. Ann. Surg., 213:473–481, 1991.
138. Salisbury, R.E., Wilmore, D.W., Silverstein, P., and Pruitt, B.A., Jr.: Biological Dressings for Skin Graft Donor Sites. Arch. Surg., 106:705–706, 1973.
139. Salter, R.B., Simmonds, D.F., Malcolm, B.W., Rumble, E.J., MacMichael, D., and Clements, N.D.: The Biological Effect of Continuous Passive Motion on the Healing of Full-Thickness Defects in Articular Cartilage. J. Bone Joint Surg., 62A:1232–1251, 1980.
140. Sanders, R., Jesinovich, I., Angle, J., Pasquale, D., and Herscovici, D.: The Treatment of Open Tibial Shaft fractures Using Interlocked Intramedullary Nail Without Reaming. J. Orthop. Trauma, 8:504–510, 1994.
141. Sanders, R., Koval, K.J., DiPasquale, T., Helfet, D., and Frankle, M.: Retrograde Reamed Femoral Nailing. J. Orthop. Trauma, 7:293–302, 1993.
142. Sanders, R., Pappas, J., Mast, J., and Helfet, D.: The Salvage of Open Grade 3B Ankle and Talus Fractures. J. Orthop. Trauma, 6:201–208, 1992.
143. Sarmiento, A.: A Functional Below-the-Knee Cast for Tibial Fractures. J. Bone Joint Surg., 49A:855–875, 1967.
144. Sarmiento, A., Sobol, P.A., Sem Hoy, A.L., Ross, S.D.K., Racette, W.L., and Tarr, M.S.: Prefabricated Functional Braces for the Treatment of Fractures of the Tibial Diaphysis. J. Bone Joint Surg., 66A:1328–1339, 1984.
145. Schandelmaier, P., Krettek, C., and Tscherne, H.: Superior Results of Un-reamed Tibial Nailing Compared to External Fixation In Tibial Shaft Fractures With Severe Soft Tissue Injury. Presented before the Orthopaedic Trauma Association, New Orleans, 1993.
146. Schenk, R., Stamer, D., and Aurori, B.: Complex Tibial Plateau Fractures Treated With a Hybrid Ring External Fixator. Presented before the Orthopaedic Trauma Association, Los Angeles, 1994.
147. Scully, R.E., Artz, C.P., and Sako, Y.: An Evaluation of the Surgeon's Criteria for Determining the Viability of Muscle During Debridement. Arch. Surg., 73:1031–1035, 1956.
148. Seibel, R., LaDuca, J., Hassett, J., Babikian, G., Mills, B., Border, D.O., and Border, J.R.: Blunt Multiple Trauma (ISS36),

Femur Traction, and the Pulmonary Failure-Septic State. Ann. Surg., 202:283–295, 1985.

149. Seligson, D.: Antibiotic-Impregnated Beads in Orthopaedic Infectious Problems. J. Ky. Med. Assoc., 82:25–29, 1984.
150. Shires, G.T.: Care of the Injured: The Surgeons Responsibility. Tenth Annual Scudder Oration. Bull. Am. Coll. Surg., 58:7–21, 1973.
151. Schemitsch, E., Kowalski, M., Swiontkowski, M., and Harrington, R.: Effects of Reamed vs. Un-reamed Locked Nailing on Callus Blood Flow and Early Strength of Union in a Fracture Sheep Tibia Model. J. Orthop. Trauma, 8:373–382, 1994.
152. Schemitsch, E., Waddell, J., Kellam, J., and Powell, J.: Results of Immediate Internal Fixation of Open Supracondylar Fractures of the Femur. Orthop. Trauma Association, Toronto, Canada, 1990.
153. Slauterbeck, J.R., Briton, C., Noneim, M.S., and Clevenger, F.W.: Mangled Extremity Severity Score: An Accurate Guide to Treatment of the Severely Injured Lower Extremity. J. Orthop. Trauma, 8:282–285, 1994.
154. Small, J.O., and Mollan, R.A.: Management of the Soft Tissues in Open Tibial Fractures. Br. J. Plast. Surg., 45:571–577, 1992.
155. Spiegel, J., Bray, T., Chapman, M., and Swanson, T.: The Lottes Nail Versus AO External Fixation in Open Tibia Fractures (abstract). Orthop. Trans., 12(3):656, 1988.
156. Südkamp, N., Haas, N., Flory, P.,J., Tscherne, H., and Berger, A.: Kriterien der Amputation, Rekonstruktion, und Replantation von Extremitaten bei Mehrfachverletzen. Chirurg, 60:774–781, 1989.
157. Südkamp, N., and Tscherne, H.: Fraktur und Weichteilschaden: Offen Frakturan, thesis for Doctorate of Medicine at the Medizinischen Hochschule Hannover, 1991.
158. Swiontkowski, M.F.: Criteria for Bone Debridement in Massive Lower Limb Trauma. Clin. Orthop. Rel. Res., 243:41–47, 1989.
159. Swiontkowski, M.F., Ganz, R., Schlegel, U., and Perren, S.M.: Laser Doppler Flowmetry for Clinical Evaluation of Femoral Head Osteonecrosis: Preliminary Experience. Clin. Orthop., 218:181–185, 1987.
160. Tanner, J.C., Jr., Vandeput, J., and Olley, J.F.: The Mesh Skin Graft. Plast. Reconstr. Surg., 34:287–292, 1964.
161. Templeman, D.C., Larson, C., Varecka, T.F., and Kyle, R.F.: Decision Making Errors in the Use of Interlocking Tibial Nails. Presented before the Orthopaedic Trauma Association, Los Angeles, 1994.
162. Templeman, D.C., Thomas, M., Varecka, T.F., and Kyle, R.F.: Results of Exchange Reamed Intramedullary Nails for Severe Tibial Shaft Fractures Initially Treated by Non-reamed Nails. Presented before the Orthopaedic Trauma Association, Minneapolis, 1992.
163. Trafton, P.G.: Tibial Shaft Fractures. *In* Skeletal Trauma. Philadelphia, W.B. Saunders, 1992.
164. Tornetta, P., Bergman, M., Watnik, N., Berkowitz, G., and Steuer, J.: Treatment of Grade 3B Open Tibial Fractures: A Prospective Randomized Comparison of External Fixation to Non-reamed Locked Nailing. J. Bone Joint Surg., 76B:13–19, 1994.
165. Tscherne, H.: The Management Of Open Fractures. *In* Fractures With Soft Tissue Injuries. New York, Springer-Verlag, 1984.
166. Trueta, J.: The Principles and Practice of War Surgery With Reference to the Biological Method of the Treatment of War Wounds and Fractures. St. Louis, C.V. Mosby, 1943.
167. Trunkey, D.D., Chapman, M.W., Lim, R.C., Jr., and Dunphy, E.: Management of Pelvic Fractures in Blunt Trauma Injury. J. Trauma, 14:912–923, 1974.
168. Vander Griend, R., Tomasin, J., and Ward, E.F.: Open Reduction and Internal Fixation of Humeral Shaft Fractures: Results Using AO Plating Techniques. J. Bone Joint Surg., 68A:430–433, 1986.
169. van Winkle, B.A., and Neustein, J.: Management of Open Fractures With Sterilization of Large, Contaminated, Extruded Cortical Fragments. Clin. Orthop., 223:275–281, 1987.
170. Wade, P.A., and Campbell, R.D., Jr.: Open Versus Closed Methods in Treating Fractures of the Leg. Am. J. Surg., 95:599–616, 1958.
171. Walker, M.L., Poindexter, J.M., and Stovall, I.: Principles of Management of Shot Gun Wounds. J. Surg. Gynecol Obstet., 170:97–105, 1990.
172. Wangensteen, O.H., and Wangensteen, S.D.: The Rise of Surgery From Empiric Craft to Scientific Discipline. The Minneapolis, University of Minnesota Press, 1978, as cited in Behrens, F.: Fractures With Soft Tissue Injuries. *In* Skeletal Trauma. Philadelphia, W.B. Saunders, 1992.
173. Waterman, N.G., Howell, R.S., and Babich, M.: The Effect of a Prophylactic Antibiotic (Cephalothin) on the Incidence of Wound Infection. Arch. Surg., 97:365–370, 1968.
174. Watson, J.T.: High Energy Fractures of the Tibial Plateau. Orthop. Clin. North Am., 25:723–752, 1994.
175. Watson, J.T., Morandi, M., Buckle, R, Blake, R., and Browner, B.D.: Treatment of Complex Tibial Plateau Fractures With the Circular External Fixator. Orthop. Trans., 18:8, 1994.
176. Wilkins, J., and Patzakis, M.: Choice and Duration of Antibiotics in Open Fractures. Orthop. Clin. North Am., 22:433–437, 1991.
177. Whittle, A.P., Russell, T.A., Taylor, J.C., and Lavelle, P.G.: Treatment of Open Fractures of the Tibial Shaft With the Use of Interlocking Nailing Without Reaming. J. Bone Joint Surg., 74A:1162–1171, 1992.
178. Wiss, D.A.: Flexible Medullary Nailing of Acute Tibial Shaft Fractures. Clin. Orthop., 212:122–132, 1986.
179. Wiss, D.A., Brien, W.W., and Becker, V.: Interlocking Nailing for the Treatment of Femoral Fractures Due to Gun Shot Wound. J. Bone Joint Surg., 73A:598–606, 1991.
180. Wiss, D.A., Segal, D., Gumbs, V.L., and Salter, D.: Flexible Medullary Nailing of Tibial Shaft Fractures. J. Trauma, 26:1106–1112, 1986.
181. Worlock, P., Slack, R., Harvey, L., and Mawhinney, R.: The Prevention of Infection in Open Fractures: An Experimental Study of the Effect of Antibiotic Therapy. J. Bone Joint Surg., 70A:1341–1347, 1988.
182. Worlock, P., Slack, R., Harvey, L., and Mawhinney, R.: The Prevention of Infection in Open Fractures: An Experimental Study of the Effect of Fracture Stability. Injury, 25:31–38, 1994.
183. Wu, C.C., and Shih, C.H.: Complicated Open Fractures of the Distal Tibia Treated by Secondary Interlocking Nailing. J. Trauma, 34:792–796, 1993.
184. Wu, C.C., and Shih, C.H.: The Treatment of Open Femoral and Tibial Shaft Fractures: Preliminary Report On External Fixation and Secondary Intramedullary Nailing. J. Formos. Med. Assoc., 90:1179–1185, 1991.
185. Yokoyama, K., Shindo, M., Itoman, M., Yamamoto, M., and Sasamota, N.: Immediate Internal Fixation for Open Fractures of the Long Bones of the Upper and Lower Extremities. J. Trauma, 37:230–236, 1994.

Rockwood and Green's Fractures in Adults, Fourth Edition,
edited by Charles A. Rockwood, David P. Green, Robert W. Bucholz and James D. Heckman.
Lippincott-Raven Publishers, Philadelphia © 1996.

CHAPTER 7

Bone and Soft-Tissue Reconstruction

William C. Pederson and William E. Sanders

In the past 20 years revolutionary changes have occurred in the approach to complex injuries of the bony skeleton and soft-tissue envelope. Open fractures have long been the bane of the orthopaedic surgeon, and the many articles in the literature attest to the high incidence of complications that accompany open musculoskeletal injuries. Management of the soft-tissue component of complex injuries has been advanced by refinement of older techniques and development of newer ones. Microsurgical composite tissue transfer has made reconstruction of almost any defect possible, whereas systematic study of the vascular supply to the skin has prompted the development of better-vascularized (and thus more reliable) local flaps.[748] In this chapter we provide a philosophy of management for these types of injuries and give the reader a variety of reconstructive options.

TERMINOLOGY

A *graft* is any piece of tissue that is transferred from one site to another and relies on the recipient site for ingrowth of vascularity. Almost any type of tissue can be transferred as a graft, but the larger the graft the less likely that the recipient site can regenerate adequate vascular supply to retain viability of the graft. This is particularly true of soft-tissue grafts, but less of a problem with large bone grafts because stability may be imparted if enough revascularization occurs for the margins to heal. Bone grafts may be autografts (from the same individual) or allografts (cadaver bone transplants). Autogenous bone grafts may be cortical, cancellous, or both and may be transferred without vascular supply (conventional bone graft) or as a vascularized bone graft either on a pedicle or as a free graft.[870]

A *flap* is any piece of tissue that is transferred to another site and retains its own vascularity, thus not relying on the recipient site for blood supply. Flaps are classified by the tissue type (ie, skin, muscle, bone) or types (myocutaneous, osteocutaneous) transferred. Skin flaps are classified by their blood supply: cutaneous or random (from the surrounding skin), arterial or axial (based on a known arterial pedicle), and island (based on an arteriovenous pedicle).[166] A free flap is composed of any type of tissue (or several in the case of a composite flap) that can be transferred by microvascular anastomosis of its vascular pedicle.[6,347,348,404,608,734,801]

HISTORICAL REVIEW OF FLAPS

Tubed Pedicle Flaps

Historically, soft-tissue loss with exposed bone was treated with local soft-tissue rotation flaps.[70,151,356,358] If the local tissues were inadequate for coverage, then some type of distant pedicle flap would have to be used. So-called tubed pedicle flaps were first described in 1917 for use in the head and neck and were reported for coverage of the leg in 1922.[859] These flaps required up to five operations over a total of 5 to 8 months for completion and carried a 9% to 20% failure rate.[769,775] A flap was first raised from the abdomen or chest and attached by means of a "tube" of tissue to the forearm.[109] After a period of time to allow growth of vascular connections from the arm to the tubed flap, it would be divided from the torso. This flap was then placed over the wound (usually the leg) while still attached to the arm for vascularity. After another waiting period to allow the flap to become vascularized from the leg, the tube was divided from its attachment to the arm with the flap now covering the leg wound. This approach is obviously far from ideal and relied heavily on the ability of the soft tissues of the arm and leg to revascularize the transferred flap.[735]

Cross-Leg Flaps

Another flap previously used in lower extremity reconstruction but now primarily of historical interest is the cross-leg flap. Although first described in 1854 by Hamilton, this flap first became widely used in the 1940s[262,626] and continued to find indications through the 1970s.[152,181,396] The cross-leg flap is indicated for defects in the lower leg[152,396] and foot[262,419,768] and involves raising a flap of skin and subcutaneous tissue from the contralateral noninjured leg. Flaps may be raised from either the thigh or lower leg,[626,768] and cross-leg flaps for foot reconstruction from the contralateral plantar foot have also been described.[567] After it is raised, the flap is then partially sewn into the soft-tissue defect on the injured limb and the legs left attached together for a period long enough to provide vascularity to the flap from capillary ingrowth from the wound surface. After 3 to 5 weeks, the base of the flap on the donor leg is divided and used to cover the remaining wound. The cross-leg flap has many problems associated with its use, including obvious problems with positioning, the potential for venous thrombosis in the leg, and failure rates of up to 20%.[181,879]

The philosophical problem with both of these techniques of wound management is that neither tube-pedicle nor cross-leg flaps import any vascularity into the wounded area. In fact, they are both in essence parasites in that they require ingrowth of vessels from the damaged area to survive. Most open fractures, particularly in the lower leg, are the result of high-energy injuries. A significant part of the damage is from devascularization of the surrounding soft tissues, either from crushing or direct vascular injury. Thus, the ideal flap for coverage of soft-tissue defects would carry its own blood supply and not rely on the injured tissue for survival.

Pedicled Muscle Flaps

The management of open fractures or soft-tissue defects underwent profound change with the advent of local pedicled muscle flaps.[662] Much of the early work with this type of coverage came from Ger, who proved the utility of muscle flaps in management of wounds and ulcers of the lower extremity.[254,256,259] Systematic study of the vasculature of muscles by Mathes,[523,525,528] among others, gave the surgeon a wide supply of donor muscles that could be used to cover almost any wound.[18,36,37,68,401,409,416,450,484,548,648,817,894] This type of flap has a number of advantages over the older-styled pedicled skin flaps: (1) the procedure can be performed as a single stage, without having to connect two extremities together[37,254,256,648]; (2) the muscle imports vascularity into the wound, rather than acting as a parasite[386,484,548,683]; and (3) as confirmed by many later studies, muscle placed in a contaminated wound bed can actually decrease the bacterial count, as opposed to simple skin flaps.[119,410,519–521,695]

Free Tissue Flaps

Despite the development of pedicled muscle flaps, some wounds remained problematic. This was particularly true of areas of the body without a large amount of muscle tissue (ie, the distal extremities). Experience gained in microvascular surgery from replantation was extrapolated to the experimental "free" transfer of vascularized tissue from the late 1960s through the early 1970s.[172,777,791] This research experience was brought to clinical fruition in 1973 in Melbourne, Australia, when Taylor and Daniels reported the first successful microvascular free tissue transfer in the English literature.[170] A rash of successful case reports followed, but the number of available donor tissues remained limited.[6,27,45,84,169,241,346,347,434,607,608,611,684,734,796,800,801] Further systematic study of the vascularity of skin and muscle has led to a wide variety of tissues becoming available for microvascular transfer.[69,88,343,348,378,527,533,582,591,646,740,804,805]

The ability to transfer a living piece of bone was first described in dogs by Ostrup in 1975,[621] and microvascular bone reconstruction is now commonly practiced.[264,390,446,461,605,794,795,797,862,863,865,868–870,872,893] These developments of the past 20 years have totally changed the practice of orthopaedic surgery, and advancing knowledge should continue to improve our ability to deal with difficult problems.

PHILOSOPHY OF MANAGEMENT OF COMPLEX MUSCULOSKELETAL INJURIES

The long-accepted attitude of just "getting the wound closed" has radically changed in today's practice. Open fractures in particular are multisystem injuries, and the management of the soft tissues is an important aspect of treatment.[830] Before appropriate soft-tissue reconstruction was possible, the soft-tissue defect often determined the outcome of the fracture. Carpenter stated, "If the soft tissues overlying the tibia are not preserved, hope of primary healing of the underlying fracture is gone forever."[110] Although this statement originally referred to a specific area, it is applicable to any fracture with damage or loss of the soft-tissue envelope. If early soft-tissue reconstruction is successful, the bone becomes the problematic area, and the final result then depends on the extent of bone devascularization and contamination (Table 7-1).[323]

Orthopaedic surgeons in earlier years had to temper wound debridement by the ability for the soft tissues to be reconstructed.[185,598,617] Fear of not being able to cover a wound often made surgeons hesitant or fearful of doing adequate debridement. Complex wounds were therefore sometimes treated expectantly, with the attitude that the wound would either heal properly

TABLE 7-1
Complications in Various Categories of Type III Open Fractures, 1976–1979

Category	Number	Wound Infection	Chronic Infection	Delayed Union or Nonunion	Amputation
Gunshot wound	12	0	0	0	0
Farm injury	4	4 (100%)	3 (75%)	2 (50%)	1 (25%)
Segmental fracture	11	2 (18.18%)	0	2 (18.18%)	1 (9.09%)
Vascular injury	12	5 (41.66%)	2 (16.66%)	2 (16.66%)	5 (41.66%)
Extensive soft-tissue injury	21	13 (61.90%)	8 (30.09%)	6 (28.57%)	4 (19.04%)

Gustilo, R.B., Mendoza, R.M., and Williams, D.N.: Problems in the Management of Type III (Severe) Open Fractures: A New Classification of Type III Open Fractures. J. Trauma 24:742–746, 1984.

or not, given enough time and dressing changes. If adequate soft-tissue coverage was not provided by wound contraction or epithelialization, the extremity could be amputated. Unfortunately, this attitude of "expectant" soft-tissue management prevails in some surgeons' minds today. The advent of pedicled muscle flaps and free tissue transfer has obviated these concerns. For this reason, the early management of the wound should include thorough wound debridement to remove *all devitalized structures* (short of major neurovascular pedicles). In the presence of a difficult wound problem, early involvement of orthopaedic or plastic surgeons capable of appropriate soft-tissue reconstruction is optimum.[295,756,903] Even if the primary treating orthopaedic surgeon is not trained in microsurgical techniques, knowledge of the prerequisites, timing, and availability of soft-tissue and bone reconstruction will affect the initial treatment plan.[295] Collaboration in the management of the bone and soft tissues can lead to early appropriate wound coverage and primary healing of all injured structures.

Even with the wide variety of techniques available, debate continues as to the most appropriate coverage in many wounds. In general, the reconstructive ladder should proceed from the simplest technique that will close the wound to the most complex. This attitude should be tempered with the caveat that *the selected reconstruction should also be the best* for the purposes of coverage and performance of later procedures. We are no longer required by reconstructive limitations to treat the soft tissues inadequately. Although an open tibial fracture with soft-tissue loss *can* be treated with repeated dressing changes and skin grafting once the periosteum has granulated,[578,884] this is certainly *not* the best treatment available. This is arguably not even the simplest technique for wound closure, although it may appear so on the surface. The multiple (and usually inadequate) debridement and "wait for granulation" approach is time intensive and may subject the patient to unnecessary sequelae (Fig. 7-1).[93,209,884] This type of reconstruction frequently leads to infection,[154] long-term instability of the soft tissue over the bone,[83,819] and poor coverage if the need for osteotomy or bone grafting arises. Secondary coverage procedures, if necessary, may be more difficult than if done early, owing to scarring or chronic infection of the soft tissues. Thus, an early, definitive approach to wound management in open fractures may in fact be simpler for the surgeon and safer for the patient in light of the final results (Table 7-2).[317,532,874]

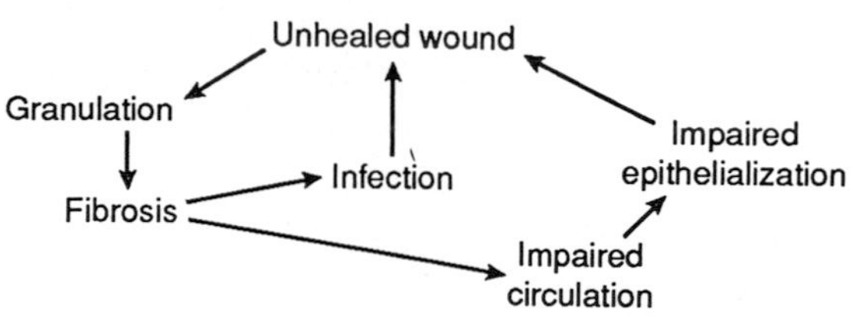

FIGURE 7-1. The hazards of open wound treatment.

OPEN FRACTURES—EVOLUTION OF SOFT-TISSUE MANAGEMENT

In 1976, Gustilo reported on a large personal series of open fractures and described a classification system for these injuries that is still in use today (with modification by various authors).[315] In this report, he stated that soft-tissue loss, instability, and large areas of exposed bone remained unsolved problems. In a second review of his experience with over 1400 open fractures in 1982,[317] he noted that the final outcome depended on five factors:

1. Degree of soft-tissue injury
2. Adequacy of debridement
3. Appropriate use of antibiotics
4. Fracture stability
5. Early soft-tissue coverage

To understand the place of muscle flaps and free tissue transfers in the management of open fractures, we need to trace the important advances in treatment during the past 200 years. The best historical reviews of the treatment of open fractures are given by Saad,[701] Wangensteen,[852] Gustilo,[307,319] and Brown.[83] Brown advocated early soft-tissue coverage in 1965, but lacked the techniques to accomplish it. Understanding the history of management of open fractures lets us appreciate that early soft-tissue coverage is not a radically new concept but a *technique* allowing us to take another step in the development of a treatment plan for open fractures; one that has gradually changed over time and through three wars, but always in the direction of the earliest possible closure of the *adequately debrided* open fracture.

Before aseptic wound management and antibiotics, abscess formation and granulation ("laudable pus") indicated a favorable outcome, whereas a watery, brown discharge was usually fatal. Therefore, the goal of treatment was to *produce* pus, a line of reasoning inappropriate today.[397] The modern era of wound surgery began in the 1700s when Desault first recommended debridement. Before the invention of the motorcycle and automobile, severe soft-tissue loss associated with open fractures was almost always secondary to battlefield casualties. Amputation was the standard treatment for severe extremity injury,[204] and history records that Larrey, Napoleon's battle surgeon, supervised more than 200 amputations in a 24-hour period during the battle of Borodino. The mortality

TABLE 7-2
Open Fractures: Compiled Complication Rates of Series With Early Versus Delayed Soft-Tissue Reconstruction

	No. of Fractures	Treatment/ Coverage	Infection	Osteo-myelitis	Delayed Union or Nonunion	Amputation	Hospital-ization
Gustilo[318]	60	Open	40%	22%	20%	18%	—
Byrd	38	Open	—	41%	29%	29%	—
		Acute flap	—	5%	14%	5%	—
Hallock[323]							
Cierny[140]	36	Delayed	67%	0%	17%	33%	9 weeks
		Early	12%	0%	4%	4%	4.2 weeks
Jones[426]	8	Early	—	—	0%	0%	—
Yaremchuk[903]	22	Delayed	14%	0%	0%*	9%	—
Godina[268]		By 72 hours	1.5%	—†	—†	—†	27 days
		3 days–3 months	17.5%				130 days
		After 3 months	6%				256 days
Caudle[112]							
IIIA	11		0	—	27%	0	—
IIIB	42		29%	—	43%	17%	—
Group 1	24	By 1 week	8%	—	23%	24%	—
Group 2	17	After 1 week	59%	—	77%	24%	—
IIIC	9			—	100%	78%	—

* All healed after six had cancellous graft.
† Not clearly stated; article implies that none of these complications occurred.

rate was as high as 75% during that time, but Larrey lowered this to 25% by applying his technique of early amputation, a radical but effective method of *early closure of an adequately debrided open fracture.* Despite this approach, mortality from open fractures remained significant into the early 1900s.[204]

During World War I, the standard treatment for open fractures was either amputation or debridement followed by plaster immobilization with healing by secondary intention (granulation). Orr advocated antisepsis, wide drainage by wound packing, and plaster immobilization but did not stress debridement. Trueta advocated debridement and stated that "sepsis will not follow if all devitalized tissue is removed."[823,824] Limb salvage was much greater than in the Napoleonic wars, but postfracture osteomyelitis was as high as 80%.[83] Unfortunately, the necessity of adequate debridement has had to be relearned time and again.[82,296]

Better transportation of the injured, better surgical facilities, mandated debridement, and the arrival of antibiotics further improved the statistics during World War II.[145] During this period, the World War I treatment of plaster and granulation changed gradually to plaster and secondary closure, and later to plaster and delayed primary closure.[87,93,145,213,335] Flaps were occasionally used, and the importance of good soft-tissue coverage in obtaining fracture healing was better understood.[688] The practice of a "second look" at 4 to 7 days to assess the potential for delayed primary wound closure or coverage was established.[93] The essential change during this time was conversion of the contaminated open fracture to a clean closed one as early as possible. As a result, the incidence of osteomyelitis and nonunion decreased to approximately 25%.[97]

Gradually, the importance of the soft-tissue envelope as a determinant of the final outcome was better appreciated,[110,206] and guidelines for debridement were established.[766] After adequate debridement, significant bone and soft-tissue defects may be present, and if these are not closed, they may lead to chronic osteomyelitis and nonunion.[625] During the Vietnam era, radical debridement was practiced, and the fact that uncovered bone, fascia, and tendon would become necrotic was understood. Primary and delayed primary closure were used when possible.[336]

In 1956, Connelly noted that "everyone recognizes the value of immediate coverage in hand cases, but why we neglect immediate coverage in leg and foot problems is hard to understand"[152]—an observation echoed by others.[396] Inadequate debridement was identified as the major error in early wound closure.[93,175,396,847] This may explain the increased incidence of infection reported with closed wound management in some series.[209] Primary or secondary wound closure is an elective procedure that should only be done when the wound has been adequately debrided and is surgically clean.[93] Soft-tissue reconstruction by pedicle, rotation, or free flap transfer enables the surgeon to be more radical and thorough in debridement.[573]

The last step in this direction was taken by Marko Godina of Yugoslavia, whose series of early microsurgical reconstructions of complex extremity trauma was published posthumously in 1986.[268] He divided the wounds into those covered within 72 hours (group I), 3 days to 3 months (group II), and after 3 months (group III). The flap loss rate and postoperative infection rate was lowest in wounds covered immediately and highest in those covered between 3 days and 3 months (Table 7-3).

Unfortunately, most patients needing free tissue transfer for coverage are initially treated expectantly. This results in most wounds falling into Godina's group II when first seen in our experience. Godina found earlier operations easier to do because there was less fibrosis of adjacent tissues (especially vessels) and because bone fragments could be retained and would revascularize from the soft-tissue envelope. Eighty percent of his transfers were done on the day of injury, and the low 1.5% infection rate in this group attests to his skill in radical debridement. Duration of hospital stay was lowest in this group as well.

Thus, we see that the goals of treatment have changed with the passage of time: initially life preservation, then preservation of function, and now avoidance of osteomyelitis.[830] Recognition of the role of soft-tissue reconstruction has been slow; and except in certain centers, the application of these techniques has not been routine. A 1983 textbook discussion of the management of infected nonunions did not mention free tissue transfer as an option[312] (10 years after the introduction of the free flap!) Ironically, the pendulum is still swinging, and the initial infatuation with complex staged reconstruction is tempered by the financial and economic costs when compared with early amputation—also a function-preserving option.[316,537]

This experience has shown that the two most important principles in management of open fractures are (1) achievement of fracture stability and (2) improvement of the vascular environment around the fracture site. The methods and benefits of enhancement of the vascular environment are the subject of this chapter. Fracture stabilization is covered elsewhere in this text.

BONE RECONSTRUCTION

VASCULARITY OF BONE

The blood supply of an adult long bone comes from three sources: (1) the nutrient artery, (2) the metaphyseal arteries, and (3) the periosteal arterioles.[78,159,681,682] In an immature long bone, the epi-

TABLE 7-3
Complex Extremity Trauma: Effect of Delay in Closure on Complication Rate

Early Closure	Delayed Closure	Late Closure	Totals
No. of patients (%) 134 (25.2)	167 (31.4)	231 (43.4)	532 (100)
No. of microsurgical procedure failures (%) 1 (0.75)	20 (12)	22 (9.5)	43 (8)
No. of postoperative infections (%) 2 (1.5)	29 (17.5)	14 (6)	45 (8.45)
Bone healing time (average) 6.8 months (n = 33)	12.3 months (n = 95)	29 months (n = 78)	17.7 months (n = 206)
Hospitalization time (average) 27 days	130 days	256 days	159 days
No. of anesthesias (average) 1.3	4.1	7.8	5

Godina, M. Early Microsurgical Reconstruction of Complex Trauma of the Extremities. Plast. Reconstr. Surg., 78:285–292, 1986.

physis has a separate supply. Bone necrosis (loss of vascularity) is of great significance in both fracture healing and osteomyelitis.[851] The effect of various internal fixation devices on bone blood supply, and the ability of the blood supply to adapt by collateral circulation, have been studied by several authors. The consensus is as follows[282,372,681,682]:

1. Afferent blood flow is normally from medullary to periosteal (ie, centrifugal).
2. The periosteal vessels are mainly efferent and normally supply only the outer third of the cortex.
3. In fracture healing, the callus is supplied with an extraosseous supply from the periosseous tissues.
4. Drainage occurs through an efferent venous system.
5. Intramedullary reaming and rod placement damage the medullary supply (from the nutrient and metaphyseal arteries). Until these vessels regenerate (10 days to 4 weeks), only the periosteal circulation is available.[282]
6. Fractures with displacement may tear the nutrient artery or its branches and effectively devascularize a segment of cortex.[204]

Other studies have suggested that collaterals from the metaphyseal arteries fill the medullary circulation after loss of the nutrient artery.[826] Experimental studies in dogs suggest that the periosteal network can reverse flow and supply the entire cortex and medullary area.[864]

PRIMARY BONE HEALING

Many factors affect the healing of fractures and bone grafts.[160] Fractures can heal by external or endosteal callus, but both types of healing require viable fragments. Like all tissues, bone requires adequate vascularity to heal properly, which can be supplied from intrinsic or extrinsic sources. Callus formation relies on the presence of the multipotential mesenchymal cells that can transform into viable osteocytes. Poorly oxygenated and malnourished mesenchymal cells are unlikely to undergo this necessary osteogenic induction.[42,370]

True endosteal callus forms from the medullary (intrinsic) vascular supply of bone.[682,825] In addition to this intrinsic source of blood supply, fractures have an external vascularized callus supplied by extraosseous vessels, mainly from surrounding muscle.[97,895] The blood supply of fracture fragments is inversely proportional to the degree of initial displacement. Stripping of the periosteum by displacement or open reduction of the fracture may destroy the periosteal blood supply. Intramedullary nailing can further damage the vascularity at the fracture site by compromise of the nutrient artery and medullary supply.[83,281,499] Avascular fragments require replacement by "creeping substitution" of bone from surrounding vascularized segments. Even without comminution, the site of fracture can lose all intrinsic vascularity owing to the nature of the fracture or technique of stabilization. In these instances, the extrinsic blood supply is all important for fracture healing.

Experimentally, ischemic bone will not revascularize until the surrounding soft-tissue envelope has done so. Therefore, in open fractures, the vascularity of the remaining soft-tissue envelope is of great importance. Experimentally, muscle tissue is the primary source of bone revascularization; therefore, absence or destruction of a viable muscular or soft-tissue envelope delays bone healing.[386] In several clinical series of nonunited fractures with soft-tissue defects treated by flaps, fracture union occurred after soft-tissue reconstruction without the need for bone grafting.[109,151,419,575] Both parasitic and vascularized flaps can have this effect,[109,151,419] although intuitively one would assume that a flap with its own vascularity would fare better.

Decreased oxygen tension slows fracture healing and favors cartilage formation instead of bone, whereas increased tissue oxygen stimulates fracture healing.[599,898] Systemic hypoxia delays fracture healing and decreases its eventual strength.[372] Because the ingrowth of vessels into fracture callus relies on the surrounding soft tissues (mainly muscle), areas not normally enveloped by muscle (eg, the distal third of the tibia) have lower healing potential.[281]

REVASCULARIZATION OF BONE

The ability of bone that has lost its intrinsic or extrinsic blood supply to revascularize has been a subject of much interest in the past decade. This technique has potential applications both in fracture management and in avascular disease of various bones (eg, aseptic necrosis of the femoral head and lunate).[427] These two problems do not offer the same parameters for revascularization, and the approaches have been different, as discussed later.

Bone that has been acutely devascularized offers an excellent opportunity for revascularization. This is the case in many open fractures, and muscle is the best tissue for revascularization of bone.[20,119,683] Although cutaneous tissue (skin and subcutaneous fat) may offer stable coverage, it is inferior in terms of its ability to provide vascular ingrowth to bone. Muscle also offers better control of subflap bacterial levels and may improve delivery of antibiotics to the bone.[119,695] Cutaneous flaps containing well-vascularized fascia also offer excellent properties for infection control, but are probably inferior in terms of revascularization. Omentum, with its well-know ability to revascularize ischemic soft tissue, also revascularizes bone well.[27,343,411,613]

The use of an arteriovenous pedicle for implantation into bone with the potential for revascularization of the bone has been attempted in cases of avascular necrosis of the proximal carpal bones (Kienbock's and Preiser's diseases).[74,790] Although some success has been reported with this technique, it has not been widely accepted. Vascularized bone grafts placed within ischemic bone have also shown promise in the ability to revascularize the recipient, particularly in the case of ischemic necrosis of the femoral head.[85,240,481,836]

MANAGEMENT OF BONE LOSS

Bone Grafting

Many articles have been published on the history of bone grafting, revascularization of autogenous and allograft bone, and vascularized bone grafts.[55,862,863,875] Several other thorough and well-referenced review articles on the fate of bone grafts have also been written.[81,94,95,124,373,400,663] The exact mechanism of incorporation is not known, but the graft depends on the host bed for revascularization.

Two theories have been proposed. The first suggests that osteogenic cells survive transplantation and contribute to new bone formation.[61,650] However, because only a small percentage of osteogenic cells survive, a second theory suggests that bone is formed as the bone graft induces the surrounding connective tissue to undergo metaplasia into bone.[160,840] Both mechanisms are probably involved.

Conventional Autogenous Bone Grafts

Conventional bone grafts depend on diffusion of nutrients from the surrounding tissue for viability of the osteogenic cells. Cancellous bone has an open structure that permits diffusion and vessel ingrowth with rapid incorporation, whereas cortical bone is relatively impenetrable and may never be completely revascularized.[90,91] Despite this, nonvascularized cortical grafts have been used with success, especially after tumor resection.[206] In either case, if the cells do not survive, the dead bone must first be resorbed and then replaced by new bone—the process known as "creeping substitution."[205,650,840] Obviously, a stable vascular recipient bed is necessary for this to occur,[94,370,862,867] and the rate of revascularization correlates strongly with clinical "success" of the graft. Autogenous cancellous grafts 5 mm thick are completely revascularized in 20 to 25 days.[160,779] Autogenous bone grafts replaced by creeping substitution are weaker structurally from 6 weeks to 6 months but may be normal by 1 year.[205] For maximum osteocyte survival, bone grafts should be kept in chilled blood or a sponge moistened with chilled saline and not exposed to air.[56,61,663]

In general, cancellous grafts are useful for short defects (<6 cm) in a well-vascularized, noninfected bed (Fig. 7-2).[597,858] These grafts have a higher success rate

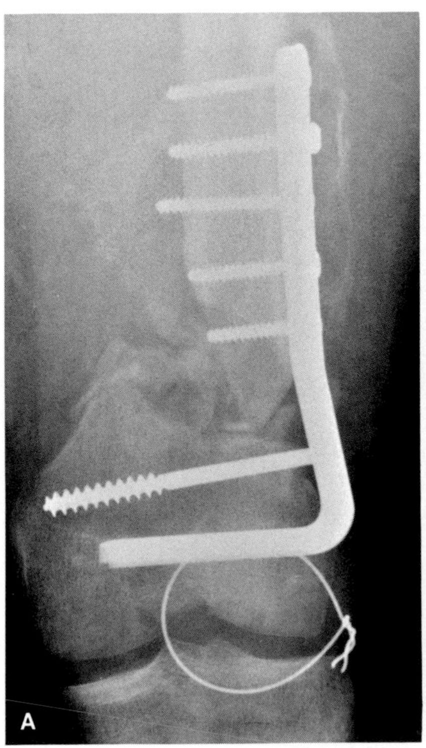

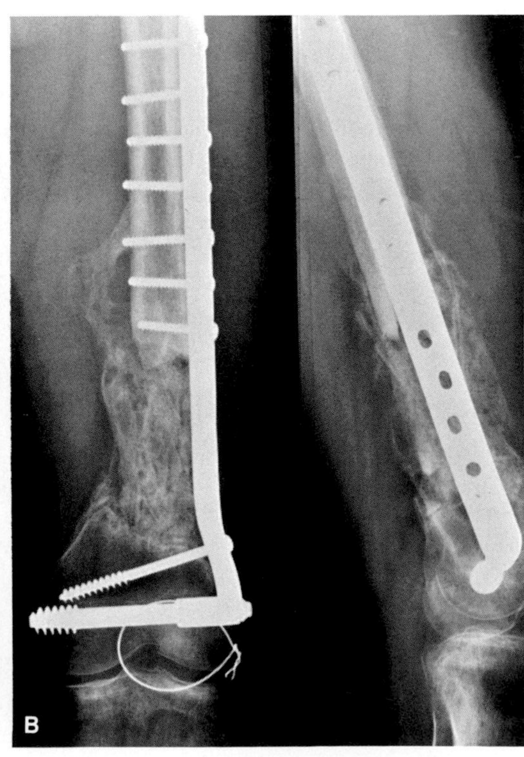

FIGURE 7-2. (**A**) A 25-year-old man with a segmental femoral defect treated elsewhere by shortening of 8 to 9 cm and plating in external rotation. (**B**) The result following leg lenthening, secondary internal fixation, and cancellous grafting from both posterior iliac crests.

and are more completely revascularized than cortical grafts, which always contain areas of necrotic bone.[71,90,91] Defects larger than 9 cm in length, however, may exceed the supply of cancellous bone graft available.[293] Direct cancellous grafting of infected fractures with a healthy layer of granulation (Papineau technique) is an option when soft-tissue coverage is absent (Fig. 7-3).[100,148,310] Papineau grafts are excellent for filling large open metaphyseal defects in long bones.[203] The posterolateral approach, which avoids the anterior area of soft-tissue loss, is superior to Papineau grafts in diaphyseal areas.[201,203,236,351,674] Larger segmental defects may be treated with cortical grafting,[624] and Enneking's report of results with this technique serves as a basis for comparison with vascularized free bone grafting.[206]

Allografts

Allografts do not stimulate osteogenesis to the extent autografts do. Revascularization is slower and less complete than in autografts,[875] and, at least in freeze-dried grafts, no cells survive. However, allografts do not have the size limitations of autogenous grafts, and a joint or joint surface may be transferred.[623,624] Although they are especially useful in tumor surgery,[91,505] their application to post-traumatic injury is limited owing to potential infection and loss of the graft.

Bone Transport (Ilizarov Technique)

The ability to bridge bony gaps by the process now known as bone transport was originally worked out in the 1950s and 1960s by Ilizarov in Russia.[407] Since this early experience, the technique has found wide application for both restoring gaps in bone and bone lengthening.[165,590,627,630] Bone transport may also be used in the management of difficult fractures, particularly in the lower extremity,[731,831] and in the presence of infected nonunions.[577,630,638]

In clinical application, an open or closed corticotomy is performed on the bone segment to be lengthened. In the case of a defect in a long bone, the osteotomy is made several centimeters above or below the site of the defect.[628] A previously placed halo external fixator connected to crossed transosseous pins allows for distraction of the bone at the site of the osteotomy.[292] Slow distraction (0.5 to 1 mm/day) of the segments on either side of the corticotomy will result in new bone formation at the site of distraction.[23] This occurs by means of "bone transport" of progenitor cells from the medullary canal on either side of the corticotomy. In experiments on dogs, Ilizarov demonstrated the importance of maintenance of medullary and periosteal blood supply when performing the bony osteotomy. He found that a properly performed osteotomy (osteoclasis) could preserve medullary blood supply, which he demonstrated with arteriograms. In animals with such an osteotomy, osteogenesis at the site of distraction was very rapid and could, in fact, cause early consolidation of the bone if the rate of distraction was too slow.[405] On the other hand, damage to the medullary and periosteal blood supply could lead to poor bone regeneration in both experimental and clinical cases.

This type of bone regeneration has been generally used for traumatic defects of up to 6 to 7 cm, with successful healing reported in the greater than 90% range.[165,590,831] In cases of limb lengthening with the

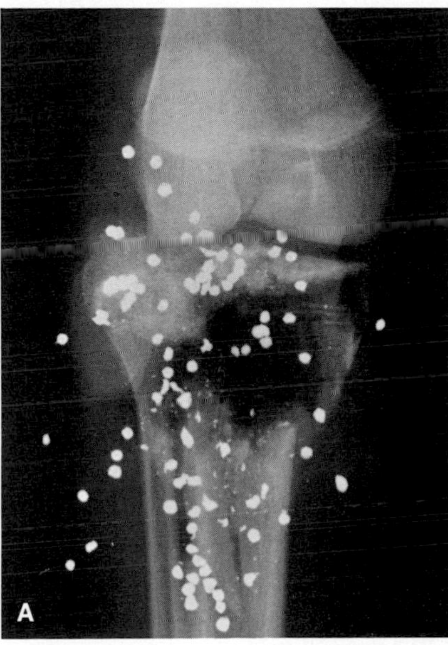

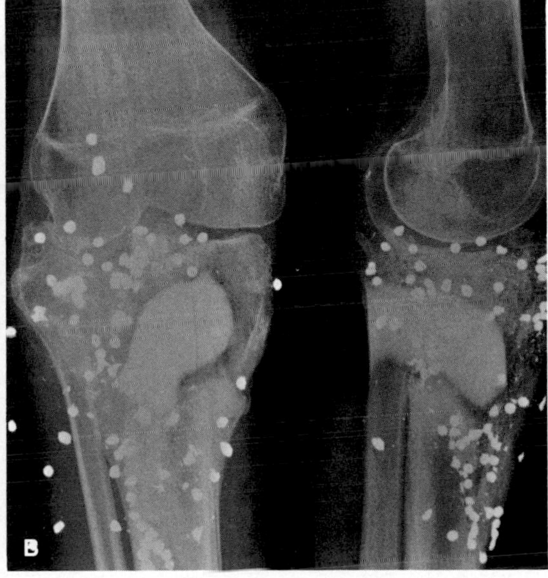

FIGURE 7-3. (**A**) Radiograph of the knee joint of a 16-year-old boy after a shotgun wound to the popliteal area. Revascularization was accomplished by vein bypass graft. The fractures were managed by an external fixator and healed, but a large cavity persisted in the proximal tibia. (**B**) Sinograms showing a large metaphyseal defect. Healing was accomplished by Papineau graft, done in two stages because of the size of the defect.

Ilizarov device, discrepancies of up to 20 cm have been overcome, but most series deal with lengthenings in the 5- to 10-cm range.[627] The ability to make up these gaps is not without morbidity, however. Some of the problems associated with bone transport include neurologic injury, joint subluxation, joint stiffness, and nonunion.[629]

One of the purported advantages of the Ilizarov technique in the management of open fractures is the potential for adequate soft-tissue management without the need for flap coverage. The ability of the soft tissues to tolerate stress and in fact generate new cells while undergoing distraction is well documented.[405,406] It has been our experience, however, that in the case of a severe complex extremity injury, the Ilizarov technique alone cannot usually make up for marked soft-tissue loss. Management of such injuries by primary soft-tissue free flap transfer followed by bone transport for the osseous defect has been proposed as an alternative to microvascular bone transfer.[431,832]

Vascularized Bone Grafting

Pedicled Grafts

The first vascularized bone graft was a pedicled fibula transfer to an ipsilateral tibial defect reported by Huntington in 1905.[398] This proved to be a viable technique, and more recent reports confirm high success rates in the management of difficult nonunions of the tibia with pedicled fibulae.[106,117,128,174,190,398,428,632,858] The fibula may be also used as a living "strut" to reconstruct the lower leg by tibiofibular synostosis (Fig 7-4).[104,266,300,550,560] The iliac crest pedicled on the tensor fascia lata or iliopsoas muscle has also been used for acetabular reconstruction and hip fusion.[116,177,178,182,561] The osteogenic potential, vascularity, and strength of these grafts is thought to be greater than conventional bone grafts.

Free Vascularized Bone Grafts

Ostrup and Frederickson performed the first reported experimental vascularized bone transfer in 1974.[620] Using the canine rib as a model, they demonstrated rapid union of transferred bone with microsurgical anastomosis of the rib's vascular pedicle. Based on the success of this experimental procedure, Taylor reported the first clinical application of free vascularized bone transfer in 1975.[802] His group transferred a vascularized fibula from the contralateral leg to repair a large tibial defect in a young man that had failed attempts at conventional bone grafting. The potential for microsurgical transfer of complex tissue consisting of soft

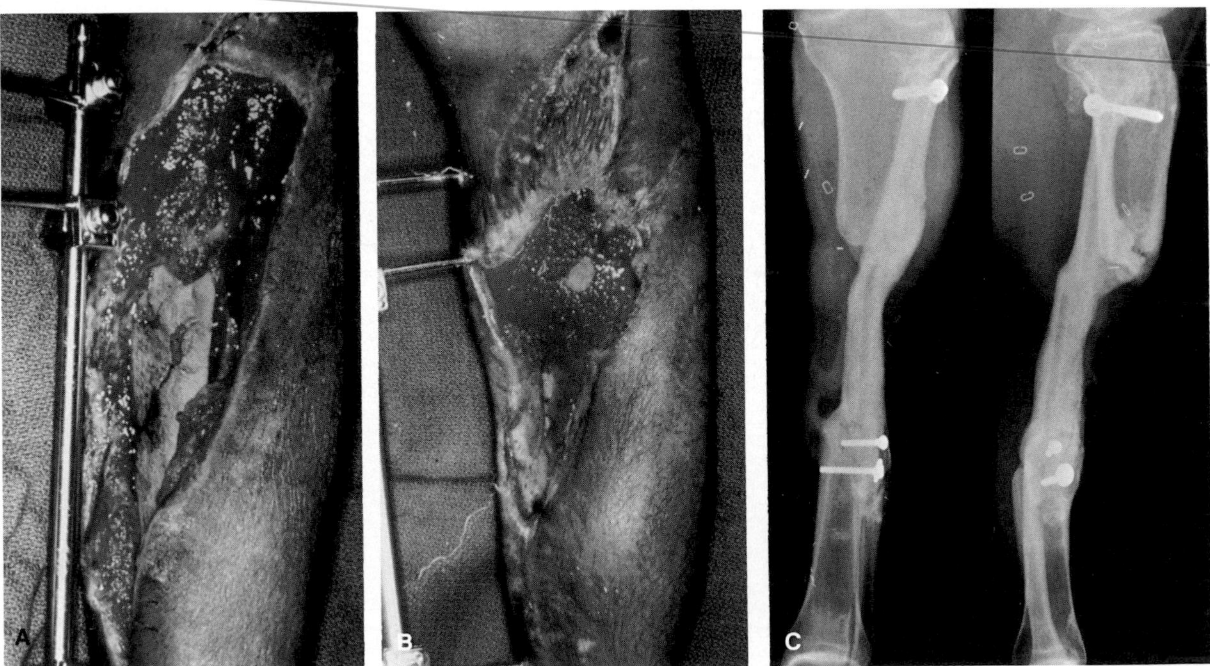

FIGURE 7-4. (**A**) Clinical photo of a 25-year-old patient 3 weeks after a severe crush injury of both legs sustained while cleaning a commercial meat grinder. The AO frame was applied at another hospital and a butterfly fragment with no soft tissue attachment was left in place. (**B**) A latissimus dorsi free flap was done, but infection occurred and the distal half of the flap was lost. The cause of this was thought to be the retained necrotic bone fragment, and this fragment was subsequently removed. Once the wound had been redebrided and infection controlled, a second free tissue transfer was done using a rectus abdominis, and ultimately coverage was obtained. (**C**) Bone construction by fibular transfer resulted in healing, and the patient is now ambulatory on both legs.

tissue and bone was realized in 1977, when Buncke's group reported the successful transfer of a portion of rib and overlying skin for treatment of a tibial pseudarthrosis.[88] Although these and later studies have proven the clinical applicability of vascularized bone grafts, some controversy exists as to the nature of the contribution of the intact vascular pedicle.

Fate of Vascularized Bone Grafts

Some early studies of vascularized bone grafts demonstrated nonviable elements in the marrow and empty lacunae in the transferred segments.[620,621] Experimental work with canine vascularized bone transfers suggested that cutting a bone and thus disrupting its intrinsic vascular channels may cause some osteocyte loss and bone death.[272,767] These studies also showed that periosteal circulation alone may not be sufficient to maintain the viability of osteocytes in the haversian system. These findings have been disputed by others, who maintain that a vascularized bone graft can remain totally viable through the periosteal circulation alone.[53,57,744] There is no argument that some osteogenic cells survive,[15,54,191] however, and repair is by the usual process of fracture healing between the graft and the recipient bone, rather then by creeping substitution.[622,865] Free bone grafts and segmental fractures appear to heal in the same manner in experimental models.[887] Even if vascularized bone grafts do not heal exactly like fractures, they have the advantage over conventional grafts of more rapid healing and hypertrophy of the transferred bone.[162,361,445,474,478,811]

Donor Sites

A number of potential donor sites for vascularized bone have been described. The rib was among the first described,[88,167,513,798] but it is rarely used today owing to its difficult dissection and morbidity.[16]

Vascularized Iliac Crest Graft. A systematic study of the vascular anatomy of bones led to the description of the vascularized iliac crest, which was first taken with the skin of a groin flap based on the superficial circumflex iliac vascular system.[806] The primary blood supply, however, was later shown by Taylor to come from the deep circumflex iliac artery and this is now the preferred vascular pedicle for microvascular transfer of this graft.[804,805] This source of vascularized graft gives an excellent segment of corticocancellous bone with good vascularity and can be taken with overlying skin.[665,722,888,892] The primary disadvantage of this donor site is that the longest straight segment that can be taken is limited to 5 to 6 cm.[765,797,806,865] Likewise, the dissection is demanding, the skin paddle is relatively thick, and potential donor site morbidity is relatively high.[264,302,604,706,781,838] Although the iliac crest will hypertrophy and remodel with time, this happens more slowly than with the free fibula, and up to a third of patients will require secondary cancellous grafting for adequate healing.[765,863] With the description and better understanding of the anatomy of the vascularized fibula, this donor site has likewise found fewer applications in recent years.

Free Fibular Graft. The free fibula, first described in 1975,[802] has become the donor site of choice for most microvascular bone transfers. The fibula receives its vascularity from both the nutrient artery (a branch of the peroneal) and periosteal supply from the adjacent peroneal vessels.[549] This allows for osteotomy of the fibula for certain indications, as discussed further later. This piece of donor bone is the best available for reconstruction of long defects of the tubular bones of the extremities. It has been used extensively for reconstruction of segmental defects in the diaphyseal area of the tibia (Fig. 7-5).[129,302,413,433,461] It can be taken with or without a skin paddle, although some reports have questioned the reliability of the skin when based on the peroneal perforators.[730] The fibula can also be harvested with a portion of the soleus muscle,[47] which may aid in reconstruction of complex defects. A total length of bone approximately 20 cm can be taken, with a reliable vascular anatomy and minimal morbidity. The fibula can be doubled over to provide two struts of live bone for pelvic reconstruction, vertebral fusion,[394] and femur reconstruction.

Donor site morbidity from free vascularized fibular transfer is minimal in most patients. Moderate gait changes have been noted before 10 months postoperatively, but the changes are minimal after this period.[908] Likewise, some decreased calf muscle strength is noted in all patients, and the more fibula harvested, the greater the loss of ankle eversion strength.[908] We have noted some problems with contracture of the toe flexors after fibula harvest, but this has responded well to physical therapy. Significant weakness in the motor function of the peroneal nerve was noted in 3 of 60 patients in one study,[893] but we have found this to be transient unless direct injury to the nerve occurs.

Other Donor Sites. Although several other donor sites for vascularized bone have been described, the amount of bone that can be transferred is limited. These sites include the radius, humerus, and lateral scapula. The primary indication for use of these donor sites is in reconstruction of specific types of problems in the hand, which is discussed further later.

Free Bony Epiphyseal Graft. The ability to transfer a bony epiphysis to allow growth in immature individuals has been the subject of several experimental and clinical studies.[72,192,595] Although the nonrevascularized transfer of an epiphyseal plate was first reported in 1929,[776] enthusiasm for this procedure has remained low because of unpredictable results.[237,667,881] Early results with transfer of the fibular epiphysis in clinical cases gave poor results when revascularized solely on the peroneal vessels.[829] Anatom-

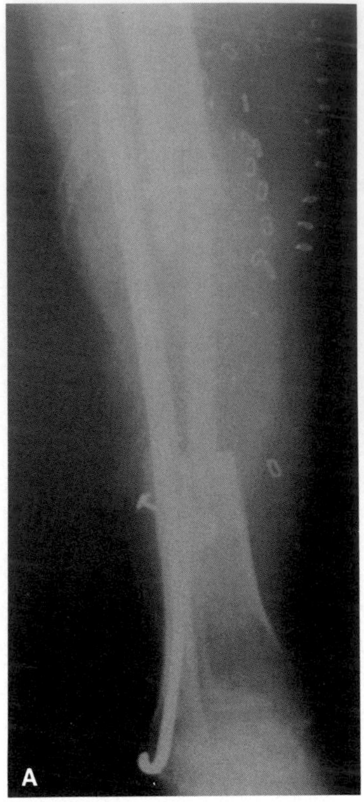
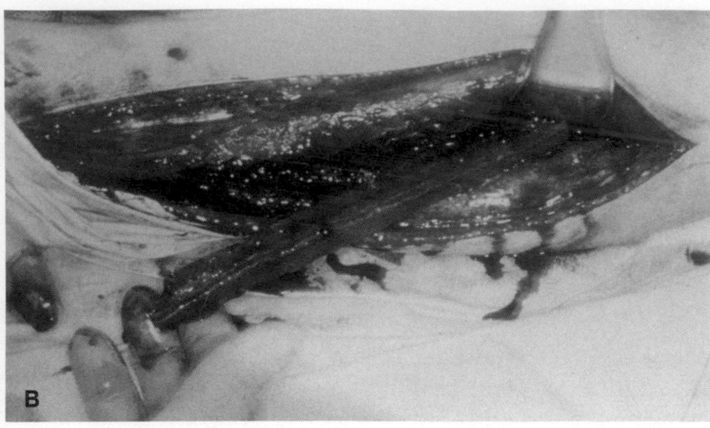

FIGURE 7-5. (**A**) A segmental defect of the tibial shaft treated by free fibular bone graft. Note that length and alignment of the leg were maintained by Rush rod fixation of the fibular fracture. (**B**) The free fibula graft after its dissection from a lateral approach before division of the pedicle.

ical studies of the vascularity of the epiphysis showed that this area relies on branches of the anterior tibial artery and lateral inferior genicular artery.[679,807] The clinical results of microsurgical transfer of the fibular epiphysis based on its anterior tibial blood supply have improved results,[651,807,829] although there are no large series yet to properly evaluate this procedure.

MANAGEMENT OF SPECIFIC SITES (BONE LOSS)

General Indications for Vascularized Bone Transfer

The standard dictum is that any defect in a long bone of greater than 6 to 8 cm is best handled by vascularized bone transfer.[862,863,893] This is particularly true in cases in which the surrounding soft tissue has inadequate vascularity due to trauma, tumor resection, or irradiation.[1,574,729] Another indication is in cases of congenital pseudarthrosis, which has proven difficult to manage with standard techniques.[65,125,183,280,529,752,761,866] As with most microvascular tissue transfers, the indications for vascularized bone transfer have broadened over the past decade, owing to improved techniques and better donor sites. As discussed earlier, understanding of the physiology of bone healing and specifically of the behavior of bone transferred with microsurgical revascularization has also improved.[272,273] Thus, defects of less than 6 cm are often treated with vascularized bone transfer if there has been failure of traditional grafting or if the vascularity of the surrounding soft-tissue bed is severely compromised.[186,399,705] Patients with chronic osteomyelitis or infected nonunion are also often considered for vascularized bone grafting, because the living piece of transferred bone probably resists reinfection better than a nonliving graft.[891] Application of the Ilizarov technique has decreased some of the need for vascularized bone transfers over the past several years but has not entirely usurped microsurgical techniques in long-bone reconstruction.

Complex injuries with loss of bone and soft-tissue coverage can present many challenges to the reconstructive surgeon. The approach to these problems depends on the experience of the surgeon, and both primary reconstruction of bone and soft tissue or staged reconstruction are viable options (Table 7-4). Vascularized bone transfer can be used as either a primary

TABLE 7-4
Methods of Reconstruction for Combined Soft-Tissue and Bone Defects

IMMEDIATE RECONSTRUCTION
Composite bone and soft-tissue flap
Iliac
Fibula
Soft-tissue flap and cancellous graft
Double flap
STAGED RECONSTRUCTION
Soft-tissue coverage
Delayed cancellous graft
Conventional
Papineau
Posterolateral bone graft
Delayed free vascularized bone graft
Fibula transposition
Papineau graft and later split-thickness skin graft or soft-tissue flap

procedure or at a later date after adequate soft-tissue coverage has been obtained.

Upper Extremity

Most areas of bone loss in the upper extremity can be managed with standard bone grafting techniques, either cancellous or corticocancellous.[289,564,597,600] The exceptions to this rule are encountered in cases of tumor extirpation[305,306,654,702] and in the presence of infection or recalcitrant nonunion (often seen with infection).[261,380,869,871] Although indications for vascularized bone transfer in the hand are decidedly unusual, they do occur in cases of massive bone loss, infection, and nonunion.[129,186,390,391,399,460,619,655,705,870,907]

The primary donor sites for these cases are the distal radius,[58] humerus,[58] and scapula.[173] All three of these donor sites are used with the overlying skin paddle of the radial forearm flap, lateral arm flap, and scapular flap, respectively.

Because of the dual-bone anatomy of the forearm, indications for grafting of long segments for gross instability are unusual. In cases with significant loss of bone in the forearm, an accepted technique such as conversion to a one-bone forearm is often used.[321,496,589] On rare occasions, however, the option of vascularized bone transfer may be considered in the forearm. The bone most frequently used in these cases would be the free vascularized fibula, owing to its similar size and shape to the bones of the forearm. The peroneal artery can be taken with this transfer to restore continuity to the radial or ulnar artery by arterial anastomoses at both ends as a "flow-through" flap.[186,870] It has been suggested that the periosteal-muscular envelope around the fibula may decrease the incidence of synostosis as well.[399] In the case of loss of a significant portion of both bones, the fibula can be fashioned into a "double-barrel" configuration to reconstruct both bones[425] or as a single strut to the radius to "reconstruct" a one-bone forearm.[460] Vascularized bone transfer is also used in difficult nonunions with or without infection.[186,399,705] The fibula has found particular application in reconstruction of the distal radius after tumor resection, and the possibility for growth exists if the epiphysis is revascularized by means of the anterior tibial vessels.[652–654,702]

In management of significant bone loss in the humerus, a different set of problems occurs. Although some shortening is well-tolerated, resection of major humeral segments in the course of tumor excision or for infected nonunions may leave defects that need to be reconstructed. In the case of proximal humeral resections involving the humeral head, an appropriate-sized allograft may be used with reasonable success.[207] Long defects of the shaft of the humerus may also be managed with allograft transfer, but the procedure of choice in most patients with bone loss due to trauma is vascularized fibular transfer. This procedure has been proven effective for segmental losses of greater than 6 to 8 cm[80,261,888] and in the presence of complex nonunions.[429,889] The fibula vascularized on both its peroneal and anterior tibial pedicles has been used for reconstruction of the humeral head in adolescents, with growth of the arm reported in the postoperative period.[807]

Femur

The two primary indications for vascularized bone transfer to the femur are avascular necrosis of the femoral head and infected nonunion with bone loss.[427,430,619] The use of a segment of revascularized fibula placed into the femoral head has shown promise for revascularization of the avascular segment.[240,836] Long-term studies have shown reasonable results after vascularized fibula transfer in treatment of this difficult problem.[85,905] The iliac crest can be used as a pedicled vascularized graft for problem nonunions of the hip.[722] Although infected nonunion of the femur is a relatively infrequent problem, it can be difficult to manage when combined with loss of length.[121] A single strut of vascularized fibula can be used for reconstruction in such cases,[430] but the stresses placed on this thin segment of bone can lead to a high refracture rate.[899] This problem has been addressed by placing a "folded" double strut of fibula in the femoral defect, surrounded by cancellous graft.[425,606] Results with this technique show a lower refracture rate, and this is our preferred procedure for difficult femoral reconstructions.[388]

Tibia

Bone loss due to trauma and infection is frequently seen after high-energy injuries to the tibia. One third of the tibial circumference is subcutaneous, directly anterior where it is most susceptible to injury.[284,842] Although conventional closed or open techniques of grafting have given reasonable results in the past, free vascularized bone transfer has proven its advantages in this situation.[279,604,892] Both the iliac crest[393,703,722,806,892] and fibula[129,337,413,604,780,789,792] have been used in this situation, but most authors now prefer the fibula.[263,565,765,863,893] A recent series from the Mayo Clinic found that 32% of patients undergoing iliac crest transfer required a secondary procedure to obtain final healing, whereas only 17% of patients undergoing free fibula transfer needed secondary surgery.[337] A large skin paddle (10–20 cm) can be harvested with the free fibula, which can be used to manage soft-tissue defects.[111,129,353,907] In our hands the fibula offers the best option for reconstruction of lengthy (>7 cm) defects in the tibia, and although the ipsilateral fibula may be used in some instances, it is often unavailable because of fracture or vascular damage (Fig. 7-6).

SOFT-TISSUE RECONSTRUCTION

PRINCIPLES IN THE MANAGEMENT OF SOFT-TISSUE LOSS

Assessment of the Soft Tissues

The ability of a wound to heal is predicated primarily on the vascularity of the surrounding tissue. Although other factors such as bacterial count in the tissue may have some effect on wound healing, the capacity for a wound to manage a bacterial inoculum and finally heal is dependent solely on its blood supply. Any factor that decreases the blood flow to the wound can impede healing. These factors may include vascular disease or injury, trauma to soft tissues, and tension on the wound edges at closure. An important concept in dealing with open fractures was outlined by Rhinelander, who stated that "vascularity is the biological basis, and stability the biomechanical basis, of . . . healing."[284] In the management of open fractures, biological considerations should always take precedence over biomechanical ones. Stabilizing dead bone will not necessarily lead to healing. On the other hand, stabilizing a fracture prevents further damage to the soft-tissue envelope.

In evaluation of the pathophysiology of soft-tissue healing associated with fractures, Oestern and Tscherne[610] listed five important points:

1. All injuries, whether open or closed, lead to hypoxia in the damaged tissue.
2. Hypoxia and acidosis cause a further increase in vascular permeability.
3. The increased permeability leads to interstitial edema, swelling, and, by raising the interstitial pressure, amplification of the hypoxia and acidosis.
4. In severely injured patients with general hypoxia and acidosis, this tissue damage becomes protracted in the periphery.
5. Any mechanical constriction, whether caused by fascia or skin, causes further deterioration of the metabolic state in the injured tissue, predisposing to infection and hampering wound repair.

An accurate evaluation of the soft-tissue injury is essential to the primary care of any wound. Soft tissues in hypoxic areas heal poorly and are more susceptible to infection, and tissue hypoxia decreases the effectiveness of intravenous antibiotics.[850] The ability to assess the vascularity of a wound takes some experience, but surgeons dealing with musculoskeletal trauma must learn this skill. The first parameter to look at is the adequacy of macrovascular inflow. This is done by palpation of proximal and distal pulses and may be aided by use of a Doppler ultrasound device.[717] The absence of palpable or Doppler pulses in the major vessels proximal to and distal to a wound should alert the examiner to a high likelihood of poor wound perfusion. In the case of absent palpable or Doppler pulses, arteriography should probably be done before reconstructive attempts to delineate the extent and nature of vascular trauma. The routine use of arteriography in limbs with palpable pulses in the presence of severe trauma remains controversial,[745] but some authors believe that a vascular dye study is indicated if free tissue transfer is contemplated.[452]

The area surrounding the wound should then be visually examined. Surrounding skin should have normal color and capillary refill. Skin that is too light (pale) or too dark (hyperemic or congested) is often ischemic or traumatized. Any trauma to the skin should be noted, especially bruising, abrasion, or blistering. Although "fracture blisters" have often been considered a normal sequelae of fractures, this sign is always an indication of ischemic damage to the skin if it is otherwise intact. Blistering frequently occurs from tension on the skin, whether it is from underlying swelling or a too-tight wound closure, and is a sign of ischemia secondary to tension. In the case of bruising, evaluation of the skin may be difficult, because color and refill will not be normal.

The wound itself is then examined. Areas of subcu-

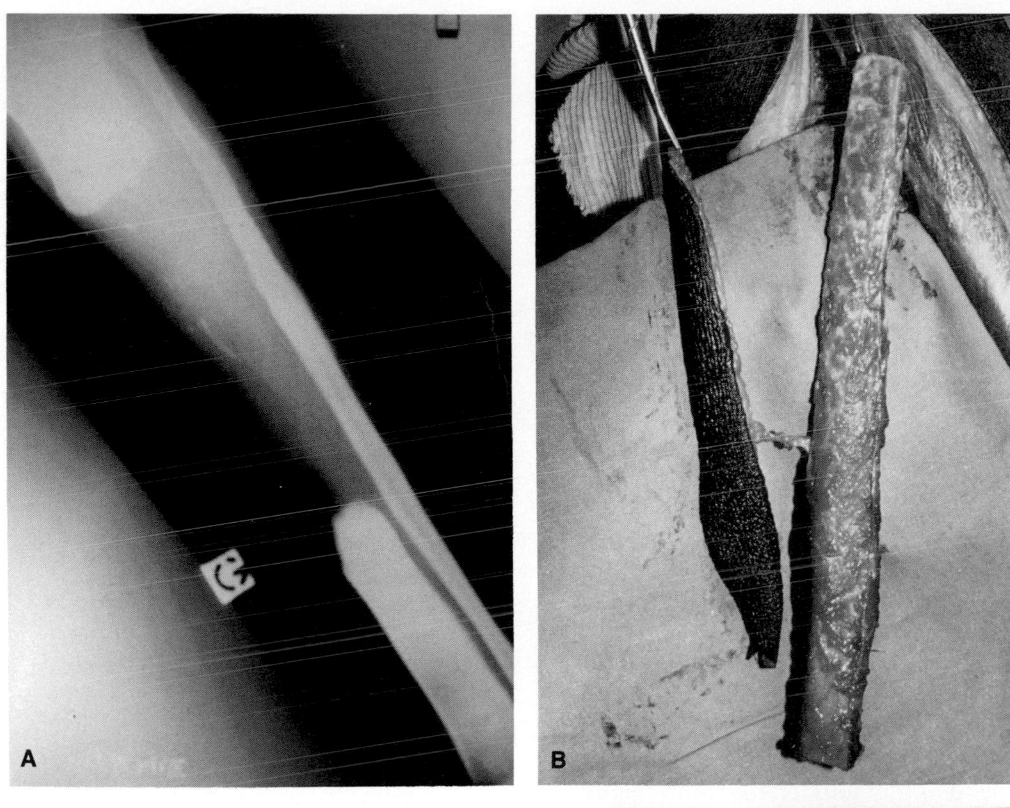

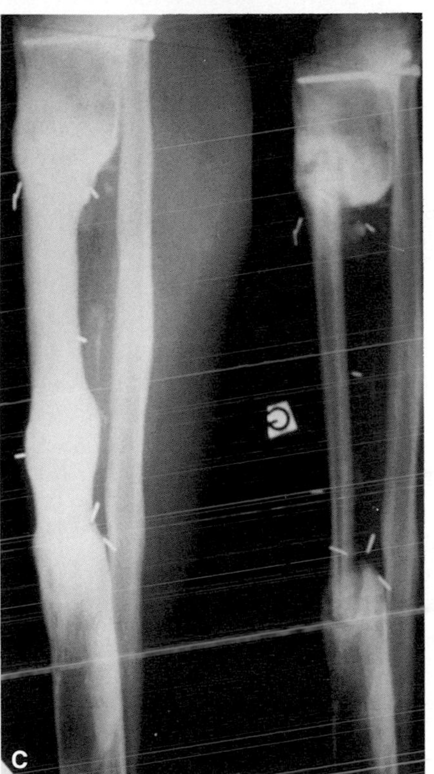

FIGURE 7-6. (**A**) Radiograph of the lower leg in a 28-year-old man with chronic osteomyelitis after radical debridement of an infected tibia. (**B**) A free fibula graft raised with a skin island. (**C**) Immediate and 18-month postoperative radiographs showing graft hypertrophy. (*Case courtesy of Alain Gilbert, M.D., Paris, France.*)

taneous fat should be moist and healthy looking, rather than dry and blood stained. Exposed fascia and muscle should be moist and glistening, with a pinkish hue. Damaged muscle will be bruised or darkened, and purplish muscle is probably not viable. All exposed soft tissues should bleed when abraded or cut with a knife.

Debridement

Debridement of the wound is a matter that often receives too little attention in discussions of wound management. This subject may seem mundane and obvious, but attitudes toward debridement have changed significantly in the past 20 years. Before the advent of microsurgical free tissue transfer, surgeons were often reluctant to adequately debride a wound for fear of inability to provide coverage. Although this attitude is unacceptable by today's standards, it is still practiced by many. Simple debridement of the wound margins ignores the extended "zone of injury." Tissue with marginal vascularity heals with extensive fibrosis and may eventually fail to provide adequate coverage. Hypoxic tissue likewise has poor resistance to infection and if left in a wound constitutes a nidus for infection. Inadequate debridement is the most common cause of wound complications,[151,610,743] with multiple studies attesting to the problems caused by skin and soft-tissue necrosis in and around the wound (Fig. 7-7).[48,204,355,374,417,819]

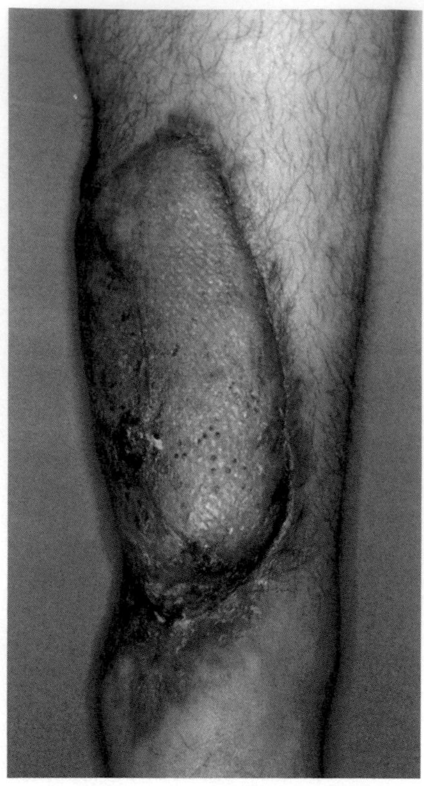

FIGURE 7-7. Despite a successful free flap, inadequate excision of surrounding scar tissue resulted in a persistent sinus tract at the distal edge.

Adequate debridement consists of removal of all nonviable and marginal tissue to establish a clean surgical wound. The basis of Godina's outstanding results with early flap closure of traumatic wounds was radical debridement of all necrotic and contaminated tissues, a procedure that he called "necrectomy."[270] His concept was to remove any questionable tissue (exclusive of intact major nerves) in preparation for wound closure. Much of the tissue surrounding an open wound may not be viable, although it may appear so on initial inspection. Large degloved areas of tissue with no connection to the underlying fascia are usually nonviable,[122,578,903] as are free fragments of bone. All of these tissues (with the possible exception of some bone fragments) should be debrided if in question. In acute injuries, this type of debridement prepares the fracture for conversion from an open injury to a closed one with reconstruction of the soft-tissue envelope.[319,532,680,692,743] In general, radical debridement should not be undertaken unless the surgeon is prepared to close the wound expeditiously. If one is unsure about the remaining wound margins, a second look at 24 to 48 hours allows identification and debridement of further nonviable tissues.[66,98,99,115,140,141,201,302,311,426,441,588,830] With experience, radical initial debridement can be followed immediately by coverage without a second look.[268] In any event, most debrided wounds should not be left open beyond 72 hours to prevent potential infection and increasing wound fibrosis.

The decision as to which tissues to debride is based on experience, and techniques for obtaining an adequately debrided wound differ. Any tissue that is severely crushed or contaminated with foreign material should obviously be removed, with the usual exception of major neurovascular structures. Many authors prefer debridement without a tourniquet, to allow visualization of bleeding from tissue edges.[66,98,296,636,780] Although this technique will definitively allow assessment of tissue circulation, it may cause undue blood loss. Arterial injection of fluorescein has been used to evaluate the viability of skin flaps[545] and has been advocated for evaluation of degloving injuries,[547] but this technique has not found wide application in wound debridement.

Muscle debridement is done on the basis of Sculley's "four *C*s": color, capacity to bleed, contractibility, and consistency (see Chapter 6).[732] It is more difficult to determine which bone fragments should be left in place and which should be removed. Retaining bone fragments that are potentially vascularized by soft-tissue attachment has been recommended, whereas contaminated fragments with no attachment should generally be removed.[255,540,787] One must also remember that bone segments that are not loose or free may also be devascularized by loss of their intramedullary blood supply or periosteal covering. Godina suggested leaving loose bone fragments that are not grossly contaminated in place at the time of debridement and flap coverage.[270]

We prefer to debride extremity wounds under tourniquet control, which is the technique advocated by Godina.[270] With experience, one can accurately determine the viability of wound margins by assessing the color and consistency of the tissues. All tissues in question are debrided, but major neurovascular structures are simply trimmed of surrounding nonviable tissue and left in situ. Sharp debridement with a knife is supplemented by gentle irrigation with warm antibiotic-containing solution. The use of devices that forcibly pump high-pressure irrigation fluid is to be avoided on freshly debrided wound edges, because the force used can further damage soft tissue and insufflates the tissue with fluid. Once the field appears to be adequately debrided, the tourniquet is deflated. The viability of the wound margins can then be further assessed by observing bleeding from the debrided edges. Areas of soft tissue that do not bleed well should undergo further debridement. At this point, the wound is ready for closure and the chances for uncomplicated healing are maximized.

A secondary aim of debridement is to provide a wound that can be covered without leaving significant areas of dead space under the flap. One goal of flap placement is to obliterate dead space within the wound. To this end, the wound after debridement should present a three-dimensional space that can be easily filled with the chosen flap. Any open spaces remaining under the flap after it is placed in the wound are potential breeding grounds for bacteria. Godina went so far as to advocate removal of some normal tissue at the margins of the wound if this would give a more uniform surface for flap placement.[270] Although we usually stop short of total "saucerization" of the wound, this principle of obliteration of dead space is basic to successful wound management.

Antibiotics

Antibiotics are "therapeutic" (as contrasted with "prophylactic") when used in the treatment of open fractures, because all open wounds are by definition contaminated.[66,634,637] If antibiotic therapy is continued beyond 48 to 72 hours, the emergence of resistant strains is enhanced.[313,635,689,880] However, antibiotics never reach devascularized bone and soft tissue[700] and are never a substitute for adequate debridement.[308] Reconstruction of the soft-tissue envelope brings blood supply and with it antibiotics to the injured area.[519]

Options for Reconstruction

Secondary Healing

The capacity for healing in the normal human is enormous, and most wounds will contract and close given adequate vascularity and enough time. This type of wound healing, or *healing by secondary intention*, has been allowed (or tolerated) by surgeons throughout history. It is still appropriate treatment in certain types of soft-tissue defects but has many disadvantages in the management of complex musculoskeletal injury. Among these disadvantages are the following:

1. The open wound acts as a portal for the entry of secondary pathogens.[105,355,497]
2. Desiccation of bone and tendon occurs.
3. Fibrosis constricts vascularity on both macroscopic and microscopic levels, leading to hypoxia. Wound hypoxia is detrimental to leukocyte and phagocyte function.[153,213,426,519]

The usual index for a healthy wound healing by secondary intention is "good granulation tissue." We believe that this is an oxymoron in terms of proper management of the complex wound. The presence of granulation tissue simply implies that there is adequate vascularity of the wound margins. Granulation tissue consists of fibroblasts and capillaries, which ultimately translates into scar. Granulation tissue can be full of bacteria on the microscopic level, and granulating wounds covered in a sea of pus are not uncommon. Although skin grafts are commonly placed directly on nondebrided granulating wound beds, this is, in fact, a poor bed for grafting.[153] The optimum management of a granulating wound is to debride the granulations and scar bed and place a skin graft directly on fresh tissue. The ultimate test of wound coverage, however, that of long-term stability, is often poor with skin-grafted granulations. It was recognized many years ago that wounds managed in this fashion would often require later debridement and flap coverage.[396]

Primary Healing

Primary soft-tissue reconstruction in complex extremity trauma has many proven advantages.[66,98,99,140,204,258,302,319,426,450,903] With early well-vascularized coverage, open fractures are converted to closed injuries.[99,123,692] Earlier bone fixation or reconstruction is possible with stable soft-tissue coverage. Bone grafts may be placed directly underneath a flap raised secondarily on its pedicle, obviating the need for posterior or posterolateral approaches. Tissue with its own vascularity, independent of the state of the wound, resists necrosis, has a higher oxygen level, and imports host defense mechanisms.[521] As noted in the previous discussion, the ability to import vascular tissue allows *total* debridement of the wound, resulting in a decreased rate of wound healing complications.[842]

Flap Selection

The selection of type of tissue for coverage depends to a certain extent on the nature of the wound. The force of wounding determines the amount of surrounding soft-tissue damage, and this varies depending on the cause of injury (Table 7-5).[223] Very clean low-energy wounds covered in the first 72 hours can often be managed with cutaneous or fasciocutaneous flaps. Although cutaneous flaps offer excellent stability, their potential for revascularization of the surrounding tissue and to resist infection is limited. Muscle flaps, on the other hand, have a greater potential for importing vascularity. Muscle and fasciocutaneous flaps have been shown not only to tolerate subflap infection better but also to actually decrease the bacterial count beneath the flap.[119,519,520] Based on these facts, muscle offers a better choice for the management of higher-energy wounds and in cases of greater soft-tissue loss.

A wide variety of flap transfer techniques are available to the surgeon performing soft-tissue reconstruction, from local rotation flaps to flaps transferred from distant sites by microvascular surgery. The selection of the most appropriate technique for coverage ultimately depends on the training and experience of the surgeon, but certain circumstances dictate the use of one technique over another. Clean, low-energy wounds with minimal soft-tissue loss can be managed with local tissue from the extremity, whether cutaneous or muscle. High-energy wounds or those with increased contamination should probably always be reconstructed with muscle, for the reasons listed earlier. It is these complex wounds that often present a problem in terms of the selection of donor muscle. In the case of open tibial fractures, proximal or middle-third defects *can* be covered with local muscle rotation flaps. The problem in high-energy injuries is that the donor muscles are in the field of injury and may suffer vascular compromise when rotated. Successful coverage in these cases is largely dependent on the expertise of the surgeon, and either local tissue or free tissue transfer may be appropriate.

One area of wounding that is believed to present an absolute indication for free tissue transfer is in the distal tibia and ankle. Although techniques of lower leg coverage with distally pedicled muscle flaps[816,820] or fasciocutaneous flaps[228] are available, the morbidity of these flaps is generally excessive compared to free flaps. Some of the earliest free flaps reported were done to cover complex wounds of the ankle, in limbs that would have probably undergone amputation otherwise.[170,607] The value of this technique was recognized early, and studies documented the advantages of free tissue transfer over local flaps in distal lower extremity reconstruction (Fig. 7-8).[735,737]

The question of which free muscle flap to select (when microsurgical reconstruction is undertaken) is also partially a function of the surgeon's experience, but increasing sophistication in free tissue transfer has placed a greater emphasis on selection of the *appropriate* muscle.[603] Placement of the entire latissimus dorsi muscle on any and every wound is no longer considered appropriate.[269] The aim of reconstruction should be to provide adequate stable coverage that does not interfere with function due to excessive bulk. Even though most flaps can be safely debulked at a later stage, current philosophy aims at single-stage reconstruction whenever possible. Although the latissimus dorsi remains the gold standard in management of large wounds, smaller muscles such as the rectus abdominus, gracilis, and serratus anterior have wide application in microsurgical management of smaller wounds. The actual selection of donor tissue is discussed in more detail in the following sections.

TABLE 7-5
Energy Level to the Tibia From Various Mechanisms of Injury

Mechanism	Energy Level
Fall from a sidewalk	100 ft-lb
Skiing injury	300–500 ft-lb
High-velocity gunshot wound	2000 ft-lb
Motorcycle injury	80,040 ft-lb
Bumper injury at 20 mph	100,000 ft-lb

Data from references 223, 268, and 270.

Flap Loss

The proper approach to soft-tissue reconstruction should bear in mind the relative loss rates of various types of flaps. Unfortunately, many surgeons still believe that pedicle muscle flaps have advantage over free flaps owing to the potential for loss of free flaps.[108] Mathes and Nahai reviewed a large series of conventional pedicled muscle flaps and found approximately 10% loss rate of a significant portion of the flap.[526] Microsurgical free flap transfer has a well-established overall failure rate of around 5%,[79,141,341,345] and even series of lower extremity flaps in the presence of severe injury have success rates of 90% to 98%.[168,268,828,902] Free flaps have also been shown to be safe and effective for extremity reconstruction in children[747] and elderly patients.[245,271] These data support current thinking that free flap transfer by experienced surgeons is as safe as, if not safer than, local muscle transfer.

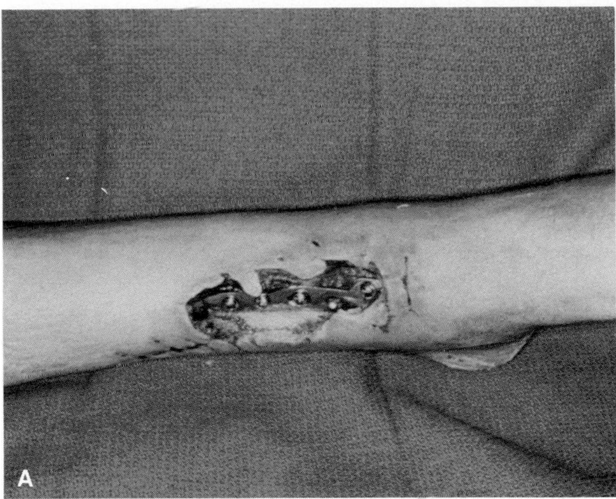

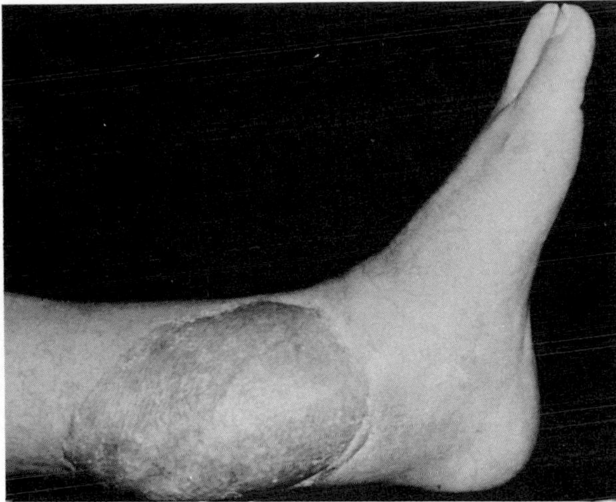

FIGURE 7-8. (**A**) The leg of a 50-year-old patient who suffered necrosis of skin and overlying subcutaneous tissue after open reduction and internal fixation of a severe tibial plafond fracture. Coverage had to be delayed for 6 weeks because of a pulmonary embolus and the patient's consequent medical status. The wound was managed by local dressing changes, and a flap was applied at 6 weeks. (**B**) The latissimus dorsi free flap and split-thickness skin graft healed without incident, and there has been no subsequent drainage from the tibia over 3 years. The plafond fracture healed after one subsequent bone grafting procedure, approached by lifting the posterior margin of the flap.

Tissue Expansion

The use of implantable devices to expand skin has found wide application in reconstructive surgery. These devices rely on the ability of the epidermis and dermis to stretch, and studies have demonstrated the actual production of new cellular material in the expanded tissue.[26] Although this technique has proven value with low complication rates in the scalp and torso, expansion of extremity skin remains problematic. Most series report complication rates of around 30% with elective extremity expansion, primarily infection and extrusion of the expander.[557,910] Authors experienced with this technique generally reserve it for secondary reconstruction when there are no open wounds,[64] or for expansion of distant skin flaps before microsurgical transfer to the limb.[571]

Hyperbaric Oxygenation

Effect on Bone

Adjunctive hyperbaric oxygenation may aid in the differentiation of viable and nonviable bone and experimentally results in faster bone healing.[599,898] In one large series of patients with osteomyelitis, 34 of 38 patients who were treated with hyperbaric oxygenation and allowed to heal had no drainage at an average of 34 months after treatment ended. An average of 6.1 operations was required, but the authors concluded that hyperbaric oxygenation prolonged the infection-free interval.[180] Others have confirmed the potential benefit of hyperbaric oxygen treatment in chronic osteomyelitis.[179,214,215] This treatment has found application in management of osteoradionecrosis of the mandible as well[218] and might be helpful in similar situations in the extremities.

Effect on Soft Tissue

Although the use of hyperbaric oxygen treatment in the management of difficult soft-tissue wounds has found many advocates,[332,856] there are little scientific data to support this application. Hyperbaric oxygenation is definitely indicated in cases of clostridial myonecrosis[382] and has been shown to increase the rate of angiogenesis in wound margins.[476,559] Experimental studies have also demonstrated increased survival of muscle in the case of compartment syndromes treated with hyperbaric oxygen.[778] Hyperbaric oxygenation has not proven to be beneficial in the treatment of failing skin flaps[102] and in fact has been demonstrated in one study to have toxic effects on capillary endothelium.[369]

Despite the proven and unproven benefits of hyperbaric oxygen therapy, this treatment is prolonged and very expensive. It may increase granulation tissue and epithelialization of wounds, but it cannot provide stable coverage for bone, particularly if later procedures are required.[82,99,143,209,296,477] We therefore believe that it has little place in the management of acute complex extremity injury.

Amputation Versus Salvage

Timely amputation is indicated for a severely injured limb that, after successful soft-tissue and bone reconstruction, would be less functional than a prosthesis. In the upper extremity, prosthetic replacement is usually a poor substitute for even a marginally functional hand. Lower limb amputees, on the other hand, are usually quite functional, and thus this discussion focuses on lower extremity salvage.

The problem in mangling lower extremity injuries is in determining early what the ultimate outcome will be with or without attempts at salvage. We have treated several patients in whom multiple reconstructive attempts were made, and it was only obvious after some time that the limb was not as functional as would have been obtained by early amputation. Therefore, the decision to attempt salvage or to amputate is difficult. This depends on many factors, not the least of which is the expertise and judgment of the trauma surgeon.[62,112,158,297,338,468,471,472,497] With current techniques, salvage of a functional limb in a reasonable time span and at reasonable cost is possible.[640] The following guidelines represent the consensus of authors who have studied this problem.[98,112,115,274,432]

Salvage should be attempted in children, even if replantation is necessary.[251,581] If amputation is performed in a child, bony overgrowth through the soft-tissue envelope is a common problem.[466,483] If the ischemia time has not been too great, epiphyses generally stay open and growth of the limb after replantation should be expected.[242,385,449] If limb-length discrepancy develops, equalizing can be done later by lengthening or by contralateral epiphysiodesis.[392,841]

In adults, entire limb reconstruction or salvage requires a sensate foot (intact posterior tibial nerve) that is or can be made viable.[208,314,316,389,472,540] Restoration of sensation by nerve repair after replantation of the foot has been reported and is worth consideration in a patient with a sharp injury.[485,500] An intact fibula or other reasonable method of maintaining nominal length (eg, external fixator) is necessary.[117,673,692,784] Treatment of the fibula is often neglected, but if the fibula is aligned early by a Rush rod, maintenance of length and limb alignment is enhanced (see Fig. 7-5). A healed fibula will preserve length and alignment, may allow earlier removal of the external fixator, and is often used for later bone reconstruction, especially in the "single-vessel" leg.[117,383,673,692,784,785] An intact or healed fibula greatly simplifies management. Limb shortening of 2 cm or less is well tolerated and may obviate the need for skeletal and even soft-tissue reconstruction.

Limb salvage in the Gustilo grade III tibial fracture remains somewhat controversial. Although many of these limbs can be successfully reconstructed, long-term function and socioeconomic factors must be considered.[62,339] Early enthusiasm for microsurgical reconstruction of these injuries (particularly the Gustilo grade IIIC) has been tempered by critical appraisal of long-term function and late amputation rates. Despite successful flap transfer, these patients may have significant problems with osteomyelitis, nonunion, degenerative joint problems, and chronic venous insufficiency with skin ulceration.[900] The reconstructive process is lengthy, and many patients are not able to return to work for up to 2 years. Amputation rates after "successful" reconstruction of the mangled leg have ranged from 12% to 61%,[62,112,472,857,900] with the higher rate being seen in patients suffering combined major vascular injury. Recent long-term functional evaluation of reconstructed patients compared with those undergoing early amputation has shown mixed results. One enthusiastic report on reconstruction found that 67% of patients with salvaged limbs returned to work,[233] but a matching rate has been reported for a similar group of patients after below-knee amputation.[639] In terms of overall functional impairment, some authors believe that rates are better with limb salvage.[440] Others disagree, citing a prolonged time to full weight bearing, decreased ankle and subtalar mobility, limb swelling, and problems with return to occupational and recreational activities in the reconstructed group.[234,252,475] Despite these problems with limb salvage, our experience is similar to those authors who have found a high overall level of patient satisfaction with their reconstructed legs.[234,640]

Attempts to predict the ability to salvage mangled extremities have been made using injury severity scoring systems. A score of more than 7 using the Mangled Extremity Severity Score (MESS) has been reported to be 100% predictive for eventual need for amputation (Table 7-6).[367,551] Advocates of this system propose early amputation in patients with such scores. Others have found that the predictive value of injury severity scoring and other variables relative to the need for early amputation is poor.[659] Further work in this area may lead to better decision making in the salvage of limbs with complex injuries.

Salvage of Useful Parts

The goals of limb salvage can be modified in some instances to reconstruct sufficient length to allow fitting of a below-knee rather than an above-knee prosthesis. In lieu of discarding the distal tissue entirely, it can be used to salvage a below-knee stump and avoid higher amputation.[230,762] The entire distal portion of the extremity can be replanted to the proximal stump to provide length and soft-tissue coverage,[131] or soft-tissue flaps alone can be harvested from the distal limb.[150] The sole or dorsum of the foot has been used

TABLE 7-6
Mangled Extremity Severity Score

Injury Severity Score (ISS)	
0–25	1
25–50	2
>50	3
Integument	
Guillotine	1
Crush/burn	2
Avulsion/degloving	3
Nerve	
Contusion	1
Transection	2
Avulsion	3
Vascular	
Artery	
Transected	1
Thrombosed	2
Avulsed	3
Vein damage	1
Bone	
Simple fracture	1
Segmental fracture	2
Segmental comminuted fracture	3
Segmental comminuted fracture with bone loss < 6 cm*	4
Segmental fracture, intra- or extra-articular, with bone loss < 6 cm	5
Segmental fracture, intra- or extra-articular, with bone loss > 6 cm	6
Lag time	1 point for every hour > 6
Age (years)	
40–50	1
50–60	2
60–70	3
Preexisting disease	1
Shock	2
A score of less than 7 points suggests that salvage should be attempted. Conversely, amputation should be considered if the score is more than 20 points.	

* Add 1 point for bone loss > 6 cm.
Helfet, D.L. Howey, T., Sanders, R., and Johansen, K.: Limb salvage versus amputation: Preliminary results of the Mangled Extremity Severity Score. Clin. Orthop. Rel. Res., 256:80–86, 1990.

in this manner both as a pedicled flap and as free flaps to preserve a below-knee stump (Fig. 7-9).[149,304] Although distant free flaps also have utility in reconstruction of amputation stumps, use of the amputated part to avoid other donor site morbidity should be considered.

External Versus Internal Fixation

Hippocrates first used a crude external fixation device of padded rings about the knee and ankle, with bent tree branches for distraction. More recently, fracture immobilization was by plaster or traction until trials of external fixation devices began during World War II. The incidence of infection and nonunion was so high that their use was forbidden by the armed forces.[145,477] With better understanding of the principles of their use, external fixators have enjoyed a rebirth in recent years. They are an extremely valuable adjunct to the treatment of open fractures,[50,122,308,435,480] especially when combined with current wound coverage techniques.[117,201–203,216,318,342,426,830]

Advantages of external fixation in complex injury include the following:

1. Avoidance of additional soft-tissue stripping or injury[48,284,878]
2. Protection of vascular repairs
3. Decreased incidence of infection and nonunion in grade III injury[29,44,105,123,315,355,468,615,685,694,847]
4. Ease of dressing change, redebridement, and soft-tissue care and reconstruction[216,342]
5. Prevention of contractures of the foot and ankle[66,203]
6. Less disruption of intramedullary blood supply than with intramedullary nailing[281,282,313,681]
7. Use in infected nonunions to maintain length while allowing bone and soft-tissue debridement[291,309]
8. Ease of realignment, removal, and replacement[202]

Ideally, pin placement requires early cooperation between the orthopaedist and the surgeon doing the soft-tissue reconstruction.[334] In most cases, a single frame placed directly anterior will allow access for most rotational and free tissue transfers and will not impale vascular structures or potential muscle flap donor sites (Fig. 7-10).[29,50,66,911] Studies have demonstrated that most external fixators do not interfere with either local rotational muscle flaps or free flap transfers.[845,846]

Use of intramedullary rods has been recommended for high-energy injuries to the tibia,[359,495] but has the disadvantage of damage to the medullary circulation.[29,281,282,313,681,682,826] The use of small, nonreamed nails might be expected to preserve some blood supply while maintaining length and alignment. Some studies suggest that the use of nonreamed nails offers equivalent results to external fixators in grade IIIB tibial fractures when covered with muscle flaps.[821] Infection rates in this study were low, but the potential for pandiaphyseal infection remains a serious drawback to intramedullary nailing.[468]

Plating of high-grade open fractures is usually not recommended because of the additional soft-tissue stripping necessary. However, if the bone is already exposed, no additional trauma is caused by plate application.[12] Plating has a higher infection rate, but an

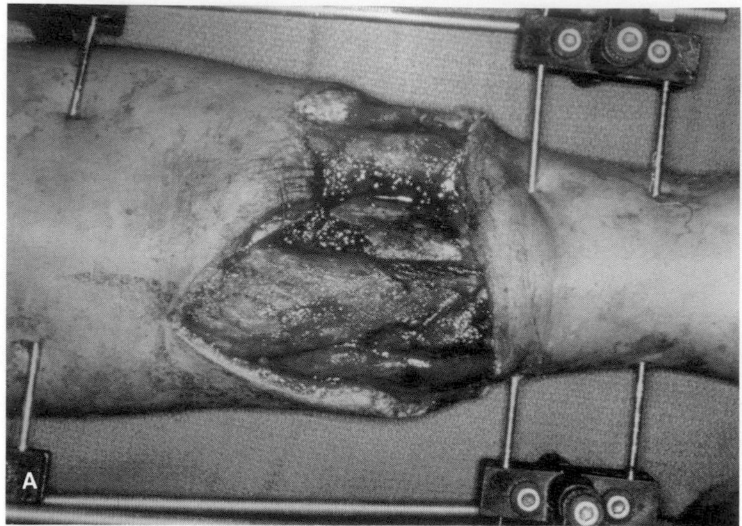

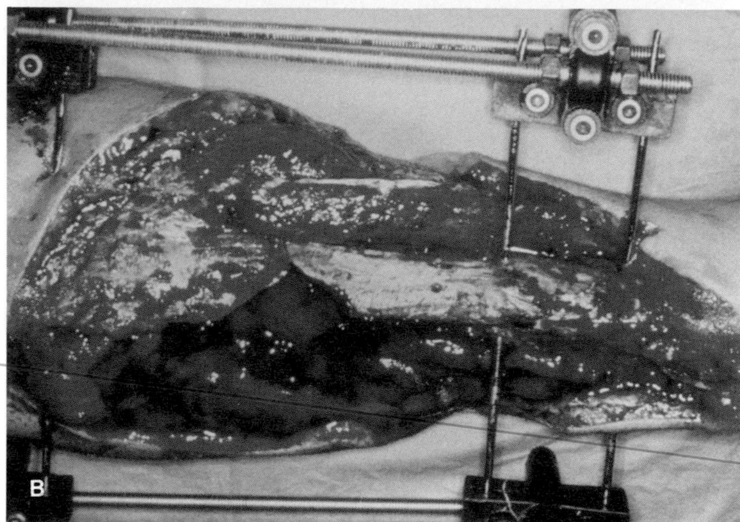

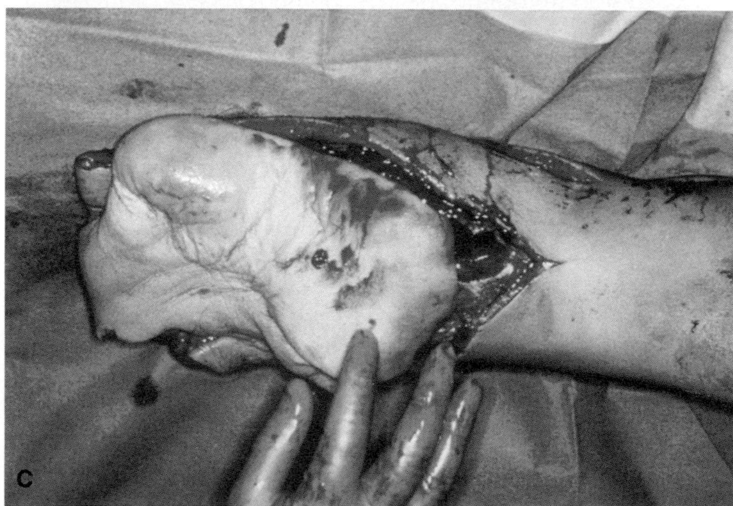

FIGURE 7-9. (**A**) The leg of an 18-year-old patient 5 days after an open fracture of the tibia. The limb was severely contaminated with dirt, and a limited debridement and application of external fixation device had been performed at another hospital. The patient developed fever and foul-smelling drainage and was transferred for definitive care. (**B**) Appearance of the leg after radical debridement of the zone of injury and necrotic muscle and bone. Cultures subsequently grew clostridia. The patient was treated in a hyperbaric chamber, and the infection was controlled. A bone scan showed significant devascularization of the exposed tibia and the only muscles to the foot were the posterior group. Therefore, amputation was elected. However, because there was inadequate soft tissue to cover the stump, an elective fillet flap of the foot was performed. (**C**) The posterior tibial artery was the only vessel intact to the foot. The perforating branch between the first and second metatarsals was preserved, and the entire foot was filleted from the bone. It was then folded up to cover the stump.

continues

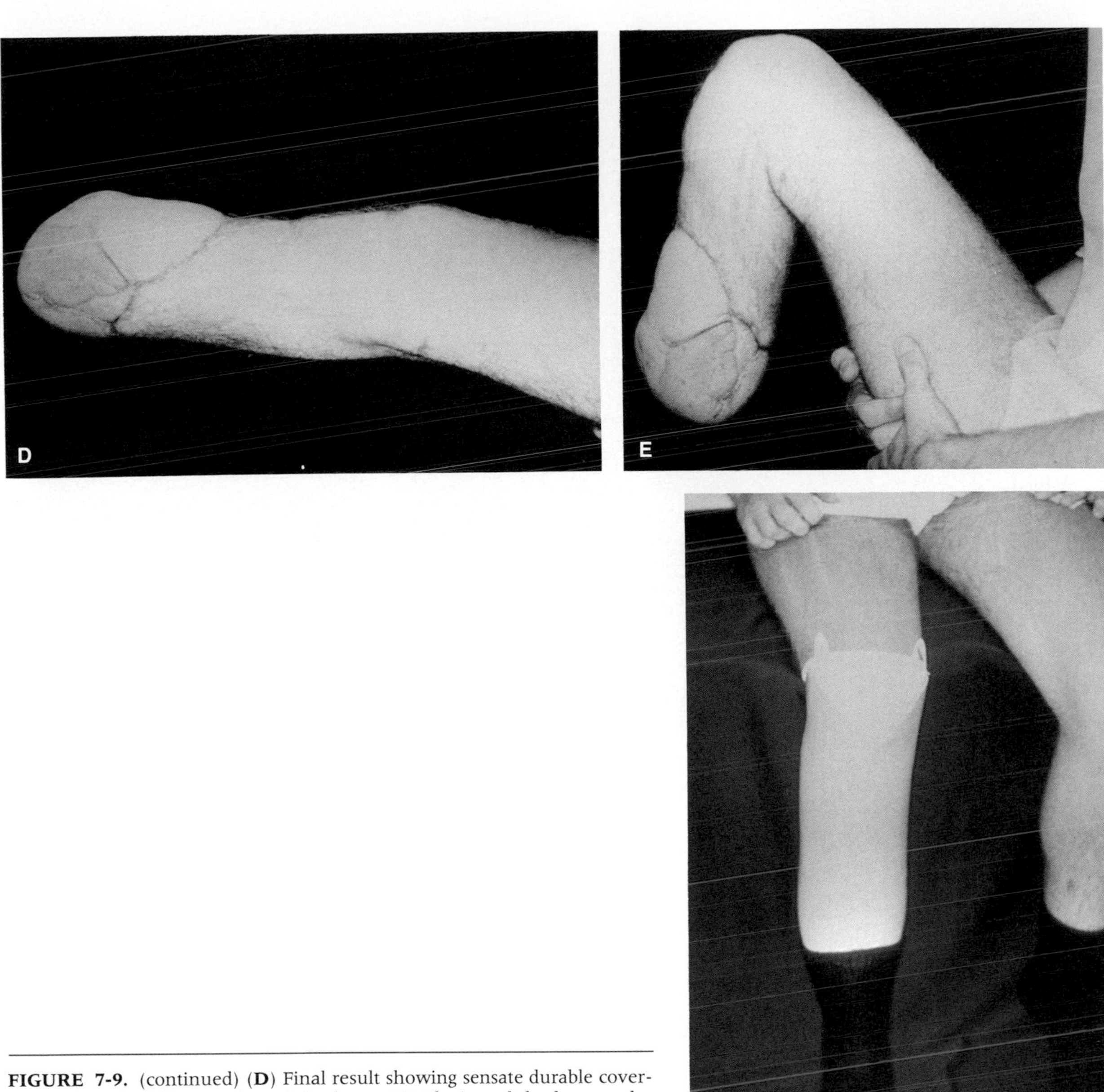

FIGURE 7-9. (continued) (**D**) Final result showing sensate durable coverage and nearly full extension of the knee. (**E**) Flexion of the knee and a lateral view of the stump. (**F**) The patient fitted with his prosthesis.

infected plate that has maintained fracture stability should be retained and covered with a well-vascularized flap. This frequently results in control of the infection. Some patients tolerate exposed hardware remarkably well, and we have covered plates exposed for more than 6 weeks with free flaps, with no further drainage (see Fig. 7-8). In some cases of an unavoidable delay in flap coverage of a complex wound, the incidence of subflap infection may be increased secondary to colonization of the wound. If a question exists as to the potential for infection under a fresh flap, skin grafting is delayed and the patient can be returned to the operating room in a few days with subflap irrigation and debridement as necessary.[890] When the flap becomes adherent to the underlying tissue, it can be sutured down and covered with a split-thickness skin graft. Likewise, if the fixation is solid and the bone appears to be healing, the subflap area can be drained periodically if fluid collections occur. When the bone is healed, the hardware can be removed and the infection will usually resolve.

SOFT-TISSUE FLAPS

Classification of Flaps Based on Anatomy of Circulation

Skin Flaps

Skin receives its vascularity from a number of sources, and some areas of skin have more than one blood supply. The vascularity of the skin was

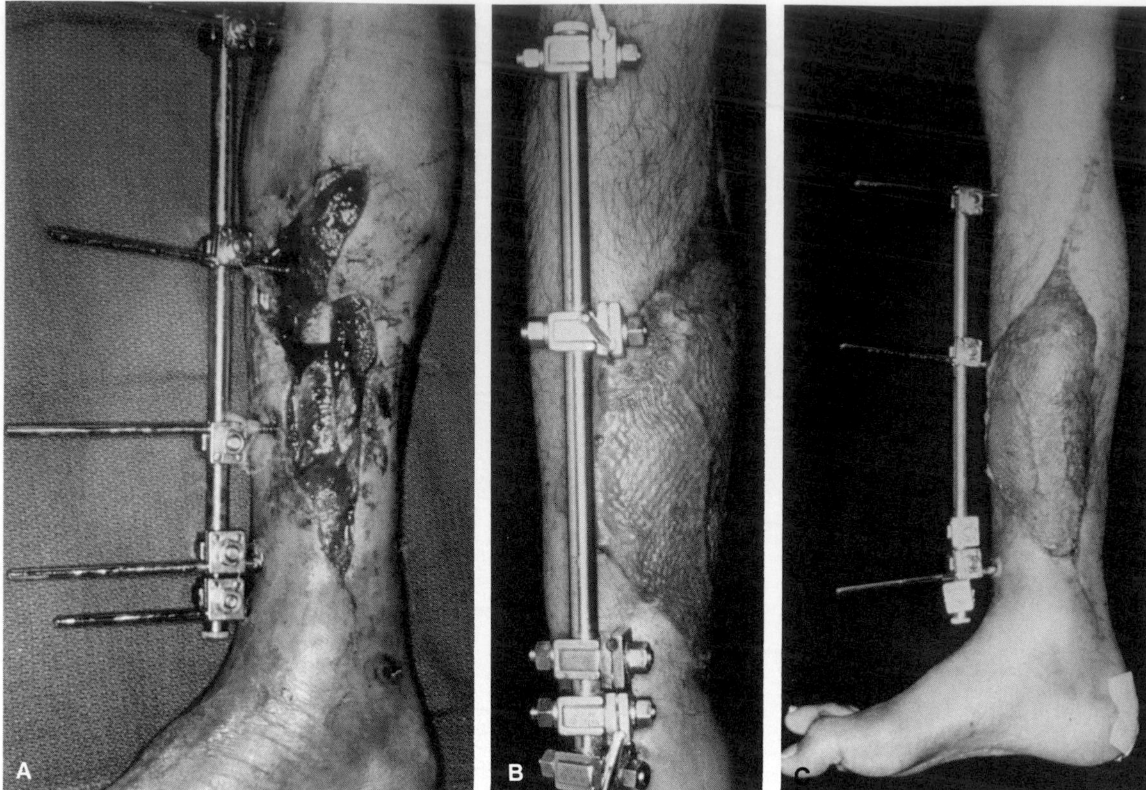

FIGURE 7-10. (**A**) A 1-week-old open fracture of the tibia treated by debridement and a single anterior AO external fixator. (**B**) The result 6 weeks after coverage by a latissimus dorsi free flap plus a split-thickness skin graft. (**C**) Lateral view.

extensively studied and mapped in the late 1800s and early 1900s,[503,712,713] although clinical application of this information was delayed until recently. Elegant studies in the past several years by Taylor have confirmed[714,715] and expanded[799,803] on this work and will be the benchmark for skin flap design in the future. Most skin of the body receives its blood supply directly from the underlying muscles or from vascular perforators lying in the enveloping fascia. A few areas of skin that do not overlie muscle or fascial vessels have direct axial vessels (eg, the groin flap).

Skin flaps are generally classified based on the anatomy of their circulation.[142] The final common pathway in skin circulation is the subdermal plexus of vessels, which as the name implies lies between the dermis and subcutaneous fat. *Random pattern* skin flaps are those local flaps based solely on this subdermal plexus, which receive their blood supply from vascular perforators at the base of the flap. These types of skin flaps usually cannot be longer than they are wide (1:1 ratio). *Axial pattern* skin flaps contain an axial vascular pedicle within the flap that is usually a named vessel or a branch of a named vessel. The length of these flaps depends solely on the length of the axial vessels, although they can be lengthened by adding a *random portion* to their distal end. Some axial pattern flaps can be transferred as free flaps if their vessels are large enough to allow microvascular anastomosis. The prototype of this flap is the groin flap, which is based on the superficial circumflex iliac vessels[546] and was one of the first flaps transferred by microsurgical techniques.[170]

Fasciocutaneous Flaps

Fasciocutaneous flaps are cutaneous flaps that receive their blood supply from perforators arising from the underlying fascia.[818] The vessel supplying the fascia is a named regional vessel and usually runs between muscle groups. The primary vascular pedicle supplies branches to the fascia, which then supply the skin. Fasciocutaneous flaps whose vessels lie in a muscular septum are referred to as *septocutaneous flaps.* These flaps have been categorized into several different groups, depending on the nature of their primary intrafascial vascular supply.[156,467] The size of a fasciocutaneous flap depends on the vascular supply to the fascia and the local anatomy.[33] An example of this type of flap is the radial forearm flap, in which the forearm skin is raised with the muscular fascia that envelops the radial artery.[231,763] Fasciocutaneous flaps that are raised with a discrete vascular pedicle and rotated into a wound are called *island pedicle flaps.* This type of flap can also be transferred to another site with microvascular anastomoses after division of the primary vascular pedicle.[169,239,697]

Myocutaneous Flaps

When a skin flap receives its vascularity from an attached underlying piece of muscle it is called a *myocutaneous flap.* Muscles that are transferred without their overlying skin are called simply *muscle flaps.* For a muscle to be transferred, it must have vascular anatomy that will allow elevation of all or a portion of the muscle so that it can be moved and survive on its own vascular pedicle.[542] Muscles available for transfer by rotation or as free flaps are classified by their vascular supply (Table 7-7). Mathes and Nahai described five patterns of muscle circulation based on (1) the regional source of the pedicle(s), (2) the size of the pedicle(s), (3) the number of pedicles, (4) the location of the pedicle(s), and (5) the angiographic pattern of internal vessels.[524,525] Within a muscle, the vessels of the pedicle arborize into a very rich capillary plexus.[519] Most muscles that can be reliably transferred have a primary vessel or vessels that allow elevation of a majority of the muscle. This type of muscle can also be transferred to a distant site with microsurgical techniques. A muscle with ideal characteristics for local or distant transfer is the latissimus dorsi, which can survive in its entirety on the thoracodorsal vascular pedicle alone.[533,751]

Prefabricated Flaps

Experience with microsurgical tissue transfer has led to the development of the so-called *prefabricated flap.* This type of flap undergoes manipulation at its original site before transfer to improve the results of reconstruction. Prefabricated flaps may simply be expanded before transfer to increase the area of coverage.[444] Experimental work has shown that soft tissue revascularized by implantation of a vascular pedicle can be microsurgically transferred and survive.[210,211,217,901] This technique has been applied clinically to provide "custom-made" flaps for certain applications of soft-tissue reconstruction.[661] Further extension of this principle has allowed the construction of composite tissue flaps at the donor site, although these have been of limited size.[46]

TABLE 7-7
Classification of Muscle Flaps by Vascularity

Type I	One vascular pedicle
Type II	Dominant vascular pedicles plus minor pedicles
Type III	Two dominant pedicles
Type IV	Segmental vascular pedicles
Type V	One dominant vascular pedicle and secondary segmental vascular pedicles

Commonly Used Flaps for Soft-Tissue Reconstruction

Muscle Flaps

Latissimus Dorsi

The latissimus dorsi was first used as a myocutaneous flap for coverage of the chest after mastectomy by Tansini in 1906[793] and reported by other authors in 1912.[163] These were the first reports of a myocutaneous flap for wound reconstruction, but the attributes of the latissimus dorsi as a valuable muscle for wound coverage were not fully appreciated until the 1970s.[616,664] It rapidly became the muscle of choice for free transfer owing to its reliable vascular anatomy,[39,535,693] ease of dissection, size, and minimal donor site morbidity (Fig. 7-11).[60,465,696] The latissimus dorsi has also found wide application in coverage and functional reconstruction of the shoulder[147,771] and upper arm.[470,751]

The latissimus dorsi has been classified by Mathes and Nahai as a type V muscle, having one dominant pedicle and secondary segmental pedicles.[518,525] This muscle will support a large skin paddle overlying nearly the entire muscle, although the distal portion (over the fascial origin) is less reliable. The primary pedicle is the thoracodorsal artery and vein, which enters the muscle with the thoracodorsal nerve about 10 cm below its tendon of insertion. This vascular pedicle is a branch of the subscapular artery and arises distal to the circumflex scapular vessels (Fig. 7-12). The thoracodorsal system gives a branch to the serratus anterior,[693] and in fact the muscle can be rotated based on retrograde flow from the serratus branch if the thoracodorsal has been divided proximally.[225] This serratus branch will also allow elevation of one or multiple slips of the serratus anterior with the latissimus dorsi on the same vascular pedicle if more muscle mass is required to complete the reconstruction.[350] The secondary pedicles are perforators entering the muscle medially from the thoracic and lumbar area through the paraspinous muscles. The entire muscle can be rotated either on the primary pedicle or the secondary pedicles, depending on the area of coverage required. The arc or rotation of the muscle

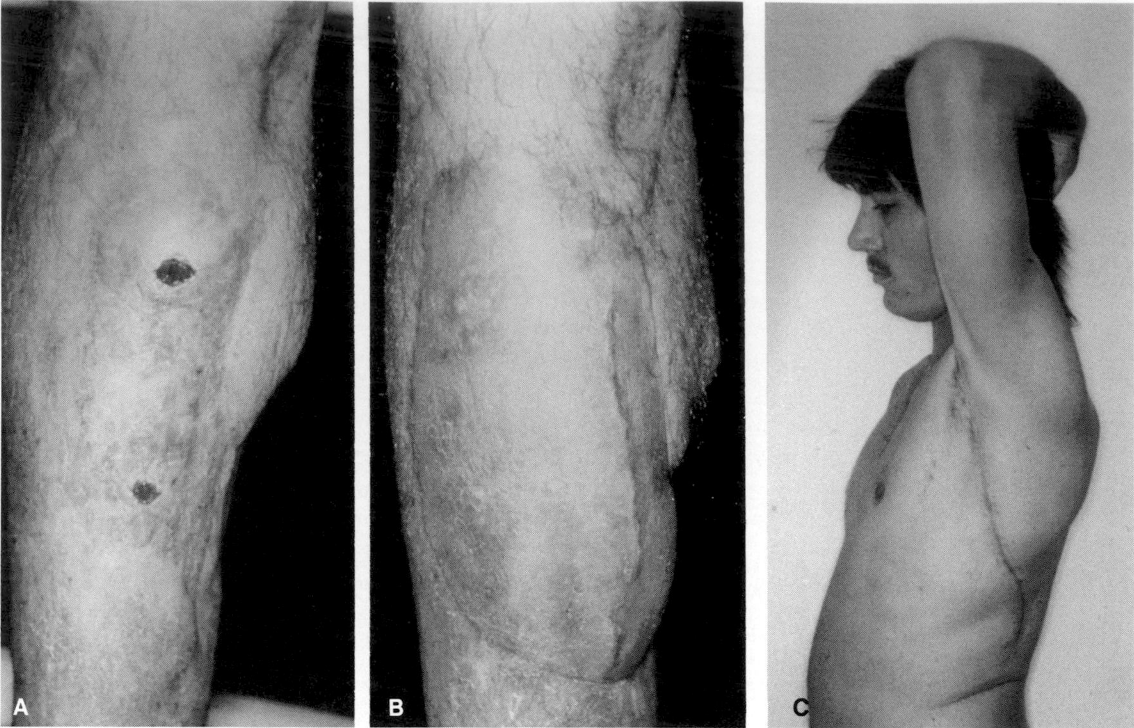

FIGURE 7-11. (**A**) The leg of a 23-year-old patient after an open fracture of the tibia, which healed with some shortening and external rotation. The patient complained of continued breakdown of the nondurable epithelialized granulation tissue anteriorly because he frequently climbed a ladder in his occupation as a carpenter. (**B**) At 8 weeks after cover with a latissimus dorsi free flap and a split-thickness skin graft, durable full-thickness soft tissue reconstruction has been obtained. (**C**) The patient has full range of motion of the shoulder, and the donor scar is acceptable.

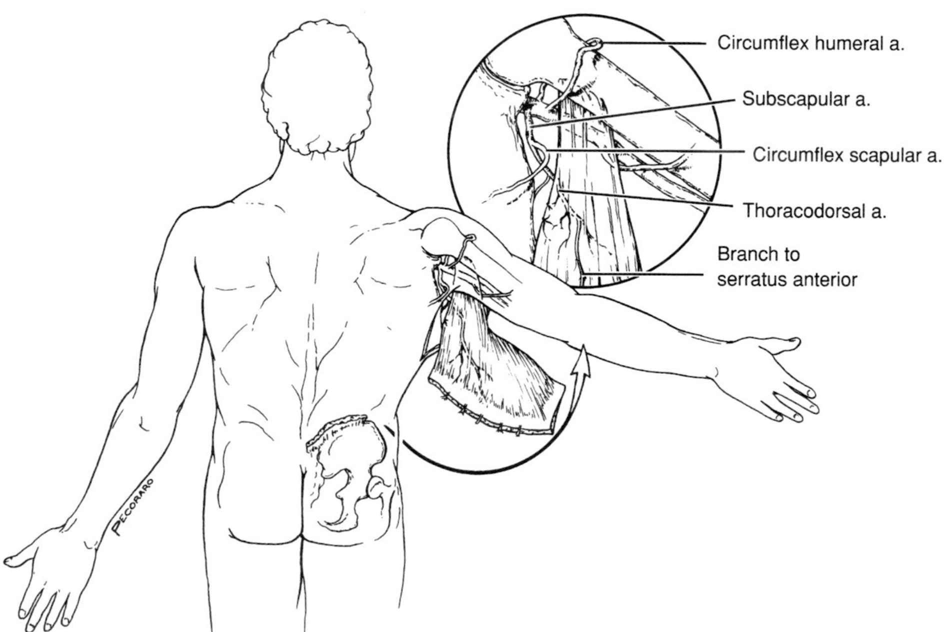

FIGURE 7-12. Arc of rotation and arterial pedicle anatomy of the latissimus dorsi muscle flap.

based on the thoracodorsal system will allow coverage of the shoulder,[147,771] axilla,[5] or upper arm to the level of the elbow (Fig. 7-13).[2,518,751] When based on the medial perforators, the muscle will afford coverage of the middle and lower back.[67,772] Because the thoracodorsal nerve enters the muscle with the primary vascular pedicle, the muscle has found application as a pedicled transfer for functional reconstruction of the deltoid,[414] biceps,[127,381,686,771] and finger flexor muscles[498] by means of rotation on the pedicle.[470,788] The thoracodorsal vessel and nerve split once they enter the muscle in the majority of patients, which allows division of the muscle down its long axis. This tech-

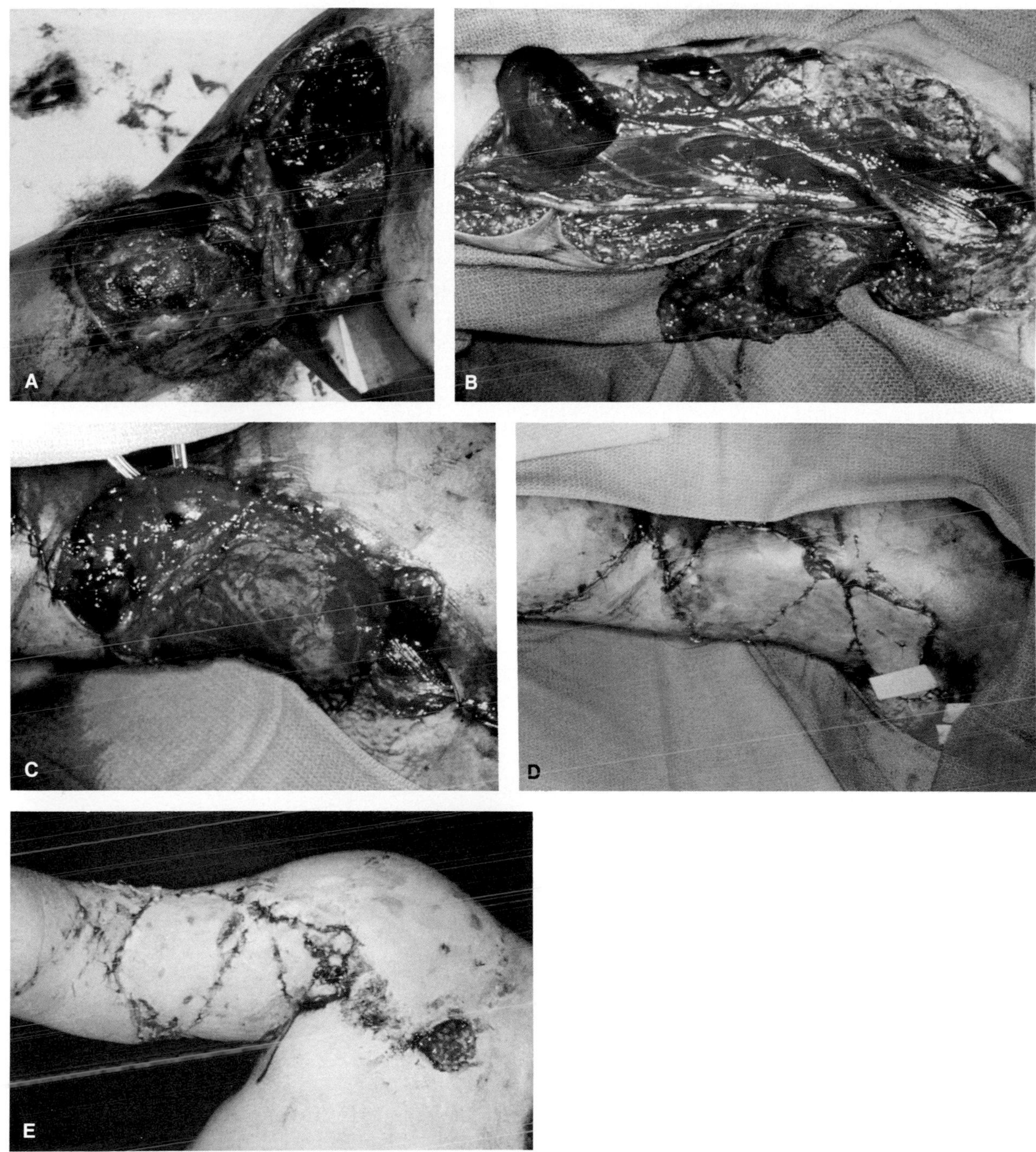

FIGURE 7-13. (**A**) A severe crush injury to the right axilla and upper arm after a fall into a rock crusher. The arm was devascularized and the biceps completely avulsed. (**B**) After debridement and vein grafting with the latissimus dorsi raised as a rotational flap. (**C**) Transposition of the flap for coverage of the defect. (**D**) Immediate application of split-thickness skin graft. (**E**) The wound at 3 weeks.

nique is useful for covering smaller defects in the arm or shoulder and leaves a functional portion of latissimus dorsi intact.

Authors' Preferred Technique of Latissimus Dorsi Elevation

The patient is placed in the lateral decubitus position and the arm is prepped into the surgical field. We prefer to have the arm free so that the shoulder can be moved during the dissection to improve visualization of the pedicle proximally. In no case should the arm be abducted during the entire operative procedure; we have seen postoperative cases of global brachial plexus palsy from this positioning. Placement of the arm in an abducted position causes pressure on the superior portion of the brachial plexus against the clavicle.[494] The muscle is approached through an incision at about the level of the anterior edge of the muscle, with a zigzag as it crosses the posterior aspect of the axilla. After the skin is elevated off the muscle, the anterior border of the muscle is elevated off the chest. At the lower anterior muscular insertion, the latissimus dorsi may be interdigitated with the serratus anterior, and care should be taken to avoid elevation of this muscle as well. Once the anterior border is sharply elevated, the pedicle can easily be identified as it enters the proximal third of the muscle. Once the pedicle is visualized, the undersurface of the muscle is freed from the chest wall. A number of large secondary perforators will be found entering the muscle near its medial origin, and these should be divided between ligatures or surgical clips. The dissection of the undersurface proceeds quickly, because this is a natural gliding plane. The distal portion of the muscle at its origin is dissected sharply and, depending on the size or length requirements, is divided. One must remember that the distal fascial portion of the latissimus dorsi may not have adequate vascularity for support of overlying skin or a skin graft, but this distal portion can be taken in functional reconstructions to aid in attachment to distal tendons.

After the muscle has been elevated off the chest, the pedicle is dissected. This should be done with loupe magnification to avoid damaging the vessels and nerve. A large branch to the serratus is present in nearly all patients, and this is divided between ligatures or clips. As the dissection proceeds proximally, the circumflex scapular vessels will be encountered 8 to 9 cm from the muscular insertion of the vessels.[693] These are likewise divided, which allows another 2 to 3 cm in pedicle length to be obtained. We usually leave the tendon attached during pedicle dissection to avoid too much traction on the vessels.

Once the pedicle has been dissected, the muscle can be rotated to cover the shoulder or arm or the pedicle and tendon can be divided to allow free transfer of the muscle. The reader is referred to more detailed descriptions of actual reconstructions as the technique varies with the reconstructive requirements.[2,5,127,147,381,414,470,518,686,751,771] The back wound is closed over several large suction drains, which should be left in for 4 to 5 days in most cases, or at least until the patient is moving about, because seromas are relatively common in this large donor site.

Rectus Abdominis

The rectus abdominis muscle is another versatile muscular unit for reconstruction of the extremities. It is classified as a type III muscle with two dominant pedicles: the superior epigastric system and deep inferior epigastric system.[518] The entire skin overlying the muscle can be raised with it, and transverse or oblique skin extensions can be safely taken to increase the bulk or coverage area of the muscle.[572] It is segmentally innervated by means of distal intercostal nerves, and thus cannot be transferred as a functional muscle. Its dominant pedicle is the deep inferior epigastric artery for most purposes of this discussion, although the muscle can be pedicled superiorly on the superior epigastric arteries. This technique has been proposed for coverage of difficult hand and arm wounds, where the rectus abdominis is pedicled to the arm and later divided.[299,660] Based on the inferior arterial supply, the pedicled rectus abdominis will easily reach the groin, anterior hip, and pelvic regions.[594,657,849] Further dissection or creation of tunnels in and around the pelvis allows coverage of the lateral hip, inferior and posterior pelvis, and lower back.[52,363,568,645] This muscle has also found application in the treatment of osteomyelitis of the hip.[408,424]

The rectus abdominus also has ideal characteristics for free muscle transfer and has become the muscle of choice by some surgeons for reconstruction of extremity wounds.[657,882] It has the advantage over the latissimus dorsi in that it can be harvested with the patient in the supine position. Although most microsurgeons would consider prior lower abdominal surgery a contraindication to its use (owing to potential damage to the inferior epigastric vessels), the rectus abdominis has been transferred as a free flap based on the superior system.[107] It has been used in both the upper extremity[232,660,904] and lower extremity for free flap reconstructions.[594,657,672,882] It can be taken in combination with a free vascularized iliac crest graft for bone and soft-tissue reconstruction of the lower extremity as well.[454] If care is taken in closure of the donor site, minimal morbidity can be expected,[594,657] although herniation has been reported if dehiscence of the anterior rectus sheath fascia occurs.[328]

Rectus Femoris

The rectus femoris muscle has found application for reconstruction of many wounds around the thigh and pelvic region.[522] This muscle is categorized as type I based on its single dominant vascular pedicle from the lateral circumflex femoral artery.[518] The neurovascular pedicle enters the muscle in its superior third and is reliably present.[14] It has the widest arc of motion of any muscle in the thigh and is thus very useful in coverage of wounds in this region.[649] Although not offering much bulk, the muscle has been found to be very useful in providing vascularized tissue to fill the dead space left after removal of a failed total hip arthroplasty.[20,553,642] If more tissue is required, the rectus femoris muscle can be used in combination with other local muscles.[718] Although it has good characteristics for potential microvascular transfer both for coverage and functional reconstruction, its application in this area has been limited.[726] The relatively limited use of this muscle for free transfer may be related to potential donor site morbidity from loss of knee extension. We have found that suturing the vastus medialis and lateralis together in the area just above the knee after harvest of the rectus femoris minimizes functional morbidity, which has been confirmed by postoperative dynamic testing.[113]

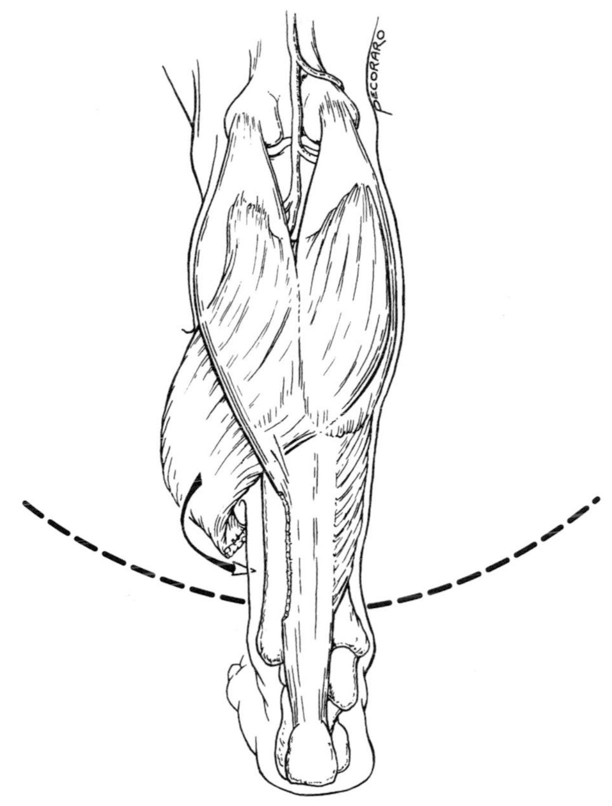

FIGURE 7-14. Arc of rotation of the soleus muscle for coverage of defects of the middle third of the tibia.

Soleus

The soleus was one of the first muscles used for extremity reconstruction,[770] and its usefulness was proven in cases of pretibial skin loss and chronic ulceration by Ger.[253,254] He later expanded the use of the soleus to reconstruct cases of open fracture[255] and improve the treatment of osteomyelitis.[256,258,259] Based on his experience, he was also the first to suggest specific muscle transposition for wounds of the tibia based on location of the defect, dividing the tibia into proximal, middle, and distal thirds.[256] The soleus is classified as a type II muscle, having dominant pedicles based on muscular branches of the popliteal vessels, posterior tibial vessels, and peroneal vessels.[518] The posterior tibial artery supplies several minor pedicles as it runs deep to the medial surface of the muscle. The entire muscle can be safely rotated as a pedicle flap on either of its primary proximal pedicles (popliteal or peroneal) and can be split longitudinally into medial and lateral halves up to the insertion of the pedicle.[324] As it lies deep to the gastrocnemius muscle, it cannot be rotated with a skin paddle. The soleus is the primary local muscle used for coverage of defects in the middle third of the tibia (Fig. 7-14).[98,450,523,528,648,844]

The muscle can be lengthened somewhat and *may* cover some distal third injuries by making transverse cuts in the fascia and epimysium,[897] but one must be careful to avoid damage to the underlying vessels. The use of the soleus as a distally based flap for coverage of the distal tibia and ankle has been reported,[219,820] but the vascular supply based solely on leaving a muscular connection is not always reliable.[30,593] The use of the soleus as a distally based island flap on the posterior tibial vessels has also been described,[320] but this technique requires division of the posterior tibial artery proximally, which is probably not wise in trauma patients. The entire soleus has not been used for microvascular transfer, primarily because of the severe donor morbidity due to the need for transfer of a portion of the popliteal vessels to ensure viability. A portion of the soleus can be transferred by microsurgery in cases of complex reconstruction where the lateral portion of the muscle is taken along with a portion of the fibula, both based on peroneal perforators.[47,137]

Gastrocnemius

This muscle, which lies just superficial to the soleus, has also found wide application in lower extremity coverage.[21,36,187,301,543,710] It is classified as a type I muscle based on its single dominant pedicle, the sural artery and vein. The anatomy of the circulation to this muscle allows use of either one of the heads separately, because the sural vessels divide and vascularize the medial and lateral heads individually.[523] The arc of rotation of the gastrocnemius allows coverage of defects over the proximal third of the tibia[187,255,543] and the entire knee (Fig. 7-15).[36,298,656] The medial head of the muscle will reach the anterior knee better in most patients,[220] because the lateral head must come around the proximal fibula to reach the knee, and this decreases the effective length of the muscle. The overlying skin is reliably vascularized by the gastrocnemius, and the soft tissue available for coverage can be effectively lengthened by using a fasciocutaneous skin extension distally.[132] The reach of the medial or lateral heads can be increased by dividing the proximal muscle and tendon and making it an island pedicle flap on the sural vessels (Fig. 7-16).[457] With bony defects of the proximal tibia, the muscle can actually be placed within the tibial plateau to provide well-vascularized tissue to close the dead space.[579]

The gastrocnemius has become the workhorse in soft-tissue reconstruction around the knee. It is the flap of choice for reconstruction of the popliteal fossa, whether for trauma or scar contracture.[212,585] It has also found particular applicability for repair of soft-tissue defects associated with total knee replacement.[260,368,716] If wound breakdown occurs after prosthetic replacement of the knee, early coverage with the gastrocnemius may salvage the prosthesis.[294,298,644,704] It is widely used after bone and soft-tissue sarcoma resection around the knee and proximal tibia as well.[8,501,504] In a technical variation, the muscle can be divided at its origin, and based on its proximal vascular supply, advanced to cover distal defects[132,491,707] and to reconstruct the Achilles' tendon.[418] The gastrocnemius has been used as a muscular cross-leg flap in severe injuries of the contralateral leg.[244] Like the soleus, distally based flaps of gastrocnemius have been reported for reconstruction of more distal soft-tissue loss.[41,86] This modification has not been widely used, owing to the high potential for loss of this pedicled muscle and the success of free tissue transfer to this area. One report has proposed using a pedicled gastrocnemius flap for reconstruction of the quadriceps apparatus and patellar tendon in anterior knee injuries.[28] This may prove to be another worthwhile application for the gastrocnemius.

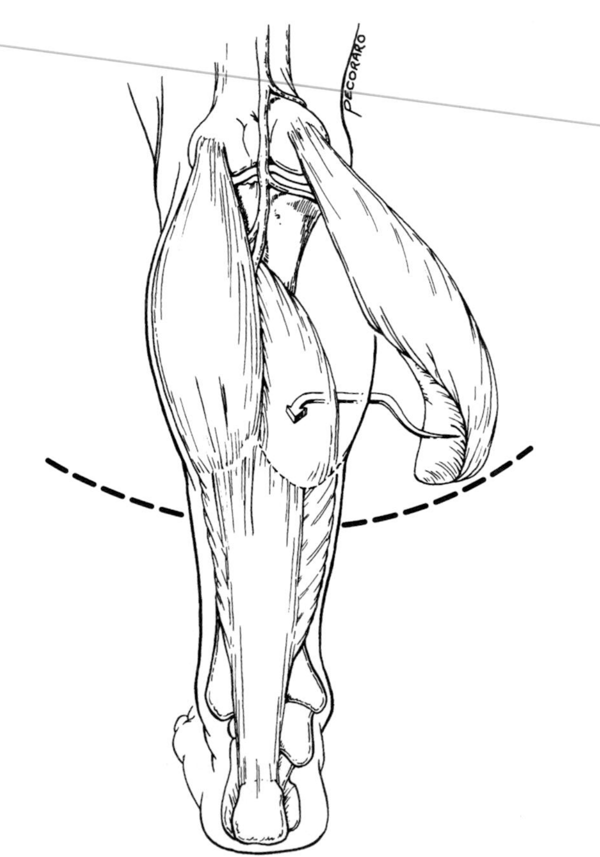

FIGURE 7-15. Arc of rotation of the gastrocnemius muscle for coverage of defects of the proximal tibia and knee.

The vascular anatomy of the gastrocnemius makes it potentially valuable as a free microsurgical transfer, although applications have been few. With the use of vein grafts placed microsurgically to "lengthen" the sural pedicle, the gastrocnemius has been used for coverage of the distal leg.[708] Another group has reported transfer of the muscle based distally and augmentation of the circulation with an arterial microanastomosis.[126] The gastrocnemius has also been transferred to the arm as a functional muscle for the reconstruction of Volkmann's contracture.[493] Although these reports show the potential microsurgical versatility of the gastrocnemius, its primary value lies in reliable pedicled muscle coverage about the knee.

Authors' Preferred Technique of Soleus or Gastrocnemius Transfer

The appropriate choice of one of these muscles to use for transfer is based on the area of coverage required, which is discussed elsewhere. Dissection of these muscles is always done with a proximal tourniquet inflated, and we generally approach the calf muscles with a straight medial or lateral incision. If the gastrocnemius is to be rotated pedicled only on its vascular structures, a straight posterior incision can be useful. A skin paddle may be taken over the gastrocnemius, but usually the flap is lifted without skin. The skin in these cases is sharply dissected off the gastrocnemius. The space between the gastrocnemius and soleus can usually be dissected with blunt finger dissection because there are no major vascular structures in this interval. In the case of harvest of either muscle, the distal insertion into the conjoined Achilles' tendon must be sharply divided. Care must be taken to not divide the tendon entirely during division of the distal muscle chosen.

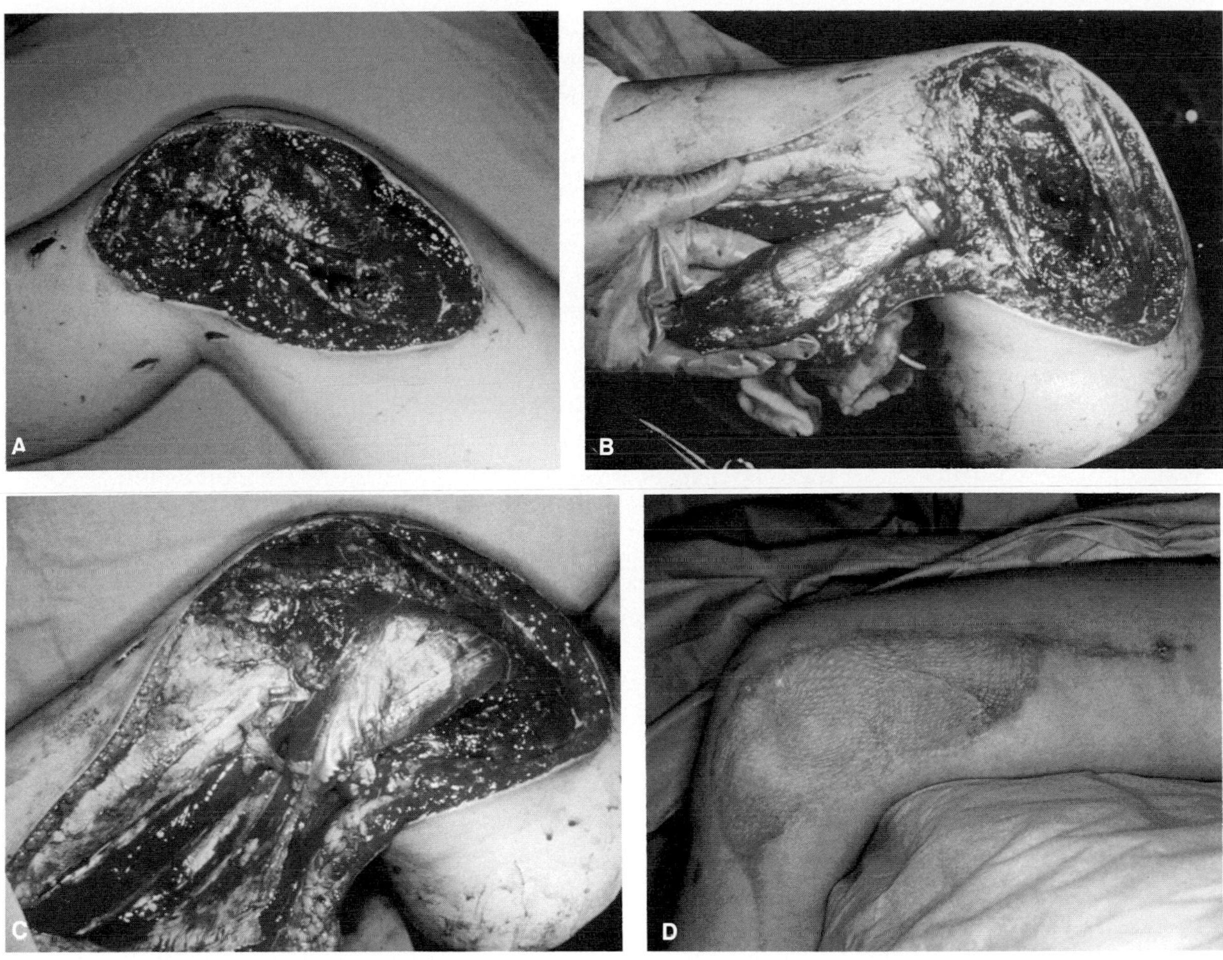

FIGURE 7-16. (**A**) The knee joint of a 16-year-old girl with a segmental femur fracture at the midshaft and supracondylar levels. The joint was exposed and was treated elsewhere by tight closure of the lateral capsule and extensor mechanism. This tight closure resulted in lateral subluxation of the patella. Coverage of the knee joint and restoration of alignment of the extensor mechanism was planned with intramedullary nailing of the segmental femur fracture. (**B**) A lateral gastrocnemius rotation flap was developed, the tendon and epimysium were removed, and the origin divided to allow a better arc of rotation. When the wound was debrided, the defect in the lateral joint capsule could be appreciated. (**C**) The defect is well covered by the muscle flap. (**D**) Final appearance of the wound following split-thickness skin grafting.

In the case of the gastrocnemius, one head may be left attached at this tendon and the muscle split longitudinally. This must be done sharply with scissors or knife, and a few interconnecting vessels may be encountered between the heads. The sural nerve should be left intact if at all possible; it passes from laterally over the distal gastrocnemius to lie between the heads near the knee. The split is continued proximally until enough muscle to cover the soft-tissue defect has been dissected free. The skin incision may need to be carried in an "S" fashion posteriorly into the area of the popliteal fossa for more proximal dissection of the gastrocnemius and pedicle. If the muscle will not reach the defect with its origin intact, this can be divided, but only after identifying the sural pedicle entering the deep surface of the muscle at about the level of the joint. The gastrocnemius is elevated off the soleus, and the pedicle is sought with careful sharp and blunt dissection, entering the muscle in the popliteal fossa. Once identified, the proximal muscle can be divided with the pedicle protected. If the motor nerve can be identified running in the pedicle it should be divided, because this will help avoid the muscle pulling loose from the recipient bed.[656] The gastrocnemius should then easily reach most parts of the knee without difficulty. If the muscle appears to be too bulky, it can be trimmed superficially to improve its aesthetic appearance without damage to its vascularity.[458]

The soleus muscle, on the other hand, is usually left attached at its origin. It is generally raised from the medial aspect of the calf and rotated over the tibia. As noted earlier with the gastrocnemius, the fibula decreases the arc of anterior rotation if the soleus is raised from the lateral aspect of the leg. After the muscle is divided from the common distal tendon, dissection proceeds proximally on the deep surface. The posterior tibial vessels and nerve must be protected and left on the posterior surface of the flexor hallucis and flexor digitorum muscles and not elevated with the soleus. A number of perforators from this vascular pedicle will be encountered as the soleus is elevated and must be carefully divided between ligatures of vascular clips to avoid damage to the posterior tibial vessels. The lateral aspect of the soleus must be sharply divided from its fibular attachments, and this is usually done with the electrocautery. For most applications, the proximal pedicles will not be directly visualized, because the bulk of the soleus can reach across the tibia without very proximal dissection. Caution is advised if one proceeds with proximal muscle dissection, because a number of perforators may be encountered and the vascularity of the muscle can be compromised if these are damaged.

The tourniquet should be let down before final insetting of the muscle to judge vascularity, particularly of the distal end of the muscle transferred. If the muscle fails to "pink up" after 10 or 15 minutes, the very distal portion should be debrided and the quality of bleeding assessed. If the proximal portion of the muscle has a healthy color, the distal end will *usually* be viable. Problems in vascularity of the entire muscle can occur in cases of high-energy trauma to the leg, in which case damage to the muscle may compromise more distal portions when it is rotated as a flap. Closed suction drains are always left in place to decrease the dead space from muscle rotation and the access incisions closed primarily. The muscles are usually covered with split-thickness skin grafts, which we prefer to do at the time of muscle transfer.

Cutaneous Flaps

Scapular Flap

The potential for a skin flap to be raised from the area of the scapula was first recognized by Dos Santos from Brazil in 1980.[193,194] Appreciation of its value both as a pedicled flap for coverage of the proximal upper extremity and as a microvascular transfer soon followed.[40,265,331,539,837] Its vascular basis is the cutaneous branch of the circumflex scapular artery, which provides excellent perfusion to nearly half of the skin of the upper back.[812] This vessel enters the parascapular skin after traversing the *triangular* space between the teres major, teres minor, and long head of the triceps just lateral to the border of the scapula.[247] Before exiting this space, it gives branches to the lateral border of the scapula. It then forms a rich plexus in the fascia that supplies the overlying skin. Flaps based on this pedicle can be designed either vertically,[415] transversely,[40,43] or obliquely down the back (the "parascapular" flap).[331,453,592] The pedicle is reliably present, and with dissection down to the subscapular system can be lengthened to about 6 cm.[837] This pedicle will support the transfer of a large flap of skin in the range of at least 12 × 24 cm,[331] and reports have shown that the entire skin of the upper back can be used as a free transfer if both circumflex scapular systems are used for revascularization.[43]

When rotated locally, the pedicled scapular cutaneous flap will easily reach the axilla, making it useful for coverage and release of contractures.[189,511,808,809] We have found that it will also reliably cover the superior aspect of the shoulder, and others[275] have used it for soft-tissue reconstruction of the posterior neck.[275] Studies have shown that the skin paddle of transverse flaps can be taken across the midline safely to provide more skin.[812] The territories of the scapular and parascapular flaps can be combined to provide very large pieces of tissue for transfer, although the donor site usually requires skin grafting.[453]

The vascular anatomy of the scapular flap makes it ideal for free flap transfer, and thus it has become one of the flaps of choice for cutaneous coverage of the extremities.[267] Smaller flaps raised on the circumflex scapular system have been used for reconstruction of the hand[633] and foot.[669] Larger flaps like those just described are very useful in coverage of lower extremity defects such as degloving injuries.[453,774] The cutaneous area of the scapular flap can be expanded even farther with tissue expanders before transfer, which increases the available tissue and may allow primary closure of the donor site.[464]

Because the vascularity enters the skin from the underlying fascia, flaps based only on the fascia have also been reported.[421] This type of flap provides thin tissue for coverage of the hand or foot but must be covered with a skin graft. The vascular anatomy in the triangular space allows inclusion of a portion of the lateral scapula with the skin flap, which can be used for complex defects requiring a relatively small portion of vascularized bone.[173,733] Although the lateral scapula has been used without a skin flap for bony reconstruction of the lower extremity,[9] its size limitations compared with other vascularized bone donor sites relegate it to secondary choice for this application in our practice.

Radial Forearm Flap

The radial forearm flap was first used for hand reconstruction by the Chinese in 1978 and is still referred to as the Chinese flap by many. It was first reported in the English literature in 1982,[120,587,763] and since that time it has become one of the workhorses in reconstruction of the upper extremity. For quality coverage of hand and forearm wounds, this flap has little competition. Because the radial forearm flap is a skin flap that receives its vascularity from septal perforators of the radial artery and venae comitantes that arborize in the deep fascia of the forearm, it is a *septocutaneous* flap. Due to the supply of the radial artery to various tissues of the forearm, many different types of composite flaps can be raised for reconstruction of difficult defects. Nearly the entire skin of the forearm can be elevated with the radial artery, along with segments of the palmaris longus tendon,[764] radius,[155] lateral antebrachial cutaneous nerve,[329] and muscle.[276,330] Because of the wide variety of tissue available, this flap has been called a "reconstructive chameleon."[596]

The flap can be designed proximally based on a distal reverse-flow vascular pedicle for coverage of the hand, which was the initial description of the flap. Although reverse flow through the radial artery is understandable if the patient has an intact arch, the ability for venous blood to flow backward through the venae comitantes has been the cause of much discussion.[114,283,442,490,773,813,860] Most authors now believe that the ability for this to occur is due to the dual nature of the venae comitantes, which have many interconnections as they wrap around the radial artery. These interconnections allow the venous blood to bypass the valves, thus effectively reversing the flow in the veins. Others believe that elevation of the pedicle denervates it, which renders the valves incompetent under the effects of increased back-pressure.

Regardless of the physiology that allows for reverse flow in the veins, the distally based pedicled radial forearm flap provides excellent, reliable coverage of many hand defects (Fig. 7-17).[49,114,287,530,764] It is particularly useful for dorsal hand defects and can be taken with a small portion of the radius and palmaris longus tendon for reconstruction of complex dorsal injuries. It is also one of the best options for covering the first web space after release of contractures. The fascia alone can be raised with the radial vascular pedicle and covered with a skin graft, which decreases the cosmetic deformity on the forearm but supplies excellent vascularized fascia for coverage.[92,133] This fascia also has utility for decreasing scar adhesion after flexor tenolysis, in that a reversed fascial flap can be "tubed" around the flexor tendons at the wrist after tenolysis in the face of severe scarring.[759] Coverage of the elbow can be accomplished by basing the pedicle of the flap on the proximal radial artery, and this technique has been used for reconstruction of difficult wounds in this area.[554,711] Using the pedicled radial forearm flap for such defects has the advantages of not requiring microsurgical expertise and of avoiding the morbidity of pedicled flaps from the torso.

Because of the large vascular pedicle provided by the radial vessels, this flap has also found wide application in microsurgical transfer. It is useful for transfer to the opposite hand for coverage[287,764] and can in fact be used for both repair of soft-tissue defects and revascularization of the distal extremity by anastomosis of both ends of the radial artery.[157] Because this flap provides very thin skin, it is also a very good choice for free flap reconstruction of defects around the ankle,[827] posterior heel/Achilles region,[853] and foot.[329] When used as a free flap, it is generally taken based on the proximal vascular pedicle, but it can be based on the distal pedicle.[49,643] The distally based free flap is bothersome to most reconstructive microsurgeons, because the potential for poor flow through the reversed veins might lead to anastomotic thrombosis.[773]

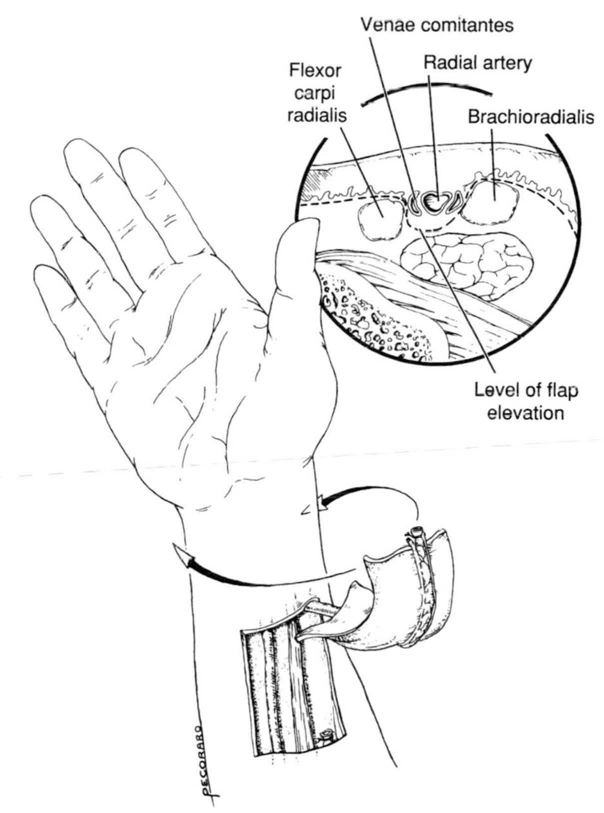

FIGURE 7-17. Vascular anatomy and arc of rotation of the distally based radial forearm flap.

Notwithstanding the exceptional qualities that this flap possesses for soft-tissue and complex reconstructions, it remains somewhat controversial because of two problems: (1) a major limb artery must be sacrificed to use the flap and (2) the donor site can be cosmetically unsightly.[814] Obviously, one must perform an Allen's test before raising a radial forearm flap and sacrificing the radial artery.[199] In our experience, there are very few patients in whom this flap cannot be used, although cases of acute hand ischemia after radial forearm flap elevation have been reported.[423] This problem can be avoided by careful preoperative examination of the patient by Allen's testing and acoustical Doppler examination, which is our routine. Early on in our experience with this flap we routinely reconstructed the radial artery with a vein graft, but we have not done so in the past 5 years without any adverse sequelae, an experience borne out by other authors.[35]

Concern has also been raised about the long-term effect on the hand of loss of the vascular contribution of the radial artery. Although studies have documented an increased warming time (on cold stress testing) in the radial digits of patients' hands after radial forearm flap transfer, these same patients have generally been clinically asymptomatic in this regard.[448,555] Recently, modification in the technique of harvest of this flap to include only distal fascial perforators has been proposed to avoid the necessity of including the radial artery.[877] Although this adaptation does not allow as wide an arc of rotation as a standard pedicle flap, it may prove useful for coverage of more proximal hand injuries.

In terms of the cosmetic defect, it is generally acceptable with the use of smaller flaps. When large flaps are taken the defect can become unsightly, particularly in women, in whom cosmesis may be more important.[482] The donor site defect can also be problematic if loss of the split-thickness skin graft occurs over the distal flexor tendons, particularly the flexor carpi radialis. Our preference, and that of others, is to use a full-thickness skin graft (taken from the groin) to cover the forearm defect, which obviates many of the aforementioned problems.[250,489,755] Because the lateral antebrachial cutaneous nerve is usually included in the flap, numbness is common, and neuromas have been reported after radial forearm flap harvest,[482,782] but these problems are usually not significant. If bone is harvested from the volar radius, late fractures have been reported. This complication can usually be prevented by avoiding right-angled osteotomies at the ends of the harvest site.[558]

Despite the reported donor site morbidity of the radial forearm flap, it remains one of the flaps of choice for reconstruction of the hand and foot. Most authors believe that the advantages of this flap outweigh the disadvantages, and clinical series report a low incidence of patient complaints secondary to the donor site problems.[63,556]

Groin Flap

The groin flap was one of the first *axial pattern* flaps described,[546,758] and receives its vascularity from the superficial circumflex iliac artery and vein.[344,611,647] This flap was initially reported as a pedicled flap for coverage of the hand and forearm, and later was used for early free flap transfers.[45,170,607,608,739] Before the anatomy and advantages of muscle transfer were understood, this flap was the workhorse for microsurgical extremity reconstruction.[6,84,96,222,249,434,719,734,796] Although application of multiple other free flap donor sites has eclipsed the widespread use of the groin flap, it remains an excellent choice for pedicled coverage of hand injuries.

The groin flap has the advantages of supplying a rather large area of skin for coverage with a (relatively) concealed donor site. All but the very largest flaps allow primary closure of the donor site. As a pedicled flap, it can be used for coverage of large defects of the hand,[340] and it may be combined with other flaps from the torso or thigh if necessary.[437,447] The use of bilateral simultaneous or staged pedicled groin flaps has been reported for degloving injuries of the hand.[365,412] The skin area taken can be further enlarged by either including some of the lower abdominal skin (with the superficial inferior epigastric vessels)[757] or by preexpanding the flap with tissue expanders.[184] A portion of the iliac crest may be taken with a pedicled groin flap, which allows reconstruction of composite hand defects without the need for microsurgery.[4,96,677]

The use of the pedicled groin flap for primary hand coverage has had somewhat of a resurgence in recent years, despite the reliability of free flap coverage.[492] This is primarily due to its minimal donor site morbidity, and the fact that later microsurgical reconstruction (ie, toe transfer) is somewhat easier if no prior microvascular anastomoses have been performed. Many authors still believe that the pedicled groin flap is the primary choice for hand coverage.[38,136,235,303,382] We agree that the groin flap offers superior coverage to that of free flaps in many instances, particularly if delayed microsurgical reconstruction is contemplated. One must be aware of the potential problems with use of this pedicled flap, however.

Care must be taken with the design and insetting of the flap to avoid healing problems.[728] Most favor making the flap longer than necessary to allow tubing of the proximal portion.[136,728] This allows a bit more mobility of the hand and may decrease the risk of inadvertent detachment from the hand. Others have proposed attaching the wrist to the iliac crest with an external fixator to avoid pulling the flap loose,[197] but we believe that this is unnecessary. Although the flap can usually be safely divided by 3 weeks, partial necrosis of the flap after division of the pedicle has been reported to be as high as 18%.[896] This may be decreased by performing a *delay* of the base of the flap (ie, partial division of the base) several days to 1 week before final division to allow reorientation of blood supply from the pedicle to the hand.[896] One should probably not inset the flap primarily after division, because the portion nearest the division point may not be viable. Allowing this area to demarcate before final insetting avoids further wound problems. Dissection of the lateral portion of the flap must likewise be done carefully to avoid damage to the lateral femoral cutaneous nerve, which can lead to painful neuroma formation.[584] High complication rates in patients older than the age of 50 have been reported with use of the pedicled groin flap, primarily due to the position required. This positioning can lead to stiffness, pneumonia, and pulmonary embolus in older patients.[17,290]

Although microvascular transfer of the groin flap has lost some of its appeal, it continues to have some indications. When taken based on the deep circumflex iliac system rather than the superficial system, a large portion of vascularized iliac crest and skin can be taken for osseocutaneous reconstructions.[229,278,783,804,805] It has found special application for some difficult reconstructive problems. The skin, iliac crest, and aponeurosis of the tensor fascia lata can be used for reconstruction of complex defects involving the calcaneus and Achilles tendon.[861] Skin taken with the aponeurosis of the external oblique can be used for reconstruction of avulsions of the dorsum of the foot, in which the aponeurosis is used for extensor tendon reconstruction.[420] Some authors continue to prefer this donor site for cutaneous reconstructions, primarily due to the minimal cosmetic donor site deformity.[139,322] The variable vascular anatomy and short pedicle lead to reliability problems with this flap, however, and even those surgeons still using this flap report failure rates with microvascular transfer from 8%[139] to 28%.[322] These loss rates are too high to consider the groin flap a first choice for free transfer in most instances.

MANAGEMENT OF SPECIFIC SOFT-TISSUE PROBLEMS

Upper Extremity

In the upper extremity, except the elbow, wrist, and hand, there is thick muscle coverage over the skeleton. Soft-tissue loss around the humerus, radius, and ulna can usually be managed by standard plastic surgery techniques, using skin grafting or pedicle flaps from the trunk and groin.[699,843] Free tissue transfer is an option for the wrist and hand, as are local fasciocutaneous flaps.

Shoulder and Humerus

Small soft-tissue defects can be managed by standard plastic surgery methods. Large degloving injuries as far distal as the elbow can be managed by a rotation or pedicled latissimus dorsi flap (see Fig. 7-13)[576,751] or scapular flap. The arc of rotation of either flap may be extended by vein grafts,[709] but this requires microvascular expertise. The latissimus dorsi may be used to simultaneously restore elbow flexion or extension and provide soft-tissue coverage.[69,470,909] Other applications for the latissimus dorsi include defects with dead space in the shoulder area from infected prostheses or gunshot wounds (Fig. 7-18).[69] The pectoralis major can also be rotated into this area and has been used to treat sternoclavicular osteomyelitis.[77] Larger defects with extensive damage to the soft tissues of the shoulder may mandate free tissue transfer. This occurs with avulsion injuries and nearly complete amputations, and usually a large flap such as the opposite latissimus dorsi is required. Vascular injury is often seen in such cases, and restoration of arterial flow and coverage may be required. One option in this instance is a fasciocutaneous flap based on the posterior tibial artery, which has been used to provide both soft-tissue coverage and reconstruct a brachial artery defect.[614]

Complex injuries with loss of skin and bone can usually be managed by traditional bone grafts covered with the previously mentioned pedicled flaps. In the case of severe injuries, composite free flaps may be indicated. Short defects can be repaired by vascularized iliac crest transfer (osseocutaneous groin flap),[380] and larger defects with the free fibula osseocutaneous flap.[566,586] Further description of techniques for vascularized bone transfer to the humerus are discussed in the previous section.

Elbow

Loss of the thin skin covering the posterior aspect of the elbow may occur from burns,[711] "sideswipe" injuries,[25,377,750,886] or olecranon bursa infections.[554] Attempts to treat open elbow wounds without flap coverage have not been particularly successful.[176,377] Release of severe elbow flexion contractures may also mandate flap coverage.[563] Small defects can be covered by rotation of the brachioradialis anteriorly or laterally,[463] although this muscle is small and has had reliability problems. The flexor carpi ulnaris may be rotated proximally to cover the olecranon[552] but suffers from the same problems as the brachioradialis. The lateral arm flap can be rotated distally on the recurrent radial artery for elbow coverage,[146,161,479] although we have had problems with reliability of this distally based flap. Most small defects of the elbow can be reliably covered with a pedicled radial forearm flap,[554,711] which is our usual preference.

Free groin flaps,[130,249] free latissimus dorsi muscle,[402] and free scapular flaps[40,331] have all been used for coverage of larger defects of the elbow. A pedicled latissimus dorsi muscle can also cover many large defects and avoids the need for microsurgery (Fig. 7-19). The pedicled latissimus can also be used to simultaneously replace posterior soft-tissue and triceps function,[470] but the distal end can be unreliable and may not afford adequate elbow coverage. Pedicled flaps from the chest[3] and abdomen[224,299,723] have been reported, but we believe that these flaps

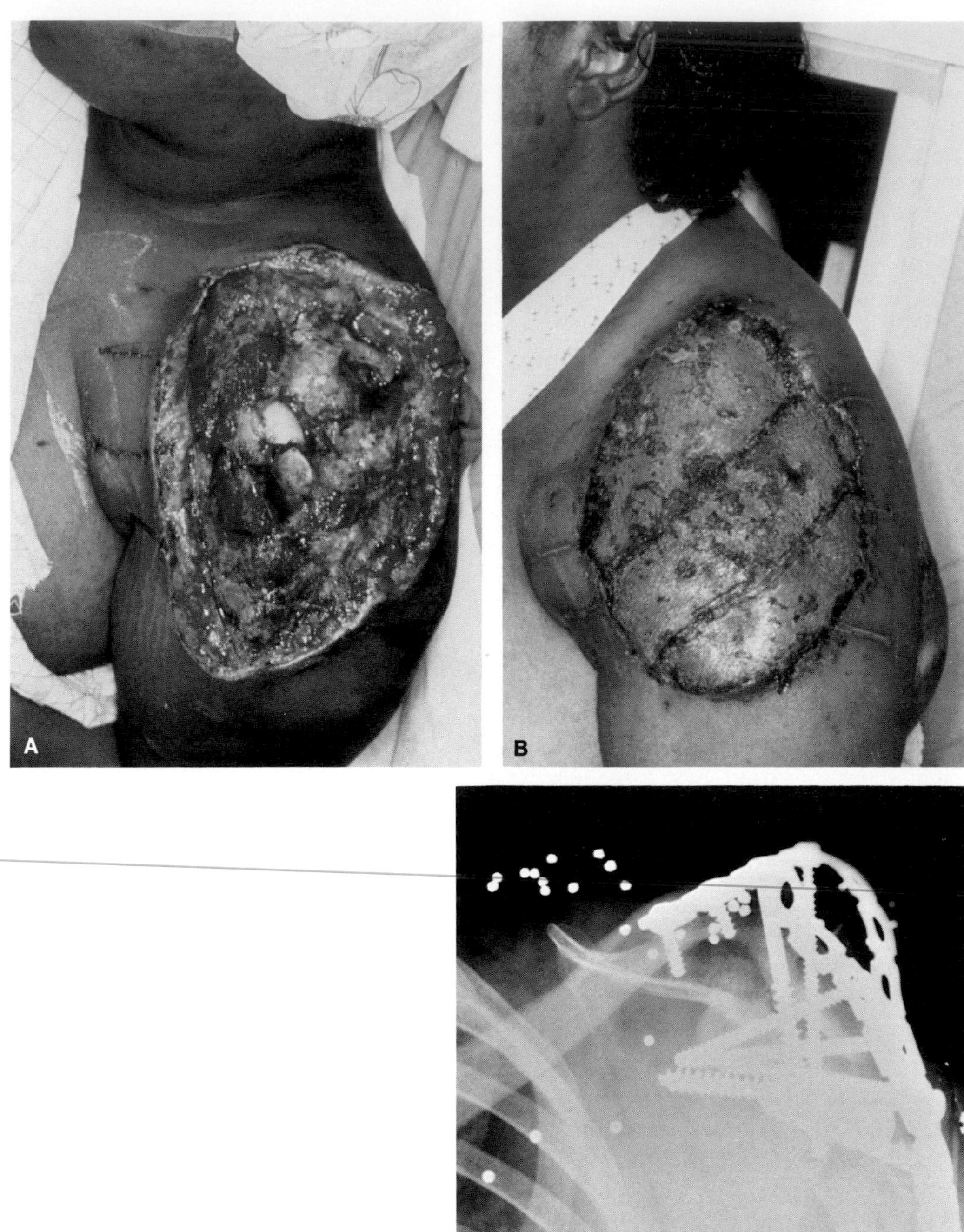

FIGURE 7-18. (**A**) A close-range gunshot wound to the anterior aspect of the left shoulder with destruction of the glenohumeral joint. (**B**) Debridement and closure of the wound by rotational latissimus dorsi muscle flap and split-thickness skin graft coverage. (**C**) Subsequent reconstruction of bone accomplished by scapulohumeral arthrodesis.

lack any advantage over pedicled flaps from the arm or shoulder.

Forearm and Wrist

Most soft-tissue defects in the forearm or wrist are manageable by standard coverage techniques. Exposed muscle in the proximal forearm can be adequately covered by split-thickness skin grafts. The distal forearm, however, is similar anatomically to the lower third of the leg in that tendon, bone, and joint are often exposed and local muscle flaps are not available. Although pedicle flaps from the chest and groin can be used for coverage of the distal arm,[108,138] this type of flap has inherent disadvantages. Local island pedicled fasciocutaneous flaps

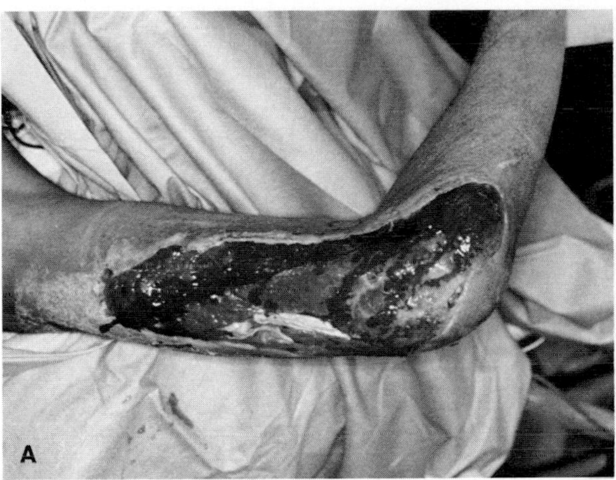

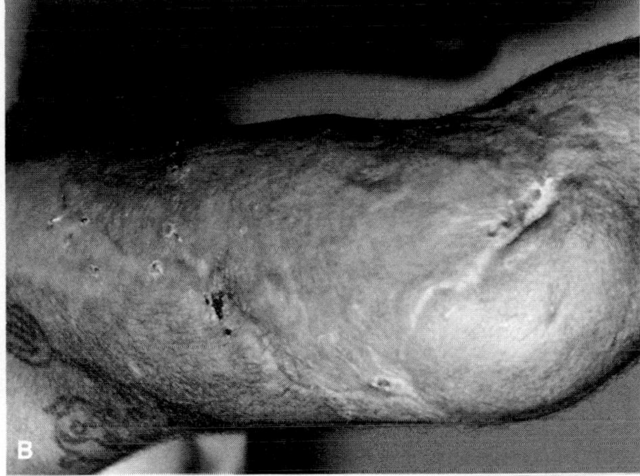

FIGURE 7-19. (**A**) A degloving injury of the posteromedial arm and elbow treated by a large rotational latissimus dorsi flap. (**B**) These flaps will reach below the elbow for coverage.

such as the radial forearm flap have many advantages over flaps from the torso and can cover most defects in this area. We prefer to use the distally pedicled radial forearm flap for management of most smaller wounds of the hand if no vascular compromise is present.

Free flaps offer many advantages for closure of difficult wounds in this area, including

1. Coverage for larger defects
2. Reconstruction of composite bone and soft-tissue defects
3. Ability to elevate the upper extremity, decreasing edema and scarring
4. Earlier motion

Cutaneous free flaps from the shoulder and upper extremity have the advantage that they provide a cosmetic match for the forearm and, if taken from the ipsilateral limb, decrease the overall morbidity to the patient. The scapular free flap is ideal for coverage of larger defects in the forearm,[206] and the underlying soft tissue or fascia may be wrapped around tendons to decrease scar formation and to promote tendon gliding.[40,705] The lateral arm free flap has found wide application for coverage of smaller defects in the forearm and hand[438,439,725,854] and may be harvested from the ipsilateral arm (Fig. 7-20).[724] This flap can be taken with a small portion of the lateral humerus for bony reconstruction[238] and is of use in repair of complex defects of the dorsal hand.[238,438] The radial forearm flap taken as a free flap from the ipsilateral or contralateral limb also offers a good choice in hand reconstruction.[114,287]

Larger defects, or those involving recalcitrant osteomyelitis, may be better managed by free muscle transfer. The latissimus dorsi has been the gold standard for large wound coverage[171,402] and is the flap of choice in severe degloving injuries (Fig. 7-21). Smaller defects can be adequately covered with the rectus abdominus[699,764] or gracilis[348,527] free flaps.

Functional Muscle Transfer

Experimental functional free muscle transfers in dogs were first reported in the early 1970s.[459,791] The first clinical case reported was from China in 1974, where a portion of the pectoralis major was transferred with microneurovascular anastomoses to restore finger flexion.[678] Further experience added applications for functional muscle transfer in the management of Volkmann's ischemic contracture[403,507] and facial paralysis.[349,609] Experimentally, the success rates of functional recovery of muscle fibers in innervated free flaps range from 25%[810] to as high as 60% to 80%[401] and may take from 6 to 24 months to occur.

Functional reconstruction of forearm injuries has been reported with the rectus femoris,[726,727] pectoralis major,[402,403,507,508,510] latissimus dorsi,[498,834] and gracilis.[403,506,507,510] Studies of forearm muscles have emphasized the use of appropriate transfers in terms of size and excursion for functional reconstruction,[73] and therefore the gracilis and latissimus dorsi have become the muscles of choice for functional forearm reconstruction.[641] The transfer of a free innervated muscle should be considered in the case of severe injury to the forearm in which significant loss of extensor or flexor muscles occur. If coverage of such an injury is required, the use of an innervated muscle may decrease the need for later functional reconstruction.[641]

Although injuries to the forearm are the usual indication for functional muscle transfer, this tech-

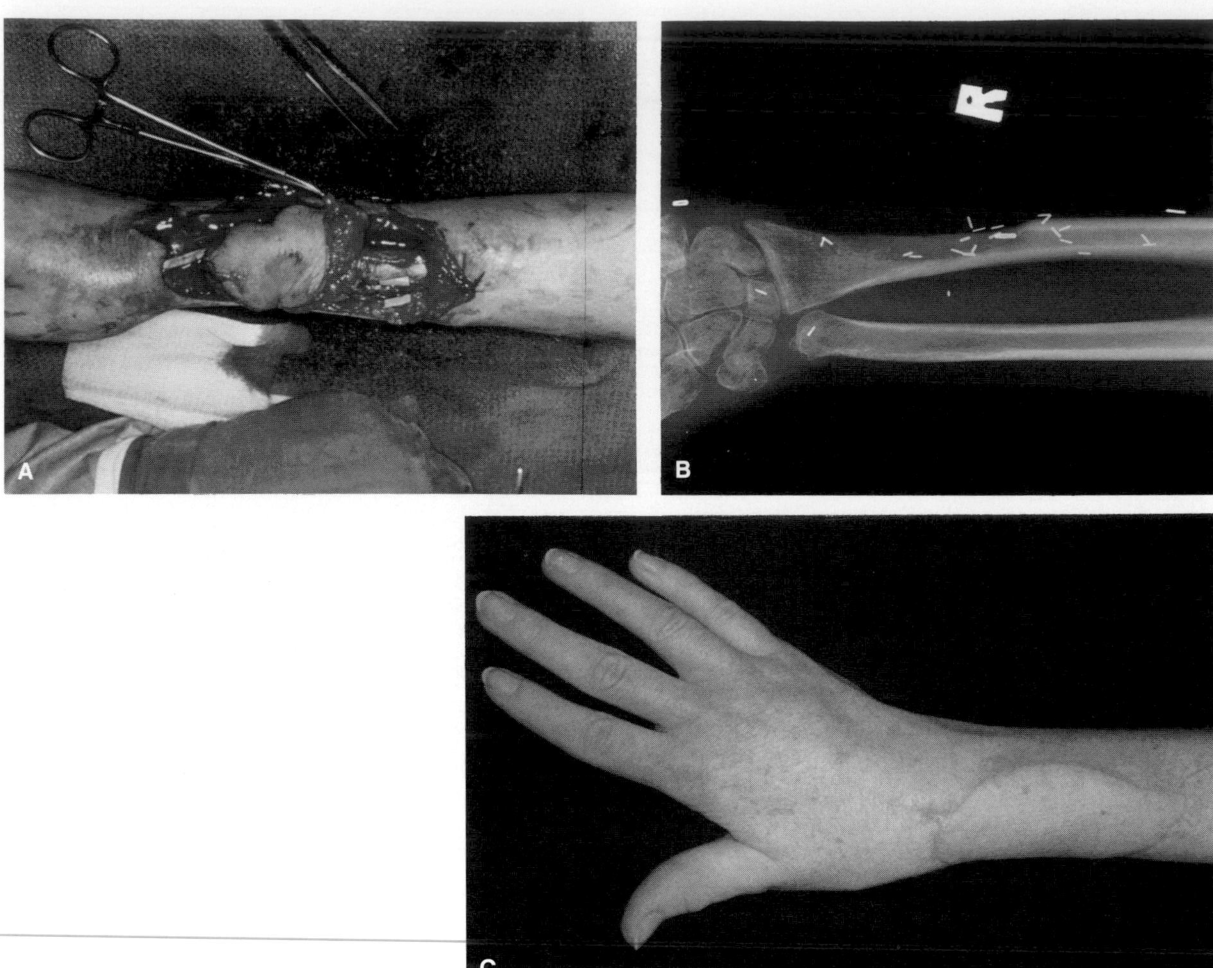

FIGURE 7-20. (**A**) A 55-year-old woman with epithelioid sarcoma of the first dorsal compartment. (**B**) Compartmental resection with 2-cm margins. An x-ray after compartmental resection of the first and second dorsal compartments and saucerization of the radius. (**C**) Healed lateral arm flap, with excellent function.

nique may also have application in the upper arm,[509] in cases of brachial plexus injury,[7] and in certain cases of lower extremity injury (particularly loss of anterior compartment muscles). The particulars of this technique are covered in detail in other texts.[506]

Femur

Wounds of the thigh rarely lead to the need for additional soft-tissue coverage, owing to the large enveloping muscle mass. On occasion, especially in the presence of bone loss or the need for internal fixation, local coverage may be inadequate. In these cases, local muscle rotation flaps from the thigh will almost always suffice for wound management.[227] The primary muscles for this purpose are the rectus femoris, vastus lateralis, and vastus medialis.[20,642] The use of the rectus femoris has been discussed earlier, and its primary use is for coverage of the lateral thigh. The vastus medialis can be based either superiorly or inferiorly on its segmental pedicles and used for anterior coverage of the thigh.[518] This muscle is especially useful if left attached proximally and used for pedicled coverage of the distal anterior thigh.[815] If taken with its distal tendon, the vastus medialis is also useful for coverage and functional reconstruction of knee extension. In this application, a distal portion of the tendon and fascia is taken with the muscle, and this is then attached to the patellar tendon.[22] The vastus lateralis can also be used for anterior reconstruction, but it is primarily indicated for lateral thigh and hip coverage. Although it has been primarily used in paraplegics,[360] reports have shown minimal morbidity if it is used in ambulatory patients.[195] The ipsilateral rectus abdominus muscle will reach the proximal thigh as well and may be the flap of choice in some patients (see p. 7-28). Free flap cov-

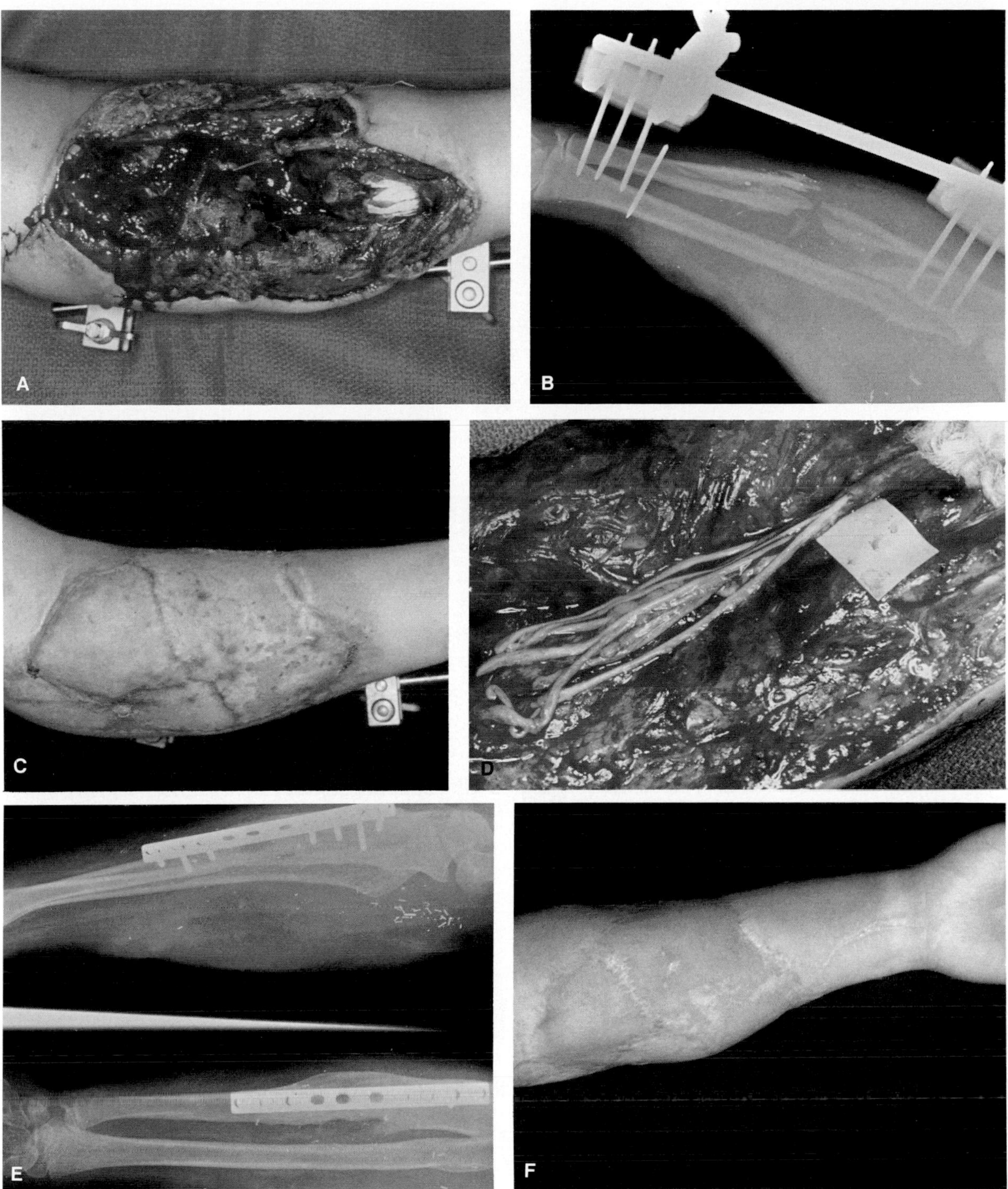

FIGURE 7-21. (**A**) The arm of a 13-year-old boy who suffered a .270-caliber, high-velocity gunshot wound to the forearm resulting in an 8-cm loss of the median nerve. (**B**) Associated segmental fracture of the ulna. (**C**) Coverage by latissimus dorsi free flap and split-thickness skin graft. (**D**) Delayed interfascicular nerve graft of the median nerve 8 weeks later. The patient ultimately regained 6-mm, two-point discrimination. (**E**) The ulnar defect was bone grafted and healed without difficulty. (**F**) The final clinical result; note the atrophy of the flap—no defatting was done.

erage of the femur is rarely indicated, but in the case of severe defects and in instances of bone loss or infection, it may be necessary to afford adequate soft tissue.[642]

Knee

The anterior knee has minimal overlying soft tissue and is frequently involved in trauma. For these reasons, the knee frequently requires some type of flap coverage for wound management. In the case of an exposed joint, treatment by the open technique requires a reasonable soft-tissue envelope.[176] Most knee wounds can be managed by the medial or lateral gastrocnemius muscles as discussed on page 381 (Fig. 7-22).[21,36,37,220,248,294,298,543,656] The vastus lateralis muscle has also been used as a distally pedicled muscle flap for management of wounds around the knee.[786] Interest in the application of fasciocutaneous flaps has led to the development of a number of flaps for use around the knee.[487,583] These flaps can be based on the lateral sural cutaneous vessels,[488] lateral genicular vessels,[362] or posterior popliteal perforators.[512] Knowledge of the vascular anatomy of these (and all) flaps and experience in their elevation is vital to avoid complications, however. For these reasons, we prefer local muscle flaps for knee coverage in most cases. Larger wounds may require free tissue transfer, and the rectus abdominus[239] or latissimus dorsi[666] are the muscles of choice. This type of wound is frequently seen after tumor resection or knee fusion for complex injury. Vascular access can be difficult in this location, espe-

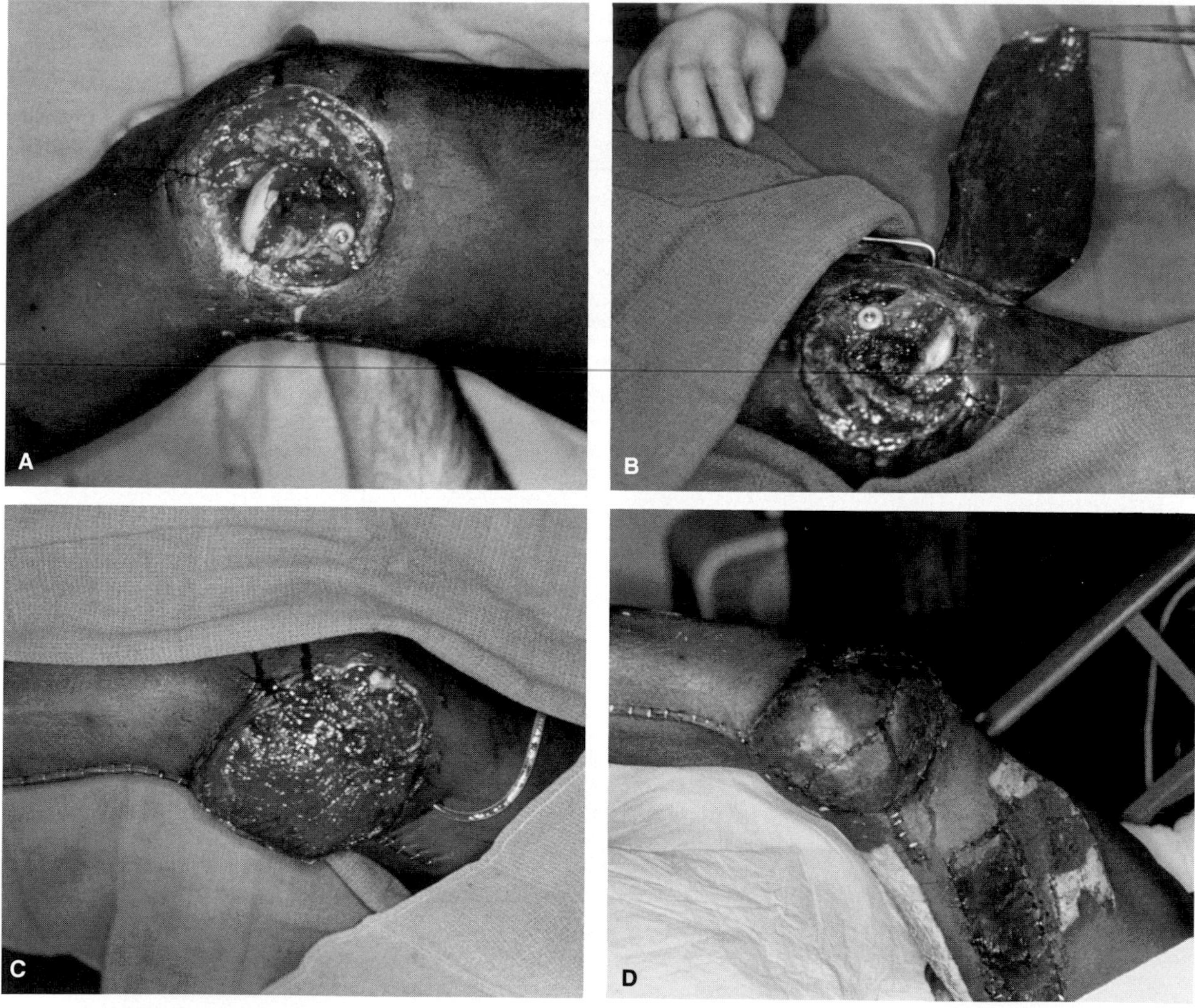

FIGURE 7-22. (**A**) A close-range gunshot wound to the medial aspect of the knee with an open intra-articular fracture of the femoral condyles treated by AO lag-screw fixation. The joint was widely exposed. (**B**) An elevated medial gastrocnemius muscle rotation flap. (**C**) Coverage of the joint was obtained by removal of the deep tendon and epimysium and spreading of the muscle flap. A split-thickness skin graft was then applied. (**D**) Appearance of the flap and split-thickness skin graft coverage 2 weeks postoperatively. The patient had started knee range of motion.

cially after severe trauma or multiple prior procedures,[422] and microsurgical reconstruction should be approached with care.

Tibia

Open fractures of the tibia have long been problematic to the orthopaedic surgeon, with high rates of soft-tissue loss,[83,110,255,355,688,819] bone loss,[417] nonunion,[48,383,692,839] and infection.[259,300,375] Reconstruction of the soft-tissue envelope is paramount to decrease bony complications,[110,839] and muscle flap coverage is considered the gold standard.[24,37,279,475,683,743] For purposes of soft-tissue coverage, the tibia is generally divided into thirds: proximal, middle, and distal.[256] The proximal and middle thirds are usually covered with local muscle rotation flaps, while the distal third is considered territory for free muscle transfer. As with the knee, the proximal tibia is best managed by the gastrocnemius muscle if it is available.[21,220,255,301,543,710] The soleus may reach proximal defects, but its arc of rotation is limited compared with the gastrocnemius. Middle-third tibial defects are the classic indication for the soleus rotation flap (Fig. 7-23).[30,255,387] The tibialis anterior muscle and toe extensor muscles can be used in very small wounds without surrounding soft-tissue damage, but the indications for use of these muscles is very limited.[687] High-energy injuries to the middle third of the tibia will often result in significant injury to the soleus or its vascularity, however, which can limit its reliability.[593] In this situation and in injuries to the distal third of the tibia, microvascular muscle transfer is indicated.[6,89,98,200,302,533,534,737,741] Fasciocutaneous flaps have also been suggested as a solution for many defects of the lower leg.[33,228,467,658,818] The problem with these flaps is that their vascular supply is often in the area of wounding, and they have reported complication rates of up to 71% in the management of post-traumatic wounds.[188] Early application of these flaps, before the onset of infection, and raising them as "bipedicled" flaps may improve their relative reliability.[188,327] Reports emphasize the reliability and value of small (~6 × 5 cm) fasciocutaneous flaps based on the medial or lateral midcalf for anterior tibial coverage.[364]

Free flap coverage of the tibia has evolved from one of "salvage" to the procedure of first choice in compound distal injuries. Early series of free flaps to the lower leg had high failure rates owing to the timing of transfer and a generally poor understanding of the pathophysiology of complex musculoskeletal injury.[249,347,737] Although the groin flap was used first, it

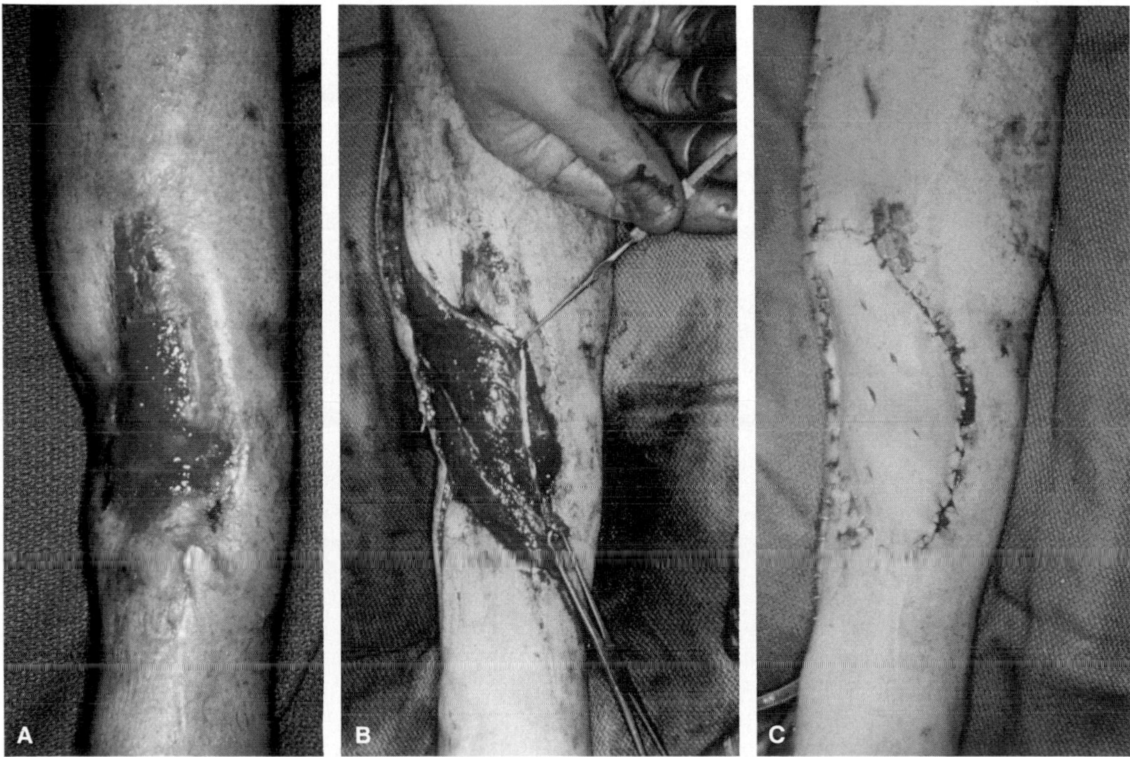

FIGURE 7-23. (**A**) Open fracture of the tibia with a relatively small soft-tissue defect in the middle third. Attempts at healing by granulation had this result at 8 weeks. (**B**) A soleus rotation flap was used to cover the wound. (**C**) Appearance of the flap after split-thickness skin grafting. The wound healed uneventfully without further drainage.

has been largely replaced by muscle flaps and other more reliable free skin flaps. Wounds with minimal contamination that are covered early can be safely managed with free skin flaps.[239,827,837,911] The omentum has also been used for coverage of open tibial fractures,[19,27,343,411,612,613] and while it offers excellent ability to revascularize the surrounding tissue, this flap suffers from the necessity to perform an intra-abdominal procedure (with attendant morbidity). Most authors prefer muscle, however, for its ability to resist infection,[119] deliver antibiotics,[695] and revascularize bone.[683] Although any of a number of muscles are suitable for microvascular transfer, the latissimus dorsi[98,239,533,534,737,741,743] and rectus abdominis[89,657,671,882] are the primary muscles used for tibial coverage (Fig. 7-24). Myocutaneous flaps were used early on,[473] but most reconstructive surgeons prefer to use a free muscle flap covered with split-thickness skin grafts because the latter are less bulky and contour to the leg better.[277,538] Free muscle flaps are also preferred for late reconstruction and in the management of osteomyelitis.[13,24,76,279,409,410,519,521,873,876,890]

In certain rare instances, cross-leg flaps may still be indicated in the management of soft-tissue defects of the tibia. These cases are primarily those of soft-tissue loss combined with significant vascular injury that would make free tissue transfer potentially dangerous to the distal limb (due to the need for vascular anastomosis to the remaining vessel).[11] These flaps have much less morbidity from positioning in younger patients and are still advocated by some for treatment of tibial defects in children.[384,395] They may also be indicated after failure of free tissue transfer to provide adequate coverage.[34] In these instances, use of a cross-leg muscle flap such as the gastrocnemius is probably more appropriate than skin flaps.[243,244,618] Another adaptation of the cross-leg flap is the cross-leg free flap. This technique is applicable in patients who have poor or inadequate vascularity in the area of the wound to support free tissue transfer. Vascular anastomoses are performed to the contralateral leg at the level of injury and the flap is placed across to the injured leg.[75,742,833] The pedicle can usually be safely divided by 3 to 4 weeks with survival of the flap over the wound.

Subsequent Operations Beneath a Flap

In terms of free tissue transfer to the tibia, the question of the long-term necessity of the vascular pedicle has often been raised.[59] This is an important factor in considerations of later elevation of the flap for bone grafting, which is frequently necessary to complete lower leg reconstruction.[24,279,743] Any transferred flap will gain new vascularity from the surrounding soft-tissue bed, which is the basis for distant pedicle flap coverage (ie, groin flap or cross-leg flap). Free flaps are no exception to this physiologic rule and will generally receive a certain amount of vascularity from the soft-tissue margins of the wound.[738] Although reports have documented the survival of free flaps placed into soft-tissue beds after division of the pedicle as early as 10 days,[443] loss of a muscle flap placed over the tibia at 7 months, owing to trauma to the pedicle, has been documented as well.[226] Studies from Scandinavia on patients after free flap transfer to the tibia have documented significant decreases in flap blood flow at up to 48 months postoperatively with compression of the vascular pedicle.[455,456]

Although secondary elevation of free flaps placed over the tibia for bone grafting is considered routine, certain guidelines should be followed. The surgeon elevating the flap should be aware of the position of the vascular pedicle and elevate the margin of the flap most distal to the pedicle. The plane of dissection should be deep to the flap muscle fibers if at all possible, to avoid damage to the vessels within the flap. At least one half of the healed margin of the flap should be left intact. Leaving this margin of flap attached should provide adequate vascularity to the tissue if the pedicle is inadvertently damaged during elevation.

Flap Coverage of Amputation Stumps

Flap coverage of the lower leg after amputation may be a consideration in cases in which the level of soft-tissue damage is proximal to the usual site of division of the tibia for below-knee amputation. In these cases, some type of flap coverage of the distal bone may be required to allow knee salvage and below-knee prosthesis fitting.[855] If the vasculature is intact, the sole of the foot may be transferred through the posterior tibial vessels as an island flap to the below-knee stump (the "fillet of sole").[640,698] One option that is often overlooked is use of a portion of the amputated (or to be amputated) leg as a free flap.[149,432] The dorsal foot may be transferred on its anterior tibial vascular supply and the plantar surface on the posterior tibial vessels (Fig. 7-25). The amputated limb must have been properly treated (ie, kept on ice) for this to be a viable option. Early or late coverage problems with below-knee stumps can be managed with either local muscles (gastrocnemius)[8,298] or free flap transfer.[134,436,774]

Ankle

Coverage of defects of the ankle is limited by the lack of expendable skin and muscle mass in the area. Although some wounds of the ankle region can be managed with skin grafts, many full-thickness skin losses lead to exposure of bone or the Achilles tendon, which will require flap transfer. Large wounds of the ankle

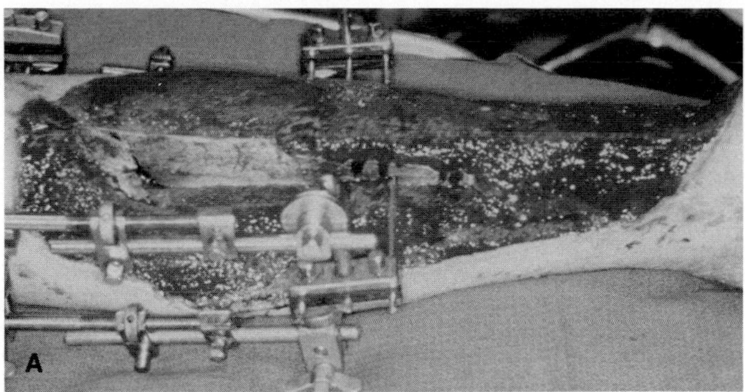

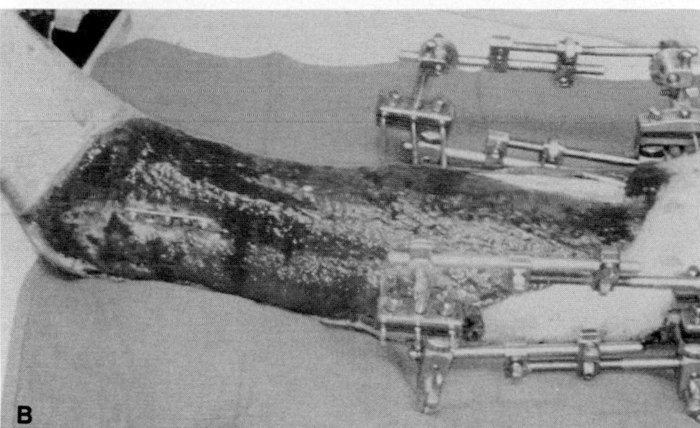

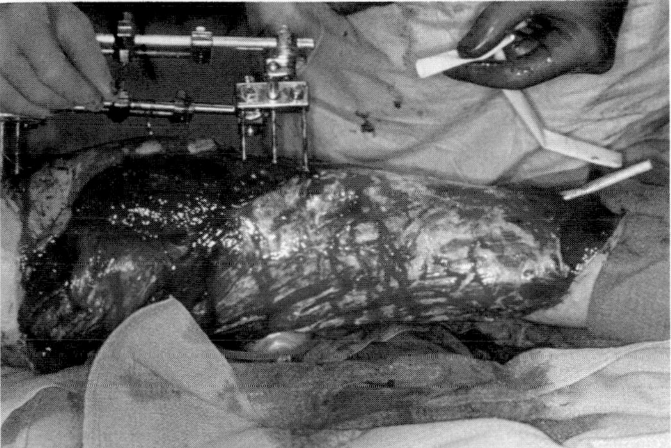

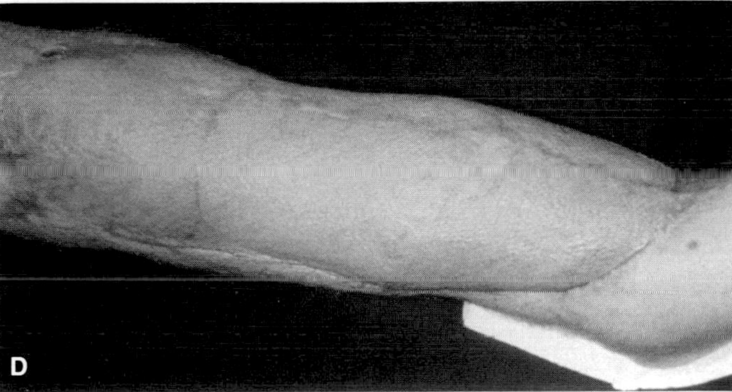

FIGURE 7-24. (**A**) The right tibia 4 weeks after a degloving injury. A significant segment of the bone was exposed, and the only treatment had been debridement and hyperbaric oxygen. (**B**) Lateral view showing a plate on the fibula, which was also exposed. (**C**) This is the largest defect ever covered by of the authors (WES), and coverage required a combined medial gastrocnemius rotational flap and a latissimus dorsi free flap wrapped around to cover both the inferior exposed tibia and the exposed fibular plate. (**D**) The healed soft tissue envelope reconstruction.

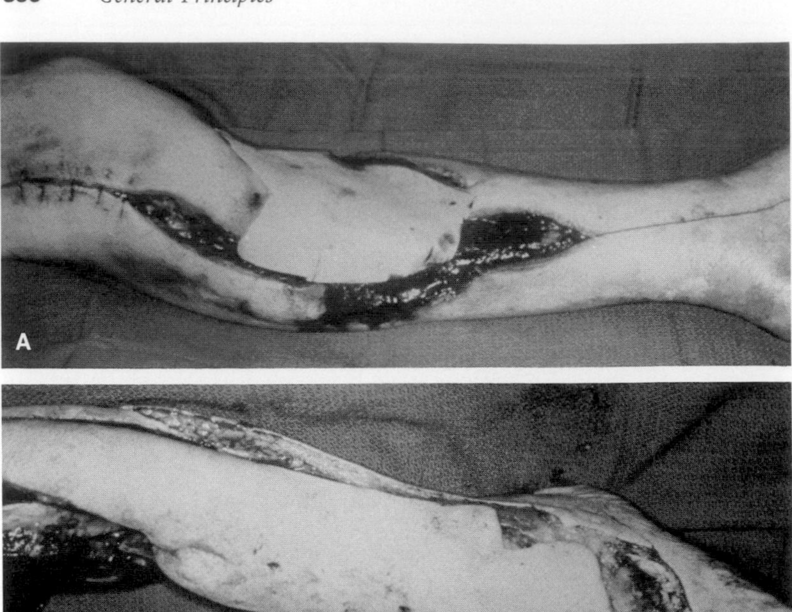

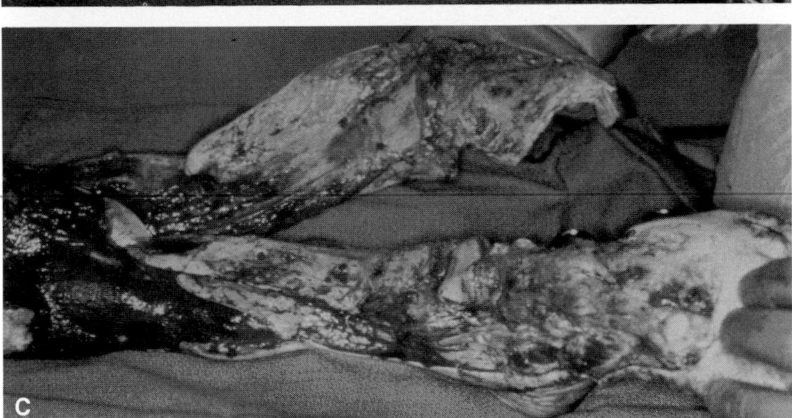

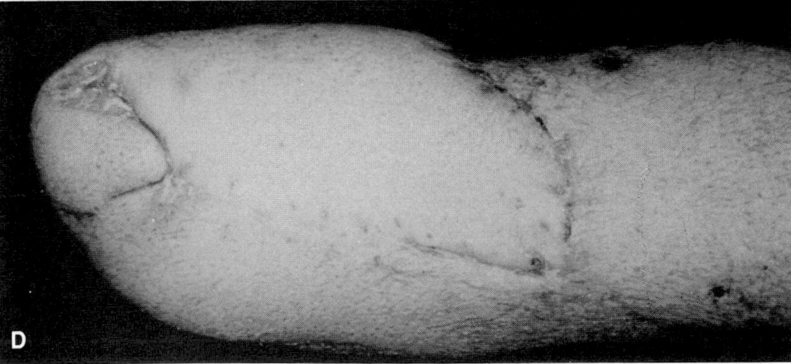

FIGURE 7-25. (**A**) A large anterior soft-tissue defect and segmental tibial defect. Amputation has been selected as definitive treatment. To provide durable sensate coverage to the stump, the dorsal skin of the foot will be filleted based on the anterior tibial artery—the only remaining blood supply to the foot. Note the posterior skin defect, which prevents use of a standard posterior flap. (**B**) After application of the template to the dorsum of the foot, a flap exactly matching the defect is raised. (**C**) The flap has been raised, the deep surface is shown, and the amputation can be completed. (**D**) Appearance of the leg 8 weeks after amputation showing the full-thickness sensate coverage of the medial and anterior aspects of the tibial stump.

dictate distant flap coverage,[37,51,262] but smaller defects may be managed by local flaps in certain instances.

The primary local flaps used for ankle coverage are based on the distal perforators of the peroneal vessels and are the lateral supramalleolar flap or lateral calcaneal flap. The lateral supramalleolar flap is based on the first cutaneous branch of the peroneal artery after it penetrates the interosseous membrane about 5 cm above the lateral malleolus.[514] This flap is reportedly reliable when designed up to 9 cm in width and 12 to 18 cm in length. It has been used for coverage of the posterior heel/Achilles region and can be distally based. The lateral calcaneal flap is based on the distal continuation of the peroneal vessels (the lateral calcaneal) and is a shorter flap based just posterior to the lateral malleolus.[288] This flap is innervated by the sural nerve and can be used for coverage of the lateral malleolus. Both of these flaps require skin grafting of their donor sites. Although these two flaps may have limited indications, we believe that problems with reliability and potential morbidity (neuroma formation of the sural nerve stump) outweigh their usefulness in most cases.[144] A number of smaller local fasciocutaneous flaps have been described for ankle coverage, but we believe that they are rarely indicated because of the need for multiple stages[462] and potential complications.[325,326]

Island pedicle flaps of tissue from the foot offer options for malleolar coverage, in particular. The extensor digitorum brevis muscle may be rotated on its nutrient vessels from the anterior tibial system,[379,469,517] although this muscle is thin and small in area. Malleolar coverage with this muscle requires distal ligation of the dorsalis pedis artery and division of the extensor retinaculum to allow mobilization of the anterior tibial vessels.[246] Although there is no discernible morbidity from harvesting of this muscle, care must be taken with its use in patients with vascular trauma or disease, because one of the major vessels supplying the foot must be ligated. It has the advantage that the donor site can be closed primarily, rather than requiring a skin graft.

Another coverage option that will reach the malleoli or posterior ankle is the dorsalis pedis island pedicle flap (Fig. 7-26).[285,502] This is a fasciocutaneous flap taken from the dorsum of the foot with vascularity derived from fascial perforators from the dorsalis pedis artery.[544] It may be taken as a sensate flap if branches of the superficial peroneal nerve are raised with the soft-tissue component. This neurosensory flap has application in coverage of the posterior heel because insensate flaps in this area have a tendency to break down from shoe pressure.[690] Although this flap provides excellent thin coverage for ankle defects, it has the morbidity of division of the dorsalis pedis artery and deep peroneal nerve. This can obviously lead to problems with distal foot vascularity and neuroma formation. The other problem with this donor site is potential loss of the skin graft, which is necessary for closure. We believe that the dorsalis pedis pedicled flap is valuable in certain situations, but the donor site must be *meticulously* managed to avoid long-term wound healing problems on the dorsum of the foot. This involves the use of a full-thickness skin graft for coverage and elevation of the foot for at least 3 full weeks to allow complete take of the graft. If this is not done, the patient may trade one problem wound for another, which negates the advantages of the dorsalis pedis for ankle reconstruction.

Larger defects and those secondary to complex injury generally require free tissue transfer for proper management. This was appreciated early on, as the first two reports of free tissue transfer were for anterior ankle defects.[170,607] Although a number of flaps have been used around the ankle,[84,249,451,672,883] the most appropriate are those that afford thin coverage. For this reason, the radial forearm flap,[144,516,643,827] lateral arm flap,[749] and scapular flap[676] are frequently used. The radial forearm and lateral arm flaps have the advantage that they can be transferred as sensate flaps by suturing the lateral antebrachial cutaneous or lateral cutaneous nerves of the arm to sensory nerves in the ankle. The dorsalis pedis flap can also be transferred from the ipsilateral foot as a sensate free flap,[198,668] and has the advantage of limiting distant donor site morbidity.[103] Deeper defects and those with bone loss or osteomyelitis should be covered with free muscle (Fig. 7-27). The donor site should generally be one of the smaller muscles, such as the gracilis or rectus abdominus, to avoid problems with excess bulk at the ankle.[672,822] The posterior ankle/Achilles region poses special problems, especially with damage or loss of the distal tendon and calcaneus. Soft-tissue coverage of this area should be thin and sensate if possible, with the radial forearm flap and lateral arm flap offering good options.[853] If reconstruction of skin, Achilles tendon, and calcaneus is necessary, the groin flap with iliac crest and fascia[861] and tensor fascia lata myocutaneous flap with iliac crest[591] have been proposed. The tensor fascia lata flap has the advantage that it can be reinnervated by connecting a sensory nerve at the ankle to the lateral femoral cutaneous nerve of the thigh.

Foot

Coverage of complex foot wounds presents many challenges, compounded by the need for the transferred tissue to withstand dependency and the pressures of ambulation. Superficial losses are best managed by skin grafting, especially on the dorsum. Although skin loss *alone* on the plantar surface is well managed by

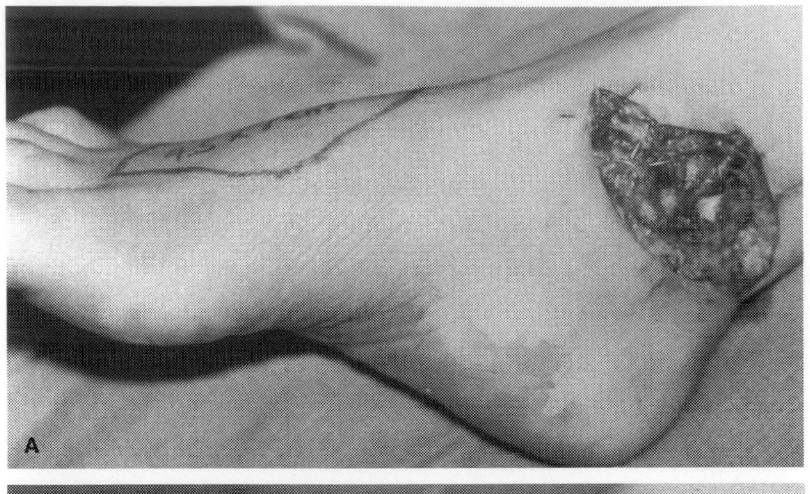

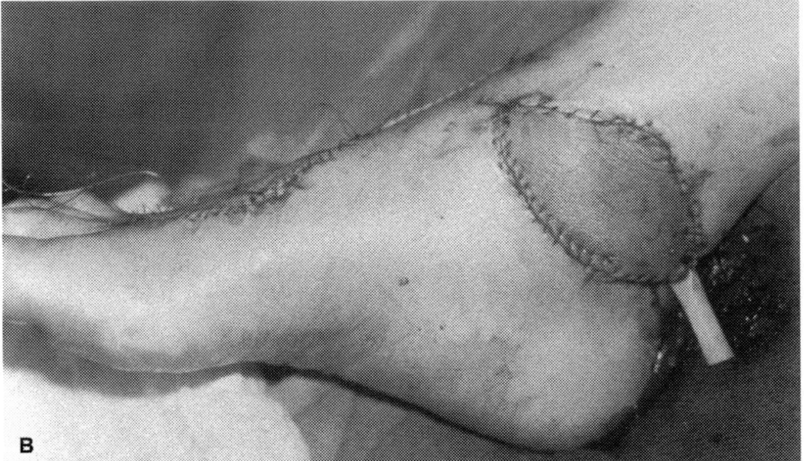

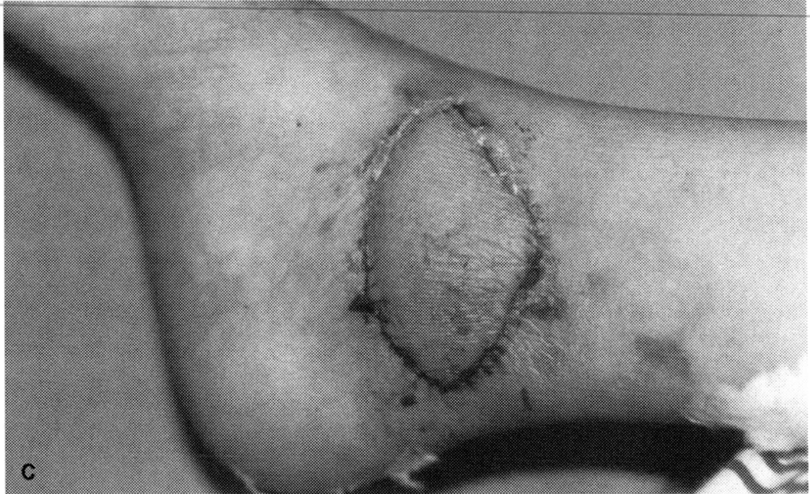

FIGURE 7-26. (**A**) The ankle of a patient after an open fracture and soft-tissue loss over the medial malleolus. Note exposed hardware and markings on the dorsum of the foot for dorsalis pedis island pedicle flap. (**B**) View after wound debridement and flap rotation. Note that the pedicle runs through the subcutaneous tunnel and the donor wound is covered with full-thickness skin graft. (**C**) The flap at 3 weeks.

continues

split-thickness skin grafts,[885] deeper wounds or those with tendon or bone exposure usually require flap coverage.[286] The requirements for coverage of the dorsal and plantar surfaces are completely different, however, and the surgeon undertaking foot reconstruction should be aware of these. The dorsal surface needs coverage that is thin enough to avoid problems with footwear yet stable enough to stand up to shear forces in shoes from walking (Fig. 7-28). Stability of coverage is probably the most important aspect of plantar coverage, although sensation may be just as important in avoiding breakdown of the flap from shear forces and pressure.[118,736]

In many instances, local flaps raised from adjacent areas of the foot offer an excellent choice for reconstruction, but one must be aware of the vascular anat-

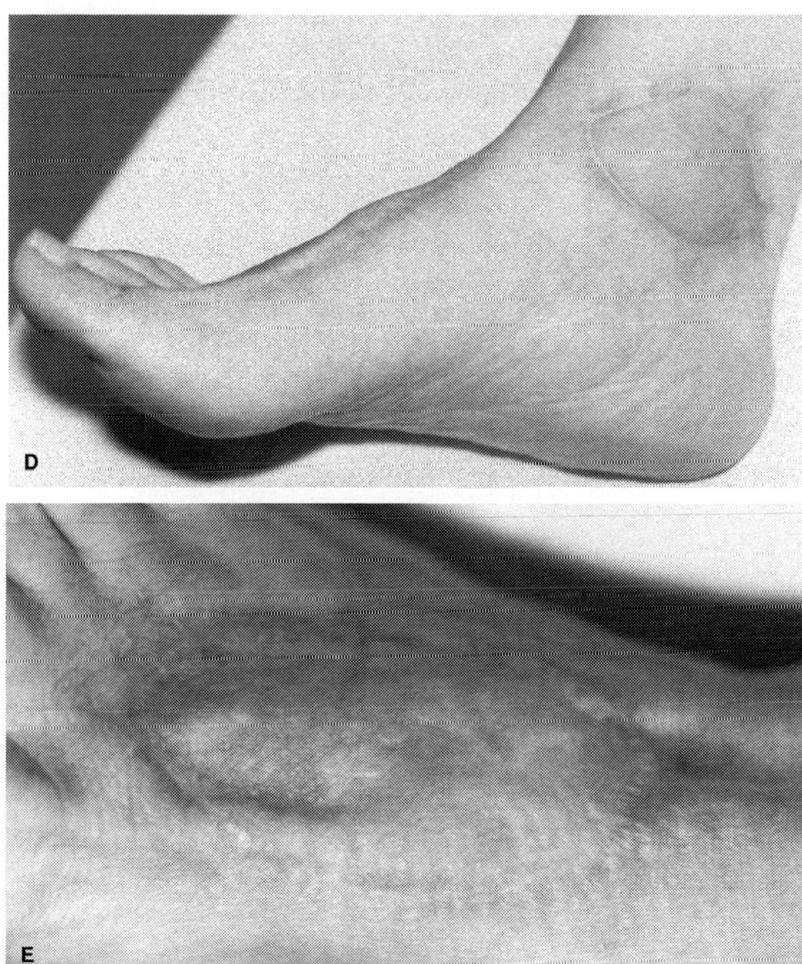

FIGURE 7-26. (continued) (**D**) The flap at 6 months. (**E**) The dorsum of the foot at 6 months. Note excellent coverage provided by the full-thickness skin graft with motion of the extensor hallucis longus.

omy to avoid compromising such flaps.[326,376] These small flaps can be used for coverage of smaller defects on the dorsum or weight-bearing surface. In distal foot injuries, the toes can be used as "fillet" flaps to cover wounds and provide sensation, particularly on the plantar surface.[541,760] The dorsalis pedis flap can be used for coverage of many foot and ankle wounds, as discussed earlier.[144,285] It has the advantage of the potential for sensate flap coverage[198] and may be used as a pedicled flap or free flap for this purpose. The dorsal foot skin can also be taken based on the distal dorsalis pedis/first dorsal metatarsal circulation. This flap is then used for coverage of distal defects in the manner of the distally pedicled radial forearm flap.[720,848] In the severely traumatized foot, the dorsalis pedis flap should be used selectively to avoid further compromise to the circulation.

The small muscles of the plantar aspect of the foot can also be used to provide padding and a well-vascularized base for skin grafting. The abductor hallucis can be rotated proximally based on the medial plantar artery and will cover smaller defects of the heel.[257] The muscles of the little toe (primarily the abductor digiti minimi) can also be used as proximally[631] or distally[257] based flaps for lateral foot coverage. For heel coverage, the flexor digitorum brevis can be based proximally and used as a "turn-over" flap for coverage.[68] This muscle is vascularized by the medial plantar vessels and can be taken with a skin paddle to improve stability of coverage.[357,754] Although all of these flaps have some usefulness in soft-tissue reconstruction of the foot, they are generally only useful for smaller defects. Their inappropriate use can lead to further morbidity in the foot, and we have treated patients who had local foot muscle flaps who required later free flap transfer for management of donor site complications.

Although there are few instances in the body where an "ideal" reconstruction can be accomplished, the patient with intact circulation and a heel wound may offer this opportunity. The skin from the arch of the foot can be transferred to the heel on the medial plantar vasculature, and inclusion of branches of the medial plantar nerve going to the arch skin offers a sensate flap.[569] This flap offers the ideal tissue in terms of heel reconstruction, in that it is glabrous and has

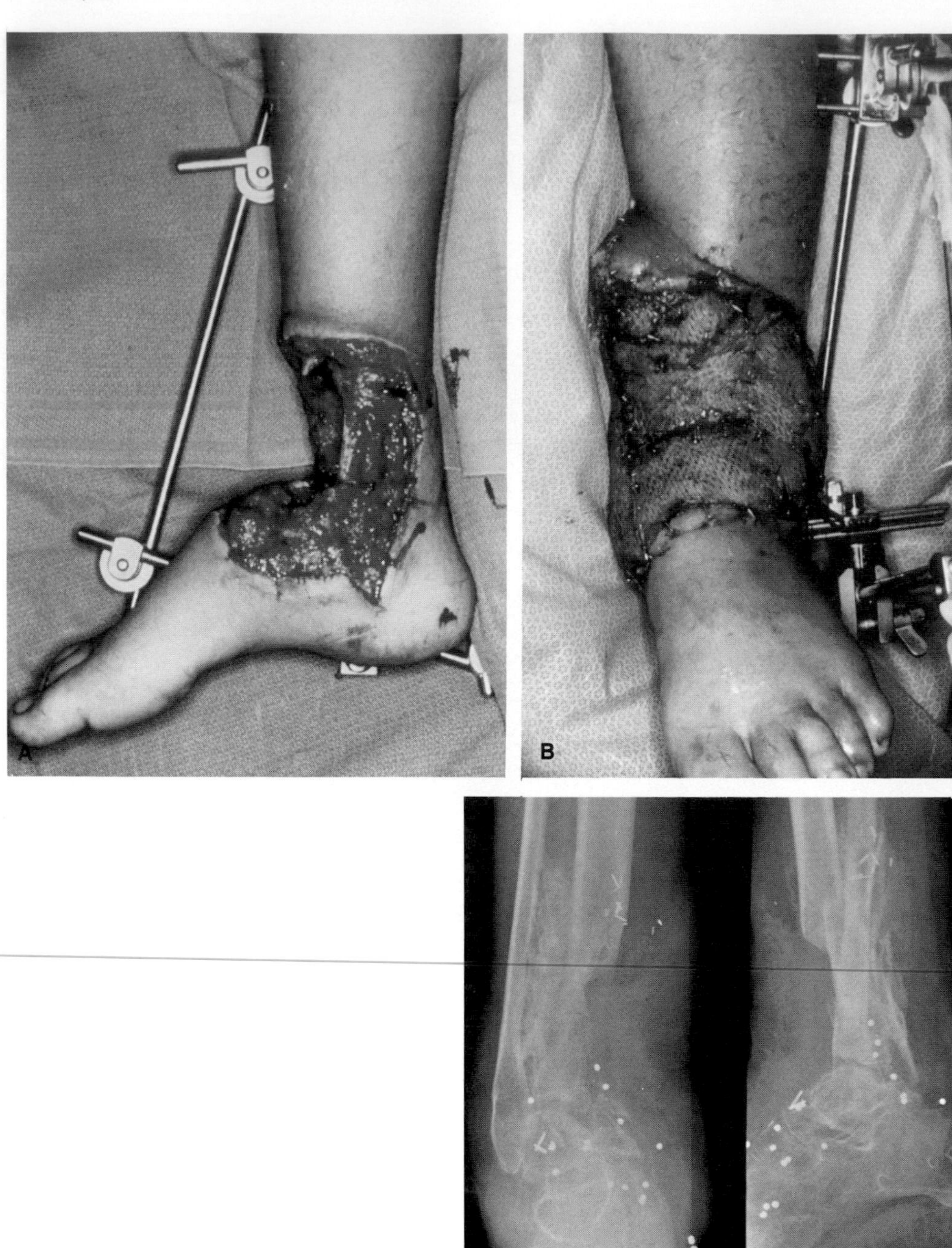

FIGURE 7-27. (**A**) The foot of a 23-year-old woman who suffered a close-range shotgun wound with loss of the talar dome and distal 2 inches of the tibia. The posterior tibial neurovascular bundle was intact, but there was a large anterior soft-tissue defect. (**B**) Anterior view of a latissimus flap and split-thickness skin graft 3 weeks postoperatively. (**C**) A posterolateral bone graft was performed, which healed proximally but not distally. Further grafting is planned.

appropriate sensibility. Some authors have proposed taking the skin with the underlying abductor hallucis muscle,[354,602,675] but the inclusion of muscle is unnecessary for flap survival. The added muscle under the skin can also lead to problems of bulk and instability of the flap, with the potential for increased breakdown. If taken as a fasciocutaneous flap alone, the "instep" flap will cover nearly the entire heel and offers excellent coverage in terms of sensation and stability.[31,746] To preserve distal sensation, the cutaneous branches to the flap must be carefully dissected free from the main body of the medial plantar nerve.[580] Although this intrafascicular dissection of the nerve is technically demanding, it is necessary to allow adequate rotation of

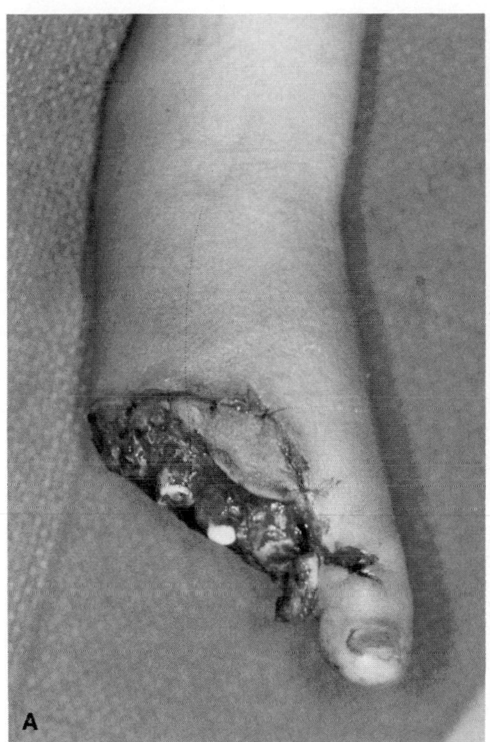

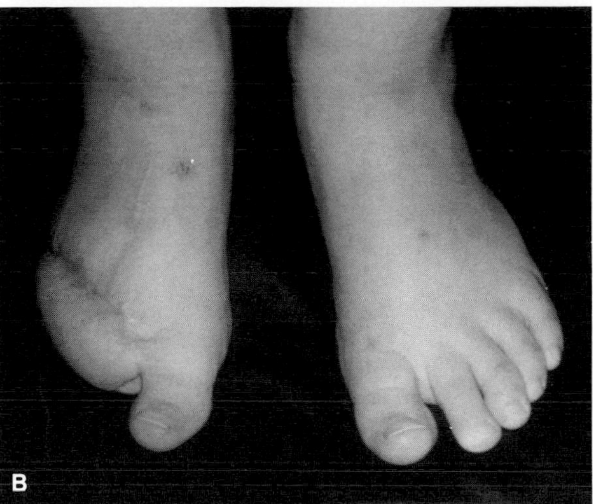

FIGURE 7-28. (**A**) A 10-year-old with loss of all four lateral toes and adjacent soft tissue. (**B**) Durable coverage and maintenance of metatarsal length by a lateral arm free flap (1 year postoperatively). (*Case courtesy of Robert N. Hotchkiss, M.D., New York, NY.*)

the flap to cover the heel. This flap can also be distally based and used for coverage of difficult wounds of the metatarsal heads.[10] Although it has been proposed as an island pedicle flap for coverage of the ankle,[32] we believe that the potential morbidity of the donor site dictates the use of other flaps for areas other than the plantar foot. The medial plantar flap has also been used as a free flap to cover the contralateral heel,[580,602] but we prefer to avoid imparting potential morbidity to an otherwise normal foot. Despite these reservations, we believe that this flap offers the best reconstruction available for heel defects. The donor site is covered with a split-thickness skin graft, which has been shown to have minimal morbidity in terms of overall foot function (Fig. 7-29).[31,486]

In terms of distant flaps, a number have been proposed for foot reconstruction. Skin flaps raised from the ipsilateral thigh or buttock have been used as pedicle flaps for foot coverage.[196,384,570] These require the knee to be acutely flexed for the flap to reach and obviously are limited in their use to children to avoid severe joint contracture. Cross-leg flaps are still advocated by some and may be indicated where vascular damage to the leg limits access for free tissue transfer.[384,393,531,835] The contralateral foot can be used to provide a glabrous "cross-foot" pedicle flap from the mid-sole to resurface plantar injuries,[567] but potential donor site problems make this flap undesirable.[44] Distally based island pedicle flaps on the posterior tibial or peroneal vessels have also been described for plantar coverage,[721,906] but the need to divide a major vessel to the foot makes this type of flap a secondary choice in most hands.

The "state of the art" for reconstruction of most deep plantar wounds has become free tissue transfer.[221,239,371,451,562,601,668,676,753,911] This technique offers the ability to provide adequate coverage without further morbidity to the injured limb. Technical success of free tissue transfer to the foot has to be tempered by the appreciation that complex plantar wound reconstruction remains problematic in most hands. The two most important parameters for plantar reconstruction are *flap stability* and *flap sensation*.[736] Underlying bony abnormalities that are not corrected before flap placement also predispose the patient to breakdown of the coverage. A "perfect" free flap placed on a foot with abnormal bony architecture or poor surrounding sensation cannot be expected to stand up to the rigors of ambulation, and thus these problems must be corrected before flap transfer if at all possible.[366]

Long-term studies of free flaps placed on the plantar foot have proven the benefit of this approach but have also shown the shortcomings of distant flaps placed on the weight-bearing foot surface. The need for a stable

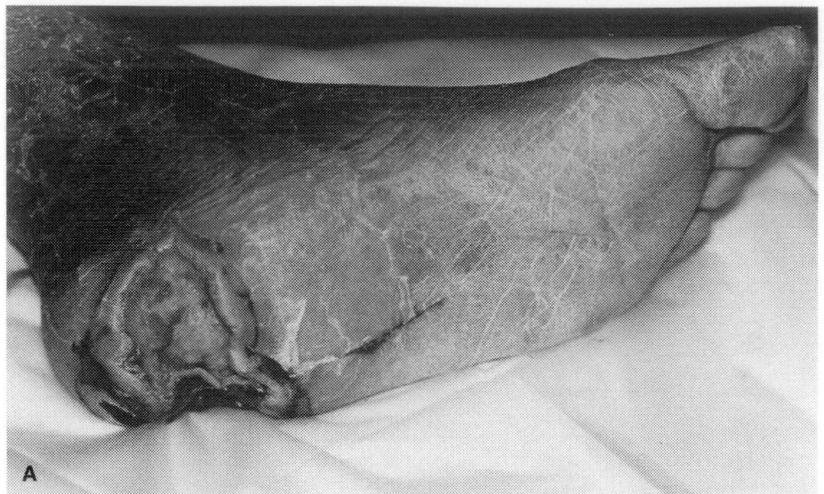

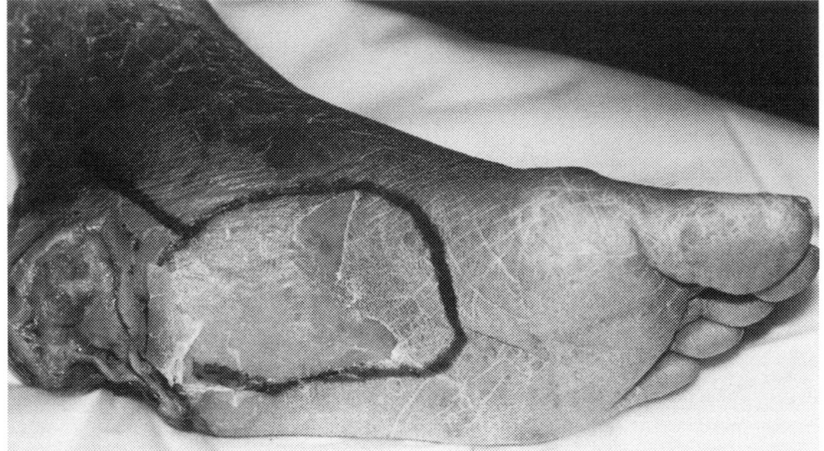

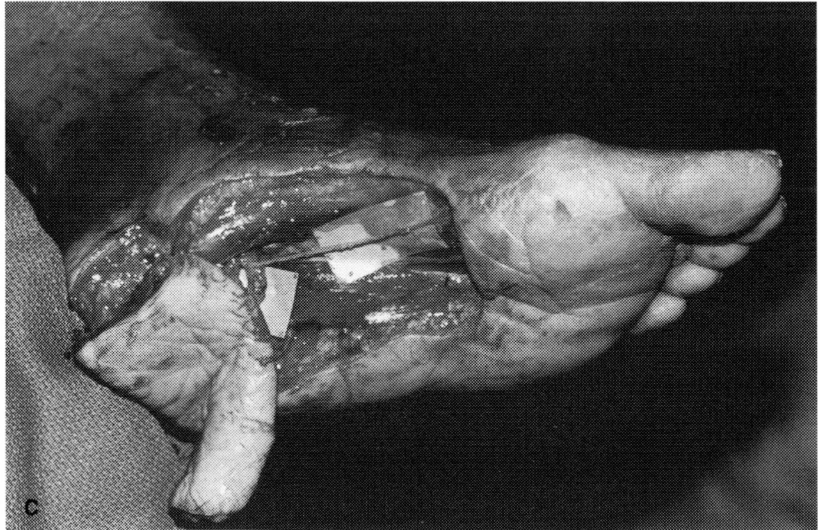

FIGURE 7-29. (**A**) The heel of 45-year-old diabetic after necrosis from infection. The patient had intact plantar sensation and excellent palpable pulses. (**B**) View of the foot after outlining the medial plantar artery flap. The vessel is followed with Doppler examination from the posterior tibial artery. (**C**) The flap after elevation, rotated into the defect. The structure running distally is the medial plantar nerve to the distal foot.

continues

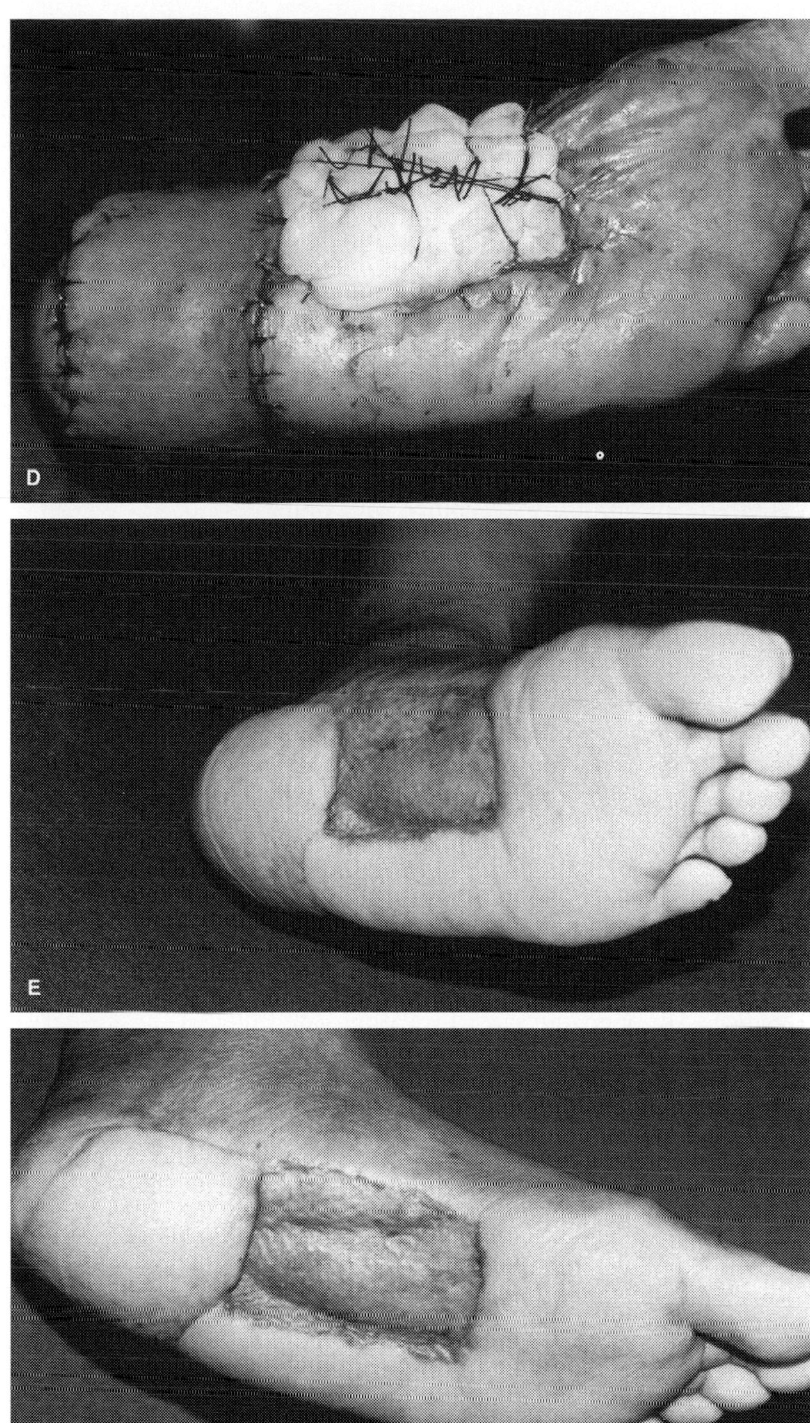

FIGURE 7-29. (continued) (**D**) The foot after insetting of the flap and placement of a split-thickness skin graft on donor site. Note the tie-over bolster to hold the graft down. (**E** and **F**) The foot at 4 months. The patient has excellent sensation in the transferred flap and subsequently had no further breakdown at 18 months.

flap that would tolerate ambulation with little shear was recognized early on, and May[536] was one of the earliest authors to propose the use of thin free muscle flaps covered with split-thickness skin grafts. His study of 18 cases showed that patients reconstructed in this manner could return to ambulation in normal footwear with little or no flap breakdown. Other authors have found that even well-contoured muscle flaps can break down over time with ambulation, however.[352,753] Most studies have found that insensate *free skin flaps* have a tendency to be too wobbly and break down over time due to shear stress between the flap and bony structures of the foot.[562,668,670,719,753] This breakdown occurs despite the fact that free skin flaps (transferred without sensory nerve reconstruction) will often develop some sensibility with time.[670]

The ability to reconstruct the plantar surface of the foot with a free flap containing a sensory nerve with its territory was recognized early on as a desirable option in this area.[101,118,164,515] The problem with this concept is that many of the donor tissues with appropriate sensory nerve supply are either too bulky or cannot provide adequate padding for walking.[101] Likewise, reinnervation of the transferred flap takes at least several months, and during this period the patient is at risk for "walking through" the flap. Experience in the application of sensory free flaps has further refined the role of these flaps in plantar reconstruction. Management of smaller plantar wounds with reinnervated flaps from the lateral arm[333,672,676,749] and radial forearm[135,329,587] has proven to provide long-term stable coverage. Although the use of an innervated medial plantar artery flap as a free flap from the contralateral foot has been proposed,[580,602] we believe that the potential morbidity of harvesting this flap from a normal foot should be avoided.

A number of free flaps have been proposed for plantar wound reconstruction,[451,670,691,848] but the consensus of most authors today is to use muscle flaps covered with split-thickness skin grafts for larger wounds and one of the thin innervated cutaneous flaps for smaller wounds. We agree with this approach, but we have seen long-term difficulties with breakdown in both types of coverage, which mirrors the experience of other authors.[352,562,668,670,753] Regardless of the type of flap chosen for plantar reconstruction, postoperative care must be coordinated in terms of appropriate shoe wear and adequate patient instruction and follow-up to decrease the incidence of late problems.

REFERENCES

1. Aberg, M., Rydholm, A., Holmberg, J. and Wieslander, J.B.: Reconstruction With a Free Vascularized Fibular Graft for Malignant Bone Tumor. Acta. Orthop. Scand., 59:430–437, 1988.
2. Abu Jamra, F.N., Akel, S.R., and Shamma, A.R.: Repair of Major Defect of the Upper Extremity With a Latissimus Dorsi Myocutaneous Flap: A Case Report. Br. J. Plast. Surg., 34:121–123, 1981.
3. Abu-Dalu, K., Muggia, M., and Schiller, M.: A Bipedicled Chest Wall Flap to Cover an Open Elbow Joint in a Burned Infant. Injury, 13:292–293, 1982.
4. Acarturk, S., and Ozmen, E.: Composite Osteo-cutaneous Groin Flap for the Reconstruction of Wrist and Forearm Defects. Br. J. Plast. Surg., 37:388–393, 1984.
5. Achauer, B.M., Spenler, C.W., and Gold, M.E.: Reconstruction of Axillary Burn Contractures With the Latissimus Dorsi Fasciocutaneous Flap. J. Trauma, 28:211–213, 1988.
6. Acland, R. and Smith, P.: Microvascular Surgical Techniques Used to Provide Skin Cover Over an Ununited Tibial Fracture. J. Bone Joint Surg., 58B:471–473, 1976.
7. Akasaka, Y., Hara, T., and Takahashi, M.: Free Muscle Transplantation Combined With Intercostal Nerve Crossing for Reconstruction of Elbow Flexion and Wrist Extension in Brachial Plexus Injuries. Microsurgery, 12:346–351, 1991.
8. Albers, G.H., van der Eijken, J.W., and Bras, J.: Through Knee Amputation With Gastrocnemius Musculocutaneous Flap: 6 Cases of Tibial Osteosarcoma Followed for 3 (1–6) Years. Acta Orthop. Scand., 65:67–70, 1994.
9. Allen, R.J., Dupin, C.L., Dreschnack, P.A., Glass, C.A., and Mahon-Deri, B.: The Latissimus Dorsi/Scapular Bone Flap (the Latissimus/Bone Flap). Plast. Reconstr. Surg., 94:988–996, 1994.
10. Amarante, J., Martins, A., and Reis, J.: A Distally Based Median Plantar Flap. Ann. Plast. Surg., 20:468–470, 1988.
11. Ambroggio, G., Oberto, E., and Teich-Alasia, S.: Twenty Years' Experience Using the Cross-Leg Flap Technique. Ann. Plast. Surg., 9:152–163, 1982.
12. Anderson, J.T., and Gustilo, R.B.: Immediate Internal Fixation in Open Fractures. Orthop. Clin. North Am., 11:569–578, 1980.
13. Anthony, J.P., Mathes, S.J., and Alpert, B.S.: The Muscle Flap in the Treatment of Chronic Lower Extremity Osteomyelitis: Results in Patients Over 5 Years After Treatment. Plast. Reconstr. Surg., 88:311–318, 1991.
14. Arai, T., Ikuta, Y., and Ikeda, A.: A Study of the Arterial Supply in the Human Rectus Femoris Muscle. Plast. Reconstr. Surg., 92:43–48, 1993.
15. Arata, M.A., Wood, M.B., and Cooney, W.P.I.: Revascularized Segmental Diaphyseal Bone Transfers in the Canine: An Analysis of Viability. J. Reconstr. Microsurg., 1:11–19, 1984.
16. Ariyan, S., and Finseth, F.J.: The Anterior Chest Approach for Obtaining Free Osteocutaneous Rib Grafts. Plast. Reconstr. Surg., 62:676–685, 1978.
17. Arner, M., and Moller, K.: Morbidity of the Pedicled Groin Flap: A Retrospective Study of 44 Cases. Scand. J. Plast. Reconstr. Surg. Hand Surg., 28:143–146, 1994.
18. Arnold, P.G., and Hodgkinson, D.: Extensor Digitorum Turndown Muscle Flap. Plast. Reconstr. Surg., 66:599–604, 1980.
19. Arnold, P.G., and Irons, G.B.: The Greater Omentum: Extensions in Transposition and Free Transfer. Plast. Reconstr. Surg., February 167:169–176, 1981.
20. Arnold, P.G., and Irons, G.B.: Lower-Extremity Muscle Flaps. Orthop. Clin. North Am., 15:441–449, 1984.
21. Arnold, P.G., and Mixter, R.C.: Making the Most of the Gastrocnemius Muscles. Plast. Reconstr. Surg., 72:38–48, 1983.
22. Arnold, P.G., and Pruner-Carrillo, F.: Vastus Medialis Muscle Flap for Functional Closure of the Exposed Knee Joint. Plast. Reconstr. Surg., 68:69, 1981.
23. Aronson, J., Johnson, E., and Harp, J.H.: Local Bone Transportation for Treatment of Intercalary Defects by the Ilizarov Technique: Biomechanical and Clinical Considerations. Clin. Orthop. Rel. Res., 243:71–79, 1989.
24. Asko-Seljavaara, S., Slatis, P., Kannisto, M., and Sundell, B.: Management of Infected Fractures of the Tibia With Associated Soft Tissue Loss: Experience With External Fixation, Bone Grafting and Soft Tissue Reconstruction Using Pedicle Muscle Flaps or Microvascular Composite Tissue Grafts. Br. J. Plast. Surg., 38:546–555, 1985.
25. Aufranc, O.E., Jones, W.N., and Harris, W.H.: Sideswipe Injury to Right Elbow. J.A.M.A. 187:1017–1019, 1964.

26. Austad, E.D., Pasyk, K.A., McClatchey, K.D., and Cherry, G.W.: Histomorphologic Evaluation of Guinea Pig Skin and Soft Tissue After Controlled Tissue Expansion. Plast. Reconstr. Surg., 70:704–710, 1982.
27. Azuma, H., Kondo, T., Mikami, M., and Harii, K.: Treatment of Chronic Osteomyelitis by Transplantation of Autogenous Omentum with Microvascular Anastomosis. Acta Orthop. Scand., 47:271–275, 1976.
28. Babu, N.V., Chittaranjan, S., Abraham, G., Bhattacharjee, S., Prem, H., and Korula, R.J. Reconstruction of the Quadriceps Apparatus Following Open Injuries to the Knee Joint Using Pedicled Gastrocnemius Musculotendinous Unit as Bridge Graft. Br. J. Plast. Surg., 47:190–193, 1994.
29. Bach, A.W., and Hansen, S.T., Jr.: Plates Versus External Fixation in Severe Open Tibial Shaft Fractures: A Randomized Trial. Clin. Orthop. Rel. Res., 241:89–93, 1989.
30. Badasivan, K.K., Ogden, J.T., and Albright, J.A.: Anatomic Variations of the Blood Supply of the Soleus Muscle. Orthopedics, 14:679–683, 1991.
31. Baert, C., and Monballiu, G.: The Treatment of Heel Skin Defects Using a Medial Plantar Skin Flap. Acta Chir. Belg., 90:262–266, 1990.
32. Baker, G.L., Newton, E.D., and Franklin, J.D.: Fasciocutaneous Island Flap Based on the Medial Plantar Artery: Clinical Applications for Leg, Ankle, and Forefoot (see Comments). Plast. Reconstr. Surg., 85:47–58; discussion, 1990.
33. Barclay, T.L., Cardoso, E., Sharpe, D.T., and Crockett, D.J.: Repair of Lower Leg Injuries with Fascio-cutaneous Flaps. Br. J. Plast. Surg., 35:127–132, 1982.
34. Barclay, T.L., Sharpe, D.T., and Chisholm, E.M.: Cross-leg Fasciocutaneous Flaps. Plast. Reconstr. Surg., 72:843–846, 1983.
35. Bardsley, A.F., Soutar, D.S., Elliot, D., and Batchelor, A.G.: Reducing Morbidity in the Radial Forearm Flap Donor Site. Plast. Reconstr. Surg., 86:287–92; discussion, 1990.
36. Barfod, B., and Pers, M.: Gastrocnemius-plasty for Primary Closure of Compound Injuries of the Knee. J. Bone Joint Surg., 52:124–127, 1970.
37. Barfred, T., and Reumert, T.: Myoplasty for Covering Exposed Bone or Joint on the Lower Leg. Acta Orthop. Scand., 44:532–538, 1973.
38. Baron, J.L., Benichou, M., Louchahi, N., Gomis, R., Reynaud, J.P., and Allieu, Y.: Current Techniques and Indications of Pedicled Groin Flap for Hand Surgery: Apropos of 100 Cases. Ann. Chir. Plast. Esthet., 36:31–44, 1991.
39. Bartlett, S.P., May, J.W., Jr., and Yaremchuk, M.J.: The Latissimus Dorsi Muscle: A Fresh Cadaver Study of the Primary Neurovascular Pedicle. Plast. Reconstr. Surg., 67:631–636, 1981.
40. Barwick, W.J., Goodkind, D.J., and Serafin, D.: The Free Scapular Flap. Plast. Reconstr. Surg., 69:779–785, 1982.
41. Bashir, A.H.: Inferiorly-based Gastrocnemius Muscle Flap in the Treatment of War Wounds of the Middle and Lower Third of the Leg. Br. J. Plast. Surg., 36:307–309, 1983.
42. Bassett, C.A.L.: Current Concepts of Bone Formation. J. Bone Joint Surg., 44A:1217–1244, 1962.
43. Batchelor, A.G., and Bardsley, A.F.: The Bi-scapular Flap. Br. J. Plast. Surg., 40:510–512, 1987.
44. Batten, R.L., Donaldson, L.J., and Aldridge, M.J.: Experience With the AO-Method in the Treatment of 142 Cases of Fresh Fractures of the Tibial Shaft Treated in the United Kingdom. Injury 10:108–114, 1978.
45. Baudet, J., LeMaire, J., and Guimberteau, J.: Ten Free Groin Flaps. Plast. Reconstr. Surg., 57:577–595, 1976.
46. Baudet, J., Martin, D., and Cullen, K.: Maximizing Donor Tissue Use While Minimizing Donor Site Morbidity. Prob. Plast. Reconstr. Surg., 1:64–124, 1991.
47. Baudet, J., Panconi, B., Caix, P., Schoofs, M., Amarante, J., and Kaddoura, R.: The Composite Fibula and Soleus Free Transfer. Int. J. Microsurg., 4:10–26, 1982.
48. Bauer, G.C., Edwards, P., and Widmark, P.H.: Shaft Fractures of the Tibia: Etiology of Poor Results in a Consecutive Series of 173 Fractures. Acta Chir. Scand., 124:386–393, 1962.
49. Bauland, C.G., van Twisk, R., Bos, M.Y., and Nicolai, J.P.: Impossible Reversed Radial Forearm Free Flap in Microsurgical Reconstruction. Microsurgery, 14:601–604, 1993.
50. Behrens, F.: General Theory and Principles of External Fixation. Clin. Orthop. Rel. Res., 241:15–23, 1989.
51. Bennett, J.E., and Kahn, R.A.: Surgical Management of Soft Tissue Defects of the Ankle-Heel Region. J. Trauma., 12:696–703, 1972.
52. Bentivegna, P.E., and Greenberg, B.M.: Use of an inferiorly based rectus muscle flap in flank wound coverage. Ann. Plast. Surg., 29:261–262, 1992.
53. Berggren, A., Weiland, A.J., and Dorfman, H.: Free Vascularized Bone Grafts: Factors Affecting Their Survival and Ability to Heal to Recipient Bone Defects. Plast. Reconstr. Surg., 69:19–29, 1982.
54. Berggren, A., Weiland, A.J., and Dorfman, H.: The Effect of Prolonged Ischemia Time on Osteocyte and Osteoblast Survival in Composite Bone Grafts Revascularized by Microvascular Anastomoses. Plast. Reconstr. Surg., 69:290–298, 1982.
55. Berggren, A., Weiland, A.J., and Ostrup, L.T.: Bone Scintigraphy in Evaluating the Viability of Composite Bone Grafts Revascularized by Microvascular Anastomoses, Conventional Autogenous Bone Grafts and Free Non-Vascularized Periosteal Grafts. J. Bone Joint Surg., 64A:799–809, 1982.
56. Berggren, A., Weiland, A.J., Ostrup, L.T., and Dorfman, H.: The Effects of Storage Media and Perfusion on Osteoblast and Osteocyte Survival in Free Composite Bone Grafts. J. Microsurg., 2:273–282, 1981.
57. Berggren, A., Weiland, A.J., Ostrup, L.T., and Dorfman, H.: Microvascular Free Bone Transfer with Revascularization of the Medullary and Periosteal Circulation or the Periosteal Circulation Alone. J. Bone Joint Surg., 64A:73–87, 1982.
58. Biemer, E., and Stock, W.: Total Thumb Reconstruction: A One-Stage Reconstruction Using an Osteocutaneous Forearm Flap. Br. J. Plast. Surg., 36:52–55, 1983.
59. Black, M.J.M., Chait, L., O'Brien, B.M., Sykes, P.J., and Sharzer, L.A.: How Soon May the Axial Vessels of a Surviving Free Flap Be Safely Ligated: A Study in Pigs. Br. J. Plast. Surg. 31:295–299, 1978.
60. Bochdansky, T., Utku, Y., Zauner-Dungl, A., Schemper, M., and Piza-Katzer, H.: Evaluation of Shoulder Function After Removal of the Latissimus Dorsi Muscle for Surgical Flap. Handchir. Mikrochir. Plast. Chir., 22:321–325, 1990.
61. Bohr, H., Ravn, H.O., and Werner, H.: The Osteogenic Effect of Bone Transplants in Rabbits. J. Bone Joint Surg., 50B:866–873, 1968.
62. Bondurant, F.J., Cotler, H.B., Buckle, R., Miller-Crotchett, P., and Browner, B.D.: The Medical and Economic Impact of Severely Injured Lower Extremities. J. Trauma, 28:1270–1273, 1988.
63. Bootz, F., and Biesinger, E.: Reduction of Complication Rate at Radial Forearm Flap Donor Sites. O.R.L. J. Otorhinolaryngol. Relat. Spec., 53:160–164, 1991.
64. Borges Filho, P.T., Neves, R.I., Gemperli, R., et al.: Soft-tissue expansion in lower extremity reconstruction. Clin. Plast. Surg., 18:593–599, 1991.
65. Bos, K.E., Besselaar, P.P., Van der Eyken, J.W., Taminiau, A.H., and Verbout, A.J.: Reconstruction of Congenital Tibial Pseudarthrosis by Revascularized Fibular Transplants. Microsurgery, 14:558–562, 1993.
66. Bosse, M.J., Burgess, A.R., and Brumback, R.J.: Evaluation and Treatment of the High-Energy Open Tibia Fracture. Adv. Orthop. Surg., 8:3–17, 1984.
67. Bostwick, J., Scheflan, M., Nahai, F., and Jurkiewicz, M.J.: The Reverse Latissimus Dorsi Muscle and Musculocutaneous Flap: Anatomical and Clinical Applications. Plast. Reconstr. Surg., 65:395–399, 1980.
68. Bostwick, J., III.: Reconstruction of the Heel Pad by Muscle Transposition and Split Skin Graft. Surg. Gynecol. Obstet. 143:973–974, 1976.
69. Bostwick, J., III, Nahai, F., Wallace, J.G., and Vasconez, L.O.: Sixty Latissimus Dorsi Flaps. Plast. Reconstr. Surg., 63:31–41, 1979.
70. Bowen, J., and Meares, A.: Delayed Local Leg Flaps. Br. J. Plast. Surg., 27:167–170, 1974.
71. Boyd, H.B.: The Treatment of Difficult and Unusual Non-

Unions: With Special Reference to the Bridging of Defects. J. Bone Joint Surg., 25:535–552, 1943.

72. Boyer, M.I., Bray, P.W., and Bowen, C.V.A.: Epiphyseal Plate Transplantation: An Historical Review. Br. J. Plast. Surg., 47:563–569, 1994.
73. Brand, P.W., Beach, R.B., and Thompson, D.E.: Relative Tension and Potential Excursion of Muscles in the Forearm and Hand. J. Hand Surg., 6A:209–219, 1981.
74. Braun, R.M.: Viable Pedicle Bone Grafting in the Wrist. *In* Urbaniak, J.R. (ed.): Microsurgery for Major Limb Reconstruction, pp 220–229. St. Louis, C.V. Mosby, 1987.
75. Brenman, S.A., Barber, W.B., Pederson, W.C., and Barwick, W.J.: Pedicled Free Flaps: Indications in Complex Reconstruction. Ann. Plast. Surg., 24:420–426, 1990.
76. Briggs, J.G., Jr., Huang, T.T., and Lewis, S.R.: Use of Muscle Flaps in Treatment of Osteomyelitis of the Tibia. Tex. Med., 74:82–87, 1978.
77. Broadwater, J.R., and Stair, J.M.: Sternoclavicular Osteomyelitis: Coverage With a Pectoralis Major Muscle Flap. Surg. Rds. Orthop., September:47–50, 1988.
78. Brookes, M.: The Blood Supply of Bone, pp. 1–22. London, Butterworths, 1971.
79. Brown, K., Marie, P., Lyszakowski, T., Daniel, R., and Cruess, R.: Epiphysial Growth After Free Fibular Transfer With and Without Microvascular Anastomosis: Experimental Study in the Dog. J. Bone Joint Surg., 65B:493–501, 1983.
80. Brown, K.L.: Limb Reconstruction With Vascularized Fibular Grafts After Bone Tumor Resection. Clin. Orthop. Rel. Res., 262:64–73, 1991.
81. Brown, K.L., and Cruess, R.L.: Bone and Cartilage Transplantation in Orthopaedic Surgery: A Review. J. Bone Joint Surg., 64A:270–279, 1982.
82. Brown, P.W.: The Prevention of Infection in Open Wounds. Clin. Orthop. Rel. Res., 96:42–50, 1973.
83. Brown, R.F.: The Management of Traumatic Tissue Loss in the Lower Limb, Especially When Complicated by Skeletal Injury. Br. J. Plast. Surg., 18:26–50, 1965.
84. Brownstein, M.L., Gordon, L., and Buncke, H.J., Jr.: The Use of Microvascular Free Groin Flaps for the Closure of Difficult Lower Extremity Wounds. Surg. Clin. North Am., 57:977–985, 1977.
85. Brunelli, G.: Free Microvascular Fibular Transfer for Idiopathic Femoral Head Necrosis: Long-Term Follow-up. J. Reconstr. Microsurg., 7:285–295, 1991.
86. Bruns, J., and Holtje, W.J.: Inferior Pedicled Gastrocnemius Flap in the Treatment of Soft Tissue Defects of the Distal Lower Leg (Case Report). Handchir. Mikrochir. Plast. Chir., 19:191–194, 1987.
87. Buchman, J., and Blair, J.E.: The Surgical Management of Chronic Osteomyelitis by Saucerization, Primary Closure, and Antibiotic Control: Preliminary Report on Use of Aureomycin. J. Bone Joint Surg., 33A:107–118, 1951.
88. Buncke, H.J., Jr., Furnas, D.W., Gordon, L., and Achauer, B.M.: Free Osteocutaneous Flap From a Rib to the Tibia. Plast. Reconstr. Surg., 59:799–805, 1977.
89. Bunkis, J., Walton, R.L., and Mathes, S.J.: The Rectus Abdominis Free Flap for Lower Extremity Reconstruction. Ann. Plast. Surg., 11:373–380, 1983.
90. Burchardt, H.: The Biology of Bone Graft Repair. Clin. Orthop. Rel. Res., 174:28–42, 1983.
91. Burchardt, H., and Enneking, W.F.: Transplantation of Bone. Surg. Clin. North Am., 58:403–427, 1978.
92. Burkhalter, E.W.: The Fascial Radial Flap. J. Hand Surg., 13A:432–437, 1988.
93. Burkhalter, W.E.: Open Injuries of the Lower Extremity. Surg. Clin. North Am., 53:1439–1457, 1973.
94. Burri, C.: Chronic Post-Traumatic Osteomyelitis. *In* Post-Traumatic Osteomyelitis, pp 163–243. Bern, Hans Huber, 1975.
95. Burwell, R.G.: The Fate of Bone Grafts. *In* Apley, A.G. (ed.): Recent Advances in Orthopaedics, pp 115–207. London, J & A Churchill, 1969.
96. Button, M., and Stone, E.J.: Segmental Bony Reconstruction of the Thumb by Composite Groin Flap: a Case Report. J. Hand Surg., 5A:488–491, 1980.
97. Byrd, H.S.: Lower Extremity Reconstruction: Selected Readings. Plast. Surg., 1:1–26, 1982.
98. Byrd, H.S., Cierny, G.I., and Tebbetts, J.B.: The Management of Open Tibial Fractures With Associated Soft-Tissue Loss: External Pin Fixation With Early Flap Coverage. Plast. Reconstr. Surg., 68:73–79, 1981.
99. Byrd, H.S., Spicer, T.E., and Cierny, G., III.: The Management of Open Tibial Fractures. Plast. Reconstr. Surg., 76:719–728, 1985.
100. Cabanela, M.E.: Open Cancellous Bone Grafting of Infected Bone Defects. Orthop. Clin. North Am., 15:427–440, 1984.
101. Caffee, H.H., and Asokan, R.: Tensor Fascia Lata Musculocutaneous Free Flaps. Plast. Reconstr. Surg., 68:195–200, 1981.
102. Caffee, H.H., and Gallagher, T.J.: Experiments on the Effects of Hyperbaric Oxygen on Flap Survival in the Pig. Plast. Reconstr. Surg., 81:751–754, 1988.
103. Caffee, H.H., and Hoefflin, S.M.: The Extended Dorsalis Pedis Flap. Plast. Reconstr. Surg., 64:807, 1979.
104. Campanacci, M., and Zanoli, S.: Double Tibiofibular Synostosis (Fibula Pro Tibia) for Non-union and Delayed Union of the Tibia. J. Bone Joint Surg., 48A:44–56, 1966.
105. Campbell, R.D., Jr.: Treatment of Tibial Shaft Fractures. *In* Wade, P.A. (ed.): Surgical Treatment of Trauma, pp. 635–672. New York, Grune & Stratton, 1960.
106. Campbell, W.C.: Transference of the Fibula as an Adjunct to Free Bone Graft in Tibial Deficiency: Report of Three Cases. J. Orthop. Surg., 7:625–631, 1979.
107. Canales, F.L., Furnas, H., Glafkides, M., Davis, J.W., and Lineaweaver, W.C.: Microsurgical Transfer of the Rectus Abdominis Muscle Using the Superior Epigastric Vessels. Ann. Plast. Surg., 24:534–537, 1990.
108. Cannon, B.: Flaps Old and New. J. Hand Surg., 6A:1–2, 1981.
109. Cannon, B., Lischer, C.E., Davis, W.B., et al.: The Use of Open Jump Flaps in Lower Extremity Repairs. Plast. Reconstr. Surg., 2:336–341, 1947.
110. Carpenter, E.B.: Management of Fractures of the Shaft of the Tibia and Fibula. J. Bone Joint Surg., 48A:1640–1646, 1966.
111. Carr, A.J., MacDonald, D.A., and Waterhouse, N.: The Blood Supply of the Osteocutaneous Free Fibular Graft. J. Bone Joint Surg., 70:319–321, 1988.
112. Caudle, R.J., and Stern, P.J.: Severe Open Fractures of the Tibia. J. Bone Joint Surg., 69-A:801–807, 1987.
113. Caulfield, W.H., Curtsinger, L., Powell, G., and Pederson, W.C.: Donor Leg Morbidity After Pedicled Rectus Femoris Muscle Flap Transfer for Abdominal Wall and Pelvic Reconstruction. Ann. Plast. Surg., 32:377–382, 1994.
114. Cavanagh, S., and Pho, R.W.: The Reverse Radial Forearm Flap in the Severely Injured Hand: An Anatomical and Clinical Study. J. Hand Surg., 17B:501–503, 1992.
115. Chacha, P.B.: Salvage of Severe Open Fractures of the Tibia That Might Have Required Amputation. Injury, 6:154–172, 1973.
116. Chacha, P.B.: Vascularized Pedicular Bone Grafts. Int. Orthop., 8:117–138, 1984.
117. Chacha, P.B., Ahmed, M., and Daruwalla, J.S.: Vascular Pedicle Graft of the Ipsilateral Fibula for Nonunion of the Tibia With a Large Defect: An Experimental and Clinical Study. J. Bone Joint Surg., 63B:244–253, 1981.
118. Chang, K.N., and Buncke, H.J.: Sensory Reinnervation in Reconstruction of the Foot. Foot Ankle, 7:124–132, 1986.
119. Chang, N., and Mathes, S.J.: Comparison of the Effect of Bacterial Inoculation in Musculocutaneous and Random-Pattern Flaps. Plast. Reconstr. Surg., 70:1–10, 1982.
120. Chang, T.S., and Wang, W.: Application of Microsurgery in Plastic and Reconstructive Surgery. J. Reconstr. Microsurg., 1:55–63, 1984.
121. Chapman, M.W.: Closed Intramedullary Bone-Grafting and Nailing of Segmental Defects of the Femur. J. Bone Joint Surg., 62A:1004–1008, 1980.
122. Chapman, M.W., and Hansen, S.T., Jr.: Open Fractures: II. Current Concepts in the Management of Open Fractures. *In*

Rockwood, C.A., Jr., and Green, D.P. (eds.): Fractures in Adults, pp 199–218. Philadelphia, J.B. Lippincott, 1984.

123. Chapman, M.W., and Mahoney, M.: The Role of Early Internal Fixation in the Management of Open Fractures. Clin. Orthop. Rel. Res., 138:120–131, 1979.
124. Chase, S.W., and Herndon, C.H.: The Fate of Autogenous and Homogenous Bone Grafts: A Historical Review. J. Bone Joint Surg., 37:809–885, 1955.
125. Chen, C.W., Yu, Z.J., and Wang, Y.: A New Method of Treatment of Congenital Tibial Pseudoarthrosis using Free Vascularized Fibular Graft: A Preliminary Report. Ann. Acad. Med. Singapore, 8 No. 4:465–473, 1979.
126. Chen, H.C., Tang, Y.B., and Noordhoff, M.S.: Distally Based Gastrocnemius Myocutaneous Flap Augmented With an Arterial Anastomosis: A Combination of Myocutaneous Flap and Microsurgery. J. Trauma, 28:110–114, 1988.
127. Chen, W.S.: Restoration of Elbow Flexion by Latissimus Dorsi Myocutaneous or Muscle Flap. Arch. Orthop. Trauma Surg., 109:117–120, 1990.
128. Chen, Z.W., Chen, L.E., Zhang, G.J., and Yu, H.L.: Treatment of Tibial Defect With Vascularized Osteocutaneous Pedicled Transfer of Fibula. J. Reconstr. Microsurg., 2:199–203, 205, 1986.
129. Chen, Z.W., and Yan, W.: The Study and Clinical Application of the Osteocutaneous Flap of Fibula. Microsurgery, 4:11–16, 1983.
130. Chen, Z.W., Yang, D.Y., and Chang, D.S.: Free Skin Flap Transfer. *In* Microsurgery, pp. 198–231. Berlin, Springer-Verlag, 1982.
131. Chen, Z.W., and Yu, H.L.: Lower-Limb Replantation. *In* Urbaniak, J.R. (ed.): Microsurgery for Major Limb Reconstruction, pp. 67–73. St. Louis, C.V. Mosby, 1987.
132. Cheng, H.H., Rong, G.W., Yin, T.C., Wang, H.Y., and Jiao, Y.C.: Coverage of Wounds in the Distal Lower Leg by Advancement of an Enlarged Medial Gastrocnemius Skin Flap. Plast. Reconstr. Surg., 73:671–677, 1984.
133. Cherup, L.L., Zachary, L.S., Gottlieb, L.J., and Petti, C.A.: The Radial Forearm Skin Graft-Fascial Flap. Plast. Reconstr. Surg., 85:898–902, 1990.
134. Chicarilli, Z.N.: Free-Flap Salvage of a Traumatic Below-Knee Amputation. Plast. Reconstr. Surg., 79:968–973, 1987.
135. Chicarilli, Z.N., and Price, G.J.: Complete Plantar Foot Coverage With the Free Neurosensory Radial Forearm Flap. Plast. Reconstr. Surg., 78:94–101, 1986.
136. Chow, J.A., Bilos, Z.J., Hui, P., Hall, R.F., Seyfer, A.E., and Smith, A.C.: The Groin Flap in Reparative Surgery of the Hand. Plast. Reconstr. Surg., 77:421–426, 1986.
137. Chuang, D.C., Chen, H.C., Wei, F.C., and Noordhoff, M.S.: Compound Functioning Free Muscle Flap Transplantation (Lateral Half of Soleus, Fibula, and Skin Flap). Plast. Reconstr. Surg., 89:335–339, 1992.
138. Chuang, D.C., Colony, L.H., Chen, H.C., and Wei, F.C.: Groin Flap Design and Versatility. Plast. Reconstr. Surg., 84:100–107, 1989.
139. Chuang, D.C., Jeng, S.F., Chen, H.T., Chen, H.C., and Wei, F.C.: Experience of 73 Free Groin Flaps. Br. J. Plast. Surg., 45:81–85, 1992.
140. Cierny, G., III, Byrd, H.S., and Jones, R.E.: Primary Versus Delayed Soft Tissue Coverage for Severe Open Tibial Fractures: A Comparison of Results. Clin. Orthop. Rel. Res., 178:54–63, 1983.
141. Cierny, G.I., Mader, J.T., and Pennick, J.J.: A Clinical Staging System for Adult Osteomyelitis. Contemp. Orthop., 10:17–37, 1985.
142. Ciresi, K.F., and Mathes, S.J.: The Classification of Flaps. Orthop. Clin. North Am., 24:383–391, 1993.
143. Clancey, G.J., and Hansen, S.T., Jr.: Open Fractures of the Tibia: A Review of One Hundred and Two Cases. J. Bone Joint Surg., 60A:118–122, 1978.
144. Clark, N., and Sherman, R.: Soft-Tissue Reconstruction of the Foot and Ankle. Orthop. Clin. North Am., 24:489–503, 1993.
145. Coates, J.B., Jr., Cleveland, M., and McFetridge, E.M.: Orthopedic Surgery in the European Theater of Operations, pp. 322–353. Washington, D.C., Office of the Surgeon General, Department of the Army, 1956.
146. Coessens, B., Vico, P., and De Mey, A.: Clinical Experience with the Reverse Lateral Arm Flap in Soft-Tissue Coverage of the Elbow. Plast. Reconstr. Surg., 92:1133–1136, 1993.
147. Cohen, B.E.: Shoulder Defect Correction With Island Latissimus Dorsi Flap. Plast. Reconstr. Surg., 74:650–656, 1984.
148. Coleman, H.M., Bateman, J.E., Dale, G.M., and Starr, D.E.: Cancellous Bone Grafts for Infected Bone Defects: A Single Stage Procedure. Surg. Gynecol. Obstet., 83:392–398, 1946.
149. Colen, S.R., Romita, M.C., Godfrey, N.V., and Shaw, W.W.: Salvage Replantation. Clin. Plast. Surg., 10:125–131, 1983.
150. Comtet, J.J., Saint Cast, Y., and Remy, D.: Emergency Knee Joint Salvage Utilizing a Free Musculofasciocutaneous Flap Based on the Anterior Tibial Artery: Case Report. Microsurgery, 10:302, 1989.
151. Connelly, J.R.: Pedicle Coverage in Non-union of Fractures. Plast. Reconstr. Surg., 3:727–739, 1948.
152. Connelly, J.R.: Plastic Surgery in Bone Problems. Plast. Reconstr. Surg., 17:129–167, 1956.
153. Converse, J.M.: Early Skin Grafting in War Wounds of the Extremities. Ann. Surg., 115:321–335, 1942.
154. Copeland, C.X., Jr., and Enneking, W.F.: Incidence of Osteomyelitis in Compound Fractures. Am. Surg., 31:156–158, 1965.
155. Cormack, G.C., Duncan, M.J., and Lamberty, B.G.H.: The Blood Supply of the Bone Component of the Compound Osteo-cutaneous Radial Artery Forearm Flap: An Anatomical Study. Br. J. Plast. Surg., 39:173–175, 1986.
156. Cormack, G.C., and Lamberty, B.G.H.: A Classification of Fascio-cutaneous Flaps According to Their Patterns of Vascularization. Br. J. Plast. Surg., 37:80–87, 1984.
157. Costa, H., Guimaraes, I., Cardoso, A., Malta, A., Amarante, J., and Guimaraes, F.: One-staged Coverage and Revascularisation of Traumatised Limbs by a Flow-through Radial Midforearm Free Flap. Br. J. Plast. Surg., 44:533–537, 1991.
158. Crenshaw, A.H.: Delayed Union and Nonunion of Fractures. *In* Crenshaw, A.H. (ed.): Campbell's Operative Orthopaedics, pp. 2053–2118. St. Louis, C.V. Mosby, 1987.
159. Crock, H.V.: The Shafts of the Tibia and the Fibula. *In* The Blood Supply of the Lower Limb Bones in Man, pp 64–71. Edinburgh, E & S Livingstone, 1967.
160. Cruess, R.L.: Healing of Bone, Tendon, and Ligament. *In* Rockwood, C.A., Jr., and Green, D.P. (eds.): Fractures in Adults, pp 147–167. Philadelphia, J.B. Lippincott, 1984.
161. Culbertson, J.H., and Mutimer, K.: The Reverse Lateral Upper Arm Flap for Elbow Coverage. Ann. Plast. Surg., 18:62–68, 1987.
162. Cutting, C.B., and McCarthy, J.G.: Comparison of Residual Osseous Mass Between Vascularized and Nonvascularized Onlay Bone Transfers. Plast. Reconstr. Surg., 72:672–674, 1983.
163. d'Este, S.: La Technique de l'Amputation de la Mammelle Pour Carcinome Mammaire. Rev. Chir., 45:164, 1912.
164. Dabb, R.W., and Conklin, W.T.: A Sensory Innervated Latissimus Dorsi Musculocutaneous Free Flap: Case Report. J. Microsurg., 3:289–293, 1981.
165. Dagher, F., and Roukoz, S.: Compound Tibial Fractures With Bone Loss Treated by the Ilizarov Technique. J. Bone Joint Surg., 73B:316–321, 1991.
166. Daniel, R.K.: Toward an Anatomical and Hemodynamic Classification of Skin Flaps. Plast. Reconstr. Surg., 56:330–332, 1975.
167. Daniel, R.K.: Free Rib Transfer by Microvascular Anastomoses. Plast. Reconstr. Surg., 59:737–738, 1977.
168. Daniel, R.K., and Lidman, D.: Vascular Complications in Free Flap Transfer. *In* Buncke, H.J., and Furnas, D.W. (eds.): Symposium on Clinical Frontiers in Reconstructive Microsurgery, pp. 387–396. St. Louis, C.V. Mosby, 1984.
169. Daniel, R.K., and May, J.W., Jr.: Free Flaps: An Overview. Clin. Orthop. Rel. Res., 133:122–131, 1978.
170. Daniel, R.K., and Taylor, G.I.: Distant Transfer of an Island Flap by Microvascular Anastomoses: A Clinical Technique. Plast. Reconstr. Surg., 52:111–117, 1973.

171. Daniel, R.K., and Weiland, A.J.: Free Tissue Transfers for Upper Extremity Reconstruction. J. Hand Surg., 7A:66–76, 1982.
172. Daniel, R.K., and Williams, H.B.: The Free Transfer of Skin Flaps by Microvascular Anastomoses: An Experimental Study and a Reappraisal. Plast. Reconstr. Surg., 52:16–31, 1973.
173. Datiashvili, R.O., Shibaev, E.Y., Chichkin, V.G., and Oganesian, A.R.: Reconstruction of a Complex Defect of the Hand With Two Distinct Segments of the Scapula and a Scapular Fascial Flap Transferred as a Single Transplant (see Comments). Plast. Reconstr. Surg., 90:687–694, 1992.
174. Davis, A.G.: Fibular Substitution for Tibial Defects. J. Bone Joint Surg., 25:229–237, 1944.
175. Davis, A.G.: Primary Closure of Compound-Fracture Wounds With Immediate Internal Fixation, Immediate Skin Graft, and Compression Dressings. J. Bone Joint Surg., 30A:405–415, 1948.
176. Davis, G.L.: Management of Open Wounds of Joints During the Vietnam War: A Preliminary Study. Clin. Orthop. Rel. Res., 68:3–9, 1970.
177. Davis, J.B.: The Muscle-Pedicle Bone Graft in Hip Fusion. J. Bone Joint Surg., 36A:790–799, 1954.
178. Davis, J.B., and Taylor, A.N.: Muscle Pedicle Bone Grafts—Experimental Study. Arch Surg., 65:330–336, 1952.
179. Davis, J.C.: Adjuctive Hyperbaric Oxygen in Chronic Refractory Osteomyelitis: Long-Term Follow-up Results (Letter). Clin. Orthop. Rel. Res. 4:310, 1986.
180. Davis, J.C., Heckman, J.D., DeLee, J.C., and Buckwold, F.J.: Chronic Non-Hematogenous Osteomyelitis Treated With Adjuvant Hyperbaric Oxygen. J. Bone Joint Surg., 68A:1210–1217, 1986.
181. Dawson, R.L.: Complications of the Cross-leg Flap Operation. Proc. R. Soc. Med., 65:2–5, 1972.
182. Day, B., and Shim, S.S.: Increased Femoral Head Vascularity After an Iliopsoas Muscle Pedicle Bone Graft. Surg. Forum, 30:494–496, 1979.
183. de Boer, H.H., Verbout, A.J., Nielsen, H.K., and van der Eijken, J.W.: Free Vascularized Fibular Graft for Tibial Pseudarthrosis in Neurofibromatosis. Acta Orthop. Scand., 59:425–429, 1988.
184. DeHaan, M.R., Hammond, D.C., and Mann, R.J.: Controlled Tissue Expansion of a Groin Flap for Upper Extremity Reconstruction. Plast. Reconstr. Surg., 86:979–982, 1990.
185. Dehne, E., Deffer, P.A., Hall, R.M., Brown, P.W., and Johnson, E.V.: The Natural History of the Fractured Tibia. Surg. Clin. North Am., 41:1495–1513, 1961.
186. Dell, P.C., and Sheppard, J.E.: Vascularized Bone Grafts in the Treatment of Infected Forearm Nonunions. J. Hand Surg., 9A:653–658, 1984.
187. Dibbell, D.G., and Edstrom, L.E.: The Gastrocnemius Myocutaneous Flap. Clin. Plast. Surg., 7:45–50, 1980.
188. Dickson, W.A., Dickson, M.G., and Roberts, A.H.: The Complications of Fasciocutaneous Flaps. Ann. Plast. Surg., 19:234–237, 1987.
189. Dimond, M., and Barwick, W.: Treatment of Axillary Burn Scar Contracture Using an Arterialized Scapular Island Flap. Plast. Reconstr. Surg., 72:388–390, 1983.
190. Doherty, J.H., and Patterson, R.L., Jr.: Fibular By-Pass Operation in the Treatment of Non-union of the Tibia in Adults. J. Bone Joint Surg., 49A:1470–1471, 1967.
191. Doi, K., Tominaga, S., and Shibata, T.: Bone Grafts with Microvascular Anastomoses of Vascular Pedicles: An Experimental Study in Dogs. J. Bone Joint Surg., 54A:809–815, 1977.
192. Donski, P.K., and O'Brien, B.M.: Free Microvascular Epiphyseal Transplantation: An Experimental Study in Dogs. Br. J. Plast. Surg., 33:169–178, 1980.
193. dos Santos, L.F.: Retalho Escapular: Um Novo Retalho Livre Microcirurgico. Rev. Bras. Cir., 70:133–144, 1980.
194. dos Santos, L.F.: The Vascular Anatomy and Dissection of the Free Scapular Flap. Plast. Reconstr. Surg., 73:599–603, 1984.
195. Dowden, R.V., and McCraw, J.B.: The Vastus Lateralis Muscle Flap: Technique and Application. Ann. Plast. Surg., 4:396, 1980.
196. Drabyn, G.A., and Avedian, L.: Ipsilateral Buttock Flap for Coverage of a Foot and Ankle Defect in a Young Child. Plast. Reconstr. Surg., 63:422–423, 1979.
197. Drabyn, G.A., Porterfield, H.W., Mohler, L.R., and Nappi, J.F.: Wrist-Iliac Crest Fixation for Groin Flap-Thumb Immobilization. Plast. Reconstr. Surg., 70:98–99, 1982.
198. Duncan, M.J., Zuker, R.M., and Manktelow, R.T.: Resurfacing Weight Bearing Areas of the Heel: The Role of the Dorsalis Pedis Innervated Free Tissue Transfer. J. Reconstr. Microsurg., 1:201, 1985.
199. Dunet, E., Leyder, P., Devauchelle, B., Levy, B., Oliki, J.M., and Bourquelot, P.: Neurovascular Sequelae Related to the Removal of Forearm Fasciocutaneous Free Flaps With Radial Pedicle: Preliminary Study. Ann. Chir. Plast. Esthet., 35:307–312, 1990.
200. Ecker, J., and Sherman, R.: Soft-Tissue Coverage of the Distal Third of the Leg and Ankle. Orthop. Clin. North Am., 24:481–488, 1993.
201. Edwards, C.C.: Staged Reconstruction of Complex Open Tibial Fractures Using Hoffman External Fixation. Clin. Orthop. Rel. Res., 178:130–161, 1983.
202. Edwards, C.C., and Jaworski, M.F.: Hoffmann External Fixation in Open Tibial Fractures With Tissue Loss. J. Bone Joint Surg. Orthop. Trans., 3:261–262, 1979.
203. Edwards, C.C., Simmons, S.C., Browner, B.D., and Weigel, M.C.: Severe Open Tibial Fractures: Results Treating 202 Injuries with External Fixation. Clin. Orthop. Rel. Res., 230:98–115, 1988.
204. Edwards, P.: Fracture of the Shaft of the Tibia: 492 Consecutive Cases in Adults: Importance of Soft Tissue Injury. Acta Orthop. Scand. Suppl. 76:9–59, 1965.
205. Enneking, W.F., Burchardt, H., Puhl, J.J., and Piotrowski, G.: Physical and Biological Aspects of Repair in Dog Cortical-Bone Transplants. J. Bone Joint Surg., 57A:237–252, 1975.
206. Enneking, W.F., Eady, J.L., and Burchardt, H.: Autogenous Cortical Bone Grafts in the Reconstruction of Segmental Skeletal Defects. J. Bone Joint Surg., 62A:1039–1058, 1980.
207. Enneking, W.F., and Mindell, E.R.: Observations on Massive Retrieved Human Allografts. J. Bone Joint Surg., 73A:1123–1142, 1991.
208. Epps, C.H., Jr.: Principles of Amputation Surgery in Trauma. *In* Evarts, C.M. (ed.): Surgery of the Musculoskeletal System, vol 4, pp. 7—23. New York, Churchill Livingstone, 1983.
209. Epps, C.H., Jr., and Adams, J.P.: Wound Management in Open Fractures. Am. Surg., 27:766–769, 1961.
210. Erol, O.O.: The Transformation of a Free Skin Graft Into a Vascularized Pedicled Flap. Plast. Reconstr. Surg., 58:470–477, 1976.
211. Erol, O.O., and Spira, M.: Development and Utilization of a Composite Island Flap Employing Omentum: Experimental Investigation. Plast. Reconstr. Surg., 65:405–417, 1980.
212. Ersek, R.A., Abell, J.M., Jr., and Calhoon, J.H.: The Island Pedicle Rotation Advancement Gastrocnemius Musculocutaneous Flap for Complete Coverage of the Popliteal Fossa. Ann. Plast. Surg., 12:533–536, 1984.
213. Essex-Lopresti, P.: The Open Wound in Trauma. Lancet, 258:745–751, 1950.
214. Esterhai, J.L., Jr., Pisarello, J., Brighton, C.T., Heppenstall, R.B., Gellman, H., and Goldstein, G.: Adjunctive Hyperbaric Oxygen Therapy in the Treatment of Chronic Refractory Osteomyelitis. J. Trauma, 27:763–768, 1987.
215. Esterhai, J.L., Jr., Pisarello, J., Brighton, C.T., Heppenstall, R.B., Gelman, H., and Goldstein, G.: Treatment of Chronic Refractory Osteomyelitis With Adjunctive Hyperbaric Oxygen. Orthop. Rev., 17:809–815, 1988.
216. Etter, C., Burri, C., Claes, L., Kinzl, L., and Raible, M.: Treatment by External Fixation of Open Fractures Associated With Severe Soft Tissue Damage of the Leg. Clin. Orthop. Rel. Res., 178:80–88, 1983.
217. Falco, N.A., Pribaz, J.J., and Eriksson, E.: Vascularization of Skin Following Implantation of an Arteriovenous Pedicle: Implications in Flap Prefabrication. Microsurgery, 13:249–254, 1992.
218. Fattore, L., and Strauss, R.A.: Hyperbaric Oxygen in the Treatment of Osteoradionecrosis: A Review of Its Use and Efficacy. Oral Surg. Oral Med. Oral Pathol., 63:280–286, 1987.
219. Fayman, M.S., Orak, F., Hugo, B., and Berson, S.D.: The Dis-

tally Based Split Soleus Muscle Flap. Br. J. Plast. Surg., 40:20–26, 1987.
220. Feldman, J.J., Cohen, B.E., and May, J.W., Jr.: The Medial Gastrocnemius Myocutaneous Flap. Plast. Reconstr. Surg., 61:531–539, 1978.
221. Ferreira, M.C., Besteiro, J.M., Monteiro Junior, A.A., and and Zumiotti, A.: Reconstruction of the Foot With Microvascular Free Flaps. Microsurgery, 15:33–36, 1994.
222. Ferreira, M.C., Monteiro, A.A., and Besteiro, J.M.: Free Flaps for Reconstruction of the Lower Extremity. Ann. Plast. Surg., 6:475–481, 1981.
223. Findlay, J.A.: The Motor-cycle Tibia. Injury, 4:75–78, 1972.
224. Fisher, J.: External Oblique Fasciocutaneous Flap for Elbow Coverage. Plast. Reconstr. Surg., 75:51–61, 1985.
225. Fisher, J., Bostwick, J., and Powell, R.W.: Latissimus Dorsi Blood Supply After Thoracodorsal Vessel Division: The Serratus Collateral. Plast. Reconstr. Surg., 72:502–508, 1983.
226. Fisher, J., and Wood, M.B.: Late Necrosis of a Latissimus Dorsi Free Flap. Plast. Reconstr. Surg., 74:274–281, 1984.
227. Fitzgerald, R.H., Jr., Ruttle, P.E., Arnold, P.G., Kelly, P.J., and Irons, G.B.: Local Muscle Flaps in the Treatment of Osteomyelitis. J. Bone Joint Surg., 67:175–185, 1985.
228. Fix, R.J., and Vasconez, L.O.: Fasciocutaneous Flaps in Reconstruction of the Lower Extremity. Clin. Plast. Surg., 18:571–582, 1991.
229. Fogdestam, I., Hamilton, R., and Markhede, G.: Microvascular Osteocutaneous Groin Flap in the Treatment of an Ununited Tibial Fracture With Chronic Osteitis: A Case Report. Acta Orthop. Scand., 51:175–179, 1980.
230. Foster, R.J., Barry, R.J., Holloway, A., and Burney, D.W.I.: A 50-cm Fillet Flap for Preservation of Maximal Lower Extremity Residual Limb Length. Clin. Orthop. Rel. Res., 178:216–219, 1983.
231. Foucher, G., van Genechten, F., Merle, N., and Michon, J.: A Compound Radial Artery Forearm Flap in Hand Surgery: An Original Modification of the Chinese Forearm Flap. Br. J. Plast. Surg., 37:139–148, 1984.
232. Foulkes, G.D., Floyd, W.E., and McLendon, C.L.: Utilization of the Extended Rectus Abdominis Myofasciocutaneous Free Flap in Upper Extremity Reconstruction. J. Hand Surg., 16A:590–593, 1991.
233. Francel, T.J.: Improving Reemployment Rates After Limb Salvage of Acute Severe Tibial Fractures by Microvascular Soft-Tissue Reconstruction. Plast. Reconstr. Surg., 93:1028–1034, 1994.
234. Francel, T.J., VanderKolk, C.A., Hoopes, J.E., Manson, P.N., and Yaremchuk, M.J.: Microvascular Soft-Tissue Transplantation for Reconstruction of Acute Open Tibial Fractures: Timing of Coverage and Long-Term Functional Results. Plast. Reconstr. Surg., 89:478–487, 1992.
235. Freedlander, E., Dickson, W.A., and McGrouther, D.A.: The Present Role of the Groin Flap in Hand Trauma in the Light of a Long-Term Review. J. Hand Surg., 11B:187–190, 1986.
236. Freeland, A.E., and Mutz, S.B.: Posterior Bone-Grafting for Infected Ununited Fracture of the Tibia. J. Bone Joint Surg., 58A:653–657, 1976.
237. Freeman, B.S.: The Results of Epiphyseal Transplants by Flap and by Free Graft: A Brief Survey. Plast. Reconstr. Surg., 36:227–230, 1965.
238. Friedman, J.D., and Sherman, R.: Options for Vascularized Bone Transfer in the Upper Extremity. Prob. Plast. Reconstr. Surg., 3:312–326, 1993.
239. Frykman, G.K., and Leung, V.C.: Free Vascularized Flaps for Lower Extremity Reconstruction. Orthopedics, 9:841–848, 1986.
240. Fujimaki, A., and Yamauchi, Y.: Vascularized Fibular Grafting for Treatment of Aseptic Necrosis of the Femoral Head: Preliminary Results in Four Cases. Microsurgery, 4:17–22, 1983.
241. Fujino, T., and Harashina, T.: Vascularized Free Flap Transfers. Clin. Orthop. Rel. Res., 133:154–157, 1978.
242. Furnas, D.W.: Growth and Development in Replanted Fore Limbs. Plast. Reconstr. Surg., 46:445, 1970.
243. Furnas, D.W., and Anzel, S.H.: Two Consecutive Repairs of the Lower Limb with a Single Gastrocnemius Cross-leg Flap. Plast. Reconstr. Surg., 66:137–140, 1980.
244. Furnas, D.W., and Anzel, S.H.: Two Consecutive Repairs of the Lower Limb with a Single Gastrocnemius Musculocutaneous Cross-leg flap. Plast. Reconstr. Surg., 66:137–140, 1980.
245. Furnas, H., Canales, F., Lineaweaver, W., Buncke, G.M., and Buncke, H.J.: Microsurgical Tissue Transfer in Patients More Than 70 Years of Age. Ann. Plast. Surg., 26:133–139, 1991.
246. Gahhos, F.N., Jaquith, M., and Hidalgo, R.: The Extended Digitorum Brevis Muscle Flap. Ann. Plast. Surg., 23:255–262, 1989.
247. Gahhos, F.N., Tross, R.B., and Salomon, J.C.: Scapular Free-Flap Dissection Made Easier. Plast. Reconstr. Surg., 75:115–118, 1985.
248. Galumbeck, M., and Colen, L.B.: Coverage of Lower Leg: Rotational Flap. Orthop. Clin. North Am., 24:473–480, 1993.
249. Garrett, J.C., and Buncke, H.J., Jr.: Free Groin Flap Transfer for Skin Defects Associated With Orthopaedic Problems of the Extremities. Am. Surg., 45:597–601, 1979.
250. Gaukroger, M.C., Langdon, J.D., Whear, N.M., and Zaki, G.A.: Repair of the Radial Forearm Flap Donor Site With a Full-Thickness Graft. Int. J. Oral Maxillofac. Surg., 23:205–208, 1994.
251. Gayle, L.B., Lineaweaver, W.C., Buncke, G.M., et al.: Lower Extremity Replantation. Clin. Plast. Surg., 18:437–447, 1991.
252. Georgiadis, G.M., Behrens, F.F., Joyce, M.J., Earle, A.S., and Simmons, A.L.: Open Tibial Fractures With Severe Soft-Tissue Loss: Limb Salvage Compared With Below-the-Knee Amputation. J. Bone Joint Surg., 75A:1431–1441, 1993.
253. Ger, R.: The Operative Treatment of the Advanced Stasis Ulcer: A Preliminary Communication. Am. J. Surg., 111:659, 1966.
254. Ger, R.: The Management of Pretibial Skin Loss. Surgery, 63:757–763, 1968.
255. Ger, R.: The Management of Open Fractures of the Tibia With Skin Loss. J. Trauma, 10:112–121, 1970.
256. Ger, R.: The Technique of Muscle Transposition in the Operative Treatment of Traumatic and Ulcerative Lesions of the Leg. J. Trauma, 11:502–510, 1971.
257. Ger, R.: The Surgical Management of Ulcers of the Heel. Surg. Gynecol. Obstet., 140:909, 1975.
258. Ger, R.: Muscle Transposition for Treatment and Prevention of Chronic Post-Traumatic Osteomyelitis of the Tibia. J. Bone Joint Surg., 59A:784–791, 1977.
259. Ger, R., and Efron, G.: New Operative Approach in the Treatment of Chronic Osteomyelitis of the Tibial Diaphysis: A Preliminary Report. Clin. Orthop. Rel. Res., 70:165–169, 1970.
260. Gerwin, M., Rothaus, K.O., Windsor, R.E., Brause, B.D., and Insall, J.N.: Gastrocnemius Muscle Flap Coverage of Exposed or Infected Knee Prostheses. Clin. Orthop. Rel. Res., 286:64–70, 1993.
261. Gerwin, M., and Weiland, A.J.: Vascularized Bone Grafts to the Upper Extremity: Indications and Technique. Hand Clin., 8:509–523, 1992.
262. Ghormley, R.K., and Lipscomb, P.R.: The Use of Untubed Pedicle Grafts in the Repair of Deep Defects of the Foot and Ankle. Technique and Results. J. Bone Joint Surg., 26:483–488, 1944.
263. Gilbert, A.: Vascularized Transfer of the Fibular Shaft. Int. J. Microsurg., 1:100–102, 1979.
264. Gilbert, A.: Free Vascularized Bone Grafts. Int. Surg., 66:27–31, 1981.
265. Gilbert, A., and Teot, L.: The Free Scapula Flap. Plast. Reconstr. Surg., 69:601–604, 1982.
266. Girdlestone, G.R., and Foley, W.B.: Extensive Loss of Tibial Diaphysis: Tibio-fibular Grafting. Br. J. Surg., 20:467–471, 1933.
267. Godina, M.: Discussion: The Free Scapula Flap. Plast. Reconstr. Surg., 69:786–787, 1982.
268. Godina, M.: Early Microsurgical Reconstruction of Complex Trauma of the Extremities. Plast. Reconstr. Surg., 78:285–292, 1986.
269. Godina, M.: The Tailored Latissimus Dorsi Free Flap. Plast. Reconstr. Surg., 80:304–306, 1987.
270. Godina, M.: Wound Care and Timing of Microvascular Flap Transfer to the Lower Leg. *In* Godina, M. (ed.): A Thesis on

the Management of Injuries to the Lower Extremity, pp 77–84. Ljubljana, Presernova Druzba, 1991.

271. Goldberg, J.A., Alpert, B.S., Lineaweaver, W.C., and Buncke, H.J.: Microvascular Reconstruction of the Lower Extremity in the Elderly. Clin. Plast. Surg., 18:459–465, 1991.
272. Goldberg, V.M., Shaffer, J.W., Field, G., and Davy, D.R.: Biology of Vascularized Bone Grafts. Orthop. Clin. North Am., 18:197–205, 1987.
273. Goldberg, V.M., and Stevenson, S.: Natural History of Autografts and Allografts. Clin. Orthop. Rel. Res., 225:7–16, 1987.
274. Goldstrohm, G.L., Mears, D.C., and Swartz, W.M.: The Results of 39 Fractures Complicated by Major Segmental Bone Loss and/or Leg Length Discrepancy. J. Trauma, 24:50–58, 1984.
275. Gopinath, K.S., Chandrashekar, M., Kumar, M.V., and Bhargava, A.: The Scapular Fasciocutaneous Flap: A New Flap for Reconstruction of the Posterior Neck. Br. J. Plast Surg., 46:508–510, 1993.
276. Gordon, D.J., and Small, J.O.: The Addition of Muscle to the Lateral Arm and Radial Forearm Flaps for Wound Coverage. Plast. Reconstr. Surg., 89:563–566, 1992.
277. Gordon, L., Buncke, H.J., and Alpert, B.S.: Free Latissimus Dorsi Muscle Flap With Split-Thickness Skin Graft Cover: A Report of 16 Cases. Plast. Reconstr. Surg., 70:173–178, 1982.
278. Gordon, L., Buncke, H.J., Alpert, B.S., Wilson, C., and Koch, R.A.: Free Vascularized Osteocutaneous Transplant From the Groin for Delayed Primary Closure in the Management of Loss of Soft-Tissue and Bone in the Hand and Wrist: Report of Two Cases. J. Bone Joint Surg. [Am.], 67:958–964, 1985.
279. Gordon, L., and Chiu, E.J.: Treatment of Infected Non-unions and Segmental Defects of the Tibia With Staged Microvascular Muscle Transplantation and Bone-grafting. J. Bone Joint Surg., 70A:377–386, 1988.
280. Gordon, L., Weulker, N., and Jergesen, H.: Vascularized Fibular Grafting for the Treatment of Congenital Pseudarthrosis of the Tibia. Orthopedics, 9:825–832, 1986.
281. Gothman, L.: Arterial Changes in Experimental Fractures of the Rabbit's Tibia Treated With Intramedullary Nailing: A Microangiographic Study. Acta Chir. Scand., 120:289–302, 1960.
282. Gothman, L.: The Arterial Pattern of the Rabbit's Tibia After the Application of an Intramedullary Nail: A Microangiographic Study. Acta Chir. Scand., 120:211–220, 1961.
283. Gottlieb, L.J., Tachmes, L., and Pielet, R.W.: Improved Venous Drainage of the Radial Artery Forearm Free Flap: Use of the Profundus Cubitalis Vein. J. Reconstr. Microsurg., 9:281–4; discussion, 1993.
284. Gotzen, L., and Haas, N.: The Operative Treatment of Tibial Shaft Fractures With Soft Tissue Injuries. *In* Tscherne, H., and Gotzen, L. (eds.): Fractures With Soft Tissue Injuries, pp. 46–74. New York, Springer-Verlag, 1984.
285. Gould, J.S.: The Dorsalis Pedis Island Pedicle Flap for Small Defects of the Foot and Ankle. Orthopedics, 9:867–871, 1986.
286. Gould, J.S.: Management of Soft-Tissue Loss on the Plantar Aspect of the Foot. Instr. Course Lect., 39:121–126, 1990.
287. Govila, A., and Sharma, D.: The Radial Forearm Flap for Reconstruction of the Upper Extremity. Plast. Reconstr. Surg., 86:920–927, 1990.
288. Grabb, W.C., and Argenta, L.C.: The Lateral Calcaneal Artery Skin Flap. (The Lateral Calcaneal Artery, Lesser Saphenous Vein, and Sural Nerve Flap). Plast. Reconstr. Surg., 68:723, 1981.
289. Grace, T.G., and Eversmann, W.W.: The Management of Segmental Bone Loss Associated With Forearm Fractures. J. Bone Joint Surg., 62:1150–1159, 1980.
290. Graf, P., and Biemer, E.: Morbidity of the Groin Flap Transfer: Are We Getting Something for Nothing? Br. J. Plast. Surg., 45:86–88, 1992.
291. Green, S.A.: Septic Nonunion. *In* Uhthoff, H. (ed.): Current Concepts of External Fixation of Fractures, pp. 221–233. New York, Springer-Verlag, 1982.
292. Green, S.A.: Ilizarov External Fixation Technical and Anatomic Considerations. Bull. Hosp. Jt. Dis. Orthop. Inst., 48:28–35, 1988.
293. Green, S.A., and Dlabal, T.A.: The Open Bone Graft for Septic Nonunion. Clin. Orthop. Rel. Res., 180:117–124, 1983.
294. Greenberg, B., LaRossa, D., Lotke, P.A., Murphy, J.B., and Noone, R.B.: Salvage of Jeopardized Total-Knee Prosthesis: The Role of the Gastrocnemius Muscle Flap. Plast. Reconstr. Surg., 83:85–9, 97–9, 1989.
295. Green, T.L., and Beatty, M.E.: Soft Tissue Coverage for Lower-Extremity Trauma: Current Practice and Techniques: A Review. J. Orthop. Trauma, 2:158–173, 1988.
296. Gregory, C.F.: Open Fractures: I. *In* Rockwood, C.A., Jr., and Green, D.P. (eds.): Fractures in Adults, pp. 169–198. Philadelphia, J.B. Lippincott, 1984.
297. Gregory, R.T., Gould, R.J., Peclet, M., et al.: The Mangled Extremity Syndrome (M.E.S.): A Severity Grading System for Multisystem Injury of the Extremity. J. Trauma, 25:1147–1150, 1985.
298. Greminger, R.F., and Leather, R.P.: Knee Salvage Utilizing the Myocutaneous Principle. Plast. Reconstr. Surg., 73:131–136, 1984.
299. Grenga, T.E.: Elbow Joint Salvage With Transverse Rectus Island Flap. Plast. Reconstr. Surg., 85:830–831, 1990.
300. Griffiths, J.C.: Defects in Long Bones From Severe Neglected Osteitis. J. Bone Joint Surg., 50B:813–821, 1968.
301. Gryskiewicz, J.M., Edstrom, L.E., and Dibbell, D.G.: The Gastrocnemius Myocutaneous Flap in Lower-Extremity Injuries. J. Trauma, 24:539–543, 1984.
302. Guba, A.M., Jr.: The Use of Free Vascular Tissue Transfers in Lower Extremity Injuries. Adv. Orthop. Surg., 7:60–68, 1983.
303. Guiga, M., Fourati, M.K., Meherzi, A., Belhassine, H., Nahali, N., and Darghouth, M.: Our Experiences With Pedicled Groin Flaps: Apropos of 80 Cases. Ann. Chir. Main., 7:79–84, 1988.
304. Gumley, G.J., MacLeod, A.M., and Thistlethwaite, S.: Case Report: Total Cutaneous Harvesting From an Amputated Foot: Two Free Flaps Used for Acute Reconstruction. Br. J. Plast. Surg., 40:313, 1987.
305. Guo, F., and Ding, B.F.: Vascularized Free Fibula Graft in Bone Tumors: Report of 3 Cases. Chin. Med. J., 93:745–752, 1980.
306. Guo, F., and Ding, B.F.: Vascularized Free Fibula Transfer in the Treatment of Bone Tumours: Report of Three Cases. Arch. Orthop. Trauma Surg., 98:209–215, 1981.
307. Gustilo, R.B.: Management of Open Fractures: An Analysis of 673 Cases. Minn. Med., 54:185–189, 1971.
308. Gustilo, R.B.: Use of Antimicrobials in the Management of Fractures. Arch. Surg., 114:805–808, 1979.
309. Gustilo, R.B.: Management of Infected Fractures. *In* Sledge, C.B. (ed.): Management of Open Fractures and Their Complications, pp. 133–158. Philadelphia, W.B. Saunders, 1982.
310. Gustilo, R.B.: Management of Infected Nonunion. *In* Sledge, C.B. (ed.): Management of Open Fractures and Their Complications, pp. 159–182. Philadelphia, W.B. Saunders Co., 1982.
311. Gustilo, R.B.: Principles of the Management of Open Fractures. *In* Sledge, C.B. (ed.): Management of Open Fractures and Their Complications, pp. 15–54. Philadelphia, W.B. Saunders, 1982.
312. Gustilo, R.B.: Management of Infected Nonunion. *In* Evarts, C.M. (eds.): Surgery of the Musculoskeletal System, vol 4, pp. 135–151. New York, Churchill Livingstone, 1983.
313. Gustilo, R.B.: Management of Infected Fractures. *In* Evarts, C.M. (ed.): Surgery of the Musculoskeletal System, vol. 4, pp. 105–134. New York: Churchill Livingstone, 1983.
314. Gustilo, R.B.: Management of Chronic Osteomyelitis. *In* Gustilo, R.B., Bruninger, R.P., and Tsukayama, D.T. (eds.): Orthopaedic Infection: Diagnosis and Treatment, pp. 155–165. Philadelphia, W.B. Saunders, 1989.
315. Gustilo, R.B., and Anderson, J.T.: Prevention of Infection in the Treatment of One Thousand and Twenty-Five Open Fractures of Long Bones. J. Bone Joint Surg., 58A:453–458, 1976.
316. Gustilo, R.B., Gruninger, R.P., and Davis, T.: Classification of Type III (Severe) Open Fractures Relative to Treatment and Results. Orthopedics, 10:1781–1788, 1987.
317. Gustilo, R.B., and Mendoza, R.M.: Results of Treatment of 1400 Open Fractures. *In* Gustilo, R.B. (ed.): Management of Open Fractures and Their Complications, pp. 202–208. Philadelphia, W.B. Saunders, 1982.
318. Gustilo, R.B., Mendoza, R.M., and Williams, D.N.: Problems in the Management of Type III (Severe) Open Fractures: A

New Classification of Type III Open Fractures. J. Trauma, 24:742–746, 1984.
319. Gustilo, R.B., Simpson, L., Nixon, R., Ruiz, A., and Indeck, W.: Analysis of 511 Open Fractures. Clin. Orthop. Rel. Res., 66:148–154, 1969.
320. Guyuron, B., Dinner, M.I., Dowden, R.V., and Labandter, H.P.: Muscle Flaps and the Vascular Detour Principle: The Soleus. Ann. Plast. Surg., 8:132–140, 1982.
321. Haddad, R.J., Jr., and Drez, D.: Salvage Procedure for Defects in the Forearm Bones. Clin. Orthop. Rel. Res., 104:183–190, 1974.
322. Hahn, S.B., and Kim, H.K.: Free Groin Flaps in Microsurgical Reconstruction of the Extremity. J. Reconstr. Microsurg., 7:187–95; discus, 1991.
323. Hallock, G.: Severe Lower-Extremity Injury: The Rationale for Microsurgical Reconstruction. Orthop. Rev., 15:77–92, 1986.
324. Hallock, G.G.: Function Preservation With the Soleus Muscle Flap. Orthop. Rev., 14:472–477, 1985.
325. Hallock, G.G.: Distal Lower Leg Local Random Fasciocutaneous Flaps. Plast. Reconstr. Surg., 86:304–311, 1990.
326. Hallock, G.G.: Local Fasciocutaneous Flap Skin Coverage for the Dorsal Foot and Ankle. Foot Ankle, 11:274–281, 1991.
327. Hallock, G.G.: Bipedicled Fasciocutaneous Flaps in the Lower Extremity. Ann. Plast. Surg., 29:397–401, 1992.
328. Hallock, G.G.: Identical Rectus Abdominis Donor-Site Morbidity in Compromised and Healthy Patients. J. Reconstr. Microsurg., 10:339–343, 1994.
329. Hallock, G.G., Rice, D.C., Keblish, P.A., and Arangio, G.A.: Restoration of the Foot Using the Radial Forearm Flap. Ann. Plast. Surg., 20:14–25, 1988.
330. Hamilton, R.B., and Proudman, T.W.: The Radial Forearm—Flexor Carpi Radialis Myocutaneous Flap: Case Report (see Comments). Br. J. Plast. Surg., 45:322–323, 1992.
331. Hamilton, S.G., and Morrison, W.A.: The Scapular Free Flap. Br. J. Plast. Surg., 35:2–7, 1982.
332. Hammarlund, C., and Sundberg, T.: Hyperbaric Oxygen Reduced Size of Chronic Leg Ulcers: A Randomized Double-Blind Study. Plast. Reconstr. Surg., 93:829–33; discussion, 1994.
333. Hammer, H., and Bugyi, I.: Free Transfer of a Lateral Upper Arm Flap. Handchir. Mikrochir. Plast. Chir., 20:20–26, 1988.
334. Hammer, R., Lidman, D., Nettelblad, H., and Ostrup, L.: Team Approach to Tibial Fracture: 37 Consecutive Type III Cases Reviewed After 2–10 years. Acta Orthop. Scand., 63:471–476, 1992.
335. Hampton, O.P., Jr.: Delayed Internal Fixation of Compound Battle Fractures in the Mediterranean Theater of Operations: A Follow-Up Study in the Zone of Interior. Ann. Surg., 123:1–26, 1946.
336. Hampton, O.P., Jr.: Basic Principles in Management of Open Fractures. J.A.M.A., 159:417–419, 1955.
337. Han, C.-S., Wood, M.B., Bishop, A.T., and Cooney, W.P.: Vascularized Bone Transfer. J. Bone Joint Surg., 74A:1441–1449, 1992.
338. Hansen, S.T., Jr.: The Type-IIIC Tibial Fracture: Salvage or Amputation (Editorial). J. Bone Joint Surg., 69A:799–800, 1987.
339. Hansen, S.T., Jr.: Overview of the Severely Traumatized Lower Limb: Reconstruction Versus Amputation. Clin. Orthop. Rel. Res., 243:17–19, 1989.
340. Hanumadass, M., Kagan, R., and Matsuda, T.: Early Coverage of Deep Hand Burns With Groin Flaps. J. Trauma, 27:109–114, 1987.
341. Harashina, T.: Analysis of 200 Free Flaps. Br. J. Plast. Surg., 41:33–36, 1988.
342. Hardaker, W.T., Jr., Ward, W.T., and Goldner, J.L.: External Fixation in the Management of Severe Musculoskeletal Trauma. Orthopedics, 5:437–444, 1981.
343. Harii, K.: Clinical Application of Free Omental Flap Transfer. Clin. Plast. Surg., 5:273–281, 1978.
344. Harii, K.: The Groin Flap. *In* Microvascular Tissue Transfer, pp. 48–57. Tokyo, Igaku-Shoin, 1983.
345. Harii, K., Daniel, R., Finseth, F., and Ferreira, M.C.: Report of the Subcommittee on Microvascular Flaps. J. Hand Surg., 8:734–735, 1983.
346. Harii, K., and Ohmori, K.: Direct Transfer of Large Free Groin Skin Flaps to the Lower Extremity Using Microvascular Anastomoses. Chir. Plast., 3:1–14, 1975.
347. Harii, K., and Ohmori, K.: Free Skin Flap Transfer. Clin. Plast. Surg., 3:111–127, 1976.
348. Harii, K., Ohmori, K., and Sekiguchi, J.: The Free Musculocutaneous Flap. Plast. Reconstr. Surg., 57:294–303, 1976.
349. Harii, K., Ohmori, K., and Torii, S.: Free Gracilis Muscle Transplantation, With Microneurovascular Anastomoses for the Treatment of Facial Paralysis: A Preliminary Report. Plast. Reconstr. Surg., 57:133–143, 1976.
350. Harii, K., Yamada, A., Ishihara, K., Miki, Y., and Itoh, M.: A Free Transfer of Both Latissimus Dorsi and Serratus Anterior Flaps With Thoracodorsal Vessel Anastomoses. Plast. Reconstr. Surg., 70:620–629, 1982.
351. Harmon, P.H.: A Simplified Surgical Approach to the Posterior Tibia for Bone-Grafting and Fibular Transference. J. Bone Joint Surg., 27:496–498, 1945.
352. Harris, P.G., Letrosne, E., Caouette-Laberge, L., and Egerszegi, E.P.: Long-Term Follow-up of Coverage of Weight Bearing Surface of the Foot With Free Muscular Flap in a Pediatric Population. Microsurgery, 15:424–429, 1994.
353. Harrison, D.H.: The Osteocutaneous Free Fibular Graft. J. Bone Joint Surg., 68:804–807, 1968.
354. Harrison, D.H., and Morgan, B.D.: The Instep Island Flap to Resurface Plantar Defects. Br. J. Plast. Surg., 34:315–318, 1981.
355. Harrison, S.H.: Fractures of the Tibia Complicated by Skin Loss. Br. J. Plast. Surg., 21:262–276, 1968.
356. Harrison, S.H., and Saad, M.N.: The Sliding Transposition Flap: Its Application to Leg Defects. Br. J. Plast. Surg., 30:54–58, 1977.
357. Hartrampf, C.R., Jr., Scheflan, M., and Bostwick, J.I.: The Flexor Digitorum Brevis Muscle Island Pedicle Flap: A New Dimension in Heel Reconstruction. Plast. Reconstr. Surg., 66:264–270, 1984.
358. Hartwell, S.W., and Evarts, C.M.: Secondary Coverage of Pretibial Skin Defects: Report of Four Representative Cases. Plast. Reconstr. Surg., 46:39–42, 1970.
359. Harvey, F.J., Hodgkinson, A.H.T., and Harvey, P.M.: Intramedullary Nailing in the Treatment of Open Fractures of the Tibia and Fibula. J. Bone Joint Surg., 57A:909–915, 1975.
360. Hauben, D.J., Smith, A.R., and Sonneveld, G.J.: The Use of the Vastus Lateralis Musculocutaneous Flap for the Repair of Trochanteric Pressure Sores. Ann. Plast. Surg., 10:359, 1983.
361. Haw, C.S., O'Brien, B.C., and Kurata, T.: The Microsurgical Revascularization of Resected Segments of Tibia in the Dog. J. Bone Joint Surg., 60B:266–269, 1978.
362. Hayashi, A., and Maruyama, Y.: The Lateral Genicular Artery Flap. Ann. Plast. Surg., 24:310–317, 1990.
363. Hayashi, A., and Maruyama, Y.: Transiliac and retroperitoneal approach for coverage of sacrogluteal defects with inferiorly based rectus abdominis musculocutaneous flaps. Plast. Reconstr. Surg., 90:1096–1101, 1992.
364. Healy, C., Tiernan, E., Lamberty, B.G.H., and Campbell, R.C.: Rotation Fasciocutaneous Flap Repair of Lower Limb Defects. Plast. Reconstr. Surg., 95:243–251, 1995.
365. Heath, P.M., Jackson, I.T., Cooney, W.P., and Morgan, R.G.: Simultaneous Bilateral Staged Groin Flaps for Coverage of Mutilating Injuries of the Hand. Ann. Plast. Surg., 11:462–468, 1983.
366. Heckman, J.D., and Champine, M.J.: New Techniques in the Management of Foot Trauma. Clin. Orthop. Rel. Res., 105–114, 1989.
367. Helfet, D.L., Howey, T., Sanders, R., and Johansen, K.: Limb Salvage Versus Amputation: Preliminary Results of the Mangled Extremity Severity Score. Clin. Orthop. Rel. Res., 256:80–86, 1990.
368. Hemphill, E.S., Ebert, F.R., and Muench, A.G.: The Medial Gastrocnemius Muscle Flap in the Treatment of Wound Complications Following Total Knee Arthroplasty. Orthopedics, 15:477–480, 1992.
369. Heng, M.C., and Kloss, S.G.: Endothelial Cell Toxicity in Leg

Ulcers Treated With Topical Hyperbaric Oxygen. Am. J. Dermatopathol., 8:403–410, 1986.
370. Hentz, V.R., and Pearl, R.M.: The Irreplaceable Free Flap: I. Skeletal Reconstruction by Microvascular Free Bone Transfer. Ann. Plast. Surg., 10:36–42, 1983.
371. Hentz, V.R., and Pearl, R.M.: Application of Free Tissue Transfers to the Foot. J. Reconstr. Microsurg., 3:309–320, 1987.
372. Heppenstall, R.B., Goodwin, C.W., and Brighton, C.T.: Fracture Healing in the Presence of Chronic Hypoxia. J. Bone Joint Surg., 58A:1153–1156, 1976.
373. Heslop, B.F., Zeiss, I.M., and Nisbet, N.W.: Studies on Transference of Bone: I. A Comparison of Autologous and Homologous Bone Implants With Reference to Osteocyte Survival, Osteogenesis and Host Reaction. Br. J. Exp. Pathol., 441:269–287, 1960.
374. Hicks, J.H.: Amputation in Fractures of the Tibia. J. Bone Joint Surg., 46B:388–392, 1964.
375. Hicks, J.H.: Long-Term Follow-Up of a Series of Infected Fractures of the Tibia. Injury, 7:2–7, 1975.
376. Hidalgo, D.A., and Shaw, W.W.: Reconstruction of Foot Injuries. Clin. Plast. Surg., 13:663–680, 1986.
377. Highsmith, L.S., and Phalen, G.S.: Sideswipe Fractures. Arch. Surg., 52:513–522, 1946.
378. Hill, H., Nahai, F., and Vasconez, L.O.: The Tensor Fascia Lata Myocutaneous Free Flap. Plast. Reconstr. Surg., 61:517–522, 1978.
379. Hing, D.N., Buncke, H.J., and Alpert, B.S.: Applications of the Extensor Digitorum Brevis Muscle for Soft Tissue Coverage. Ann. Plast. Surg., 19:530–537, 1987.
380. Hirayama, T., Suematsu, N., Inoue, K., Baitoh, C., and Takemitsu, Y.: Free Vascularized Bone Grafts in Reconstruction of the Upper Extremity. J. Hand Surg., 10B:169–175, 1985.
381. Hirayama, T., Takemitsu, Y., Atsuta, Y., and Ozawa, K.: Restoration of Elbow Flexion by Complete Latissimus Dorsi Muscle Transposition. J. Hand Surg., 12B:194–198, 1987.
382. Hirn, M., Niinikoski, J., and Lehtonen, O.P.: Effect of Hyperbaric Oxygen and Surgery on Experimental Multimicrobial Gas Gangrene. Eur. Surg. Res., 25:265–269, 1993.
383. Hoaglund, F.T., and States, J.D.: Factors Influencing the Rate of Healing in Tibial Shaft Fractures. Surg. Gynecol. Obstet., 124:71–76, 1967.
384. Hodgkinson, D.J., and Irons, G.B.: Newer Applications of the Cross-Leg Flap. Ann. Plast. Surg., 4:381–390, 1980.
385. Hoehn, J.G., Jacobs, R.L., and Karmody, A.: Replantation of the Foot. Surg. Rounds, 1:53–60, 1978.
386. Holden, C.E.: The Role of Blood Supply to Soft Tissue in the Healing of Diaphyseal Fractures. J. Bone Joint Surg., 54A:993–1000, 1972.
387. Horowitz, J.H., Nichter, L.S., Kenney, J.G., and Morgan, R.F.: Lawnmower Injuries in Children: Lower Extremity Reconstruction. J. Trauma, 25:1138–1146, 1985.
388. Hou, S.M., and Liu, T.K.: Reconstruction of Skeletal Defects in the Femur With 'Two-Strut' Free Vascularized Fibular Grafts. J. Trauma, 33:840–845, 1992.
389. Howe, H.R., Jr., Poole, G.V., Jr., Hansen, K.J., et al.: Salvage of Lower Extremities Following Combined Orthopedic and Vascular Trauma: A Predictive Salvage Index. Am. Surg., 53:205–208, 1987.
390. Hu, C.T., Chang, C.W., Su, K.L., Shen, C.C., and Shen, S. Free Vascularised Bone Graft using Microvascular Technique. Ann. Acad. Med. Singapore, 8:459–464, 1979.
391. Hu, Q., Jiang, Q., Su, G., Shen, J., and Shen, X.: Free Vascularized Bone Graft. Chin. Med. J., 93:753–757, 1980.
392. Huang, C.T., Li, P.H., and Kong, G.T.: Successful Restoration of a Traumatic Amputated Leg. Chin. Med. J, [Engl] 84:641–645, 1965.
393. Huang, G.K., Liu, Z.Z., Shen, Y.L., Hu, R.Q., Miao, H., and Yin, Z.Y.: Microvascular Free Transfer of Iliac Bone Based on the Deep Circumflex Iliac Vessels. J. Microsurg., 2:113–120, 1980.
394. Hubbard, L.F., Herndon, J.H., and Buonanno, A.R.: Free Vascularized Fibula Transfer for Stabilization of the Thoracolumbar Spine: A Case Report. Spine, 10:891–893, 1985.
395. Hudson, D.A., and Millar, K.: The Cross-Leg Flap: Still a Useful Flap in Children. Br. J. Plast. Surg., 45:146–149, 1992.
396. Hueston, J.T., and Gunter, G.S.: Primary Cross-Leg Flaps. Plast. Reconstr. Surg., 40:58–62, 1967.
397. Hunt, T.K., and Halliday, B.: Inflammation in Wounds: From "Laudable Pus" to Primary Repair and Beyond. *In* Hunt, T.K. (ed.): Wound Healing and Wound Infection: Theory and Surgical Practice, pp. 281–293. New York, Appleton-Century-Crofts, 1980.
398. Huntington, T.W.: A Case of Bone Transference: Use of a Segment of Fibula to Supply a Defect in the Tibia. Ann. Surg., 41:249–251, 1905.
399. Hurst, L.C., Mirza, M.A., and Spellman, W.: Vascularized Fibular Graft for Infected Loss of the Ulna: Case Report. J. Hand Surg., 7:498–501, 1982.
400. Hutchinson, J.: The Fate of Experimental Bone Autografts and Homografts. Br. J. Surg., 39:552–561, 1952.
401. Ikuta, Y.: Skeletal Muscle Transplantation in the Severely Injured Upper Extremity. *In* Serafin, D., and Buncke, H.J., Jr. (eds.): Microsurgical Composite Tissue Transplantation, pp. 587–604. St. Louis, C.V. Mosby, 1979.
402. Ikuta, Y.: Vascularized Free Flap Transfer in the Upper Limb. Hand Clin., 1:297–307, 1985.
403. Ikuta, Y., Kubo, T., and Tsuge, K.: Free Muscle Transplantation by Microsurgical Technique to Treat Severe Volkmann's Contracture. Plast. Reconstr. Surg., 58:407–411, 1976.
404. Ikuta, Y., Watari, S., Kawamura, K., et al.: Free Flap Transfers by End-to-Side Arterial Anastomosis. Br. J. Plast. Surg., 28:1–7, 1975.
405. Ilizarov, G.A.: The Tension-Stress Effect on the Genesis and Growth of Tissues: I. The Influence of Stability of Fixation and Soft-Tissue Preservation. Clin. Orthop. Rel. Res., 283:249–281, 1989.
406. Ilizarov, G.A.: The Tension-Stress Effect on the Genesis and Growth of Tissues: II. The Influence of the Rate and Frequency of Distraction. Clin. Orthop. Rel. Res., 239:263–285, 1989.
407. Ilizarov, G.A., and Ledyaev, V.I.: The Classic: The Replacement of Long Tubular Bone Defects by Lengthening Distraction Osteotomy of One of the Fragments. Clin. Orthop. Rel. Res., 280:7–10, 1992.
408. Irons, G.B.: Rectus Abdominus Muscle Flaps for Closure of Osteomyelitis Hip Defects. Ann. Plast. Surg., 11:469–473, 1983.
409. Irons, G.B., Arnold, P.G., Masson, J.K., and Woods, J.E.: Experience With 100 Muscle Flaps. Ann. Plast. Surg., 4:2–6, 1980.
410. Irons, G.B., Fisher, J., and Schmitt, E.H.I.: Vascularized Muscular and Musculocutaneous Flaps for Management of Osteomyelitis. Orthop. Clin. North Am., 15:473–480, 1984.
411. Irons, G.B., Witzke, D.J., Arnold, P.G., and Wood, M.B.: Use of the Omental Free Flap for Soft-Tissue Reconstruction. Ann. Plast. Surg., 11:501–507, 1983.
412. Isenberg, J.S., Nguyen, H., and Salomon, J.: Bilateral Simultaneous Groin Flaps in the Salvage of a Pediatric Blast-Injured Hand. Ann. Plast. Surg., 33:415–417, 1994.
413. Ito, T., Kohno, T., and Kojima, T.: Free Vascularized Fibular Graft. J. Trauma, 24:756–760, 1984.
414. Itoh, Y., Sasaki, T., Ishiguro, T., and Uchinishi, K.: Transfer of Latissimus Dorsi to Replace a Paralysed Anterior Deltoid: A New Technique Using an Inverted Pedicled Graft. J. Bone Joint Surg., 69:647–651, 1987.
415. Iwahira, Y., and Maruyama, Y.: Free ascending scapular flap. Ann. Plast. Surg., 28:565–572, 1992.
416. Jackson, I.T., and Scheker, L.: Muscle and Myocutaneous Flaps on the Lower Limb. Injury, 13:324–330, 1982.
417. Jackson, R.W., and MacNab, I.: Fractures of the Shaft of the Tibia: A Clinical and Experimental Study. Am. J. Surg., 97:543–557, 1959.
418. Jastrzebski, J., and Huber, P.: Reconstruction in Achilles Tendon Rupture and Simultaneous Covering of a Skin and Soft Tissue Defect Using the Myocutaneous Gastrocnemius Sliding Flap. Handchir. Mikrochir. Plast. Chir., 19:281–283, 1987.
419. Jayes, P.H.: Cross-leg Flaps: A Review of Sixty Cases. Br. J. Plast. Surg., 3:1–5, 1950.
420. Jeng, S.F.: Free Composite Groin Flap and Vascularized Exter-

nal Oblique Aponeurosis for Traumatic Avulsion Injuries of the Foot. J. Trauma, 35:71–74, 1993.

421. Jin, Y.T., Cao, H.P., and Chang, T.S.: Clinical Application of the Free Scapular Fascial Flap. Ann. Plast. Surg., 23:170–177, 1989.

422. Johnson, P.E., Harris, G.D., Nagle, D.J., and Lewis, V.L.: The Sural Artery and Vein as Recipient Vessels in Free Flap Reconstruction About the Knee. J. Reconstr Microsurg., 3:233–241, 1987.

423. Jones, B.M., and O'Brien, C.J.: Acute Ischemia of the Hand Resulting From Elevation of a Radial Forearm Flap. Br. J. Plast. Surg., 38:396–397, 1985.

424. Jones, N.F., Eadie, P., Johnson, P.C., and Mears, D.C.: Treatment of Chronic Infected Hip Arthroplasty Wounds by Radical Debridement and Obliteration With Pedicled and Free Muscle Flaps. Plast. Reconstr. Surg., 88:95–101, 1991.

425. Jones, N.F., Swartz, W.M., Mears, D.C., Jupiter, J.B., and Grossman, A.: The Double Barrel: Free Vascularized Fibular Bone Graft. Plast. Reconstr. Surg., 81:378–385, 1988.

426. Jones, R.E., and Cierny, G.C.I.: Management of Complex Open Tibial Fractures with External Skeletal Fixation and Early Myoplasty or Myocutaneous Coverage. Can. J. Surg., 23:242–244, 1980.

427. Judet, H., Judet, J., and Gilbert, A.: Vascular Microsurgery in Orthopaedics. Int. Orthop., 5:61–68, 1981.

428. Judet, P.R., and Patel, A.: Muscle Pedicle Bone Grafting of Long Bones by Osteoperiosteal Decortication. Clin. Orthop. Rel. Res., 87:74–79, 1972.

429. Jupiter, J.B.: Complex Nonunion of the Humeral Diaphysis: Treatment With a Medial Approach, an Anterior Plate, and a Vascularized Fibular Graft. J. Bone Joint Surg., 72A:701–707, 1990.

430. Jupiter, J.B., Bour, C.J., and May, J.W., Jr.: The Reconstruction of Defects in the Femoral Shaft With Vascularized Transfers of Fibular Bone. J. Bone Joint Surg., 69A:365–374, 1987.

431. Jupiter, J.B., Kour, A.K., Palumbo, M.D., and Yaremchuk, M.J.: Limb Reconstruction by Free-Tissue Transfer Combined With the Ilizarov Method. Plast. Reconstr. Surg., 88:943–951, 1991.

432. Jupiter, J.B., Tsai, T.M., and Kleinert, H.E.: Salvage Replantation of Lower Limb Amputations. Plast. Reconstr. Surg., 69:1–8, 1982.

433. Kalb, B.: Medicine—Making Bones as Good as New. Time, January 14:62, 1985.

434. Karkowski, J., and Buncke, H.J.: A Simplified Technique for Free Flap Transfer of Groin Flaps, by Use of a Doppler Probe. Plast. Reconstr. Surg., 55:682–686, 1975.

435. Karlstrom, G., and Olerud, S.: Percutaneous Pin Fixation of Open Tibial Fractures. J. Bone Joint Surg., 57A:915–924, 1975.

436. Kasabian, A.K., Colen, S.R., Shaw, W.W., and Pachter, H.L.: The Role of Microvascular Free Flaps in Salvaging Below-Knee Amputation Stumps: a Review of 22 Cases. J. Trauma, 31:495–500; discu, 1991.

437. Katsaros, J., Gilbert, D., and Russell, R.: The Use of a Combined Latissimus Dorsi-Groin Flap as a Direct Flap for Reconstruction of the Upper Extremity. Br. J. Plast. Surg., 36:67–71, 1983.

438. Katsaros, J., Schusterman, M., Beppu, M., Banis, J.C., Jr., and Acland, R.D.: The Lateral Upper Arm Flap: Anatomy and Clinical Applications. Ann. Plast. Surg., 12:489–500, 1984.

439. Katsaros, J., Tan, E., and Zoltie, N.: The Use of the Lateral Arm Flap in Upper Limb Surgery. J. Hand Surg., 16A:598–604, 1991.

440. Kemp, A.G., van Niekerk, J.L., and van Meurs, P.A.: Impairment Scores of Type III Open Tibial Fractures. Injury, 24:161–162, 1993.

441. Kenmore, P.I., and Garagusi, V.F.: Complications of Musculoskeletal Infections. *In* Epps. C.H., Jr. (ed.): Complications in Orthopaedic Surgery, pp. 179–205. Philadelphia: J.B. Lippincott, 1986.

442. Khashaba, A.A., and MacGregor, I.A.: Haemodynamics of the Radial Forearm Flap. Br. J. Plast. Surg., 39:441–450, 1986.

443. Khoo, C.T., and Bailey, B.N.: The Behaviour of Free Muscle and Musculocutaneous Flaps After Early Loss of Axial Blood Supply. Bri. J. Plast. Surg., 35:43–46, 1982.

444. Khouri, R.K., Upton, J., and Shaw, W.W.: Principles of Flap Prefabrication. Clin. Plast. Surg., 19:763–771, 1992.

445. Klein, L., Stevenson, S., Shaffer, J.W., Davy, D., and Goldberg, V.M.: Bone Mass and Comparative Rates of Bone Resorption and Formation of Fibular Autografts: Comparison of Vascular and Nonvascular Grafts in Dogs. Bone, 12:323–329, 1991.

446. Kleinert, H.E.: Bone and Osteocutaneous Microvascular Free Flaps. J. Hand Surg., 8A:735–737, 1983.

447. Kleinman, W.B., and Dustman, J.A.: Preservation of Function Following Complete Degloving Injuries to the Hand: Use of Simultaneous Groin Flap, Random Abdominal Flap, and Partial-Thickness Skin Graft. J. Hand Surg., 6A:82–89, 1981.

448. Kleinman, W.B., and O'Connell, S.J.: Effects of the Fasciocutaneous Radial Forearm Flap on Vascularity of the Hand. J. Hand Surg., 18A:953–958, 1993.

449. Kline, S.C., Hotchkiss, R.N., and Randolph, M.A.: Study of Growth Kinetics and Morphology in Limbs Transplanted Between Animals of Different Ages. Plast. Reconstr. Surg., 85:273, 1990.

450. Kojima, T., Kohno, T., and Ito, T.: Muscle Flap With Simultaneous Mesh Skin Graft for Skin Defects of the Lower Leg. J. Trauma, 19:724–729, 1979.

451. Koman, L.A.: Free Flaps for Coverage of the Foot and Ankle. Orthopedics, 9:857–862, 1986.

452. Koman, L.A., Pospisil, R.F., Nunley, J.A., and Urbaniak, J.R.: Value of Contrast Arteriography in Composite Tissue Transfer. Clin. Orthop. Rel. Res., 172:195–206, 1983.

453. Koshima, I., and Soeda, S.: Repair of a Wide Defect of the Lower Leg With the Combined Scapular and Parascapular Flap. Br. J. Plast. Surg., 38:518–521, 1985.

454. Koshima, I., Soeda, S., Nakayama, Y., and Ishii, M.: A Combined Rectus Abdominis Musculocutaneous Flap and Vascularized Iliac Bone Graft With Double Vascular Pedicles. Plast. Reconstr. Surg., 88:492–496, 1991.

455. Krag, C., Hesselfeldt-Nielsen, J., and Gothgen, I.: Late Patency of Clinical Microvascular Anastomoses to Free Composite Tissue Transplants: II. Hemodynamic Aspects. Scand. J. Plast. Reconstr. Surg., 19:73–79, 1985.

456. Krag, C., and Lavendt, E.: Late Patency of Clinical Microvascular Anastomoses to Free Composite Tissue Transplants: I. Angiographical Aspects. Scand. J. Plast. Reconstr. Surg., 19:65–72, 1985.

457. Kroll, S.S.: Radical Thinning of the Pedicle of a Gastrocnemius Musculocutaneous Flap. Ann. Plast. Surg., 23:363–368, 1989.

458. Kroll, S.S., and Marcadis, A.: Aesthetic Considerations of the Medial Gastrocnemius Myocutaneous Flap. Plast. Reconstr. Surg., 79:67–71, 1987.

459. Kubo, T., Ikuta, Y., and Tsuge, K.: Free Muscle Transplantation in Dogs by Microneurovascular Anastomoses. Plast. Reconstr. Surg., 57:495–501, 1976.

460. Kumar, V.P., Satku, K., Helm, R., and Pho, R.W.: Radial Reconstruction in Segmental Defects of Both Forearm Bones. J. Bone Joint Surg., 70B:815–817, 1988.

461. Kutz, J.E., and Thomson, C.B.: Free Vascularized Bone Grafts. *In* Urbaniak, J. R. (ed.): Symposium on Microsurgery: Practical Use in Orthopaedics, pp. 254–278. St. Louis, C.V. Mosby, 1979.

462. Lagvankar, S.P.: Distally-Based Random Fasciocutaneous Flaps for Multi-staged Reconstruction of Defects in the Lower Third of the Leg, Ankle and Heel. Br. J. Plast. Surg., 43:541–545, 1990.

463. Lai, M.F., Krishna, B.V., and Pelly, A.D.: The Brachioradialis Myocutaneous Flap. Br. J. Plast. Surg., 34:431–434, 1981.

464. Laitung, J.K., and Batchelor, A.G.: Successful Preexpansion of a Free Scapular Flap. Ann. Plast. Surg., 25:205–207, 1990.

465. Laitung, J.K.G., and Peck, F.: Shoulder Function Following the Loss of the Latissimus Dorsi Muscle. Br. J. Plast. Surg., 38:375–379, 1985.

466. Lambert, C.N.: Amputation Surgery in the Child. Orthop. Clin. North Am., 3:473–482, 1972.

467. Lamberty, B.G., and Cormack, G.C.: Fasciocutaneous Flaps. Clin. Plast. Surg., 17:713–726, 1990.

468. Lancaster, S.J., Horowitz, M., and Alonso, J.: Open Tibial Fractures: Management and Results. South. Med. J., 79:39, 1986.
469. Landi, A., Soragni, O., and Monteleone, M.: The Extensor Digitorum Brevis Muscle Island Flap for Soft-Tissue Loss Around the Ankle. Plast. Reconstr. Surg., 75:892, 1985.
470. Landra, A.P.: The Latissimus Dorsi Musculocutaneous Flap Used to Resurface a Defect on the Upper Arm and Restore Extension to the Elbow. Br. J. Plast. Surg., 32:275–277, 1979.
471. Lange, R.H.: Limb Reconstruction Versus Amputation Decision Making in Massive Lower Extremity Trauma. Clin. Orthop. Rel. Res., 243:92–99, 1989.
472. Lange, R.H., Bach, A.W., Hansen, S.R., Jr., and Johansen, K.H.: Open Tibial Fractures With Associated Vascular Injuries: Prognosis for Limb Salvage. J. Trauma, 25:203–208, 1985.
473. LaRossa, D., Mellissinos, E., Matthews, D., and Hamilton, R.: The Use of Microvascular Free Skin-Muscle Flaps in Management of Avulsion Injuries of the Lower Leg. J. Trauma, 20:545–550, 1980.
474. Lau, R.S.F., and Leung, P.C.: Bone Graft Viability in Vascularized Bone Graft Transfer. Br. J. Radiol., 55:325–329, 1982.
475. Laughlin, R.T., Smith, K.L., Russell, R.C., and Hayes, J.M.: Late Functional Outcome in Patients With Tibia Fractures Covered With Free Muscle Flaps. J. Orthop. Trauma, 7:123–129, 1993.
476. LaVan, F.B., and Hunt, T.K.: Oxygen and Wound Healing. Clin. Plast. Surg., 17:463–472, 1990.
477. Lawyer, R.B., Jr., and Lubbers, L.M.: Use of the Hoffman Apparatus in the Treatment of Unstable Tibial Fractures. J. Bone Joint Surg., 62A:1264–1273, 1980.
478. Lazar, E., Rosenthal, D.I., and Jupiter, J.: Free Vascularized Fibular Grafts: Radiographic Evidence of Remodeling and Hypertrophy. A.J.R., 161:613–615, 1993.
479. Lazarou, S.A., and Kaplan, I.B.: The Lateral Arm Flap for Elbow Coverage. Plast. Reconstr. Surg., 91:1349–1354, 1993.
480. Leach, R.E.: Fractures of the Tibia and Fibula. *In* Rockwood, C.A., Jr., and Green, D.P. (eds.): Fractures in Adults, pp. 1593–1663. Philadelphia, J.B. Lippincott, 1984.
481. Lee, C.K., and Rehmatullah, N.: Muscle-Pedicle Bone Graft and Cancellous Bone Graft for the "Silent Hip" of Idiopathic Ischemic Necrosis of the Femoral Head in Adults. Clin. Orthop. Rel. Res., 158:185–194, 1981.
482. Legre, R., Kevorkian, B., and Magalon, G.: Analysis of Sequelae Secondary to the Radial Forearm Flap: A Study of Twenty-Six Cases. Ann. Chir. Main, 5:208–212, 1986.
483. Lembert, C.N.: Amputation Surgery in the Child. Orthop. Clin. North Am., 3:473–482, 1972.
484. Lentz, M.W., Noyes, F.R., and Neale, H.W.: Muscle Flap Transposition for Traumatic Soft Tissue Defects of the Lower Extremity. Clin. Orthop. Rel. Res., 143:200–210, 1979.
485. Lesavoy, M.A.: Successful Replantation of Lower Leg and Foot, With Good Sensibility and Function. Plast. Reconstr. Surg., 64:760–765, 1979.
486. Leung, P.C., Hung, L.K., and Leung, K.S.: Use of the Medial Plantar Flap in Soft Tissue Replacement Around the Heel Region. Foot Ankle, 8:327–330, 1988.
487. Lewis, V.L., Jr., Mossie, R.D., Stulberg, D.S., Bailey, M.H., and Griffith, B.H.: The Fasciocutaneous Flap: a Conservative Approach to the Exposed Knee Joint. Plast. Reconstr. Surg., 85:252–257, 1990.
488. Li, Z., Liu, K., Lin, Y., and Li, L.: Lateral Sural Cutaneous Artery Island Flap in the Treatment of Soft Tissue Defects at the Knee. Br. J. Plast. Surg., 43:546–550, 1990.
489. Liang, M.D., Swartz, W.M., and Jones, N.F.: Local Full-Thickness Skin-Graft Coverage for the Radial Forearm Flap Donor Site. Plast. Reconstr. Surg., 93:621–625, 1994.
490. Lin, S.D., Lai, C.S., and Chiu, C.C.: Venous Drainage in the Reverse Forearm Flap. Plast. Reconstr. Surg., 74:508–512, 1984.
491. Linton, P.C.: The Combined Medial and Lateral Gastrocnemius Musculocutaneous V-Y Island Advancement Flap. Plast. Reconstr. Surg., 70:490–493, 1982.
492. Lister, G.D.: Letter #1989-41. A.S.S.H. Newsl., April:130–140, 1989.
493. Liu, X.Y., Ge, B.F., Win, Y.M., and Jing, H.: Free Medial Gastrocnemius Myocutaneous Flap Transfer With Neurovascular Anastomosis to Treat Volkmann's Contracture of the Forearm (see Comments). Br. J. Plast. Surg., 45:6–8, 1992.
494. Logan, A.M., and Black, M.J.M.: Injury to the Brachial Plexus Resulting From Shoulder Positioning During Latissimus Dorsi Flap Pedicle Dissection. Br. J. Plast. Surg., 38:380–382, 1985.
495. Lottes, J.O., Hill, L.J., and Key, J.A.: Closed Reduction, Plate Fixation, and Medullary Nailing of Fractures of Both Bones of the Leg: A Comparative End-Result Study. J. Bone Joint Surg., 34A:861–877, 1952.
496. Lowe, H.G.: Radio-ulnar Fusion for Defects in the Forearm Bones. J. Bone Joint Surg., 45B:351–359, 1962.
497. Lucas, K., Fitzgibbon, G.M., and Evans, E.M.: Discussion on Amputation in Relation to Severe Compound Fractures of the Tibia. J. Bone Joint Surg., 39B:158, 1957.
498. MacKinnon, S.E., Weiland, A.J., and Godina, M.: Immediate Forearm Reconstruction With a Functional Latissimus Dorsi Island Pedicle Myocutaneous Flap. Plast. Reconstr. Surg., 71:706–710, 1983.
499. MacNab, I. and De Haas, W.G. The Role of Periosteal Blood Supply in the Healing of Fractures of the Tibia. Clin. Orthop. Rel. Res., 105:27–33, 1974.
500. Magee, H.R., and Parker, W.R.: Replantation of the Foot: Results After Two Years. Med. J. Aust., 1:751–755, 1972.
501. Malawer, M.M., and Price, W.M.: Gastrocnemius Transposition Flap in Conjunction With Limb-Sparing Surgery for Primary Bone Sarcomas Around the Knee. Plast. Reconstr. Surg., 73:741–750, 1984.
502. Man, D., and Acland, R.D.: The Microarterial Anatomy of the Dorsalis Pedis Flap and Its Clinical Applications. Plast. Reconstr. Surg., 65:419–423, 1980.
503. Manchot, C.: The Cutaneous Arteries of the Human Body. New York: Springer-Verlag, 1983.
504. Manfrini, M., Capanna, R., Caldora, P., and Gaiani, L.: Gastrocnemius Flaps in the Surgical Treatment of Sarcomas of the Knee. Chir. Organi. Mov., 78:95–104, 1993.
505. Mankin, H.K., Doppelt, S., and Tomford, W.: Clinical Experience With Allograft Implantation: The First Ten Years. Clin. Orthop. Rel. Res., 174:69–86, 1983.
506. Manktelow, R.T.: Free Muscle Transfers. *In* Green, D.P. (ed.): Operative Hand Surgery, pp.1215–1244. New York, Churchill Livingstone, 1988.
507. Manktelow, R.T., and McKee, N.H.: Free Muscle Transplantation to Provide Active Finger Flexion. J. Hand Surg., 3:416–426, 1978.
508. Manktelow, R.T., McKee, N.H., and Vettese, T.: An Anatomical Study of the Pectoralis Major Muscle as Related to Functioning Free Muscle Transplantation. Plast. Reconstr. Surg., 65:610–615, 1980.
509. Manktelow, R.T., and Zuker, R.M.: The Principles of Functioning Muscle Transplantation: Applications to the Upper Arm. Ann. Plast. Surg., 22:275–281, 1989.
510. Manktelow, R.T., Zuker, R.M., and McKee, N.H.: Functioning Free Muscle Transplantation. J. Hand Surg., 9:32–39, 1984.
511. Maruyama, Y.: Ascending Scapular Flap and its Use for the Treatment of Axillary Burn Scar Contracture. Br. J. Plast. Surg., 44:97–101, 1991.
512. Maruyama, Y., and Iwahira, Y.: Popliteo-posterior Thigh Fasciocutaneous Island Flap for Closure Around the Knee. Br. J. Plast. Surg., 42:140–3; discussion, 1989.
513. Maruyama, Y., Onishi, K., Iwahira, Y., Okajima, Y., and Motegi, M.: Free Compound Rib–Latissimus Dorsi Osteomusculocutaneous Flap in Reconstruction of the Leg. J. Reconstr. Microsurg., 3:8–13, 1986.
514. Masquelet, A.C., Beveridge, J., Romana, C., and Gerber, C.: The Lateral Supramalleolar Flap. Plast. Reconstr. Surg., 81:74–81, 1988.
515. Masquelet, A.C., Rinaldi, S., Mouchet, A., and Gilbert, A.: The Posterior Arm Free Flap. Plast. Reconstr. Surg., 76:908–913, 1985.
516. Masser, M.R.: The Preexpanded Radial Free Flap (see Comments). Plast. Reconstr. Surg., 86:295–301; discussion, 1990.
517. Massin, P., Romana, C., and Masquelet, A.C.: Anatomic Basis of a Pedicled Extensor Digitorum Brevis Muscle Flap. Surg. Radiol. Anat., 10:267–272, 1988.

518. Mathes, S., and Nahai, F.: Clinical Application for Muscle and Musculocutaneous Flaps. St. Louis, C.V. Mosby, 1982.
519. Mathes, S.J.: The Muscle Flap for Management of Osteomyelitis. N. Engl. J. Med., 306:294–295, 1982.
520. Mathes, S.J., Alpert, B.S., and Chang, N.: Use of Muscle Flap in Chronic Osteomyelitis: Experimental and Clinical Correlation. Plast. Reconstr. Surg., 69:815–829, 1982.
521. Mathes, S.J., Feng, L.J., and Hunt, T.K.: Coverage of the Infected Wound. Ann. Surg., 198:420–429, 1983.
522. Mathes, S.J., and Hurwitz, D.J.: Repair of Chronic Radiation Wounds of the Pelvis. World J. Surg., 10:269–280, 1986.
523. Mathes, S.J., McCraw, J.B., and Vasconez, L.O.: Muscle Transposition Flaps for Coverage of Lower Extremity Defects—Anatomic Considerations. Surg. Clin. North Am., 54:1337–1354, 1974.
524. Mathes, S.J., and Nahai, F.: Clinical Atlas of Muscle and Musculocutaneous Flaps. St. Louis, C.V. Mosby, 1979.
525. Mathes, S.J., and Nahai, F: Classification of the Vascular Anatomy of Muscles: Experimental and Clinical Correlation. Plast. Reconstr. Surg., 67:177–187, 1981.
526. Mathes, S.J., and Nahai, F.: Muscle and Musculocutaneous Flaps. *In* Goldwyn, R. (ed.): The Unfavorable Result in Plastic Surgery: Avoidance and Treatment, pp. 99–122. Boston, Little, Brown & Co, 1984.
527. Mathes, S.J., Nahai, F., and Vasconez, L.O.: Myocutaneous Free-Flap Transfer: Anatomical and Experimental Considerations. Plast. Reconstr. Surg., 62:162–166, 1978.
528. Mathes, S.J., Vasconez, L.O., and Jurkiewicz, M.J.: Extension and Further Application of Muscle Flap Transposition. Plast. Reconstr. Surg., 60:6, 1977.
529. Mathoulin, C., Gilbert, A., and Azze, R.G.: Congenital Pseudarthrosis of the Forearm: Treatment of Six Cases With Vascularized Fibular Graft and a Review of the Literature. Microsurgery, 14:252–259, 1993.
530. Matthews, R.N., Fatah, F., Davies, D.M., Eyre, J., Hodge, R.A., and Walsh-Waring, G.P.: Experience With the Radial Forearm Flap in 14 Cases. Scand. J. Plast. Reconstr. Surg., 18:303–310, 1984.
531. Mavili, M.E., Erk, Y., and Gursu, G.: Use of a Subfascial Pocket on the Contralateral Calf for Salvage of an Avulsed Foot. Plast. Reconstr. Surg., 92:147–150, 1993.
532. Maxwell, G.P., and Hoopes, J.E.: Management of Compound Injuries of the Lower Extremity. Plast. Reconstr. Surg., 63:176–185, 1979.
533. Maxwell, G.P., Manson, P.N., and Hoopes, J.E.: Experience With Thirteen Latissimus Dorsi Myocutaneous Free Flaps. Plast. Reconstr. Surg., 64:1–8, 1979.
534. May, J.W., Jr., Gallico, G.G., and Lukash, F.N.: Microvascular Transfer of Free Tissue for Closure of Bone Wounds of the Distal Lower Extremity. N. Engl. J. Med., 306:253–257, 1982.
535. May, J.W., Jr., Gallico, G.G.I., Jupiter, J., and Savage, R.C.: Free Latissimus Dorsi Muscle Flap With Skin Graft for Treatment of Traumatic Chronic Bony Wounds. Plast. Reconstr. Surg., 73:6411–649, 1984.
536. May, J.W., Jr., Halls, M.J., and Simon, S.R.: Free Microvascular Muscle Flaps With Skin Graft Reconstruction of Extensive Defects of the Foot: A Clinical and Gait Analysis Study. Plast. Reconstr. Surg., 75:627–639, 1985.
537. May, J.W., Jr., Jupiter, J.B., Weiland, A.J., and Byrd, H.S.: Clinical Classification of Post-Traumatic Tibial Osteomyelitis. J. Bone Joint Surg., 71A:1422–1428, 1989.
538. May, J.W., Jr., Lukash, F.N., and Gallico, G.G.: Latissimus Dorsi Free Muscle Flap in Lower Extremity Reconstruction. Plast. Reconstr. Surg., 68:603–607, 1981.
539. Mayou, B.J., Whitby, D., and Jones, B.M.: The Scapular Flap—An Anatomical and Clinical Study. Br. J. Plast. Surg., 35:8–13, 1982.
540. McAndrew, M.P., and Lantz, B.A.: Initial Care of Massively Traumatized Lower Extremities. Clin. Orthop. Rel. Res., 243:20–29, 1989.
541. McCraw, J.B.: Selection of Alternative Local Flaps in the Leg and Foot. Clin. Plast. Surg., 6:227–246, 1979.
542. McCraw, J.B., Dibbell, D.G., and Carraway, J.H.: Clinical Definition of Independent Myocutaneous Vascular Territories. Plast. Reconstr. Surg., 60:341–352, 1977.
543. McCraw, J.B., Fishman, J.H., and Sharzer, L.A.: The Versatile Gastrocnemius Myocutaneous Flap. Plast. Reconstr. Surg., 62:15–23, 1978.
544. McCraw, J.B., and Furlow, L.T., Jr.: The Dorsalis Pedis Arterialized Flap: A Clinical Study. Plast. Reconstr. Surg., 55:177–185, 1975.
545. McCraw, J.B., Myers, B., and Shanklin, K.D.: The Value of Fluorescein in Predicting the Viability of Arterialized Flaps. Plast. Reconstr. Surg., 60:710–719, 1977.
546. McGregor, I.A., and Jackson, I.T.: The Groin Flap. Br. J. Plast. Surg., 25:3–16, 1972.
547. McGrouther, D.A., and Sully, L.: Degloving Injuries of the Limbs: Long-Term Review and Management Based on Whole-Body Fluorescence. Br. J. Plast. Surg., 33:9–24, 1980.
548. McHugh, M., and Prendiville, J.B.: Muscle Flaps in the Repair of Skin Defects over the Exposed Tibia. Br. J. Plast. Surg., 28:205–209, 1975.
549. McKee, N.H., Haw, P., and Vettese, T.: Anatomic Study of the Nutrient Foramen in the Shaft of the Fibula. Clin. Orthop. Rel. Res., 184:141–144, 1984.
550. McMaster, P.E., and Hohl, M.: Tibiofibular Cross-peg Grafting: A Salvage Procedure for Complicated Ununited Tibial Fractures. J. Bone Joint Surg., 47A:1146–1158, 1965.
551. McNamara, M.G., Heckman, J.D., and Corley, F.G.: Severe Open Fractures of the Lower Extremity: A Retrospective Evaluation of the Mangled Extremity Severity Score (MESS). J. Orthop. Trauma, 8:81–87, 1994.
552. Meals, R.A.: The Use of a Flexor Carpi Ulnaris Muscle Flap in the Treatment of an Infected Nonunion of the Proximal Ulna: A Case Report. Clin. Orthop. Rel. Res., 240:168–172, 1989.
553. Meland, B., Arnold, P.G., and Weiss, H.C.: Management of the Recalcitrant Total-Hip Arthroplasty Wound. Plast. Reconstr. Surg., 88:681–685, 1991.
554. Meland, N.B., Clinkscales, C.M., and Wood, M.B.: Pedicled Radial Forearm Flaps for Recalcitrant Defects About the Elbow. Microsurgery, 12:155–159, 1991.
555. Meland, N.B., Core, G.B., and Hoverman, V.R.: The Radial Forearm Flap Donor Site: Should We Vein Graft the Artery? A Comparative Study. Plast. Reconstr. Surg., 91:865–70; discussion, 1993.
556. Meland, N.B., Lincenberg, S.M., Cooney, W.P., Wood, M.B., and Hentz, V.R.: Experience With the Island Radial Forearm Flap in Local Hand Coverage. J. Trauma, 29:489–493, 1989.
557. Meland, N.B., Loessin, S.J., Thimsen, D., and Jackson, I.T.: Tissue Expansion in the Extremities Using External Reservoirs. Ann. Plast. Surg., 29:36–39, 1992.
558. Meland, N.B., Maki, S., Chao, E.Y., and Rademaker, B.: The Radial Forearm Flap: A Biomechanical Study of Donor-Site Morbidity Utilizing Sheep Tibia. Plast. Reconstr. Surg., 90:763–773, 1992.
559. Meltzer, T., and Myers, B.: The Effect of Hyperbaric Oxygen on the Bursting Strength and Rate of Vascularization of Skin Wounds in the Rat. Am. Surg., 52:659–662, 1986.
560. Meyerding, H.W., and Cherry, J.H.: Tibial Defects with Nonunion Treated by Transference of the Fibula and Tibiofibular Fusion. Am. J. Surg., 52:397–404, 1941.
561. Meyers, M.H.: The Role of Posterior Bone Grafts (Muscle-Pedicle) in Femoral Neck Fractures. Clin. Orthop. Rel. Res., 152:143–146, 1980.
562. Milanov, N.O., and Adamyan, R.T.: Functional Results of Microsurgical Reconstruction of Plantar Defects. Ann. Plast. Surg., 32:52–56, 1994.
563. Millard, D.R., Jr., and Ortiz, A.C.: Correction of Severe Elbow Contractures. J. Bone Joint Surg., 47A:1347–1354, 1965.
564. Miller, R.C., and Phalen, G.S.: The Repair of Defects of the Radius With Fibular Bone Grafts. J. Bone Joint Surg., 29:629–636, 1947.
565. Minami, A., Kaneda, K., Itoga, H., and Usui, M.: Free Vascularized Fibular Grafts. J. Reconstr. Microsurg., 5:37–43, 1989.
566. Minami, A., Usui, M., Ogino, T., and Minami, M.: Simultaneous Reconstruction of Bone and Skin Defects by Free Fibular Graft With a Skin Flap. Microsurgery, 7:38–45, 1986.

567. Mir y Mir, L.: Functional Graft of the Heel. Plast. Reconstr. Surg., 14:444–450, 1954.
568. Mixter, R., Wood, W.A., and Dibbell, D.G.: Retroperitoneal Transposition of the Rectus Abdominis Myocutaneous Flaps to the Perineum and Back. Plast. Reconstr. Surg., 85:437–441, 1990.
569. Miyamoto, Y., Ikuta, Y., Shigeki, S., and Yamura, M.: Current Concepts of Instep Island Flap. Ann. Plast. Surg., 19:97–102, 1987.
570. Mladick, R.A., Pickrell, K.L., Thorne, F.L., and Royer, J.R.: Ipsilateral Thigh Flap for Total Plantar Resurfacing: Case Report. Plast. Reconstr. Surg., 43:198–200, 1969.
571. Moghari, A., Emami, A., Sheen, R., and O'Brien, B.M.: Lower Limb Reconstruction in Children Using Expanded Free Flaps. Br. J. Plast. Surg., 42:649–652, 1989.
572. Moon, H.K., and Taylor, G.I.: The Vascular Anatomy of Rectus Abdominis Musculocutaneous Flaps Based on the Deep Superior Epigastric System. Plast. Reconstr. Surg., 82:815–832, 1988.
573. Moore, J.R., and Weiland, A.J.: Free Vascularized Bone and Muscle Flaps for Osteomyelitis. Orthopedics, 9:819–824, 1986.
574. Moore, J.R., Weiland, A.J., and Daniel, R.K.: Use of Free Vascularized Bone Grafts in the Treatment of Bone Tumors. Clin. Orthop. Rel. Res., 175:37–44, 1983.
575. Morain, W.D.: Soft-Tissue Reconstruction of Below-Knee Defects. Am. J. Surg., 139:495–502, 1980.
576. Morain, W.D.: Flaps of the Latissimus Dorsi Muscle in Difficult Wounds of the Trunk and Arm. Am. J. Surg., 145:520–525, 1983.
577. Morandi, M., Zembo, M.M., and Ciotti, M.: Infected Tibial Pseudarthrosis. A 2-Year Follow Up on Patients Treated by the Ilizarov Technique. Orthopedics, 12:497–508, 1989.
578. Morley, G.H.: Application of Plastic Surgery to the Care of the Injured. Br. Med. J., 1:823–827, 1966.
579. Morris, D.J., and Pribaz, J.J.: Transtibial Transposition of Gastrocnemius Muscle and Musculocutaneous Flaps. Br. J. Plast. Surg., 45:59–61, 1992.
580. Morrison, W.A., Crabb D.M., O'Brien, B.M., and Jenkins, A.: The Instep of the Foot as a Fasciocutaneous Island and as a Free Flap for Heel Defects. Plast. Reconstr. Surg., 72:56–63, 1983.
581. Morrison, W.A., O'Brien, B.M., and MacLeod, A.M.: Major Limb Replantation. Orthop. Clin. North Am., 8:343–348, 1977.
582. Morrison, W.A., O'Brien, B.M., and MacLeod, A.: Clinical Experiences in Free Flap Transfer. Clin. Orthop. Rel. Res., 133:132–139, 1978.
583. Moscona, A.R., Govrin-Yehudain, J., and Hirshowitz, B.: The Island Fasciocutaneous Flap: A New Type of Flap for Defects of the Knee. Br. J. Plast. Surg., 38:512–514, 1985.
584. Moscona, A.R., and Hirshowitz, B.: Meralgia Paresthetica as a Complication of the Groin Flap. Ann. Plast. Surg., 4:161–163, 1980.
585. Moscona, A.R., Keret, D., and Reis, N.D.: The Gastrocnemius Muscle Flap in the Correction of Severe Flexion Contracture of the Knee. Arch. Orthop. Trauma Surg., 100:139–142, 1982.
586. Moss, A.L., Waterhouse, N., and Townsend, P.: Free Vascularized Fibular Graft to Reconstruct Early a Traumatic Humeral Defect. Injury, 16:41–46, 1984.
587. Muhlbauer, W., Herndl, E., and Stock, W.: The Forearm Flap. Plast. Reconstr. Surg., 70:336–342, 1982.
588. Muhr, G.: Early Complications of Fractures with Soft Tissue Injuries. *In* Tscherne, H., and Gotzen, L. (eds.): Fractures with Soft Tissue Injuries, pp. 131–138. New York, Springer-Verlag, 1984.
589. Murray, R.A.: The One-Bone Forearm: A Reconstructive Procedure. J. Bone Joint Surg., 37A:366–370, 1955.
590. Naggar, L., Chevalley, F., Blanc, C.H., and Livio, J.J.: Treatment of Large Bone Defects With the Ilizarov technique. J. Trauma, 34:390–393, 1993.
591. Nahai, F., Hill, H., and Hester, T.R.: Experiences With the Tensor Fascia Lata Flap. Plast. Reconstr. Surg., 63:788–799, 1979.
592. Nassif, T.M., Vidal, L., Bovet, J.L., and Baudet, J.: The Parascapular Flap: A New Cutaneous Microsurgical Free Flap. Plast. Reconstr. Surg., 69:591–600, 1982.
593. Neale, H.W., Stern, P.J., Kreilein, J.G., Gregory, R.O., and Webster, K.L.: Complications of Muscle-Flap Transposition for Traumatic Defects of the Leg. Plast. Reconstr. Surg., 72:512–515, 1983.
594. Nesmith, R.L., Marks, M.W., DeFranzo, A.J., and Meredith, W.: Inferiorly Based Rectus Abdominis Flaps in Critically Ill and Injured Patients. Ann. Plast. Surg., 30:35–40, 1993.
595. Nettelblad, H., Randolph, M.A., and Weiland, A.J.: Free Microvascular Epiphyseal Plate Transplantation: An Experimental Study in Dogs. J. Bone Joint Surg., 66A:1421–1429, 1984.
596. Niazi, Z.B., McLean, N.R., and Black, M.J.: The Radial Forearm Flap: A Reconstructive Chameleon. J. Reconstr. Microsurg., 10:299–304, 1994.
597. Nicoll, E.A.: The Treatment of Gaps in Long Bones by Cancellous Insert Grafts. J. Bone Joint Surg., 38B:70–82, 1956.
598. Nicoll, E.A.: Fractures of the Tibial Shaft: A Survey of 705 Cases. J. Bone Joint Surg., 46B:373–387, 1964.
599. Niinikoski, J., and Hunt, T.K.: Oxygen Tensions in Healing Bone. Surg. Gynecol. Obstet. 134:746–750, 1972.
600. Noellert, R.C., and Louis, D.S.: Long-Term Follow-up of Nonvascularized Fibular Autografts for Distal Radial Reconstruction. J. Hand Surg., 10A:335–340, 1985.
601. Noever, G., Bruser, P., and Kohler, L.: Reconstruction of Heel and Sole Defects by Free Flaps. Plast. Reconstr. Surg., 78:345–352, 1986.
602. Nohira, K., Shintomi, Y., Sugihara, T., and Ohura, T.: Replacing Losses in Kind: Improved Sensation Following Heel Reconstruction Using the Free Instep Flap. J. Reconstr. Microsurg., 5:1–6, 1989.
603. Nunley, J.A.: Elective Microsurgery for Orthopaedic Reconstruction: I. Donor Site Selection for Cutaneous and Myocutaneous Free Flaps. Instr. Course Lect. 33:417–460, 1984.
604. Nusbickel, F.R., Dell, P.C., McAndrew, M.P., and Moore, M.M.: Vascularized Autografts for Reconstruction of Skeletal Defects Following Lower Extremity Trauma: A Review. Clin. Orthop. Rel. Res., 243:65–70, 1989.
605. O'Brien, B.M.: Microvascular Free Bone and Joint Transfer. *In* Microvascular Reconstructive Surgery, pp. 267–289. Edinburgh, Churchill-Livingstone, 1977.
606. O'Brien, B.M., Gumley, G.J., Dooley, B.J., and Pribaz, J.J.: Folded Free Vascularized Fibula Transfer. Plast. Reconstr. Surg., 82:311–318, 1988.
607. O'Brien, B.M., MacLeod, A.M., Hayhurst, J.W., and Morrison, W.A.: Successful Transfer of a Large Island Flap from the Groin to the Foot by Microsurgical Anastomoses. Plast. Reconstr. Surg., 52:271–278, 1973.
608. O'Brien, B.M., Morrison, W.A., Ishida, H., MacLeod, A.M., and Gilbert, A.: Free Flap Transfers with Microvascular Anastomoses. Br. J. Plast. Surg., 27:220–230, 1974.
609. O'Brien, B.M., Pederson, W.C., Khanzanchi, R.K., Morrison, W.A., MacLeod, A.M., and Kumar, V.: Results of management of facial palsy with microvascular free-muscle transfer. Plast. Reconstr. Surg., 86:12–20, 1990.
610. Oestern, H.-J.. and Tscherne, H.: Pathophysiology and Classification of Soft Tissue Injuries Associated With Fractures. *In* Tscherne. H. and Gotzen, L. (eds.): Fractures With Soft Tissue Injuries, pp. 1–9. New York, Springer-Verlag, 1984.
611. Ohmori, K., and Harii, K.: Free Groin Flaps; Their Vascular Basis. Br. J. Plast. Surg., 28:238–243, 1975.
612. Ohtsuka, H., and Shioya, N.: The Fate of Free Omental Transfers. Br. J. Plast. Surg., 38:478–482, 1985.
613. Ohtsuka, H., Torigai, K., and Itoh, M.: Free Omental Transfer to the Lower Limbs. Ann. Plast. Surg., 4:71–78, 1980.
614. Okada, T., Yasuda, Y., Kitayama, Y., and Tsukada, S.: Salvage of an Arm by Means of a Free Cutaneous Flap Based on the Posterior Tibial Artery. J. Reconstr. Microsurg., 1:25–29, 1984.
615. Olerud, S., and Karlstrom, G.: Tibial Fractures Treated by AO Compression Osteosynthesis: Experiences From a Five-Year Material. Acta Orthop. Scand., 59:1–104, 1972.
616. Olivari, N.: The Latissimus Flap. Br. J. Plast. Surg., 29:126, 1976.

617. Orr, H.W.: Compound Fractures: With Special Reference to the Lower Extremity. Am. J. Surg., 46:733–737, 1939.
618. Orticochea, M.: Immediate (Undelayed) Musculocutaneous Island Cross Leg Flaps. Br. J. Plast. Surg., 31:205–209, 1978.
619. Osterman, A.L., and Bora, F.W.: Free Vascularized Bone Grafting for Large-Gap Nonunion of Long Bones. Orthop. Clin. North Am., 15:131–142, 1984.
620. Ostrup, L.T., and Frederickson, J.M.: Distant Transfer of a Free, Living Bone Graft by Microvascular Anastomoses: An Experimental Study. Plast. Reconstr. Surg., 54:274–285, 1974.
621. Ostrup, L.T., and Frederickson, J.M.: Reconstruction of mandibular defects after radiation using a free living bone graft transferred by microvascular anastomosis. Plast. Reconstr. Surg., 55:563–572, 1975.
622. Ostrup, L.T., and Tam, C.S.: Bone Formation in a Free, Living Bone Graft Transferred by Microvascular Anastomoses. Scand. J. Plast. Reconstr. Surg., 9:101–106, 1975.
623. Ottolenghi, C.E.: Massive Osteoarticular Bone Grafts: Transplant of the Whole Femur. J. Bone Joint Surg., 48B:646–659, 1966.
624. Ottolenghi, C.E.: Massive Osteo and Osteo-articular Bone Grafts: Technic and Results of 62 Cases. Clin. Orthop. Rel. Res., 87:156–164, 1972.
625. Overton, L.M., and Tully, W.P.: Surgical Treatment of Chronic Osteomyelitis in Long Bones. Am. J. Surg., 126:736–741, 1973.
626. Padgett, E.C., and Gaskins, J.H.: The Use of Skin Flaps in the Repair of Scarred or Ulcerative Defects Over Bone and Tendons. Surgery, 18:287–298, 1945.
627. Paley, D.: Current Techniques of Limb Lengthening. J. Pediatr. Orthop., 8:73–92, 1988.
628. Paley, D.: Bone Transport: The Ilizarov Treatment of Bone Defects. Surg. Rds. Orthop., 3(11):17–29, 1989.
629. Paley, D.: Problems, Obstacles, and Complications of Limb Lengthening by the Ilizarov Technique. Clin. Orthop. Rel. Res., 250:81–104, 1990.
630. Paley, D., Catagni, M.A., Argnani, F., Villa, A., Benedetti, G.B., and Cattaneo, R.: Ilizarov Treatment of Tibial Nonunions With Bone Loss. Clin. Orthop. Rel. Res., 241:146–165, 1989.
631. Papp, C.T., and Hasenohrl, C.: Small Toe Muscles for Defect Coverage. Plast. Reconstr. Surg., 86:941–945, 1990.
632. Parisien, V.: Fibular Transfer for Tibial Defect. Bull. Hosp. Joint Dis., 24:142–146, 1963.
633. Park, C., and Shin, K.S.: Total Palmar Resurfacing With Scapular Free Flap in a 26-Year Contracted Hand. Ann. Plast. Surg., 26:183–187, 1991.
634. Patzakis, M.J., Harvey, J.P., Jr., and Ivler, D.: The Role of Antibiotics in the Management of Open Fractures. J. Bone Joint Surg., 56A:532–541, 1974.
635. Patzakis, M.J., and Wilkins, J.: Factors Influencing Infection Rate in Open Fracture Wounds. Clin. Orthop. Rel. Res., 243:36–40, 1989.
636. Patzakis, M.J., Wilkins, J., and Moore, T.M.: Considerations in Reducing the Infection Rate in Open Tibial Fractures. Clin. Orthop. Rel. Res., 178:36–41, 1983.
637. Patzakis, M.J., Wilkins, J., and Moore, T.M.: Use of Antibiotics in Open Tibial Fractures. Clin. Orthop. Rel. Res., 178:31–35, 1983.
638. Pearson, R.L., and Perry, C.R.: The Ilizarov Technique in the Treatment of Infected Tibial Nonunions. Orthop. Rev., 18:609–613, 1989.
639. Pedersen, P., and Damholt, V.: Rehabilitation After Amputation Following Lower Limb Fracture. J. Trauma, 36:195–197, 1994.
640. Pederson, W.C.: Limb Salvage. Prob. Plast. Reconstr. Surg., 1:125–155, 1991.
641. Pederson, W.C.: Functional Muscle Transfer to the Forearm. Prob. Plast. Reconstr. Surg., 3:410–425, 1993.
642. Pederson, W.C.: Coverage of Hips, Pelvis, and Femur. Orthop. Clin. North Am., 24:461–472, 1993.
643. Pederson, W.C., Eades, E., Occhialini, A., Schuster, J., and Demas, C.: The Distally-Based Radial Forearm Free Flap With Valvulotomy of the Cephalic Vein: A Preliminary Report. Br. J. Plast. Surg., 43:140–144, 1990.
644. Peled, I.J., Frankl, U., and Wexler, M.R.: Salvage of Exposed Knee Prosthesis by Gastrocnemius Myocutaneous Flap Coverage. Orthopedics, 6:1320–1322, 1983.
645. Pena, M.M., Drew, G.S., Smith, S.J., and Given, K.S.: The Inferiorly Based Rectus Abdominis Myocutaneous Flap for Reconstruction of Recurrent Pressure Sores. Plast. Reconstr. Surg., 89:90–95, 1992.
646. Pennington, D.G., Lai, M.F., and Pelly, A.D.: The Rectus Abdominis Myocutaneous Free Flap. Br. J. Plast. Surg., 33:277, 1980.
647. Penteado, C.V.: Venous Drainage of the Groin Flap. Plast. Reconstr. Surg., 71:678–684, 1983.
648. Pers, M., and Medgyesi, S.: Pedicle Muscle Flaps and Their Application in the Surgery of Repair. Br. J. Plast. Surg., 26:313, 1973.
649. Peters, W., Cartotto, R., Morris, S., and Jewett, M.: The Rectus Femoris Myocutaneous Flap for Closure of Difficult Wounds of the Abdomen, Groin, and Trochanteric Areas. Ann. Plast. Surg., 26:572–576, 1991.
650. Phemister, D.B.: The Fate of Transplanted Bone and Regenerative Power of its Various Constituents. Surg. Gynecol. Obstet., 19:303–333, 1914.
651. Pho, R.W., Patterson, M.H., Kour, A.K., and Kumar, V.P.: Free Vascularised Epiphyseal Transplantation in Upper Extremity Reconstruction. J. Hand Surg., 13B:440–447, 1988.
652. Pho, R.W.H.: Free Vascularized Fibular Transplant for Replacement of the Lower Radius. J. Bone Joint Surg., 61B:362–365, 1979.
653. Pho, R.W.H.: Malignant Giant-Cell Tumor of the Distal End of the Radius Treated by a Free Vascularized Fibular Transplant. J. Bone Joint Surg., 63A:877–884, 1981.
654. Pho, R.W.H., Levack, B., Satku, K., and Patradul, A.: Free Vascularized Fibular Graft in the Treatment of Congenital Pseudarthrosis of the Tibia. J. Bone Joint Surg., 67B:64–70, 1985.
655. Pho, R.W.H., Vajara, R., and Satku, K.: Free Vascularized Bone Transplants in Problematic Nonunions of Fractures. J. Trauma, 23:341–349, 1983.
656. Pico, R., Luscher, N.J., Rometsch, M., and de Roche, R.: Why the Denervated Gastrocnemius Muscle Flap Should Be Encouraged. Ann. Plast. Surg., 26:312–324, 1991.
657. Piza-Katzer, H., and Balogh, B.: Experience With 60 Inferior Rectus Abdominis Flaps. Br. J. Plast. Surg., 44:438–443, 1991.
658. Ponten, B.: The Fasciocutaneous Flap: Its Use in Soft Tissue Defects of the Lower Leg. Br. J. Plast. Surg., 34:215–220, 1981.
659. Poole, G.V., Agnew, S.G., Griswold, J.A., and Rhodes, R.S.: The Mangled Lower Extremity: Can Salvage Be Predicted? Am. Surg., 60:50–55, 1994.
660. Press, B.H., Chiu, D.T., and Cunningham, B.L.: The Rectus Abdominis Muscle in Difficult Problems of Hand Soft Tissue Reconstruction. Br. J. Plast. Surg., 43:419–425, 1990.
661. Pribaz, J.J., Maitz, P.K., and Fine, N.A.: Flap Prefabrication Using the Vascular Crane Principle: An Experimental Study and Clinical Application. Br. J. Plast. Surg., 47:250–256, 1994.
662. Prigge, E.K.: The Treatment of Chronic Osteomyelitis by the Use of Muscle Transplant or Iliac Graft. J. Bone Joint Surg., 28:576–593, 1946.
663. Puranen, J.: Reorganization of Fresh and Preserved Bone Transplants: An Experimental Study in Rabbits Using Tetracycline Labelling. Acta Orthop. Scand. [Suppl.], 92:1–75, 1966.
664. Quillan, C.G., Shearin, J.C., and Georgiade, N.G.: Use of the Latissimus Dorsi Myocutaneous Island Flap for Reconstruction of the Head and Neck Area. Plast. Reconstr. Surg., 62:113, 1976.
665. Quillen, C.G., Wiener, B., Mendoza, L., and Giampapa, V. Experiences in the Use of Eight Cutaneous and Osteocutaneous Superficial and Deep Circumflex Iliac Free Flaps. J. Reconstr. Microsurg., 1:269–281, 1985.
666. Radici, G., Donati, L., Fox, U., Candiani, P., Signorini, M., and Klinger, M.: Latissimus Myocutaneous Free Flap in the Reconstruction of Lower Limb Defects—Three Clinical Cases. Ann. Plast. Surg., 9:4–9, 1982.
667. Rank, B.J.: Long-Term Results in Epiphyseal Transplants in

Congenital Deformities of the Hand. Plast. Reconstr. Surg., 61:321–329, 1978.

668. Rautio, J., Asko-Seljavaara, S., Harma, M., and Sundell, B.: Reconstruction of the Foot Using Free Flaps. Handchir. Mikrochir. Plast. Chir., 21:227–234, 1989.
669. Rautio, J., Asko-Seljavaara, S., Laasonen, L., and Harma, M.: Suitability of the Scapular Flap for Reconstructions of the Foot. Plast. Reconstr. Surg., 85:922–928, 1990.
670. Rautio, J., Hamalainen, H., and Kekoni, J.: Covering the Foot Sole and Heel With Pedicled and Free Transplants. Handchir. Mikrochir. Plast. Chir., 24:182–186, 1992.
671. Reath, D.B., and Taylor, J.W.: Free Rectus Abdominis Muscle Flap: Advantages in Lower Extremity Reconstruction. South. Med. J., 82:1143–1146, 1989.
672. Reath, D.B., and Taylor, J.W.: The Segmental Rectus Abdominis Free Flap for Ankle and Foot Reconstruction. Plast. Reconstr. Surg., 88:824–828, 1991.
673. Reckling, F.W., and Roberts, M.D.: Primary Closure of Open Fractures of the Tibia and Fibula by Fibular Fixation and Relaxing Incisions. J. Trauma, 10:835–866, 1970.
674. Reckling, F.W., and Waters, C.H., III: Treatment of Non-Unions of Fractures of the Tibial Diaphysis by Posterolateral Cortical Cancellous Bone-Grafting. J. Bone Joint Surg., 62A:936–941, 1980.
675. Reiffel, R.S., and McCarthy, J.G.: Coverage of Heel and Sole Defects: A New Subfascial Arterialized Flap. Plast. Reconstr. Surg., 66:250–260, 1980.
676. Reigstad, A., Hetland, K.R., Bye, K., Waage, S., Rokkum, M., and Husby, T.: Free Flaps in the Reconstruction of Foot Injury: 4 (1–7) Year Follow-up of 24 Cases. Acta Orthop. Scand., 65:103–106, 1994.
677. Reinisch, J.F., Winters, R., and Puckett, C.L.: The Use of the Osteocutaneous Groin Flap in Gunshot Wounds of the Hand. J. Hand Surg., 9A:12–17, 1984.
678. Research Laboratory for Replantation of Severed Limbs, S.S., Shanghai. Free Muscle Transplantation by Microsurgical Neurovascular Anastomoses: Report of a Case. Chin. Med. J., 2:47–50, 1976.
679. Restrepo, J., Katz, D., and Gilbert, A.: Arterial Vascularization of the Proximal Epiphysis and the Diaphysis of the Fibula. Int. J. Microsurg., 2:49–54, 1980.
680. Reynolds, F.C.: Open Fractures and War Wounds. *In* Conwell, H.E. and Reynolds, F.C. (eds.): Key and Conwell's Management of Fractures, Dislocations, and Sprains, pp. 158–182. St. Louis, C.V. Mosby, 1961.
681. Rhinelander, F.W.: Effects of Medullary Nailing on the Normal Blood Supply of Diaphyseal Cortex. Instr. Course Lect., 22:161–187, 1973.
682. Rhinelander, F.W.: Tibial Blood Supply in Relation to Fracture Healing. Clin. Orthop. Rel. Res., 105:34–81, 1974.
683. Richards, R.R., Orsini, E.C., Mahoney, J.L., and Verschuren, R.: The Influence of Muscle Flap Coverage on the Repair of Devascularized Tibial Cortex: An Experimental Investigation in the Dog. Plast. Reconstr. Surg., 79:946–956, 1987.
684. Rigg, B.M.: Transfer of a Free Groin Flap to the Heel by Microvascular Anastomoses. Plast. Reconstr. Surg., 55:36–40, 1975.
685. Rittmann, W.W., Schibli, M., Matter, P., and Allgower, M.: Open Fractures: Long-Term Results in 200 Consecutive Cases. Clin. Orthop. Rel. Res., 138:132–140, 1979.
686. Rivet, D., Boileau, R., Saiveau, M., and Baudet, J.: Restoration of Elbow Flexion Using the Latissimus Dorsi Musculocutaneous Flap. Ann. Chir. Main, 8:110–123, 1989.
687. Robbins, T.H.: Use of Fascio-muscle Flaps to Repair Defects in the Leg. Plast. Reconstr. Surg., 57:460–462, 1976.
688. Robinson, D.W.: Coverage Problem in Fractures of the Tibia. Arch. Surg., 63:53–59, 1951.
689. Rojczyk, M.: Results of the Treatment of Open Fractures, Aspects of Antibiotic Therapy. *In* Tscherne, H., and Gotzen, L. (eds.): Fractures With Soft Tissue Injuries, pp. 33–38. New York, Springer-Verlag, 1984.
690. Rooks, M.D.: Coverage Problems of the Foot and Ankle. Orthop. Clin. North Am., 20:723–736, 1989.
691. Rose, E.H., and Norris, M.S.: The Versatile Temporoparietal Fascial Flap: Adaptability to a Variety of Composite Defects. Plast. Reconstr. Surg., 85:224–232, 1990.
692. Rosenthal, R.E., MacPhail, J.A., and Ortiz, J.E.: Non-Union in Open Tibial Fractures: Analysis of Reasons for Failure of Treatment. J. Bone Joint Surg., 59A:244–248, 1977.
693. Rowsell, A.R., Davies, D.M., Eisenberg, N., and Taylor, G.I.: The Anatomy of the Subscapular-thoracodorsal Arterial System: Study of 100 Cadaver Dissections. Br. J. Plast. Surg., 37:574–576, 1984.
694. Ruedi, T., Webb, J.K., and Allgower, M.: Experience with the Dynamic Compression Plate (DCP) in 418 Recent Fractures of the Tibial Shaft. Injury, 7:252–257, 1976.
695. Russell, R.C., Graham, D.R., Feller, A.M., Zook, E.G., and Mathur, A.: Experimental Evaluation of the Antibiotic Carrying Capacity of a Muscle Flap into a Fibrotic Cavity. Plast. Reconstr. Surg., 81:162–168, 1988.
696. Russell, R.C., Pribaz, J., Zook, E.G., Leighton, W.D., Eriksson, E., and Smith, C.J.: Functional Evaluation of the Latissimus Dorsi Donor Site. Plast. Reconstr. Surg., 78:336–344, 1986.
697. Russell, R.C., Upton, J., and Merrell, J.C.: Free Flap Donor Sites: Anatomical, Functional, and Technical Considerations. *In* Riley, W.B., Jr. (ed.): Plastic Surgery Educational Foundation: Instructional Courses, vol. 1, pp. 316–360. St. Louis, C.V. Mosby, 1988.
698. Russell, R.C., Vitale, V., and Zook, E.C.: Extremity Reconstruction Using the "Fillet of Sole" Flap. Ann. Plast. Surg., 17:65–72, 1986.
699. Russell, R.C., and Zamboni, W.A.: Coverage of the Elbow and Forearm. Orthop. Clin. North Am., 24:425–434, 1993.
700. Ruttle, P.E., Kelly, P.J., Arnold, P.G., Irons, G.B., and Fitzgerald R.H., Jr.: Chronic Osteomyelitis Treated With a Muscle Flap. Orthop. Clin. North Am., 15:451–459, 1984.
701. Saad, M.N.: The Problems of Traumatic Skin Loss of the Lower Limbs, Especially When Associated With Skeletal Injury. Br. J. Surg., 57:601–615, 1970.
702. Salenius, P., Santavirta, S., Kiviluoto, O., and Koskinen, E.V.: Application of Free Autogenous Fibular Graft in the Treatment of Aggressive Bone Tumors of the Distal End of the Radius. Arch Orthop. Trauma Surg., 98:285–287, 1981.
703. Saliban, A.H., Anzel, S.H., and Salyer, W.A.: Transfer of Vascularized Grafts of Iliac Bone to the Extremities. J. Bone Joint Surg., 69A:1319–1327, 1987.
704. Salibian, A.H., and Anzel, S.H.: Salvage of an Infected Total Knee Prosthesis With Medial and Lateral Gastrocnemius Muscle Flaps: A Case Report. J. Bone Joint Surg., 65A:681–684, 1983.
705. Salibian, A.H., Anzel, S.H., Mallerich, M.M., and Tesoro, V.E.: Microvascular Reconstruction for Close-Range Gunshot Injuries to the Distal Forearm. J. Hand Surg., 9A:799–804, 1984.
706. Salibian, A.H., Anzel, S.H., and Salyer, W.A.: Transfer of Vascularized Grafts of Iliac Bone to the Extremities. J. Bone Joint Surg., 69A:1319–1327, 1987.
707. Salibian, A.H., and Menick, F.J.: Bipedicle Gastrocnemius Musculocutaneous Flap for Defects of the Distal One-Third of the Leg. Plast. Reconstr. Surg., 70:17–23, 1982.
708. Salibian, A.H., Rogers, F.R., and Lamb, R.C.: Microvascular Gastrocnemius Muscle Transfer to the Distal Leg Using Saphenous Vein Grafts. Plast. Reconstr. Surg., 73:302–307, 1984.
709. Salibian, A.H., Tesoro, V.R., and Wood, D.L.: Staged Transfer of a Free Microvascular Latissimus Dorsi Myocutaneous Flap Using Saphenous Vein Grafts. Plast. Reconstr. Surg., 71:543–547, 1983.
710. Salimbeni-Ughi, G., Santoni-Rugiu, P., and de Vizia, G.P. The Gastrocnemius Myocutaneous Flap (GMF): An Alternative Method to Repair Severe Lesions of the Leg. Arch. Orthop. Trauma Surg., 98:195–200, 1981.
711. Salinas Velasco, V.M., Garcia-Morato, V., and Fregenal Garcia, F.J.: Burn of the Elbow: The Role of the Radial Forearm Island Flap. Burns, 18:71–73, 1992.
712. Salmon, M.: Les Arteres des Muscles des Membres et du Tronc. Paris, Masson, 1933.
713. Salmon, M: Les Voies Anastomotiques Arterielles des Membres. Paris, Masson, 1939.

714. Salmon, M: Arteries of the Skin. London, Churchill Livingstone, 1988.
715. Salmon, M: Anatomic Studies. St. Louis, Quality Medical Publishing, 1994.
716. Sanders, R., and O'Neill, T.: The Gastrocnemius Myocutaneous Flap Used as a Cover for the Exposed Knee Prosthesis. J. Bone Joint Surg., 63B:383–386, 1981.
717. Sanders, W.E., and Godsey, J.B.: Non-Invasive Vascular Testing in Candidates for Reconstructive Microsurgery. J. Vasc. Technol., 11:40–43, 1987.
718. Santanelli, F., Berlin, O., and Fogdestam, I.: The Combined Tensor Fasciae Latae/Rectus Femoris Musculocutaneous Flap: A Possibility for Major Soft Tissue Reconstruction in the Groin, Hip, Gluteal, Perineal, and Lower Abdominal Regions. Ann. Plast. Surg., 31:168–174, 1993.
719. Santoni-Rugiu, P.: Review of 33 Free Groin Flaps in the Repair of Complicated Defects of the Lower Limbs. Ann. Plast. Surg., 9:10–17, 1982.
720. Satoh, K., and Kaieda, K.: Resurfacing the Distal Part of the Foot With a Dorsal Foot Skin Island Flap Pedicled on the Plantar Vasculature. Plast. Reconstr. Surg., 95:176–180, 1995.
721. Satoh, K., Sakai, M., Hiromatsu, N., and Ohsumi, N.: Heel and Foot Reconstruction Using Reverse-Flow Posterior Tibial Flap. Ann. Plast. Surg., 24:318–327, 1990.
722. Satoh, T., Tsuchiya, M., Kobayaski, M., et al.: Experience With Free Composite Tissue Transplantation Based on the Deep Circumflex Iliac Vessels. J. Microsurg., 3:77–84, 1981.
723. Sbitany, U., and Wray, R.C., Jr.: Use of the Rectus Abdominis Muscle Flap to Reconstruct an Elbow Defect. Plast. Reconstr. Surg., 77:988–989, 1986.
724. Scheker, L.R., Kleinert, H.E., and Hanel, D.P.: Lateral Arm Composite Tissue Transfer to Ipsilateral Hand Defects. J. Hand Surg., 12A:665–672, 1987.
725. Scheker, L.R., Lister, G.D., and Wolff, T.W.: The Lateral Arm Free Flap in Releasing Severe Contracture of the First Web Space. J. Hand Surg., 13B:146–150, 1988.
726. Schenck, R.R.: Free Muscle and Composite Skin Transplantation by Microneurovascular Anatomoses. Orthop. Clin. North Am., 8:367–375, 1977.
727. Schenck, R.R.: Rectus Femoris Muscle and Composite Skin Transplantation by Microneurovascular Anastomoses for Avulsion of Forearm Muscles: A Case Report. J. Hand Surg., 3:60–69, 1978.
728. Schlenker, J.D.: Important Considerations in the Design and Construction of Groin Flaps. Ann. Plast. Surg., 5:353–357, 1980.
729. Schuind, F., Burny, F., and Lejeune, F.J.: Microsurgical Free Fibula Bone Transfer: A Technique for Reconstruction of Large Skeletal Defects Following Resection of High-Grade Malignant Tumors. World J. Surg., 12:310–317, 1988.
730. Schusterman, M.A., Reece, G.P., Miller, M.J., and Harris, S.: The Osteocutaneous Free Fibula Flap: Is the Skin Paddle Reliable? Plast. Reconstr. Surg., 90:787–93; discussion, 1992.
731. Schwartsman, V., Martin, S.N., Ronquist, R.A., and Schwartsman, R.: Tibial Fractures. The Ilizarov Alternative. Clin. Orthop. Rel. Res., 278:207–216, 1992.
732. Scully, R.E., Artz, C.P., and Sako, Y.: An Evaluation of the Surgeon's Criteria for Determining the Viability of Muscle During Debridement. Arch. Surg., 73:1031–1035, 1956.
733. Sekiguchi, J., Kobayashi, S., and Ohmori, K.: Use of the Osteocutaneous Free Scapular Flap on the Lower Extremities. Plast. Reconstr. Surg., 91:103–112, 1993.
734. Serafin, D., and Georgiade, N.G.: Microsurgical Composite Tissue Transplantation: A New Method of Immediate Reconstruction of Extensive Defects. Am. J. Surg., 133:752–757, 1977.
735. Serafin, D., Georgiade, N.G., and Smith, D.H.: Comparison of Free Flaps With Pedicled Flaps for Coverage of Defects of the Leg or Foot. Plast. Reconstr. Surg., 59:492–499, 1977.
736. Serafin, D., and Pederson, W.C.: Philosophy of Restoration of Weight Bearing Area. *In* Brunelli, G. (ed.): Textbook of Microsurgery. Milan, Masson, 1988.
737. Serafin, D., Sabatier, R.E., Morris, R.L., and Georgiade, N.G.: Reconstruction of the Lower Extremity With Vascularized Composite Tissue: Improved Tissue Survival and Specific Indications. Plast. Reconstr. Surg., 66:230–241, 1980.
738. Serafin, D., Shearin, J.C., and Georgiade, N.G.: The Vascularization of Free Flaps. Plast. Reconstr. Surg., 60:233–241, 1977.
739. Serafin, D., Villarreal Rios, A., and Georgiade, N.: Fourteen Free Groin Flap Transfers. Plast. Reconstr. Surg., 57:707–715, 1976.
740. Serafin, D., Villarreal-Rios, A., and Georgiade, N.G.: A Rib-Containing Free Flap to Reconstruct Mandibular Defects. Br. J. Plast. Surg., 30:263–266, 1977.
741. Serafin, D., and Voci, V.E.: Reconstruction of the Lower Extremity: Microsurgical Composite Tissue Transplantation. Clin. Plast. Surg., 10:55–72, 1983.
742. Serra, J.M., Ballesteros, A., Paloma, V., and Mesa, F.: Simultaneous Reconstruction of Both Feet With a Vascularized Latissimus Dorsi Free Flap. J. Reconstr. Microsurg., 6:353–356, 1990.
743. Seyfer, A.E., and Lower, R.: Late Results of Free-Muscle Flaps and Delayed Bone Grafting in the Secondary Treatment of Open Distal Tibial Fractures. Plast. Reconstr. Surg., 83:77–84, 1989.
744. Shaffer, J.W., Field, G.A., Goldberg, V.M., and Davy, D.T.: Fate of Vascularized and Nonvascularized Autografts. Clin. Orthop. Rel. Res., 197:32–43, 1985.
745. Shah, D.M., Corson, J.D., Karmody, A.M., Fortune, J.B., and Leather, R.P.: Optimal Management of Tibial Arterial Trauma. J. Trauma, 28:228–234, 1988.
746. Shanahan, R.E., and Gingras, R.P.: Medial Plantar Sensory Flap for Coverage of Heel Defects. Plast. Reconstr. Surg., 64:295, 1979.
747. Shapiro, J., Akbarnia, B.A., and Hanel, D.P.: Free Tissue Transfer in Children. J. Pediatr. Orthop., 9:590–595, 1989.
748. Shaw, W.W.: Microvascular Free Flap—The First Decade. Clin. Plast. Surg., 10:3–20, 1983.
749. Shenaq, S.M.: Pretransfer Expansion of a Sensate Lateral Arm Free Flap. Ann. Plast. Surg., 19:558–562, 1987.
750. Shorbe, H.B.: Car Window Elbows. South. Med. J., 34:372–376, 1941.
751. Silverton, J.S., Nahai, F., and Jurkiewicz, M.J.: The Latissimus Dorsi Myocutaneous Flap to Replace a Defect on the Upper Arm. Br. J. Plast. Surg., 31:29–31, 1978.
752. Simonis, R.B., Shirali, H.R., and Mayou, B.: Free Vascularised Fibular Grafts for Congenital Pseudarthrosis of the Tibia. J. Bone Joint Surg., 73B:211–215, 1991.
753. Sinha, A.K., Wood, M.B., and Irons, G.B.: Free Tissue Transfer for Reconstruction of the Weight-bearing Portion of the Foot. Clin. Orthop. Rel. Res., 242:269–271, 1989.
754. Skef, Z., Ecker, H.A., Jr., and Graham, W.P.I.: Heel Coverage by a Plantar Myocutaneous Island Pedicle Flap. J. Trauma, 23:466–472, 1983.
755. Sleeman, D., Carton, A.T., and Stassen, L.F.: Closure of Radial Forearm Free Flap Defect Using Full-Thickness Skin from the Anterior Abdominal Wall. Br. J. Oral Maxillofac. Surg., 32:54–55, 1994.
756. Smith, D.J., Jr., and Coyler, R.A.: An Aggressive Treatment Approach for Adult Osteomyelitis. Am. Surg., 51:363–366, 1985.
757. Smith, P.J.: The Y-shaped Hypogastric—Groin Flap. Hand, 14:263–270, 1982.
758. Smith, P.J., Foley, B., McGregor, I.A., and Jackson, I.T.: The Anatomical Basis of the Groin Flap. Plast. Reconstr. Surg., 49:41–47, 1972.
759. Smith, P.J., and Ross, D.A.: Tubed Radial Fascial Flap and Reconstruction of the Flexor Apparatus in the Forearm. J. Hand Surg., 18A:959–962, 1993.
760. Snyder, G.B., and Edgerton, M.T., Jr.: The Principle of the Island Neurovascular Flap in the Management of Ulcerated Anesthetic Weightbearing Areas of the Lower Extremity. Plast. Reconstr. Surg., 36:518–528, 1965.
761. Solonen, K.A.: Free Vascularized Bone Graft in the Treatment of Pseudarthrosis. Int. Orthop., 6:9–13, 1982.
762. Song, E.K., Moon, E.S., Rowe, S.M., Chung, J.Y., and Yoon, T.R.: Below Knee Stump Reconstruction by Turn-Up Tech-

nique: Report of 2 Cases. Clin. Orthop. Rel. Res., 307:229–234, 1994.
763. Song, R., Gao, Y., Song, Y., and Yu, Y.: The Forearm Flap. Clin. Plast. Surg., 9:21–26, 1982.
764. Soucacos, P.N., Beris, A.E., Xenakis, T.A., Malizos, K.N., and Touliatos, A.S.: Forearm Flap in Orthopaedic and Hand Surgery. Microsurgery, 13:170–174, 1992.
765. Sowa, D.T., and Weiland, A.J.: Clinical Applications of Vascularized Bone Autografts. Orthop. Clin. North Am., 18:257–273, 1987.
766. Speed, K.: A Textbook of Fractures and Dislocations Covering Their Pathology, Diagnosis and Treatment, pp. 79–83; 848–850. Philadelphia, Lea & Febiger, 1935.
767. Springfield, D.S.: Massive Autogenous Bone Grafts. Orthop. Clin North Am., 18:249–256, 1987.
768. Stark, R.B.: Cross-leg Flap Procedure. Plast. Reconstr. Surg., 39:173–204, 1952.
769. Stark, R.B., and Kernahan, D.A.: Reconstructive Surgery of the Leg and Foot. Surg. Clin. North Am., 39:469–490, 1959.
770. Stark, W.J.: The Use of Pedicled Muscle Flaps in the Surgical Treatment of Chronic Osteomyelitis Resulting from Compound Fractures. J. Bone Joint Surg., 28:343–350, 1946.
771. Stern, P.J., and Carey, J.P.: The Latissimus Dorsi Flap for Reconstruction of the Brachium and Shoulder. J. Bone Joint Surg., 70:526–535, 1988.
772. Stevenson, T.R., Rohrich, R.J., Pollock, R.A., Dingman, R.O., and Bostwick, J.: More Experience With the "Reverse" Latissimus Dorsi Musculocutaneous Flap: Precise Location of Blood Supply. Plast. Reconstr. Surg., 74:237–243, 1984.
773. Stewart, D.H., and Puckett, C.L.: Is Reversed Venous Flow Safe in Free-Flap Transfer? A Dilemma With the Radial Forearm Flap. Plast. Reconstr. Surg., 89:237–242, 1992.
774. Stokes, R., Whetzel, T.P., and Stevenson, T.R.: Three-Dimensional Reconstruction of the Below-Knee Amputation Stump: Use of the Combined Scapular/Parascapular Flap. Plast. Reconstr. Surg., 94:732–736, 1994.
775. Stranc, M.F., Labandter, H., and Roy, A.: A Review of 196 Tubed Pedicles. Br. J. Plast. Surg., 28:54–58, 1975.
776. Straub, G.F.: Anatomical Survival, Growth and Physiological Function of an Epiphyseal Bone Transplant. Surg. Gynecol. Obstet., 48:687–690, 1929.
777. Strauch, B., and Murray, D.E.: Transfer of Composite Graft With Immediate Suture Anastomosis of Its Vascular Pedicle Measuring Less Than 1 mm. in External Diameter Using Microsurgical Techniques. Plast. Reconstr. Surg., 40:325–329, 1967.
778. Strauss, M.B., Hargens, A.R., Gershuni, D.H., et al.: Reduction of Skeletal Muscle Necrosis Using Intermittent Hyperbaric Oxygen in a Model Compartment Syndrome. J. Bone Joint Surg., 65A:656–662, 1983.
779. Stringa, G.: Studies of the Vascularisation of Bone Grafts. J. Bone Joint Surg., 39B:395–420, 1957.
780. Sudasna, S., Thienprasit, P., Poneprasert, S., and Chiang-Thong, K.: Treatment of Massive Tibial Diaphyseal Defect With Free Fibular Transfer. J. Med. Assoc. Thai., 63:478–486, 1980.
781. Suematsu, N., Hirayama, T., Atsuta, Y., and Takemitsu, Y.: Postoperative Course of Patients Treated With Iliac Osteocutaneous Free Flaps: A Two- to Five-Year Follow-up Study. Clin. Orthop. Rel. Res., 223:257–264, 1987.
782. Swanson, E., Boyd, J.B., and Manktelow, R.T.: The Radial Forearm Flap: Reconstructive Applications and Donor-Site Defects in 35 Consecutive Patients. Plast. Reconstr. Surg., 85:258–266, 1990.
783. Swartz, W.M.: Immediate Reconstruction of the Wrist and Dorsum of the Hand With a Free Osteocutaneous Groin Flap. J. Hand Surg., 9A:18–21, 1984.
784. Swartz, W.M.: Discussion: Late Results of Free-Muscle Flaps and Delayed Bone Grafting in the Secondary Treatment of Open Distal Tibial Fractures. Plast. Reconstr. Surg., 83:83–84, 1989.
785. Swartz, W.M., and Mears, D.C.: The Role of Free-Tissue Transfers in Lower-Extremity Reconstruction. Plast. Reconstr. Surg., 76:364–373, 1985.
786. Swartz, W.M., Ramasastry, S.S., McGill, J.R., and Noonan, J.D.: Distally Based Vastus Lateralis Muscle Flap for Coverage of Wounds About the Knee. Plast. Reconstr. Surg., 80:255–265, 1987.
787. Swiontkowski, M.F.: Criteria for Bone Debridement in Massive Lower Limb Trauma. Clin. Orthop. Rel. Res., 243:41–47, 1989.
788. Takamai, H., Takahashi, S., and Ando, M.: Latissimus Dorsi Transplantation to Restore Elbow Flexion to the Paralysed Limb. J. Hand Surg., 9B:61–63, 1984.
789. Takami, H., Doi, T., Takahashi, S., and Ninomiya, S.: Reconstruction of a Large Tibial Defect With a Free Vascularized Fibular Graft. Arch Orthop. Trauma Surg., 102:203–205, 1984.
790. Tamai, S., Hori, Y., and Fujiwara, H.: Treatment of Avascular Necrosis of Lunate and Other Bones by Vascular Bundle Transplantation. *In* Urbaniak, J.R. (ed.): Microsurgery for Major Limb Reconstruction, pp. 209–219. St. Louis, C.V. Mosby, 1987.
791. Tamai, S., Komatsu, S., Sakamoto, H., et al.: Free Muscle Transplants in Dogs With Microsurgical Neurovascular Anastomoses. Plast. Reconstr. Surg., 46:219–225, 1970.
792. Tamai, S., Sakamoto, H., Hori, Y., et al.: Vascularized Fibula Transplantation: A Report of 8 Cases in the Treatment of Traumatic Bony Defect or Pseudarthrosis of Long Bones. Int. J. Microsurg., 2:205–212, 1980.
793. Tansini, I.: Sopra il Mio Nuovo Processo di Amputazione della Mammella. Reforma Med. (Palermo, Napoli), 12:757, 1906.
794. Taylor, G.I.: Free Bone Transfer. *In* Daniel, R. K., Terzis, J. K. (eds.): Reconstructive Microsurgery, pp. 275–280. Boston: Little, Brown & Co, 1977.
795. Taylor, G.I.: Microvascular Free Bone Transfer: A Clinical Technique. Orthop. Clin. North Am., 8:425–447, 1977.
796. Taylor, G.I.: Tissue Defects in the Limbs: Replacement with Free Vascularized Tissue Transfers. Aust. N.Z. J. Surg., 47:276–284, 1977.
797. Taylor, G.I.: The Current Status of Free Vascularized Bone Grafts. Clin. Plast. Surg., 10:185–209, 1983.
798. Taylor, G.I., Buncke, H.J., Jr., Watson, N., and Murray, W.: Vascularized Osseous Transplantation for Reconstruction of the Tibia. *In* Serafin, D., and Buncke, H.J. (eds.): Microsurgical Composite Tissue Transplantation, pp. 713–742. St. Louis, C.V. Mosby, 1979.
799. Taylor, G.I., Caddy, C.M., Watterson, P.A., and Crock, J.A.: The Venous Territories (Venosomes) of the Human Body: Experimental Study and Clinical Implications. Plast. Reconstr. Surg., 86:185–213, 1990.
800. Taylor, G.I., and Daniel, R.K.: The Free Flap: Composite Tissue Transfer by Vascular Anastomosis. Aust. N.Z. J. Surg., 43:1–3, 1973.
801. Taylor, G.I., and Daniel, R.K.: The Anatomy of Several Free Flap Donor Sites. Plast. Reconstr. Surg., 56:243–253, 1973.
802. Taylor, G.I., Miller, G.D.H., and Ham, F.J.: The Free Vascularized Bone Graft: A Clinical Extension of Microvascular Techniques. Plast. Reconstr. Surg., 55:533–544, 1975.
803. Taylor, G.I., and Palmer, J.H.: The vascular Territories (Angiosomes) of the Body: Experimental Study and Clinical Applications. Br. J. Plast. Surg., 40:113–141, 1987.
804. Taylor, G.I., Townsend, P., and Corlett, R.: Superiority of the Deep Circumflex Iliac Vessels as the Supply for Free Groin Flaps: Experimental Work. Plast. Reconstr. Surg., 64:595–604, 1979.
805. Taylor, G.I., Townsend, P., and Corlett, R.: Superiority of the Deep Circumflex Iliac Vessels as the Supply for Free Groin Flaps—Clinical Work. Plast. Reconstr. Surg., 64:745–759, 1979.
806. Taylor, G.I., and Watson, N.: One-Stage Repair of Compound Leg Defects With Free, Revascularized Flaps of Groin Skin and Iliac Bone. Plast. Reconstr. Surg., 61:494–506, 1978.
807. Taylor, G.I., Wilson, K.R., Rees, M.D., Corlett, R.J., and Cole, W.G.: The Anterior Tibial Vessels and Their Role in Epiphyseal and Diaphyseal Transfer of the Fibula: Experimental Study and Clinical Applications. Br. J. Plast. Surg., 41:451–469, 1988.
808. Teot, L., and Bosse, J.P.: The Use of Scapular Skin Island Flaps in the Treatment of Axillary Postburn Scar Contractures. Br. J. Plast. Surg., 47:108–111, 1994.

809. Teot, L., Martinetto, J.P., Griffe, O., and Souyris, F.: Treatment of Axillary Burn Scars by a Scapular Island Flap With a Vascular Pedicle. Ann. Chir. Plast. Esthet., 36:507–13; discussion, 1991.
810. Terzis, J.K., Sweet, R.C., Dykes, R.W., and Williams, H.B.: Recovery of Function in Free Muscle Transplants Using Microneurovascular Anastomoses. J. Hand Surg., 3:37–59, 1978.
811. Tessier, J., Bonnel, F., and Allieu, Y.: Vascularization, Cellular Behavior, and Union of Vascularized Bone Grafts: Experimental Study in the Rabbit. Ann. Plast. Surg., 14:494–505, 1985.
812. Thoma, A.. and Heddle, S.: The Extended Free Scapular Flap. Br. J. Plast. Surg., 43:709–712, 1990.
813. Timmons, M.J.: The Vascular Basis of the Radial Forearm Flap. Plast. Reconstr. Surg., 77:80–92, 1986.
814. Timmons, M.J., Missotten, F.E.M., and Roole, M.D.: Complications of Radial Forearm Flap Donor Sites. Br. J. Plast. Surg., 39:176–178, 1986.
815. Tobin, G.R.: Vastus Medialis Myocutaneous and Myocutaneous Tendinous Composite Flaps. Plast. Reconstr. Surg., 75:677, 1985.
816. Tobin, G.R.: Hemisoleus and Reversed Hemisoleus Flaps. Plast. Reconstr. Surg., 76:87, 1985.
817. Tolhurst, D.E.: "Skin and Bone": The Use of Muscle Flaps to Cover Exposed Bone. Br. J. Plast. Surg., 33:99–114, 1980.
818. Tolhurst, D.E., Haeseker, B., and Zeeman, R.J.: The Development of the Fasciocutaneous Flap and its Clinical Applications. Plast. Reconstr. Surg., 71:597–605, 1983.
819. Tonnesen, P.A., Heerfordt, J., and Pers, M.: 150 Open Fractures of the Tibial Shaft—The Relation Between Necrosis of the Skin and Delayed Union. Acta Orthop. Scand., 46:823–835, 1975.
820. Townsend, P.L.G.: An Inferiorly Based Soleus Muscle Flap. Br. J. Plast. Surg., 31:210, 1978.
821. Trabulsy, P.P., Kerley, S.M., and Hoffman, W.Y.: A Prospective Study of Early Soft Tissue Coverage of Grade IIIB Tibial Fractures. J. Trauma, 36:661–668, 1994.
822. Tropet, Y., Najean, D., Brientini, J.M., Elias, B.E., and Vichard, P.: Treatment of Extensive Traumatic Loss of Substance of the Foot and Ankle by Free Flaps: Apropos of 7 Clinical Cases. Ann. Chir. Plast. Esthet., 38:584–9; discussion, 1993.
823. Trueta, J.: Treatment of War Wounds and Fractures with Special Reference to the Closed Method as Used in the War in Spain, pp. 1–150. London, W. Hamilton, 1939.
824. Trueta, J.: "Closed" Treatment of War Fractures. Lancet 1:1452–1455, 1939.
825. Trueta, J.: Blood Supply and the Rate of Healing of Tibial Fractures. Clin. Orthop. Rel. Res., 105:11–26, 1974.
826. Trueta, J., and Caladias, A.X.: A Study of the Blood Supply of the Long Bones. Surg. Gynecol. Obstet., 118:485–498, 1964.
827. Trumble, T.E., Benirschke, S.K., and Vedder, N.B.: Use of Radial Forearm Flaps to Treat Complications of Closed Pilon Fractures. J. Orthop. Trauma, 6:358–365, 1992.
828. Tsai, T.M., Bennett, D.L., Pederson, W.C., and Matiko, J.: Complications and Vascular Salvage of Free-Tissue Transfers to the Extremities. Plast. Reconstr. Surg., 82:1022–1026, 1988.
829. Tsai, T.M., Ludwig, L., and Tonkin, M.: Vascularized Fibular Epiphyseal Transfer: A Clinical Study. Clin. Orthop. Rel. Res., 210:228–234, 1986.
830. Tscherne, H.: The Management of Open Fractures. *In* Tscherne, H., and Gotzen, L. (eds.): Fractures With Soft Tissue Injuries, pp. 10–32. New York, Springer-Verlag, 1984.
831. Tucker, H.L., Kendra, J.C., and Kinnebrew, T.E.: Management of Unstable Open and Closed Tibial Fractures Using the Ilizarov Method. Clin. Orthop. Rel. Res., 280:125–135, 1992.
832. Tukiainen, E., and Asko-Seljavaara, S.: Use of the Ilizarov Technique After a Free Microvascular Muscle Flap Transplantation in Massive Trauma of the Lower Leg. Clin. Orthop. Rel. Res., 297:129–134, 1993.
833. Tvrdek, M., Kletensky, J., Pros, Z., and Stehlik, J.: An Extensive Defect on the Tibia Covered by a Free Cross Flap Using M. Latissimus Dorsi. Acta Chir. Plast., 34:143–147, 1992.
834. Uhm, K.I., Shin, K.S., Lee, Y.H., and Lew, J.D.: Restoration of Finger Extension and Forearm Contour Utilizing a Neurovascular Latissimus Dorsi Free Flap. Ann. Plast. Surg., 21:74–76, 1988.
835. Uhm, K.I., Shin, K.S., and Lew, J.D.: Crane Principle of the Cross-Leg Fasciocutaneous Flap: Aesthetically Pleasing Technique for Damaged Dorsum of Foot. Ann. Plast. Surg., 15:257–261, 1985.
836. Urbaniak, J.R.: Aseptic Necrosis of the Femoral Head Treated by Vascularized Fibular Graft. *In* Urbaniak, J.R. (ed.): Microsurgery for Major Limb Reconstruction, pp. 178–184. St. Louis, C.V. Mosby, 1987.
837. Urbaniak, J.R., Koman, L.A., Goldner, R.D., Armstrong, N.B., and Nunley, J.A.: The Vascularized Cutaneous Scapular Flap. Plast. Reconstr. Surg., 69:772–778, 1982.
838. Urbaniak, J.R., and Richards, R.R.: Complications in Microvascular Surgery. *In* Epps, C.H., Jr. (ed.): Complications in Orthopaedic Surgery, pp. 845–864. Philadelphia, J.B. Lippincott, 1986.
839. Urist, M.R., Mazet, R., Jr., and McLean, F.C.: The Pathogenesis and Treatment of Delayed Union and Nonunion: A Survey of Eighty-five Ununited Fractures of the Shaft of the Tibia and One Hundred Control Cases With Similar Injuries. J. Bone Joint Surg., 36:931–967, 1954.
840. Urist, M.R., and McLean, F.C.: Osteogenic Potency and New-Bone Formation by Induction in Transplants to the Anterior Chamber of the Eye. J. Bone Joint Surg., 34A:443–467, 1952.
841. Usui, M., Minami, M., and Ishii, S.: Successful Replantation of An Amputated Leg in a Child. Plast. Reconstr. Surg., 63:613–617, 1979.
842. Varecka, T.F.: Soft Tissue Coverage in Open Fractures. *In*: Gustilo, R.B., Gruninger, R. P., and Tsukayama, D. T. (eds.): Orthopaedic Infection: Diagnosis and Treatment, pp. 118–122. Philadelphia, W.B. Saunders, 1989.
843. Vasconez, H.C., and Oishi, S.: Soft-Tissue Coverage of the Shoulder and Brachium. Orthop. Clin. North Am., 24:435–448, 1993.
844. Vasconez, L.O., Bostwick, J., III, and McCraw, J.: Coverage of Exposed Bone by Muscle Transposition and Skin Grafting. Plast. Reconstr. Surg., 53:526–530, 1974.
845. Velazco, A., and Fleming, L.L.: Open Fractures of the Tibia Treated by the Hoffmann External Fixator. Clin. Orthop. Rel. Res., 180:125–132, 1983.
846. Velazco, A., Fleming, L.L., and Nahai, F.: Soft Tissue Reconstruction of the Leg Associated With the Use of the Hoffmann External Fixator. J. Trauma, 23:1052–1057, 1983.
847. Veliskakis, K.P.: Primary Internal Fixation in Open Fractures of the Tibial Shaft: The Problem of Wound Healing. J. Bone Joint. Surg., 41B:342–354, 1959.
848. Vergote, T., Revol, M., Martinaud, C., Le Fourn, B., Servant, J.M., and Banzet, P.: Use of Parascapular Semi-free Flap in the Covering of Substance Loss of the Lower Third of the Leg and Foot: Apropos of 3 Cases. Ann. Chir. Plast. Esthet., 38:192–197, 1993.
849. Vergote, T., Revol, M., Servant, J.M., and Banzet, P.: Use of the Inferiorly Based Rectus Abdominis Flap for Inguinal and Perineal Coverage—Low Venous Pressure Zone Concept. Br. J. Plast. Surg., 46:168–172, 1993.
850. Verklin, R.M., Jr., and Mandell, G.L.: Alteration of Effectiveness of Antibiotics by Anaerobiosis. J. Lab. Clin. Med., 80:65–71, 1977.
851. Waldvogel, F.A., and Vasey, H.: Osteomyelitis: The Past Decade. N. Engl. J. Med., 303:360–370, 1980.
852. Wangensteen, O.H., Wangensteen, S.D., and Klinger, C.F.: Wound Management of Ambroise Paré and Dominique Larrey, Great French Military Surgeons of the 16th and 19th Centuries. Bull. Hist. Med., 46:207–234, 1972.
853. Waris, T.H., Kaarela, O.I., Raatikainen, T.K., Teerikangas, H.E., and Heikkinen, E.S.: Microvascular Flaps From the Lateral Arm and Radial Forearm for the Repair of Defects of the Achilles Tendon Region: Case Report. Scand. J. Plast. Reconstr. Surg. Hand. Surg., 25:87–89, 1991.
854. Waterhouse, N., and Healy, C.: The Versatility of the Lateral Arm Flap. Br. J. Plast. Surg., 43:398–402, 1990.
855. Waters, R.L., Perry, J., Antonelli, D., and Hislop, H.: Energy

Cost of Walking of Amputees: The Influence of Level of Amputation. J. Bone Joint Surg., 58A:42–46, 1976.

856. Wattel, F., Mathieu, D., Coget, J.M., and Billard, V.: Hyperbaric Oxygen Therapy in Chronic Vascular Wound Management. Angiology, 41:59–65, 1990.

857. Weaver, F.A., Rosenthal, R.E., Waterhouse, G., and Adkins, R.B.: Combined skeletal and vascular injuries of the lower extremities. Am. Surg., 50:189–197, 1984.

858. Weber, B.G., and Cech, O.: Pseudarthrosis: Pathophysiology, Biomechanics, Therapy, Results, pp. 1–60. New York, Grune & Stratton, 1976.

859. Webster, J.P.: The Early History of the Tubed Pedicle Flap. Surg. Clin. North Am., 39:261–275, 1959.

860. Wee, J.T.: Reversed Venous Flow in the Distally Pedicled Radial Forearm Flap: Surgical Implications. Handchir. Mikrochir. Plast. Chir., 20:119–123, 1988.

861. Wei, F.C., Chen, H.C., Chuang, C.C., and Noordhoff, M.S.: Reconstruction of Achilles Tendon and Calcaneus Defects With Skin-Aponeurosis-Bone Composite Free Tissue From the Groin Region. Plast. Reconstr. Surg., 81:579–589, 1988.

862. Weiland, A.J.: Current Concepts Review: Vascularized Free Bone Transplants. J. Bone Joint Surg., 63A:166–169, 1981.

863. Weiland, A.J.: Elective Microsurgery for Orthopaedic Reconstruction: III. Vascularized Bone Transfers. Instr. Course Lect., 33:446–460, 1984.

864. Weiland, A.J., Berggren, A., and Jones, L.: The Acute Effects of Blocking Medullary Blood Supply on Regional Cortical Blood Flow in Canine Ribs as Measured by the Hydrogen Washout Technique. Clin. Orthop. Rel. Res., 165:265–272, 1982.

865. Weiland, A.J., and Daniel, R.K.: Microvascular Anastomoses for Bone Grafts in the Treatment of Massive Defects in Bone. J. Bone Joint Surg., 61A:98–104, 1979.

866. Weiland, A.J., and Daniel, R.K.: Congenital Pseudarthrosis of the Tibia: Treatment With Vascularized Autogenous Fibular Grafts: A Preliminary Report. Johns Hopkins Med. J., 147(3):89–95, 1980.

867. Weiland, A.J., and Daniel, R.K.: Clinical Techniques of Segmental Autogenous Bone Grafting on Vascular Pedicles. *In* Mears, D. C. (ed.): External Skeletal Fixation, pp. 656–679. Baltimore, Williams & Wilkins, 1983.

868. Weiland, A.J., Daniel, R.K., and Riley, L.H., Jr.: Application of the Free Vascularized Bone Graft in the Treatment of Malignant or Aggressive Bone Tumors. Johns Hopkins Med. J., 140(3):85–96, 1977.

869. Weiland, A.J., Kleinert, H.E., Kutz, J.E., and Daniel, R.K.: Vascularized Bone Grafts in the Upper Extremity. *In* Serafin, D., and Buncke, H. (eds.): Microsurgical Composite Tissue Transplantation, pp. 605–625. St. Louis, C.V. Mosby, 1979.

870. Weiland, A.J., Kleinert, H.E., Kutz, J.E., and Daniel, R.K.: Free Vascularized Bone Grafts in Surgery of the Upper Extremity. J. Hand Surg., 4:129–144, 1979.

871. Weiland, A.J., and Moore, J.R.: Vascularized Bone Grafts. *In* Green, D. P. (ed.): Operative Hand Surgery, pp. 1245–1269. New York, Churchill Livingstone, 1988.

872. Weiland, A.J., Moore, J.R., and Daniel, R.K.: Vascularized Bone Autographs: Experience With 41 Cases. Clin. Orthop. Rel. Res., No. 174:87–95, 1983.

873. Weiland, A.J., Moore, J.R., and Daniel, R.K.: The Efficacy of Free Tissue Transfer in the Treatment of Osteomyelitis. J. Bone Joint Surg., 66A:181–193, 1984.

874. Weiland, A.J., Moore, J.R., and Hotchkiss, R.N.: Soft Tissue Procedures for Reconstruction of Tibial Shaft Fractures. Clin. Orthop. Rel. Res., 178:42–53, 1983.

875. Weiland, A.J., Phillips, T.W., and Randolph, M.A.: Bone Grafts: A Radiologic, Histologic, and Biomechanical Model Comparing Autographs, Allografts, and Free Vascularized Bone Grafts. Plast. Reconstr. Surg., 74:368–379, 1984.

876. Weiland, A.J.: Symposium: The Use of Muscle Flaps in the Treatment of Osteomyelitis in the Lower Extremity. Contemp. Orthop., 10:127–159, 1985.

877. Weinzweig, N., Chen, L., and Chen, Z.W.: The Distally Based Radial Forearm Fasciosubcutaneous Flap With Preservation of the Radial Artery: An Anatomic and Clinical Approach. Plast. Reconstr. Surg., 94:675–684, 1994.

878. Weller, S.: The External Fixator for the Prevention and Treatment of Infections. *In* Uhthoff, H.: Current Concepts of External Fixation of Fractures, pp. 215–220. New York, Springer-Verlag, 1982.

879. White, W.L., Dupertuis, S.M., Gaisford, J.C., Musgrave, R.H., and Hanna, D.C.: Evaluation of 114 Cross-leg Flaps. *In* Skoog, T., and Ivy, R. H. (eds.): Transactions of the First Congress of the International Society of Plastic Surgeons, pp. 516–524. Baltimore, Williams & Wilkins, 1955.

880. Williams, D.N.: Antibiotic Penetration Into Bones and Joints. *In* Gustilo, R.B., Gruninger, R.P., and Tsukayama, D.T. (eds.): Orthopaedic Infection: Diagnosis and Treatment, pp. 52–59. Philadelphia, W.B. Saunders, 1989.

881. Wilson, J.N.: Epiphyseal Transplantation: A Clinical Study. J. Bone Joint Surg., 48A:245–256, 1966.

882. Wiss, D.A., Sherman, R., and Oechsel, M.: External Skeletal Fixation and Rectus Abdominis Free-Tissue Transfer in the Management of Severe Open Fractures of the Tibia. Orthop. Clin. North Am., 24:549–556, 1994.

883. Withers, E.H., Bishop, J.O., and Tullos, H.S.: Microvascular Free Flap Transfers to Foot and Ankle. Orthop. Rev., 14(9):33–38, 1985.

884. Witschi, T.H., and Omer, G.E., Jr.: The Treatment of Open Tibial Shaft Fractures From Vietnam War. J. Trauma, 10:105–111, 1970.

885. Woltering, E.A., Thorpe, W.P., and Reed, J.K.: Split Thickness Skin Grafting of the Plantar Surface of the Foot After Wide Excision of Neoplasms of the Skin. Surg. Gynecol. Obstet., 149:229, 1979.

886. Wood, C.F.: Traffic Elbow. Kentucky Med. J., 39:78–81, 1941.

887. Wood, M.B.: Comparison of Microsurgically Revascularized Diaphyseal Bone Grafts to Viable Segmental Long-Bone Fractures in the Canine: Blood Flow and Fluorochrome Uptake Quantitation. Orthop. Trans., 8:301–302, 1984.

888. Wood, M.B.: Free Vascularized Bone Transfers for Nonunions, Segmental Gaps and Following Tumor Resection. Orthopedics, 9(6):810–816, 1986.

889. Wood, M.B.: Upper Extremity Reconstruction by Vascularized Bone Transfers: Results and Complications. J. Hand Surg., 12A:422–427, 1987.

890. Wood, M.B.: Utility of Free Muscle Flap Transfer in Chronic Osteomyelitis. *In* Urbaniak, J.R. (ed.): Microsurgery for Major Limb Reconstruction, pp. 162–169. St. Louis, C.V. Mosby, 1987.

891. Wood, M.B., and Cooney, W.P., III.: Vascularized Bone Segment Transfers for Management of Chronic Osteomyelitis. Orthop. Clin. North Am., 15:461–472, 1984.

892. Wood, M.B., Cooney, W.P., III, and Irons, G.B.: Posttraumatic Lower Extremity Reconstruction by Vascularized Bone Graft Transfer. Orthopedics, 7:255–262, 1984.

893. Wood, M.B., Cooney, W.P.I., and Irons, G.B.: Skeletal Reconstruction by Vascularized Bone Transfer: Indications and Results. Mayo Clin. Proc. 60:729–734, 1985.

894. Woods, J.E., Irons, G.B., Jr., and Masson, J.K.: Use of Muscular, Musculocutaneous, and Omental Flaps to Reconstruct Difficult Defects. Plast. Reconstr. Surg., 59:191–199, 1977.

895. Wray, J.B.: Factors in the Pathogenesis of Nonunion. J. Bone Joint Surg., 47A:168–173, 1965.

896. Wray, R.C., Wise, D.M., Young, V.L., and Weeks, P.M.: The Groin Flap in Severe Hand Injuries. Ann. Plast. Surg., 9:459–462, 1982.

897. Wright, J.K., and Watkins, R.P.: Use of the Soleus Muscle Flap to Cover Part of the Distal Tibia. Plast. Reconstr. Surg., 68:957–958, 1981.

898. Yablon, I.G., and Cruess, R.L.: The Effect of Hyperbaric Oxygen on Fracture Healing in Rats. J. Trauma, 8:186–202, 1969.

899. Yajima, H., Tamai, S., Mizumoto, S., and Ono, H.: Vascularised Fibular Grafts for Reconstruction of the Femur. J. Bone Joint Surg., 75B:123–128, 1993.

900. Yakuboff, K.P., Stern, P.J., and Neale, H.W.: Technical Successes and Functional Failures After Free Tissue Transfer to the Tibia. Microsurgery, 11:59–62, 1990.

901. Yao, S.T.: Vascular Implantation Into Skin Flap: Experimental

Study and Clinical Application: A Preliminary Report. Plast. Reconstr. Surg., 68:404–410, 1981.

902. Yaremchuk, M.J.: Acute Management of Severe Soft-Tissue Damage Accompanying Open Fractures of the Lower Extremity. Clin. Plast. Surg., 13:621–629, 1986.
903. Yaremchuk, M.J., Brumback, R.J., Manson, P.N., Burgess, A.R., Poka, A., and Weiland, A.J.: Acute and Definitive Management of Traumatic Osteocutaneous Defects of the Lower Extremity. Plast. Reconstr. Surg., 80:1–12, 1987.
904. Yim, K.K., Hui, K.C., Ramos, D., and Lineaweaver, W.C.: Use of Intercostal Nerves as Nerve Grafts in Hand Reconstruction With Rectus Abdominis Flaps. J. Hand Surg., 19:238–240, 1994.
905. Yoo, M.C., Chung, D.W., and Hahn, C.S.: Free Vascularized Fibula Grafting for the Treatment of Osteonecrosis of the Femoral Head. Clin. Orthop. Rel. Res., 277:128–138, 1992.
906. Yoshimura, M., Shimada, T., Imura, S., Shimamura, K., and Yamauchi, S.: Peroneal Island Flap for Skin Defects in the Lower Extremity. J. Bone Joint Surg., 67A:935–941, 1985.
907. Yoshimura, M., Shimamura, K., Iwai, Y., Yamauchi, S., and Ueno, T.: Free Vascularized Fibular Transplant: A New Method for Monitoring Circulation of the Grafted Fibula. J. Bone Joint Surg., 65:1295–1301, 1983.
908. Youdas, J.W., Wood, M.B., Cahalan, T.D., and Chao, E.Y.: A Quantitative Analysis of Donor Site Morbidity After Vascularized Fibula Transfer. J. Orthop. Res., 6:621–629, 1988.
909. Zancolli, E., and Mitre, H.: Latissimus Dorsi Transfer to Restore Elbow Flexion. J. Bone Joint Surg., 55A:1265–1275, 1973.
910. Zoltie, N., Chapman, P., and Joss, G.: Tissue Expansion: A Unit Review of Non-scalp, Non-breast Expansion. Br. J. Plast. Surg., 43:325–327, 1990.
911. Zook, E.G., Russell, R.C., and Asaadi, M.: A Comparative Study of Free and Pedicle Flaps for Lower Extremity Wounds. Ann. Plast. Surg. 17(1):21–33, 1986.

Rockwood and Green's Fractures in Adults, Fourth Edition,
edited by Charles A. Rockwood, David P. Green, Robert W. Bucholz and James D. Heckman.
Lippincott-Raven Publishers, Philadelphia © 1996.

CHAPTER 8

Complications

Vincent D. Pellegrini, Jr., J. Spence Reid,
C. McCollister Evarts

SYSTEMIC COMPLICATIONS OF INJURY

Complications of musculoskeletal trauma can jeopardize life or limb depending on the severity of the local injury and the nature of the resultant systemic response. Even a "simple" femoral shaft fracture can trigger a life-threatening cascade of events culminating in multisystem failure, underscoring the fact that rarely does there exist a truly "isolated" long-bone extremity fracture.

Shock

Shock is defined as a clinical state in which there is poor tissue perfusion with resultant tissue hypoxia threatening damage to vital organs. Simeone stated that, "shock is a clinical condition in which, because of insufficient effective circulating blood volume or because of abnormal partitioning of cardiac output, the capillary blood flow in the vital tissues or in all tissues is reduced to levels below the minimum requirements for oxidative metabolism."[108]

For centuries, shock has been recognized as a clinical entity. In 1872, Gross defined shock as "a manifestation of root unhinging of the machinery of life."[47] Many experimental studies have been performed to investigate the pathophysiologic mechanisms of shock.* Wiggers characterized shock as "a state of low cardiac output with decrease in total peripheral resistance."[122] However, more recent investigators have shown that low cardiac output is not always present and that the hemodynamic pattern is directly related to the etiology of shock.[103,104,119]

Classification

In 1934, Blalock suggested four categories of shock[13]:

1. Hematogenic (oligemia)
2. Neurogenic (caused primarily by nervous influences)
3. Vasogenic (initially decreased vascular resistance and increased vascular capacity)
4. Cardiogenic (caused by either failure of the heart

* References 14, 15, 20, 21, 24, 27, 32, 49, 50, 77, 78, 86, 111, 122.

as a pump or diminished cardiac output from various causes)

Shires and coworkers believed that shock invariably results from the loss of one or more of four separate but interrelated functions (ie, the heart, the volume of blood, the arteriolar resistance vessels, and the capacitance vessels).[102] More recently, the American College of Surgeons Committee on Trauma categorized shock as either hemorrhagic or nonhemorrhagic. Shock states not associated with volume loss (nonhemorrhagic) are subdivided further by etiology (cardiogenic, tension pneumothorax, neurogenic, or septic).[4]

Hemorrhagic (Hypovolemic) Shock

Hemorrhagic (hypovolemic) shock is the most common type of shock occurring in patients with multiple trauma and skeletal injury. With acute bleeding, the blood volume and central venous pressure are reduced, and early circulatory responses are compensatory. Progressive vasoconstriction of cutaneous and muscle tissue begins in an attempt to maintain adequate diastolic cardiac filling and preserve renal, cardiac, and cerebral perfusion. The earliest manifestation of shock is tachycardia. If the hemorrhage is of sufficient magnitude, peripheral vasoconstriction, increased myocardial contractility, and tachycardia are insufficient to maintain blood pressure, and hypotension develops. The amount of blood loss required to provoke a given physiologic response is somewhat variable given the hydration status and cardiac reserve of the individual. In evaluating a patient with acute blood loss, it is helpful to remember that the circulating blood volume of the average adult is about 7% of body weight (8% to 9% in children). Thus, a 70-kg man has a circulating blood volume of about 5 L. The American College of Surgeons Committee on Trauma has subdivided hemorrhagic shock into four classes based on the amount of circulating blood volume loss.[4] These classifications and their physiologic responses are listed in Table 8-1.

This classification system has clinical relevance for orthopaedic surgeons. The incidence of hypovolemic shock (class III or IV) in a blunt trauma population has been estimated at between 13% and 18%.[62,88] Pedestrian injuries are significantly above this average at 38%.[88] The contribution of orthopaedic injuries as a cause of shock has been estimated by Pedowitz and Shackford.[88] In their study, 55.7% of hypotensive patients had only noncavitary sources of blood loss, and of this subgroup, 50% had a long-bone fracture and 32.4% sustained a pelvis fracture. This underscores the fact that multiple orthopaedic injuries can produce hypovolemic shock in the absence of a major abdominal or thoracic injury.[88]

Ostrum and colleagues evaluated 100 patients with closed isolated femoral shaft fractures and noted that no patient presented in (or progressed to) class III or IV shock.[87] In these patients, bleeding from the femur fracture was insufficient to produce hypotension. Thus, a diligent search for a second source of blood loss must be performed in the hypotensive patient with a closed femoral shaft fracture. Pelvic ring injuries are associated with other injuries in more than 90% of cases.[91] Although notorious for hemorrhage, bleeding from a pelvic ring injury is the major cause of death in only 7% to 18% of fatal cases.[38,65,79,91,115] In the remainder, the pelvic fracture either is not a factor in the fatal outcome or plays a contributory role as a source of volume loss.[28,92] Dalal and associates have shown that hemorrhage from pelvic fractures is strongly dependent on fracture type, and that fractures

TABLE 8-1
Classes of Acute Hemorrhage

	Class I	Class II	Class III	Class IV
Blood loss (mL)	750	1000–1250	1500–1800	2000–2500
Blood loss (units)	1–2	2–3	3–4	5
Blood loss* (%)	15	20–25	30–35	40–50
Pulse rate† (bpm)	72–84	>100	>120	>140
Blood pressure‡ (mm Hg)	118/82	110/80	70–90/50–60	<50–60 systolic
Pulse pressure (mm Hg)	36	30	20–30	10–20
Capillary blanch test	Normal	Delayed	Delayed	Delayed
Respiratory rate	14–20	20–30	30–40	>35
Urine output (mL/h)	30–35	25–30	5–15	Negligible
Central nervous system—mental status	Slightly anxious	Mildly anxious	Anxious and confused	Confused-lethargic
Fluid replacement	Crystalloid	Crystalloid	Crystalloid + Blood	Crystalloid + Blood

* Percentage of blood volume in a standard 70-kg man.
† Assume normal of 72 bpm.
‡ Assume normal of 120/80 mm Hg.
(Alexander, R.H., and Proctor, H.J.: Shock. *In* Committee on Trauma (eds): *Advanced Trauma Life Support Manual—Program for Physicians,* p. 86. Chicago, American College of Surgeons, 1993.)

associated with complete dissociation of the posterior pelvis have the highest blood loss and mortality from shock.[30]

Treatment. The goal of treatment of hypovolemic shock is to restore safely adequate intravascular volume and oxygen-carrying capacity. Thus, the goal of fluid resuscitation should be to restore adequate tissue perfusion rather than to correct empirically an estimated specific deficit.[16,18,51,104] It is widely accepted that the initial resuscitation fluid should be crystalloid. This is both physiologic, because it provides at least transient intravascular expansion, and practical, because fully crossmatched or type-specific whole blood rarely is immediately available. In an elegant animal model, Traverso and coworkers determined that Ringer's lactate was the crystalloid of choice because of its decreased chloride load compared with normal saline. The higher chloride concentration in normal saline was found to displace bicarbonate and result in a dilutional hyperchloremic acidosis.[113] Studies also have shown that Ringer's lactate does *not* aggravate lactic acidosis when it is used to treat patients in shock.[11,101,114] Lactate levels actually have been shown to decrease as cellular perfusion is increased and the shock state resolves.[22,99] The critical factor is restoration of volume to enhance the microcirculation.

The Committee on Trauma of the American College of Surgeons recommends an initial rapid fluid bolus of 1 to 2 L of lactated Ringer's solution in the adult patient and 20 mL/kg in the pediatric patient. Further therapeutic and diagnostic decisions are based on the response of the patient to this initial bolus. Patients who respond rapidly to the initial fluid bolus and remain stable represent class I shock, without ongoing blood loss. Acute transfusions rarely are required in this subgroup. Most trauma patients have some response to the initial fluid bolus but then deteriorate as fluid administration is slowed. Sources of ongoing hemorrhage must be determined, and transfusion therapy probably is indicated. Acute surgical intervention is likely in this group. A smaller group presents in profound (class IV) shock with a greater than 40% loss of circulating volume and minimal response to a crystalloid bolus. The need for transfusion is clear and immediate. It is this group of patients who are candidates for immediate surgery to control exsanguinating hemorrhage. Occasionally, primary pump failure coexists with volume loss, as in the case of myocardial contusion or tamponade, and measurement of the central venous pressure aids in the differential diagnosis.[4]

Crystalloid Versus Colloid. In severe hypovolemic shock, both the oxygen-carrying capacity and the extracellular fluid deficit need to be replenished. There has been a long-standing debate regarding the best asanguineous fluid for use in acute resuscitation. The term *crystalloid* in clinical practice refers to a balanced salt solution. The term *colloid* refers to the class of solutions that contains a balanced salt solution in addition to a suspension of particles or macromolecules. The molecular weights of the macromolecules are too small to settle under the influence of gravity, but too large to pass through an *intact* semipermeable membrane. The concentration of macromolecules on one side of a semipermeable membrane generates an "oncotic pressure" that is related directly to their concentration.

Crystalloid administration expands the entire extracellular space, and acute restoration of intravascular volume requires about a 1:3 volume ratio of blood lost to crystalloid administered to allow replenishment of both interstitial and intracellular volume.[4,66] In contrast, colloid preferentially expands the intravascular volume without simultaneously expanding the interstitial water.[43] The blood volume and the cardiorespiratory system show a much greater response to colloid administration than to crystalloid administration.[59,73,74,106,107] Theoretically, colloid solutions may minimize interstitial edema in the lung by maintaining the intravascular oncotic pressure.

The clinically available colloids are balanced salt solutions containing either 5% albumin, dextran 40, or hydroxyethyl starch (Hespan) as the osmotically active molecule. Contrary to the theoretic advantage of albumin, a large body of experimental and clinical evidence contraindicates the use of supplemental albumin therapy for hemorrhagic shock. Albumin has been found to extravasate into the lungs, heart, kidneys, and liver, thus increasing the likelihood of edema formation.[56] Although albumin can restore such levels as total serum protein and serum albumin to normal, it also can have a decidedly negative inotropic effect on the heart.[29] The administration of albumin also probably leads to impaired salt and water excretion and may contribute to central volume overload, respiratory failure, and acute renal failure.[68] Albumin has a detrimental effect on pulmonary function that may be caused by reduced saline diuresis, increased interstitial pulmonary water from trapped albumin, or impaired left ventricular function. Clinical trials examining the addition of albumin to the usual regimen of whole blood and balanced electrolyte solution for resuscitation from hypovolemic shock have been added to the experimental evidence in the indictment against the use of albumin in such situations. In addition, supplemental albumin added to standard resuscitative measures for hypovolemic shock increases the total serum protein and serum albumin levels to almost normal, while producing a relative reduction in the globulins and other fractions. This results in decreased plasma fibrinogen levels and a prolonged prothrombin time (PT), which may lead to significantly impaired coagulation in albumin-treated patients. The mild reduction in serum albumin concentration that occurs when shock is treated with blood and crystalloid solution actually may be desirable. Therefore, it can be concluded that supplemental albumin is contraindicated for patients in hypovolemic shock.[66,67,69]

Low–molecular-weight dextran (in the range of 35 to 45 kilodaltons) received initial enthusiasm as a plasma expander because of observations that it lowered blood viscosity and prevented red blood cell clumping in a low-flow state.[34] Subsequent work indicates that the effect on blood viscosity may be due entirely to hemodilution.[94] In addition, dextran 40 may produce serious defects in the clotting mechanism.[101]

In an attempt to clarify the conflicting data on colloid and crystalloid use in hemorrhagic shock, Poole and associates in 1982 reviewed the available literature and concluded, "There appears to be no justification for the use of albumin or other colligative solutions during resuscitation from hemorrhagic shock."[90] They further stressed the need to use physiologic end points of resuscitation such as cardiac output. In this review, pulmonary edema was not increased in patients resuscitated with crystalloid, and the initially decreased levels of serum oncotic pressure seen in that group were short lived and well tolerated. In 1989, Velanovich performed a meta-analysis of eight randomized clinical trials comparing crystalloid versus colloid resuscitation from 1977 to 1984.[117] When the data from the trauma patients were pooled, there was a 12.3% difference in mortality in favor of crystalloid therapy. In the nontrauma patients, there was a 7.8% difference in mortality in favor of colloid therapy. The author hypothesized that the difference between trauma and nontrauma patients resulted from altered pulmonary capillary permeability in the trauma group (possibly secondary to sepsis), negating the theoretic benefit of the colloid. The use of crystalloids in the acute resuscitation of trauma patients is justified further on a cost basis. One liter of 5% albumin (Albumisol) is about 40 to 50 times more costly on a patient-charge basis than 1 L of Ringer's lactate (less than $10.00).

Nagy and colleagues compared lactated Ringer's solution with a relatively new plasma expander, pentastarch, in resuscitation from hemorrhagic shock.[83] This material is clinically similar to hetastarch but has a shorter half-life (12 hours) and produces a volume expansion of 1.5 times the administered volume. They concluded that significantly less pentastarch than lactated Ringer's solution was required to achieve the same blood pressure and urine output. No coagulation abnormalities or deleterious pulmonary effects were noted. The role of this new material awaits further investigation.

The use of small-volume (less than 12 mL/kg) hypertonic solutions (3% to 7.5% NaCl) in severe hypovolemia has been reported intermittently over the past 30 years.[10,39,118] Holcroft and coworkers compared a hypertonic/hyperoncotic fluid (7.5% NaCl/dextran 70) with lactated Ringer's solution in a randomized, double-blind trial of severely injured patients during prehospital transport and found a significant increase in both blood pressure and survival in the hypertonic group.[57] The theoretic risks of hypertonic solutions, including phlebitis, hypokalemia, arrhythmias, and mental status changes, were not encountered in this study. Some authors suggest that hypertonic solutions have a role in patients with shock who have elevated intracranial pressures.[75] The indications for the use of hypertonic fluids and their optimal formulation and dosage have yet to be fully elucidated but appear to warrant further investigation.[61]

Transfusion Therapy. Fresh whole blood or packed red blood cells are appropriate in the resuscitation of the trauma victim needing restoration of oxygen-carrying capacity. Because of concerns regarding the transmission of hepatitis and the human immunodeficiency virus (HIV), transfusion typically is delayed until the isovolemic hematocrit falls to less than 25 in the otherwise healthy person.[43] A standard type and crossmatch, screening for ABO grouping, Rh typing, and antibody screening requires about 1 hour to process. The total elapsed time between sending the sample to the laboratory and starting a fully matched transfusion is about $1\frac{1}{2}$ hours. The safety factor against reaction is 99.9%. An abbreviated emergency crossmatch requires 15 minutes and offers 99.8% safety. In an emergency, major grouping and Rh typing can be done in 10 minutes and offers 99% safety. The use of universal donor or group O Rh-negative blood is no quicker and somewhat less safe than specific blood and should be avoided whenever possible.[54]

Controversy remains over the choice between packed red blood cells and whole blood as transfusion therapy for hemorrhagic shock.[5,100,104] In an effort to maximize the use of blood products, most blood banks increasingly encourage the use of component therapy in the hypotensive patient.[4,55] Chaplin believes that 80% of transfusion therapy needs in the United States can be met with packed red blood cells.[24] Some clinicians contend that the only legitimate reason to use whole blood is for acute blood loss, and even then, specific component therapy directed at correction of the particular problem is preferred. Supporting this recommendation, many patients and laboratory animals have withstood acute blood loss with only crystalloid solutions administered for replacement.[35,45,46,112] In the absence of preexisting cardiopulmonary disease, the hematocrit should be maintained between 25% and 30% to create a satisfactory balance between adequate oxygen transport capacity and reduced viscosity to allow unimpeded flow in the microcirculation.[35,37,81,84,112]

However, the use of stored blood for patients in profound shock carries several risks and potential complications, including depression of the oxygen-carrying capacity of the red blood cells, coagulation changes with secondary bleeding, increased acid load, and introduction of cellular aggregates and debris causing pulmonary microemboli.

The oxygen affinity of hemoglobin increases when red blood cells lose their 2,3-diphosphoglycerate. This left shift in the hemoglobin dissociation curve impedes oxygen transfer at the tissue level. When the cells are stored in citrate-phosphate-dextrose solution, this shift occurs after about 10 to 12 days of storage. In the patient receiving a nonemergency transfusion, this rarely is a problem because 2,3-diphosphoglycerate is resynthesized within 24 hours of transfusion. However, in the massively transfused trauma patient, the use of red blood cell concentrates that are less than 10 days old may be advantageous.[55,101]

Previous teaching held that the massively transfused patient receiving more than 10 units of red blood cells or whole blood every 24 hours also should receive 1 to 2 units of fresh frozen plasma, 10 units of platelets, and 2 ampules of calcium.[26,53,116] These recommendations were empiric and directed at reversing the "washout" effect of massive transfusion on coagulation proteins, as well as correcting qualitative and quantitative platelet defects. The clinical need for platelet concentrates in the massively transfused patient was critically evaluated by Harrigan and coworkers in 22 seriously injured patients.[53] They found that in the absence of platelet administration, the platelet count was low during surgery and continued to fall until the second postoperative day. Platelet aggregation was depressed during surgery and remained depressed. Bleeding times were abnormal through the fourth postoperative day. Despite these abnormalities, no patient had clinical "oozing." These authors concluded that *prophylactic* administration of platelet concentrates in the absence of a clinically detectable bleeding abnormality was not warranted.

Hemorrhagic shock and resuscitation have been shown to cause a significant fall (20% to 40%) in the level of coagulation factor proteins and an increase in all clotting times. This reflects dilution as well as increased hemostatic demands and acutely decreased hepatic synthesis.[52] Resuscitation with fresh frozen plasma has been shown to have a minimal effect on the decline of coagulation factor proteins when compared with lactated Ringer's solution.[70] Thus, fresh frozen plasma should *not* be used routinely in massive transfusion and should be used only in patients who have clinical oozing and a defined defect in the coagulation cascade.[82,110]

The use of macropore filters (160 μm) is recommended when stored whole blood or red blood cells are being administered. These in-line devices remove platelet aggregates and debris that otherwise might become trapped in the pulmonary microcirculation. Olcott and Lim have shown that when whole blood is administered through a macropore filter, 20% to 40% of the functioning platelets can be removed.[85]

Some blood banks routinely remove the buffy coat layer in whole blood, which effectively removes 80% of the microaggregates from the red blood cell unit and reduces by 60% the incidence of febrile transfusion reactions. The use of a microaggregate filter with this preparation is a special situation and can yield a reaction-free transfusion even when recipients have leukocyte antibodies.[55]

Whole blood stored for up to 21 days in acid citrate dextrose at 4°C contains all the components necessary for opsonization, with only a slight reduction of activity as compared with fresh whole blood.[71,72] Reconstituted packed red blood cells, however, contain only 30% of their volume as plasma components and, consequently, have a markedly reduced content of plasma opsonins.[25,71] Evidence suggests that low levels of opsonic proteins predispose a host to infection,[3,6,7,44,76] pulmonary dysfunction,[42] and multisystem organ failure[17]; impaired opsonization may be one of the most common causes of dysfunction of host defense mechanisms against infection.[24,80,121] The use of cryoprecipitate as an opsonin-rich solution has been reported in the successful treatment of postburn sepsis[63] and the pulmonary dysfunction of severe adult respiratory distress syndrome.[96,97] Opsonic activity is important in the response to shock and trauma, and on this basis, whole blood may be preferable to packed red blood cells for resuscitation in acute hemorrhagic shock when the effect on repletion of circulating opsonic elements is considered. In the setting of severe shock, a significant decrease in host reticuloendothelial clearance occurs, and the failure of large-volume transfusion of packed red blood cells to reverse this deficiency in opsonic activity may have a considerable negative effect on ultimate survival.[12,13]

Hypothermia. Hypothermia in the patient with shock can develop secondary to massive transfusion of room temperature fluids as well as exposure during resuscitation. In profound hypothermia (less than 33°C), coagulation defects can develop that respond only to rewarming.[89] Cardiac irritability also increases as core temperature falls. In cases of massive transfusion, special attention should be given to preventing hypothermia by prewarming the infused fluids.[98] Crystalloids can be kept at 39° to 40°C in a warming closet before administration, and the remaining fluids can be passed through an in-line warmer.[4] Several devices are commercially available that can both prewarm and

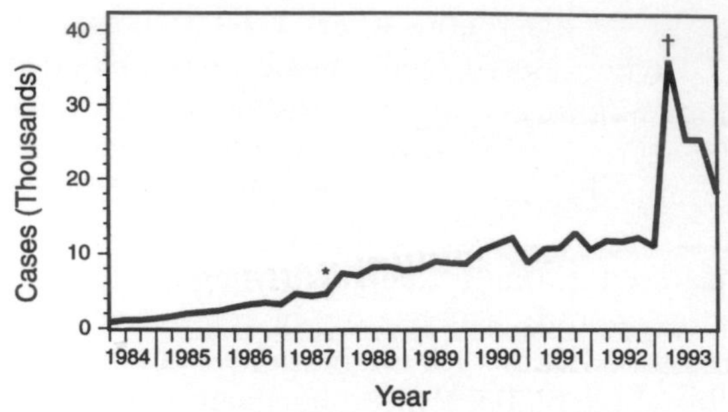
Cases (Thousands)
Year
*Case definition revised in October 1987 to include additional illnesses and to revise diagnostic criteria (3).
†Case definition revised in 1993 to include CD4+ criteria and three illnesses (pulmonary tuberculosis, recurrent pneumonia, and invasive cervical cancer) (1).

FIGURE 8-1. AIDS cases, by quarter year of report in the United States, 1984–1993.

infuse fluid at a rate of more than 500 mL/min, and their use is recommended (Rapid Infusion System, Haemometics Corporation, Braintree, Mass.; Level One Technology, Marshfield, Mass.).[33,43]

Transmission of Disease. *Surgeon Risk.* Human immunodeficiency virus and hepatitis B and C remain significant occupational hazards for the orthopaedic surgeon. As of 1993, about 240,000 cases of clinical acquired immunodeficiency syndrome (AIDS) had been reported to the Centers for Disease Control (Fig. 8-1). An additional 1 million individuals are estimated to be HIV positive (Fig. 8-2). Blood-soiled wounds, especially those with the sharp bone ends encountered in open fractures, should be handled using universal precautions to protect against direct contact with blood and other body fluids. Data from urban trauma centers suggest that the seroprevalence for HIV infection ranges from 2% to 8.9%,[109] and may be as high as 15% in the penetrating trauma population.[36] About 40 cases of AIDS have been documented from occupational transmission in the healthcare setting. The risk of seroconversion after a hollow-bore needlestick is about 1:500.[41] The risk to an operating surgeon probably is substantially less because solid needles are used that must pass through surgical gloves before entering the skin. Popejoy and Fry reviewed 684 surgical procedures over a 1-month period and found that at least one member of the operative team had a blood contact event in 28% of the cases.[93] In 8% of the cases, a percutaneous exposure occurred. Trauma and cardiothoracic surgeons were at particularly high risk (Fig. 8-3). In 1991, the Centers for Disease Control conducted an anonymous survey of 3420 orthopaedic surgeons at the annual meeting of the American Academy of Orthopaedic Surgeons. HIV serology was performed on all volunteers and an anonymous questionnaire was completed. In this study, only two surgeons had positive HIV serology and both reported high-risk personal behavior. These findings underscore the low rates of seroconversion from the multitude of blood exposure events that must have occurred in this group over the years.[41]

Hepatitis B and C (non-A, non-B) represent a larger risk statistically to the surgeon than does HIV. In one study, the rate of seropositivity for HBsAg in an urban trauma population was shown to be 3.1%.[109] The Centers for Disease Control estimates that up to 250 healthcare workers per year die as a result of hepatitis

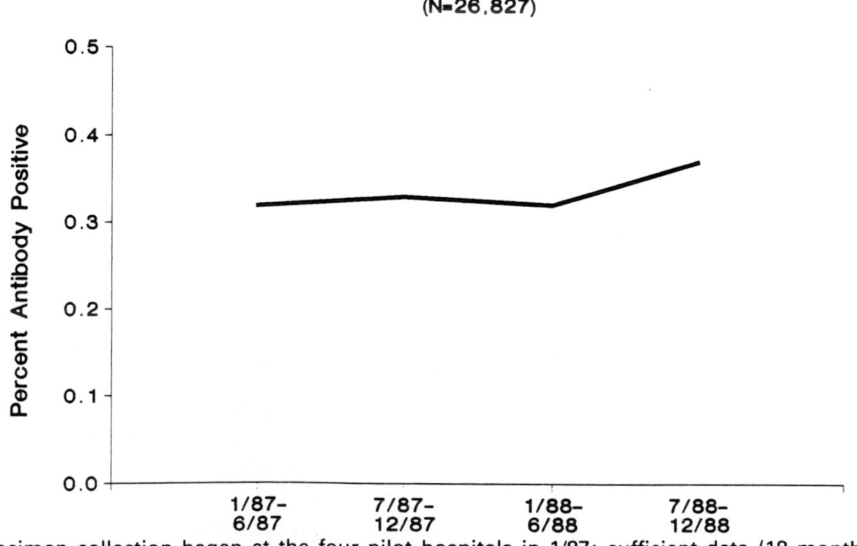
(N=26,827)
Percent Antibody Positive
1/87–6/87
7/87–12/87
1/88–6/88
7/88–12/88
*Specimen collection began at the four pilot hospitals in 1/87; sufficient data (18 months or more) for trend analysis are expected from the next five hospitals by 9/89 and for the remaining 31 hospitals by 3/90.

FIGURE 8-2. HIV antibody prevalence in patients at four pilot sentinel hospitals,* from January 1987 to December 1988.[2]

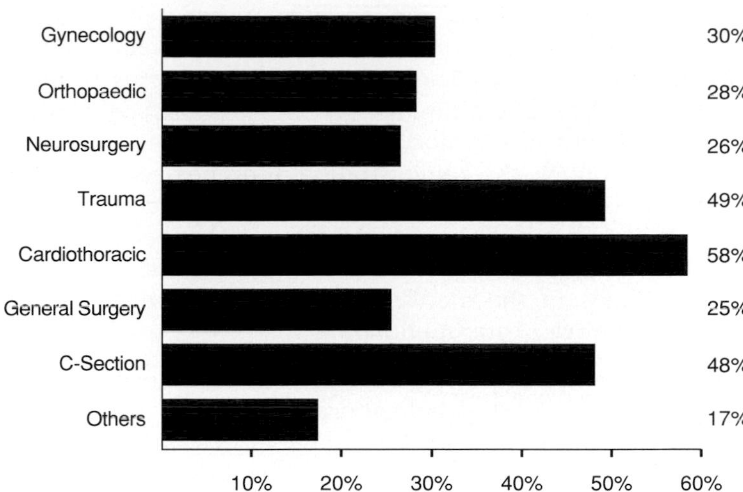

FIGURE 8-3. The relative frequency by surgical specialty of blood contact that is sustained by operating room personnel during the conduct of operative procedures (C-Section—cesarean section). (*Fry, D.E.: Occupational Risks of Infection in the Surgical Management of Trauma Patients. Am. J. Surg., 165 (Suppl 2A):30S, 1993.*)

B infection. The etiology of these deaths is divided between fulminant hepatitis and liver failure, cirrhosis and secondary liver failure, and hepatocellular carcinoma, and they may occur 20 or more years after the acute infection.[23] Despite these statistics, it has been estimated that up to 50% of surgeons have not been vaccinated against hepatitis B. The current hepatitis B vaccine is manufactured from recombinant technology, and is safe and effective. Seroconversion should be confirmed after the three-dose series is completed, but can be expected in 95% of cases. Unfortunately, there is no vaccine for non-A, non-B hepatitis, and current estimates are that more than 500,000 individuals in the United States may be chronic carriers. This disease remains a significant risk to healthcare workers. Like HIV, prevention rests in the control of exposure events.[39]

Patient Risk. Despite improvements in the screening of blood donors, the risk of disease transmission to the patient through transfusion remains real.[2,48,58] Non-A, non-B hepatitis, HIV, and cytomegalovirus infection continue to occur at relatively constant rates. Current estimates of the risk of contracting HIV infection from a unit of transfused blood range from 1:40,000 to 1:250,000 (Fig. 8-4). Since 1990, the rate of transfusion-associated HIV infection has remained constant at about 640 to 760 new cases per year. This mode of transmission accounts for about 2.3% of HIV-infected patients.[120] The increased risk of HIV transmission through pooled blood products from multiple donors generally should restrict their use to life-threatening situations.[35,84,112] The risk of contracting non-A, non-B hepatitis is about 1% to 2%, with a subsequent chronic carrier rate of 30% to 50%.[19,35,40,48]

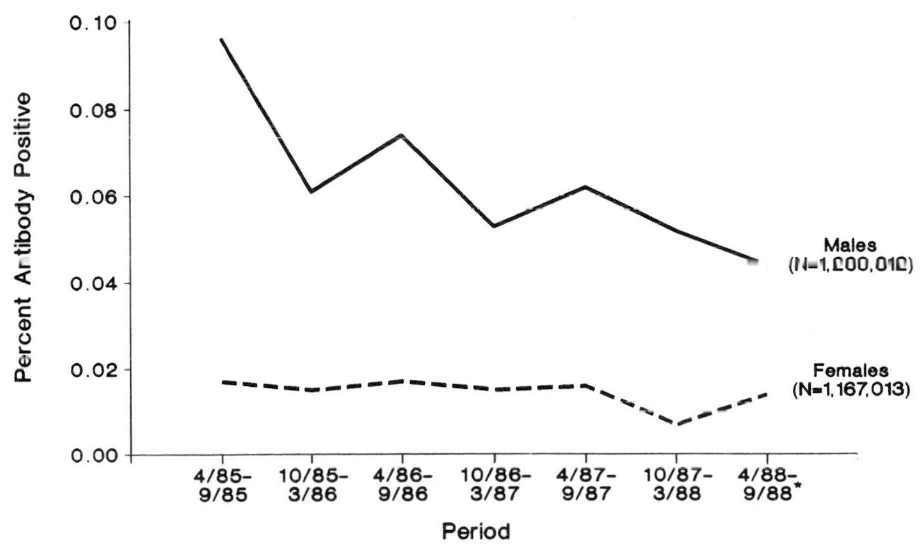

FIGURE 8-4. HIV antibody prevalence in first-time blood donors, by sex, as reported by the American Red Cross, from April 1985 to September 1988.[2]

Other Agents. Vasopressors, hydrocortisone, and vasodilators are of questionable value in the treatment of hemorrhagic shock.[9] The response to these agents has been variable and unpredictable.[102,105] For the patient with hypovolemic shock who has open fractures and large wounds, the administration of prophylactic antibiotics is advisable.[59,76] Unless a patient has Addison's disease, has had an adrenalectomy, or has been receiving long-term corticosteroid therapy, the use of corticosteroids in the management of hypovolemic shock is otherwise contraindicated.

Monitoring the Patient in Shock. In the patient being resuscitated, arterial blood pressure, pulse, central venous pressure, and urinary output must be monitored closely. These all are indirect measurements to help ascertain the patient's intravascular volume. Adequate venous access should be obtained through the placement of several peripheral lines. An arterial line may be useful for continuous monitoring of blood pressure and frequent checks of arterial blood oxygenation. A central venous pressure line, inserted through the internal jugular vein or the subclavian vein, should be placed so that the catheter tip is in or near the right atrium. A normal pressure is 5 to 10 cm H_2O; the central venous pressure normally should not exceed 15 cm H_2O. More accurate monitoring of intravascular volume and cardiac output can be obtained from a Swan-Ganz catheter. Data obtained from this device may be essential to the differentiation of cardiogenic from noncardiogenic pulmonary edema during fluid resuscitation.

Renal function must be monitored closely. The average adult should have a urinary output of 50 mL/h as monitored by an indwelling Foley catheter, placed only after adequate rectal examination to investigate the possibility of urethral disruption.[4] Renal function may be decreased by hemorrhagic shock, hyponatremia, urinary tract injury, or the use of pressors.

Post-shock Complications. Tissue in shock is, by definition, ischemic to some degree. Resulting tissue damage can be minimized by restoring tissue perfusion and oxygenation as rapidly as possible. Several studies have shown that tissue oxygen debt can persist in certain vascular beds if only hemodynamic parameters of resuscitation are measured. Some researchers advocate increasing oxygen delivery until oxygen consumption has peaked—usually at 50% above the normal level. The splanchnic circulation is particularly vulnerable to inadequate resuscitation, which may predispose it to increased permeability to both bacteria and endotoxin.[152] This process appears to be mediated by hydroxyl radicals derived from xanthine oxidase.[31] Bacterial translocation from the gut may be the initiating event in post-shock multisystem organ failure. The concept of bacterial translocation from the gut during shock is supported by both animal studies and clinical series.[31,60] Rush and coworkers have shown that the incidence of positive blood culture results is correlated with the severity of shock.[95] Fifty-six percent of their patients with a systolic pressure of less than 80 mm Hg had positive blood culture results, 22% with gram-negative organisms.

There is increasing evidence that oxidants play an important role in the post-shock events that may lead to generalized inflammation by altering membrane permeability. These oxidants may impair cellular function even when tissue delivery appears to be optimized. Pharmacologic antioxidants such as dobutamine, deferoxamine-hetastarch, 21-aminosteroids, pentoxifylline, and ibuprofen are being studied intensely as they relate to shock injury. The optimal role of nutritional antioxidants such as β-carotene and vitamins C and E has yet to be determined.[152]

Cardiopulmonary Arrest

Standards and guidelines for cardiopulmonary resuscitation and emergency cardiac care have been set by the American Heart Association.[142,143] The major impetus for this was an increasing appreciation of premature cardiovascular mortality and morbidity. Resuscitation by cardiopulmonary resuscitation outside the hospital, followed by advanced measures in the hospital, has been an effective lifesaving intervention in 40% to 60% of select subgroups of patients.[141,146,147]

The American Heart Association has recommended that competence in cardiopulmonary resuscitation be mandatory for physician reappointment to faculty.[143] Reviews of in-hospital resuscitation efforts show poor results, with a success rate of about 20%.[131] The practice of orthopaedic surgery encompasses numerous situations in which cardiac arrest can occur.[†] Our patient population includes many elderly, infirm patients who may have accompanying cardiopulmonary, renal, and metabolic diseases that predispose them to cardiac arrest.[136] Moreover, trauma frequently affects young people, who may suffer significant cardiopulmonary insult in addition to musculoskeletal injuries.[123,140] For these reasons, the orthopaedic surgeon should be capable of instituting care in the management of cardiac arrest and must be proficient in the techniques of cardiopulmonary resuscitation and advanced cardiac life support. Because it is beyond the scope of this text to cover this material in detail, the reader is referred to several excellent references for further study.[‡]

† References 124, 126, 129, 130, 137, 148, 149, 151.
‡ References 125, 127, 128, 132, 135, 138, 139, 142, 145, 150.

Fat Embolism Syndrome/Acute Respiratory Distress Syndrome

The fat embolism syndrome is a major cause of morbidity and mortality after fractures in the patient with multiple injuries. For more than a century, the puzzling features of this entity have interested many. Its relationship to skeletal and soft-tissue injury is well recognized, and many cases have been reported.[183,184,252] Fat embolism is an important cause of acute respiratory distress syndrome.[170,190,258,282] However, the fat embolism syndrome is not necessarily seen as a sequel of trauma and is being recognized increasingly after any surgical instrumentation of the medullary canal. It has been reported in association with a variety of nontraumatic entities, including hemoglobinopathy,[208] collagen disease,[216] diabetes,[187] burns,[189] severe infection,[236] inhalation anesthesia,[295] metabolic disorders,[217] neoplasms, osteomyelitis,[176,197] blood transfusion,[234] cardiopulmonary bypass,[242] renal infarction,[180] decompression from altitude,[215] and renal homotransplantation.[220] Since the mid-1960s, a better understanding of the underlying pathophysiologic mechanisms of the fat embolism syndrome has developed,[182,193,207] and its relationship to acute respiratory distress syndrome has been clarified. Sproule and colleagues identified the role of fat embolization in post-traumatic respiratory insufficiency.[277] They established that fat embolism must be recognized as one of the acute respiratory distress syndromes. With prompt recognition, the treatment of the fat embolism syndrome has become more specific and less empiric, resulting in decreased morbidity and mortality. In more recent years, prevention of the fat embolism syndrome by early fracture fixation and patient mobilization has become the focus of a wave of clinical investigation.[§]

Historical Review

In 1861, Zenker described fat droplets in the lung capillaries of a railroad worker who sustained a fatal thoracoabdominal crush injury.[300] In 1865, Wagner described the pathologic features of fat embolism.[290] However, in 1873, Bergmann became the first to establish the clinical diagnosis of fat embolism syndrome in a 38-year-old patient who sustained a comminuted fracture of the distal femur.[168] Postmortem examination revealed a large amount of pulmonary fat. In 1875, Czerny called attention to the symptoms associated with cerebral fat embolism and noted the importance of a funduscopic examination.[188] In 1879, Fenger and Salisbury from Cook County Hospital made the first clinical diagnosis of fat embolism syndrome in the United States in a patient who had a proximal femoral fracture.[196] Autopsy examination revealed massive fat emboli in the lungs and brain.

In 1879, Scriba reviewed and correlated the clinical, pathologic, and experimental observations of the fat embolism syndrome.[268] In 1911, Benestad[164] and Grondahl[210] first described the characteristic petechial rash seen with the fat embolism syndrome. Warthin in 1913,[292] Gauss in 1916,[201] Lehman and Moore in 1927,[229] Vance in 1931,[288] and Scuderi in 1941[269] presented review papers and experimental evidence on the origin and nature of intravenous fat globules, the frequency and importance of fat embolism, and the clinical entity of cerebral fat embolism. In 1957, 1969, and 1971, Peltier appraised the problem of fat embolism and established the importance of pulmonary fat embolism.[251,253,254] Sproule and associates were the first to report severe arterial hypoxemia in three patients with the fat embolism syndrome.[277] In 1966, Ashbaugh and Petty first described the use of corticosteroids in the treatment of the respiratory complications of fat embolism syndrome.[158]

In 1973, Beck and Collins[163] published an extensive review of the theoretic and clinical aspects of the post-traumatic fat embolism syndrome, and in 1982, Gossling and Pellegrini[207] reexamined the pathophysiology and physiologic basis of treatment of the fat embolism syndrome.

Incidence

The exact incidence of and mortality caused by the fat embolism syndrome are not known; it is difficult to accumulate the data necessary to determine these statistics. Suffice it to say that, historically, we consistently have underestimated the importance of this syndrome in post-traumatic fatalities. Sutton stated that 10% of battle casualties in World War I suffered fat emboli.[279] In World War II, a postmortem study of 60 patients who died of battle wounds revealed a 65% incidence of fat emboli.[298] In a study of 6250 civilian accident victims, fat emboli occurred in 855 and contributed to death in more than half.[200] In Britain, an estimated 80 deaths resulting from highway accidents occur because of the fat embolism syndrome.[244] Clinical studies,[‖] including a review of post-traumatic fat embolism in children,[191,296] have documented the frequent occurrence of this syndrome as a sequela to trauma, especially in patients with multiple fractures. It is apparent that rises in automobile, motorcycle, and snowmobile accidents, as well as other types of trauma, will lead to an increased frequency of the fat

§ References 172, 173, 195, 204, 206, 219, 235, 259, 261, 263, 264, 270, 280, 283, 299.

‖ References 153, 169, 175, 237, 243, 263, 285, 297.

embolism syndrome. In addition, the greatest risk of the fat embolism syndrome occurs with multiple fractures.[192] The mortality has been estimated to be as high as 50%. The fat embolism syndrome has become a frequent, serious, and often fatal complication of trauma, both on the battlefield and in civilian life. It has been estimated that more than 5000 deaths annually are the result of the fat embolism syndrome.

The clinical signs and symptoms associated with the fat embolism syndrome are evident in 0.5% to 2% of patients with long-bone fractures and in nearly 10% of those with multiple skeletal fractures associated with unstable pelvic injuries.[207] Given the subjective clinical criteria essential for diagnosis of the syndrome, its exact incidence is difficult to define from the various reports in the literature. However, systemic embolization of marrow fat as a subclinical event occurs with nearly all fractures of long bones, and its direct clinical effect is measured most readily by monitoring the arterial blood gas level.[159] Therefore, the clinically apparent fat embolism syndrome is rare compared with the subclinical fat embolization that is seen after nearly all lower extremity and pelvic trauma.[257] Clinical manifestations develop in children almost 100 times less frequently than they do in adults with comparable injuries, presumably because of a differing marrow fat content with a higher proportion of hematopoietic elements in children.[232] Myelodysplastic disorders, collagen vascular disease, osteoporosis, and extremity immobilization all cause medullary cavity enlargement and an increased liquid marrow fat content, thereby constituting an increased risk for the development of the fat embolism syndrome. Fat embolism after intramedullary reaming and nailing of long bones has been documented, especially when performed in situ for an impending pathologic fracture.[213,238,249,250,280,294] It also has been reported after fractures of the hip treated with prosthetic hemiarthroplasty.[207] In one controlled series of 854 patients with hip fractures treated without operation, the frequency of fat embolism syndrome ranged from 4% to 7%.[273] The clinical syndrome also has been reported after total hip and knee replacement, especially with bilateral sequential total knee arthroplasty and cementing of the femoral component of a total hip arthroplasty.[165,228,257] We have had unfortunate experiences with acute fatal respiratory failure developing immediately after cemented total hip arthroplasty and intramedullary rod fixation of the intact femur with metastatic lytic lesions for impending pathologic fracture.[250] Postmortem examination revealed extensive embolization of marrow elements to the pulmonary capillary bed and embolic fat with small infarcts in the capillary bed of the brain.

Pathogenesis

The pathogenesis of the fat embolism syndrome is the subject of conjecture and controversy. The source of the embolic fat is thought by most to be the bone marrow.[204] Bone marrow elements have been demonstrated in lung sections, indicating that mechanical fat embolization does occur.[157,214,240,293] The physicochemical theory of fat embolism postulates that changes that occur in lipid stability after trauma and the alteration of microcirculatory flow patterns combine to cause inadequate tissue perfusion, subsequent tissue hypoxia, and the fat embolism syndrome.[230,231,266,291] More than one possibility exists for the source of embolic fat, and the causes are not mutually exclusive.

However, most investigators agree that bone marrow is the source of embolic fat seen in the lungs.[#] Considerably fewer agree on the exact role of this fat in the production of the clinical fat embolism syndrome.** Few investigators subscribe to Peltier's original hypothesis that lipase endogenous to the lung converts neutral fat to toxic free fatty acids.[251,254,255] Recent work by Barie and colleagues demonstrates that free fatty acids are bound rapidly by albumin and transported through the bloodstream and lymphatic channels in this benign form.[162] However, conversion to free fatty acids need not be implicated to produce the clinically apparent respiratory failure seen in this syndrome.[207] An abundance of tissue thromboplastin is released with the marrow elements after long-bone fracture. This activates the complement system and the extrinsic coagulation cascade through direct activation of factor VII.[165,212,226,265,276,284] Intravascular coagulation by-products such as fibrin and fibrin degradation products then are produced. These blood elements, along with leukocytes, platelets, and fat globules, combine to increase pulmonary vascular permeability, both by their direct actions on the endothelial lining and through the release of numerous vasoactive substances.[186,207] In addition, these same substances activate platelet aggregation. Suppression of the fibrinolytic system in the injured patient then may aggravate an ongoing accumulation of cellular aggregates, fat macroglobules, and clotting factors that are concentrated in the lung by virtue of its filtering action on venous blood before it is recycled to the systemic circulation.[186] It has become increasingly apparent that embolic marrow fat and other elements may only represent the catalyst for a single early step in a long chain of events leading to the final common pathway of increased pulmonary vascular permeability in response to many forms of systemic injury.

Clinical Findings

The clinician must distinguish between the clinical entity of the fat embolism syndrome as the cause of acute respiratory insufficiency and the presence of intravas-

References 157, 201, 218, 224, 225, 240, 266.

** References 162, 167, 212, 222, 231, 239, 284.

cular fat emboli, which have been described in various conditions, including pancreatitis, osteomyelitis, diabetes, burns, and prolonged corticosteroid therapy. The signs and symptoms of the fat embolism syndrome are predominantly those of the adult respiratory distress syndrome.

The most common etiologic factor associated with the fat embolism syndrome is a high-energy long-bone fracture in a patient in the second or third decade of life, when tibial or femoral fractures are likely to occur, or in a patient in the sixth or seventh decade of life, when low-energy fractures of the hip are frequent. The onset of clinical symptoms may be immediate or may not occur for 2 or 3 days after trauma.[194] Sevitt stated that of 100 patients with fat embolism, 25 showed symptoms within the first 12 hours after injury, 75 showed symptoms within 36 hours, and 85 demonstrated symptoms within 48 hours.[271] In the earlier literature, however, emphasis was placed on the lucid interval; this interval may be more apparent than real. It may be difficult to diagnose a fulminating and rapidly progressing case that terminates in death and is associated with multiple fractures. Coma develops rapidly and is accompanied by marked respiratory distress. Occasionally, the patient demonstrates hemoptysis, and pulmonary edema becomes manifest. Often, the symptoms and signs of fat embolism syndrome are masked by shock or coma, or by an anesthetized state in a patient undergoing early operative treatment.

It also is likely that many cases of mild fat embolism syndrome are overlooked. The phenomenon called fracture fever, or hematoma fever, in the early postinjury state may be an unrecognized, mild variety of fat embolism syndrome.[194]

The enigma of the clinical fat embolism syndrome remains that, although early diagnosis is extremely important in the management of the life-threatening pulmonary failure, the recognition of the fat embolism syndrome remains a diagnosis of exclusion dependent on the clinician's high index of suspicion. Certain features of the fat embolism syndrome assist in its early clinical recognition. Symptoms are shortness of breath, which may begin relatively suddenly, followed by restlessness and confusion. The patient often becomes obstreperous and difficult to manage. Arterial hypoxemia is the hallmark. Other clinical signs associated with the fat embolism syndrome involve a flat temperature elevation to 39° to 40°C; tachypnea, with rates of 30 breaths per minute or higher; and tachycardia, with rates of 140 beats per minute or higher. Blood pressure does not vary widely and usually remains within normal limits. Another striking feature is the changing neurologic picture: the onset of restlessness, disorientation followed by marked confusion, stupor, or coma.[227] Long-tract signs may be present, with occasional extensor posturing and decerebrate rigidity, and even focal seizures. These neurologic signs can change rapidly. Urinary incontinence may occur despite the patient's apparent well-being. In a young, healthy patient with a fracture, such a situation may indicate the onset of the fat embolism syndrome. Recovery may take several months, and permanent neurologic deficits have been reported, including severe mental retardation. Furthermore, it may be difficult to distinguish these neurologic manifestations of the fat embolism syndrome from those of primary craniocerebral trauma (Table 8-2).

The second or third day after injury, petechiae may be seen, characteristically located across the chest, the axilla, and the root of the neck and in the conjunctivae (Fig. 8-5). This distribution is in contrast to the petechial rash seen in patients with subacute bacterial endocarditis. The petechial rash is fleeting and may last only a short while, fading rapidly (Fig. 8-6). It may occur periodically, with accompanying attacks of coma. The conjunctival lesions are sharp and distinct and can be seen by rolling back the eyelids (Fig. 8-7). Retinal lesions can be identified by funduscopic examination and appear as microinfarcts at the ends of the retinal arterioles.[223] There may be permanent changes in the optic nerve center after the fat embolism syndrome.

The clinical manifestations as described result from a reduced blood flow to vital organs, such as the lungs, with dyspnea and cyanosis; the cerebral cortex, with dyspnea, disorientation, and restlessness; and, occasionally, the kidneys, with resultant oliguria. Many injuries other than multiple fractures are associated with the fat embolism syndrome. The more common are intrathoracic, intra-abdominal, intracranial, and major arterial injuries. It is most important to identify all associated injuries, to institute corrective measures for their treatment, and to not overlook the blood loss that occurs with an associated injury as well as with the fracture.

TABLE 8-2
Comparison of Features of Cerebral Fat Embolism and Craniocerebral Trauma

Signs and Symptoms	Cerebral Fat Embolism	Craniocerebral Trauma
Lucid interval	18–24 h	6–10 h
Confusion	Severe	Moderate
Pulse rate	Rapid (140–160)	Slow
Respiration rate	Rapid	Slow
Onset of coma	Rapid	Slow
Localizing signs	Usually absent	Usually present
Decerebrate rigidity	Early	Terminal

(Evarts, C.M.: Diagnosis and Treatment of Fat Embolism. *J.A.M.A.*, 194:899–901, 1965.)

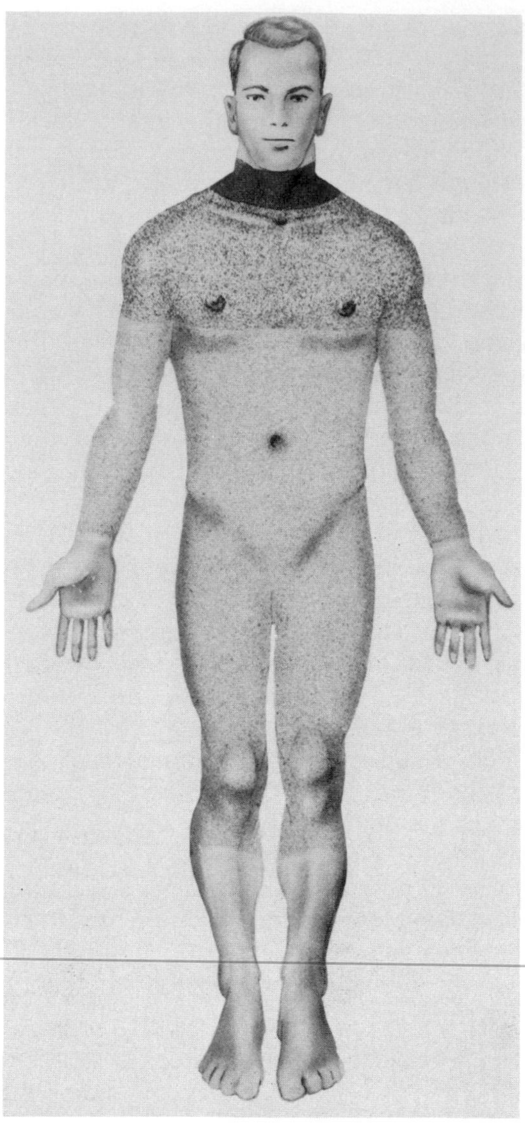

FIGURE 8-5. Sites of petechial rash in the fat embolism syndrome. (*Evarts, C.M.: The Fat Embolism Syndrome: A Review. Surg. Clin. North Am., 50:493–507, 1970.*)

Laboratory Findings

Unfortunately, a pathognomonic laboratory test for fat embolism syndrome does not exist, but arterial hypoxemia is the hallmark of this condition and should be sought immediately after injury. It is most important to obtain serial arterial blood gas measurements in patients suspected of having fat embolism syndrome with pulmonary insufficiency.[160,166,179,248] The measurement of arterial hypoxemia is a sensitive index of the degree of pulmonary fat embolism and monitors the response to treatment. Po_2 values of less than 60 mm Hg indicate significant pulmonary hypoxemia. More sophisticated studies, such as the alveolar-arterial oxygen difference ($AaDo_2$) measured after the inhalation of 100% oxygen for 10 minutes, help determine physiologic shunting and also identify the presence of pulmonary embolization. Serial determinations of the arterial Po_2 values can provide an index of the effectiveness of the treatment of the hypoxic state associated with pulmonary insufficiency accompanying the fat embolism syndrome. It has become clear that inapparent hypoxemia can occur in a patient without other clinical aspects of fat embolism. Symptoms directly referable to the respiratory system often are not present until the Po_2 falls below 65 mm Hg; tachypnea and cyanosis are present much less frequently and are seen only in the presence of severe oxygen desaturation.

In the early stages, thrombocytopenia may occur with platelet values of less than 150,000/mm^3. The hematocrit value often decreases, sometimes with startling drops.[256]

Serial chest x-ray films should be obtained, because they demonstrate progressive snowstorm-like pulmonary infiltrations in patients with the fat embolism syndrome. The changes in chest x-ray films are characteristic but not specific[239] (Fig. 8-8). They frequently occur after the fat embolism syndrome is well under way.

Electrocardiographic changes may occur, demonstrating prominent S waves, arrhythmias, inversion of T waves, and a right bundle-branch block. However, these changes are not specific and reflect cardiac strain. Another helpful laboratory technique used to identify the fat embolism syndrome is a cryostat-frozen section of clotted blood, which reveals the presence of fat. Pathologic fat in the venous circulating blood can be measured by filtering the blood through a microfilter with a pore size of 10 microns, allowing filtration of smaller fat globules but retaining the larger fat globules

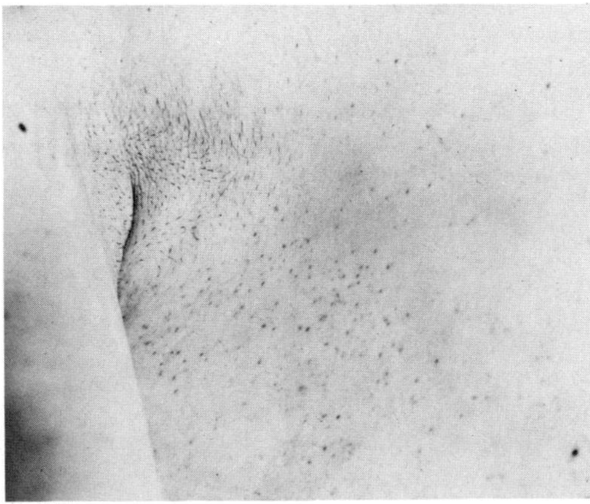

FIGURE 8-6. Axillary petechiae. (*Evarts, C.M.: The Fat Embolism Syndrome: A Review. Surg. Clin. North Am., 50:493–507, 1970.*)

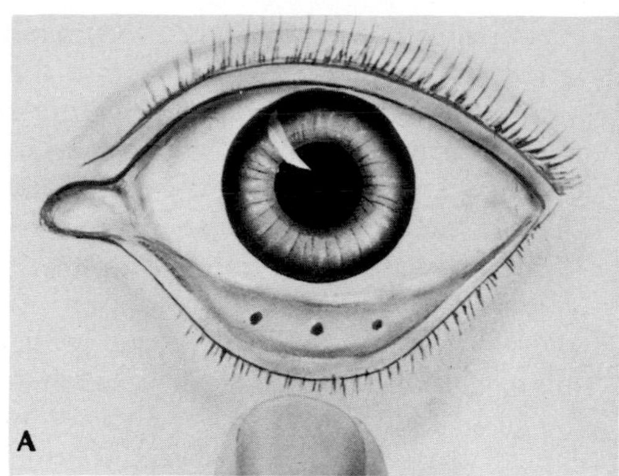

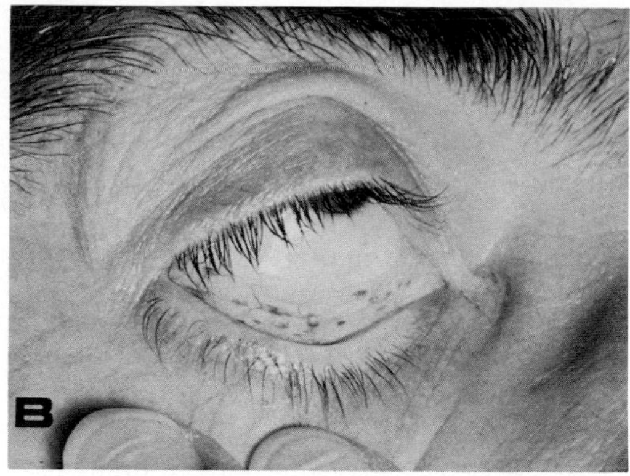

FIGURE 8-7. (**A**) Diagram of conjunctival petechiae. (**B**) Clinical appearance of conjunctival petechiae. (*Evarts, C.M.: The Fat Embolism Syndrome: A Review. Surg. Clin. North Am., 50:493–507, 1970.*)

for staining. Gurd reported this test to be of some value in the identification of the fat embolism syndrome.[211]

If coma persists and there is no means of identifying the patient's problem, one author has suggested renal biopsy as a diagnostic aid in differentiating between coma that has occurred from cerebral trauma and coma that is the result of fat embolism.[271] Lung biopsy has been suggested for the same reason, but its risk does not justify its widespread use. Biopsy of a skin petechial lesion can reveal the presence of embolic intravascular fat.[274] Analysis of the sputum or urine for fat has not proved to be accurate,[171] nor has the sizzle test of Scuderi.[269] Neither spinal fluid examination nor electroencephalography is specifically diagnostic for fat embolism.[198,281]

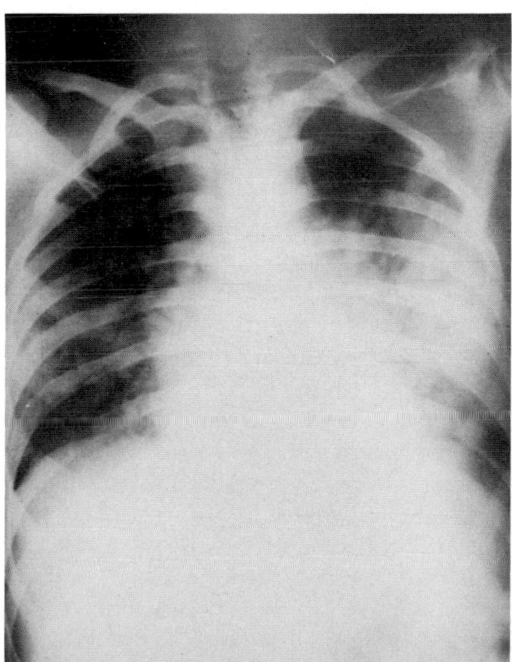

FIGURE 8-8. Radiograph showing pulmonary infiltrate in a patient with the fat embolism syndrome.

Treatment

Many forms of treatment have been suggested for patients with the fat embolism syndrome[194,253,254,272]; unfortunately, many of these modes of therapy are derived from anecdotal studies without control subjects. Treatment can be considered in two categories: nonspecific, general measures and specific measures. As with all patients who have sustained multiple injuries, the following general management principles should be followed: the airway must be maintained, blood volume should be restored, fluid and electrolyte balance must be maintained, and unnecessary transportation should be avoided. The injured part or parts should be immobilized before any transportation is considered, because excess movement may cause further fat embolization.

Treatment of Hypoxemia

The initial (and perhaps the only specific) treatment of fat embolism is directed at decreasing the hypoxemia that occurs as a result of the respiratory distress. Oxygen should be administered immediately on admission to the emergency department. Accurate monitoring of blood gases is critical in the management of pulmonary insufficiency. The arterial oxygen tension should be maintained at 90 mm Hg or higher. If the degree of hypoxemia is relatively mild, oxygen can be given by mask or nasal catheter, but this can be expected to deliver only a 40% or 50% oxygen concentration. If the degree of hypoxemia is severe and respiratory failure is impending, prompt mechanical ventilatory assistance is mandatory. Endotracheal intubation is the preferred method, because it provides suction and prevents aspiration. It has the disadvantage of causing tracheal necrosis when required for long-term use. A volume-cycled ventilator is used for mechanical ventilatory support in conjunction with positive end-expiratory pressure of 5 to 10 cm H_2O to assist in maintaining the patency of small airways. The utmost caution should be taken in treating patients with hypoxemia; vigilance and meticulous attention to details are required if treatment is to be successful.

Specific Drug Therapy

The mystique of management and prevention of the fat embolism syndrome surrounds the issues of specific drug therapy and the role and timing of definitive fracture fixation. Our vague understanding of the pathology of this process and difficulty in making an early clinical diagnosis have led to the development of a host of empiric therapies with a paucity of clinical and experimental justification for their use.[††]

Ethanol. Ethanol initially was proposed as an emulsifying agent and later was shown to function as a lipase inhibitor in suppressing the rise of free fatty acids in trauma patients. There has been some suggestion that intoxicated patients fare better after multiple skeletal injuries than do those without a measurable blood alcohol level. Although Meyers and Taljaard have demonstrated a significant reduction in the incidence of the fat embolism syndrome with a blood alcohol level of 20 mg%, there have been no prospective controlled investigations of this agent.[241]

Heparin. Heparin initially was used for its ability to stimulate a circulating lipase that would break down the embolic neutral fats from the marrow. After free fatty acids were shown to be toxic to the lung parenchyma, the rationale for continued use of this agent relied on its anticoagulant effects in decreasing platelet aggregation. No clinical trials have demonstrated any benefit, however, and some have proven harmful effects.[155] Again, potential bleeding complications in the acutely injured patient and the demonstration of acute renal failure with this agent in hypovolemic laboratory animals have considerably tempered its use. No laboratory investigations have demonstrated its therapeutic value in this setting.

Hypertonic Glucose. Hypertonic glucose has been suggested as an alternative metabolic fuel that would block the post-traumatic mobilization of free fatty acids.[275,278] Prospective clinical trials have demonstrated a significant improvement in levels of arterial oxygenation; when compared with control agents, however, hypertonic glucose has not been shown to be effective in preventing the full-blown fat embolism syndrome. Although numerous other treatment protocols have been followed, none has demonstrated efficacy in reducing the incidence of pulmonary failure after multiple fractures.

Corticosteroids. Although few prospective studies exist, accumulating evidence supports the use of methylprednisolone in the treatment of the acute respiratory failure of fat embolism syndrome.[‡‡] Ashbaugh and Petty first used 100-mg doses of cortisone intramuscularly in 1966, when they reported two successful cases of reversal of acute respiratory insufficiency after drug treatment.[158] Numerous laboratory investigations have demonstrated efficacy in the prevention of pulmonary failure when animals were pretreated before fatty acid injection to create a fat embolism model. Detailed study has revealed that methylprednisolone does not alter the acute hemodynamic effects of fat embolization to the lung; in a mongrel dog model, increases in pulmonary artery pressure and pulmonary vascular resistance were unaffected by corticosteroid pretreatment.[177] Similarly, systemic thromboxane and prostaglandin levels, as mediators of lung injury, were comparably elevated in both pretreated and control groups.[178] However, the delayed fall in oxygen saturation was blunted by methylprednisolone, and similar protective effects on oxygenation have been demonstrated in human studies.

In 1971, Fischer and associates documented a consistent pattern of improvement in respiratory failure after the administration of methylprednisolone (Solu-Medrol) in an uncontrolled series of 13 human patients.[198] Arterial hypoxemia cleared within 12 hours, pulmonary compliance improved within 72 hours, and neurologic deficits resolved by 3 days after the start of methylprednisolone treatment. Rokkanen and associates were the first to administer corticosteroids prophylactically in dosages of 10 mg/kg of body weight every 8 hours starting in the emergency department.[262] They noted a reduction in the incidence of the fat embolism syndrome from 6 of 15 patients in the control group to 1 of 14 patients in the treatment group.

In 1977, Shier and colleagues reported on a series comparing fluid loading, hypertonic glucose, aspirin, corticosteroid, and control groups.[275] Methylprednisolone was used in dosages of 30 mg/kg of body weight every 6 hours beginning at the time of hospital admission. No patients in the series demonstrated clinical fat embolism syndrome requiring respiratory support; however, the corticosteroid-treated group had consistently better arterial oxygenation when compared with all other groups. Hypertonic glucose, methylprednisolone, and control groups also were compared in a study by Stoltenberg and Gustilo in 1979 in which treatment commenced at the time of hospital admission.[278] Methylprednisolone was given in empiric dosages of 1 g every 8 hours. Of 64 patients, clinical fat

†† References 163, 169, 194, 203, 207, 254, 272.

‡‡ References 154, 158, 181, 198, 199, 221, 233, 262, 267, 275, 278, 289.

embolism syndrome developed in 3 in the glucose group and 2 in the control group after femoral shaft fractures. The syndrome did not develop in any patient in the corticosteroid group; however, the study size was too small to prove statistical significance. There was statistically significant improvement in arterial oxygenation in all patients in the corticosteroid group when compared with the glucose and control groups. Alho and associates in 1978[154] and Schonfeld and colleagues in 1983[267] were the first to prove statistical significance in the protection offered by prophylactic administration of methylprednisolone in a dosage of 7 to 10 mg/kg of body weight four times daily. In the latter series, clinical fat embolism syndrome developed in 9 of 41 patients in the placebo group as compared with 0 of 21 patients in the corticosteroid group. A petechial rash was found in 5 of the 9 patients with the fat embolism syndrome and was the only diagnostic criterion in this series that was specific for this condition. Complement activation as determined by C5a levels was found to be a nonspecific indicator of the syndrome, with a positive predictive value of only 41%.

In 1987, Lindeque and associates demonstrated improved arterial oxygenation in a methylprednisolone-treated group given 30 mg/kg of body weight twice on the day of hospital admission.[233] The definition of fat embolism syndrome in this study was based largely on hypoxemia of less than 60 mm Hg without consideration of adjunctive physical findings. Petechial rash was seen in only 39% of the patients with arterial hypoxemia of less than 60 mm Hg. Again, serum C5a levels were elevated in almost all patients with long-bone fractures, regardless of the development of fat embolism syndrome. Similar efficacy of methylprednisolone in blunting hypoxemia after fat embolism has been observed at intermediate doses of 9 to 10 mg/kg; the frequency of occurrence of the full-blown fat embolism syndrome, the severity of hypoxemia, and the prevalence of hypoxemia all were decreased under the influence of corticosteroid treatment.[221]

Although it is clear that methylprednisolone does not alter the direct hemodynamic consequences of fat embolization on the lung, it does appear to modify the pulmonary response to this injury as manifest by a relative preservation of arterial oxygenation in both the laboratory and the patient. The mechanism of action of this effect remains the subject of discussion. A general anti-inflammatory action is hypothesized to protect the capillary endothelium and preserve vascular integrity, stabilize granulocyte lysosomal membranes, reduce complement system activation, retard platelet aggregation and release of serotonin, and minimize transudation of interstitial edema. It likewise has been postulated that blockade of vasoactive substances relieves pulmonary vascular spasm and allows a rapid partial correction of ventilation-perfusion mismatch, thereby improving oxygenation. The late improvement in lung compliance and oxygenation is attributed to a gradual clearance of interstitial edema after the ongoing inflammatory process has been controlled by the corticosteroids. Stabilization of the complement system may minimize the contribution of complement-mediated neutrophil activation to the production of increased pulmonary alveolar capillary permeability. Perhaps most important, methylprednisolone has been shown to stimulate the proliferation and maturation of type II pneumocytes in laboratory animals, resulting in increased surfactant production and restoration of a new cellular permeability barrier lining the alveolus.[181] Despite the multiplicity of potential sites of action of methylprednisolone, the safety and relative efficacy of the escalation of corticosteroid dosages in published series has been largely untested in controlled trials. Therefore, a measured approach to the use of these agents, in a dosage range of 10 mg/kg, in the prophylaxis and treatment of fat embolism syndrome is appropriate pending further clinical investigation.

The Role of Fracture Stabilization

The second and most hotly contested issue in the management of the fat embolism syndrome is the role of operative fracture stabilization in the multiply injured patient. A large body of evidence has accumulated over the past decade in support of early fracture fixation within 24 hours after injury based on a demonstrated decrease in the incidence of the fat embolism syndrome and an improvement in pulmonary function. However, this philosophy notably evolved from a more conservative original posture of delayed fracture fixation, which has attracted renewed interest in the discussion of the optimum timing of fracture stabilization.

Analysis of comparative series of multiply injured patients is facilitated by the use of a common system of injury severity assessment. The Abbreviated Injury Scale was first proposed in 1971 by the Committee on Medical Aspects of Automotive Safety and graded nonfatal injury to five body areas based on a rating system from 0 (no injury) to 5 (critical).[185] Baker and associates then observed that overall mortality increased in the presence of associated injury to a second or third body system, but injury to a fourth system had little effect on survival.[161] Based on this information, the Injury Severity Score (ISS) was devised, consisting of the sum of the squares of the three highest Abbreviated Injury Scale grades, with the maximum score being $3 \times (5)^2$, or 75. In 1980, the American College of Surgeons Committee on Trauma modified the Abbreviated Injury Scale and adopted the Hospital Trauma Index by adding evaluation of cardiovascular injury and substituting objective diagnoses for subjective impressions in determining a specific injury grade in each body system.[156] Currently, the Hospital Trauma Index includes injury assessment of six body systems: respiratory, cardiovascular, nervous, abdominal, extremity, and skin/subcutaneous tissues. The specific grading system applied to extremity trauma is included in Table 8-3. Subsequent application of the ISS to various series of multiply injured patients has confirmed the correlation between ISS and mortality rates, and has demonstrated the consistency of mortality figures for different ISS levels among the various studies. Although the ISS has significant shortcomings in predicting injury survival by omitting age or patient-specific risk factors, it remains the best available system by which the efficacy and appropriateness of different treatments can be evaluated in the multiply injured patient.

The Finnish experience with the care of long-bone fractures in multiply injured patients documents a progressive decline in the incidence of the fat embolism syndrome with the adoption in 1969 of a policy of rigid internal fracture fixation in these patients.[259,261] In the 3 years before 1970, 203 patients were seen with pelvis or long-bone fractures, 24% underwent operative treatment of their fractures, and there was a 29% overall incidence of the fat embolism syndrome. In contrast, in the 5 subsequent years from 1970 to 1974, 425 patients were seen with pelvic or long-bone fractures, 46.2% had their fractures treated with early internal fixation, and the fat embolism syndrome developed in only 7.8%. By 1974, two thirds of all patients with fractures underwent operative treatment of their skeletal injuries, and no cases of the fat embolism syndrome were seen in 73 patients. During this same 5-year period, there were 47 patients with multiple injuries who had at least two long-bone fractures treated by early internal fixation. In this subset, the fat embolism syndrome developed in 9 patients (19%), and 8 of these patients demonstrated this complication before the surgical intervention, which always was undertaken within 2 weeks of the injury. In no patient was the respiratory status worsened by the surgery, which was done while the syndrome was still present. Overall, from 1967 through 1974, the incidence of the clinical fat embolism syndrome was 22% in patients with fractures treated by nonoperative means compared with 4.5% in patients with fractures that were surgically fixed. These data prompted Riska to adopt a more aggressive stance toward early operative fixation of fractures in multiply injured patients.[260,261] During the ensuring 4 years from 1975 to 1978, 211 patients with multiple injuries and long-bone fractures were treated by "emergency surgery" with internal fixation in a primary stage. The resulting incidence of the clinical fat embolism syndrome was only 1.4%. The syndrome always appeared after surgery, petechiae were noted in 21 of 22 patients, only 3 patients required specific respiratory treatment because of hypoxemia, and only 1 patient died. In 1979, Hansen and Winquist provided similar data regarding the chronology of the fat embolism syndrome.[213] In reporting their first 300 cases of closed intramedullary rod fixation of femoral fractures, they noted the clinical fat embolism syndrome requiring respiratory support in 9% of patients. In that study population, patients spent a minimum of 5 to 7 days in preoperative traction after the injury and all cases of fat embolism syndrome occurred during this interval. In no instance was the syndrome caused or, when already present, exacerbated by the operative procedure.

Subsequent research in dogs has demonstrated a significantly greater neutral fat release after intramedullary reaming of an intact femur compared with a fractured femur.[238] Neutral fat recovered from blood specimens from the ipsilateral femoral vein increased 500% in the intact bone compared with 25% in the fractured femur. In addition, intramedullary pressure in the intact bone approached 200 mm Hg in contrast to a level of only 50 mm Hg reached in the fractured bone during reaming. In 1983, Talucci and coworkers from Seattle compared patients in whom immediate intramedullary nailing of femoral shaft fractures was done within 24 hours of hospital admission with patients in whom femoral rod fixation was delayed a minimum of 5 days.[280] The fat embolism syndrome was not seen in the 57 patients who underwent immediate nailing; however, the 5 patients (11%) who underwent delayed nailing had this complication, and the syndrome was diagnosed during the preoperative interval in 4 of them. Even greater significance is attached to these data when one considers that, ac-

TABLE 8-3
Hospital Trauma Index Extremity Injury

Injury	Class	Index
No injury	No injury	0
Minor sprains and fractures—no long bones	Minor	1
Simple fractures: humerus, clavicle, radius, ulna, tibia, fibula, single nerve	Moderate	2
Fractures: multiple moderate, compound moderate, femur (simple), pelvic (stable), dislocation major, major nerve	Major	3
Fractures: two major, compound femur, limb crush or amputation, unstable pelvic	Severe	4
Fractures: two severe, multiple major	Critical	5

American College of Surgeons: Hospital Trauma Index. Bull. Am. Coll. Surg., 65:31–33, 1980.

cording to Baker, the average ISS in the group with immediate nailing was nearly twice that in the group with delayed nailing. However, "critical hypoxemia" was seen in 20% of patients in the former group as compared with 14% in the latter group; adult respiratory distress syndrome not related to fat embolism occurred in 7% of patients who had immediate nailing and 5% of those who had delayed nailing. The total incidence of pulmonary complications was 30% in both study groups. Although this is cause to consider the contribution of intramedullary nailing in the production of significant hypoxemia without the other classic findings of the fat embolism syndrome, the authors noted that a 27.8% incidence of critical hypoxemia was found in another group of 40 trauma patients without fractures who had ISSs similar to those found in the group undergoing immediate nailing. They concluded that early intramedullary femoral nailing can be accomplished in severely injured patients without increasing the risk of the fat embolism syndrome.

In 1985, Johnson and coworkers reported retrospectively on the occurrence of the adult respiratory distress syndrome in 132 multiply injured patients who had undergone operative fracture stabilization at different intervals from the time of injury.[219] Injury to the central nervous system, overall ISS using the Hospital Trauma Index, and the time to operative stabilization all were found to be significant in predicting the incidence of adult respiratory distress syndrome. The overall incidence of adult respiratory distress syndrome was increased more than fivefold in the group in whom pelvic and major long-bone fracture stabilization was delayed more than 24 hours after injury, increasing from 7% in the group receiving early fixation to 39% in the group receiving delayed fixation. The strength of this association increased, as did the severity of the injury. In patients with an ISS of less than 30, no adult respiratory distress syndrome was seen in the group that underwent early stabilization as compared with an 8% incidence when orthopaedic surgery was delayed more than 24 hours. In patients with an ISS exceeding 30, the adult respiratory distress syndrome was found in 17% of those who underwent early fracture stabilization and in 75% of those who had a delay in operative fracture fixation. These data have been statistically significant for both the overall study group and the subset with an ISS of greater than 40.

Several other investigators have demonstrated the efficacy of early internal fracture stabilization in decreasing the duration of mechanical ventilatory support in multiply injured patients.[264,287,299] The main cause of death in victims of multiple trauma who survive 1 week beyond injury remains remote organ failure caused by sepsis.[205] Performing early internal fracture fixation, optimizing pulmonary function and the mechanics of breathing by eliminating the enforced supine position, decompressing the fracture hematoma as an ongoing source of fat emboli and retained necrotic debris, and eliminating the pain and physiologic stress associated with continued fracture motion all likely contribute to reduced ventilatory dependence and, in turn, improve late survival. It has been shown that the pulmonary failure state after blunt multiple trauma lasts 48 to 72 hours on average, and that prolongation of respiratory compromise is determined largely by the subsequent selection of specific therapy for the injured parts.[270] In addition, planned postoperative mechanical ventilation used in conjunction with positive end-expiratory pressure has been effective in preventing as well as treating adult respiratory distress syndrome in patients with multiple trauma.[204,206,264,299] Goris developed a prevention scale for adult respiratory distress syndrome (Table 8-4) by which the need for prophylactic ventilatory assistance was assessed; a score of 10 correlated with an ISS of 25 or two major fractures and identified patients receiving postoperative mechanical ventilation.[204] When considering the two variables of early internal fracture stabilization and prophylactic ventilatory support, both were found to reduce independently the incidence and severity of adult respiratory distress syndrome complicating the course of patients with fractures and multiple injuries. In a cohort of patients receiving planned mechanical ventilation, those with early operative treatment of fractures (ISS 39.4) had an 11% incidence of adult respiratory distress syndrome, whereas those who underwent nonoperative treatment (ISS 54.6) had a 75% incidence of this complication.[206] When these two

TABLE 8-4
Prevention Scale for Adult Respiratory Distress Syndrome

Injury	Value Points*
Simple fracture of foot, ankle, wrist, rib, and mandible	1
Forearm, Le Fort II	2
Humerus, tibia, vertebra, LeFort IV	3
Femur, pelvis	5
Ruptured spleen	3
Ruptured liver	4
Transfusion > 4 units of blood	3
Initial blood pressure < 80 mm Hg	4
Pao_2 < 60 mm Hg	5
Flail chest, aspiration	10
Intestinal perforation	6
Contusio cerebri	4

* Total score of 10 or more points indicates the need for mechanical ventilation prophylactically to reduce the risk of adult respiratory distress syndrome.

Goris, R.J.A.: The Injury Severity Score. World J. Surg., 7:12–18, 1983.

groups were normalized for injury severity and only those with scores greater than 50 were considered, the mortality rate was 8% and the incidence of adult respiratory distress syndrome was 15% in the group treated with surgery (ISS 56) compared with 50% and 80%, respectively, in the group treated without surgery (ISS 58). Furthermore, among patients with an ISS greater than 30, mortality from late sepsis was 6% and the mean duration of ventilation was 6 days in those treated with surgery compared with 55% and 11 days, respectively, in those treated without surgery.[204,206] The independent value of prophylactic mechanical ventilation was evidenced by an 11% incidence of adult respiratory distress syndrome in the ventilated, operatively treated fracture group as compared with a 50% incidence in the nonventilated, operatively treated fracture group; this was especially noteworthy in view of the higher average ISS of 39.4 in the ventilated group compared with the ISS of 29.6 in the nonventilated group.[206]

Also addressing the question of prophylactic mechanical ventilation, Ruedi and Wolff reported a study group of 57 multiply injured patients, all of whom were treated by early fracture stabilization. Two percent of those who received prophylactic postoperative ventilation acquired adult respiratory distress syndrome, in contrast to 67% of those who did not receive postoperative ventilation.[264] In a similar investigation, Seibel and associates found that in comparison with multiply injured patients with operatively treated femur fractures, 10 days of skeletal traction for a fractured femur doubled the duration of ventilatory failure, increased the number of positive blood cultures by a factor of 10, and nearly quadrupled the number of fracture complications.[270] Thirty days of skeletal traction had proportionately greater detrimental effects: up to 5 times the duration of pulmonary failure, a 74-fold increase in positive blood culture results, and nearly 20 times the number of fracture complications. They concluded that traction for femoral shaft fractures in patients with blunt multiple trauma should be avoided because it greatly increases the risk of multiple system organ failure and the cost of care. In 1986, Lozman and associates reported that immediate fixation of all fractures in multiply injured patients resulted in a significantly lower intrapulmonary shunt and a significant increase in the cardiac index in the 4 days after injury.[235] Other significant changes were a lower platelet count and a greater fibrinogen concentration in the group receiving immediate fixation. Interestingly, the ability to demonstrate fat globules in pulmonary capillary blood samples was no different between the two groups. In a prospective series, Bone and coworkers noted a 43% incidence of adult respiratory distress syndrome in patients with multiple injuries who had a femoral fracture stabilized more than 48 hours after injury, in contrast to a 3.3% incidence of adult respiratory distress syndrome in those who had a femoral fracture stabilized within 24 hours.[173]

More recently, Tscherne, Pape, and colleagues identified a subset of multiply injured patients with severe thoracic injury in whom early reamed intramedullary femoral nailing was associated with significantly higher rates of adult respiratory distress syndrome (33% versus 8%) and mortality (21% versus 4%) when compared with patients having similar injuries and delayed fracture stabilization.[247] The previously stated benefits of fewer septic pulmonary complications and improved pulmonary function were still apparent in the multiply injured group without pulmonary injury when fracture stabilization was completed early. In a subsequent prospective investigation of multiply injured patients without pulmonary contusion, a transient increase in pulmonary artery pressure and worsening of pulmonary gas exchange was observed during reaming of the femoral canal. In contrast, a subset of patients who underwent *unreamed* nailing of the femoral shaft demonstrated no increase in pulmonary artery pressure and no compromise of gas exchange during the operative procedure. These authors suggested that unreamed nailing may be a preferable approach to femoral fixation in multiply injured patients with pulmonary contusion.[174,245–247]

This growing body of evidence seems to construct an almost compelling case for early orthopaedic intervention in the care of multiply injured patients. The mechanism of this beneficial effect from surgical fracture stabilization likely is dependent on improved patient positioning and better mechanics of breathing afforded during the postoperative period. In addition, it long has been observed that the incidence of fat embolism syndrome is considerably less after open fractures than closed injuries. Surgical decompression of the fracture hematoma may diminish intramedullary pressure sufficiently to reduce the escape of fat and thromboplastic material from the medullary canal into the systemic circulation. More likely, marrow contents routinely escape to the lung and go unnoticed clinically despite minor changes in pulmonary gas exchange. However, recent information suggests that in the setting of additional direct trauma to the chest wall resulting in pulmonary contusion, unreamed nailing may be prudent to reduce the embolic debris collecting in the lungs.[174,247,286] Despite the intuitive appeal of this strategy, the necessary clinical studies comparing methods of long-bone stabilization have yet to be done to address systematically the pulmonary effects of fat embolization during reaming of the femoral canal.

In any event, although this approach to fracture management contributes constructively to patient care, there are some shortcomings to be considered. In addition to logistical problems in maintaining access to the operating theater and having skilled orthopaedic surgeons available to perform "immediate" fracture stabilization, the question of skeletal infection must be addressed. In 1977, Riska and associates noted that, in a group of 47 patients treated with rigid skeletal fixation, there were nine (19%) wound infections, which equaled the incidence of fat embolism syndrome in this same population.[261] Four cases were deep infection and five were superficial in nature, with three in each group occurring in open fractures. In 1985, Johnson and colleagues noted a 2.5-fold increase in the rate of "major orthopaedic infection" in the early fracture stabilization group (21%) as compared with the late or nonoperative group (8%).[219] Although these data were not statistically significant, they resurrect at least a theoretic cause for concern. Goris and associates reported a 7.7% incidence of "posttraumatic osteitis" in patients surviving multiple injury after early operative fracture stabilization.[206] Until there are convincing data refuting an increased risk of deep infection with early operative fracture fixation, it appears that this philosophy of management of skeletal injuries in the multiply injured patient still must be tempered by the traditional concern over osteomyelitis, which, even in the current era of medical care, frequently remains a lifelong disease.

Prognosis

The prognosis for recovery from the fat embolism syndrome is poor in patients who have marked pulmonary failure and coma. Mortality is high with these complications. Mild cases often go undetected, and mortality is low in patients without severe pulmonary insufficiency or cerebral manifestations. It is virtually impossible to perform a controlled prospective study to determine true mortality and morbidity. In patients with severe, fulminating, and progressive fat embolism syndrome, treatment as outlined should begin early and promptly; without it, the condition may be fatal.

In summary, embolization of marrow fat is a common complication of multiple skeletal injuries, and it may present as a clinical variant of the adult respiratory distress syndrome. The clinical fat embolism syndrome is noted by the characteristic manifestations of fever, tachycardia, and confusion in association with arterial hypoxemia and other pertinent laboratory findings. Modern techniques in the management of respiratory distress have led to decreased mortality and morbidity. Recent clinical research suggests that early corticosteroid administration may aid in the treatment of fat embolism syndrome.[207] Early fracture fixation providing for rapid mobilization of the patient with multiple injuries provides hope for preventing the respiratory failure associated with the fat embolism syndrome in the setting of multiple injury, in which multiple organ system failure often is fatal.

Hemorrhagic Complications[§§]

Hemorrhagic problems facing the orthopaedic surgeon usually fall into one of two categories. First, there are the problems related to the treatment, operative or conservative, of orthopaedic complications of congenital bleeding disorders, such as hemophilia. Second, there are those failures in the hemostatic mechanism that may arise during or after major surgical procedures or trauma. A detailed discussion of complex hemostatic disorders is beyond the scope of this section, which reviews three topics: the normal hemostatic mechanism, the diagnosis of the more common hemorrhagic disorders, and the principles of their treatment.[308]

Normal Hemostasis

When a blood vessel is pierced or damaged, a series of events occurs to prevent loss of blood and repair the wound. This series consists of adhesion of platelets at the site of injury, aggregation of additional platelets to form a hemostatic plug, formation of fibrin to stabilize the platelet plug and form a clot, and removal of the clot and repair of damaged tissue. The events are described sequentially but overlap considerably. There is, of course, a limit to the size of the wound and the size of the vessel beyond which the normal hemostatic mechanism is ineffective without the addition of local pressure or mechanical closure.

Platelet and Vascular Phase

Local vasoconstriction occurs promptly after vascular damage, slowing or even stopping blood flow in the vessel and facilitating clot formation. Vessel wall damage also disrupts the normal endothelial cell lining, resulting in adherence of platelets to components of the subendothelium.[322,328] Release of adenosine diphosphate, thrombin, and other humoral agents causes the aggregation of additional platelets at the injury site. This enlarging platelet mass may be sufficient to initially stop the flow of blood from smaller vessels and to facilitate activation of the coagulation system to stabilize the hemostatic plug and form a fibrin clot.

Blood Coagulation

Activation of the coagulation system results in the formation of the proteolytic enzyme thrombin, which converts soluble fibrinogen to an insoluble fibrin clot.

[§§] Charles W. Francis, M.D., Professor of Medicine, Division of Hematology, University of Rochester School of Medicine and Dentistry, contributed to the production of this section.

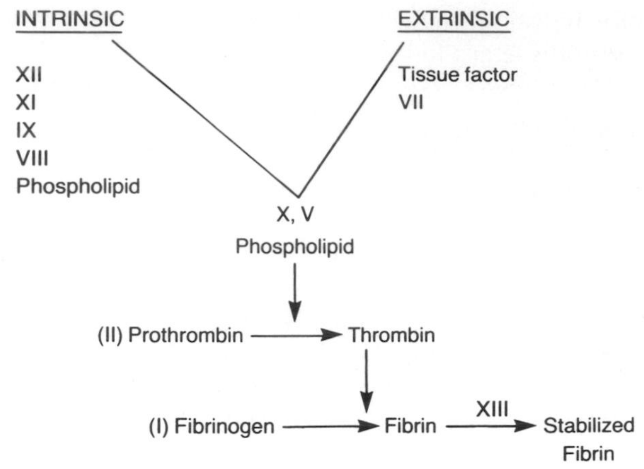

FIGURE 8-9. A simplified scheme of the coagulation pathway.

Local vascular damage initiates the extrinsic coagulation pathway (Fig. 8-9), which is activated through factor VII by exposure of blood to tissue factor, the one coagulation factor that is not present in the blood but is expressed on the membranes of many cells.[321] The intrinsic system functions solely with elements present in the blood. It is activated by the interaction of factor XII with components of the subendothelium, which are exposed to the blood when the vessel is damaged. Both pathways must function for normal hemostasis to occur; this is evident from the fact that an individual who is deficient in factor VIII bleeds, despite having a normal extrinsic pathway, and conversely, factor VII deficiency results in a hemorrhagic diathesis, despite the presence of a normal intrinsic pathway. There are important connections between the two pathways. For example, in addition to activating factor X directly, factor VII and tissue factor can activate factor IX.[320] The components of the intrinsic system are required for a normal partial thromboplastin time, and the PT is used to assess the extrinsic system. Clotting normally is restricted to the local site of need by the combination of local activation at the site of vascular damage, binding of activated coagulation factors to platelets, and systemic inhibition of any activated coagulation factors by circulating inhibitors. These include antithrombin III (AT III), which inhibits the enzymatic activities of coagulation factors in reactions accelerated by heparin.[325] Protein C is a circulating zymogen converted by thrombin to activated protein C, a coagulation inhibitor that acts on factors V and VIII.[306] A lipoprotein-associated inhibitor of the extrinsic system also has been described.[324]

Fibrinolysis and Repair

After the leakage of blood has stopped, repair begins. The clot first must be removed by the fibrinolytic system (Fig. 8-10). The basic framework of this system is similar to that of coagulation, with a series of linked enzymatic reactions resulting in the production of the proteolytic enzyme plasmin.[307] Physiologic activators include tissue-type plasminogen activator and urokinase-like plasminogen activator, which differ in biochemical and immunologic properties.[301] Plasminogen activators are readily available at sites of clot formation or tissue damage, because they are present in most blood and in endothelial cells. Urokinase, a plasminogen activator normally found in the urine; streptokinase, an enzyme produced by bacteria; and tissue plasminogen activator, produced by recombinant DNA techniques, are available for systemic administration to treat thrombotic disorders by activation of the fibrinolytic system. As in coagulation, the fibrinolytic system is restricted to a local area through mechanisms of local activation, specific binding of plasminogen and plasmin to the fibrin clot, and systemic inhibition of fibrinolysis both by the plasmin inhibitor-$_2^-$ antiplasmin and by inhibitors of plasminogen activators. Repair of the vessel wall also involves the coagulation mechanisms, because factor XIII (fibrin-stabilizing factor) not only converts fibrin to a cross-linked, stabilized form, but also plays a role in local growth of fibroblasts.

Preoperative Evaluation

The best defense against unexpected, excessive operative bleeding resulting from hemorrhagic disorders is an adequate preoperative evaluation.[303,323] The history is the single most useful element to evaluate. Most adult patients have had major challenges to the integrity of the hemostatic system, such as tooth extraction, prior surgery, or trauma. A history of normal hemostasis with such procedures makes the presence of a significant congenital bleeding disorder unlikely, whereas a history of abnormal bleeding necessitates a more thorough hemostatic evaluation. The preoperative evaluation also reveals serious illnesses, such as liver

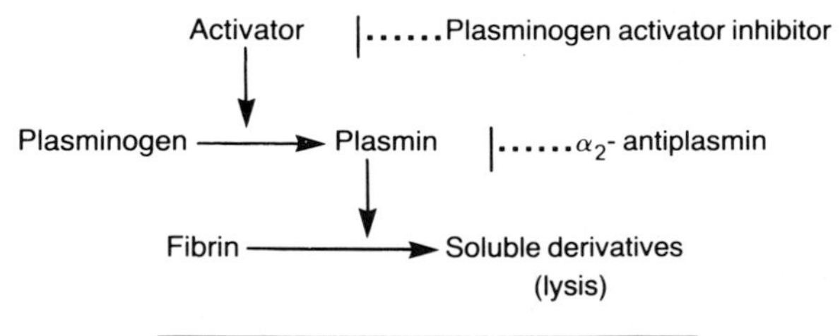

FIGURE 8-10. The fibrinolytic system.

or kidney disease, that may have important effects on hemostatic competence. Laboratory testing is a useful supplement to this evaluation and is particularly important in patients in whom an adequate history cannot be obtained. An activated partial thromboplastin time (aPTT), to test the coagulation system, and an examination of a blood smear or a platelet count, to rule out thrombocytopenia, are the most useful tests. A PT is less useful, but occasionally detects unsuspected liver disease or oral anticoagulant use. If the history or the screening laboratory tests suggest an abnormality, more extensive evaluation is required.

Hemorrhagic Disorders and Laboratory Testing

A derangement of any phase of hemostasis may lead to excessive bleeding. It is important to bear this in mind when considering the possible factors contributing to a hemorrhagic diathesis and the laboratory tests that may be used to elucidate its cause. In view of the complexity of the hemostatic process, the long list of causes of excessive bleeding should not be surprising. Discussion of each entity is beyond the scope of this section, but the common causes of hemorrhage and the more useful laboratory tests are considered as they relate to the several phases of hemostasis.

Platelet and Vascular Phase

Thrombocytopenia is the most common cause of a defect in the platelet and vascular phase. A general correlation exists between the degree of thrombocytopenia and the occurrence of hemorrhage. Hemostasis usually is normal at platelet counts above 100,000/mm^3. Below this level, progressive impairment of hemostasis can be expected. When the platelet count is less than 20,000/mm^3, spontaneous bleeding can occur, typically taking the form of bleeding into the skin and mucous membranes (eg, petechiae, purpura, bruising). The more common causes of thrombocytopenia include reactions to drugs, idiopathic thrombocytopenic purpura, systemic lupus erythematosus, and the administration of cytotoxic drugs. The transfusion of large amounts of stored blood can be expected to lower the platelet count and can contribute to bleeding during surgery.[310]

Abnormal platelet function also can cause bleeding disorders. These conditions are associated with a normal platelet count but a prolonged bleeding time. The most common congenital disorder of this type is von Willebrand's disease, in which a prolonged bleeding time is caused by abnormal platelet function resulting from deficiency or abnormality in a plasma protein known as von Willebrand's factor. (von Willebrand's disease is discussed further in a later section.) Uremia and severe liver disease often are associated with clinically significant platelet dysfunction, and many drugs, including aspirin and other nonsteroidal anti-inflammatory agents, interfere with platelet function and can prolong the bleeding time. It is important to distinguish the antiplatelet effects of aspirin, which last for the entire 5- to 10-day lifespan of the irreversibly acetylated platelet, from those of the nonsteroidal anti-inflammatory agents, which are reversible in the time necessary to clear the drug from the system, depending on its specific pharmacokinetics.

Simple laboratory tests can be used to ensure normal platelet number and function. Platelet number can be evaluated by examination of the blood smear, or a platelet count can be obtained. The bleeding time, an excellent screening test of the integrity of this phase of hemostasis, usually is normal with platelet counts of more than 100,000/mm^3 and is increasingly prolonged with greater degrees of thrombocytopenia.[314] In the presence of a normal platelet count, a prolonged bleeding time generally is indicative of abnormal platelet function, which can be evaluated further by specialized tests performed in a coagulation laboratory.

Blood Coagulation

Failure of normal coagulation can result from either a deficiency of one or more clotting factors or the presence of anticoagulant (inhibitor), which interferes with the function of the clotting factors. Deficiencies can be inherited or acquired. Inherited deficiencies usually involve a single factor, whereas most acquired abnormalities affect several factors. Hemophilia A, the most common hereditary hemorrhagic diathesis, is a sex-linked disorder caused by deficiency of factor VIII (antihemophilic factor).[316,317] The severity of the clinical manifestations is related to the level of circulating factor VIII, with severe disease occurring in the presence of a factor VIII level less than 1% of normal, resulting in frequent, apparently spontaneous bleeding into the joints and deep tissues. A level greater than 5% results in mild disease, with few spontaneous bleeding problems, but can cause serious hemorrhage after surgery or trauma. Factor VIII levels between 1% and 5% are associated with moderate disease of intermediate severity. Hemarthrosis is the major orthopaedic complication. It occurs almost invariably in the severe form of the disease but rarely in the mild form. After surgery or trauma, hemostasis may appear to be normal in hemophilia because platelet function is essentially normal. Excessive bleeding typically is delayed, beginning several hours after the operation.

Factor IX deficiency (Christmas disease, hemophilia B) is less common than hemophilia A but is clinically identical and also is inherited as a sex-linked disorder. von Willebrand's disease, the second most common hereditary hemorrhagic disorder, is inherited as an autosomal dominant trait and has two associated abnormalities: deficiency of factor VIII and a prolonged bleeding time.[326] Both abnormalities are caused by a decreased plasma concentration or abnormal function of von Willebrand's factor. This high-molecular-weight plasma protein is synthesized in endothelial cells and is essential for normal platelet adherence to damaged subendothelium. Factor VIII circulates in plasma in association with von Willebrand's factor and is variably low in von Willebrand's disease as a result of the von Willebrand's factor abnormality. A wide spectrum of clinical syndromes can be seen. In the most severe form, spontaneous bleeding and hemarthrosis occur; in mild cases, hemostasis may be normal except after major surgery.

Acquired deficiencies of clotting factors usually are multiple. Deficiency of the vitamin K–dependent factors, II (prothrombin), VII, IX, and X, can result from lack of intake of vitamin K (in newborns), malabsorption, liver disease, and administration of coumarin-containing drugs. Orthopaedic complications are rare. Deficiencies of several clotting factors, including platelets, factor VIII, and fibrinogen, can result from disseminated intravascular coagulation (DIC). This complex disorder of diverse etiology in which excessive activation of coagulation results in consumption of clotting factors is dealt with in more detail in another section.

Circulating anticoagulants (inhibitors) cause bleeding by interfering with the action of one or more coagulation factors.[327] The most common inhibitor is an antibody that develops in about 10% of patients with hemophilia and inactivates transfused factor VIII, greatly complicating therapy.[316,318] Spontaneous factor VIII inhibitors also occur occasionally in individuals without hemophilia. They can develop in the elderly without other apparent systemic disease, in the postpartum state, or in association with other immunologic disorders. The lupus anticoagulant is an antibody that interferes with the lipid used in coagulation testing in vitro and does not result in abnormal bleeding. Identification of a lupus inhibitor is important both as an explanation for the prolonged coagulation test results and because it is associated with an increased risk of thrombotic disease.[302] Heparin is used so commonly as an anticoagulant in hospitalized patients that it is a frequent cause of abnormal coagulation test results.

Laboratory evaluation of the coagulation system is simplified by the availability of screening tests, which are useful in identifying the presence of an abnormality and providing a basis for further investigation. The overall strategy is to begin with preliminary, screening-type tests and to use the results as a guide for more specific evaluation. The most useful screening tests are the aPTT and the PT. The aPTT involves adding a contact-activating substance, such as kaolin, and a platelet substitute (phospholipid) to the patient's plasma and measuring the clotting time after adding calcium. It provides a sensitive evaluation of the intrinsic clotting pathway. The PT evaluates the extrinsic pathway and measures the time required for the patient's plasma to clot after the addition of tissue thromboplastin and calcium. The aPTT and PT evaluate both coagulation pathways and are sensitive to clinically significant abnormalities. Correction studies distinguish between a deficiency state and the presence of an anticoagulant and also can be used to identify the specific deficiency present. Their correct use and interpretation are predicated on the results of the preliminary studies.

Fibrinolysis and Repair

Excessive fibrinolysis can be primary or can occur as a secondary physiologic response to intravascular coagulation, or it can result from the therapeutic administration of plasminogen activators such as urokinase, streptokinase, or tissue plasminogen activator.[311,312] Primary fibrinolysis is an uncommon disorder but can lead to a hemorrhagic diathesis in patients with cirrhosis of the liver or carcinoma of the prostate. In DIC, widespread microvascular thrombi form, and the fibrinolytic system is activated in response to maintain vascular patency. Laboratory testing may reveal evidence of heightened fibrinolysis, but this usually is of secondary clinical importance to the hemostatic derangements that result from the consumption of coagulation factors. Hemorrhagic complications occur during fibrinolytic therapy, but normal hemostasis can be restored by discontinuing the drug and replacing consumed factors.

Laboratory evaluation can identify excessive fibrinolysis and help in distinguishing primary and secondary forms. In primary fibrinolysis, the euglobulin lysis time is shortened, reflecting excess circulating plasminogen activator, and serum fibrinogen degradation products are elevated as a result of fibrinogen and fibrin breakdown. In secondary fibrinolysis, the results of these tests also are abnormal, and there is further evidence of consumption of coagulation factors, especially platelets.

Treatment

Hemorrhagic problems in orthopaedic disorders most frequently occur in two situations: (1) the orthopaedic problems associated with congenital hemorrhagic disorders, such as hemophilia; and (2) bleeding disorders occurring as a complication of operative procedures.

The hemostatic abnormality in hemophilia A is caused by a deficiency of factor VIII. This can be corrected reliably with appropriate replacement therapy using cryoprecipitate, factor VIII concentrates, or recombinant factor VIII.[304,317] Cryoprecipitate is the factor VIII–rich, cold-insoluble portion of a single unit of plasma. Its factor VIII content is somewhat variable, but usually is between 70 and 100 units. The advantage of cryoprecipitate over factor VIII concentrate in replacement therapy is that the risk of transmission of hepatitis and other diseases is less, because there is exposure to fewer donors. Disadvantages include the inconvenience of administering multiple units, the problem of refrigerated storage, and less certainty regarding the amount of factor VIII infused. Commercial concentrates are prepared from large pools of donor blood. Their factor VIII content is assayed, and they are easy to store and can be reconstituted quickly for administration. Contamination of the blood supply with HIV led to a high incidence of HIV infection and AIDS in hemophiliacs because of their frequent use of pooled plasma products and exposure to many blood donors. Improved methods of preparation that inactivate HIV have made the use of concentrates safer, but the availability of genetically engineered recombinant factor VIII has revolutionized replacement therapy for hemophilia. Although it is more costly than other sources, recombinant factor VIII all but eliminates the risk of disease transmission and effectively ends the epidemic of HIV associated with replacement therapy for this disease. Finally, desmopressin (DDAVP) causes the release of von Willebrand's factor and factor VIII from storage sites and raises plasma concentrations. In selected patients with mild to moderate hemophilia A, it is the treatment of choice for limited surgical procedures because it has few adverse effects.[305,313]

Many hemophiliacs are on home transfusion programs that result in rapid treatment of bleeding episodes, less morbidity, and fewer hospital visits. Surgical procedures in hemophiliacs must be performed with adequate replacement therapy. The optimum factor VIII plasma level to ensure hemostasis is dependent on the extent of the surgical procedure.[317] Hemophiliacs with circulating inhibitors pose special problems, because they usually cannot be treated with factor VIII replacement alone. No completely adequate treatment is available, although plasmapheresis, cytotoxic agents, and prothrombin complex concentrates have been used successfully.[319] The administration of factor VII also has been effective in a few patients.[315]

The treatment of von Willebrand's disease requires the replacement of von Willebrand's factor. In most cases, this is accomplished best with the use of cryoprecipitate that is especially rich in high–molecular-weight, functional von Willebrand's factor. Therapy normally can be guided by the level of factor VIII coagulant activity, but more frequent transfusion to correct the bleeding time sometimes is necessary. Replacement therapy in von Willebrand's disease is modified further by the prolonged rise in factor VIII coagulant activity that occurs after transfusion in these patients. DDAVP has been used successfully to manage surgery and represents the treatment of choice in appropriate patients.[313]

Hemophilia B must be treated with factor IX replacement, using either plasma or prothrombin complex concentrates.[317] Replacement with plasma is difficult, because the large volumes that must be transfused can result in fluid overload. Prothrombin complex concentrates are convenient to use, but are prepared from large donor pools and, therefore, carry a high risk of hepatitis and other disease transmission.

The treatment of complex, multifactorial, acquired hemostatic abnormalities is more complicated than that of congenital deficiencies. Vitamin K is specific therapy for deficiencies of this vitamin and can be used to correct overdoses of coumarin drugs. Deficiencies of vitamin K–dependent factors caused by liver disease rarely respond to vitamin K administration and are treated best with plasma. The treatment of DIC must be tailored to the individual patient, but the most effective treatment is aimed at correcting the underlying cause. Bleeding resulting from deficiencies of coagulation factors and platelets is treated best initially with plasma and platelet concentrates, but heparin administration may be required to stop the intravascular coagulation, especially when tissue ischemia from microvascular thrombosis becomes a problem.

Platelet concentrates for the treatment of thrombocytopenia are available through most blood banks. They are especially effective in patients who have low platelet counts as a result of defective production (eg, after cytotoxic drug therapy) or who have thrombocytopenia after massive transfusion.[309] They generally are ineffective in patients who have immunologically mediated thrombocytopenia (eg, idiopathic thrombocytopenic purpura), because the transfused platelets are destroyed rapidly.

In summary, normal function of the hemostatic system involves several elements acting in concert. Initial hemostasis is provided by platelets, which adhere to a site of vascular injury and aggregate to form a hemostatic plug. Activation of the coagulation system results in fibrin formation, which stabilizes the plug and provides a firm clot. The fibrinolytic system aids in remodeling the clot and eventually restores vascular patency. Defects in each of these phases of the hemostatic system can result in different bleeding problems and require separate laboratory evaluation.

In preoperative evaluation of the hemostatic system, the patient's history is paramount. Laboratory testing is used to supplement the history and should include, as a minimum, an evaluation of platelet count, PT, and aPTT. More extensive investigation is required in the patient with a history suggestive of a bleeding disorder.

Accurate diagnosis of and specific therapy for most congenital bleeding disorders are now available. Complex acquired hemostatic abnormalities resulting from systemic disease or occurring after trauma or surgery usually are caused by deficient production or excessive consumption of platelets and multiple coagulation factors. A logical sequence of laboratory investigation of these disorders, beginning with screening tests and proceeding with more specific assays in consultation with a coagulation laboratory, is essential for optimum management. Successful management demands an understanding of underlying pathophysiology, laboratory evaluation to identify specific abnormalities, and familiarity with the products available for replacement therapy.

Disseminated Intravascular Coagulation[§§]

Disseminated intravascular coagulation is a syndrome of diverse etiology resulting in a complex derangement of hemostasis, with elements of vascular obstruction, consumption of coagulation factors, and heightened fibrinolysis, often leading to excessive bleeding.[336] It is not a primary diagnosis, but develops as a manifestation of a serious underlying clinical condition that provides the inciting stimulus for activation of the coagulation system. The presentation and laboratory manifestations of DIC are modified by the wide variety of associated clinical conditions, such as those shown subsequently.[336,342,354,355] Several of these conditions, including malignancy, massive trauma, and septicemia, may be seen in routine orthopaedic practice. The surgeon must be prepared to recognize the manifestations, initiate laboratory investigations, and assist in difficult management decisions.

Widespread damage to the endothelium, such as occurs in endotoxemia, and entry of procoagulant proteins into the circulation, as can occur in disseminated malignancy or trauma, may be important inciting stimuli in DIC. The resultant excessive intravascular activation of coagulation results in varying degrees of microvascular obstruction, consumption of coagulation factors, and activation of fibrinolysis. The clinical and laboratory findings reflect these pathogenic processes. Vascular obstruction results in tissue ischemia and necrosis, with organ dysfunction. Consumption of coagulation factors results in thrombocytopenia and low levels of fibrinogen and other consumable coagulation proteins, leading to a bleeding tendency. The intense action of fibrinolysis that may occur can result in further consumption of coagulation factors and high circulating levels of fibrinogen or fibrin degradation products, which have anticoagulant properties that can exacerbate the hemostatic abnormality.[343]

Clinical Findings

The clinical manifestations of DIC are microvascular thrombosis and bleeding superimposed on the underlying primary disorder. Platelet-fibrin thrombi occlude small blood vessels, resulting in tissue ischemia and organ dysfunction of variable extent and severity. Findings related to the skin, kidneys, and brain are recognized most often. Sharply demarcated hemorrhagic skin infarctions are recognized easily and give the dramatic picture of purpura fulminans in their most severe form. Renal involvement usually presents as oliguria and acute renal failure, which may be worsened by coexisting shock. Nonspecific neurologic findings, such as delirium, convulsions, or coma, are more common than focal findings. Other organ systems frequently involved with severe DIC are the lungs, gastrointestinal tract, and adrenal glands.

The complex hemostatic dysfunction associated with DIC often results in a serious bleeding diathesis, possibly in the form of hemorrhage at the operative site during or after surgery. However, bleeding frequently occurs at nonoperative sites as well, and this usually is the first clear indication of the presence of a bleeding disorder. Thrombocytopenia and platelet dysfunction may result in petechiae and purpura. Bleeding from venipuncture sites, bleeding from gums, hematuria, and epistaxis often occur, as well as serious hemorrhage from arteriotomies. Gastrointestinal bleeding may complicate the course.

Laboratory Evaluation

Laboratory findings in DIC reflect the consumption of platelets and coagulation factors as well as heightened fibrinolysis.[354,355] Unfortunately, no single laboratory abnormality is diagnostic for DIC, and the diagnosis depends on a pattern of findings. In addition, the degree of abnormality in coagulation test results is variable, depending on the severity of the process. In acute severe DIC, gross hemostatic abnormalities are identified easily; in the chronic form, findings are subtle.[350,353]

A common feature in DIC is the consumption of platelets, and some degree of thrombocytopenia is found in nearly all cases. A good estimate of platelet number can be readily obtained by examination of the peripheral blood smear, or a more precise platelet count can be performed. The results of screening coagulation tests, such as the PT, aPTT, and thrombin clotting time, typically are prolonged, reflecting decreased coagulation factors and the anticoagulant effect of circulating fibrin(ogen) degradation products. The plasma concentration of fibrinogen usually is decreased in severe cases; however, fibrinogen is an acute-phase reactant, so that a normal level in an acutely ill patient may indicate a substantial decrease from the expected level. Serum fibrin(ogen) degradation products generally are elevated, sometimes to a striking degree.

Many additional abnormalities can be found in DIC, and some provide useful diagnostic help, particularly in difficult cases. Factor assays can be performed to verify the depression of consumable coagulation factors. AT III is consumed in the process of inactivating thrombin and often is low.[331,332,355] Heightened fibrinolysis is reflected by a decreased concentration of plasminogen and shortened euglobulin lysis time. Red blood cells may be damaged by their interaction with microvascular thrombi, and variable numbers of histocytes or red blood cell fragments are found on examination of the peripheral blood smear,[352] a finding that is not sensitive or specific for DIC.

On the basis of laboratory findings, it may be difficult to distinguish DIC, liver disease, and primary fibrinolysis. The presence of liver disease usually is evident from the typical clinical and laboratory findings; however, the hemostatic abnormalities can closely mimic those of DIC. Primary fibrinolysis occurs less commonly than DIC, and the laboratory abnormalities reflect marked activation of fibrinolysis. In contrast to DIC, the platelet count usually is normal, whereas the fibrinogen level may be markedly decreased with higher levels of circulating fibrin(ogen) degradation products.[333,346]

Treatment

The most effective therapy for DIC is correction of the inciting disorder. If this can be done, the hemostatic abnormalities will improve without specific therapy. Because patients with DIC often are critically ill with shock and multiple organ dysfunction, aggressive supportive therapy usually is a critical factor in their successful treatment.

Therapy specifically designed for DIC is necessary when the underlying disorder cannot be reversed rapidly or when the hemostatic abnormalities assume major clinical significance. Treatment decisions should focus on the clinical manifestations and not aim solely to correct laboratory abnormalities. If microvascular thrombosis with tissue ischemia or organ dysfunction is the principal clinical finding, anticoagulation with heparin is the treatment of choice.[337] Therapy is difficult to manage, because the usual laboratory tests used to monitor its progress show abnormal results before therapy. In addition, heparin may exacerbate any coexisting bleeding.[337] In addition to assessing the effect of heparin on the clinical abnormalities, monitoring the fibrinogen level, platelet counts, and serum fibrin(ogen) degradation products is useful. With successful treatment, consumption should decrease, resulting in a rise in fibrinogen and platelet levels and a fall in degradation product levels. Heparin should be given in the smallest dose that will improve tissue ischemia and hemostatic abnormalities. The necessary dose varies widely, but an infusion of 8 to 15 units/kg/h often is successful.

If the primary manifestation of DIC is bleeding due to consumption of platelets and coagulation functions, then replacement therapy is the most appropriate first choice of treatment. In addition to plasma, cryoprecipitate can be given to replace fibrinogen and factor VIII, and platelet concentrates should be used to improve thrombocytopenia. If the underlying disorder cannot be corrected, replacement is unlikely to be adequate therapy, because consumption will continue or increase in intensity. A logical approach in this situation is first to stop the consumption by administration of heparin and then to replace the necessary coagulation factors and platelets by transfusion.

In summary, DIC is a complex hemostatic disorder resulting from microvascular thrombosis, consumption of coagulation factors, and heightened fibrinolysis. The clinical manifestations are variable and include organ dysfunction and a generalized bleeding diathesis. Laboratory abnormalities include thrombocytopenia, prolonged screening coagulation test results, low fibrinogen levels, and increased fibrinogen degradation products. Prompt treatment of the underlying disorder and aggressive supportive therapy are critical in the management of DIC. The administration of heparin and appropriate transfusion therapy to replace coagulation factors and platelets may help correct the hemostatic abnormalities.

Crush Syndrome

The term *crush syndrome,* or *traumatic rhabdomyolysis,* refers to the sequela of prolonged continuous pressure on muscle tissue. This clinical entity often is seen in earthquake victims who are rescued from beneath rubble after several hours or days of entrapment.[344] It also is seen in motor vehicle accident victims who require prolonged extrication or in patients who have compressed their own extremity during a drug-induced stupor. In addition, the condition has been reported as a potential complication associated with the use of a fracture table[341] and as a result of the prolonged application of military antishock trousers.[338,357] In contrast, the term *crush injury* refers to a variety of local trauma to muscle such as occurs in a pedestrian tibia fracture or injury of a limb in a press.[358] A crush injury may exhibit variable amounts of direct muscle injury, but the prolonged period of compression unique to the crush syndrome is absent. Compartment syndrome can occur in either injury as a secondary event.

Pathophysiology

Treatment of the victims of the 1940 to 1941 London bombing provided the description of rhabdomyolysis, myoglobinuria, and subsequent renal failure classically associated with crush syndrome.[334] Intramuscular pressure in a crushed limb can reach as high as 240 mm Hg, initiating muscle breakdown resulting from direct pressure (pressure-stretch myopathy) that is initially independent of ischemia.[348] The basic defect proposed by Knochel is impairment of sarcolemmic sodium-potassium-adenosine triphosphate activity.[340] Neutral proteases are activated as a result of the increase in cytosolic calcium, which then break down myofibrils.[335] Entrapped patients may be relatively protected from the systemic effects of rhabdomyolysis because the ischemic muscle cannot be accessed by the circulation. Much like the situation with prolonged tourniquet application, limbs may have flaccid paralysis and anesthesia.[330] Extrication and the resulting reperfusion of necrotic and ischemic muscle with oxygenated blood leads to a second insult termed *reperfusion myopathy*. This reperfusion injury is felt to result largely from the formation of reactive oxygen metabolites. During ischemia and early in reperfusion, xanthine oxidase is produced in skeletal muscle. One of its two substrates, hypoxanthine, also appears. The second substrate, molecular oxygen, is delivered during reperfusion and results in the rapid production of superoxide radicals and hydrogen peroxide.[347] As a result of both injuries, there is failure of ion pumps and increased membrane permeability of both myocytes and the microvasculature. Systemically, the resulting fluid shifts can produce shock quickly when an extensive amount of muscle is involved. Large amounts of intracellular potassium, phosphorus, lactic acid, and myoglobin are released into the circulation. The rapidly rising potassium level can cause cardiac irritability and even cardiac arrest soon after reperfusion.[329] Locally, in susceptible regions such as the calf or forearm, compartment pressures can rise above arteriolar perfusion pressure and produce a secondary compartment syndrome.[345] Thus, adequate treatment of this entity involves attention to management of the local injury, treatment and prevention of shock and acidosis, and prevention of renal failure.

Systemic Treatment

Hyperkalemia, hyperphosphatemia, hypocalcemia, myoglobinuria, and metabolic acidosis may begin within hours of rescue in the extricated and untreated patient. Treatment should begin at the time of extrication and anticipate the onset of this syndrome. In the adult, a saline infusion of 1500 mL/h should be initiated during extrication.[330] When a urine flow has been established, a forced mannitol-alkaline diuresis of up to 8 L/d should be maintained (urine pH greater than 6.5). Alkalinization increases the urine solubility of acid hematin and aids in its excretion.[339] This may protect against renal failure and should be continued until myoglobin no longer is detectable in the urine.[351] In addition to its protective effect as an osmotic diuretic, mannitol also is an effective scavenger of oxygen free radicals and may help reduce the reperfusion component of this injury by this mechanism.[347] Loop diuretics generally are contraindicated, but acetazolamide may be helpful if arterial blood pH rises above 7.45 as a result of the bicarbonate infusion. Calcium salts usually are not required.[330,351] In addition, allopurinol may help limit reperfusion injury by inhibiting xanthine oxidase activity. It also is effective in limiting the hyperuricemia often found in this syndrome and aiding in renal protection. Renal failure generally can be averted with the aggressive treatment outlined earlier.

Local Treatment

Treatment of the local injury remains difficult. In the absence of an open wound or a compartment syndrome sufficient to threaten distal tissue, most authors recommend conservative management.[330] Reis and Michaelson have stressed that the skin has an extraordinary ability to withstand compression and, even if contused, may still act as a bacterial barrier and should not be excised.[349] Better and Stein stated that, "The urge to surgically explore limbs with traumatic rhabdomyolysis should be resisted unless there is an overriding reason to do so."[330] Exposing a large volume of necrotic muscle carries a substantial risk of severe limb-threatening infection.

Fasciotomy to treat a documented compartment syndrome complicating a crush syndrome is a valid surgical indication. Some authors suggest that early fasciotomy (less than 12 h) preserves muscle tissue, but this is controversial.[339] Most authors contend that fasciotomy will not cure the necrotic muscle in the incised compartment and the goal in these cases is to preserve perfusion to a viable distal extremity. Detection of a compartment syndrome superimposed on a crush syndrome may be difficult by physical examination alone because of the anesthesia and paralysis that often are present as a result of the rhabdomyolysis. The threshold and indicators for compartment release in this clinical setting are markedly different than in the usual evaluation of a compartment at risk.[330] Reis and Michaelson state, "The only rational indication for performing a fasciotomy in a patient with a crush injury of a limb is absence of distal pulses for several hours due to high compartment pressures."[349] Because the physical examination is so unreliable, documentation of high compartment pressures should be done by direct measurement.[330] If fasciotomy is required, it generally is agreed that debridement of necrotic muscle should be radical to minimize infection risk. Bleeding alone is not an accurate indicator of viable muscle, and the response to mechanical or electrical stimuli should be included in the debridement decisions.[349] In this clinical setting, if muscle viability is questionable, it is much safer to remove it than to leave it as a culture medium.

Treatment of the open crush injury is difficult and requires radical debridement as well as fasciotomy. Despite such therapy, amputation through healthy tissue occasionally is required to control sepsis or bleeding.[349,356]

Thromboembolism

Thromboembolic disease is one of the most common and dangerous of all complications in patients sustaining skeletal trauma and undergoing elective musculoskeletal surgery.[‖] Despite some dissenting opinions, evidence exists that the incidence of pulmonary embolism is increasing and that a genuine rise in fatal pulmonary emboli has occurred.[402,458,479] Pulmonary embolism is the leading cause of hospital admissions for respiratory disease, excluding pneumonia. The threat of thromboembolism increases with the age of the patient, the extent and duration of the surgical procedure, the degree and length of immobilization, and the severity of the underlying systemic disease.[##] As more older patients undergo major joint replacements, the prevalence of this disease will rise. Trauma to or instrumentation of the skeleton triggers a systemic hypercoagulability, which probably is secondary to the release of tissue thromboplastin from the marrow fat and medullary sinusoids into the systemic circulation. It is important for the orthopaedist to recognize that patients undergoing musculoskeletal operations are at greater risk of thromboembolic disease than are their general surgical counterparts.

Ascertaining the true incidence of thromboembolic disease is difficult. It probably is higher in most European countries and North America than in Africa, Asia, and South America.[453,509] The frequency of the problem also varies within regions of the United States. Clinical investigators, particularly those using retrospective analysis, have grossly underestimated the incidence of thromboembolic disease. Orthopaedic surgeons have tended to deny that thromboembolic disease is a major problem. Such an outlook is not only incorrect but also dangerous. In one autopsy study of 161 patients who died after hip fractures, 38% died of pulmonary emboli.[391,516] In direct contrast, pulmonary embolism was thought to be the cause of death in only 2% of 87 patients with hip fractures who were evaluated on clinical grounds only, without autopsy. Table 8-5 illustrates the high incidence of thromboembolism associated with fractures of the hip or lower extremities and pelvis. To be both accurate and sensitive, any clinical study undertaken on the incidence, treatment, and prophylaxis of thromboembolic disease must be prospective, and the diagnosis must be established by phlebography. Far more studies with such venographic documentation of deep vein thrombosis have been completed on patients undergoing elective joint replacement than on those with skeletal trauma. One recent investigation of 349 multiply injured patients identified deep vein thrombosis in 58% and proximal vein thrombosis in 18% of all patients; only 1.5% of patients with a positive venogram result had clinical findings suggestive of venous thrombosis before venography.[419] Skeletal injury was a particularly strong risk factor. Three patients suffered fatal pulmonary embolism before venography was performed. Deep vein thrombosis was identified in 61% of patients with pelvic fractures,

[‖] References 389, 391, 398, 403, 406, 431, 523, 535.
[##] References 374, 383, 384, 386, 417, 453, 515, 519.

TABLE 8-5
Thromboembolism Associated With Fractures of the Hip, Lower Extremities, or Pelvis

Author	Injury	Number of Patients	Thromboembolism (%)
Sevitt and Gallagher[511]	Hip fractures	319	39.3
Tubiana and Duparc[523]	Hip fractures	389	15.0
Fagan[405]	Hip fractures	162	28.7
Solonen[517]	Fractures of lower extremities	178	21.3
Neu and associates[483]	Fractures of pelvis, lower extremities	100	20.0
Salzman and associates[507]	Hip fractures	184	26.0
Freeark and associates[414]	Hip fractures	70	42.0*
Hamilton and associates[427]	Hip fractures	38	48.0*
Sevitt and Gallagher[512]	Fractures	468	20.3
Golodner and associates[422]	Hip fractures	25	36.0

* Diagnosis of venous thrombosis confirmed by venography.

62% of those with spinal injuries, 77% of those with tibial fractures, and 80% of those with femoral shaft fractures. On balance, the magnitude of the problem is considerable. Deep vein thrombosis develops in at least 50% of patients undergoing joint replacement surgery or having sustained fractures of the lower extremity; 10% of these patients run the risk of pulmonary emboli, and unless adequate protection is provided, 2% will die of fatal pulmonary emboli.[432,515] Of all patients with a confirmed diagnosis of pulmonary embolism, 11% do not survive beyond 1 hour from the onset of symptoms. Of the remaining patients, 8% die despite appropriate anticoagulation, and mortality rises to 30% for those in whom the diagnosis is not made and no therapy is instituted.[490,503,525]

Preventing thromboembolism is much preferable to treating it. Therapeutic anticoagulation beginning after the diagnosis of deep vein thrombosis may not significantly decrease the incidence of pulmonary emboli and adds a considerable risk of bleeding in the multiply injured patient.[468] Clearly, the most effective intervention is prophylactic rather than therapeutic.[417,443,485,491] The National Institutes of Health (NIH) Consensus Conference concluded that venous thromboembolic disease in orthopaedic patients "can be significantly reduced by prophylactic regimens, which should be used more extensively."[485] Despite the NIH conclusion that aspirin prophylaxis "has not been shown to be beneficial,"[485] a recent survey of practicing orthopaedic surgeons found aspirin to be the most popular agent for prophylaxis in adults undergoing elective hip surgery or repair of hip fracture.[491] Of some concern, this same survey also revealed that 15% to 25% of all orthopaedic surgeons do not use prophylaxis in all patients undergoing hip surgery, and 5% to 10% never use any form of prophylaxis, even in "high-risk" patients.[491] The accumulating evidence is compelling that prevention of pulmonary embolism through prophylaxis of deep vein thrombosis is cost-effective and reduces mortality from embolic complications.[485,490]

Thromboembolic disease has many enigmatic features: the initiating mechanisms are obscure, clinical recognition is elusive, the recurrence rate is high, and mortality is unpredictable.

Thrombogenesis

The basis for understanding thrombosis began more than a century ago, when Virchow provided a conceptual framework for thrombogenesis.[527] He stated that thrombosis may result from changes in the vessel wall, changes in the blood composition, or changes in blood flow promoting stasis. Early research emphasized the role of plasma coagulation factors in thrombus formation.[392] Two types of thrombi were proposed, each with a different pathogenesis: first, the red thrombus, which was composed primarily of erythrocytes and fibrin, and characteristically formed in areas of venous stasis or retarded flow; and second, the white thrombus, which was composed primarily of platelets and fibrin, was relatively poor in erythrocytes, and was found almost exclusively in areas of rapid arterial flow. The role of the platelet was thought to be secondary in the formation of the red (venous) thrombus. Controversy existed as to whether the activation of a clotting mechanism preceded or followed the development of a mural platelet thrombus as the first stage of thrombus formation, not only in the arterial system but also in the venous system.[400] In addition, several studies have demonstrated abnormalities of platelet adhesiveness and survival time as well as alterations in fibrinolysis in patients with postoperative thromboemboli.[379,438,451,467] The available evidence suggests that the activation of the venous thrombus may occur after the formation of a small platelet nidus, thereby providing a common pathogenesis with its arterial counterpart.[445]

In the past decade, circulating vitamin K–dependent *anticoagulant* factors, protein C and protein S, have been recognized as playing a critical role in preventing unwanted thrombosis.[501] Hereditary deficiencies of these factors may contribute to a genetically determined increased risk of thrombosis in some patients.[455,458] However, deficiencies of protein C, protein S, or AT III have been shown to occur in only about 5% of patients with familial thrombosis.[363,426] More recently, a hereditary defect in factor V has been identified that results in the substitution of a single amino acid in the protein C cleavage area, rendering activated factor V resistant to physiologic inactivation by protein C. This mutation, known as factor V Leiden, has been demonstrated in nearly 50% of patients with recurrent familial thrombosis and greatly increases the likelihood of deep vein thrombosis in patients exposed to other risk factors such as skeletal trauma or operation.[363,423,426,520] Among the general population at large, factor V Leiden is significantly more prevalent in men who previously have had deep vein thrombosis or pulmonary embolism. This mutation was found in more than 25% of men older than 60 years of age with *primary* deep vein thrombosis and is the most common heritable factor predisposing patients to deep vein thrombosis.[502]

The cascade, or waterfall, mechanism for thrombus formation begins with adhesion of platelets to the exposed collagen in the damaged vessel wall. A series of morphologic and biochemical changes occur through a chain of enzymatic steps. Adenosine diphosphate is released, causing further platelet aggregation, and tissue factor lipoprotein in the endothelial cell membrane activates the extrinsic cascade. The clotting process then proceeds to thrombus formation (see Fig. 8-9).

The sequence of events leading to thrombus formation after trauma or musculoskeletal procedures is not completely understood. Little is known about the types of thrombi that are prone to pulmonary emboli or that cause valvular damage and the postphlebitic syndrome. The pathogenesis of thrombosis remains elusive, despite extensive experimental work. More inquiry is required into the dynamics of peripheral clot formation.[364] The results of a study of 132 patients undergoing elective orthopaedic surgery showed that postoperative venous thrombosis developed in 40 patients.[451] Of the 40 clots, 14 disappeared within 72 hours of surgery and 26 persisted. All clots in the latter group originated with activity in the calf veins; 9 demonstrated proximal extension to the popliteal or femoral veins, and 4 of these resulted in pulmonary emboli. Venography, autopsy studies, and ^{125}I-labeled fibrinogen studies help to substantiate the viewpoint that thromboses primarily begin in the calf and later propagate into the popliteal and femoral veins. Flanc and associates have shown that venous thrombosis is present in patients returning from elective surgery, strongly suggesting that the thrombotic process actually begins during surgery.[408] In their study of 96 patients, the ^{125}I-labeled fibrinogen technique was used for diagnosis, and the results were confirmed by venography. Thromboses developed in 35% of patients; 50% of the thromboses developed during the operative procedure. This indicates that greater attention should be given to the administration of prophylactic agents before—and certainly during—the operative procedure. It is known that changes in platelet adhesiveness occur after elective hip surgery as well as after trauma. In view of the primary role of platelet adhesion and aggregation in thrombus formation, an attempt can be made to alter these factors and suppress the development of thrombi. The usual anticoagulants, heparin and dicumarol, do not effectively suppress platelet surface reactions or adenosine diphosphate–induced platelet aggregation. These agents theoretically should be effective only in preventing the growth phase of the thrombus and in decreasing the diffuse clotting effect.[367,370,416,481]

Detection of Venous Thrombosis

Because the clinical signs and symptoms of deep vein thrombosis are notoriously unreliable, the detection of venous thrombosis cannot be based on clinical findings alone.[404] However, accurate evaluation of possible clot formation requires careful clinical observation, including a daily examination of the calf and the remainder of the lower extremity for pain, swelling, and tenderness, accompanied by an increase in temperature and pulse rate. Such signs, if present, cannot be ignored; they are an indication for further investigation of the possibility of deep vein thrombosis. At least half of all cases of deep vein thrombosis cannot be diagnosed clinically.[385]

Venography

Venography remains the standard of detection.[374,385,388] The lesser saphenous veins or subcutaneous veins of the foot provide excellent portals of entry to the venous system for the injection of the opaque medium used in venography. Current techniques allow for the identification of the soleal veins as well as the other calf veins and vessels of the lower extremity. The diagnosis of venous thrombosis depends on certain signs: (1) constant filling defects, (2) abrupt termination of the opaque contrast medium column occurring at a constant site, (3) nonfilling defects of the entire deep system, and (4) diversion of flow.[466] Rabinov and Paulin believe that the most direct sign of thrombosis is demonstration of the thrombus itself.[500] The other three signs reflect obstruction to venous flow and are indirect signs.[391] The artifacts that occur with phlebography include underfilling, dilution, and streamlining. A loose, potentially movable thrombus is thought to produce a ground-glass type of shadow, and the contrast medium can be seen between the thrombus and the vein wall. If the thrombus is old and fixed, the affected vein disappears on x-ray film and dilated collateral veins often appear more prominent. One study revealed that, despite careful clinical examination by members of the peripheral vascular disease department, 30 of 37 cases (81%) of postoperative venous thrombosis were overlooked.[404] It remained for venography to demonstrate the presence of venous thrombosis in these patients. It should be recognized that there is a slight risk (less than 5%) of inducing thrombosis by venography with conventional ionic contrast medium; the availability of nonionic contrast agents has reduced this frequency (less than 1% to 2%). This test cannot be repeated on a daily basis and, therefore, is not useful for frequent longitudinal follow-up examination. However, it reveals the position and extent of thrombus formation, particularly in the calf, where other screening modalities are notoriously insensitive, which in turn aids in the selection of therapeutic agents for treatment.

Radioactive Iodine–Labeled Fibrinogen

Another technique for the detection of venous thrombosis in the lower extremity uses radioactive iodine–labeled fibrinogen.[361,449,482,488] This method is based on the principle that if labeled fibrinogen is injected intravenously, it behaves in vivo as unlabeled fibrinogen and is converted into fibrin in any thrombotic process. The ^{125}I-labeled fibrinogen accumulates in the thrombus and can be detected by a scintillation counter placed over the affected area. However, this technique may give false-positive or false-negative results in the area of a femoral artery or venous pooling in the calf. It cannot be used in the vicinity of a large wound and, hence, is impractical after major hip surgery. It cannot detect thrombosis in the upper thigh, iliac, or deep pelvic veins, which is a significant drawback. The risk of transmitting serum hepatitis is largely avoided in part by obtaining the human fibrinogen from a restricted pool of donors who are screened by laboratory testing to nearly eliminate the possibility of the presence of viral hepatitis.[375] The accuracy of the method in detecting thrombi in the legs, below the popliteal space, compares favorably with that of venography (90% to 95%). It has been used widely in Great Britain for the detection of venous thrombosis.

Ultrasound

Another screening test for the detection of deep vein thrombosis is based on the use of an ultrasound flowmeter using the Doppler effect, a noninvasive technique for detecting blood flow.[513,514] The patency of major veins can be examined. However, the obvious disadvantage is that small thrombi beginning in the calf or extending to the popliteal veins in the region of the adductor hiatus cannot be detected. The test also is inaccurate for the diagnosis of deep vein thrombosis in the large hip wound. Great sophistication is required in the technical aspects of its use, and the good results obtained by certain authors are not easily duplicated. The ultrasound technique is 76% to 93% accurate in the thigh, as recorded by various studies. Compression ultrasonography is not useful for detecting clots below the popliteal space, but has been shown to have high specificity and sensitivity in detecting those in the thigh.[409,415,459,498] Color flow ultrasonography is a significant recent advance in ultrasound technology, but it remains sufficiently insensitive in detecting thrombus in the calf and is so highly technician dependent as to preclude its widespread routine use as a screening tool for deep vein thrombosis.[387,530,532]

Impedance Plethysmography

Impedance plethysmography is another method that has been suggested for the diagnosis of deep vein thrombosis.[439,534] This technique has been found to be inaccurate when compared with venography, particularly in identifying thrombi in the calf. It is most efficacious in detecting proximal disease above the knee, but is technically difficult to perform on patients with hip pain and with a restricted range of hip motion. The combined use of ^{125}I-fibrinogen scanning and impedance plethysmography has been suggested.[493] The impedance technique is only 53% to 88% accurate, even in the hands of proponents, and has fallen from favor in recent years.[530]

Magnetic Resonance Imaging

Magnetic resonance venography is the most recent addition to the diagnostic armamentarium for deep vein thrombosis. As a noninvasive screening test, it possesses some important theoretic advantages over contrast venography; namely, the ability to perform serial studies, the lack of any risk of induced thrombophlebitis, and the ability to image more reliably the deep veins of the pelvis.[399] Early experience with this modality has suggested a high sensitivity in the calf and pelvis, as well as the thigh.[399,528] Other advantages include identification of concomitant contributory mass or traumatic lesions,[396] posterior compartment muscle edema associated with deep vein thrombosis,[425] and upper extremity deep vein thrombosis,[396] and assessment of the acute or chronic nature of venous thrombi.[396] However, as in other areas where magnetic resonance technology has been newly applied, false-positive results have reduced its positive predictive value because of the high, but nonspecific, sensitivity of this imaging technique.[380] The lack of widespread experience with the technology of magnetic resonance venography, coupled with the logistical challenge of studying the multiply injured patient within the confines of the magnetic resonance imaging (MRI) gantry, make this technique more suited to investigational use than to commonplace application as a routine tool for deep vein thrombosis screening.

Diagnosis of Pulmonary Embolism

As the techniques for the diagnosis of deep vein thrombosis have become more sophisticated, it has been recognized that the detection of pulmonary embolism is equally inaccurate when based on the usual clinical, x-ray, biochemical, and electrocardiographic criteria.[394,494,529] The diagnosis of pulmonary embolism during life often is impossible because of the lack of characteristic signs and symptoms or the explanation of certain signs and symptoms by alternative diagnoses. Smith and coworkers estimated that pulmonary embolism is diagnosed accurately before death in less than 50% of cases.[516] A retrospective study showed that many deaths occurring from pulmonary embolism could have been prevented by anticoagulation.[499] Results of retrospective studies on pulmonary embolism are grossly inconsistent because of the inaccurate methods of routine autopsy. In 136 cases, Morrell and Dunnill reported a 52% incidence of pulmonary emboli in 263 right lungs.[478] In the same study, they found that the incidence of pulmonary embolism increased with age and that there was a distinct association between pulmonary embolism and operation. In 14% of the total number, death was entirely attributable to the embolism. The reported incidence in retrospective studies is about 10% to 18%. Hildner and

Ormand stated that most cases of pulmonary embolism were not identified by symptoms, physical findings, electrocardiographic examinations, serum enzyme determinations, or chest x-ray films.[434]

Lung Scanning

Radioisotope lung scanning has been used to investigate the regional pulmonary blood flow to help determine the presence of perfusion defects.[381,465,474] However, it is difficult to differentiate the causes of such perfusion defects. If a perfusion defect is combined with a normal plain chest x-ray film, as well as the symptoms and signs of a decrease in Pao_2 values, dyspnea, tachypnea, chest pain, cough, hemoptysis, cyanosis, tachycardia, fever, and early heart failure, pulmonary embolism is highly suggested. However, even in "low"- and "high"-probability scans, there remains an error rate approaching 15%, resulting in a significant number of false-negative and false-positive interpretations, respectively, when confirmed by pulmonary angiography.[465] Although changes in serial perfusion scans are accurate in identifying pulmonary embolism, a single ventilation-perfusion scan without a baseline study can be misleading in any individual patient.

Pulmonary Angiography

Pulmonary angiography remains the most accurate method of detecting pulmonary embolism.[372] The primary positive signs are the trailing edges of vascular occlusions within an arterial network of the lung and intraluminal defects outlined by contrast material within the pulmonary vasculature. There are associated secondary signs, including nonfilling of vessels, areas of slow perfusion, vascular tortuosity, and delayed clearance of contrast medium.

Greater emphasis must be placed on the definitive identification of the presence of a pulmonary embolus. Blood gas studies should be obtained routinely. Chest x-ray films should be performed in all patients suspected of having deep vein thrombosis or in patients with positive results on venography or fibrinogen scanning. If the chest x-ray films are normal, scintigrams of the lungs should be obtained in an attempt to detect silent pulmonary emboli. If the diagnosis of pulmonary embolism then can be made in conjunction with the clinical picture, no further testing is necessary. If the chest x-ray films are abnormal, pulmonary angiography can be requested to detect the presence of pulmonary emboli. Angiography and lung scanning are complementary studies; both should be performed when necessary and correlated with the plain chest x-ray films. However, although it is an invasive procedure, the risks associated with performing a pulmonary angiogram for the diagnosis of pulmonary embolism are less than the risks of a significant bleeding episode associated with the use of therapeutic heparin in the postoperative or multiply injured patient population.[495]

Prophylaxis and Treatment of Deep Vein Thrombosis

The hallmark of the treatment of thromboembolic disease is prevention. A profile of the orthopaedic patient in whom thromboembolic disease is likely to develop should be established. The archetype is an obese, elderly person with multiple injuries or operations, a history of associated cardiovascular or pulmonary disease, and a prior episode or family history of deep vein thrombosis, who is about to undergo major musculoskeletal surgery.

Sodium Warfarin (Coumadin)

It has been statistically proven that crystalline sodium warfarin (Coumadin), an anticoagulant, can reduce the risk of thromboembolic disease when given prophylactically.[404,545] Two regimens of sodium warfarin use are followed, and both require meticulous attention to detail.[359,410,432,521] Ten milligrams of sodium warfarin can be administered the evening before surgery. The PT must be obtained after surgery, and sodium warfarin is given the night after surgery at a usual dosage of 5 to 10 mg. The daily maintenance dosage ranges from 2 to 10 mg, administered orally. Previously, it was believed that the PT should be maintained at 2 to 2.5 times the control value; however, recent data suggest that prolongation of the PT by 3 to 5 seconds over the control value (ratio of 1.3 to 1.6; International Normalized Ratio [INR] 2.0 to 2.5) is equally effective in preventing thrombus propagation.[436,437,440,489,530] In their studies of thromboembolism in orthopaedic surgery, many authors have shown that this method is effective in reducing the frequency of thromboembolic disease.[359,432] Alternatively, sodium warfarin can be administered at a low dosage 7 to 10 days before an elective procedure to deplete essential vitamin K–dependent factors while maintaining the PT at no more than 14 seconds until after the planned procedure. However, this regimen has been shown to be associated with a greater likelihood of perioperative bleeding complications and has fallen from favor.[410,496,521]

The use of sodium warfarin is contraindicated in patients with hemorrhagic disorders, peptic ulceration, active liver disease, hematuria, melena, hemoptysis, cerebral insufficiency, or a history of infarct. Closed head injury, spinal fracture, and liver or spleen contusions pose a particular risk in multiply injured patients. An increased risk of major bleeding has been demonstrated in patients older than 65 years of age.[455] Many drugs decrease the effectiveness of sodium warfarin, including phenylbutazone and barbiturates. Several other drugs (eg, aspirin, chloral hydrate) increase the PT by effectively displacing sodium warfarin from the plasma proteins that act as the intravascular transport vehicle. After the administration of sodium warfarin, it is essential to obtain stool guaiac examinations periodically, hematocrit values three times per week, and PTs each day. Such complications as hemorrhage at the wound site, gastrointestinal bleeding, renal bleeding, and cerebral bleeding have occurred, along with the difficulty of administration and monitoring of sodium warfarin anticoagulation. The incidence of major bleeding complications associated with outpatient warfarin therapy is 4% for the first month and 10% to 15% over 1 year; the risk of major hemorrhage increases 80% for every 1.0 increase in the PT-to-control ratio.[456]

Dextran

The primary role of platelet adhesiveness and aggregation in thrombus formation has been emphasized previously. There is much to suggest that platelet activity underlies the initiation and propagation of certain venous thrombi.[393] In a search for safer and more reliable agents to prevent thromboembolism, attention was directed toward the dextran solutions. In 1944, Gronwall and Ingleman developed fractionated dextran as a plasma volume expander.[424] Bull and associates[376] confirmed the clinical value of dextran, and Bloom[371] prepared the first dextran in the United States and demonstrated its value as a blood volume expander. The dextrans represented a group of polysaccharides containing D-glucose units with predominantly 1:6 linkage. Clinical dextrans are glucose polymers containing a broad molecular weight distribution composed of average molecular weight fractions, either low–molecular-weight dextran (average molecular weight 40,000 daltons) or clinical dextran (average molecular weight 70,000 daltons).

The antithrombotic actions of dextran have been studied extensively, both experimentally[360,373,397,447] and clinically.[366,454,505,536] Dextran decreases thrombus formation after arterial surgery. In experimentally damaged large veins, dextran decreases the incidence of thrombosis.[401] Low–molecular-weight dextran has been shown to increase cardiac output and reduce the mean transit time.[392] These changes are the result of plasma volume expansion and the reduction of blood viscosity from hemodilution. Low–molecular-weight dextran causes a significant reduction in platelet adhesiveness, partly as a result of adsorption to platelets and the alteration of their membranes, interaction of the plasma proteins, and coating of the endothelial walls. After intravenous administration of low–molecular-weight dextran, a change in electrophoretic mobility of the platelet occurs.[377,378] There appears to be no difference between the antithrombotic effects of low–molecular-weight dextran in comparison with clinical dextran. The relative efficacy of low–molecular-weight dextran as a prophylactic agent against thromboemboli has been studied frequently in clinical trials.[368,369,404,457,508,522] Efficacy less than that found with sodium warfarin coupled with frequent complications related to volume expansion and fluid overload have all but eliminated the routine use of dextran as a prophylactic agent.[369,490]

Absolute contraindications to the use of low–molecular-weight dextran are pulmonary edema, congestive heart failure, renal failure, severe dehydration, and allergic manifestations. Hypersensitivity reactions can range from mild cutaneous eruptions to generalized urticaria, nausea and vomiting, wheezing, and (rarely) anaphylactic shock. Such reactions almost always develop in the first few minutes after the initiation of therapy. Therefore, the patient should be observed closely during the initial infusion. If any adverse symptoms or signs appear, the infusion should be stopped immediately. Therapy to counteract anaphylactic shock, including epinephrine, corticosteroids, and antihistamines, should be started promptly. If large amounts are given in the face of decreased urinary output, congestive heart failure and pulmonary edema may occur. A renal profile must be obtained before surgery, and if chronic renal dysfunction is suspected, dextran administration should be avoided. Renal failure has occurred after the administration of low–molecular-weight dextran, and renal dialysis has been required in some patients.[404]

Aspirin

Other antiplatelet drugs, including aspirin, have been suggested to prevent thromboembolic disease.[392,487,531] Certain case reports and retrospective studies have suggested a beneficial action of aspirin.[429,446] Stamatakis and associates found that aspirin failed to prevent postoperative deep vein thrombosis in patients undergoing total hip replacement.[518] On the basis of published data, there is no persuasive evidence that aspirin is reliably effective in the prophylaxis of venous thromboembolism in patients undergoing musculoskeletal surgery.*** Its efficacy has not been proved for high-risk patients, especially women, and its effects are not readily reversible after discontinuation of the drug, lasting about 10 days for the lifetime of the acetylated platelet.[429]

Heparin

Renewed attention has been given to the role of heparin in the prevention of thromboembolic disease.[418,452,461,484] After the identification of a potent, naturally occurring inhibitor, AT III, to activated factor X and the recognition of the potentiated response of such a factor to minidose heparin, it was suggested that minidose heparin might prevent thrombus formation.[533] The anticoagulant effect of the inhibitor to activated factor X is markedly influenced by trace amounts

*** References 390, 395, 429, 430, 435, 446, 504, 510, 526.

of heparin in vitro. One microgram of the inhibitor, by neutralizing 32 units of activated factor X, indirectly prevents the generation of 1600 NIH units of thrombin. Indeed, activated factor X may be a more potent thrombogenic agent than thrombin itself. However, in a study in which 5000 international units (IU) of heparin was given subcutaneously 2 hours before surgery, on the night after surgery, and every 12 hours for the next 7 to 10 days, venous thrombosis developed in 7 of 25 patients.[403] Pulmonary embolism occurred in 6 of these patients who were undergoing total hip replacement. It was believed that the blood levels of heparin were not sufficiently high to exert a prophylactic effect.[463] In another study, low-dose heparin did not prevent deep vein thrombosis in 100 patients undergoing total hip replacement.[428] In contrast to the conclusions of individual reports such as these, a controversial statistical review of previously published studies of heparin prophylaxis in orthopaedic surgery subsequently suggested that collective consideration of all available data demonstrated a significant effect in the prevention of deep vein thrombosis.[382]

Furthermore, recent studies of heparin administered in conjunction with AT III after total hip and knee replacement have yielded incidences of venographically documented clots comparable to the best results previously reported with sodium warfarin.[411,412] Laboratory investigations suggest that musculoskeletal trauma results in a physiologic consumption of AT III, the naturally occurring antithrombotic substance to which heparin binds to produce its anticoagulant effect. Depletion of AT III after orthopaedic surgery may explain the apparent previous ineffectiveness of heparin in this setting without concurrent administration of AT III to restore normal levels of this circulating factor X antagonist.[421] Dihydroergotamine-heparin combination therapy has demonstrated efficacy in the prevention of orthopaedic thromboembolic disease comparable to other regimens, but its attendant risks of vasospasm in the elderly population with preexisting vascular disease make it an unattractive choice for most patients.[365,450,471]

Most recently, the use of a low–molecular-weight heparin has shown promise in the prevention of thrombosis after orthopaedic procedures.[477,524] This fractionated heparin produces an anticoagulant effect by more specifically binding to activated factor Xa in the clotting cascade, allowing the administration of higher doses of active drug. Well-designed studies have demonstrated decided efficacy of low–molecular-weight heparin, which may be superior to that of warfarin, in both prevention and treatment of deep vein thrombosis in patients undergoing elective orthopaedic procedures.[442] However, bleeding complications have been more frequent with this regimen, ranging from 4% to 12%, and may present a significant deterrent to the broad application of low–molecular-weight heparin in multiply injured patients.[442,460] With this renewed interest in heparin and its derivatives, additional controlled studies with varying dosages and in vivo measurement of both heparin and AT III levels are necessary before the safety and efficacy of this agent in the prevention of orthopaedic thromboembolism ultimately can be determined.

Pneumatic External Compression Devices

Pneumatic external compression devices have been the focus of considerable interest in the prevention of thromboembolic disease because of their noninvasive nature and lack of associated drug-induced adverse effects.[433,492] Although this approach is particularly attractive because the risk of associated bleeding complications is entirely avoided, several studies have demonstrated a lack of efficacy in preventing proximal venous thrombosis in patients undergoing total hip arthroplasty despite significant reductions in calf deep vein thrombosis.[413,448] Other noninvasive mechanical methods of thrombosis prophylaxis, such as continuous passive motion, have yet to be proven efficacious.[464]

Prophylaxis and Treatment of Pulmonary Embolism

The initial management of pulmonary embolism is contingent on *definitive* diagnosis of the embolic condition, especially in acute multiply injured or postoperative patients, in whom the risk of bleeding from therapeutic heparin anticoagulation often exceeds that of death from recurrent pulmonary emboli. As already mentioned, in this situation, the confidence of diagnosis by pulmonary angiography outweighs the disadvantages associated with the invasive nature of this procedure. Once the diagnosis is established, treatment is begun with intravenous heparin to prolong the partial thromboplastin time to 2 to 2.5 times the control value. Full anticoagulation of this intensity has been shown to be necessary to reduce the risk of recurrent pulmonary emboli.

Intraluminal interruption of the inferior vena cava has been used for the *treatment* of pulmonary embolism in high-risk patients who demonstrate recurrent pulmonary embolism in the face of full-intensity heparin anticoagulation, or those with known deep vein thrombosis or pulmonary embolism and contraindications to anticoagulation.[475] Alternatively, placement of a Greenfield filter can be considered as a means of *prophylaxis* against pulmonary embolism in the trauma patient with contraindications to even low-level prophylactic anticoagulation for deep vein thrombosis by virtue of intracranial, abdominal, or skeletal injury at high risk of bleeding in the face of any anticoagulation. It should be noted that the placement of an intraluminal vena cava filter ideally is coupled with low-level anticoagulation, in those patients who can tolerate it, to discourage thrombosis around the prosthetic device.

 *Authors' Preferred Method of Treatment*

A confirmed diagnosis of deep vein thrombosis warrants serious consideration for further anticoagulant treatment.[462,476,480] Although virtually all clinically evident pulmonary emboli arise from proximal vein thrombi, 20% to 25% of all calf vein thrombi propagate to the proximal veins, from which embolic events then may originate.[364,451,480,506] Because of documented clinically significant embolic complications from untreated deep system thrombosis distal to the knee,[497] we recommend treatment of all deep system thromboembolic disease after orthopaedic injury and elective surgery. As soon as the diagnosis of deep vein thrombosis or pulmonary embolism is established, treatment should commence promptly. Deep system thrombi of the calf distal to the popliteal vein are well managed by warfarin anticoagulation to prolong the PT index to 1.5 times control; treatment is continued for 6 weeks or until normal activity is resumed, whichever is longer. Excellent prevention of pulmonary embolism has been documented with this regimen. Intravenous heparin is reserved for proximal thrombi of the thigh veins or documented pulmonary emboli. However, intravenous heparin should be used only if the diagnosis is *certain;* although it is rare, heparin-induced hemorrhage, thrombocytopenia, and thrombosis can be life-threatening.[362] Given the limitations of most diagnostic studies, as previously described, contrast venography of the lower extremities or pulmonary angiography generally is required. Treatment should begin with 10,000 to 15,000 IU of heparin (aqueous heparin sodium injection) administered intravenously as a loading dose.[420] The administration of heparin then is converted to a continuous drip delivering 1000 IU/h, and is adjusted to maintain the partial thromboplastin time at 2 to 2.5 times normal. This is continued for the next 72 hours, and sodium warfarin (5 to 15 mg/d) administration is begun. The heparin is discontinued after 5 days or when the PT has been prolonged to 1.3 to 1.6 times normal under the influence of sodium warfarin, whichever is longer.[436,437,440] During this initial period of anticoagulation, all physical therapy should be suspended and the patient should be maintained on bed rest. Sodium warfarin is continued for 3 to 6 months in doses sufficient to maintain the PT at 3 to 6 seconds greater than normal. Slightly greater prolongation to 1.6 to 1.8 times normal is indicated in the treatment of recurrent systemic embolism.[437] Infrequently, there are certain indications for pulmonary embolectomy, such as persistent hypotension, persistent cyanosis, and pulmonary arteriographic evidence of massive pulmonary embolism.[466,506] The initial treatment of a massive acute pulmonary embolism involves closed chest cardiac massage, fluid resuscitation, and the immediate administration of heparin, positive-pressure ventilation, and vasopressors. If the patient survives, pulmonary embolectomy may be indicated. Again, although they are infrequent, there are certain indications for surgical venous interruption.[470,473] These involve suppurative venous thromboembolism, microembolic clots with cor pulmonale, and failure of anticoagulants to control thromboembolic episodes. In addition, when anticoagulants and antiplatelet agents are contraindicated or pulmonary emboli recur despite adequate anticoagulation, surgical interruption of the vena cava by an intraluminal filter may be necessary.

In summary, it is imperative that the orthopaedic surgeon dealing with skeletal trauma and related disorders recognize the magnitude of the problem of thromboembolic disease. It is the most common disease occurring after trauma or surgical procedures. Deep vein thrombosis develops in at least 50% of patients, and 2% of all untreated patients die of pulmonary embolism after elective hip surgery, including total hip replacement. A much higher percentage die of pulmonary embolism after trauma. A diagnosis of thromboembolism is confirmed best by venography or pulmonary angiography.

Prophylaxis remains the cornerstone of treatment. The prevention of thromboembolism depends on maintaining mobility and activity in injured or postoperative patients, using graduated elastic compression stockings, elevating the lower limbs, and prescribing appropriate prophylactic anticoagulant therapy. The severity of thromboembolism is of great concern; appropriate attention should be given to using the most effective methods available to eliminate the occurrence of life-threatening complications. Meanwhile, the search continues for a noninvasive technique of identifying those patients whose blood is likely to clot and develop emboli, as well as identifying a safe oral agent that is uniformly effective in preventing thromboembolic disease.

REGIONAL COMPLICATIONS OF EXTREMITY INJURY

Gas Gangrene

Gas gangrene is one of the most serious complications of traumatic wounds. Generally regarded as a disease associated with battlefield casualties, the high incidence of highway accidents and regional prevalence of farm injuries has refocused the attention of orthopaedic surgeons on this devastating problem. MacLennan has stated, "While true gas gangrene is an uncommon disease in civilian life, it is by no means so rare as is generally believed."[565] Several authors have described the recognition and management of gas gangrene and have commented on the use of hyperbaric oxygen as an adjunct in the treatment of anaerobic infections.[546,559] In addition, postoperative clostridial infections are being reported with increasing frequency.[548] Many anaerobic bacteria thought to be commensal organisms have become invasive and produced gas gangrene in the face of host changes induced by extensive surgery or therapy with corticosteroids, cytotoxic agents, or antibiotics.[543,578]

Although the historical accounts of gas gangrene date to the Middle Ages, accurate descriptions of this entity became available beginning in the 18th century.[560] In 1871, Bottini recognized the bacterial nature of the disease but did not isolate the invading organism.[544] Further descriptions separated the various disease states, but these were somewhat ignored until World War I. World War II brought forth the recognition that the term *gas gangrene* should be limited to those invasive anaerobic infections of muscle that are characterized by profound toxemia, extensive edema, massive tissue necrosis, and gas production.[563] In 1945, Robb-Smith proposed the name *anaerobic myonecrosis* to emphasize that the basic lesion is necrotic rather than inflammatory.[572]

Bacteriology and Pathogenesis

The most important species in the etiology of gas gangrene is *Clostridium perfringens.* This agent is identified on the basis of its morphology, patterns of fermentation, toxin production, and neutralization.[582] *C perfringens* is a nonmotile, gram-positive, anaerobic bacillus without spores that produces marked milk fermentation with a lecithinase activity inhibited by *C perfringens* antitoxin on a Nagler plate.[555,581] Such organisms are obligate anaerobes and cannot multiply in healthy tissues with high oxygen reduction potentials. Clostridia are found widely distributed in fecal matter. *C perfringens* is regarded as a ubiquitous organism also found in operating rooms, emergency departments, and hospital corridors, as well as on cart wheels and shoes. It is a saprophytic commensal of the alimentary tract and can be isolated from the skin in about 20% of patients.[570] The risk of clostridial contamination always is present in the operating room. The significant toxins associated with the clostridia are listed later. When the cell wall (a lipoprotein complex containing a lecithin) is attacked by the toxin, a dermonecrotizing lecithinase, cell wall destruction and cell death occur.

Clostridial infections are caused not by the extra virulence of the organism, but rather by unique local conditions. Oakley discussed the factors required to establish a clostridial infection and pointed out that with ischemia and necrosis of muscle, a decreased oxidation reduction potential promotes the rapid advance of a highly lethal infection.[567] The exact mechanism that converts the saprophytic state to the fulminating gangrenous state is not known. An unidentified lethal factor may contribute to the invasiveness and the toxemia that accompany gas gangrene.[566]

It is easy to understand how such factors as trauma from the injury itself, surgery, and tight casts can lower the oxidation reduction potential values and create the proper environment for clostridial infection. Dirty wounds, especially those closed primarily without appropriate debridement, provide an ideal setting for the onset of gas gangrene.

The clinical course of gas gangrene depends on the spread of lethal toxins produced by clostridial organisms in a local lesion of dead tissue. The local lesion arises when toxicogenic clostridia are introduced into a deep wound of muscle, where, under favorable conditions, they multiply and produce toxins that diffuse into the surrounding tissues and devitalize them, allowing further colonization by the clostridial organisms.[547] Figure 8-11 illustrates the mode of action of clostridia with the production and diffusion of the tissue toxins. This vicious cycle promotes astonishingly rapid growth of the organisms and diffusion of the toxins. Although the activities of some of the toxins produced have been defined, the toxemia associated with gas gangrene is not clearly understood and has been attributed to release of the products of tissue necrosis, interference with cell enzyme systems, and acidosis.[579]

Classification

MacLennan has provided a classification of the histotoxic infections in humans.[565]

It is important to recognize the different categories

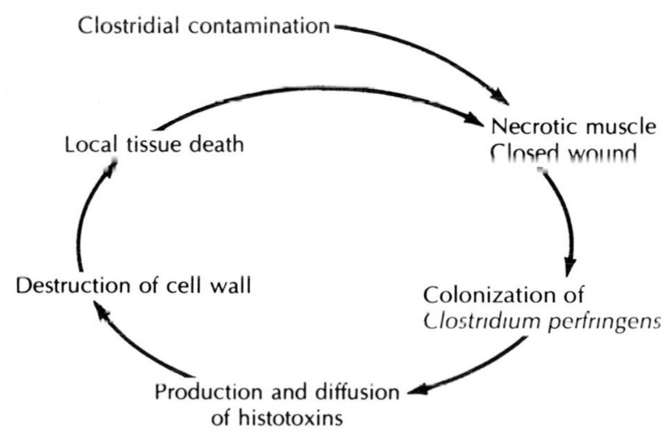

FIGURE 8-11. Pathogenesis of clostridial myonecrosis.

of traumatic wound infections. The mere presence of anaerobic organisms in the wound and their multiplication do not cause pain or a systemic reaction, and such an infection often is not recognized. In a few instances, the wound appears ragged and deep, with a watery, brown, seropurulent discharge. This represents simple contamination of a wound, and the surgeon need only remove the necrotic debris.

Anaerobic cellulitis or necrotizing fasciitis is a clostridial infection of ischemic tissue, usually occurring after several days, in an inadequately debrided wound. Altemeier and Culbertson commented on the rapidly spreading emphysematous infection along the fascial planes with extensive gas formation.[538] Altemeier and Fullen outlined the causes of crepitation in a wound.[539]

Other common gas-forming organisms include the coliform bacteria, anaerobic streptococci, and anaerobic *Bacteroides*. In anaerobic cellulitis, the onset is gradual and the toxemia is slight. The exudate is brown and seropurulent.[543,549,565] The gas formation is foul-smelling and abundant, but there remains no actual muscle invasion. There have been many needless amputations for anaerobic cellulitis, because it can be confused with gas gangrene. Table 8-6 presents the differential features.

The nontraumatic infections have been classified as idiopathic and infected vascular gangrene.[554] It is doubtful that true idiopathic gas gangrene occurs in humans, although it is well documented in veterinary medicine. It is more likely that the clostridial spores remain dormant in scar tissue for years after the original injury.

Infected vascular gangrene is a specific histotoxic infection of humans in which gas-producing anaerobes are found proliferating in gangrenous but anatomically intact muscle.[547] The organisms are saprophytes, not invaders in a limb that is ischemic. A line of demarcation is seen, and bacterial spread is limited. A foul smell and gas production occur, but the signs and symptoms of acute toxemia rarely are observed. Although it is a relatively benign form of infection, vascular gangrene, if neglected, can develop into a true clostridial myonecrosis.

Incidence

The incidence of gas gangrene is not known. Reports have emphasized the continuing problem of clostridial myonecrosis in civilian practice.[568,570] The presence of clostridial organisms in a wound has been reported to be as high as 18% to 46%.[575] Anaerobic cellulitis may develop in about 5% of traumatic wounds. In a total series of 187,936 traumatic wounds, the overall incidence of gas gangrene was 1.76%.[540] The incidence of gas gangrene is related to the interval between injury and surgical treatment. In addition, the site of injury is significant. Clostridial myonecrosis occurs most frequently in wounds of the buttocks and thigh, then in the shoulder, and, finally, in the lower extremity. The mortality rate varied from more than 50% in World War I to less than 25% in World War II.[562] Treatment modalities, including the use of antibiotics and hyperbaric oxygen, have helped reduce the morbidity and mortality.

Clinical Findings

The third category of traumatic wound infection in MacLennan's classification is anaerobic myonecrosis, separated into clostridial and streptococcal myonecrosis.[550,553] Almost without exception, the original wound involves injury to muscle—a deep, penetrating wound sealed off from ready access to the surface. The incubation period of clostridia is not long, about 12 to 24 hours after injury. The initial symptom is pain or a sense of heaviness in the affected area, followed by local edema and exudation of a thin, dark fluid. There is a dissociation between tachycardia and temperature

TABLE 8-6
Histotoxic Infections—Differential Diagnosis

Features	Anaerobic Cellulitis	Streptococcal Myonecrosis	Clostridial Myonecrosis
Incubation	>3 d	3–4 d	<3 d
Onset	Gradual	Subacute	Acute
Toxemia	Slight	Severe (late)	Severe
Pain	Absent	Variable	Severe
Swelling	Slight	Severe	Severe
Skin	Little change	Tense, copper colored	Tense, white
Exudate	Slight	Seropurulent	Serous, hemorrhagic
Gas	Abundant	Slight	Rarely abundant
Smell	Foul	Slight	Variable, "mousy"
Muscle	No change	Moderate	Severe

(DeHaven, K.E., and Evarts, C.M.: The Continuing Problem of Gas Gangrene: A Review and Report of Illustrative Cases. *J. Trauma*, 11:983–991, 1971.)

elevation; the pulse rate is elevated but the temperature is not high initially. The progress of the disease is rapid and spectacular, with an increase in toxemia and local spread of the infection. Profound shock can occur. A peculiar bronze discoloration develops in the wound, along with a musty odor and a slight amount of gas production. A symptom characteristic of gas gangrene is the mental awareness marked by a terror of death in the face of profound toxemia. Shortly before death, the patient usually becomes apathetic and coma ensues. It is difficult to determine the actual extent of muscle invasion and necrosis without surgical exploration. When examined, the muscle appears edematous, gray or dark red, and ischemic. Contractility is absent, and gas bubbles froth from the muscle fiber bundles.[552] Muscle involvement is invariably greater than the skin changes might indicate.

The other form of anaerobic myonecrosis is secondary to anaerobic streptococcal infection.[553,564] Most streptococcal myonecrosis infections have been located in either the perirectal or inguinal regions. Recent studies have indicated changes in the pattern of this illness, with a higher mortality reflecting increased longevity.[537] Superficially, this infection resembles clostridial gas gangrene; however, there is a slightly longer incubation period and the characteristic pain of clostridial myonecrosis is not present. Gas formation is slight, but there is a large amount of seropurulent discharge, in direct contrast to the discharge found in clostridial myonecrosis. Toxemia is less at the outset, and marked pain and septicemia do not occur except as terminal events. Important differential features of anaerobic cellulitis, streptococcal myonecrosis, and clostridial myonecrosis are listed in Table 8-6.

Diagnosis

The diagnosis of clostridial myonecrosis can be established by its clinical features. The most important are severe local pain and swelling associated with extensive tissue destruction and marked systemic toxemia. Gas formation is not a pathognomonic feature and in some instances may be scant.[541] Occasionally, jaundice, hemoglobinemia, and hemoglobinuria occur. Other differential features are listed in Table 8-6. Detection of gas may be obscured by the massive edema. Modern-day trauma can produce infections by other types of gas-forming organisms.

The radiographic interpretation of gas in the tissues is not specific for clostridial myonecrosis. Although it can detect the presence of gas in the tissues, it cannot identify the specific organism.[561]

The bacteriologic demonstration of pathogenic clostridia in infected tissues also is of limited significance, because the organisms, as previously mentioned, are commensal and widespread.[556] Type-specific identification takes a relatively long period—too long for lifesaving treatment to be delayed. However, a Gram stain of the exudate should be made. The common identifying features are listed in Table 8-7.

Prophylaxis

The initial measure of prophylaxis is to recognize the predisposing causes of clostridial myonecrosis. These include deep penetrating wounds of the buttock and thigh, tight plaster casts, and loss of blood supply. The greatest problem in prophylaxis is delay of effective treatment. The fact that clostridial infections are caused not by uniquely pathologic strains, but rather by uniquely local circumstances requires reemphasis. The most important prophylactic step is early surgical treatment, which consists of meticulous and complete removal of any necrotic tissue.[583] The nonviable muscle must be removed; tight packing should be avoided, as should immediate primary suture if any possibility of clostridial infection remains. The prophylactic use of antibiotics for the prevention of postoperative gas gangrene has been suggested in those patients thought to be at high risk for the development of this complication.[569] Penicillin is the antibiotic of choice. However, there is no evidence that penicillin alone will prevent the onset of clostridial myonecrosis in humans without proper surgical debridement and cleansing.

Although immunologic prophylaxis would be most desirable, no consistently effective preparation has been found for active immunization against *C perfringens*. The use of antitoxin for passive immunization has largely been abandoned.[584]

TABLE 8-7
Analysis of Gram Stain of Exudate From Histotoxic Infections

Features	Anaerobic Cellulitis	Streptococcal Myonecrosis	Clostridial Myonecrosis
Leukocytes	Present	Present	±
Gram-positive rods	Present	Absent	Present
Flora	Varied	*Streptococcus*	Varied

Treatment

The success of the treatment of gas gangrene depends on early diagnosis and prompt surgical decompression and debridement. Surgery remains the cornerstone of therapy for clostridial myonecrosis.[547,559] Multiple incisions and fasciotomy for decompression and drainage of the fascial compartments, excision of the involved muscles, and open amputation constitute appropriate operative management.[565] Arrest of the infection can be accomplished without amputation if the diagnosis is made early in the course of the disease.

Resuscitation must include careful scrutiny of fluid, blood, and electrolyte requirements; prompt replacement is mandatory. Fluid loss is marked, more so than with third-degree burns. Central venous pressure monitoring and urinary output measurements aid fluid replacement therapy.

Large intravenous dosages of penicillin, 3 million units every 3 hours, should be administered. In most patients who are allergic to penicillin, a cephalosporin or clindamycin would be effective treatment.[574] A second antibiotic, such as an aminoglycoside, often is given because of the common presence of organisms other than clostridial species.[557] Vigorous antibiotic therapy is an important adjunct to operative treatment.

A promising adjunct in the treatment of clostridial myonecrosis is the use of hyperbaric oxygen. In 1961, Boerema developed a hyperbaric chamber and subsequently treated two patients with advanced gas gangrene, who recovered dramatically.[542] Then, Brummelkamp and coworkers reported its use in gas gangrene.[545] The mechanism underlying the action of oxygen at high pressure appears complex. Experimental studies in vitro have demonstrated both bacteriostatic and bactericidal effects of high oxygen tension on *C perfringens.* Inhibition of toxin production and improvement of tissue oxygenation also may play a role.[539] Three atmospheric pressures are recommended for obtaining arterial oxygen tensions from 1200 to 1700 mm Hg. The patient should be placed in a hyperbaric chamber for 60 to 90 minutes every 8 to 12 hours as necessary. Usually, 4 to 6 exposures result in maximum effect. There are distinct hazards in the use of hyperbaric oxygen therapy, including barotrauma, decompression sickness, convulsions, otitis media, claustrophobia, and oxygen poisoning.[577] Lung damage has been reported in animals. If a large hyperbaric oxygen chamber is available, the surgical treatment can be performed during the initial hyperbaric oxygen exposure. Few such chambers are available in the United States, and for most hospitals, the cost of such a large chamber is prohibitive. Vital time may be lost transferring patients to facilities with hyperbaric oxygen.

Several reports have illustrated the efficacy of hyperbaric oxygenation in the treatment of clostridial myonecrosis.[551,557,558,573,576,580] It has been instrumental in arresting the progress of the clostridial infection and allows amputation at the most distal level possible. In patients with fulminating clostridial myonecrosis and those in whom ablative surgery is not feasible, the use of hyperbaric oxygen may be lifesaving.

The treatment regimen consists of four phases beginning immediately after the clinical diagnosis is made: (1) fluid and electrolyte replacement, (2) antibiotic administration, (3) meticulous surgical debridement and decompression, and (4) hyperbaric oxygenation. This regimen has resulted in a striking reduction of morbidity and mortality.

Illustrative Case[547]

A 10-year-old girl fell while horseback riding and sustained open fractures of both bones of her right forearm. Initial treatment consisted of blind surgical pinning of the ulna, primary suture of the open wound of the forearm, reduction, application of a long-arm cast, and administration of ampicillin and chloramphenicol.

Twenty-four hours after the injury, the patient began to have severe pain in the forearm, followed by swelling of the hand and low-grade fever. Splitting the cast gave no relief, and the cast was removed. The forearm wound was foul and discolored, and a hemorrhagic exudate was present. Smear of the exudate showed gram-positive rods. The patient was given a large dose of penicillin and was transferred to a tertiary care facility.

On admission to the hospital, 90 hours after injury, she was in a toxic condition with a temperature of 40.6°C and tachycardia of 140 beats per minute. She was fearful of dying. Her right hand was white, swollen, anesthetic, and paralytic. The forearm wound was foul and necrotic, with a thin hemorrhagic exudate and bubbling gas. Smear of the exudate again revealed gram-positive rods, and cultures subsequently grew *C perfringens.*

Treatment consisted of immediate debridement and decompression. There was extensive necrosis affecting all muscles of the volar aspect of the forearm, with associated thrombosis of major vessels, and there were pockets of gas within the muscle substance up to the level of the antecubital fossa. The wound was packed open, and the patient was placed in the hyperbaric oxygen chamber. In addition, she was given penicillin and polyvalent antitoxin intravenously. Three treatments with hyperbaric oxygen were administered.

Within 6 hours, the patient's temperature was essentially normal and the toxemia cleared. It subsequently was necessary to perform an amputation below the elbow, after which she made an uneventful recovery.

The history of falling off a horse is significant and must not be disregarded; barnyard contamination is a real threat. Internal fixation of a forearm fracture in a 10-year-old child is not indicated in the presence of an open wound that is grossly contaminated from a barnyard accident. Debridement and drainage of the wound were inadequate, and primary suturing of such a wound is ill advised. Delayed primary suture or healing by secondary intention is safer and provides a satisfactory cosmetic result. A circular cast should be used during the first 48 to 72 hours only if necessary and should be bivalved immediately to allow for swelling. There was only a slight delay in recognition of the development of gas gangrene, but there was a significant delay in definitive treatment because of geographic separation from a hyperbaric oxygen treatment facility.

In conclusion, the incidence of anaerobic infections ranging from simple contamination to massive necrotizing muscle involvement is significant and may be increasing. The orthopaedic surgeon must be familiar with the diagnosis and management of the infections caused by the histotoxic anaerobic bacteria.

Tetanus

Tetanus is a potentially fatal disease but, unlike gas gangrene, one that is preventable by appropriate immunization. It is a severe, infectious complication of wounds, especially lacerations, abrasions, or open fractures. In contrast to clostridial myonecrosis, which occurs in the patient with a neglected deep wound, tetanus can occur in the patient with a superficial wound or in the patient with no demonstrable wound.[609] Tetanus toxin must be produced by *Clostridium tetani* organisms for tetanus to occur. In contrast to clostridial myonecrosis, tetanus immunization is available and effective, and complete primary immunization with tetanus toxoid provides a long-lasting protective antitoxin level.

Accurate descriptions of tetanus (lockjaw) are found in the works of Hippocrates[603] and Aretaeus.[586] In 1884, Carle and Rattone produced the disease in rabbits.[589] Kitasato obtained a pure culture of *C tetani* in 1889 and described the toxins produced by this organism in 1890.[608] The concept and use of tetanus toxoid for active immunization were presented by Ramon and Zoeller in 1927.[620] By 1946, tetanus immune globulin (human) was available from fractionated plasma. In 1966, 250 units of tetanus immune globulin (human) was established as the routine prophylactic dose for passive immunization.[610,613]

Bacteriology

C tetani organisms and spores are widespread in the fecal matter of both domestic animals and humans. Soil fertilized with manure contains these anaerobes, whose function is to convert organic waste material into fertile soil. *C tetani* are resistant and can be dormant for years, sealed in scar tissue. With subsequent injury, infection may occur. In direct distinction to *C perfringens*, the tetanus organism is noninvasive and tends to remain localized. *C tetani* is a large, gram-positive, motile bacillus that is strictly anaerobic.[631] Spores cannot germinate in the presence of small amounts of oxygen.[622] *C tetani* produces two exotoxins: tetanolysin and tetanospasmin.[634] Tetanolysin, a hemolysin, may contribute to the manifestations of clinical tetanus.[601] Tetanospasmin, a neurotoxin, is extremely toxic, and a small amount can be lethal. Spores are resistant, and 1 to 4 hours of boiling is necessary to kill the organism. Autoclaving for about 10 minutes at 120°C provides satisfactory sterilization.

The skin of humans, especially outdoor workers, frequently is contaminated, and any wound, however small, can carry *C tetani* deep into the tissues. Three factors favor progression of the infection: (1) deep wounds without exposure to air, (2) wounds containing ischemic tissues, and (3) wounds infected with other organisms. Once *C tetani* begin to grow, the exotoxin tetanospasmin is produced and carried through the peripheral nerves to the central nervous system. In both the central and peripheral nervous tissues, the toxin is bound with high affinity to the gangliosides.[607] The exact mechanism and site of action are not known, but experimental studies in the mouse demonstrate that tetanus toxin causes a presynaptic blockade of neuromuscular transmission and functional denervation of muscle.[592] Voluntary muscle is more sensitive to the toxic effects than is involuntary smooth muscle.

Muscle spasm in humans is caused by hyperactivity of spinal motor neurons.[587] There is considerable evidence that tetanus toxin impairs cholinergic transmission in both the voluntary and autonomic nervous systems.[602,606,615,629] Morphologically, no tissue damage is done by the tetanus toxin; however, a critical feature of tetanus infection is the inability of the antitoxin to neutralize tissue-bound toxin.

Incidence

Tetanus has been a major problem during wars. Despite the availability and widespread use of a highly effective toxoid vaccine, tetanus continues to be a serious health problem in the United States.[593] After decreasing continuously from 1955 through 1976, the number of reported cases of tetanus has remained stable (Fig. 8-12), a situation most likely related to inade-

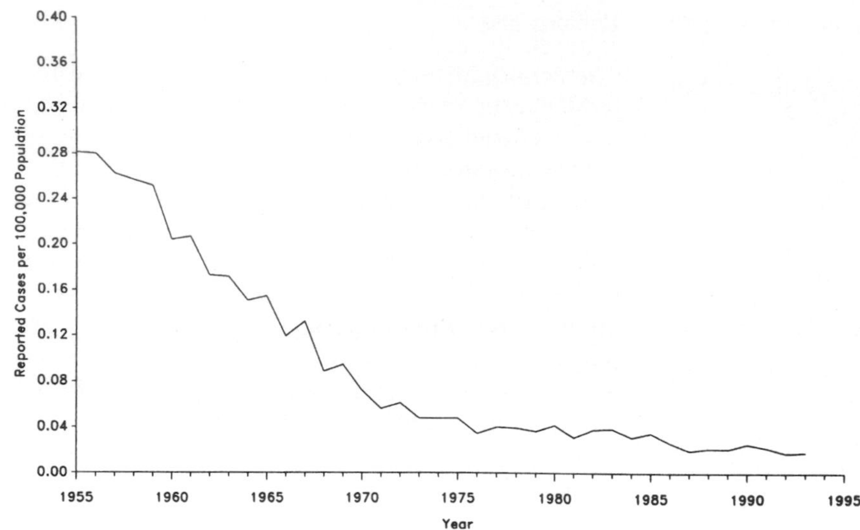

FIGURE 8-12. Tetanus by year in the United States, 1955–1993.

quate vaccination levels in a portion of the population.[598] Figure 8-13 shows that people older than 60 years of age have the highest incidence of tetanus, which again may result from inadequate vaccination coverage.[598,621] The incidence is highest in the lower Mississippi Valley and the Southeast. Recently, the case-to-fatality ratio has remained at about 60%. The hands and feet are the most common sites of injury, and injuries occurring at home account for more than 70% of all cases of tetanus infection.[609] The mean incubation period is about 1 week, and in one series of studies, 88% of the cases began within 14 days of injury. The length of the incubation period has been considered an indication of the prognosis of tetanus, with a short period indicating a poor prognosis.[626] Tetanus involves all age groups but is more serious and often fatal in neonates and the elderly.

Clinical Findings

Glenn stated, "In my clinical experience I have never seen such a terrifying disease as tetanus."[597] Tetanus may appear either locally or in a general form. Local spasm at the site of injury may be the first sign associated with this infection. The local form tends to be less serious.

The symptoms of generalized involvement are most commonly trismus, risus sardonicus, and difficulty in swallowing. The trismus is caused by muscle spasm, and the sustained contraction of the facial muscles pro-

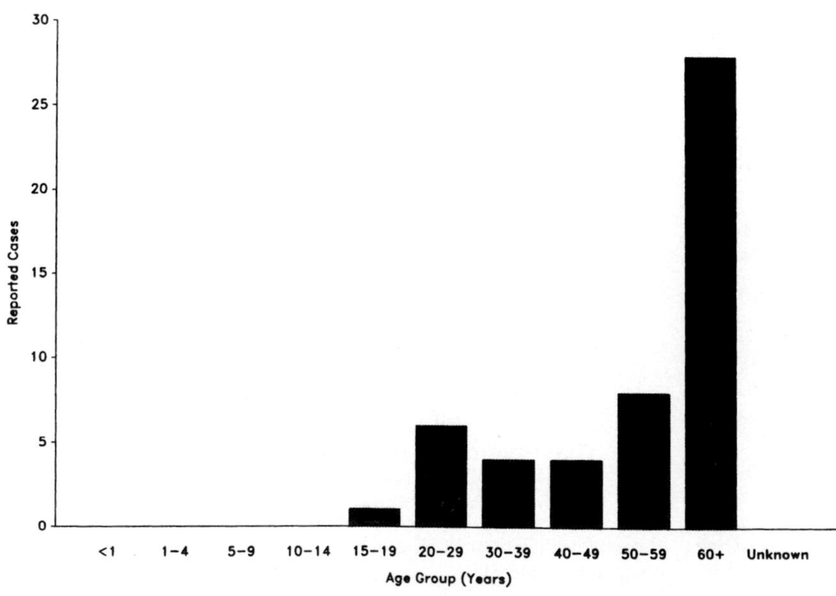

FIGURE 8-13. Tetanus by age group in the United States, 1993.

duces a wry expression. Some patients have prodromal symptoms of restlessness and headaches. If the pharyngeal muscles are in spasm, swallowing is difficult. Opisthotonos is common, especially in patients with severe tetanus. Other muscle groups become progressively involved, and muscle hyperirritability occurs.[617] Frequent toxic convulsions are part of the picture of *C tetani* infection and are produced by minimal stimuli.[596] Death from tetanus infection may occur from the asphyxia associated with unremitting spasm of the laryngeal and respiratory muscles. During the disease, the patient remains mentally clear. There is an associated tachycardia and often marked perspiration from hyperparasympathetic activity. The deep tendon reflexes are hyperactive, but no sensory changes are observed in tetanus. Death usually occurs within 2 weeks of the onset of the *C tetani* infection. The mortality rate, although difficult to determine, is about 60%.

Diagnosis of *C tetani* infection must be made from its clinical features. In one series of 160 cases, only 32% of the cultures were positive for *C tetani.*[609] This finding is related to the specific anaerobic growth requirements of *C tetani.* Occasionally, bacterial overgrowth is thought to decrease the chance of recovery of the organism. Despite the lack of bacteriologic confirmation, the dramatic and characteristic symptoms and signs of tetanus in the presence of a wound or site of infection make possible the diagnosis. Other common laboratory studies are nonspecific in establishing the diagnosis of tetanus.

Prophylaxis

Satisfactory active immunization exists for tetanus and, therefore, the disease can be prevented. Progress has been made internationally in developing a standard tetanus toxoid.[604] Tetanus toxoid has been administered by intramuscular or subcutaneous injection. The experience in World War II demonstrates the efficacy of tetanus toxoid as a prophylactic agent.[611] Once the toxoid is administered, the immune reactions are sensitized so that subsequent doses of tetanus toxoid booster result in the production of circulating serum tetanus antitoxin. Allergic reactions to tetanus toxoid are unusual; when they occur, they most often are manifest as local edema and tenderness.[605,632] Hypersensitivity reactions to tetanus immune globulin (human) are rare.[594]

Tetanus toxoid is highly effective, and its administration results in excellent protection. The National Health Service Immunization Practices Advisory Committee has suggested that primary immunization with DTP—diphtheria, tetanus toxoid, and pertussis vaccine—should be given to children aged 6 weeks to 6 years. It should be given intramuscularly four times: three doses at 6-week intervals and a fourth dose 1 year after the first injection. For schoolchildren, a single DTP injection is recommended. After the initial immunization, it is recommended that one dose of adult tetanus-diphtheria toxoid be given every 10 years provided wound management is not required.[621]

The success of the prophylaxis of tetanus depends on early recognition and prompt surgical wound management. All wounds must be meticulously debrided and cleaned. The tissue care should be gentle, and wounds should not be closed primarily if there are questions about anaerobic conditions deep within the wound.

The Committee on Trauma of the American College of Surgeons has published a guide to prophylaxis.[585]

Prophylaxis Against Tetanus in Wound Management

General Principles

I. The attending physician must determine for each patient with a wound, individually, what is required for adequate prophylaxis against tetanus.

II. Regardless of the active immunization status of the patient, meticulous surgical care, including removal of all devitalized tissue and foreign bodies, should be provided immediately for all wounds. Such care is essential as part of the prophylaxis against tetanus.

III. Each patient with a wound should receive adsorbed tetanus toxoid[†††] intramuscularly at the time of injury, either as an initial immunizing dose or as a booster for previous immunization, unless he or she has received a booster or has completed the initial immunization series within the past 5 years. Because the antigen concentration varies in different products, specific information on the volume of a single dose is provided on the label of the package.

IV. Whether to provide passive immunization with tetanus immune globulin (human) must be decided individually for each patient. The characteristics of the wound, the conditions under which it was incurred, its treatment, its age, and the previous active immunization status of the patient must be considered.

V. To every wounded patient, a written record of the immunization should be provided, with instructions to carry the record at all times, and, if indicated, to complete active immunization.

[†††] In 1981, the Public Health Service Immunization Practices Advisory Committee recommended DTP for basic immunization in infants and children from 6 weeks through the sixth year of age, and Td (combined tetanus and diphtheria toxoids: adult type) for basic immunization of those over 6 years of age. For the latter group, Td toxoid is recommended for routine or wound boosters, but if there is any reason to suspect hypersensitivity to the diphtheria component, tetanus toxoid (T) should be substituted for Td.

For precise tetanus prophylaxis, an accurate and immediately available history regarding previous active immunization against tetanus is required.

VI. Basic immunization with adsorbed tetanus toxoid requires three injections. A booster of adsorbed tetanus toxoid is indicated 10 years after the third injection or 10[‡‡‡] years after an intervening wound booster. All individuals, including pregnant women, should have basic immunization and indicated booster injections.

Specific Measures for Patients With Wounds

I. Previously immunized individuals.
   A. When the patient has been actively immunized within the past 10[‡‡‡] years:
      1. To the great majority, give 0.5 mL of adsorbed tetanus toxoid[†††] as a booster unless it is certain that the patient has received a booster within the previous 5 years.
      2. To those with severe, neglected, or old (more than 24 hours) tetanus-prone wounds, give 0.5 mL of adsorbed tetanus toxoid[†††] unless it is certain that the patient has received a booster within the previous year.
   B. When the patient has been actively immunized more than 10[‡‡‡] years previously:
      1. To the great majority, give 0.5 mL of adsorbed tetanus toxoid.[†††]
      2. To those with severe, neglected, or old (more than 24 hours) tetanus-prone wounds:
         a. Give 0.5 mL of adsorbed tetanus toxoid.[††† §§§]
         b. Give 250 units of tetanus immune globulin (human).[§§§]
         c. Consider providing oxytetracycline or penicillin.
II. Individuals not previously immunized.
   A. With clean minor wounds in which tetanus is most unlikely, give 0.5 mL of adsorbed tetanus toxoid[†††] (initial immunizing dose).
   B. With all other wounds:
      1. Give 0.5 mL of adsorbed tetanus toxoid[†††] (initial immunizing dose).[§§§]
      2. Give 250 units[‖‖] of tetanus immune globulin (human).[§§§]
      3. Consider providing oxytetracycline or penicillin.

Precautions Regarding Passive Immunization With Tetanus Antitoxin (Equine)

I. If the patient is not sensitive to tetanus antitoxin (equine), and if the decision is made to administer it for passive immunization, give at least 3000 units.
II. Do not administer tetanus antitoxin (equine) except when tetanus immune globulin (human) is not available within 24 hours, and only if the possibility of tetanus outweighs the danger of reaction to heterologous tetanus antitoxin.
III. Before using tetanus antitoxin (equine), question the patient for a history of allergy and test for sensitivity. If the patient is sensitive to tetanus antitoxin (equine), do not use it, because the danger of anaphylaxis probably outweighs the danger of tetanus; rely on penicillin or oxytetracycline. Do not attempt desensitization, because it is not worthwhile.

There is no proof that the administration of antibiotics is effective in the prophylaxis of tetanus; antibiotics are known to have no effect against the toxin produced.[617] Antibiotics, especially penicillin and tetracycline, given immediately after injury may have a deterrent action against *C tetani* infection by influencing the organisms that have not been removed surgically.[596] However, antibiotics cannot be used as a substitute for active or passive immunization.

Treatment

The treatment of tetanus involves both general supportive therapy and the specifics of wound care, passive immunization, sedation, and pulmonary ventilation.[###]

Patients with marked hyperirritability should be kept in a quiet, dark room, avoiding as many external stimuli as possible. Intensive nursing care should be provided. Proper fluid and electrolyte balance must be maintained.

A combination of penicillin, 2 million units intravenously every 6 hours, and streptomycin, 0.5 g intramuscularly every 12 hours, helps to decrease secondary invasive wound infections. The use of intrathecal injections of tetanus immune globulin has shown some promise.[599]

The management of the wound is important. If the tissues have been crushed, all devitalized tissue should be completely removed, and every attempt must be

‡‡‡ Some authorities advise 6 rather than 10 years, particularly for patients with severe, neglected, or old (more than 24 hours) tetanus-prone wounds.

§§§ Use different syringes, needles, and sites of injection.

‖‖ In severe, neglected, or old (more than 24 hours) tetanus-prone wounds, 500 units of tetanus immune globulin (human) are advisable.

References 588, 590, 591, 594, 595, 600, 619, 627, 628.

made to convert the wound from dirty to clean in every sense of the word.

Tetanus immune globulin (human) should be given early in doses of 500 to 1000 units until a total dosage of 6000 to 10,000 units has been received.[612,614,618] Sedation is one of the keystones in the management of tetanus. Mild cases can be treated with phenobarbital, secobarbital, or paraldehyde.[626] In more severe cases, thiopental sodium should be given by intravenous drip to quiet the patient and to lessen the number of convulsive attacks. The administration of muscle relaxants (D-tubocurarine and succinylcholine) should be supervised by an anesthesiologist, because improper administration can result in respiratory arrest.[630,633]

Maintaining an open airway and preventing the complications associated with tracheostomy are a challenge for the surgeon. Proper emphasis on the prevention of respiratory problems is a recent advance in the management of tetanus.[623,625] Smythe presented a series of infants in whom the mortality rate was decreased to less than 20%.[624] The good results were thought to be related to the proper use of tracheostomy and intubation in the infant, the control of intermittent positive-pressure ventilation monitoring the CO_2 level, and the improvement in control of infection after the instillation of penicillin and colistin into the tracheostomy tube.

If pharyngospasm or laryngospasm develops in a patient, tracheostomy should be performed promptly and assisted mechanical ventilation should be instituted. Careful, continuous observation and monitoring of blood gases are vital in the treatment of respiratory infections.

Other measures, such as hyperbaric oxygen therapy, have been tried in the treatment of tetanus, but these have not been helpful in preventing the toxemic state of an acute *C tetani* infection.[616,617]

In summary, although the incidence of tetanus has decreased in the United States, it is a major potential problem for the orthopaedic surgeon dealing with traumatic wounds. Advances in the past century have made tetanus a preventable disease. It is the physician's responsibility to be aware of the prophylaxis and treatment of infections of all degrees caused by *C tetani.*

Osteomyelitis

There remains a significant failure rate in the treatment of bone infections despite advances in antibiotic therapy; thus, osteomyelitis remains a great challenge to the orthopaedic surgeon. Continued interest and research have led to a better understanding of its etiology, pathogenesis, diagnosis, and treatment. A change in the character of osteomyelitis was suggested by Waldvogel and associates in a comprehensive review in 1971.[780] Most of the 248 cases reviewed were diagnosed as nonhematogenous osteomyelitis and occurred in an older age group, in contrast to a few cases of acute hematogenous osteomyelitis. The widespread use of appropriate antibiotics in the treatment of acute infections of bone has reduced dramatically the mortality from acute hematogenous osteomyelitis.[658,681,688,698] The increase in injury to bone secondary to vehicular accident trauma, with subsequent infection, and the increase in major reconstructive orthopaedic surgical procedures have contributed to a definite rise in the incidence of nonhematogenous osteomyelitis.[646] The most effective treatment of osteomyelitis remains its prevention, by meticulous wound care and debridement after open fractures. Appropriate antibiotic treatment and early soft-tissue coverage should further lower the incidence of this complication. Unfortunately, the emergence of resistant bacterial strains has complicated treatment. In many patients with chronic osteomyelitis, the infections developed before the availability of microvascular techniques and bone transport, thus placing a practical limitation on the ability of the initial treating surgeons to aggressively debride the disease.

Classification

Simply stated, bacterial osteomyelitis is a suppurative process in bone caused by a pyogenic organism. During the course of osteomyelitis, inflammation of the osteocytes and osteoblasts, their neurovascular components, and supportive connective tissue occurs within the confines of a mineral matrix. Bone matrix is destroyed by proteolytic enzymes, decalcified by hyperemia, and resorbed by osteoclasts.[636] Initially, osteomyelitis was classified as acute or chronic, according to the duration and severity of the infection. Clinically, the distinction between acute and chronic osteomyelitis can be difficult. Patients with acute osteomyelitis may have indolent, subclinical, chronic bone infection, whereas patients with chronic bone infections often experience acute exacerbations.

A classification modified from that of Waldvogel and associates separates osteomyelitis into three groups on the basis of the pathogenesis of the lesion[780]: (1) hematogenous osteomyelitis, (2) osteomyelitis secondary to a contiguous focus of infection, and (3) osteomyelitis from direct inoculation of bacteria at the time of injury or surgery. Unfortunately, this classification system provides no information on the anatomic extent of the disease.

May and colleagues presented a five-part classification system for post-traumatic tibial osteomyelitis based on the size of the tibial defect after complete debridement and on the status of the fibula.[732] This classification system is focused on the osseous and soft-tissue reconstructive needs of the limb.

In 1985, Cierny and associates reported on an extensive experience in the treatment of 240 adult patients with osteomyelitis.[652] They identified four factors that had a direct effect on treatment and outcome: (1) the condition of the host, (2) the site of involvement, (3) the extent of bony necrosis, and (4) the degree of impairment caused by the disease. A classification system combining these four anatomic types of disease with three physiologic classes of host was created to define 12 clinical stages of disease (Table 8-8).

In *medullary* osteomyelitis (type I), the nidus is endosteal. The soft-tissue component usually is minimal, but there may be secondary sinus tracts. *Superficial* osteomyelitis (type II) involves the surface of the bone secondary to a defective soft-tissue covering. *Localized* osteomyelitis (type III) involves a well-marginated sequestra of cortical bone. There is local soft-tissue involvement and, usually, a well-defined sinus. Complete excision is possible without causing segmental instability. *Diffuse* osteomyelitis (type IV) is a permeative process involving the entire segment of bone and has characteristics of types I, II, and III. This category typically is unstable both before and after debridement (Fig. 8-14).

In the Cierny-Mader classification, the patient (host) also is stratified according to his or her physiologic capacity to withstand the infection and the treatment protocol. A-hosts are normal, healthy patients. B-hosts have some degree of compromise that will affect treatment and are subdivided according to local (B^L) or systemic (B^S) factors, or a combination of both ($B^{L,S}$). The various local and systemic factors are listed in Table 8-9. Class C hosts are those in whom the treatment or the results of treatment may be more compromising than the disease itself.[651]

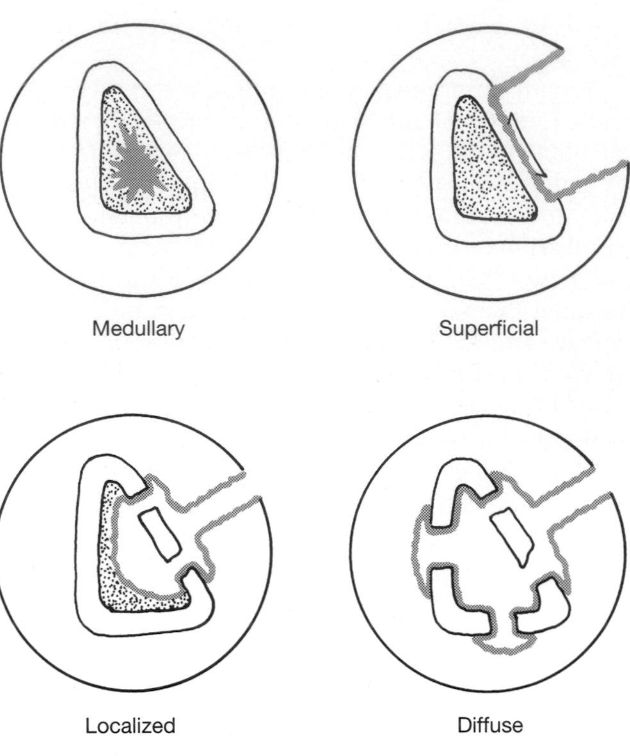

FIGURE 8-14. The anatomic classification of adult osteomyelitis. Medullary and superficial lesions are limited to the inner and outer surfaces of the bone, respectively. In the localized type, the segment remains stable after debridement. A diffuse lesion is unstable both before and after debridement. (*Cierny III, G.: Chronic Osteomyelitis: Results of Treatment. (Review) Instr. Course Lect., 39:495, 1990.*)

TABLE 8-8
Cierny-Mader Classification for Adult Osteomyelitis*

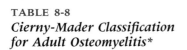

ANATOMIC TYPE
Type I: Medullary osteomyelitis
Type II: Superficial osteomyelitis
Type III: Localized osteomyelitis
Type IV: Diffuse osteomyelitis
PHYSIOLOGIC CLASS
A-Host: Good immune system and delivery
B-Host: Compromised locally (B^L) or systemically (B^S)
C-Host: Requires suppressive or no treatment; minimal disability; treatment worse than disease; not a surgical candidate
CLINICAL STAGE
Type + Class = Clinical Stage
Example: Stage IVB^S osteomyelitis = a diffuse lesion in a systemically compromised host

* The four anatomic types are combined with the physiologic status of the host to define 12 clinical stages of disease.

(Cierny, III, G., Mader, J.T., Penninck, J.J.: A Clinical Staging System for Adult Osteomyelitis. *Contemp. Orthop.,* 10:17, 1985.)

Pathophysiology

Acute/Hematogenous

Acute bone infection is a complex process that depends on many factors. The bacteria must be localized, and the environment must support bacterial growth. The localization of acute hematogenous osteomyelitis has been outlined according to patient age by Kahn and Pritzker.[709] In childhood, the infectious process usually is localized in the metaphyseal portion of the long bones.[751] Hobo studied the vascularity adjacent to the metaphyseal side of the growth plate and demonstrated that branches of the nutrient arteries in the metaphysis have straight, narrow capillaries, which in turn twist sharply back on themselves at the growth plate and terminate in veins with a much wider caliber than the capillaries.[702] Trueta believed that a decrease in blood flow occurred at the junction between the capillary side of the circulation and the larger-caliber

TABLE 8-9
Systemic and Local Factors That Affect Immune Surveillance, Metabolism, and Local Vascularity in the Treatment of Chronic Osteomyelitis

Systemic	Local
Malnutrition	Chronic lymphedema
Renal, hepatic failure	Venous stasis
Alcohol abuse	Major vessel compromise
Immune deficiency	Arteritis
Chronic hypoxia	Extensive scarring
Malignancy	Radiation fibrosis
Diabetes mellitus	
Extremes of age	
Corticosteroid therapy	
Tobacco abuse	

(Cierny, III, G., Mader, J.T., Penninck, J.J.: A Clinical Staging System for Adult Osteomyelitis. *Contemp. Orthop.*, 10:20, 1985.)

veins on the venous side.[776] He postulated that a relative stasis would increase the susceptibility to osteomyelitis. The combination of bacteremia and metaphyseal trauma has been shown in an animal model to be pathogenic for osteomyelitis.[743] Once a focus of infection in bone is established, the initial response is that of increased vascularity, leukocyte infiltration, and edema of the surrounding tissues. As the suppurative process continues within a rigid-walled structure, the resultant accumulation of pus exerts significant pressure on the surrounding tissues. The bacterial organisms liberate exotoxins, causing cell death and necrosis; these necrotic tissues serve in turn as a culture medium.[671,715] The infection may spread from the metaphysis along the path of least resistance into either the medullary canal or the subperiosteal space.[701] The nutrient artery supplying the inner two thirds of the cortex is compromised by the advancing infection. As the suppurative process spreads beneath the periosteum, the blood supply to the outer one third of the cortex is destroyed. Thus, it can be appreciated that untreated acute hematogenous osteomyelitis may extend to involve the entire bone. Furthermore, if the anatomic location of the metaphysis is intracapsular, the infection rapidly can become intra-articular, causing a secondary septic arthritis (eg, the proximal femur).[679,709,751]

Chronic/Nonhematogenous

Nonhematogenous osteomyelitis is secondary to a contiguous focus of infection. The pathophysiology of this type is different from that of acute hematogenous osteomyelitis. The bacterial organisms enter the bone directly through interrupted tissue planes as a result of fractures or surgical procedures. The mere presence of bacteria in bone is insufficient to produce osteomyelitis.[709] The surgical or traumatic insult sets the stage for the secondary infection.[744] Periosteum and muscle are injured, creating regions of cortical bone that no longer are perfused adequately. Devitalized bone presents a collagen protein matrix and acellular crystal regions to which bacteria can bind directly.[693] Bacterial receptors also can bind to bone sialoprotein.[692,761] Hematoma formation and necrotic muscle creates an ideal additional culture medium. In adult bone, the periosteum is bound firmly to a thick cortex and extensive periosteal elevation is uncommon.[709] Large regions of the intramedullary canal may become involved by direct extension, provoking little periosteal response. Sequestration and involucrum formation are much less pronounced than that seen in acute pediatric osteomyelitis. Low-virulence organisms may produce only a local chronic inflammation manifested as delayed union or nonunion of a fracture.[734]

The presence of metallic internal fixation devices also changes the milieu for bacterial adherence and pathogenesis. Studies have shown that when bacteria adhere to a surface, they become more resistant to antibiotics and the effect is specific to the type of biomaterial.[691,692,748] Initially, it was thought that the mechanism of increased antibiotic resistance was due to the diffusion barrier of the mucoid biofilm. Subsequently, this resistance has been observed in bacteria that are devoid of biofilm. It now is believed that adherent bacteria manifest a lower metabolic rate and are physiologically altered from their free-floating counterparts.[691,748] Thus, eradication of osteomyelitis in the face of a biomaterial ultimately may require its removal.

The fundamental problem in chronic osteomyelitis is infection of the skeleton that devascularizes a segment of bone, leaving protected pockets of necrotic material to support bacterial growth in relative seclusion from systemic antibiotic therapy. The peculiar blood supply to bone leaves trabeculae more vulnerable to vascular isolation and necrosis than their soft-tissue counterparts.

Clinical Findings and Diagnosis

Signs and Symptoms

If a patient has severe pain, bone tenderness, high fever, headache, and vomiting, the diagnosis of this classic form of acute hematogenous osteomyelitis is not difficult.[655] However, this is a clinical picture not frequently observed. Often, patients have vague symptoms and signs with an insidious onset.[698] Slight fever, few constitutional symptoms, and minimal complaints of pain may be present. A history of upper respiratory tract infection or mild trauma may be elicited. If a high index of suspicion is not maintained, further examination of the musculoskeletal system will not be performed, and the diagnosis of osteomyelitis will be missed. Inappropriate use of antibiotics often obscures the clinical signs and symptoms, and the usual course of events associated with osteomyelitis is altered.

The clinical characteristics of osteomyelitis secondary to an infection occurring with an open fracture or a reconstructive orthopaedic procedure are somewhat different. The symptoms and signs are not those of severe sepsis. The patient may complain of pain or have a low-grade fever. The wound usually becomes edematous and erythematous, and it drains in most cases. The diagnosis often is obscure. Any attempt at aspiration of the involved area should be performed under sterile precautions and fluoroscopic control.

The history and physical examination remain the keystones in the diagnosis of osteomyelitis. They at least should raise the suspicion of an inflammatory process and instigate an effort to locate the site of infection and determine the offending organism. Early identification is of utmost importance because early treatment (within 72 hours) drastically reduces the incidence of subsequent chronic osteomyelitis and osseous destruction.[781]

Laboratory Examination

Routine laboratory investigations are of only modest help in the diagnosis of acute osteomyelitis. Markedly elevated body temperature and white blood cell count no longer are common. Rather, some degree of leukocytosis, with a shift to the left, and mild anemia often are present. In a study by Morrey and Peterson, only 25% of children with osteomyelitis had a white blood cell count above normal for their age, and only 65% had an abnormal differential.[742] Serum calcium, phosphate, and alkaline phosphatase levels typically are normal. The erythrocyte sedimentation rate usually is elevated but is a nonspecific finding. It may be helpful in assessing activity during treatment; however, it has been shown to remain elevated for some time, even at the end of a course of adequate treatment, when the adjacent joint has been involved.[667] Antibodies to teichoic acid, a component of the cell wall of *Staphylococcus aureus,* are present in high titers in nearly all patients with endocarditis. They are present in low titers in some patients with staphylococcal osteomyelitis. Their determination may be helpful in equivocal cases.[777]

In chronic osteomyelitis, blood culture results usually are negative unless a contained secondary abscess develops, which then can mimic an acute infection. Blood culture results in acute hematogenous osteomyelitis have been shown to be positive in about 50% of untreated cases.[657,750,757]

Radiographic Evaluation

Diagnostic radiography is not effective in the early management of acute osteomyelitis.[647] The bone changes seen on x-ray films are delayed, first appearing 10 to 21 days after the onset of symptoms.[721] Soft-tissue swelling with a loss of well-defined muscle planes and a diffuse haziness usually are the first radiographic signs. The earliest bone changes are hyperemia and demineralization. Actual changes in bone structure, such as lysis, are not visible on x-ray films until 40% of the bone substance has been destroyed. It is not common to observe massive periosteal reactive bone, although periosteal elevation appears simultaneously with the loss of bone. Bone sclerosis is a late radiographic sign and indicates chronicity of the osteomyelitis.[712] Antibiotic therapy given for the various forms of osteomyelitis has changed the radiographic features: the onset of bone changes is delayed, bone destruction is less, and multiple lytic defects are rare. The most common radiographic sign of early bone infection is rarefaction, representing diffuse demineralization secondary to inflammatory hyperemia.

Radionuclide Imaging

The diagnosis of osteomyelitis usually can be made by clinical, radiographic, and laboratory evaluation. Precise localization of the site and extent of disease, however, can be difficult with plain radiographs alone. ^{99m}Tc is perhaps the most widely used bone imaging nuclide.[772] These compounds bind to the surface of the hydroxyapatite crystal. There is evidence to suggest that the technetium phosphates bind to both the organic and the inorganic matrix. They have particular affinity for demineralized bone and immature collagen, and this explains their increased uptake in regions of osteoblastic activity.[737]

The three-phase bone scan is the routine nuclear medicine procedure for the diagnosis of osteomyelitis. This technique consists of a radionuclide angiogram, an immediate postinjection blood pool image, and a delayed image made at 3 hours, when urinary excretion has decreased the soft-tissue activity. Classically, cellulitis has increased activity in the first two phases but minimal focal increase in the delayed image. Osteomyelitis has increased activity in the first two phases and focal uptake in the third phase. In the absence of other lesions that cause increased bone turnover (eg, fractures, tumors, implants), the three-phase bone scan is highly sensitive (94%) and specific (95%) for osteomyelitis.[760,762] False-positive images also can occur in the diabetic foot, septic arthritis,[730] inflammatory bone disease, and adjacent to decubitus ulcers.[695] Diagnostic aspiration of bone has been shown *not* to affect the accuracy of a subsequent bone scan.[650] Some authors have proposed the addition of a 24-hour image to create a "four-phase" bone scan.[695,705,762,763] Uptake of ^{99m}Tc stops at about 4 hours in mature lamellar bone, but continues for up to 24 hours in immature woven bone. The lesion:background ratio should increase in the fourth phase in cases of osteomyelitis.[763]

This four-phase technique has been reported to improve the specificity of the three-phase study in differentiating osteomyelitis from other conditions that cause increased bone turnover. It also may aid in the subsequent interpretation of an ^{111}In-white blood cell (^{111}In-WBC) scan.[694,695] The four-phase bone scan is not widely used, however, possibly because of the logistical difficulty in having patients return for the 24-hour study.[762]

The increased concentration of ^{67}Ga at the site of inflammation is believed to be caused by the exudation of in vivo labeled serum protein (transferrin, haptoglobin, and albumin) and its accumulation in granulocytes, primarily neutrophils.[703,720] Although originally intended as a bone-scanning nuclide, the sensitivity and specificity for osteomyelitis were found to be unacceptably low (81% and 69%, respectively) when ^{67}Ga was used as a single agent.[762] When it was combined as a sequential scan with ^{99m}Tc, the sensitivity increased but the specificity decreased and the overall accuracy did not change.[737,759] In one study of complex cases, the addition of ^{67}Ga imaging failed, in 67% of cases, to add useful information beyond that obtained in the three-phase bone scan.[765] Although it is highly sensitive (up to 100%), sequential ^{99m}Tc and ^{67}Ga imaging suffers from low specificity (25%). Given the availability of ^{111}In-WBC imaging, its usefulness in the evaluation of osteomyelitis is limited.[762,763,765]

The use of ^{111}In-WBC imaging has increased significantly the specificity of diagnosis of osteomyelitis in complicated situations involving trauma, previous surgery, or fracture[736,789] (see Case 2). Esterhai and coworkers reported prospectively on a series of fracture nonunions evaluated with radiographs and ^{111}In-WBC imaging, and concluded that this technique could detect the presence but not the extent of infection.[674] Seabold and associates prospectively compared sequential ^{99m}Tc-MDP/^{67}Ga imaging with ^{99m}Tc-MDP/^{111}In-WBC imaging in 50 fracture nonunions.[766] Using open biopsy as the benchmark for infection, they noted that the ^{99m}Tc-MDP/^{111}In-WBC combination yielded a sensitivity of 84%, a specificity of 97%, and an overall accuracy of 88% in detecting osteomyelitis complicating nonunion. The accuracy of ^{99m}Tc-MDP/^{67}Ga scanning was only 39%. In diabetic foot ulcers, the combined ^{99m}Tc-MDP/^{111}In-WBC scan has been shown to yield an accuracy of 89% in the differentiation of osteomyelitis from soft-tissue infection, and is significantly better than the ^{111}In-WBC scan alone.[731,764] Disadvantages of ^{111}In-WBC imaging include a relatively tedious preparation procedure, an 18- to 24-hour delay in obtaining images, and a relatively high radiation dose to the spleen.[773] Detection of vertebral osteomyelitis with ^{111}In-WBC scanning has been shown to be significantly less reliable than in the appendicular skeleton. Whalen and colleagues noted a false-negative rate of 83% when this modality was used to image vertebral infection that had been treated with antibiotics, and suggested that MRI be used in this clinical setting.[784]

Magnetic Resonance Imaging and Computed Tomography

Although radionuclide scans have a high sensitivity and specificity in detecting osteomyelitis, they lack the spatial resolution necessary to evaluate accurately the extent of the infection in preparation for surgical treatment.[640] In addition, differentiating between infected bone and involved adjacent soft-tissue structures such as sinus tracts and tendon sheaths is difficult when only nuclide scans are evaluated. Because of its superior soft-tissue resolution and exquisite sensitivity to changes in fat and water content, the use of MRI in the evaluation of osteomyelitis has received extensive attention. Its utility is enhanced further by the fact that images can be acquired in any orientation and there is no radiation exposure.[745] The initial screening technique for suspected osteomyelitis includes standard T1- and T2-weighted images in the orientation best suited to the anatomy of interest. The classic finding in established infection is a relatively dark marrow signal on the T1 image coupled with a bright or mixed signal in the area of inflammation on the T2 image (Fig. 8-15). These findings are caused by the replacement of normal marrow fat with granulation tissue having a high water content.[763] In chronic osteomyelitis, the cortex can become markedly thickened and will appear as an area of low signal intensity on all scans.[745] In cellulitis, the edema is confined to the soft tissue and not associated with marrow changes. The use of MRI is not contraindicated by the presence of metal in the area of interest, but there may be a loss of detail due to absorption of the radiofrequency.[739] Other pathologic processes, such as occult fracture, infarction, and neoplasm, can mimic the marrow changes described,[773] and for this reason, MRI may have a lower specificity than radionuclide imaging.[640,728] However, the sensitivity of MRI in acute and chronic osteomyelitis approaches or exceeds that of a three-phase ^{99m}Tc-MDP scan.[640,689] Depending on the series reviewed, MRI has a sensitivity of 92% to 100% and a specificity of 89% to 100% in the detection of osteomyelitis.[763] MRI accurately delineates soft-tissue extension of infection, allowing sinus tracts to be visualized as a bright T2 image from the skin to the medullary cavity (Fig. 8-16).

Gadolinium-DTPA has been introduced as an injectable contrast agent for use with MRI. In the appendicular skeleton, gadolinium enhancement with a T1 sequence has proved useful in the detection of soft-tissue changes such as cellulitis and abscess.[773] It does not aid in the detection of pus.

MRI is extremely valuable in the evaluation of vertebral osteomyelitis. It has been shown to have high

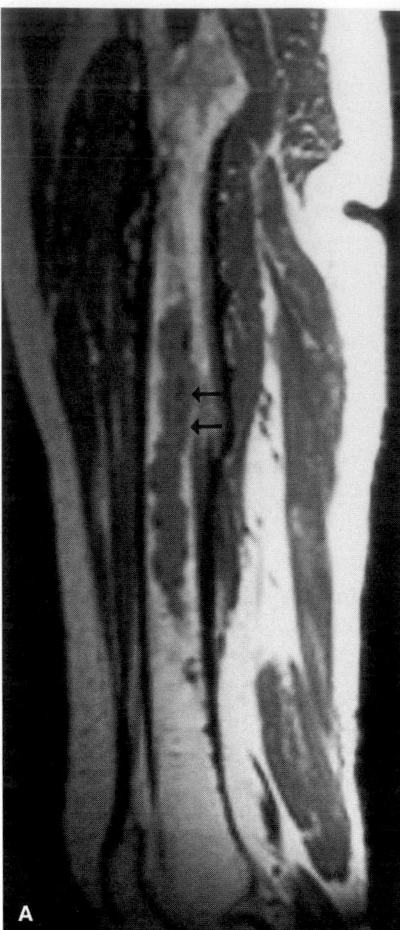

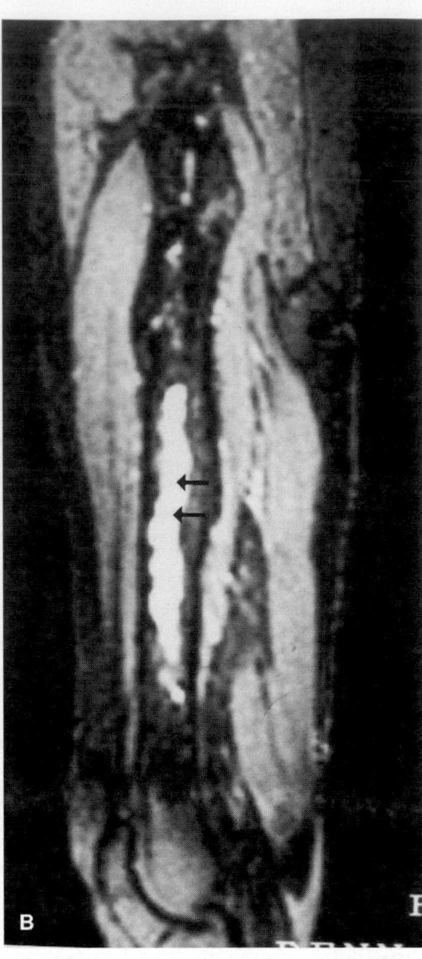

FIGURE 8-15. Characteristic sagittal MRI images in chronic osteomyelitis of the femur. (**A**) A T1-weighted scan showing the low-intensity signal (*arrow*) in the involved portion of the medullary cavity. (**B**) A T2-weighted image with a high-intensity marrow signal (*arrows*) consistent with edematous granulation tissue.

sensitivity (96%), specificity (92%), and accuracy (94%) in the diagnosis of spine infection.[739] MRI yields more accurate anatomic detail than do radionuclide images, particularly regarding the thecal sac, intervertebral disc, and paravertebral structures. Gadolinium-DTPA enhancement has particular utility in MRI imaging of disc space infections and epidural abscesses.[773]

Computed tomography has assumed a lesser role in the evaluation of osteomyelitis with the widespread use of MRI. It remains unsurpassed, however, in the imaging of cortical and cancellous bone. It is especially useful in delineating the cortical details in chronic osteomyelitis, such as sequestra and foreign bodies[763,773] (see Case 2). It also is useful in evaluating the adequacy of cortical debridement in the staged treatment of chronic osteomyelitis.

Aspiration and Biopsy

Identification of the offending organism is crucial to a successful outcome in the management of both acute and chronic osteomyelitis. In *acute* cases, aspiration remains the diagnostic treatment of choice.[668,756] It generally is not difficult or time-consuming and often can be done under local anesthesia. Under fluoroscopic guidance, a large-bore needle is advanced to the subperiosteal space. Pus in this location denotes an abscess. If no pus is encountered, the needle is advanced into the metaphyseal bone. Aspiration of the marrow is performed and sent for Gram's staining and bacterial culture. Bone aspiration may have up to a 10% to 15% false-negative rate.[668,689a]

In chronic osteomyelitis, identification of the causative organisms can be more difficult. Blood culture results rarely are positive. In the presence of a draining sinus tract, Mackowiak and associates have shown that the isolation of gram-negative organisms from the sinus tract bears no relation and the isolation of *S aureus* bears little relation to the results of cultures obtained during surgery.[723] More recently, Gentry has reported an overall specificity for sinus tract cultures of 86% and a sensitivity of 76%.[684] He further noted that *S aureus* and *Enterococcus* present in bone are recovered from the sinus tract less than 70% of the time in the face of significant gram-negative overgrowth. Conversely, he found only a 30% chance that *Pseudomonas aeruginosa* isolated in the sinus tract also would be isolated from bone. Thus, sinus tract cultures *should not*

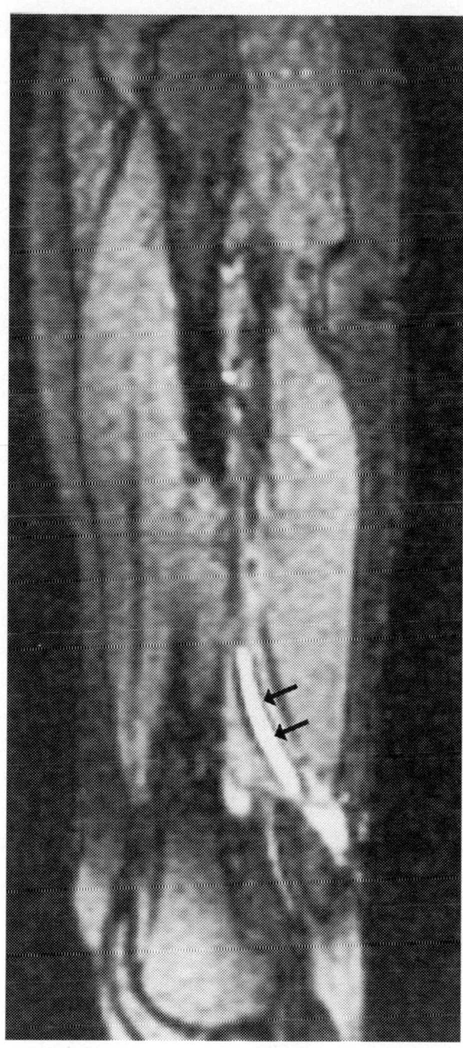

FIGURE 8-16. Sagittal MRI T2-weighted image showing a sinus tract (*arrows*) extending from the posterior skin to the cortex of the femur.

be used to guide antibiotic treatment. Bone biopsy remains the preferred diagnostic procedure in chronic osteomyelitis.[667,684,733,749] The high incidence of multiple pathogens in chronic osteomyelitis has been stressed by several authors.[652,753]

Microbiology

Acute/Hematogenous

S aureus remains the most frequent etiologic agent, being responsible for more than 90% of cases.[742,756,767,781] In children younger than 3 years of age, *Haemophilus influenzae* type b is responsible for 5% to 30% of cases.[680] Other organisms play a role in certain patient populations. *Salmonella* osteomyelitis may develop in children with sickle-cell anemia.[727] In infants less than 1 year of age, group B *Streptococcus* and enteric organisms (eg, *Escherichia coli*) must be considered.[668] Osteomyelitis associated with a foot puncture wound is likely to be secondary to *P aeruginosa*.[707,756] Acute hematogenous osteomyelitis in adults is unusual and may be secondary to indwelling catheters or intravenous drug use.[685]

Chronic/Nonhematogenous

In 1971, Waldvogel and associates presented a comprehensive review of osteomyelitis and noted that most cases were associated with trauma and caused by susceptible strains of *S aureus*.[780] Over the past 20 years, there has been a significant change in the organisms responsible for chronic osteomyelitis (Table 8-10). The incidence of gram-negative infections has increased by twofold to threefold, with particular emergence of *P aeruginosa* as the responsible pathogen.[684,685] The incidence of pure *S aureus* infection has fallen to about 25%. Coagulase-negative staphylococci now are widely recognized as virulent pathogens. More than 70% are methicillin resistant and require parenteral vancomycin. Methicillin-resistant *S aureus*, however, is an unusual pathogen in cortical bone.[684] Review of the available data[652,684,685] reinforces the concept that chronic osteomyelitis is polymicrobial in more than 30% of cases and may contain up to five identifiable organisms, including anaerobes.[747] Thus, adequate treatment requires accurate identification and antibiotic coverage of all pathogens.

Treatment

Acute/Hematogenous

In early acute hematogenous osteomyelitis, antibiotic therapy without surgical intervention may result in cure, provided the blood supply has not yet been compromised and adequate antibiotic levels in bone can be obtained.[645,687,740] The mainstay of treatment remains rapid identification of the responsible pathogen and the initiation of appropriate antibiotic therapy. In patients with the appropriate clinical presentation, there

TABLE 8-10
The Bacterial Pathogens in Adult Osteomyelitis Over the Past 10 Years*

Pathogen	1980 (%)	1990 (%)
Staphylococcus aureus	60.1	25.0
Pseudomonas aeruginosa	0.6	21.3
Enterobacteriaceae	35.2	36.3
Other	4.1	17.4

* Excludes infected prostheses.
(Gentry, L.O.: Newer Concepts in Antimicrobial Therapy. (Review) *Clin. Orthop.*, 261:24, 1990.)

should be no delay between the acquisition of blood cultures and bone aspirates and the initiation of empiric antibiotic coverage. An antistaphylococcic agent always must be used. Table 8-11 displays the recommended empiric antibiotic and dosage based on the most likely pathogen.

Historically, acute *S aureus* osteomyelitis required 4 to 8 weeks of intravenous therapy.[756] Subsequent studies have shown that early conversion to oral therapy can be equally effective.[713,758,775] The decision to convert to oral therapy is based on clinical factors. Typically, fever, pain, swelling, and local inflammation begin to resolve after 4 to 10 days of appropriate intravenous therapy. If an appropriate oral agent is available and the patient is compliant, the remainder of therapy can be completed on an outpatient basis. The duration of treatment depends on the pathogen. *S aureus* or enteric gram-negative organisms require a minimum of 4 weeks of treatment. Infections caused by *H influenzae, Neisseria meningitidis,* or streptococci may require only 14 days of treatment. The decision to discontinue treatment should be based on both the clinical response of the patient and a falling erythrocyte sedimentation rate.[661] Regardless of the method of antibiotic administration, it appears that maintaining a peak serum bactericidal titer of greater than 1:8[757] or a trough level of greater than 1:2[783] is predictive of successful therapy.

Indications for surgical drainage or debridement must be individualized and include the presence of a subperiosteal abscess, a coexistent septic arthritis, and failure to respond to appropriate antibiotic therapy after 36 to 48 hours.[656,661]

Chronic/Nonhematogenous

The classification system of chronic osteomyelitis described by Cierny and Mader is rational and functional, and was presented earlier[652] (see Table 8-8; see Fig. 8-14). Treatment decisions stem directly from the clinical stage of the disease. The anatomic extent of the disease and the physiologic status of the host and the local tissues must be understood completely before surgical planning and patient counseling can begin. Previous treatment history should be documented thoroughly, including adverse reactions to antibiotics. Physical examination should include the location of sinus tracts, previous scars, and a thorough neurovascular evaluation. Laboratory testing should include a sedimentation rate and an assessment of nutritional status if this is questionable. Imaging adequate to define the extent of the lesion and the goals of debridement should be performed. Plastic surgery consultation should be considered if soft-tissue coverage is a

TABLE 8-11
Likely Pathogens and Empiric Antibiotic Therapy for Acute Hematogenous Osteomyelitis

Host Factor	Likely Pathogens	Antibiotic Selection	Dosage	
			mg/kg/d	*Doses/d*
Older than 3 years of age	*Staphylococcus aureus*	Nafcillin, clindamycin, or cefazolin	150 30–40 100	4 3 3
Younger than 3 years of age	*Staphylococcus aureus* *Haemophilus influenzae* type b	Cefuroxime, nafcillin, and cefotaxime, or ceftriaxone	120 150 100 50	4 4 4 2
Neonate	Group B streptococci Enteric organisms	Nafcillin and gentamicin or nafcillin and cefotaxime	100 5–7.5 100 150	4 3 4 4
Child with sickle-cell anemia	*Salmonella* sp. *Staphylococcus aureus*	Cefuroxime or nafcillin and cefotaxime	120 150 100	4 4 4
After puncture wound to foot	*Pseudomonas aeruginosa*	Ceftazidime with or without gentamicin	150 5–7.5	3 3

(Prober, C.G.: Current Antibiotic Therapy of Community-Acquired Bacterial Infections in Hospitalized Children: Bone and Joint Infections. Pediatr. Infect. Dis. J., 11:157, 1992.)

concern. Optimization of host factors may be considered.

The cornerstone of the successful treatment of chronic osteomyelitis is the complete removal of all involved bone and soft tissue. The goal is to convert a necrotic, hypoxic, infected wound to a contaminated live wound that can be sterilized by appropriate antibiotic therapy. The precise debridement necessary depends on the anatomic type (see Fig. 8-14). In general, debridement should be direct and atraumatic. Sinus tracts present for more than 1 year should be excised[652a] and sent for pathologic examination to rule out an occult carcinoma.[683] Soft-tissue retraction should be minimal, and flaps should not be created. All suspicious soft tissue and bone should be sent for operative culture. Bone debridement with a pneumatic bur is atraumatic and can be performed until uniform haversian canal or cancellous bleeding is observed throughout the wound. At the conclusion of the debridement, the extremity is assessed for stability and external fixation is placed if necessary.[708] Segmental resection occasionally is appropriate, particularly in diffuse lesions (type IV), and the need for stabilization can be anticipated. If bone transport is the selected method of osseous reconstruction, an appropriate external frame can be placed.[689b] The wound typically is packed open at the conclusion of the debridement.[652]

Although satisfactory results in chronic osteomyelitis have been reported with a single-stage procedure,[638] most authors advocate a two-stage technique. The first step consists of thorough debridement and culture, and the initiation of empiric antibiotic coverage. Definitive soft-tissue reconstruction generally is performed in 3 to 9 days.[651,753] This interval allows time for final culture results from the initial debridement to be obtained and specific antibiotic therapy directed against all cultured pathogens to be initiated. The term *dead space* refers to the combined osseous and soft-tissue defect that is present after complete debridement.[753] Depending on the anatomy and stage of the disease, reconstruction often involves bone grafting or bone transport as well as the transfer of local or free muscle flaps. A prerequisite for proceeding with reconstruction is the presence of a live surgical wound.

Because the goal of treatment is to maintain a durable, well-vascularized soft-tissue envelope, healing by secondary intention generally is not used because the resulting soft-tissue coverage is relatively avascular.[652] If structural augmentation is not necessary and the osseous segment is stable, dead-space management with local or transferred muscle alone suffices. Studies over the past decade have increased our understanding of how muscle flaps aid in the healing of osteomyelitic wounds. Macroscopically, muscle flaps are pliable enough to completely fill dead space within the debridement cavity with vascularized tissue. They also serve as a vascular bed for immediate skin grafting. Because of the markedly increased blood supply of muscle compared with skin, local oxygen tension, delivery of leukocytes, and antibiotic levels all have been shown to increase in the presence of a muscle flap.[637] The success of bone grafting also appears to be enhanced by these same factors. These flaps appear to be effective for at least 5 years.[638] In post-traumatic tibial osteomyelitis, Koval and coworkers reported significantly better results with flap coverage (80% success) than with primary closure and suction/irrigation (46%) or open cancellous bone grafting (40%).[714] Other authors have reported success rates of 80% to 100% in the use of muscle flaps to cover osteomyelitic wounds.[638,729,733,782]

If structural augmentation is required (greater than 30% to 50% volume loss) or nonunion is present, autogenous cancellous bone grafts usually are indicated. In a noncompromised (A-host) patient with a clean wound, these grafts can be placed directly beneath local or transferred muscle at the time of wound closure. Cierny reported a success rate of 93% using this approach and recommended the addition of powdered, pathogen-specific antibiotic to the cancellous grafts at the time of insertion.[651] Some authors recommend staged bone grafting in B-hosts, in the presence of internal fixation, or when massive grafting is required (greater than 50 mL).[651,735] In the interim, the osseous dead space can be maintained with antibiotic-impregnated polymethylmethacrylate (PMMA) beads (see Antibiotics: Local Administration). Using this technique, the patient is brought back at a later date (2 to 6 weeks) for removal of beads and definitive grafting when the infection is arrested and the host factors are optimized.[735]

Segmental defects can be reconstructed using massive cancellous grafting in a staged reconstruction,[651] free bone transfer,[787] or the bone transport techniques of Ilizarov.[689b] The method of Ilizarov offers unique, comprehensive solutions to the problems associated with treating a large, infected bone segment. Using the established techniques of stable external fixation, atraumatic corticotomy, and appropriate delay before distraction, large skeletal defects can be spanned (see Case 1). This reconstructive ability permits radical segmental debridement of infected regions. Instead of using necrotic cancellous bone, the dead space is slowly replaced with highly vascular regenerate bone, which has been shown to increase global blood flow to the entire extremity.[704] Some authors suggest that muscle flaps appropriate for the soft-tissue defect be used before initiating transport.[682] Ilizarov has shown that this may not be necessary because the skin and soft tissue will move with the transporting segment and close the soft-tissue defect as the bone gap closes.[689b,704] Functional use of the limb during treatment is encouraged.

Problems with this technique are numerous. External frames must be in place for extended periods. The patient must be compliant and motivated. Many outpatient visits and adjustments are required, and pin-tract infections are common. Using this technique, Greene reported an average regenerate length of 5.7 cm in a small series.[689b] Cierny reported an overall complication rate of 28% to 38% using this method, but noted that this was lower than the complication rate encountered when conventional bone grafting was used in a compromised host (62%).[651]

Antibiotics: New Developments

Several excellent reviews have been published regarding antibiotic therapy in osteomyelitis[684,685,726,771] (Table 8-12). One of the most important recent developments in antimicrobial therapy has been the introduction of the oral quinolones. Oral ciprofloxacin has a broad spectrum of activity against both gram-positive and gram-negative organisms. It has a long half-life, low toxicity, and excellent penetration into bone. In randomized trials, ciprofloxacin was as safe and effective as parenteral therapy against a wide variety of organisms, particularly *P aeruginosa,* with a 2-year success rate of 77%.[684] Its efficacy against *S aureus* is controversial, and some authors suggest the use of combination therapy for the treatment of gram-positive infections.[684,779] The problem of emerging antibiotic resistance also is under investigation.[666] This agent is not approved for use in skeletally immature patients.[726]

Most coagulase-negative staphylococci are methicillin resistant,[684] and are recognized as virulent pathogens. Teicoplanin is a new glycopeptide antibiotic with activity similar to vancomycin.[716] It has a sufficiently long half-life to allow once-daily dosing. It also can be administered by intramuscular injection or rapid intravenous infusion. In several trials, teicoplanin was as effective as vancomycin against all gram-positive organisms and had a low rate of adverse events. The prospect of once-daily intramuscular dosing and low toxicity may make this agent attractive for the outpatient treatment of methicillin-resistant gram-positive infections.

Antibiotics: Local Administration

The local deposition of antibiotics has received increased attention in recent years.**** These techniques use a space-filling carrier agent that elutes high concentrations of antibiotic into the local tissue. Advantages include local levels of antibiotics that surpass the minimal inhibitory concentration for most pathogens with minimal systemic levels or complications. In the treatment of chronic osteomyelitis, local antibiotic deposition can be considered adjuvant therapy after a complete surgical debridement. The carrier agent can be either biological, as in the case of bone graft, demineralized bone matrix, or calcium hydroxyapatite, or biologically inert, such as PMMA or plaster of Paris.[662] Selection of the appropriate carrier agent depends on the biological needs of the wound. In cases where dead-space management is to be staged, an inert carrier agent (eg, PMMA beads) can be placed and subsequently removed at the time of application of autogenous bone graft. Permanent implantation of inert carrier agents remains controversial.[644] If staged management is not necessary, then a biological agent may be more appropriate. It is important to remember that the elution characteristics of each antibiotic/carrier agent combination are unique and should be understood before it is used. The antibiotic should be water soluble, nontoxic to tissue, bactericidal, available in powder form, and heat stable if used in PMMA.[755]

**** References 643, 644, 676, 738, 755, 769.

TABLE 8-12

Infected Bone Concentrations After Antibiotic Administration in Experimental* Staphylococcus aureus *Osteomyelitis

Antibiotic	Dose (mg/kg)	Serum (μg/mL)	Infected Bone (μg/g)	Serum Percentage (%)
Clindamycin	70	12.1 ± 0.6	11.9 ± 1.9	98.3
Vancomycin	30	36.4 ± 4.6	05.3 ± 0.8	14.5
Nafcillin	40	21.8 ± 4.6	02.1 ± 0.3	9.6
Moxalactam	40	65.2 ± 5.2	06.2 ± 0.7	9.5
Tobramycin	5	14.3 ± 1.3	01.3 ± 0.1	9.1
Cefazolin	15	67.2 ± 2.6	04.1 ± 0.7	6.1
Cefazolin	5	45.6 ± 3.2	02.6 ± 0.2	5.7
Cephalothin	40	34.8 ± 2.8	01.3 ± 0.2	3.7

(Mader, J.T., Landon, G.C., Calhoun, J.: Antimicrobial Treatment of Osteomyelitis. Clin. Orthop. 295:93, 1993.)

TABLE 8-13
Tobramycin Eluted From Various Carrier Agents as a Function of Time From Implantation

	Tobramycin eluted (μg/g pellet)					
	Day 1	*Day 2*	*Day 4*	*Day 7*	*Day 14*	*Day 21*
Bone graft	17,047 ± 1,952	703 ± 214	163 ± 31	35 ± 26	0	0
Demineralized bone matrix	11,437 ± 2,610	291 ± 215	123 ± 42	0	0	0
Plaster of Paris	4,294 ± 347	65 ± 13	43 ± 29	0	29 ± 7	29 ± 6
Polymethylmethacrylate	1,670 ± 875	75 ± 15	65 ± 32	32 ± 21	20 ± 16	2 ± 4
	$r^2 = 0.95$	$r^2 = 0.73$	$r^2 = 0.6$	$r^2 = 0.6$	$r^2 = 0.79$	$r^2 = 0.93$

(Miclau, T., Dahners, L.E., Lindsey, R.W.: In Vitro Pharmacokinetics of Antibiotic Release From Locally Implantable Materials. J. Orthop. Res., 11:629, 1993.)

Miclau and associates performed a direct comparison of the elution rate of tobramycin from bone graft, demineralized bone matrix, plaster of Paris, and PMMA.[738] Their results are summarized in Table 8-13. Cancellous bone graft released 70% of its antibiotic load in the first 24 hours. Demineralized bone matrix showed a similar elution, with 45% total release in the first 24 hours. Neither agent was detectable at 14 days. Thus, it is important to adjust the dose of antibiotic mixed with bone graft and demineralized bone matrix to prevent a potentially toxic serum level secondary to rapid absorption. Plaster of Paris released 17% of its antibiotic load over the first 24 hours, with measurable elution at 21 days. PMMA eluted only 7% during the first 24 hours, with trace amounts detectable at 14 days.

The most commonly used carrier agent in the past has been PMMA. Combinations of antibiotics and PMMA have been used extensively in the treatment of infected total joint replacements, and the elution characteristics of many antibiotics from this material have been studied thoroughly.[746] Commercial preparations of the material are available in Europe (Septopal, Merck, Darmstadt, Germany) but not yet in the United States.[643,644] Therefore, surgeons must custom formulate their own product before use. Typically, high doses of the appropriate antibiotics are mixed thoroughly with the PMMA powder. While this mixture is in the dough stage, it is formed into small beads that subsequently are laced onto a length of surgical wire or heavy suture and placed into the bone defect. Several authors have published recommendations for the appropriate mixing ratio for various antibiotic and PMMA combinations[651,755] (Table 8-14). The limiting factor appears to be the volume of the antibiotic powder, and it is suggested that no more than 24 mL of powder should be mixed in a standard 40-g pack of PMMA.[651]

The use of antibiotic-impregnated PMMA beads in the treatment of chronic osteomyelitis has been reported in several series. Blaha and colleagues conducted an eight-center trial comparing the use of PMMA/gentamicin beads (Septopal) and short-duration antibiotic therapy (5 days) with conventional 4- to 6-week intravenous antibiotic therapy in a matched set.[643] The authors noted no statistical difference in treatment success between the two groups, but the conventionally treated group had a higher rate of adverse reactions (54%) than did the Septopal group (30%), largely because of the systemic effects of the intravenous antibiotics (elevated renal and liver function test results). The Septopal group averaged 20% fewer days in the hospital, with a significant cost savings. In a rabbit model, Evans and Nelson found a trend toward higher cure rates when Septopal beads were implanted *and* conventional antibiotic therapy was used compared with either modality alone.[676]

The use of calcium hydroxyapatite ceramic as a biocompatible carrier for antibiotics has been investi-

TABLE 8-14
Amount of Antibiotic Added to 40 g of Palacos Bone Cement During Fabrication of Antibiotic-Impregnated Beads

Antibiotic	Grams (Powder)
Tobramycin	3
Amikacin*	1
Vancomycin	5
Gentamicin†	3
Cefazolin	6
Cefamandole	6
Cefotaxime	6
Ticarcillin	7
Nafcillin	6
Clindamycin*	6
Erythromycin	6
Primaxin	4

* Unavailable in the United States in powder form for clinical use.
† Available only in nonsterile powder in the United States.
(Popham, G.J., Mangino, P., Seligson, D., Henry, S.L.: Antibiotic–Impregnated Beads: Part II, Factors in Antibiotic Selection. *Orthop. Rev.*, 20:332, 1991.)

gated.[769] Calcium hydroxyapatite ceramic previously has been shown to have excellent biocompatibility[672] and mechanical properties.[717] Removal is not necessary because the material is slowly resorbed. This material showed elution characteristics significantly more prolonged than those of either PMMA or plaster of Paris. Gentamicin concentrations reached a peak 8 days after implantation but still showed bactericidal concentrations after 90 days, with 30% of the drug remaining. Further research is necessary, but this class of materials may have significant utility in the adjuvant treatment and dead-space management of chronic osteomyelitis.

Hyperbaric Oxygen

Hyperbaric oxygen has been used as adjunctive therapy for difficult cases of osteomyelitis for more than 30 years.[770] Recently, the mechanism of action of this modality and the appropriate indications for its use have been refined. The direct effect of hyperbaric oxygenation is to increase oxygen tension to tissue beds. Several investigators have shown in an animal model that normal intramedullary bone has an oxygen tension of about 32 to 45 mm Hg under ambient conditions.[673,725] In osteomyelitis, the oxygen tension falls to about 17 to 23 mm Hg, rendering the bone hypoxic. When these animals are placed at 2 atm of pressure on 100% oxygen, the intramedullary oxygen tensions increase to greater than 100 mm Hg in the osteomyelitic bone and greater than 300 mm Hg in the normal bone.

High tissue oxygen levels appear to be directly toxic to strictly anaerobic bacteria.[724] These organisms lack the enzyme superoxide dismutase and are sensitive to the superoxide radicals present in highly oxygenated tissue. In contrast, aerobic bacteria can degrade superoxide radicals rapidly by increasing their superoxide dismutase levels in an oxygen-rich environment.[690] It appears that hyperbaric oxygen may be effective in the treatment of aerobic infections by increasing the oxygen-dependent intercellular killing of the polymorphonuclear leukocytes.[649] Fibroblast proliferation, collagen production, and angiogenesis also are suboptimal in hypoxic conditions and appear to be enhanced by hyperbaric oxygen therapy.[724] Mader and coworkers showed that the phagocytic killing of *S aureus* was markedly decreased under hypoxic conditions (23 mm Hg), improved significantly as the oxygen tension was increased to 45 mm Hg, and continued to improve up to an oxygen tension level of 1500 mm Hg in an animal model.[725] In addition, hyperbaric oxygen has been demonstrated to augment the bactericidal action of the aminoglycoside class of antibiotics, which perform poorly in hypoxic conditions.[778]

Despite the theoretically beneficial effects of hyperbaric oxygen and the promising results of animal studies, convincing evidence of its efficacy in human series has been lacking. In two uncontrolled studies, Morrey and colleagues[741] and Davis and associates[663] reported encouraging results in chronic nonhematogenous osteomyelitis using similar protocols of 2.4 atm—100% oxygen—90 min/d for about 45 days, with remission rates of greater than 85%. In both these studies, the hyperbaric oxygen was adjunctive treatment because aggressive debridement and appropriate antibiotics also were used. In one of the few prospective, randomized, controlled studies evaluating hyperbaric oxygen therapy, Esterhai and associates attempted to match patients by clinical stage of disease and, after debridement, assigned the matched pairs to receive either hyperbaric oxygen therapy and antibiotics or conventional antibiotic therapy alone.[652,675] These authors failed to show any effect on the recurrence rate, rate of wound healing, and length of hospitalization by the addition of hyperbaric oxygen to the treatment regimen. Unfortunately, this study was hampered by small patient numbers (14 per group). The current role of hyperbaric oxygen in the treatment of chronic osteomyelitis remains undefined. Clearly, the use of radical debridement to remove hypoxic bone and the ability to cover and reconstruct nearly all wounds with well-perfused tissue decreases the theoretic indications for hyperbaric oxygen therapy. Additional research is needed to determine whether hyperbaric oxygen has a role in cases where either the debridement or the patient is compromised.

Illustrative Cases

Case 1. A 14-year-old boy sustained a grade IIIB fracture of his distal tibia in a farm accident. Initial treatment consisted of immediate wide debridement and irrigation with pulsed saline. Stabilization was achieved with unilateral external fixation. Initial antibiotic coverage consisted of a first-generation cephalosporin, gentamicin, and penicillin G. After two additional debridements, soft-tissue coverage was achieved on day 6 with a soleus flap. Antibiotic therapy was discontinued 48 hours after flap coverage.

The patient was seen 5 weeks after the injury with a mild increase in pain at the fracture site but no fever. Radiographs obtained at that time are shown in Figure 8-17**A**. His soleus flap was elevated and *Enterobacter cloacae* was cultured. The periosteum of the intermediate bone segment had been partially stripped by the injury and, at the time of reexploration, the segment was found to be nonviable and was removed (see Fig. 8-17**B**). After a second debridement, a 10-cm segmental bone defect was present and wound closure was achieved with a free flap over tobramycin-impregnated PMMA beads to manage the dead space (see Fig. 8-17**C**). After 6 weeks of intravenous antibiotic therapy, the beads were removed, a unilateral

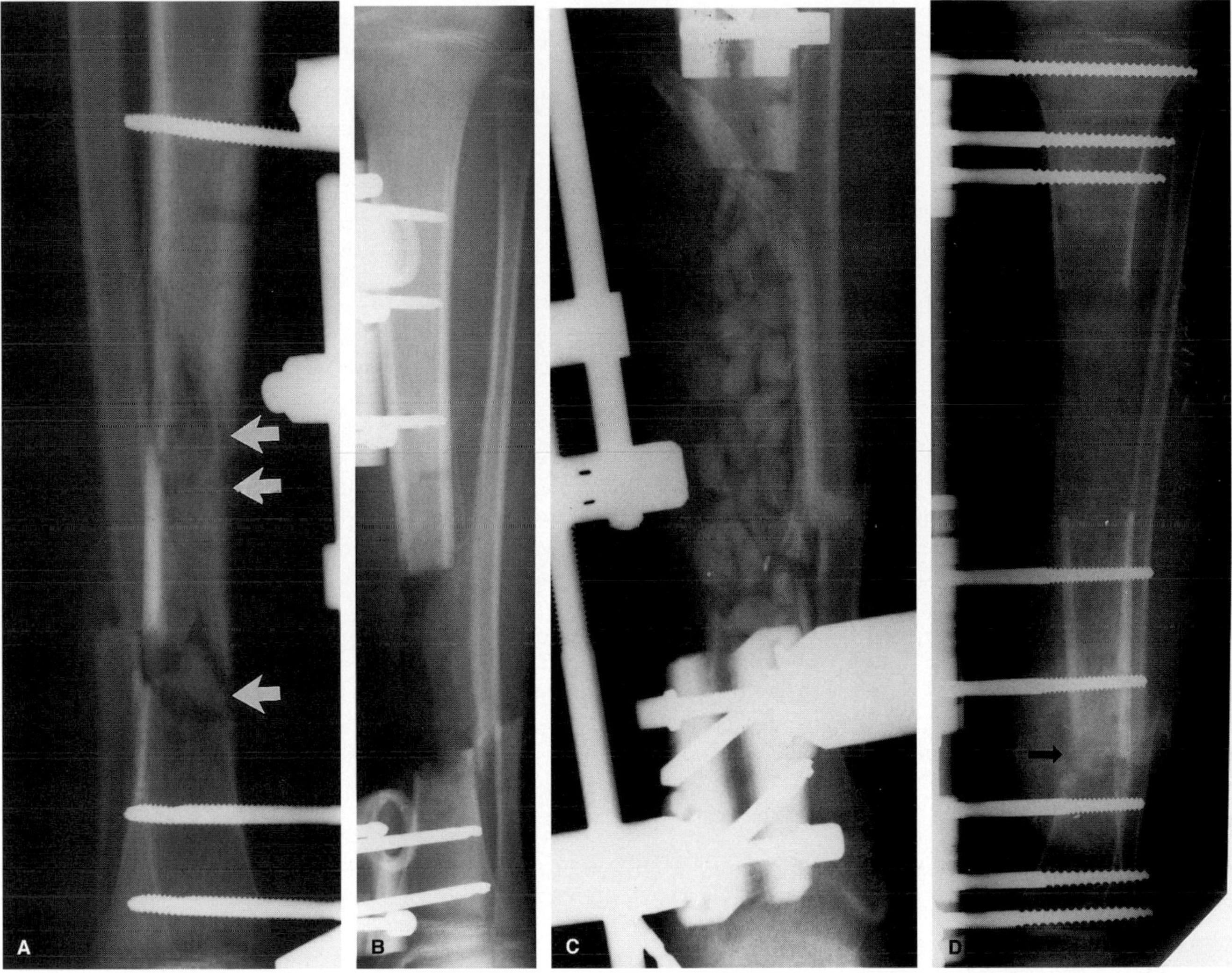

FIGURE 8-17. Case 1: Lateral radiograph of the tibia of a 15-year-old boy 5 weeks after a grade IIIB open fracture (**A**). The original fracture can be seen (*single arrow*). An early post-traumatic gram-negative osteomyelitis developed (*double arrows*), rendering the intervening segment necrotic. After serial debridement, a 10-cm segmental defect resulted (**B**). The dead space was managed in a staged fashion with placement of tobramycin-impregnated PMMA beads under a latissimus dorsi free flap (**C**). After 6 weeks of intravenous antibiotics, the beads were removed and bone transport was initiated with a unilateral frame. The appearance at the completion of transport and after bone grafting of the docking site (*arrow;* **D**).

transport frame (Orthofix-EBI) was placed, and a metaphyseal corticotomy was performed. Transport at 1 mm/d was initiated after a 12-day latent period.

After 100 days, the transport segment docked with the distal fragment and a small posterolateral bone graft was placed to ensure union of the docking site (see Fig. 8-17**D**). The patient progressed in his weight bearing in the frame as the regenerate bone consolidated. The frame was removed 12 months after the original injury. Both the proximal and the distal physis remained open and he grew 2 in during the year of treatment. The patient returned to competitive swimming and equestrian events.

Case 2. An 83-year-old man had a 60-year history of chronic distal tibia osteomyelitis after an episode of meningococcemia. He suffered with chronic foul-smelling drainage from an anterolateral sinus tract (Fig. 8-18**B**). The patient desired surgical treatment because of increased pain and drainage despite oral antibiotic suppression with ciprofloxacin. In addition to plain radiographs (see Fig. 8-18**A**), the evaluation consisted of a sequential ^{99m}Tc-MDP/^{111}In-WBC (see Fig. 8-18**C**) scan as well as MRI and computed tomography. Computed tomography revealed complex medullary sequestra as well as significant thickening of the cortical bone in the involved segment (see Fig. 8-18**E**). MRI was particularly helpful in delineating the exten-

(text continues on page 482)

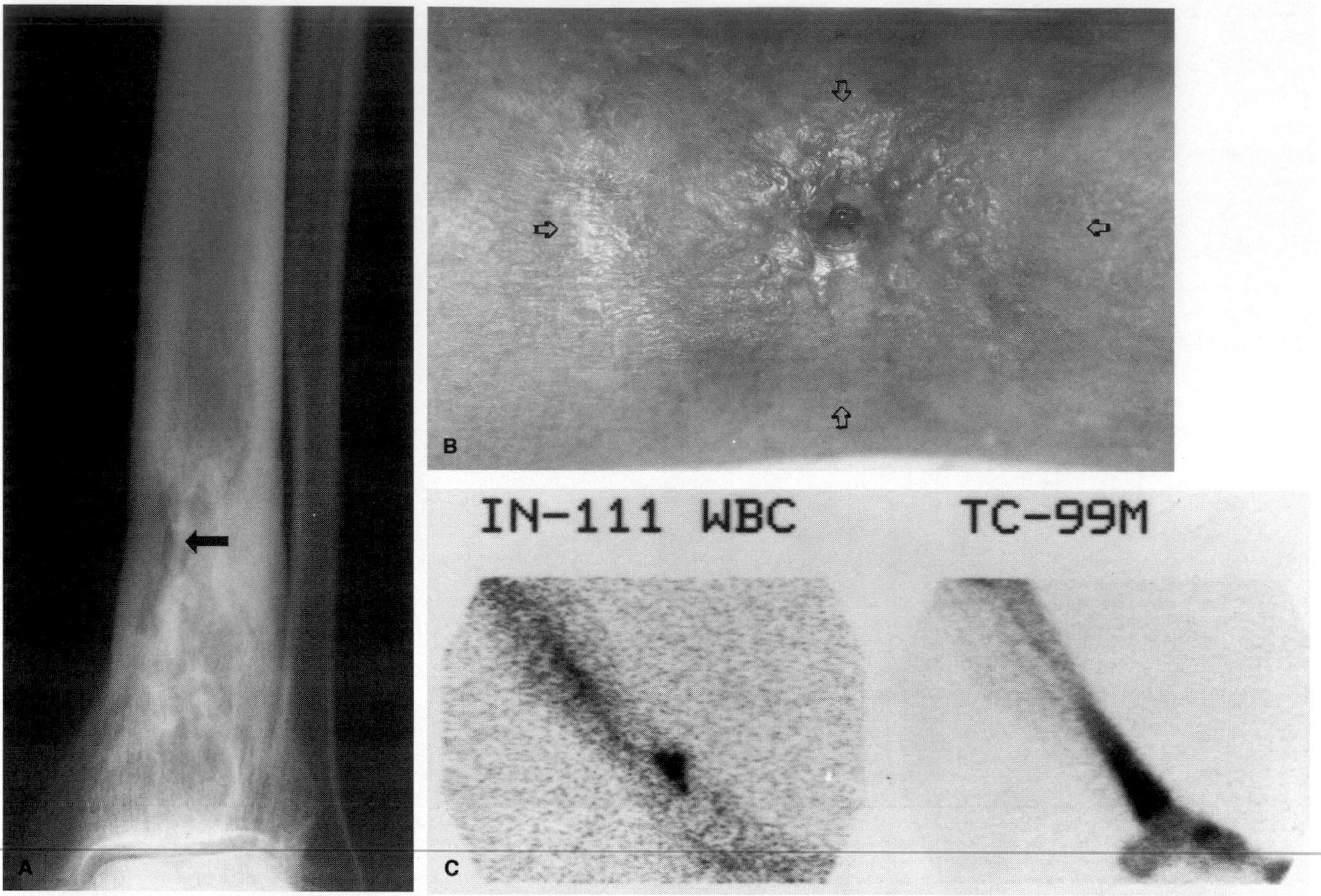

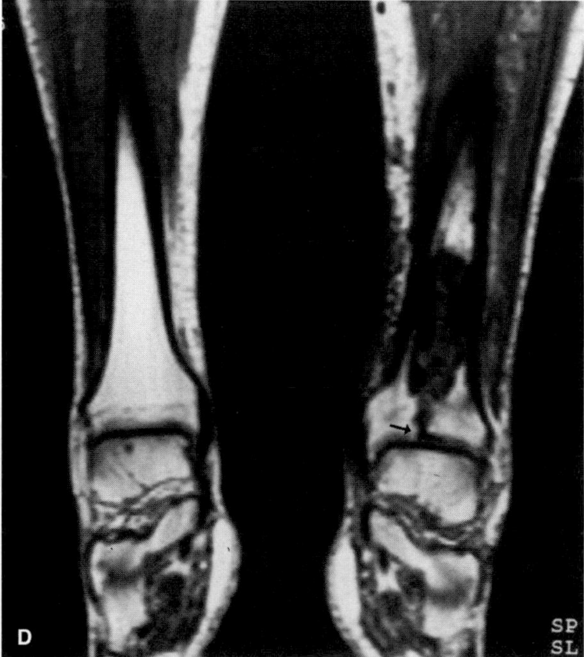

FIGURE 8-18. Case 2: Chronic distal tibial osteomyelitis in an 83-year-old man. An anteroposterior radiograph of the tibia with a medial cortical sinus (*arrow;* **A**). The sinus tract and surrounding indurated skin (*arrows;* **B**). Staging studies included sequential ^{99m}Tc and ^{111}In white blood cell scans (**C**), an MRI scan (T1-weighted image; **D**) showing that the granulation tissue extended to the subchondral bone of the ankle joint (*arrow*), and a CT scan

continues

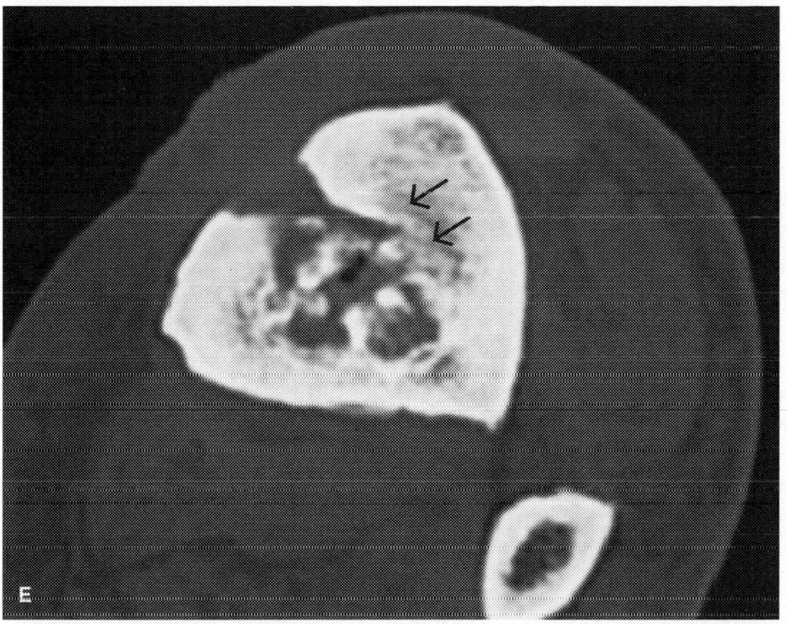
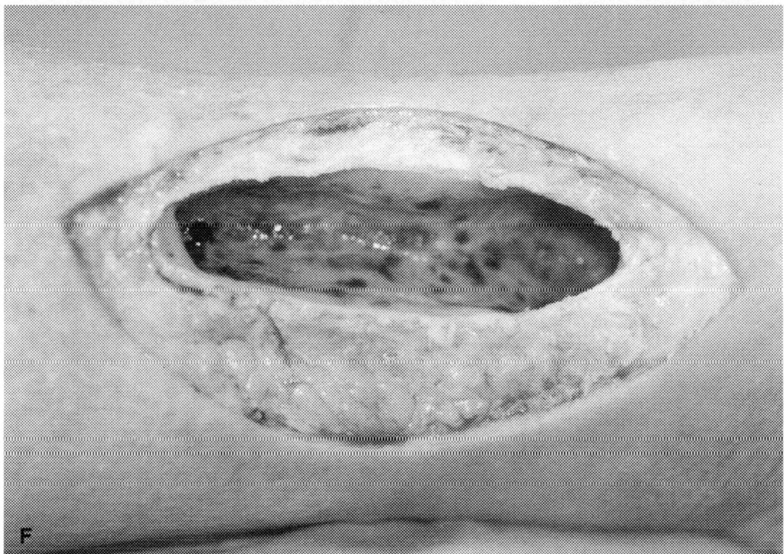
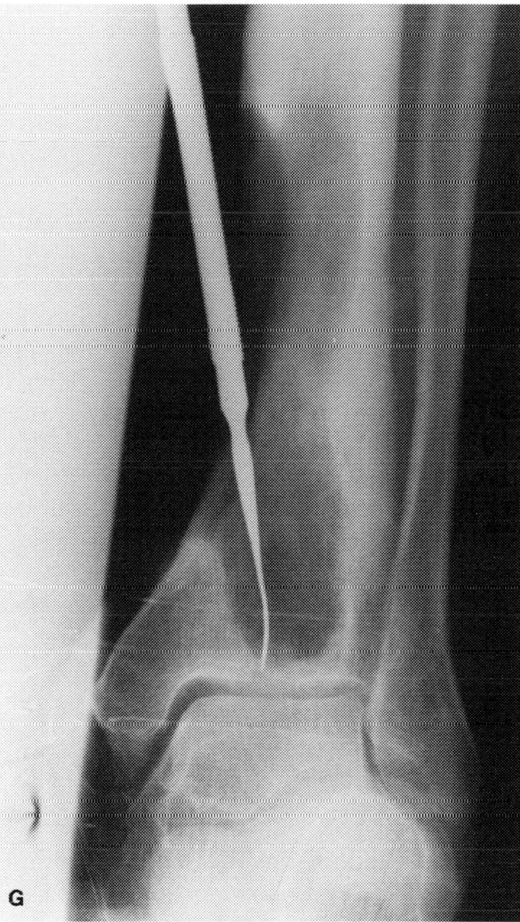
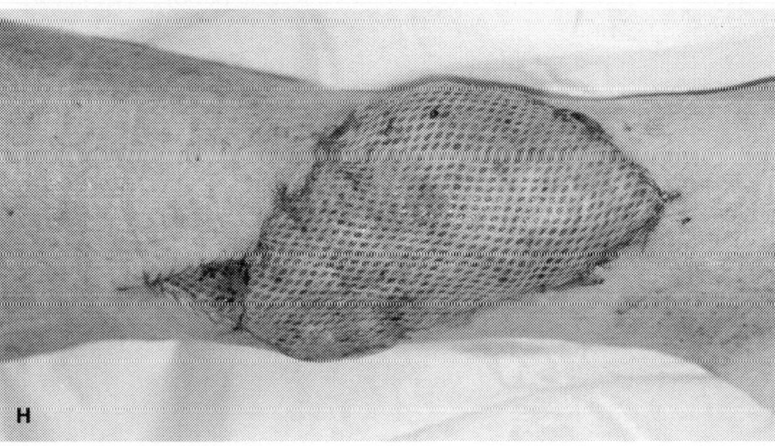

FIGURE 8-18. (continued) (at the level of the cortical sinus; **E**) showing the extensive cortical remodeling and sequestra within the medullary canal. An en bloc resection of the sinus tract and surrounding skin was performed (**F**). The intraoperative radiograph after the first debridement is shown (**G**). A rectus abdominis free flap was placed after a second debridement (**H**).

sion of the marrow involvement to the subchondral bone of the ankle (see Fig. 8-18**D**). The radionuclide imaging suggested that the medullary infection was more localized than the MRI scan indicated.

A wide debridement was performed with excision of all the scarred and nonmobile skin. The cortical cloaca was exposed and a pneumatic bur was used to enlarge the cortical defect until the full extent of the infection as outlined on the MRI scan could be accessed (see Fig. 8-18**F**). Curettage and culture of the medullary contents was performed, followed by debridement with the bur until normal haversian canal bleeding was observed over the entire bone surface. An intraoperative radiograph (see Fig. 8-18**G**) was obtained to verify the extent of distal debridement. The defect was packed with tobramycin/PMMA beads and the wound was left open.

Cultures from the medullary canal grew *P aeruginosa, Bacteroides fragilis,* and microaerophilic *Streptococcus.* On the fourth postoperative day, the patient was returned to the operating room and the beads were removed. The bone was debrided lightly throughout until haversian canal bleeding returned. A rectus abdominis free flap was placed into the bone defect and covered with an immediate skin graft (see Fig. 8-18**H**). The patient received 4 weeks of intravenous tobramycin and combined ticarcillin sodium and clavulanate potassium (Timentin). Partial weight bearing was allowed in a windowed short-leg cast. He remains free of infection at 1 year.

Post-traumatic Reflex Sympathetic Dystrophy

For many years, certain vague, ill-defined, widespread, painful conditions have been observed after trauma, infection, or thrombophlebitis of the extremities.[808] A variety of terms, such as *minor causalgia, major causalgia,*[797] *causalgia-like states, post-traumatic painful osteoporosis, Sudeck's atrophy,*[876,877] *reflex dystrophy, post-traumatic dystrophy,*[848] and *shoulder-hand syndrome,*[851,879] have been used to designate these conditions. Several theories regarding the pathogenesis of these conditions have been proposed, but no single theory has been proven. In this section, the individual characteristics of reflex sympathetic dystrophy (RSD), the shoulder-hand syndrome, and causalgia are considered. The orthopaedic surgeon is expected to recognize and manage these problems, which often are caused by fractures and dislocations, with associated soft-tissue, nerve, and vascular injury. More recently, RSD has been discussed after arthroscopic procedures around the knee, especially when performed in the treatment of patellofemoral pain syndromes.[806,839]

Pathogenesis

de Takats has suggested a holistic concept under the heading of post-traumatic reflex dystrophy and has characterized this syndrome by chronic sensory stimulus, persistent vasomotor response, motor response, and eventual atrophy of tissue, bone, tendon, and muscle, with joint contractures, chronic edema, and fibrosis.[808] It remains to be demonstrated how a minor injury can cause severe, persistent pain after the injured tissues have healed. A series of reflexes dependent on cross-stimulation between sympathetic efferent and damaged demyelinated sensory fibers may account for the underlying pathophysiology.[810] Livingston proposed that three factors caused a circle of reflexes.[843] He believed that chronic irritation of a peripheral sensory nerve led to an abnormal state of activity in the internuncial neuron center, which in turn led to a continuum of increased stimulation of efferent motor and sympathetic neurons. Figure 8-19 illustrates the factors that may be involved in a reflex dystrophic state. No single concept of pathogenesis has been proven[805,825,853,881,885]; the fact that there is an abnormal sympathetic reflex is well established.[801,829,858,860,879,880]

Clinical Findings

Pain, hyperesthesia, and tenderness out of proportion to the physical findings are the predominant features in a patient with RSD.[790,817] The pain may vary in severity and character, and may be accompanied by swelling and decreased range of motion in the involved extremity. The skin color, texture, and temperature may vary, depending on the stage of the disease. The diagnosis can be confusing, because these variations may be completely opposite, such as hot or cold, pale or red, sweaty or dry. Early on, increased sweating (hyperhidrosis), redness,[840] warmth, and swelling are more common. In the later stages, pallor, with dry and shiny skin, and coolness of the involved part become the predominant features (Fig. 8-20).

Most authors have separated the clinical findings into three stages: early, dystrophic, and atrophic. The first stage is that which occurs within 3 months of onset of symptoms and is identified by constant burning or aching pain in the extremity. The pain is increased by external stimuli or motion and is out of proportion to the severity of the injury and related physical findings. The stimuli that trigger the pain response can vary from peculiar noises, height, and excitement to emotional upset, vibration, arguments, deep breathing, laughter, or the use of certain words.[808,856]

The second stage develops in about 3 months and extends until 1 year after the onset of symptoms. At this stage, most patients have significant edema; cold,

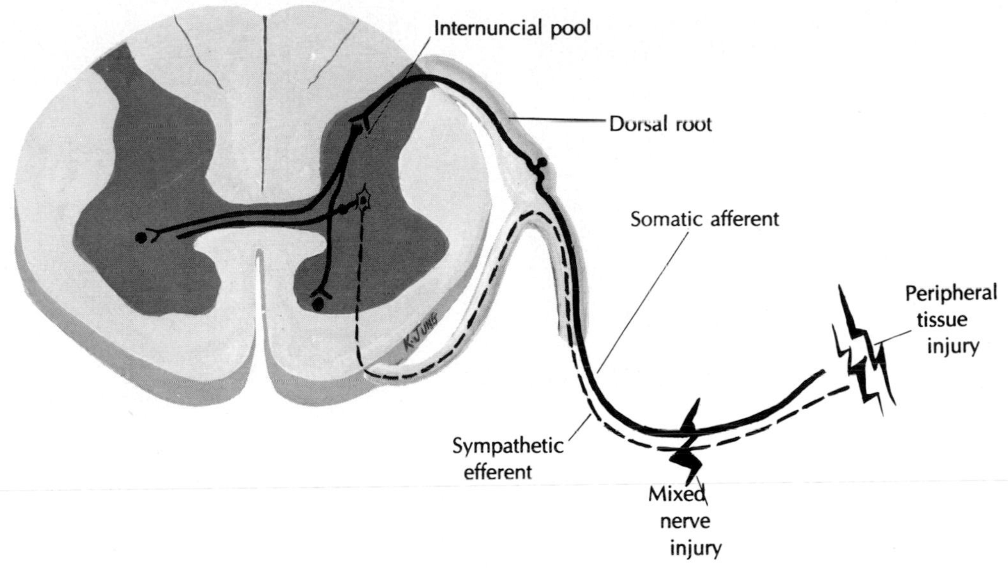

FIGURE 8-19. Neural pathways in reflex dystrophy.

glossy skin; and a limited range of joint motion. X-ray films often reveal a diffuse osteopenia.

The third, or atrophic, stage occurs 12 months to many years after the onset of symptoms and is marked by a progressive atrophy of the skin and muscle, joint motion that is severely limited by evolving fibrosis, and contractures that may be irreversible. Marked, diffuse osteopenia is seen on the x-ray films. The pain may involve the whole limb and approach intractability.

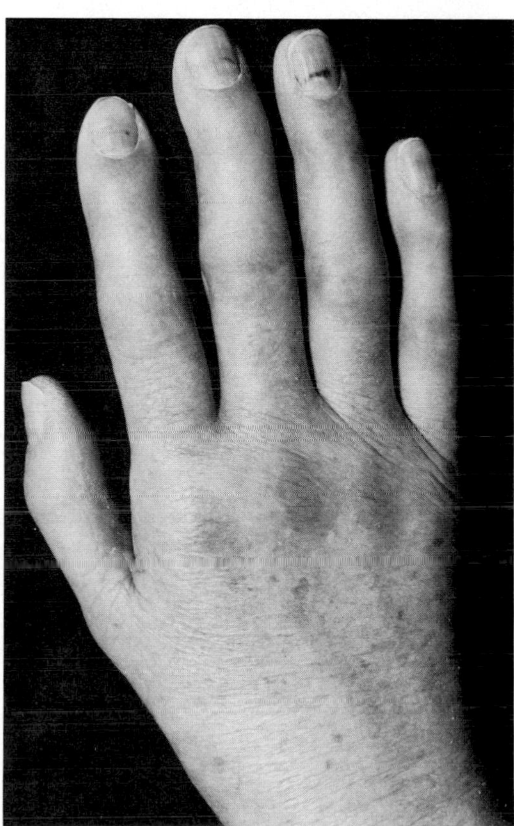

FIGURE 8-20. Swollen, pale, stiff fingers in a patient with post-traumatic reflex dystrophy.

In 1900, Sudeck described acute bony atrophy, relating the onset to "inflammation."[876] Subsequently, Sudeck expanded his concept to include trauma or infection as causes of bone atrophy.[877] He believed that the clinical features of pain, muscle atrophy, cyanosis, and edema developed secondary to the bone atrophy. He also stated that the changes did not take place if a reflex arc was broken, as occurs in such diseases as syringomyelia or poliomyelitis. Lenggenhager has suggested that aseptic inflammation around an involved joint is responsible for the mottled osteodystrophy and has recommended forced mobilization, under anesthesia, of the stiffened joints.[841]

The term *Sudeck's atrophy* should not be used if the characteristic radiographic appearance is not present[812,857,865] (Fig. 8-21). Spotty rarefaction, present in the involved bones, is different from the generalized ground-glass appearance seen with disuse atrophy of bone.[830,831] The radiographic features occur about 6 to 8 weeks after the onset of symptoms.[793,799]

Diagnosis

Hartley listed several clinical entities that may cause confusion in the diagnosis of post-traumatic reflex dystrophy: tenosynovitis, disuse atrophy, senile osteoporosis, peripheral neuritis, and peripheral vascular disease states.[828] It often is necessary to determine whether the patient's condition is caused by a major functional overlay in conjunction with a minor organic problem.

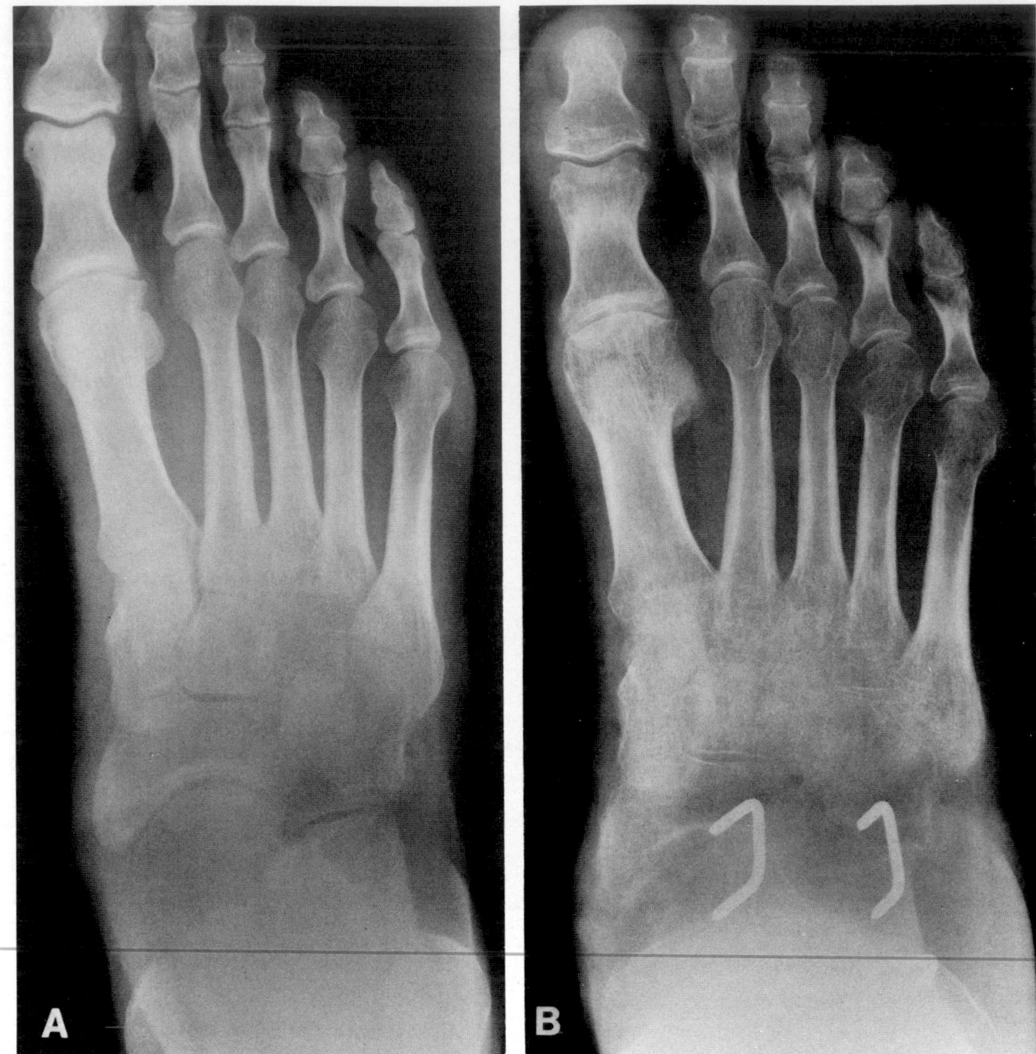

FIGURE 8-21. (**A**) Anteroposterior radiograph of the right foot before operation. (**B**) Anteroposterior radiograph of the right foot after operation showing spotty rarefaction, characteristic of Sudeck's atrophy.

Plain radiographs are an important initial study to evaluate the possibility of a sympathetic dystrophy diagnosis. The classic appearance of diffuse spotty osteopenia is not apparent for several weeks, but the radiographs allow investigation of possible underlying causes of pain in the extremity that may be remediable. Despite a clear clinical diagnosis of RSD, up to one third of patients have normal plain radiographs.[847]

Digital temperature recording and thermography may be helpful in the objective diagnosis of a sympathetic dystrophy.[819] Although no absolute criteria exist to establish the diagnosis on these grounds, a consistent and reproducible elevation of temperature in the digits of the affected extremity constitutes the primary pathologic alteration. Venous congestion likewise may elevate the skin temperature independent of RSD, whereas peripheral vascular disease has the opposite effect.[794]

Scintigraphic patterns of uptake on a three-phase bone scan constitute the best objective, strictly diagnostic test. Although several investigators have advocated the bone scan in this setting, MacKinnon and Holder have adopted the strictest criteria for diagnosis and consequently have demonstrated the greatest predictive value of a favorable response to treatment.[809,822,838,844,861,868] They require a diffuse increase in delayed periarticular tracer uptake in *all* joints of the affected hand, and have reported positive and negative predictive values of 88% and 99%, respectively.[844]

A local anesthetic block of the appropriate sympathetic ganglia represents the best practical combined diagnostic and prognostic test in the management of the patient being evaluated for a suspected RSD.[813] Successful achievement of a sympathetic blockade, as evidenced by a Horner's syndrome (miosis, ptosis, and anhidrosis) and warming of the affected extremity, in conjunction with relief of the chief complaint of pain confirms the diagnosis of RSD. Although failure of pain relief does not rule out the diagnosis of RSD, a positive response with relief of symptoms all but assures the diagnosis and, more importantly, predicts a favorable response to a series of therapeutic sympathetic blocks.

Treatment

Elimination of the responsible noxious stimulus, if identifiable, that perpetuates the pathologic sympathetic reflex arc is the ideal goal of treatment. Stated in more practical terms, to interrupt the vicious cycle of pain is the focus of any intervention, even when the offending source is not readily apparent, as is often the case. Occasionally, prompt immobilization of the injured part obviates further treatment.[836] Many patients with mild forms of post-traumatic RSD recover spontaneously after the institution of a directed program of functional use, or "stress loading," of the affected limb.[884] It is equally important to provide emotional support for patients during this stage of impending or early reflex dystrophy.[827,888]

If conservative measures fail, some form of sympathetic interruption is used most frequently. Interrupting the sympathetic reflex has been attempted by several modalities,[806,839] including sympatholytic drugs, given both orally[814,821,869,882] and regionally,[796,803,804,818,823,859] somatic nerve blocks, periodic perineural infusions,[842,854] and stellate ganglion blocks.[867] Serial sympathetic ganglion blocks with local anesthetic have been the most reliable and successful intervention for established RSD. If the patient demonstrates a favorable response to the initial block, a series of as many as 20 blocks may be required to achieve a long-lasting response using longer-acting anesthetic drugs. Alternatively, sufentanil stellate ganglion blockade has provided good results in cases refractory to conventional anesthetic blockade, suggesting the presence of opiate receptors in the sympathetic ganglia.[792]

For RSD that does not respond to sympathetic ganglion blockade, intravenous regional blockade is a reasonable next intervention. Classically, guanethidine and reserpine have demonstrated good results in RSD by effecting a pharmacologic sympathectomy by interfering with norepinephrine metabolism at the synapse. Although both drugs have a demonstrated efficacy in up to 90% of patients by providing good long-term pain relief,[800,816,863] 83% of placebo group patients obtained pain relief for up to 4 weeks in one study.[800] However, neither drug is available in the United States for parenteral use. Bretylium tosylate, an antihypertensive agent with a similar mechanism of action by inhibiting the synaptic release of norepinephrine, has been tested in this setting and has produced good initial results, with pain relief lasting longer than 6 months.[819,834] Intravenous corticosteroids also have been used in this setting to specifically counteract postmanipulation edema after a regional anesthetic.[811] Similarly, smoking has been implicated in RSD by increasing the local and systemic effects of the sympathetic nervous system, and cessation of tobacco use is a rational recommendation during treatment.[791]

Various other medications, including corticosteroids[797,812,814,874] and calcitonin,[862,886] have been used in the treatment of this problem, the former with frequently good results and the latter with only minimal improvement over control agents.[798,824] Other popular oral medications have included amitriptyline, which assists in the relief of burning paresthesias and improves sleep when given as a bedtime dose; nifedipine, a calcium channel blocker that likely acts through peripheral vasodilation; and phenytoin, which may act centrally to limit regional sympathetic system activity and reduce pain.[802] Several other adjunctive forms of treatment,[883] including transcutaneous nerve stimulation, biofeedback with thermal self-regulation,[826] trigger point injections, and splinting, are helpful and should be considered. Infrequently, the abnormal sympathetic reflex requires permanent interruption by surgical sympathectomy,[807,815,817,870,872] but such intervention should be reserved for only the most refractory of cases that have a good, albeit transient, response to anesthetic blockade of the sympathetic ganglia.

A final imperative note is that all the preceding treatment alternatives often do no more than allow the initiation of a program of functional physical exercise free of pain, which is the real cornerstone of treatment in the recovery of a useful extremity afflicted with RSD.

Shoulder-Hand Syndrome

Steinbrocker and Argyros stated that the shoulder-hand syndrome is a distinctive and severe symptom complex with specific features that allow its identification.[873] It can result from external injuries or from internal disorders, such as coronary occlusion or a cerebrovascular accident. However, it is a syndrome that can be classified as a form of reflex dystrophy.[835,852,855,866] The term *shoulder-hand* refers to the chief features of the syndrome—a painful, disabled shoulder associated with painful disability of the hand and fingers. Stiffness is characteristic in both locations.

The syndrome occurs more frequently in older age groups and after cardiac dysfunction.[832,835] It can occur after cervical spondylitis, all types of fractures, a cerebrovascular accident, coronary occlusion, or any visceral, musculoskeletal, vascular, or neural process that involves reflex neurovascular responses. The syndrome characteristically evolves through three stages (Table 8-15).

As with other forms of RSD, the severity of the shoulder-hand syndrome is not proportional to the extent of the underlying disorder. A mild contusion of the shoulder might be followed by severe reflex dystrophy. Some authors believe that prompt recognition leads to more effective treatment.[795,887] No drug is specific for the treatment of the shoulder-hand syndrome; however, it is obvious that the underlying disorders require treatment before any resolution can be expected. Local injections with lidocaine (Xylocaine) and corticosteroids may be both diagnostic and therapeutic.[797,874]

It is inadvisable to manipulate the shoulder under anesthesia. Gentle but progressive active, assisted exercises of the shoulder and hand have been most helpful. Contractures are gradually lessened, and pain is decreased. Repeated sympathetic blocks may be effective. The administration of oral corticosteroids is of indefinite value in the management of the shoulder-hand syndrome.

The shoulder-hand syndrome may be prevented by early recognition.[873,875] Casts and manipulation should be avoided, and gentle, graduated exercises should be encouraged. Injection of trigger points with lidocaine may prove beneficial.

Causalgia

Causalgia, by definition, means burning pain. In 1864, Mitchell and coworkers were the first to describe this clinical syndrome.[849] It is associated with a lesion of a peripheral nerve containing sensory fibers and is characterized by extreme pain in the affected extremity. Richards has listed the features of causalgic pain: spontaneous, hot, burning, intense, diffuse, persistent, and intermittent.[862] It is elicited by stimuli that do not necessarily produce physical change and leads to profound alterations in the mental state of the patient. Chuinard and colleagues have stated, "We consider causalgia to be a clinical syndrome associated with a lesion of a peripheral nerve containing sensory fibers manifested by pain in the affected extremity. This pain is usually of a burning character and is usually located in an area corresponding to the cutaneous distribution of the involved nerve. An integral characteristic of this pain, one whose presence is necessary in order to make the diagnosis, is its accentuation by certain disturbing features of the affected individual's environment."[803]

The incidence of causalgia depends on the criteria accepted for diagnosis. In the Civil War, it was estimated to occur in 38% of patients with nerve injuries.[850,871] White and coworkers stated that causalgia occurs in about 5% of wounds of major nerves, especially in those associated with injuries to the median and sciatic nerves.[885] In wartime, it was seen most frequently after a high-velocity missile injury with incomplete division of the tibial portion of the sciatic nerve. Incised or lacerated wounds of nerves rarely are complicated by causalgia. It is not a frequent problem in civilian practice.

The exact etiology of causalgia remains uncertain, but it appears that crossover effects at the areas of injury permit interaction between efferent sympathetic and afferent sensory fibers.[846,862,878]

The clinical picture is one of excruciating, unbearable pain, with superimposed stabbing, crushing sensations. The pain begins immediately after injury in about one third of cases and within a week in the remaining cases. The duration of the pain is extremely variable, reaching maximum intensity 1 or 2 months after injury and, in some cases, persisting for 20 years or more. The pain may regress spontaneously. The area of sensory involvement usually is more than the cutaneous distribution of a single nerve. The extreme guarding of the patient against external stimuli makes

TABLE 8-15
Clinical Manifestations of Shoulder-Hand Syndrome

	Shoulder	Hand	Fingers	Vasomotor Changes	Radiographic Changes
Stage I	Pain Limitation of motion Diffuse tenderness	Pain Diffuse marked tenderness Dorsal swelling	Swelling Incomplete painful flexion	Vasodilation Vasospasm (occasionally)	Spotty osteoporosis
Stage II	Pain Early atrophy	Induration of skin	Firm induration Shiny atrophic skin	Vasospasm Hyperhidrosis	Progressive diffuse osteoporosis
Stage III	Slight residual pain occurs Limitation of motion	Residual dystrophy and contractures	Diffuse atrophy Residual contractures	Usually absent with dystrophic changes	Generalized osteoporosis

(Modified from Steinbrocker, O., and Argyros, T.G.: The Shoulder-Hand Syndrome; Present Status as a Diagnostic and Therapeutic Entity. Med. Clin. North Am., 42:1533–1553, 1958.)

motor evaluation of the involved limb difficult, but if the pain is relieved temporarily, the extent of sensory and motor involvement appears to be no greater than that expected from a peripheral nerve lesion without causalgia.[862] Many stimuli aggravate the pain, among them movement, examination, dependence, noise, excitement, touching dry objects, hearing certain words, and laughter. Often the patients are referred for psychological evaluation and are thought to be emotionally unstable. The image of the patient with severe causalgia holding the involved limb wrapped in a moist towel, anxiously avoiding all contact with external forces, is dramatic and not easily forgotten. Skin changes, such as glossiness, atrophy, moistness, and mottling, reflect the underlying vasomotor instability manifest by either vasoconstriction or dilation.

Operation on the peripheral nerve or its scar has not been effective treatment.[849] Neurolysis does not relieve pain. Alcohol injections have been tried to no avail.[841] Other operations, such as periarterial sympathetic section of the posterior nerve roots and arterial ligation, have not proved helpful in the management of causalgia. In 1930, Spurling described a complete cure of causalgia by cervicothoracic sympathetic ganglionectomy.[872] The World War II experience with this lesion showed that interruption of the appropriate sympathetic nerve fibers is almost always successful in the treatment of causalgia. Sympathetic blocks often provide temporary relief and, in some instances, complete relief after a series of treatments.[862,864] If a sympathetic block is to be done, it should be performed soon after the injury and the onset of symptoms. A satisfactory response to anesthetic sympathetic blockade may be a useful predictor of the anticipated effect of surgical sympathectomy.

In his centennial review of causalgia, Richards stated that certain facts are well established in regard to this syndrome[862]: "(1) True causalgia is rarely seen, except in missile wounds; (2) the nerve injury is usually proximal in the limb and is multiple; (3) the nerve injury is usually incomplete; (4) the anatomic lesions of the nerve are similar to noncausalgic nerve lesions; (5) surgical removal of the involved sympathetic ganglion is an effective mode of treatment."

Although rare, this syndrome represents a challenge in treatment when encountered by the orthopaedic surgeon.

Compartment Syndromes

One of the most devastating complications after a limb injury is ischemic muscle necrosis and subsequent contracture. More than a century ago, Richard von Volkmann reported the first account of a post-traumatic muscle contracture of acute onset, with increasing deformity despite splinting and passive exercises.[928] In his classic paper of 1881, he enumerated his reasons for believing that the paralysis and contracture of limbs "too tightly bandaged" resulted from ischemic changes of the muscles.[929] Since that time, physicians have become increasingly aware of the many varied circumstances in which increased tissue pressure can compromise the microcirculation. Jepson was the first investigator to prove that paralysis and contracture could be prevented by prompt decompression.[904] He showed in laboratory animals that contracture deformity is caused by a combination of factors, the most important of which are impairment of venous flow, extravasation of blood and serum, and swelling of the tissues, with resulting increased extravascular pressure compromising local tissue perfusion.

The compartment syndrome is a significant clinical problem, causing major functional losses after a wide variety of traumatic, vascular, hematologic, neurologic, surgical, pharmacologic, renal, and iatrogenic conditions.[909] Although it should be familiar to all clinicians, its common characteristics are obscured by the many names and descriptions used to identify it. A compartment syndrome is defined as a condition in which the circulation and function of tissues within a closed space are compromised by an increased pressure within that space. Matsen proposed that there be a unified concept with which to consider all compartment syndromes because the underlying features of all the syndromes are essentially the same, irrespective of etiology or location.[914] The names of some conditions in which compartment syndrome plays a central role are as follows:

1. Volkmann's ischemia[890,896,916,927]
2. Compartment syndrome[891,917,918,920,930]
3. Impending ischemic contractures[924]
4. Rhabdomyolysis[908]
5. Crush syndrome[922]
6. Exercise ischemia[906]
7. Local ischemia[912]
8. Traumatic tension ischemia in muscles[903]
9. Acute ischemic infarction[910]
10. Ischemic necrosis[893]
11. Anterior tibial syndrome[894,913,925]
12. Peroneal nerve palsy[923]
13. Calf hypertension[899]
14. Phlegmasia cerulea dolens[895]

Essentially, any cause of increased compartmental pressure can result in a compartment syndrome. Matsen suggested the following list of etiologies[914]:

I. Decreased compartment size
   A. Closure of fascial defects
   B. Tight dressings
   C. Localized external pressure
II. Increased compartment content

- A. Bleeding
  1. Major vascular injury
  2. Bleeding disorder
- B. Increased capillary permeability
  1. Postischemic swelling
  2. Exercise
  3. Seizure and eclampsia
  4. Trauma (other than major vascular)
  5. Burns
  6. Intra-arterial drugs
  7. Orthopaedic surgery
- C. Increased capillary pressure
  1. Exercise
  2. Venous obstruction
  3. Long-leg brace
- D. Muscle hypertrophy
- E. Infiltrated infusion
- F. Nephrotic syndrome

Pathophysiology

Although the common inciting pathogenic factor in compartment syndromes is increased tissue pressure, three theories have been proposed to explain the development of tissue ischemia found in this pathologic state:

1. Arterial spasm may result from increased intracompartmental pressure.[889,896]
2. The theory of critical closing pressure states that because of the small luminal radius and the high mural tension of arterioles, a significant transmural pressure difference (arteriolar pressure minus tissue pressure) is required to maintain their patency. If tissue pressure rises or if arteriolar pressure drops significantly so that this critical pressure difference does not exist (ie, critical closing pressure is reached), the arterioles close.[892]
3. Because of their thin walls, veins will collapse if tissue pressure exceeds venous pressure. If blood continues to flow from capillaries, the venous pressure will rise until it again exceeds tissue pressure and patency is reestablished. The augmentation of venous pressure reduces the arteriovenous gradient and, as a result, the tissue blood flow.[907,916]

Ashton studied the effect of increased tissue pressure on regional blood flow and concluded that at least two mechanisms appear to be involved[889]: (1) active closure of small arterioles under the influence of vasomotor tone when transmural pressure is lowered, either by falls in intravascular pressure or by rises in tissue pressure; and (2) passive collapse of soft-walled capillaries when tissue pressure rises above intracapillary pressure. These mechanisms were thought to become particularly important when tissues were surrounded by noncompliant fascial compartments.

The response of skeletal muscle to ischemia or trauma is similar regardless of the mechanism of injury.[921] When muscles become anoxic, histamine-like substances are released that dilate the capillary bed and increase the endothelial permeability. Subsequently, intramuscular transudation of plasma occurs, with erythrocyte sludging and a decrease of the microcirculatory flow.[902] The muscle gains weight in proportion to the duration of ischemia and has increased as much as 30% to 50% in net weight.[901] The necrosis of muscle is not immediate, because some arterial blood flow often continues, but the intramuscular edema is progressive.[896] It is now known beyond all controversy that after muscle ischemia and direct trauma, muscle has considerable ability to regenerate by the formation of new muscle cells. When only part of the length of a muscle cell succumbs or when some muscle cells disintegrate and others remain viable, marked regeneration can take place. Therefore, it is extremely important to decompress ischemic muscle as early as possible.[921]

Neural tissues also require a continuous and adequate supply of oxygen. Experimental studies on the effects of temporary ischemia, with special reference to intraneural microvascular pathophysiology, have shown that the microvessels of nerves possess an excellent capacity to recover function, even after long periods of ischemia.[911]

Diagnosis

Signs and Symptoms

The clinical presentation of compartment syndromes often is indefinite and confusing, and delays in diagnosis occur even when physicians are aware of the signs and symptoms. The classic signs of impending compartment syndromes are pain, pallor, paresthesias, paralysis, and pulselessness. The prognosis is better if these are *not* always present, because by the time these classic findings have evolved, especially pulselessness, the limb is neither viable nor salvageable. Each sign must be evaluated, separated, and interpreted within the overall clinical picture.

Pain. Pain is perhaps the earliest and most important and consistent sign. Unfortunately, it is variable, and its presence cannot always be relied on. Compartment syndromes often are associated with inherently painful conditions such as crush injuries and fractures. However, the pain of tissue ischemia typically is described as deep, unremitting, and poorly localized. It is not the type of pain generally associated with a fracture, and it is difficult to control with the usual mild analgesic measures used for fractures. In upper extremity fractures, passive finger extension exacerbates the pain and is an early physical finding of a deep forearm compartment syndrome. In children, restlessness and pain that continue after a fracture reduction should raise suspicion.[926]

Pallor. Pallor may or may not be present. The extremity may appear cyanotic or mottled early in the course of events. Cyanosis is present early, whereas marked pallor in the distal extremity occurs late, after major arterial occlusion has occurred. Neither pallor nor cyanosis should be considered a sign that is necessary for the diagnosis of compartment syndrome.

Paresthesia. Paresthesias in the cutaneous distribution of the peripheral nerve coursing through the affected compartment usually are an early sign of impending, but still reversible, compartment syndrome. Sensory disturbance generally precedes motor dysfunction; however, fixed hypoesthesia or anesthesia is a relatively late finding. The presence of true paresthesias, often experienced as a burning or prickling sensation, warrants at least close observation and, in the appropriate clinical context, may dictate a need for definitive treatment of an established compartment syndrome.

Paralysis. When a physician waits for obvious motor deficits to occur or for pulses to be obliterated, ischemia usually has been well established for some time and permanent damage may have occurred. Motor function is the first nerve function to be lost when a limb is rendered ischemic. Irreversible muscle fiber changes occur as early as 6 hours after the onset of tissue ischemia. Bradley reported that fasciotomy for anterior compartment syndrome resulted in complete recovery in only 13% of those patients who had footdrop at the time of diagnosis.[891]

Pulselessness. The loss of palpable pulses has been shown to occur late, or sometimes not at all, in the course of compartment syndromes.[932] Clinical experience and experimental evidence verify that irreversible tissue damage can occur in a patient with palpable pulses.[915,933]

Intracompartmental Pressures

If a developing compartment syndrome is suspected, constricting casts or circular dressings must be removed immediately. Garfin and associates have presented experimental evidence to substantiate the adverse effects on intracompartmental pressure caused by the most common offending dressing—the circular cast.[898] With dry Webril cast padding, the average intracompartmental pressure fell 30% after the cast was split on one side, and by 65% after the cast was spread. Splitting of the padding led to only a 10% further reduction in compartmental pressure. Complete removal of the cast reduced the pressure by another 15%, for a total decrease of 85% from baseline measurement. With a cast in place, it was found that about 40% less fluid, infused into the anterolateral compartment of the leg, was needed to elevate the compartment pressure to levels equivalent to those of limbs not in casts.

Because increased intracompartmental pressure has been incriminated as the primary pathogenic factor in compartment syndromes, and because the diagnosis of these syndromes often is so difficult to make on clinical grounds alone, the measurement of intracompartmental tissue pressures has become a valuable clinical tool. Reneman and Jagenean described a method for determining total intramuscular pressure, but their technique was rather cumbersome.[919] Whitesides and associates advocated the use of a simple pressure-measuring device consisting of a needle and plastic tubing filled with saline solution and air attached to a mercury manometer; they established tissue pressure measurement criteria as determinants of the need for fasciotomy[931,932] (Fig. 8-22).

The technique of Whitesides and associates requires only a few items that are readily available in most offices and hospitals. Both experimental and clinical experience have demonstrated that normal tissue pressure within closed compartments is about 0 mm Hg. This pressure increases markedly in compartment syndromes. There is inadequate perfusion and relative ischemia when the tissue pressure within a closed compartment rises to within 10 to 30 mm Hg of a patient's diastolic blood pressure. Whitesides and coworkers believed that fasciotomy usually is indicated when the tissue pressure rises to 40 to 45 mm Hg in a patient who has a diastolic blood pressure of 70 mm Hg and any signs or symptoms of a compartment syndrome. There is no effective tissue perfusion within a closed compartment when the tissue pressure equals or exceeds the patient's diastolic blood pressure. A fasciotomy is definitely indicated in this circumstance, even though distal pulses still may be present. Using their criteria, Whitesides and colleagues had no deficits develop in patients after the physician elected not to perform a fasciotomy on the basis of tissue pressures. Conversely, all patients showed conclusive evidence of a compartment syndrome at operation when the suggested tissue pressures were used as an adjunct in making the decision for fasciotomy.[932]

Previously available commercial kits for the determination of intracompartmental pressures have been fraught with technical problems and difficulty in reproducibility of pressure measurements; use of a homemade manometer setup has proven to be more reliable. In our institution, we have assembled kits for the measurement of intracompartmental pressures. Each kit contains the following items:

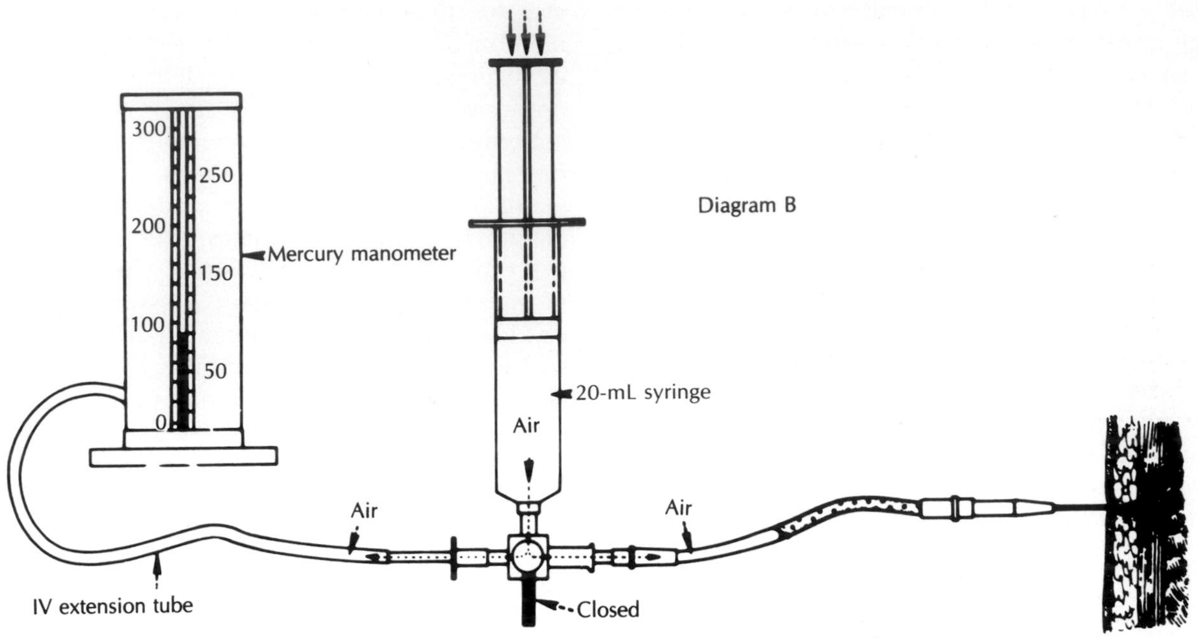

FIGURE 8-22. A device for measuring compartment pressures, made up of materials present in most hospitals, has been advocated by Whitesides. (*Whitesides, T.E., Jr., Haney, T.C., Morimoto, K., Harada, H.: Tissue Pressure Measurements as a Determinant for the Need of Fasciotomy. Clin. Orthop., 113:43, 1975.*)

1 sterile 20-mL syringe with Luer-Lok tip
1 four-way stopcock
1 18-gauge, 1 $^1/_4$-in Angiocath intravenous catheter
2 89-cm-long (35-in) extension tube sets
2 18-gauge needles
1 Telfa adhesive dressing pad
1 set of instructions and diagram (Fig. 8-23)

More recently, diminished tibial venous blood flow, as assessed noninvasively by Doppler identifying loss of normal phasic patterns, accurately predicted the need for surgical fasciotomy.[905] Although pressure measurement and other objective methods of assessment are invaluable adjuncts in the evaluation of impending compartment syndrome, especially in the obtunded or comatose patient, careful physical examination remains the cornerstone to early diagnosis and expedient treatment.

Treatment (Fasciotomy)

Jepson's early work proved that the treatment of choice for compartment syndrome is early decompression.[877] Delay in adequately decompressing the offending compartment can result in permanent damage to underlying tissues. Nerves have been found to demonstrate functional abnormalities (paresthesias and hypoesthesias) within 30 minutes of the onset of ischemia. Irreversible functional loss begins after 12 to 24 hours of total ischemia.[914,916] Muscle shows functional changes after 2 to 4 hours of ischemia, with irreversible functional loss beginning after 4 to 12 hours.[904,931] Ischemia lasting 4 hours gives rise to significant myoglobinuria, which reaches a maximum about 3 hours after the circulation is restored but persists for as long as 12 hours. Contractures are produced after 12 hours of total ischemia.[908,922,924] Capillary endothelium permeability is pathologically altered after 3 hours, resulting in postischemia swelling of 30% to 60%.

Initial decompression should be done by immediate splitting or removal of casts or other compromising circular dressings. A pneumatic pump providing intermittent mechanical compression of the plantar plexus of the foot has attracted interest as a potentially valuable adjunct in the management of compartment syndromes. By augmenting venous flow through the affected limb, reductions in soft-tissue swelling and intracompartmental pressures have been observed. The place, if any, of this device in the treatment of the spectrum of compartment syndromes remains to be defined. If the tissue pressure remains elevated in a patient with any other signs or symptoms of a compartment syndrome, adequate decompressive fasciotomy must be performed as an emergency procedure. (Using the criteria of Whitesides and associates, elevation means that the tissue pressure rises to within 30 mm Hg of the diastolic pressure.)

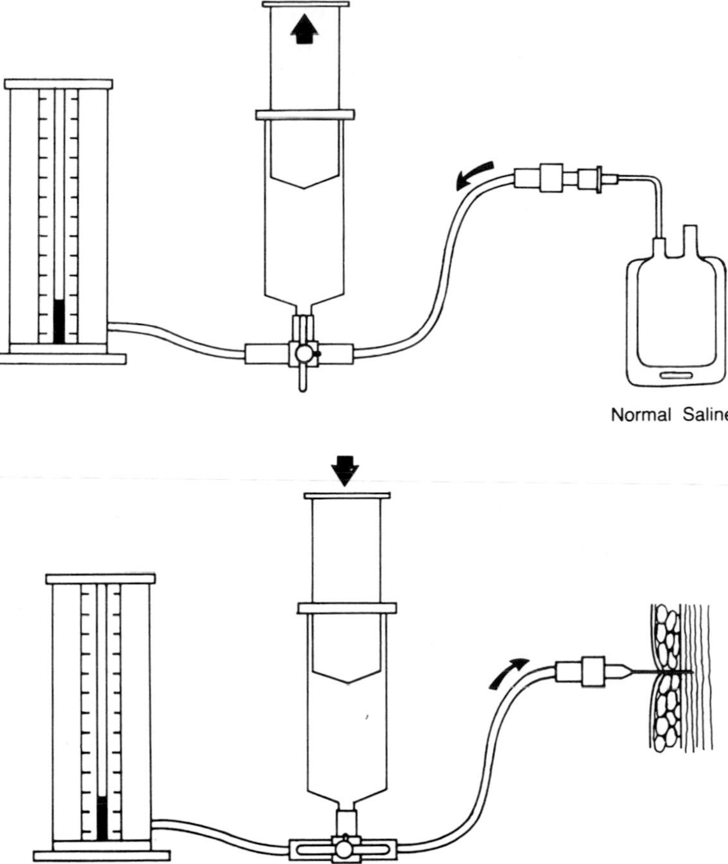

FIGURE 8-23. Instructions for measuring intracompartmental pressure.
1. Clean and prepare the area of the extremity to be evaluated.
2. Assemble the 20-mL syringe with the plunger at the 15-mL mark and connect it to an open end of the four-way stopcock (see diagram).
3. Connect the sterile plastic IV extension tube and an 18-gauge needle on one end of the stopcock and a second IV extension tube to the opposite end of the stopcock (see diagram) to a blood pressure manometer.
4. Insert the tip of the 18-gauge needle into the saline bag and open the stopcock to allow flow through the needled IV tubing only. Aspirate the saline solution without bubbles into about half the length of the extension tube. Turn the four-way stopcock to close off this tube so that the saline solution is not lost during transfer of the needle.
5. Insert the 18-gauge needle into the muscle of the compartment in which the tissue pressure is to be measured.
6. Turn the stopcock so that the syringe is open to both extension tubes, forming a "T" connection, as shown in the diagram. This produces a closed system in which the air is free to flow into both extension tubes as the pressure within the system is increased.
7. Increase the pressure in the system gradually by slowly depressing the plunger of the syringe while watching the saline/air meniscus. The mercury manometer will rise as the pressure within the system rises. When the pressure in this system has just surpassed the tissue pressure surrounding the needle, a small amount of saline solution will be injected into the tissue and the meniscus will be seen to move. When the column moves, stop the pressure on the syringe plunger and read the level of the manometer. The manometer reading at the time the saline column moves is the tissue pressure in millimeters of mercury.

The technique of fasciotomy is a matter of surgical choice. It can be done either subcutaneously or through limited or extensive skin incisions. However, the surgical goal is salvage of a viable and functional extremity; in no way should the adequacy of decompression be compromised by misdirected concerns over cosmesis and the number or lengths of incisions. It is essential to decompress all tight compartments. The skin must be considered a potentially significant limiting structure.[900]

The classic lower extremity fasciotomy does not provide adequate decompression of all four muscle compartments of the leg. Often, the deep posterior compartment has been neglected in discussions or descriptions of fasciotomy, access to which is obtained best behind the posteromedial border of the tibia in the distal third of the leg where the belly of the flexor digitorum longus muscle is exposed. Ernst and Kaufer described fibulectomy-fasciotomy as a way to decompress adequately all four compartments of the leg through one incision.[897] Mubarak and Owen advocated the double-incision fasciotomy, which permits access through two incisions to any or all of the four compartments of the leg when they are involved with acute or chronic compartment syndromes.[915] The technique of double-incision fasciotomy is as follows.

Anterolateral Incision

The anterolateral incision, used for an approach to the anterior or lateral compartment, is 15 to 20 cm long and placed halfway between the fibular shaft and the tibial crest, allowing easy access to both compartments. A smaller incision, or two short incisions, also can be used for chronic compartment syndromes. The skin edges are undermined to allow adequate exposure of the fascia. A short longitudinal incision is made just through the fascia overlying the muscle bellies, allowing a gloved finger to palpate the intermuscular septum that separates the anterior compartment from the lateral compartment. A longitudinal exploratory incision minimizes risk to the nerve until it is visualized. Identification of the septum is helpful in locating the superficial peroneal nerve that lies in the lateral compartment, adjacent to the septum where it crosses at the junction of the middle and distal thirds of the leg.

With 12-in Metzenbaum scissors, the *anterior compartment* fascia is opened through the length of the leg by extending the exploratory incision. The scissors are pushed gently with the tips opened slightly. Visualization is aided by the use of Army-Navy retractors, and the superficial peroneal nerve is protected in the distal third of the wound. If there is any question of whether the tip of the scissors has strayed from the fascia, the instrument is left in place and a small incision is made over its tip. If the fasciotomy is incomplete, further release can be performed through this small incision.

The *lateral compartment* fasciotomy is made in line with the fibular shaft posterior to the intermuscular septum. The scissors are directed proximally toward the fibular head and distally toward the lateral malleolus, remaining posterior to the superficial peroneal nerve. At the completion of this portion of the procedure, both compartments have been widely decompressed and the superficial peroneal nerve should remain intact and uninjured.

Posteromedial Incision

The posteromedial incision, used for an approach to the superficial or deep posterior compartments, is 15 to 20 cm long, slightly distal to the previous incision, and 2 cm posterior to the medial tibial margin. Placing the incision in this location prevents injury to the saphenous nerve and vein that course along the posterior margin of the tibia in this locale. Once again, the skin edges are undermined. The saphenous nerve and vein are retracted anteriorly. It usually is easiest to first decompress the *superficial posterior compartment*. Fasciotomy is extended proximally as far as possible and then distally behind the medial malleolus. The Achilles tendon in the superficial posterior compartment and the tendon of the flexor digitorum longus in the deep posterior compartment are identified. The deep posterior compartment then is released distally to proximally under the bridge created by the soleus origin attachment to the medial border of the tibia.

The wounds are left open, and delayed primary closure is anticipated in 7 to 10 days. Skin grafting may be necessary if, after a full week, sufficient swelling remains to preclude direct closure of the wound margins.

ACKNOWLEDGMENT

The authors gratefully acknowledge the assistance of Debra M. Bennett in the preparation of this chapter.

REFERENCES

HYPOVOLEMIA (SHOCK)

1. AIDS Diagnosis and Reporting Under the Expanded Surveillance Definition for Adolescents and Adults—United States, 1993. 1994 Update. M.M.W.R., 43, 1994.
2. AIDS and HIV Infection in the United States: 1988 Update. M.M.W.R., 38(Suppl. 4):36, 1989.
3. Alexander, J.W., McClellan, M.A., Ogle, C.K., Ogle, J.D.: Consumptive Opsoninopathy: Possible Pathogenesis in Lethal and Opportunistic Infections. Ann. Surg., 184:672–678, 1976.
4. Alexander, R.H., and Proctor, H.J.: Shock. *In* Committee on Trauma (eds.): Advanced Trauma Life Support Manual—Program for Physicians, pp. 75–94. Chicago, American College of Surgeons, 1993.
5. Allen, J.G.: Response to Blood Replacement and Volume Expanders in Acute Hemorrhagic Index Hypovolemia. *In* Mills, L.C., and Moyer, J.H. (eds.): Shock and Hypotension: Pathogenesis and Treatment, pp. 397–400. New York, Grune & Stratton, 1965.
6. Alper, C.A., Abramson, N., Block, K.J., Johnston, R.B., Rosen, F.S.: Increased Susceptibility to Infection Associated With Abnormalities of Complement Mediated Functions and of the Third Component (C3). N. Engl. J. Med., 282:349–354, 1970.
7. Altermeier, W.A., Todd, J.C., Inge, W.W.: Gram-Negative Septicemia: A Growing Threat. Ann. Surg., 166:530–542, 1967.
8. American College of Surgeons, Committee on Trauma. Advanced Trauma Life Support Course. Student Manual. 1981.
9. Aviado, D.M.: Pharmacologic Approach to the Treatment of Shock. Ann. Intern. Med., 62:1050–1059, 1965.
10. Baue, A.E., Tragus, E.T., Parkins, W.M.: A Comparison of Isotonic and Hypertonic Solutions and Blood on Blood Flow and Oxygen Consumption in the Initial Treatment of Hemorrhagic Shock. J. Trauma, 7:743–756, 1967.
11. Baue, A.E., Tragus, E.T., Wolfson, S.K., Jr., Cary, A.L., Parkins, W.M.: Hemodynamic and Metabolic Effects of Ringer's Lactate Solution in Hemorrhagic Shock. Ann. Surg., 166:29–38, 1967.
12. Beiting, C.V., Kozak, K.J., Kozak, B.A., Dreffer, R., Stinnett, J.D., Alexander, J.W.: Whole Blood vs. Packed Red Blood Cells for Resuscitation of Hemorrhagic Shock: An Examination of Host Defense Parameters in Dogs. Surgery, 84:194–200, 1978.
13. Blalock, A.: Shock. Further Studies With Particular Reference to the Effects of Hemorrhage. Arch. Surg., 29:837–857, 1934.
14. Blalock, C.V.: Principles of Surgical Care, Shock, and Other Problems, pp. 1–325. St. Louis, C.V. Mosby, 1940.
15. Boba, A., and Converse, J.G.: Ganglionic Blockage and Its Protective Action in Hemorrhage: A Review. Anesthesiology, 18:559–572, 1957.
16. Border, J.R.: Advances and Newer Concepts in Shock. *In* Cooper Surgery Annual, pp. 69–123. New York, Appleton-Century-Crofts, 1969.
17. Border, J.R., Chenier, R., McMenamy, R.H., et al.: Multiple Systems Organ Failure: Muscle Fuel Deficit With Visceral Protein Malnutrition. Surg. Clin. North Am., 56:1147–1167, 1976.
18. Border, J.R., LaDuca, J., Seibel, R.: Priorities in the Management of the Patient With Polytrauma. Prog. Surg., 14:84–120, 1975.
19. Bove, J.: Transfusion-Associated Hepatitis and AIDS. What Is the Risk? N. Engl. J. Med., 317:242–245, 1987.
20. Byrne, J.J.: Symposium on Shock. Am. J. Surg., 110:293–297, 1965.
21. Cahill, J.M., Jouasset-Strieder, D., Byrne, J.J.: Lung Function in Shock. Am. J. Surg., 110:324–329, 1965.
22. Canizaro, P.C., Prager, M.D., Shires, G.T.: The Infusion of Ringer's Lactate Solution During Shock. Am. J. Surg., 122:494–501, 1971.
23. Centers for Disease Control: Guidelines for Prevention of Transmission of Human Immunodeficiency Virus and Hepatitis B Virus to Health-Care and Public Safety Workers. M.M.W.R., 38:1–37, 1989.
24. Chaplin, H.: Packed Red Blood Cells. N. Engl. J. Med., 281:364–367, 1969.
25. Cloutier, C.T.: The Effect of Hemodilutional Resuscitation on Serum Protein Levels in Humans in Hemorrhagic Shock. J. Trauma, 9:514–521, 1969.
26. Collins, J.A.: Problems Associated With Massive Transfusion of Stored Blood. Surgery, 75:274–295, 1974.
27. Crile, G.W.: Blood Pressure in Surgery: An Experimental and Clinical Research. Philadelphia, J.B. Lippincott, 1903.
28. Cryer, H.M., Miller, F.B., Evers, B.M., Rouben, L.R., Seligson, D.L.: Pelvic Fracture Classification: Correlation With Hemorrhage. J. Trauma, 28:973–980, 1988.
29. Dahn, M.S., Lucas, C.E., Ledgerwood, A.M., Higgins, R.F.: Negative Inotropic Effect of Albumin Resuscitation for Shock. Surgery, 86:235–241, 1978.
30. Dalal, S.A., Burgess, A.R., Siegel, J.H., et al.: Pelvic Fracture

in Multiple Trauma: Classification by Mechanism Is Key to Pattern of Organ Injury, Resuscitative Requirements, and Outcome. J. Trauma, 29:981–1002, 1989.

31. Deitch, E.A., Bridges, W., Li, M., Berg, R., Specian, R.D., Granger, D.N.: Hemorrhagic Shock-Induced Bacterial Translocation: The Role of Neutrophils and Hydroxyl Radicals. J. Trauma, 30:942–946, 1990.
32. Duff, J.H., Scott, H.M., Peretz, D.I., Mulligan, G.W., and MacLean, L.D.: The Diagnosis and Treatment of Shock in Man Based on Hemodynamic and Metabolic Measurements. J. Trauma, 6:145–156, 1966.
33. Dunham, C.M., Belzberg, H., Lyles, R., et al.: The Rapid Infusion System: A Superior Method for the Resuscitation of Hypovolemic Trauma Patients. Resuscitation, 21:207–227, 1991.
34. Evarts, C.M.: Low Molecular Weight Dextran. Med. Clin. North Am., 51:1285–1299, 1967.
35. FDA Drug Bulletin: Use of Blood Components. FDA Drug Bull., 14–15, 1989.
36. Flynn, N.: AIDS: Risk and Treatment. South Pasadena, Calif., Orthopaedic Audio-Synopsis Foundation, 1989.
37. Fortune, J., Feustel, P., Saifi, J., Stratton, H., Newell, J., Shah, D.: Influence of Hematocrit on Cardiopulmonary Function After Acute Hemorrhage. J. Trauma, 27:243–249, 1987.
38. Fox, M.A., Mangiante, E.C., Fabian, T.C., Voeller, G.R., Kudsk, K.A.: Pelvic Fractures: An Analysis of Factors Affecting Prehospital Triage and Patient Outcome. South. Med. J., 83:785–788, 1990.
39. Frey, L., Kesel, K., Pruckner, S., Pacheco, A., Welte, M., Messmer, K.: Is Sodium Acetate Dextran Superior to Sodium Chloride Dextran for Small Volume Resuscitation From Traumatic Hemorrhagic Shock? Anesth. Analg., 79:517–524, 1994.
40. Friedland, G., and Klein, R.: Transmission of the Human Immunodeficiency Virus. N. Engl. J. Med., 317:1125–1135, 1987.
41. Fry, D.E.: Occupational Risks of Infection in the Surgical Management of Trauma Patients. Am. J. Surg., 165(Suppl. 2A):26S–33S, 1993.
42. Fulton, R.L., and Jones, C.E.: The Cause of Post-traumatic Pulmonary Insufficiency in Man. Surg. Gynecol. Obstet., 140:179–185, 1975.
43. Giesecke, A.H., Jr., Grande, C.M., Whitten, C.W.: Fluid Therapy and the Resuscitation of Traumatic Shock. Crit. Care Clin., 6:61–72, 1990.
44. Gleckman, R., Gleckman, R., Esposito, A.: Gram-Negative Bacteremic Shock: Pathophysiology, Clinical Features, and Treatment. South. Med. J., 74:335–341, 1981.
45. Gollub, S., and Bailey, C.P.: Management of Major Surgical Blood Loss Without Transfusions. J.A.M.A., 198:1171–1174, 1966.
46. Gollub, S., Svigals, R., Bailey, C.P., Hirose, T., Shaefer, C.: Electrolyte Solution in Surgical Patients Refusing Transfusion. J.A.M.A., 215:2077–2083, 1971.
47. Gross, S.G.: A System of Surgery: Pathological, Diagnostic, Therapeutique, and Operative, pp. 1–1098. Philadelphia, Lea & Febiger, 1872.
48. Hamilton, S.M.: The Use of Blood in the Resuscitation of the Trauma Patient. Can. J. Surg., 36:21–27, 1993.
49. Hamit, H.F.: Current Trends of Therapy and Research in Shock. Surg. Gynecol. Obstet., 120:835–851, 1965.
50. Hardaway, R.M., III: Microcoagulation in Shock. Am. J. Surg., 110:298–301, 1965.
51. Hardaway, R.M., III: Intensive Study and Treatment of Shock in Man. Vascular Diseases, 4:53–58, 1967.
52. Harrigan, C., Lucas, C.E., Ledgerwood, A.M.: The Effect of Hemorrhagic Shock on the Clotting Cascade in Injured Patients. J. Trauma, 29:1416–1421, 1989.
53. Harrigan, C., Lucas, C.E., Ledgerwood, A.M., Walz, D.A., Mammen, E.F.: Serial Changes in Primary Hemostasis After Massive Transfusion. Surgery, 98:836–844, 1985.
54. Henry, S.B., and Boral, L.I.: The Type and Screen: A Safe Alternative and Supplement in Selected Surgical Procedures. Transfusion, 17:163–168, 1977.
55. Hogman, C.F., Bagge, L., Thoren, L.: The Use of Blood Components in Surgical Transfusion Therapy. World J. Surg., 11:2–13, 1987.
56. Holcroft, J.W., Trunkey, D.D., Lim, R.D.: Further Analysis of Lung Water in Baboons Resuscitated From Hemorrhagic Shock. J. Surg. Res., 20:291–297, 1976.
57. Holcroft, J.W., Vasser, M.J., Turner, J.E., Derlet, R.W., Kramer, G.C.: 3% NaCl and 7.5% NaCl/Dextran 70 in the Resuscitation of Severely Injured Patients. Ann. Surg., 206:279–288, 1987.
58. Human Immunodeficiency Virus Infection in the United States: A Review of Current Knowledge. U.S. Department of Health and Human Services. M.M.W.R., 36(Suppl. 6): 1987.
59. Jones, R.C., and Blotchy, M.J.: Initial Management of the Severely Injured Patient. South. Med. J., 62:260–265, 1969.
60. Koziol, J.M., Rush, B.F., Smith, S.M., Machiedo, G.W.: Occurrence of Bacteremia During and After Hemorrhagic Shock. J. Trauma, 28:10–15, 1988.
61. Krausz, M.M.: Controversies in Shock Research: Hypertonic Resuscitation—Pros and Cons. Shock, 3:69–72, 1995.
62. Lane, P.L., McLellan, H.A., Johns, P.D.: Etiology of Shock in Blunt Trauma. Can. Med. Assoc. J., 133:199–201, 1985.
63. Lanser, M., and Saba, R.: Correction of Serum Opsonic Defects After Burn and Sepsis by Opsonic Fibronectin Administration. Arch. Surg., 118:338–342, 1983.
64. Litwin, M.S.: Blood Viscosity in Shock. Am. J. Surg., 110:313–316, 1965.
65. Looser, K.G., and Crombie, H.D., Jr.: Pelvic Fractures: An Anatomic Guide to Severity of Injury. Review of 100 Cases. Am. J. Surg., 132:638–642, 1976.
66. Lucas, C.E.: Update on Trauma Care in Canada. 4. Resuscitation Through the Three Phases of Hemorrhagic Shock After Trauma. (Review) Can. J. Surg., 33:451–456, 1990.
67. Lucas, C.E., Bouwman, D.L., Ledgerwood, A.M., Higgins, R.: Differential Serum Protein Changes Following Supplemental Albumin Resuscitation for Hypovolemic Shock. J. Trauma, 20:47–51, 1980.
68. Lucas, C.E., Ledgerwood, A.M., Higgins, R.F.: Impaired Salt and Water Excretion After Albumin Resuscitation for Hypovolemic Shock. Surgery, 86:544–549, 1978.
69. Lucas, C.E., Ledgerwood, A.M., Higgins, R.F.: Impaired Pulmonary Function After Albumin Resuscitation from Shock. J. Trauma, 20:446–451, 1980.
70. Martin, D.J., Lucas, C.E., Ledgerwood, A.M., Hoschner, J., McGonigal, M.D., Grabow, D.: Fresh Frozen Plasma Supplement to Massive Red Cell Transfusion. Ann. Surg., 202:505–511, 1985.
71. McClellan, M.A., and Alexander, J.W.: The Opsonic Activity of Stored Blood. Transfusion, 17:227–232, 1977.
72. McCullough, J.: Preservation of Opsonic Activity Against *S. aureus* and *E. coli* in Banked Blood. J. Lab. Clin. Med., 79:886–892, 1972.
73. Matsuda, H., and Shoemaker, W.C.: Cardiorespiratory Responses to Dextran 40. Arch. Surg., 110:296–300, 1975.
74. Matsuda, H., and Shoemaker, W.C.: Survivors' and Nonsurvivors' Response to Dextran 40. Arch. Surg., 110:301–305, 1975.
75. Mattar, J.A.: Hypertonic and Hyperoncotic Solutions in Patients. (Editorial) Crit. Care Med., 17:297–298, 1989.
76. Miller, R.M., Polakavetz, S.H., Hornick, R.B., Cowley, R.A.: Analysis of Infections Acquired by the Severely Injured Patient. Surg. Gynecol. Obstet., 137:7–10, 1973.
77. Moncrief, J.A.: Shock in the Multiple-Injury Patient. J. Bone Joint Surg., 49A:540–546, 1967.
78. Moore, F.D.: Metabolic Care of the Surgical Patient, pp. 1–1011. Philadelphia, W.B. Saunders, 1959.
79. Mucha, P., Jr., and Farnell, M.B.: Analysis of Pelvic Fracture Management. J. Trauma, 24:379–386, 1984.
80. Munster, A.M., Hoagland, H.D., Pruitt, B.A., Jr.: The Effect of Thermal Injury on Serum Immunoglobulins. Ann. Surg., 172:965–969, 1970.
81. Murray, D.: Complications of Treatment of Fractures and Dislocations: General Considerations. *In* Epps, C. (ed.): Complications in Orthopaedic Surgery, pp. 3–55. Philadelphia, J.B. Lippincott, 1978.

82. Murray, D.J., Olson, J., Strauss, R.: Coagulation Changes During Packed Red Cell Replacement of Major Blood Loss. Anesth, 69:839–845, 1988.
83. Nagy, K.K., Davis, J., Duda, J., Fildes, J., Roberts, R., Barrett, J.: A Comparison of Pentastarch and Lactated Ringer's Solution in the Resuscitation of Patients With Hemorrhagic Shock. Circ. Shock, 40:289–294, 1993.
84. Office of Medical Applications of Research, National Institutes of Health: Perioperative Red Cell Transfusion. J.A.M.A., 260:2700–2703, 1988.
85. Olcott, C., IV, and Lim, R.C., Jr.: Specialized Blood Filters and Fresh Whole Blood. J. Am. Coll. Emerg. Phys., 5:510–511, 1976.
86. Ollodart, R., and Mansberger, A.R.: The Effect of Hypovolemic Shock on Bacterial Defense. Am. J. Surg., 110:302–307, 1965.
87. Ostrum, R.F., Verghese, G.B., Santner, T.J.: The Lack of Association Between Femoral Shaft Fractures and Hypotensive Shock. J. Orthop. Trauma, 7:338–342, 1993.
88. Pedowitz, R.A., and Shackford, S.R.: Non-cavitary Hemorrhage Producing Shock in Trauma Patients: Incidence and Severity. J. Trauma, 29:219–222, 1989.
89. Phillips, G.R., Kauder, D.R., Schwab, C.W.: Massive Blood Loss in Trauma Patients. The Benefits and Dangers of Transfusion Therapy. Postgrad. Med., 95:61, 1994.
90. Poole, G.V., Meredith, J.W., Pennell, T., Mills, S.A.: Comparison of Colloids and Crystalloids in Resuscitation From Hemorrhagic Shock. Surg. Gynecol. Obstet., 154:577–586, 1982.
91. Poole, G.V., and Ward, E.F.: Causes of Mortality in Patients With Pelvic Fractures. Orthopedics, 17:691–696, 1994.
92. Poole, G.V., Ward, E.F., Muakkassa, F.F., Hsu, H.S.H., Griswold, J.A., Rhodes, R.S.: Pelvic Fracture From Major Blunt Trauma—Outcome Is Determined by Associated Injuries. Ann. Surg., 213:532–539, 1991.
93. Popejoy, S.L., and Fry, D.E.: Blood Contact and Exposure in the Operating Room. Surg. Gynecol. Obstet., 172:480–483, 1991.
94. Rcploglc, R.L., Kundler, H., Gross, R.E.: Studies in the Hemodynamic Importance of Blood Viscosity. J. Thorac. Cardiovasc. Surg., 50:658, 1965.
95. Rush, B.F., Jr., Sori, A.J., Murphy, T.F., Smith, S., Flanagan, J.J., Jr., Machiedo, G.W.: Endotoxemia and Bacteremia During Hemorrhagic Shock. The Link Between Trauma and Sepsis? Ann. Surg., 207:549–554, 1988.
96. Saba, T.M., Blumenstock, F.A., Scovill, W.A., Bernard, H.: Cryoprecipitate Reversal of Opsonic-2 Surface Binding Glycoprotein Deficiency in Septic Surgical and Trauma Patients. Science, 201:622–624, 1978.
97. Saba, T.M., and Jaffe, E.: Plasma Fibronectin (Opsonic Glycoprotein): Its Synthesis by Vascular Endothelial Cells and Role in Cardiopulmonary Integrity After Trauma as Related to Reticuloendothelial Function. Am. J. Med., 68:577–594, 1980.
98. Satiani, B., Fried, S.J., Zeeb, P., Falcone, R.E.: Normothermic Rapid Volume Replacement in Traumatic Hypovolemia. A Prospective Analysis Using a New Device. Arch. Surg., 122:1044–1047, 1987.
99. Schumer, W., Moss, G.S., Nyhus, L.M.: Metabolism of Lactic Acid in the Macacus Rhesus Monkey in Profound Shock. Am. J. Surg., 118:200–205, 1969.
100. Shires, G.T. (ed.): Care of the Trauma Patient, pp. 3–677. New York, McGraw-Hill, 1966.
101. Shires, G.T.: Principles and Management of Hemorrhagic Shock. *In* Shires, G.T. (ed.): Principles of Trauma Care, pp. 3–42. New York, McGraw-Hill, 1985.
102. Shires, G.T., Carrico, L.J., Canizaro, P.C.: Shock, Major Problems in Clinical Surgery, pp. 1–162. Philadelphia, W.B. Saunders, 1973.
103. Shoemaker, W.C.: Sequential Hemodynamic Patterns in Various Etiologies of Shock. Surg. Gynecol. Obstet., 132:411–423, 1971.
104. Shoemaker, W.C.: Comparison of the Relative Effectiveness of Whole Blood, Transfusions and Various Types of Fluid Therapy in Resuscitation. Crit. Care Med., 4:71, 1976.
105. Shoemaker, W.C., and Brown, R.S.: The Dilemma of Vasopressors and Vasodilators in the Therapy of Shock. Surg. Gynecol. Obstet., 132:51–57, 1971.
106. Shoemaker, W.C., Elwyn, D.H., Levine, H., Rosen, A.L.: Use of Nonparametric Analysis of Cardiorespiratory Variables as Early Predictors of Death and Survival in Postoperative Patients. J. Surg. Res., 17:301–314, 1974.
107. Shoemaker, W.C., Montgomery, E.S., Kaplan, E., Elwyn, D.H.: Use of Sequential Physiologic Patterns of Surviving and Nonsurviving Shock Patients for Defining Criteria for Therapeutic Goals and Early Warning of Death. Arch. Surg., 106:630–636, 1973.
108. Simeone, F.A.: Shock. *In* Sabiston, D. (ed.): Davis–Christopher's Textbook of Surgery, pp. 65–94. Philadelphia, W.B. Saunders, 1964.
109. Sloan, E.P., McGill, B.A., Zalenski, R., et al.: Human Immunodeficiency Virus and Hepatitis B Virus Seroprevalence in an Urban Trauma Population. J. Trauma, 38:736–746, 1995.
110. Swisher, S.N.: Overview of Fresh Frozen Plasma. *In* NIH Consensus Development Conference (eds.): Fresh Frozen Plasma: Indications and Risks, pp. 13–18. 1984.
111. Thal, A.P., and Sardesai, V.M.: Shock and the Circulating Polypeptides. Am. J. Surg., 110:308–312, 1965.
112. Transfusion Alert: Indications for the Use of Red Blood Cells, Platelets, and Fresh Frozen Plasma. Bethesda, Md., U.S. Department of Health and Human Services, Public Health Service, National Institutes of Health, 1989.
113. Traverso, L.W., Lee, W.P., Langford, M.J.: Fluid Resuscitation After an Otherwise Fatal Hemorrhage: I. Crystalloid Solutions. J. Trauma, 26:168–175, 1986.
114. Trinkle, J.K., Rush, B.E., Eiseman, B.: Metabolism of Lactate Following Major Blood Loss. Surgery, 63:782, 1968.
115. Trunkey, D.D., Chapman, M.W., Lim, R.C., Jr., Dunphy, J.E.: Management of Pelvic Fractures in Blunt Trauma Injury. J. Trauma, 14:912–923, 1974.
116. Valeri, C.R.: Blood Components in the Treatment of Acute Blood Loss: Use of Freeze Preserved Red Cells, Platelets, and Plasma Proteins. Anesth. Analg., 54:1–14, 1975.
117. Velanovich, V.: Crystalloid Versus Colloid Fluid Resuscitation: A Meta-analysis of Mortality. Surgery, 105:65–71, 1989.
118. Velasco, I.T., Pontieri, V., Rocha e Silva, M., Jr., Lopes, O.U.: Hyperosmotic NaCl and Severe Hemorrhagic Shock. Am. J. Physiol., 239:664–673, 1980.
119. Villazon, S.A., Sierra, V.A., Lopez, S.F., Rolando, M.A.: Hemodynamic Patterns in Shock and Critically Ill Patients. Crit. Care Med., 3:215–221, 1975.
120. Ward, J.W.: Transfusion-Associated (T-A)-AIDS in the United States. Developments in Biologic Standardization. 81:41–43, 1993.
121. Weinstein, R.J., and Young, L.S.: Neutrophil Function in Gram-Negative Bacteremia. J. Clin. Invest., 58:190–199, 1976.
122. Wiggers, C.J.: The Present Status of the Shock Problem. Physiol. Rev., 22:74–123, 1942.

CARDIOPULMONARY ARREST

123. Briggs, B.A., and Hayes, H.R.: Cardiopulmonary Resuscitation. *In* Wilkins, E.W., et al. (eds.): MGH Textbook of Emergency Medicine, pp. 27–37. Baltimore, Williams & Wilkins, 1979.
124. Brown, D.L., Brown, D.L., Parmley, C.L.: Second Degree Atrioventricular Block After Methylmethacrylate. Anesthesiology, 56:391–392, 1982.
125. The Closed-Chest Method of Cardiopulmonary Resuscitation—Revised Statement. (Editorial) Circulation 31:641–642, 1965.
126. Deyerle, W., Crossland, S., Sullivan, H.: Methylmethacrylate: Uses and Complications. A.O.R.N. J., 29:696, 1979.
127. Drugs of Choice From the Medical Letter: Cardiac Arrhythmias. Med. Lett. Drugs Ther., 21–23, 1981.
128. Eisenberg, M., Hallstrom, A., Bergner, L., et al.: The ACLS Score. J.A.M.A., 246:50–52, 1981.
129. Frank, N., van Ackern, K., Plane, R., et al.: Circulatory Complications Caused by Bone Cement. Effect of Polymethyl-

methacrylate on Circulation Parameters of Elderly Patients. M.M.W.R., 121:1601–1602, 1979.
130. Gatch, G.: Cardiac Arrest in the O.R. A.O.R.N. J., 32:983–993, 1980.
131. Gross, P.: Drugs to Start the Heart. Emerg. Med. Clin. North Am., 11:79–87, 1979.
132. Johnson, J.D.: A Plan of Action in Cardiac Arrest. J.A.M.A., 186:468–472, 1963.
133. Jude, J.R.: Cardiac Arrest and Resuscitation. *In* Management of Surgical Complications, 3rd ed., p. 108. Philadelphia, W.B. Saunders, 1975.
134. Jude, J.R.: Cardiac Arrest and Resuscitation. *In* Complications in Surgery and Their Management, pp. 114–125. Philadelphia, W.B. Saunders, 1981.
135. Jude, J.R., Kouwenhoven, W.B., Knickerbocker, G.G.: A New Approach to Cardiac Resuscitation. Ann. Surg., 154:311–319, 1961.
136. Kallina, C.: Morbidity and Mortality in Elderly Orthopaedic Patients. Surg. Clin. North Am., 62:297–300, 1982.
137. Keret, D., Reis, N.D., Zinman, C., et al: Cardiac Arrest and Death in Hip Replacement. Harefuah, 98(3):119–121, 1980.
138. Kouwenhaven, W.B., Jude, J.R., Knickerbocker, G.G.: Closed Chest Cardiac Massage. J.A.M.A., 173:1064–1067, 1960.
139. Landau, I.: New Legal Risks in Cardiac Arrest. Hospital Physician, 2:80–91, 1966.
140. Levison, M., and Trunkey, D.D.: Initial Assessment and Resuscitation. Surg. Clin. North Am., 62:3–8, 1982.
141. Lund, I., and Skulberg, A.: Cardiopulmonary Resuscitation by Lay People. Lancet, 2:702–704, 1976.
142. McIntyre, K.M., Lewis, A.J., et al.: Textbook of Advanced Cardiac Life Support. New York, American Heart Association, 1981.
143. McIntyre, K.M., Parker, M.R., Guildner, C.W., et al.: Standards and Guidelines for Cardiopulmonary Resuscitation (CPR) and Emergency Cardiac Care. J.A.M.A., 244:453–509, 1980.
144. MacKenzie, G.J., Taylor, S.H., McDonald, A.H., McDonald, K.W.: Haemodynamic Effects of External Cardiac Compression. Lancet, 1:1342–1345, 1964.
145. Messer, J.V.: Cardiac Arrest. N. Engl. J. Med., 275:35–39, 1966.
146. Myerberg, R.J., Conde, C.A., Sung, R.J., et al.: A Clinical Electrophysiologic and Hemodynamic Profile of Patients Resuscitated From Prehospital Cardiac Arrest. Am. J. Med., 68:568–576, 1980.
147. Myerberg, R.J., Kessler, K.M., Zaman, L., et al.: Survivors of Prehospital Cardiac Arrest. J.A.M.A., 247(10):1485–1490, 1982.
148. Newens, A.F., and Volz, R.G.: Severe Hypotension During Prosthetic Hip Surgery With Acrylic Bone Cement. Anesthesiology, 36:298–300, 1972.
149. Powell, J.N., McGrath, D.J., Lahiri, S.K., Hill, P.: Cardiac Arrest Associated With Bone Cement. B.M.J., 3:326, 1970.
150. Safar, P., Brown, T.C., Holtey, W.J., Wilder, R.J.: Ventilation and Circulation With Closed Chest Cardiac Massage in Man. J.A.M.A., 176:574–576, 1961.
151. Schuh, F.T., Schuh, S.M., Viguera, M.G., Terry, R.N.: Circulatory Changes Following Implantation of Methylmethacrylate Bone Cement. Anesthesiology, 39:455–457, 1973.
152. Youn, Y.K., LaLonde, C., Demling, R.: Use of Antioxidant Therapy in Shock and Trauma. Circ. Shock, 35:245–249, 1991.

FAT EMBOLISM SYNDROME

153. Aach, R., and Kissane, J. (eds.): Clinicopathologic Conference. Fat Embolism. Am. J. Med., 51:258–268, 1971.
154. Alho, A., Saikku, K., Eerola, P., Koskinen, M., Hamaleinen, M.: Corticosteroids in Patients With a High Risk of Fat Embolism Syndrome. Surg. Gynecol. Obstet., 147:358–362, 1978.
155. Allardyce, D.B.: The Adverse Effect of Heparin in Experimental Fat Embolism. Surg. Forum, 22:203–205, 1971.
156. American College of Surgeons: Hospital Trauma Index. Bull. Am. Coll. Surg., 65:31–33, 1980.
157. Armin, J., Jr., and Grant, R.T.: Observations on Gross Pulmonary Fat Embolism in Man and the Rabbit. Clin. Sci., 10:441–469, 1951.
158. Ashbaugh, D.G., and Petty, T.L.: The Use of Corticosteroids in the Treatment of Respiratory Failure Associated With Massive Fat Embolism. Surg. Gynecol. Obstet., 123:493–500, 1966.
159. Bagg, R.J., Stein, S., Urban, R.T., McKay, D.: Parameters of the Fat Emboli Syndrome (F.E.S.). Orthop. Trans., 3:278, 1979.
160. Baker, P.L., Kuenzig, M.C., Peltier, L.F.: Experimental Fat Embolism in Dogs. J. Trauma, 9:577–586, 1969.
161. Baker, S., O'Neill, B., Haddon, W., Long, W.: The Injury Severity Score: A Method for Describing Patients With Multiple Injuries and Evaluating Emergency Care. J. Trauma, 14:187–196, 1974.
162. Barie, P., Minnear, F., Malik, A.: Increased Pulmonary Vascular Permeability After Bone Marrow Injection in Sheep. Am. Rev. Respir. Dis., 123:648–653, 1981.
163. Beck, J.P., and Collins, J.A.: Theoretical and Clinical Aspects of Posttraumatic Fat Embolism Syndrome. Instr. Course Lect. 22:38–87, 1973.
164. Benestad, G.: Falle von Fettembolie mit punktformigen Blutungen in der Haut. Dtsch. Zentralbl. Chir., 112:194–205, 1911.
165. Bengston, A., Larsson, M., Gammer, W., Heideman, M.: Anaphylatoxin Release in Association With Methylmethacrylate Fixation of Hip Prostheses. J. Bone Joint Surg., 69A:46–49, 1987.
166. Benoit, P.R., Hampson, L.G., Burgess, J.H.: Value of Arterial Hypoxemia in the Diagnosis of Pulmonary Fat Embolism. Ann. Surg., 175:128–137, 1972.
167. Bergentz, S.E.: Studies on the Genesis of Posttraumatic Fat Embolism. Acta. Chir. Scand. Suppl., 282:1–72, 1961.
168. Bergmann, E.B.: Ein Fall todlicher Fettembolie. Klin. Wochenschr., 10:385–387, 1873.
169. Bivins, B.A., Madauss, W.C., Griffen, W.O., Jr.: Fat Embolism Syndrome: A Clinical Study. South. Med. J., 65:937–940, 1972.
170. Blaisdell, F.W., and Lewis, F.R.: Respiratory Distress Syndrome of Shock and Trauma. Major Problems in Clinical Surgery, 21:1–237, 1977.
171. Blath, R.A., and Collins, J.A.: The Relationship of Lipuria to Fat Embolism in Rabbits. J. Trauma, 10:901–904, 1970.
172. Bone, L., and Bucholz, R.: Current Concepts Review: The Management of Fractures in the Patient With Multiple Trauma. J. Bone Joint Surg., 68A:945–949, 1986.
173. Bone, L., Johnson, K., Weigelt, J., Scheinberg, R.: Early Versus Delayed Stabilization of Femoral Fractures. A Prospective Randomized Study. J. Bone Joint Surg. 71A:336–340, 1989.
174. Bone, R.C., Maunder, R., Slotman, G., et al.: An Early Test of Survival in Patients With the Adult Respiratory Distress Syndrome. Chest, 94:849–851, 1989.
175. Bradford, D.S., Foster, R.R., Nossel, H.L.: Coagulation Alterations, Hypoxemia, and Fat Embolism in Fracture Patients. J. Trauma, 10:307–321, 1970.
176. Broder, G., and Ruzumna, L.: Systemic Fat Embolism Following Acute Primary Osteomyelitis. J.A.M.A., 199:1004–1006, 1967.
177. Byrick, R.J., Mullen, J.B., Wong, P.Y., Kay, J.C., Wigglesworth, D., Doran, R.J.: Prostanoid Production and Pulmonary Hypertension After Fat Embolism Are Not Modified by Methylprednisolone. Can. J. Anaesth., 38:660–670, 1991.
178. Byrick, R.J., Mullen, J.B., Wong, P.Y., Wigglesworth, D., Kay, J.C.: Corticosteroids Do Not Inhibit Acute Pulmonary Response to Fat Embolism. Can. J. Anaesth., 37.5130, 1990.
179. Cahill, J.M., Daly, B.F.T., Byrne, J.J.: Ventilatory and Circulatory Response to Oleic Acid Embolus. J. Trauma, 14:73–76, 1974.
180. Carver, G.M., Jr.: Traumatic Renal Infarction Concurrent With Massive Fat Embolism. J. Urol., 66:331–339, 1951.
181. Cheney, F., Huang, T., Gronka, R.: Effects of Methylprednisolone on Experimental Pulmonary Injury. Ann. Surg., 190:236–242, 1979.

182. Cobb, C.A., Jr., and Hillman, J.W.: Fat Embolism. Instr. Course Lect., 18:122–129, 1961.
183. Collins, J.A., Gordon, W.C., Jr., Hudson, T.L., Irvin, R.W., Jr., Kelly, T., Hardaway, R.M., III: Inapparent Hypoxemia in Casualties With Wounded Limbs: Pulmonary Fat Embolism? Ann. Surg., 167:511–520, 1968.
184. Collins, J.A., Hudson, T.L., Hamacher, W.R., Rokous, J., Williams, G., Hardaway, R.M., III: Systemic Fat Embolism in Four Combat Casualties. Ann. Surg., 167:493–499, 1968.
185. Committee on Medical Aspects of Automotive Safety: Rating the Severity of Tissue Damage. J.A.M.A., 215:277–280, 1971.
186. Crocker, S.H., Eddy, D.O., Obenauf, R.N., Wismar, B.L., Lowery, B.D.: Bacteremia: Host-Specific Lung Clearance and Pulmonary Failure. J. Trauma, 21:215–220, 1981.
187. Cuppage, F.E.: Fat Embolism in Diabetes Mellitus. Am. J. Clin. Pathol., 40:270–275, 1963.
188. Czerny, V.: Ueber die klinische Bedeutung der Fettembolie. Klin. Wochenschr., 12:593, 1875.
189. Derian, P.S.: Fat Embolization—Current Status. J. Trauma, 5:580–586, 1965.
190. Divertie, M.B.: The Adult Respiratory Distress Syndrome. Mayo Clin. Proc., 57:371–378, 1982.
191. Drummond, D.S., Salter, R.B., Boone, J.: Fat Embolism in Children: Its Frequency and Relationships to Collagen Disease. Can. Med. Assoc. J., 101:200–203, 1969.
192. Evarts, C.M.: Emerging Concepts of Fat Embolism. Clin. Orthop., 33:183–193, 1964.
193. Evarts, C.M.: Diagnosis and Treatment of Fat Embolism. J.A.M.A., 194:899–901, 1965.
194. Evarts, C.M.: The Fat Embolism Syndrome: A Review. Surg. Clin. North Am., 50:493–507, 1970.
195. Fabian, T., Hoots, A., Stanford, D., Patterson, C., Mangiante, E.: Fat Embolism Syndrome: A Prospective Evaluation in 92 Fracture Patients. J. Trauma, 27:820, 1987.
196. Fenger, G., and Salisbury, J.H.: Diffuse Multiple Capillary Fat Embolism of the Lungs and Brain in a Fatal Complication in Common Fractures, Illustrated by a Case. Chicago Medical Journal, 39:587–595, 1879.
197. Field, M.: Fat Embolism From a Chronic Osteomyelitis. J.A.M.A., 59:2065–2066, 1912.
198. Fischer, J.F., Turner, R.H., Herndon, J.H., Riseborough, E.J.: Massive Steroid Therapy in Severe Fat Embolism. Surg. Gynecol. Obstet., 132:667–672, 1971.
199. Flick, M., and Murray, J.: High Dose Corticosteroid Therapy in the Adult Respiratory Distress Syndrome. J.A.M.A., 251:1054, 1984.
200. Fuschsig, P., Brucke, P., Blumel, G., Gottlob, R.: A New Clinical and Experimental Concept of Fat Metabolism. N. Engl. J. Med., 276:1192–1193, 1967.
201. Gauss, H.: Studies in Cerebral Fat Embolism: With Reference to the Pathology of Delirium and Coma. Arch. Intern. Med., 18:76–102, 1916.
202. Gauss, H.: The Pathology of Fat Embolism. Arch. Surg., 9:593–605, 1924.
203. Gerbershagen, H.U.: Fettembolie: Therapie mit niedrig viscosem Dextran. Anaesthesist, 21:23–25, 1972.
204. Goris, R.J.A.: The Injury Severity Score. World J. Surg., 7:12–18, 1983.
205. Goris, R.J.A., and Draaisma, J.: Causes of Death After Blunt Trauma. J. Trauma, 22:141, 1982.
206. Goris, R.J.A., Gimbrere, J.S.F., Van Niekerk, J.L.M., Schoots, F.J., Body, L.H.D.: Early Osteosynthesis and Prophylactic Mechanical Ventilation in the Multitrauma Patient. J. Trauma, 22:895–903, 1982.
207. Gossling, H.R., and Pellegrini, V.D., Jr.: Fat Embolism Syndrome: A Review of the Pathophysiology and Physiological Basis of Treatment. Clin. Orthop., 165:68–82, 1982.
208. Graber, S.: Fat Embolization Associated With Sickle Cell Crisis. South Med. J., 54:1395–1398, 1961.
209. Gresham, G.A., Kuxzynski, A., Rosborough, D.: Fatal Fat Embolism Following Replacement Arthroplasty for Transcervical Fractures of Femur. B.M.J., 2:617–619, 1971.
210. Grondahl, N.B.: Utersuchungen uber Fettembolie. Dtsch. Z. Chir., 111:56–124, 1911.
211. Gurd, A.R.: Fat Embolism: An Aid to Diagnosis. J. Bone Joint Surg., 52B:732–737, 1970.
212. Hammerschmidt, D., Weaver, L., Hudson, L., Craddock, P., Jacob, H.: Association of Complement Activation and Elevated Plasma C5a With Adult Respiratory Distress Syndrome. Lancet, 1:947–949, 1980.
213. Hansen, S., and Winquist, R.: Closed Intramedullary Nailing of the Femur: Kuntscher Technique With Reaming. Clin. Orthop., 138:56–61, 1979.
214. Hausberger, F.X., and Whitenack, S.H.: Effect of Pressure on Intravasation of Fat From the Bone Marrow Cavity. Surg. Gynecol. Obstet., 134:931–936, 1972.
215. Haymaker, W., and Davison, C.: Fatalities Resulting From Exposure to Simulated High Altitudes in Decompression Chambers, Clinico-pathologic Study of 5 Cases. J. Neuropathol. Exp. Neurol., 9:29–59, 1950.
216. Hill, R.B., Jr.: Fatal Fat Embolism From Steroid-Induced Fatty Liver. N. Engl. J. Med., 265:318–320, 1961.
217. Immelman, E.J., Bank, S., Krige, H., Marks, I.N.: Roentgenologic and Clinical Features of Intramedullary Fat Necrosis in Bones in Acute and Chronic Pancreatitis. Am. J. Med., 36:96–105, 1964.
218. Jacobs, R.R., Wheeler, E.J., Jelenko, C., III, McDonald, T.F., Bliven, F.E.: Fat Embolism: A Microscopic and Ultrastructure Evaluation of Two Animal Models. J. Trauma, 13:980–993, 1973.
219. Johnson, K., Cadambi, A., Seibert, B.: Incidence of Adult Respiratory Distress Syndrome in Patients With Multiple Musculoskeletal Injuries: Effect of Early Operative Stabilization of Fractures. J. Trauma, 25:375–384, 1985.
220. Jones, J.P., Jr., Engleman, E.P., Najarian, J.S.: Systemic Fat Embolism After Renal Homotransplantation and Treatment With Corticosteroids. N. Engl. J. Med., 273:1453–1458, 1965.
221. Kallenbach, J., Lewis, M., Zaltzman, M., Feldman, C., Orford, A., Zwi, S.: "Low-Dose" Corticosteroid Prophylaxis Against Fat Embolism. J. Trauma, 27:1173–1176, 1987.
222. Kaplan, J.E., and Saba, T.M.: Humoral Deficiency and Reticuloendothelial Depression After Traumatic Shock. Am. J. Physiol., 230:7–14, 1976.
223. Kearns, T.P.: Fat Embolism of the Retina Demonstrated by Flat Retinal Preparation. Am. J. Ophthalmol., 41:1–2, 1956.
224. Kerstell, J.: Pathogenesis of Posttraumatic Fat Embolism. Am. J. Surg., 121:712–715, 1971.
225. Kerstell, J., Hallgren, B., Rudenstam, C.M., Svanborg, A.: 1. The Chemical Composition of the Fat Emboli in the Postabsorptive Dog. Acta Med. Scand. Suppl., 499:3–18, 1969.
226. King, E.G., Weily, H.S., Genton, E., Ashbaugh, D.G.: Consumption Coagulopathy in the Canine Oleic Acid Model of Fat Embolism. Surgery, 69:533–541, 1971.
227. Kraus, K.A.: Ueber Fettembolie des Gehirns nach Unfallen. Montasschr. Unfallheilkunde, 58:353–361, 1955.
228. Lachiewicz, P.F., and Ranawat, C.S.: Fat Embolism Syndrome Following Bilateral Total Knee Replacement With Total Condylar Prosthesis: A Report of Two Cases. Clin. Orthop., 160:106–108, 1981.
229. Lehman, E.P., and Moore, R.M.: Fat Embolism Including Experimental Production Without Trauma. Arch. Surg., 14:621–622, 1927.
230. LeQuire, V.S., Hillman, J.W., Gray, M.E., Snowden, R.T.: Clinical and Pathologic Studies of Fat Embolism. Instr. Course Lect., 19:12–35, 1970.
231. LeQuire, V.S., Shapiro, J.L., LeQuire, C.B., Cobb, C.A., Jr., Fleet, W.F., Jr.: A Study of the Pathogenesis of Fat Embolism Based on Human Necropsy Material and Animal Experiments. Am. J. Pathol., 35:999–1016, 1959.
232. Limbird, T.J., and Ruderman, R.J.: Fat Embolism in Children. Clin. Orthop., 136:267–269, 1978.
233. Lindeque, B., Schoeman, H., Dommisse, G., Boeyens, M., Vlok, A.: Fat Embolism and the Fat Embolism Syndrome: A Double-Blind Therapeutic Study. J. Bone Joint Surg., 69B:128–131, 1987.
234. Love, J., and Stryker, W.S.: Fat Embolism: A Problem of Increasing Importance to the Orthopedist and the Internist. Ann. Intern. Med., 46:342–351, 1957.

235. Lozman, J., Deno, C., Fenstel, P., et al.: Pulmonary and Cardiovascular Consequences of Immediate Fixation or Conservative Management of Long Bone Fractures. Arch. Surg., 121:992–999, 1986.
236. Lynch, M.J.: Nephrosis and Fat Embolism in Acute Hemorrhagic Pancreatitis. Arch. Intern. Med., 94:709–717, 1964.
237. McCarthy, B., Mammen, E., Leblanc, L.P., Wilson, R.F.: Subclinical Fat Embolism: A Prospective Study of 50 Patients With Extremity Fractures. J. Trauma, 13:9–16, 1973.
238. Manning, J., Bach, A., Herman, C., Carrico, C.J.: Fat Release After Femur Nailing in the Dog. J. Trauma, 23:322–326, 1983.
239. Maruyama, Y., and Little, J.B.: Roentgen Manifestations of Traumatic Pulmonary Fat Embolism. Radiology, 79:945–952, 1962.
240. Meek, R.N., Woodruff, B., Allardyce, D.B.: Source of Fat Macroglobules in Fractures of the Lower Extremity. J. Trauma, 12:432–434, 1972.
241. Meyers, R., and Taljaard, J.J.F.: Blood Alcohol and Fat Embolism Syndrome. J. Bone Joint Surg., 59A:878–880, 1977.
242. Miller, J.A., Fonkalsrud, E.W., Latta, H.L., Maloney, J.V., Jr.: Fat Embolism Associated With Extra-corporeal Circulation and Blood Transfusion. Surgery, 51:448–451, 1962.
243. Motamed, H.A.: Fundamental Aspects of Post-Multiple Injury Fat Embolism. Clin. Orthop., 82:169–181, 1972.
244. O'Driscoll, M., and Powell, F.J.: Injury, Serum, Lipids, Fat Embolism, and Clofibrinate. B.M.J., 4:149–151, 1967.
245. Pape, H.-C., Auf'm'Kolk, M., Paffrath, T., et al: Primary Intramedullary Fixation in Polytrauma Patients With Associated Lung Contusion: A Cause of Posttraumatic ARDS? J. Trauma, 34:540–547, 1993.
246. Pape, H.-C., Dwenger, A., Regel, G., et al.: Pulmonary Damage Due to Intramedullary Femoral Nailing in Severe Trauma in Sheep: Is There an Effect From Different Nailing Methods? J. Trauma, 33:574–581, 1992.
247. Pape, H.-C., Regel, G., Dwenger, A., et al.: The Risk of Early Intramedullary Nailing of Long Bone Fractures in Multiply Traumatized Patients. Complications in Orthopaedics, Spring:15–23, 1995.
248. Parker, F.B., Jr., Wax, S.D., Kusajima, K., Webb, W.R.: Hemodynamic and Pathological Findings in Experimental Fat Embolism. Arch. Surg., 108:70–74, 1974.
249. Pellegrini, V.D. Jr., and Evarts, C.M.: The Fat Embolism Syndrome. *In* Evarts, C.M. (ed.): Surgery of the Musculoskeletal System, 2nd ed., pp. 37–54. New York, Churchill Livingstone, 1989.
250. Pellegrini, V.D., Jr., and Evarts, C.M.: The Fat Embolism Syndrome Revisited: Acute Respiratory Failure Complicating Elective Orthopaedic Surgery, in progress.
251. Peltier, L.F.: Collective Review: An Appraisal of the Problem of Fat Embolism. Int. Abstr. Surg., 104:313–324, 1957.
252. Peltier, L.F.: The Diagnosis of Fat Embolism. Surg. Gynecol. Obstet., 121:371–379, 1965.
253. Peltier, L.F.: Fat Embolism. A Current Concept. Clin. Orthop., 66:241–253, 1969.
254. Peltier, L.F.: The Diagnosis and Treatment of Fat Embolism. J. Trauma, 11:661–667, 1971.
255. Peltier, L.F., Adler, F., Lai, S.P.: Fat Embolism: The Significance of an Elevated Serum Lipase After Trauma to Bone. Am. J. Surg., 99:821–826, 1960.
256. Pipkin, G.: The Early Diagnosis and Treatment of Fat Embolism. Clin. Orthop., 12:171–182, 1958.
257. Renne, J., Wurthier, R., House, E., Cancro, J.C., Hoaglund, F.T.: Fat Macroglobulemia Caused by Fractures or Total Hip Replacement. J. Bone Joint Surg., 60A:613–618, 1978.
258. Rinaldo, J.E., and Rogers, R.M.: Adult Respiratory Distress Syndrome. N. Engl. J. Med., 306:900–909, 1982.
259. Riska, E., and Myllynen, P.: Fat Embolism in Patients With Multiple Injuries. J. Trauma, 22:891, 1982.
260. Riska, E., Von Bonsdorff, H., Hakkinen, S., Jaroma, H., Kiviluoto, O., Paavilainen, T.: Prevention of Fat Embolism by Early Internal Fixation of Fractures in Patients With Multiple Injuries. Injury, 8:110, 1976.
261. Riska, E., Von Bonsdorff, H., Hakkinen, S., Jaroma, H., Kiviluoto, O., Paavilainen, T.: Primary Operative Fixation of Long Bone Fractures in Patients With Multiple Injuries. J. Trauma, 17:111–121, 1977.
262. Rokkanen, P., Alho, A., Avikainen, V., et al.: The Efficacy of Corticosteroids in Severe Trauma. Surg. Gynecol. Obstet., 138:69–73, 1974.
263. Rokkanen, P., Lahdensuu, M., Kataja, J., Julkunen, H.: The Syndrome of Fat Embolism: Analysis of Thirty Consecutive Cases Compared to Trauma Patients With Similar Injuries. J. Trauma, 10:299–306, 1970.
264. Ruedi, T., and Wolff, G.: Vermeidung Postraumatischer Komplikationen Durch Fruhe Definitive Versorgung Von Polytraumatisierten mit Frakturen des Bewegungsapparats. Helv. Chir. Acta, 42:507, 1975.
265. Saldeen, T.: Fat Embolism and Signs of Intravascular Coagulation in Posttraumatic Autopsy Material. J. Trauma, 10:273–286, 1970.
266. Schnaid, E., Lamprey, J., Viljoen, M., Joffe, B., Seftel, H.: The Early Biochemical and Hormonal Profile of Patients With Long Bone Fractures at Risk of Fat Embolism Syndrome. J. Trauma, 27:309–311, 1987.
267. Schonfeld, S., Ploysongsang, Y., Dilisio, R., et al.: Fat Embolism Prophylaxis With Corticosteroids: A Prospective Study in High Risk Patients. Ann. Intern. Med., 99:438, 1983.
268. Scriba, J.: Untersuchungen uber die Fettembolie. Leipzig, J.B. Hirschfeld, 1879.
269. Scuderi, C.S.: Fat Embolism: A Clinical and Experimental Study. Surg. Gynecol. Obstet., 72:732–746, 1941.
270. Seibel, R., Laduca, J., Hassett, J., et al.: Blunt Multiple Trauma (ISS 36), Femur Traction, and the Pulmonary Failure-Septic State. Ann. Surg., 202:283–295, 1985.
271. Sevitt, S.: The Significance and Classification of Fat Embolism. Lancet, 2:825–828, 1960.
272. Sevitt, S.: Fat Embolism. London, Butterworth, 1962.
273. Sevitt, S.: Fat Embolism in Patients With Fractured Hips. B.M.J., 2:257–262, 1972.
274. Sevitt, S., Clarke, R., Badger, F.G.: Modern Trends in Accident Surgery and Medicine. London, Butterworth, 1959.
275. Shier, M., Wilson, R., James, R., Riddle, J., Mammen, E., Pedersen, H.: Fat Embolism Prophylaxis: A Study of Four Treatment Modalities. J. Trauma, 17:621–629, 1977.
276. Soloway, H.B., and Robinson, E.F.: The Coagulation Mechanism in Experimental Pulmonary Fat Embolism. J. Trauma, 12:630–631, 1972.
277. Sproule, B.J., Brady, J.L., Gilbert, J.A.L.: Studies on the Syndrome of Fat Embolization. Can. Med. Assoc. J., 90:1243–1247, 1964.
278. Stoltenberg, J.J., and Gustilo, R.B.: The Use of Methylprednisolone and Hypertonic Glucose in the Prophylaxis of Fat Embolism Syndrome. Clin. Orthop., 143:211–221, 1979.
279. Sutton, G.E.: Pulmonary Fat Embolism and Its Relation to Traumatic Shock. B.M.J., 2:368–370, 1918.
280. Talucci, R., Manning, J., Lampard, S., Bach, A., Carrico, A.: Early Intramedullary Nailing of Femoral Shaft Fractures: A Cause of Fat Embolism Syndrome. Am. J. Surg., 146:107–111, 1983.
281. Tedeschi, C.G., Walter, C.E., Lepore, T., Tedeschi, L.G.: An Assessment of the Cerebrospinal Fluid and Choroid Plexus in Relation to Systemic Fat Embolism. Neurology, 19:386–590, 1969.
282. Tedeschi, C.G., Walter, C.E., Tedeschi, L.G.: Shock and Fat Embolism: An Appraisal. Surg. Clin. North Am., 48:431–452, 1968.
283. Ten Duis, H., Nijsten, M., Klasen, H., Binnendijk, B.: Fat Embolism in Patients With an Isolated Fracture of the Femoral Shaft. J. Trauma, 28:383–390, 1988.
284. Tennenberg, S., Jacobs, M., Solomkin, J.: Complement-Mediated Neutrophil Activation in Sepsis- and Trauma-Related Adult Respiratory Distress Syndrome. Arch. Surg., 122:26–32, 1987.
285. Thomas, J.E., and Ayyar, D.R.: Systemic Fat Embolism: A Diagnostic Profile in 24 Patients. Arch. Neurol., 26:517–523, 1972.

286. Trafton, P.G.: ARDS and IM Nailing: To Ream or Not to Ream? Complications in Orthopaedics, Spring:5, 1995.
287. Trentz, O., Oesteru, H.J., Hempelmann, G., et al.: Kriterien fur die Operabilitat von Polytraumatisierten. Unfallheilkunde, 81:451, 1978.
288. Vance, B.M.: The Significance of Fat Embolism. Arch. Surg., 23:426–465, 1931.
289. Van Der Merwe, C., Louw, A., Welthagen, D., Schoeman, H.: Adult Respiratory Distress Syndrome in Cases of Severe Trauma—The Prophylactic Value of Methylprednisolone Sodium Succinate. South Afr. Med. J., 67:279–284, 1985.
290. Wagner, E.: Die Fettembolie der Lungencapillaren. Arch. Heilk., 6:369–381, 1865.
291. Warner, W.A.: Release of Free Fatty Acids Following Trauma. J. Trauma, 9:692–699, 1969.
292. Warthin, A.S.: Traumatic Lipaemia and Fatty Embolism. Int. Clin., 4:171–227, 1913.
293. Weinberg, H., and Finsterbush, A.: Fat Embolism: Vascular Damage to Bone Due to Blunt Trauma. Intraosseous Phlebography Study. Clin. Orthop., 83:273–278, 1972.
294. Weisz, G.M.: Fat Embolism: Current Problems in Surgery. Chicago, Year Book Medical Publishing, 1974.
295. Weisz, G.M., and Barellai, A.: Nonfulminant Fat Embolism: Review of Concepts on Its Genesis and Orthophysiology. Anesth. Analg., 52:303–309, 1973.
296. Weisz, G.M., Rang, M., Salter, R.B.: Posttraumatic Fat Embolism in Children: Review of the Literature and of Experience in the Hospital for Sick Children, Toronto. J. Trauma, 13:529–534, 1973.
297. Weisz, G.M., and Steiner, E.: The Cause of Death in Fat Embolism. Chest, 59:511–516, 1971.
298. Wilson, J.V., and Salisbury, C.V.: Fat Embolism in War Surgery. Br. J. Surg., 31:384–392, 1944.
299. Wolff, G., Dittman, M., Ruedi, T., et. al.: Koordination von Chirurgie und Intenvismedizin zur Vermeidung der Posttraumatischen Respiratorische Insuffizienze. Unfallheilkunde, 81:425, 1978.
300. Zenker, F.A.: Beitrage zur Anatomie und Physiologie der Lunge. Dresden, J. Braunsdorf, 1861.

HEMORRHAGIC COMPLICATIONS

301. Bachman, F.: Plasminogen Activators. *In* Colman, R.W., Hirsh, J., Marder, V.J., Salzman, E.W. (eds.): Hemostasis and Thrombosis. Basic Principles and Clinical Practice, 2nd ed., pp. 318–339. Philadelphia, J.B. Lippincott, 1987.
302. Boey, M.L., Colaco, C.B., Gharavi, A.E., Elkon, K.B., Loizou, E., Hughes, G.R.V.: Thrombosis in Systemic Lupus Erythematosus: Striking Association With the Presence of Circulating Lupus Anticoagulant. B.M.J., 287:1021–1023, 1983.
303. Bowie, E.J., and Owen, C.A., Jr.: The Significance of Abnormal Preoperative Hemostatic Tests. *In* Spaet, T.H. (ed.): Progress in Hemostasis and Thrombosis, vol. 5, pp. 179. New York, Grune & Stratton, 1980.
304. Brettler, D.B., and Levine, P.H.: Factor Concentrates for Treatment of Hemophilia: Which One to Choose? Blood, 73:2067–2073, 1989.
305. Centers for Disease Control: Update on Acquired Immune Deficiency Syndrome (AIDS) Among Patients With Hemophilia. M.M.W.R., 31:644–652, 1982.
306. Clouse, L.H., and Comp, P.C.: The Regulation of Hemostasis: The Protein C System. N. Engl. J. Med., 314:1298–1304, 1986.
307. Collen, D.: On the Regulation and Control of Fibrinolysis. Thromb. Haemost., 43:77–89, 1980.
308. Colman, R.W., Hirsh, J., Marder, V.J., Salzman, E.W. (eds.): Hemostasis and Thrombosis: Basic Principles and Clinical Practice, 2nd ed., pp. 1–65. Philadelphia, J.B. Lippincott, 1987.
309. Consensus Development Conference: Platelet Transfusion Therapy. J.A.M.A., 257:1777–1780, 1987.
310. Counts, R.B., Haisch, C., Simon, T.L., Maxwell, N.G., Heimbach, D.M., Carrico, C.J.: Hemostasis in Massively Transfused Trauma Patients. Ann. Surg., 190:91–99, 1979.
311. Francis, C.W., and Marder, V.J.: Physiologic Regulation and Pathologic Disorders of Fibrinolysis. Hum. Pathol., 18:263–274, 1987.
312. Francis, C.W., and Marder, V.J.: Physiologic Regulation and Pathologic Disorders of Fibrinolysis. *In* Colman, R.W., Hirsh, J., Marder, V.J., Salzman, E.W. (eds.): Hemostasis and Thrombosis. Basic Principles and Clinical Practice, 2nd ed., pp. 358–379. Philadelphia, J.B. Lippincott, 1987.
313. Fuente, (de la) B., Kasper, C.K., Rickles, F.R., Hoyer, L.W.: Response of Patients With Mild and Moderate Hemophilia A and von Willebrand's Disease to Treatment With Desmopressin. Ann. Intern. Med., 103:6–14, 1985.
314. Harker, L.A., and Slichter, S.J.: The Bleeding Time as a Screening Test for Evaluation of Platelet Function. N. Engl. J. Med., 287:155–159, 1972.
315. Hedner, U., and Kisiel, W.: Use of Human Factor VIIa in the Treatment of Two Hemophilia A Patients With High-Titer Inhibitors. J. Clin. Invest., 71:1836–1841, 1983.
316. Hoyer, L.W.: Review: The Factor VIII Complex: Structure and Function. Blood, 58:1–13, 1981.
317. Levine, P.H.: The Clinical Manifestations and Therapy of Hemophilias A and B. *In* Colman, R.W., Hirsh, J., Marder, V.J., Salzman, E.W. (eds.): Hemostasis and Thrombosis: Basic Principles and Clinical Practice, 2nd ed., pp. 97–111. Philadelphia, J.B. Lippincott, 1987.
318. Lusher, E.B.: Factor VIII Inhibitors: Etiology, Characterization, Natural History and Management. Ann. N. Y. Acad. Sci., 509:89–102, 1987.
319. Lusher, J.M., Shapiro, S.S., Palaszak, J.E., Rao, A.J., Levine, P.H., Blatt, P.M.: Efficacy of Prothrombin-Complex Concentrates in Hemophiliacs With Antibodies to Factor VIII: A Multicenter Therapeutic Trial. N. Engl. J. Med., 303:421–425, 1980.
320. Marlar, R.A., Kleiss, A.J., Griffin, J.H.: An Alternative Extrinsic Pathway of Human Blood Coagulation. Blood, 60:1353–1358, 1982.
321. Nemerson, Y.: Tissue Factor and Hemostasis. Blood, 71:1–8, 1988.
322. Packham, M.A., and Mustard, J.F.: Platelet Adhesion. Prog. Hemost. Thromb., 7:211–288, 1984.
323. Rapaport, S.: Preoperative Hemostatic Evaluation: Which Tests, If Any? Blood, 61:229–231, 1983.
324. Rapaport, S.I.: Inhibition of Factor VIIa/Tissue Factor-Induced Blood Coagulation: With Particular Emphasis Upon a Factor Xa-Dependent Inhibitory Mechanism. Blood, 73:359–365, 1989.
325. Rosenberg, R.D.: Actions and Interactions of Antithrombin and Heparin. N. Engl. J. Med., 292:146–151, 1975.
326. Ruggeri, Z.M., and Zimmerman, T.S.: von Willebrand Factor and von Willebrand Disease. Blood, 70:895–904, 1987.
327. Shapiro, S.S., and Hultin, M.: Acquired Inhibitors to the Blood Coagulation Factors. Semin. Thromb. Hemost., 1:336–385, 1975.
328. Weiss, H.J.: Platelet Physiology and Abnormalities of Platelet Function. N. Engl. J. Med., 293:531–541, 1975.

DISSEMINATED INTRAVASCULAR COAGULATION

329. Allister, C.: Cardiac Arrest After Crush Injury. B.M.J., 287:531–532, 1983.
330. Better, O.S., and Stein, J.H.: Early Management of Shock and Prophylaxis of Acute Renal Failure in Traumatic Rhabdomyolysis. N. Engl. J. Med., 322:825–829, 1990.
331. Bick, R.: Clinical Relevance of Antithrombin III. Semin. Thromb. Hemost., 8(4):276–287, 1982.
332. Bick, R.L., Bick, M.D., Fekete, L.F.: Antithrombin III Patterns in Disseminated Intravascular Coagulation. Am. J. Clin. Pathol., 73:577–583, 1980.
333. Breen, F.A., and Tullis, J.L.: Ethanol Gelatin: A Rapid Screening Test for Intravascular Coagulation. Ann. Intern. Med., 69:1197–1206, 1968.
334. Bywaters, E.G.L., and Beall, D.: Crush Injuries With Impairment of Renal Function. B.M.J., 1:427–432, 1941.
335. Cheung, J.Y., Bonventure, J.V., Malis, C.D., Leaf, A.: Calcium and Ischemic Injury. N. Engl. J. Med., 314:1670–1676, 1982.
336. Colman, R.W., Robboy, S.J., Minna, J.D.: Disseminated Intra-

vascular Coagulation: A Reappraisal. Annu. Rev. Med., 30:359–374, 1979.
337. Feinstein, D.I.: Diagnosis and Management of Disseminated Intravascular Coagulation: The Role of Heparin Therapy. Blood, 60:284–287, 1982.
338. Godbout, B., Burchard, K.W., Slotman, G.J., Gann, D.S.: Crush Syndrome With Death Following Pneumatic Antishock Garment Application. J. Trauma, 24:1052–1056, 1984.
339. Kikta, M.J., Meyer, J.P., Bishara, R.A., Goodson, S.F., Schuler, J.J., Flanigan, P.: Crush Syndrome Due to Limb Compression. Arch. Surg., 122:1078–1081, 1987.
340. Knochel, J.P.: Rhabdomyolysis and Myoglobinuria. *In* Suki, W.N., and Eknoyan, G. (eds.): The Kidney in Systemic Disease, pp. 263–284. New York, John Wiley, 1981.
341. McLaren, A.C., Ferguson, J.H., Miniaci, A.: Crush Syndrome Associated With Use of the Fracture-Table. A Case Report. J. Bone Joint Surg., 69A:1447–1449, 1987.
342. Marder, V.J., Martin, S.E., Francis, C.W., Colman, R.W.: Consumptive Thrombohemorrhagic Disorders. *In* Colman, R.W., Hirsh, J., Marder, V.J., Salzman, E.W. (eds.): Hemostasis and Thrombosis: Basic Principles and Clinical Practice, 2nd ed., pp. 975–1015. Philadelphia, J.B. Lippincott, 1987.
343. Marder, V.J., and Shulman, N.R.: High Molecular Weight Derivatives of Human Fibrinogen Produced by Plasmin, II. Mechanism of Their Anticoagulant Activity. J. Biol. Chem., 244:2120–2124, 1969.
344. Michaelson, M., Taitelman, U., Bursztein, S.: Management of Crush Syndrome. Resuscitation, 12:141–146, 1984.
345. Mubarek, S., and Owen, C.A.: Compartment Syndrome and Its Relation to the Crush Syndrome. A Spectrum of Disease. A Review of 11 Cases of Prolonged Limb Compression. Clin. Orthop., 113:81–89, 1975.
346. Niewiarowski, S., and Gurewich, V.: Laboratory Identification of Intravascular Coagulation: The Serial Dilution Protamine Sulfate Test for the Detection of Fibrin Monomer and Fibrin Degradation Products. J. Lab. Clin. Med., 77:665–676, 1971.
347. Odeh, M.: The Role of Reperfusion-Induced Injury in the Pathogenesis of the Crush Syndrome. N. Engl. J. Med., 324:1417–1421, 1991.
348. Owen, C.A., Mubarak, S.J., Hargens, A.R., Rutherford, L., Garetto, L.P., Akeson, W.H.: Intramuscular Pressures With Limb Compression: Clarification of the Pathogenesis of the Drug-Induced Muscle-Compartment Syndrome. N. Engl. J. Med., 300:1169–1172, 1979.
349. Reis, N.D., and Michaelson, M.: Crush Injury to the Lower Limbs. Treatment of the Local Injury. J. Bone Joint Surg., 68A:414–418, 1986.
350. Rickles, F.R., and Edwards, R.L.: Activation of Blood Coagulation in Cancer: Trousseau's Syndrome Revisited. Blood, 62: 14–31, 1983.
351. Ron, D., Taitelman, U., Michaelson, M., Bar-Joseph, G., Bursztein, S., Better, O.S.: Prevention of Acute Renal Failure in Traumatic Rhabdomyolysis. Arch. Intern. Med., 144:277–280, 1984.
352. Rubenberg, M.L., Regoeczi, E., Bull, B.S., Dacie, J.V., Brain, M.C.: Microangiopathic Haemolytic Anaemia: The Experimental Production of Haemolysis and Red-Cell Fragmentation by Defibrination in Vivo. Br. J. Haematol., 14:627–642, 1968.
353. Sack, G.H., Levin, J., Bell, W.R.: Trousseau's Syndrome and Other Manifestations of Chronic Disseminated Coagulopathy in Patients With Neoplasms: Clinical, Pathologic and Therapeutic Features. Medicine (Baltimore), 56:1–37, 1977.
354. Siegal, T., Seligsohn, U., Aghai, E., Modan, M.: Clinical and Laboratory Aspects of Disseminated Intravascular Coagulation (DIC). A Study of 118 Cases. Thromb. Haemost., 39:122–134, 1978.
355. Spero, J.A., Lewis, J.H., Hasiba, U.: Disseminated Intravascular Coagulation. Findings in 346 Patients. Thromb. Haemost., 43:28–33, 1980.
356. Stewart, I.P.: Major Crush Injury. (Editorial) B.M.J., 294:854–855, 1987.
357. Taylor, D.C., Salvian, A.J., Shackleton, C.R.: Crush Syndrome Complicating Pneumatic Antishock Garment (PASG) Use. Injury, 19:43–44, 1988.
358. Ziv, I., Zeligowski, A.A., Elyashuv, O., Mosheiff, R., Lilling, M., Segal, D.: Immediate Care of Crush Injuries and Compartment Syndromes With the Split-Thickness Skin Excision. Clin. Orthop., 256:224–228, 1990.

THROMBOEMBOLISM

359. Amstutz, H., Friscia, D., Dorey, F., Carney, B.: Warfarin Prophylaxis to Prevent Mortality From Pulmonary Embolism After Total Hip Replacement. J. Bone Joint Surg., 71A:321–326, 1989.
360. Arfors, K.E., Hint, H.C., Dhall, D.P., Matheson, N.A.: Counteraction of Platelet Activity at Sites of Laser-Induced Endothelial Trauma. B.M.J., 4:430–431, 1968.
361. Atkins, P., and Hawkins, L.A.: The Diagnosis of Deep-Vein Thrombosis in the Leg Using ^{125}I-Fibrinogen. Br. J. Surg., 55:825–830, 1968.
362. Barber, F.A., Burton, W., Guyer, R.: The Heparin-Induced Thrombocytopenia and Thrombosis Syndrome. Report of a Case. J. Bone Joint Surg., 69A:935–937, 1987.
363. Bauer, K.A.: Hypercoagulability—A New Cofactor in the Protein C Anticoagulant Pathway. N. Engl. J. Med., 330:566–567, 1994.
364. The Behavior of Thrombi. Arch. Surg., 105(5):681–682, 1972.
365. Beisaw, N., Comerota, A., Groth, H., et al.: Dihydroergotamine/Heparin in the Prevention of Deep Vein Thrombosis After Total Hip Replacement. A Controlled Prospective Randomized Multicenter Trial. J. Bone Joint Surg., 70A:2–10, 1988.
366. Bergentz, S.E.: Dextran in the Prophylaxis of Pulmonary Embolism. World J. Surg., 2:19–25, 1978.
367. Bergentz, S.E., Gelin, L.E., Rudenstam, C.M.: Fats and Thrombus Formation. An Experimental Study. Thromb. Diath. Haemorrh., 5:474–479, 1961.
368. Bergqvist, D., Efsing, H.L., Hallbook, T., Hendlund, T.: Thromboembolism After Elective and Post-traumatic Hip Surgery—A Controlled Prophylactic Trial With Dextran 70 and Low Dose Heparin. Acta Chir. Scand., 145:213–218, 1979.
369. Bergqvist, D.: Dextran in the Prophylaxis of Deep-Vein Thrombosis. J.A.M.A., 258:324, 1987.
370. Berman, H.J.: Anticoagulant-Induced Alterations in Hemostasis, Platelet Thrombosis, and Vascular Fragility in the Peripheral Vessels of the Hamster Cheek Pouch. *In* Macmillan, R.L., and Mustard, J.F. (eds.): International Symposium: Anticoagulants and Fibrinolysins, pp. 95–107. Philadelphia, Lea & Febiger, 1961.
371. Bloom, W.L.: Present Status of Plasma Volume Expanders in the Treatment of Shock. Clinical Laboratory Studies. Arch. Surg., 63:739–741, 1951.
372. Bookstein, J.J.: Segmental Arteriography in Pulmonary Embolism. Radiology, 93:1007–1012, 1969.
373. Borgstrom, S., Gelin, L., Zederfeldt, B.: The Formation of Vein Thrombi Following Tissue Injury: An Experimental Study in Rabbits. Acta Chir. Scand. Suppl., 247:1–36, 1959.
374. Borow, M., and Goldson, H.: Postoperative Venous Thrombosis. Am. J. Surg., 141:245–251, 1981.
375. Browse, N.L.: The ^{125}I-Fibrinogen Uptake Test. Arch. Surg., 104:160–163, 1972.
376. Bull, J.P., Ricketts, D., Squire, J.R., et al.: Dextran as a Plasma Substitute. Lancet, 1:134–143, 1949.
377. Bydgeman, S., and Eliasson, R.: Effect of Dextrans on Platelet Adhesiveness and Aggregation. Scand. J. Clin. Lab. Invest., 20:17–23, 1967.
378. Bydgeman, S., Eliasson, R., Gullbring, B.: Effect of Dextran Infusion on the Adenosine Diphosphate Induced Adhesiveness and the Spreading Capacity of Human Blood Platelets. Thromb. Diath. Haemorrh., 15:451–456, 1966.
379. Bydgeman, S., Eliasson, R., Johnson, S.R.: Relationship Between Postoperative Changes in Adenosine Diphosphate Induced Platelet Adhesiveness and Venous Thrombosis. Lancet, 1:1301–1302, 1966.

380. Carpenter, J.P., Holland, G.A., Baum, R.A., Owen, R.S., Carpenter, J.T., Cope, C.: Magnetic Resonance Venography for the Detection of Deep Venous Thrombosis: Comparison With Contrast Venography and Duplex Doppler Ultrasonography. J. Vasc. Surg., 18:734–741, 1993.
381. Cheely, R., McCartney, W.H., Perry, J.R., et al.: The Role of Noninvasive Tests Versus Pulmonary Angiography in the Diagnosis of Pulmonary Embolism. Am. J. Med., 70:17–22, 1981.
382. Collins, R., Scrimgeour, A., Yusuf, S., Peto, R.: Reduction in Fatal Pulmonary Embolism and Venous Thrombosis by Perioperative Administration of Subcutaneous Heparin. Overview of Results of Randomized Trials in General, Orthopaedic, and Urologic Surgery. N. Engl. J. Med., 318:1162–1173, 1988.
383. Coon, W.W., and Coller, F.A.: Some Epidemiologic Considerations of Thromboembolism. Surg. Gynecol. Obstet., 109:487–501, 1959.
384. Coon, W.W., and Willis, P.W., III: Deep Venous Thrombosis and Pulmonary Embolism. Prediction, Prevention and Treatment. Am. J. Cardiol., 4:611–621, 1959.
385. Couch, N.P.: Guest Editor's Introduction. A.M.A. Archives Symposium on Diagnostic Techniques in Phlebothrombosis. Arch. Surg., 104:132–133, 1972.
386. Crandon, A.J., Peel, V.R., Anderson, J.A., Thompson, V., McNicol, G.P.: Postoperative Deep Vein Thrombosis. Identifying High Risk Patients. B.M.J., 281:343–344, 1980.
387. Cronan, J., Dorfman, G., Grusmark, J.: Lower Extremity Deep Venous Thrombosis: Further Experience With and Refinements of Ultrasound Assessment. Radiology, 168:101–107, 1988.
388. Culver, D., Crawford, J.S., Gardiner, J.H., Wiley, A.M.: Venous Thrombosis After Fractures of the Upper End of the Femur. A Study of Incidence and Site. J. Bone Joint Surg., 52B:61–69, 1970.
389. Davis, F.M., and Qunice, M.: Deep Vein Thrombosis and Anaesthetic Technique in Emergency Hip Surgery. B.M.J., 281:1528–1529, 1980.
390. DeLee, J.C., and Rockwood, C.A., Jr.: Current Concepts Review. The Use of Aspirin in Thromboembolic Disease. J. Bone Joint Surg., 62A:149–152, 1980.
391. DeWeese, J.A., and Rogoff, S.M.: Clinical Uses of Functional Ascending Phlebography of the Lower Extremity. Angiology, 9:268–278, 1958.
392. Deykin, D.: Thrombogenesis. N. Engl. J. Med., 276:622–628, 1967.
393. Deykin, D.: Emerging Concepts of Platelet Function. N. Engl. J. Med., 290:144–151, 1974.
394. Dorfman, G., Cronan, J., Tupper, T., Messersmith, R., Denny, D., Lee, C.: Occult Pulmonary Embolism: A Common Occurrence in Deep Venous Thrombosis. Am. J. Radiol., 148:263–266, 1987.
395. Effect of Aspirin on Postoperative Venous Thrombosis. Lancet, 2:441–444, 1972.
396. Erdman, W.A., Jayson, H.T., Redman, H.C., Miller, G.L., Parkey, R.W., Peshock, R.W.: Deep Venous Thrombosis of Extremities: Role of MR Imaging in the Diagnosis. Radiology, 174:425–431, 1990.
397. Ernst, C.B., Fry, W.J., Fraft, R.O., DeWeese, M.S.: The Role of Low Molecular Weight Dextran in the Management of Venous Thrombosis. Surg. Gynecol. Obstet., 119:1243–1247, 1964.
398. Eskeland, G., Solheim, K., Skjorten, F.: Anticoagulant Prophylaxis, Thromboembolism and Mortality in Elderly Patients With Hip Fractures. Acta Chir. Scand., 131:16–29, 1966.
399. Evans, A.J., Sostman, H.D., Kuelson, M.H., et al.: 1992 ARRS Executive Council Award. Detection of Deep Venous Thrombosis: Prospective Comparison of MR Imaging With Contrast Venography. A.J.R. Am. J. Roentgenol., 161:131–139, 1993.
400. Evans, G., and Mustard, J.F.: Platelet-Surface Reaction and Thrombosis. Surgery, 64:273–280, 1968.
401. Evarts, C.M.: Low Molecular Weight Dextran. Med. Clin. North Am., 51:1285–1299, 1967.
402. Evarts, C.M.: Thromboembolic Disease. Instr. Course Lect., 28:67–71, 1979.
403. Evarts, C.M., and Alfidi, R.J.: Thromboembolism After Total Hip Reconstruction. Failure of Low Doses of Heparin in Prevention. J.A.M.A., 225:515–516, 1973.
404. Evarts, C.M., and Feil, E.I.: Prevention of Thromboembolic Disease After Elective Surgery of the Hip. J. Bone Joint Surg., 53A:1271–1280, 1971.
405. Fagan, D.G.: Prevention of Thromboembolic Phenomena Following Operations on the Neck of the Femur. Lancet, 1:846–848, 1964.
406. Fahmy, N., and Patel, D.: Hemostatic Changes and Postoperative Deep Vein Thrombosis Associated With Use of a Pneumatic Tourniquet. J. Bone Joint Surg., 63A:461–465, 1981.
407. Fitts, W.T., Jr., Lehr, H.B., Bitner, R.L., Spelman, J.W.: An Analysis of 950 Fatal Injuries. Surgery, 56:663–668, 1964.
408. Flanc, C., Kakkar, V.V., Clarke, M.B.: The Detection of Venous Thrombosis of the Legs Using ^{125}I-Labeled Fibrinogen. Br. J. Surg., 55:742–747, 1968.
409. Flinn, W., Sandager, G., Cerullo, L., Havey, R., Yao, R.: Duplex Venous Scanning for the Prospective Surveillance of Perioperative Venous Thrombosis. Arch. Surg., 124:901–905, 1989.
410. Francis, C.W., Marder, V.J., Evarts, C.M., Yaukoolbodi, S.: Two Step Warfarin Therapy. Prevention of Postoperative Venous Thrombosis Without Excessive Bleeding. J.A.M.A., 249:374–378, 1983.
411. Francis, C.W., Pellegrini, V.D., Jr., Harris, C., Marder, V.: Antithrombin III Prophylaxis of Venous Thromboembolic Disease After Total Hip or Knee Replacement. Am. J. Med., 87:615–665, 1989.
412. Francis, C.W., Pellegrini, V.D., Marder, V., et al.: Prevention of Venous Thrombosis After Total Hip Arthroplasty. Antithrombin III and Low-Dose Heparin Compared With Dextran 40. J. Bone Joint Surg., 71A:327–335, 1989.
413. Francis, C.W., Pellegrini, V.D., Marder, V., et al.: Comparison of Warfarin and External Pneumatic Compression in the Prevention of Venous Thrombosis after Total Hip Replacement. JAMA 267:2911–2922, 1992.
414. Freeark, R.J., Bostwick, J., Fardin, R.: Posttraumatic Venous Thrombosis. Arch. Surg., 95:567–575, 1967.
415. Froehlich, J., Dorfman, G., Cronan, J., Urbanek, P., Herndon, J., Aaron, R.: Compression Ultrasonography for the Detection of Deep Venous Thrombosis in Patients Who Have a Fracture of the Hip. A Prospective Study. J. Bone Joint Surg., 71A:249–256, 1989.
416. Fulton, G.P., Akers, R.P., Lutz, B.R.: White Thromboembolism and Vascular Fragility in the Hamster Cheek Pouch After Anticoagulants. Blood, 8:140–152, 1953.
417. Gallus, A.S., and Hirsh, J.: Prevention and Treatment of Venous Thromboembolism. Semin. Thromb. Hemost., 11:291–331, 1976.
418. Gallus, A.S., Hirsh, J., Tuttle, R.J., et al.: Small Subcutaneous Doses of Heparin in Prevention of Venous Thrombosis. N. Engl. J. Med., 288:545–551, 1973.
419. Geerts, W., Code, K., Jay, R., Chen, E., Szalai, J.: A Prospective Study of Venous Thromboembolism After Major Trauma. N. Engl. J. Med., 24:1601–1606, 1994.
420. Genton, E.: Management of Venous Thromboembolism. Adv. Cardiol., 27:305–312, 1980.
421. Gitel, S.N., Salvati, E.A., Wessler, S., Robinson, H.J., Jr., Worth, M.N.: The Effect of Total Hip Replacement and General Surgery on Antithrombin III in Relation to Venous Thrombosis. J. Bone Joint Surg., 61A:653–656, 1979.
422. Golodner, H., Morse, L.J., Angrist, A.: Pulmonary Embolism in Fractures of the Hip. Surgery, 18:418–423, 1945.
423. Greengard, J.S., Eichinger, S., Griffin, J., Bauer, K.: Brief Report: Variability of Thrombosis Among Homozygous Siblings With Resistance to Activated Protein C Due to an Arg-Gln Mutation in the Gene for Factor V. N. Engl. J. Med., 331:1559–1561, 1994.
424. Gronwall, A., and Ingleman, B.: Dextran as a Volume Expander. Acta Physiol. Scand., 7:97–107, 1944.
425. Haaverstad, R., Nilsen, G., Myhre, H.O., Saether, O.D., Rink,

P.A.: The Use of MRI in the Investigation of Leg Oedema. Eur. J. Vasc. Surg., 6:124–129, 1992.

426. Hajjar, K.A.: Factor V Leiden—An Unselfish Gene? N. Engl. J. Med., 331:1585–1587, 1994.
427. Hamilton, H.W., Crawford, J.S., Gardiner, J.H., Wiley, A.M.: Venous Thrombosis in Patients With Fracture of the Upper End of the Femur. A Phlebographic Study of the Effect of Prophylactic Anticoagulation. J. Bone Joint Surg., 52B:268–289, 1970.
428. Hampson, W.G.J., Lucas, H.K., Harris, F.C., et al.: Failure of Low-Dose Heparin to Prevent Deep-Vein Thrombosis After Hip Replacement Arthroplasty. Lancet, 2:795–797, 1974.
429. Harris, W.H., Athanasoulis, C., Waltman, A., Salzman, E.: High and Low Dose Aspirin Prophylaxis Against Venous Thromboembolic Disease in Total Hip Replacement. J. Bone Joint Surg., 64A:63–66, 1982.
430. Harris, W.H., Salzman, E.W., Athanasoulis, C.A., Waltman, A.C., DeSanctis, R.W.: Aspirin Prophylaxis of Venous Thromboembolism. N. Engl. J. Med., 297:1246–1248, 1977.
431. Harris, W.H., Salzman, E.W., DeSanctis, R.W.: The Prevention of Thromboembolic Disease by Prophylactic Anticoagulation. A Controlled Study in Elective Hip Surgery. J. Bone Joint Surg., 49:81–89, 1967.
432. Harris, W.H., Saltzman, E.W., DeSanctis, R.W., Coutts, R.D.: Prevention of Venous Thromboembolism Following Total Hip Replacement. J.A.M.A., 220:1319–1322, 1972.
433. Hartman, J.T., Pugh, J., Smith, R., Robertson, W., Yost, R., Janssen, H.: Cyclic Sequential Compression of the Lower Limb in Prevention of Deep Venous Thrombosis. J. Bone Joint Surg., 64A:1059–1062, 1982.
434. Hildner, F.J., and Ormand, R.S.: Accuracy of the Clinical Diagnosis of Pulmonary Embolism. J.A.M.A., 202:567–570, 1967.
435. Hirsh, J.: The Clinical Role of Antiplatelet Agents. Drug Ther., 6:63–74, 1981.
436. Hirsh, J.: Therapeutic Range for the Control of Oral Anticoagulant Therapy. Arch. Intern. Med., 145:1187–1188, 1985.
437. Hirsh, J.: The Optimal Intensity of Oral Anticoagulant Therapy. J.A.M.A., 258:2723–2726, 1987.
438. Hirsh, J., and McBride, J.A.: Increased Platelet Adhesiveness in Recurrent Venous Thrombosis and Pulmonary Embolism. B.M.J., 2:797–799, 1965.
439. Huisman, M., Buller, H., Ten Cate, J., Vreeken, J.: Serial Impedance Plethysmography for Suspected Deep Venous Thrombosis in Outpatients. The Amsterdam General Practitioner Study. N. Engl. J. Med., 314:823–828, 1986.
440. Hull, R., Hirsch, J., Jay, R., et al.: Different Intensities of Oral Anticoagulant Therapy in the Treatment of Proximal Vein Thrombosis. N. Engl. J. Med., 307:1676–1681, 1982.
441. Hull, R., Raskob, G., Hirsh, J., et al.: Continuous Intravenous Heparin Compared With Intermittent Subcutaneous Heparin in the Initial Treatment of Proximal Vein Thrombosis. N. Engl. J. Med., 315:1109–1114, 1986.
442. Hull, R., Raskob, G., Pineo, G., et al.: A Comparison of Subcutaneous Low Molecular Weight Heparin with Warfarin Sodium Prophylaxis against Deep Vein Thrombosis after Hip or Knee Implantation. N. Engl. J. Med., 329:1370–1376, 1993.
443. Hull, R.D., and Raskob, G.E.: Current Concepts Review. Prophylaxis of Venous Thromboembolic Disease Following Hip and Knee Surgery. J. Bone Joint Surg., 68A:146–150, 1986.
445. Hume, M., Sevitt, S., Thomas, D.P.: Venous Thrombosis and Pulmonary Embolism, pp. 1–447. Cambridge, Mass., Harvard University Press, 1970.
446. Jennings, J.J., and Harris, W.H.: A Clinical Evaluation of Aspirin Prophylaxis of Thromboembolic Disease After Total Hip Arthroplasty. J. Bone Joint Surg., 58A:926–927, 1976.
447. Just-Viera, J.O., and Yeager, G.H.: Protection From Thrombosis in Large Veins. Surg. Gynecol. Obstet., 118:354–360, 1964.
448. Imperiale, T., and Speroff, T.: A Meta-Analysis of Methods to Prevent Venous Thromboembolism Following Total Hip Replacement. J.A.M.A., 271:1780–1785, 1994.
449. Kakkar, V.: The Diagnosis of Deep Vein Thrombosis Using the ^{125}I-Fibrinogen Test. Arch. Surg., 104:152–159, 1972.
450. Kakkar, V., Fok, P., Murray, W., et al.: Heparin and Dihydroergotamine Prophylaxis Against Thromboembolism After Hip Arthroplasty. J. Bone Joint Surg., 67B:538–542, 1985.
451. Kakkar, V.V., Howe, C.T., Flanc, C., Clarke, M.B.: Natural History of Postoperative Deep Vein Thrombosis. Lancet, 2:230–232, 1969.
452. Kakkar, V.V., Spindler, J., Flute, P.T., et al.: Efficacy of Low Doses of Heparin in Prevention of Deep Vein Thrombosis After Major Surgery. Lancet, 2:101–106, 1972.
453. Kim, Y.H., and Suh, J.-S.: Low Incidence of Deep Vein Thrombosis After Cementless Total Hip Replacement. J. Bone Joint Surg., 70A:878–882, 1988.
454. Koekenberg, L.J.L.: Experimental Use of Macrodex as a Prophylaxis Against Postoperative Thromboembolism. Bull. Soc. Int. Chir., 21:501–512, 1962.
455. Landefeld, C.S., and Goldman, L.: Major Bleeding in Outpatients Treated With Warfarin: Incidence and Prediction by Factors Known at the Start of Outpatient Therapy. Am. J. Med., 87:144–152, 1989.
456. Landefeld, C.S., Rosenblatt, M., Goldman, L.: Bleeding in Outpatients Treated With Warfarin: Relation to Prothrombin Time and Important Remediable Lesions. Am. J. Med., 87:153–159, 1989.
457. Langsjoen, P., and Murray, R.A.: Treatment of Postsurgical Thromboembolic Complications. J.A.M.A., 218:855–860, 1971.
458. Laufman, H.: Deep Vein Thrombophlebitis. Current Status of Etiology and Treatment. Arch. Surg., 99:489–493, 1969.
459. Lensing, A., Prandoni, P., Brandjes, D., et al.: Detection of Deep Vein Thrombosis by Real Time B-Mode Ultrasonography. N. Engl. J. Med., 320:342–345, 1989.
460. Levine, M.N., Hirsh, J., Gent, M., et al: Prevention of Deep Vein Thrombosis After Elective Hip Surgery: A Randomized Trial Comparing Low Molecular Weight Heparin with Standard Unfractionated Heparin. Ann. Intern. Med., 114:545–551, 1991.
461. Leyvraz, P., Richard, J., Bachmann, F., et al.: Adjusted Versus Fixed Dose Subcutaneous Heparin in the Prevention of Deep Vein Thrombosis After Total Hip Replacement. N. Engl. J. Med., 309:954–958, 1983.
462. Lotke, P., Ecker, M., Alavi, A., Berkowitz, H.: Indications for the Treatment of Deep Venous Thrombosis Following Total Knee Replacement. J. Bone Joint Surg., 66A:202–208, 1984.
463. Lowe, L.L.: Venous Thrombosis and Embolism. J. Bone Joint Surg., 63B:155–167, 1981.
464. Lynch, A., Bourne, R., Rorabeck, C., Rankin, R., Donald, A.: Deep Vein Thrombosis and Continuous Passive Motion After Total Knee Arthroplasty. J. Bone Joint Surg., 70A:11–14, 1988.
465. McBride, K., LaMorte, W., Menzoian, J.: Can Ventilation-Perfusion Scans Accurately Diagnose Acute Pulmonary Embolism? Arch. Surg., 121:754–757, 1986.
466. MacLean, L.D., Shibara, H.R., McLean, A.P.H., Skinner, G.B., Gutelius, J.R.: Pulmonary Embolism, the Value of Bedside Scanning, Angiography and Pulmonary Embolectomy. Can. Med. Assoc. J., 97:991–1000, 1967.
467. Mansfield, A.O.: Alteration in Fibrinolysis Associated With Surgery and Venous Thrombosis. Br. J. Surg., 59:754–757, 1972.
468. Marks, J., Truscott, B.M., Withycombe, J.F.R.: Treatment of Venous Thrombosis With Anticoagulants. Review of 1135 Cases. Lancet, 2:787–791, 1954.
469. Matsuda, M., Sugo, T., Sakata, Y., et al.: A Thrombotic State Due to an Abnormal Protein C. N. Engl. J. Med., 319:1265–1268, 1988.
470. Mavor, G.E., and Galloway, J.M.: Iliofemoral Venous Thrombosis. Pathological Considerations and Surgical Management. Br. J. Surg., 56:45–49, 1969.
471. Medical Letter, The: Dihydroergotamine-Heparin to Prevent Postoperative Deep Vein Thrombosis. Med. Lett. Drugs Ther., 27:45–46, 1985.
472. Miletich, J., Sherman, L., Broze, G.: Absence of Thrombosis in Subjects With Heterozygous Protein C Deficiency. N. Engl. J. Med., 317:991–996, 1987.

473. Miller, G.A.H.: The Diagnosis and Management of Massive Pulmonary Embolism. Br. J. Surg., 59:837–839, 1972.
474. Mishkin, F.: Lung Scanning: Its Use in Diagnosis of Disorders of the Pulmonary Circulation. Arch. Intern. Med., 118:65–69, 1966.
475. Mobin-Uddin, K., McLean, R., Bolloki, H., Jude, J.R.: Caval Interruption for Prevention of Pulmonary Embolism. Arch. Surg., 99:711–715, 1969.
476. Mohr, D., Ryu, J., Litin, S., Rosenow, E.: Recent Advances in the Management of Venous Thromboembolism. Mayo Clin. Proc., 63:281–290, 1988.
477. Monreal, M., LaFoz, E., Navarro, A., et al.: A Prospective Double-Blind Trial of a Low Molecular Weight Heparin Once Daily Compared With Conventional Low-Dose Heparin Three Times Daily to Prevent Pulmonary Embolism and Venous Thrombosis in Patients With Hip Fracture. J. Trauma, 29:873–875, 1989.
478. Morrell, M.T., and Dunnill, M.S.: The Post Mortem Incidence of Pulmonary Embolism in a Hospital Population. Br. J. Surg., 55:347–352, 1968.
479. Morrell, M.T., Truelove, S.C., Barr, A.: Pulmonary Embolism. B.M.J., 2:830–835, 1963.
480. Moser, K., and LeMoine, J.: Is Embolic Risk Conditioned by Location of Deep Venous Thrombosis? Ann. Intern. Med., 94:439–444, 1987.
481. Murphy, E.A., Mustard, J.F., Rowsell, H.C., Downie, H.G.: Quantitative Studies on the Effect of Dicumarol on Experimental Thrombosis. J. Lab. Clin. Med., 61:935–943, 1963.
482. Negus, D., Pinto, D.J., LeQuesne, L.P., Brown, N., Chapman, M.: ^{125}I-Labelled Fibrinogen in the Diagnosis of Deep Vein Thrombosis and Its Correlation With Phlebography. Br. J. Surg., 55:835–839, 1968.
483. Neu, L.T., Jr., Waterfield, J.R., Ash, C.J.: Prophylactic Anticoagulant Therapy in the Orthopaedic Patient. Ann. Intern. Med., 62:463–467, 1965.
484. Nicolaides, A.N., Desai, S., Douglas, J.N., et al.: Small Doses of Subcutaneous Sodium Heparin in Preventing Deep Venous Thrombosis After Major Surgery. Lancet, 2:890–893, 1972.
485. NIH Consensus Conference: Prevention of Venous Thrombosis and Pulmonary Embolism. J.A.M.A., 256:744–749, 1986.
486. Nylander, G.: Phlebographic Diagnosis of Acute Deep Leg Thrombosis. Acta. Chir. Scand. Suppl., 387:30–34, 1968.
487. O'Brien, J.R.: Effects of Salicylates on Human Platelets. Lancet, 1:779–783, 1968.
488. O'Brien, J.R.: Detection of Thrombosis With Iodine^{125} Fibrinogen. Data Reassessed. Lancet, 2:396–398, 1970.
489. O'Reilly, R., and Kearns, P.: Variation in the Prothrombin-Time Ratio During Oral Anticoagulation. Letter to the Editor. N. Engl. J. Med., 330:509–510, 1994.
490. Oster, G., Tuden, R., Colditz, G., A Cost-Effectiveness Analysis of Prophylaxis Against Deep Vein Thrombosis in Major Orthopaedic Surgery. J.A.M.A., 257:203–208, 1987.
491. Paiement, G., Wessinger, S., Harris, W.: Survey of Prophylaxis Against Venous Thromboembolism in Adults Undergoing Hip Surgery. Clin. Orthop., 223:188–193, 1987.
492. Paiement, G., Wessinger, S., Waltman, A., Harris, W.: Low-Dose Warfarin Versus External Pneumatic Compression for Prophylaxis Against Venous Thromboembolism Following Total Hip Replacement. J. Arthroplasty, 2:23–26, 1987.
493. Paiement, G., Wessinger, S., Waltman, A., Harris, W.: Surveillance of Deep Vein Thrombosis in Asymptomatic Total Hip Replacement Patients. Impedance Phlebography and Fibrinogen Scanning Versus Roentgenographic Phlebography. Am. J. Surg., 155:400–404, 1988.
494. Parker, B.M., and Smith, J.R.: Pulmonary Embolism and Infarction. A Review of the Physiologic Consequences of Pulmonary Arterial Obstruction. Am. J. Med., 24:402–427, 1958.
495. Patterson, B., Marchand, R., Ranawat, C.: Complications of Heparin Therapy After Total Joint Arthroplasty. J. Bone Joint Surg., 71A:1130, 1989.
496. Pellegrini, V.D., Francis, C.W., Harris, C.M., Totterman, S., Marder, V.: Comparison of Night Before and Two-Step Warfarin for Prevention of Deep Venous Thrombosis Following Total Knee Replacement. Orlando, Fla., American Association of Orthopaedic Surgeons, J. Bone Joint Surg., in press.
497. Pellegrini, V.D., Langhans, M., Totterman, S., Marder, V., Francis, C.: Embolic Complications of Calf Thrombosis Following Total Hip Arthroplasty. J. Arthroplasty, 8:449–457, 1993.
498. Persson, A., Jones, C., Zide, R., Jewell, E.: Use of the Triplex Scanner in Diagnosis of Deep Venous Thrombosis. Arch. Surg., 124:593–596, 1989.
499. Pollak, E.W., Sparks, F.C., Barker, W.F.: Pulmonary Embolism. An Appraisal of Therapy in 516 Cases. Arch. Surg., 107:66–68, 1973.
500. Rabinov, K., and Paulin, S.: Roentgen Diagnosis of Venous Thrombosis in the Leg. Arch. Surg., 104:134–144, 1972.
501. Rick, M.E.: Protein C and Protein S. Vitamin K-Dependent Inhibitors of Blood Coagulation. J.A.M.A., 263:701–703, 1990.
502. Ridker, P., Hennekens, C., Lindpaintner, K., Stampfer, M., Eisenberg, P., Miletich, J.: Mutation in the Gene Coding for Coagulation Factor V and the Risk of Myocardial Infarction, Stroke, and Venous Thrombosis in Apparently Healthy Men. N. Engl. J. Med., 332:912–917, 1995.
503. Rosenow, E.C., III, Osmundson, P.J., Brown, M.L.: Pulmonary Embolism. Mayo Clin. Proc., 56:161–178, 1981.
504. Rothman, R.H., and Booth, R.E.: Prevention of Pulmonary Embolism: A Comparison of ASA and Low Dose Coumadin Regimens. Clin. Orthop., 154:309, 1981.
505. Russell, H.E., Jr., Bradham, R.R., Lee, W.H., Jr.: An Evaluation of Infusion Therapy (Including Dextran) for Venous Thrombosis. Circulation, 33:839–846, 1966.
506. Sabiston, D.C., Jr.: Pathophysiology, Diagnosis and Management of Pulmonary Embolism. Am. J. Surg., 138:384–391, 1979.
507. Salzman, E.W., Harris, W.H., DeSanctis, R.W.: Anticoagulation for Prevention of Thromboembolism Following Fractures of the Hip. N. Engl. J. Med., 275:122–130, 1966.
508. Salzman, E.W., Harris, W.H., DeSanctis, R.W.: Reduction in Venous Thromboembolism by Agents Affecting Platelet Function. N. Engl. J. Med., 284:1287–1292, 1971.
509. Sandritter, W.: Die pathologische Anatomie der Thrombose und Lung en Embolie. Son Derdruck aus Behring-werk-Mitteilungen, 4:37–54, 1962.
510. Schondorf, T.H., Weber, U., Lasch, H.G.: Niedrig dosierts heparin und acetylsalicylsaure nach elektiven operationem am huftgelenk. Dtsch. Med. Wochenschr., 102:1314–1318, 1977.
511. Sevitt, S., and Gallagher, N.G.: Prevention of Venous Thrombosis and Pulmonary Embolism in Injured Patients. A Trial Anticoagulant Prophylaxis With Phenindione in Middle Aged and Elderly Patients With Fractured Necks of Femur. Lancet, 2:981–989, 1959.
512. Sevitt, S., and Gallagher, N.G.: Venous Thrombosis and Pulmonary Embolism: A Clinicopathological Study in Injured and Burned Patients. Br. J. Surg., 48:475–489, 1961.
513. Sigel, B., Popky, G.L., Mapp, E.M., Feigl, P., Felix, W.R., Jr., Ipsen, J.: Evaluation of Doppler Ultrasound Examination. Its Use in Diagnosis of Lower Extremity Venous Disease. Arch. Surg., 100:535–540, 1970.
514. Sigel, B., Popky, G.L., Wagner, D.K., Boland, J.P., Mapp, E.M., Feigl, P.: A Doppler Ultrasound Method for Diagnosing Lower Extremity Venous Disease. Surg. Gynecol. Obstet., 127:339–350, 1968.
515. Sikorski, J.M., Hampson, W.G., Staddon, G.E.: The Natural History and Aetiology of Deep Vein Thrombosis After Total Hip Replacement. J. Bone Joint Surg., 63B:171–177, 1981.
516. Smith, G.T., Dammin, G.J., Dexter, L.: Postmortem Arteriographic Studies of the Human Lung in Pulmonary Embolization. J.A.M.A., 188:143–151, 1964.
517. Solonen, K.A.: Prophylactic Anticoagulant Therapy in the Treatment of Lower Limb Fractures. Acta. Orthop. Scand., 33:329–341, 1963.
518. Stamatakis, J.D., Kakkar, V.V., Lawrence, D., Bently, P.G., Naim, D., Ward, V.: Failure of Aspirin to Prevent Postopera-

tive Deep Vein Thrombosis in Patients Undergoing Total Hip Replacement. B.M.J., 1:1031–1032, 1978.

519. Stulberg, B., Insall, J., Williams, G., Ghelman, B.: Deep-Vein Thrombosis Following Total Knee Replacement. An Analysis of 638 Arthroplasties. J. Bone Joint Surg., 66A:194–201, 1984.
520. Svensson, P.J., and Dahlback, B.: Resistance to Activated Protein C as a Basis for Venous Thrombosis. N. Engl. J. Med., 330:517–521, 1994.
521. Swierstra, B., Stibbe, J., Schouten, H.: Prevention of Thrombosis After Hip Arthroplasty. A Prospective Study of Preoperative Oral Anticoagulants. Acta. Orthop. Scand., 59:139–143, 1988.
522. Swierstra, B., Van Oosterhout, F., Ausema, B., Bakker, W., Van Der Pompe, W., Schouten, H.: Oral Anticoagulants and Dextran for Prevention of Venous Thrombosis in Orthopaedics. Acta Orthop. Scand., 55:251–253, 1984.
523. Tubiana, R., and Duparc, J.: Prevention of Thromboembolic Complications in Orthopaedic and Accident Surgery. J. Bone Joint Surg., 43B:7–15, 1961.
524. Turpie, A., Levine, M., Hirsh, J., et al.: A Randomized Controlled Trial of a Low Molecular Weight Heparin (Enoxaparin) to Prevent Deep Vein Thrombosis in Patients Undergoing Elective Hip Surgery. N. Engl. J. Med., 315:925–929, 1986.
525. Viamonte, M., Jr., Koolpe, H., Janowitz, W., Hildner, F.: Pulmonary Thromboembolism—Update. J.A.M.A., 243:2229–2234, 1980.
526. Vinazzer, H., Loew, D., Simma, W., Brucke, P.: Prophylaxis of Postoperative Thromboembolism by Low Dose Heparin and by Acetylsalicylic Acid Given Simultaneously. A Double Blind Study. Thromb. Res., 17:177–184, 1980.
527. Virchow, R.: Die verstopfung den lungenarterie und ihre folgen. Beitr. Exper. Path. Physiol., 2:1–12, 1846.
528. Vukov, L.F., Berquist, T.H., King, B.F.: Magnetic Resonance Imaging for Calf Deep Venous Thrombophlebitis. Ann. Emerg. Med., 20:497–499, 1991.
529. Wacker, W.E.C., Rosenthal, M., Snodgrass, P.J., Amador, E.A.: A Triad for the Diagnosis of Pulmonary Embolism and Infarction. J.A.M.A., 178:8–13, 1961.
530. Weinmann, E., and Salzman, E.: Deep-Vein Thrombosis. N. Engl. J. Med., 331:1630–1641, 1994.
531. Weiss, J.H., Aledort, L.M., Kochwa, S.: The Effect of Salicylates on the Hemostatic Properties of Platelets in Man. J. Clin. Invest., 48:2169–2180, 1968.
532. Wells, P., Lensing, A., Davidson, B., Prins, M., Hirsh, J: Accuracy of Ultrasound for the Diagnosis of Deep Venous Thrombosis in Asymptomatic Patients After Orthopedic Surgery. A Meta-Analysis. Ann. Intern. Med., 122:47–53, 1995.
533. Wessler, S., and Yin, E.T.: Theory and Practice of Minidose Heparin in Surgical Patients. Circulation, 47:671–676, 1973.
534. Wheeler, H.B., Pearson, D., O'Connell, D., Mullick, S.C.: Impedance Phlebography. Technique, Interpretation and Results. Arch. Surg., 104:164–169, 1972.
535. Wiley, A.M.: Venous Thrombosis in Orthopaedic Patients: An Overview. Orthop. Surg., 2:388–400, 1979.
536. Winfrey, E.W., III, and Foster, J.H.: Low Molecular Weight Dextran in Small Artery Surgery. Antithrombogenic Effect. Arch. Surg., 88:78–82, 1964.

GAS GANGRENE

537. Aitken, D.R., Mackett, M.C.T., Smith, L.L.: The Changing Pattern of Hemolytic Streptococcal Gangrene. Arch. Surg., 117:561–567, 1982.
538. Altemeier, W.A., and Culbertson, W.R.: Acute Nonclostridial Crepitant Cellulitis. Surg. Gynecol. Obstet., 87:206–212, 1948.
539. Altemeier, W.A., and Fullen, W.D.: Prevention and Treatment of Gas Gangrene. J.A.M.A., 217:806–813, 1971.
540. Altemeier, W.A., and Furste, W.L.: Studies in Virulence of *Clostridium welchii.* Surgery, 25:12–19, 1949.
541. Aufranc, O.E., Jones, W.N., Bierbaum, B.E.: Gas Gangrene Complicating Fracture of the Tibia. J.A.M.A., 209:2045–2047, 1969.
542. Boerema, I.: An Operating Room With High Atmospheric Pressure. Surgery, 49:291–298, 1961.
543. Bornstein, D.L., Weinberg, N., Swartz, M.N., Kunz, L.J.: Anaerobic Infections—Review of Current Experience. Medicine (Baltimore), 43:207–232, 1964.
544. Bottini, E.: La Gangrena Traumatica Invadente. Contribuzione Sperimentali ed Illustrazioni Cliniche. Giorn. Reale Accad. Med., 10:1121–1138, 1871.
545. Brummelkamp, W.H., Boerema, I., Hoogendyk, L.: Treatment of Clostridial Infections With Hyperbaric Oxygen Drenching: A Report of 26 Cases. Lancet, 1:235–238, 1963.
546. Colwill, M.R., and Maudsley, R.H.: The Management of Gas Gangrene With Hyperbaric Oxygen Therapy. J. Bone Joint Surg., 50B:732–742, 1968.
547. DeHaven, K.E., and Evarts, C.M.: The Continuing Problem of Gas Gangrene: A Review and Report of Illustrative Cases. J. Trauma, 11:983–991, 1971.
548. Eickhoff, T.C.: An Outbreak of Surgical Wound Infections Due to *Clostridium perfringens.* Surg. Gynecol. Obstet., 114: 102–108, 1962.
549. Filler, R.M., Griscom, N.T., Pappas, A.: Posttraumatic Crepitation Falsely Suggesting Gas Gangrene. N. Engl. J. Med., 278:758–761, 1968.
550. Fisher, A.M., and McKusick, V.A.: Bacteriodes Infections: Clinical, Bacteriological and Therapeutic Features of 14 Cases. Am. J. Med. Sci., 225:253–273, 1953.
551. Giuidi, M.L., Proietti, R., Carducci, P., Magalini, S.I., Pelosi, G.: The Combined Use of Hyperbaric Oxygen, Antibiotics and Surgery in the Treatment of Gas Gangrene. Resuscitation, 9:267–273, 1981.
552. Govan, A.D.T.: An Account of the Pathology of Some Cases of *C. welchii* Infection. J. Pathol. Bacteriol., 58:423–430, 1946.
553. Grossman, M., and Silen, W.: Serious Post-Traumatic Infections With Special Reference to Gas Gangrene, Tetanus and Necrotizing Fasciitis. Postgrad. Med., 32:110–118, 1962.
554. Gye, R., Rountree, P.M., Lowenthal, J.: Infection of Surgical Wounds With *Clostridium welchii.* Med. J. Aust., 48:761–764, 1961.
555. Hayward, N.J.: The Rapid Identification of *C. welchii* by Nagler Tests in Plate Cultures. J. Pathol. Bacteriol., 55:285–293, 1943.
556. Hayward, N.J., and Gray, J.A.B.: Haemolysin Tests for the Rapid Identification of *C. oedematiens* and *C. septicum.* J. Pathol. Bacteriol., 58:11–20, 1946.
557. Holland, J.A., Hill, G.B., Wolfe, W.G., Osterhout, S., Saltzman, H.A., Brown, I.W., Jr.: Experimental and Clinical Experience With Hyperbaric Oxygen in the Treatment of Clostridial Myonecrosis. Surgery, 77:75–85, 1975.
558. Hunt, T., Halliday, B., Knighton, D., et al.: Impairment of Microbicidal Function in Wounds: Correction With Oxygenation. *In* Hunt, T.K., Heppenstall, R.B., Pines, E., Rovee, D. (eds.): Soft and Hard Tissue Repair, Biological and Clinical Aspects, pp. 455–468. New York, Praeger, 1984.
559. Jeffrey, J.S., and Thomson, S.: Gas Gangrene in Italy: A Study of 33 Cases Treated With Penicillin. Br. J. Surg., 32:159–167, 1944.
560. Kellett, C.E.: The Early History of Gas Gangrene. Ann. Med. Hist., 1:452–459, 1939.
561. Kemp, F.H.: X-rays in Diagnosis and Localization of Gas Gangrene. Lancet, 1:332–336, 1945.
562. Langley, F.H., and Winkelstein, L.B.: Gas Gangrene: A Study of 96 Cases Treated in an Evacuation Hospital. J.A.M.A., 128:783–792, 1945.
563. MacLennan, J.D.: Anaerobic Infections of War Wounds in the Middle East. Lancet, 2:63–66, 1943.
564. MacLennan, J.D.: Streptococcal Infection of Muscle. Lancet, 1:582–584, 1943.
565. MacLennan, J.D.: Histotoxic Clostridial Infections in Man. Bacteriol. Rev., 26:177–276, 1962.
566. MacLennan, J.D., and MacFarlane, R.G.: Toxin and Antitoxin Studies of Gas Gangrene in Man. Lancet, 2:301–305, 1945.
567. Oakley, C.L.: Gas Gangrene. Br. Med. Bull., 10:52–58, 1954.
568. Pappas, A.M., Filler, R.M., Eraklis, A.J., Bernhard, W.F.: Clos-

tridial Infections (Gas Gangrene). Diagnosis and Early Treatment. Clin. Orthop., 76:177–184, 1971.
569. Parker, M.T.: Postoperative Clostridial Infections in Britain. B.M.J., 3:671–676, 1969.
570. Qvist, G.: Anaerobic Cellulitis and Gas Gangrene. B.M.J., 2:217–221, 1941.
571. Rifkind, D.: The Diagnosis and Treatment of Gas Gangrene. Surg. Clin. North Am., 43:511–517, 1963.
572. Robb-Smith, A.H.T.: Tissue Changes Induced by *Clostridum welchii* Type A Filtrates. Lancet, 2:362–368, 1945.
573. Roding, B., Groeneveld, P.H.A., Boerema, I.: Ten Years of Experience in the Treatment of Gas Gangrene With Hyperbaric Oxygen. Surg. Gynecol. Obstet., 134:579–585, 1972.
574. Schwartzman, J.D., Reller, L.B., Wang, W.L.: Susceptibility of *Clostridium perfringens* Isolated From Human Infections to Twenty Antibiotics. Antimicrob. Agents Chemother., 11:695–697, 1977.
575. Smith, L., and DeSpain: Clostridia in Gas Gangrene. Bacteriol. Rev., 13:233–254, 1949.
576. Tonjum, S., Digranes, A., Alho, A., Gjengsto, H., Eidsvik, S.: Hyperbaric Oxygen Treatment in Gas-Producing Infections. Acta Chir. Scand., 146:235–241, 1980.
577. Trippel, O.H., Ruggie, A.N., Staley, C.J., Van Elk, J.: Hyperbaric Oxygenation in the Management of Gas Gangrene. Surg. Clin. North Am., 47:17–27, 1967.
578. Van Beek, A., Zook, E., Yaw, P., Gardner, R., Smith, R., Glover, J.L.: Nonclostridial Gas-Forming Infections. A Collective Review and Report of Seven Cases. Arch. Surg., 108:552–557, 1974.
579. Weinstein, L., and Barza, M.A.: Gas Gangrene. N. Engl. J. Med., 289:1129–1131, 1973.
580. Welsh, F., Matos, L., deTreville, R.T.P.: Medical Hyperbaric Oxygen Therapy. 22 Cases. Aviat. Space Environ. Med., 51:611–614, 1980.
581. Willis, A.T., and Gowland, G.: Some Observations on the Mechanism of the Nagler Reaction. J. Pathol. Bacteriol., 83:219–226, 1962.
582. Willis, A.T., and Hobbs, G.: Some New Media for the Isolation and Identification of Clostridia. J. Pathol. Bacteriol., 77:511–521, 1959.
583. Wilson, T.S.: Significance of *Clostridium welchii* Infections and Their Relationship to Gas Gangrene. Can. J. Surg., 4:35–42, 1960.
584. Wolinsky, E.: Clostridial Myonecrosis. *In* Wyngaarden, J.B., and Smith, L.H. (eds.): Textbook of Medicine, 16th ed. Philadelphia, W.B. Saunders, 1982.

TETANUS

585. American College of Surgeons Committee on Trauma: A Guide to Prophylaxis Against Tetanus in Wound Management. Bulletin of the American College of Surgeons, 57:32–33, 1972.
586. Aretaeus the Cappadocian: On Tetanus. *In* Adams, F. (ed.): The Extant Works. London, 1856.
587. Brooks, V.B., Curtis, D.R., Eccles, J.C.: The Action of Tetanus Toxin on the Inhibition of Motoneurons. J. Physiol., 135:655–672, 1957.
588. Brown, H.: Tetanus. J.A.M.A., 204:614–616, 1968.
589. Carle, A., and Rattone, G.: Studio Experimentale Sull' Eziologia del Tetano. Geordr. Accad. Med. Torino, 32:174–180, 1884.
590. Christensen, M.A.: Important Concepts of Tetanus That Form the Basis for Current Treatment. *In* Eckmann, L. (ed.): Principles on Tetanus. 2nd Proceedings of the International Conference on Tetanus, pp. 455–467. Bern, Hans Huber, 1967.
591. Christensen, N.A.: Treatment of the Patient With Severe Tetanus. Surg. Clin. North Am., 49:1183–1193, 1969.
592. Duchen, L.W., and Tonge, D.A.: The Effects of Tetanus Toxin on Neuromuscular Transmission and on the Morphology of Motor End-Plates in Slow and Fast Skeletal Muscle of the Mouse. J. Physiol., 228:157–172, 1973.
593. Eckmann, L. (ed.): Principles on Tetanus. 2nd Proceedings of the International Conference on Tetanus, pp. 1–577. Bern, Hans Huber, 1967.
594. Furste, W.: Third International Conference on Tetanus: A Report. J. Trauma, 11:721–724, 1971.
595. Furste, W.: Four Keys to 100 Per Cent Success in Tetanus Prophylaxis. Am. J. Surg., 128:616–623, 1974.
596. Furste, W., and Wheeler, W.L.: Tetanus: A Team Disease. Curr. Probl. Surg., 1–72, 1972.
597. Glenn, F.: Tetanus—A Preventable Disease: Including an Experience With Civilian Casualties in the Battle for Manila (1945). Ann. Surg., 124:1030–1040, 1946.
598. Graphs and Maps for Selected Notifiable Diseases in the United States. M.M.W.R., 42, 1994.
599. Gupta, P.S., Kapoor, R., Goyal, S., Batra, V.K., Jain, B.K.: Intrathecal Human Tetanus Immunoglobulin in Early Tetanus. Lancet, 2:439–440, 1980.
600. Habermann, E.: Tetanus. *In* Vinkin, P.J., and Bruyn, G.W. (eds.): Handbook of Clinical Neurology, vol. 33, part I, pp. 491–547. New York, North Holland Publishing, 1978.
601. Hardegee, M.C., Palmer, A.E., Duffin, N.: Tetanolysin: In Vivo Effects in Animals. J. Infect. Dis., 123:51–60, 1971.
602. Helting, T.B., Zwisler, O., Wiegandt, H.: Structure of Tetanus Toxin II. Toxin Binding to Ganglioside. J. Biol. Chem., 252:194–198, 1977.
603. Hippocrates: With an English Translation by W.H.S. Jones. vol. 1, pp. 165. Cambridge, Mass., Harvard University Press, 1923.
604. International Comments Guide Lines Regarding Tetanus. J.A.M.A., 198:687–688, 1966.
605. Jacobs, R.L., Lowe, R.S., Lanier, B.Q.: Adverse Reactions to Tetanus Toxoid. J.A.M.A., 247:40–42, 1982.
606. Kaeser, H.E., and Saner, A.: The Effect of Tetanus Toxin on Neuromuscular Transmission. Eur. Neurol., 3:193–205, 1970.
607. Kerr, J.H., Corbett, J.L., Prys-Roberts, C., Smith, A.C., Spalding, J.M.K.: Involvement of the Sympathetic Nervous System in Tetanus. Studies on 82 Cases. Lancet, 2:236–241, 1968.
608. Kitasato, S.: Uber den tetanuserreger. Ztschr. Hyg., 7:225–234, 1889.
609. LaForce, F.M., Young, L.S., Bennett, J.V.: Tetanus in the United States (1965–1966). Epidemiologic and Clinical Features. N. Engl. J. Med., 280:569–574, 1969.
610. Levine, L., McComb, J.A., Dwyer, R.C., Latham, W.C.: Active-Passive Tetanus Immunization. Choice of Toxoid, Dose of Tetanus Immune Globulin and Timing of Injections. N. Engl. J. Med., 274:186–190, 1966.
611. Long, A.: The Army Immunization Program, vol. III. Preventive Medicine in World War II. Washington, D.C., U.S. Government Printing Office, 1955.
612. McComb, J.A.: The Combined Use of Homologous Tetanus Immune Globulin and Toxoid in Man. *In* Eckmann, L. (ed.): Principles on Tetanus and Proceedings of the International Conference on Tetanus, pp. 359–367. Bern, Hans Huber, 1967.
613. McComb, J.A., and Dwyer, R.C.: Passive-Active Immunization With Tetanus Immune Globulin (Human). N. Engl. J. Med., 268:857–862, 1963.
614. McCracken, G.H., Jr., Dowell, D.L., Marshall, F.N.: Double-Blind Trial of Equine Antitoxin and Human Immune Globulin in Tetanus Neonatorum. Lancet, 1:1146–1149, 1971.
615. Mellanby, J.H.: Presynaptic Effect of Tetanus Toxin at the Neuromuscular Junction. J. Physiol., 218:68P–69P, 1971.
616. Milledge, J.S.: Hyperbaric Oxygen Therapy in Tetanus. J.A.M.A., 203:875–876, 1968.
617. Murphy, K.J.: Fatal Tetanus With Brain-Stem Involvement and Myocarditis in an Ex-Serviceman. Med. J. Aust., 2:542–544, 1970.
618. Nation, N.S., Pierce, N.F., Adler, S.J., Chinnock, R.F., Wehrle, P.F.: Tetanus: The Use of Human Hyperimmune Globulin in Treatment. California Med., 98:305–307, 1963.
619. Pessi, T., Honkola, H., Liikala, E.: Results of Treatment of Patients With Severe Tetanus. Ann. Chir. Gynaecol., 70:182–186, 1981.
620. Ramon, G., and Zoeller, C.: l'Anatoxine tetanique et l'Im-

munisation Active de l'Homme vis-a-vis du Tetanos. Ann. Inst. Pasteur., 41:803–833, 1927.

621. Recommendation of the Immunization Practices Advisory Committee. Diphtheria, Tetanus and Pertussis: Guidelines for Vaccine Prophylaxis and Other Preventive Measures. M.M.W.R., 30:3927, 1981.
622. Smith, A.: Tetanus. *In* Beeson, P.B., and McDermott, W. (eds.): Textbook of Medicine, 14th ed. Philadelphia, W.B. Saunders, 1975.
623. Smythe, P.M.: Studies on Neonatal Tetanus, and on Pulmonary Compliance of the Totally Relaxed Infant. B.M.J., 1:565–571, 1963.
624. Smythe, P.M.: The Problem of Detubating an Infant With a Tracheostomy. J. Pediatr., 65:446–453, 1964.
625. Smythe, P.M.: Treatment of Tetanus in Neonates. Lancet, 1:335, 1967.
626. Spaeth, R.: Therapy of Tetanus. A Study of Two Hundred and Seventy-Six Cases. Arch. Intern. Med., 68:1133–1160, 1941.
627. Trujillo, M.J., Castillo, A., Espana, J.V., Guevara, P., Eganez, H.: Tetanus in the Adult: Intensive Care and Management Experience With 233 Cases. Crit. Care Med., 8:419–423, 1980.
628. Tsueda, K., Oliver, P.B., Richter, R.W.: Cardiovascular Manifestations of Tetanus. Anesthesiology, 40:588–592, 1974.
629. Van Heyningen, W.E., and Messanby, J.: Tetanus Toxin. *In* Kadis, S., Montie, T.C., Ajl, S.J. (eds.): Microbial Toxins, vol. 2A. New York, Academic Press, 1971.
630. Weed, M.R., Purvis, D.F., Warnke, R.D.: D-Tubocurarine in Wax and Oil: For Control of Muscle Spasm in Tetanus. J.A.M.A, 138:1087–1090, 1948.
631. Wessler, S., and Avioli, L.A.: Tetanus. J.A.M.A., 207:123–127, 1969.
632. White, W.G.: Reactions to Tetanus Toxoid. J. Hyg. (Lond.), 17:283–297, 1973.
633. Woolmer, R., and Cates, J.E.: Succinylcholine in the Treatment of Tetanus. Lancet, 2:808–809, 1952.
634. Wright, G.P.: The Neurotoxins of *Clostridium botulinum* and *Clostridium tetani.* Pharmacol. Rev., 7:413–465, 1955.

OSTEOMYELITIS

635. Alexander, J.W., Sykes, N.S., Mitchell, M.M., Fisher, M.W.: Concentration of Selected Intravenously Administered Antibiotics in Experimental Surgical Wounds. J. Trauma, 13:423–434, 1973.
636. Anderson, W.A.D.: Pathology, 4th ed. St. Louis, C.V. Mosby, 1961.
637. Anthony, J.P., and Mathes, S.J.: Update on Chronic Osteomyelitis. Clin. Plast. Surg., 18:515–523, 1991.
638. Anthony, J.P., Mathes, S.J., Alpert, B.S.: The Muscle Flap in the Treatment of Chronic Lower Extremity Osteomyelitis: Results in Patients Over 5 Years After Treatment. Plast. Reconstr. Surg., 88:311, 1992.
639. Bajpai, J., Chaturvedi, S.N., Khanuja, S.P.S.: Chemotherapy of Acute Bone and Joint Infections. Int. Surg., 62:172–174, 1977.
640. Beltran, J., McGhee, R.B., Shaffer, P.B., et al.: Experimental Infections of the Musculoskeletal System: Evaluation With MR Imaging and Tc-99m MDP and Ga-67 Scintigraphy. Radiology, 167:167–172, 1988.
641. Beltran, J., Noto, A.M., McGhee, R.B., Freedy, R.M., McCalla, M.S.: Infections of the Musculoskeletal System: High-Field-Strength MR Imaging. Radiology, 164:449–454, 1987.
642. Bernhard, W.F., and Filler, R.M.: Hyperbaric Oxygenation: Current Concepts. Am. J. Surg., 115:661–668, 1968.
643. Blaha, J.D., Calhoun, J.H., Nelson, C.L., et al.: Comparison of the Clinical Efficacy and Tolerance of Gentamicin PMMA Beads on Surgical Wire Versus Combined and Systemic Therapy for Osteomyelitis. Clin. Orthop., 295:8–12, 1993.
644. Blaha, J.D., Nelson, C.L., Frevert, L.F., et al.: The Use of Septopal (Polymethylmethacrylate Beads With Gentamicin) in the Treatment of Chronic Osteomyelitis. (Review) Instr. Course Lect., 39:509–514, 1990.
645. Blockey, N.J., and McAllister, T.A.: Antibiotics in Acute Osteomyelitis in Children. J. Bone Joint Surg., 54B:299–309, 1972.
646. Brown, P.W.: The Prevention of Infection in Open Wounds. Clin. Orthop., 96:42–50, 1973.
647. Butt, W.P.: The Radiology of Infection. Clin. Orthop., 96:20–30, 1973.
648. Caldwell, J.R., and Cluff, L.E.: The Real and Present Danger of Antibiotics. Ration. Drug Ther., 7:1–6, 1973.
649. Calhoun, J.H., Cobos, J.A., Mader, J.T.: Does Hyperbaric Oxygen Have a Place in the Treatment of Osteomyelitis? (Review) Orthop. Clin. North Am., 22:467–471, 1991.
650. Canale, S.T., Harkness, R.M., Thomas, P.A., Massie, J.D.: Does Aspiration of Bones and Joints Affect Results of Later Bone Scanning? J. Pediatr. Orthop., 5:23–26, 1985.
651. Cierny III, G.: Chronic Osteomyelitis: Results of Treatment. (Review) Instr. Course Lect., 39:495–508, 1990.
652. Cierny III, G., Mader, J.T., Penninck, J.J.: A Clinical Staging System for Adult Osteomyelitis. Contemp. Orthop., 10:17–37, 1985.
653. Clawson, D.K.: Common Bacterial Infections of Bone. G.P., 32:125–133, 1965.
654. Clawson, D.K., David, F.J., Hansen, S.T.: Treatment of Chronic Osteomyelitis With Emphasis on Closed Suction-Irrigation Techniques. Clin. Orthop., 96:88–97, 1973.
655. Cluff, L.E., and Reynolds, R.C.: Management of Staphylococcal Infections. Am. J. Med., 39:812–825, 1965.
656. Cole, W.G.: The Management of Chronic Osteomyelitis. (Review) Clin. Orthop., 264:84–89, 1991.
657. Cole, W.G., Dalziel, R.E., Leitl, S.: Treatment of Acute Osteomyelitis in Childhood. J. Bone Joint Surg., 64B:218–223, 1982.
658. Collins, D.H.: *In* Dodge, O.G. (ed.): Pathology of Bone. London, Butterworths, 1966.
659. Compere, E.L., Metzger, W.I., Mitra, R.N.: The Treatment of Pyogenic Bone and Joint Infections by Closed Irrigation (Circulation) With a Non-Toxic Detergent and One or More Antibiotics. J. Bone Joint Surg., 49A:614–624, 1967.
660. Curtis, P.: The Pathophysiology of Joint Infections. Clin. Orthop., 96:129–135, 1973.
661. Dagan, R.: Management of Acute Hematogenous Osteomyelitis and Septic Arthritis in the Pediatric Patient. Pediatr. Infect. Dis. J., 12:88–93, 1993.
662. Dahners, L.E., and Funderburk, C.H.: Gentamicin-Loaded Plaster of Paris as a Treatment of Experimental Osteomyelitis in Rabbits. Clin. Orthop., 219:278–282, 1987.
663. Davis, J., Heckman, J., DeLee, J., Buckwold, F.: Chronic Non-Hematogenous Osteomyelitis Treated With Adjuvant Hyperbaric Oxygen. J. Bone Joint Surg., 68A:1210–1217, 1986.
664. Dellinger, E., Caplan, E., Weaver, L., et al.: Duration of Preventive Antibiotic Administration for Open Extremity Fractures. Arch. Surg., 123:333–339, 1988.
665. Dellinger, E., Miller, S., Wertz, M., Grypma, M., Droppert, B., Anderson, P.: Risk of Infection After Open Fracture of the Arm or Leg. Arch. Surg., 123:1320–1327, 1988.
666. Desplaces, N., and Acar, J.F.: New Quinolones in the Treatment of Joint and Bone Infections. (Review) Rev. Infect. Dis., 10(Suppl. 1):S179–S183, 1988.
667. Dich, V.Q., Nelson, J.D., Haltalin, K.C.: Osteomyelitis in Infants and Children. Am. J. Dis. Child., 129:1273–1278, 1975.
668. Dirschl, D.R.: Acute Pyogenic Osteomyelitis in Children. Orthop. Rev., 23(4):305–312, 1994.
669. Dombrowski, E.T., and Dunn, A.W.: Treatment of Osteomyelitis by Debridement and Closed Wound Irrigation-Suction. Clin. Orthop., 43:215–231, 1965.
670. Drancourt, M., Stein, A., Argenson, J., Zannier, A., Curvale, G., and Raoult, D.: Oral Rifampin plus Ofloxacin for Treatment of Staphylococcus-Infected Orthopaedic Implants. Antimicrob. Agents Chemother., 37:1214–1218, 1993.
671. Edwards, M.S., Baker, C.J., Wagner, K.H., Taber, L.H., Barrett, F.F.: An Etiologic Shift in Infantile Osteomyelitis: The Emergence of the Group B Streptococcus. J. Pediatr., 93:578–583, 1978.
672. Eggli, P.S., Muller, W., Schenk, R.K.: Porous Hydroxyapatite and Tricalcium Phosphate Cylinders With Two Different Pore

Size Ranges Implanted Into the Cancellous Bone of Rabbits. Clin. Orthop., 232:127–138, 1988.
673. Esterhai, J.L., Clark, J., Morton, H.E., et al.: The Effect of Hyperbaric Oxygen on Oxygen Tension Within the Medullary Canal in the Rabbit Tibia Osteomyelitis Model. J. Orthop. Res., 4:330–336, 1986.
674. Esterhai, J.L., Goll, S.R., McCarthy, K.E., et al.: Indium-111 Leukocyte Scintigraphic Detection of Subclinical Osteomyelitis Complicating Delayed and Nonunion of Long Bone Fractures: A Prospective Study. J. Orthop. Res., 5:1–6, 1987.
675. Esterhai Jr., J.L., Pisarello, J., Brighton, C.T., Heppenstall, R.B., Gellman, H., Goldstein, G.: Adjunctive Hyperbaric Oxygen Therapy in the Treatment of Chronic Refractory Osteomyelitis. J. Trauma, 27:763–768, 1987.
676. Evans, R.P., and Nelson, C.L.: Gentamicin-Impregnated Polymethylmethacrylate Beads Compared With Systemic Antibiotic Therapy in the Treatment of Chronic Osteomyelitis. Clin. Orthop., 295:37–42, 1993.
677. Evarts, C.M.: Endoprosthesis as the Primary Treatment of Femoral Neck Fractures. Clin. Orthop., 92:69–76, 1973.
678. Evaskus, D.S., Laskin, D.M., Kroeger, A.V.: Penetration of Lincomycin, Penicillin, and Tetracycline Into Serum and Bone. Proc. Soc. Exp. Biol. Med., 130:89–91, 1969.
679. Eyre-Brook, A.L.: Septic Arthritis of the Hip and Osteomyelitis of the Upper End of the Femur in Infants. J. Bone Joint Surg., 42B:11–20, 1960.
680. Faden, H., and Grossi, M.: Acute Osteomyelitis in Children: Reassessment of Etiologic Agents and Their Clinical Characteristics. Am. J. Dis. Child., 154:65–69, 1991.
681. Ferguson, A.B.: Osteomyelitis in Children. Clin. Orthop., 96:51–56, 1973.
682. Fiebel, R.J., Olivia, A., Jackson, R.L., Louie, K., Buncke, H.J.: Simultaneous Free-Tissue Transfer and Ilizarov Distraction Osteosynthesis in Lower Extremity Salvage: Case Report and Review of the Literature. (Review) J. Trauma, 37:322–327, 1994.
683. Fitzgerald, R.H., Jr., Brewer, N.S., Dahlin, D.C.: Squamous Cell Carcinoma Complicating Chronic Osteomyelitis. J. Bone Joint Surg., 58A:1146–1148, 1976.
684. Gentry, L.O.: Antibiotic Therapy for Osteomyelitis. (Review) Infect. Dis. Clin. North Am., 4:485–499, 1990.
685. Gentry, L.O.: Newer Concepts in Antimicrobial Therapy. (Review) Clin. Orthop., 261:23–26, 1990.
686. Ger, R.: Muscle Transposition for Treatment and Prevention of Chronic Post-traumatic Osteomyelitis of the Tibia. J. Bone Joint Surg., 59A:784–791, 1977.
687. Gillespie, W.J., and Mayo, K.M.: The Management of Acute Hematogenous Osteomyelitis in the Antibiotic Era. J. Bone Joint Surg., 63B:126–131, 1981.
688. Gilmour, W.N.: Acute Haematogenous Osteomyelitis. J. Bone Joint Surg., 44B:841–853, 1962.
689. Gold, R.H., Hawkins, R.A., Katz, R.D.: Bacterial Osteomyelitis: Findings on Plain Radiography, CT, MR, Scintigraphy. A.J.R. Am. J. Roentgenol, 157:365, 1991.
689a. Green, N.E., and Edwards, K.: Bone and Joint Infections in children. Orthopedic Clinics of North America, 18:555–576, 1987.
689b. Green, S.A.: Osteomyelitis: The Ilizarov Perspective. [Review] Orthopedic Clinics of North America, 22:515–521, 1991.
690. Gregory, E.M., and Fridovich, I.: Introduction of Superoxide Dismutase by Molecular Oxygen. J. Bacteriol., 114:543–548, 1973.
691. Gristina, A.G., Jennings, R.A., Naylor, P.T., et al.: Comparative In-Vitro Antibiotic Resistance of Surface Colonizing Coagulase-Negative Staphylococci. Antimicrob. Agents Chemother., 33:813–816, 1989.
692. Gristina, A.G., Naylor, P.T., Myrvik, Q.N.: Mechanisms of Musculoskeletal Sepsis. (Review) Orthop. Clin. North Am., 22:363–371, 1991.
693. Gristina, A.G., Oga, M., Webb, L.X., et al.: Bacterial Colonization in the Pathogenesis of Osteomyelitis. Science, 228:990–993, 1985.
694. Gupta, N.C., Lama, P., Prezio, J.A.: Comparative Efficacy of Tc-99m MDP Four Phase Bone Scan and In-111 Leucocyte Imaging in Osteomyelitis. (Abstract) J. Nucl. Med., 28:586, 1987.
695. Gupta, N.C., and Prezio, J.A.: Radionuclide Imaging in Osteomyelitis. (Review) Semin. Nucl. Med., 18:287–299, 1988.
696. Gustilo, R., and Anderson, J.: Prevention of Infection in the Treatment of One Thousand Twenty Five Open Fractures of Long Bones. Retrospective and Prospective Analyses. J. Bone Joint Surg., 58A:453–458, 1976.
697. Hamblen, D.L.: Hyperbaric Oxygenation: Its Effect on Experimental Staphylococcal Osteomyelitis in Rats. J. Bone Joint Surg., 50A:1129–1141, 1968.
698. Harris, N.H.: Some Problems in the Diagnosis and Treatment of Acute Osteomyelitis. J. Bone Joint Surg., 42B:535–541, 1960.
699. Harris, N.H., and Kirkaldy-Willis, W.H.: Primary Subacute Pyogenic Osteomyelitis. J. Bone Joint Surg., 47B:526–532, 1965.
700. Hart, V.L.: Acute Hematogenous Osteomyelitis in Children. J.A.M.A., 108:524–528, 1937.
701. Hermans, P., and Wilhelm, M.: Vancomycin. Mayo Clin. Proc., 62:901–905, 1987.
702. Hobo, T.: Zur Pathogenese der akuten haematogen Osteomyelitis, mit Berucksichtigung der Vitalfar beng Shehre. Acta School Medicine Univ. Kioto, 4:1–29, 1921–1922.
703. Hoffer, P.: Gallium: Mechanisms. (Abstract) J. Nucl. Med., 21:282–285, 1980.
704. Ilizarov, G.A.: The Treatment of Pseudarthroses Complicated by Osteomyelitis and the Elimination of Purulent Cavities. Transosseous Osteosynthesis. *In* Transosseous Osteosynthesis, pp. 495–547. Springer-Verlag, 1992.
705. Israel, O., Gips, S., Jerushalmi, J., Frenkel, A., Front, D.: Osteomyelitis and Soft Tissue Infection: Differential Diagnosis With 24 Hour/4 Hour Ratio of Tc99m MDP Uptake. Radiology, 163:725–726, 1987.
706. Jackson, R.W., and Parson, C.J.: Distention-Irrigation Treatment of Major Joint Sepsis. Clin. Orthop., 96:160–164, 1973.
707. Jacobs, R.F., McCarthy, R.E., Elser, J.M.: Pseudomonas Osteochondritis Complicating Puncture Wounds of the Foot in Children: A Ten Year Evaluation. J. Infect. Dis., 160:657–661, 1989.
708. Jupiter, J.B., First, K., Gallico III, G.G., May, J.W.: The Role of External Fixation in the Treatment of Posttraumatic Osteomyelitis. J. Orthop. Trauma, 2:79–93, 1988.
709. Kahn, D.S., and Pritzker, P.H.: The Pathophysiology of Bone Infection. Clin. Orthop., 96:12–19, 1973.
710. Kanyuck, D.O., Welles, J.S., Emmerson, J.L., Anderson, R.C.: The Penetration of Cephalosporin Antibiotics Into Bone. Proc. Soc. Exp. Biol. Med., 136:997–999, 1971.
711. Kelly, P.J.: Osteomyelitis in the Adult. Orthop. Clin. North Am., 6:983–989, 1975.
712. King, D.M., and Mayo, K.M.: Subacute Hematogenous Osteomyelitis. J. Bone Joint Surg., 51B:458–463, 1969.
713. Kolyvas, E., Ahronheim, G., Marks, M.I., Gledhill, R., Owen, H., Rosenthall, L.: Oral Antibiotic Therapy of Skeletal Infections in Children. Pediatrics, 65:867–871, 1980.
714. Koval, K.J., Meadows, S.E., Rosen, H., et al.: Post-traumatic Tibial Osteomyelitis: A Comparison of Three Treatment Approaches. Orthopedics, 15:455, 1992.
715. Lazarus, G.S., Brown, R.S., Daniels, J.R., Fullmer, H.M.: Human Granulocyte Collagenase. Science, 159:1483–1485, 1968.
716. LeFrock, J.L., Ristuccia, A.M., Ristuccia, P.A., et al.: Teicoplanin in the Treatment of Bone and Joint Infections. Teicoplanin Bone and Joint Cooperative Study Group, USA. Eur. J. Surg. Suppl., 567:9–13, 1992.
717. Lemons, J.E.: Hydroxyapatite coatings. Clin. Orthop., 235:220–223, 1988.
718. Letts, R.M., and Wong, E.: Treatment of Acute Osteomyelitis in Children by Closed-Tube Irrigation: A Reassessment. Can. J. Surg., 18:60–63, 1975.
719. Lhowe, D., and Hansen, S.: Immediate Nailing of Open Fractures of the Femoral Shaft. J. Bone Joint Surg., 70A:812–820, 1988.
720. Lisbona, R., and Rosenthall, L.: Observations on the Sequen-

tial Use of ^{99m}Tc-Phosphate Complex and ^{67}Ga Imaging in Osteomyelitis, Cellulitis, and Septic Arthritis. Radiology, 123:123–129, 1977.

721. Lodwick, G.S.: The Bones and Joints. Atlas of Tumour Radiology. Chicago, Year Book Medical Publishers, 1971.
722. McHenry, M.C.: Antibacterial Therapy. Cleve. Clin. Q., 37:43–58, 1970.
723. Mackowiak, P.A., Jones, S.R., Smith, J.W.: Diagnostic Value of Sinus Tract Culture in Chronic Osteomyelitis. J.A.M.A., 239:2722, 1978.
724. Mader, J.T., Adams, K.R., Wallace, W.R., Calhoun, J.H.: Hyperbaric Oxygen as Adjunctive Therapy for Osteomyelitis. (Review) Infect. Dis. Clin. North Am., 4:433–440, 1990.
725. Mader, J.T., Brown, G.L., Guckian, J.C., et al.: A Mechanism for the Amelioration by Hyperbaric Oxygen of Experimental Staphylococcal Osteomyelitis in Rabbits. J. Infect. Dis., 142:915–922, 1980.
726. Mader, J.T., Landon, G.C., Calhoun, J.: Antimicrobial Treatment of Osteomyelitis. Clin. Orthop., 295:87–95, 1993.
727. Mallouh, A., and Talab, Y.: Bone and Joint Infection in Patients With Sickle Cell Disease. J. Pediatr. Orthop., 5:158–162, 1985.
728. Mason, M.D., Zlatkin, M.B., Esterhai, J.L., Dalinka, M.K., Velchik, M.G., Kressel, H.Y.: Chronic Complicated Osteomyelitis of the Lower Extremity: Evaluation With MR Imaging. Radiology, 173:355–359, 1989.
729. Mathes, S.J.: The Muscle Flap for Management of Osteomyelitis. N. Engl. J. Med., 306:294, 1984.
730. Maurer, A.H., Chen, D.C.P., Camargo, E.E., Wong, D.F., Wagner, H.N., Anderson, P.O.: Utility of Three-Phase Skeletal Scintigraphy in Suspected Osteomyelitis: Concise Communication. J. Nucl. Med., 22:941–949, 1981.
731. Maurer, A.H., Millmond, H., Knight, L.C., et al.: Infection in Diabetic Osteoarthropathy: Use of Indium-Labeled Leukocytes for Diagnosis. Radiology, 161:221–225, 1986.
732. May, J.W., Jr., Jupiter, J.B., Weiland, A.J., Byrd, H.S.: Clinical Classification of Post-traumatic Tibial Osteomyelitis. (Review) J. Bone Joint Surg., 71A:1422–1428, 1989.
733. Mayhall, C.G., Medoff, G., Marr, J.J.: Variation in the Susceptibility of Strains of *Staphylococcus aureus* to Oxacillin, Cephalothin and Gentamicin. Antimicrob. Agents Chemother., 10: 707–712, 1976.
734. McGuire, M.H.: The Pathogenesis of Adult Osteomyelitis. (Review) Orthop. Rev., 18:564–570, 1989.
735. McNally, M.A., Small, J.O., Tofighi, H.G., Mollan, R.A.B.: Two-Stage Management of Chronic Osteomyelitis of the Long Bones: The Belfast Technique. J. Bone Joint Surg., 75B:375–380, 1993.
736. Merkel, K., Brown, M., Dewanjee, M., Fitzgerald, R.: Comparison of Indium-Labelled-Leukocyte Imaging With Sequential Technetium-Gallium Scanning in the Diagnosis of Low-Grade Musculoskeletal Sepsis. J. Bone Joint Surg., 67A:465–476, 1985.
737. Merkel, K.D., Fitzgerald, R.H., Jr., Brown, M.L.: Scintigraphic Evaluation in Musculoskeletal Sepsis. (Review) Orthop. Clin. North Am., 15:401–416, 1984.
738. Miclau, T., Dahners, L.E., Lindsey, R.W.: In Vitro Pharmacokinetics of Antibiotic Release From Locally Implantable Materials. J. Orthop. Res., 11:627–632, 1993.
739. Modic, M.T., Pflanze, W., Freiglin, D.H., Belhobek, G.: Magnetic Resonance Imaging of Musculoskeletal Infections. Radiol. Clin. North Am., 24:247–258, 1986.
740. Mollan, R.A.B., and Piggott, J.: Acute Osteomyelitis in Children. J. Bone Joint Surg., 59B:2–7, 1977.
741. Morrey, B.F., Dunn, J.M., Heimbach, R.D., Davis, J.: Hyperbaric Oxygen and Chronic Osteomyelitis. Clin. Orthop., 144:121–127, 1979.
742. Morrey, B.F., and Peterson, H.A.: Hematogenous Pyogenic Osteomyelitis in Children. Orthop. Clin. North Am., 6:935–951, 1975.
743. Morrissy, R.T., and Haynes, D.W.: Acute Hematogenous Osteomyelitis. J. Pediatr. Orthop., 9:447–456, 1989.
744. Morrissy, R.T., Haynes, D.W., Nelson, C.L.: Acute Hematogenous Osteomyelitis: The Role of Trauma in a Reproducible Model. Trans. Orthop. Res. Soc., 5:324, 1980.
745. Munk, P.L., Vellet, A.D., Hilborn, M.D., Crues, J.V., Helms, C.A., Poon, P.Y.: Musculoskeletal Infection: Findings on Magnetic Resonance Imaging. (Review) Can. Assoc. Radiol. J., 45:355–362, 1994.
746. Nelson, C.L., Griffin, F.M., Harrison, B.H., Gooper, R.E.: In Vitro Elution Characteristics of Commercially and Noncommercially Prepared Antibiotic PMMA Beads. Clin. Orthop., 284:303, 1992.
747. Nettles, J.L., Kelly, P.J., Martin, W.J., Washington, J.A.: Musculoskeletal Infections Due to Bacteroides. A Study of Eleven Cases. J. Bone Joint Surg., 51A:230–238, 1969.
748. Nichols, W.W., Evans, J.J., Slack, M.P.E., et al.: The Penetration of Antibiotics Into Aggregates of Mucoid and Nonmucoid Pseudomonas aeruginosa. J. Gen. Microbiol., 135: 1291–1301, 1989.
749. Niekerk, J.P.: Hand Infections: Management and Results Based on a New Classification. A Study of More Than 1,000 Cases. S. Afr. Med. J., 40:316–319, 1966.
750. O'Brien, T., McManns, F., MacAuley, P.H., Ennis, J.T.: Acute Hematogenous Osteomyelitis. J. Bone Joint Surg., 64B:450–453, 1982.
751. Ogden, J.A.: Pediatric Osteomyelitis and Septic Arthritis: The Pathology of Neonatal Disease. Yale J. Biol. Med., 52:423–448, 1979.
752. Overton, L.M., and Tully, W.P.: Surgical Treatment of Chronic Osteomyelitis in Long Bones. Am. J. Surg., 126:736–741, 1973.
753. Patzakis, M.J., Abdollahi, K., Sherman, R., Holtom, P.D., Wilkins, J.: Treatment of Chronic Osteomyelitis With Muscle Flaps. Orthop. Clin. North Am., 24:505–509, 1993.
754. Patzakis, M.J., Harvey, J.P., Jr., Ivler, D.: The Role of Prophylactic Antibiotics in the Management of Open Fractures. J. Bone Joint Surg., 56A:532–541, 1974.
755. Popham, G.J., Mangino, P., Seligson, D., Henry, S.L.: Antibiotic-Impregnated Beads: Part II, Factors in Antibiotic Selection. Orthop. Rev., 20:331–337, 1991.
756. Prober, C.G.: Current Antibiotic Therapy of Community-Acquired Bacterial Infections in Hospitalized Children: Bone and Joint Infections. Pediatr. Infect. Dis. J., 11:156–159, 1992.
757. Prober, C.G., and Yeager, A.S.: Use of the Serum Bactericidal Titer to Assess the Adequacy of Oral Antibiotic Therapy in the Treatment of Acute Hematogenous Osteomyelitis. J. Pediatr., 95:131–135, 1979.
758. Prober, G.C.: Oral Antibiotic Therapy for Bone and Joint Infections. Pediatr. Infect. Dis. J., 1:8–10, 1982.
759. Rosenthal, L., Kloiber, R., Damtew, B., Al-Majid, H.: Sequential Use of Radiophosphate and Radiogallium Imaging in the Differential Diagnosis of Bone, Joint, and Soft Tissue Infection: Quantitative Analysis. Diagn. Imaging, 51:249–258, 1982.
760. Rosenthall, L.: Radionuclide Investigation of Osteomyelitis. (Review) Curr. Opin. Radiol., 4:62–69, 1992.
761. Ryden, C., Maxe, I., Franzen, A., et al.: Selective Binding of Bone Matrix Sialoprotein to Staphylococcus aureus in Osteomyelitis. Lancet, 29:515, 1987.
762. Schauwecker, D.S.: The Scintigraphic Diagnosis of Osteomyelitis. (Review) A.J.R. Am. J. Roentgenol., 158:9–18, 1992.
763. Schauwecker, D.S., Braunstein, E.M., Wheat, L.J.: Diagnostic Imaging of Osteomyelitis. (Review) Infect. Dis. Clin. North Am., 4:441–463, 1990.
764. Schauwecker, D.S., Park, H.M., Burt, R.W., Mock, B.H., Wellman, H.N.: Combined Bone Scintigraphy and Indium-111 Leukocyte Scans in Neuropathic Foot Disease. J. Nucl. Med., 29:1651–1655, 1988.
765. Schauwecker, D.S., Park, H.M., Mock, B.H., et al.: Evaluation of Complicating Osteomyelitis with Tc-99m MDP, In-111 Granulocytes, and Ga-67 Citrate. J. Nucl. Med., 25:849–853, 1984.
766. Seabold, J.E., Nepola, J.V., Conrad, G.R., et al.: Detection of Osteomyelitis at Fracture Nonunion Sites: Comparison of

Two Scintigraphic Methods. A.J.R. Am. J. Roentgenol., 152:1021–1027, 1989.
767. Shandling, B.: Acute Hematogenous Osteomyelitis: A Review of 300 Cases Treated During 1952–1959. S. Afr. Med. J., 34:520–524, 1960.
768. Shannon, J.B., Woolhouse, F.M., Eisinger, P.J.: The Treatment of Chronic Osteomyelitis by Saucerization and Immediate Skin Grafting. Clin. Orthop., 96:98–107, 1973.
769. Shinto, Y., Uchida, A., Korkusuz, F., Araki, N., Ono, K.: Calcium Hydroxyapatite Ceramic Used as a Delivery System for Antibiotics. J. Bone Joint Surg., 74B:600–604, 1992.
770. Slack, W.K., Thomas, D.A., Perrins, D.J.D.: Hyperbaric Oxygenation in Chronic Osteomyelitis. Lancet, 1:1093–1094, 1965.
771. Stiefeld, S.M., Graziani, A.L., MacGregor, R.R., Esterhai, J.L., Jr.: Toxicities of Antimicrobial Agents Used to Treat Osteomyelitis. (Review) Orthop. Clin. North Am., 22:439–465, 1991.
772. Subramanian, G., and McAfee, J.G.: A New Complex of ^{99m}Tc for Skeletal Imaging. Radiology, 99:192–196, 1971.
773. Tehranzadeh, J., Wang, F., Mesgarzadeh, M.: Magnetic Resonance Imaging of Osteomyelitis. (Review) Crit. Rev. Diagn. Imaging, 33:495–534, 1992.
774. Tetzlaff, T.R., Howard, J.B., McCracken, G.H., Calderon, E., Larrondo, J.: Antibiotic Concentrations in Pus and Bone of Children With Osteomyelitis. J. Pediatr., 92:135–140, 1978.
775. Tetzlaff, T.R., McCracken, G.H., Nelson, J.D.: Oral Antibiotic Therapy for Skeletal Infections of Children. J. Pediatr., 92:485–490, 1978.
776. Trueta, J.: The Three Types of Acute Haematogenous Osteomyelitis: A Clinical and Vascular Study. J. Bone Joint Surg., 41B:671–680, 1959.
777. Tuazon, C.U., and Sheagren, J.N.: Teichoic Acid Antibodies in the Diagnosis of Serious Infections With *Staphylococcus aureus*. Ann. Intern. Med., 84:543–546, 1976.
778. Verklin, R.M., and Mandell, G.L.: Alteration of Effectiveness of Antibiotics by Anaerobiosis. J. Lab. Clin. Med., 80:65–71, 1977.
779. Waldvogel, F.A.: Use of Quinolones for the Treatment of Osteomyelitis and Septic Arthritis. (Review) Rev. Infect. Dis., 11(Suppl 5):S1259–S1263, 1989.
780. Waldvogel, F.A., Medoff, G., Swartz, M.N.: Osteomyelitis. Clinical Features, Therapeutic Considerations, and Unusual Aspects, pp. 1–101. Springfield, Ill., Charles C. Thomas, 1971.
781. Waldvogel, F.A., and Vasey, H.: Osteomyelitis: The Past Decade. N. Engl. J. Med., 303:360–370, 1980.
782. Weiland, A.J., Moore, J.R., Daniel, R.K.: The Efficacy of Free Tissue Transfer in the Treatment of Osteomyelitis. J. Bone Joint Surg., 66A:181, 1984.
783. Weinstein, M.P., Stratton, C.W., Hawley, H.B., Ackley, A., Reller, L.B.: Multicenter Collaborative Evaluation of Standardized Serum Bactericidal Test as a Predictor of Therapeutic Efficacy in Acute and Chronic Osteomyelitis. Am. J. Med., 83:218–222, 1987.
784. Whalen, J.L., Brown, M.L., McLeod, R., Fitzgerald, R.H.: Limitations of Indium Leukocyte Imaging for the Diagnosis of Spine Infections. Spine, 16:193–197, 1991.
785. Widmer, A., Gaechter, A., Ochsner, P., Zimmerli, W.: Antimicrobial Treatment of Orthopedic Implant-Related Infections With Rifampin Combinations. Clin. Infect. Dis., 14:1251–1253, 1992.
786. Wilson, F.C., Worcester, J.N., Coleman, P.D., Byrd, W.E.: Antibiotic Penetration of Experimental Bone Hematomas. J. Bone Joint Surg., 53A:1622–1628, 1971.
787. Wood, M.B., Cooney, W.P., III, Irons, G.B., Jr.: Skeletal Reconstruction by Vascularized Bone Transfer: Indications and Results. Mayo Clin. Proc., 60:729–734, 1985.
788. Worlock, P., Slack, R., Harvey, L., MaWhinney, R.: The Prevention of Infection in Open Fractures. An Experimental Study of the Effect of Antibiotic Therapy. J. Bone Joint Surg., 70A:1341–1347, 1988.
789. Wukich, D., Abreu, S., Callaghan, J., et al.: Diagnosis of Infection by Preoperative Scintigraphy With Indium-Labelled White Blood Cells. J. Bone Joint Surg., 69A:1353–1360, 1987.

POST-TRAUMATIC REFLEX SYMPATHETIC DYSTROPHY

790. Amadio, P.: Current Concepts Review. Pain Dysfunction Syndromes. J. Bone Joint Surg., 70A:944–949, 1988.
791. An, H.S., Hawthorne, K.B., Jackson, W.T.: Reflex Sympathetic Dystrophy and Cigarette Smoking. J. Hand Surg., 13A:458, 1988.
792. Arias, L.M., Schwartzman, R.J., Bartkowski, R., et al.: Sufentanil Stellate Ganglion Injection in the Treatment of Refractory Reflex Sympathetic Dystrophy. Reg. Anaesth., 14:90–92, 1989.
793. Ascherl, R., and Blumel, G.: Clinical Picture in Sudeck's Dystrophy. Fortschr. Med., 99:712–720, 1981.
794. Awerbuch, M.S.: Thermography: Its Current Diagnostic Status in Musculoskeletal Medicine. Med. J. Aust., 154:441–444, 1991.
795. Bayles, T.B., Judson, W.E., Potter, T.A.: Reflex Sympathetic Dystrophy of the Upper Extremity (Hand-Shoulder Syndrome). J.A.M.A., 144:537–542, 1950.
796. Benzon, H.T., Chomka, C.M., Brunner, E.A.: Treatment of Reflex Sympathetic Dystrophy With Regional Intravenous Reserpine. Anesth. Analg., 59:500–502, 1980.
797. Berger, H.: The Treatment of Postmyocardial Infarction Shoulder-Hand Syndrome With Local Hydrocortisone. Postgrad. Med., 15:508–511, 1954.
798. Bickerstaff, D.R., and Kanis, J.A.: The Use of Nasal Calcitonin in the Treatment of Posttraumatic Algodystrophy. Br. J. Rheumatol., 30:291–294, 1991.
799. Birkenfeld, B.: Erfahrungen mit der Echinacin-Therapie beim Sudeckschen Syndrom. Ther. Ggw., 93:425, 1954.
800. Blanchard, J., Ramamurthy, S., Walsh, N., et al.: Intravenous Regional Sympatholysis: A Double-Blind Comparison of Guanethidine, Reserpine, and Normal Saline. Journal of Pain and Symptom Management, 5:357, 1990.
801. Chapman, L.F., Ramos, A.O., Goodell, H., Wolff, H.G.: Neurohumoral Features of Afferent Fibers in Man. Arch. Neurol., 4:617–650, 1961.
802. Chaturvedi, S.K.: Phenytoin in Reflex Sympathetic Dystrophy. Pain, 36:379–380, 1989.
803. Chuinard, R.G., Dabezies, E.J., Goud, J.S., Murphy, G.A., Matthews, R.E.: Intravenous Reserpine for Treatment of Reflex Sympathetic Dystrophy. South. Med. J., 74:1481–1484, 1981.
804. Coffman, J.D., and Davies, W.T.: Vasospastic Diseases: A Review. Prog. Cardiovasc. Dis., 18:123–146, 1975.
805. Collins, W.F., and Randt, C.T.: Evoked Central Nervous System Activity to Peripheral Unmyelinated or "C" Fibers in Cat. J. Neurophysiol., 21:345–352, 1958.
806. Cooper, D., DeLee, J., Ramamurthy, S.: Reflex Sympathetic Dystrophy of the Knee. Treatment Using Continuous Epidural Anesthesia. J. Bone Joint Surg., 71A:365–369, 1989.
807. de Takats, G.: The Technic of Lumbar Sympathectomy. Surg. Clin. North Am., 26:56–69, 1946.
808. de Takats, G.: Sympathetic Reflex Dystrophy. Med. Clin. North Am., 49:117–129, 1965.
809. Doury, P., Grainer, R., Pattin, S.: The Use of Bone Scintigraphy With Technetium 99m Pyrophosphates in the Diagnosis of Algodystrophies. A Report of 74 Observations. Ann. Med. Interne (Paris), 130:553–557, 1979.
810. Drucker, W.R., Hubay, C.A., Holden, W.D., Bukovnic, J.A.: Pathogenesis of Posttraumatic Sympathetic Dystrophy. Am. J. Surg., 97:454–465, 1959.
811. Duncan, K.H., Lewis, R.C., Racz, G., et al.: Treatment of Upper Extremity Reflex Sympathetic Dystrophy With Joint Stiffness Using Sympatholytic Bier Blocks and Manipulation. Orthopedics, 11:883–886, 1988.
812. Dwyer, A.F.: Sudeck's Atrophy and Cortisone. Med. J. Aust., 2:265–268, 1952.
813. Dzwierzynski, W.W., and Sanger, J.R.: Reflex Sympathetic Dystrophy. Hand Clin., 10:29–44, 1994.
814. Edmondson, A.S., and Calandruccio, R.A.: Drug Therapy for Causalgia Syndrome. Mississippi Doctor, 34:239–241, 1957.
815. Erdemir, H., Gelman, S., Galbraith, J.G.: Prediction of the Needed Level of Sympathectomy for Posttraumatic Reflex Sympathetic Dystrophy. Surg. Neurol., 17:353–354, 1982.

816. Eulry, F., Lechevalier, D., Pats, B., et al.: Regional Intravenous Guanethidine Blocks in Algodystrophy. Clin. Rheumatol., 10:377–383, 1991.
817. Evans, J.A.: Reflex Sympathetic Dystrophy. Surg. Gynecol. Obstet., 82:36–43, 1946.
818. Farcot, J.M., Mangin, P., Laugner, B., Thiebaut, J.B., Foucher, G.: Regional Intravenous Guanethidine for Sympathetic Block Algodystrophic Syndromes. Anesth. Analg., 38:383–385, 1981.
819. Feldman, F.: Thermography of the Hand and Wrist: Practical Applications. Hand Clin., 7:99–112, 1991.
820. Ford, S.R., Forrest, W.H., Eltherington, L.: The Treatment of Reflex Sympathetic Dystrophy With Intravenous Regional Bretylium. Anesthesiology, 68:137–140, 1988.
821. Fowler, F.D., and Moser, M.: Use of Hexamethonium and Dibenzyline in Diagnosis and Treatment of Causalgia. J.A.M.A., 161:1051–1053, 1956.
822. Gaucher, A., Columb, J.N., Naoun, A., et al.: Scintigraphic Characteristics of Coxopathies: Etiologic Importance. Rev. Rhum. Mal. Osteoartic., 45:641–648, 1978.
823. Glynn, C.J., Basedow, R.W., Walsh, J.A.: Pain Relief Following Post-ganglionic Sympathetic Blockage With IV Guanethidine. Br. J. Anesth., 53:1297–1302, 1981.
824. Gobelet, C., Waldburger, M., Meier, J.L.: The Effect of Adding Calcitonin to Physical Treatment on Reflex Sympathetic Dystrophy. Pain, 48:171–175, 1992.
825. Granit, R., Leksell, L., Skoglund, C.R.: Fibre Interaction in Injured or Compressed Region of Nerve. Brain, 67:125–140, 1944.
826. Grunert, B.K., Devine, C.A., Sanger, J.R., et al.: Thermal Self-Regulation for Pain Control in Reflex Sympathetic Dystrophy Syndrome. J. Hand Surg., 15A:615–618, 1990.
827. Hardy, M.A., Merritt, W.H.: Psychological Evaluation and Pain Assessment in Patients With Reflex Sympathetic Dystrophy. Journal of Hand Therapy, 3:155–164, 1988.
828. Hartley, J.: Reflex Hyperemic Deossification (Sudeck's Atrophy). Journal of the Mount Sinai Hospital, 22:268–277, 1955.
829. Helms, C.A., O'Brien, E.T., Katzberg, R.W.: Segmental Reflex Sympathetic Dystrophy Syndrome. Radiology, 135:67–68, 1980.
830. Herrmann, L.G., and Caldwell, J.A.: Diagnosis and Treatment of Posttraumatic Osteoporosis. Am. J. Surg., 51:630–640, 1941.
831. Herrmann, L.G., Reineke, H.G., Caldwell, J.A.: Posttraumatic Painful Osteoporosis. A Clinical and Roentgenological Entity. A.J.R. Am. J. Roentgenol., 47:353–361, 1942.
832. Hilker, A.W: The Shoulder-Hand Syndrome. A Complication of Coronary Artery Disease. Ann. Intern. Med., 31:303–311, 1949.
833. Homans, J.: Minor Causalgia. A Hyperesthetic Neurovascular Syndrome. N. Engl. J. Med., 222:870–874, 1940.
834. Hord, A.H., Rooks, M.D., Stephens, B.O., et al.: Intravenous Regional Bretylium and Lidocaine for Treatment of Reflex Sympathetic Dystrophy: A Randomized, Double-Blind Study. Anesth. Analg., 74:818–821, 1992.
835. Johnson, A.C.: Disabling Changes in the Hand Resembling Sclerodactylia Following Myocardial Infarction. Ann. Intern. Med., 19:433–456, 1943.
836. Johnson, E.W., and Pannozzo, A.N.: Management of Shoulder Hand Syndrome. J.A.M.A, 195:108–110, 1966.
837. Kirklin, J.W., Chenoweth, A.I., Murphey, F.: Causalgia: A Review of Its Characteristics, Diagnosis and Treatment. Surgery, 21:321–342, 1947.
838. Kozin, F., Soin, J.S., Ryan L.M., Carrera, G.F., Wortmann, R.L.: Bone Scintigraphy in the Reflex Sympathetic Dystrophy Syndrome. Radiology, 138:437–443, 1981.
839. Ladd, A.L., DeHaven, K.E., Thanik, J., Patt, R., Feuerstein, M.A.: Reflex Sympathetic Imbalance: Response to Epidural Blockade. Am. J. Sports Med., 17:660–668, 1989.
840. Lankford, L.L.: Reflex Sympathetic Dystropy. *In* Omer, G.E., Jr., and Spinner, M. (eds.): Management of Peripheral Nerve Problems, pp. 216–244. Philadelphia, W.B. Saunders, 1980.
841. Lenggenhager, K.: Sudeck's Osteodystrophy: Its Pathogenesis, Prophylaxis, and Therapy. Minn. Med., 54:967–972, 1971.
842. Lewis, D., and Gatewood, W.: Treatment of Causalgia: Results of Intraneural Injection of 60 per Cent Alcohol. J.A.M.A., 74:1–4, 1920.
843. Livingston, W.K.: Pain Mechanism: A Physiologic Interpretation of Causalagia and Its Related State, pp. 1–248. New York, Macmillan, 1943.
844. MacKinnon, S., and Holder, L.: The Use of Three-Phase Radionuclide Bone Scanning in the Diagnosis of Reflex Sympathetic Dystrophy. J. Hand Surg., 9A:556–563, 1984.
845. Marti, T.: Wesen und Behandlung des Sudeckschen Syndroms. Praxis, 43:742, 1954.
846. Mayfield, F.H., and Devine, J.W.: Causalgia. Surg. Gynecol. Obstet., 80:631–635, 1945.
847. McDougall, I.R., and Keeling, C.A.: Complications of Fractures and Their Healing. Semin. Nucl. Med., 18:113–125, 1988.
848. Miller, D.S., and de Takats, G.: Post-traumatic Dystrophy of the Extremities: Sudeck's Atrophy. Surg. Gynecol. Obstet., 75:558–582, 1942.
849. Mitchell, S.W.: Injuries of Nerves, pp. 1–164. Philadelphia, J.B. Lippincott, 1864.
850. Mitchell, S.W.: The Medical Department in the Civil War. J.A.M.A., 62:1445–1450, 1914.
851. Moberg, E.: The Shoulder-Hand-Finger Syndrome. Acta. Chir. Scand., 109:284–292, 1955.
852. Munch-Peterson, C.U.: The So-Called Shoulder-Hand Syndrome. Nord. Med., 51:291–293, 1954.
853. Nathan, P.W.: On Pathogenesis of Causalgia in Peripheral Nerve Injuries. Brain, 70:145–170, 1947.
854. Omer, G.E., Jr., and Thomas, S.: Treatment of Causalgia: Review of Cases at Brooke General Hospital. Tex. Med., 67:93–96, 1971.
855. Oppenheimer, A.: The Swollen Atrophic Hand. Surg. Gynecol. Obstet., 67:446–454, 1938.
856. Pak, T.J., Martin, G.M., Magness, J.L., Kavanaugh, G.J.: Reflex Sympathetic Dystrophy, Review of 140 Cases. Minn. Med., 53:507–512, 1970.
857. Plewes, L.W.: Sudeck's Atrophy in the Hand. J. Bone Joint Surg., 38B:195–203, 1956.
858. Pool, J.L., and Brabson, J.A.: Pain on Stimulating the Distal Segment of Divided Peripheral Nerves. J. Neurosurg., 3:468–473, 1946.
859. Porter, J.M., Lindell, T.D., Leung, B.S., Reiney, C.G.: Effect of Intra-arterial Injection of Reserpine on Vascular Wall Catecholamine Content. Surg. Forum, 23:183–195, 1972.
860. Procacci, P., Francini, F., Maresca, M., Zoppi, M.: Skin Potentials and EMG Changes Induced by Cutaneous Electrical Stimulation. II. Subjects With Reflex Sympathetic Dystrophies. Appl. Neurophysiol., 42:125–134, 1979.
861. Reiner, J.C., Moreau, R., Bernat, M., Basle, M., Jallet, P., Minier, J.F.: Contribution of Dynamic Isotopic Tests in the Study of Algodystrophies. Rev. Rhum. Mal. Osteoartic., 46:235–251, 1979.
862. Richards, R.L.: Causalgia: A Centennial Review. Arch. Neurol., 6:339–350, 1967.
863. Rocco, A.G., Kaul, A.F., Reisman, R.M., et al.: A Comparison of Regional Intravenous Guanethidine and Reserpine in Reflex Sympathetic Dystrophy: A Controlled, Randomized, Double-Blind Crossover Study. Clin. J. Pain, 5:205–209, 1989.
864. Roland, O.: Unsere Erfahrungen mit Depot-Padutin. Zentralbl. Chir., 77:1–147, 1942.
865. Rose, T.F.: Sudeck's Post-traumatic Osteodystrophy of Limbs. Med. J. Aust., 1:185–188, 1953.
866. Rosen, P.S., and Graham, W.: The Shoulder-Hand Syndrome. Can. Med. Assoc. J., 77:86–91, 1957.
867. Schutzer, S., and Gossling, H.: Current Concepts Review. The Treatment of Reflex Sympathetic Dystrophy Syndrome. J. Bone Joint Surg. 66A:625–629, 1984.
868. Simon, H., and Carlson, D.H.: The Use of Bone Scanning in the Diagnosis of Reflex Sympathetic Dystrophy. Clin. Nucl. Med., 5:116–121, 1980.

869. Simson, G.: Propranolol for Causalgia and Sudeck Atrophy. (Letter) J.A.M.A., 227:327, 1974.
870. Smithwick, R.H.: The Value of Sympathectomy in the Treatment of Vascular Disease. N. Engl. J. Med., 216:414, 1937.
871. Speigel, I.J., and Milowsky, J.L.: Causalgia. J.A.M.A., 127:9–15, 1945.
872. Spurling, R.G.: Causalgia of the Upper Extremity: Treatment by Dorsal Sympathetic Ganglionectomy. Arch. Neurol. Psychiatr., 23:784–788, 1930.
873. Steinbrocker, O., and Argyros, T.G.: The Shoulder-Hand Syndrome, Present Status as a Diagnostic and Therapeutic Entity. Med. Clin. North Am., 42:1533–1553, 1958.
874. Steinbrocker, O., Neustadt, D., Lapin, L.: The Shoulder-Hand Syndrome. Sympathetic Block Compared With Corticotropin and Cortisone Therapy. J.A.M.A, 153:788–791, 1953.
875. Steinbrocker, O., Spitzer, N., Friedman, H.H.: The Shoulder-Hand Syndrome in Reflex Dystrophy of the Upper Extremity. Ann. Intern. Med., 29:22–52, 1948.
876. Sudeck, P.: Ueber die akute entzundlicke knocke Atrophie. Arch. Klin. Chir., 62:147–156, 1900.
877. Sudeck, P.: Ueber die akute (trophoneurotische) Knockenatrophie nach Entzundungen und Traume der Extremitaten. Dtsch. Med. Wochenschr., 28:336–338, 1902.
878. Sunderland, S.: Pain Mechanisms in Causalgia. J. Neurol. Neurosurg. Psychiatry, 39:471–480, 1976.
879. Swan, D.M.: Shoulder-Hand Syndrome Following Hemiplegia. Neurology, 4:480–482, 1954.
880. Threadgill, F.D.: Afferent Conduction Via the Sympathetic Ganglia Innervating the Extremities. Surgery, 21:569–594, 1947.
881. Toumey, J.W.: Occurrence and Management of Reflex Sympathetic Dystrophy (Causalgia of the Extremities). J. Bone Joint Surg., 30A:883–894, 1948.
882. Visitsunthorn, U., and Prete, P.: Reflex Sympathetic Dystrophy of the Lower Extremity: A Complication of Herpes Zoster With Dramatic Response of Propranolol. West. J. Med., 135:62–66, 1981.
883. Walker, A.E., and Nulsen, F.: Electrical Stimulation of the Upper Thoracic Portion of the Sympathetic Chain in Man. Arch. Neurol. Psychiatr., 59:559–560, 1948.
884. Watson, H.K., and Carlson, L.: Treatment of Reflex Sympathetic Dystrophy of the Hand With an Active "Stress Loading" Program. J. Hand Surg., 12A:779–785, 1987.
885. White, J.C., Heroy, W.W., Goodman, E.N.: Causalgia Following Gunshot Injuries of Nerves. Ann. Surg., 128:161–183, 1948.
886. William, E.: Treatment of Reflex Sympathetic Dystrophy by Calcitonin. Rev. Med. Brux., 1:457–461, 1980.
887. Young, J.H., and Pearson, A.T.: The Shoulder-Hand Syndrome. Med. J. Aust., 1:776–780, 1952.
888. Zucchini, M., Alberti, G., Moretti, M.P.: Algodystrophy and Related Psychological Features. Funct. Neurol., 4:153–156, 1989.

COMPARTMENT SYNDROMES

889. Ashton, H.: The Effect of Increased Tissue Pressure on Blood Flow. Clin. Orthop., 113:15–26, 1975.
890. Benjamin, A.: The Relief of Inflatable Plastic Splints on Blood Flow. B.M.J., 2:1427–1430, 1966.
891. Bradley, E.L.: The Anterior Tibial Compartment Syndrome. Surg. Gynecol. Obstet., 136:289–297, 1973.
892. Burton, A.C.: On the Physical Equilibrium of Small Blood Vessels. Am. J. Physiol., 164:319–329, 1951.
893. Caldwell, R.K.: Ischemic Necrosis of the Anterior Tibial Muscle: Case Report With Autopsy Findings and Review of Literature. Ann. Intern. Med., 46:1191–1199, 1957.
894. Carter, A.B., Richards, R.L., Zachary, R.: The Anterior Tibial Syndrome. Lancet, 2:928–934, 1949.
895. Cywes, S., and Louw, J.H.: Phlegmasia Cerula Dolens: Successful Treatment by Relieving Fasciotomy. Surgery, 51:169–176, 1962.
896. Eaton, R.G., and Green, W.T.: Epimysiotomy and Fasciotomy in the Treatment of Volkmann's Ischemic Contracture. Orthop. Clin. North Am., 3:175–186, 1972.
897. Ernst, C.B., and Kaufer, H.: Fibulectomy-Fasciotomy: An Important Adjunct in the Management of Lower Extremity Arterial Trauma. J. Trauma, 11:365–380, 1971.
898. Garfin, S., Mubarak, S., Evans, K., Hargens, A., Akeson, W.: Quantification of Intracompartmental Pressure and Volume Under Plaster Casts. J. Bone Joint Surg., 63A:449–453, 1981.
899. Gaspard, D.J., Cohen, S.L., Gaspard, M.R.: Decompression Dermotomy: A Limb Salvage Adjunct. J.A.M.A., 220:831–833, 1972.
900. Gaspard, D.J., and Kohl, R.D.: Compartmental Syndromes in Which the Skin Is the Limiting Boundary. Clin. Orthop., 113:65–68, 1975.
901. Harman, J.W., and Gwinn, R.P.: The Significance of Local Vascular Phenomena in the Production of Ischemic Necrosis in Skeletal Muscle. Am. J. Pathol., 24:625–638, 1948.
902. Harman, J.W., and Gwinn, R.: The Recovery of Skeletal Muscle Fibers From Acute Ischemia as Determined by Histologic and Chemical Methods. Am. J. Pathol., 25:741–755, 1949.
903. Holden, C.E.A.: Traumatic Tension Ischaemia in Muscles. Injury, 5:223, 1973.
904. Jepson, P.N.: Ischemic Contracture, Experimental Study. Ann. Surg., 84:785–795, 1926.
905. Jones, W., Perry, M., Bush, H.: Changes in Tibial Venous Blood Flow in the Evolving Compartment Syndrome. Arch. Surg., 124:801–804, 1989.
906. Kirby, N.G.: Exercise Ischaemia in the Fascial Compartment of the Soleus: Case Report. J. Bone Joint Surg., 52B:738–740, 1970.
907. Kjellmer, I.: An Indirect Method for Estimating Tissue Pressure With Special Reference to Tissue Pressure in Muscle During Exercise. Acta Physiol. Scand., 62:31–40, 1964.
908. Klock, J.C., and Sexton, M.J.: Rhabdomyolysis and Acute Myoglobinuric Renal Failure Following Heroin Use. Calif. Med., 119:5–8, 1973.
909. Lewis, T.: Vascular Disorders of the Limbs, 1–107. London, McMillan, 1936.
910. Lowenberg, E.L.: Acute Ischemic Infarction of the Gastrocnemius Muscle Simulating Deep Vein Phlebitis. J. Cardiovasc. Surg., 6:104–110, 1965.
911. Lundborg, G.: Limb Ischemia and Nerve Injury. Arch. Surg., 104:631–632, 1972.
912. McQuillan, W.M., and Nolan, B.: Ischaemia Complicating Injury. J. Bone Joint Surg., 50B:482–492, 1968.
913. Manson, I.W.: Post-Partum Eclampsia Complicated by the Anterior Tibial Syndrome. B.M.J., 2:1117–1118, 1964.
914. Matsen, F.A., III: Compartmental Syndrome: A Unified Concept. Clin. Orthop., 113:8–14, 1975.
915. Mubarak, S.J., and Owen, C.A.: Double-Incision Fasciotomy of the Leg for Decompression in Compartment Syndromes. J. Bone Joint Surg., 59A:184–187, 1977.
916. Parkes, A.R.: Traumatic Ischemia of Peripheral Nerves With Some Observations on Volkmann's Ischemic Contracture. Br. J. Surg., 32:403–413, 1944.
917. Reneman, R.S.: The Anterior and the Lateral Compartment Syndrome of the Leg. The Hague, Mouton, 1968.
918. Reneman, R.S.: The Anterior and the Lateral Compartment Syndrome of the Leg Due to Intensive Use of Muscles. Clin. Orthop., 113:69–80, 1975.
919. Reneman, R.S., and Jagenean, A.H.: The Influence of Weighted Exercise on Tissue (Intramuscular) Pressure in Normal Subjects and Patients With Intermittent Claudication. Scand. J. Clin. Lab. Invest. Suppl., 128:37, 1973.
920. Reszel, P.A., Jones, J.M., Spittell, J.A.: Ischemic Necrosis of the Peroneal Musculature, A Lateral Compartment Syndrome: A Report of a Case. Mayo Clin. Proc., 38:130, 1963.
921. Sanderson, R.A., Foley, R.K., McIvor, G., Kirkaldy-Willis, W.H.: Histological Response on Skeletal Muscle to Ischemia. Clin. Orthop., 113:27–35, 1975.
922. Schreiber, S., Liebowitz, M., Berstein, L.: Limb Compression and Renal Impairment (Crush Syndrome) Following Narcotic Overdose. J. Bone Joint Surg., 54A:1683–1692, 1972.
923. Schrock, R.D.: Peroneal Nerve Palsy Following Derotation Osteotomies for Tibial Torsion. Clin. Orthop., 62:172–177, 1969.

924. Spinner, M., Mache, A., Silver, L., Barsky, A.J.: Impending Ischemic Contracture of the Hand. Plast. Reconstr. Surg., 50:341–349, 1972.
925. Sweeney, H.E., and O'Brien, G.F.: Bilateral Anterior Tibial Syndrome in Association With the Nephrotic Syndrome: Report of a Case. Arch. Intern. Med., 116:487–490, 1965.
926. Tachdjian, M.O.: Pediatric Orthopaedics, pp. 1–766. Philadelphia, W.B. Saunders, 1972.
927. Thomson, S.A., and Mahoney, L.J.: Volkmann's Ischaemic Contracture and Its Relationship to Fracture of the Femur. J. Bone Joint Surg., 33B:336–347, 1951.
928. Volkmann, R.: Die Krankheiten der Bewegung surgane. *In* Pitha, R.V., and Billroth, W.M. (eds.): Handbuch der Chirurgie, vol. 2. Stuttgart, Ferdinand Enke, 1872.
929. Volkmann, R.: Die ischaemischem Muskellamungen und Kontrakturen. Zentralbl. Chir., 8:801, 1881.
930. Weitz, E.M., and Carson, G.: The Anterior Tibial Compartment Syndrome in a Twenty-Month-Old Infant: A Complication of the Use of a Bow Leg Brace. Bull. Hosp. Jt. Dis. Orthop. Inst., 30:16, 1969.
931. Whitesides, T.E., Harada, H., Morimoto, K.: The Response of Skeletal Muscle to Temporary Ischemia: An Experimental Study. J. Bone Joint Surg., 53A:1027–1028,1971.
932. Whitesides, T.E., Jr., Haney, T.C., Morimoto, K., Harada, H.: Tissue Pressure Measurements as a Determinant for the Need of Fasciotomy. Clin. Orthop., 113:43–51, 1975.
933. Willhoite, D.R., and Moll, J.H.: Early Recognition and Treatment of Impending Volkmann's Ischemia in the Lower Extremity. Arch. Surg., 100:11–16, 1970.

Rockwood and Green's Fractures in Adults, Fourth Edition,
edited by Charles A. Rockwood, David P. Green, Robert W. Bucholz and James D. Heckman.
Lippincott-Raven Publishers, Philadelphia © 1996.

CHAPTER 9

Pathologic Fractures

Dempsey Springfield and Candace Jennings

A pathologic fracture is a fracture of abnormal bone. Typically, the fracture occurs during normal activity or with minor trauma, and the failure of bone under these circumstances should alert the surgeon to the presence of a predisposing pathologic condition. The orthopaedic surgeon must do more than just treat the broken bone because successful management of the patient requires recognition, diagnosis, and treatment of the underlying process. The management of the fracture may be dramatically altered by the associated pathologic condition, and failure to adjust the fracture management may lead to unnecessary additional difficulties. Osteoporosis is the most common pathologic condition associated with pathologic fracture, and the management of fractured osteoporotic bone may require special techniques to achieve adequate internal fixation.[4] This chapter discusses only briefly the management of fractures of osteoporotic bone. What is usually thought of when pathologic fractures are discussed is carcinoma metastatic to bone with a fracture or "impending fracture," and this chapter concentrates on the management of patients with these fractures. Other associated conditions, however, include underlying metabolic disorders, primary benign tumors, and primary malignant tumors. It is also important to remember that the management of patients with pathologic fractures demands more of the orthopaedic surgeon than the management of similar fractures in normal bone. Initial management, well planned and well executed, dramatically improves a patient's life, whereas treatment that is not planned and done well condemns the patient to far more difficulty.

INITIAL EVALUATION

History and Physical

A patient who presents with a fracture occurring spontaneously or after minor trauma, who has an unusual fracture pattern, has had several recent fractures, is older, or has a history of a primary malignancy should alert the physician to the possibility of an associated pathologic process. A complete history must be obtained from the patient, beginning with the circumstances surrounding the current injury; the degree of trauma provides information about the strength of the bone. Patients must be asked specifically about previously diagnosed or treated malignancies because they may consider themselves to be "cured" and no longer at risk for recurrence or metastases. Standard questions regarding general health, including recent weight loss, fevers, night sweats, and fatigue, are important. Questions about relevant risk factors such as smoking, dietary habits, and environmental exposures should be asked, and a careful review of systems is essential.

The physical examination should be thorough, with careful palpation for lymphadenopathy in the neck, supraclavicular fossa, axilla, and inguinal region; thyroid nodules; breast masses; prostate nodules; rectal masses; and rectal tone. A stool guaiac test is always performed. Because common things occur commonly, the history and physical examination should be considered to be a search for the most likely causes of pathologic fractures (ie, metastatic malignancy and osteoporosis). An adequate evaluation requires a careful and thorough examination of the patient. This can be done by an internist in consultation or by the treating orthopaedist.

Radiography

Radiographs of the symptomatic extremity should be obtained and carefully reviewed, with attention to specific lesions and overall bone quality. The pathologic lesion may be obvious, and frequently a diagnosis can be made from the initial radiographs, history, and physical examination. If the diagnosis is not obvious after the initial evaluation, the radiographs should be examined for diagnostic clues, such as generalized osteopenia, periosteal reaction, thinning of the cortices, abnormal radiodensity in the bone or soft tissue, Looser's lines, calcification of the small vessels, and abnormal soft-tissue shadows.

Osteopenia is the term used to indicate either inadequate bone (osteoporosis) or inadequately mineralized bone (osteomalacia). Using only plain radiographs, the physician usually cannot distinguish between these two disorders but there are suggestive differential clues. Looser's lines (compression-side radiolucent lines), calcification of small vessels, and phalangeal periosteal reaction are features of osteomalacia or hyperparathyroidism. Thin cortices and loss of the normal trabecular pattern without other abnormalities are most suggestive of osteoporosis.

The plain radiographs should be carefully and systematically examined. Initially, the focus should be on the not so obvious; ignore the fracture for a moment. Look at the remainder of the bone. Are there other lesions? Does the bone have an apparent abnormal density? Are there any extraosseous masses or abnormalities? Now look at the lesion. Its location in the bone is an important diagnostic clue. Metastatic deposits in bone are usually eccentric, with involvement of the cortex. Most commonly, they occur at the diaphyseal/metaphyseal junction but they can be located anywhere in any bone. Look for densities within the lesion. Bone formation suggests an osteosarcoma, whereas calcification suggests a chondrosarcoma. How well-developed is the reaction? The more developed the reaction (periosteal or endosteal), the less likely the lesion is malignant. How permeative is the lesion? How well can you identify the border between the normal bone and the lesion? The appearance of this interface (lesion and normal bone) is another clue to the biologic activity of the lesion. The more easily the border is seen and the sharper the transition from lesion to normal bone, the less active the lesion and the less likely it is to be malignant. Radiologists often refer to this relation as the "border of transition," and it has been suggested that the broader the border of transition, the more likely the lesion is to be malignant.

Often, careful examination of the plain radiograph provides sufficient information for a specific diagnosis.[83,84] For example, giant cell tumor of bone is almost always recognizable by its appearance (a radiolucent lesion; narrow border of transition, involving the metaphysis and epiphysis to the subchondral bone) and when a patient presents with a pathologic fracture through a clinically apparent giant cell tumor of bone, an immediate biopsy is rarely necessary. Another example of a lesion that can be diagnosed from the plain radiograph is nonossifying fibroma. These lesions are so typical (eccentric, radiolucent, narrow border of transition, metaphyseal/diaphyseal, rimmed with a thin reactive shell of bone) that when a patient presents with a pathologic fracture through a nonossifying fibroma, biopsy is not necessary. When an accurate specific diagnosis cannot be made from the plain radiograph and especially when a primary malignancy is in the differential diagnosis, a biopsy needs to be performed early. Before the biopsy, the patient's lesion must be thoroughly evaluated. A thorough evaluation is one that permits definitive treatment immediately after obtaining a specific histologic diagnosis.

When there is an identifiable specific lesion within otherwise normal bone, the initial decision is whether the lesion is inactive (most likely benign) or aggressive (most likely malignant). Small radiolucent lesions that are surrounded by a rim of reactive bone without endosteal or periosteal reaction are inactive or minimally active (ie, usually benign) primary bone tumors. Lesions that erode the cortex but are contained by a well-developed periosteal reaction are usually active benign or a low-grade malignant primary bone tumor but a metastatic deposit can also have this appearance. Large lesions that destroy the cortex and are not contained by the periosteum are aggressive lesions and usually malignant, either primary or metastatic. A permeative or "moth-eaten" pattern of cortical destruction is most suggestive of a malignancy. Most destructive bone lesions in adults are metastatic carcinoma; however, a solitary bone lesion should be initially considered to be a primary sarcoma until a primary carcinoma is found or a biopsy reveals metastatic carcinoma or myeloma. Primary bone tumors are most common in patients younger than 50 years of age and usually arise in the metaphysis of a long bone. Some lesions are essentially pathognomonic for metastatic carcinoma; for example, an avulsion fracture of the lesser trochanter is almost always pathologic, and this specific injury should arouse suspicion of occult metastatic disease (Fig. 9-1).[11,111] Cortical lesions in adults are usually metastases.[29,53]

When a metastasis is suspected, the remainder of the skeleton should be evaluated for other sites of disease. Few things should be as embarrassing for an orthopaedic surgeon as missing an impending fracture at another site in a patient being treated for a pathologic fracture due to metastatic carcinoma.

The most common sites of carcinoma metastatic to bone are the spine, ribs, pelvis, femur, and humerus; only rarely do they occur distal to the knees or elbows.[2,10,81,107,109,112,143,146] Therefore, plain radiographs should be obtained of the bones at most risk. Plain radiographs of any tender bone also should be examined. A whole-body technetium 99m (^{99m}Tc) scan is a useful screen for the entire skeleton[27,31] but we recommend plain radiographs of both humeri, the pelvis, and both femurs in addition to the bone scan. These bones are at risk for pathologic fracture, and plain radiographic assessment can be done easily and safely. Finding an impending fracture in a patient having a pathologic fracture can significantly reduce a patient's morbidity. In a study of patients having breast carcinoma, 24% of the patients with a small primary lesion, an otherwise normal physical examination, normal findings from serum chemistries, and normal plain radiographs had a bone scan that revealed skeletal metastases. The prognostic value of the bone scan was also demonstrated because 100% of patients with an abnormal bone scan on initial staging had recurrent disease at 5 years, whereas only 26% of those with a normal scan had evidence of disease at the same follow-up interval.[27]

We agree with Steckel and Kagan,[130] who recommend a limited search for the unknown primary carcinoma. Carcinoma of the breast and carcinoma of the lung are the source of most metastases to bone; therefore, a chest radiograph, breast examination, and mammogram are recommended.[1,2,146] Renal, thyroid, and prostate carcinomas are the other three tumors that frequently go to bone, and these organs should be examined. Abdominal ultrasound is the most appropriate method of evaluating the kidneys, palpation of the thyroid is an adequate screen for this organ, and a serum prostate-specific antigen (PSA) and digital examination of the prostate is sufficient for the prostate. Myeloma should be considered, and skull radiographs (in addition to serum and urine immunoelectrophoresis) are recommended. Finally, any organ system implicated by the initial review of systems should be carefully evaluated. More thorough evaluations rarely uncover the primary carcinoma and even if an occult primary carcinoma is found, the management of the patient is rarely altered.

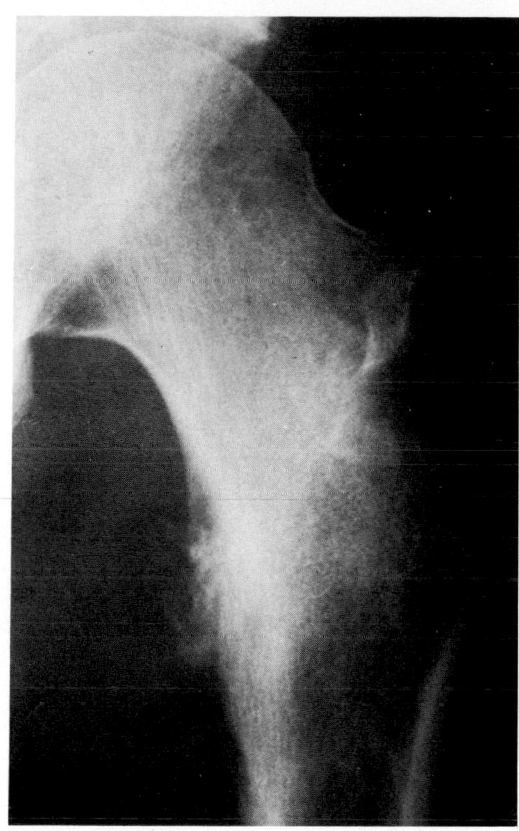

FIGURE 9-1. An anteroposterior x-ray of the proximal femur in a patient with known breast cancer. She complained of pain in the groin that worsened with weight bearing on the extremity. The subtle changes in the lesser trochanter are diagnostic of a metastasis to the proximal femur. This lesion is easy to miss and if not treated results in a pathologic fracture. A computed tomography scan is recommended to evaluate the amount of bone destruction, and a bone scan should be performed to look for other bone metastases. Prophylactic internal fixation should be considered because of the risk of fracture in this part of the femur.

Laboratory Studies

Disturbances in hematologic or metabolic parameters can aid in the diagnosis of a primary or secondary disorder associated with pathologic fractures. In all patients in whom a pathologic process is suspected, a baseline laboratory profile should be obtained, including a complete blood count with a manual differential, peripheral blood smear, and sedimentation rate; serum chemistries and enzymes should include blood urea nitrogen (BUN), serum glucose, liver function tests, albumin, calcium, phosphorus, and alkaline phosphatase. A standard urinalysis is necessary to look for microhematuria, and a 24-hour urine collection is necessary if a complete metabolic evaluation is planned. Serum and urine immunoelectrophoresis is the laboratory test of choice as a screen for myeloma. Few laboratories conduct a Bence-Jones protein analysis as originally described. When a Bence-Jones test for urinary protein is requested by the physician, the laboratory performs an immunoelectrophoresis of the urine.

Patients with osteoporosis have normal values for all the aforementioned laboratory tests, whereas patients with osteomalacia have low serum calcium, low serum phosphorus, high serum alkaline phosphatase, high urinary phosphorus, and high urinary hydroxyproline values. Patients with primary hyperparathyroidism have high serum calcium, alkaline phosphatase, and parathormone; low serum phosphorus; and high urinary calcium, phosphorus, and hydroxyproline. Those patients with renal osteodystrophy have low serum calcium, high serum phosphorus, high serum alkaline phosphatase, and an elevated BUN. When secondary hyperparathyroidism develops in these patients, the serum calcium increases to normal or above normal values and the parathormone is also elevated (Table 9-1). Urinary determinations are difficult to assess because of the abnormal glomerular filtration in patients having secondary hyperparathyroidism. Patients with Paget's disease have normal values for serum calcium and phosphorus but markedly elevated levels of alkaline phosphatase and urinary hydroxyproline. Acid phosphatase is usually elevated in patients having prostatic carcinoma, particularly when the disease has metastasized, but a PSA study has essentially replaced acid phosphatase as a screen for prostate cancer. PSA is a glycoprotein and is a sensitive measurement of prostatic cancer. A PSA of more than 20 ng/mL is associated with a significant risk of bone metastasis, whereas a PSA of less than 10 ng/mL essentially excludes the presence of bone metastasis.[27]

It should be remembered that the serum calcium is a measurement of the unbound calcium in the serum; therefore, determination of serum protein is important. If the serum protein is lower than normal, the normal range of serum calcium is lowered. Also, patients having a high intake of phosphate have a spuriously low serum calcium level.

Hypercalcemia of Malignancy

As many as 75,000 cases of hypercalcemia are diagnosed in the United States each year; most of these patients have primary hyperparathyroidism but about 40% have a malignancy causing the elevated serum calcium.[115] Rarely, the two causes occur simultaneously. The orthopaedic surgeon managing a metastatic carcinoma to bone must be aware of the risk of hypercalcemia, its symptoms, and its management. The malignancies most commonly associated with hypercalcemia are of the lung, breast, kidney, and genitourinary tract. Multiple myeloma and lymphoma may cause hypercalcemia but they comprise fewer than 10% of all cases.[30,50,120] In every patient with metastatic carcinoma to bone, the serum calcium and protein levels should be measured concurrently. Hypercalcemia can kill a patient and should be diagnosed early and treated.

Although hypercalcemia occurs frequently enough

TABLE 9-1
Disorders Producing Osteopenia

	Laboratory Values			
Disorder	*Serum Calcium*	*Serum Phosphorous*	*Serum Alkaline Phosphatase*	*Urine*
Osteoporosis	Normal	Normal	Normal	Normal Ca
Osteomalacia	Normal	Normal	Normal	Low Ca
Hyperparathyroidism	Normal to high	Normal to low	Normal	High Ca
Renal osteodystrophy	Low	High	High	—
Paget's disease	Normal	Normal	Very high	Hydroxyproline
Myeloma*	Normal	Normal	Normal	Protein

* Abnormal serum and/or urine immunoelectrophoresis.

to be a constant concern to any physician treating patients who have malignant diseases, it is rarely the presenting clinical feature of a previously undiagnosed malignancy.[43] When hypercalcemia occurs in malignancy, it is a poor prognostic sign for the patient; as many as 60% of those patients do not survive longer than 3 months and only 20% survive for 1 year. The signs and symptoms are myriad and often vague but they classically include nocturia, polydipsia, polyuria, fatigue, irritability, confusion, constipation, urinary tract infections, muscle weakness (especially of proximal muscle groups), joint and bone pain, anorexia, weight loss, nausea, vomiting, abdominal pain, unsteady gait, headache, and blurred vision. Often the signs are of nonspecific deterioration without any focal clues. None of these symptoms is specific, and it is better to diagnose the problem by measuring the serum calcium directly.

There does not appear to be a reliable correlation between the severity of the hypercalcemia and the degree of skeletal involvement.[9,50] There is, however, some relation between the type of malignant disease and concurrence of bone metastases and hypercalcemia. For example, lung cancer is likely to cause hypercalcemia without apparent bone metastases, whereas hypercalcemia in multiple myeloma or breast carcinoma and the extent of bone metastases correlate strongly.[123] Histologic evidence suggests that the presence of metastatic disease in bone is not essential for the observation of diffuse osteoclastic activity associated with clinical hypercalcemia.[52]

Once the patient with hypercalcemia is identified, a treatment plan must be established. Outpatient treatment of these patients is unsatisfactory if any long-term effect is expected. The patient with acute hypercalcemia may benefit from vigorous volume repletion; however, this is only a temporizing measure, and the hypercalcemia will recur, often more severely, unless an effort is made to reduce the degree of bone resorption. This reduction can be accomplished in some cases by treating the primary neoplasm directly or by using agents that reduce osteoclastic activity, such as phosphate, mithramycin, calcitonin, indomethacin, or glucocorticoids. Aminohydroxypropylidene diphosphonate (ADP) has been effective in producing sustained remissions of hypercalcemia secondary to malignancy. In a trial of ADP among patients with metastatic breast cancer, hypercalcemia was prevented and there was a significant reduction in bone pain and pathologic fractures.[138] Pamidronate is the most potent bisphosphonate available to control hypercalcemia.[13,14,54] A single infusion of 60 mg over 4 hours provides a dramatic reduction in the serum calcium for 6 to 11 days.[54] If needed, 1.5 mg/kg of pamidronate can be given.[14]

DIAGNOSIS OF THE PATHOLOGIC PROCESS

The preliminary evaluation may be sufficiently convincing of a diagnosis or at least a category of disease that a biopsy occasionally can be foregone. This should be the case only when absolute histologic confirmation of the diagnosis will not alter the clinical management of the patient or in any way affect the successful outcome of the patient's treatment. This is true only for self-healing benign tumors, fibrous dysplasia, and Paget's disease. Categorizing the underlying process into systemic skeletal disease, primary benign disease, primary malignant bone tumor, or metastatic carcinoma allows selection of the proper treatment plan. If a biopsy is indicated, it should be performed only after careful planning and without interfering with subsequent treatment of the patient. A good rule of thumb to remember when performing a biopsy is that any lesion may need to be widely resected and the biopsy track must be included in the resected specimen.

Indications for the Methods of Biopsy

A histologic diagnosis is required for all lesions unless the lesion can be identified without histology and needs no treatment. When the pathologic process associated with the fracture is thought to be a metastatic deposit, some of the tumor should be given to the pathologist during the operative procedure and a frozen section confirmation obtained. When the patient has a known malignancy, this is not as critical as when there is no known primary cancer. It is almost always a mistake to assume that a lesion is a metastatic deposit and treat it as such without histologic confirmation. The management of a pathologic fracture through a lesion suspected of being a primary sarcoma is the most difficult, and the patient is best treated by a team of oncologists familiar with all facets of sarcoma care. A biopsy will need to be performed but fixation of the fracture will need to be carefully considered, so that it does not significantly alter the ultimate treatment of the sarcoma. It is unfortunate when the internal fixation of a pathologic fracture secondary to a primary sarcoma is the principle reason a patient has to undergo an amputation. Usually, a minimally displaced pathologic fracture through a primary sarcoma can undergo biopsy with a needle or limited incisional exposure, treated nonoperatively initially, and then resected. Most patients with a grossly displaced pathologic fracture through a primary sarcoma probably should have an amputation. When the pathologic process has the appearance of a benign tumor, it is usually best to treat the fracture nonoperatively until it has healed and then address the tumor. Most fractures through a giant cell tumor of bone are exceptions to this rule. In the past, displaced intraarticular pathologic fractures through giant cell tumors of bone were allowed to heal, even when grossly displaced, and the lesion and adjacent articular surface were then resected; but now we recommend early operative intervention.[105] The giant cell tumor of bone with fracture is treated with an immediate aggressive curettage, open reduction, and internal fixation of the fractured articular surface. This is a difficult operation that requires technical expertise.

Technique of Biopsy

The biopsy must obtain adequate histologic material for diagnosis, contaminate as little local tissue as possible (tissue in contact with the postbiopsy hematoma must also be considered to be contaminated by tumor cells), and not adversely affect the treatment of the fracture.[126] Consultation with the pathologist before biopsy can be helpful in determining the best area from which to obtain tissue. When possible, the tissue should be obtained from a site unaffected by the fracture because the bone's reaction to the fracture produces a confusing histologic picture. (A biopsy obtained from a lesion associated with a pathologic fracture can be exceedingly difficult to interpret because of the fracture callus in-grafted on the underlying tumor.) A fine-needle (21-gauge or smaller) aspirate biopsy, a core-needle biopsy, or an open incisional biopsy can be used to obtain material for a histologic diagnosis. The fine-needle aspirate is simple and safe. It provides only cells, and the pathologist must be familiar with cytologic interpretations to make an accurate diagnosis. A core-needle biopsy is easier than an open incisional biopsy but provides limited tissue. It is best done with the aid of a computed tomography (CT) scanner. When a limited amount of tissue is likely to be sufficient for making an accurate diagnosis, a core-needle biopsy is appropriate. An open incisional biopsy is the most difficult biopsy. It requires an operating room and anesthesia but it also provides the best material for the pathologist. An open biopsy is best for the difficult cases. The needle track or incision should be positioned so that it can be excised if a subsequent resection needs to be done. With an open biopsy, minimal spreading is best, neurovascular bundles should not be exposed, and muscle should be split rather than using the standard dissection between muscles. After pathologic tissue has been obtained and a diagnosis made (or it has been confirmed that adequate tissue has been obtained), thorough hemostasis should be obtained before closing the wound. Postoperative hematomas contain tumor cells and have to be treated just like the primary tumor. If a definitive diagnosis can be made on frozen section, the treatment of the tumor and fracture may be completed at the time of the biopsy; if no diagnosis can be made, it is inappropriate to proceed with treatment of the tumor or fracture unless the treatment can be done without contamination of additional uninvolved tissue. No biopsy procedure is complete until cultures have been obtained.

SPECIFIC TREATMENT

Remembering the rule of common occurrences and assuming a normal distribution of patients, the most common pathologic fracture is due to osteoporosis. Under nearly all circumstances, these fractures should be managed as recommended in the accompanying chapters of this text. Adjustments may be necessary because of the weakened bone. Pathologic fractures due to metastatic carcinoma, the second most common cause of pathologic fracture, and the patients in whom they occur demand special considerations (Fig. 9-2).

Life expectancy after the diagnosis of metastatic carcinoma continues to increase, and those patients who have skeletal metastases require the most careful considerations. In 1990, 505,322 new cases of primary malignancy were reported in the United States; at least 50% of those patients are alive 5 years later.[15] These data suggest that there are about 2 million people in the United States with a cancer at risk for metastasis. Many of these patients will have carcinoma metastatic to bone, especially those having a primary tumor arising from the breast, prostate, lung, kidney, or thyroid. There are about 145,000 new cases of breast cancer and 155,000 cases of lung cancer diagnosed each year in the United States.[15] Among these patients, survival with metastatic disease may be several years to a decade. These numbers indicate the frequency of the problem of metastatic disease to bone.

The survival of patients with malignant disease is being improved by advances in early diagnosis and treatment. During the last decade, the philosophy of management has changed from one of simply providing comfort in anticipation of an early demise to one of trying to provide pain-free maintenance of normal daily function for the remainder of the patient's life.[47,110] Many routine techniques used to treat nonpathologic fractures are inadequate in the management of pathologic fractures secondary to metastatic carcinoma, and more complex approaches are often necessary. Accurately predicting the length of a patient's life is impossible. Patients with liver failure due to multiple liver metastases, pulmonary compromise due to lungs full of tumor, mental status changes due to brain metastasis, or metabolic imbalances (especially hypercalcemia) have a life expectancy of a few months; internal fixation of their pathologic fractures may not be warranted. Even in some of these cases, however, the quality of the remaining time can be

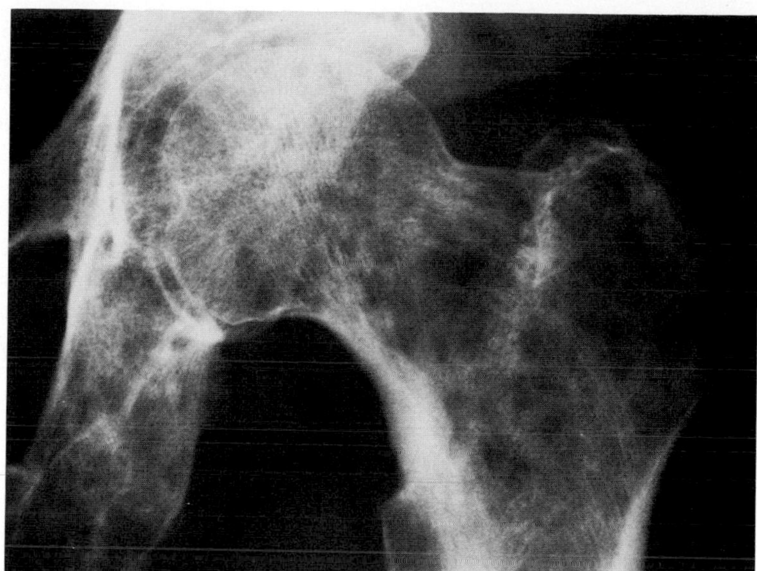

FIGURE 9-2. An anteroposterior x-ray of the proximal femur in a patient with known breast cancer. The permeative destruction of the bone is most likely due to metastatic deposits of breast cancer. Disuse osteoporosis may have a similar appearance, and the x-ray diagnosis should be confirmed by biopsy unless the diagnosis of metastatic disease in the patient has already been confirmed at another site. This permeative destruction of the proximal femur is the most common type of destruction leading to a pathologic fracture. For patients with this type of destruction, we suggest prophylactic internal fixation of the femoral neck and subtrochanteric region.

improved with operative stabilization. Recovery from an uncomplicated internal fixation takes about 2 weeks and even if the patient only has a month of life afterwards, the benefits are probably worth the operation.

Most patients with a pathologic fracture from metastatic carcinoma have been treated previously for the primary malignancy, and the diagnosis is only occasionally in question. Patients presenting with a pathologic fracture suspected to be secondary to metastatic carcinoma but without prior diagnosis should be evaluated, so that the primary tumor may also be managed. As outlined in the first section of this chapter, a thorough history and physical examination with attention to lymph nodes, thyroid, breast, rectum, and prostate; chest radiograph; and baseline laboratory values are requisite in each new patient. Additional studies may include CT scan of the lung, renal ultrasound or intravenous pyelogram, ^{99m}Tc bone scan, mammography, and special chemistries as previously outlined. If the primary tumor is not apparent from these tests, it is probably not necessary to continue to search for it.[130] Finding it is unlikely, and if it is found, knowledge of the primary tumor would not lead to a significant difference in the management of the patient. Specifically, it is not necessary to obtain a gastrointestinal series, liver–spleen scan, or CT scans of the head and abdomen unless the patient's history, review of systems, or physical examination suggests an abnormality in one of these locations.

Impending Fractures

Not infrequently, a patient is seen who has a metastatic deposit in a bone without a fracture. The orthopaedist is usually asked to decide if the bone is at risk of fracture from minimal trauma (to decide whether there is an impending fracture). It is agreed that an impending fracture should be treated with internal fixation before it breaks because the patients do better in all aspects.[20,34,133] The problem is the difficulty in determining those criteria that are reliable for making the decision. The term "impending fracture" is used throughout the literature on metastatic disease but the criteria for what constitutes an impending fracture are arbitrary. Several studies have formulated guidelines to indicate when prophylactic fixation is necessary but they are limited by the use of plain two-dimensional radiographs, subjective information from the patient, and an inadequate understanding of the biomechanical compromise of the bone by the metastatic carcinoma. Although experienced orthopaedic surgeons may think they have an intuitive sense for which lesions are at risk for fracture, considerable controversy exists regarding what constitutes an impending fracture and little reliable data are available; more definitive guidelines are needed.

Pain is the primary concern of the patient and the major indication for treatment of a bone metastasis, and it has been purported by some authors to be predictive of fracture.[100,109] Although pain is probably not a reliable indicator of impending fracture and is not reason enough for prophylactic fixation, it is the most important reason for some type of treatment, whether that is surgical stabilization, radiation therapy, chemotherapy, or a combination of modalities (Fig. 9-3).[40,121,134] Not only does pain interfere with a patient's quality of life and indicate a local problem but it is also cause of disuse osteopenia, increasing the likelihood of a fracture. Prophylactic internal fixation is a successful method of relieving pain from a meta-

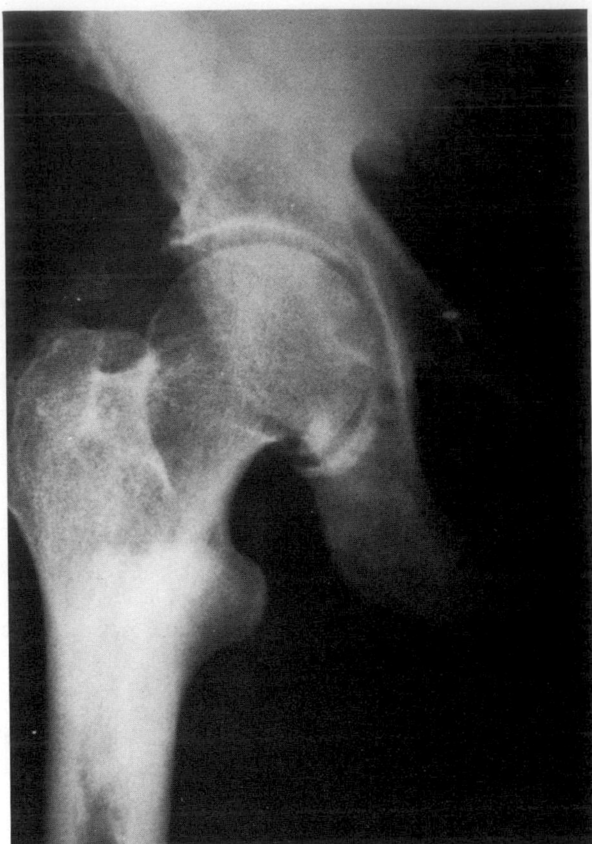

FIGURE 9-3. An anteroposterior x-ray of the proximal femur in a patient with known metastatic prostate cancer. Pathologic fractures through lesions having increased density are rare. The lesion should be irradiated if the patient has pain, and internal fixation is indicated only if the pain persists after completion of the irradiation and no other cause is found. Bone metastases that produce increased density are most likely to be due to carcinoma of the prostate; metastatic breast cancer and metastatic lung cancer also have a significant incidence of lesions that produce increased density in the bone. About 90% of prostate metastases cause increased density of the bone, whereas only 60% of breast metastases and 30% of lung metastases produce increased density.

static deposit. If the patient continues to have pain after the metastasis has been treated with irradiation, prophylactic fixation is indicated. Fidler[40] assessed preoperative and postoperative pain in patients having impending fractures and found that among patients with 50% to 75% cortical involvement, all had moderate to severe pain preoperatively and no pain or only slight pain after prophylactic internal fixation.

The accepted indications for prophylactic internal fixation of impending fractures are the presence of a destructive, painful lesion 2.5 cm in diameter or loss of 50% or more of the cortex of a long bone.[7,8,39,40,74,75,114,127] All of the available studies that use measurements of cortical destruction to predict the risk of fracture due to pathologic lesions have used plain radiographic images. These radiographs are available, making retrospective studies possible, but they are limited in several ways: no standardized position or view is used, so that radiographs are difficult to compare; permeative lesions probably have the highest fracture risk but accurate measurements of size cannot be made by any of the contemporary methods; some bone metastases produce increased density, with obscure margins; nearly all metastatic lesions have poorly defined edges, causing considerable error in calculating the percentage of cortical destruction; and the relative risk of different locations in the bone is not considered nor are the demands placed on the bone in question. Moreover, as Menck and associates[90] noted, there are biomechanical factors still to be defined (eg, bone strength, shape of the lesion, premorbid osteopenia) that all contribute to the overall fracture risk. In an investigation of bone strength reduction published by McBroom and colleagues,[89] the authors predicted the reduction in flexural strength of their model canine femurs having specifically created defects. Their predictions were based on either of two measurements of defect size: the ratio of hole diameter to bone diameter or the ratio of the defect-reduced cross-sectional area to the intact bone area. They were able to demonstrate variations in the hole-to-bone diameter ratio of up to 10%, using plain radiographs. They suggested that CT scans be used to measure cortical destruction, that CT scans are more accurate than plain radiographs, and that CT scans are more accurate in predicting the strength reduction caused by metastatic lesions.

In another series of experiments to determine the strength reduction of metastatic lesions, it was suggested that the criteria used are not accurate predictors.[25,64,65,66] The degree of porosity of the bone immediately adjacent to the defect is one of the more important variables that determine the risk of a fracture. The activity level of the patient is a particularly important factor. These experiments suggest that after 60% reduction in strength of the proximal femur, the bone is likely to fracture during normal gait.[66] It is clear that there is not a reliable method of determining when to internally fix an impending fracture. We prophylactically internally fix impending fractures in patients having a painful lower extremity destructive lesion without a reactive rim and larger than 2.5 cm or greater than 50% of the bone diameter when 6 weeks or more of life are expected. We also internally fix any bone with a destructive lesion that remains painful after a course of irradiation.

There are several advantages of prophylactic fixation of an impending fracture. These include decreased morbidity, shorter hospital stay, easier rehabilitation, more immediate pain relief, faster and less complicated surgery, and less blood loss during surgery.[22] In an animal study of prophylactic fixation of bone metastases, Bouma and associates[16] reported a decrease in the incidence of fractures and in lung metastases in patients with prophylactically fixed bone lesions.

The specific methods of surgical treatment for impending fractures are not significantly different from those for completed pathologic fractures. The operations are easier, surgical and postoperative complications are fewer, and rehabilitation is rapid. One critical caveat when treating patients who have impending lesions is that fracture risk is greatest during the surgical positioning, preparation, and draping while the patient is under anesthesia. Anesthetized patients cannot protect their own extremities and must rely on the surgical team to do this.

General Concepts in the Treatment of Pathologic Fractures

Internal fixation of pathologic fractures is temporary, and the fixation device eventually fails if the bone does not heal.[60] Loss of fixation is the most significant complication of treating pathologic fractures. Healing is slower than for fractures through normal bone, particularly when irradiation is part of the patient's preoperative or postoperative management.[12,19,21,36,48,56,121,142] All patients with metastatic carcinoma to bone with an impending fracture or completed fracture should receive irradiation as part of their treatment. Postoperative irradiation alters bone healing[21] but in our experience, postoperative irradiation of up to 50 Gy begun 3 weeks after the operation has not produced a noticeable incidence of nonunions.

Poor bone quality is not a contraindication to fixation but demands consideration when selecting the method of fixation. Polymethylmethacrylate (PMMA) improves the bending strength of a fixation construct and the outcome of fixation in both animal and human studies.* PMMA does not affect the use of therapeutic irradiation nor are the properties of the PMMA affected adversely by the radiation.[38,99] PMMA should not be used to replace missing segments of cortical bone. It is used to improve the fixation of the hardware to the bone, increasing the strength of the fixation and reducing the risk of the hardware cutting out of the bone. This approach allows early mobilization of the patient without the fear of failure of the fixation. When PMMA is used, care should be taken to avoid interposing it between fracture fragments. The fixation should be done with the intention of eventual fracture healing. If the fracture does not heal, even the most rigid fixation will fail. Only the early demise of the patient prevents fixation failure in an ununited fracture. Patients with metastatic pathologic fracture may live a few years, and a nonunion can be a significant complication. Autogenous bone graft should be used if there is inadequate local bone for healing.

The most important initial evaluation of a patient with a pathologic fracture is an examination of the remainder of the skeleton for other sites of involvement and impending fractures.[49] A ^{99m}Tc bone scan of the entire skeleton is the most efficient screen for occult bone metastasis. Before obtaining the bone scan, palpation of the skeletal system should be done and radiographs of any tender bones and both humeri, the pelvis, and both femurs should be obtained.

Patients with metastatic cancer often have significant other medical problems that affect their operative risk. The orthopaedist should assess the patient carefully and obtain assistance when necessary. The extent of the patient's disease should be determined. The sites of metastatic disease that are most important in determining the patient's prognosis are brain, lung, and liver. Patients with any localized neurologic abnormalities or changes in mentation should have a head CT or magnetic resonance imaging (MRI) scan. A plain chest radiograph is adequate to evaluate the lung. Liver function serum tests are probably all that is needed to evaluate the liver, although both ultrasound and CT can be done and should be requested if the serum values are abnormal.

Nutrition is of particular concern; it needs to be assessed by measuring serum albumin and maintained or improved, even if doing so requires the addition of enteral or parenteral hyperalimentation perioperatively. Clinically significant hypercalcemia can be induced by the bed rest necessitated by the fracture, and serum calcium levels should be monitored. Patients with metastatic cancer are at risk of having an elevated serum uric acid level; therefore, the uric acid level should be determined and if it is elevated, prophylaxis for an acute attack of gout should be instituted. Nearly all of these patients have relative bone marrow suppression and need adequate replacement of blood products. Remember to find out when the patient had their most recent chemotherapy and whether it will make them neutropenic. A minimum absolute granulocyte count of 500 is suggested before performing surgery. These patients are likely to suffer larger than usual blood losses at operation because of the hypervascularity of many lesions, thereby demanding greater intraoperative and postoperative replacement. In some circumstances, excessive blood loss can be avoided by preoperative angiographic embolization; this is especially useful for metastatic hypernephroma, in which even an open biopsy can lead to life-threatening blood loss (Fig. 9-4).[17,24] Other standards of orthopaedic care apply essentially without change (i.e., perioperative antibiotic coverage, anticoagulation or other prophylaxis for deep vein thrombosis and pulmonary

* References 2, 4, 32, 38, 55, 62, 68, 77, 82, 93, 99, 113, 123, 124, 131, 141.

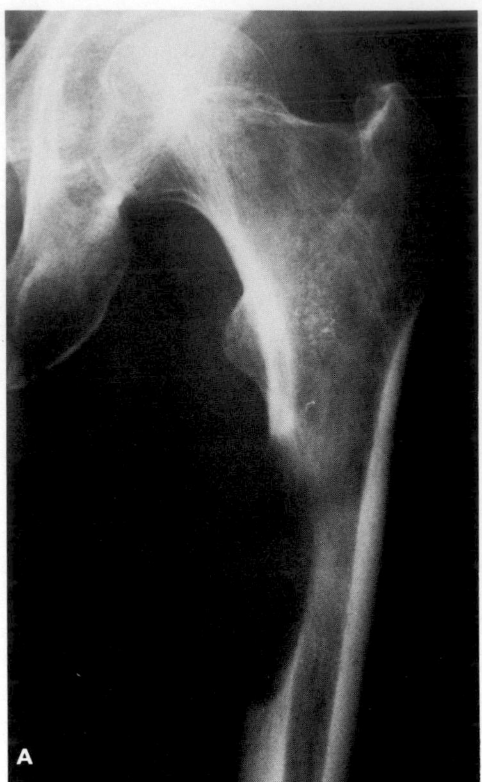

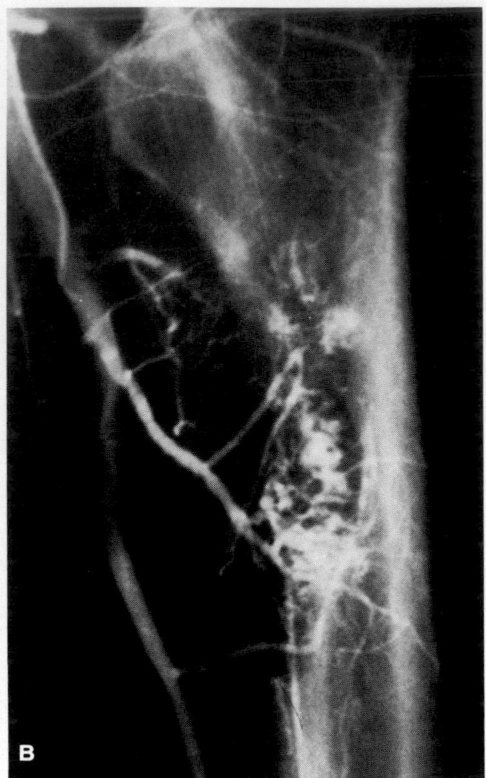

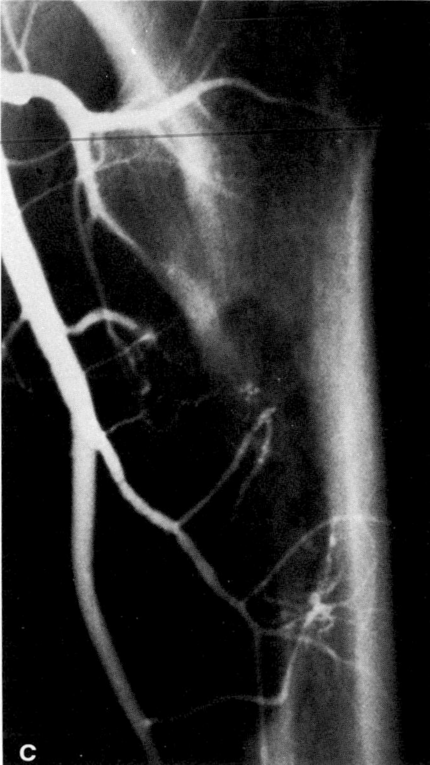

FIGURE 9-4. (**A**) An anteroposterior x-ray of the proximal femur in a patient who had carcinoma of the kidney 13 years ago. He complained of groin pain and had been treated for a "pulled muscle" for 6 weeks before this x-ray was taken. This is a typical metastatic lesion. It is in the metaphyseal/diaphyseal junction, has destroyed the cortex, and has an extra-osseous soft-tissue component. Despite the long time since the original kidney malignancy, this lesion should be suspected of being a metastasis from the hypernephroma. (**B**) On this early phase of the angiogram, the arteriovenous shunting and pooling of dye typical of metastatic hypernephroma can be seen. An operative procedure on this lesion can produce life-threatening hemorrhage. Preoperative embolization is recommended. (**C**) On the postembolization angiogram, marked reduction in vascularity can be seen.

embolus, aggressive postoperative pulmonary toilet, early mobilization). Increased weight bearing and progressive resisted exercises should be delayed until there is evidence of fracture healing; however, joint mobilization and assisted ambulation should not wait, and most patients can be out of bed not later than 2 days postoperatively.

Upper Extremity Fractures

Metastatic lesions involving the humeral shaft that have not fractured usually are treated initially with irradiation.[2,26,32,44,92] Prophylactic fixation of an impending humeral fracture is indicated when the patient has persistent pain after irradiation. While the patient is receiving irradiation, standard splinting techniques are used to reduce the risk of a fracture.

Contractures of the shoulder and elbow are common, and these joints should be kept moving. Gentle pendulum exercises can maintain motion in the shoulder and, with appropriate precautions against using torsion, are safe for most humeral shaft, neck, and head defects. (Fig. 9-5). Gravity-assisted elbow flexion and extension exercises can also be done safely by most patients.

Humeral head fractures and large humeral head lesions that remain painful after irradiation or have completely destroyed the bone should be treated by standard cemented hemiarthroplasty. Replacement of the glenoid surface is not necessary. The goal of humeral head replacement is pain relief and preservation of existing function; range of motion of the joint should not be expected to improve. Postoperative care is routine, with the addition of irradiation, if not already done. When bone destruction or involvement of the glenoid and humeral head is extensive, a resection arthroplasty of the shoulder (Tikoff-Lindberg resection) is suggested.[67]

The surgical treatment of humeral shaft fractures and impending fractures has changed during the past few years but it is still not clear which fixation method is best.[78,116,136,143a] The development of rigid, interlocked humeral rods offers the advantages of adequate internal fixation of the entire humerus, with a limited exposure. Some reports suggest that these devices are useful in the treatment of both impending fractures or completed fractures of the humerus. Humeral rod placement is technically demanding, and care should be used when placing the rod in the weakened humerus. It probably is best to be satisfied with a smaller-diameter rod than to try to ream up to the maximal diameter possible. A common side effect of using a humeral rod is persistent shoulder pain at the site of insertion. We do not recommend the use of flexible rods (eg, Enders and Rush) for prophylactic fixation of impending humeral fractures.

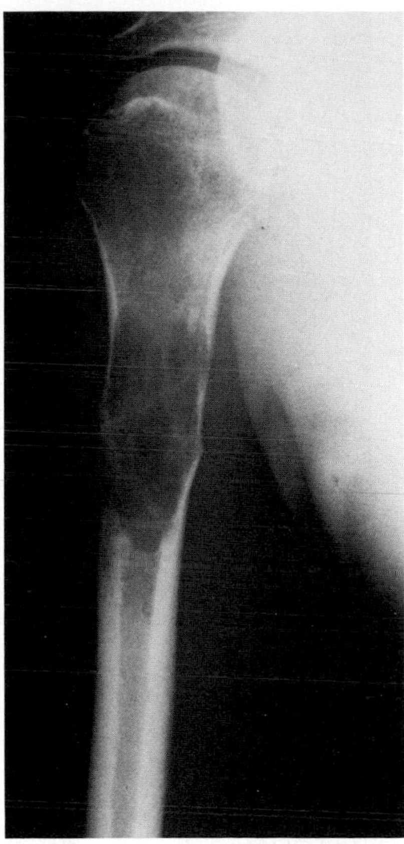

FIGURE 9-5. An anteroposterior x-ray of the proximal humerus in a patient with a plasmacytoma of the proximal humerus. He was treated with irradiation, without stabilizing the humerus, and a sling and pendulum exercises were used to keep his shoulder moving. If the bone fractures, a resection or stabilization can be performed but if the bone heals without surgery, the patient has better function. Surgery before irradiation delays the irradiation and makes surgical stabilization more difficult.

The best advice is to use the device that is most familiar. The advantage of the intramedullary device is the limited dissection required to strengthen the whole humerus—often a major advantage because of the high incidence of multiple lesions in the same bone. The disadvantage is its relative lack of rigid immobilization, compared with a compression plate. Rigid fixation is important for both pain relief and eventual healing, and compression plating is recommended when the intramedullary device cannot achieve adequately rigid fixation. This situation usually occurs secondary to loss of a large portion of cortical bone or in a patient with a particularly large medullary canal. When a large segment of the humerus has been destroyed by the lesion, compression plate fixation is recommended. We use the 4.5-mm compression plates, with screw fixation of six cortices on either side of the bone defect whenever possible (Fig. 9-6). As mentioned, PMMA can be used to improve the fixation of the intramedullary rod or compression plate

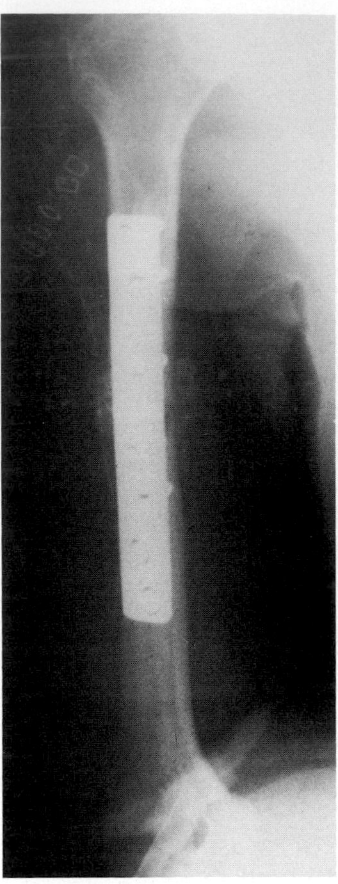

FIGURE 9-6. An anteroposterior x-ray of the humerus in a patient with a metastasis to the humeral diaphysis that had been treated with irradiation but fractured. The lesion was exposed and curetted. The humerus was shortened to obtain adequate bone contact. A plate was used to provide immediate solid stabilization.

but should not be used to replace bone. In those rare cases in which adequate bone-to-bone apposition cannot be achieved, a bone graft, allograft, or autograft, can be used. Another option is to shorten the humerus to obtain adequate bone contact (see Fig. 9-6). In our experience, the humerus can be shortened at least 4 cm without compromising the function of the extremity.

Metastases distal to the elbow are unusual but they pose problems of rotational and angular control similar to those of proximal lesions of the upper extremity. As with the humeral pathologic fractures, closed treatment is unlikely to succeed and early internal fixation is recommended. The 3.5-mm compression plate system securing six cortices on each side of the lesion, with or without cement augmentation, provides appropriate fixation in most cases. Fractures of the radial head can be treated by radial head resection. These distal upper extremity lesions are rare but they deserve the same aggressive approach as lesions elsewhere because the patient's survival does not vary from that of patients having proximal or axial disease.

Metastatic carcinoma to the hand is unusual.[81] Most cases are secondary to lung cancer, although occasionally other primary carcinomas can spread to a bone in the hand. Surgical resection of these metastases is usually the best management.

Lower Extremity Fractures

More than half of all pathologic fractures occur in the proximal part of the femur; thus, they are the most frequently treated and studied lesions.[91,118,139,145] Perhaps because of the weight-bearing demands of the lower extremity, metastatic disease of the femur is the most likely lesion to cause disabling pain. Pathologic fractures of the femur suddenly alter the quality of a patient's life and significantly threaten an individual's level of independence. Without proper surgical attention, the patient with a pathologic fracture of the femur is confined to bed—a situation that is medically and psychologically devastating.

As discussed in other sections, the early diagnosis of primary malignancies, improved treatment of many diseases and their complications, and extended life expectancy of many patients with metastatic disease create a greater incentive for improved surgical management of impending or completed pathologic fractures. In all cases, the goal of surgical intervention is to achieve maximum protection of the bone or stabilization of the fracture, with the least extensive exposure. There is virtually no place for nonoperative treatment of completed pathologic fractures of the femur. Lesions of the femoral neck, intertrochanteric area, and subtrochanteric area should almost always be prophylactically fixed whenever found because of the high incidence of subsequent fracture and the ease of the operation when performed before fracture, compared with the difficulties and complications of surgery after a fracture has occurred.

Lesions within the femoral head are successfully treated with replacement arthroplasty, either hemiarthroplasty or total hip replacement.[32,79,82] Total hip replacement is indicated when the acetabulum has lost its strength due to a metastatic focus or when the patient has significant degenerative disease. Routine use of total hip replacement is not necessary. We palpate the acetabulum at the time of the operation and replace the acetabulum only if it is ballottable. A long-stem endoprosthesis is recommended when there are lesions in the proximal femur. We use PMMA fixation of endoprosthetic replacements in patients who have metastatic disease. Patients with bone metastasis seem to have a greater risk of developing intraoperative acute pulmonary distress.[77] It is our practice to thoroughly curet and lavage the involved bone and to be sure that the patient does not have volume depletion when the PMMA is injected and the endoprosthetic stem is pushed into place. Acute respiratory distress can occur in patients who have metastatic cancer during internal fixation with an intramedullary device even without PMMA, and care should be exercised during reaming and implantation of these devices. Adequate fluid balance and oxygenation are important, and the orthopaedist should discuss this with the anesthesiologist before the operation.

Impending fractures of the femoral neck can be treated with prophylactic fixation. We prefer to use a sliding hip screw device unless the patient has other lesions within the femur, in which case a locked intramedullary rod that allows screw fixation of the femoral neck is preferred.[137] The results of treating completed femoral neck fractures by pinning techniques have been unsatisfactory, with a high rate of nonunion and failure of fixation.[92] Therefore, this approach is not recommended. Endoprosthetic replacement is best for the completed fracture of the femoral neck.

Solitary intertrochanteric fractures can be managed with a sliding screw and side plate if bone loss is minimal and solid bone-to-bone contact can be achieved. If there is loss of much bone or if solid bone-to-bone contact cannot be achieved, it is better to replace the proximal femur with an endoprosthesis. Usually, a calcar replacement device is adequate. Building up the bone with PMMA to support a standard endoprosthesis is not recommended. The postoperative recovery is quickest when the patient can bear weight early, which requires either rigid internal fixation or endoprosthetic reconstruction.

Fractures in the subtrochanteric region of the femur are more difficult to treat. As with fractures in the intertrochanteric region, internal fixation is adequate, usually with a locked intramedullary device, if solid bone-to-bone contact can be achieved. The availability of modular proximal femoral endoprostheses to replace the proximal femur makes them an attractive alternative to internal fixation, and they are recommended whenever solid internal fixation cannot be achieved.

Fractures of the femoral shaft are treated most effectively with an intramedullary device, with or without PMMA.[35,77,93,95] Although compression plates provide excellent rigid internal fixation (experimentally attaining as much as 75% of the normal torsional strength of the bone),[3] their use requires a wide surgical exposure, results in increased blood loss, and provides strength only to the bone under the plate. Intramedullary rod fixation, although not as rigid, is technically simple (especially when used as prophylactic fixation of an impending fracture), can be done through a limited exposure, and reinforces the entire bone. The development of intramedullary nails with proximal and distal interlocking screws has made the use of these devices our preferred method in nearly all patients having impending and completed pathologic fractures of the femoral shaft. When intramedullary rods are used, the canal is overreamed 1 to 1.5 mm to avoid high impaction forces during rod placement. The ability to fix the bone both proximally and distally eliminates the complication of telescoping and provides excellent control of length and rotation of the femur. Intramedullary rods are available with the proximal screws directed proximally through the central portion of the femoral neck into the femoral head, thus allowing good fixation for subtrochanteric lesions or the fractured femur with an associated femoral neck lesion, both of which have been difficult to manage in the past. With both proximal and distal interlocking screws, intramedullary rods can be employed to treat lesions and fractures involving most parts of the femur.

When there is a completed fracture and extensive bone destruction, exposure of the fracture, removal of the metastatic tumor, and bone grafting may be useful. In this situation, PMMA can be used to improve the fixation of the femur but should not be relied on to replace a segment of missing bone. If a gap is present, an intercalary allograft is recommended (Fig. 9-7). If bone contact is minimal, an autogenous bone graft should be used. When there is an impending fracture, an intramedullary rod inserted from the proximal end is sufficient. The rod should be locked with fixation screws proximally or distally if the lesion is proximal or distal, or the entire rod can be encased in PMMA. The use of an intramedullary rod and PMMA is most helpful when the patient has multiple lesions or a lesion in the distal metaphysis. When the lesion is in the distal metaphysis, the rod can be introduced from distal to proximal.

The technique developed for the retrograde instillation of low-viscosity cement through a fluted intramedullary rod was described by Miller and associates.[93] A small diameter (11-mm), closed-section, fluted intramedullary rod is introduced at the piriformis fossa or through the knee. When an intramedullary rod is introduced into the femur from the distal end, a standard knee arthrotomy is used and the femoral canal is opened through the articular surface of the intercondylar notch, just anterior to the femoral origin of the anterior cruciate ligament. The femoral canal is reamed to 15 or 16 mm. The 11-mm rod is used as a cannula through which the low-viscosity cement is injected, with retrograde filling of the femoral canal (Fig. 9-8). Biomechanical testing of this system and comparison with another rod and cement construct showed a significant improvement in torsional strength. In a clinical trial of this technique, successful results were achieved, except in three patients having completed fractures and extensive bone destruction.[93] Although this system can be used in treating comp-

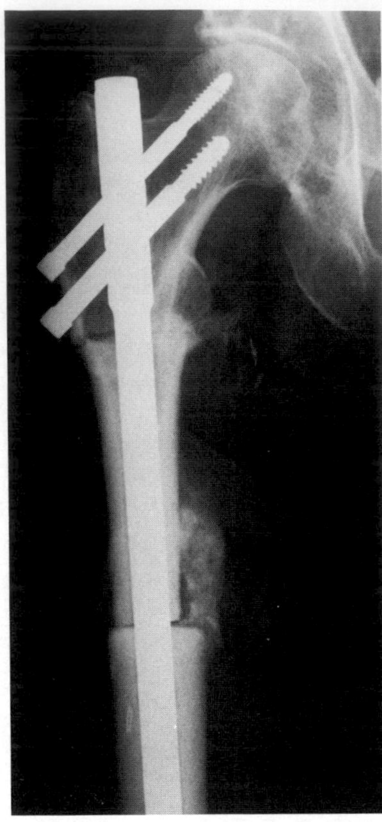

FIGURE 9-7. An anteroposterior x-ray of the proximal femur in a patient who had an intercalary allograft to reconstruct the femur after the resection of a metastatic renal cell carcinoma. This was his first metastasis, 13 years after the initial diagnosis. Metastases first found more than 2 years after the initial tumor are often best treated by resection. This is especially true of metastases from renal or thyroid carcinomas.

leted fractures, we recommend it only for prophylactic fixation.

Supracondylar fractures, as are intertrochanteric fractures, are managed well by standard devices such as blade plates but augmentation with PMMA to improve screw fixation in the weakened metaphyseal bone may be needed.

Occasionally, the entire distal femur is destroyed by metastatic cancer. As with proximal femoral destructive lesions, the distal femur can be replaced with a modular endoprosthesis. These devices are inherently stable and, when cemented in place, permit the patient a rapid recovery to normal activities (Fig. 9-9).

Pelvic and Acetabular Lesions

Many metastatic deposits in the bony pelvis do not affect weight-bearing functions and consequently do not need surgical intervention unless an open biopsy is necessary. Periacetabular lesions, particularly in the medial and superior segments of the acetabulum, present a particularly difficult problem (Fig. 9-10). The loss of function may be gradual, and the patient may remain relatively asymptomatic (or the symptoms may be attributed to an adjacent femoral head or neck lesion), so that when the patient is seen, extensive destruction has already occurred.[58] Surgical reconstruction is difficult and can cause considerable perioperative morbidity, particularly blood loss. Preoperative arteriography is suggested and if possible, embolization of the tumor should be done.[24] This procedure is safe and can significantly reduce the operative blood loss and risk of intraoperative exsanguination. The periacetabular lesions are best seen on CT scan, on which the extent of tumor destruction can be clearly appreciated.[114] When the lesion is small and the acetabular subchondral bone is intact or has only a small defect, curettage and packing with PMMA are recommended. This usually relieves the patient's symptoms, and irradiation will control the remaining microscopic disease. When a major portion of the acetabular bone is destroyed, a total hip replacement is preferred. It is not possible to accurately determine the point at which curettage and PMMA packing will no longer be adequate and a total hip replacement must be performed. Certainly, if the acetabulum is fractured, even with only minimal displacement, a total hip replacement is indicated. A routine acetabular component is usually adequate but the surgeon must be careful that the acetabular components are adequately supported. A protrusio cup is often all that is necessary, although occasionally, a large-fragment bone graft (allograft or autograft) is needed (Fig. 9-11). Rarely, a combination of PMMA and Steinmann pins is required to reconstruct the pelvis.[58,69] This demanding surgery is probably best undertaken by someone with extensive experience.

Spinal Fractures

A compression fracture of a vertebral body presents a diagnostic challenge. Most spinal compression fractures not associated with a neurologic deficit are secondary to osteoporosis. These require minimal treatment: usually a short period of bracing (4 to 6 weeks) and management of the underlying osteoporosis. The other three causes of a spinal compression fracture in an adult that must be considered are osteomalacia, myeloma, and metastatic cancer. They can be excluded relatively easily. Osteomalacia can be excluded if the history is negative for renal, gastrointestinal, or dietary abnormalities and the serum calcium, serum phosphorus, serum alkaline phosphatase, BUN, and urinary calcium are normal. Myeloma is excluded (for all practical purposes) with a normal serum and urine immunoelectrophoresis. The search for a primary cancer includes taking a history for prior diagnosis of a cancer;

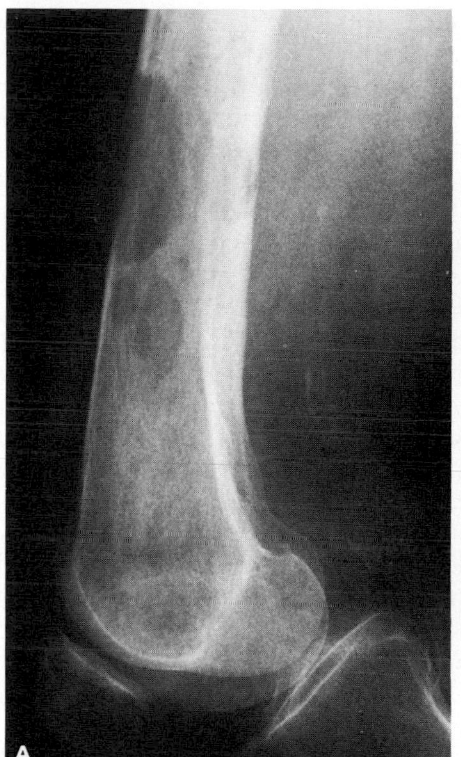

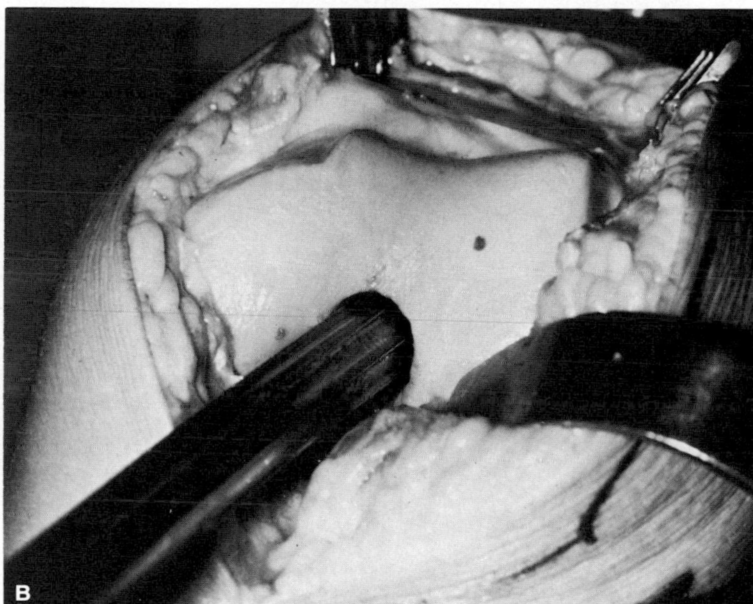

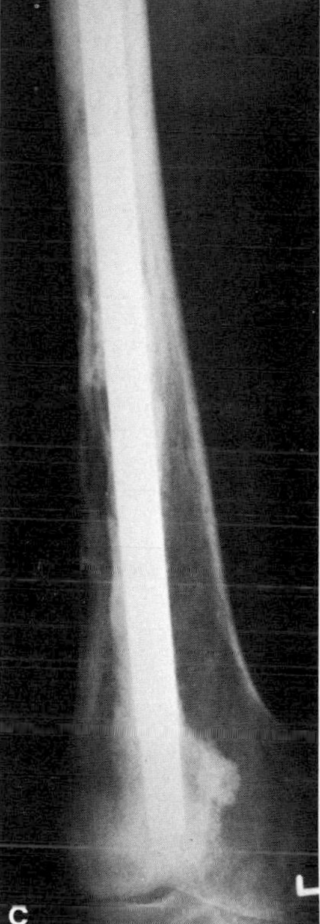

FIGURE 9-8. (**A**) A lateral x-ray of the femur in a woman with known metastatic breast cancer. Metastatic lesions in the distal femur, especially when a large segment of the femur is involved, can be difficult to stabilize. (**B**) In a technique we have used, the intramedullary rod is introduced through the intercondylar notch of the distal femur. An interlocking nail can be used or methylmethacrylate can be injected through the rod for additional fixation. (**C**) The intramedullary rod is pushed up entirely into the femoral canal before the methylmethacrylate hardens. This method has been successful in stabilizing impending femoral fractures in the distal half of the femur.

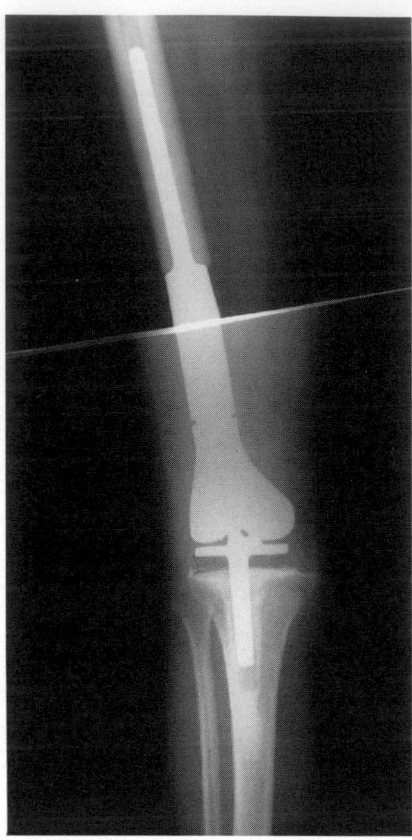

FIGURE 9-9. An anteroposterior x-ray of the distal femur and proximal tibia of a patient who had a modular endoprosthetic replacement of his distal femur for metastatic colon cancer. Preoperatively, the patient had a fractured distal femur, with involvement of both condyles. He was ambulating within 2 days of his surgery, and the endoprosthesis functioned well for the remaining 12 months of his life.

a physical examination, especially of the rectum, thyroid, and breast or prostate gland; a stool guaiac; a chest radiograph; and ultrasound of the kidney. A whole-body ^{99m}Tc bone scan also should be done. If these examinations are normal, a diagnosis of an osteoporotic compression fracture can be made. The evaluation should be repeated if the patient does not have pain relief within 6 to 8 weeks or if a neurologic deficit develops.

If the patient has a fracture and a neurologic deficit, it is more likely that the patient has myeloma, a metastasis, or rarely, a primary sarcoma. Extraosseous masses can be seen on a CT scan or MRI. If a diagnosis cannot be made without a biopsy, the biopsy can usually be performed easily with a needle, using CT for localization. If an open biopsy of a vertebral body is necessary, we prefer the transpedicular approach. The patient is positioned prone on the operating table. For thoracic vertebrae, the tip of the transverse process is identified; for lumbar vertebrae, the superior facet is used as the landmark. The pedicle is just medial to each of these structures. The cortical bone is removed, and the pedicle is found with a small curet and followed into the vertebral body. A core biopsy or curet biopsy is then taken. A cross-table lateral radiograph can be taken in the operating room to confirm the position of the instrument. Bone wax or a small amount of PMMA should be used to close the biopsy hole, so that tumor does not escape into the soft tissues.

Skeletal metastases occur most commonly in the spine, affecting the vertebral body more often than the posterior elements.[59,102] These lesions may remain asymptomatic for months to years and may be appreciated only when a bone scan is obtained during a routine metastatic workup. The classic plain radiograph finding is the loss of a pedicle on a plain anteroposterior view of the spine (Fig. 9-12). This sign should be sought carefully in all patients who have metastatic disease to bone. As the lesion progresses, the patient feels moderate to severe pain that can persist for

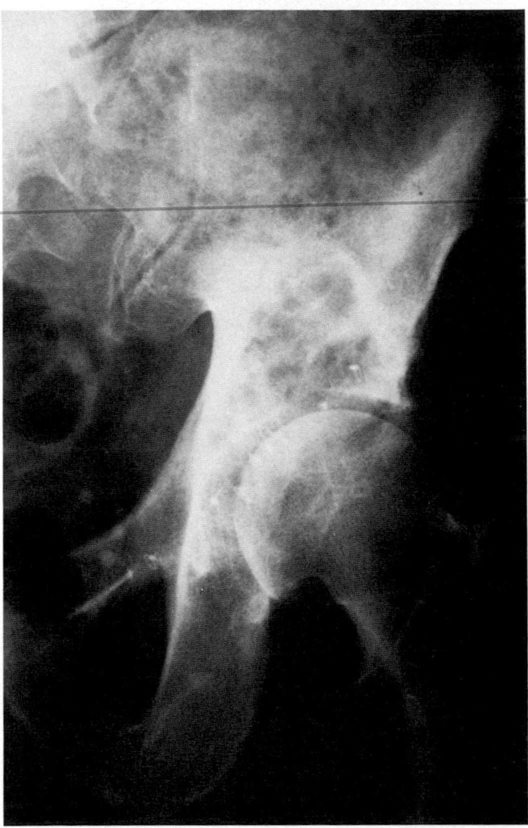

FIGURE 9-10. An anteroposterior x-ray of the pelvis in a man with metastatic prostate carcinoma to the ilium just above the acetabulum. Most metastases from prostate carcinoma are "blastic" and do not require stabilization but this defect in the ilium weakens the acetabulum and should be surgically treated. As long as the subchondral bone is uninvolved or only minimally resorbed, curettage and packing with polymethylmethacrylate is sufficient. Steinmann pins can be used to increase the strength of the reconstruction.

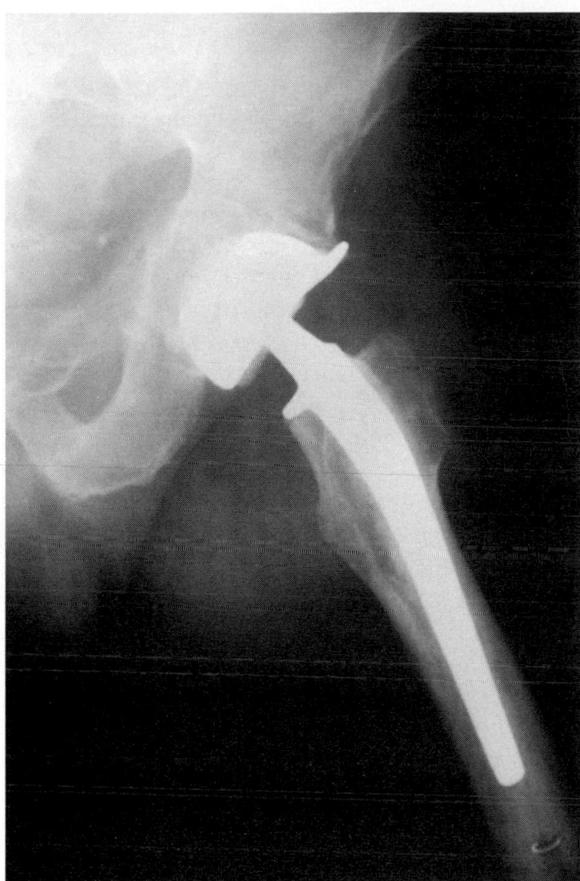

FIGURE 9-11. An anteroposterior x-ray of the hip of a patient who had a metastatic deposit from a breast cancer in her acetabulum. She had intractable pain, a destroyed medial acetabular wall, and protrusio of her femoral head. She had this total hip replacement, with her femoral head used to fill the acetabular defect and a protrusio ring used for additional strengthening of the acetabulum.

months before the onset of focal neurologic deficits. Occasionally, the onset of pain is sudden, after a pathologic compression fracture. Impingement of the cord or nerve roots occurs by direct extension of the tumor but can be secondary to spinal instability and deformity.[132] Early recognition and management by bracing and irradiation before neurologic deficit occurs usually results in pain relief, making an operation unnecessary. When the patient has compression of the spinal cord secondary to metastatic cancer, decompression and stabilization are required; this can usually be accomplished through a posterior approach. A wide laminectomy of each involved level should be done. Removal of both pedicles provides adequate exposure for removal of the anterior offending disease. The spine should be stabilized with rigid internal fixation. Anterior decompression is reserved for patients having primary disease or whose spinal cord cannot be decompressed by a posterior approach.[96,106] When the spine is kyphotic with anterior collapse of the vertebrae and anterior compression of the spinal cord, the patient should be treated by an anterior decompression and stabilization. When the posterior elements are involved and the cord is compressed anteriorly, the patient should have a posterior stabilization and an anterior decompression (Fig. 9-13). Techniques for anterior and posterior decompression and stabilization, including the use of many instrumentation systems, are described in the literature, and the interested reader is referred there for more detailed information.[41,42,57,61,85,88,96,98,103,117,119] The literature strongly supports early decompression and stabilization of patients having any neurologic compromise and vertebral collapse, and we agree. When there is minimal or no bone destruction and cord compression is due to the soft-tissue extension of the metastasis, emergent irradiation is recommended. The patient should also be treated with a short course of high-dose corticosteroids, with a rapid taper to reduce the edema that

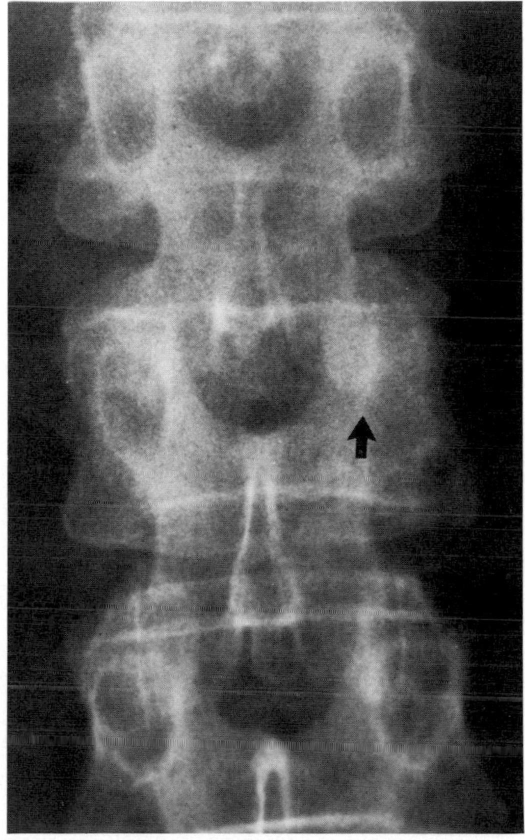

FIGURE 9-12. This anteroposterior x-ray of the lumbar spine in a patient who complained of back pain shows a subtle finding that is often called the "winking owl." The cortical bone of the pedicles is seen at the upper outer corners of the vertebral bodies as dense round structures because we are looking at it in cross section. When metastatic deposits involve the vertebrae, the cortices of the pedicles are usually thinned and therefore cannot be seen on the plain film. This "missing" pedicle (*arrow*) is the closed or "winked" eye and is almost pathognomonic of metastatic disease but we have also seen it in a patient who had a lymphoma of bone.

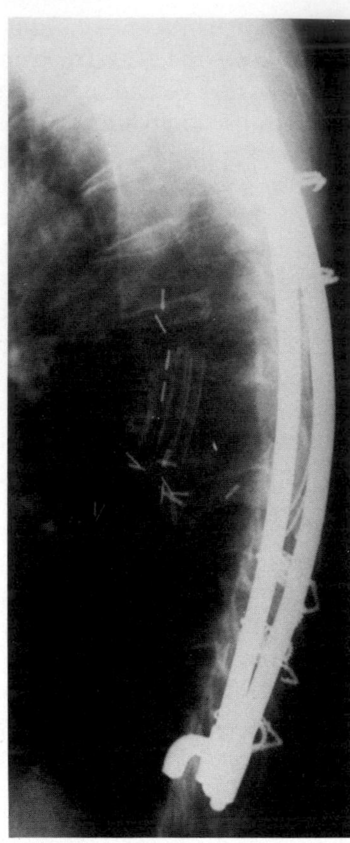

FIGURE 9-13. A lateral x-ray of the thoracic spine in a woman with a metastasis to the seventh thoracic vertebra, with extensive destruction of both the posterior elements and the body. She was treated first with posterior decompression and stabilization and then anterior decompression, with the rib used as bone graft.

adds to the compression and neurologic damage. Our recommendation is 30 mg/kg of methylprednisolone, given intravenously over 1 hour, then 5.4 mg/kg/hour, given intravenously for the next 23 hours and then discontinued.

Resection and Allograft Reconstruction

There is an occasional indication for definitive surgical resection of a metastatic focus. A patient with a solitary metastasis from any origin who has been tumor-free for more than a couple of years should be considered to be a candidate for a resection. Renal cell carcinoma and follicular cell thyroid carcinoma are the two tumors most likely to produce isolated bone metastasis years after therapy for the primary tumor.[2]

Reconstruction methods are similar to the methods used to reconstruct an extremity after the resection of a primary bone tumor. Because many metastatic deposits are diaphyseal or at the diaphyseal/metaphyseal junction, intercalary allografts are often used to replace the resected segment of bone.

Primary Benign Disease of Bone

As a general rule, benign lesions associated with a pathologic fracture eventually require surgical management, although unicameral bone cyst is an exception.[5,76] Spontaneous healing of a pathologic fracture through benign tumor has been observed but it does not occur regularly. There is no evidence that the fracture stimulates healing of even the least active lesions. Often, the fracture callus temporarily obscures the tumor but on radiographs taken after the fracture callus has remodeled, the lesion is usually still present.

Nonetheless, surgery is not always required. In a child with a fracture through a unicameral bone cyst, the fracture should be allowed to heal and the patient observed. If the cyst does not heal spontaneously by the time the fracture callus has remodeled, corticosteroid injection is recommended. Curettage is probably best reserved for those unicameral bone cysts that do not heal after three or four corticosteroid injections. A solitary enchondroma in the hand is another example.[101] The fracture heals but the lesion does not. If the patient had no symptoms before the fracture occurred and the injury that produced the fracture resulted in a significant force to the bone, surgery is not necessary. Conversely, if the patient had symptoms before the fracture or the fracture occurred with minimal or no trauma, it is probably best to curet and bone graft the enchondroma because another fracture is liable to occur in the future. Most other benign tumors should be operated on but surgery usually is possible and easier when delayed until after the fracture has healed. Closed treatment of the pathologic fracture associated with a benign tumor is usually best and is recommended.

When surgery for a benign bone lesion is necessary, we recommend intralesional excision (simple curettage) for those that usually heal spontaneously (eg, nonossifying fibroma, unicameral bone cyst, enchondroma). Those tumors that do not heal spontaneously (eg, chondroblastoma, osteoblastoma, ossifying fibroma, chondromyxofibroma) should be treated with more aggressive surgery. An en bloc wide surgical excision (eg, fibular head excision) is the treatment of choice for locally aggressive benign tumors if the resulting function will be normal. Usually, this is not technically possible, and curettage is the initial treatment. If curettage is selected, it should include removal of the reactive bone surrounding the lesion.

Giant cell tumor of bone is a common benign tumor associated with a pathologic fracture in young adults. Our management of this fracture has changed dramatically in the past few years.[23,37,104] It was previously believed that those patients who had a pathologic fracture through a giant cell tumor of bone had a particularly aggressive tumor and that they should be treated with a primary resection. The routine management of a patient with a pathologic fracture through a giant cell tumor of bone was to allow the fracture, usually grossly displaced, to heal, and then the tumor was widely excised. This excision required removal of the entire end of the bone. Although it is recognized that curettage may be inadequate and that the patient has a 25% chance of local recurrence, we have elected to treat the patient with a thorough and extended curettage, open reduction of the fracture, packing of the cavity with PMMA, and internal fixation of the reconstructed fracture. Only when the bone has been destroyed beyond reconstruction do we believe that it is necessary to do a primary excision.

Primary Malignant Disease of Bone

Primary malignant bone tumors include those treated primarily by irradiation (eg, myeloma, and non-Hodgkin's lymphoma of bone) and those treated primarily by surgical resection and adjuvant chemotherapy or radiation therapy (eg, osteosarcoma, Ewing's sarcoma, chondrosarcoma, fibrosarcoma, malignant fibrous histiocytoma). The prognosis for patients presenting with a pathologic fracture through a primary malignant bone tumor is believed to be worse than that for patients who do not have a pathologic fracture.[80] The presence of a pathologic fracture through a primary sarcoma changes the appropriate treatment only when the fracture is grossly displaced. Those patients having minimally displaced fractures can be treated as patients without a fracture but those having a grossly displaced fracture probably should have an early amputation.

Whole-lung tomography or CT scan of the lung and ^{99m}Tc bone scan are recommended as initial screening tests for possible metastasis from a primary bone sarcoma. Because metastases to the brain, liver, and spleen from sarcoma are rare, it is not necessary to routinely evaluate these organs beyond physical examination and routine laboratory tests. For those patients with no evidence of neurologic dysfunction on physical examination, no further evaluation is believed to be needed; however, if the patient has clinical evidence of mental dysfunction (eg, memory abnormalities, seizure, confusion), a CT scan of the brain is indicated. For patients without hepatic or splenic enlargement and in whom results of the serum liver function tests (ie, serum glutamic-oxaloacetic transaminase, SGPT, albumin, alkaline phosphatase, total protein, total bilirubin) and peripheral blood smear are normal, no further investigation is indicated with respect to the liver or spleen. If any of these results are abnormal, an abdominal CT scan is required.

Biopsy of a bone sarcoma with an associated pathologic fracture is especially difficult. The healing process alters the histology and may confuse the pathologist. Whenever possible, the surgeon should perform a biopsy on tissue at a distance from the fracture. The pathologist should always be told that there is a pathologic fracture. When a soft-tissue mass is associated with the tumor, a needle biopsy is usually adequate but when there is limited extraosseous tissue and the fracture callus has had an opportunity to develop (5 days or more), an open biopsy provides better material and is preferred.[86]

Internal fixation of a pathologic fracture due to a primary sarcoma is not appropriate; when surgical resection of the sarcoma is not required (Ewing's sarcoma, myeloma, lymphoma of bone), the fracture should still be treated closed. If the fracture cannot be treated closed, surgical resection is recommended. Resection without an amputation is more difficult, more likely to be inadequate, and therefore only occasionally recommended.

A radical amputation is the best oncologic treatment of the sarcoma requiring surgical resection (osteosarcoma, chondrosarcoma, fibrosarcoma, malignant fibrous histiocytoma) and usually the best treatment for the patient having a primary bone sarcoma and a grossly displaced pathologic fracture.

Those patients with a primary malignancy of bone and pathologic fracture require the carefully coordinated care of an oncology team, including the medical oncologist, radiation therapist, pathologist, radiologist, and orthopaedic surgeon; only with the full complement of care can these patients achieve the best quality of life and maximum life expectancy.

Systemic Skeletal Disease

When the surgeon is planning the management of a pathologic fracture in a patient with a systemic skeletal disease, it is best to separate the systemic skeletal diseases into those that can be corrected and those that cannot. The former include renal osteodystrophy, hyperparathyroidism, osteomalacia (Fig. 9-14), and disuse osteoporosis; examples of the latter include osteogenesis imperfecta, polyostotic fibrous dysplasia, postmenopausal osteoporosis, Paget's disease, and osteopetrosis. As a category, these disorders have in common bones that are weak and predisposed to fracture or plastic deformation. The fracture callus usually does not form normally, and healing occurs slowly. Patients with Paget's disease of bone have an increased incidence of fracture, and delayed union or nonunion is likely when these fractures are treated without internal fixation.[73] There is no evidence that open reduction and internal fixation is associated with increased blood loss or other operative complications.[70,140] Systemic treatment is not necessary. Displaced fractures of the femoral neck should be treated with a replacement endoprosthesis rather than internal fixation.[140]

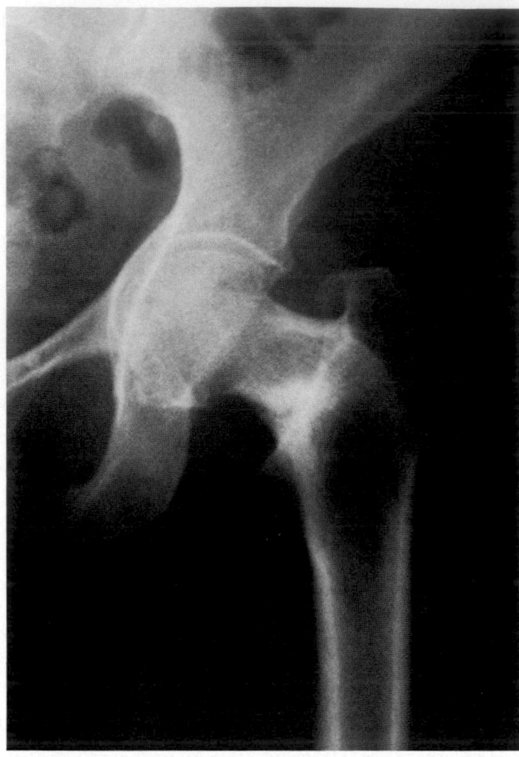

FIGURE 9-14. An anteroposterior x-ray of the proximal femur in a woman with osteomalacia. The femoral neck is in varus because of the bone's inability to withstand the forces of weight bearing. The bone may need the temporary additional support of an internal fixation device but more importantly, the cause of the osteomalacia must be determined and corrected so that the bone can repair itself.

Because the entire skeleton is affected by systemic skeletal disease, the treatment of the fracture must be accomplished without adversely affecting the remainder of the skeleton while the fracture unites. If the underlying process is correctable, treatment of the underlying process should be started, and the fracture should then be treated as a nonpathologic fracture. If the underlying process cannot be corrected, the condition of the remainder of the skeleton must be considered when planning treatment of the fracture. Most femoral neck fractures and intertrochanteric fractures are in patients with osteoporosis, and the strength of the bone expected to hold screws or a prosthesis must be considered when planning the surgical fixation technique. Although the bone usually is strong enough to hold the fixation device, occasionally PMMA must be used to secure the screws in the bone. A primary goal in the management of patients with any systemic skeletal disease is to prevent disuse osteoporosis, which may lead to additional pathologic fractures. A secondary goal is to provide long-term mechanical support for the weakened bone. Reduction and internal fixation are indicated, so that the patient can remain active. Intramedullary rods provide prolonged support for the bone. PMMA is used if needed for adequate fixation of the device.[4]

SUMMARY

In summary, any abnormality of the bone that reduces the strength of the bone predisposes it to mechanical failure during normal activity or with minimal trauma. The mechanical failure manifests itself as a fracture, and this fracture must be recognized as a pathologic fracture if the patient is to be treated properly. Often, the underlying pathologic process is obvious but occasionally it is overlooked if not specifically sought. When the fracture is recognized as being a pathologic fracture, the underlying pathologic process should be determined. When the clinical setting makes the diagnosis obvious, it is not always necessary to biopsy the lesion. When there is a significant possibility that the underlying process is a primary sarcoma, a biopsy should be done before definitive treatment is instituted.

Fatigue Fractures

Fatigue fractures are fractures due to fatigue of the bone caused by repeated strain.[33,125] It is strain, not stress, that produces the conditions of fracture. Under normal conditions, bone that is strained hypertrophies (Wolfe's law) and rather than failing becomes stronger. Fatigue fractures occur under abnormal or pathologic conditions. The most common pathologic condition is in the patient's activity, not in the patient's bone (eg, runners who overtrain, military recruits who are pushed too hard). Less commonly, the bone is weak due to osteoporosis or osteomalacia and fractures occur from the normal strains of everyday activities.

The patient with a fatigue fracture usually presents with complaints of pain, most commonly only with activity. Many athletes have pain only with their training or competitive activities. The radiographic findings are usually diagnostic or at least strongly suggestive (Fig. 9-15). The most important part of the evaluation is the history. The patient with normal bones should give a history of a change in their physical activity within the 4 weeks before the onset of their symptoms. Scully and Besterman[122] studied military personnel going through basic training and discovered that fatigue fractures occurred during the third week of basic training and that by decreasing the physical activities of basic training during the third week, the incidence of fatigue fracture was essentially eliminated. This is the best evidence of how long it usually takes the bone to be strained beyond its capacity to hypertrophy. If strained less, it will hypertrophy; if strained more, it will acutely fail. If the patient gives a history of a

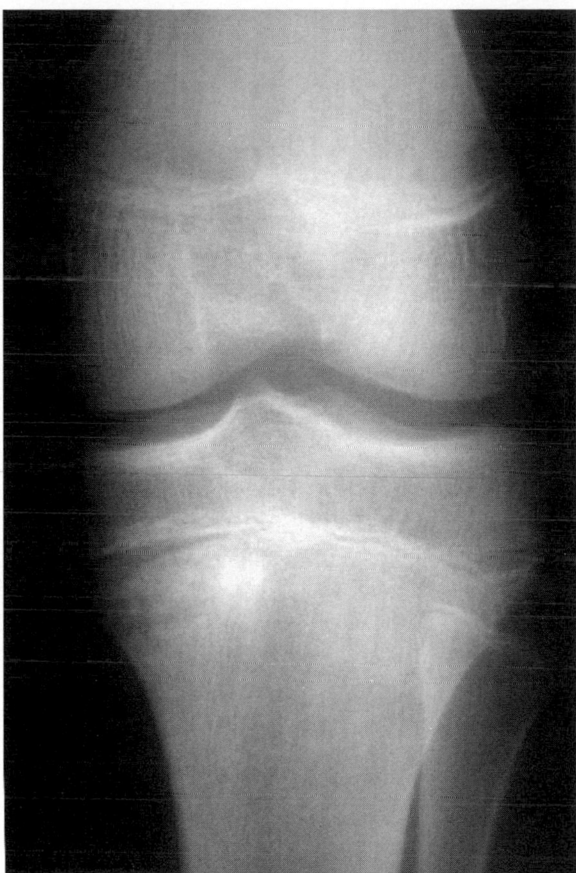

FIGURE 9-15. An anteroposterior x-ray of a 13-year old's knee. The patient was a soccer player who had started practice 6 weeks before this x-ray was taken. The patient had had pain in the medial plateau for 3 weeks and until the x-ray was taken was thought to have bursitis in the pes bursa. The patient's activities were restricted for 1 month and the patient then allowed to begin resumption of physical activities, slowly.

change in activity consistent with causing a fatigue fracture (eg, beginning an exercise program, increasing the intensity of an exercise program, beginning organized practice, adding hills to a training regimen), further evaluation for a cause is unnecessary. If there is no such history, the quality of the bone should be evaluated.

Bone weakened due to osteoporosis or osteomalacia fails because of fatigue under situations of normal activities. A compression fracture of the spine in a patient with senile osteoporosis is probably not a fatigue fracture but many femoral neck fractures in this age group are likely due to fatigue of the bone. Tountas[135] reviewed a few documented fatigue fractures of the femoral neck in the older patient and discovered that if they were not found and internally fixed, they would usually go on to fail completely and the patient would present with a displaced femoral neck fracture. These are probably the group of patients who say that their hip gave way and they fell rather than the fall being the cause the fracture. This is one of the most important fatigue fractures to recognize before the patient develops a completed fracture. Another group of common fatigue fractures in this older group of patients occurs in the posterior ilium.[52] The patients with weakened bone need treatment of their underlying bone disorder. If bone strength can be improved, fatigue fractures are less likely. If the bone cannot be improved, healing is difficult but internal fixation is complicated by the weakened bone.

The basic pathophysiology of fatigue fractures is not fully understood. Frankel and Burstein[46] have stated that when the muscles fatigue, the muscles are not able to protect the bone from excessive strain. This leads to the bone being overstrained and failing. Johnston says that based on his observations of biopsy material from early fatigue fractures, the initial finding is localized osteoporosis.[71] This suggests that the pathologic strain stimulates bone resorption, as opposed to the bone apposition associated with physiologic strain. Biomechanical studies have been done in vitro and although the fatigue characteristics of in vivo bone are probably not completely explained by these studies, an understanding of the mechanical behavior is useful. The fatigue mechanism is similar to that of artificial, oriented, short-fiber composite materials.[125] There are three stages. The primary stage is crack initiation, the second stage is crack propagation, and the tertiary stage is rapid failure of the bone. It is clear that the bone can repair itself quickly if the pathologic strain is removed before stage three occurs, and this is the basis of treatment.

Numerous bones have been reported to have fatigue fractures but those of the metatarsals, calcaneus, and tibia comprise the majority.[97] The metatarsals are implicated in more than half of all clinical fatigue fractures, whereas the calcaneus comprises another fourth and the tibia almost 20%. The femur is the next most common but is found in less than 5%, and the fibula is involved in about 1%. The tarsal navicular has been reported as a site of fatigue fracture in athletes.[72]

The clinical presentation and radiographic findings are usually sufficient for a diagnosis but occasionally the patient's presentation is not so clear. The most common confusing aspect of the presentation is a normal radiograph. If the patient is seen early (first week or two) after the pain is first noticed, the plain radiograph is likely to be normal. ^{99m}Tc bone scans are accurate in the detection of the occult fatigue fracture.[45,51,94,108] The bone with a fatigue fracture imaged with magnetic resonance is abnormal.[18,87,128,129] The abnormal findings are not specific for a fatigue fracture and can be alarming if the clinician does not consider fatigue fracture in the differential diagnosis. Patients with the clinical presentation of a fatigue fracture who have a typical radiograph do not need further evaluation; however, those with a normal radiograph can have a ^{99m}Tc bone scan for a more immediate determination. Another option is to treat the patient with a presumptive diagnosis of a fatigue fracture and repeat the radiograph in a week or two. At that time, the usual radiographic findings should be evident.

Fatigue fractures are treated with a decrease in activity. Usually, this means only a reduction in the patient's exercise program and only rarely is it necessary for the patient to eliminate activities of daily living. The reduction in activities should be sufficient for the patient to have minimal or no pain. If the patient continues to have pain, further reduction is necessary. The bone should be able to heal within a month and allow resumption of activities. During the reduction of activities, it is usually best to allow the patient to remain as active as possible for two reasons. First, the continued activity reduces the risk of disuse osteoporosis and second, most of the patients who sustain fatigue fractures enjoy their physical activity and resist complete elimination of them.

Clancy[28] has outlined a specific program for runners with fatigue fractures of the lower extremities. He recommends immediate cross-training activities, using aerobic activities such as bicycling or rowing. If the patient can tolerate roller-blading or cross-country skiing activities, these are allowed. Pool running is allowed. Once the pain is minimal, the patient begins a graduated return to running. The patient starts with every-other-day runs of half the pre-injury distance and progresses at weekly intervals if there is no progression of pain. The patient is usually back to full activities within 6 to 8 weeks of their initial symptoms.

Mid-shaft anterior cortical tibial fatigue fractures do not behave like most fatigue fractures.[6] This unique fatigue fracture most commonly occurs in the competitive jumping athlete. The radiographic appearance is of a partial or complete radiolucent line in the anterior cortex of the tibial diaphysis, usually having reactive periosteum both proximal and distal to it. This fatigue fracture is slow to heal, and prolonged rest or surgical excision and bone grafting is necessary. Strenuous activities should be avoided until the radiolucent line has completely filled in because a completed fracture can occur when jumping is resumed, even if the patient has no symptoms.

Fatigue fractures are rarely a source of treatment difficulty, with the exception of the most competitive athletes. The difficulty arises from making the diagnosis. The patients may present with pain and not provide a typical history, and their radiograph may still be normal. The orthopaedist must remember to keep fatigue fracture in the differential diagnosis for these patients. This is increasingly true as more individuals of all ages are involved in strenuous physical activities.

REFERENCES

1. Abrams, H., Spiro, R., and Goldstein, N.: Metastasis in Carcinoma: Analysis of 1000 Autopsied Cases. Cancer 3:74–85, 1950.
2. Albright, J.A., Gillespie, T.E., and Butaud, T.R.: Treatment of Bone Metastases. Semin. Oncol. 7(4):418–434, 1980.
3. Anderson, J.T., Erickson, J.M., Thompson, R.C. Jr., and Chao, E.Y.: Pathologic Femoral Shaft Fractures Comparing Fixation Techniques Using Cement. Clin. Orthop. 131:273–277, 1978.
4. Bartucci, E.J., Gonzalez, M.H., Cooperman, D.R., Freedberg, H.I., Barmada, R., and Laros, G.S.: The Effect of Adjunctive Methylmethacrylate on Failures of Fixation and Function in Patients With Intertrochanteric Fractures and Osteoporosis. J. Bone Joint Surg. 67A:1094–1107, 1985.
5. Baschang, A., von Laer, L.: Indication and Procedure of the Operative Treatment of Benign Bone Cyst in Children and Adolescents. European J. Ped. Surg. 1:207–209, 1991.
6. Beals, R.K., and Cook, R.D.: Stress Fractures of the Anterior Tibial Diaphysis: Review. Orthopedics 14:869–875, 1991.
7. Beals, R.K., Lawton, G.D., and Snell, W.E.: Prophylactic Internal Fixation of the Femur in Metastatic Breast Cancer. Cancer 28:1350–1354, 1971.
8. Behr, J.T., Doboz, W.R., and Badrinath, K.: The Treatment of Pathologic and Impending Pathologic Fractures of the Proximal Femur in the Elderly. Clin. Orthop. 198:173–178, 1985.
9. Bender, R.A., and Hansen, H.: Hypercalcemia in Bronchogenic Carcinoma. A Prospective Study of 200 Patients. Ann. Intern. Med. 80:205–208, 1974.
10. Berretton, B.A., and Carter, J.R.: Current Concepts Review: Mechanisms of Cancer Metastasis to Bone. J. Bone Joint Surg. 68A:308–312, 1986.
11. Bertin, K.C., Horstman, J., and Coleman, S.S.: Isolated Fractures of the Lesser Trochanter in Adults: An Initial Manifestation of Metastatic Malignant Disease. J. Bone Joint Surg. 66A:770–773, 1984.
12. Blake, D.D.: Radiation Treatment of Metastatic Bone Disease. Clin. Orthop. 73:89–100, 1970.
13. Body, J.J.: Medical Treatment of Tumor-induced Hypercalcemia and Tumor-induced Osteolysis: Challenges for Future Research. Support. Care Cancer 1:26033, 1993.
14. Body, J.J., and Dumon, J.C.: Treatment of Tumour-induced Hypercalcemia With Bisphosphonate Pamidronate: Dose-response Relationship and Influence of Tumour Type. Ann. Oncol. 5:359-363, 1994.
15. Boring, C.C., Squires, T.S., Tong, T., and Montgomery, S.: Cancer Statistics. CA Cancer J. Clin. 44:7–26, 1994.
16. Bouma, W.H., Mulder, J.H., and Hop, C.J.: The Influence of Intramedullary Nailing Upon the Development of Metastasis in the Treatment of an Impending Pathologic Fracture: An Experimental Study. Clin. Exp. Metastasis 1:205–212, 1983.
17. Bowers, T.A., Murray, J.A., Channsangarej, C., Soo, C.S., Chuang, V.P., and Wallace, S.: Bone Metastasis From Renal Carcinoma. J. Bone Joint Surg. 64A:749–754, 1982.
18. Brahme, S.K., Cervilla, V., Vint, V., Cooper, K., Kortman, K., Resnick, D.: Magnetic Resonance Appearance of Sacral Insufficiency Fractures. Skeletal Radiol. 19:489–493, 1990.
19. Brener, R.A., and Jelliffe, A.M.: The Management of Pathological Fracture of the Major Long Bones From Metastatic Cancer. J. Bone Joint Surg. 40B:652–659, 1958.
20. Broos, P., Reynders, P., van den Bogert, W., and Vanderschot, P.: Surgical Treatment of Metastatic Fracture of the Femur Improvement of Quality of Life. Acta Orthop. Belg. 59(Suppl.1):52–56, 1993.
21. Brown, R.K., Pelker, R.R., Friedlaender, G.E., Peschel, R.E., and Panjabi, M.M.: Postfracture Irradiation Effects on the Biomechanical and Histologic Parameters of Fracture Healing. J. Orthop. Res. 9:876–882, 1991.
22. Bunting, R.W., Boublik, M., Blevins, F.T., Dame, C.C., Ford, L.A., and Lavine, L.S.: Functional Outcome of Pathologic Fracture Secondary to Malignant Diseases in a Rehabilitation Hospital. Cancer 69:98–102, 1992.
23. Campanacci, M., Baldini, N., Boriani, S., and Sudanese, A:

Giant Cell Tumor of Bone. J. Bone Joint Surg. 69A:106–114, 1987.

24. Carpenter, P.R., Ewing, J.W., Cook, A.J., and Kuster, A.H.: Angiographic Assessment and Control of Potential Operative Hemorrhage With Pathologic Fractures Secondary to Metastases. Clin. Orthop. 123:6–8, 1977.
25. Cheal, E.J., Hipp, J.A., and Hayes, W.C.: Evaluation of Finite Element Analysis for Prediction of the Strength Reduction Due to Metastatic Lesions in the Femoral Neck. J. Biomech. 26: 251–264, 1993.
26. Cheng, D.S., Seitz, C.B., and Eyre, H.J.: Nonoperative Management of Femoral, Humeral, and Acetabular Metastasis in Patients With Breast Carcinoma. Cancer 45:1533–1537, 1980.
27. Chybowski, F.M., Larson-Keller, J.J., Bergstralh, E.J., and Desterlung, J.E.: Predicting Radionucleotide Bone Scan Finding in Patients With Newly Diagnosed Untreated Prostatic Cancer: Prostate Specific Antigen is Sperior to All Other Clinical Parameters. J. Urol. 145:313–318, 1991.
28. Clancy, W.G. Jr.: Specific Rehabilitation for the Injuried Recreational Runner. Instr. Course Lect. 38:483–486, 1989.
29. Coerkamp, E.G., and Kroon, H.M.: Cortical Bone Metastasis. Radiology. 169:525–528, 1988.
30. Coggeshall, J., Merrill, W., Hande, K., and DesPrez, R.: Implications of Hypercalcemia With Respect to Diagnosis and Treatment of Lung Cancer. Am. J. Med. 80:325–328, 1986.
31. Coleman, R.E., Mashiter, G., Whitaker, K.B., Moss, D.W., Rubens, R.D., and Folgelman, I.: Bone Scan Flare Predicts Successful Systemic Therapy for Bone Metastases. J. Nucl. Med. 29:1354–1359, 1988.
32. Cornell, C.N., and Lane, J.M.: Management of Pathologic Fractures in Patients With Breast Cancer. Surgical Rounds 9:25–41, 1986.
33. Courtenay, B.G., Bowers, D.M.: Stress Fractures: Clinical Features and Investigation. Med. J. Aust. 153:155–156, 1990.
34. Dijkstra, S., Wiggers, T., van Geel, B.N., and Boxma, H.: Impending and Actual Pathological Fractures in Patients With Bone Metastases of the Long Bones. Eur. J. Surg. 160: 535–542, 1994.
35. Dobozi, W.R., Dvonch, V.M., Saltzman, M.L., Beigler, D.F., and Belich, P.: Treatment of Impending Pathological Fractures of the Femur With Flexible Intramedullary Nails. Orthopedics 7:1682–1688, 1984.
36. Douglass, H.O. Jr., Shukla, S.K., and Mindell, E.: Treatment of Pathological Fractures of Long Bones Excluding Those Due to Breast Cancer. J. Bone Joint Surg. 58A:1055–1061, 1976.
37. Eckardt, J.J., and Grogan, T.J.: Giant Cell Tumor of Bone. Clin. Orthop. Rel. Res. 204:45–58, 1986.
38. Eftekhar, N.S., and Thurston, C.W.: Effect of Irradiation on Acrylic Cement With Special Reference to Fixation of Pathological Fractures. J. Biomech. 8:53–56, 1975.
39. Fidler, M.: Incidence of Fracture Through Metastasis in Long Bones. Acta Orthop. Scand. 52:623–627, 1981.
40. Fidler, M.: Prophylactic Internal Fixation of Secondary Neoplastic Deposits in Long Bones. Br. Med. J. 1:341–343, 1973.
41. Fidler, M.W.: Anterior Decompression and Stabilization of Metastatic Spinal Fractures. J. Bone Joint Surg. 68B:83–90, 1986.
42. Fidler, M.W.: Pathological Fractures of the Cervical Spine: Palliative Surgical Treatment. J. Bone Joint Surg. 67B:352–357, 1985.
43. Fisken, R.A., Heath, D.A., Somers, S., and Bold, A.M.: Hypercalcemia in Hospital Patients. Lancet 1:202–207, 1981.
44. Flemming, J.E., and Beals, R.K.: Pathologic Fracture of the Humerus. Clin. Orthop. 203:258–260, 1986.
45. Floyd, W.M. Jr., Butler, J.E., Clanton, T., Kim, E.E., and Pjura, G.: Roentgenologic Diagnosis of Stress Fractures and Stress Reaction. South. Med. J. 80:433–439, 1987.
46. Frankel, V.H., and Burstein, A.H.: Orthopaedic Biomechanics. Philadelphia, Lea & Febiger, 1970.
47. Frassica, F.J., Gitelis, S., and Sims, F.H.: Metastatic Bone Disease: General Principles, Pathophysiology, Evaluation, and Biopsy. Instr. Course Lect. 61:293–300, 1992.
48. Gainor, B.J. and Buchert, P.: Fracture Healing in Metastatic Bone Disease. Clin. Orthop. 178:297–302, 1983.
49. Galasko, C.S.B.: Skeletal Metastases. Clin. Orthop. 210:18–30, 1986.
50. Galasko, C.S.B., and Bunn, J.I.: Hypercalcemia in Patients With Advanced Mammary Cancer. Br. Med. J. 3:573–577, 1971.
51. Gotis-Graham, I., McGuigan, L., Diamond, T., et al.: Sacral Insufficiency Fractures in the Elderly. J. Bone Joint Surg. 76A:882–886, 1984.
52. Graham, W.P. III., Gardner, B., Thomas, A.N., Gordon, G.S., Loken, H.F., and Goldman, L.: Hypercalcemia in Carcinoma of the Female Breast. Surg. Gynecol. Obstet. 117:709–714, 1963.
53. Greenspan, A., and Norman, A.: Osteolytic Cortical Destruction: An Unusual Pattern of Skeletal Metastases. Skeletal Radiol. 17:402–406, 1988.
54. Gucalp, R., Theriault, R., Gill, I., et al.: Treatment of Cancer-Associated Hypercalcemia. Double Blind Comparison of Rapid and Slow Intravenous Infusion Regimens of Pamidronate Disodium and Saline Alone. Arch. Intern. Med. 154:1935–1944, 1994.
55. Habermann, E.T.: Review of 125 Cases of Pathological Fractures Secondary to Breast Metastases Treated With and Without the Use of Methylmethacrylate. Orthop. Trans. 4:346, 1980.
56. Habermann, E.T., Sachs, R., Stern R.E., Hirsh, D.M., and Anderson, W.J.: The Pathology and Treatment of Metastatic Disease of the Femur. Clin. Orthop. 169:70–82, 1982.
57. Harrington, K.D.: Anterior Decompression and Stabilization of the Spine as a Treatment for Vertebral Collapse and Spinal Cord Compression From Metastatic Malignancy. Clin. Orthop. 233:177–197, 1988.
58. Harrington, K.D.: The Management of Acetabular Insufficiency Secondary to Metastatic Malignant Disease. J. Bone Joint Surg. 63A:653–664, 1981.
59. Harrington, K.D.: Current Concepts Review: Metastatic Disease of the Spine. J. Bone Joint Surg. 68A:1110–1115, 1986.
60. Harrington, K.D.: Problems of Pathologic Fractures. Complications in Orthopedics, 2(1):4, 1987.
61. Harrington, K.D.: The Use of Methylmethacrylate for Vertebral Body Replacement and Anterior Stabilization of Pathologic Fracture-Dislocation of Spine Due to Metastatic Malignant Disease. J. Bone Joint Surg. 63A:36–46, 1981.
62. Harrington, K.D., Sim, F.H., Enis, J.E., Johnston, J.O., Dick, H.M., and Gristina, A.G.: Methylmethacrylate as an Adjunct in Internal Fixation of Pathologic Fractures. J. Bone Joint Surg. 58A:1047–1055, 1976.
63. Heisterberg, L., and Johansen, T.S.: Treatment of Pathologic Fractures. Acta Orthop. Scand. 50:787–790, 1979.
64. Hipp, J.A., McBroom, R.J., Cheal, E.J., and Hayes, W.C.: Structural Consequences of Endosteal Metastatic Lesions in Long Bone. J. Orthop. Res. 7:828–837, 1989.
65. Hipp, J.A., Rosenberg, A.E., and Hayes, W.C.: Mechanical Properties of Trabecular Bone Within and Adjacent to Osseous Metastases. J. Bone Mineral Res. 7:1165–1171, 1992.
66. Hipp, J.A., Springfield, D.S., Hayes, W.C.: Predicting Pathologic Fracture Risk in the Management of Metastatic Bone Defects. Clin. Orthop. In press.
67. Jacobsen, K.D., Folleras, G., and Fossa, S.D.: Metastases From Renal Cell Carcinoma to the Humerus or the Shoulder Girdle. Br. J. Urol. 73:124–128, 1994.
68. Jensen, T.M., Dillon, W.L., and Reckling, F.W.: Changing Concepts in the Management of Pathologic and Impending Pathologic Fractures. J. Trauma 16:496–502, 1976.
69. Johnson, J.T.H.: Reconstruction of Pelvic Ring Following Tumor Resection. J. Bone Joint Surg. 60A:747–751, 1978.
70. Johnston, C.C. Jr., Altman, R.D., Canfield, R.E., Finerman, G.A.M., Taulbee, J.D., and Ebert, M.L.: Review of Fracture Experience During Treatment of Paget's Disease of Bone With Etidronate Disodium (EHDP). Clin. Orthop. 172:186–194, 1983.
71. Johnston, L.: personal communication, Armed Forces Institute of Pathology, 1978.

72. Khan, K.M., Fuller, P.J., Brukner, P.D., Kearney, C., Burry, H.C.: Outcome of Conservative and Surgical Management of Navicular Stress Fractures in Athletes. Eighty-six Cases Proven With Computerized Tomography. Am. J. Sports Med. 20:657–666, 1992.
73. Kaplan, F.S.: Paget's Disease of Bone: Orthopaedic Complications. Semin. Arth. Rheum. 23:250–252, 1944.
74. Keene, J.S., Sellinger, D.S., McBeath, A.A., and Englser, W.D.: Metastatic Breast Cancer in the Femur: A Search for the Lesion at Risk of Fracture. Clin. Orthop. 203:282–288, 1986.
75. Krebs, H.: Management of Pathologic Fractures of Long Bones in Malignant Disease. Arch. Orthop. Trauma. Surg. 92:133–137, 1978.
76. Kruls, H.S.A.: Pathological Fractures in Children Due to Solitary Bone Cyst. Reconstr. Surg. Traumatol. 17:133, 1979.
77. Kunec, J.R., and Lewis, R.J.: Closed Intramedullary Rodding of Pathologic Fractures With Supplemental Cement. Clin. Orthop. 188:183–186, 1984.
78. Lancaster, J.M., Koman, L.A., Gristine, A.G., et al.: Pathologic Fractures of the Humerus. South. Med. J. 81: 52–55, 1989.
79. Lane, J.M., Sculco, T.P., and Zolan, S.: Treatment of Pathological Fractures of the Hip by Endoprosthetic Replacement. J. Bone Joint Surg. 62A:954–959, 1980.
80. Larsson, S.E., Lorentzon, R., Warden, H., and Boquist, L.: The Prognosis in Osteosarcoma. Int. Orthop. 5:305–310, 1981.
81. Leeson, M.C., Makley, J.T., and Carter, J.R.: Metastatic Skeletal Disease Distal to the Elbow and Knee. Clin. Orthop. 206:94–99, 1986.
82. Levy, R.N., Sherry, H.S., and Siffert, R.S.: Surgical Management of Metastatic Disease of Bone at the Hip. Clin. Orthop. 169:62–69, 1982.
83. Lodwick, G.S., Wilson, A.J., Farrell, C., Virtama, P., and Dittrich, F.: Determining Growth Rates of Focal Lesions of Bone From Radiographs. Radiology 134:577–583, 1980.
84. Lodwick, G.S., Wilson, A.J., Farrell, C., Virtama, P., Smeltzer, F.M., and Dittrich, F.: Estimating Rate of Growth in Bone Lesions Observer Performance and Error. Radiology 134:585–590, 1980.
85. Lord, C.F., and Herndon, J.H.: Spinal Cord Compression Secondary to Kyphosis Associated With Radiation Therapy for Metastatic Disease. Clin. Orthop. 210:120–127, 1986.
86. Mankin, H.J., Lange, T.A., and Spanier, S.S.: The Hazards of Biopsy in Patients With Malignant Primary Bone and Soft-tissue Tumors. J. Bone Joint Surg. 64A:1121–1127, 1982.
87. Martin, S.D., Healey, J.H., and Horowitz, S.: Stress Fracture MRI. Orthopedics 16:75–78, 1993.
88. McAfee, P.C., Bohlman, H.H., Ducker, T., and Eismont, F.S.: Failure of Stabilization of the Spine With Methylmethacrylate. J. Bone Joint Surg. 68A:1145–1157, 1986.
89. McBroom, R.J., Cheal, E.J., and Hayes, W.C.: Strength Reductions From Metastatic Cortical Defects in Long Bones. J. Orthop. Res. 6:369–378, 1988.
90. Menck, H., Schulze, S., and Larsen, E.: Metastasis Size in Pathologic Femoral Fractures. Acta Orthop. Scand. 59:151–154, 1988.
91. Mikelson, M.R., and Bonfiglio, M.: Pathologic Fractures in the Proximal Part of the Femur Treated by Zickel-Nail Fixation. J. Bone Joint Surg. 58A:1067–1070, 1976.
92. Miller, F., and Whitehill, R.: Carcinoma of the Breast Metastatic to the Skeleton. Clin. Orthop. 184:121–127, 1984.
93. Miller, G.J., Vander Griend, R.A., Blake, W.P., and Springfield, D.S.: Performance Evaluation of a Cement-Augmented Intramedullary Fixation System for Pathologic Lesions of the Femoral Shaft. Clin. Orthop. 221:246–254, 1987.
94. Mills, G.Q., Marymont, J.H. 3rd., and Murphy, D.A.: Bone Scan Utilization in the Differential Diagnosis of Exercise Induced Lower Extremity Pain. Clin. Orthop. Rel. Res. 149: 207–210, 1980.
95. Moehring, H.D.: Closed Flexible Intramedullary Fixation for Pathologic Lesions in Long Bones. Orthopedics 7:829–834, 1984.
96. Moran, J.M., Berg, W.S. Berry, J.L. Geiger, J.M., and Steffee, A.D.: Transpedicular Screw Fixation. J. Orthop. Res. 7:107–114, 1989.
97. Morris, J.M., Blickenstaff, L.D.: Fatigue Fractures: A Clinical Study. Springfield, IL, Charles C. Thomas, 1967.
98. Murray, J.A.: Metastasis to Spine (letter). J. Bone Joint Surg. 69A:633–634, 1987.
99. Murray, J.A., Bruels, M.C., and Lindberg, R.D.: Irradiation of Polymethylmethacrylate in vitro Gamma Radiation Effect. J. Bone Joint Surg. 56A:311–312, 1974.
100. Murray, J.A., and Parrish, F.F.: Surgical Management of Secondary Neoplastic Fractures About the Hip. Orthop. Clin. North Am. 5:887–901, 1974.
101. Newhouse, K.E., El-Khoury, G.Y., and Buckwalter, J.A.: Occult Sacral Fractures in Osteopenic Patients. J. Bone Joint Surg. 74A:1472–1477, 1992.
102. Nicholas, J.A., Wilson, P.D., and Freiberger, R.: Pathological Fractures of the Spine: Etiology and Diagnosis. J. Bone Joint Surg. 42A:127–137, 1960.
103. Nicholls, P.J., and Jarecky, T.W.: The Value of Posterior Decompression by Laminectomy for Malignant Tumors of the Spine. Clin. Orthop. 201:210–213, 1985.
104. Noble, J., and Lamb, D.W.: Enchondromata of Bones of the Hand, A Review of 40 Cases. Hand 6:275, 1974.
105. O'Donnell, R.J., Springfield, D.S., Motwani, H.K., Ready, J.E., Gebhardt, M.C., and Mankin, H.J.: Recurrence of Giant-Cell Tumors of the Long Bones after Curettage and Packing With Cement. J. Bone Joint Surg. 76A:1827–1833, 1994.
106. Olerud, C., Sjostrom, L., Jonsson, H. Jr., and Karlstrom, G.: Posterior Reduction of a Pathologic Spinal Fracture. Acta. Orthop. Scand. 63:345–346, 1992.
107. Oni, O.O.A.: Mechanics of Cancer Metastatic to Bone (Letter). J. Bone Joint Surg. 69A:309–310, 1987.
108. Park, C.H., Kapadis, F., O'Hara, A.E.: Three Phase Bone Scan Findings in Stress Fracture. Clin. Nucl. Med. 6:587–588, 1981.
109. Parrish, F.F., and Murray, J.A.: Surgical Treatment for Secondary Neoplastic Fractures. J. Bone Joint Surg. 52A:665–686, 1970.
110. Perez, G.A., Bradfield, J.S., and Morgan, H.C.: Management of Pathologic Fractures. Cancer 29:684–693, 1972.
111. Phillips, C.D., Pope, T.L., Jones, J.E., Keats, T.E., and MacMillan, R.H.: Nontraumatic Avulsion of the Lesser Trochanter: A Pathognomonic Sign of Metastatic Disease? Skeletal Radiol. 17:106–110, 1988.
112. Price, J.E.: The Biology of Metastatic Breast Cancer. Cancer 66(6 Suppl):1313-1320, 1990.
113. Pugh, J., Sherry, H.S., Futterman, B., and Frankel, V.H.: Biomechanics of Pathologic Fractures. Clin. Orthop. 169:109–114, 1982.
114. Rafii, M., Firooznia, H., Kramer, E., Golimbu, C., and Sanger, J.: The Role of Computed Tomography in Evaluation of Skeletal Metastasis. Journal of Computed Tomography 12:19–24, 1988.
115. Ralston, S., Fogelman, I., Gardner, M.D., and Boyle, I.T.: Hypercalcemia and Metastatic Bone Disease: Is There a Causal Link? Lancet 2:903–905, 1982.
116. Riemer, B.L., Butterfield, S.L., D'Ambrosia, R. and Kellam, J.: Seidel Intramedullary Nailing of Humeral Diaphyseal Fractures. A preliminary Report. Orthopedics 14:239–246, 1991.
117. Roy-Camille, R., Saillant, G., and Mazel, C.: Internal Fixation of the Lumbar Spine With Pedicle Screw Plating. Clin. Orthop. 203:7–17, 1986.
118. Ryan, T.R., Rowe, D.E., and Salciccioli, G.G.: Prophylactic Internal Fixation of the Femur for Neoplastic Lesions. J. Bone Joint Surg. 58A:1071–1074, 1976.
119. Santori, F.S., Ghera, S., dePalma, F., and de Chiara, N.: Treatment of Pathological Fractures and Impending Pathological Fractures of the Femur With Ender Nails. Orthopedics 7:269–274, 1984.
120. Schechter, G.P., Jaffe, E.S., Cossman, J., Horton, J.E., and Whitcomb, C.C.: Malignant Lymphoma With Hypercalcemia. N. Engl. J. Med. 306:995, 1982.
121. Schocker, J.D., and Brady, L.W.: Radiation Therapy for Bone Metastasis. Clin. Orthop. 169:38–43, 1982.

122. Scully, T.J., Besterman, G.: Stress Fractures. A Preventable Training Injury. Mil. Med. 147:285–287, 1982.
123. Sherry, M.M., Greco, F.A., Johnson, D.H., and Hainsworth, J.D.: Metastatic Breast Cancer Confined to the Skeletal System: An Indolent Disease. Am. J. Med. 81:381–386, 1986.
124. Sim, F.H., Daugherty, T.W., and Ivins, J.C.: The Adjunctive Use of Methylmethacrylate in Fixation of Pathological Fractures. J. Bone Joint Surg. 56A:40–48, 1974.
125. Simon, S.R. (ed.): Orthopaedic Basic Science. Chicago, American Academy of Orthopaedic Surgeons 1994:151–153.
126. Smith, D.G., Behr, J.T., Hall, R.F., and Dobozi, W.R.: Closed Flexible Intramedullary Biopsy of Metastatic Carcinoma. Clin. Orthop. 229:162–164, 1988.
127. Snell, W., and Beals, R.K.: Femoral Metastases and Fractures From Breast Carcinoma. Surg. Gynecol. Obstet. 119:22–24, 1964.
128. Stabler, A., Beck, R., Bartl, R: Schmidt, D., and Reiser, M.: Vacuum Phenomena in Insufficiency Fractures of the Sacrum. Skeletal Radiol. 24:31–35, 1995.
129. Stafford, S.A., Rosenthal, D.A., Gebhardt, M.C., Brady, T.J., and Scott, J.A.: MRI in Stress Fractures. Am. J. Roentgenol. 147:553–556, 1986.
130. Steckel, R.J., and Kagan, A.R.: Diagnostic Persistence in Working Up Metastatic Cancer With an Unknown Primary Site. Radiology 134:367–369, 1980.
131. Sterling, J.C., Edelstein, D.W., Calvo, R.D., Webb, R. 2nd.: Stress Fracture in the Athlete. Diagnosis and Management. Sports Med. 14:336–346, 1992.
132. Tabbara, I.A., Sibley, D.S., and Quesenberry, P.J.: Spinal Cord Compression Due To Metastatic neoplasm. South. Med. J. 83:519–523, 1990.
133. Thompson, R.C. Jr.: Impending Fracture Associated With Bone Destruction. Orthopedics 15:547-550, 1992.
134. Tong, D., Gillick, L., and Hendrickson, F.R.: The Palliation of Symptomatic Osseous Metastases. Cancer 50:893–899, 1982.
135. Tountas, A.A.: Insufficiency Stress Fractures of the Femoral Neck in Elderly Women. Clin. Orthop. Rel. Res. 292:202–209, 1993.
136. Vail, T.P. and Harrelson, J.M.: Treatment of Pathologic Fractures of the Humerus. Clin. Orthop. 268:197–202, 1991.
137. van der Hulst, R.R.W., van den Wildenberg, F.A.J.M., Vroemen, J.P.A.M., and Greve, J.W.M.: Intramedullary Nailing of (Impending) Pathologic Fractures. J. Trauma 36:211–215, 1994.
138. van Holten-Verzantvoort, A.Th., Bijvoet, O.L.M., Hermans, J., et al.: Reduced Morbidity From Skeletal Metastases in Breast Cancer Patients During Long-Term Bisphosphonate (ADP) Treatment. Lancet 2:983–985, 1987.
139. Vaughn, P.B., and Brindley, H.H.: Pathologic Fractures of Long Bones. South. Med. J., 72:788–794, 1979.
140. Verinder, D.G.R. and Burke, J.: The Management of Fractures in Paget's Disease of Bone. Injury 10:276–280, 1979.
141. Wang, G.J., Reger, S.I., Maffeo, C., McLaughlin, R.E., and Stamp, W.G.: The Strength of Metal Reinforced Methylmethacrylate Fixation of Pathologic Fractures. Clin. Orthop. 135:287–290, 1978.
142. Widmann,R.F., Pelker,R.R., Friedlaender, G.E., Panjabi, M.M., and Peschel,R.E.: Effects of Prefracture Irradiation on the Biomechanical Parameters of Fracture Healing. J. Orthop. Res. 11:422–428, 1993.
143. Wirth, C.R.: Metastatic Bone Cancer. Curr. Probl. Cancer 3:1–36, 1979.
143a. Yazaway, Y., Frassica, F.J., Chao, E.Y., Pritchard, D.J., Sim, F.H., and Shives, T.C.: Metastatic Bone Disease: A Study of the Surgical Treatment of 166 Pathologic Humeral and Femoral Fractures. Clin. Orthop. 251:213-219, 1990.
144. Yuh, W.T.C., Zacharck, C.K., Barloon, T.J., Satoy, Y., Sickels, W.J., and Hawes, O.R.: Vertebral Compression Fractures: Distinction Between Benign and Malignant Causes With MR Imaging. Radiology 172:215–218, 1989.
145. Zickel, R.E., and Mouradian, W.H.: Intramedullary Fixation of Pathological Fractures and Lesions of the Subtrochanteric Region of the Femur. J. Bone Joint Surg. 58A:1061–1066, 1976.
146. Zimskind, P.D., and Surver, J.M.: Metastasis to Bone From Carcinoma of the Breast. Clin. Orthop. 11:202–215, 1958.

Rockwood and Green's Fractures in Adults, Fourth Edition,
edited by Charles A. Rockwood, David P. Green, Robert W. Bucholz and James D. Heckman.
Lippincott-Raven Publishers, Philadelphia © 1996.

CHAPTER 10

Periprosthetic Fractures

Jay D. Mabrey and Michael A. Wirth

In seeking absolute truth we aim at the unattainable and must be content with finding broken portions.
- Sir William Osler

Part I. Periprosthetic Fractures of the Upper Extremity

Michael A. Wirth

PERIPROSTHETIC FRACTURES OF THE SHOULDER

HISTORICAL REVIEW

The complications associated with prosthetic shoulder arthroplasty are unequivocally tied to the early prototypic constrained variety of shoulder replacement devices that were designed for the dual purpose of restoring stability in the face of an irreparable rotator cuff deficiency and replacing an arthritic joint. Most of the complications encountered with these prostheses involved implant failure, mechanical loosening due to failure of scapular fixation, and periprosthetic fractures of the adjacent humerus or scapula.[9,12,13,19,23,26,32] These failures reflected not only an error in design, but also an underestimation of the forces involved in glenohumeral mechanics. This was attributable to the fact that the early designers of shoulder implants did not appreciate the major loading to which the joint is subjected with normal activity. It was not until much later that investigators determined that the glenohumeral joint reactive force approaches the patient's body weight during simple unrestricted active shoulder elevation.[25] An awareness of these potentially tremendous forces led to further investigation of shoulder kinematics and the evolution of constrained shoulder implants to more anatomically and physiologically unconstrained and semiconstrained prostheses.

It is apparent from a historical perspective of complications, a comprehensive understanding of shoulder biomechanics, and survivorship data, that the indications for constrained shoulder prostheses are exceedingly rare. Therefore, this section is devoted to periprosthetic fractures associated with unconstrained and semiconstrained shoulder replacements.

PERIPROSTHETIC FRACTURES OF UNCONSTRAINED AND SEMICONSTRAINED SHOULDER IMPLANTS

Prevalence

Early and mid-range follow-up studies of total shoulder arthroplasty have been encouraging, with good and excellent results reported in more than 90% of shoulders.[2,3,9,24] Despite this success, the overall prevalence of complications is about 14% and includes the following factors in order of frequency: instability, rotator cuff tear, ectopic ossification, glenoid loosening, periprosthetic fracture, nerve injury, infection, and humeral loosening.[9] Fractures involving the glenoid or humerus account for only a fraction of these problems, constituting less than 2% of all complications (Fig. 10-1).

In Neer's 1982 report,[24] four postoperative fractures of the ipsilateral extremity occurred. Of these injuries,

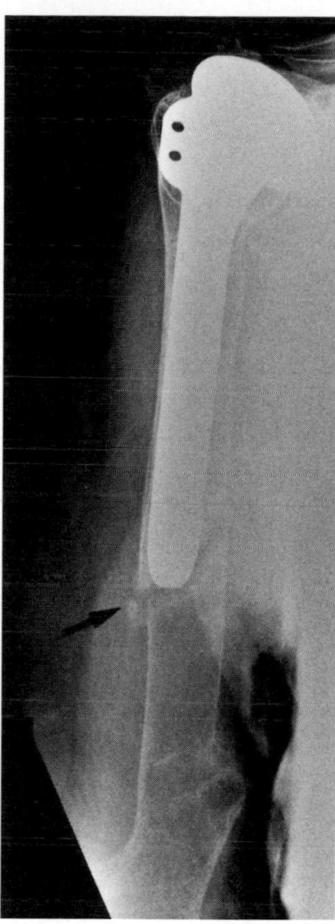

FIGURE 10-1. Postoperative radiograph demonstrating a short oblique fracture at the tip of a Neer humeral prosthesis (*arrow*).

one involved an obese woman who fell from a ladder, fracturing the humerus and dislodging the humeral component. Definitive treatment necessitated a revision procedure. In 1987, Barrett and colleagues[1] noted two intraoperative fractures (4%) in their series of shoulder replacements. One fracture was attributed to excess torque placed on the humerus during preparation of the humeral canal in a patient with rheumatoid arthritis. The other fracture also occurred in a patient with rheumatoid arthritis and involved the greater tuberosity. Both fractures healed clinically and the patients were asymptomatic, although the humeral shaft fracture did not demonstrate obvious callus formation on radiography. In 1989, Hawkins and associates[17] reported two humeral shaft fractures and two glenoid fractures in a series of 70 total shoulder arthroplasties, all of which were sustained during surgery. The humeral shaft fractures occurred in elderly patients with rheumatoid arthritis. Overzealous reaming, impaction of the humeral component, and excess torque of the humerus were listed as plausible causes of fracture. The humeral shaft fractures were treated initially with cerclage wiring and postoperative immobilization, but both required reoperation. One was treated successfully with a long-stem revision humeral component and the second was treated with compression plating. This last patient subsequently refractured the humerus distal to the plate, but was treated successfully with a humeral fracture brace. In 1990, Boyd and colleagues[6] described two intraoperative fractures of the humerus in their series of 146 Neer total shoulder arthroplasties and 64 Neer hemiarthroplasties. The mechanism by which these fractures occurred and their subsequent treatment and final outcome were not discussed.

In 1992, Bonutti and Hawkins[4] presented four patients with humeral shaft fractures associated with total shoulder arthroplasty. Two patients had intraoperative fractures that were recognized at surgery and were treated with open reduction and internal fixation. One patient had an intraoperative fracture that was diagnosed 3 days after surgery, and one patient sustained a traumatic fracture 1 year after the index procedure. The fractures were immobilized with a simple sling, shoulder immobilizer, or Orthoplast splint. All the fractures failed to heal and required reoperation using several techniques, including bone grafting, cerclage wiring, component revision with a long-stem humeral component, and postoperative immobilization with a shoulder spica cast for up to 6 weeks. The authors concluded that these fractures were prone to delayed union and generally required aggressive surgical treatment.

In the same year, Boyd and coworkers[5] described seven patients who had humeral fractures after either total shoulder replacement or shoulder hemiarthroplasty. Trauma after a fall was the cause of fracture in six patients; the final patient was injured in a motor vehicle accident. The fracture configuration was characterized by a spiral pattern in four patients, an oblique pattern in two patients, and a transverse pattern in one patient. Common to all injuries was a fracture pattern that involved the humeral shaft at the tip of the prosthesis. The initial treatment in four patients consisted of an Orthoplast or sugar-tong splint, whereas two patients were immobilized with only a sling-and-swathe bandage. Both of these last patients had progressive loss of radial nerve function that necessitated early operative intervention. Surgical management of the fractures consisted of open reduction and internal fixation with a dynamic compression plate in two patients and revision shoulder arthroplasty with a long-stem humeral component in three patients. All operatively treated fractures healed at an average time to union of about 5 months after surgery. Of the two patients treated nonoperatively, one had a nonunion but refused further treatment for medical reasons and one eventually required revision surgery unrelated to the humeral fracture. In the last patient, the humeral fracture united with the tip of the prosthesis protruding outside the humeral shaft.

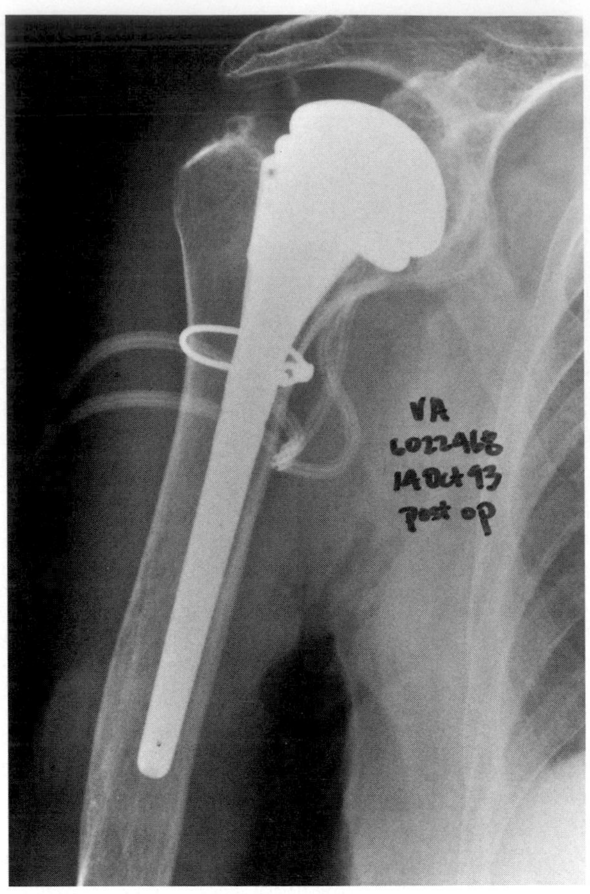

FIGURE 10-2. Radiograph of a nondisplaced proximal humerus fracture that was secured with a single cerclage wire. The fracture occurred during broaching of the proximal humerus.

Apparently, persistent symptoms were attributed to glenoid component loosening and the humeral malunion was asymptomatic. The authors noted a decrease in shoulder motion from preinjury levels in five of six patients, but the extent of this was unclear because information specifying the range of shoulder motion before injury was not available. In their conclusion, Boyd and colleagues[5] emphasized several factors that influenced the natural history of fractures adjacent to humeral prostheses, including the advanced age of many of the patients and the presence of osteopenia or reduced bone quality, rheumatoid arthritis, and associated deficiencies of the soft tissues. They also stressed that only one of seven fractures healed with immobilization alone, but the results of conservative fracture management could not be assessed in two patients because of the development of a radial nerve palsy that prompted subsequent operative intervention. Moreover, by admission of the investigators, these seven cases probably did not represent all the periprosthetic fractures that occurred during the 15-year period of their study.

In 1994, we presented the results of our experience at the University of Texas Health Science Center at San Antonio in the treatment of fractures adjacent to humeral prostheses.[14] The series consisted of 12 humeral fractures, 8 of which occurred as intraoperative complications and 4 of which resulted from postoperative trauma. Of the 8 intraoperative humeral fractures, 6 occurred during primary shoulder arthroplasty and 2 occurred during revision procedures. In the primary arthroplasty group of 6 patients, fractures occurred during manipulation of the limb in 2 patients, reaming of the intramedullary canal in 1 patient, broaching of the canal in 1 patient, and insertion of the prosthesis in 2 patients (Fig. 10-2). Both revision procedures were performed for aseptic prosthetic loosening. One fracture occurred during distal cement removal and the second occurred during seating of the revision implant. Severe cortical thinning of the humerus was noted in both revision procedures. In both cases, fractures occurred in areas of moderate to severe cortical thinning. Intraoperative fractures were managed with open reduction and internal fixation with simple cerclage wiring or a long-stem prosthesis in conjunction with cerclage wiring (Fig. 10-3). All intraoperative fractures healed at an average of 8 weeks with a mean forward elevation at final follow-up of 122°.

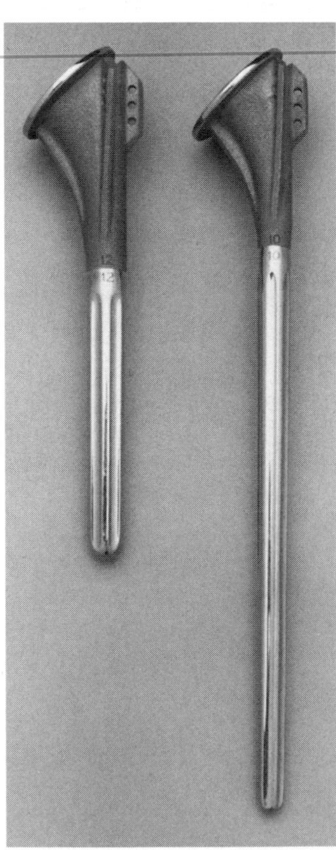

FIGURE 10-3. Photograph of modular humeral components available in standard and revision stem lengths.

Four postoperative fractures occurred at an average of 14 months after the index arthroplasty. All these injuries were managed with a fracture orthosis and resulted in bony union at an average of 9 weeks after injury (Fig. 10-4). At final evaluation, the average forward elevation was 121°.

Classification

A simple classification of periprosthetic shoulder fractures is important for proper evaluation and management of these injuries. At the University of Texas Health Science Center at San Antonio, we have adopted a workable classification of periprosthetic shoulder fractures modified from that of Johansson and colleagues.[18] This classification scheme is based on the location of the fracture in relationship to the prosthesis and is offered here as a means of managing these potentially difficult injuries (Fig. 10-5).

Type I: Fractures occurring proximal to the tip of the humeral prosthesis

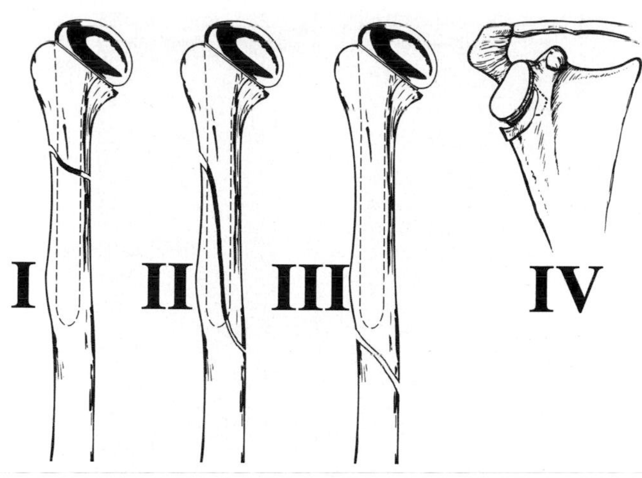

FIGURE 10-5. Classification of periprosthetic shoulder fractures. Type I: Fractures occurring proximal to the tip of the prosthesis. Type II: Fractures occurring in the proximal portion of the humerus with distal extension beyond the tip of the prosthesis. Type III: Fractures occurring entirely distal to the tip of the prosthesis. Type IV: Fractures occurring adjacent to the glenoid prosthesis.

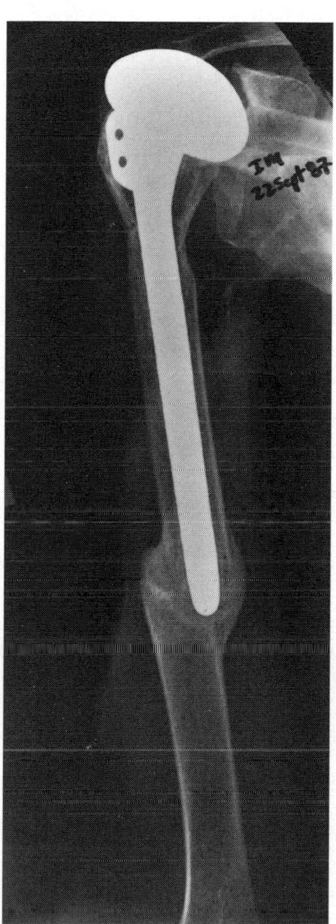

FIGURE 10-4. Bony union is apparent in this periprosthetic fracture of the humeral shaft. The injury occurred after surgery and healed uneventfully with expectant treatment.

Type II: Fractures occurring in the proximal portion of the humerus with distal extension beyond the tip of the humeral prosthesis

Type III: Fractures occurring entirely distal to the tip of the humeral prosthesis

Type IV: Fractures occurring adjacent to the glenoid prosthesis

Treatment

The treatment of periprosthetic shoulder fractures is divided into two seemingly divergent schools of thought. Bonutti and Hawkins[4] advocated aggressive treatment of these injuries, including open reduction and internal fixation, bone grafting, and postoperative immobilization in a spica cast for a minimum of 6 weeks. Similarly, Boyd and associates[5] reported an increased likelihood of nonunion after nonoperative treatment and suggested that fractures treated operatively would fare better.

Although uniform treatment guidelines would be expected based on the 11 patients in the reports of Bonutti and Hawkins,[4] and Boyd and colleagues,[5] the results of our series of 12 patients[14] suggest an alternative and perhaps more conservative approach to the management of these fractures. Three patients in our series with fractures that extended distal to the tip of the prosthesis (type II) were treated with a fracture orthosis and healed uneventfully. In all, there were five fractures that progressed to bony union that were managed with an Orthoplast fracture brace, isometric exercises, and early range-of-motion rehabilitation. We were more aggressive

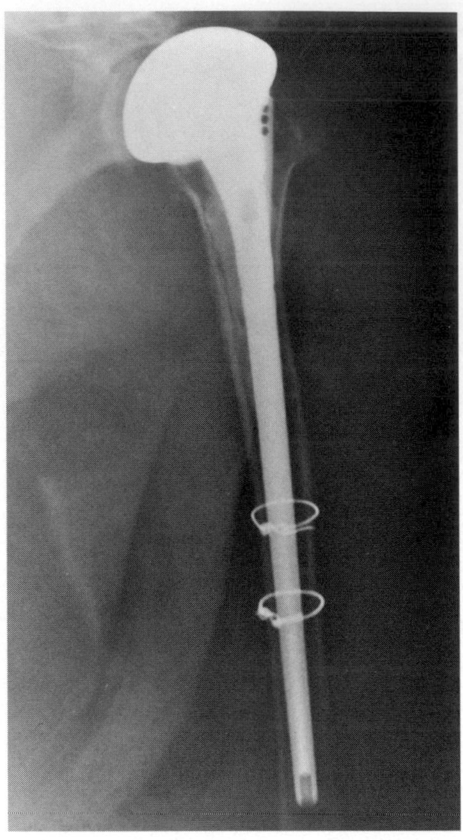

FIGURE 10-6. Radiograph of a type II intraoperative fracture that was treated with a long-stem humeral component and cerclage wires.

with intraoperative fractures; most of these injuries were treated with open reduction and internal fixation using cerclage wire. Four intraoperative fractures also were managed by replacing the primary prosthesis with a long-stem revision component (Fig. 10-6). Bony union was achieved in all cases without supplemental bone grafting or postoperative shoulder spica cast immobilization.

In summary, the treatment of each patient was individualized, with the goal of maintaining or obtaining a stable fracture that would allow early motion without having to deviate from the standardized shoulder arthroplasty rehabilitation program advocated by Rockwood.[27]

Author's Preferred Method of Treatment

Fewer than 40 cases of periprosthetic shoulder fracture have been reported in the literature[3–6,14,17,24] (Table 10-1). In many of these reports, specific fracture management was not discussed in any detail, or recommendations were so diverse that it precluded meaningful conclusions. Nonetheless, a review of the available information suggests that both nonoperative and operative treatment can be successful in the treatment of these complications.[30]

INTRAOPERATIVE PERIPROSTHETIC FRACTURES

Although a meaningful comparison of various treatment modalities is difficult because of the small number of reported cases, I prefer to manage all intraoperative fractures by whatever means necessary to obtain a stable surgical construct. The purpose of this treatment is to restore stability to the limb, to create an environment that is favorable to fracture healing, and to allow unimpeded postoperative rehabilitation so that the functional result is not compromised by prolonged immobilization.

For the most part, intraoperative fractures of the humerus or glenoid stem from errors in surgical technique, many of which are preventable.[30] These surgical errors include inadvertent reaming, overzealous impaction, and manipulation of the upper extremity during exposure of the glenoid, and several points deserve empha-

TABLE 10-1
Periprosthetic Fractures of the Shoulder

Author	Year	Number of Fractures	Type of Fracture		Fracture Occurrence	
			Humeral	*Glenoid*	*Intraoperative*	*Postoperative*
Neer et al.[24]	1982	4	4			4
Barrett et al.[3]	1987	2	2		2	
Hawkins et al.[17]	1989	4	2	2	4	
Boyd et al.[6]	1990	2	2		2	
Bonutti et al.[4]	1992	4	4		3	1
Boyd et al.[5]	1992	7	7			7
Curtis et al.[14]	1994	12	12		8	4
Total		35	33	2	19	16

sis. To this end, a brief discussion of intraoperative technical considerations as emphasized by Rockwood and Wirth[28] is presented. First, spiral fractures of the humerus usually are observed when the shoulder is externally rotated by using the upper extremity as a lever arm. This places the humerus at risk for fracture because of the magnitude of torsional stress generated by this maneuver (Fig. 10-7). The torsional force imparted to the humerus can be minimized by performing a complete anterior and inferior capsular release, and by using a bone hook on the humeral neck to deliver the proximal humerus out of the glenoid fossa (Fig. 10-8). Occasionally, exposure is still less than optimal, but this can be improved by continuing the inferior soft-tissue release to the posteroinferior and posterior capsular structures. Meticulous attention must be paid to detail while releasing the capsule from the glenoid in this region of the glenohumeral joint because of the proximity of the axillary nerve as it passes through the quadrangular space (Fig. 10-9). Second, if the arm is not extended off the side of the operating table, it is difficult to insert the trial prosthesis or medullary reamers, and this can result in perforation or complete fracture of the proximal humerus (Fig. 10-10). Third, after humeral head resection, the entry point of the trial stem or reamer should be superolateral in an eccentric location on the cancellous surface of the proximal humerus. This assures that the reamer will pass directly down into the medullary canal rather than medially, where it can perforate the humeral neck or medial cortex (Fig. 10-11). Finally, hand reaming is preferable to power instrumentation because the latter can remove too much cancellous bone or increase the likelihood of perforating osteoporotic bone.

The shoulder arthroplasty system that I use allows

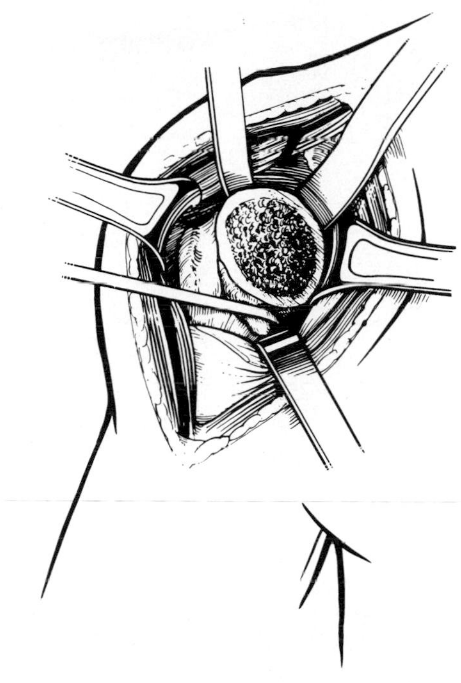

FIGURE 10-8. A bone hook or similar device is used to deliver the proximal humerus into the operative field as the limb is gently externally rotated and extended.

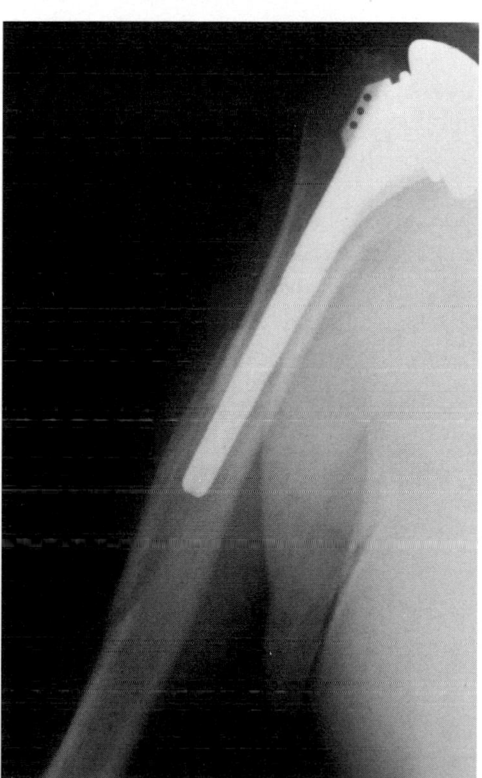

FIGURE 10-7. Anteroposterior radiograph of a healed type II spiral fracture of the humerus. The fracture occurred during manipulation of the limb and was treated with a postoperative fracture brace.

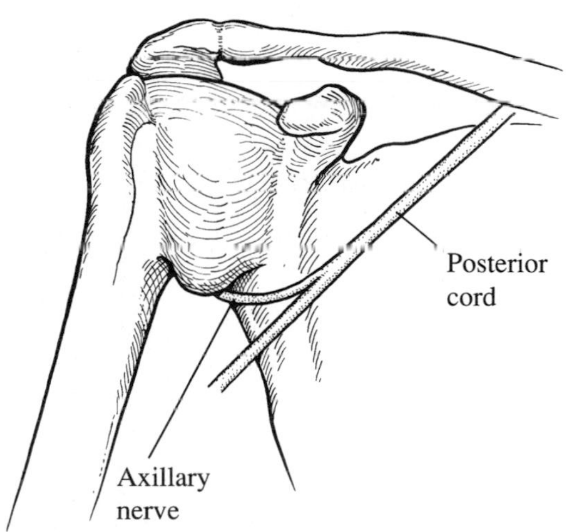

FIGURE 10-9. The axillary nerve is close to the inferior capsule as it passes beneath the glenohumeral joint.

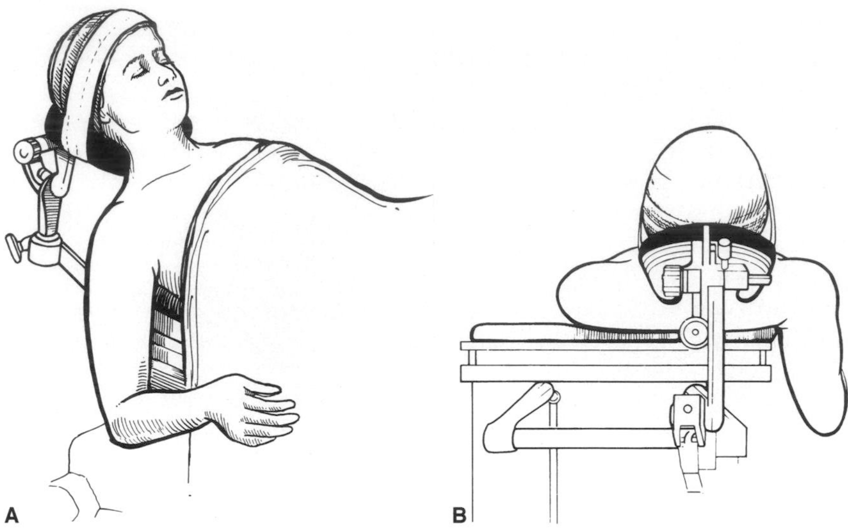

FIGURE 10-10 . (**A** and **B**) Careful positioning of the patient near the edge of the operating table allows the involved limb to be externally rotated and extended off the table.

for careful graded medullary reaming of the humerus and employs a unique humeral body-sizing osteotome (Fig. 10-12). This osteotome, or "cookie cutter," performs two important functions: first, it cuts the lateral, medial, anterior, and posterior fin tracts before broaching or trial prosthetic placement; and second, it outlines the area of cancellous bone that will be displaced by the prosthesis. If the cancellous bone of the proximal humerus is osteoporotic, then minimal bone will be removed. However, if the patient is young and the cancellous bone is substantial, it is important to remove some of the bone outlined by the osteotome so that broaching or impaction does not create a wedge effect that could fracture the humerus (Fig. 10-13).

Should intraoperative fractures occur, I have been pleased with the results of cerclage wiring and the use of a long-stem prosthesis if the situation warrants. For most type I fractures, simple cerclage wiring of the proximal humerus and implantation of a standard size prosthesis is appropriate. Autogenous bone graft from the humeral head is used to make a slurry of cancellous bone, which is placed into the metaphyseal por-

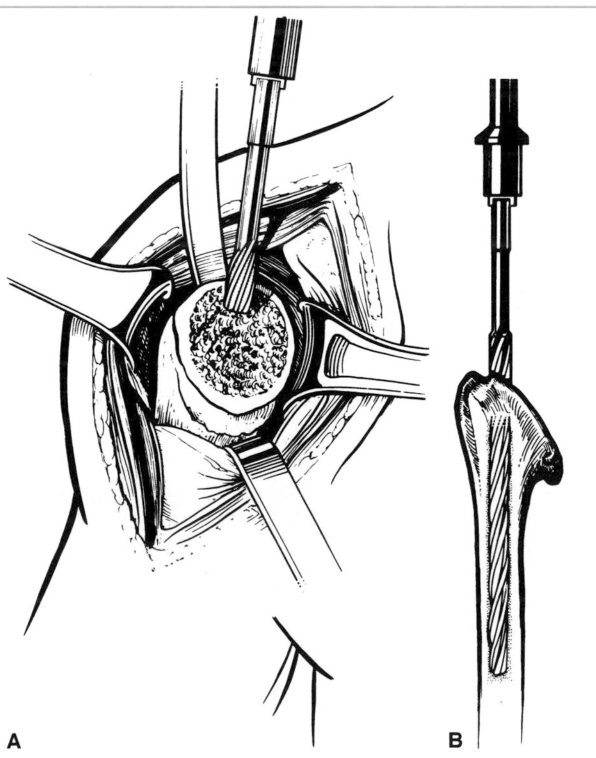

FIGURE 10-11. (**A** and **B**) A superolateral entry point of the reamer or broach facilitates subsequent passage.

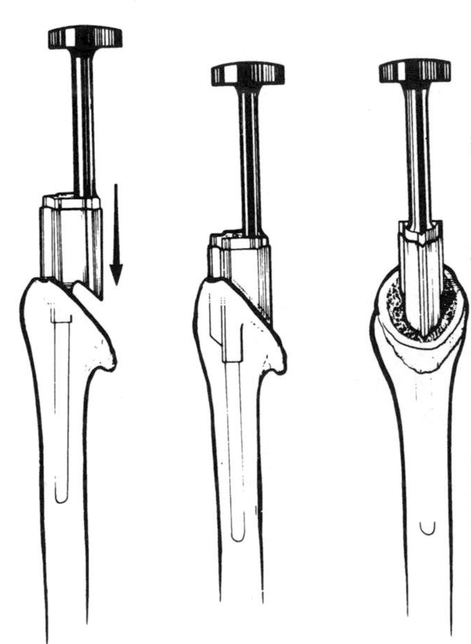

FIGURE 10-12. Seating of the body-sizing osteotome in the cancellous bone of the proximal humeral metaphysis.

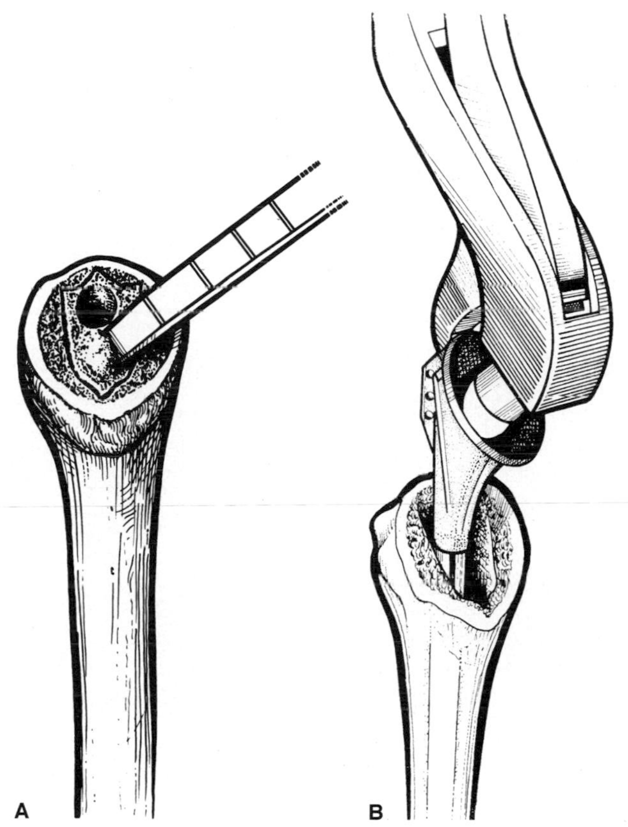

FIGURE 10-13. (**A**) Cancellous bone from within the boundaries outlined by the body-sizing osteotome can be removed easily with a curet, rongeur, or small osteotome. (**B**) Diagram illustrating the implantation of a humeral prosthesis. Note the cancellous bone that has been removed from the proximal humerus to accommodate the body of the prosthesis.

tion of the proximal humerus after the stem of the prosthesis is inserted to the level of the metaphyseal–diaphyseal junction. The trial prosthesis then is used in a pistoning fashion to work the slurry of autogenous bone into the fracture site or other areas of bony deficiency before seating of the final prosthesis. For type II and type III fracture patterns, I prefer to use a long-stem prosthesis that extends at least two humeral cortical diameters beyond the most distal extent of the fracture (Fig. 10-14). This is accomplished by extending the deltopectoral incision into an extensile anterolateral approach to the humerus. The relatively straight, cylindrical anatomy of the humeral diaphysis is ideal for this method of intramedullary fracture fixation. There are several advantages of this form of treatment over dynamic compression plating or cerclage wiring alone. First, the need for secure screw purchase in bone that often is of poor quality is obviated. Second, bending and torsional loads are better tolerated, which decreases the risk of implant failure. Third, a rigid and biomechanically sound surgical construct usually is ensured. Fourth, the extensile exposure and soft-tissue dissection needed for plate fixation is avoided. Finally, the ever-present concern for stress shielding is minimized.

The issue of whether to use bone cement is unresolved. In general, the use of cement is reserved for those situations in which the implant stability is less than optimal because of compromised metaphyseal or diaphyseal support. In this situation, a protective sheeting is placed around the humeral shaft in the region of the fracture to prevent the potentially harmful extravasation of cement into the soft tissues, as advocated by Miller and Bigliani.[20]

In regard to the extremely rare type IV fractures, glenoid component stability is affected by glenoid preparation, soft-tissue balancing, and the availability of uncompromised glenoid bone stock for prosthetic fixation.[29] Scapular fractures adjacent to glenoid components can compromise implant stability and lead to symptomatic loosening (Fig. 10-15). Bone grafting or revision glenoid components that are built up with a wedge to accommodate the defect can be used, but if bony support cannot be ensured, resurfacing of the glenoid should not be performed. In this situation, the remaining glenoid is sculpted with a hand bur or glenoid reamer to match the radius of curvature on the head of the humeral component and the glenoid component is omitted.

POSTOPERATIVE PERIPROSTHETIC FRACTURES

My initial approach to the management of postoperative periprosthetic fractures of the shoulder generally is more conservative than the usual methods of treatment recommended for similar fractures that occur during surgery. If a trial of expectant management is not contraindicated by the development of a radial nerve palsy or other ominous complication, a simple regimen can be instituted consisting of an Orthoplast fracture brace, isometric exercises for the entire upper extremity, and early motion as pain and swelling subside. In our experience at the University of Texas Health Science Center at San Antonio, satisfactory results often are obtained with this simple form of initial treatment. However, the treating physician must do whatever is necessary to ensure that early functional rehabilitation is not delayed, because prolonged immobilization has been associated with poor results (Fig. 10-16).

SPECIAL CONSIDERATIONS

One of the greatest pitfalls in the surgical management of periprosthetic shoulder fractures is underestimation of the technical demands and substantial complica-

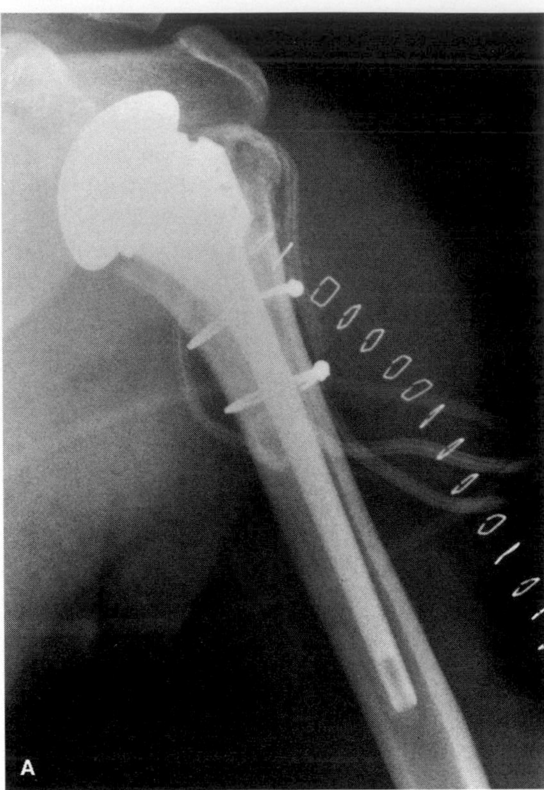

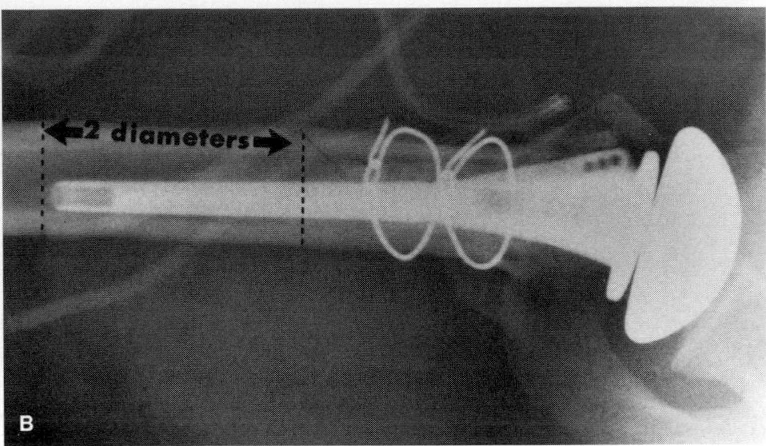

FIGURE 10-14. (**A**) This patient sustained a comminuted three-part fracture dislocation of the proximal humerus that extended distally for several centimeters. Treatment consisted of a cemented hemiarthroplasty augmented with cerclage wires. (**B**) Note that the humeral stem bypasses the distal extent of the fracture by about two cortical diameters.

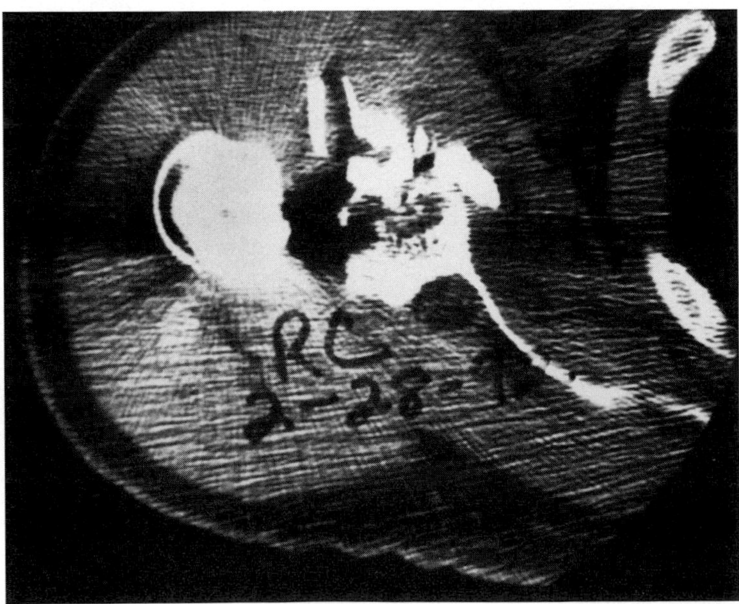

FIGURE 10-15. CT scan of a patient with a total shoulder arthroplasty who sustained an anterior glenoid fracture after a traumatic dislocation of the shoulder. This injury severely compromised the glenoid component stability and necessitated a revision procedure. (*Courtesy of Gerald R. Williams, M.D., Philadelphia, PA*)

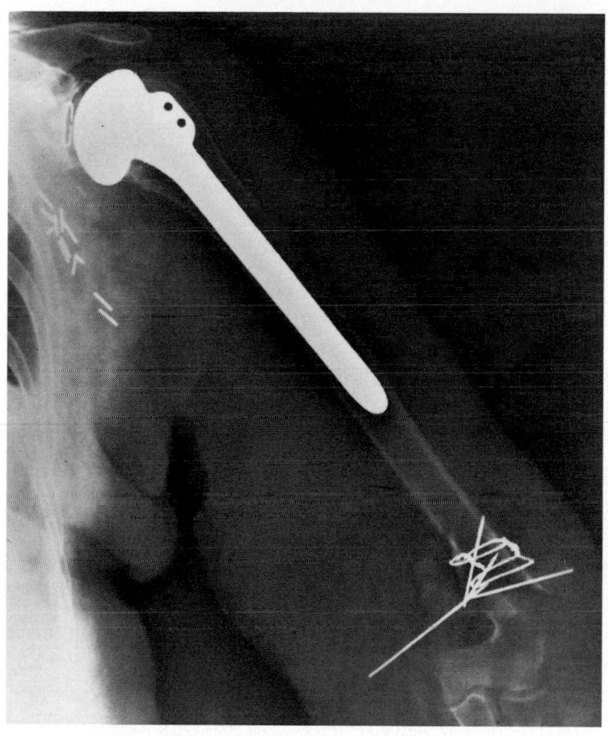

FIGURE 10-16. This difficult type III periprosthetic fracture of the humerus was treated with several unsuccessful attempts at open reduction and internal fixation. Successful management ultimately required a cemented total elbow arthroplasty. (*Courtesy of Eugene T. O'Brien, M.D., San Antonio, TX*)

tions that can occur with revision surgery of this magnitude. The literature reflects revision rates after shoulder arthroplasty of 0% to 17%,[1,6,17,21,24] but publications specifically addressing revision shoulder surgery are rare, especially in regard to the treatment of fracture complications (Table 10-2).[8,23]

In 1982, Neer and Kirby[23] reported the causes of failure and approaches to treatment in a series of 37 unconstrained total shoulder and humeral head arthroplasties. The authors reviewed their results and analyzed the major causes of failure of the previous replacements. They concluded that revision arthroplasty was the most technically difficult of reconstructive shoulder procedures, and that overall results were inferior when compared with other diagnostic categories.

We reviewed 38 consecutive unconstrained shoulder arthroplasty revisions performed at our institution between 1977 and 1993.[32] The initial indication for arthroplasty was acute trauma in 19 shoulders, osteoarthritis in 12 shoulders, postreconstruction arthropathy in 5 shoulders, and rheumatoid arthritis in 2 shoulders. An analysis of the reason for failure was performed in all patients and an evaluation of the success of revision was performed for 25 patients with more than 2 years of follow-up. Reasons for failure were multifactorial, making it difficult to assign one specific cause of failure in about 68% of cases. Satisfactory pain relief and improvement in activity was reliably achieved in more than 70% of patients; however, similar to the findings of Neer and Kirby,[23] overall results were inferior compared with primary arthroplasty procedures.

The preceding discussion is not intended to discourage revision surgery as a worthy treatment option, but to emphasize the importance of careful patient selection, comprehensive preoperative planning, and surgical expertise. Although I agree in principle with the concepts of aggressive fracture management, the choice between revision surgery and expectant treatment depends on the symptoms, functional limitations, age, activity level, and life expectancy of the patient. If an elderly patient with limited activity goals is experiencing minimal to no pain and can function in simple activities of daily living such as caring for personal hygiene and eating, then surgery is not recommended.

Once the decision for surgery has been made, several important factors must be considered to minimize complications and ensure a successful outcome. Careful preoperative planning and the anticipation of potential complications represent an investment with considerable dividends. Of primary importance are good-quality preoperative imaging studies. Shoulder radiographs must be of sufficient quality to detect nondisplaced longitudinal extensions of the more obvious fracture as well as subtle comminution of the supporting metaphyseal bone. Often, it is difficult to assess the geometry and dimensions of the involved humerus because of the severe comminution and anatomic distortion that accompany many of these injuries. To circumvent this difficulty, preoperative radiographs of the contralateral humerus with a magnification marker are recommended. With this technique, problems associated with radiographic magnification are minimized, and both the ideal size of the revision prosthesis and its position relative to the fracture site are easily determined by template silhouetting (Fig. 10-17). Moreover, this technique minimizes inadvertent lengthening or shortening of the humerus, which Neer,[22,23] Rockwood,[27,30–32] and others[7,9,11,16,23] have emphasized as an important complication to prevent. Minimizing this problem ensures the

TABLE 10-2
Unconstrained Shoulder Arthroplasty Revision

Results	Neer & Kirby[23]	Caldwell et al.[8]	Wirth et al.[32]
Number of shoulders	37	13	38
Mean follow-up (mo)	42	36	35
Instability (%)	49	23	43
Loosening (%)	0	15	26
Deltoid denervation (%)	14	0	11

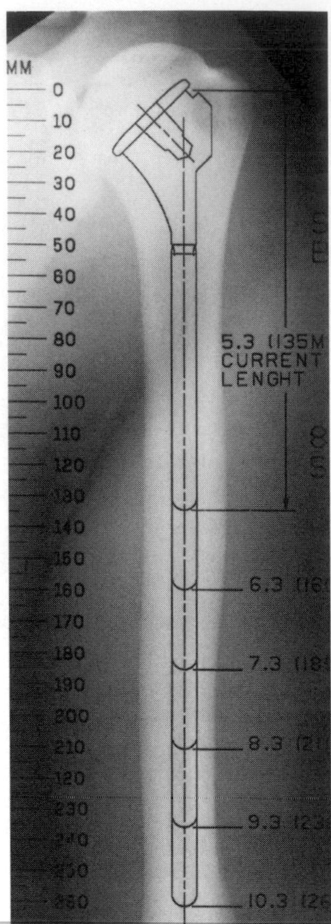

FIGURE 10-17. When revision surgery is anticipated, the proper size and length of a prosthesis is determined by careful preoperative template silhouetting of the contralateral humerus.

restoration of anatomic humeral length and reestablishes the resting tension of the deltoid that is so vital to shoulder strength and function.

Revision shoulder arthroplasty procedures that involve the removal of a cemented prosthesis can be challenging unless the prosthesis is grossly loose. Long-stem power burs, cement osteotomes, Moreland revision instrumentation, and slap-hammer extraction devices are useful for this arduous task (Fig. 10-18). A good light source and a high-quality image intensifier are important adjuncts that help to minimize cortical perforation during cement extraction and canal preparation. Occasionally, an ultrasonic transducer is useful in facilitating the removal of a cemented prosthesis, but difficulties usually are encountered with this device because of the inability to reach the proximal cement mantle, which is sheltered by the collar of the humeral component (Fig. 10-19). Although distal access to an implant through a cortical window created in the femoral shaft has been shown to be an effective means of facilitating the removal of an obstinate femoral component, the application of this technique when extrapolated to the humerus has not been as helpful in my experience. Alternatively, the operative technique that I have favored for the past several years was learned from my teacher and associate, Dr. Charles A. Rockwood, Jr. This is a simple, yet effective, method of extracting a cemented humeral component that entails the removal of fibrous tissue and extruded cement from around the humeral collar followed by the creation of a controlled longitudinal osteotomy of the metaphysis and proximal humeral shaft. The nondisplaced fracture created by the osteotomy is gently pried open and the implant is removed using a Ring prosthesis extractor, slap-hammer, punch, or other device (Fig. 10-20). After cement and implant removal,

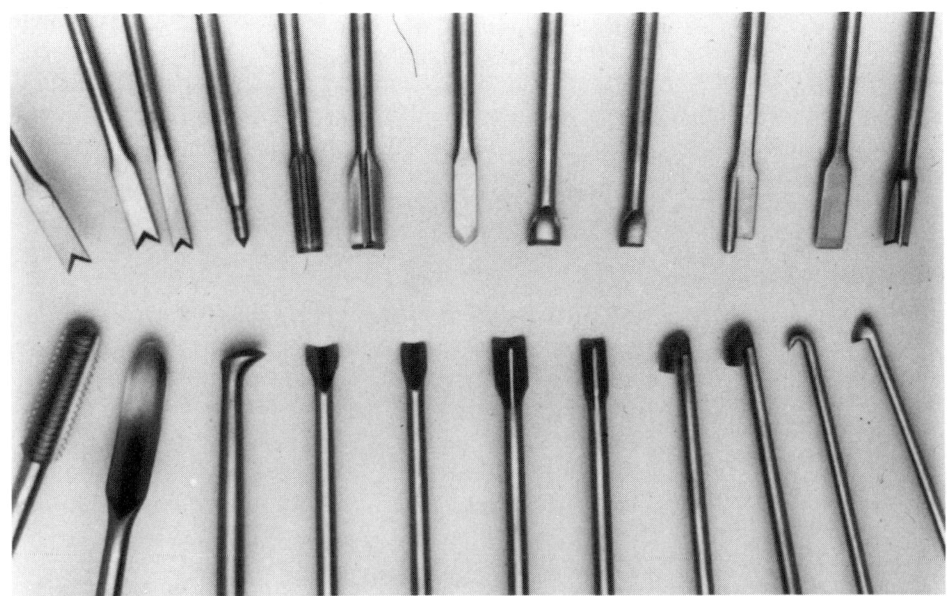

FIGURE 10-18. A wide selection of revision instruments is helpful for implant removal and cement extraction.

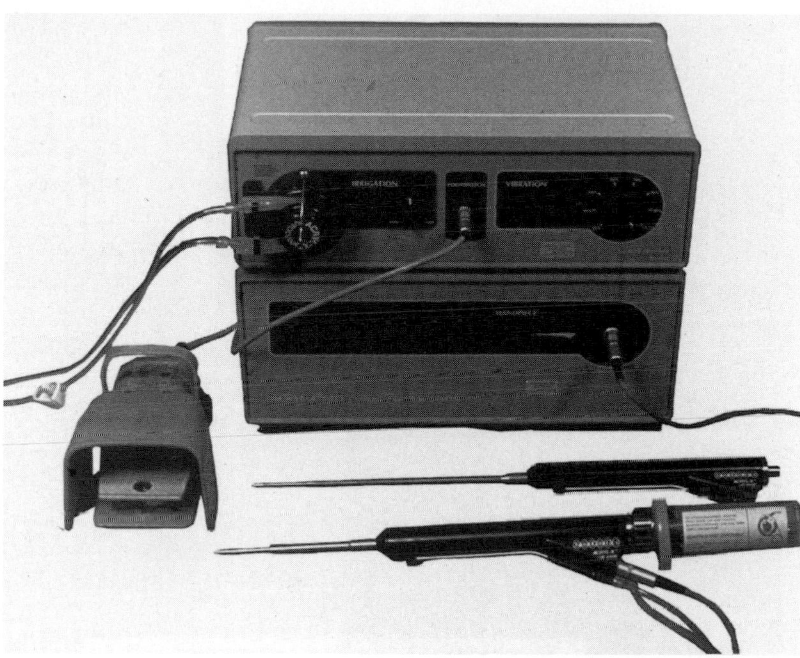

FIGURE 10-19. Ultrasonic bone cement removal system for removal of cemented prostheses.

the fracture is reduced and stabilized around a long-stem revision prosthesis using cerclage cables or wires.

Occasionally, reconstructive surgery of the humerus after a periprosthetic fracture is complicated by the loss of endosteal or cortical bone stock (Fig. 10-21). When these structural defects are substantial, the loss of supporting bone significantly complicates revision surgery. The American Academy of Orthopaedic Surgeons Committee on the Hip has introduced a comprehensive classification system of bone deficiencies and other abnormalities.[15] The proposed classification system is comprised of two basic categories that include segmental and cavity defects, and is useful in the preoperative planning of shoulder revision cases. When a stable surgical construct cannot be achieved because of insufficient or otherwise compromised host bone, a structural fibular strut graft secured over morselized bone graft with cerclage cable or wires is recommended. If the entire proximal humerus is deficient or severely damaged during implant and cement removal, an allograft–prosthesis composite may be necessary to reconstruct the segmental or cavitary defect. This is a technique that I learned from my associate, Dr. Ronald P. Williams, while performing limb-salvage procedures in patients with musculoskeletal tumors (Fig. 10-22*A*).

If the entire proximal humerus requires replacement, preoperative radiographs of the contralateral humerus are analyzed to determine the dimensions of an appropriate sized allograft. The head of the humeral allograft is resected using the same surgical technique that is used for a primary shoulder arthroplasty (see Fig. 10-22*B*). Using a humeral osteotomy template for this step minimizes error in the varus/valgus plane of resection and ensures proper support of the humeral prosthesis. After the proximal resection is complete, the allograft is resected to an appropriate length by a step-cut osteotomy of the shaft. After completion of the step-cut osteotomy, the prosthesis is cemented within the allograft to form a composite before being cemented into the remaining host bone (see Fig. 10-22*C* and *D*). Before final implantation and cementing, the proximal portion of the remaining distal humeral shaft is osteotomized in a step-cut 180° inverted mirror image of the allograft. This increases the contact surface area between the host bone and the allograft, and maximizes rotational stability of the final construct. Cerclage cables or wires are used as supplemental fixation when necessary (see Fig. 10-22*E*). A more complete treatise on the use of humeral allografts is beyond the scope of this chapter, but I have been satisfied with the results of this technique in carefully selected patients.

PERIPROSTHETIC FRACTURES OF THE ELBOW

The successful management of fractures of the humerus or ulna adjacent to a total elbow arthroplasty can be challenging. In a review of 16 total elbow arthroplasty series (852 implant procedures) in the literature, complications included 67 documented periprosthetic fractures with an overall prevalence of 8%* (Table 10-3). Frequently, these are complicated injur-

*References 33, 39, 40, 42, 44–46, 48, 49, 51, 52, 54, 56–58, 61.

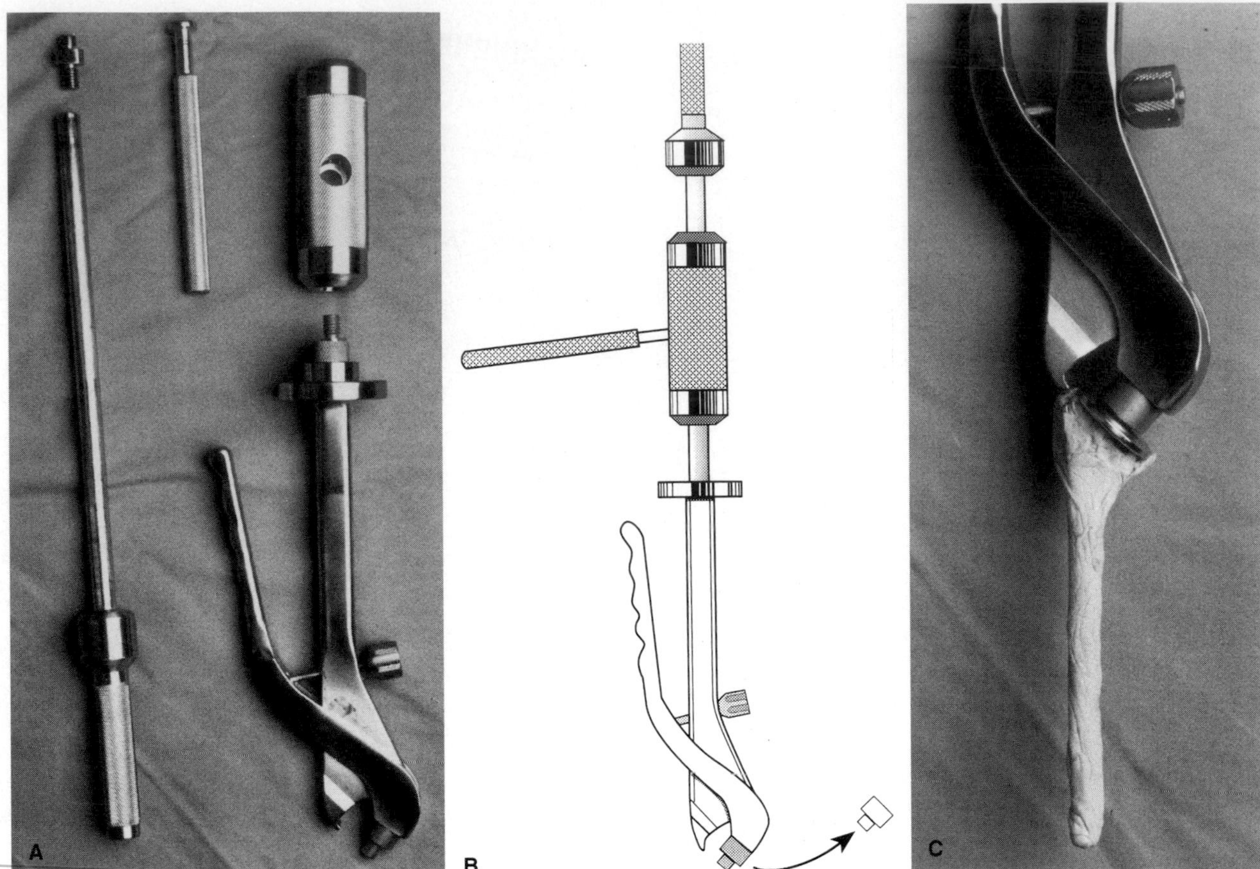

FIGURE 10-20. (**A**) Extraction instrumentation for removal of a cemented Global humeral prosthesis. (**B**) Diagram depicting assembled extraction instrumentation. Note that the Delrin tip on the driver-extractor has been exchanged for a steel tip. (**C**) Driver-extractor device attached to a cemented humeral component.

ies that can result in loss of elbow motion, poor function, and disability, even for simple activities of daily living (Fig. 10-23). To optimize functional outcome, it is imperative to assess all pathology accurately, because successful treatment is related directly to the accuracy of diagnosis. Not only must the diagnosis be correct, but the treating physician must be able to distinguish those fractures that respond best to surgery from those that can be managed without surgery in a timely fashion, because unnecessary delays in treatment can compromise the functional result.

HISTORICAL REVIEW

In 1967, Silva[59] described distal humeral replacement using a Teflon prosthesis. Before this report, there was little in the literature regarding prosthetic arthroplasty of the elbow joint, although many investigators already were developing implants for hemiarthroplasty or total arthroplasty of the elbow using a variety of materials, including Silastic, high-density polyethylene, acrylic polymers, and various alloys.[60] Many of the early designs were based on experience with hinge-type knee arthroplasties and constrained total shoulder replacements. The myriad of elbow arthroplasties that followed were diverse, but could be categorized broadly into one of three groups: (1) constrained (fixed fulcrum), (2) semiconstrained, and (3) unconstrained (capitellocondylar).

The early progress of total elbow arthroplasty was impeded primarily by mechanical loosening of constrained implants and instability of unconstrained implants. Although these were the two most common problems noted in the literature, complications such as sepsis, neurovascular injury, implant failure, triceps insufficiency, ankylosis, and periprosthetic fractures also were described.

CONSTRAINED TOTAL ELBOW REPLACEMENT

Only a few reports on early hinged total elbow replacements appear in the literature, and there is even less information regarding fractures around these fully constrained devices (Table 10-4). In a review of 74

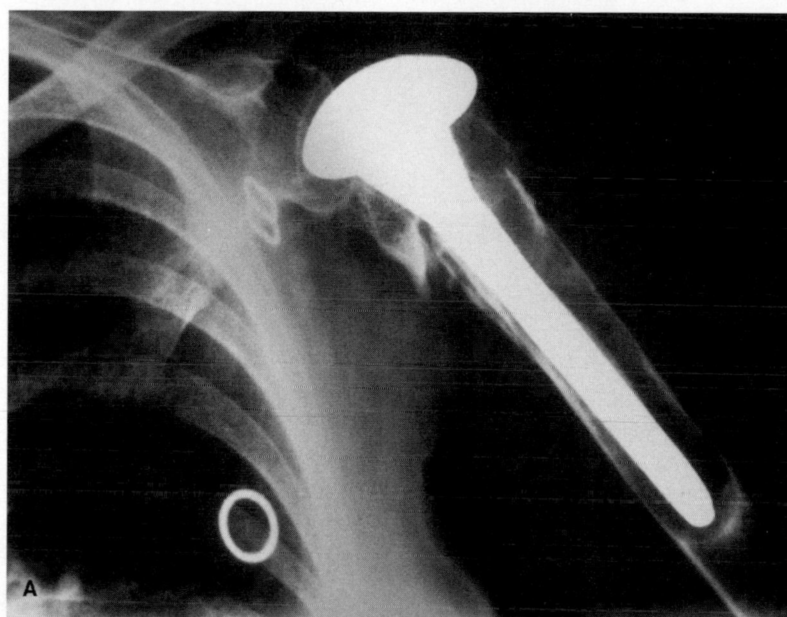

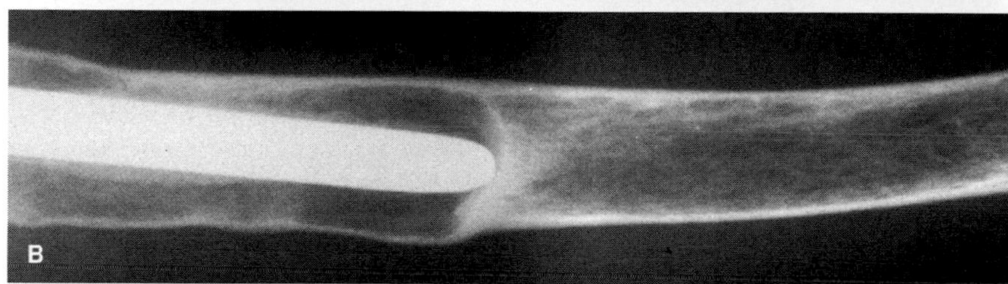

FIGURE 10-21. (**A**) Progressive loosening of a humeral prosthesis associated with endosteal erosion and cortical thinning. Note the metaphyseal fracture of the humerus and the abnormal version of the prosthesis. (**B**) Lateral radiograph revealing endosteal scalloping of the humerus secondary to the windshield wiper effect of the loose humeral component.

constrained elbow replacements described in three reports, complications were numerous and included an 11% prevalence of ipsilateral fractures of the humerus or ulna.[36,49,60] Some of these fractures probably were the result of design constraints, because many of the original prototype metallic hinge prostheses were large and insertion of these devices into patients of small stature was difficult or impossible without fracture of the humerus or ulna. Another explanation for the occurrence of periprosthetic fractures around fully constrained total elbow replacements involves the long lever arm and the considerable rotational forces that are present when the ulnar and humeral components are linked directly in a single-axis hinged mechanism. The constrained total elbow design essentially eliminates the restraint to varus/valgus angulation provided by the soft tissue and transfers it directly to the bone–cement interface, resulting in an increased propensity for loosening or fracture.[53] As suggested by Ewald,[37] the lever arm for this moment becomes the entire length of the forearm and the resultant normal forces around the elbow give way to abnormal torques that are transmitted directly to the bone–cement interface. For many reasons, including the considerations listed, the overall failure rate of constrained total elbow arthroplasties has been unacceptably high and the use of these implants seldom is indicated.

In 1973, Dee[36] reported his experience with 30 single-axis-of-rotation, chromium-cobalt total elbow prostheses. With less than 2 years of follow-up in many cases, one humeral fracture was reported when a patient fell 3 months after surgery. The prosthesis subsequently was revised, but the patient had symptomatic loosening at 12 months and the component eventually was removed at a second revision procedure. Also in 1973, Souter[60] reported 25 hinged elbow arthroplasties (McKee and Dee implants) in 20 patients with rheumatoid arthritis. With a follow-up period that ranged from 4 months to 2 $^1/_2$ years, two intraoperative fractures and one postoperative fracture were noted. In one of the intraoperative fractures, the ulnar shaft was split when the tip of the prosthesis penetrated the posterior cortex of the ulna, but the fracture healed uneventfully. The second intraoperative fracture involved the anterior cortex of the humerus and resulted in progressive loosening of the prosthesis that required revision arthroplasty. The solitary postoperative fracture occurred at the junction of the olecranon with the shaft of the ulna and was noted

(text continues on page 556)

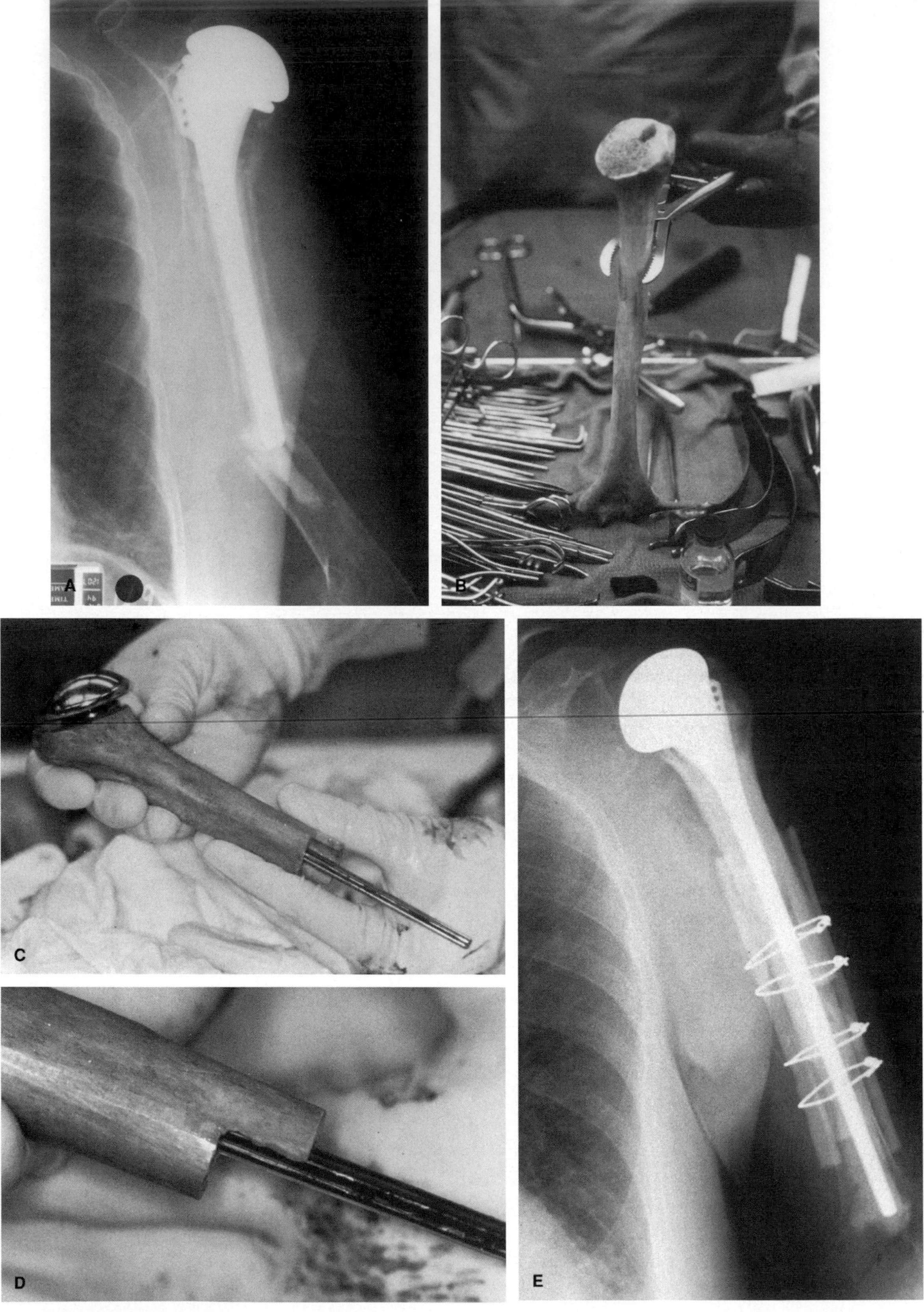

FIGURE 10-22. (**A**) Anteroposterior radiograph demonstrating a periprosthetic fracture of the humerus. Note the rotatory instability of the prosthesis, endosteal bone erosion, and severe cortical thinning. (**B**) Intraoperative photograph after resection of the allograft humeral head. (**C**) Cemented prosthetic-allograft composite. (**D**) Enlarged photograph demonstrating the step-cut osteotomy of the allograft. (*Courtesy of Ronald P. Williams, M.D., Ph.D., San Antonio, TX*) (**E**) Postoperative radiograph of the completed construct. Note the fibular strut grafts that were used to enhance further the overall stability.

TABLE 10-3

Periprosthetic Fractures of Total Elbow Replacement Surgery

Author	Year	Mean Follow-up (y)	Diagnosis	Type of Implant	Number of Elbows	Periprosthetic Fractures (%)	Revisions Related to Fractures	Fractures						Fracture Occurrence		
								Condylar Medial	Supracondylar Lateral	Shaft	Humeral	Ulnar	Unspecified	Intraoperative	Postoperative	Unspecified
Ewald et al.	1980	3.5	RA	Ewald*	69	4	1		1			2		1	2	
Inglis et al.	1980	3.7	RA (71%) PTA (29%)	Pritchard-Walker & triaxial†	36	8	1				2	1			1	2
Brumfield et al.	1981	2.2	RA (93%) OA (7%)	Mayo & AHSC†	28	11	0	3						2	1	
Morrey et al.	1981	4.1	RA (74%) PTA (26%)	Mayo & Coonrad†	80	15	3		9	2		1		11	1	
Rosenfield & Anzel	1982	2.6	RA	Pritchard*	17	29	1				4	1		1	2	2
Pritchard	1983	1.5	RA (92%) PTA (8%)	Pritchard*	13	8	1	1							1	
Rosenberg & Turner	1982	2.9	RA	Ewald*	28	4	0					1			1	
Lowe et al.	1984	3	RA (84%) PTA (16%)	Northwick*	47	4	N/A	1			1				2	
Morrey & Bryan	1987	5.1	Failed TEA	Multiple*†‡ TEA designs	33	21	0					4	3			7
Trancik et al.	1987	5.6	RA (97%) PTA (3%)	Capitellocondylar*	35	9	1	2			1			2	1	
Gschwend et al.	1988	4.1	RA (81%) PTA (16%)	GSB†	71	3	0	1				1		2		
Figgie et al.	1989	5.7	Ankylosis of elbow	Multiple designs†	19	5	0					1			1	
Morrey et al.	1991	6.3	PTA	Coonrad (original & modified)*‡	55	7	3					1	3			4
Ruth & Wilde	1992	6.5	RA (95%) PTA (5%)	Ewald*	51	14	1	2	1		2		2	2	5	
Morrey & Adams	1992	3.8	RA	Modified Coonrad†	68	12	0	4	2	N/A		2		4	4	
Ewald et al.	1993	5.6	RA	Ewald*	202	3	1				1	3	1	2	3	

RA—rheumatoid arthritis; *OA*—osteoarthritis; *PTA*—Post-traumatic arthritis; *N/A*—not available; *TEA*–total elbow arthroplasty; *GSB*–Gschwend-Scheier-Bähler; *AHSC*–Arizona Health Science Center.

* Unconstrained.

† Semiconstrained.

‡ Constrained.

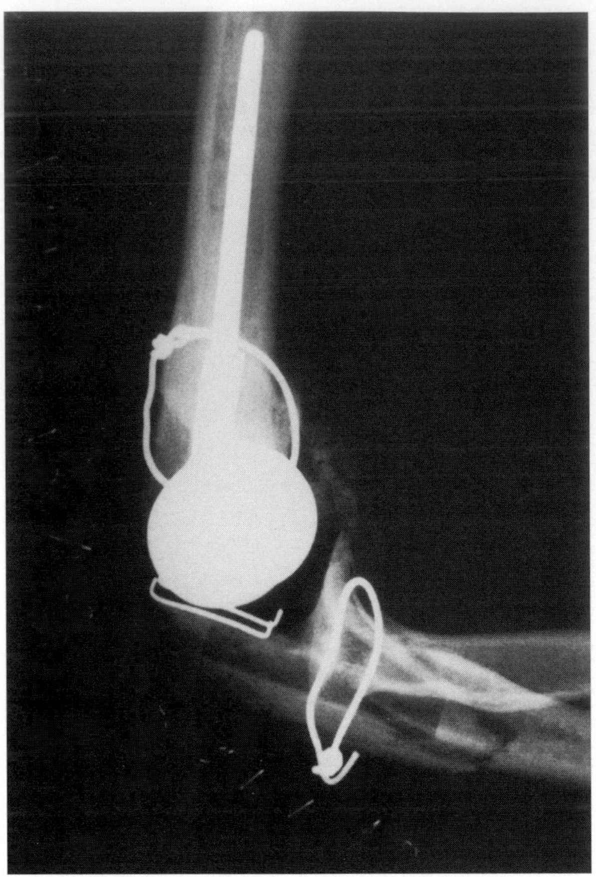

FIGURE 10-23. Lateral radiograph demonstrating fixation of both humeral and ulnar intraoperative fractures with cerclage wire. Note the minimally displaced ulnar fracture at the nonarticulating end of the ulnar component. (*Courtesy of Eugene T. O'Brien, M.D., San Antonio, TX*)

1 year after surgery as an incidental finding. The patient apparently had no symptoms. In 1991, Morrey and colleagues[49] described their experience with total elbow replacement for posttraumatic arthritis. From 1973 to 1978, during the initial phase of their study, a constrained titanium implant with a high-density polyethylene hinge was used in 19 elbow arthroplasties. At an average follow-up of nearly 10 years, the prevalence of periprosthetic fractures was 21% and included three humeral fractures and one fracture of the ulna. All elbow arthroplasties associated with a fracture of the humerus were graded as an unsatisfactory result and eventually required revision.

SEMICONSTRAINED TOTAL ELBOW REPLACEMENT

Periprosthetic fractures constitute about 20% of the complications reported for semiconstrained total elbow replacements. In a review of the literature pertaining to this type of implant, the prevalence of intraoperative or postoperative fractures of the humerus or ulna ranged from 0% to 29%.† The propensity for fracture associated with the use of semiconstrained prostheses is attributable to numerous risk factors, including osteoporosis, the paucity of bone between the medial and lateral columns of the distal humerus, abnormal humeral bowing in the sagittal plane, the size and angulation of the humeral and ulnar medullary canals, the amount of bone that must be resected to accommodate the prosthesis, and previous injuries or surgery that may alter the bony architecture or integrity.

In 1980, Inglis and Pellicci[45] reported 36 semiconstrained total elbow prostheses that were followed up for a minimum of 2 years. The overall complication rate was 53%, and 19% of these problems were related to fractures of the humerus or ulna. In 1982, Rosenfeld and Anzel[57] retrospectively reviewed 17 elbow arthroplasties in 13 patients with a mean follow-up of 2.6 years. Complications included four fractures of the humerus above the prosthesis (three of which were in one patient) and an intraoperative fracture of the ulna.

Intraoperative Periprosthetic Fractures of the Elbow

Intraoperative fractures that were contiguous with or in proximity to a total elbow prosthesis accounted for about 50% of periprosthetic fracture complications noted in four series containing 247 semiconstrained elbow prostheses.[33,44,48,52]

In 1981, Brumfield and coworkers[33] noted two intraoperative fractures of the humeral condyles that were treated by immobilization for 3 to 6 weeks without loss of motion or other complications. Also in 1981, Morrey and colleagues[52] reported 55 complications after 80 Mayo and Coonrad total elbow arthroplasties. Of these 55 complications, 20% were intraoperative supracondylar fractures that involved the medial column in nine elbows and the lateral column in two elbows. With the exception of one elbow that was excluded because of postoperative infection, analysis of these fractures revealed no progressive loosening in five elbows, 1- to 2-mm progressive radiolucency at the bone–cement interface in two elbows, and symptomatic loosening necessitating revision surgery in three elbows. In 1988, Gschwend and associates[44] described two intraoperative fractures in a series of 71 semiconstrained Gschwend-Scheier-Bähler components. In one case, a humeral condyle fracture occurred, and in a second case, the ulna was fractured. Both elbows were treated successfully with internal fixation. In 1992, Morrey and Adams[48] reported a

†References 33, 41, 42, 44, 45, 48, 51, 52, 57.

TABLE 10-4
Comparison of Constrained, Semiconstrained, and Nonconstrained Elbow Replacements

	Number of Operations	Average Follow-Up (y)	Periprosthetic Fracture (%)
CONSTRAINED			
Dee (1973)	30	N/A	3
Souter (1973)	25	N/A	12
Morrey et al. (1991)	19	9.8	21
Total	74	N/A	11
SEMICONSTRAINED			
Inglis et al. (1980)	36	3.7	8
Brumfield et al. (1981)	28	2.2	11
Morrey & Anzel (1981)	80	4.1	15
Rosenfield et al. (1982)	17	2.6	29
Gschwend & Adams (1988)	71	4.1	3
Morrey et al. (1992)	68	3.8	12
Total	300	3.7	11
NONCONSTRAINED			
Ewald et al. (1980)	69	3.5	4
Pritchard (1983)	13	1.5	8
Rosenberg & Turner (1984)	28	2.9	4
Lowe et al. (1984)	47	3	4
Trancil et al. (1987)	35	5.6	9
Ruth & Wilde (1982)	51	6.5	14
Total	243	4.2	7

N/A—not available.

complication rate of 22% in 58 semiconstrained modified Coonrad prostheses. Half the complications noted in this series were related to periprosthetic fractures, and half of these occurred at the time of surgery. All four intraoperative fractures involved the humeral condyles; in two elbows, a painless nonunion developed, and in the remaining two elbows, the fragment was excised at the time of surgery without adversely affecting implant stability or the final result.

Postoperative Periprosthetic Fractures of the Elbow

A review of several large series in the literature reveals a 7% prevalence of postoperative fractures adjacent to semiconstrained total elbow prostheses.[33,42,44,48,52,54] The time of occurrence of these injuries was noted in only 17% of cases, making it difficult to determine the temporal relationship of these fractures to the time of surgery in most cases. In the six elbows in which this complication was temporally defined, the mean time to fracture was about 10 months (range, 1 to 25 months).[42,48,52]

One postoperative fracture involving the humeral condyle was noted by Brumfield and colleagues[33] in their series of 28 Mayo and Voltz total elbow prostheses. As with two intraoperative humeral condyle fractures also reported by these authors, this fracture was treated by immobilization for several weeks without significant loss of motion. Morrey and colleagues[52] reported only 1 postoperative fracture involving the ulna in contrast to 11 intraoperative supracondylar fractures of the humerus. The ulnar fracture occurred more than 1 year after surgery and was treated by immobilization in plaster. The fracture united uneventfully and subsequent radiographic examinations revealed a nonprogressive radiolucent line at the bone–cement interface. Figgie and associates[42] described one fracture complication in a series of 19 semiconstrained total elbow replacements that were performed for complete ankylosis of the elbow. This complication occurred 3 months after surgery and was described as a nondisplaced fracture at the tip of the olecranon. The patient's elbow function was not affected by this injury and the diagnosis was delayed until radiographs were obtained at a routine subsequent follow-up visit. In a study by Morrey and Adams[48] involving 58 semiconstrained modified Coonrad elbow implants for patients with rheumatoid arthritis, four postoperative fractures were noted. These four injuries occurred between 3 weeks and 25 months after the operation and included two supracondylar humeral column fractures and two nondisplaced ulnar fractures distal to the prosthesis. All fractures healed after immobilization of the extremity in a cast for an unspecified period. Pritchard[54] reviewed the results of 100 orthopaedic surgeons' experience with a semiconstrained hinge prosthesis (Pritchard Mark I and Mark II types). Information from 269 cases was analyzed from a standardized questionnaire, which revealed 28 periprosthetic fractures (10%). Although the specific time of fracture was not reported, 13% of Mark I implants and 5% of Mark II implants were associated with fractures of the humerus at some point after surgery. Most transverse fractures were located in the midshaft of the humerus close to the proximal end of the prosthesis and healed without incident after sling-and-swathe bandage immobilization. Comminuted fractures and displaced spiral fractures of the distal humerus that involved fixation of the component required revision surgery, but the number of these cases was not specified.

Fracture of Semiconstrained Total Elbow Prostheses

Failure of semiconstrained total elbow prostheses as a result of fractured components is relatively uncommon, with a prevalence of less than 3%.[‡,47] The frequency with which this complication occurs ranges from 0% to 12%, although this figure appears to be declining because most fractured prostheses involved the humeral component of early prototypic elbow implants.[45,48,51,54,57] Fractures of the humeral component of semiconstrained elbow prostheses account for more than 80% of fractured implants, but fractures of the ulnar component and axle or linkage pin also have been described[45,48] (Fig. 10-24).

In the series by Inglis and Pellicci,[45] two broken components accounted for 10% of the overall complication rate of 53%. One of these failures was the result of a fracture in an implant that occurred at the site where it had been machined to accommodate bony geometry. The second implant failure was due to a broken axle. Both these fractured implants required revision surgery, with one good and one poor result. Rosenfeld and Anzel[57] described two patients whose postoperative courses were complicated by humeral component fractures above the articulation in Pritchard Mark I semiconstrained total elbow prostheses. Similar to the patients in the study of Inglis and Pellicci,[45] both these failed implants required revision surgery. In a report of revision total elbow arthroplasty by Morrey and Bryan,[51] the indication for revision in 3 of 33 cases was a failed prosthetic device. One of these failures was a semiconstrained Mayo prosthesis that fractured at the humeral stem. The other two failed devices included the ulnar component in an early unconstrained capitellocondylar prosthesis and a Swanson Silastic implant. In another series by Morrey and Adams,[48] 1 fractured implant was reported from a series of 58 semiconstrained modified Coonrad elbow implants. In this prosthesis, the ulnar component fractured at 27 months after surgery. The patient was a 65-year-old man who had returned to unrestricted activity against medical advice and was injured while building a stone fence and lifting buckets of water that weighed up to 23 kg. Pritchard[54] reviewed 177 semiconstrained total elbow prostheses (Pritchard Mark I design) implanted by numerous practicing orthopaedic surgeons across the United States. Fracture of the polyethylene humeral component was noted in eight cases. In reviewing the postoperative radiographs of these cases, the author concluded that insufficient bony support secondary to the absence of one or both epicondyles or surgical error leading to a subsequent stress fracture of the polyethylene was the cause of this complication.

‡References 33, 41, 42, 44, 45, 48, 51, 52, 54, 57.

UNCONSTRAINED TOTAL ELBOW REPLACEMENT

With the exception of elbow instability, the introduction of metal-on-plastic capitellocondylar arthroplasty for unconstrained resurfacing of the elbow joint has been associated with relatively few complications. However, in a review of 455 capitellocondylar elbow arthroplasties reported in the literature, the frequency of fractures around unconstrained implants varied between 0% and 14%, with an overall prevalence of about 5%. As with semiconstrained total elbow prostheses, postoperative fractures of the humerus or ulna usually occur as a result of trauma, whereas intraoperative fractures commonly are associated with reaming or broaching of the medullary canal, impaction of the prosthesis, or extraction of the cement mantle and implant in revision procedures.

Intraoperative Periprosthetic Fractures of the Elbow

Intraoperative fractures adjacent to unconstrained total elbow prostheses occur with a prevalence of less than 2%,[§] and are outnumbered by postoperative fractures by a 2:1 ratio.

In 1980, Ewald and associates[39] reported 27 complications in a 2-to 5-year follow-up series of 69 unconstrained capitellocondylar total elbow prostheses in 64 patients with rheumatoid arthritis. The 39% complication rate was based on the total number of prostheses and included only one intraoperative fracture. This injury involved the medial epicondyle; healing was uneventful, but the management of this fracture was not discussed. In 1987, Trancik and coworkers[61] noted a complication rate of 57% for their 2- to 8-year follow-up series of 35 capitellocondylar elbow arthroplas-

§References 35, 39, 40, 43, 46, 55, 56, 58, 61.

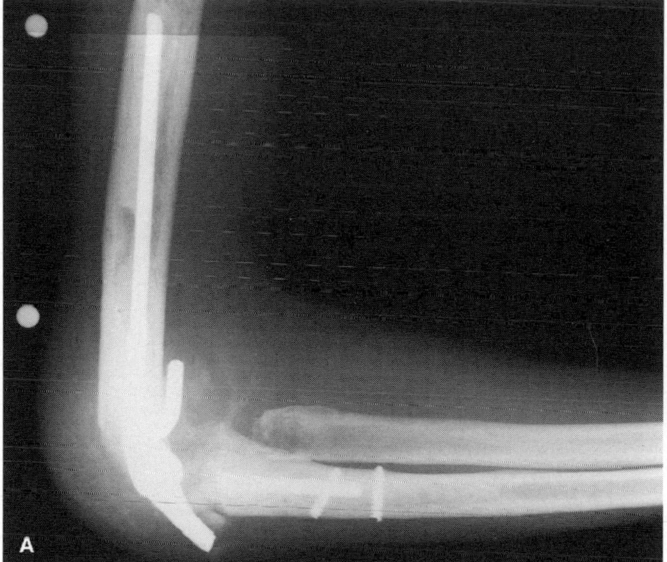

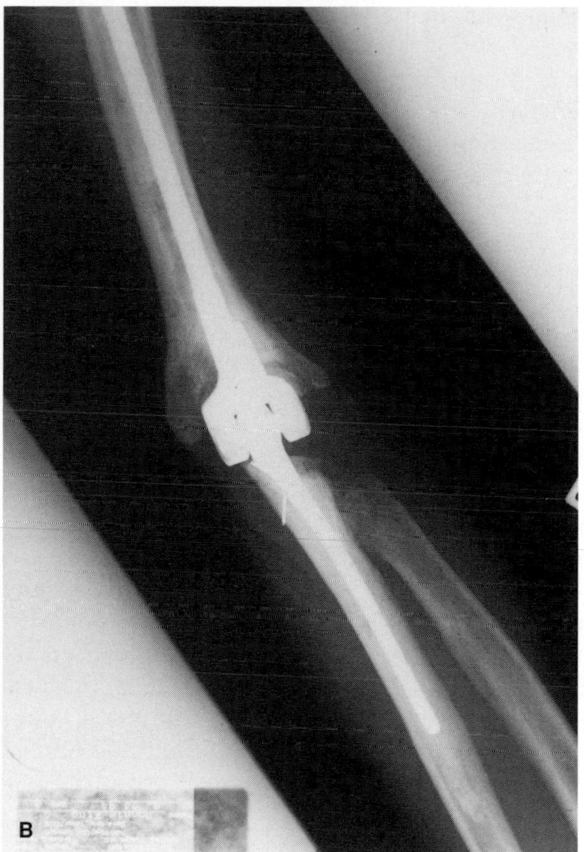

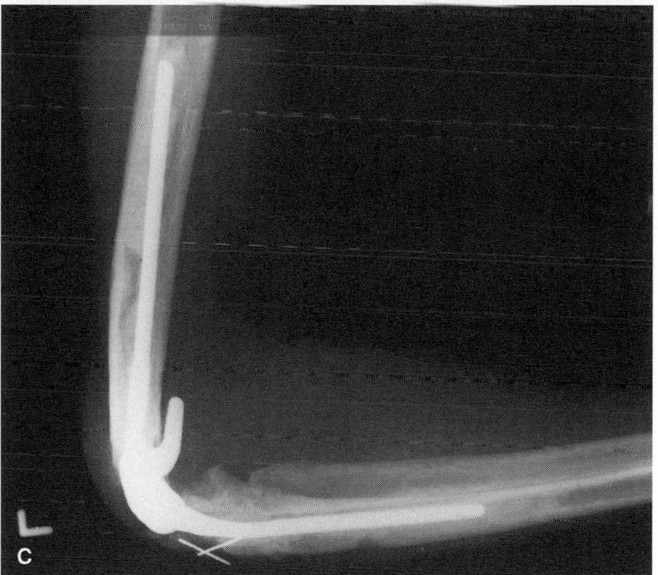

FIGURE 10-24. (**A**) Postoperative radiograph revealing an obvious fracture of the ulnar component of a semiconstrained total elbow implant. (**B** and **C**) Anteroposterior and lateral radiographs after revision elbow arthroplasty with a long-stem ulnar component. *(Courtesy of Eugene T. O'Brien, M.D., San Antonio, TX)*

ties. Complications included three infections, three dislocations, nine transient ulnar nerve palsies, one perforation of the ulnar cortex, and two intraoperative fractures. Perforation of the ulna occurred while rasping in an area of osteoporotic cortex and was managed with bone grafting of the defect before cement fixation of the ulnar component. The other two intraoperative fractures involved the medial condyle of the humerus; one occurred during extraction of a Street humeral prosthesis and one during trial reduction of the implant. In both cases, the fractured medial condyle was treated with internal fixation at the time of surgery and subsequent healing was uneventful. In 1992, Ruth and Wilde[58] described two intraoperative fractures and one perforation of the ulnar cortex in a series of 51 capitellocondylar elbow replacements. Both fractures were treated with internal fixation, but in neither case was the involved bone or postoperative treatment specified. In 1993, Ewald and colleagues[40] reported a large series of more than 200 unconstrained capitellocondylar total elbow replacements with a mean follow-up of 69 months. Only two intraoperative complications were noted and both of these involved fractures. There was one fracture each of the humerus and ulna, and both were stabilized at the time of surgery before insertion of the prosthesis.

Postoperative Periprosthetic Fractures of the Elbow

Postoperative periprosthetic fractures adjacent to unconstrained total elbow implants occur with about twice the frequency of intraoperative fractures.[39,40,55,56,58,61] These injuries occur at an average of 5 years after replacement surgery (range, 1 to 8 years) but a review of several series revealed that the time of postoperative fracture was noted in only 50% of cases.[55,56,58,61]

In a 2- to 5-year follow-up study of 69 unconstrained capitellocondylar metal-on-plastic total elbow arthroplasties, Ewald and associates[39] noted two postoperative fracture complications. Both fractures involved the olecranon and probably occurred in areas weakened by bony resorption around loose ulnar components. One patient did well with splint immobilization, and the other had revision of the ulnar component with excision of the fracture fragment and advancement of the triceps tendon. In a preliminary report of 13 cases with a mean follow-up of 18 months, Pritchard[55] described a fracture dislocation of the distal humerus in a patient with rheumatoid arthritis who fell 1 year after surgery. This postoperative complication required revision of the nonstemmed humeral component to a stemmed design. In a study by Lowe and colleagues,[46] two cases of postoperative humeral fracture occurred after falls, one in a patient with a nonstemmed humeral component and one in a patient with a stemmed design. Fracture healing proceeded uneventfully around the stemmed humeral component, but there was a malunion of the distal humerus associated with implant loosening with the nonstemmed humeral implant. Rosenberg and Turner[56] reported one postoperative fracture from their series of 28 capitellocondylar elbow arthroplasties. The patient fractured her ulna and the all-plastic ulnar component when she fell on her elbow about 3 years after surgery. Revision surgery was offered because of persistent discomfort and decreased motion, but the patient declined. In a study by Trancik and colleagues,[61] one of three periprosthetic fractures occurred in the postoperative period. This injury involved a fracture of the humerus in a patient who fell 3 years after the index arthroplasty procedure. Subsequent management included revision of the unconstrained implant to a semiconstrained Gschwend-Scheier-Bähler prosthesis. Ruth and Wilde's[58] analysis of 51 capitellocondylar total elbow replacements included a 10% incidence of postoperative fractures among an overall complication rate of 80%. All five postoperative fractures involved the humerus and included the condyles or epicondyles in three cases and the metaphysis and shaft in one case each. The fractures occurred at an average of 6.4 years after the index procedure and only one required revision surgery. In this patient, the humeral shaft fracture failed to unite and the prosthesis was revised with a long-stem semiconstrained implant at another hospital. Ewald and associates[40] recorded a total of five periprosthetic fractures from a large series of 202 condylar total elbow arthroplasties. Three of these fractures were late complications that occurred in the postoperative period. These injuries included two fractures of the ulna and a fracture of the humeral shaft. The ulnar fractures were managed without surgery, in contrast to the humeral fracture, which required open reduction and internal fixation.

Fracture of Unconstrained Total Elbow Prostheses

Failure of unconstrained capitellocondylar total elbow prostheses secondary to implant fracture is rare.[‖] The incidence of this complication is less than 1%, and about three fourths of the failures reported in the literature involved an early design, non–metal-backed polyethylene ulnar component.[40,51,56,58]

CLASSIFICATION

Desirable features of any fracture classification system include a high coefficient of intraobserver reproducibility and interobserver reliability. These elements should occupy a central role in the development of any classification scheme, including a system for classifying fractures adjacent to a total elbow arthroplasty. The importance of such a system seems intuitively obvious because of the implications for both treatment and prognosis, yet no such system exists for the elbow. Pursuant to this, a fundamental classification system for periprosthetic elbow fractures is proposed as follows (Fig. 10-25):

- Type I: Fracture of the humerus proximal to the humeral component
- Type II: Fracture of the humerus or ulna in any location along the length of the prosthesis (including those fractures that extend proximal and distal to the humeral and ulnar components, respectively)
- Type III: Fracture of the ulna distal to the ulnar component
- Type IV: Fracture of the implant

TREATMENT

Fracture of the ipsilateral elbow in a patient with a total elbow arthroplasty is an uncommon but potentially serious complication that can jeopardize an otherwise successful implant and impose severe functional limitations on the patient.

Based on the results of more than 850 total elbow arthroplasty procedures from 16 series in the literature, the overall (intraoperative and postoperative) prevalence of periprosthetic fractures is about 8%, and up to 20% of these require reoperation. Although

‖References 35, 39, 40, 43, 46, 55, 56, 58, 61.

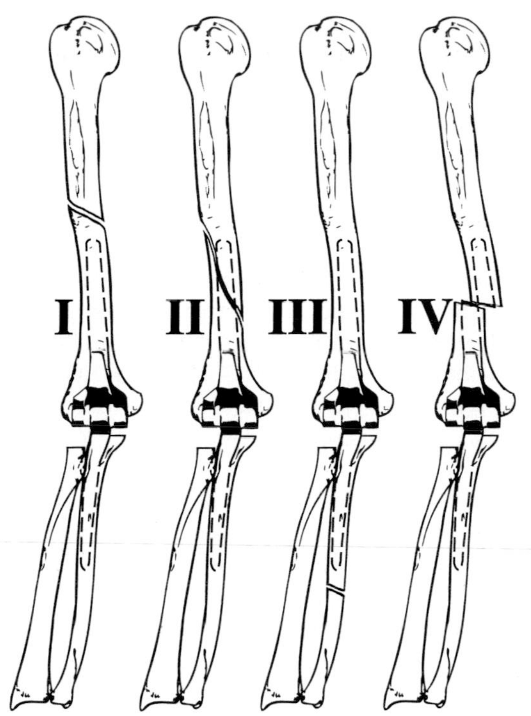

FIGURE 10-25. Classification of periprosthetic elbow fractures. Type I: Fracture of the humerus proximal to the humeral component. Type II: Fracture of the humerus or ulna in any location along the length of the prosthesis (including those fractures that extend proximal and distal to the humeral and ulnar components, respectively). Type III: Fracture of the ulna distal to the ulnar component. Type IV: Fracture of the implant.

complications of total elbow arthroplasties are widely publicized, periprosthetic fractures per se have not received much attention. Furthermore, there are no reports that describe the treatment of these injuries in any detail and there is little objective documentation of long-term results.

Intraoperative Fractures

Intraoperative fractures of the humerus or ulna associated with total elbow replacement surgery occur for numerous reasons, including the amount of bony resection required to accommodate the prosthesis, overzealous reaming or broaching, seating or impaction of oversized components, poor-quality bone, implant design limitations, inadequate exposure, and inappropriate or overzealous manipulation.

For intraoperative fractures that compromise implant stability or would otherwise adversely affect postoperative rehabilitation, the usual method of treatment is secure internal fixation using AO principles such as tension band wiring or lag screw fixation. For small condylar or epicondylar fractures, the fragment can be left in place or resected.

Postoperative Fractures

Periprosthetic elbow fractures of the humerus and ulna occur more commonly in the postoperative period. Factors contributing to the incidence of these injuries include overuse, osteoporosis, trauma, component loosening, intraoperative complications such as cortical perforations, and underestimation of the forces involved in elbow kinematics. As with intraoperative fractures, postoperative fractures can occur at any location around the elbow and often are the result of stress concentration created by the elastic modulus gradient between the cemented component and the adjacent host bone. Fractures that occur during the postoperative period usually are managed expectantly with a short period of immobilization. With the exception of fractures that are markedly displaced, grossly comminuted, or transverse in nature, many of these injuries progress to uneventful healing with acceptable function.

For those fractures that demonstrate persistent displacement, functional limitations, and obvious symptoms, open reduction and internal fixation often is the treatment of choice. In addition, fractures that cannot be immobilized satisfactorily and comfortably or those associated with implant failure, loosening, or instability may require revision arthroplasty. Closed methods of treatment that require prolonged immobilization or extremes of positioning are inappropriate because they can result in a functionally disabling arthrofibrosis.

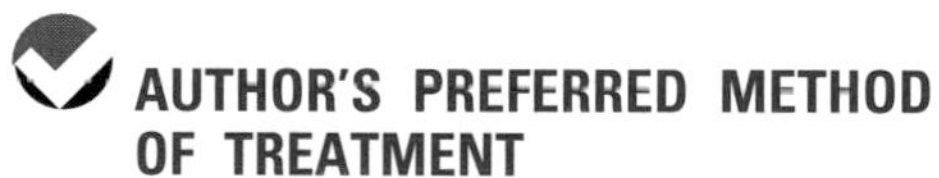

AUTHOR'S PREFERRED METHOD OF TREATMENT

Most published reports on the treatment of complications after elbow replacement surgery have focused on common problems such as recurrent elbow instability, implant loosening, sepsis, and peripheral nerve injury. In contrast, little has been written about the treatment of periprosthetic elbow fractures. This may be at least partially explained by the fact that total elbow arthroplasty is uncommon in comparison to arthroplasty of other joints, coupled with the knowledge that periprosthetic elbow fractures are exceedingly rare. Nevertheless, it is difficult to recommend treatment based on a dearth of experience. Deciding on the proper treatment for these uncommon injuries also can be difficult because there are no set standards to apply. Consequently, successful management of these fractures requires an accurate diagnosis, a healthy measure of clinical acumen, and a good bit of experience. In general, each case must be treated individually based on fundamental orthopaedic principles.

Intraoperative Periprosthetic Fractures of the Elbow

The guidelines for the treatment of intraoperative periprosthetic elbow fractures are based predominantly on the degree of displacement, the characteristics of the fracture, the potential for complications, and the stability of the implant. There are numerous approaches to the treatment of fractures occurring at the time of total elbow arthroplasty procedures, and I believe that optimal management must take into account the type of fracture and the considerable magnitude of torsional stress that is transmitted across the elbow. Walker,[62] and Davis and associates[35] have estimated that, under certain conditions, shoulder abduction increases the torsional load of the forearm up to 6 times body weight or 10 to 20 times the amount of weight held in the hand. The magnitude of these forces emphasizes the necessity of secure fracture fixation that permits early rehabilitation while avoiding the problems associated with prolonged immobilization.

Type I

With rare exception, type I fractures of the humeral shaft that occur during total elbow replacement surgery should be rigidly fixed to provide a stable surgical construct. This is especially applicable to short oblique or transverse fracture patterns, which are at risk for further displacement, shortening, and nonunion. The means by which an unstable fracture can be rendered stable vary, but popular methods include plate fixation with or without supplemental autogenous bone grafting, intramedullary techniques, and simple cerclage wiring. When using a plate and screw technique, the plate should be long enough so that it extends proximal and distal to the fracture site by several cortical diameters. When possible, the plate should be secured to the bone with bicortical screws. Unicortical screws or cerclage wires are used in the bony region that encloses the implant. An alternative method involves the placement of a long-stem component that functions as a means of intramedullary fixation. Previous experience with periprosthetic fractures around the hip and shoulder have emphasized this technique, and it can be used effectively in the elbow as well. Although a component with a larger stem that extends beyond the fracture site by at least two cortical diameters may provide sufficient stability, adjunctive cerclage wire or cables can be used to supplement the fixation.

Type II

Nondisplaced or minimally displaced fractures of the humerus or ulna that are located along the length of the prosthesis can be treated with postoperative bracing if there is no compromise of implant stability. The type II injuries that are most amenable to this type of management include epicondylar fractures, proximal olecranon fractures, and longitudinal splitting fractures of the metaphysis or shaft that occur during reaming, broaching, or component insertion and do not propagate beyond the tip of the humeral or ulnar components.

Insignificant fractures of the supracondylar ridge that do not affect implant stability or a substantial area of forearm muscle origin can be excised. Conversely, large epicondylar or metaphyseal fragments should be secured with AO screws, Kirschner wires, tension band wires, or 1-mm Dacron ligature so that postoperative rehabilitation can proceed without substantial deviation from the usual protocol (Fig. 10-26). Occasionally, the treatment of epicondylar or supracondylar ridge fractures results in fibrous union, but these patients usually do not demonstrate significant pain, weakness, or functional difficulty.

Type II fracture patterns characterized by displacement, comminution, or extension beyond the tip of the component should be managed with supplemental fixation such as Parham bands or cerclage wires. Occasionally, a long-stem prosthesis that bypasses the fracture site also is required. When using this technique, isolation and protection of the ulnar, radial, and musculocutaneous nerves is imperative while passing circumferential devices around the humerus.

Intraoperative type II fractures involving the distal humerus or proximal ulna can impose restrictions on the choice of implant, specifically precluding the use of unconstrained total elbow components in many situations. According to Ewald,[38] the strategy for securing unconstrained implants is based on three-point bony fixation in both humeral and ulnar components. In the humerus, these fixation points include the capitellum, trochlea, and medullary canal. For the ulna, three-point fixation is mediated by the medial and lateral facets of the trochlear notch and the medullary canal. Because the stability of unconstrained total elbow implants is vitally dependent on soft-tissue restraints and bony support, unstable fractures involving these fixation points require rigid fixation (Fig. 10-27). If rigid fixation cannot be obtained intraoperatively to the satisfaction of the surgeon, consideration should be given to a more constrained total elbow prosthesis.

Type III fractures of the ulna occurring distal to the tip of the ulnar component usually are the result of surgical error at the time of medullary broaching or reaming and are managed easily with cerclage wiring.

POSTOPERATIVE CARE AND REHABILITATION

The upper extremity is placed in a bulky compressive dressing and elevated for 24 to 48 hours. During this time, cryotherapy is used for the elbow and active use

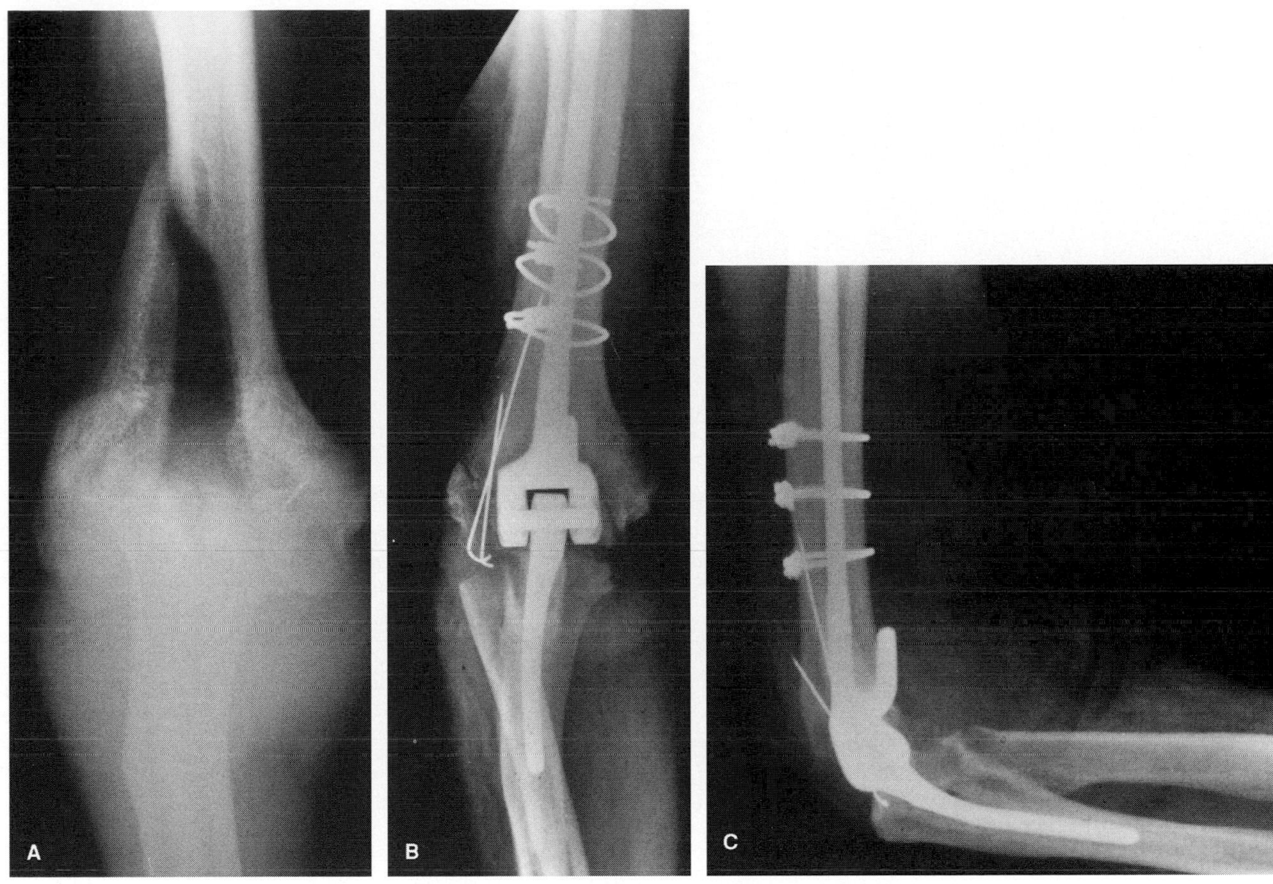

FIGURE 10-26. (**A**) Anteroposterior radiograph of a patient seen several months after sustaining a posterior intercondylar fracture dislocation of the distal humerus. Marked destruction of the elbow joint precluded open reduction and internal fixation. (**B** and **C**) Postoperative radiographs after successful reconstruction with a long-stem revision total elbow implant. Note the intraoperative lateral condyle fracture that was stabilized with Kirschner wires. (*Courtesy of Eugene T. O'Brien, M.D., San Antonio, TX*)

of the hand and wrist is encouraged. Drains generally are removed by the second postoperative day and a light dressing and removable posterior splint are applied. Sutures are removed at 7 to 10 days and the posterior splint is exchanged for a hinged Orthoplast fracture brace that permits gentle active and active-assisted elbow motion. Patients are instructed to use this brace until clinical and radiographic evidence of fracture healing is apparent. These simple guidelines must be tailored for individual cases.

POSTOPERATIVE PERIPROSTHETIC FRACTURES OF THE ELBOW

Postoperative periprosthetic fractures of the elbow that do not compromise implant stability generally can be managed expectantly at first with a fracture brace and early isometric exercises of the upper extremity. The obvious goal of this treatment is to obtain uneventful fracture healing without compromising the functional result through prolonged immobilization. In a biomechanical study of elbow motion, Morrey and associates[50] found that most activities of daily living required an elbow range of motion from 30° of extension to 130° of flexion and a range of pronation and supination of 100°. To obtain or maintain this range of motion after careful and judicious immobilization ensures an acceptable outcome in the absence of other associated complications such as implant failure or loosening, neurovascular injury, or symptomatic nonunion.

The preferred treatment of postoperative fractures that occur in proximity to a total elbow prosthesis depends on many factors, including displacement, implant stability, fracture pattern, functional impairment, and patient demographics. In general, my initial approach to the management of these injuries is more conservative than the usual methods of treatment that are used for similar fractures that occur during surgery.

When feasible, a trial of immobilization is recommended as initial management. Many of these injuries can be managed by the usual methods of expectant

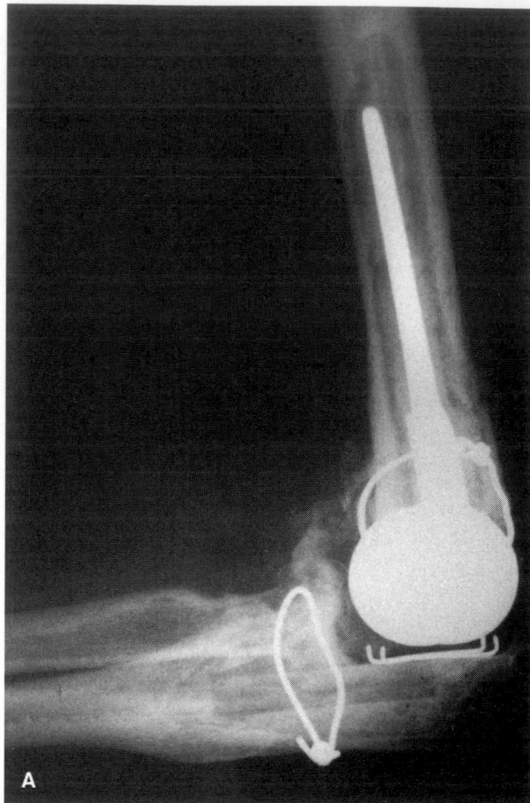

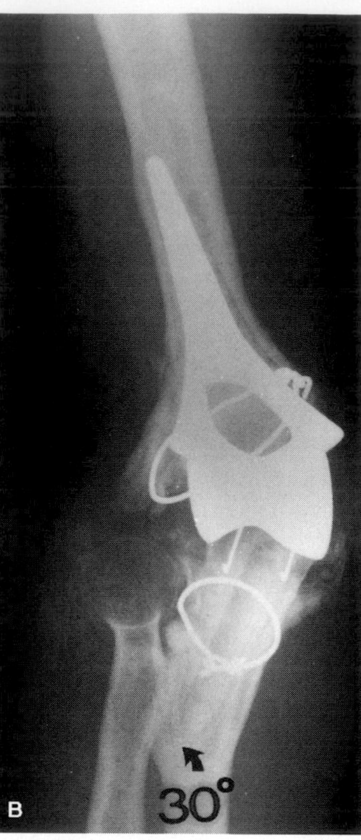

FIGURE 10-27. (**A** and **B**) Radiographs of a 43-year-old patient with an unconstrained total elbow replacement. The arthroplasty procedure was complicated by an intraoperative fracture of the ulna that healed in 30 degrees of angulation. The patient did well for several years but eventually required revision surgery because of progressive pain; elbow motion was limited to a range of 25 degrees. (*Courtesy of Eugene T. O'Brien, M.D., San Antonio, TX*)

therapy for similar fractures not associated with a total elbow arthroplasty. This initial approach to treatment usually is satisfactory for spiral or oblique fracture patterns, minimally displaced fractures, and fractures that have not affected implant stability. Conservative treatment generally includes a short period of immobilization with the elbow splinted at 90° until swelling subsides. Following the general principles of musculoskeletal healing, motion of the elbow is initiated at 3 to 6 weeks as the inflammatory phase of healing subsides and the reparative phase increases. Immobilization for this period usually is not associated with a significant loss of motion. During this time, the patient should be warned of the possibilities of further fracture displacement, nonunion, and the need for revision surgery.

Although patients with periprosthetic elbow fractures do not always have clinical symptoms, the risk of progressive implant loosening, fracture displacement, and other complications must be considered. As mentioned earlier, fractures that are not amenable to an initial trial of closed treatment include irreducible fractures, fractures that cannot be adequately maintained by closed methods, fractures that are associated with implant instability or failure, and open injuries. These injuries must be evaluated carefully and undivided attention given to meticulous preoperative planning, because poorly executed or ill-advised surgery can leave the patient in a far worse condition than if surgery had never been performed. The prepared surgeon is well versed in a variety of techniques for fracture management, but also is equipped to manage a revision procedure requiring cement extraction and reimplantation of a new or custom prosthesis (Fig. 10-28). Surgical precision, fracture management expertise, and a thorough understanding of elbow anatomy and biomechanics enhance the likelihood of a successful outcome. The fact that complications are common with surgical reconstructions of this magnitude underscores the importance of investing ample time in preoperative counseling of both the patient and the family.

Once the decision to operate has been made, it is imperative that the method of fixation be rigid enough to allow early motion. I prefer the Bryan-Morrey posterior approach to the elbow, which is a true triceps-sparing exposure.[34] This is a modification of various triceps-releasing approaches that provides excellent exposure and preserves the extensor mechanism of the triceps. Without exception, the ulnar nerve should be identified and protected. Frequently, it is prudent to identify and protect the radial nerve as well.

For fractures associated with a stable implant, the same methods of internal fixation are applied that were described earlier for intraoperative fractures. In the case of an unstable prosthesis, the original implant and cement are removed (Fig. 10-29). Cement re-

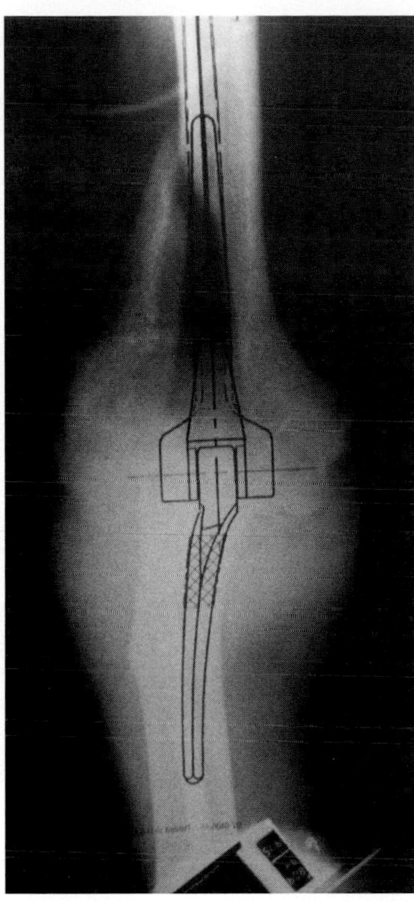

FIGURE 10-28. Preoperative planning is facilitated by template silhouetting, which ensures the availability of a proper-sized component.

moval is facilitated by revision instrumentation, including long-stem power burs, reamers, curets, and osteotomes. A good light source and a high-quality image intensifier are important adjuncts that help minimize the chance of cortical perforation during cement extraction (Fig. 10-30). For cases in which cement removal is difficult and bone quality is poor, the use of an ultrasonic transducer can be helpful. Once the cement has been removed, the fracture is reduced and stabilized around a long-stem elbow prosthesis using cerclage cables or wires. Less commonly, an AO or Ogden-type plate is used to bridge the fracture site. The plate is secured with unicortical or tangential screws in the region of the implant and with bicortical screws where the medullary canal is free of the prosthetic stem. Circumferential wire is an alternative method of plate fixation in the region of the implant. However, the surgeon must be careful not to place cerclage wire or cable at the tip of the prosthesis because it can function as a stress riser in a region that already is predisposed to fracture. Before cementing the new prosthesis, the component can be carefully removed and a slurry of cancellous bone graft introduced into the medullary canal of the humerus and ulna. The stem of a trial prosthesis is inserted into the canal and used in a pistoning fashion to work the bone graft into the fracture site or other areas of bony deficiency.

Periprosthetic elbow fractures that occur after progressive bony resorption secondary to aseptic loosening are especially difficult to manage. Because the integrity of the distal humerus and proximal ulna are critical to component fixation, the bone loss and destruction commonly associated with these injuries preclude reconstruction unless an allograft and custom prosthesis are available for a composite replacement. Although this is a viable option, there is limited information on this technique and it should be reserved for those with considerable expertise in revision elbow arthroplasty.

PERIPROSTHETIC FRACTURES OF THE WRIST AND HAND

PERIPROSTHETIC FRACTURES OF THE WRIST

Total wrist arthroplasty accounts for less than 1% of all arthroplasty procedures performed annually in the United States.[108] Accordingly, there is a paucity of literature regarding wrist replacement surgery in comparison to the number of reports detailing the results of arthroplasty in other joints, such as the hip, knee, and shoulder.

The complications commonly associated with total wrist arthroplasty are similar to those of shoulder or elbow replacement surgery in that component loosening and instability are among the most frequent problems encountered (Fig. 10-31). In contrast to the complications of component loosening and instability, periprosthetic wrist fractures are uncommon and treatment recommendations are not well defined.

Prevalence

The true incidence of periprosthetic wrist fractures is not known. The reason may lie in reporting methods, difficulties in differentiating complete but stable fractures from simple perforations, or simple omissions because the investigators know that the clinical consequences often are insignificant. Regardless of these considerations, a higher frequency of fractures would be expected than is generally reported because the tensile force needed to fracture a metacarpal possessing a cortical thickness of about 0.5 mm is only

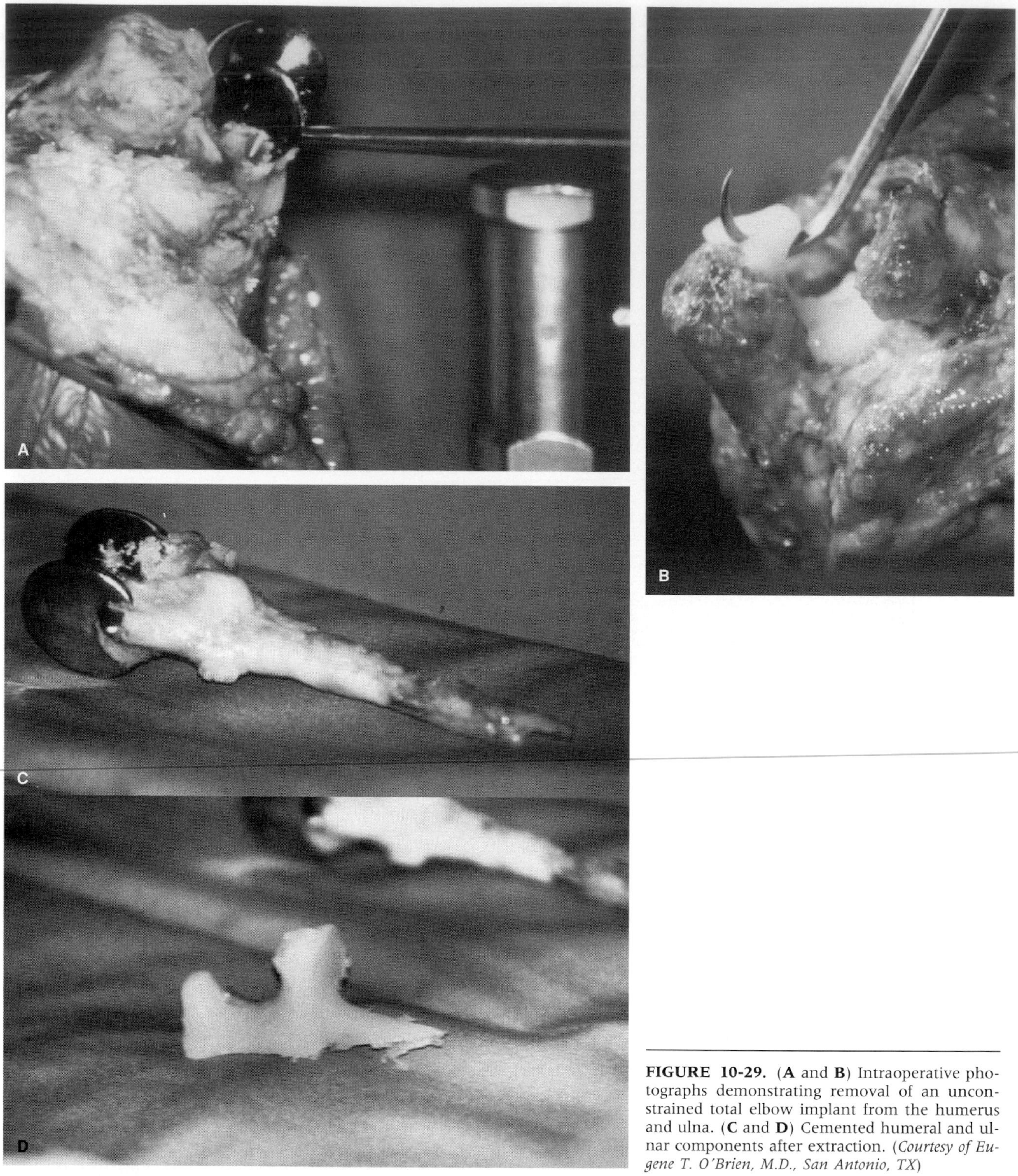

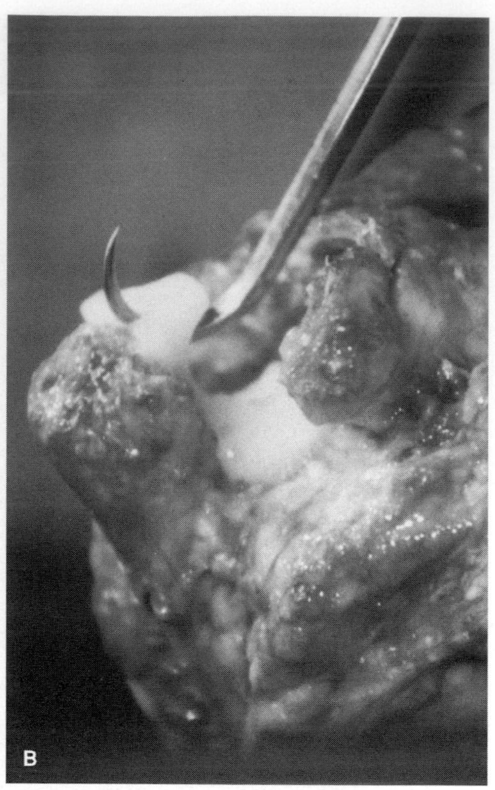

FIGURE 10-29. (**A** and **B**) Intraoperative photographs demonstrating removal of an unconstrained total elbow implant from the humerus and ulna. (**C** and **D**) Cemented humeral and ulnar components after extraction. (*Courtesy of Eugene T. O'Brien, M.D., San Antonio, TX*)

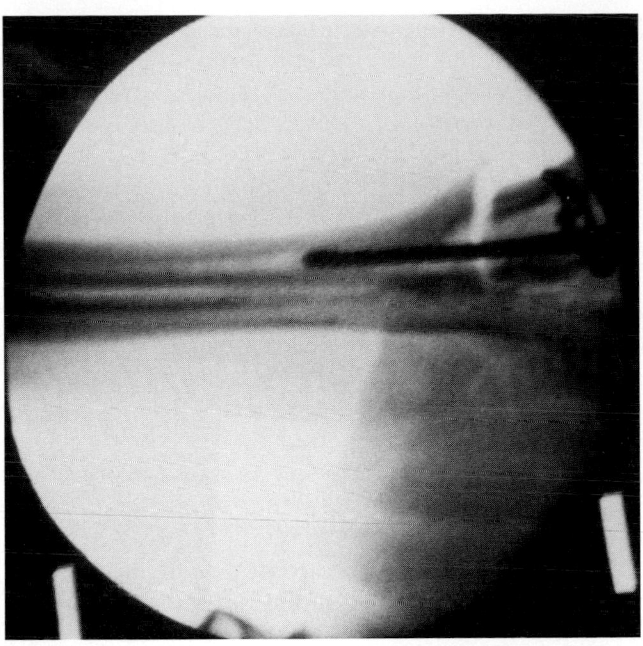

FIGURE 10-30. The risk of cortical perforation is decreased substantially by using intraoperative image intensification.

about 3 kg more than the same force required to disrupt the metal stem–cement interface of a distal total wrist component.[120]

Historical Review

In the 1970s, Meuli[96–98] and Volz[121] independently developed a cemented total wrist arthroplasty device and reported their preliminary results. Experience with the use of both these implants has shown uniformly good results in regard to pain relief, but numerous complications related to an inability to balance the forces across the wrist have been noted.[68,82,99,121] Among these complications are periprosthetic fractures of the distal radius or metacarpals. Although frequently difficult to identify, the factors associated with these fractures include trauma, surgical technique, bone quality, implant stability, and wrist kinematics.

Cemented Total Wrist Arthroplasty

In a review of 148 total wrist arthroplasties at the Mayo Clinic, Linscheid and colleagues[93] identified numerous technical difficulties associated with total wrist replacement procedures. Many of these difficulties resulted in periprosthetic wrist and hand fractures, and were related to technical problems such as eccentric intramedullary reaming of the metacarpal canal, inaccurate bending of the implant stems, incomplete cementing techniques, difficulty with reinsertion of the prostheses after the introduction of cement, and improper alignment of the implants. The authors noted several instances of stem perforation through the metacarpals at the time of prosthetic insertion, as well as perforation of a metacarpal in a patient with aseptic loosening of the prosthesis (Fig. 10-32). The overall incidence of these fractures was not reported. Beckenbaugh and Linscheid[67] presented a preliminary report of 26 Meuli total wrist arthroplasties in 1977. Evaluation at 7 to 17 months after surgery revealed that 92% of wrists were relieved of pain, but reoperation was necessary in 35% of the 26 wrists. Although intraoperative or postoperative periprosthetic fractures were not included among the complications, two of four radiographically illustrated cases revealed perforation of the metacarpals by the stem of the distal component. Similar to another report by these same authors,[93] the consequences of this finding were presumably negligible, although follow-up was limited.

More recently, Rettig and Beckenbaugh[109] reviewed their series of 13 revision total wrist arthroplasties and reported a 38% incidence of intraoperative complica-

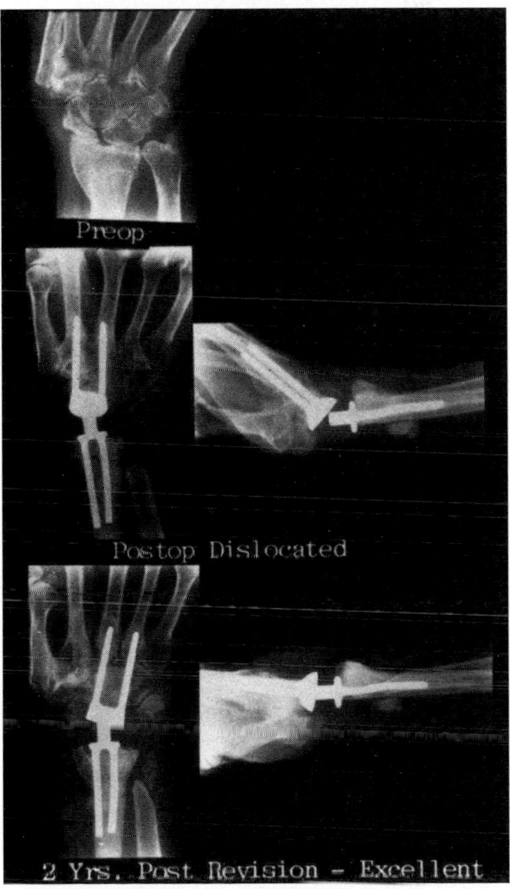

FIGURE 10-31. Radiographs of a Meuli prosthesis revealing a postoperative disassociation of the proximal and distal components. Two-year postoperative revision radiographs reveal a concentric relationship between the wrist components. The clinical result was excellent. (*Courtesy of James H. Dobyns, M.D., Rochester, MN*)

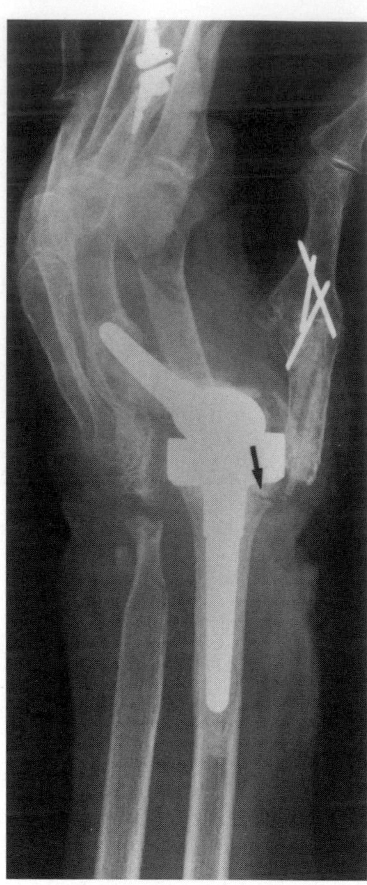

FIGURE 10-32. Radiograph of a Mayo total wrist prosthesis demonstrating erosion of the third metacarpal and a fracture of the bone-cement mantle of the distal radius (*arrow*). (*Courtesy of David P. Green, M.D., San Antonio, TX*)

tions, all of which were secondary to fractures. In one case, the patient sustained a longitudinal fracture of the radius that permitted cement to extrude dorsally into the extensor compartment. This complication led to symptoms on the dorsal surface of the wrist that necessitated an additional procedure for cement removal 2 years later. In three cases, the long-finger metacarpal was perforated during preparation of the intramedullary canal. No further complications related to these perforations were apparent at latest follow-up. In the final case, a circumferential fracture of the distal radius occurred during extraction of the primary component. This injury resulted in nonunion of the radius despite lengthy immobilization, and was revised 4 months later to a wrist arthrodesis.

Silicone Rubber Total Wrist Arthroplasty

As with any nonbiological joint implant, mechanical problems such as component loosening, instability, and fracture are bound to occur. According to Swanson and colleagues,[117] the durability of flexible-implant wrist arthroplasty has been attributed to implant shape and material, protection of the bone–implant interface, restriction of motion, surgical technique, and control of disease progression. Although fractures occurring adjacent to a flexible wrist implant are exceedingly rare, fracture of the implant itself is common. In 1991, Swanson and deGroot-Swanson[116] reviewed 25 revision procedures for fractured flexible implants. Fracture rates of 16% in 32 original silicone components and 8% in 248 second-generation elastomer components were noted. A further reduction in component fracture incidence was described after the introduction of titanium grommets.[116] In 1993, Rettig and Beckenbaugh[109] reported their experience with revision total wrist arthroplasty as a salvage procedure for 13 failed wrist replacements of various designs. The indication for 6 of these revisions was a fractured Swanson implant associated with severe pain, fixed deformity, and marked limitation of motion (Fig. 10-33).

CARPAL AND TRAPEZIOMETACARPAL IMPLANTS

The complications and risks associated with implant replacement surgery of the carpal bones and trapeziometacarpal joint are similar to those of other joint replacement procedures, although implant failure and loosening generally are more common. Since the 1970s, several total joint prostheses have been used in the treatment of trapeziometacarpal joint arthritis, including the Lewis (Howmedica),[76] Braun (Zimmer),[74,75] de la Caffiniere (Francobal),[63,77–79,92,100] and Steffee (Laure Prosthetics)[69,84] implants. Of 127 cemented total arthroplasties of the thumb trapeziometacarpal joint described in three reports,[76,84,100] only one periprosthetic fracture was noted. This case was described by Nicholas and Calderwood,[100] who reviewed 20 de la Caffiniere trapeziometacarpal arthroplasties for osteoarthritis at an average follow-up of 64 months. One of two failures was attributed to collapse of the trapezium with loosening of the implant. This complication occurred in a patient whose trapezium was perforated as a result of overzealous reaming at the time of surgery. At final follow-up, the patient had symptoms and demonstrated functional limitations.

TREATMENT

Wrist Arthroplasty

The major goals in the treatment of periprosthetic wrist fractures are to achieve bony union, prevent malunion and implant loosening, and restore hand and

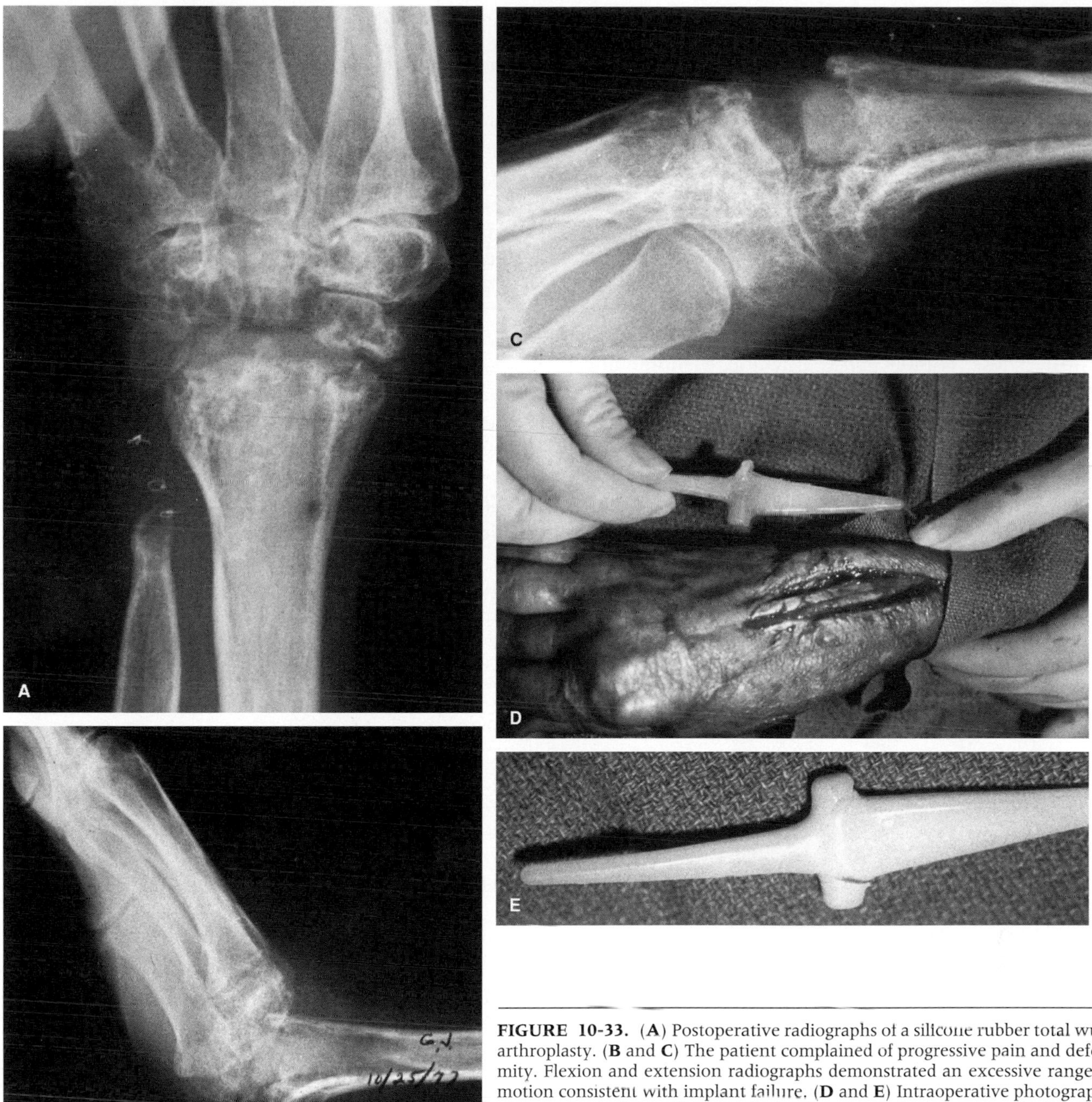

FIGURE 10-33. (**A**) Postoperative radiographs of a silicone rubber total wrist arthroplasty. (**B** and **C**) The patient complained of progressive pain and deformity. Flexion and extension radiographs demonstrated an excessive range of motion consistent with implant failure. (**D** and **E**) Intraoperative photographs after removal of the silicone wrist implant. Note the fracture at the hinge of the prosthesis. (*Courtesy of Spencer A. Rowland, M.D., San Antonio, TX*)

wrist function in a timely fashion while minimizing disability. Similar in regard to total elbow arthroplasty, total wrist arthroplasty is an exceedingly rare procedure in comparison to arthroplasty of other joints, and there is little in the literature regarding the management of fracture complications.

Most periprosthetic hand and wrist fractures occur during surgery and involve perforation of the metacarpals during reaming of the intramedullary canal or insertion of the prosthesis. Fortunately, the literature suggests that these injuries heal uneventfully after a short period of immobilization, and that most patients are satisfied with the degree of pain relief and functional improvement that is achieved.[67,93,109]

Although trauma would seem to be a common cause of periprosthetic hand and wrist fractures in the postoperative period, fractures during this time are more likely to occur indirectly as a result of component loosening. Component loosening, the major long-term complication of several wrist replacement designs, results in palmar drifting of the distal component secondary to the forces transmitted through the wrist when it is in dorsiflexion.[65,109] These forces create a "rocking-horse" effect on the distal component whereby the articulating portion of the distal component encroaches on the carpal tunnel and the stems migrate dorsally, eventually eroding through the cortex of the metacarpals (Fig. 10-34). Symptoms resulting from this complication usually are secondary to compromise of the carpal tunnel and unrelated to the metacarpal shaft involvement. Accordingly, treatment is directed to the carpal tunnel symptomatology and occasionally requires release of the transverse carpal ligament.[65]

Revision of a total wrist arthroplasty may become necessary because of failure related to fracture complications. These complications include symptomatic nonunion, progressive component loosening, functional disability, and implant failure. The treatment of these complications is relatively finite and includes resection arthroplasty, revision with a new or custom wrist arthroplasty, and wrist arthrodesis with autogenous iliac crest bone graft (Fig. 10-35).

Carpal and Trapeziometacarpal Implants

The advent of flexible silicone rubber prostheses was initiated independently in the 1960s by Niebauer and associates,[102,103] and by Swanson.[111–114,118] Although the introduction of this technology revolutionized arthroplasty of the hand for the treatment of arthritis, it also introduced new problems related to the generation of silicone wear particles and the resulting adverse histologic response.[104,105,110] Silicone implants for the hand have been voluntarily withdrawn from the marketplace by the leading manufacturer of these products. As astutely suggested by Pellegrini and Burton, this decision most likely was fueled by the medicolegal climate of increasing product liability, the emotional controversy surrounding the silicone breast implant, and reports in the orthopaedic literature.[64,66,85,90,104–107,110] As of 1992, 30% to 40% of the cost of silicone medical products in general is designated for the purpose of legal defense.[85]

With rare exception, fractures after implant surgery of the carpus primarily involve flexible silicone implants. Whether fracture failure of the implant increases the propensity for an adverse histologic reaction is unknown, but concerns for this problem are justified (Fig. 10-36). Nonetheless, there are many widely accepted methods for the treatment of this complication, including removal of the prosthesis, cancellous bone grafting and curettage of cystic defects, limited intercarpal arthrodesis, tendon interposition arthroplasty, and arthrodesis of the radiocarpal joint.

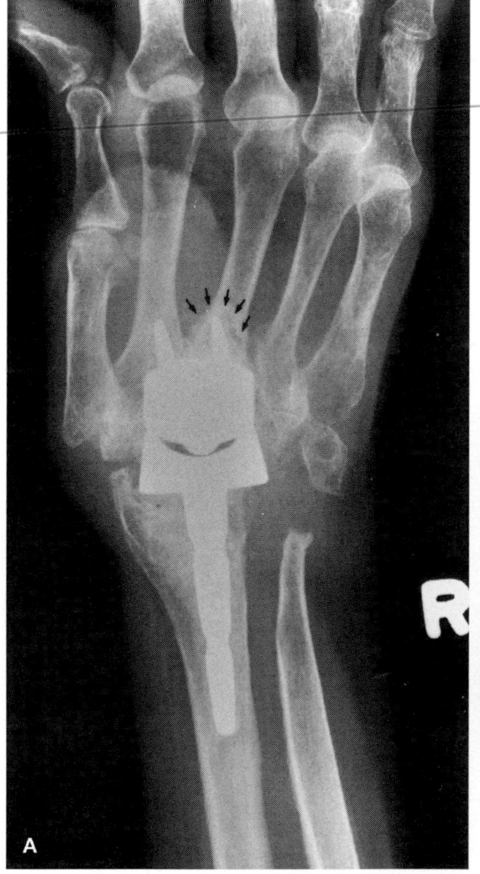

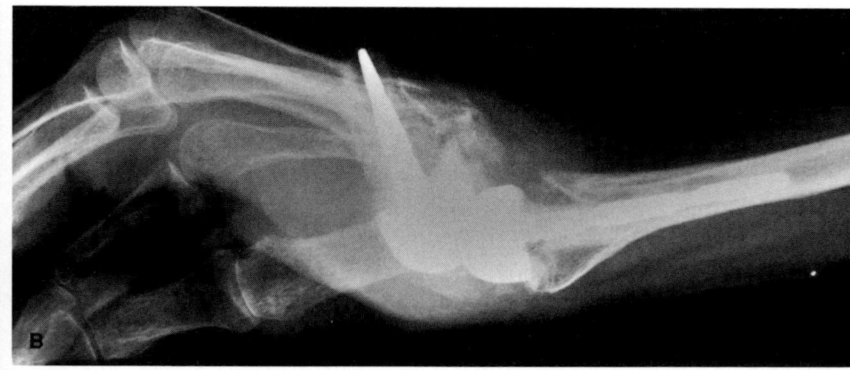

FIGURE 10-34. (**A** and **B**) Double-pronged Voltz AMC total wrist prosthesis that has eroded through the metacarpals. Note the fracture and reactive bone formation at the base of the third metacarpal (*arrows*). (*Courtesy of David P. Green, M.D., San Antonio, TX*)

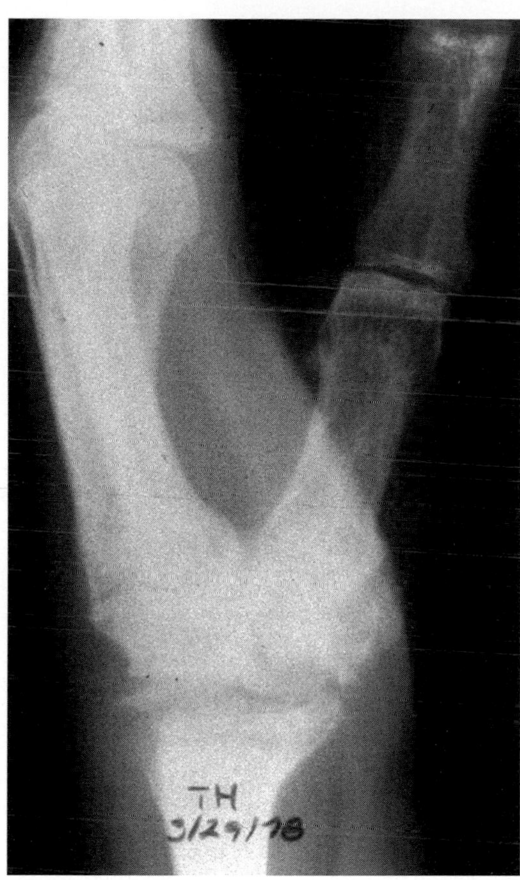

FIGURE 10-35. Lateral wrist radiograph after removal of Silastic total wrist arthroplasty. Note bony fragmentation at site of resectional arthroplasty. (*Courtesy of James H. Dobyns, M.D., Rochester, MN*)

Author's Preferred Method of Treatment

The same principles of fracture care used to manage periprosthetic fractures of other joints can be applied to the wrist. In general, minimally displaced fractures of the hand and distal radius that are reasonably stable can be managed expectantly with splinting or casting (Fig. 10-37). Although open reduction and internal fixation is a consideration for those fractures that do not meet these criteria, it often is difficult to obtain secure fixation. An explanation for this, apart from the obvious technical consideration, is the fact that most of these patients have moderate to severe rheumatoid arthritis and many are dependent on systemic corticosteroids, cytotoxic agents, and antimetabolic drugs that are known to have a detrimental effect on bone quality and healing. For this reason, every attempt is made to secure fracture healing by conservative methods before considering revision surgery. When revision surgery is deemed necessary after a fracture that fails conservative treatment, wrist arthrodesis generally is the procedure of choice because of the likelihood for successful fusion and the predictable functional outcome.

PERIPROSTHETIC FRACTURES OF THE HAND

With few exceptions, fractures associated with implants in the hand predominantly involve the prosthesis, with no compromise to the structural integ-

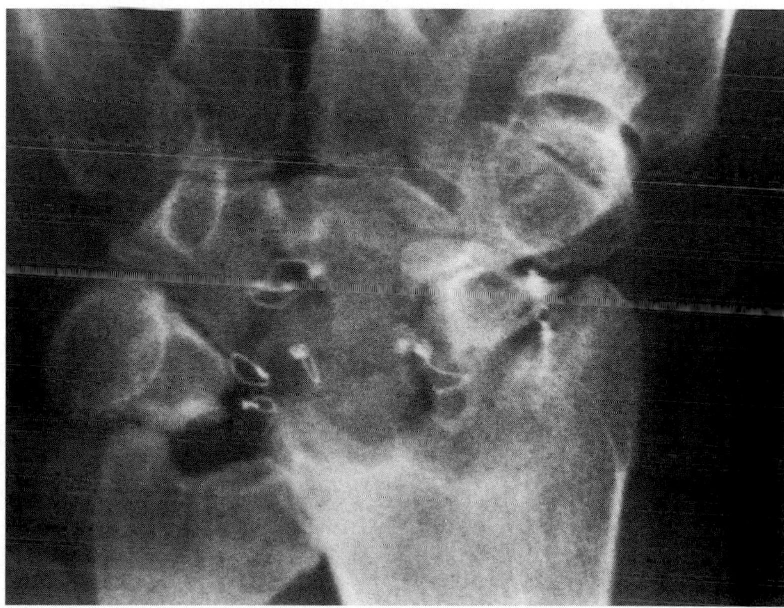

FIGURE 10-36. Destructive arthropathy after Silastic lunate implant for Kienböck's disease. Note the gross scaphoid deformity and cystic changes of the distal radius. (*Courtesy of James H. Dobyns, M.D., Rochester, MN*)

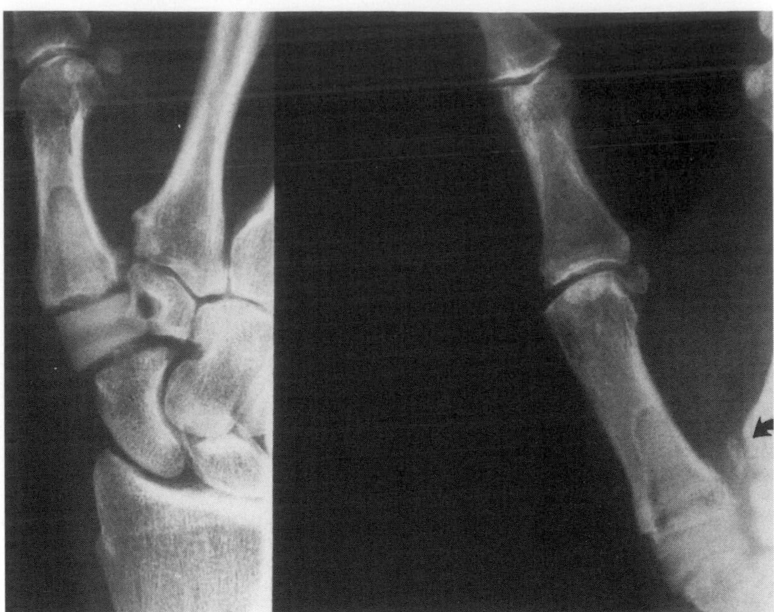

FIGURE 10-37. Silicone rubber metacarpophalangeal joint arthroplasty of the thumb. A fracture at the radial base of the index metacarpal is evident (*arrow*). This minimally displaced fracture was an incidental radiographic finding and no particular treatment was required. (*Courtesy of James H. Dobyns, M.D., Rochester, MN*)

rity of the surrounding bone. Furthermore, although much has been speculated, little is known about the etiology of implant fracture and few reports have correlated this complication with physical limitations such as the need for assistive ambulatory devices.

A diverse array of flexible silicone rubber implants, cemented hinged interphalangeal and metacarpophalangeal joint devices, and carpal bone implants have been used for joint replacement surgery.[69,74–79,92,94,100] Common to all these devices is a significant incidence of component failure secondary to fracture of the implant (Fig. 10-38). For silicone rubber and silicone Dacron implants alone, reported rates of implant fracture have ranged from 0% to 50%.[#] In contrast, fractures of the carpal, metacarpal, or phalangeal bones adjacent to these implants are rare or underreported.

Cemented or Metallic Metacarpophalangeal and Interphalangeal Implants

In 1959, Brannon and Klein[73] described a method of proximal interphalangeal and metacarpophalangeal total joint replacement using a single-axis hinged prosthesis. A tendency for migration of the prosthesis was noted after 10 to 12 months in 2 of the 12 cases with adequate follow-up. In these 2 cases, radiographs demonstrated perforation of the proximal phalanx in one and perforation of the middle phalanx with involvement of the distal interphalangeal joint in the second. Both patients reported no pain or disability at 17- and 19-month evaluations, respectively. In 1961, Flatt[86] presented an interim report on the trial of a metallic hinged prosthesis for rheumatoid arthritis of the metacarpophalangeal and proximal interphalangeal joints. The series consisted of 57 prostheses and included seemingly inevitable complications such as typical boutonnière deformities, limited motion, and infection. Also noted was a 12% incidence of intraoperative phalanx fractures that occurred during insertion of the prostheses. One of these injuries was grossly unstable and necessitated removal of the prosthesis. The remaining fractures occurred during insertion of the prosthesis and were attributed to insufficient reaming of the medullary canal. Healing was uneventful and the implants were stable at latest follow-up. In a later study by Flatt and Ellison,[87] no bony fractures were reported, but fatigue fracture of the implant occurred in the index fingers of two patients. In 1984, Dryer and colleagues[81] presented their results with 56 Flatt prostheses used for proximal interphalangeal joint reconstruction of the rheumatoid hand. Complications included cortical erosion in 80% of the implants followed up for longer than 6 years. Severe cortical erosion was associated with violation of the adjacent distal interphalangeal and metacarpophalangeal joints in an unspecified number of cases. In 1984, Blair and associates[71] published a long-term clinical study of 41 Flatt metallic hinged prostheses used to replace the metacarpophalangeal joints of ten patients with rheumatoid arthritis. With an average follow-up of more than 11 years, this

[#]References 66, 70, 72, 80, 83, 88, 89, 91, 95, 101, 115, 119.

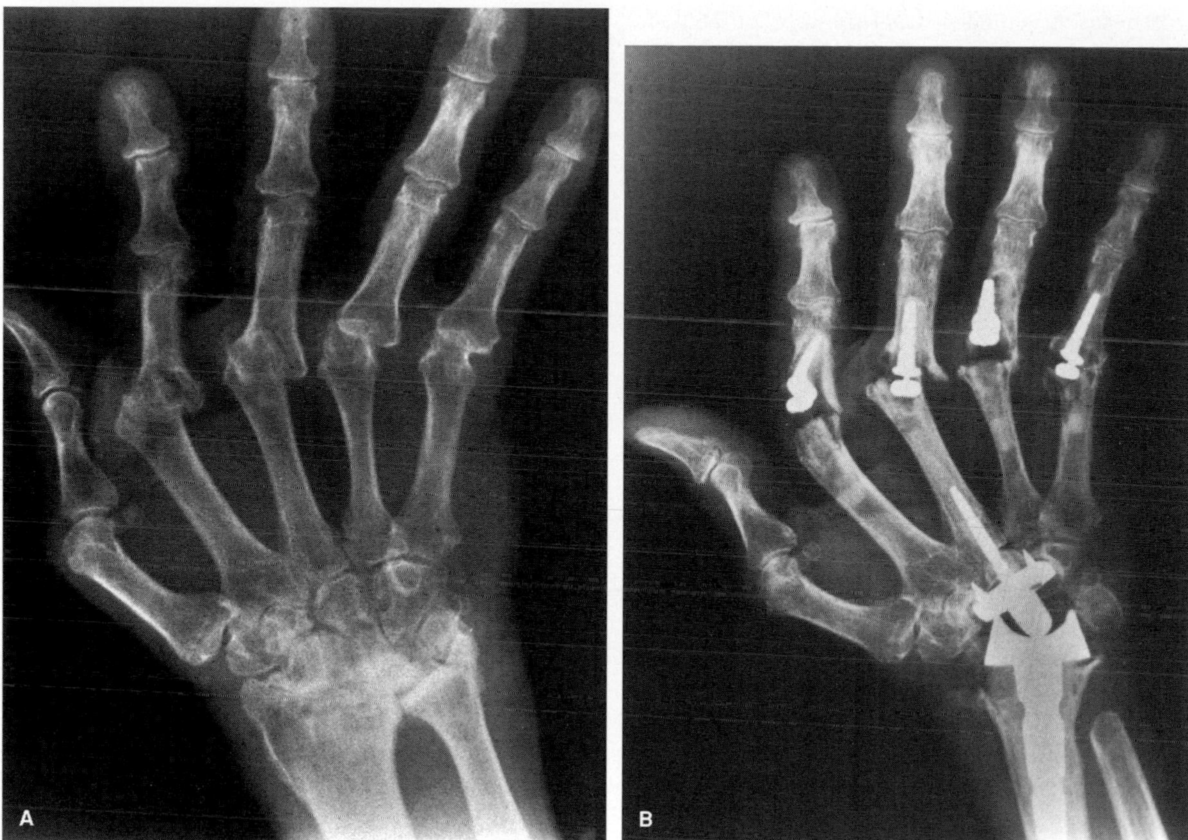

FIGURE 10-38. (**A**) Preoperative anteroposterior radiograph of a patient with long-standing rheumatoid arthritis. (**B**) Postoperative radiograph about 4 years after Voltz AMC total wrist arthroplasty and Steffe total metacarpophalangeal joint replacements. Several broken or dislocated metacarpophalangeal implants are seen in conjunction with fractures of the proximal phalanges. (*Courtesy of James H. Dobyns, M.D., Rochester, MN*)

study provides a valuable historical and clinical perspective on the use of this prosthesis. As with previous studies, migration of the prosthesis was a common complication and resulted in cortical perforation of the metacarpal or proximal phalanx in about 50% of cases. In addition, fatigue failure of the prosthetic stem was common, with an incidence of 12%. Despite the high number of additional complications, including recurrent ulnar deviation, malrotation of the digits and radiographic implant loosening, most patients were satisfied with the postoperative appearance of the hand and the degree of pain relief. Although patient satisfaction was acceptable, the high incidence of complications associated with the use of this prosthesis dissuaded the authors from recommending its further use. In 1990, Pellegrini and Burton[106] retrospectively reviewed seven hinged Biomeric implants. These cemented prostheses were preferentially implanted in the radial proximal interphalangeal joints of the hand for optimal lateral stability during pinch maneuvers. In all cases, the implant failed through the elastomer hinge connecting the titanium stems. Ultimately, all prostheses underwent revision surgery for symptomatic failure and recurrent deformity of the involved digit.

Silicone and Silicone Dacron Flexible Implants

In 1972, Swanson[115] reviewed the development, basic concepts, and techniques of flexible implant arthroplasty of the hand. Fracture of the implant was noted in early cases in which the implant had been fixed with crossed pins, cement, or a Dacron cover on the stems. Analysis of nearly 4000 improved high-performance elastomer implants from the Grand Rapids and Field Clinic study series revealed fractured implants in less than 2% of cases.

In 1976, Beckenbaugh and colleagues[66] reported a series of 530 consecutive silicone rubber metacarpophalangeal implants. Detailed clinical evaluation of

254 prostheses revealed a fracture rate of 26% for Swanson implants and 38% for Niebauer silicone rubber Dacron-impregnated implants. Both the Swanson and the Niebauer implants used for this study were of the original design. Overall, 13 joints required 19 reoperations, and 12 of these were prosthetic revisions secondary to fractured implants. Problems associated with the fractured components included the following findings in order of frequency: ulnar drift or other clinical deformity, weakness or instability, and hyperextension of the involved joint. Radiographic examination suggested that bony impingement was the cause of fracture in 29% of implants, but the authors were unable to delineate the timing of the fracture because in many cases radiographs were not obtained until 2 years after surgery. No periprosthetic fractures of the adjacent bone were reported (Fig. 10-39). In 1984, Dryer and coworkers[81] presented a long-term retrospective evaluation of 30 Swanson and 7 Niebauer prostheses with an average follow-up of 6 years. Fracture or fragmentation of the Swanson prosthesis was identified in three cases, all of which were performed before 1974. Similar to the report of Beckenbaugh and colleagues,[66] fractured implants were commonly associated with the development of a swan-neck or angular deformity of the involved digit. In 1984, Blair and colleagues[72] evaluated 115 Silastic metacarpophalangeal joint arthroplasties at an average follow-up of 54 months. Twenty-four implant fractures (21%) were noted at both the stem–hinge junction and within the hinge itself. Collapse and fragmentation of the implants also was noted frequently. Postoperative radiographic findings included a 41% incidence of bone resorption around the implant, but no perforations or fractures of the cortical bone were reported. The authors concluded that bone resorption was minimal and did not appear to represent, at least for the period of follow-up, a clinically significant finding. In 1986, Bieber and associates[70] reported their results with 210 silicone rubber implants in 46 patients with rheumatoid arthritis. No fractures of the second-generation high-performance silicone elastomer implants were recorded during the 2- to 8-year evaluation period. In 1986, Derkash and colleagues[80] reported at least four fractured silicone Dacron implants (Niebauer type) from a series of 89 metacarpophalangeal arthroplasties that were followed up for an average of 11.5 years. The authors found implant integrity difficult to assess on radiographic examination, but noted severe bone destruction around the prosthesis in 43% of joints and mild destruction in an additional 44%. Instability of the metacarpophalangeal joint with palmar subluxation was a common finding in 58% of joints. The authors were unable to attribute this complication to one specific etiology, but suggested that it was the result of a combination of factors, including fracture of the prosthesis, buckling or deformity of the prosthesis, and bony destruction (Fig. 10-40).

In 1993, Kirschenbaum and colleagues[91] reported a series of 144 improved silicone elastomer metacarpophalangeal arthroplasties with a minimum follow-up of 5 years. This is the longest reported follow-up analysis of patients with rheumatoid arthritis who underwent metacarpophalangeal joint replacement with high-performance Swanson silicone rubber prostheses. Complications were infrequent in this series, but roentgenographic evaluation revealed 15 fractured implants. Three of these failures occurred in the same hand of one patient and all required revision surgery. In this patient, the history was significant for multiple metacarpophalangeal joint steroid injections in the region of the implants. Interestingly, several needle holes were found in each prosthesis at the time of revision surgery and probably contributed to failure of the implants. Additional complications included an

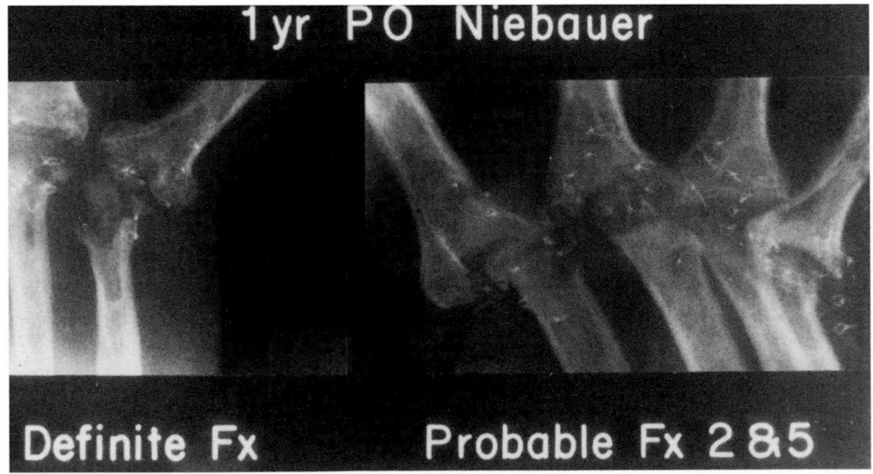

FIGURE 10-39. Radiographs obtained 1 year after the placement of Neibauer silicone rubber Dacron-impregnated metacarpophalangeal implants. Obvious implant fracture (*left*) and probable implant failures involving the index and small fingers (*right*) can be seen. Also note the proximal phalanx fracture of the index finger (ulnar base) (*right*). (*Adapted from Beckenbaugh, R.D., Dobyns, J.H., Linschied, R.L., Bryan, R.S.: Review and Analysis of Silicone-Rubber Metacarpophalangeal Implants. J. Bone Joint Surg., 58A:483, 1976.*)

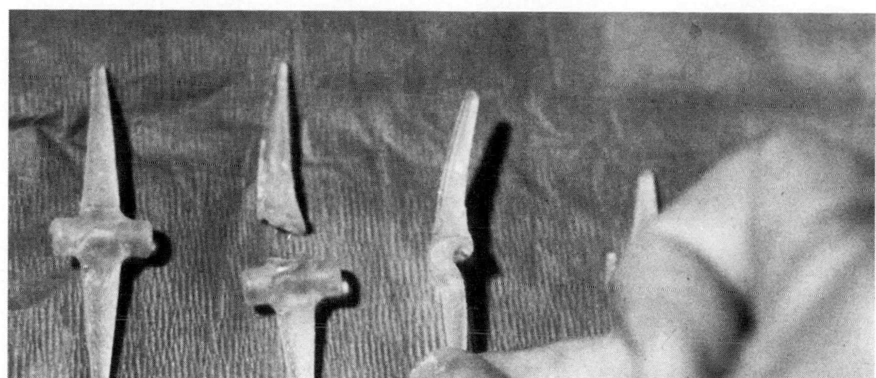

FIGURE 10-40. Fractured or deformed Silastic metacarpophalangeal implants that were removed because of progressive deformity and pain. (*Courtesy of Spencer A. Rowland, M.D., San Antonio, TX*)

intraoperative metacarpal shaft fracture that was treated successfully with cerclage wiring.

TREATMENT

Most reports discussing implant replacement surgery of the metacarpophalangeal and interphalangeal joints overwhelmingly emphasize patient satisfaction despite prosthetic failure.** Because fracture of the implant rarely causes symptoms and generally does not affect function, patients usually are unaware of the complication (Fig. 10-41). In view of these considerations, most authors would consider revision surgery only in the event of rectifiable disability, pain, or progressive periprosthetic bone erosion. Pellegrini and Burton[106] have emphasized the large torques generated by the thumb in lateral pinch and advocate arthrodesis of the proximal interphalangeal joint as an effective means of salvaging failed implants in the radial digits. In general, treatment options include prosthetic replacement in the absence of contiguous bony destruction, re-

**References 66, 70, 72, 80, 81, 91, 106, 107, 111–115, 118.

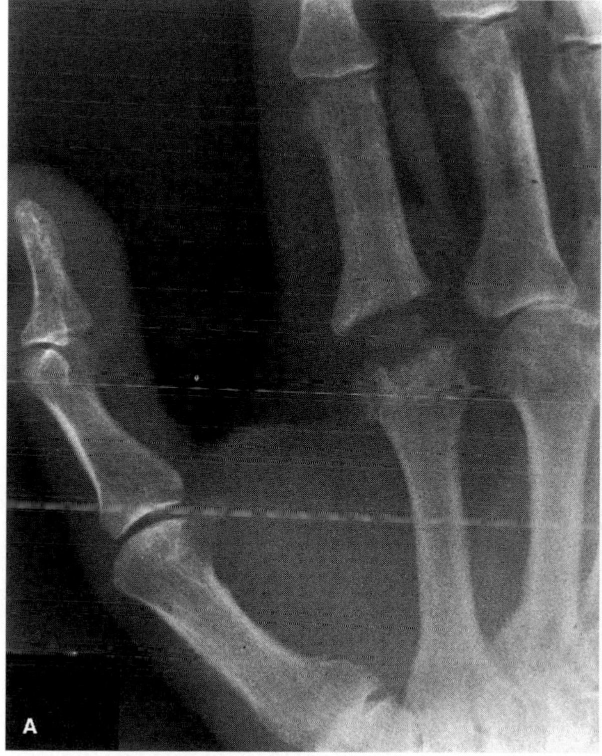

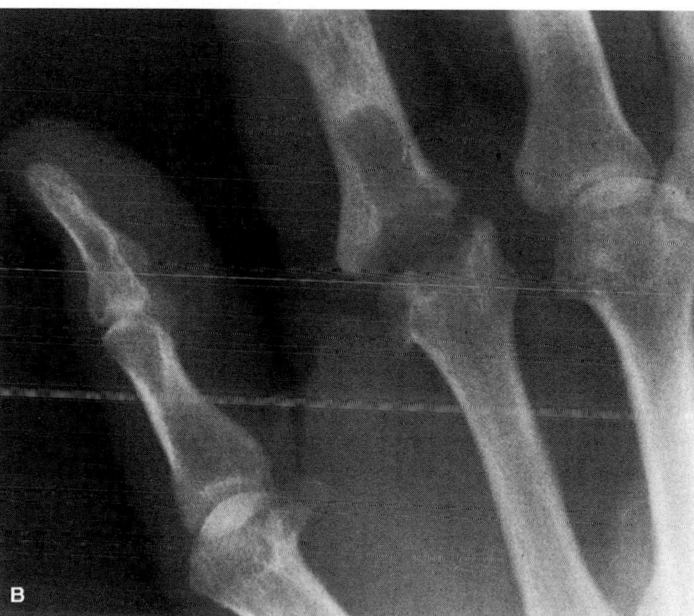

FIGURE 10-41. (**A**) Early postoperative radiograph of a noncemented, metacarpophalangeal pyrolytic carbon implant. (**B**) Eighteen-month follow-up film demonstrating deformation of both the metacarpal and proximal phalanx. (*Courtesy of James H. Dobyns, M.D., Rochester, MN*)

moval of the implant or resection arthroplasty, and arthrodesis.

Part II. Periprosthetic Fractures of the Lower Extremity

Jay D. Mabrey

PERIPROSTHETIC FRACTURES OF THE HIP

Fractures around hip arthroplasties comprise the largest group of periprosthetic fractures affecting primarily the femur and occasionally the acetabulum or pubic ramus. Half of all artificial joints are located in the hip, and two thirds of those hips are in persons 65 years of age or older.[214] In 1989, there were 63,000 primary total hip replacements, 14,000 hip revisions, and 26,000 hemiarthroplasties billed to Medicare alone.[231] With a 5% annual rate of increase in total hip replacement cases between 1985 and 1989,[231] there is an ever-expanding pool of patients at risk for periprosthetic fracture.

Periprosthetic fractures of the hip have been reported for the last four decades in association with uncemented hemiarthroplasties,[††] for the last 20 years around cemented total hip replacements,[‡‡] and for the last 10 years in association with uncemented prostheses.[§§]

FRACTURES OF THE FEMUR

Prevalence

The prevalence of periprosthetic fractures of the hip varies among prostheses and according to whether the fracture occurs during or after surgery. Intraoperative fractures associated with cemented stems have been reported since the early 1970s, averaging 1% overall, with a range of 0.3% to 6.9%.[‖‖] Later studies noted rates between 1% and 1.8%.[125,253] Scott and colleagues[242] reported an intraoperative fracture rate of only 0.4% in more than 5000 cemented arthroplasties, demonstrating the advantage of experience in preventing this complication. At the other extreme, another group reported an intraoperative fracture incidence of 27% in a population of patients undergoing surgery for chronically dislocated hips.[157]

Intraoperative fractures are more likely to occur with uncemented, press-fit components. The prevalence in these cases ranges from 2.6% to 4% for primary hip replacements,[138,172,208,241] to as high as 17.6% for uncemented revisions.[134,145,162,167,211]

With respect to postoperative fractures, Coventry[150] reported none in his review of the first 2000 cemented total hips at the Mayo Clinic, but Nolan and associates[217] later noted a 0.1% fracture rate after 1000 additional cases. Scott and coworkers[242] also reported a postoperative rate of 0.1%, and Cupic[153] noted no postoperative fractures in his long-term series of more than 400 Charnley hips. Other large series of cemented hips report rates of 0.6% to 1.6%.[168,171] The true incidence is reflected best in those studies that report on fractures around both cemented and uncemented stems, and ranges from 0.8% to 2.3%.[132,166,253,269]

Hospitalization costs are significant for periprosthetic fractures of the hip. Intraoperative fractures can extend a patient's stay from 4 to 6 weeks,[145,253] whereas postoperative fractures can require up to 7 weeks of hospitalization after surgical repair.[168,209,266] Management of these injuries with traction alone can take up to 4 months.[168,253]

Classification

The nature of periprosthetic fractures of the hip has evolved along with changes in the implantation procedure. Early reports noted that proximal fractures occurred during the insertion of blade-like hemiarthroplasty stems[176] and during reduction of the prosthesis into the acetabulum.[126] Penetration of the cortex by sharp broaches during cemented total hip implantation left stress risers that led to postoperative fracture through the defect.[252] Later, the revision of loose cemented components required the creation of cortical windows, leading to intraoperative[180] and postoperative[180,185] fractures. The current use of porous ingrowth and press-fit femoral components creates hoop stresses within the proximal femur that can easily fracture the cortex during surgery.[167,177,208,230]

Whittaker and colleagues[265] proposed one of the earliest classification schemes based primarily on their experience with hemiarthroplasties. Johansson and associates[180] presented their more familiar classification in 1981, based on both intraoperative and postoperative fractures associated with cemented total hip arthroplasties (Fig. 10-42). Type I fractures were proximal to the tip of the prosthesis with the stem remaining in the medullary canal. In type II fractures, the fracture line extended from the proximal portion of the femoral

††References 122, 126, 128, 135, 146, 174, 176, 178, 182, 188, 191, 197, 210, 221–223, 249, 257, 261, 267.

‡‡References 125, 130–132, 144, 147–150, 156, 157, 168, 169, 171, 178, 180, 183, 188, 194, 196, 197, 202, 210, 217, 220, 225, 234, 236, 242, 247, 252, 253, 255, 259, 265, 266, 268, 269.

§§References 127, 134, 138, 159, 162, 167, 172, 184, 186, 198, 200, 241, 245, 250, 258.

‖‖References 129, 133, 143, 158, 160, 161, 164, 165, 175, 190, 195, 203, 206, 216, 224, 256, 263.

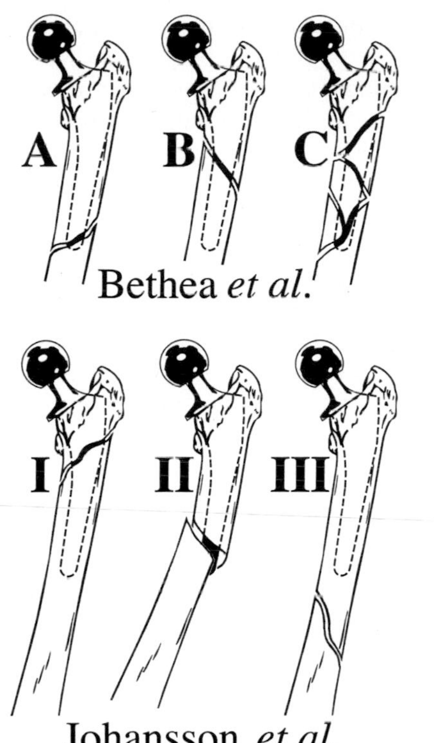

FIGURE 10-42. Comparison of classification schemes proposed by Bethea[131] and Johansson.[190]

shaft to beyond the distal portion of the prosthesis with the prosthetic stem dislodged from the medullary canal of the distal fragment, and in type III fractures, the fracture line was entirely distal to the tip of the prosthesis.[180] The next year, Bethea and colleagues[131] proposed a system that excluded all fractures distal to the tip of the prosthesis. In their scheme, type A was a fracture at the tip of the component, type B was a spiral fracture around the component, and type C was a comminuted fracture around the stem. Subsequent attempts at classification were variations of either Johansson's or Bethea's work.[##] More recently, Mont and Maar[207] proposed a six-part classification based on a review of almost 500 cases reported in the literature.

The American Academy of Orthopaedic Surgeons (AAOS) Committee on the Hip[123] proposed a six-part classification in 1990, which is outlined in Table 10-5. Similar to an earlier proposal by Van Elegem and Blaimont,[257] the scheme divides the femur into three separate regions (Fig. 10-43), with level I defined by the proximal femur distally to the lower extent of the lesser trochanter. Level II includes the 10 cm of the femur distal to level I, and level III covers the remainder of the femur distal to level II.

The six fracture types are depicted in Figure 10-44 beginning with type I, a fracture proximal to the intertrochanteric line that usually occurs during dislocation of the hip. It also can result from a partial saw cut that is completed with an osteotome. Often, this fracture requires only a revision of the neck cut, but it could become a problem for a prosthesis that relies on the femoral neck for fixation. Type II is a vertical or spiral split that does not extend past the lower extent of the lesser trochanter, whereas type III does extend past the lesser trochanter but not beyond level II, usually the junction of the middle and distal thirds of the femoral stem. Type IV fractures traverse or lie within the area of the femoral stem tip in level III, with type IVA being a spiral fracture around the tip and type IVB being a simple transverse or short oblique fracture, similar to a Bethea[131] type A or a Johansson[180] type II fracture. Type V fractures are severely comminuted fractures around the stem in level III, and type VI fractures are fractures distal to the stem tip, also in level III. The utility of the AAOS system is that it accounts for a wide variety of fracture etiologies, both during and after surgery.

TABLE 10-5
American Academy of Orthopaedic Surgeons Fractures Associated With Hip Arthroplasty (see Figs. 10-43 and 10-44)

Level	Classification	Description
Level I	Type I	Proximal to the intertrochanteric line
	Type II	Vertical split not extending past the lower portion of the lesser trochanter
Level II	Type III	Vertical or spiral split extending past the lower portion of the lesser trochanter
Level III	Type IV	Fracture in the region of the tip of the femoral stem: Type IVA: Spiral; Type IVB: Transverse or short oblique
	Type V	Severely comminuted type III or IV
	Type VI	Fracture distal to prosthesis

A.A.O.S., Committee on the Hip: Classification and Management of Femoral Defects in Total Hip Replacement. Exhibit. 57th Annual Meeting of the American Academy of Orthropaedic Surgeons; 1990; New Orleans, LA.

[##]References 147, 148, 198, 212, 244, 250, 255.

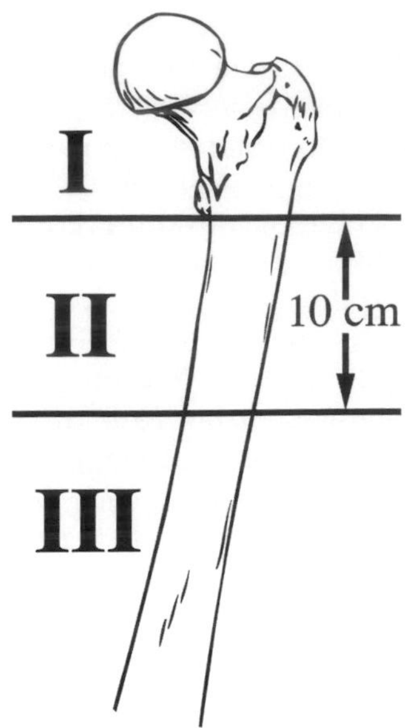

FIGURE 10-43. Levels of fractures associated with hip arthroplasty. (*Petty, W. (ed.): Total Joint Replacement, pp. 291–314. Philadelphia, W.B. Saunders, 1991.*)

Mechanism of Injury

Cortical Defects

Several authors have implicated bony abnormalities of the femur as a major cause of intraoperative and postoperative periprosthetic fractures.*** These defects can result from the removal of previous fixation devices or cement, or they can occur directly from motion of a loose implant or improper broaching and reaming techniques (Table 10-6). The AAOS Committee on the Hip has published a classification scheme of these abnormalities[155] and has standardized the nomenclature, emphasizing the need for careful preoperative planning in dealing with these defects.

***References 147, 148, 167, 180, 229, 236, 242, 244.

Periprosthetic fractures occurring less than a year after arthroplasty have a high association with surgically generated cortical defects[148,242] (Figs. 10-45 and 10-46). Primary cemented hips are not immune to this risk, with a reported intraoperative femoral perforation rate of up to 2.8% with simple broaching.[226,252] Stress risers are generated whenever a screw is removed from the femur, weakening the bone for at least 4 weeks.[136] Larger defects involving 50% of the cortical width can reduce torsional strength to 44% of the original value,[192] but bypassing such a defect with a cemented stem doubles the bone's strength.[192]

Revision Arthroplasty

Femoral fractures associated with revision arthroplasty were first reported by Charnley[144] and are associated with high morbidity and prolonged convalescence.[145] Some authors have reported either no fractures in their series of revisions[163] or no difference in fracture rates between revision and primary surgery.[241] However, many authors note that a large percentage of their periprosthetic fractures are associated with revision.[134,156,162,250] One study reported a fivefold increase in fractures during revision compared with primary arthroplasty,[167] and other studies have reported a nearly sixfold increase in fractures during uncemented revisions compared with cemented revisions.[211,212] Risk factors specific to revision arthroplasty include penetration of the cortex during cement removal,[185,244] creation of cortical windows for cement removal,[180,251] attempts to dislocate the femur in the face of a scarred joint capsule,[125,180] and sepsis.[198] It also is possible that the trauma of prior surgery to the proximal femur weakens it by disrupting its blood supply or inducing osteoporosis.[124] Previous arthroplasties, osteotomies, and fractures also can alter the geometry of the proximal femur and increase the risk of fracture.[167]

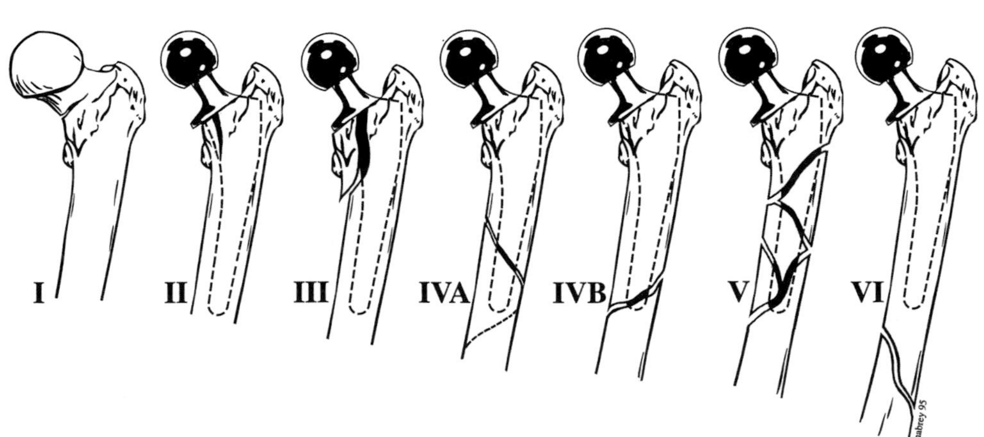

FIGURE 10-44. American Academy of Orthopaedic Surgeons classification of fractures associated with hip arthroplasty. (*Petty, W. (ed.): Total Joint Replacement, pp. 291–314. Philadelphia, W.B. Saunders, 1991.*)

TABLE 10-6
Mechanical Risk Factors Associated With Intraoperative Periprosthetic Fracture

Factor	Precautionary Measures
CORTICAL DEFECT	
Screw hole	Bypass by 2 cortical diameters; allow to remodel
Instrument penetration	Careful orientation of device; adequate operative exposure
Cortical window	Use other removal techniques*; bypass by 2 cortical diameters; cortical strut graft
Osteolysis	Bypass and bone graft
OVERSIZED BROACH/PROSTHESIS	
	Accurate preoperative template silhouetting; intraoperative radiographs; familiarity with technique; cerclage cable or wire
NONANATOMIC FEMUR	
Developmental	Custom broach/prosthesis; extra small broach/prosthesis; osteotomy/shortening; 3-D CT† reconstruction
Osteotomy or fracture	Custom broach/prosthesis; 3-D CT† reconstruction
PERICAPSULAR PATHOLOGY	
Periarticular scarring	Careful capsulectomy
Heterotopic ossification	Careful resection of heterotopic ossification

* Ultrasonic devices, high-speed/low-torque burs, segmental cement extraction devices.
† Three-dimensional computed tomography.

Mismatched Components

Fractures caused by oversized femoral broaches or prostheses are necessarily intraoperative in nature, although they may be detected only on careful review of postoperative radiographs. These fractures have been associated with cemented arthroplasty during the initial reaming for, or seating of, the component,[125,180,242,253] and with malalignment of the broaches.[196] Unusual anatomy can be a significant factor, with Dunn and Hess[177] reporting a 27% intraoperative fracture rate while seating a curved Charnley prosthesis into the relatively narrow, straight femoral shafts of patients with chronically dislocated hips. Charnley[144] has indicated that intraoperative fractures heal in the presence of fresh cement, provided it does not become interposed between the fracture surfaces.

Uncemented femoral stems require initial stability to promote proper osseous integration or bony ingrowth,[137,170,173] and any micromotion between the implant and bone can lead to the formation of fibrous tissue at the interface.[230] Thus, these implants and their broaches and reamers come into intimate contact with cortical bone and may result in increased assembly stresses during insertion that can approach the yield stress of cortical bone.[177] Components that are oversized with respect to the femur create significant assembly strains, or hoop stresses, whereas same-sized components produce only moderate strains.[177] Intraoperative fracture rates for uncemented components vary from 4.2% to 15.2% depending on the type of prosthesis[167]; according to one report,[208] three fourths of these fractures occur during preparation of the femoral canal and the remainder are noted during insertion of the component.

Experience plays a significant role in the successful implantation of these devices. Separate authors report markedly different fracture rates for the same prosthesis,[127,200] whereas others note marked reductions in fracture rates after several hundred procedures or several months of training.[241,245]

Among the latest generation of uncemented femoral components are those that use a milling or tapered reaming technique to prevent hoop stresses in the proximal femur.[139,152,264] A computer-guided milling device has been used in more than 100 human total hip replacements without any adverse events (B. Musits, PhD, personal communication, 1994). This system allows for excellent preoperative planning in complex cases using a variety of total hip prostheses, and it achieves extremely close tolerances at surgery that are not possible with manual techniques. However, the high cost of setting up the system may limit widespread application of this technology.

Pericapsular Pathology

Failure to release adequately a tight or scarred hip capsule also can lead to intraoperative fracture of the femoral neck or shaft during attempts to dislocate the femoral head. This situation can be encountered in cases of primary total hip replacement involving acetabular protrusion, ankylosing spondylitis, prior osteotomy[144] or fracture of the proximal femur, or prior fracture of the acetabulum. Fracture caused by manipulation of the femur during revision arthroplasty has been reported in several series,[145,180,241,242] with the riskiest maneuver being the initial dislocation of the femoral component from the acetabulum. Heterotopic ossification, usually arising from prior trauma, also can make dislocation hazardous.

Loose Components

Loose femoral components are associated with as many as one third to three fourths of periprosthetic fractures in some series.[131,132,156,171,178] In a general

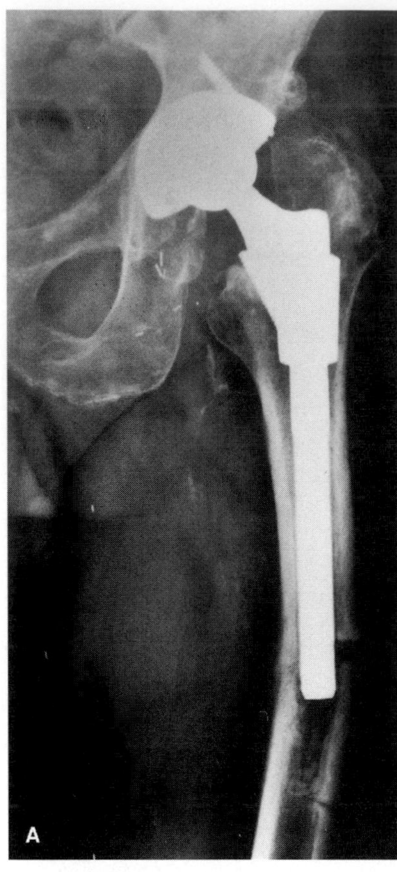

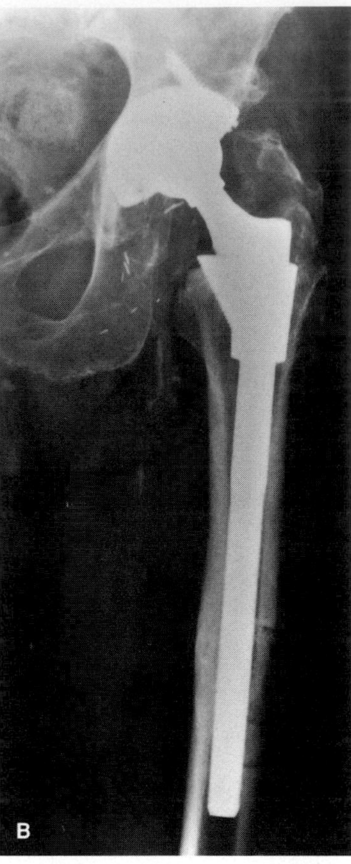

FIGURE 10-45. Radiographs of a 65-year-old man 7 months after revision of a loose cemented femoral component. A cortical window was used during an earlier revision and was clinically healed at the time of revision surgery. The patient had a 4-month history of thigh pain before the fracture. (**A**) American Academy of Orthopaedic Surgeons type IVB fracture at the tip of the modular, uncemented prosthesis. (**B**) Seven months after long-stem revision. The modularity of the prosthesis permitted easy revision by removing the stem component from the proximal fixation collar and replacing it with a long-stem revision. The fluted design of the stem provided excellent rotational control without supplementary fixation. (*Courtesy of Lorence W. Trick, M.D., San Antonio, TX*)

population of patients with total hip replacements, only 0.2% of cemented femoral components were loose at over 11 years of follow-up[153] and only 2% had been revised for loosening at 20 years of follow-up,[240] suggesting that mechanical failure plays a significant role in these fractures. Jensen and colleagues[178] noted that the loose cemented prostheses in their series were more likely to fracture around the proximal femur, whereas the well-fixed cemented components fractured around the tip. One possibility is that a loose component is more likely to transmit stress at relatively few contact points, thus overloading the femur, rather than to distribute the force over the wide contact area afforded a well-fixed component.

Osteoporosis

Mechanical risk factors allow the surgeon some degree of control over intraoperative and postoperative fractures. Osteoporosis is the one constitutional risk factor that is mentioned frequently in association with periprosthetic fracture of the hip and over which the orthopaedist has little control.[126,144,145,194,253] One Swedish group noted that more than half their cases of periprosthetic fracture occurred in patients who had undergone arthroplasty for hip fracture, yet only one in ten primary total hip arthroplasties on their service were performed for hip fracture.[124] This is not surprising, considering that patients with femoral neck fractures have more osteoporosis than do age-matched control subjects.[239]

Osteolysis

Osteolysis rarely is cited as a primary cause of periprosthetic fracture of the hip[148,225] and clinical reviews focusing on osteolysis around total hip implants do not mention fracture as a complication.[177,237] However, osteolytic lesions can leave the cortex dangerously weak and susceptible to intraoperative fracture during manipulation or instrumentation.

FRACTURES OF THE PUBIC RAMUS

The prevalence of fractures of the pubic ramus in association with arthroplasty of the hip is low (0.06%)[202] compared with the rates for femoral fractures. A review of the available case reports[151,193,201,202,218,229] reveals several common factors: (1) just as in the first reports of pubic ramus fractures in military recruits,[243] these patients experienced an unusual increase in ac-

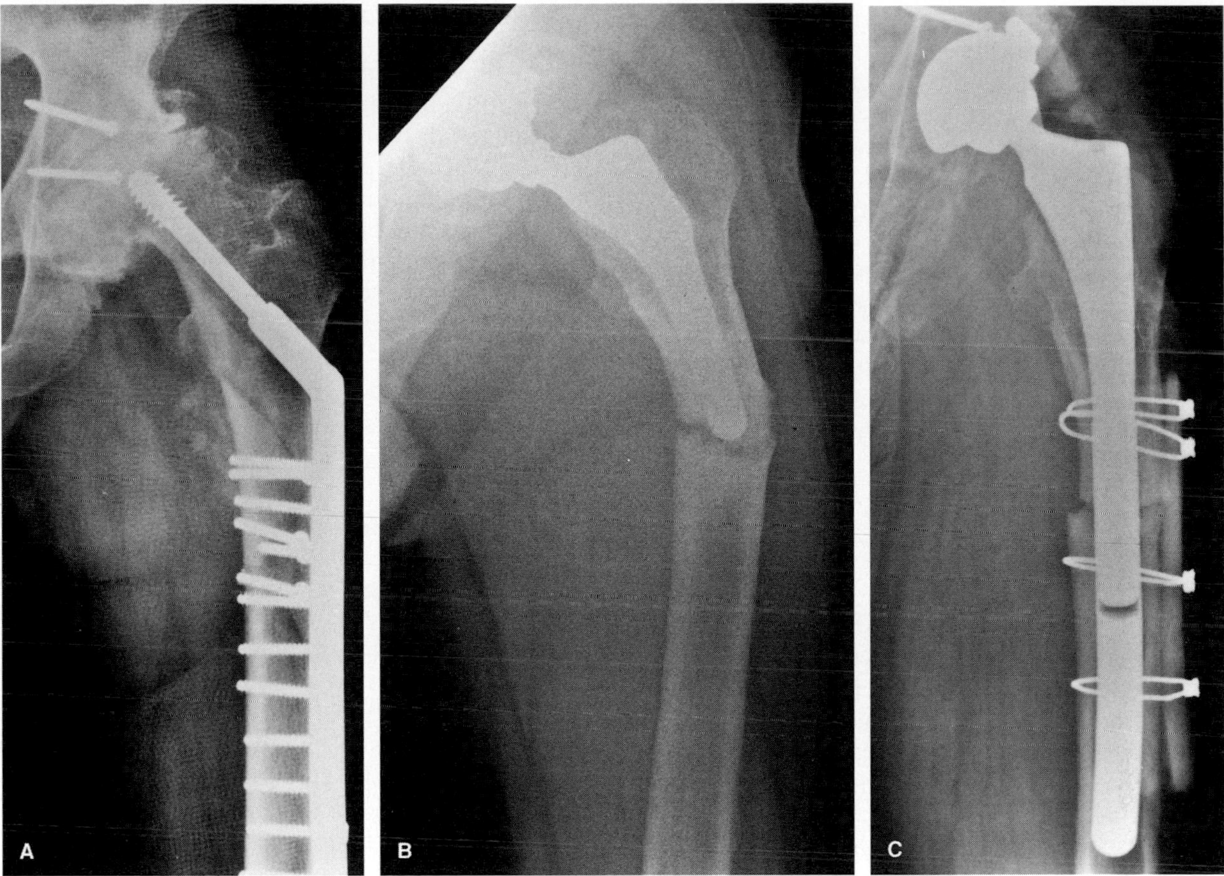

FIGURE 10-46. A 48-year-old man underwent open reduction internal fixation (ORIF) of a comminuted subtrochanteric fracture after a motor vehicle accident. The patient subsequently underwent uncemented total hip arthroplasty and was free of symptoms for 4 years until he noted the acute onset of thigh pain while walking. (**A**) Initial ORIF with sliding hip screw and long side plate. (**B**) American Academy of Orthopaedic Surgeons type IVB fracture through a previous screw hole at the tip of an undersized prosthesis. (**C**) Reduction and stabilization accomplished with revision of the femoral component to a long-stem prosthesis and supplemental extramedullary fixation with cortical strut graft and cerclage cables.

tivity; (2) the fractures often appeared within the first year or so of the arthroplasty; (3) many of the patients had osteoporosis; (4) persistent groin pain was a typical symptom; (5) symptoms in all cases resolved after 4 to 6 weeks of protected weight bearing; and (6) fracture healing often was documented on follow-up radiographs of the pelvis. Bone scan of the pelvis greatly assists in establishing the diagnosis and ruling out infection of the joint.[151]

FRACTURES OF THE ACETABULUM

Periprosthetic fractures of the acetabulum are rare and associated primarily with older metal-on-metal devices such as the McKee-Farrar and Ring prostheses.[169,205,232] Clinical studies report no fractures associated with press-fit acetabular components.[213,238] Laboratory investigations suggest that inadequately reaming the acetabulum by as much as 3 mm less than the component is safe, but that inadequately reaming it by 4 mm leads to some fractures of the pelvis.[154,189] These fractures typically occur during surgery, although they may not be noted until much later. Simple rim fractures should not affect the overall stability of the cup, but an oversized component that splits and distracts the acetabulum can lead to a painful fibrous union.

Laboratory investigations suggest that the most common pattern is a fracture of the peripheral rim of the acetabulum, and that these rim fractures occur only in larger specimens in the range of 56 to 58 mm.[187] Displaced split fractures running from the anterior to the posterior wall are seen only in smaller-sized specimens in the range of 50 to 54 mm. The authors also note that one third of the fractures are visible only on special cup oblique views.[187]

TREATMENT

An assessment of prefracture function is essential to providing the best outcome for each patient. With up to 75% of periprosthetic fracture cases demonstrating evidence of femoral loosening on prefracture radiographs,[131] there is a strong possibility that the joint will require revision in the future. It is possible for the prosthesis to become loose even if the femoral component is stable at the time of fracture stabilization. This is true for both intraoperative fractures[180,242] and those that occur after the primary arthroplasty.[124,131,148]

Although it is unlikely that the acetabulum will be compromised by fracture of the femoral component alone, the surgeon still must determine whether the acetabulum also should be revised for loosening, malposition, or wear. Dislocation is common after revision arthroplasty, and a poorly positioned cup should be revised. The modularity of current acetabular components allows the liner to be replaced without removing the metal shell. If the acetabulum is to be spared but the femoral component revised, it is important to have the proper size of femoral head available to fit the cup.

Nonunion of periprosthetic fractures places an added burden on an already compromised patient, and reoperation frequently is necessary in these cases.[131,141,246,247] Allowing a patient to ambulate with a pseudarthrosis, even if it is not painful, places a constant stress on the remaining components and can result in fracture of the stem.[244] Delayed union not only prolongs the patient's convalescence,[148,265] but also can result in fatigue failure of the component.[131]

Proximal fractures that are stable and incomplete are almost certain to heal,[241] and fractures that are stabilized by a well-fixed prosthesis also have a high union rate.[131,148,180] Fractures distal to the tip of the prosthesis, however, are inherently unstable and have a high nonunion rate when treated without surgery.[131]

Nonoperative Techniques

Indications

Absolute indications for the nonoperative management of periprosthetic fractures of the hip are few and simple. Stress fractures of the pubic ramus, as noted earlier, invariably heal without complication.[151,193,201,218] Incomplete, proximal, longitudinal split fractures (AAOS type II) that occur early after surgery, or that were missed during surgery, do not require operative fixation[241] but should be observed carefully. Relative indications include patients who are at high risk for surgical procedures and fractures that can be maintained readily with either casting or traction[148,180,229] or those in which the prosthesis provides significant stability.[180]

Observation or Protected Weight Bearing

Observation or protected weight bearing should be reserved for stable, incomplete, proximal split fractures (AAOS type II) that are identified either during surgery or soon thereafter.[124,200,241,242,265] A prosthesis that relies on distal fixation for stability is less likely to require intraoperative stabilization of a proximal split than is one that relies on proximal fit and fill.[241] Little change in the postoperative management of these cases is necessary because many protocols for uncemented devices already call for 4 to 8 weeks of protected weight bearing.

Traction

Contemplation of traction management should carry the same weight as the decision to operate. Treatment can last from 9 weeks to 4 months,[124,168,253] with the added risk that prolonged bed rest can result in increased mortality and still not prevent surgery.[171] In one series, nearly one third of the patients treated with traction required subsequent operative correction for malalignment of the fracture.[124] In other series, patients treated with traction have had to undergo revision to long-stem femoral components.[217,227] Complications associated with this modality include refracture,[168] decubitus ulcers,[174] gangrene,[124] and death.[124,174,265] Conversely, traction may be the only option in medically unstable patients (Fig. 10-47).

Certain fracture patterns around prostheses have slightly better results. Long oblique fractures[125] and fractures associated with well-fixed stems[179] fare better than do those around loose stems[179] or those located at or distal to the tip of the prosthesis.[174]

Skin traction can be used as temporary stabilization while awaiting surgery or casting, but pin traction should be considered for long-term management of unstable fractures. Careful consideration should be given to pin placement around the knee because a knee arthroplasty may be present as well and placement of a femoral pin may contaminate the femur for future procedures. The orthopaedist should consider the use of air-supported mattresses as an essential component of this technique for the prevention of decubitus ulcers.

Casting or Bracing

Casting and bracing of periprosthetic femoral fractures have been used both as adjuncts to traction and as primary modes of treatment. Preliminary traction for 4 to 7 weeks can be followed by the application of either a long leg cast[124] or a hip spica cast.[265] Primary

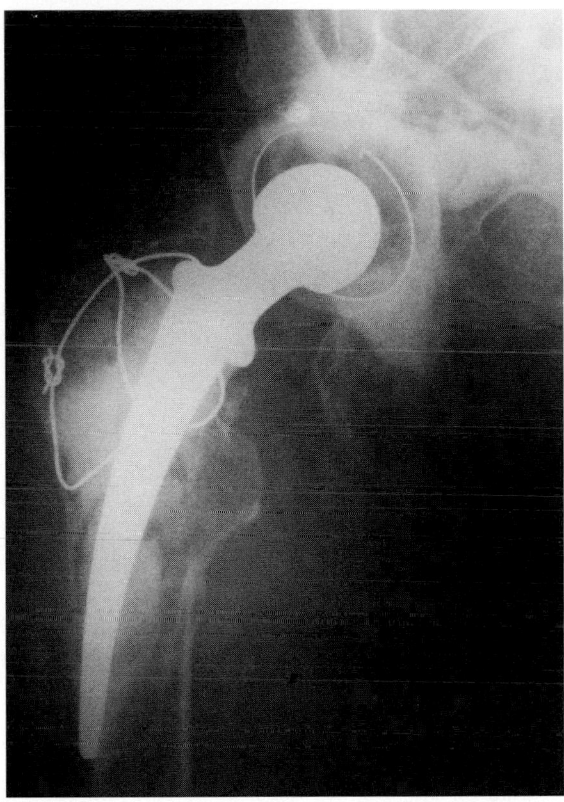

FIGURE 10-47. A 65-year-old man with ankylosing spondylitis and multiple joint replacements was severely injured in a motor vehicle accident, sustaining multiple fractures, including this type V periprosthetic fracture of the proximal femur and an ipsilateral type V periprosthetic fracture of the knee (see Fig. 10-58). He was treated initially with skin traction because of his tenuous medical status. (*Courtesy of James D. Heckman, M.D., San Antonio, TX*)

spica cast treatment works better with fractures that are minimally displaced and easily controlled.[159,241]

Operative Techniques

Indications

Intraoperative fractures are an absolute indication for the operative management of periprosthetic fractures around the femur, and may call for nothing more than a single cerclage wire. Unless there are other, more pressing circumstances, there is no better time to stabilize the femur than during the initial exposure. Strong relative indications for operative management of postoperative fractures include loose or fractured prostheses,[131,148,178] malalignment of the fracture,[124] and fractures distal to the stem tip.[131,180,267]

Intramedullary Techniques

Flexible intramedullary devices have been used successfully to treat fractures primarily around uncemented hemiarthroplasties,[146,188,222] but they also have been used in more distal fractures around cemented total hip prostheses.[188,197] Küntscher nails have been inserted antegrade around both cemented hips[125] and uncemented hemiarthroplasties.[135] In addition, rigid nails have been used as extensions of standard total hips when longer revision components were not immediately available.[197,219,220,266] This experience led Luck and colleagues[196] to suggest the development of modular stems for hip prostheses as early as 1972.

Long-stem femoral revisions account for a significant percentage of the operative treatment in several studies.[†††] In most cases, long-stem revision is used as a primary mode of treatment, but in some cases, it is used after more conservative modalities have failed.[217,227] Some authors consider revision arthroplasty to be the treatment of choice for periprosthetic fractures if the femoral component is loose[178] and the length of hospitalization is considerably shorter than with traction management[168]; however, problems with healing may require reoperation with bone grafting.[124] When these longer stems are inserted, it is important to bypass any cortical defects by at least two cortical widths to decrease stress concentrations[204] (see Fig. 10-46).

Fluted or "ribbed" stems add significant rotational control to the distal fragment and their success has been well documented in the European literature.[235,260,262,268,269] These devices eliminate the need for extramedullary stabilization in many cases. Modular, ribbed stem designs allow the insertion of a longer stem to bypass fracture sites while maintaining the integrity of a proximal fixation collar (L.W. Trick, MD, personal communication, 1994; see Fig. 10-45).

Proximal femoral replacement has been used in cases where simple revision arthroplasty was not stable enough, either for acute fractures[233,246,255] or for cases of chronic nonunion around prostheses.[246] Although the Harris Hip Scores for one series of patients undergoing proximal femoral replacement averaged 91 after surgery,[246] leg-length discrepancies ranged from 1.5 cm long to 2.5 cm short on the affected side and half the patients had moderate to marked abductor weakness.[246]

Extramedullary Techniques

Stabilization of periprosthetic fractures with metal plates allows accurate reduction and early mobilization.[244] Plate fixation around hip arthroplasty owes its popularity to the ready availability of the materials and the nearly universal familiarity of orthopaedic sur-

†††References 125, 156, 168, 171, 179, 217, 227, 253, 255, 265.

geons with the technique. Success with this modality has been reported in several series,[244,247,265,267] with union rates as high as 100%.[244] Loss of cortical bone beneath broad cerclage bands has interfered with bridging callus and led to refracture in one series.[181] Narrow cerclage cables do not appear to have this problem and are widely available.

Plate fixation is particularly useful in fractures distal to the tip of the prosthesis (AAOS type VI).[132,145] An excellent review of the subject by Serocki and colleagues[244] recommends using a broad AO dynamic compression plate with at least eight cortices of fixation on each side of the fracture. Screws occasionally need to be angled more than the 7° to 25° allowed by the AO plates to avoid the stem, leaving the screw heads incompletely seated.[244] After surgery, some authors recommend 3 months of no weight bearing followed by another 6 months of progressive weight bearing.

Cortical allograft struts also have proven successful in periprosthetic fractures[140–142,228] (Fig. 10-48*C*). Chandler and colleagues[141] reported on a series of fractures around or below well-fixed femoral components. Nearly 90% of the fractures united and the patients returned to their preinjury status within less than 5 months.[121] The fractures first are reduced and temporarily stabilized with cerclage wires (Fig. 10-49). Two equal struts of fresh frozen femoral shaft allograft from an ipsilateral femur then are contoured to fit with a high-speed bur and are held to the host with 2-mm cerclage cables at 4-cm intervals. Autograft from the pelvis always is added to the fracture site.[141] The average hospital stay is only 12 days.

Advantages of this technique include the ability to customize the graft to any femur and the low modulus of elasticity of the graft.[20] Experimental studies have shown that stiffer plates lead to a significant reduction in bone mass under the plate compared with more flexible plates.[215] In addition, the cortical plate may even stimulate healing of the periprosthetic fracture.[199] Disadvantages include the cost of the allograft as well as the possibility of disease transmission.[254] Finally, if

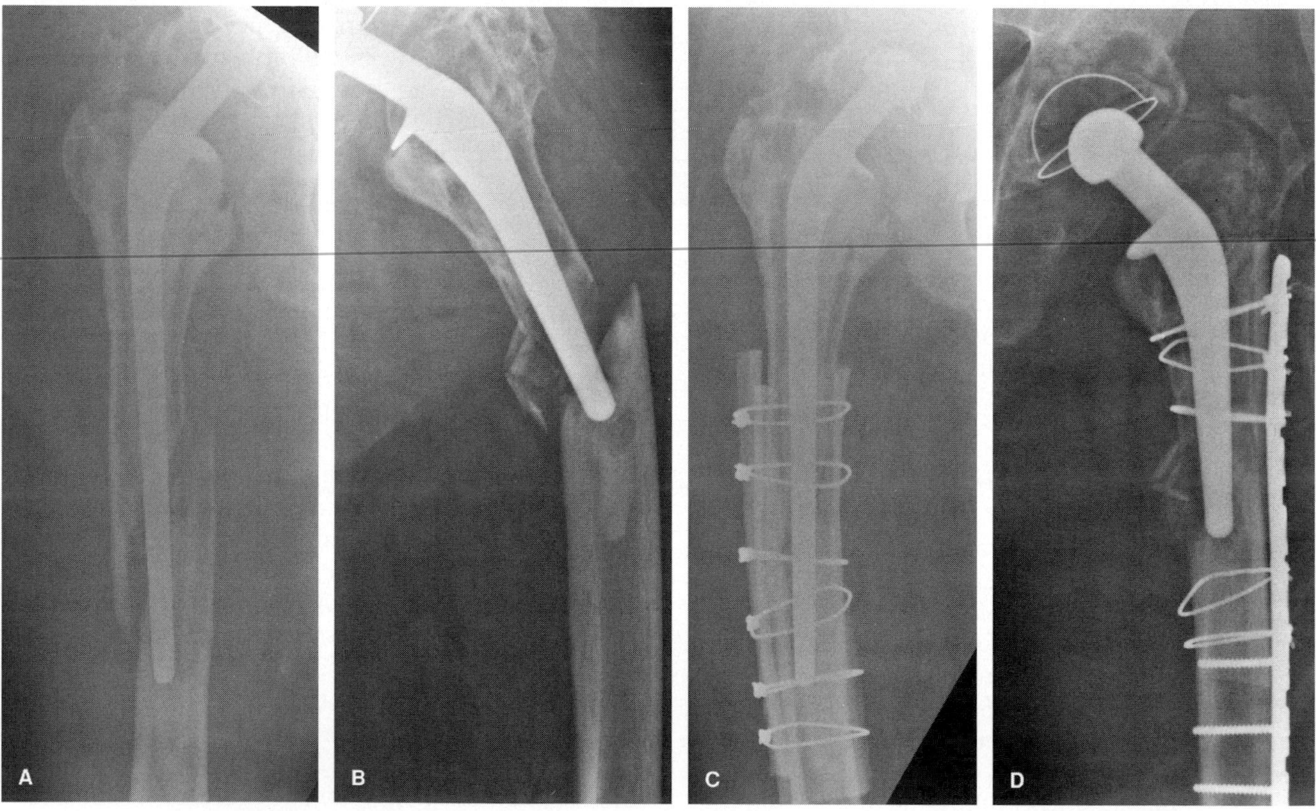

FIGURE 10-48. A 72-year-old former Canadian hockey player, with four-vessel coronary artery disease, fell on New Year's Day, sustaining bilateral periprosthetic femoral fractures. Full revision of both components at the time of injury was considered too risky given his cardiac history. (**A**) American Academy of Orthopaedic Surgeons (AAOS) type IVA fracture around a loose cemented long-stem revision on the right. (**B**) AAOS type V fracture at the tip of a loose, cemented, primary total hip on the left. (**C**) Reduction and stabilization of the right femur with contoured cortical struts and cerclage cables. (**D**) Reduction and stabilization of the left femur with a medial cortical allograft strut, cerclage cables, and a lateral plate. Stabilization of both fractures allowed early mobilization of the patient.

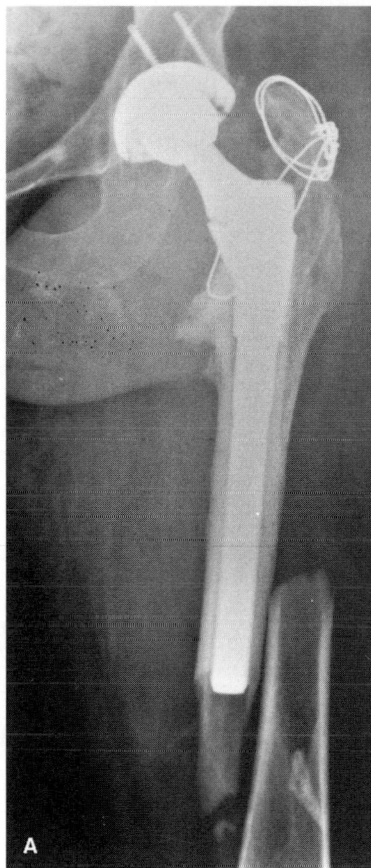

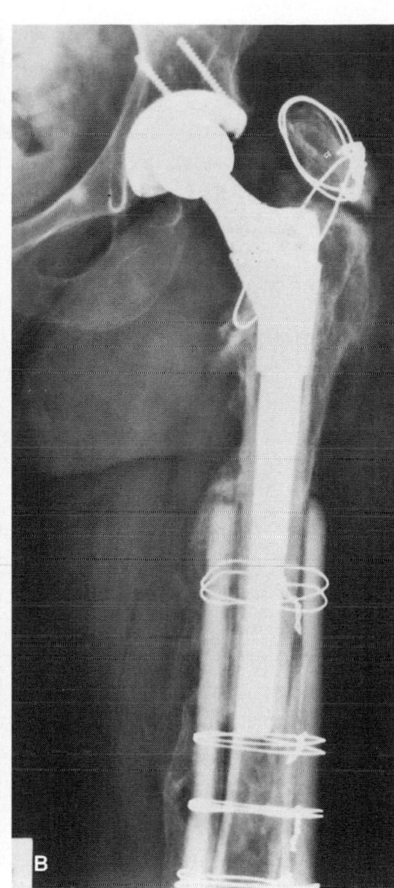

FIGURE 10-49. A 64-year-old woman noted sudden pain in the thigh while transferring from bed to chair 2 weeks after revision for an infected total hip arthroplasty. (**A**) American Academy of Orthopaedic Surgeons type IVB fracture at the tip of an uncemented modular component. (**B**) Reduction and stabilization with cortical struts and cerclage wire 7 months after revision. The patient is ambulatory and free of pain. Note bony incorporation of strut grafts and rounding of proximal edges. (*Courtesy of Lorence W. Trick, M.D., San Antonio, TX*)

there is any delay in healing, the struts can fail because they become weaker by 4 to 6 months as they incorporate into the fracture site.[248]

Combined Techniques

Several authors report success using a combination of techniques, usually a long-stem prosthesis in conjunction with cerclage fixation alone or with plates.[‡‡‡] In Johansson's series,[180] the six fractures treated with long-stem revision and either cerclage fixation or dynamic compression plating all did well, whereas only one of five of the periprosthetic fractures treated with a long-stem revision alone had a satisfactory result. Long oblique fractures treated with long-stem revision are more readily stabilized with cerclage fixation than are transverse fractures, which offer little purchase. In this situation, the addition of an extramedullary cortical strut provides additional rotational stability (see Fig. 10-46C).

Complications

Reported complications associated with operative treatment of these fractures include infection,[141,149,180] malunion,[180,259] nonunion,[141,180,247] and subsequent loosening of the prosthesis.[146,147,180] However, it is helpful to consider the usual complications associated with operating on failed total hip arthroplasties when evaluating the relative risks of surgical management of these fractures.

‡‡‡References 125, 131, 156, 168, 178, 180, 220, 242, 265.

Special Considerations

Infected Fractures

Infection has been implicated as a contributory factor in postoperative periprosthetic fractures,[148,205] in addition to being associated with intraoperative fractures occurring during revision for sepsis.[145,198] During an infected revision, the hip should be debrided of all old cement and reactive tissue, and the prosthesis should not be replaced, although it may be necessary to stabilize the fracture with internal fixation.[145] The patient then is treated in traction and with antibiotics based on culture results. A delayed reimplantation is performed at a time based on the individual surgeon's protocol.

Fractures Around Total Hip and Total Knee Combinations

Ipsilateral total hip and total knee replacements are common in patients with multiple joint involvement, such as rheumatoid arthritis. If the femoral component of the knee replacement uses an intramedullary stem (eg, Guepar, rotating hinge, modular revision stem), there is a greater concentration of stress between the tips of the hip and knee components.[149] Extramedullary fixation, with either a dynamic compression plate[149] or cortical struts, is indicated.

Bilateral Periprosthetic Fractures

Simultaneous fracture of both femora places great stress on patients in terms of blood loss, pain, and mobilization. Zuber and associates[268] reported on one case of bilateral fracture that was treated by bilateral proximal femoral replacements staged 4 days apart. This was followed by 8 weeks in a rehabilitation hospital. In the case presented in Figure 10-48, parts A through D, the plan was to mobilize the patient by stabilizing both fractures and then to revise each hip separately once the fractures had healed. The patient was transferred back to his home country before this could occur. Overall, it may be best to perform the definitive procedure on each hip separately, even if this means a delay of 1 or 2 weeks between procedures.

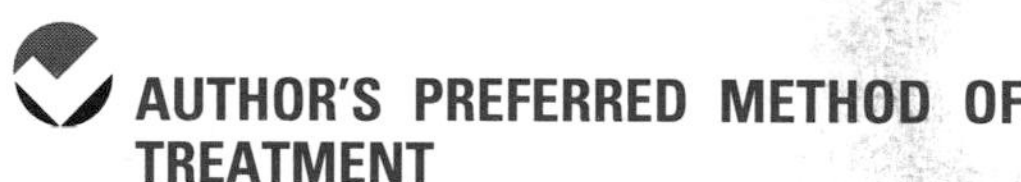

AUTHOR'S PREFERRED METHOD OF TREATMENT

Proximal Region (AAOS Level I)

Intraoperative fractures in the proximal femur are readily identified during the procedure and should be dealt with at that time. They usually are a result of using press-fit or porous ingrowth components with tight tolerances. Components that rely on an extensive porous coating and distal incorporation are reported to be stable in this situation,[241] especially with a simple vertical split, but all other noncemented components can be expected to increase the hoop stresses around the proximal femur under load and should be stabilized with a cerclage wire or cable. Cemented cases should be stabilized with wire or cable before cement injection, primarily to prevent extravasation of cement into the fracture. For stable patterns, the postoperative regimen consists of protected weight bearing while monitoring prosthesis position on radiographs.

Immediate postoperative fractures in this region usually are actually intraoperative fractures that were missed. Treatment of stable patterns involves protected weight bearing and careful observation. If the prosthesis remains loose and symptomatic, it can be revised once the fracture has healed.

Long-term postoperative fractures usually are the result of a stress riser or osteoporosis. These fractures are treated with revision of the component and may benefit from a head and neck replacement prosthesis.

Middle Region (AAOS Level II)

Fractures in the middle region often are associated with either a previous stress riser or a loose prosthesis. Intraoperative fractures typically occur during revision surgery and are treated with a long-stem prosthesis that bypasses the cortical defect by two cortical diameters.

Postoperative fractures can be associated with either a loose stem or a well-fixed component. The femoral component is revised to a long stem if it is loose and may require supplemental extramedullary fixation. Well-fixed stems can be retained, especially if they provide some stability, and extramedullary stabilization is achieved with either cortical allograft or metal plates. With a variety of cerclage systems available based on aircraft cable or wire, the surgeon should not have to rely on broad-banded systems for fixation.

Distal Region (AAOS Level III)

As noted earlier, the nonunion rate for fractures in the distal region is high.[131,180,267] If the component is well fixed, consideration is given to extramedullary stabilization alone, and if it is loose, the femoral component is revised.

Combination Fractures

Fractures involving the proximal and middle regions offer little support to the new component and warrant consideration of either a proximal femoral replacement or a long-stem component in a proximal femoral allograft. An alternative is to stabilize the femur with a contoured, split, ipsilateral femoral allograft.[142]

PERIPROSTHETIC FRACTURES OF THE KNEE

INTRODUCTION

The first report of periprosthetic fracture of a total knee arthroplasty did not appear until 1977,[317] nearly a quarter century after it had been reported around the hip.[270] However, the number of these cases should rise quickly, given that implantation of total knee arthroplasties increased at three times the annual rate of total hip arthroplasties between 1985 and 1989.[312] In 1988, there was a cumulative total of 521,000 artificial knees in the United States,[308] 69% of which were in patients 65 years of age and older.[308] In 1989, in Medicare patients alone, 80,647 primary total knee arthroplasties were performed along with an additional 6127 revision arthroplasties.[312]

INCIDENCE

Combining the results of five series[271,282,285,318,332] with a total of 2178 patients, the overall prevalence of periprosthetic knee fractures is 1.2%, although some series report rates as high as 5.6% associated with revision cases.[278] Periprosthetic knee fractures have been reported to occur anytime from during surgery to up to 10 years afterward,[275,306] and most result from minimal trauma.[281,282,292,320,326,327] Manipulation of total knee prostheses under anesthesia to improve range of motion also has led to periprosthetic fractures.[281,327] Cases resulting from motor vehicle accidents or other violent force are more difficult to treat, especially when they are bilateral.[290]

Unlike total hip prostheses, the basic design of the bone–implant interface in total knee prostheses has not changed significantly over the years. Most current total knee arthroplasties are simple resurfacings that require no more than five planar saw cuts on the distal femur. Moreover, the line-to-line fit of the original cemented implants changed little during the rush toward porous ingrowth technology. Thus, principles derived from initial designs are readily applicable to today's uncemented prostheses as well.

Fractures of the patella after total knee arthroplasty can occur in both resurfaced and unresurfaced patellae, but are more common after resurfacing.[287] The prevalence of these fractures ranges from 0.1% to 8.5%.[§§§]

CLASSIFICATION

The first formal grouping of periprosthetic knee fractures was suggested by Sisto and colleagues,[327] who classified their cases as nondisplaced, displaced, and displaced-comminuted. The next year, Merkel and Johnson[306] proposed classifying their series of fractures according to the system described by Neer and colleagues[309] for supracondylar fractures of the femur (Fig. 10-50).

The modified Neer classification of periprosthetic fractures by which many authors classify their cases consists of three groups: type I fractures are extraarticular and nondisplaced, with less than 5 mm of translation and less than 5° of angulation in any plane; type II fractures are extraarticular, with displacement of greater than 5 mm or 5° of angulation (Fig. 10-51); and type III fractures are severely comminuted, with loss of cortical contact and often significant angulation[283,285,328] (Fig. 10-52). Neer and colleagues[309] originally applied the classification only to fractures within 7.5 cm of the joint line, but later studies extend the limit to 15 cm.[283,322]

My experience with a rising number of knee revisions suggests two additions to the modified Neer classification system (Table 10-7; see Fig. 10-50). First, the modular intramedullary stems that frequently are used in total knee revisions transfer stresses into the diaphyseal region just as the one-piece Guepar stem once did. Fracture of the femur at the tip of this stem is referred to as a type IV fracture, much like the AAOS type IV fracture of the hip. Moreover, the problems encoun-

[§§§]References 274, 277, 287, 294, 313, 319, 323.

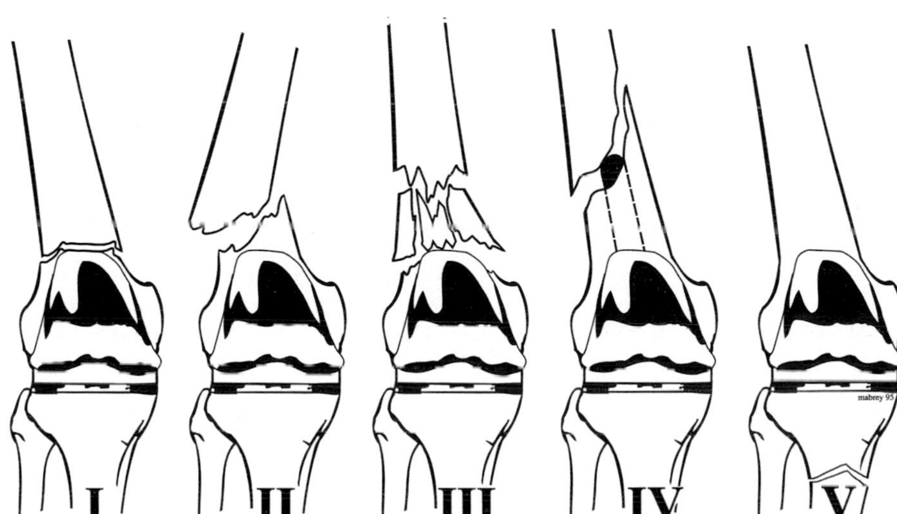

FIGURE 10-50. Classification scheme for periprosthetic fracture of the knee. (I, II, and III after Neer[309] and Merkel.[306])

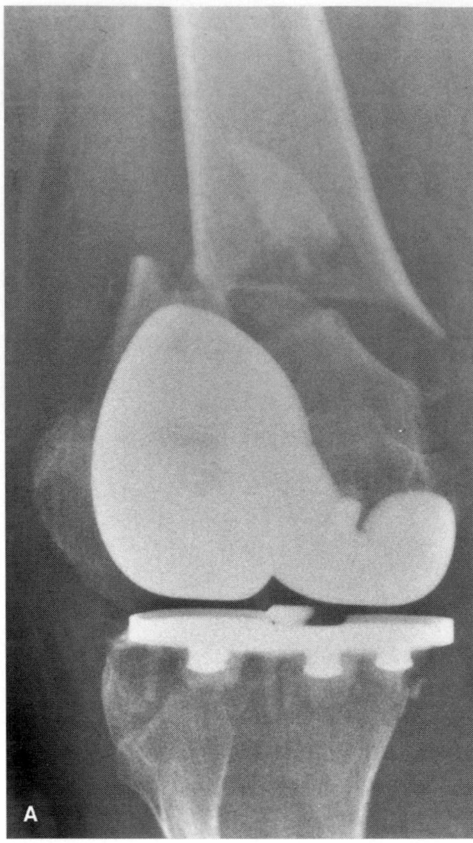

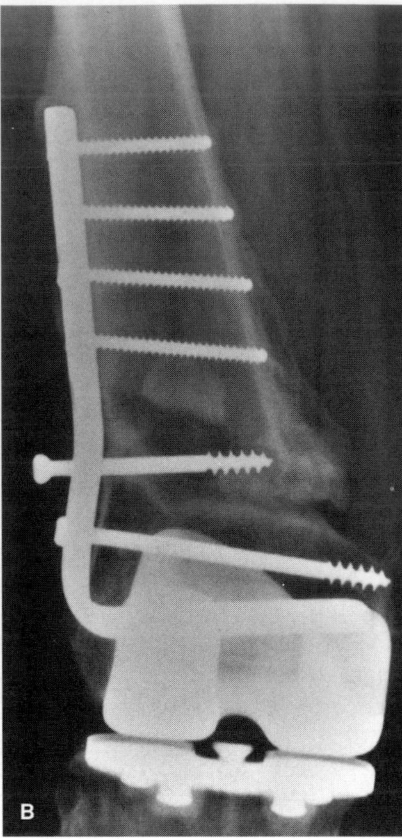

FIGURE 10-51. A 54-year-old man sustained this injury after a minor fall. (**A**) A type II fracture is seen around a well-fixed, cemented, posterior cruciate ligament (PCL)-sparing prosthesis. (**B**) The patient initially underwent ORIF of the fracture with blade plate fixation. Iliac crest bone grafting of the fracture site was performed 8 months later for nonunion. Although the fracture has healed in valgus orientation, the patient is asymptomatic and has regained preinjury function. (*Courtesy of Ronald P. Williams, Ph.D., M.D., San Antonio, TX*)

tered in the fixation of these fractures are similar to those encountered in the treatment of periprosthetic fractures of the hip. Also included in the type IV category are fractures of the femoral diaphysis that do not involve the prosthesis, similar to the AAOS type V fracture or Johansson's type III fracture. The second additional category for periprosthetic fractures of the knee includes any total knee arthroplasty with a fracture of the proximal tibia (Fig. 10-53). These are classified as type V fractures.

Goldberg and colleagues[286] proposed a five-part classification system for patellar fractures in which type I fractures have no involvement of the implant–cement composite or the extensor mechanism; type II fractures do involve the implant-cement composite or the extensor mechanism; type III fractures are inferior pole fractures, with subtype IIIA associated with patellar ligament rupture and subtype IIIB not associated with rupture; and type IV fractures are fracture dislocations of the patella.

FRACTURES OF THE FEMUR

Mechanism of Injury

Bony Defects

Surgical infringement on the anterior distal femoral cortex,[271] or notching, has been implicated as a major cause of supracondylar fracture of the femur after total knee arthroplasty.[‖‖] The incidence of fracture associated with notching is around 40% in some series[271,285] and less than 1% in others.[318]

As noted in the radiographs in Figure 10-54, several trabeculae take their origin from the progressively tapering anterior cortex. Resection of this bone to accommodate the patellar flange of the femoral component poses the risk of cutting too deep and interrupting the transfer of stress from the metaphysis to the diaphysis.[271] Anterior referencing guides will prevent this from occurring unless the intramedullary guide rod is angled too far posteriorly.

Culp and colleagues[281] calculated the effect on torsional strength of the distal femur in relation to the thickness of anterior cortex removed. Reductions in the polar moment of inertia for this region were 23.8% for a 1.5-mm loss of cortex and 29.2% for a 3-mm loss.[281]

In line with the problem of cortical defects, one study found that two of the three men in their series of periprosthetic fractures had no other risk factors for fracture except for having had a healed supracondylar fracture before their initial total knee arthroplasty.[306] The same series reported a nearly threefold increase (0.6% versus 1.6%) in the inci-

[‖‖]References 271, 275, 281, 285, 306, 307, 310.

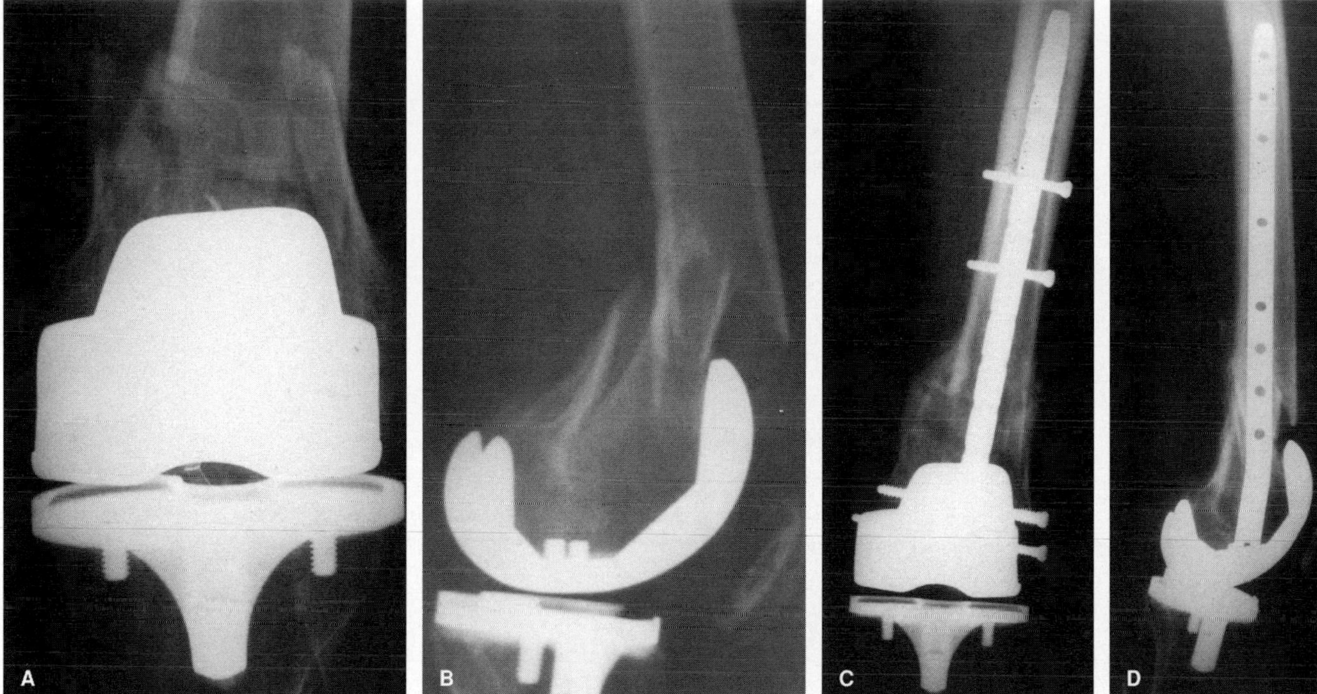

FIGURE 10-52. A 72-year-old man fell down two steps. Anteroposterior (**A**) and lateral (**B**) radiographs of a type III, comminuted periprosthetic fracture around an uncemented femoral component. The bone-prosthesis interface is intact. Anteroposterior (**C**) and lateral (**D**) radiographs 1 year after retrograde, interlocked, intramedullary nailing. The fracture has healed and the patient remains free of symptoms with a 10° flexion contracture and 110° of flexion. (*Smith, W., Mabrey, J.D., Martin, S.L.: Use of a Supracondylar Nail for Treatment of a Supracondylar Fracture of the Femur Following Total Knee Arthroplasty: A Case Report. J. Arthroplasty, in press.*)

dence of periprosthetic supracondylar fractures in patients with previous total knee arthroplasty.[306] Twenty-five percent of the patients in another series of fractures had undergone a revision arthroplasty before their periprosthetic femur fracture.[275] This may have been due in part to residual cortical defects from the earlier procedures, as well as disruption of the epiphyseal and intramedullary blood supply to the distal femur.[316]

Osteolysis, whether from polyethylene[314] or titanium (P. Jacobs and J.D. Mabrey, unpublished data, 1995) wear debris, renders the distal femur susceptible to fracture. Polyethylene liners of the appropriate thickness and the judicious use of metal-backed patellae reduce the risk.

TABLE 10-7
Classification of Periprosthetic Fractures of the Knee (see Table 10-6 for Criteria for Acceptable Alignment)

Type I	Minimally displaced supracondylar fracture
Type II	Displaced supracondylar fracture
Type III	Comminuted supracondylar fracture
Type IV	Fracture at the tip of the femoral prosthetic stem or fracture of the femoral diaphysis above the prosthesis
Type V	Any fracture of the tibia

Osteopenia

Several studies implicate osteopenia as a major contributing factor to periprosthetic fractures in total knee arthroplasty.[271,275,281,291,306] With women being at much greater risk for osteoporosis than men,[272] it is not surprising that between 75% and 100% of the patients in these series are female.[281,291,292,311] Patients with rheumatoid arthritis,[271,273,275,292,311] especially those taking corticosteroids,[275,306,310] are at increased risk for fracture. Women dominate these groups as well because they are 2 to 3 times more likely to have rheumatoid arthritis than are men.[336]

Implant Design

Several aspects of total knee implant design contribute to periprosthetic fractures. Resurfacing the distal femur with a cobalt chrome shell renders the composite

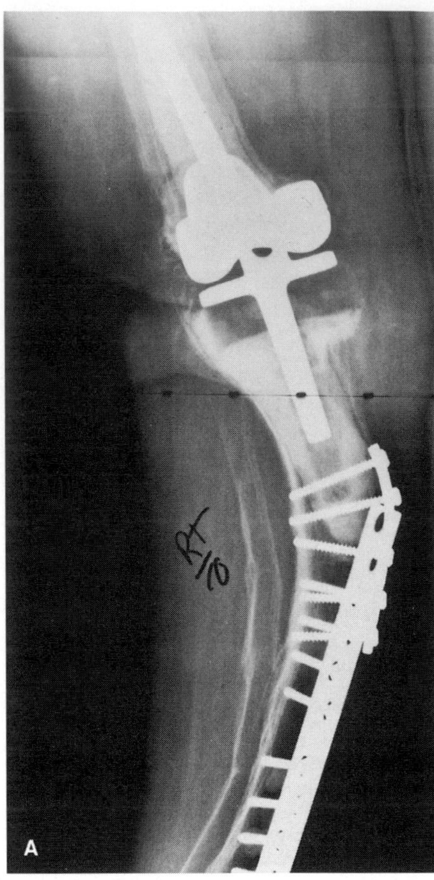
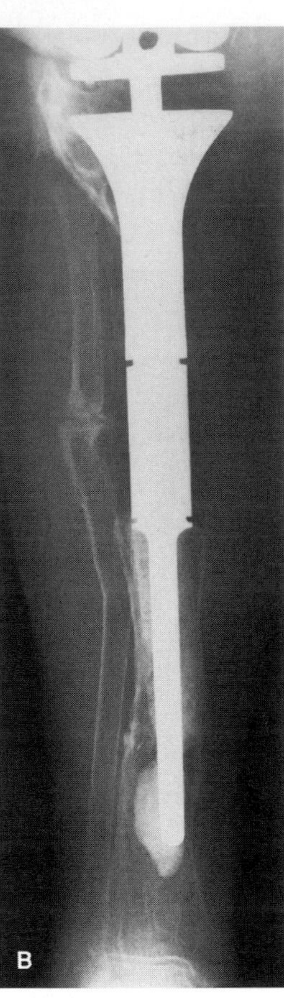

FIGURE 10-53. A 68-year-old woman with severe rheumatoid arthritis underwent a fourth knee revision with a constrained rotating hinge. (**A**) A type V fracture at the tip of the cement mantle was treated initially with 4.5-mm and 3.5-mm compression plates, with subsequent failure of the 3.5-mm plate. (**B**) The tibial component was removed, leaving a proximal shell of bone, and was replaced with an oncology management prosthesis.

structure stiffer and concentrates stress at the junction of the metaphysis and the femoral component.[273] This is the same area where notching is most likely to occur, as well as the site of origin of major metaphyseal trabeculae.

Rotational forces also are more likely to be transmitted directly to the femur through constrained or semiconstrained components.[281,310,329] Hinged devices, which make up 10% to 25% of some series,[281,310] are extremely rigid and transmit high loads to the implant–cement–bone junction instead of relying on the patient's ligaments to absorb some of the energy.[329]

Total knee arthroplasties that incorporate intramedullary stems, especially those that are cemented along their length, concentrate torsional and bending forces at the tip of that stem. Several stemmed total knee implants, such as the Waldius,[307] Guepar,[275,282,296,321] variable axis,[326,332] Gschwend-Scheier-Bähler,[288] and spherocentric,[278,329] have been associated with fractures at the tip of the femoral stem. Although most of these prostheses are no longer in use, current modular designs allow the addition of a variety of stem lengths and diameters to both the tibial and femoral components.

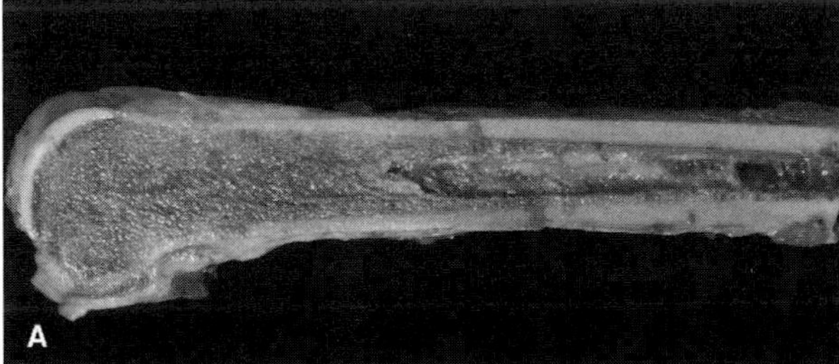
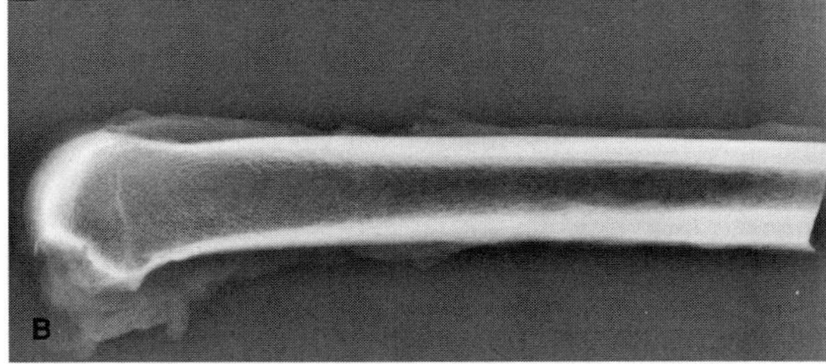

FIGURE 10-54. Sagittal section of the distal femur centered on the patellar trochlea. (**A**) Photograph demonstrating the abrupt drop-off of cancellous bone within the medullary canal. (**B**) Radiograph of adjacent slice demonstrating the gradual tapering of the anterior femoral cortex in the patellar trochlea. Note the origin of the anterior femoral trabeculae from the thin anterior cortex. The anterior cut for the patellar flange of the prosthesis terminates at this site. (*Courtesy of Christopher K. Hersh, M.D., San Antonio, TX*)

Neurologic Disorders

Culp and colleagues[281] noted that more than one third of the patients in their series had a preexisting neurologic disorder such as seizures, cerebral ataxia, or Parkinson's disease. These patients may have been predisposed to fracture secondary to disuse osteoporosis,[281] ataxic gait,[281,290] or osteoporosis resulting from prolonged phenytoin (Dilantin) use. Abnormalities in gait could subject the bone–implant interface to higher stresses or lead to an increased incidence of falls.

Ipsilateral Hip Arthroplasty

The mean energy absorption (**E**) of the femur before fracture in torsion is 35 J.[302] The addition of a total hip arthroplasty to the same side as a total knee prosthesis can increase the torsional rigidity of the femur and reduce the value of **E** in torsion,[282] resulting in fracture between the two components. The few cases reported list additional risk factors, including rheumatoid arthritis,[320] femoral total knee components with intramedullary stems,[280] and osteoporosis.[282]

TREATMENT

Maintenance of joint function and range of motion can be challenging even during primary total knee arthroplasty. With periprosthetic fractures, the orthopaedist must balance these goals against the added problem of achieving bony union. Proper alignment of components during primary knee arthroplasty is important for a good clinical result,[293,301] a maxim that also holds true for the treatment of periprosthetic fractures,[275] regardless of technique.

Nonoperative Techniques

Initial treatment of these fractures with traction has been reported in several series.[###] Typically, 2 to 8 weeks of pin traction is followed by casting or cast bracing,[285,306] or even by supplemental internal fixation and then cast bracing.[329]

Neer and colleagues,[309] after treating most of their nonprosthetic supracondylar femur fractures with traction, reported that the most common deformities were varus and internal rotation. Malunions in varus or valgus orientation are common with this technique.[273,279,285,327] In Figgie's series,[285] seven of ten fractures treated with traction followed by casting healed with the femoral component in an average of 7° of varus orientation relative to the long axis of the femur. Of particular note is that four of those seven knees developed new and progressive lucent lines around the tibial components on follow-up radiographs.[285] Overall, these patients lost 19° of motion and 13 points on their knee scores.[285] In the same series, the operative patients lost 15° of motion and 22 points on their knee scores.

Casting as an initial mode of treatment is most effective in minimally displaced fractures.[273,281,306,310,327] Culp and colleagues[281] reported a loss of 26° of motion with this technique compared with a loss of 12° in patients treated with traction followed by casting.

External Fixation

External fixation of periprosthetic fractures of the knee has been reported in a total of five cases, with mixed results.[281,285,306] One became infected and was converted to a fusion[285] and the others were reported to have either good or excellent results.[306] In the future, thin wire fixators hybridized with half-pin devices may prove useful in specific cases.

Operative Techniques

Internal Fixation

Open reduction and internal fixation of periprosthetic knee fractures is particularly challenging because of the proximity of the prosthesis to the cement mantle, as well as the lack of intramedullary support. Fixation is compromised further by the fact that many of these patients have osteoporosis and some also have rheumatoid arthritis being treated with corticosteroids. Reduction is maintained best by some type of rigid internal fixation.

Healy and colleagues[291] reported a series of 20 cases treated successfully with open reduction and internal fixation through a lateral approach, and noted that bone grafting the fracture site was a key factor in their success. On average, the patients maintained their prefracture knee scores. The authors preferred using the blade plate over the condylar screw plate because it removed less bone and provided better rotational control of the distal fragment.[291] However, they noted that placement of the blade between the anterior femoral flange and the condylar lugs could be a tight fit. Blade plates also have been used in several other series[285,292,327] and at my institution (see Fig. 10-51) with generally good results. Another reported option is fixation with buttress plates or dynamic compression plates.[****]

[###]References 273, 275, 279, 281, 282, 285, 292, 306, 311, 326, 327, 332.

[****]References 273, 275, 279, 281, 285, 306, 310, 317, 326, 332, 335.

Experience with intramedullary fixation of these fractures is limited but effective (Fig. 10-55). One series reported good results in three cases treated with an antegrade interlocking nail in which the fracture was at least 8 cm from the joint line.[290] Another group used a Huckstep intramedullary nail to engage the tip of a stemmed femoral component.[325] Retrograde nailing of certain fractures also is effective,[295,304,328] but the surgeon must check to ensure clearance of the device with the femoral component. The intercondylar distance of commonly used knee arthroplasties ranges from 12 to 20 mm,[295] whereas available supracondylar nails are available in diameters of 11 and 12 mm. Posterior stabilized devices may not allow passage of the nail. In addition, there must be adequate bone remaining distally for fixation. Flexible nails also have been used,[4,43] but proper fixation of these implants can require even more intact distal bone than do the interlocked nails to achieve adequate three-point fixation.

Revision Arthroplasty

Revision arthroplasty for the management of distal femoral periprosthetic fractures offers advantages similar to those discussed earlier for the hip. Immediate revision preserves the alignment of the extremity and allows early weight bearing.[279] Fractures secondary to osteolysis from either polyethylene[314] or metallic (P. Jacobs and J.D. Mabrey, unpublished data, 1995) debris often leave little bone behind with which to work. Multiple revision arthroplasties also can make surgical stabilization difficult, and revision arthroplasty may be the only alternative to amputation.[330] As with the hip, surgical options include stabilization of the fracture around a longer intramedullary stem,[278,279,329] replacement of the distal femur with allograft and a long-stem prosthesis,[285,300,314] and complete replacement with a distal femoral prosthesis[317,330] (P. Jacobs, R. Williams, and J.D. Mabrey, unpublished data, 1995; Fig. 10-56). Instability is a problem in some cases treated with distal femoral allograft,[300] whereas the distal prosthetic replacements must rely entirely on a mechanical linkage for stability.

Unusual Fracture Patterns

Several authors have reported fractures associated with stemmed prostheses such as the Guepar[280,282] and the variable axis.[326] Their stems are long enough to interfere with fixation in the metaphysis but rarely long enough to provide additional stabilization for the fracture. Initial treatment with casting in one series

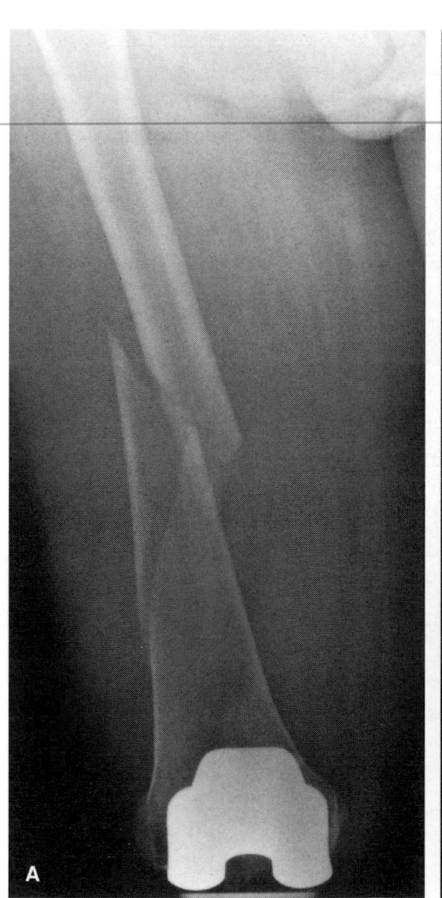

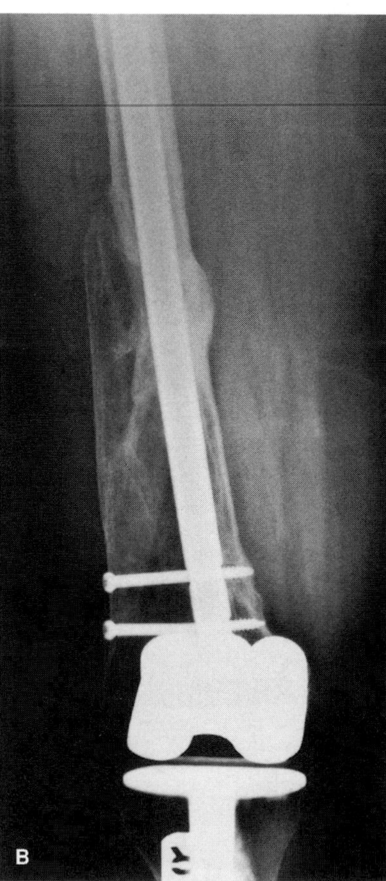

FIGURE 10-55. A 66-year-old woman sustained this injury after a minor fall. (**A**) A type IV, spiral diaphyseal fracture of the femur is seen in which the implant-bone interface remains intact. The diaphyseal location of the fracture permitted treatment independent of the presence of the total knee implant. (**B**) Eighteen months after antegrade, interlocked, intramedullary nailing, the fracture had healed and the patient remained free of symptoms with no loss of preoperative motion. If a femoral or tibial traction pin is used during intramedullary nailing, it should be inserted under fluoroscopy to avoid the implant. (*Courtesy of Joseph O. Muscat, M.D., Kingwood, TX*)

led to subsequent open reduction and internal fixation in half the fractures associated with stemmed implants.[326] Most successes come from plate fixation, with care taken to angle the screws around the stem and the cement mantle.[280]

Patients with multiple joint replacements, such as those with rheumatoid arthritis, are at risk for fracture of the femur between ipsilateral knee and hip prostheses. As noted earlier, the presence of a hip stem proximally increases the torsional rigidity of the femur and lowers its energy absorption capacity in torsion.[282] Possible treatment approaches in this situation include plate fixation,[280] Rush pin stabilization,[320] intramedullary extension of the knee component,[321] and cast treatment.[282]

Massive osteolysis of the distal femur is particularly challenging because the metaphyseal bone is essentially absent at surgery[314] (P. Jacobs and J.D. Mabrey, unpublished data, 1995; see Fig. 10-56*A*). The extensive nature of the osteolysis may not be readily apparent in the initial preoperative radiographs, so it is helpful to obtain oblique and direct lateral views of the distal femur. Distal femoral replacement with either femoral allograft[314] or an oncology management prosthesis (P. Jacobs and J.D. Mabrey, unpublished data, 1995; and P. Jacobs, R. Williams, and J.D. Mabrey, unpublished data, 1995) offers the most stable solution.

Treatment Algorithm for Femoral Fractures

Periprosthetic fractures of the knee are complex and challenging even for the most experienced surgeons. A treatment algorithm for fracture types I, II, and III is presented in Figure 10-57 and is based in large part on a comprehensive review of the subject by DiGioia and Rubash.[283] That same review defines acceptable alignment as less than 5 mm of translation, less than 5° to 10° of angulation, less than 1 cm of shortening, and less than 10° of rotation.

In cases involving patients with multiple joint involvement, it is important to consider their functional status before injury. Previous infections of the involved joint can have a bearing on the course of treatment, as can the quality of the patient's bone.

Type I, minimally displaced fractures can be treated successfully with casting or cast bracing, provided the fracture is stable and the patient can use crutches or a walker effectively. Chen and colleagues,[276] in a review of the literature, suggest that an 83% success rate is possible with nonoperative treatment in type I fractures. Type II fractures also can be treated with

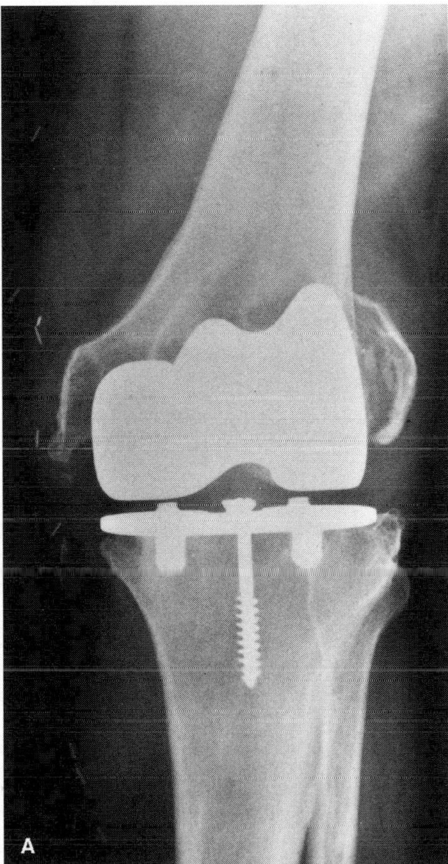

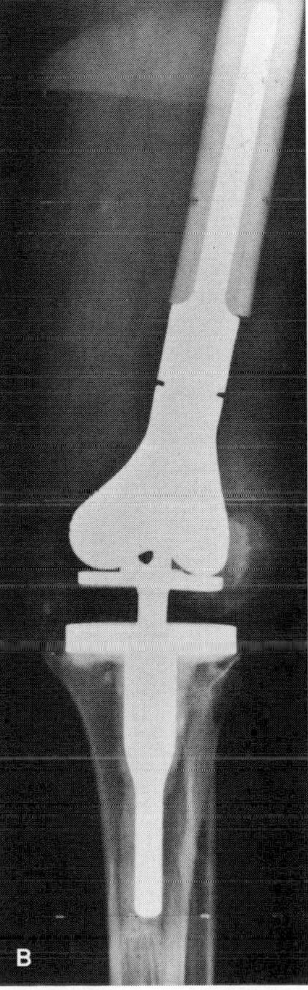

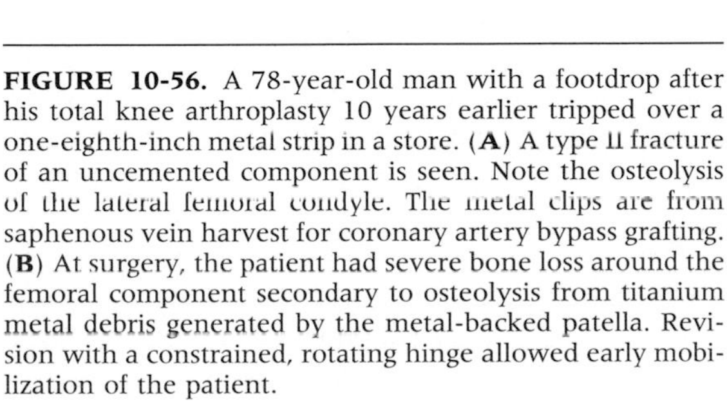

FIGURE 10-56. A 78-year-old man with a footdrop after his total knee arthroplasty 10 years earlier tripped over a one-eighth-inch metal strip in a store. (**A**) A type II fracture of an uncemented component is seen. Note the osteolysis of the lateral femoral condyle. The metal clips are from saphenous vein harvest for coronary artery bypass grafting. (**B**) At surgery, the patient had severe bone loss around the femoral component secondary to osteolysis from titanium metal debris generated by the metal-backed patella. Revision with a constrained, rotating hinge allowed early mobilization of the patient.

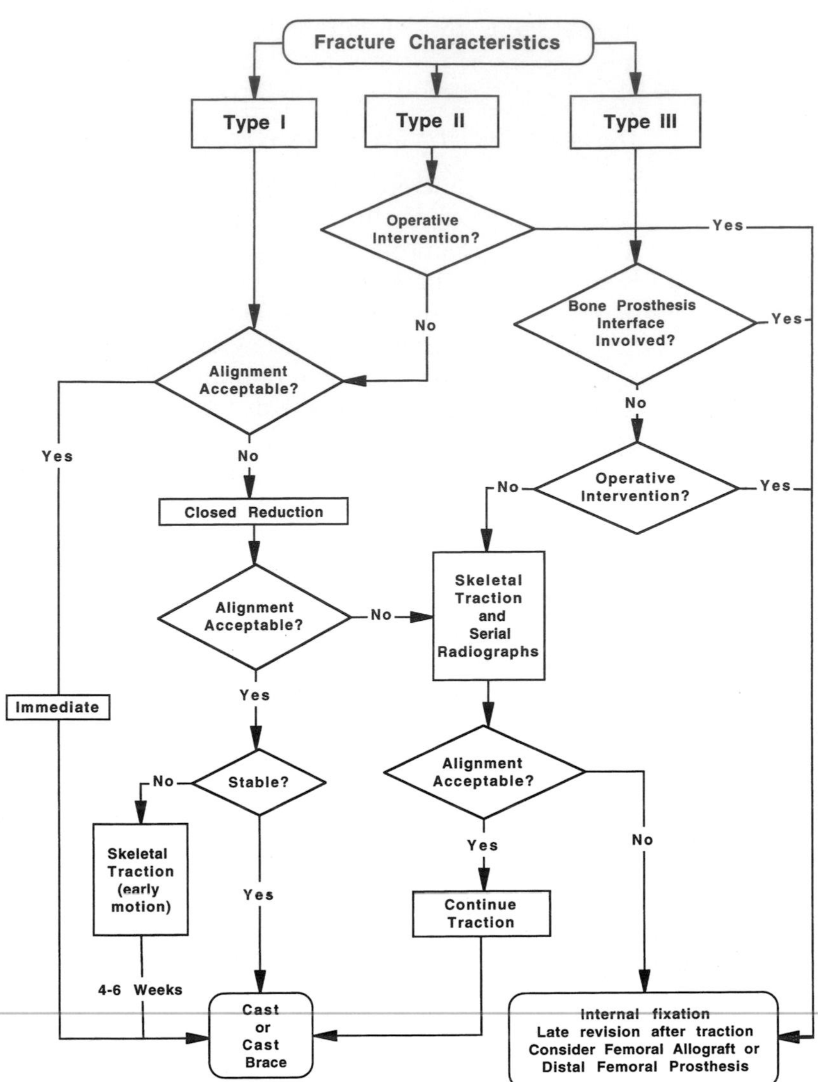

FIGURE 10-57. Treatment algorithm for types I, II, and III periprosthetic fractures of the knee.[283]

casting or bracing, provided a stable reduction is achieved; otherwise, traction or internal fixation is indicated. Type III fractures can be treated in traction if the bone–prosthesis interface is not disrupted. If it is disrupted, some type of internal fixation or revision is indicated. Type IV fractures can be treated successfully with plate fixation if the fracture is far enough from the joint line.

FRACTURES OF THE TIBIA

Two types of proximal tibial fractures in association with total knee prostheses have been reported: stress fractures of the tibial plateau[315] and fractures at the tip of the tibial cement mantle.[289] The stress fractures were a result of poorly aligned components and most of the cases underwent successful revision.[315] The fracture at the component tip followed three previous revisions in a patient with multiple joint involvement from rheumatoid arthritis (see Fig. 10-53). Her proximal tibia subsequently was replaced by the oncology management version of the rotating hinge prosthesis she already had in place.

FRACTURES OF THE PATELLA

Fractures of the patella rarely accompany periprosthetic fractures of the femur or tibia except in cases of severe trauma. They are most commonly a result of fatigue,[313] which can be related to excessive resection of bone,[277,287] malalignment,[284] or avascularity of the patella.[297,305,323,324,333] Rand[313] suggests that patellar fractures that are not associated with loosening and have an intact quadriceps mechanism are treated best without surgery. Dislocation, loosening, and disruption of the extensor mechanism are all indications for open treatment.[313]

Author's Preferred Method of Treatment

Type I fractures can be managed safely with casting or bracing provided they are observed closely for displacement. Patients who cannot follow instructions and those who have difficulty using crutches or a walker should not be considered for this modality. I prefer to manage subsequent displacement with internal fixation rather than traction to avoid the problems of prolonged bed rest.

Type II fractures almost always are managed with internal fixation because of the difficulty in obtaining and maintaining acceptable alignment after displacement. Blade plate fixation is an excellent choice because it does not remove much metaphyseal bone and provides some rotational control in the sagittal plane.[291] Bone grafting is an essential component of the procedure, preferably with autologous bone. However, the option of retrograde nailing through the notch avoids extensive exposure of the distal femur, which can destroy an already tenuous blood supply. It is important to check for proper clearance of the intramedullary device through the notch of a trial implant before proceeding.[328]

Special consideration is reserved for type II fractures through an area of distal osteolysis. With no metaphyseal bone available for fixation, my preference is to replace the entire distal femur with an oncology management prosthesis (P. Jacobs, R. Williams, and J.D. Mabrey, unpublished data, 1995). Patients treated in this way are on their feet again within days of surgery and are out of the hospital within a week.

Type III fractures are particularly suited for retrograde nailing because dissection around multiple fragments is certain to devascularize them. If the comminution is not too great and there is adequate metaphyseal bone for fixation, a blade plate also is useful. If the comminution is too extensive, I would consider a tumor replacement prosthesis. In a younger patient who could tolerate prolonged traction, it might be possible to allow the fracture to heal and then to revise it with a more conventional component later.

Type IV fractures around the diaphysis or the tip of a femoral component can be treated much like the

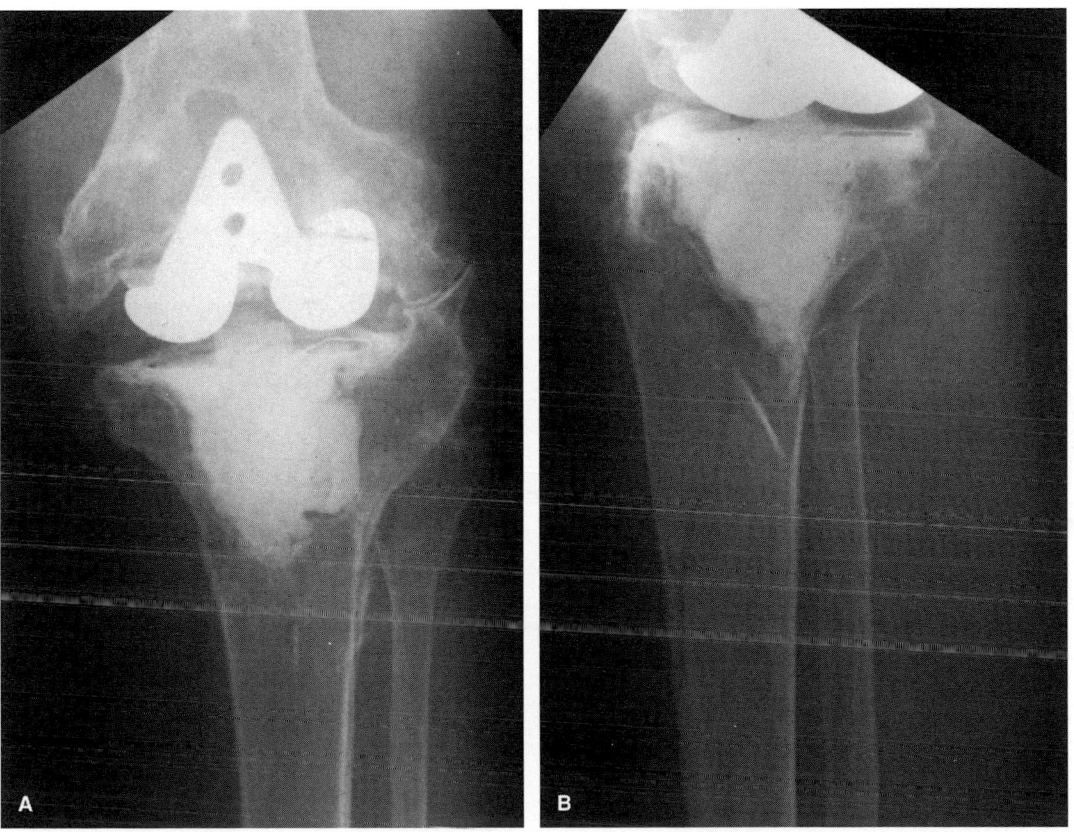

FIGURE 10-58. Anteroposterior (**A**) and lateral (**B**) radiographs of the right knee of the 65-year-old man with ankylosing spondylitis presented in the preceding section. This type V periprosthetic tibia fracture along with his ipsilateral type V femur fracture were treated initially in skin traction because he was a poor surgical candidate. (*Courtesy of James D. Heckman, M.D., San Antonio, TX*)

periprosthetic fractures of the hip. If the bone–implant interface is intact and comminution is minimal, I prefer to use cortical allograft struts and cerclage cable. A combination of dynamic compression plates and cerclage cable also could be used. Simple diaphyseal fractures without interfering intramedullary stems can be managed according to the surgeon's preference with either plates or intramedullary fixation (see Fig. 10-55).

Type V fractures of the tibia invariably involve the bone–implant interface, which makes revision of the component my procedure of choice. It might be possible to reduce and fix a split-type fracture, with the option of revising it in the future. When associated with major trauma, treatment of these fractures often must be delayed until patients recover from their other injuries (Fig. 10-58).

PERIPROSTHETIC FRACTURES OF THE ANKLE

Total ankle arthroplasty has been most successful when applied to patients with rheumatoid arthritis but is not as successful as total hip or knee arthroplasty.[289] During the same period when total ankle arthroplasty was being developed, ankle fusion techniques were improved and shown to provide excellent functional results.[289]

Because the total number of ankle arthroplasties performed is small, it is difficult to provide an overall incidence of periprosthetic fractures. Several large series have noted no fractures during follow-up periods ranging from 2 to 17 years.[298,303,331] One series reported two periprosthetic fractures: a lateral malleolar stress fracture that was treated successfully with avoidance of weight bearing, and a talar neck fracture that required subsequent fusion.[289] Another series of 36 total ankle arthroplasties reported a 22% incidence of fractures of the medial or lateral malleolus.[334] With regard to treatment, the conversion of failed total ankle arthroplasty to ankle fusion has a success rate approaching 90% using primarily external fixation and bone graft,[299] although some prefer bicortical iliac crest grafts and casting to preserve limb length.[289]

ACKNOWLEDGMENT

The authors would like to thank Kathleen Allen and Anand Masilamani, M.D., for their assistance in preparing this manuscript.

REFERENCES

PERIPROSTHETIC FRACTURES OF THE SHOULDER

1. Barrett, W.P., Franklin, J.L., Jackins, S.E., Wyss, C.R., Matsen, F.A. III: Total Shoulder Arthroplasty. J. Bone Joint Surg., 69A:865, 1987.
2. Barrett, W.P., Jackins, S.E., Wyss, C.R., Matsen, F.A. III: Total Shoulder Arthroplasty: The University of Washington Experience. Abstract. Presented at the Meeting of the American Shoulder and Elbow Surgeons; February, 1986; New Orleans, LA.
3. Barrett, W.P., Thornhill, T.S., Thomas, W.H., and colleagues: nonConstrained Total Shoulder Arthroplasty for Patients With Polyarticular Rheumatoid Arthritis. Presented at the Meeting of the American Shoulder and Elbow Surgeons; January, 1987; San Francisco, CA.
4. Bonutti, P.M., and Hawkins, R.J.: Fracture of the Humeral Shaft Associated With Total Replacement Arthroplasty of the Shoulder. J. Bone Joint Surg., 74A:617, 1992.
5. Boyd, A.D., Thornhill, T.S., Barnes, C.L.: Fractures Adjacent to Humeral Prostheses. J. Bone Joint Surg., 74A:1498, 1992.
6. Boyd, A.D. Jr., Thomas, W.H., Scott, R.D., Sledge, C.B., Thornhill, T.S.: Total Shoulder Arthroplasty Versus Hemiarthroplasty. J. Arthroplasty, 5:329, 1990.
7. Burkhead, W.Z.: Use of Porous-Coated Modular Prosthesis in the Treatment of Complex Fractures of the Proximal Humerus. Presented at the Tenth Annual Meeting of the American Shoulder and Elbow Surgeons; September, 1991; Seattle, WA.
8. Caldwell, G.L. Jr., Dines, D., Warren, R., Altchek, D., Wickiewicz, T.: Revision Shoulder Arthroplasty. Abstract. Presented at the Annual Meeting of the American Shoulder and Elbow Surgeons; February, 1993; San Francisco, CA.
9. Cofield, R.H.: Total Shoulder Arthroplasty With the Neer Prosthesis. J. Bone Joint Surg., 66A:899, 1984.
10. Cofield, R.H.: Complications of Shoulder Arthroplasty. Instructional Course Lecture Number 317. Presented at the American Academy of Orthopaedic Surgeons Annual Meeting; February, 1993; San Francisco, CA.
11. Cofield, R.H., and Edgerton, B.C.: Total Shoulder Arthroplasty: Complications and Revision Surgery. *In* Greene, W.B. (ed.): Instructional Course Lectures, pp. 449–462. Vol. 39. Park Ridge, IL, American Academy of Orthopaedic Surgeons, 1990.
12. Cofield, R.H., and Stauffer, R.N.: The Bickel Glenohumeral Arthroplasty. *In* Institute of Mechanical Engineering Conference Publications, pp. 15–19. London, Mechanical Publications Limited for the Institution of Mechanical Engineers, 1977.
13. Copeland, S.A., Lettin, A.W.F., Scales, J.T.: The Stanmore Total Shoulder Replacement—A Clinical Review. J. Bone Joint Surg., 60B:144, 1978.
14. Curtis, R.J., Groh, G.I., Heckman, M.M., Wirth, M.A., Rockwood, C.A. Jr.: Treatment of Fractures Adjacent to Humeral Prostheses. Presented at the 61st Annual Meeting of the American Academy of Orthopaedic Surgeons; February 1994; New Orleans, LA.
15. D'Antonio, J., McCarthy, J., Bargar, J.C., and colleagues: Classification of Femoral Abnormalities in Total Hip Arthroplasty. Clin. Orthop., 296:133, 1993.
16. Frich, L.H., Sojbjerg, J.O., Sneppen, O.: Shoulder Arthroplasty in Complex Acute and Chronic Proximal Humeral Fractures. Orthopedics 14:949, 1991.
17. Hawkins, R.J., Bell, R.H., Jallay, B.: Total Shoulder Arthroplasty. Clin. Orthop., 242:188, 1989.
18. Johansson, J.E., McBroom, R., Barrington, T.W., Hunter, G.A.: Fracture of the Ipsilateral Femur in Patients With Total Hip Replacement. J. Bone Joint Surg., 63A:1435, 1981.
19. Lugli, T.: Artificial Shoulder Joint by Péan (1893). The Facts of an Exceptional Intervention and the Prosthetic Method. Clin. Orthop., 133:215, 1978.
20. Miller, S.R, and Bigliani, L.U.: Complications of Total Shoulder Replacement. *In* Bigliani, L. (ed.): Complications of Shoulder Surgery, p. 59. Baltimore, Williams & Wilkins, 1993.
21. Neer, C.S.: Displaced Proximal Humeral Fractures. Part II. Treatment of Three-Part and Four-Part Displacement. J. Bone Joint Surg., 52A:1090, 1970.
22. Neer, C.S. II: Replacement Arthroplasty for Glenohumeral Osteoarthritis. J. Bone Joint Surg., 56A:1, 1974.
23. Neer, C.S. II, and Kirby, R.M.: Revision of Humeral Head and Total Shoulder Arthroplasties. Clin. Orthop., 170:189, 1982.
24. Neer, C.S. II, Watson, K.C., Stanton, F.J.: Recent Experience

in Total Shoulder Replacement. J. Bone Joint Surg., 64A:319, 1982.
25. Poppen, N.K., and Walker, P.S.: Normal and Abnormal Motion of the Shoulder. J. Bone Joint Surg., 58A:195, 1976.
26. Post, M., Haskell, S.S., Jablon, M.: Total Shoulder Replacement With a Constrained Prosthesis. J. Bone Joint Surg., 62A:327, 1980.
27. Rockwood, C.A. Jr.: The Technique of Total Shoulder Arthroplasty. *In* Green, W.B. (ed.): Instructional Course Lectures, p. 437. Vol. 39. Park Ridge, IL, American Academy of Orthopaedic Surgeons, 1990.
28. Rockwood, C.A. Jr., and Wirth, M.A.: *Global Total Shoulder Arthroplasty—Parts I & II* [videotape]. AAOS Individual Orthopaedic Instruction Video Award Winner. Park Ridge, IL, American Academy of Orthopaedic Surgeons, 1992.
29. Wirth, M.A., Basamania, C., Rockwood, C.A. Jr.: Fixation of Glenoid Component: Keel Versus Pegs. Op Tech Orthop, 4:218, 1994.
30. Wirth, M.A., and Rockwood, C.A. Jr.: Complications of Shoulder Arthroplasty. Clin. Orthop., 307:47, 1994.
31. Wirth, M.A., and Rockwood, C.A. Jr.: Complications of Treatment of Injuries to the Shoulder. *In* Epps, C.H. (ed.): Complications in Orthopaedic Surgery, pp. 229–255. 3rd ed. Philadelphia, J.B. Lippincott, 1994.
32. Wirth, M.A., Seltzer, D.G., Senes, H.R., Pannone, A., Lee, J., Rockwood, C.A. Jr.: An Analysis of Failed Humeral Head and Total Shoulder Arthroplasty. Presented at the American Shoulder and Elbow Surgeons 10th Open Meeting; February, 1994; New Orleans, LA.

PERIPROSTHETIC FRACTURES OF THE ELBOW

33. Brumfield, R.H., Volz, R.G., Green, J.F.: Total Elbow Arthroplasty: A Clinical Review of 30 Cases Employing the Mayo and AHSC Prostheses. Clin. Orthop., 158:137, 1981.
34. Bryan, R.S., and Morrey, B.F.: Extensile Posterior Exposure of the Elbow. A Triceps-Sparing Approach. Clin. Orthop., 166:188, 1982.
35. Davis, R.F., Weiland, A.J., Hungerford, D.S., Moore, J.R., Volenec-Dowling, S.: Non-constrained total elbow arthroplasty. Clin. Orthop., 171:156, 1982.
36. Dee, R.: Total Replacement of the Elbow Joint. Orthop. Clin. North Am., 4:415, 1973.
37. Ewald, F.C.: Total Elbow Replacement. Orthop. Clin. North Am., 6:685, 1975.
38. Ewald, F.C.: Capitellocondylar Total Elbow Arthroplasty. *In* Morrey, B.F. (ed.): Master Techniques in Orthopaedic Surgery, The Elbow, p. 209. New York, Raven Press, 1994.
39. Ewald, F.C., Scheinberg, R.D., Poss, R., Thomas, W.H., Scott, R.D., Sledge, C.B.: Capitellocondylar Total Elbow Arthroplasty. J. Bone Joint Surg., 62A:1259, 1980.
40. Ewald, F.C., Simmons, E.D. Jr., Sullivan, J.A., and colleagues: Capitellocondylar Total Elbow Replacement in Rheumatoid Arthritis: Long-Term Results. J. Bone Joint Surg., 75A:498, 1993.
41. Figgie, H.E. III, Inglis, A.E., Ranawat, C.S., Rosenberg, G.M.: Results of Total Elbow Arthroplasty as a Salvage Procedure for Failed Elbow Reconstructive Operations. Clin. Orthop., 219:185, 1987.
42. Figgie, M.P., Inglis, A.E., Mow, C.S., Figgie, H.E. III.: Total Elbow Arthroplasty for Complete Ankylosis of the Elbow. J. Bone Joint Surg., 71A:513, 1989.
43. Friedman, R.J., Lee, D.E., Ewald, F.C.: Nonconstrained Total Elbow Arthroplasty: Development and Results in Patients With Functional Class IV Rheumatoid Arthritis. J. Arthroplasty, 4:31, 1989.
44. Gschwend, N., Loehr, J., Ivosevic-Radovanovic, D., Scheier, H., Munzinger, U.: Semiconstrained Elbow Prostheses With Special Reference to the GSB III Prosthesis. Clin. Orthop., 232:104, 1988.
45. Inglis, A.E., and Pellicci, P.M.: Total Elbow Replacement. J. Bone Joint Surg., 62A:1252, 1980.
46. Lowe, L.W., Miller, A.J., Allum, R.L., Higginson, D.W.: The Development of an Unconstrained Elbow Arthroplasty. J. Bone Joint Surg., 66B:243, 1984.
47. Morrey, B.F.: Semiconstrained Total Elbow Replacement. *In* Morrey, B.F. (ed.): Master Techniques in Orthopaedic Surgery, The Elbow, p. 231. New York, Raven Press, 1994.
48. Morrey, B.F., and Adams, R.A.: Semiconstrained Arthroplasty for the Treatment of Rheumatoid Arthritis of the Elbow. J. Bone Joint Surg., 74A:479, 1992.
49. Morrey, B.F., Adams, R.A., Bryan, R.S.: Total Replacement for Post-Traumatic Arthritis of the Elbow. J. Bone Joint Surg., 73B:607, 1991.
50. Morrey, B.F., Askew, J.N., An, K.N., Chao, E.Y.: A Biomechanical Study of Normal Elbow Motion. J. Bone Joint Surg., 63A:872, 1981.
51. Morrey, B.F., and Bryan, R.S.: Revision Total Elbow Arthroplasty. J. Bone Joint Surg., 69A:523, 1987.
52. Morrey, B.F., Bryan, R.S., Dobyns, J.H., Linscheid, R.L.: Total Elbow Arthroplasty—A Five-Year Experience at the Mayo Clinic. J. Bone Joint Surg., 63A:1050, 1981.
53. O'Driscoll, S.W., An, K.-N., Korinek, S., Morrey, B.F.: Kinematics of Semi-Constrained Total Elbow Arthroplasty. J. Bone Joint Surg., 74B:297, 1992.
54. Pritchard, R.W.: Long-Term Follow-Up Study: Semi-Constrained Elbow Prosthesis. Orthopedics, 4:151, 1981.
55. Pritchard, R.W.: Anatomic Surface Elbow Arthroplasty—A Preliminary Report. Clin. Orthop., 179:223, 1983.
56. Rosenberg, G.M., Turner, R.H.: Nonconstrained Total Elbow Arthroplasty. Clin. Orthop., 187:154, 1984.
57. Rosenfeld, S.R., and Anzel, S.H.: Evaluation of the Pritchard Total Elbow Arthroplasty. Orthopedics, 5:713, 1982.
58. Ruth, J.T., and Wilde, A.H.: Capitellocondylar Total Elbow Replacement: A Long-Term Study. J. Bone Joint Surg., 74A:95, 1992.
59. Silva, J.F.: Arthroplasty of the Elbow. Singapore Med J, 8:222, 1967.
60. Souter, W.A.: Arthroplasty of the Elbow—With Particular Reference to Metallic Hinge Arthroplasty in Rheumatoid Patients. Orthop. Clin. North Am., 4:395, 1973.
61. Trancik, T., Wilde, A.H., Borden, L.S.: Capitellocondylar Total Elbow Arthroplasty: Two-to Eight-Year Experience. Clin. Orthop., 223:175, 1987.
62. Walker, P.S.: Human Joints and Their Artificial Replacements, p. 190. Springfield, IL, CC Thomas, 1977.

PERIPROSTHETIC FRACTURES OF THE WRIST AND HAND

63. Alnot, J.Y., Saint Laurent, Y.: Total Trapeziometacarpal Arthroplasty. Report on 17 Cases of Degenerative Arthritis of the Trapeziometacarpal Joint. Ann. Chir. Main., 4:11, 1985.
64. Angell, M.: Breast Implants—Protection or Paternalism? N. Engl. J. Med., 326:1695, 1992.
65. Beckenbaugh, R.D.: Total Wrist Arthroplasty. *In* Gelberman, R.H. (ed.): Master Techniques in Orthopaedic Surgery, The Wrist, p. 253. New York, Raven Press, 1994.
66. Beckenbaugh, R.D., Dobyns, J.H., Linscheid, R.L., Bryan, R.S.: Review and Analysis of silicone rubber Metacarpophalangeal Implants. J. Bone Joint Surg., 58A:483, 1976.
67. Beckenbaugh, R.D., and Linscheid, R.L.: Total Wrist Arthroplasty: A Preliminary Report. J. Hand. Surg., 2:337, 1977.
68. Beckenbaugh, R.D., and Linscheid, R.L.: Arthroplasty in the Hand and Wrist. *In* Green, D.P. (ed.): Operative Hand Surgery, 2nd ed., pp. 167–214. Vol. I. New York, Churchill Livingstone, 1982.
69. Beckenbaugh, R.D., and Steffe, A.D.: Total Joint Arthroplasty for the Metacarpophalangeal Joint of the Thumb. A Preliminary Report. Orthopedics, 4:298, 1981.
70. Bieber, E.J., Weiland, A.J., Volenec-Dowling, S.: silicone rubber Implant Arthroplasty of the Metacarpophalangeal Joints for Rheumatoid Arthritis. J. Bone Joint Surg., 68A:206, 1986.
71. Blair, W.F., Shurr, D.G., Buckwalter, J.A.: Metacarpophalangeal Joint Arthroplasty With a Metallic Hinged Prosthesis. Clin. Orthop., 184:156, 1984.
72. Blair, W.F., Shurr, D.G., Buckwalter, J.A.: Metacarpophalangeal Joint Implant Arthroplasty With a Silastic Spacer. J. Bone Joint Surg., 66A:365, 1984.

73. Brannon, E.W., Klein, G.: Experiences With a Finger-Joint Prosthesis. J. Bone Joint Surg., 41A:87, 1959.
74. Braun, R.M.: Total Joint Replacement for Arthritis of the Base of the Thumb. Presented at the Annual Meeting of the American Society for Surgery of the Hand; 1978; San Francisco, CA.
75. Braun, R.M.: Total Joint Replacement at the Base of the Thumb—Preliminary Report. J. Hand. Surg., 7:245, 1982.
76. Cooney, W.P., Linscheid, R.L., Askew, L.J.: Total Arthroplasty of the Thumb Trapeziometacarpal Joint. Clin. Orthop., 220:35, 1987.
77. de la Caffiniere, J.: Long-Term Results of Total Trapeziometacarpal Prosthesis in Osteoarthritis of the Thumb. French J. Orthop. Surg, 5:263, 1991.
78. de la Caffiniere, J.Y.: Prothese Totale Trapezo-Metacarpienne. Rev. Chir. Orthop. Reparatrice. Appar. Mot., 60:299, 1974.
79. de la Caffiniere, J.Y., and Aucoutorier, P.: Trapeziometacarpal Arthroplasty by Total Prosthesis. Hand, 11:41, 1979.
80. Derkash, R.S., Niebauer, J.J., Lane, C.S.: Long-Term Follow-Up of Metacarpal Phalangeal Arthroplasty With Silicone Dacron Prostheses. J. Hand. Surg., 11A:553, 1986.
81. Dryer, R.F., Blair, W.F., Shurr, D.G., Buckwalter, J.A.: Proximal Interphalangeal Joint Arthroplasty. Clin. Orthop., 185:187, 1984.
82. Ferlic, D.C., and Clayton, M.L.: Total Joint Arthroplasty of the Large Joints of the Upper Extremities, as Relief for Degeneration and Rheumatoid Arthritis. Colo. Med., 78:262, 1981.
83. Ferlic, D.C., Clayton, M.L., Holloway, M.: Complications of Silicone Implant Surgery in the Metacarpophalangeal Joint. J. Bone Joint Surg., 57A:991, 1975.
84. Ferrari. B., and Steffe, A.D.: Trapeziometacarpal Total Joint Replacement Using the Steffe Prosthesis. J. Bone Joint Surg., 68A:1177, 1986.
85. Fisher, J.: The Silicone Controversy—When Will Science Prevail? N. Engl. J. Med., 326:1696, 1992.
86. Flatt, A.E.: Restoration of Rheumatoid Finger-Joint Function. J. Bone Joint Surg., 43A:753, 1961.
87. Flatt, A.E., and Ellison, M.R.: Follow Up Notes on Articles Previously Published in The Journal of Restoration of Rheumatoid Finger Joint Function. III. J. Bone Joint Surg., 54A:1317, 1972.
88. Hagert, C.-G., Eiken, O., Ohlsson, N.-M., Aschan, W., Movin, A.: Metacarpophalangeal Joint Implants. I. Roentgenographic Study on the Silastic Finger Joint Implant, Swanson Design. Scand. J. Plast. Reconstr. Surg., 9:147, 1975.
89. Kay, A.G.L., Jeffs, J.V., Scott, J.T.: Experience With Silastic Prostheses in the Rheumatoid Hand. A 5-Year Follow-Up. Ann. Rheum. Dis., 37:255, 1978.
90. Kessler, D.: The Basis for the FDA's Decision on Breast Implants. N. Engl. J. Med., 326:1713, 1992.
91. Kirschenbaum, D., Schneider, L.H., Adams, D.C., Cody, R.P.: Arthroplasty of the Metacarpophalangeal Joints With Use of silicone rubber Implants in Patients Who Have Rheumatoid Arthritis. J. Bone Joint Surg., 75A:3, 1993.
92. Linscheid, R., Cooney, W., Dobyns, J.: Metacarpotrapezial Arthroplasty. *In* Inglis, A. (ed.): AAOS Symposium on Total Joint Replacement of the Upper Extremity, p. 289. St. Louis, Mosby, 1982.
93. Linscheid, R.L., Beckenbaugh, R.D., Dobyns, J.H.: Total Wrist Arthroplasty. *In* Inglis, A.E. (ed.): American Academy of Orthopaedic Surgeons. Symposium on Total Joint Replacement of the Upper Extremity, pp. 255–264. St. Louis, Mosby, 1982.
94. Linscheid, R.L., and Dobyns, J.H.: Total Joint Arthroplasty—The Hand. Mayo Clin. Proc., 54:516, 1979.
95. Mannerfelt, L., and Andersson, K.: Silastic Arthroplasty of the Metacarpophalangeal Joints in Rheumatoid Arthritis. Long-Term Results. J. Bone Joint Surg., 57A:484, 1975.
96. Meuli, H.C.: Reconstructive Surgery of the Wrist Joint. Hand, 4:88, 1972.
97. Meuli, H.C.: Arthroplastie due poignet. Ann. Chir., 27:527, 1973.
98. Meuli, H.C.: Alloarthroplastik des Handegelenks. Z. Orthop. Ihre. Grenzgeb., 113:476, 1975.
99. Meuli, H.C.: Arthroplasty of the Wrist. Clin. Orthop., 149:118, 1980.
100. Nicholas, R.M., and Calderwood, J.W.: De La Caffiniere Arthroplasty for Basal Thumb Joint Osteoarthritis. J. Bone Joint Surg., 74B:309, 1992.
101. Nicolle, F.V., Stephen, G.: Assessment of Past Results and Current Practice in the Treatment of Rheumatoid Metacarpophalangeal Joints. Five Year Review. Hand, 11:151, 1979.
102. Niebauer, J.J., and Landry, R.M.: Dacron-Silicone Prosthesis for the Metacarpophalangeal and Interphalangeal Joints. Hand, 3:55, 1971.
103. Niebauer, J.J., Shaw, J.L., Doren, W.W.: Silicone-Dacron Hinge Prosthesis. Design, Evaluation, and Application. Ann. Rheum. Dis., 28(Suppl.):56, 1969.
104. Peimer, C., Medige, J., Eckert, B., Wright, J.: Reactive Synovitis After Silicone Arthroplasty. J. Hand. Surg., 11A:624, 1986.
105. Pellegrini, V.D., and Burton, R.I. Jr.: Surgical Management of Basal Joint Arthritis of the Thumb. Part I. Long-Term Results of Silicone Implant Arthroplasty. J. Hand Surg., 11A:309, 1986.
106. Pellegrini, V.D., and Burton, R.I.: Osteoarthritis of the Proximal Interphalangeal Joint of the Hand: Arthroplasty or Fusion? J. Hand Surg., 15A:194, 1990.
107. Pellegrini, V.D. Jr., and Burton, R.I.: Complications of Implant Surgery in the Hand. *In* Epps, C.H. Jr. (ed.): Complications in Orthopaedic Surgery, p. 997. 3rd ed. Philadelphia, JB Lippincott, 1994.
108. Praemer, A., Furner, S., Rice, D.: Medical Implants and Major Joint Procedures. *In* Musculoskeletal Conditions in the United States, p. 125. 1st ed. Chicago, American Academy of Orthopaedic Surgeons, 1992.
109. Rettig, M.E., and Beckenbaugh, R.D.: Revision Total Wrist Arthroplasty. J. Hand Surg., 18A:798, 1993.
110. Smith, R., Atkinson, R., Jupiter, J.K.: Silicone Synovitis of the Wrist. J. Hand Surg., 10A:47, 1985.
111. Swanson, A.B.: A Flexible Implant for Replacement of Arthritic or Destroyed Joints in the Hand. New York University, Post-Graduate Medical School Inter-Clin Inform Bull, 6:16, 1966.
112. Swanson, A.B.: Silicone Rubber Implants for Replacement of Arthritic or Destroyed Joints in the Hand. Surg. Clin. North Am., 48:1113, 1968.
113. Swanson, A.B.: Finger Joint Replacement by Silicone Rubber Implants and the Concept of Implant Fixation by Encapsulation. International Workshop on Artificial Finger Joints. Ann. Rheum. Dis., 28(Suppl.):47, 1969.
114. Swanson, A.B.: Silicone Rubber Implant Arthroplasty in Trapeziometacarpal Joint Arthritis. J. Bone Joint Surg., 51A:799, 1969.
115. Swanson, A.B.: Flexible Implant Arthroplasty for Arthritic Finger Joints. J. Bone Joint Surg., 54A:435, 1972.
116. Swanson, A.B., and deGroot-Swanson, G.: Flexible Implant Arthroplasty of the Radiocarpal Joint. Sem. Arthrop., 2:78, 1991.
117. Swanson, A.B., deGroot-Swanson, G., Herndon, J.H.: Complications of Arthroplasty and Joint Replacement at the Wrist. *In* Epps, C.H. Jr. (ed.): Complications in Orthopaedic Surgery, p. 957. 3rd ed. Philadelphia, JB Lippincott, 1994.
118. Swanson, A.B., and Yamauchi, Y.: Silicone Rubber Implants for Replacement of Arthritic or Destroyed Joints. J. Bone Joint Surg., 50A:1272, 1968.
119. Vahvanen, V., and Vijakka, T.: Silicone Rubber Implant Arthroplasty of the Metacarpophalangeal Joints in Rheumatoid Arthritis: A Follow-Up Study of 32 Patients. J. Hand Surg., 11A:333, 1986.
120. Volz, R.G.: The Development of a Total Wrist Arthroplasty. Clin. Orthop., 116:209, 1976.
121. Volz, R.G.: Total Wrist Arthroplasty. A New Approach to Wrist Disability. Clin. Orthop., 128:180, 1977.

PERIPROSTHETIC FRACTURES OF THE HIP

122. A.A.O.S., Committee on Scientific Investigation: Preliminary Survey on Femoral Head Prostheses. J. Bone Joint Surg., 35A:489–494, 1953.
123. A.A.O.S., Committee on the Hip: Classification and Management of Femoral Defects in Total Hip Replacement. Exhibit.

57th Annual Meeting of the American Academy of Orthopaedic Surgeons; Feb. 8–13, 1990; New Orleans, LA.

124. Adolphson, P., Jonsson, U., Kalén, R.: Fractures of the Ipsilateral Femur After Total Hip Arthroplasty. Arch. Orthop. Trauma Surg., 106:353–357, 1987.
125. Ali Khan, M.A., and O'Driscoll, M.: Fractures of the Femur During Total Hip Replacement and Their Management. J. Bone Joint Surg., 59B:36, 1977.
126. Anderson, L.D., Hamsa, W.R.J., Waring, T.L.: Femoral-Head Prostheses. A Review of Three Hundred and Fifty-Six Operations and Their Results. J. Bone Joint Surg., 46A:1049–1065, 1964.
127. Andrew, T.A., Flanagan, J.P., Gerundini, M., Bombelli, R.: The Isoelastic, Noncemented Total Hip Arthroplasty. Preliminary Experience With 400 Cases. Clin. Orthop., 206:127–138, 1986.
128. Aufranc, O.E., Jones, W.N., Turner, R.H.: Femoral Shaft Fractures Below Hip Prosthesis. J.A.M.A., 194:1378, 1965.
129. Bergstrom, B., Lindberg, L., Persson, B.M., Onnerfalt, R.: Complications After Total Hip Arthroplasty According to Charnley in a Swedish Series of Cases. Clin. Orthop., 95:91–95, 1973.
130. Berman, A.T., and Levenberg, R.J.: Femur Fractures Associated With Total Hip Arthroplasty. Orthopedics, 15:751–753, 1992.
131. Bethea, J.S. III, DeAndrade, J.R., Fleming, L.L., Lindenbaum, S.D., Welch, R.B.: Proximal Femoral Fractures Following Total Hip Arthroplasty. Clin. Orthop., 170:95–106, 1982.
132. Blatter, G., Fiechter, T., Magerl, F.: Peri-Prosthesis Fractures in Total Hip Endoprostheses. [German]. Orthopade, 18:545–551, 1989.
133. Breck, L.W.: Metal to Metal Total Hip Joint Replacement Using the Wrist Socket: An End Result. Clin. Orthop., 95:38–42, 1973.
134. Brindley, G.W., Kavanagh, B.F., Fitzgerald, R.H.: Intraoperative Fractures During Uncemented Total Hip Arthroplasty. Orthopaedic Transactions, 11:463, 1987.
135. Broad, C.P., and Hamami, M.N.: Kuntscher Nailing of Femoral Fractures Associated With Austin Moore's Prosthesis. Injury, 12:252–255, 1980.
136. Burstein, A.H., Currey, J., Frankel, V.H., Heiple, K.G., Lunseth, P., Vessely, J.C.: Bone Strength: The Effect of Screw Holes. J. Bone Joint Surg., 54A:1143–1156, 1972.
137. Callaghan, J.J.: The Clinical Results and Basic Science of Total Hip Arthroplasty With Porous-Coated Prostheses. J. Bone Joint Surg., 75A:299–310, 1993.
138. Callaghan, J.J., Heekin, R.D., Savory, C.G., Dysart, S.H., Hopkinson, W.J.: Evaluation of the Learning Curve Associated With Uncemented Primary Porous-Coated Anatomic Total Hip Arthroplasty. Clin. Orthop., 282:132–144, 1992.
139. Cameron, H.U., Jung, Y.K., Noiles, D.G., McTighe, T.: Design Features and Early Clinical Results With a Modular Proximally Fixed Low Bending Stiffness Uncemented Total Hip Replacement. Presented at the 55th Annual Meeting of the American Academy of Orthopaedic Surgeons; Feb 4–9, 1988; Atlanta, GA.
140. Chandler, H.P.: Use of Allografts and Prostheses in the Reconstruction of Failed Total Hip Replacements. Orthopedics, 15:1207–1218, 1992.
141. Chandler, H.P., King, D., Limbird, R., and colleagues: The Use of Cortical Allograft Struts for Fixation of Fractures Associated With Well-Fixed Total Joint Prostheses. Seminars In Arthroplasty, 4:99–107, 1993.
142. Chandler, H.P., Penenberg, B.L. (eds.): Bone Stock Deficiency in Total Hip Replacement, pp. 103–164. Thorofore, N.J., SLACK Incorporated, 1989.
143. Chapchal, G.J., Sloof, J.J., Nollen, A.D.: Results of Total Hip Replacement: A Critical Follow-Up Study. Clin. Orthop., 95:111–117, 1973.
144. Charnley, J.: The Healing of Human Fractures in Contact With Self-Curing Acrylic Cement. Clin. Orthop., 47:157–163, 1966.
145. Christensen, C.M., Seger, B.M., Schultz, R.B.: Management of Intraoperative Femur Fractures Associated With Revision Hip Arthroplasty. Clin. Orthop., 248:177–180, 1989.
146. Clancey, G.J., Smith, R.F., Madenwald, M.B.: Fracture of the Distal End of the Femur Below Hip Implants in Elderly Patients. J. Bone Joint Surg., 65A:491–494, 1983.
147. Cooke, P.H., and Newman, J.H.: Femoral Fractures in Relation to Cemented Hip Prostheses. J. Bone Joint Surg., 66B:278, 1984.
148. Cooke, P.H., and Newman, J.H.: Fractures of the Femur in Relation to Cemented Hip Prostheses. J. Bone Joint Surg., 70B:386–389, 1988.
149. Courpied, J.P., Watin-Augouard, L., Postel, M.: Fractures du fémur chez les sujets porteurs de prosthèses totales de hanche ou de genou. Int. Orthop., 11:109–115, 1987.
150. Coventry, M.B., Beckenbaugh, R.D., Nolan, D.R., Ilstrup, D.M.: Two Thousand and Twelve Total Hip Arthroplasties: A Study of Postoperative Course and Complications. J. Bone Joint Surg., 56A:273, 1974.
151. Cracchiolo, A.: Stress Fractures of the Pelvis as a Cause of Hip Pain Following Total Hip and Knee Arthroplasty. Arthritis Rheum., 24:740–742, 1981.
152. Cuckler, J.: Richards Modular Hip System. Memphis, TN, Smith & Nephew Richards Inc., 1994.
153. Cupic, Z.: Long Term Follow-Up of Charnley Arthroplasty of the Hip. Clin. Orthop., 141:28–43, 1979.
154. Curtis, M.J., Jinnah, R.H., Wilson, V.D., Hungerford, D.S.: The Initial Stability of Uncemented Acetabular Components. J. Bone Joint Surg. [Br.], 74:372–376, 1992.
155. D'Antonio, J., McCarthy, J.C., Bargar, W.L., and colleagues: Classification of Femoral Abnormalities in Total Hip Arthroplasty. Clin. Orthop., 296:133–139, 1993.
156. De Beer, J.D.V., and Learmonth, I.D.: 'Pathological' Fracture of the Femur—A Complication of Failed Total Hip Arthroplasty. S. Afr. Med. J., 79:202–205, 1991.
157. Dunn, H.K., and Hess, W.E.: Total Hip Reconstruction in Chronically Dislocated Hips. J. Bone Joint Surg., 58A:838, 1976.
158. Dupont, J.A., and Charnley, J.: Low Friction Arthroplasty of the Hip for the Failures of Previous Operations. J. Bone Joint Surg., 54B:77, 1972.
159. Dysart, S.H., Savory, C.G., Callaghan, J.J.: Nonoperative Treatment of a Postoperative Fracture Around an Uncemented Porous-Coated Femoral Component. J. Arthroplasty, 4:187–190, 1989.
160. Eftekhar, N.S., Smith, D.M., Henry, J.H., Stinchfield, F.E.: Revision Arthroplasty Using Charnley Low Friction Arthroplasty Technique. Clin. Orthop., 95:48–59, 1973.
161. Eftekhar, N.S., and Stinchfield, F.E.: Experience With Low Friction Arthroplasty. Clin. Orthop., 95:60–68, 1973.
162. Ejested, R., and Olsen, N.J.: Revision of Failed Total Hip Arthroplasty. J. Bone Joint Surg., 69B:57–60, 1987.
163. Engh, C.A., Glassman, A.H., Griffin, W.L., Mayer, J.G.: Results of Cementless Revision for Failed Cemented Total Hip Arthroplasty. Clin. Orthop., 235:91–110, 1988.
164. Evanski, P.M., Waugh, T.R., Orofino, C.F.: Total Hip Replacement With the Charnley Prosthesis. Clin. Orthop., 95:69–72, 1973.
165. Evarts, C.M., DeHaven, K.E., Nelson, C.L., Collins, H.R., Wilde, A.H.: Interim Results of Charnley-Muller Total Hip Arthroplasty. Clin. Orthop., 95:193–200, 1973.
166. Federici, A., Carbone, M., Sanguineti, F.: Intraoperative Fractures of the Femoral Diaphysis in Hip Arthroprosthesis Surgery. Ital. J. Orthop. Traumatol., 14:311–321, 1988.
167. Fitzgerald, R.H. Jr., Brindley, G.W., Kavanagh, B.F.: The Uncemented Total Hip Arthroplasty: Intraoperative Femoral Fractures. Clin. Orthop., 235:61–66, 1988.
168. Fredin, H.O., Lindberg, H., Carlsson, A.S.: Femoral Fracture after Hip Arthroplasty. Acta Orthop Scand, 58:20, 1987.
169. Freeman, P.A., Lee, P., Bryson, T.W.: Total Hip Joint Replacement in Osteoarthrosis and Polyarthritis. Clin. Orthop., 95:224–230, 1973.
170. Friedman, R.J., Black, J., Galante, J.O., Jacobs, J.J., Skinner, H.B.: Current Concepts in Orthopaedic Biomaterials and Implant Fixation. J. Bone Joint Surg., 75A:1086–1109, 1993.
171. García-Cimbrelo, E., Munuera, L., Gil-Garay, E.: Femoral Shaft Fractures After Cemented Total Hip Arthroplasty. Int. Orthop., 16:97–100, 1992.

172. Giacometti, R.C., and Pace, A.: CLS Femoral Component. Orthopedics, 12:1195–1200, 1989.
173. Haddad, R.J. Jr., Cook, S.D., Thomas, K.A.: Biological Fixation of Porous-Coated Implants. J. Bone Joint Surg., 69A:1459–1466, 1987.
174. Harrington, I.J., Tountas, A.A., Cameron, H.U.: Femoral Fractures Associated With Moore's Prosthesis. Injury, 11:23–32, 1979.
175. Harris, W.H.: Preliminary Report of Results of Harris Total Hip Replacement. Clin. Orthop., 95:168–173, 1973.
176. Hinchey, J.J., and Day, P.L.: Primary Prosthetic Replacement in Fresh Femoral Neck Fractures: A Review of 294 Consecutive Cases. J. Bone Joint Surg., 46A:223–240, 1964.
177. Jasty, M., Henshaw, R.M., O'Connor, D.O., Harris, W.H.: High Assembly Strains and Femoral Fractures Produced During Insertion of Uncemented Femoral Components. J. Arthroplasty, 8:479–487, 1993.
178. Jensen, J.S., Barfod, G., Hansen, D., and colleagues: Femoral Shaft Fracture After Hip Arthroplasty. Acta Orthop. Scand., 59:9, 1988.
179. Jensen, T.T., Overgaard, S., Mossing, N.B.: Partridge Cerclene System for Femoral Fractures in Osteoporotic Bones With Ipsilateral Hemi/Total Arthroplasty. J. Arthroplasty, 5:123—126, 1990.
180. Johansson, J.E., McBroom, R., Barrington, T.W., Hunter, G.A.: Fracture of the Ipsilateral Femur in Patients With Total Hip Replacement. J. Bone Joint Surg., 63A:1435–1442, 1981.
181. Jones, D.G.: Bone Erosion Beneath Partridge Bands. J. Bone Joint Surg., 68B:476, 1986.
182. Kallel, S., Bouillet, R.: The Use of Partridge Plates in the Treatment of Femoral Diaphysis Fractures Near a Prosthesis in Elderly Patients. French. Acta Orthop. Belg., 57:11–18, 1991.
183. Kavanagh, B.F., Fitzgerald, R.H.: Multiple Revisions for Failed Total Hip Arthroplasty Not Associated With Infections. J. Bone Joint Surg., 69A:1144, 1987.
184. Kavanagh, B.F., Fitzgerald, R.H., Ilstrup, D.: PCA Uncemented THA. Orthopaedic Transactions, 12:704, 1988.
185. Kavanagh, B.F., Ilstrup, D.M., Fitzgerald, R.H.: Revision Total Hip Arthroplasty. J. Bone Joint Surg., 67A:517–526, 1985.
186. Kim, Y.-H.: Total Arthroplasty of the Hip After Childhood Sepsis. J. Bone Joint Surg., 73B:783–786, 1991.
187. Kim, Y.S., Callaghan, J.J., Ahn, P.B., Brown, T.D.: Acetabular Fracture During Oversized Component Insertion. *In* Proceedings of the 41st Annual Meeting of the Orthopaedic Research Society, p. 245. Vol. 20, Section 1. Orlando, 1995.
188. Kolmert, L.: A Method for Fixation of Femoral Fractures Below Previous Hip Implants. J. Trauma, 27:407, 1987.
189. Kwong, L.M., O'Connor, D.O., Sedlacek, R.C., Krushell, R.J., Maloney, W.J., Harris, W.H.: A Quantitative In Vitro Assessment of Fit and Screw Fixation on the Stability of a Cementless Hemispherical Acetabular Component. J. Arthroplasty, 9:163–170, 1994.
190. Langenskiold, A., and Paavilainen, T.: Total Replacement of 116 Hips by the McKee-Farrar Prosthesis: A Preliminary Report. Clin. Orthop., 95:143–150, 1973.
191. Larsen, E., Menck, H., Rosenklint, A.: Fractures After Hemialloplastic Hip Replacement. J. Trauma, 27:72–74, 1986.
192. Larson, J.E., Chao, E.Y.S., Fitzgerald, R.H.J., and colleagues: Bypassing Femoral Cortical Defects With Cemented Intramedullary Stems. J. Orthop. Res., 9:414, 1991.
193. Launder, W.J., and Hungerford, D.S.: Stress Fracture of the Pubis After Total Hip Arthroplasty. Clin. Orthop., 159:183–185, 1981.
194. Lazansky, M.G.: Complications in Total Hip Replacement With the Charnley Technique. Clin. Orthop., 72:40, 1970.
195. Leinbach, I.S., and Barlow, F.A.: 700 Total Hip Replacements. Clin. Orthop., 95:174–192, 1973.
196. Luck, J.V., Brannon, E.W., Luck, J.V., Jr.: Total Hip Replacement Arthroplasties: Causes, Orthopaedic Management, and Prevention of Selected Problems. J. Bone Joint Surg., 54A:1569–1571, 1972.
197. Mackechnie-Jarvis, A.C.: Fractures Below a Femoral Prosthesis—A Report on Two Cases Treated by Conservative Surgery. Injury, 17:271–273, 1986.
198. Mallory, T.H., Kraus, T.J., Vaughn, B.K.: Intraoperative Femoral Fractures Associated With Cementless Total Hip Arthroplasty. Orthopedics, 12:231–239, 1989.
199. Mankin, H.J., Friedlander, G.E.: Biology of Bone Grafts. Bone Stock Deficiency in Total Hip Replacement. Thorofare, NJ, Slack, 1989.
200. Marega, T., Feroldi, G., Marega, L.: Our Experience With the Uncemented Isoelastic Total Hip Prosthesis. [Italian]. Arch. Putti Chir. Organi Mov., 37:65–75, 1989.
201. Marmor, L.: Stress Fracture of the Pubic Ramus Simulating a Loose Total Hip Replacement. Clin. Orthop., 121:103, 1976.
202. McElfresh, E.C., and Coventry, M.B.: Femoral and Pelvic Fractures After Total Hip Arthroplasty. J. Bone Joint Surg., 56A:483–492, 1974.
203. McKee, G.K., and Chen, S.C.: The Statistics of the McKee-Farrar Method of Total Hip Replacement. Clin. Orthop., 95:26–33, 1973.
204. Mihalko, W.M., Beaudoin, A.J., Cardea, J.A., Krause, W.R.: Finite-Element Modelling of Femoral Shaft Fracture Fixation Techniques Post Total Hip Arthroplasty. J. Biomech., 25:469–476, 1992.
205. Miller, A.J.: Late Fracture of the Acetabulum After Total Hip Replacement. J. Bone Joint Surg., 54B:600–606, 1972.
206. Moczynski, G., Abraham, E., Barmada, R., Ray, R.D.: Evaluation of Total Hip Replacement Arthroplasties. Clin. Orthop., 95:213–216, 1973.
207. Mont, M.A., and Maar, D.C.: Fractures of the Ipsilateral Femur After Hip Arthroplasty: A Statistical Analysis of Outcome Based on 487 Patients. J. Arthroplasty, 9:511–519, 1994.
208. Mont, M.A., Maar, D.C., Krackow, K.A., Hungerford, D.S.: Hoop-Stress Fractures of the Proximal Femur During Hip Arthroplasty: Management and Results in 19 Cases. J. Bone Joint Surg., 74B:257–260, 1992.
209. Montijo, H., Ebert, F.R., Lennox, D.A.: Treatment of Proximal Femur Fractures Associated With Total Hip Arthroplasty. J. Arthroplasty, 4:115–123, 1989.
210. Moroni, A., Ruggeri, N.: Le fratture intraoperatorie di femore in corso di protesizzazione d'anca. Chir. Organi Mov., 66:703–713, 1980.
211. Morrey, B.F., Kavanagh, B.F.: Comparison of Cemented and Uncemented Femoral Revision Total Arthroplasty: Analysis of Complications and Reoperations. Orthopaedic Transactions, 13:496, 1989.
212. Morrey, B.F., and Kavanagh, B.F.: Complications With Revision of the Femoral Component of Total Hip Arthroplasty. Comparison Between Cemented and Uncemented Techniques. J. Arthroplasty, 7:71–79, 1992.
213. Morscher, E., and Masar, Z.: Development and First Experience With an Uncemented Press-Fit Cup. Clin. Orthop., 232:96–103, 1988.
214. Moss, A.J., Hamburger, S., Moore, R.M., and colleagues: Use of Selected Medical Device Implants in the United States, 1988.
215. Moyen, B.J.-L., Lahey, P.J., Weinberg, E.H., Harris, W.H.: Effects on Intact Femora of Dogs of the Application and Removal of Metal Plates. J. Bone Joint Surg., 60A:940, 1978.
216. Murray, W.R.: Results in Patients With Total Hip Replacement Arthroplasty. Clin. Orthop., 95:80, 1973.
217. Nolan, D.R., Fitzgerald, R.H., Beckenbaugh, R.D., Coventry, M.B.: Complications of Total Hip Arthroplasty Treated by Reoperation. J. Bone Joint Surg., 57A:977, 1975.
218. Oh, I., and Hardacre, J.A.: Fatigue Fracture of the Inferior Pubic Ramus Following Total Hip Replacement for Congenital Hip Dislocation. Clin. Orthop., 147:154–156, 1980.
219. Olerud, S.: Reconstruction of a Fractured Femur Following Total Hip Replacement. J. Bone Joint Surg., 61A:937, 1979.
220. Olerud, S.: Hip Arthroplasty With Extended Femoral Stem for Salvage Procedures. Clin. Orthop., 191:64, 1984.
221. Overgaard, S., Jensen, T.T., Bonde, G., Mossing, N.B.: The Uncemented Bipolar Hemiarthroplasty for Displaced Femoral Neck Fractures. 6-Year Follow-Up of 171 Cases. Acta Orthop. Scand., 62:115–120, 1991.
222. Pankovich, A.M., Thrabishy, I., Barmada, R.: Fractures Below Non-Cemented Femoral Implants. J. Bone Joint Surg., 63A:1024, 1981.

223. Parrish, T.F., and Jones, J.R.: Fracture of the Femur Following Prosthetic Arthroplasty of the Hip. J. Bone Joint Surg., 46A:241, 1964.
224. Patterson, F.P., and Brown, C.S.: The McKee-Farrar Total Hip Replacement: Preliminary Results and Complications of 368 Operations Performed in Five General Hospitals. J. Bone Joint Surg., 54A:257, 1972.
225. Pazzaglia, U., and Byers, P.D.: Fractured Femoral Shaft Through an Osteolytic Lesion Resulting From the Reaction to a Prosthesis: A Case Report. J. Bone Joint Surg., 66B:337–339, 1984.
226. Pellici, P.M., Inglis, A.E., Salvati, E.A.: Perforation of the Femoral Shaft During Total Hip Replacement: Report of 12 Cases. J. Bone Joint Surg., 62A:234–240, 1980.
227. Pellici, P.M., Wilson, P.D.J., Sledge, C.B., and colleagues: Revision Total Hip Arthroplasty. Clin. Orthop., 170:34, 1982.
228. Penenberg, B.L.: Femoral Fractures Below Hip Implants. A New and Safe Technique of Fixation. Orthopaedic Transactions, 13:496, 1989.
229. Petty, W. (ed.): Total Joint Replacement, pp. 291–314. Philadelphia, WB Saunders, 1991.
230. Poss, R., Walker, P., Spector, M., Reilly, D.T., Robertson, D.D., Sledge, C.B.: Strategies for Improving Fixation of Femoral Components in Total Hip Arthroplasty. Clin. Orthop., 235:181–194, 1988.
231. Praemer, A., Furner, S., Rice, D.P.: Musculoskeletal Conditions in the United States, p. 199. Park Ridge, IL, American Academy of Orthopaedic Surgeons, 1992.
232. Ranawat, C.S., and Greenberg, R.: Tripartite Fracture of the Acetabulum After Total Hip Arthroplasty: A Case Report. Clin. Orthop., 155:48–51, 1981.
233. Ritschl, P., and Kotz, R.: Fractures of the Proximal Femur in Patients With Total Hip Endoprostheses. Arch. Orthop. Trauma Surg., 104:392–397, 1986.
234. Roffman, M., and Mendes, D.G.: Fracture of the Femur After Total Hip Arthroplasty. Orthopedics, 12:1067–1070, 1989.
235. Schenk, R.K., and Wehril, U.: Reaction of Bone to a Cement-Free SL Femoral Stem Used in Revision Arthroplasty. [German]. Orthopade, 18:454–462, 1989.
236. Scher, M.A.: Fractures of the Femoral Shaft Following Total Hip Replacement. J. Bone Joint Surg., 63B:472, 1981.
237. Schmalzried, T.P., Jasty, M., Harris, W.H.: Periprosthetic Bone Loss in Total Hip Arthroplasty. J. Bone Joint Surg., 74A:849–863, 1992.
238. Schmalzried, T.P., Wessinger, S.J., Hill, G.E., Harris, W.H.: The Harris-Galante Porous Acetabular Component Press-Fit Without Screw Fixation. Five-Year Radiographic Analysis of Primary Cases. J. Arthroplasty, 9:235–242, 1994.
239. Schnitzler, C.M.: Bone Formation, Bone Resorption and Bone Mineralisation in Osteoarthritis and Osteoporosis. J. Bone Joint Surg., 61B.257, 1979.
240. Schulte, K.R., Callaghan, J.J., Kelley, S.S.: The Outcome of Charnley Total Hip Arthroplasty With Cement After a Minimum Twenty Year Follow-Up. The Results of One Surgeon. J. Bone Joint Surg., 75A:961–975, 1993.
241. Schwartz, J.J., Mayer, J.G., Engh, C.A.: Femoral Fracture During Non-Cemented Total Hip Arthroplasty. J. Bone Joint Surg. [Am], 71:1135–1142, 1989.
242. Scott, R.D., Turner, R.H., Leitzes, S.M., Aufranc, O.E.: Femoral Fractures in Conjunction With Total Hip Replacement. J. Bone Joint Surg., 57A:494–501, 1975A.
243. Selakovich, W., and Love, L.: Stress Fractures of the Pubic Ramus. J. Bone Joint Surg., 36A:573–576, 1954.
244. Serocki, J.H., Chandler, R.W., Dorr, L.D.: Treatment of Fractures About Hip Prostheses With Compression Plating. J. Arthroplasty, 7:129–135, 1992.
245. Sharkey, P.F., Hozack, W.J., Booth, R.E., Rothman, R.H.: Intraoperative Femoral Fractures in Cementless Total Hip Arthroplasty. Orthop. Rev., 21:337–342, 1992.
246. Sim, F.H., Chao, E.Y.S.: Hip Salvage by Proximal Femoral Replacement. J. Bone Joint Surg., 63A:1228, 1981.
247. Sleeswijk Visser, S.V.: Accidental Femoral Shaft Fractures Following Hip Arthroplasty of the Same Leg. [Dutch]. Ned. Tijdschr. Geneesk., 124:962–964, 1980.
248. Springfield, D.S.: Massive Autogenous Bone Grafts. Orthop. Clin. North Am., 18:249–256, 1987.
249. Stern, R.E., Harwin, S.F., Kulick, R.G.: Management of Ipsilateral Femoral Shaft Fractures Following Hip Arthroplasty. Orthop. Rev., 20:779–784, 1991.
250. Stuchin, S.A.: Femoral Shaft Fracture in Porous and Press-Fit Total Hip Arthroplasty. Orthop. Rev., 19:153–159, 1990.
251. Sydney, S.V., and Mallory, T.H.: Controlled Perforation. A Safe Method of Cement Removal From the Femoral Canal. Clin. Orthop., 253:168–172, 1990.
252. Talab, Y.A., States, J.D., Evarts, C.M.: Femoral Shaft Perforation. A Complication of Total Hip Reconstruction. Clin. Orthop., 141:158–165, 1979.
253. Taylor, M.M., Meyers, M.H., Harvey, J.P.: Intraoperative Femur Fractures During Total Hip Replacement. Clin. Orthop., 137:96–103, 1978.
254. Tomford, W.W., Thongphasuk, J., Mankin, H.J., Ferraro, M.J.: Frozen Musculoskeletal Allografts: A Study of the Clinical Incidence and Causes of Infection Associated With Their Use. J. Bone Joint Surg., 72A:1137–1143, 1990.
255. Toni, A., Giunti, A., Graci, A., and colleagues: Fratture Post-Operatorie del Femore Prossimale con Protesi D'anca. Chir. Organi Mov., 70:53–65, 1985.
256. Torgerson, W.R.: Three Years Experience With Total Hip Replacement. Clin. Orthop., 95:151–157, 1973.
257. Van Elegem, P., and Blaimont, P.: Les Fractures Femorales et Cotyloidiennes sur Prostheses de la Hanche. Acta Orthop. Belg., 45:299–309, 1979.
258. Vaughn, B.K., and Mallory, T.H.: Porous Coated Anatomic Cementless Total Hip Replacement—Clinical and Roentgenographic Results With Minimum Two-Year Follow Up. Orthopaedic Transactions, 12:696, 1988.
259. Vicenzi, G., Moroni, A., Ponziani, L.: An Unusual Case of Proximal Femoral Fracture in a Patient With a Total Hip Prosthesis. [Italian]. Chir. Organi Mov., 73:161–163, 1988.
260. Wagner, H.: Revisionsprothese fur das Huftgelenk. Orthopade, 18:438–453, 1989.
261. Wang, G.J., Miller, T.O., Stamp, W.G.: Femoral Fracture Following Hip Arthroplasty. J. Bone Joint Surg., 67A:956–957, 1985.
262. Wehrli, U.: Wagner Cement-Free Revision Stem. [German]. Z. Unfallchir. Versicherungsmed., 84:216–224, 1991.
263. Welch, R.B., and Charnley, J.: Low-Friction Arthroplasty of the Hip in Rheumatoid Arthritis Patients and Ankylosing Spondylitis. Clin. Orthop., 72:22, 1972.
264. Whitesides, L.A.: Impact Modular Total Hip System. Warsaw, IN, Biomet, Inc., 1994.
265. Whittaker, R.P., Sotos, L.N., Ralston, E.L.: Fractures of the Femur About Femoral Endoprostheses. J. Trauma, 14:675, 1974.
266. Wroblewski, B.M., Browne, A.O., Hodgkinson, J.P.: Treatment of Fracture of the Shaft of the Femur in Total Hip Arthroplasty by a Combination of a Kuntscher Nail and a Modified Cemented Charnley Stem. Injury, 23:225–227, 1992.
267. Zenni, E.J., Pomeroy, D.L., Caudle, R.J.: Ogden Plate and Other Fixations for Fractures Complicating Femoral Endoprostheses. Clin. Orthop., 231.83–90, 1988.
268. Zuber, K., Jutzi, J., Ganz, R.: Bilateral Femoral Fracture at the Site of Bilateral Hip Prostheses. A Case Report. [German]. Unfallchirurg, 95:240–242, 1992.
269. Zuber, K., Koch, P., Lustenberger, A., Ganz, R.: Femoral Fractures Following Total Hip Prosthesis. [German]. Unfallchirurg, 93:467–472, 1990.

PERIPROSTHETIC FRACTURES OF THE KNEE

270. A.A.O.S., Committee on Scientific Investigation: Preliminary Survey on Femoral Head Prostheses. J. Bone Joint Surg., 35A:489–494, 1953.
271. Aaron, R.K., and Scott, R.S.: Supracondylar Fracture of the Femur After Total Knee Arthroplasty. Clin. Orthop., 219:136–139, 1987.
272. Barth, R.W., and Lane, J.M.: Osteoporosis. Orthop. Clin. North Am., 19:845–858, 1988.
273. Bogoch, E., Hastings, D., Gross, A., Gschwend, N.: Supracon-

dylar Fractures of the Femur Adjacent to Resurfacing and MacIntosh Arthroplasties of the Knee in Patients With Rheumatoid Arthritis. Clin. Orthop., 229:213–220, 1988.
274. Brick, G.W., Scott, R.D.: The Patellofemoral Component of Total Knee Arthroplasty. Clin. Orthop., 231:163–178, 1988.
275. Cain, P.R., Rubash, H.E., Wissinger, H.A., McClain, E.J.: Periprosthetic Femoral Fractures Following Total Knee Arthroplasty. Clin. Orthop., 208:205–214, 1986.
276. Chen, F., Mont, M.A., Bachner, R.S.: Management of Ipsilateral Supracondylar Femur Fractures Following Total Knee Arthroplasty. J. Arthroplasty, 9:521–526, 1994.
277. Clayton, M.L., and Thirupathi, R.: Patellar Complications After Total Condylar Arthroplasty. Clin. Orthop., 170:152–155, 1982.
278. Convery, F.R., Minteer-Convery, M., Malcom, L.L.: The Spherocentric Knee: A Re-Evaluation and Modification. J. Bone Joint Surg., 62A:320–327, 1980.
279. Cordeiro, E.N., Costa, R.C., Carazzato, J.G., Silva, J.D.S.: Periprosthetic Fractures in Patients With Total Knee Arthroplasties. Clin. Orthop., 252:182–189, 1990.
280. Courpied, J.P., Watin-Augouard, L., Postel, M.: Fractures du Femur Chez les Sujets Porteurs de Prostheses Totales de Hanche ou de Genou. Int. Orthop., 11:109–115, 1987.
281. Culp, R.W., Schmidt, R.G., Hanks, G., Mak, A., Esterhai, J.L., Heppenstall, R.B.: Supracondylar Fracture of the Femur Following Prosthetic Knee Arthroplasty. Clin. Orthop., 222:212–222, 1987.
282. Delport, P.H., Van Audekercke, R., Martens, M.: Conservative Treatment of Ipsilateral Supracondylar Femoral Fracture After Total Knee Arthroplasty. J. Trauma, 24:846–849, 1984.
283. DiGioia, A.M., and Rubash, H.E.: Periprosthetic Fractures of the Femur After Total Knee Arthroplasty: A Literature Review and Treatment Algorithm. Clin. Orthop., 271:135–142, 1991.
284. Figgie, H.E.I., Goldberg, V.M., Figgie, M.P., Inglis, A.E., Kelly, M., Sobel, M.: The Effect of Alignment of the Implant on Fractures of the Patella After Condylar Total Knee Arthroplasty. J. Bone Joint Surg., 71A:1031–1039, 1989.
285. Figgie, M.P., Goldberg, V.M., Figgie, H.E., III: The Results of Treatment of Supracondylar Fracture Above Total Knee Arthroplasty. J. Arthroplasty, 5:267–276, 1990.
286. Goldberg, V.M., Figgie, H.E. III, Inglis, A.E., and colleagues: Patellar Fracture Type and Prognosis in Condylar Total Knee Arthroplasty. Clin. Orthop., 236:115–122, 1988.
287. Grace, J.N., and Sim, F.H.: Fracture of the Patella After Total Knee Arthroplasty. Clin. Orthop., 230:168–175, 1988.
288. Grob, D., Gschwend, N.: Periprothetische Frakturen Nach Totalersatz des Kniegelenkes. Orthopade, 11:109, 1982.
289. Groth, H.E., and Fitch, H.F.: Salvage Procedures for Complications of Total Ankle Arthroplasty. Clin Orthop, 224:244–250, 1987.
290. Hanks, G.A., Mathews, H.H., Routson, G.W., Loughran, T.P.: Supracondylar Fracture of the Femur Following Total Knee Arthroplasty. J. Arthroplasty, 4:289–292, 1989.
291. Healy, W.L., Siliski, J.M., Incavo, S.J.: Operative Treatment of Distal Femoral Fractures Proximal to Total Knee Replacements. J. Bone Joint Surg., 75A:27–34, 1993.
292. Hirsh, D.M., Bhalla, S., Roffman, M.: Supracondylar Fracture of the Femur Following Total Knee Replacement: Report of Four Cases. J. Bone Joint Surg., 63A:162–163, 1981.
293. Hood, R.W., Vanni, M., Insall, J.N.: The Correction of Knee Alignment in 225 Consecutive Total Condylar Knee Replacements. Clin. Orthop., 160:94–105, 1981.
294. Insall, J.N., Lachiewicz, P.F., Burstein, A.H.: The Posterior Stabilized Condylar Prosthesis: A Modification of the Total Condylar Design. Two to Four-Year Clinical Experience. J. Bone Joint Surg., 64A:1317–1323, 1982.
295. Jabczenski, F.F., and Crawford, M.: Retrograde Intramedullary Nailing of Supracondylar Femur Fractures Above Total Knee Arthroplasty. J. Arthroplasty, 10:95–101, 1995.
296. Jahn, K., and Siegling, C.W.: Femurfrakturen bei Totalondoprosthesenplastiken. Zentralbl. Chir., 106:463–468, 1981.
297. Kayler, D.E., and Lyttle, D.: Surgical Interruption of Patellar Blood Supply by Total Knee Arthroplasty. Clin. Orthop., 229:221–227, 1988.
298. Kitaoka, H.B., Patzer, G.L., Ilstrup, D.M., Wallrichs, S.L.: Survivorship Analysis of the Mayo Total Ankle Arthroplasty. J. Bone Joint Surg., 76A:974–979, 1994.
299. Kitaoka, H.B., and Romness, D.W.: Arthrodesis for Failed Ankle Arthroplasty. J. Arthroplasty, 7:277–284, 1992.
300. Kraay, M.J., Goldberg, V.M., Figgie, M.P., Figgie H.E. III: Distal Femoral Replacement With Allograft/Prosthetic Reconstruction for Treatment of Supracondylar Fractures in Patients With Total Knee Arthroplasty. J. Arthroplasty, 7:7–16, 1992.
301. Lotke, P.A., and Ecker, M.L.: Influence of Positioning of Prosthesis in Total Knee Replacement. J. Bone Joint Surg., 59A:77–79, 1977.
302. Martens, M., van Audekercke, R., de Meester, P., Mulier, J.C.: The Mechanical Characteristics of the Long Bones of the Lower Extremity in Torsional Loading. J. Biomech., 13:667–676, 1980.
303. McGuire, M.R., Kyle, R.F., Gustilo, R.B., Premer, R.F.: Comparative Analysis of Ankle Arthroplasty Versus Ankle Arthrodesis. Clin. Orthop., 226:174–181, 1988.
304. McLaren, A.C., Dupont, J.A., Schroeber, D.C.: Open Reduction Internal Fixation of Supracondylar Fractures Above Total Knee Arthroplasties Using the Intramedullary Supracondylar Rod. Clin. Orthop., 302:194–198, 1994.
305. McMahon, M.S., Scuderi, G.R., Glashow, J.L., Scharf, S.C., Meltzer, L.P., Scott, W.N.: Scintigraphic Determination of Patellar Viability After Excision of Infrapatellar Fat Pad and/or Lateral Retinacular Release in Total Knee Arthroplasty. Clin. Orthop., 260:10–16, 1990.
306. Merkel, K.D., and Johnson, E.W.: Supracondylar Fracture of the Femur After Total Knee Arthroplasty. J. Bone Joint Surg., 68A:29–43, 1986.
307. Moreland, J.R.: Mechanisms of Failure in Total Knee Arthroplasty. Clin. Orthop., 226:49–77, 1988.
308. Moss, A.J., Hamburger, S., Moore, R.M., and colleagues: Use of Selected Medical Device Implants in the United States, 1988.
309. Neer, C., Grantom, S., Shelton, M.: Supracondylar Fracture of the Adult Femur. J. Bone Joint Surg., 49A:591, 1967.
310. Nielsen, B.F., Petersen, V.S., Varmarken, J.E.: Fracture of the Femur After Knee Arthroplasty. Acta Orthop. Scand., 59:155–157, 1988.
311. Oni, O.O.: Supracondylar Fracture of the Femur Following Attenborough Stabilized Gliding Knee Arthroplasty. Injury, 14:250–251, 1982.
312. Praemer, A., Furner, S., Rice, D.P.: Musculoskeletal Conditions in the United States, p. 199. Park Ridge, IL, American Academy of Orthopaedic Surgeons, 1992.
313. Rand, J.A.: The Patellofemoral Joint in Total Knee Arthroplasty. J. Bone Joint Surg., 76A:612–620, 1994.
314. Rand, J.A.: Supracondylar Fracture of the Femur Associated With Polyethylene Wear After Total Knee Arthroplasty. J. Bone Joint Surg., 76A:1389–1393, 1994.
315. Rand, J.A., and Coventry, M.B.: Stress Fractures After Total Knee Arthroplasty. J. Bone Joint Surg., 62A:226–233, 1980.
316. Rhinelander, F.W.: Circulation in Bone, pp. 1–77. Academic Press, 1972.
317. Rinecker, H., and Hailbock, H.: Surgical Treatment of Peri-Prosthetic Fractures After Total Knee Replacement. Arch. Orthop. Unfallchir., 87:23, 1977.
318. Ritter, M., Faris, P., Keating, E.: Anterior Femoral Notching and Ipsilateral Supracondylar Femur Fracture in Total Knee Arthroplasty. J. Arthroplasty, 3:185, 1988.
319. Ritter, M.A., and Campbell, E.D.: Postoperative Patellar Complications With or Without Lateral Release During Total Knee Arthroplasty. Clin. Orthop., 219:163–168, 1987.
320. Ritter, M.A., and Stiver, P.: Supracondylar Fracture in a Patient With Total Knee Arthroplasty: A Case Report. Clin. Orthop., 193:168–170, 1985.
321. Roscoe, M.W., Goodman, S.B., Schatzker, J.: Supracondylar Fracture of the Femur After GUEPAR Total Knee Arthroplasty: A New Treatment Method. Clin. Orthop., 222:221–223, 1989.
322. Schatzker, J., and Lambert, D.C.: Supracondylar Fractures of the Femur. Clin. Orthop., 138:77–83, 1979.
323. Scott, R.D., Turoff, N., Ewald, F.C.: Stress Fracture of the Pa-

tella Following Duopatellar Total Knee Arthroplasty With Patellar Resurfacing. Clin. Orthop., 170:147–151, 1982.

324. Scuderi, G., Scharf, S.C., Meltzer, L.P., Scott, W.N.: The Relationship of Lateral Releases to Patellar Viability in Total Knee Arthroplasty. J. Arthroplasty, 2:209–214, 1987.
325. Sekel, R., and Newman, A.S.: Supracondylar Fractures Above a Total Knee Arthroplasty: A Novel Use of the Huckstep Nail. J. Arthroplasty, 9:445–447, 1994.
326. Short, W.H., Hootnick, D.R., Murray, D.G.: Ipsilateral Supracondylar Femur Fractures Following Knee Arthroplasty. Clin. Orthop., 158:111–116, 1981.
327. Sisto, D.J., Lachiewicz, P.F., Insall, J.N.: Treatment of Supracondylar Fractures Following Prosthetic Arthroplasty of the Knee. Clin. Orthop., 196:265–272, 1985.
328. Smith, W., Mabrey, J.D., Martin, S.L.: Use of a Supracondylar Nail for Treatment of a Supracondylar Fracture of the Femur Following Total Knee Arthroplasty: A Case Report. J. Arthroplasty, in press.
329. Sonstegard, D.A., Kaufer, H., Matthews, L.S.: The Spherocentric Knee: Biomechanical Testing and Clinical Trial. J. Bone Joint Surg., 59A:602–616, 1977.
330. Steinbrink, K., Engelbrecht, E., Fenelon, G.C.C.: The Total Femoral Prosthesis. A Preliminary Report. J. Bone Joint Surg., 64B:305, 1982.
331. Takakura, Y., Tanaka, Y., Sugimoto, K., Tamai, S., Masuhara, K.: Ankle Arthroplasty. A Comparative Study of Cemented Metal and Uncemented Ceramic Prostheses. Clin Orthop, 252:209–216, 1990.
332. Webster, D.A., and Murray, D.G.: Complications of Variable Axis Total Knee Arthroplasty. Clin. Orthop., 193:160–167, 1985.
333. Wetzner, S.M., Bezreh, J.S., Scott, R.D., Bierbaum, B.E., Newberg, A.H.: Bone Scanning in the Assessment of Patellar Viability Following Knee Replacement. Clin. Orthop., 199: 215–219, 1985.
334. Wynn, A.H., and Wilde, A.H.: Long-Term Follow-Up of the Conaxial (Beck-Steffee) Total Ankle Arthroplasty. Foot Ankle, 13:303–306, 1992.
335. Zehntner, M.K.: Internal Fixation of Supracondylar Fractures After Condylar Total Knee Arthroplasty. Clin. Orthop., 293:219–224, 1993.
336. Zvaifler, N.J.: Epidemiology of Rheumatoid Arthritis. Primer on the Rheumatic Diseases. Atlanta, GA, Arthritis Foundation, 1988.

Upper Extremity

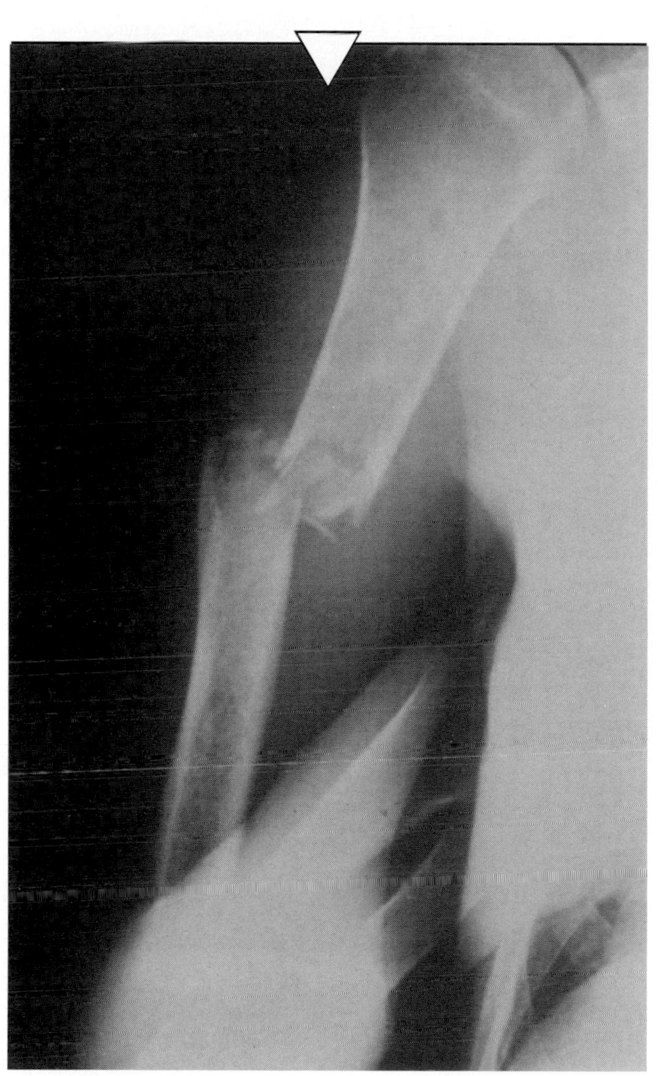

Rockwood and Green's Fractures in Adults, Fourth Edition,
edited by Charles A. Rockwood, David P. Green, Robert W. Bucholz and James D. Heckman.
Lippincott-Raven Publishers, Philadelphia © 1996.

CHAPTER 11

Fractures and Dislocations in the Hand

David P. Green and Thomas E. Butler, Jr.

Although accurate figures of relative incidence are difficult to derive, fractures of the metacarpals and phalanges are probably the most common fractures in the skeletal system. In 1962, Butt[68] reviewed 200,000 Workers' Compensation injuries and noted that fractures of the hand comprised 30% of the cases settled and were the most frequently encountered fractures. Emmett and Breck,[114] in their comprehensive review of 11,000 consecutive fractures treated in a busy private practice, found that fractures of the phalanges and metacarpals comprised 10% of the total.

Lamb[215] said that in the District General Hospitals of the British National Health Service, hand injuries were involved in one third of all injuries and 14% of all medical and surgical emergencies. In another report from a single District General Hospital,[293] 28% of all patients were seen for hand injuries.

The causes of hand injuries are as numerous as the activities man has created for work and leisure activity, but age appears to be a definite factor in the likelihood of sustaining a fracture in the hand (Table 11-1).

Perhaps because they are so common and because they occur in small bones and are therefore considered minor injuries, these fractures are often relegated for treatment to the more inexperienced members of the medical team. The results of treatment of fractures in the hand are not universally good[24] and the incidence of stiffness, malunion, and prolonged functional disability and economic loss is striking. As Quigley and Urist[309] noted, nowhere in the body are motion and function more closely related to anatomic structure than in the hand.

Who should treat hand fractures remains somewhat controversial. Maitra and Burdett-Smith[239] concluded that simple fractures of the proximal phalanges (excluding articular, oblique, comminuted, and open fractures) could be managed by accident and emergency physicians. Conversely, Davis and Stothard[96] found that the treatment of finger fractures by accident and emergency staff was inappropriate in 27% of patients in a retrospective series. Inaccurate reduction and unsatisfactory splinting were among the most common errors. Not surprisingly, the former authors were emergency room physicians, the latter orthopaedic surgeons.

TABLE 11-1
Most Common Causes of Phalangeal Fractures (From an analysis of 6,857 phalangeal fractures[97])

Age Group	Most Common Cause	% Within That Group
0–9	Compression (e.g. catching finger in a door)	41.8%
10–19	Sports related injury	43.0%
20–29	Sports related injury	27.8%
30–39	Sports related injury	21.6%
	Machinery	19.1%
40–49	Machinery	26.7%
50–59	Machinery	27.8%
60–69	Machinery	26.9%
	Accidental fall	24.3%
>70	Accidental fall	45.5%

Other causes included: motor vehicle accidents; falling/cutting object; and unspecified.

GENERAL PRINCIPLES OF MANAGEMENT

Initial Evaluation

The initial evaluation and primary care of an injured hand are critical, providing the surgeon the best opportunity to assess accurately the extent of damage and to restore the altered anatomy. Many authors have observed that the fate of the hand largely depends on the judgment of the physician who first sees the patient.

Maximum functional recovery must be the goal in every hand injury, which can be achieved only by considering the injury in relation to the patient's needs and lifestyle. His or her age, hand dominance, and occupation are critical factors, and the opening sentence of the history of any patient with an injured hand should record this information, as in the following example: "A 45-year-old right-handed electrician. . . ." Knowledge of the patient's avocations or hobbies also is important because a clerk or stockbroker may be an accomplished musician or an amateur carpenter.

Precise details about the injury should be obtained. How did it occur (ie, what was the mechanism of injury)? Was it a crushing, tearing, or twisting injury or a clean laceration? A human bite is a notoriously dangerous injury, and a short, curved laceration over a small joint in the hand must be immediately suspected of having been caused by a tooth. Where did the injury occur? Did it take place in a relatively clean environment or was it in a stable or a greasy garage? Did it occur on the job or elsewhere? This finding has important financial implications to the patient and may have significant bearing on the outcome. How much time has elapsed since the injury? What has been done in the interim? Has any treatment been given and by whom?

Physical Examination

Some fractures and dislocations may be immediately obvious because of local swelling and deformity. Angulation and displacement are often readily apparent but in fractures of the metacarpals and phalanges, it is even more important to recognize rotational malalignment.

One of the greatest pitfalls in treating injuries of the hand is to focus on the obvious fracture and overlook more subtle but often more significant damage to soft tissues. The precise area of tenderness must always be determined to accurately assess the damage to soft tissues and bone. For example, if the patient has a swollen proximal interphalangeal (PIP) joint, it is imperative to ascertain whether the maximum tenderness is over the collateral ligaments laterally or over the central slip insertion dorsally. Careful assessment must be made of an open wound regarding its precise location, its relation to skin creases, the direction and viability of skin flaps, the extent of actual skin loss, and the degree of contamination of the wound. An open wound should not be probed or handled excessively; gentle inspection with sterile instruments and gloves gives sufficient preliminary information until a thorough exploration can be done in the operating room. Damage to nerves and tendons can usually be determined by careful motor and sensory testing rather than by probing of the wound in the emergency room.

Both open and closed injuries must be examined meticulously for injury to adjacent tendons, nerves, and blood vessels. Precarious circulation may be particularly subtle in closed injuries and must be assessed by noting color and temperature, capillary filling, and patency of collateral circulation by Allen's test[1] at the wrist and in the digit.[267]

Satisfactory physical examination may not be possible without local or regional anesthesia, but the block should be postponed until an initial assessment of nerves and blood vessels has been made in the unanesthetized hand.

Radiographic Examination

Radiographs are essential in virtually all injuries of the hand, even if no bone injury is obvious on clinical examination. Many significant fractures and joint injuries are missed simply because adequate x-rays were not taken on the day of injury. At least three views are necessary: posteroanterior (PA), lateral, and oblique. Oblique films are particularly helpful in accurately assessing intra-articular fractures. For injuries involving a finger, a true lateral view of the individual digit is mandatory. Superimposition of the other fingers on a lateral view of the entire hand obscures significant details that are easily seen on a lateral view of the single digit. Throughout this chapter, many special views are mentioned that may provide additional information in specific anatomic sites.

Again, the temptation is great to concentrate on obvious abnormalities in the x-rays and overlook important but more obscure injuries. For example, one or more carpometacarpal (CMC) joints may be subluxated or dislocated when there is a displaced or angulated fracture of an adjacent metacarpal.

Foreign Bodies

It is always reasonable to suspect the presence of foreign bodies in all open or penetrating wounds. Radiographs alone cannot be relied on to identify foreign bodies because wood splinters, most types of glass, and many other foreign contaminants are not radiopaque. At one time, xerography was a favorite technique for showing foreign bodies but this modality apparently emits a high level of irradiation, and these machines have disappeared from radiology departments with the advent of more sophisticated technology.[72,399] The radiologists with whom we work recommend a low-kV mammographic film as the initial screening test in searching for a foreign body (Robert Cone, personal communication, 1995). Russell and coworkers[327] compared various methods and offered practical guidelines for detecting different types of foreign bodies:

1. If glass or gravel is suspected, a routine plain film using soft-tissue technique is the first step.
2. Plastic is only faintly seen on a computed tomography (CT) scan but may contain paint or other material that is visible on plain radiographs.
3. Glass is well seen by CT, magnetic resonance imaging (MRI), and xerography.
4. CT is the preferred method for wood and thorns.[26]
5. MRI is the final backup for all types of foreign bodies except gravel because ferromagnetic streak artifacts in gravel obscure the image.

Although probably not as accurate as MRI and CT, ultrasound offers a less costly method.[130,138,224] These various modalities should be used only when really necessary because they are expensive. In January 1995, the relative costs for these tests in our hospital were low-KV mammography, $72; ultrasound, $182; CT scan, $442; and MRI, $700 to $1500.

Anesthesia for Hand Injuries

Hand injuries cannot be treated properly without adequate anesthesia. Sometimes anesthesia may be necessary to obtain a satisfactory examination but in virtually all cases, manipulation or reduction requires complete relief of pain. General anesthesia is rarely necessary unless the patient has concomitant injuries that require it. Axillary or brachial block provides excellent anesthesia but is more than is generally required. Intravenous lidocaine (Bier block) provides good muscle relaxation and relief of pain.

We prefer to do most of our fracture manipulations and reductions under regional or digital block. Perhaps the most useful of these is a combined median and radial nerve block at the wrist, which provides excellent anesthesia for the thumb and index and long fingers. We prefer to block the ulnar nerve at the wrist, where it is necessary to add a wheal to block the dorsal sensory branch. If anesthesia of an individual finger is desired, digital block is adequate but care must be taken to avoid injecting anesthetic solution circumferentially around the base of the finger because of the likelihood of vascular impairment. A metacarpal block at the level of the palmar crease or precise injection of each of the four digital nerves from the dorsum of the finger just distal to the metacarpophalangeal (MP) joint is preferable. Epinephrine should never be used with any local anesthetic agent in the hand because vascular compromise can result. (Moore's[272] book on regional anesthesia is an excellent source of reference for reviewing the techniques of nerve blocks.)

Small wounds can be adequately anesthetized with local infiltration but we prefer not to use a local to manipulate closed fractures. When local anesthesia is employed, edema of the tissues can be minimized by adding one vial of hyaluronidase (Wydase) to each 30 mL of anesthetic solution. The addition of 10% bicarbonate solution to the local anesthetic agent neutralizes the pH and may reduce the burning sensation during injection.

Proper Use of Facilities

Closed injuries in the hand are easily treated in the emergency room, plaster room, or office if the proper precautions are taken. If any type of intravenous or regional anesthesia is used, resuscitation equipment must be immediately available, such as an airway device, Ambu bag, and intravenous drugs. Complications from the use of lidocaine and other local anesthetics are uncommon but when they occur, the physician must be prepared to provide treatment for shock, seizures, and allergic reactions.

OPEN FRACTURES

All open fractures demand appropriate wound management. This means thorough cleansing with a soap solution and irrigation—a suitable surgical prep. Extensive open fractures and other injuries that require debridement or more than minimal dissection should be treated in the operating room.

Classification of Open Fractures in the Hand

Gustillo's classification of open fractures and its subsequent modifications (see Chap. 6) has been widely accepted by orthopaedic surgeons. After reviewing a large series of patients having hand fractures, however, Swanson and coworkers[371] concluded that Gustillo's classification is not readily applicable to open fractures in the hand. Because their study indicated that the key factors influencing an increased likelihood of infection were wound contamination, delay in treatment longer than 24 hours, and systemic illness, they offered a separate classification for open fractures in the hand (Table 11-2).

In their series, the infection rate was not increased by the use of internal fixation, immediate wound closure, large wound size, associated soft-tissue injuries, or high-energy mechanism. It should be noted, however, that all of their patients were treated with careful adherence to sound principles of open fracture management.

McLain and coworkers[252] cited similar risk factors in their study of open fractures, but they concluded that extensive soft-tissue injury was a more important determinant of potential infection. Not surprisingly, many of their patients with infected wounds had prolonged convalescence and permanent impairment.

Delay in treatment has long been considered to be a risk factor. McLain and coworkers[252] found that delay of more than 12 hours did not increase the incidence of infection, but Swanson and coworkers'[371] study showed that delay of more than 24 hours was a risk factor.

Antibiotics

The need for antibiotics in the management of open fractures in the hand is controversial. Antibiotics have become such an accepted part of the management of

TABLE 11-2
Classification for Open Fractures of the Hand

TYPE I
Clean wound without significant contamination or delay in treatment
No significant systemic illness
TYPE II (ANY ONE OR MORE OF THE FOLLOWING)
Contamination with gross dirt/debris
Human or animal bites
Warm lake/river injury
Barnyard injury
Delay in treatment longer than 24 hours
Significant systemic illness (including diabetes)

Swanson, T.V., Szabo, R.M., and Anderson, D.D.: Open Hand Fractures: Prognosis and Classification. J. Hand Surg. 16A:101–107, 1991.

open fractures in other parts of the body that many orthopaedic surgeons simply assume that they should be used in the treatment of hand fractures. In an excellent prospective study, however, Suprock and coworkers[367] concluded that the routine use of antibiotics is not necessary in fingers having intact digital arteries. Peacock and coworkers[296] also concluded that perioperative antibiotics are not necessary in most open hand injuries. Both studies, however, emphasized the importance of early aggressive local wound care (ie, vigorous irrigation and debridement).

We agree strongly that local wound care is the most important factor and do not recommend antibiotics in patients having type I fractures in the Suprock classification. For type II injuries, we agree with the specific antibiotics suggested by Swanson and coworkers[371]:

All type II open fractures: cefazolin
Severe crush or massive soft-tissue injury: add an aminoglycoside
Bite wounds and barnyard injuries: add penicillin.

Wound Closure

If the wound is thoroughly scrubbed and irrigated as described earlier, wounds in association with type I open fractures can be closed primarily, as recommended by Swanson and coworkers.[371] This dictum does not apply to type II wounds and wounds with extensive soft-tissue damage (see the following section).

Massive Hand Trauma and Multiple Fractures

Most of the discussions in this chapter concern the specific management of individual fractures and dislocations in the hand, and little attention is directed toward the severely crushed or otherwise massively injured hand. In managing these difficult problems, the basic guidelines outlined throughout this chapter can be applied, but additional principles are also pertinent to this type of injury.

The ultimate goals must be to return the patient to his or her usual activities as soon as possible and to restore the structure and function of the hand to as nearly normal as possible. To achieve these goals in the severely injured hand, the surgeon must often manage concomitant injuries that seem to demand diametrically opposed methods of treatment. For example, multiple displaced fractures may create marked instability of the entire hand skeleton, yet prolonged immobilization can be disastrous. Soft-tissue damage accompanying fractures in the hand inevitably evokes marked edema. Tendons, ligaments, and intrinsic muscles become bathed in this protein-rich fluid, which rapidly becomes transformed into tough, unyielding, fibrous tissue. A bulky compressive dressing properly applied minimizes the initial edema, and early movement helps to pump the fluid out of the hand before it can become organized. Prolonged immobilization enhances its conversion into an inelastic encasement of scar.

The experience with massive hand wounds in Vietnam demonstrated conclusively that all hand wounds do not require primary closure and that some wounds in the hand actually should *not* be closed at the time of initial debridement.[61] High-velocity missile wounds, severe crush injuries, bite wounds, and open wounds that have gone untreated for longer than 24 hours are all contraindications to primary wound closure in the hand. The risk of infection is minimized by careful and adequate debridement, copious irrigation, bulky sterile dressings, and a second look in the operating room 2 to 5 days later. At the time of the second operation, delayed primary closure or skin coverage can be performed if the wound is surgically clean, or even further debridement with a third look several days hence may be necessary.

Early skeletal alignment is critical in the crushed or otherwise massively injured hand. Peacock[295] has shown how the strategic placement of a few small Kirschner wires (K-wires) at the time of the initial or subsequent operation can often provide enough stability to allow early motion and thereby minimize the stiffness that inevitably results from this type of injury. Finding the ideal compromise between stabilization and mobilization in the massively injured hand often taxes the ingenuity of even the most experienced hand surgeon.

An important detail in managing the crushed hand is maintenance of the thumb–index web space. For many years, we have stabilized the thumb metacarpal in maximum palmar abduction in any patient having a significant bone or soft-tissue injury involving the I–II web space. This should be done at the time of the initial debridement or during the second look 48 to 72 hours later. It is easily accomplished by passing one or two K-wires from the base of the thumb metacarpal into the carpus or base of second metacarpal while the thumb is held in full palmar abduction. The pins are left in for 3 to 4 weeks or until the soft tissues have healed and an appropriate therapy program is underway. This simple expedient is often all this is necessary to prevent a significant web-space contracture. Lees and coworkers[222] evaluated several different types of K-wires bent to form internal springs for accomplishing the same goal. They concluded that the strongest configuration was a V-shaped splint having unequal and offset limbs.

Delayed Primary Repair

Freeland and coworkers,[133] Jabaley and Freeland,[186] and Duncan and associates[108] have described in detail the concept of delayed primary treatment for massive hand trauma. The principle of this method is that all definitive operative repair (which may include a skin flap in addition to internal fixation of fractures and bone grafting for segmental defects) is performed several days after injury, after thorough debridement on the day of injury. One or more subsequent debridements may be required before the wound is clean enough for definitive treatment. These authors emphasize that displaced open fractures should be reduced and stabilized by the least invasive method that is commensurate with reliable biomechanical stability.[108]

We endorse the concept of early definitive treatment (delayed primary bone grafting) of segmental defects, which often also requires concomitant soft-tissue coverage. There are situations in which this is not feasible; in such cases, measures should be taken to preserve skeletal length for later reconstruction. One useful technique to maintain length in segmental skeletal defects is the "bayonet" spacer, which is easily fabricated from a 0.0625-inch K-wire by the surgeon at the operating table (Fig. 11-1). Kaplan[200] has suggested the use of carved Silastic block spacers to serve the same purpose. External fixation is another option.

In management of unequivocally irreparable segmental joint defects, the surgeon may have to consider such alternatives as a primary arthrodesis[158] or an immediate Silastic arthroplasty.[277]

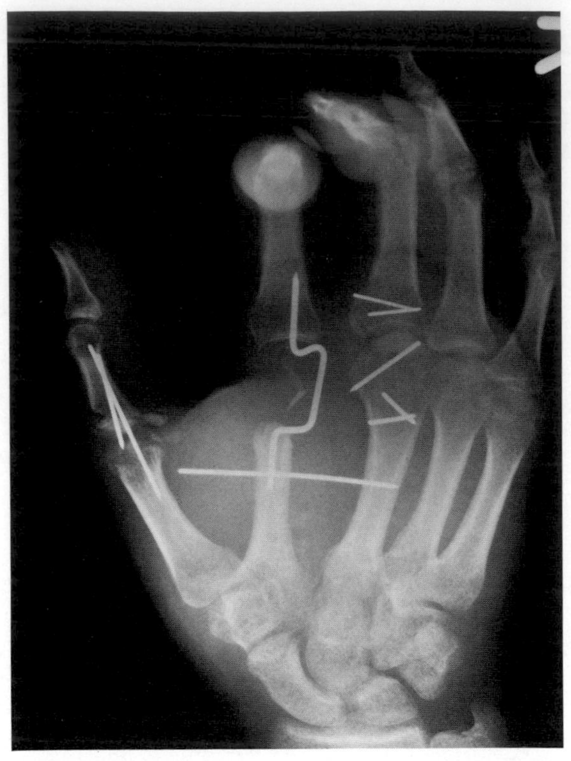

FIGURE 11-1. If delayed primary bone grafting is not performed, an effective method of maintaining length in segmental skeletal defects is with a "bayonet" spacer, shown here in the index metacarpal. The surgeon can easily fabricate these spacers at the operating table from a 0.0625-inch K-wire by using two pairs of needle-nosed pliers or large needle holders.

Tire-Explosion Injuries

A unique subset of massive trauma to the hand is caused by tire explosions. The reason for bringing special attention to these injuries is because they often have concomitant life-threatening injuries of the face, head, and eyes. The force of an exploding car tire can raise a 3000-lb car 15 feet off the ground, whereas an exploding truck tire unleases enough force to raise the same 3000-lb car 23 feet off the ground.[372] Teasdall and coworkers[372] have emphasized that these patients must be treated as polytrauma victims, treating the potentially lethal head and facial injuries first. The Occupational Safety and Health Administration (OSHA) has established standards for working with high-pressure tires[249] but the best treatment for these devastating injuries is universal education and safety training for all who perform this type of work.[372]

Gunshot Wounds

Clear distinction should be made between high-velocity and low-velocity gunshot wounds. Muzzle velocity is measured as the missile leaves the barrel of the weapon and can be classified into three groups:

1. Low-velocity (less than 1000 ft/second)—most handguns
2. Medium-velocity (1000 to 2000 ft/second)—magnum handguns and shotguns
3. High-velocity (more than 2000 ft/second)—high-powered hunting rifles and military weapons.

Bullet velocity alone, however, is not a valid predictor of wound damage.[119] Other factors that influence the amount of tissue destruction include:

Mass (weight and caliber) of the bullet. Bullet weight is usually stated in grains (1 grain = 0.065 g or 0.0014 lb). Caliber is the diameter of the bullet in 0.001 of an inch (eg, a .45 caliber pistol has a diameter of 0.455 inch).

Shape and composition of the bullet. Low-velocity weapons usually employ lead alloy bullets having low melting points. At high velocity, barrel friction causes softening of the missile, which leads to bullet deformation. Coating or "jacketing" of bullets with metals having higher melting points compensates for the effects of barrel friction.[328]

Thus, a high-velocity bullet penetrates deeper but the diameter on impact of a "soft-pointed" bullet may be 30 to 40 times greater than that of a fully jacketed nonexpandable bullet.[401] The Geneva Convention requires that all military bullets be fully jacketed and nonexpanding, but it is not required that civilian ammunition conforms to these standards.

The wound profile. Each type of weapon and bullet has a characteristic "profile," depicting its own pattern of tissue destruction.[119] A bullet carves out a "permanent cavity" of tissue destruction, but as it passes through tissue, it also creates a "temporary cavity," in which tearing and stretching of muscles and small blood vessels causes subsequent loss of blood and fluid. Increased tissue pressure resulting from swelling in a closed fascial compartment can kill more tissue than was damaged by the projectile. Wound profiles also show that even the highest-velocity military weapons may cause minimal disruption in the initial 12 cm of tissue penetration, which has significant implications in hand injuries, because the total tissue path is usually less than this distance.[119]

The distance from weapon to victim. This is most important in shotgun wounds.

Table 11-3 shows how these various factors influence the kinetic energy of a missile, which actually determines its destructive force.[32] For a more detailed discussion of bullet characteristics and wound ballistics, the reader is referred to the comprehensive review article by Russoti and Sim.[328]

Most civilian gunshot wounds in the hand are caused by low-velocity handguns, although this pattern may be changing as various types of assault weapons increasingly find their way into the hands of the population. Some authors[106,147] have noted that low-velocity gunshot wounds of the hand are relatively benign injuries, and many of these injuries can be treated in an emergency room setting. Treatment should begin with careful assessment of soft-tissue damage and appropriate x-rays to detect bone and joint injury. Minimal superficial debridement (skin edges) of the entrance and exit wounds combined with simple cleansing and copious irrigation is usually sufficient wound management.[328] When there is any question about the velocity of the missile or the

TABLE 11-3
Ballistic Properties of Common Handguns, Rifles, and Shotguns

Cartridge/Shell Type	Bullet Weight Grains	Muzzle Velocity Feet per Second	Muzzle Kinetic Energy Foot-Pounds
PISTOLS			
25 Auto	45	815	65
38 Auto	130	1040	310
9mm Federal	115	1280	420
357 Magnum	180	1145	525
44 RemMagnum	210	1495	1040
RIFLES			
22 Hornet	45	2690	723
M-16 (AR-15)	55	3240	1282
270 Winchester	100	3430	2612
30-06 Springfield	180	2700	2913
375 H&H Magnum	300	2530	4263
416 Wea. Magnum	400	2700	6474

Gauge	Shell Type	Shot Weight *ounces*	Shot Weight *grains*	Muzzle Velocity Feet per Second	Muzzle Kinetic Energy Foot-Pounds
SHOTGUNS					
20	2 3/4 inch	1	437	1165	1297
12	2 3/4 inch	1 1/2	656	1260	2278
12	3 inch Mag	2	874	1175	2640

Gun Digest 1992/46th Annual Edition DBI Books, Inc. Editor Ken Warner. Table prepared by Philip A Deffer, Jr., MD.

amount of tissue damage, the patient should be taken to the operating room for debridement. As noted, velocity alone does not fully determine the amount of tissue damage, and Dugas and D'Ambrosia[105] have emphasized the difference between low-velocity, low-caliber (.22) and low-velocity, high-caliber (.45, .357, .38) wounds, noting that the latter require more aggressive debridement. Fackler and Burkhalter[119] cautioned against overzealous excision of questionably viable tissue at the initial debridement because this may increase ultimate disability. They reemphasized the importance of the second look (ie, leaving the wound open and returning to the operating room 1 to 3 days later).

Surgeons from Cook County Hospital showed that it is safe to treat fractures of the metacarpals caused by low-velocity gunshot wounds with early (1 to 7 days) internal fixation and bone grafting.[143] Their indications for fixation were angulation greater than 15°, less than 50% bony apposition, shortening more than 5 mm, and comminution 50% or more. Their study demonstrated that interpretation of the x-rays often underestimates the degree of comminution, leading to further shortening and angulation in the nonoperatively treated fracture.

Fractures and joint damage are common but nerves and tendons often escape serious injury in low-velocity gunshot wounds. Nerve injuries are usually concussive neurapraxias and generally recover spontaneously.[105,106]

Exploration of the wound to remove bullet fragments is not necessary unless a large pellet or fragment is superficial and likely to be painful or if fragments are possibly intra-articular. Lead intoxication (plumbism, saturnism) is a theoretic complication of bullet fragments bathed in synovial fluid but probably not in the small joints of the hand.[223,328,387] Lead fragments in a joint can lead to mechanical dysfunction and eventual arthritic changes. Therefore, intra-articular fragments should probably be removed.

The most serious residual complications from low-velocity gunshot wounds in the hand are generally those involving the MP and PIP joints. Intra-articular fractures with relatively mild comminution may be amenable to the judicious use of K-wires but more severe comminution, with or without bone loss, is a prime indication for external fixation.[34,207,337] Major loss of articular surfaces requires bone grafting or subsequent arthrodesis.[133,263]

FRACTURES OF THE DISTAL PHALANX

It is not surprising that fractures of the distal phalanx comprise more than half of all hand fractures because the distal portion of the hand is the most exposed to injury.[255,257] In Butt's[67] series of fractures, the distal phalanx of the long finger was injured more than twice as often as the distal phalanx of the thumb, which was next in frequency.

Anatomy

The extensor and flexor tendons that insert on the base of the distal phalanx play no role in displacing fractures of the distal phalanx, except for avulsion injuries (which are discussed later). Fibrous septa, which radiate from bone to insert into the skin, form a dense meshwork and probably stabilize the fracture and minimize displacement.[315] Acute swelling and hematoma formation in these closed fibrous compartments undoubtedly are the cause of the severe pain that often accompanies crushing injuries of the distal phalanx.

Classification

Most distal phalangeal fractures are produced by crushing injuries; therefore, extensive soft-tissue damage and subungual hematomas are common. Kaplan[201] classified fractures of the distal phalanx into three general types: longitudinal, transverse, and comminuted (Fig. 11-2). Longitudinal fractures rarely show displacement; however, a transverse fracture close to the base of the phalanx may show a marked degree of angulation. Comminuted fractures usually involve the distal tuft of the phalanx and have been called the "crushed-eggshell type."[315] In addition to being most frequent, the crushed comminuted fracture is most commonly associated with soft-tissue damage.

Treatment

Treatment of nondisplaced fractures should be directed toward the soft-tissue damage. Dorsal or volar splints, which are frequently used for immobilization, may

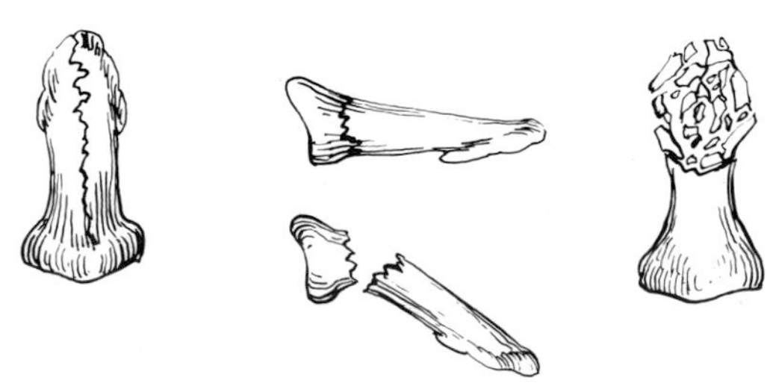

FIGURE 11-2. The three general types of fractures of the distal phalanx. (*Left*) Longitudinal fractures rarely show displacement. (*Center*) A transverse fracture may show a marked degree of angulation and may require internal or external splinting. (*Right*) The so-called crushed-eggshell–type of comminuted fracture that commonly involves the tuft. Most tuft fractures are not this severely comminuted.

cause severe pain if they are applied too tightly. A hairpin splint or fingertip guard (Fig. 11-3) provides protection without compressing the soft tissues. If such a splint is used for a prolonged period, however, one must be certain that it immobilizes only the distal interphalangeal (DIP) joint and does not block PIP flexion.

The main reason for splinting fractures of the distal phalanx is to relieve pain. Except in the displaced transverse variety, these fractures do not require immobilization to hold a reduction. The splint is provided to protect the tender fingertip from further external trauma.

Transverse angulated fractures must be reduced and held with either an external splint or a smooth K-wire. No attempt is made to reduce the displaced fragments of tuft fractures, which resemble a crushed eggshell. The fragments usually are not problematic but the finger can remain painful for many months.

Most fractures of the distal phalanx rarely require more than 3 to 4 weeks of protective splinting, but these apparently innocuous fractures can result in surprisingly prolonged morbidity, especially when there was concomitant soft-tissue crush injury.[69] In an excellent long-term follow-up article, DaCruz and colleagues[94] showed that 31% of tuft fractures had not healed radiographically and 70% of patients had bothersome symptoms at 6 months. These symptoms can be significantly lessened by a home program of desensitization modalities supervised by a hand therapist.

Nail Bed Injuries

Fractures of the distal phalanx are frequently open injuries, with significant soft-tissue damage. Associated injuries of the nail bed are often more serious and demand more attention than the fracture and yet are among the most frequently neglected of all injuries.

Evacuation of a subungual hematoma markedly relieves pain. Pressure caused by drilling a hole is unnecessarily painful. The time-honored hot paper clip is a more effective and relatively painless method of draining the hematoma, but a small battery-operated disposable cautery (Accu-Temp, Concept) is even better.

Late nail deformity is often an unavoidable complication after crush injuries of the distal phalanx, but a meticulous repair of the nail bed is the best means of minimizing such deformity.[57,235] Our practice is to repair the nail bed as carefully as possible with 7-0 chromic catgut on an ophthalmic needle under loupe magnification. If there is loss of nail bed tissue, various types of local and distant nail bed grafts[406] and even a porcine xenograft[116] can be considered.

If the nail plate has been avulsed at its base, it is carefully removed, scrubbed with povidone iodine (Betadine), and sutured back into place after repair of the nail bed (with two or three holes in the plate for drainage).[266,408] This serves not only as a protective splint but also minimizes local tenderness.[104] The old nail is pushed off gradually by growth of the new nail. If the nail plate is not available or is too badly damaged

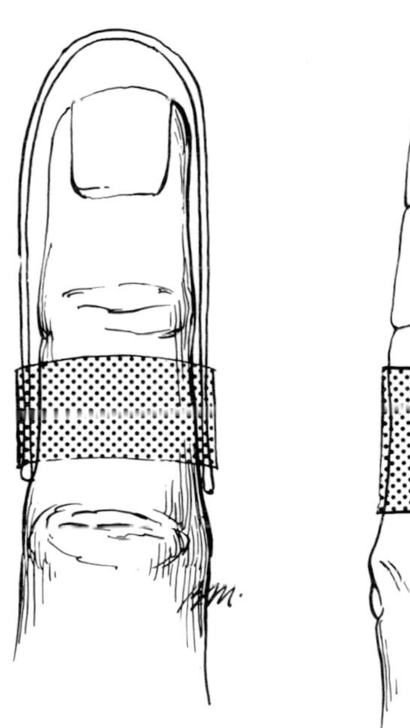

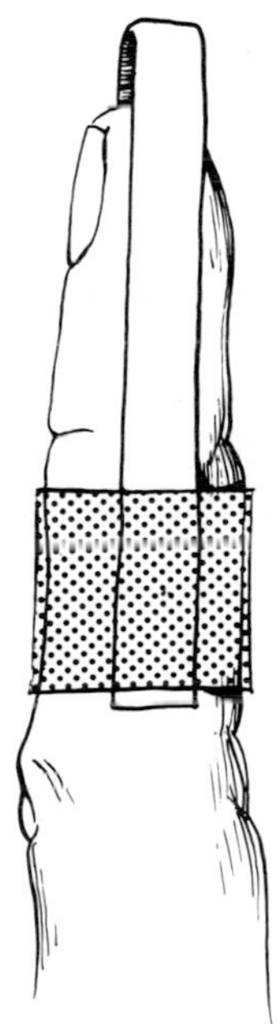

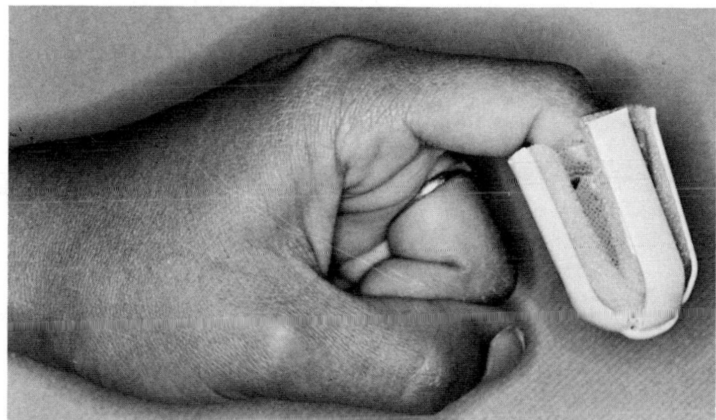

FIGURE 11-3. A hairpin splint (*left*) or fingertip guard (*right*) protects the fractured distal phalanx from further injury but allows swelling to occur without tissue compression. Both splints should be fitted so as to not block PIP flexion (*right*).

to provide adequate coverage of the matrix, a commercially available polypropylene artificial nail is a reasonable alternative.[289]

The patient should be told that some deformity of the nail is to be expected, although the full extent of the deformity will not be known until the new nail has fully regrown, a process that usually takes about 4 to 5 months.

When the nail plate has been avulsed or torn and the nail bed laceration is visible, the need for repair of the nail bed is clearly evident. When the nail plate is intact, recognition of a significant nail bed laceration is more difficult. Zook[408] has recommended exploration of the nail bed if there is a subungual hematoma involving more than 25% of the nail. Simon and Wolgin[348] attempted to correlate the association between subungual hematomas and fractures and occult nail bed lacerations. In their series, patients with a subungual hematoma greater than half the size of the nail had a 60% incidence of nail bed laceration requiring repair; when there was an associated fracture of the distal phalanx, the incidence was 95%. We do not ordinarily remove an intact nail to repair a nail bed, even if there is a large subungual hematoma. In these patients, the hematoma is drained by burning one or two holes in the nail; rarely have we seen a subsequent nail deformity in such patients. Perhaps the intact nail serves as a stent to approximate the nail bed edges in lieu of sutures. We wish to reemphasize the importance to a meticulous repair of the nail bed in all open injuries in which the nail plate has been avulsed or damaged, exposing the nail bed laceration.

Occasionally, the base of the nail bed may become entrapped in the fracture site, most commonly where the root of the nail has been avulsed from beneath the proximal nail fold. Failure to recognize this complication and extricate the nail bed from the fracture site at the time of the original wound debridement may result in nonunion of the fracture (Fig. 11-4) and a deformed finger.

Mallet Finger of Tendon Origin

By common usage, the term mallet finger has come to mean a flexion deformity of the DIP joint resulting from loss of extensor tendon continuity to the distal phalanx.[511] The same clinical picture can be caused by an intra-articular fracture involving one third or more of the dorsal lip of the distal phalanx but this entity is discussed separately under Mallet Finger of Bony Origin.

Mechanism of Injury and Classification

Forcible flexion of the DIP joint is thought to be the mechanism of injury resulting in the "mallet" or "baseball" finger. Bunnell[439] preferred the term drop finger. The injury usually occurs when the extensor tendon is taut, as in catching a ball or striking an object with the extended finger. The deformity may result

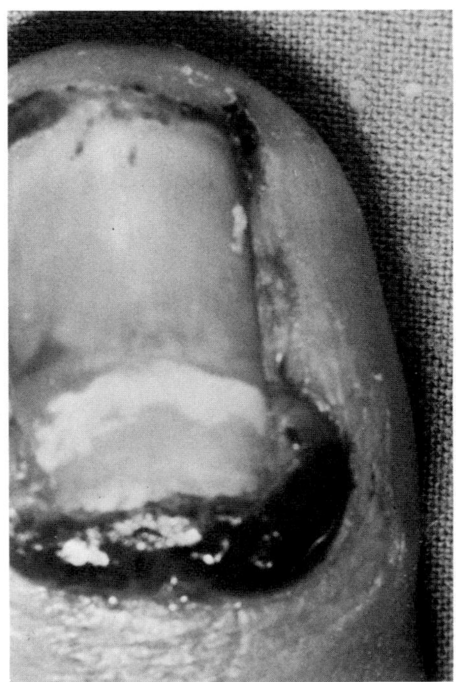

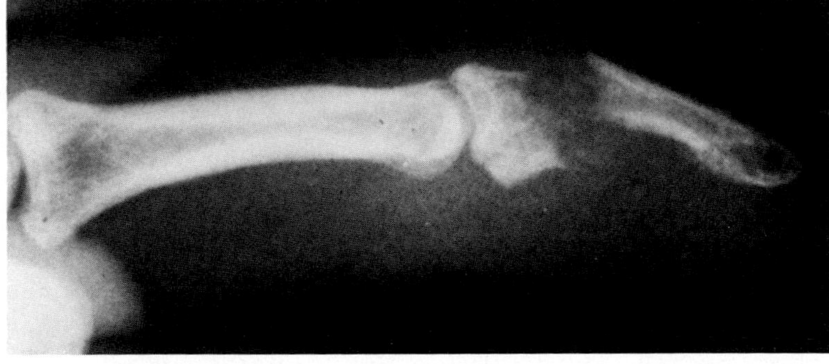

FIGURE 11-4. When the root of the nail is avulsed from beneath the cuticle (*left*), one should suspect that the nail bed may be entrapped in the fracture site. The clue to this diagnosis is widening of the fracture line (*right*) and inability to fully reduce the fracture. Failure to extricate the nail bed may result in nonunion of the fracture.

from relatively trivial trauma, and it has been suggested that a familial predisposition or an area of relative avascularity in the tendon may play a role in such patients.[465,520]

Several patterns of injury may be seen[523]:

1. The fibers of the extensor tendon over the distal joint may be stretched without completely dividing the tendon. The degree of drop of the distal phalanx is usually not pronounced—a loss of perhaps 5° to 20° extension (Fig. 11-5, *top*)—and the patient retains some weak active extension.
2. The extensor tendon may be ruptured or torn from its insertion into the distal phalanx (Fig. 11-5, *center*).[50,466] In this case, there is a greater flexion deformity (up to 60°), and the patient has complete loss of active extension at the distal joint.
3. A small fragment of the distal phalanx may be avulsed with the extensor tendon. The characteristics of this injury are identical to those of the tendon injuries previously mentioned, and the degree of drop depends not on the small fragment but on the amount of loss of continuity of the tendon mechanism. The small fragment should be ignored and these injuries should be treated as tendon injuries rather than as fractures (Figs. 11-5, *bottom* and Fig. 11-6).

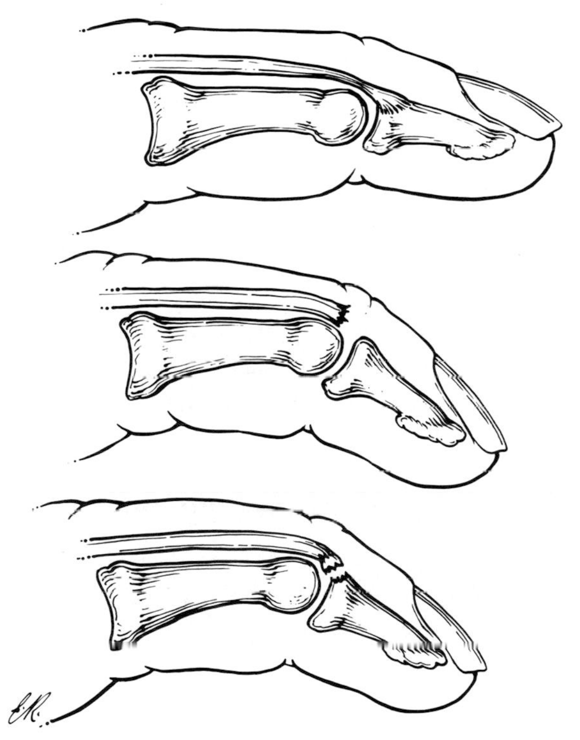

FIGURE 11-5. The three types of injury that cause a mallet finger of tendon origin. (*Top*) The extensor tendon fibers over the distal joint are stretched without complete division of the tendon. Although there is some drop of the distal phalanx, the patient retains weak active extension. (*Center*) The extensor tendon is ruptured from its insertion on the distal phalanx. There is a 30° to 60° extensor lag at the distal joint. (*Bottom*) A small fragment of the distal phalanx is avulsed with the extensor tendon. This injury has the same clinical findings as that shown in the center drawing.

In the series of Stark and coworkers,[511] 24% of the injuries were associated with small bony avulsion fractures but this finding had no effect on the final result.

If the flexion deformity of the distal joint is severe in any of these different variants of mallet finger, a secondary hyperextension deformity of the PIP joint may develop because of imbalance of the extensor mechanism, resulting in a swan-neck deformity (Fig. 11-7).

Methods of Treatment

Considerable controversy used to exist regarding whether the PIP joint need be immobilized in the treatment of mallet finger. Probably largely because such authorities as Bunnell[439] and Watson-Jones[523] recommended immobilization of the PIP joint in 60° flexion, many authors advised such treatment.* Some techniques even used K-wire fixation for both the DIP and PIP joints[493] or a combination of internal DIP fixation and external PIP immobilization.[441,442]

Most authors, however, believe that *only* the DIP joint need be immobilized.† Several types of DIP splints have been described (Fig. 11-8), including at least two modifications of the original Stack splint, one with perforations and another with larger windows, both designed to minimize skin problems.[468,510] The results of treatment with these various types of splints do not appear to be substantially different, but more minor complications were reported in one series with the dorsal aluminum splint[513]; in another series, patients preferred the Stack splint over the Abouna splint.[521] Regardless of the type of splint used, precise instructions must be given to the patient to achieve optimal results and avoid minor problems (see Authors' Preferred Method of Treatment).[444]

In the past, poor results after conservative treatment prompted some surgeons to perform immediate operative repair of the torn tendon. As early as 1930, Mason[477] recommended early operative repair of the ruptured extensor expansion. Operative treatment is aimed at freshening and approximating the

* References 233, 238, 240, 242, 243, 247, 251, 255, 269, 271, 276, 281, 283, 287, 297, 449.

† References 433, 438, 444, 447, 448, 458, 468, 482, 484, 509, 510, 513, 521.

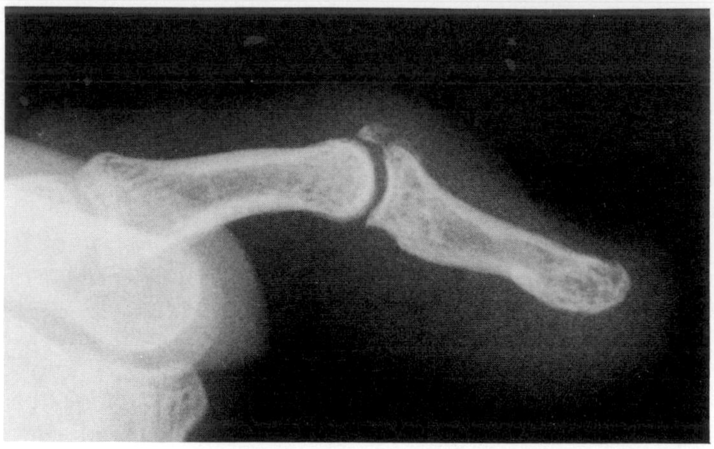

FIGURE 11-6. Mallet finger deformities with small fragments such as this should be treated as tendon injuries rather than as fractures.

edges of the tear; it is followed by immobilization of the distal and middle joints. An avulsed bone fragment can be reattached with a pull-out wire but if the fragment is small, it may be excised and the tendon reinserted by a pull-out wire through tiny drill holes. The results of operative repair of tendinous mallet fingers are not always satisfactory. Although they may give improved cosmetic results, flexion is often lost due to scarring on the dorsal aspect of the joint. The assessment of the late results in Robb's[498] series suggested that early operative repair was unnecessary and even undesirable, a viewpoint shared by most surgeons today.

The imperfect and often harmful results that followed both open and closed treatment led some to believe that the mallet deformity was being overtreated. Stiff PIP joints, pin-tract infections, and skin sloughing were severe penalties to pay for treatment of an injury that rarely caused any functional disability. Some authors[498,500] have stated that in time, practically all mallet deformities of tendon origin improve gradually to a satisfactory state of recovery without treatment. These authors believed that without treatment, the extensor tendon healed in a lengthened state and that gradual contraction of the fibrous scar tissue took place over the ensuing 6 months, resulting in a satisfactory state of recovery. For this reason, Robb[498] suggested that the only treatment necessary for most patients with mallet finger was the application of an elastic adhesive strapping or a straight spatula splint to relieve the initial discomfort from the injury.

Stark and colleagues[511] analyzed their results with 163 mallet fingers and concluded that not all patients with mallet finger should be treated in the same manner. Treatment should depend on time elapsed after injury, previous treatment, degree of loss of extension, degree of functional disability, and age of the patient. In their series, only four patients were treated surgically and none by K-wire fixation.

The results of treatment of mallet fingers are not universally good by any method. Burke[440] emphasized that assessment at the time of splint removal is valueless because subsequent recurrence of at least some of the extensor lag is likely. Flinchum[450] probably said it best when he noted that "this is a difficult injury to treat without some residual cosmetic or functional

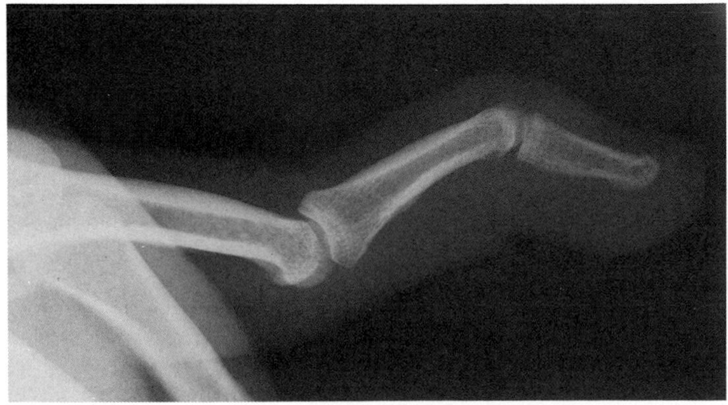

FIGURE 11-7. With severe flexion deformity of the distal joint in mallet finger injury, a secondary hyperextension deformity of the proximal interphalangeal joint may occur because of imbalance of the extensor mechanism. This produces the typical swan-neck deformity.

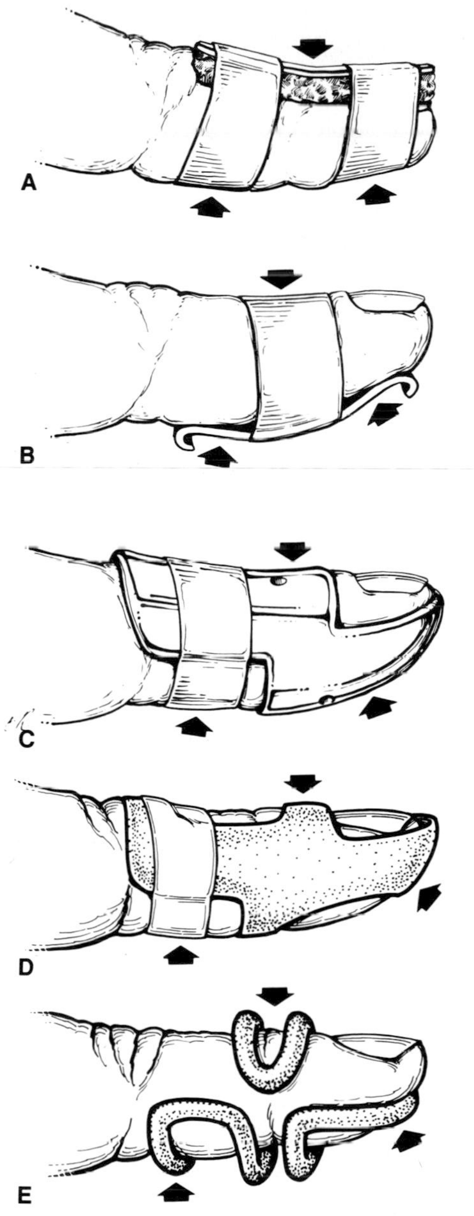

FIGURE 11-8. We prefer to immobilize only the distal interphalangeal joint in treating mallet fingers. This may be done with a dorsal padded aluminum splint (**A**), a volar unpadded aluminum splint (**B**), a Stack splint (**C**), a modified Stack splint (**D**), or an Abouna splint (**E**). Note that each of these splints uses a three-point fixation principle.

loss.'' Cold weather intolerance has been noted to be the most common late symptom and is not directly related to the amount of residual deformity.[488,519] In a follow-up study by Shankar and Goring,[504] many of their patients complained of occasional aches and cold intolerance, but 85% of the patients were satisfied with the outcome after conservative treatment.

Mikic and Helal[484] reported that although most patients are improved, only about 30% to 40% regain normal function in the DIP joint after treatment. In a comprehensive study of mallet fingers, Abouna and Brown[433] discovered that the following factors portend a poor prognosis: age older than 60 years; delay in treatment of more than 4 weeks; an initial active extensor lag greater than 50°; fewer than 4 weeks of immobilization; and patients having short, stubby fingers. Treatment of patients with associated arthritis (rheumatoid or degenerative) or peripheral vascular disease was particularly unrewarding in their experience. In our experience, patients whose mallet fingers are the result of trivial trauma also tend to have poor results from splinting.

Authors' Preferred Method of Treatment

Acute Mallet Finger. Our preferred treatment for acute mallet finger is continuous splinting of *only* the DIP joint for 6 to 10 weeks. We do not immobilize the PIP joint and have never favored operative repair of the extensor tendon in closed mallet finger injuries. (In open injuries requiring debridement, we usually approximate the tendon ends with absorbable suture.)

We prefer either a dorsal padded aluminum splint (see Fig. 11-8*A*), which tends to interfere less with the tactile pad of the finger than a volar splint, or a Stack[509] plastic mallet finger splint (see Fig.11-8*C*). Patients are often given both splints to use interchangeably because each tends to cause skin irritation and local pressure in different areas; alternating the splints may alleviate this problem. The disadvantage of the Stack splint is that it is sometimes difficult to find a size that fits perfectly; also, if swelling subsides, the splint becomes loose.

We attempt to position the DIP joint in *slight* hyperextension but the degree depends on the mobility of the patient's joints and the level of discomfort. The splint should never cause pain, and the amount of hyperextension should never cause blanching of the skin over the DIP joint. (Rayan and Mullins[497] showed that skin blanching occurs in most patients at 50% of total passive hyperextension.) The patient is shown how to take the splint off and reapply it occasionally for skin care but this requires assistance because two hands are required to hold the joint in extension and properly apply the splint.[444] At no time is the DIP joint allowed to drop into flexion. With the Stack splint, it is important to keep the tip of the finger in contact with the end of the splint, which may require an additional strip of tape placed longitudinally. If the finger does not fit any Stack splint well, Crawford[444] suggested using the smaller of the two closest sizes and cutting the splint longitudinally in the midline (a split Stack splint is now available commercially). To minimize skin irritation with the dorsal aluminum splint, Stern and Kastrup[513] suggested a layer of moleskin or gauze beneath the splint.

This method of treatment is successful only for patients who are reliable and reasonably intelligent because it requires compliance and cooperation. We make it a practice to see these patients after the initial 1 to 2 weeks of treatment to be certain that they understood the instructions and are using the splint properly. Kasdan[203] suggested that it is advisable to give written instructions to patients with mallet fingers, which is probably a good idea.

An alternative method of treatment for patients who are unreliable or unable to follow instructions is the finger cast described by Smillie[505] in 1937 (Fig. 11-9). If it is used, the PIP joint should probably not be immobilized in flexion for more than 3 to 4 weeks. We virtually never use a Smillie cast but the illustration was left in the book because it shows a clever method of making a plaster splint for a single digit if that should become necessary for any reason.

A minimum of 6 weeks continuous DIP joint immobilization is required, and some authors recommend 8 weeks.[444,524] Partial recurrence of the extensor lag is virtually inevitable, and at least 2 to 3 weeks of nighttime splinting of the DIP joint in extension is mandatory after the continuous splint has been discontinued; we prefer 4 to 6 weeks. Careful follow-up is required and this treatment must be individualized. Some patients show a greater tendency for recurrence; in these individuals, the splinting must be applied for more hours each night and for more weeks. If the recurrent extensor lag is severe, Crawford[444] suggests a second course of full-time splinting for 8 weeks. Occasionally, a patient has difficulty in regaining flexion and in this situation, less part-time splinting is indicated.

Occasionally, a patient is seen such as a dentist or a surgeon, for whom external splinting for a prolonged period would be an economic hardship. In these patients, immobilizing only the distal joint in full extension with a 0.045-inch K-wire is an acceptable method of treatment. The pin is cut off beneath the skin, and the patient can return to his or her usual activities almost immediately. We advise our patients to wear

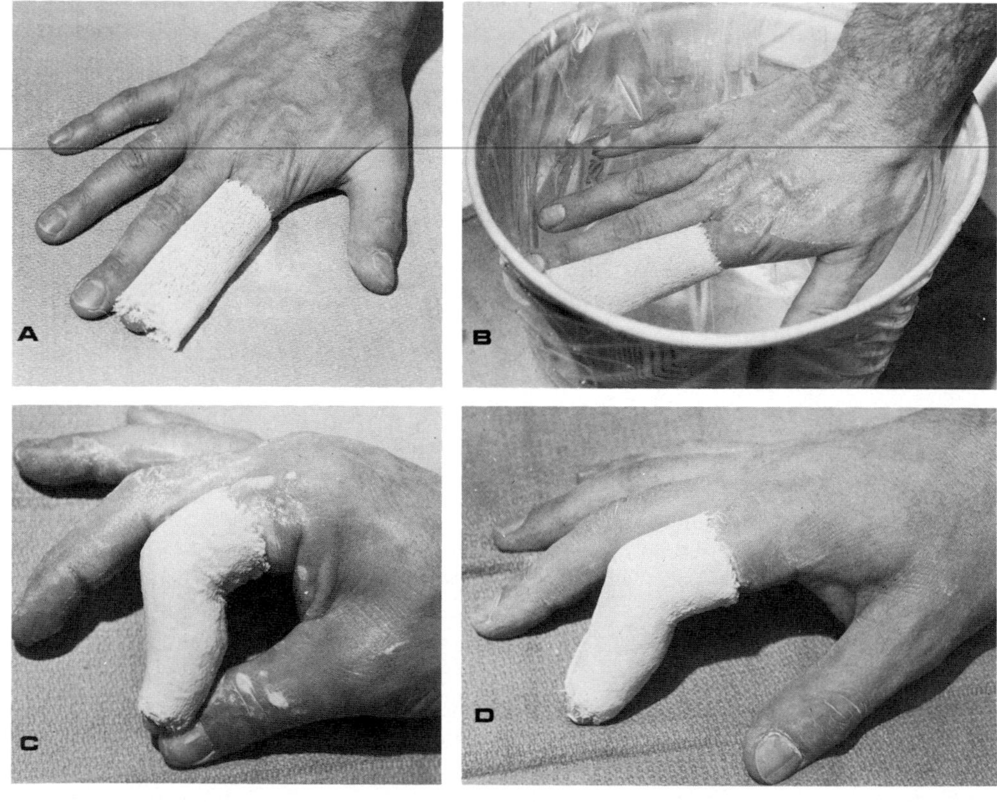

FIGURE 11-9. Smillie described a simple method of applying a mallet finger cast. (**A**) An 18-inch strip of 3- or 4-inch dry plaster is rolled into a tube and slipped over the end of the injured finger. No padding is used. (**B**) The patient dips his or her hand into a bucket of water, holding the tube of plaster in place over the finger. (**C**) The patient holds the finger in the correct position of immobilization while the physician smooths out the plaster. (**D**) The completed cast. Removal is facilitated by soaking the plaster. We virtually never use this technique, but it is a simple way to make a plaster cast for a single digit.

an external splint when not using the finger in their work. This provides some protection against bending or breakage of the pin. It is probably advisable to insert the K-wire obliquely, entering through the metaphysis of distal phalanx and penetrating the opposite cortex of middle phalanx. This has two advantages over a longitudinal K-wire: tenderness over the pin at the tip of the finger is avoided and if the wire should break, the two pieces can be removed from either end. After removal of the wire at 6 weeks, an additional 4 weeks of external night splinting is recommended. If this technique is used, the patient must be advised of the rare but dreadful complication of osteomyelitis or a septic joint.

Chronic Mallet Finger. A drop finger seen within 3 to 4 weeks should be treated as an acute injury, although the longer the delay, the less successful the result.[433,441,442,511] Mallet deformities not seen until 2 to 3 months after injury have been improved with prolonged (at least 8 weeks) splinting of the distal joint.[444,468,491] Auchincloss[434] suggested that K-wire splintage may possibly be more effective than external splinting in these patients but this is probably not necessary. Garberman and coworkers[452] reported a series in which splinting was as effective in the delayed group as it was in the early treatment population.

Many patients with late untreated mallet fingers have no functional problems and require no treatment. Shankar and Goring[504] reported a series in which even the 15% of patients who were dissatisfied with the outcome of their mallet finger treatment did not wish to have surgical correction. For those few patients who have symptoms, many different operative procedures have been proposed, including plication[509] or reefing[441,442,447] of the scarred tendon; stimulating tendon contracture by cutting and suturing the tendon, without shortening (the abbrevatio operation)[473]; tenodermodesis[464,470,519]; arthrodesis[450,511]; and even DIP disarticulation[500] (although few authors endorse Rosenzweig's recommendation for this).

The patients most likely to be symptomatic with late mallet finger are those who develop a swan-neck deformity, with a supple hyperextension posture of the PIP joint that accentuates the DIP extensor lag. Certain carefully selected patients with this problem may be candidates for Fowler's central slip release.§[457,459] As Bowers and Hurst[437] have noted, however, the indications for this procedure are strict, and the operation must be performed with meticulous care to avoid significant potential complications, including weakness of PIP joint extension. Grundberg and Reagan[454] also reported satisfactory results with this procedure but stressed that the swan-neck deformity must be due to a mallet finger and not to pathology at the PIP joint if the operation is to be successful.

Satisfactory correction of such deformities can also be achieved with the spiral oblique retinacular ligament reconstruction, although this operation is technically more demanding and requires a thorough understanding of the extensor mechanism.[469,515]

Mallet Thumb

Disruption of the extensor pollicis longus insertion into the base of distal phalanx can result in a flexion deformity of the thumb similar to that seen in the finger. Both splinting and operative repair have been shown to yield satisfactory results, although a review of the cases in these small series suggests that more limited motion in the interphalangeal (IP) joint may follow surgical treatment.[446,492,494] In reporting the largest series of mallet thumbs, Miura and coworkers[486] recommended splinting for closed injuries and operative repair for lacerations of the tendon.

Mallet Finger of Bony Origin (Mallet Fracture)

A fracture involving the dorsal articular surface of the distal phalanx produces a mallet deformity because the extensor tendon is attached to the avulsed fragment. Ordinarily, the fragment includes one third or more of the articular surface (Fig. 11-10). Displacement ranges from minimal separation to a wide gap, with tilting and malrotation of the fragment, and the remaining distal phalanx may subluxate volar to the condyles of the middle phalanx (Fig. 11-11). Several authors[443,471] believe that the mallet fracture with volar subluxation is caused by a different mechanism than that causing the usual hyperflexion injury. They suggest that these

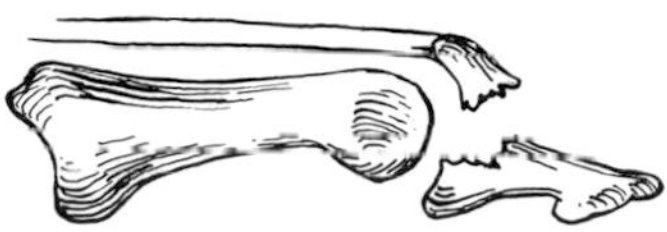

FIGURE 11-10. The mallet finger originating from bone injury (mallet fracture). The fracture fragment, which involves one third or more of the dorsal articular surface, is often tilted and malrotated and the remainder of the distal phalanx may be subluxated volar to the condyles of the middle phalanx.

§ Author's note: The origin of so-called Fowler's tenotomy is not clear in the literature.[459] In an attempt to answer this question, I called Dr. Daniel C. Riordan in September 1993. Dr. Riordan told me that during the years 1946 through 1947, he worked with Drs. J. William Littler and S. Benjamin Fowler at Valley Forge Army Hospital. In his typically concise and modest style, Dr. Riordan told me that Ben Fowler's ideas were sketched by Bill Littler, and that he (Dan Riordan) described these operations (including the central slip tenotomy) in his subsequent AAOS Instructional Course Lectures.

fractures, involving 50% or more of the articular surface, are caused by a hyperextension force and that attempted reduction by extension of the DIP joint will fail. They believe that open reduction and internal fixation (ORIF) is necessary for these fractures.

Management of mallet fractures is controversial. Several authors have cited specific indications for open reduction, including more than 2-mm displacement,[463] 3-mm displacement,[490] more than 30% involvement of the articular surface,[487,490,512] and volar subluxation of the distal phalanx.[433,444,482,487,509,511] Schneider[501,503,524] has become the champion of nonoperative treatment, however. He concluded from a large series of patients having mallet fractures that operative treatment offers no advantage over splinting of the DIP joint for 6 to 8 weeks. The only consistent "complication" was a bump over the dorsum of the joint, and this was present regardless of the method of treatment. Stern and Kastrup[513] noted a higher complication rate and more limited flexion of the DIP joint in their operated group, and even the staunchest advocates of open reduction[512] concede that "very few had normal motion" in the DIP joint after ORIF.

Inoue[462] described a unique method of treating mallet fractures with closed reduction and extension-block K-wire splinting. We have no experience with this technique.

Operative treatment of a mallet fracture is a deceptively difficult procedure, fraught with many potential problems, including fragmentation of the small dorsal lip fracture, difficulty in exposing and reducing the fragment anatomically, skin slough, loss of fixation postoperatively, and subsequent limited motion in the DIP joint.[524] Even experts in AO techniques have shown that tension-band wiring of mallet fractures has a high incidence of complications, most of which are related to soft-tissue problems.[436]

Stark and colleagues[511,512] emphasized the importance of exact anatomic reduction but noted that one collateral ligament must be divided to provide adequate exposure to see the articular surface. The technique described by Hamas and associates[455] (in which the extensor tendon is divided 5 mm proximal to the bone) provides good exposure, although at least partial division of one or both collateral ligaments is still necessary to see the articular surface. Our experience with this technique suggests that it may cause more adherence of the extensor tendon and thus limit subsequent DIP motion.

Several methods have been described for operative fixation of the fracture, each having its advantages and disadvantages.[455,512,522] Small K-wires provide better purchase and can usually be left in place longer than a pull-out wire but even the smallest (0.028-inch) K-wire may shatter the small dorsal fragment. Lubahn[476] described a technique using 0.028-inch K-wires (without having to cut the collateral ligaments), which in his patients produced results superior to closed treatment, with respect to residual extensor lag.

Damron and coworkers[445] tested several different types of fixation in the lab and concluded that tension-band suture with 2-0 Supramid was superior biomechanically to K-wire, tension-band wire, and figure-of-eight wire. Commenting on this article, Schneider[502] questioned its clinical relevance because none of the techniques provided sufficient stability of fixation to allow early unprotected motion.

Authors' Preferred Method of Treatment

Having treated many mallet fractures with open reduction and having encountered most of the complications noted in the preceding section, we have come to the conclusion that virtually all mallet fractures should be treated with splinting of the DIP joint, using the same technique as for the mallet finger of tendon origin. The main reason for this is that excellent results can be obtained in most patients with splinting alone. Moreover, nonoperative treatment avoids all of the potential complications noted previously, and even fractures having significant displacement remodel into

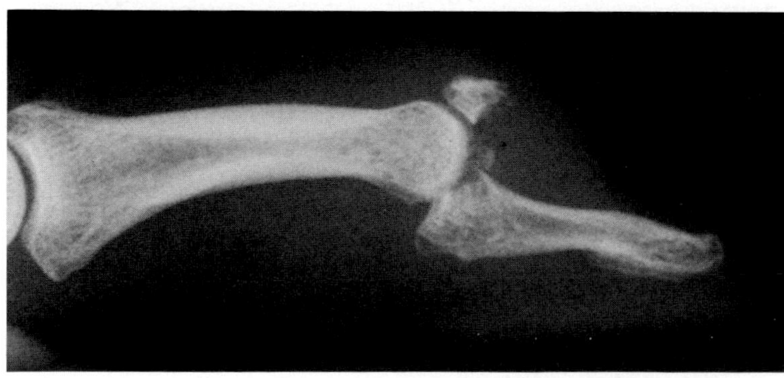

FIGURE 11-11. A mallet fracture-subluxation. Note the displacement of the avulsed fragment and the volar subluxation of the distal phalanx. This is our only indication for operative treatment. However, open reduction of a mallet fracture is technically difficult, and it is not always possible to achieve precise anatomic reduction.

a remarkably smooth articular surface (Fig. 11-12). Perhaps most important, in our experience, patients treated with splinting tend to regain better range of motion (especially flexion) of the DIP joint than those treated with ORIF.

Our only indication for open reduction is the mallet fracture with marked volar subluxation of the distal phalanx.

Flexor Digitorum Profundus Avulsion

Avulsion of the flexor digitorum profundus (FDP) tendon from its insertion into the base of the distal phalanx is a relatively uncommon injury, and the diagnosis is frequently missed.[414,421,427] A high index of suspicion and awareness of this injury are imperative because in most cases, early operative treatment is required to achieve a good result.

Mechanism of Injury

Avulsion of the FDP tendon is caused by forceful hyperextension of the DIP joint while the FDP is in maximum contraction. It occurs most commonly in sports. The classic mechanism is when a football player reaches out to tackle the ball carrier and grabs only a handful of jersey; FDP avulsion is sometimes called "jersey finger." The ring finger is involved most frequently and although the reason for this is not clearly understood, several theories have been suggested.[412,418,423,432]

The tendon may rupture directly from its insertion into the bone, or it may avulse a fragment of variable size from the base of distal phalanx. The degree of soft-tissue injury and hemorrhage is greater than that in a simple laceration of the profundus tendon, and this generally results in more extensive scarring within the flexor tendon sheath. As the avulsed tendon end re-

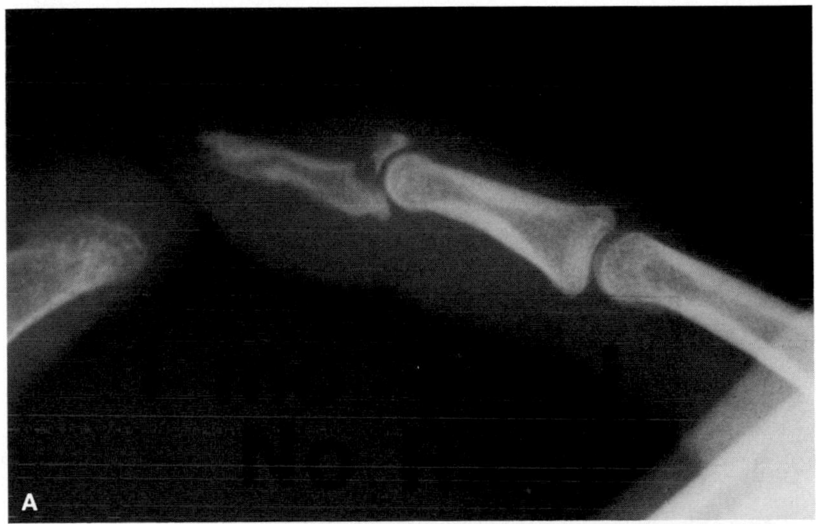

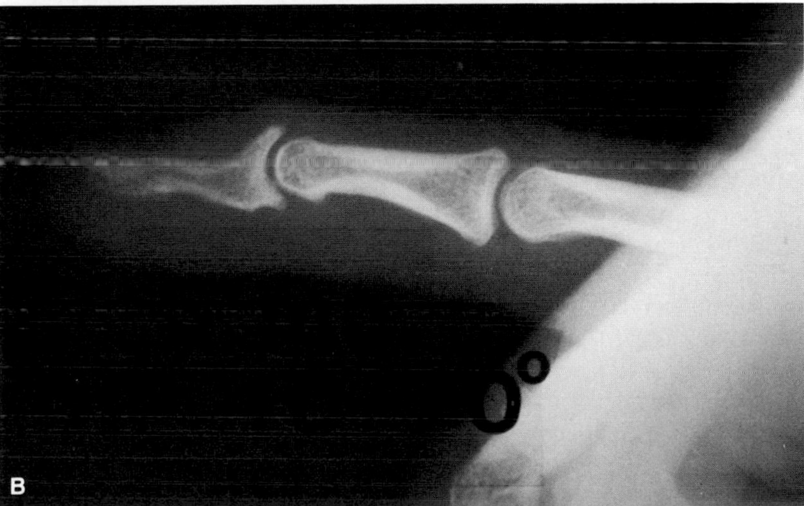

FIGURE 11-12. Mallet fractures that are moderately displaced (**A**) usually heal with reasonably good congruity (**B**). This patient had 10° to 70° of active motion in the distal interphalangeal joint and no pain 6 months after the fracture.

tracts proximally, it may become entrapped at the chiasma of the flexor digitorum superficialis (FDS) at the level of the PIP joint, and a flexion contracture may subsequently develop in that joint. More commonly, the tendon retracts to the base of the finger or to the level of the lumbrical origin in the distal palm.

Simultaneous avulsion of both flexor tendons (FDP and FDS) in the same digit was first described by Culver and associates[415] in 1981. They reported a good result in their patient by resection of the superficialis and repair of the profundus only. Other authors have treated this rare double rupture with a primary[409] or staged[420] tendon graft.

Classification

The excellent article by Leddy and Packer[422] contributed significantly to our understanding of the different types of pathology seen in this entity. They identified three distinct types of injury that have important implications in treatment:

Type I. The tendon retracts into the palm, severing all blood supply and creating extensive scarring in the tendon sheath. Repair within 7 to 10 days is required.

Type II. The tendon retracts to somewhere around the PIP joint, where it becomes entangled in the chiasma of FDS; the long vinculum remains intact. Occasionally, a small fleck of bone can be seen in a true lateral x-ray of the finger (Fig. 11-13*B*). Early treatment is advised but successful repair can be done as late as 3 months after injury. Unfortunately, not all FDP avulsions fall precisely into this neat classification because the proximal tendon stump may retract to the base of the finger—somewhere between a type I and type II. If the stump retracts proximal to the PIP joint level (Fig. 11-14), late repair without excessive tension is likely to be impossible.

Type III. A large bony fragment is avulsed by the tendon and is trapped at the level of the distal (A4) pulley (see Fig. 11-13*A*). The size and configuration of the fragment are variable.[428]

Type IV. Robins and Dobyns[428] were the first (in 1975) to note that it is possible to have both a tendon avulsion and a fracture. There is a free fragment of bone off the volar base of distal phalanx, with the FDP tendon lying somewhere more proximally in the finger. Smith[430] suggested in 1981 that this type of injury be designated type IV because it does not fit anywhere in Leddy and Packer's classification. Others[18,411,417,419,429] have reported experience with this variant. Eglseder and Russell[416] even had a patient in whom the tendon avulsion and fracture were thought to have occurred in two separate injuries 5 months apart.

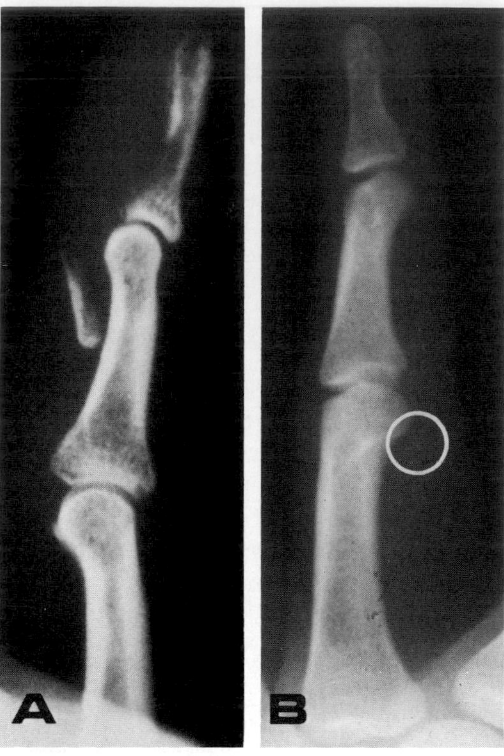

FIGURE 11-13. Rupture of the flexor digitorum profundus from its insertion into the distal phalanx may be accompanied by a fragment avulsed from the distal phalanx. (**A**) An unusually large avulsion fragment. (**B**) A tiny avulsion fragment is seen at the level of condyles of the proximal phalanx. Good-quality x-rays in true lateral and oblique views are necessary to identify the fragment. In most cases, the injury is a pure rupture of the tendon from its insertion, and no fragment is seen. (**A** *from Green, D.P.: Commonly Missed Injuries in the Hand. Am. Fam. Physician, 7:114, 1973.*)

The significance of the type IV lesion is that both injuries must be recognized and treated. Early fixation of the intra-articular fracture and reinsertion of the avulsed tendon are both required to restore function.

Diagnosis

If the injury goes unnoticed by the patient, it may not come to a physician's attention for several days or weeks. Every year at the end of high school football season in Texas, we see at least one or two players who have untreated FDP avulsion injuries that occurred several weeks to months previously. Even when the patient is seen immediately, the problem may not be obvious because there is no characteristic deformity except for a slightly decreased flexion posture of the

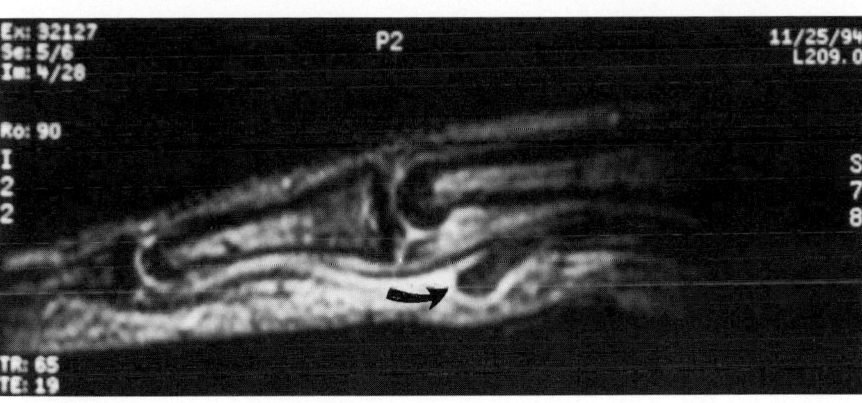

FIGURE 11-14. Sagittal magnetic resonance imaging view of the ring finger in a high school football player 3 months postinjury. The retracted end of the flexor digitorum profundus (FDP) is clearly seen (*arrow*) lying within the flexor sheath near the distal end of the A2 pulley. This would therefore be neither a true type I nor a type II injury but something in between. Myostatic contracture was such that it was not possible to bring the FDP tendon back out to length.

injured finger, so-called "hang-out." *The diagnosis is readily made by demonstrating inability to actively flex the DIP joint but this must be specifically tested.*[410,422,426] Pain and local tenderness are usually more marked over the PIP joint, where the retracted end of the tendon may have come to rest, than over the point of avulsion at the distal phalanx. If the tendon has retracted into the palm, local tenderness is present at the level of the A1 pulley. If a few days have passed since injury, there may be extensive ecchymosis, not only in the pulp but often extending proximally along the entire length of the finger.

If a fragment of bone has been avulsed from the distal phalanx by the tendon, lateral and oblique x-rays of the individual are mandatory to confirm the diagnosis. In most patients, the tendon ruptures directly from the bone and no fragment is seen radiographically.

Although the diagnosis of FDP avulsion is not difficult, it is not always possible to determine the level of the proximal stump. In the past, this determination had to be made based on only the physical examination in patients with no bony fragment. Advances in radiographic technology may have changed that. Trumble and coworkers[431] reported the use of ultrasound in locating the proximal stump, and we have found MRI to be a accurate method (see Fig. 11-14). The cost of MRI is high but in some late cases that expense may be justified if the MRI can unequivocally establish that the tendon has retracted into the palm and is therefore not reparable.

Treatment

In most cases, early operative reinsertion of the avulsed tendon is mandatory to restore active flexion of the distal joint. The success of repair is directly related to the length of delay after injury, and the most satisfactory results are obtained with immediate operative treatment. As noted, type II injuries can often be treated late but if the tendon has retracted into the palm (type I), reinsertion is difficult or impossible after only 7 to 10 days. Although Carroll and Match[413] reported successful repairs as long as 4 weeks after injury, it is usually impossible to bring the contracted tendon back out to its insertion in late cases. Even if it can be accomplished that late, the finger may develop a severe flexion deformity because of muscle contracture and scarring in the sheath.

Technique of FDP Reattachment. The finger is exposed through a Bruner zigzag incision extending from the PIP crease into the pulp. The neurovascular bundles are identified and protected throughout the procedure. In type II cases, the proximal stump of FDP is easily found in the FDS chiasma through this limited incision. For type I cases, an additional incision is made in the distal palmar crease, the A1 pulley is opened, and the proximal stump of FDP is usually found coiled on itself within the sheath. The tip of the tendon is grasped with a clamp and pulled distally outside the skin to determine whether it can be reattached to the distal phalanx without undue tension. In our experience, it is usually not possible to bring the tendon back out to length from its retracted location in the palm after more than about 10 days after the injury. Even in cases in which the tendon is somewhere in between a type I and type II (see Fig. 11-14), length often cannot be restored because of myostatic contracture of the muscle. If the muscle has not contracted excessively, the tendon is passed as atraumatically as possible distally through the sheath beneath the A2 and A3 pulleys into the distal incision. Many techniques have been described for doing this; we prefer to use a 5-French pediatric gastrostomy feeding tube (one French unit is about one-third of a mm; therefore a 5-French tube is 1.66 mm in diameter). The tube is passed easily through the sheath, and the FDP stump is then sutured side by side to the tube with a single 4-0 nylon suture. As the tube is pulled distally, the tendon is carefully passed beneath the sheath through the opening in the A1 pulley.

Repair now becomes difficult because it is not always easy to pass the tendon beneath the A4 pulley, *yet it is imperative that the integrity of the A4 pulley be maintained.* The avulsed end of the tendon is usually wider than the A4 pulley, and it may be difficult to pass this beneath the intact pulley. We prefer to narrow the tendon end by trimming off its broad lateral flares. Another method is to split the distal end of the tendon longitudinally and pass each half separately beneath the pulley. Regardless of how it is done, every effort must be made to keep the A4 pulley intact. Failure to do so will seriously impair active flexion of the DIP joint.

Reattachment of the tendon to the volar base of distal phalanx is accomplished with any of the standard techniques. Although a bone anchor such as the Mitek device can be used, we prefer a pull-out suture with 3-0 Prolene, as shown in the description of gamekeeper's thumb repair. Care should be taken to avoid passing the needles and sutures through the germinal portion of the nail matrix because this may result in subsequent nail deformity.

In the case of type III injuries (fractures), fixation may be deceptively difficult. Large fragments are fixed with either an AO minifragment screw or K-wires, taking care to not penetrate the dorsal cortex at the base of distal phalanx to avoid damaging the germinal nail matrix. Smaller fragments can be excised and the tendon reinserted with a pull-out suture, as described earlier. Some surgeons believe that bone-to-bone healing is stronger, so they retain the bone fragment and pass the pull-out suture around the sides of the fragment to approximate the fracture edges.

For the rare type IV injuries, fixation of the bone and reattachment of the tendon are both required. Most authors[416,417,425,428,430] have preferred to fix the bone fragment first and then reinsert the tendon, although it can be be done in reverse order.[419] If secure fixation of the bone or tendon is achieved, we use a standard flexor tendon protocol postoperatively, with early passive mobilization of the tendon. If fixation is less than ideal or if the patient is unreliable, the hand and fingers are immobilized for 3 weeks before beginning an active motion program under the supervision of a hand therapist.

Late Treatment

Patients with late, untreated profundus tendon avulsions seek help for one or several of the following reasons: inability to flex the DIP joint, which may result in loss of grip strength; limited motion in the PIP joint, often associated with pain; or a tender lump in the palm due to flexor tenosynovitis and the retracted stump of the tendon. The first priority in these patients is to regain full, painless PIP motion with exercise and splinting. Frequently, that is all that is needed. If the patient continues to have pain in the PIP joint or the palm, excision of the FDP stump from the palm and occasionally a volar scar release of the PIP joint may be indicated. For those people in whom DIP instability in hyperextension with pinch is the main problem, arthrodesis of the DIP joint may be the appropriate treatment. This leaves a small minority of patients who may need active flexion of the DIP joint. FDP tendon grafting through or around an intact superficialis can be performed but not without significant risk of limiting PIP motion. This is an operation that should be done only by a surgeon well versed and experienced in flexor tendon surgery.

The choice of treatment in these patients—therapy alone, arthrodesis of the DIP joint, free tendon grafting, excision of the FDP stump, or doing nothing—demands mature clinical judgment and an understanding of the consequences of each.

FRACTURES OF THE PROXIMAL AND MIDDLE PHALANGES

There is an enormous divergence of opinion regarding the treatment of phalangeal fractures. An understanding of the rationale and principles underlying many different methods of treatment is important, not merely for their historical interest but because not all fractures in the fingers can or should be treated in the same manner. McLaughlin,[424] many of whose tenets are reflected in these pages, used to say that one should not make a fracture fit a favorite treatment. The method of management should be tailored to the peculiarities of the given fracture and to the needs of the individual patient.

In the section on Methods of Treatment, we describe most of the techniques that have been advocated and attempt to put each in its proper perspective.

Anatomy

As in other long bone fractures, displacement and angulation in fracture of the phalanges are influenced by two factors: the mechanism of injury and the muscles acting as deforming forces on the fractured bone.[17] The type of injury often determines the nature of the fracture; for example, a direct blow is more likely to cause a transverse or comminuted fracture, whereas a twisting injury more often results in an oblique or spiral fracture.[380] The direction of angulation seen in

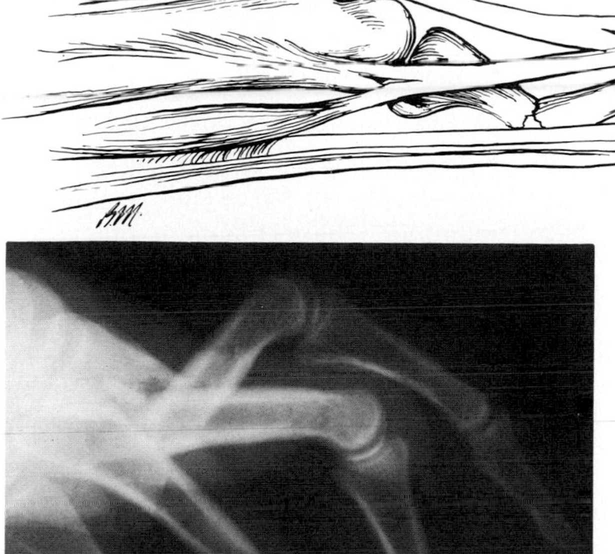

FIGURE 11-15. Unstable fractures of the proximal phalanx typically present with volar angulation. (*Top*) The proximal fragment is flexed by the bony insertion of the interossei into the base of the proximal phalanx. Once the stability of the proximal phalanx is lost, there is an accordion-like collapse at the fracture site, aggravated by further pull on the extensor hood by the extrinsic muscles. (*Right*) An x-ray, showing the typical, although somewhat exaggerated, volar angulation. More commonly, the angulation is about 30°.

fractures of the phalanges primarily depends on the muscles acting on that bone.

Unstable fractures of the proximal phalanx typically present with recurvatum-type angulation (apex volar; Fig. 11-15). The proximal fragment is flexed by the bony insertions of the interossei into the base of the proximal phalanx. Although there are no tendons inserting on the distal fragment, it tends to be pulled into hyperextension by the central slip acting on the base of the middle phalanx. Once the stability of the proximal phalanx is lost, there is an accordion-like collapse at the fracture site, aggravated by further pull on the extensor hood by the intrinsic muscles.

The middle phalanx is less commonly fractured than the proximal phalanx, and muscle forces acting on these fractures are different. The important deforming forces to be considered are the insertion of the central slip into the dorsum of the base of the middle phalanx and the insertion of the FDS volarly. The central slip has a well-defined area of insertion, and its action is to extend the middle phalanx. Although the action of the FDS is to flex the middle phalanx, its insertion is complex and is not confined to a short segment of the phalanx. Kaplan[10] described in detail the decussation of the superficialis tendon to allow the profundus tendon to pass through its two slips (see Kaplan's text for a detailed description). In essence, the superficialis divides into halves, each half turning 90° to allow the profundus to pass through and then completing another 90° rotation to insert into nearly the entire volar surface of the middle phalanx. Careful examination of a disarticulated middle phalanx reveals that there is a narrow ridge along each side of the middle two thirds of the volar aspect of the bone, into which the superficialis inserts. Many anatomic drawings depict the superficialis insertion as a precise, fixed point on the proximal aspect of the bone. A more accurate representation is illustrated in Figure 11-16, *top*, which shows the prolonged insertion of the superficialis, extending from a point just distal to the flare

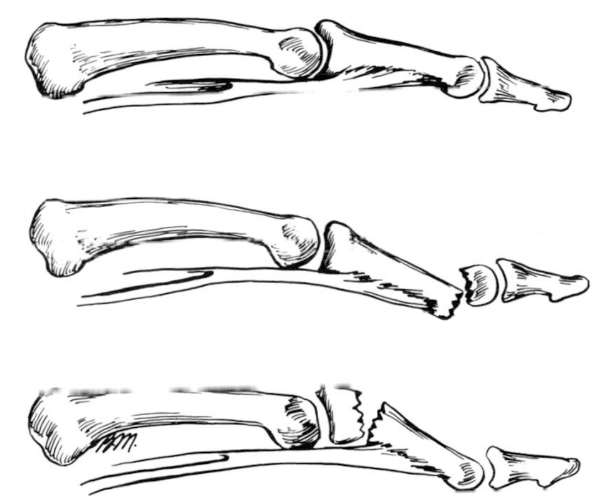

FIGURE 11-16. (*Top*) A lateral view, showing the prolonged insertion of the superficialis tendon into the middle phalanx. (*Center*) A fracture through the neck of the middle phalanx is likely to have a volar angulation because the proximal fragment is flexed by the strong pull of the superficialis. (*Bottom*) A fracture through the base of the middle phalanx is more likely to have a dorsal angulation because of the extension force of the central slip on the proximal fragment and a flexion force on the distal fragment by the superficialis.

of the base to a point only a few millimeters proximal to the neck. A fracture through the neck of the middle phalanx is likely to have volar angulation because the proximal fragment tends to be flexed by the strong pull of the superficialis (Fig. 11-16, *center*). A fracture through the base of the middle phalanx proximal to the insertion of the superficialis is more likely to be dorsally angulated because of the extending force of the central slip on the proximal fragment and a flexing force on the distal fragment by the superficialis (Fig. 11-16, *bottom*). Fractures through the middle two thirds of the bone may be angulated in either direction or not at all, and the angulation cannot always be predicted with accuracy, when based entirely on the tendon insertion.[291]

Malrotation at the fracture site is one of the most frequent complications of phalangeal fractures and can be avoided only by careful attention to anatomic detail. When the fingers are flexed, they do not remain parallel, as they are in full extension. They point generally in the direction of the scaphoid tubercle, although they do not actually converge on a single fixed point, as is sometimes depicted (Fig. 11-17). Thus, it is relatively easy to detect malrotation when the fingers are in full flexion (Fig. 11-18). With the fingers only semiflexed, it is helpful to use the planes of the fingernails as an additional guide to evaluate correct rotation. The opposite hand must be checked for comparison because often the border fingers lie in a slightly different plane of rotation as seen end on (Fig. 11-19). It may be most helpful to examine the fingernails with the palm flat and the fingers extended because flexion is usually painful for the patient with a fractured finger.[322]

Methods of Treatment

No Reduction and Early Active Motion

The method that James[190] called "garter strapping" others refer to as "buddy taping" or "dynamic splinting." The technique is simply to tape the injured finger to an adjacent normal digit and allow and actually encourage the patient to move the finger and use the hand as normally as possible while the fracture heals. The rationale is that early motion prevents stiffness in the small joints of the finger, which almost invariably results from immobilization. In a large series of patients having finger fractures, Wright[405] discovered that those treated with early active motion had less stiffness and less economic disability than those treated with immobilization. We basically agree with the idea that stiffness can be minimized and the patient can return to work sooner if the fracture is treated with buddy taping rather than immobilization. The method is not suitable for the treatment of all phalangeal fractures, however. Certain undisplaced fractures and impacted transverse fractures of the phalanges are ideally managed with buddy taping but only if two basic principles are observed. First, the fracture must truly be stable (ie, undisplaced or impacted), with no angulation in any plane. Lateral x-rays showing no displacement in both flexion and extension may help to confirm fracture stability.

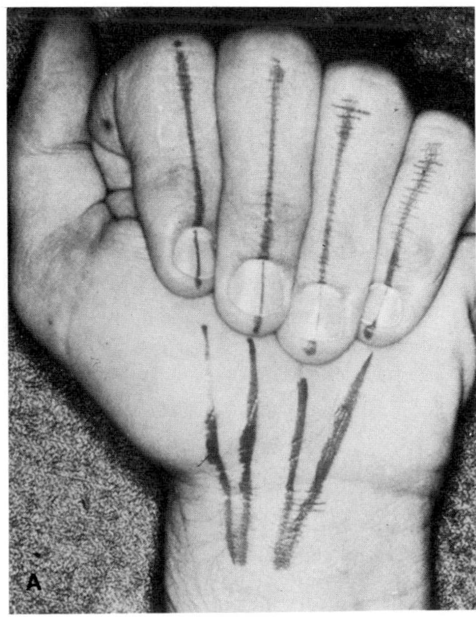

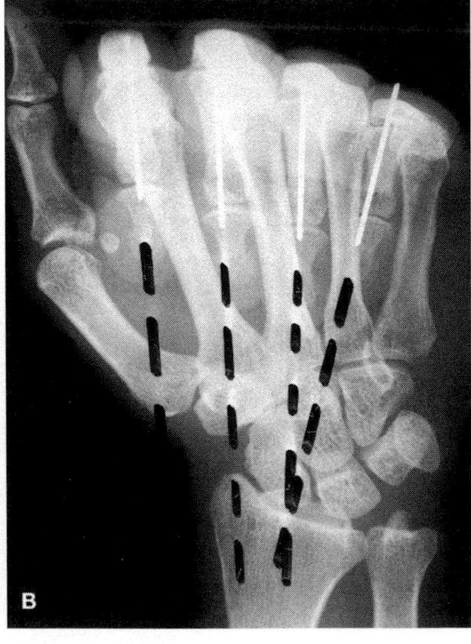

FIGURE 11-17. (**A**) When the fingers flex, they point generally in the direction of the scaphoid but they do not actually converge on a single fixed point, as is sometimes depicted. (**B**) This x-ray was made by taping K-wires on the midline dorsum of the fingers overlying the middle phalanges and positioning the hand as shown in **A**. Note that the convergence of the fingers on x-ray is even less than that seen clinically.

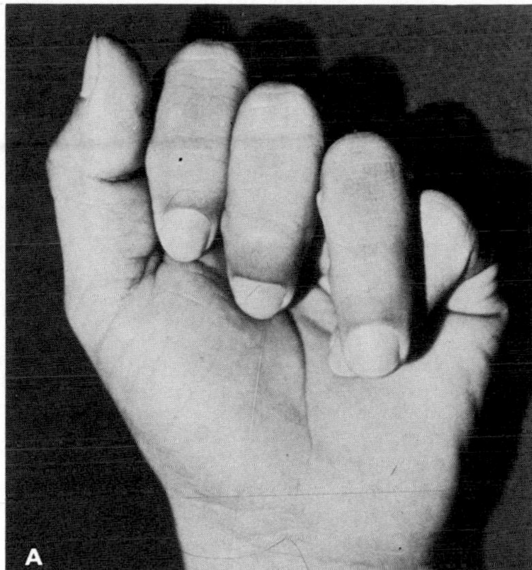

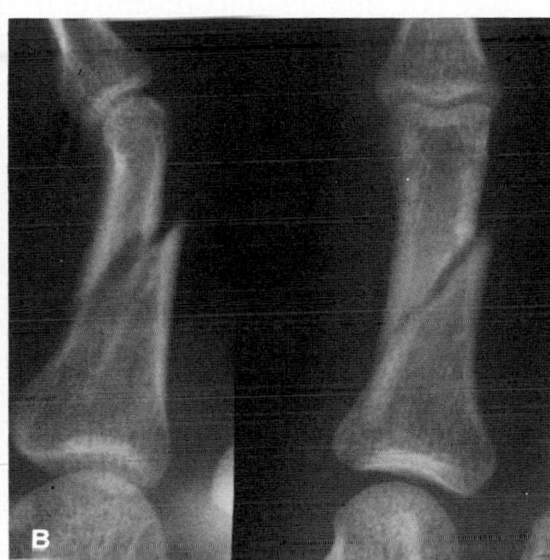

FIGURE 11-18. (**A**) Gross malalignment of the ring finger, seen in a patient in whom a fracture of the proximal phalanx was allowed to heal with rotational deformity. (**B**) Although subtle malalignment can be evaluated more critically by clinical means, rotational deformity may also be seen radiographically. The wide discrepancy in cross-sectional diameter of the proximal and distal fragments seen on the lateral view clearly demonstrates a severe rotational deformity. In the anteroposterior view, the deformity is less obvious, although any discrepancy in diameter of the two fragments should alert the physician to the possibility of rotational deformity.

Coonrad and Pohlman[82] have clearly illustrated the pitfall of misinterpreting an anteroposterior (AP) x-ray as showing an impacted fracture when the lateral view shows significant recurvatum-type angulation. Such fractures must be immobilized in flexion and are not amenable to the buddy taping technique. Second, careful clinical and radiographic follow-up of the patient during the healing phase is imperative to immediately recognize displacement or angulation at the fracture site.

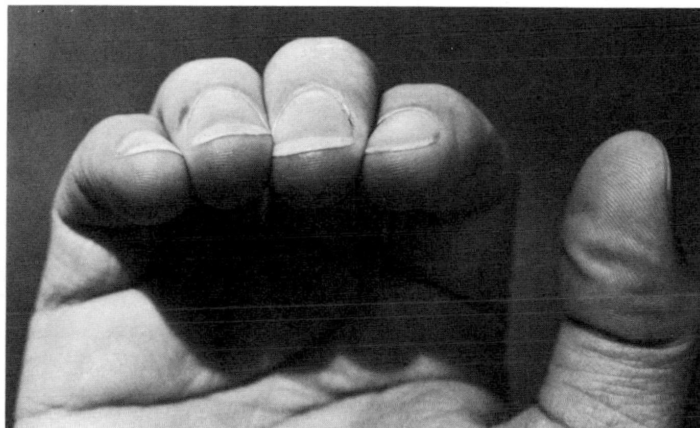

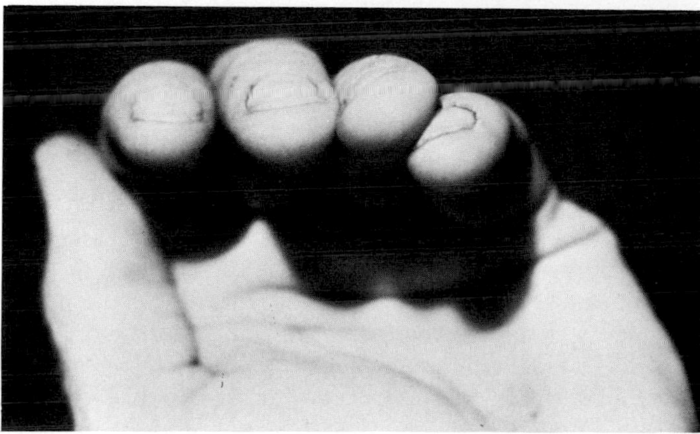

FIGURE 11-19. With the fingers only semiflexed, it is helpful to use the planes of the fingernails as an additional guide to correct rotation. The opposite hand must be checked for comparison because the border fingers frequently lie in a slightly different plane of rotation from that seen end-on (*top*). Note the significant rotational malalignment seen in the ring finger (*bottom*).

Closed Reduction and Immobilization

Many fractures of the phalanges can be satisfactorily managed by closed reduction and external immobilization, but several important principles must be followed if this method is to be successful.

1. The closed reduction maneuver must be performed before application of the cast or splint because the splint merely holds the reduction after it has been achieved. The splint must not be relied on to reduce the fracture.
2. As with fractures of any long bone, the controllable distal fragment must be brought into alignment with the uncontrollable proximal fragment.
3. The fracture must be stable after reduction for the splint to maintain the reduction. Transverse fractures generally fall into this category but spiral oblique fractures are inherently unstable, and it may be impossible to hold them reduced with any sort of splint or cast.

Types of Immobilization. A wide variety of splints and casts have been used to immobilize fractures of the phalanges. Because several muscles that act as deforming forces on the fracture originate in the forearm, it is advisable to immobilize the wrist as well as the injured finger. This is generally done with the wrist in about 30° of extension.

Circular Cast. A plaster or fiberglass short arm gauntlet cast that includes the fingers can be used. In small children, it is usually necessary to incorporate all four fingers in the cast, but the larger digits in adults may make it possible to immobilize only the fractured finger and a single adjacent finger. This method has the advantage of better stability but the disadvantage of possibly compromising the circulation if the swelling is significant.

Cast With Outrigger. A more commonly used method is to incorporate some sort of outrigger with a short arm gauntlet cast. Although different types of outriggers can be used, most are modifications of the wire finger splint described by Bohler[41] (Fig. 11-20). Because of its wide availability, the foam-padded aluminum splint is probably most commonly used in this country, although the stability that it provides leaves something to be desired, and rotational deformity may be more difficult to control. An outrigger made entirely of plaster can be used, but this is more likely to crack or break; reinforcement with a "fin," as illustrated in Figure 11-21, adds considerable strength without much additional weight or bulk.

Gutter Splints. Fractures involving the ring or small fingers can be adequately immobilized with an ulnar gutter plaster splint, leaving the radial digits completely free (Fig. 11-22*A*). A similar radial gutter splint, with a hole for the thumb, can be used for fractures in the index and long fingers (Fig. 11-23*B*). These splints are strong and easy to apply; their major disadvantage is that the plaster tends to "bunch up" in the distal palm, making it more difficult to immobilize the MP joints in flexion. This problem can be minimized by splitting the distal part of the splint and removing the volar half, making certain that the splint does not extend beyond the distal palmar crease; the dorsal half can be brought as far distally over the fingers as needed.[378] A simpler alternative is to use separate anterior and posterior splints.

Anterior and Posterior Splints. Separate well-padded anterior and posterior plaster splints are more versatile in their application than gutter splints and provide excellent stability. They have the added advantage of allowing the dressing to be split and rewrapped, without jeopardizing the reduction if the hand or fingers swell, or allowing the wrapping to be tightened if the swelling subsides.

Position of Immobilization. Unless there are local factors such as associated injuries that dictate otherwise, the preferred position of immobilization of the hand is the intrinsic plus or so-called JIP James position[191] (ie, with the MP joints in essentially full flexion and the interphalangeal [IP] joints in full extension; see Fig. 11-20*D*). The flexed position of the MP joints is desirable because of the cam effect of the metacarpal head on the collateral ligaments. As James noted, the MP joints almost never become stiff in flexion because in that position the collateral ligaments are stretched to their maximum length, whereas stiffness in extension is common because the ligaments contract if immobilized in their shortened position.

The PIP joints are more likely to become stiff in flexion but the explanation for this is not so clearcut. Although the PIP joints can occasionally become stiff in extension, that they are more likely to become stiff in flexion lends support to the concept that these joints should preferably be immobilized in minimal flexion. This dictum cannot be followed absolutely in treatment of fractures of the phalanges because of their tendency to develop volar angulation. It is imperative that the PIP joints be immobilized in sufficient flexion to correct this volar angulation unless a technique such as Burkhalter's (see later) is used that does not require immobilization of the PIP joints.

Ordinarily, it is sufficient to immobilize only the injured finger, but rotational alignment is usually easier to control if an adjacent normal finger is incorporated into the cast or splint.

Closed Reduction and Early Active Motion (Burkhalter's Technique)

Burkhalter and his colleagues[60,62,313] have described a unique method of treating phalangeal fractures, allowing early active motion of fractures that require

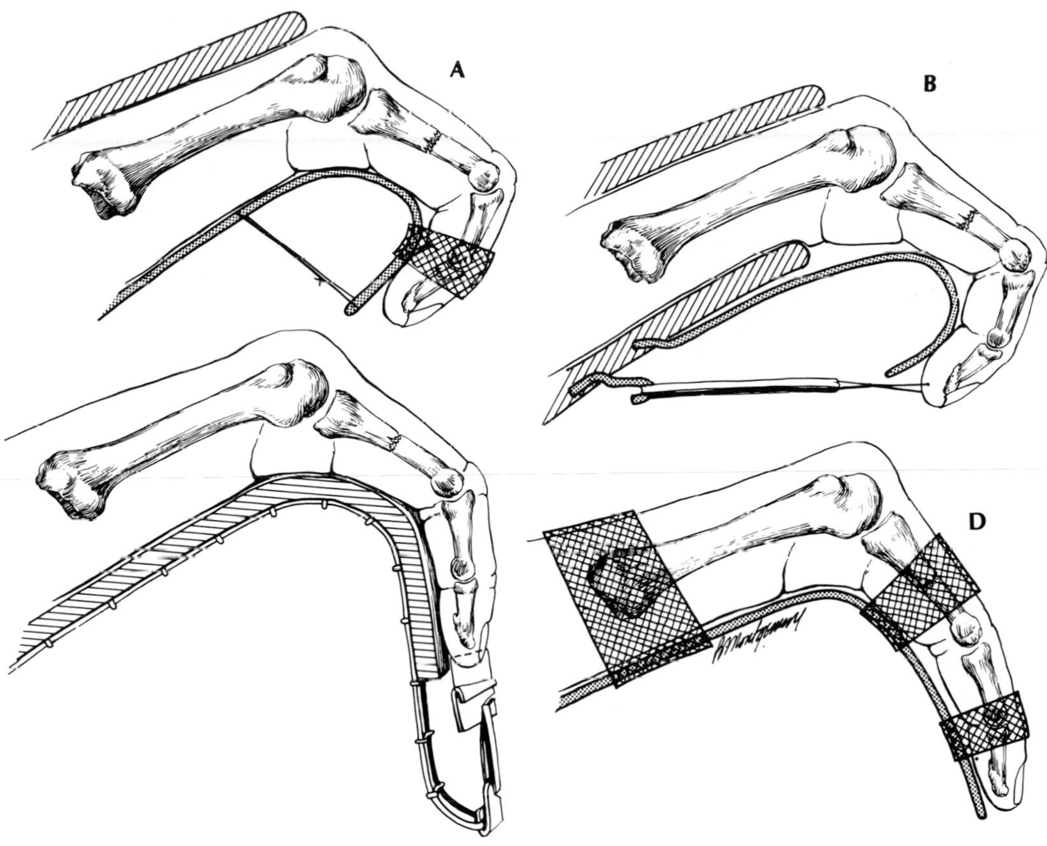

FIGURE 11-20. Several types of splinting have been described for treating fractures of the phalanges. (**A**) Böhler described the use of a wire outrigger combined with a dorsal plaster slab that immobilized the wrist. The tip of the outrigger was wired to itself to hold the finger in acute flexion. (**B**) Bunnell, and later Boyes, used a modified Böhler splint together with pulp traction, applied with sufficient tension to maintain the position obtained by manipulation. (**C**) Moberg designed a padded wire ladder that was used in conjunction with nail-pulp traction. The illustration is slightly inaccurate; the wire should pass through the periosteum at the tip of the distal phalanx. (**D**) James[190] advocated that fingers should be immobilized not in the position of function but in a position that more nearly resembles the intrinsic-plus position, in which the metacarpophalangeal joints are immobilized in at least 70° flexion and the interphalangeal joints in minimal flexion.

a closed reduction maneuver. This technique is based on the premise that with the MP joints in maximum flexion, the extensor hood is tightened to establish a dynamic tension band that provides palmar cortical compression during active flexion (Fig. 11-23*A*). After fracture reduction under digital block anesthesia, a short arm cast is applied with the wrist in 30° of extension and the MP joints in 90° of flexion (Fig. 11-23*B*). The cast extends dorsally to (but not beyond) the level of the PIP joints and is trimmed in the palm to allow full MP and PIP flexion (Fig. 11-23*C*). Simultaneous flexion of the adjacent normal digits is relied on to help control angulation and rotation.

This method is particularly effective in the treatment of transverse fractures of the phalanges with recurvatum-type angulation referred to previously, but Burkhalter[62] has emphasized that the technique requires great attention to detail on the part of the surgeon, frequent follow-up, and "enough maturity to be able to abandon the method if failure is likely."

Traction

Although it is not particularly popular in the American orthopaedic literature, traction (or extension, as it was often called) was advocated as the preferred method of treatment for finger fractures by some authors in the past.[159,261,269,271,276,315] Several types have been described, including skin traction, pulp traction, nail traction, and nail-pulp traction.[41,52,59,126,269,270,335]

Skeletal Traction. Several different variations of skeletal traction have also been described.[73,271,309] Perhaps the most serious disadvantage of skeletal traction as it was used in the past is that it severely restricts or eliminates motion in adjacent joints.

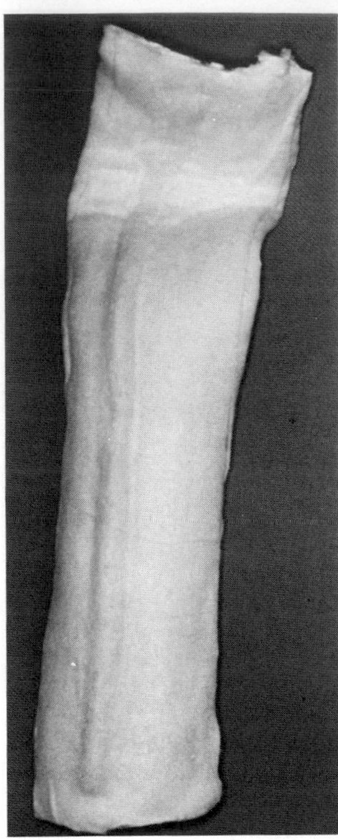

FIGURE 11-21. Plaster splints can be strengthened considerably without adding a great deal more weight by using a "fin," which is made by folding several layers of plaster longitudinally.

Dynamic Traction. In 1978, Agee[582] described a "force-couple" device that allows active motion while a simultaneous traction and reduction force is applied to the PIP joint. Agee's technique has appeared to be daunting to many and has therefore not enjoyed widespread use. (Buchanan[597] has attempted to explain Agee's force-couple concept and technique in greater detail, and the reader is encouraged to read this article before attempting to apply a force-couple device.)

Schenck[701] in 1986 introduced the term *dynamic traction*. Designed specifically for comminuted intra-articular fractures of the PIP joint, Schenck's technique provided a constant distraction force while allowing concomitant passive motion of the joint. Although sound in concept, his technique was slow to achieve widespread acceptance, mainly because of the cumbersome 10.5-inch hoop that the patient was required to wear. Schenck[333] has subsequently reduced the size of the hoop to a 6-inch diameter (Fig. 11-24*A*).

Other devices have been introduced that incorporate the dynamic traction concept of concomitant distraction and motion.[99,165,179,350,814] Hastings[165,627] has studied the problem in depth, and his articles should be read carefully to understand the indications, potential problems, and precise details in technique for application of his dynamic external fixator. Hotchkiss[171] has adapted his "compass" hinge technique (originally de-

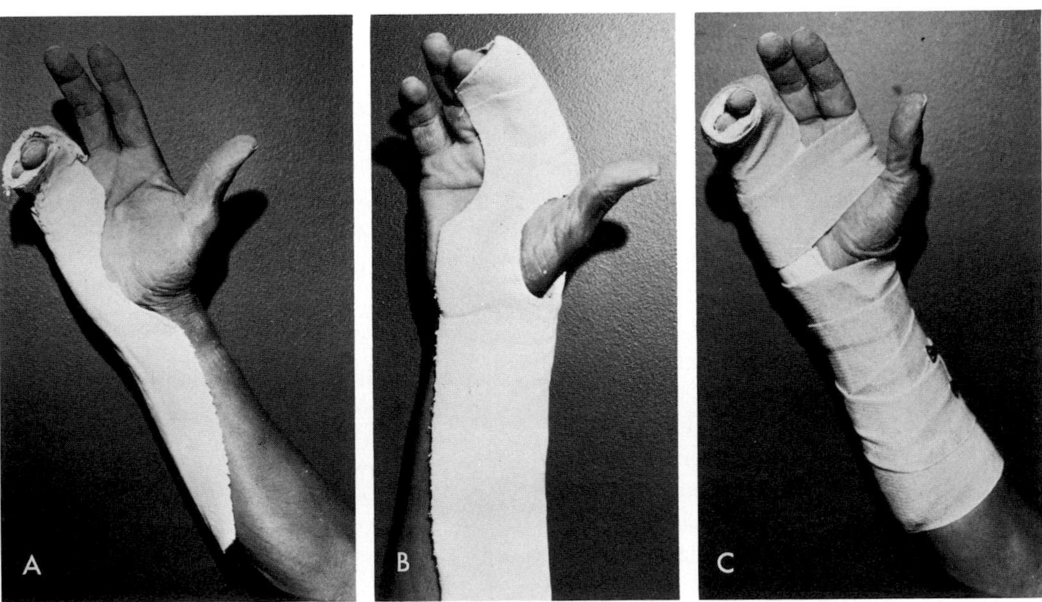

FIGURE 11-22. Gutter plaster. (**A**) Fractures involving the ring and small fingers can be adequately immobilized with an ulnar gutter splint, leaving the radial digits completely free. (**B**) A similar splint can be used on the radial side of the hand, cutting out a hole for the thumb. (**C**) The splint is held in place with an elastic bandage, wrapped securely but not tightly. We rarely use these now, preferring separate anterior and posterior splints.

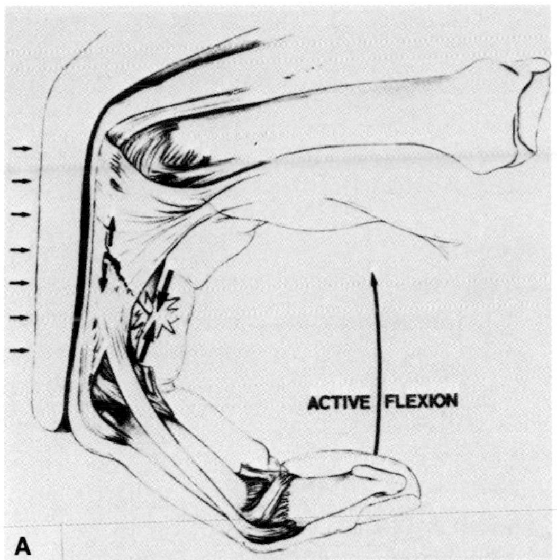

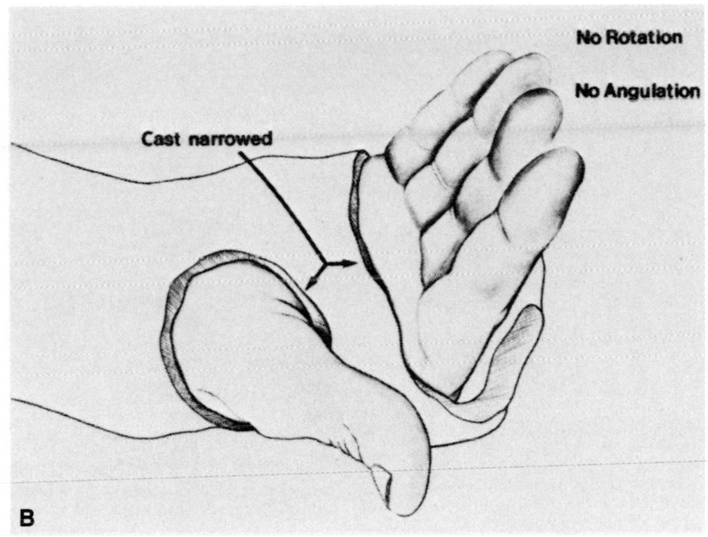

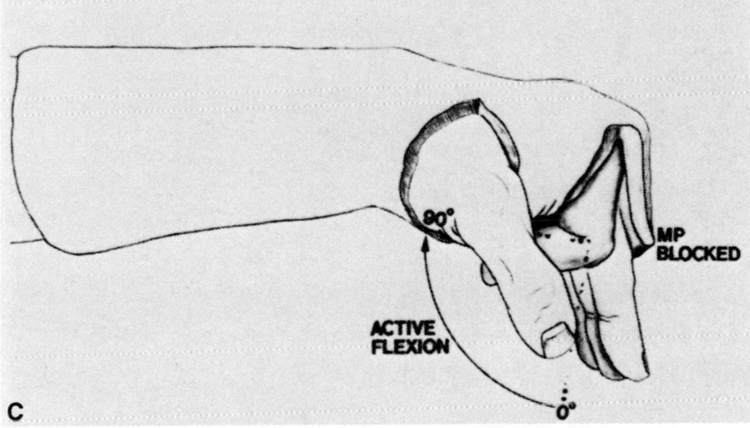

FIGURE 11-23. Burkhalter and Reyes's[62,313] method of early mobilization treatment of phalangeal fractures is based on the concept of an intact dorsal soft-tissue hinge (**A**). The metacarpophalangeal joints are flexed 70° to 90°; the cast extends dorsally to the proximal interphalangeal (PIP) joints (**B**) but is trimmed to allow full PIP flexion (**C**). (*Reyes, F.A., and Latta, L.L.: Conservative Management of Difficult Phalangeal Fractures. Clin. Orthop. 214:24, 1987.*)

signed for the elbow) to the PIP joint (Fig. 11-24*B*). His device is expensive ($795 to the hospital in early 1995) but is reusable. Inanami and coworkers[179] developed yet another type of dynamic external fixator (Fig. 11-24*C*) that is designed to apply a palmar-directing force on the middle phalanx, with concomitant distraction for PIP fracture-dislocations.

Suzuki and coworkers[369] in Japan (Fig. 11-24*D*) and Slade and coworkers[350] at Yale (Fig. 11-24*E*) have developed simpler dynamic traction systems that are fabricated by the surgeon at the operating table with K-wires and rubber bands.

Fahmy[120] has designed what he calls the "S" Quattro (Stockport Serpentine Spring System) that allows "some" motion in the involved joint, but this device should probably be considered a variant of static external fixation rather than a true dynamic fixator.

There is clearly a need for one of these various forms of dynamic traction that allows early motion in severely comminuted intra-articular fractures in the hand, especially the PIP joint. The problem is that most orthopaedic or hand surgeons encounter relatively infrequent indications for this form of treatment, and there is a fairly steep learning curve associated with the accurate application and use of these devices. It therefore behooves the surgeon to find one technique with which he or she is comfortable and try to become at least reasonably skilled in its application.

External Fixation

Techniques of external fixation in the hand evolved from a variety of homemade devices bonding percutaneous K-wires with acrylic cement (see Metacarpal Fractures). Although easily constructed from readily available supplies, these constructs had the disadvantage of not being readjustable. External fixation systems had been used in larger bones for many decades before Jaquet in 1976 developed the mini external fixator, which is applicable to fractures in the hand.[308]

The theoretic advantages of external fixation are that it:

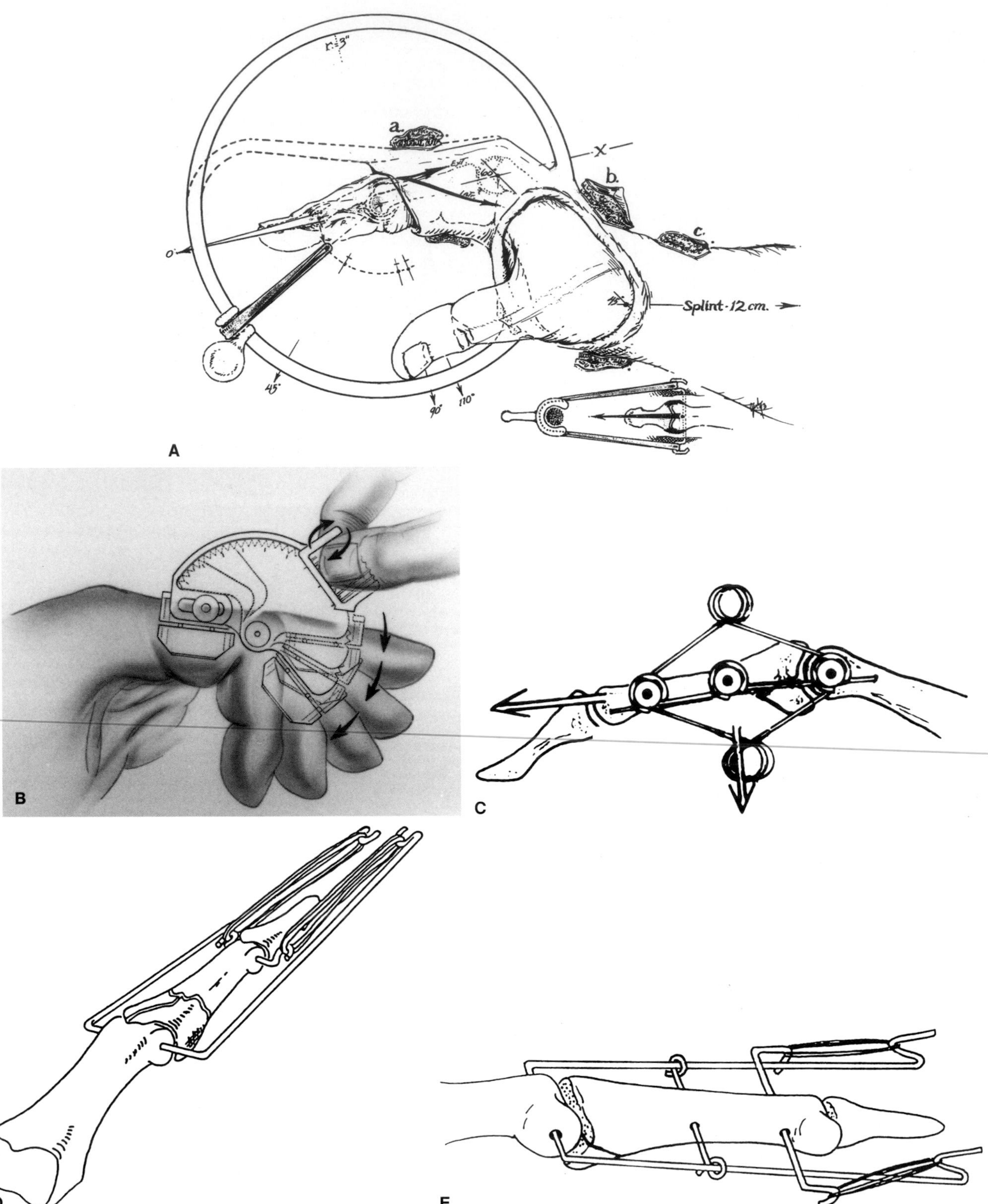

FIGURE 11-24. Several different types of "dynamic traction" devices have been introduced over the past several years. (**A**) Schenck[333] was the first to coin the term; his original device was rather cumbersome but he has subsequently reduced the diameter of the hoop from 10.5 inches to 6 inches, as shown in this drawing by Bill Littler. (**B**) Hotchkiss[171] has modified his elbow "compass" hinge to be used in the proximal interphalangeal joint. (**C**) Inanami and coworkers'[179] fixator consists of a pair of rhomboid apparatuses that apply simultaneous distraction and volarly-directed force. Suzuki and associates[369] (**D**) and Slade and colleagues[350] (**E**) have described similar devices that are constructed at the table using K-wires and rubber bands. *(Used with permission.)*

- Provides skeletal stability at a distance from the site of injury, facilitating unencumbered wound care[308]
- Immobilizes the fracture without internal hardware or conforming external splints, often with sufficient rigidity to allow early motion of adjacent joints[21,308]
- Allows postoperative adjustment of reduction in three planes (translational, rotational, and angular)[308]
- Permits compression, distraction, and lengthening.[278]

The versatility of current frame designs allows stabilization of a wide variety of fracture patterns and joint injuries.[308]

The major indications for external fixation devices in the hand are fractures with extreme comminution, particularly open fractures having severe contamination or concomitant soft-tissue injury, or segmental loss that precludes stabilization by other means.[34,131,316] In some situations, fixators may be used in conjunction with internal fixation or segmental bone grafting.[131,308]

Technique of External Fixation. The specific techniques of external fixator application vary according to the configuration of a particular fracture and the type of fixator used but there are certain general principles that form the basis for their use in all cases.

Incisions and Approaches. Behrens[27] has defined longitudinal regions, or corridors, of extremity anatomy, based on the presence of soft-tissue elements that are at risk when applying a fixator. He categorized and named these as:

- Safe corridor—the bone lies directly beneath the subcutaneous tissues that contain no neurovascular or musculotendinous structures.
- Hazardous corridor—contains musculotendinous units but no neurovascular structures.
- Unsafe corridor—both neurovascular and musculotendinous elements are at risk of injury during pin placement.

By definition, all external fixator applications in the phalanges and metacarpals will be in hazardous corridors.

In the central digits (long [III] and ring [IV] fingers), dorsolateral pin placement is necessary but lateral pin placement can be used in the border fingers (index [II] and small [V]). In the metacarpals, anatomy of the hand precludes any configuration other than dorsal pins in III and IV but lateral placement is possible (and probably preferable) in II and V.

In treating phalangeal fractures, it is virtually impossible to avoid impaling some part of the extensor apparatus with the pins; therefore, Nagy[278] advised making a generous longitudinal incision in the extensor hood at the planned pin site. In contrast, Putnam and Walsh[308] said that "care is taken to avoid the sagittal fibers at the MP joint level, and the lateral bands at the PIP level."

Pin Placement and Insertion. Most authors recommend two pins on either side of the fracture, but Parsons and coworkers[294] said that three pins are preferred, especially in the metacarpals. Ideally, only the fracture site should be bridged, sparing adjacent joints, but sometimes this is not possible.[278] Intra-articular fractures require traction across the joint, which actually may be beneficial in restoring joint congruity by ligamentotaxis.[385]

A hole for 2-mm pins should be predrilled with a 1.5-mm drill bit. Some authors have recommended that the pins be inserted either by hand or with a slow-speed power drill to minimize thermal necrosis.[294,308] Seitz and coworkers[343] believe that power should be used for drilling because it eliminates "wobble" and therefore creates better purchase for the pin. In their opinion, the most important factors in preventing thermal necrosis are: drill bit sharpness, adequate irrigation during drilling, and predrilling.

The image intensifier is useful in monitoring pin placement but plain radiographs provide a more accurate and reliable means of evaluating adequacy of reduction, especially with intra-articular fractures.

Timing. In open fractures, the fixator may be applied at the time of initial debridement and irrigation. Delayed primary wound closure or appropriate coverage can be accomplished at the time of the second look if the wound is clean or later, if indicated. Bone grafting can be also be performed as a delayed primary or secondary procedure[308] (as described in the section on Massive Trauma).

Complications. Early series of hand fractures treated with mini external fixators reported relatively high complication rates, including nonunion, pin-tract infection, and malunion. Studies have shown lower complication rates.[21,278,294]

Many of these complications can be minimized by following the important principles recommended by experienced users and briefly outlined in the preceding section.[131,278,294,308,342]

Closed Reduction and Internal Fixation (CRIF) With K-Wires

This technique is often referred to as closed reduction and percutaneous pin fixation, but Eaton's[110] acronym of CRIF (closed reduction and internal fixation) is useful because it fits with the other accepted terms commonly used in fracture treatment. The theoretic advantage of CRIF is that an unstable fracture can be rendered sufficiently stable to allow early motion, without subjecting the hand to the surgical trauma of open reduction. Excellent results can be achieved with this method but the procedure is not as easy to perform as one may anticipate.[150] Two knowledgeable surgeons facilitate the technique; one reduces and holds the fracture and the other inserts the pins (Fig. 11-25). A power-driven drill is essential, and although the image intensifier is not absolutely necessary, it makes the procedure easier (except in intra-articular fractures, where the images produced on the monitor are not clear enough to ensure precise anatomic reduction;[235] in such fractures, plain radiographs are required). Bilos[33] has developed special pins to achieve compression but we have found smooth K-wires to be entirely satisfactory and simpler to use. Several authors[70,325] have suggested the use of hypodermic needles to serve as guides for more precise pin placement; the surgeon lines up the needle and holds it in position while an assistant inserts the K-wire through the needle. (Table 11-4 lists the proper needle to use with each size K-wire.) Donahue (Paul J. Donahue, St. Paul, MN, personal communication, 1988) passed on to us Scheker's technique of using an 18-gauge angiocath as a passer for K-wires through bone. The hub is pulled and twisted off the needle, and the needle itself can then be inserted into a power drill and driven directly through the bone. The advantage of this is that it eliminates the need for the additional step of passing a K-wire but care must be taken not to crimp the blunt end of the needle while removing the hub.

Eaton and some of his former hand fellows[29,110] have been staunch advocates of percutaneous pin fixation. They recommend that the procedure be performed under local or wrist block anesthesia because allowing the patient to move the fingers painlessly through an active range of motion is the best method of assessing anatomic reduction and stability and of avoiding rotational deformity. They describe clearly two distinct methods of CRIF, both described in detail below.

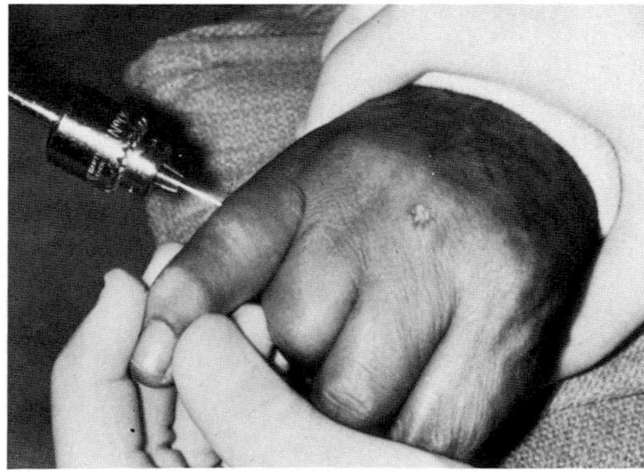

FIGURE 11-25. Closed reduction and internal fixation of unstable phalangeal fractures by direct percutaneous pinning is a useful technique but not easy to perform. (*Green, D.P., and Anderson, J.R.: Closed Reduction and Percutaneous Pin Fixation of Fractured Phalanges. J. Bone Joint Surg., 55A:1652, 1973.*)

TABLE 11-4
Hypodermic Needle Guides for Kirschner Wire Placement

Kirschner Wire	Diameter (mm)	Size Needle Required for Guide
0.028-inch	0.712	19-gauge
0.035-inch	0.889	18-gauge
0.045-inch	1.143	16-gauge
0.054-inch	1.372	16-gauge
0.0625-inch	1.588	14-gauge too small

The main disadvantages of CRIF are (1) it is difficult (especially with spiral oblique fractures), (2) reduction of the fracture may not be as precise as with open reduction, and (3) parts of the extensor mechanism may be impaled with the K-wires. However, it does avoid the considerable added surgical trauma of open reduction and is therefore an excellent alternative method of treatment for certain fractures. One disadvantage rarely mentioned is that surgeons must expose their own hands to irradiation, and Widgerow and colleagues[397] said that they rarely use CRIF for precisely this reason.

Technique of CRIF for Transverse and Short Oblique Fractures. Intramedullary pin fixation of the proximal phalanx is achieved by passing a K-wire longitudinally through the metacarpal head and across the MP joint (Fig. 11-26*C*). This method is particularly well suited for those difficult transverse fractures near the base of the proximal phalanx that tend to develop a recurvatum-type deformity. Reduction is performed by applying longitudinal traction through the middle phalanx while maximally flexing the MP joint, with the PIP joint held in least 45° flexion. A 0.045-inch K-wire is passed percutaneously into the dorsum of the metacarpal head (preferably to the side of rather than through the extensor tendon), across the flexed MP joint, and down the medullary canal of the proximal phalanx to the level of the condyles. The pin does not cross the PIP joint. A second pin can be passed parallel to the first to provide additional stability. Accuracy of reduction and correct placement of the pin are verified radiographically, and correct rotational alignment is assured by having the patient actively flex the fingers. The pins can be cut off beneath the skin but we prefer to bend them into a loop or right angle outside the skin to facilitate removal.

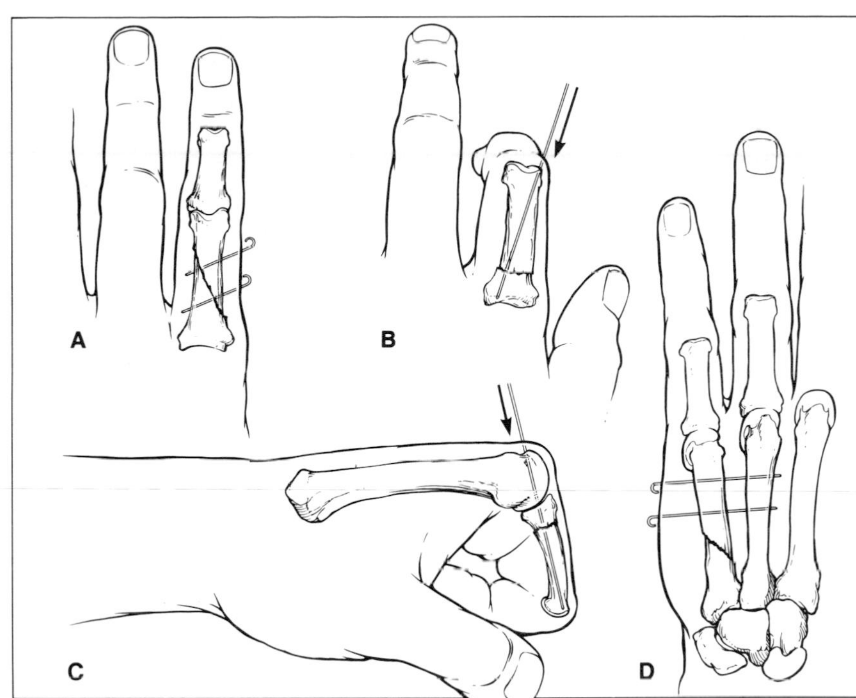

FIGURE 11-26. Four methods of closed reduction and internal fixation (CRIF). See text for details of each.

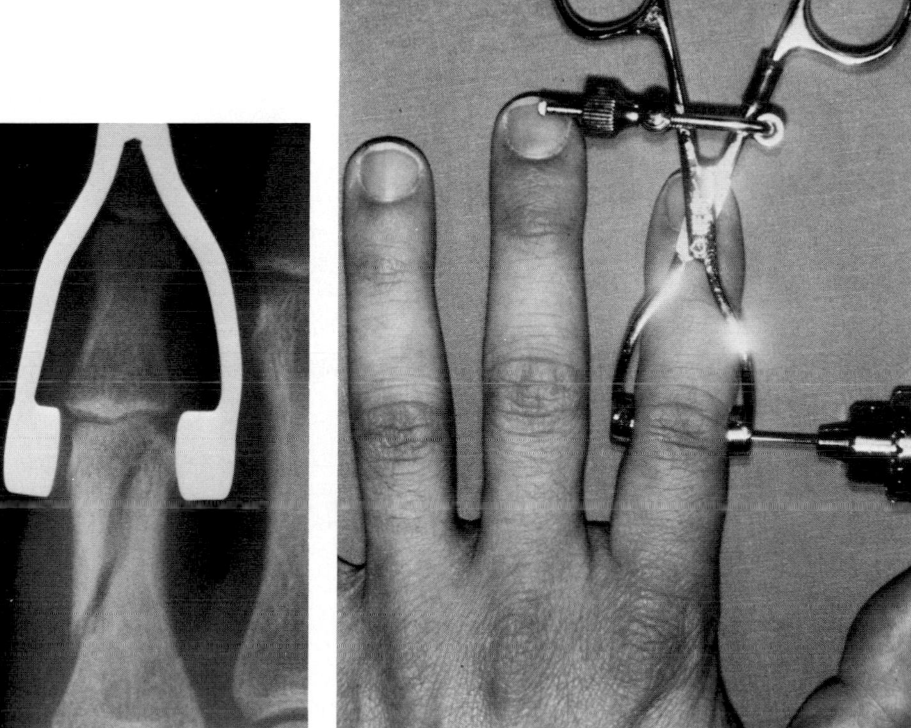

FIGURE 11-27. Fracture reduction clamps such as the Blalock are useful in closed reduction and percutaneous pin fixation of fractures of the phalanges. (*Left*) The fracture is reduced, the clamp is applied, and x-rays confirm the reduction. (*Right*) A hole in the clamp allows exact placement of the pin.

Because the wire crosses the MP joint, a short arm cast or splint that rigidly immobilizes the MP joints is imperative with this method to prevent bending or breakage of the pins. We prefer a Burkhalter-type cast that keeps the MP joints in flexion but allows full active PIP motion. Both the cast and the K-wires are removed at 3 weeks. A theoretic disadvantage of this method is the transarticular placement of the K-wire[74] but Cordrey[83] has shown that this does not necessarily result in limitation of motion if the cartilage surfaces are intact.

Technique of CRIF for Spiral and Long Oblique Fractures. Spiral oblique fractures are percutaneously pinned by direct fixation of the fracture,[29,110,151] although this technique (see Fig. 11-26*A*) is considerably more difficult than the intramedullary method used for transverse fractures, described in the previous section. There is a narrow margin for error because a few millimeters' difference in pin placement can easily result in inadequate fixation. Reduction of the fracture and pin placement are both facilitated by the use of a fracture-reduction clamp, such as the Blalock[38] (Fig. 11-27), AO,[140] or Aesculap (Fig. 11-28).

It is imperative for the surgeon to have a three-dimensional (3D) image of the fracture, and the K-wires must be inserted to accommodate this configuration. The pins probably will not gain adequate purchase on the fracture fragments if they are inserted in a purely coronal plane (ie, from the mid-axial direction). Figure 11-29, which is a 3D reconstruction of a spiral fracture made from CT scans, clearly shows that the fracture line spirals around the phalanx from dorsoulnar proximally to palmar radial distally. The K-wires must therefore be inserted in the proper plane (eg, in this case, directed from slightly palmar to dorsal if inserted from the radial side or from slightly dorsal to palmar if from the ulnar side).

At least two pins (preferably 0.045-inch) must be used, placed as far apart as possible yet providing solid purchase on both fracture fragments. Ideally, the pins should not be exactly parallel to each other because this may allow the fracture to separate. If the pins are placed properly to conform to the spiral configuration of the fracture, more stability is achieved. The further the distance between the pins at the fracture line, the more stable the fixation. Radiographic control is mandatory to ensure satisfactory reduction and pin placement.

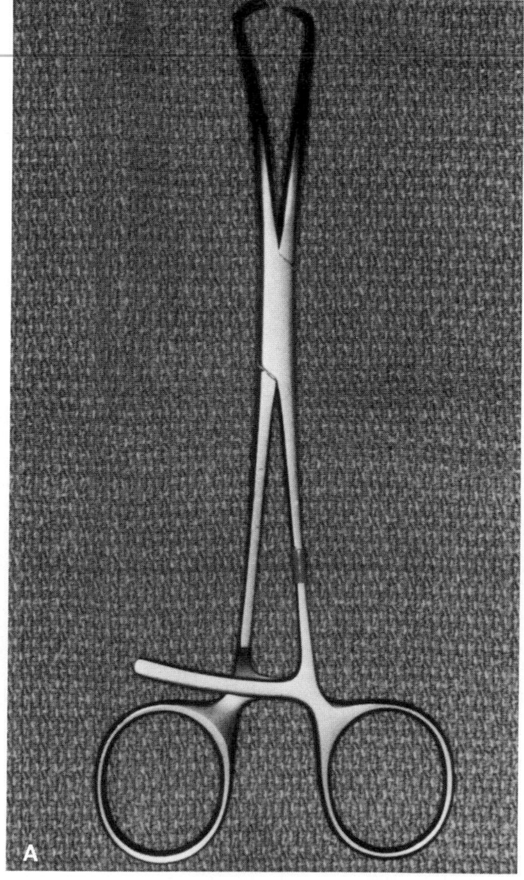

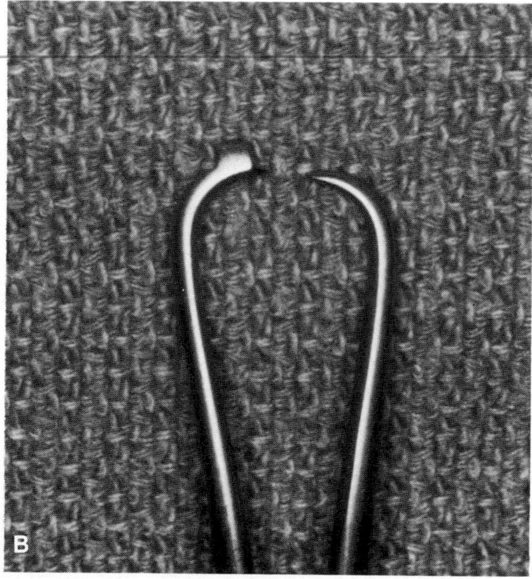

FIGURE 11-28. The Aesculap clamp (**A**) is our preferred instrument for percutaneous pin fixation. The sharp points hold the reduction achieved, and the small fenestration (**B**) allows precise placement of a K-wire.

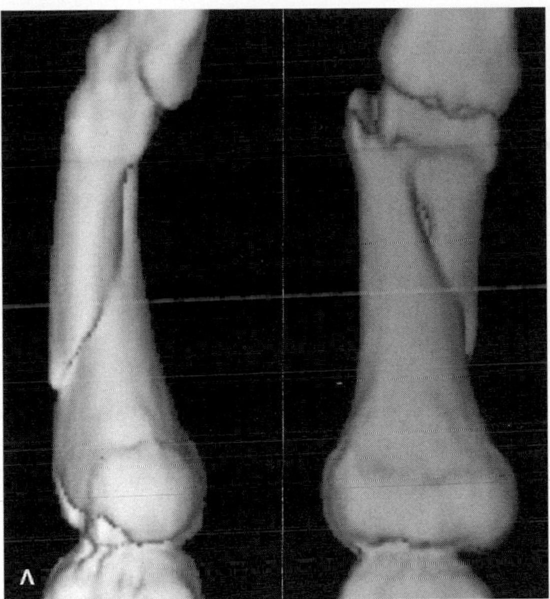

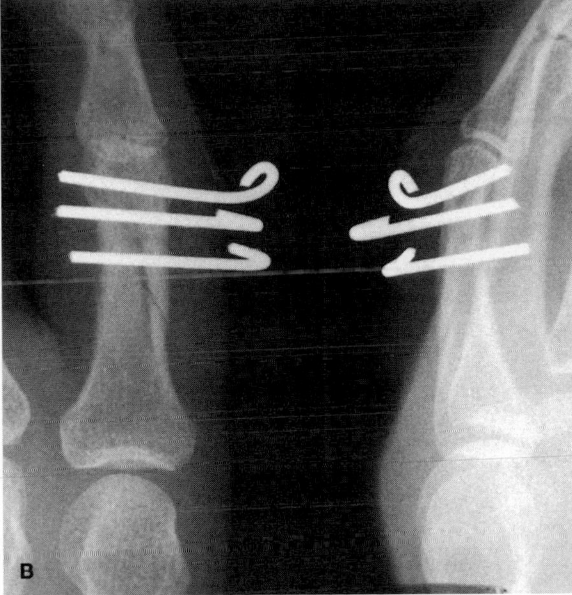

FIGURE 11-29. (**A**) Three-dimensional reconstruction from computed tomography scans shows clearly the spiral configuration of this fracture. Note that the distal spike lies palmar to the mid-axial line and the proximal spike dorsal to that line. Solid purchase (**B**) was achieved by inserting the pins along a plane from slightly palmar (distal) to slightly dorsal (proximal). Pins inserted in a purely coronal plane are less likely to be accurately placed in these narrow fracture fragments.

The pins may be cut off beneath the skin or left to protrude with the tip bent into a small loop or right angle (Fig. 11-30). To prevent loosening of the pin when it is bent, the pin must be grasped firmly with a large needle holder or needle-nosed pliers immediately adjacent to the skin. Although minimal drainage is common from percutaneous pin tracts, it usually resolves with no permanent residual problems after the pins are removed, and the ease of removing pins that have been left out through the skin makes this method our preference. If the pins are left percutaneous, patients are instructed to apply peroxide or Betadine to the pin tracts two or three times a day, and submersion of the hand in water is not allowed until the pins are removed.

With proper pin placement that provides good fracture stability, buddy taping can be instituted immediately and active range of motion encouraged from the first postoperative day. The pins are removed at 3 weeks, even though radiographically the fracture does not appear to be healed. Buddy taping is continued for another 3 weeks.

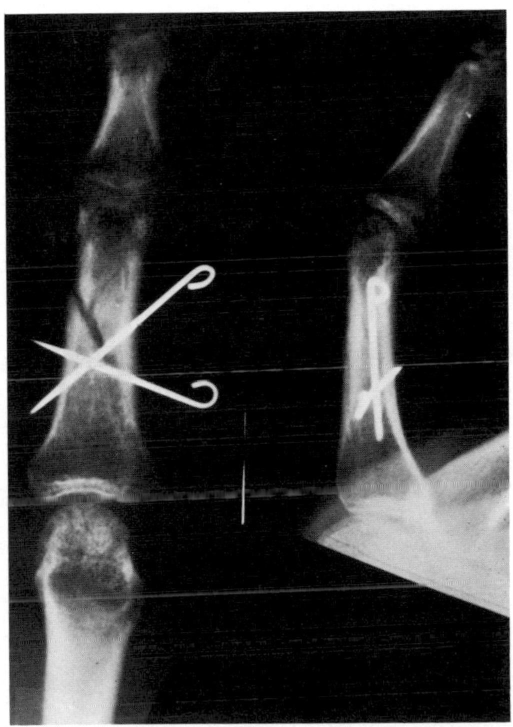

FIGURE 11-30. We prefer to leave the K-wires protruding through the skin and bent into a loop to minimize pin migration and facilitate removal later in the office.

CRIF With Screws

Freeland[134] has suggested a variation of CRIF for spiral fractures of the phalanges. He performs a closed reduction of the fracture but uses compression lag mini screws instead of K-wires. The first step of the procedure is the same as that described in the previous section, with provisional fixation achieved first with K-wires. With the fracture thus held reduced, at least two minifragment screws are inserted with lag technique through a "limited 1 cm to 2 cm incision." Freeland, who is an accomplished AO surgeon, admits that the technique is technically demanding but he believes that it combines the best attributes of both methods (CRIF and ORIF; ie, providing maximum stability with minimal dissection).

Although this method lies somewhere between CRIF and ORIF, it probably should be considered a variant of open reduction rather than closed manipulation.

Open Reduction and Internal Fixation (ORIF)

Unstable fractures that cannot be reduced by closed manipulation and maintained with external splinting require internal fixation. As noted in the preceding section, selected fractures can be reduced by closed manipulation and stabilized with percutaneously placed K-wires but in some situations, open reduction to ensure more precise anatomic reduction is warranted. Specific indications for ORIF vary widely, depending on the experience, technical skills, and judgment of the surgeon but the following are probably considered to be appropriate indications by most surgeons:

1. Most displaced intra-articular fractures involving the PIP joints and other selected intra-articular fractures—Moderate to severe comminution is a relative contraindication, again depending on the skills and experience of the surgeon
2. Multiple fractures[25,164]—The greater the number of fractures, the more desirable it is to provide stabilization of the skeleton
3. Open fractures and associated soft tissue injury—This is a somewhat radical departure from previous concepts because it was formerly suggested that open fractures were a relative contraindication to open reduction.[85]

With wider experience and more precise techniques for open reduction, some authors[164,186] believe that open injuries with severe soft-tissue injury constitute an important indication for open reduction because providing skeletal stabilization may allow the soft-tissue injury to be managed more effectively. This does not mean that internal fixation necessarily should be performed on the day of injury, and authors with wide experience have emphasized the importance of delayed primary fixation, a concept that has particular application to injuries requiring combined skeletal and soft-tissue repair and reconstruction (see Massive Hand Trauma).[133,186,260]

Once the decision has been made that internal fixation is indicated, the surgeon has an ever-increasing variety of techniques and implants from which to choose, a far cry from the situation in 1924, when Tennant[373] resorted to using a steel phonograph needle for fixation. The reader interested in the history of medicine is referred to Meals and Meuli's[259] brief but fascinating review of the evolution of internal fixation of metacarpal and phalangeal fractures.

K-Wires. K-wires have traditionally been referred to and are most recognizable by their size in English measurement (decimal fractions of inches). Because more publications are using metric units exclusively, Table 11-5 is presented to show the metric equivalents of the most familiar designations.

Smooth K-wires remain the most useful and versatile mode of fixation for fractures of the phalanges, despite numerous biomechanical studies that tend to denigrate their efficacy. Placement of the K-wires largely depends on the anatomy of the fracture (eg, long spiral fractures are more easily fixed with horizontally or obliquely directed pins, transverse fractures generally require crossed or longitudinal K-wires). Studies by Namba and colleagues[279] of Kirschner-wire configuration suggest several important technical details:

1. K-wires are not as efficient as drill bits and probably cause more thermal necrosis.[382] They are therefore best inserted at slow drilling speeds.
2. The diamond-tipped wire (two angled facets) has superior drilling properties but has a greater tendency to "walk" along the cortex before penetrating the bone.
3. The trochar-tipped wire (four angled facets) provides better holding power initially, although at

TABLE 11-5
Metric Equivalents of Kirschner Wires

0.028 inch	0.7 mm
0.035 inch	0.9 mm
0.045 inch	1.2 mm
0.054 inch	1.4 mm
0.0625 inch	1.6 mm

Sizes of Kirschner wires have traditionally been designated by their decimal fraction of an inch. Because more publications are now referring to K-wire diameters in metric units, this table is provided to show the metric equivalents of the more familiar English units. The metric equivalents have been rounded off and are therefore approximations.

3 weeks there is no difference in holding power between the trochar and diamond tips.

4. An oblique cutting tip made by the surgeon when a K-wire is shortened in the operating room is clearly inferior in both drilling and holding properties. This implies that for hand surgery, the commercially available double-ended 6-inch K-wires are to be preferred over the standard 9-inch wires.

Ruggeri and colleagues[325] and others[111] have suggested that K-wire placement can be facilitated by using a hypodermic needle as a pin guide, having the surgeon hold the needle while an assistant inserts the K-wire (see Table 11-4 for appropriate-size needles).

Alexander and coworkers[18] noted that slippage at the bone–wire interface is the most common cause of failure of K-wire fixation. This potential problem theoretically may be minimized with the Bilos compression pin, but Noyez and Verstreken[284] have recommended that the Bilos pin be predrilled with a K- wire. Viegas and coworkers[388] have done laboratory studies to compare the strength of various K-wire configurations.

Some authors have suggested that crossed K-wires may actually distract the fracture site and delay healing.[197] Despite the theoretic disadvantages, however, properly placed crossed K-wires are an excellent time-proved method of fixation of transverse fractures. O'Brien's description[111,287] of retrograde placement of K-wires is helpful in ensuring proper apposition of the fragments (Fig. 11-31).

Botte and coworkers[48] found that many complications of K-wires were associated either with poor initial pin placement or lack of patient compliance.

Whether to leave pins protruding through the skin or cut them off beneath the surface is a matter of personal preference of the surgeon. Our basic guideline is that if it is anticipated that the pins will be removed in 4 weeks or less, they are left percutaneous; if they are to be left in longer, they are buried. Based on Botte and coworkers'[48] findings in their extensive study of K-wire complications, this appears to be a reasonable rule because in their series, pin-tract infections occurred at a mean time of 10 weeks and loosening at 8 weeks. Their routine was to remove the pins "as soon as bony healing allowed," with a mean duration in their cases of 6.5 weeks.

Absorbable Pins. Relatively little has been published about the use of absorbable pins in treatment of fractures in the hand, although they have been used in other types of fractures and in maxillofacial surgery.[45,300] Several different types of materials have been tested, including sapphire (monocrystalline alumina ceramic), PGA (polyglycolic acid), and PLA (polylactic acid).[184,214,300] PLA is said to have a longer degradation time than PGA, which loses virtually all of its strength in 3 weeks. In one of the few studies in which absorbable pins were used for phalangeal and metacarpal fractures, the intramedullary PGA pin was supplemented with a wire loop in all cases.[214]

If used to penetrate the cortex, all of these absorbable pins share the common disadvantage of requiring a predrilled hole. There is also some concern about possible late inflammatory reaction.[45]

Intramedullary Fixation. Intramedullary fixation is an appealing concept but it has not achieved a high level of popularity in the fixation of hand fractures for

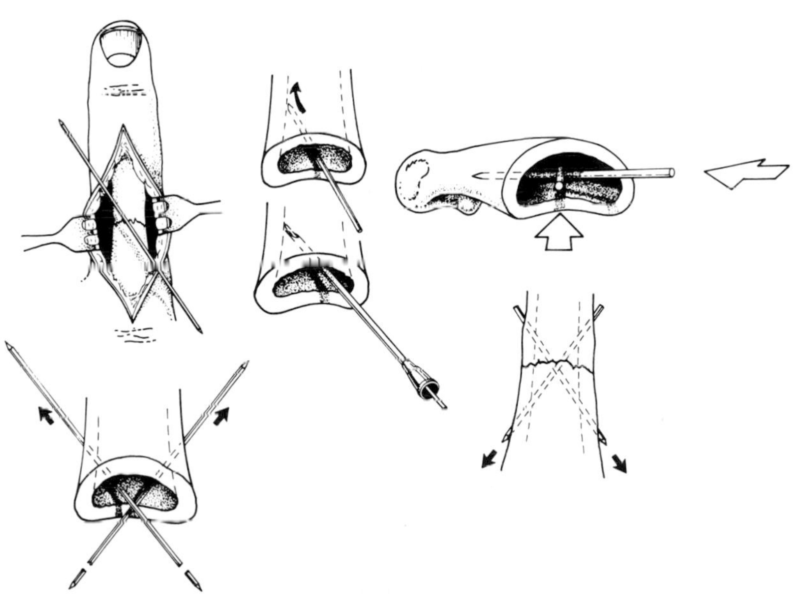

FIGURE 11-31. Retrograde placement of crossed K-wires through the fracture site ensures more accurate fixation than trying to engage both cortices with the fracture reduced. (*O'Brien, E.T.: Fractures of the Metacarpals and Phalanges. In Green, D.P. (ed.): Operative Hand Surgery, p. 615. New York, Churchill-Livingstone, 1982.*)

a variety of reasons, including difficulty of insertion, impairment of adjacent joint motion, relatively poor control of rotational alignment, and problems with removal. Grundberg[156] described an ingenious technique that obviates some of these disadvantages (Fig. 11-32). A Steinmann pin one size larger than the medullary canal is used to enlarge the proximal and distal canals by drilling first with the sharp end of the pin and then with the blunt end, so that it does not penetrate into the adjacent joint. The blunt end is then introduced into the proximal fragment, and the pin is cut off so that it protrudes 1 cm in a phalanx and 1.5 cm in a metacarpal. The fracture is then distracted and the pin is introduced into the medullary canal of the distal fragment as the fracture is reduced. We have used this method in difficult situations in which other forms of fixation would not suffice; the major problem we encountered was in obtaining adequate purchase on the distal fragment.

Hall[160,161] has described the use of Enders-type flexible intramedullary rods, which he says provides sufficiently rigid fixation to obviate a cast and is therefore a good method to employ in the noncompliant patient. The main disadvantage of Hall's method is that it requires specially made rods. Varela and Carr[384] developed a modification of Hall's technique, using standard 0.045-inch K-wires. Before insertion, the pins are bent with pliers or needle holders into a gently curved configuration to take advantage of intramedullary three-point fixation, as is done with Rush rods, and the sharp tip is dulled with a rasp. The pins are inserted by hand under direct vision through a limited incision and are "stacked" to fill the medullary canal (two to five pins are generally used).

Iselin and Thevenin[181] designed a flexible intramedullary screw that was also reported to allow early motion with no external immobilization. Lewis and colleagues[226,282] reported on an expandable intramedullary device that was shown in the laboratory to provide good fixation but long-term follow-up clinical data have never been published.

Intraosseous Wiring. The technique of intraosseous wiring was probably first used by Robertson[319] for arthrodesis of IP joints, but its application to fractures in the hand should be attributed to Lister[230] (Fig. 11-33), who noted that the method is particularly useful in transverse fractures near a joint. Biomechanical studies have shown this to be a consistently rigid method of internal fixation,[136] and Lister[230] has recommended minimal external splinting after its use. Whether this technique should be called intraosseous (within bone) or interosseous (between bones) is debatable but because Lister chose the former in his original description, we have tended to use that term.

Technique of Intraosseous Wiring. Parallel drill holes are made 5 mm distal and proximal to the fracture site with a 0.035-inch K-wire. Twenty-six–gauge stainless steel monofilament wire is then passed through the holes. Before the wire loop is tied, the 0.035-inch K-wire is driven from the fracture site out distally through the cortex of the distal fragment. With the fracture held reduced under direct vision, the obliquely oriented K-wire is driven back across the fracture site to engage the opposite cortex of the proximal fragment. The wire loop is then tied and its free end buried into a small hole in the adjacent cortex.

Several authors[139,145,258] have offered tips on the technique of intraosseous wiring. There is some latitude in the choice of wire size. Vanik and coworkers[383] concluded from their laboratory studies that 24-gauge wire is the strongest but is too stiff, and they prefer 26- or 28-gauge wire in the clinical setting. Gingrass and associates[139] recommended 30-gauge wire for comminuted fractures with small fragments, using the straight needle (0.022-inch) that comes swaged on the Ethicon 4-0 pull-out wire for drilling the holes. Passage of wire through the drill holes is facilitated by inserting a hypodermic needle through the hole.[332] (Table 11-6 lists the proper size needle required.)

Variations of intraosseous wiring include the use of an intramedullary K-wire instead of the oblique orientation described above; and 90-90 wiring.[175,407] The 90-90 wiring technique is probably more applicable to replantations, wherein circumferential bone exposure is easily obtained.

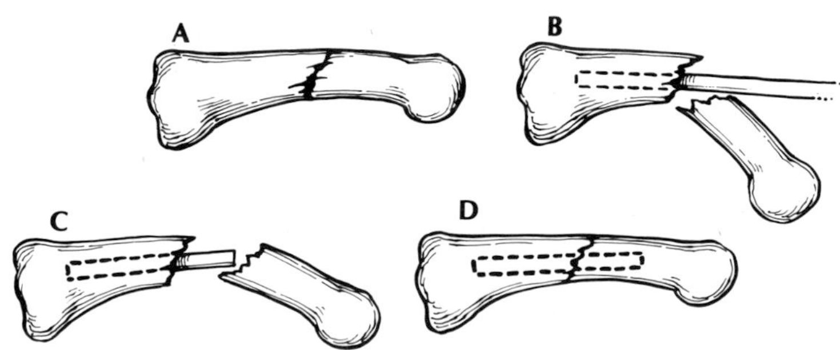

FIGURE 11-32. A method of intramedullary fixation of phalangeal and metacarpal fractures that avoids passing pins through the joints. (*Redrawn from Grundberg, A. B.: Intramedullary Fixation for Fractures of the Hand. J. Hand Surg. 6:572, 1981.*)

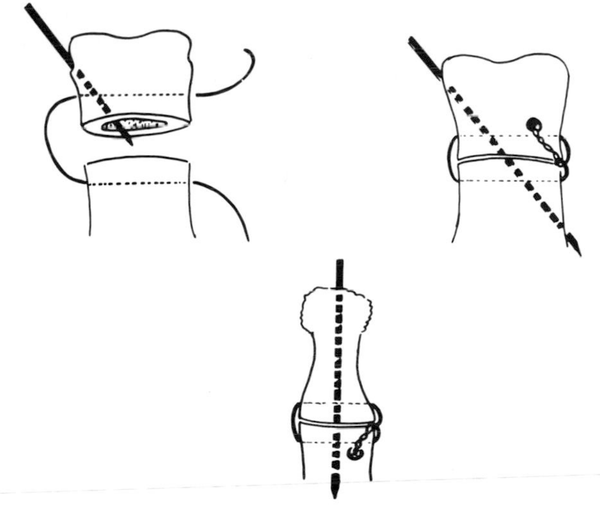

FIGURE 11-33. The intraosseous wiring technique is good for obtaining stable internal fixation of transverse fractures, especially those adjacent to a joint. (*Lister, G.: Intraosseous Wiring of the Digital Skeleton. J. Hand Surg. 33:428, 1978.*)

Rayhack and Bottke[311] used a technique they called "intraosseous compression wiring," which they recommend for comminuted intra- and periarticular fractures. This method combines the features of intraosseous wiring and tension-band wiring.

Tension-Band Wiring. The tension-band concept is a principle of fracture management that has been thoroughly documented by the AO group.[274] In the hand, the dorsal surface is generally considered to be the tension side and the palmar surface the compression side.[193] Tension-band wiring applied to the dorsal surface of a phalanx or metacarpal can thus provide good stability. Greene and associates[152] have reported good results with this technique and have also devised a variation that they call "composite wiring," using K-wires to maintain alignment and wire loops about the pins to apply compression.[153] Jupiter and Sheppard[199] use tension-band wiring mainly for avulsion-type fractures, such as those seen with mallet and gamekeeper's-type injuries. The preferred wire size for phalangeal fractures is 26-gauge, with finer (28- to 30-gauge) used for the smaller intra-articular fractures.[152,199] In a later series, several AO surgeons[35] reported good results in bony gamekeeper's and corner avulsion fractures of the phalanges but poor results in mallet fractures with tension-band wiring.

Technique of Tension-Band Wiring for Avulsion Fractures. Jupiter and his AO associates[35,198,199] have described and illustrated the technique nicely in the literature. The fracture site is exposed, with care taken not to disrupt its remaining soft-tissue attachments. Interposed hematoma is removed with gentle curettage and irrigation. The periosteum is elevated from the bone just enough to expose the fracture site, and a drill hole is made with a 0.035-inch K-wire parallel and about 1 cm distal to the fracture line (for corner fractures at the base of proximal phalanx, for example, the hole is made vertically from dorsal to volar; Fig. 11-34). A 28-gauge wire is then passed through this hole. A 20-gauge hypodermic needle is directed through the insertion of the ligament or tendon attached to the fragment to serve as a guide for passage of the wire. The wire is passed about the fragment as either a figure-of-eight or loop and then inserted into the beveled end of the needle. The needle is removed, the fragment reduced, and the wire tightened.

Postoperatively, early active motion is encouraged, although some protection (splinting for 1 to 3 weeks) may be required if the quality of fixation is not optimal.

Cerclage Wiring. One of the earliest forms of internal fixation in the hand was cerclage wiring, as described by Lambotte[217] in 1987 but it is not widely used today. Gropper and Bowen,[154] however, have found it to be

TABLE 11-6
Needle and Kirschner Wire Sizes for Placing Intraosseous Wiring

Wire Size (No.)	Suture Equivalent	Needle That Will Allow Passage of Wire	Kirschner Wire to Make Hole for Needle
20	5	18-gauge	0.054-inch
22	4	19-gauge	0.045-inch
24	2	19-gauge	0.045-inch
25	1	20-gauge	0.035-inch
26	0	20-gauge	0.035-inch
28	2-0	21-gauge	0.035-inch
30	3-0	21-gauge	0.035-inch
32	4-0	22-gauge	0.035-inch

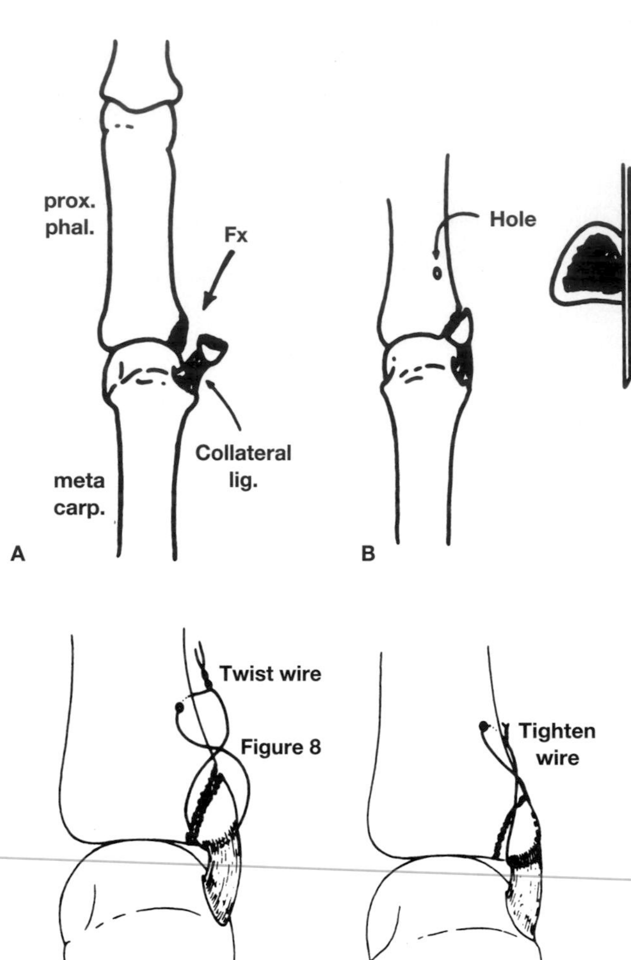

FIGURE 11-34. AO technique for tension-band wiring of small avulsion fractures. (*Bischoff, R., Buechler, U., De Roche, R., and Jupiter, J.: Clinical Results of Tension Band Fixation of Avulsion Fractures of the Hand. J Hand Surg. 19A:1019–1026, 1994.*)

an effective method of fixing oblique and spiral fractures, and Jordan and Greider[194] have described the use of an angiocathether to facilitate passage of the wire around the bone.

ASIF (AO)‡ Techniques. With increasing emphasis on rigid internal fixation techniques elsewhere in the skeleton, it is not surprising that these principles have become more popular and widely used in the hand also. It is important to note that those most experienced with AO methods emphasize that most fractures in the hand can be satisfactorily managed with other techniques.[85,110,164,168,265,360] Barton[25] has stated that only about 5% of hand fractures require internal fixation; Melone[260] postulates about 10%.

Biomechanical studies and clinical experience have shown that properly applied AO minifragment plates and screws provide the most stable form of internal fixation. This mechanical superiority, however, must be balanced by individual considerations for each fracture:

- Is rigid stabilization with plates and screws necessary for mobilization and healing of that fracture?
- Can rigid fixation of that fracture be achieved, given the fracture configuration and expertise of the surgeon?
- Do the potential disadvantages—increased soft-tissue dissection, increased operative time, and possible subsequent plate removal—outweigh the potential advantages for that fracture?

Barton[23] made an important statement about internal fixation of hand fractures when he said, "The reason for operation must be that there is good reason to believe that an operation by the surgeon in question will produce a result which is not just as good as but better than will be achieved conservatively." It is not at all clear from the literature that superior results are achieved from internal fixation of hand fractures, partly because only the more difficult fractures tend to be treated operatively. For this reason and because of the myriad associated factors involved in hand fractures and the differences in reporting results, the reader is rarely able to compare two or more series from different authors. For example, in two separate series of patients treated with AO minifragment screws and plates, excellent results were reported as 92% in one series[44] and 27% in the other.[307]

Virtually all authors having extensive experience using the AO methods stress that the technique is demanding and that the margin for error is small.[25,129,193,260,307,363,402] Before using AO techniques in a patient, the surgeon must prepare himself or herself by reading the excellent books and articles that describe the important principles and by attending the hands-on instructional courses presented by experienced AO faculty.[58,93,164,168,260,339] Beyond that, Hastings[164] has made the excellent suggestion that the surgeon gain experience with these techniques in metacarpal fractures before attempting to fix the more difficult phalangeal fractures.

Technique of Plates and Screws (AO Principles). A detailed and comprehensive description of all AO techniques is beyond the scope of this chapter but it is appropriate to list the most important and fundamen-

‡ ASIF (Association for the Study of Internal Fixation) is the English translation of AO (Arbeitsgemeinschaft für Osteosynthesefragen)

tal principles of the use of plates and screws in the hand:

Pre-operative Planning. Precise preoperative planning is absolutely essential, using drawings of the fracture fragments superimposed on the x-rays to have a clear idea of what is to be done before entering the operating room.[58,193,260] As experience is gained, the ability to "see" the fracture in three dimensions should be developed, which is the hallmark of the true AO surgeon. Alternative plans of fixation should be formulated before the operation in the event that it proves impossible to use the AO minifragment implants effectively.

Surgical Approach. The approach should be planned to minimize soft-tissue trauma. In the fingers, this usually means a mid-lateral incision, preferably on the side of the distal spike, as direct access to this spike facilitates an accurate reduction.[86,108,124,129,260] At the base of the phalanx, a mid-dorsal extensor-splitting approach is sometimes recommended but the mid-axial may be preferred even in these.[58,124] The lateral band and oblique retinacular portion of the extensor hood can be incised and repaired or even resected. Whichever approach is used, the plane between the extensor hood and the periosteum should be disturbed as little as possible, and stripping of the periosteum should be limited to that required only to see the fracture fragments well.[265]

Provisional Fixation. After the fracture has been reduced, temporary or "provisional" stabilization should be obtained with small 0.028-inch or 0.035-inch K-wires, preferably in positions that do not interfere with subsequent screw placement.[164,243] Although sometimes difficult to accomplish, this is a most important concept because it allows the surgeon to focus attention entirely on screw and plate placement, without having to hold the fracture reduced at the same time.

Screw Placement. Extreme care must be taken in screw placement, keeping in mind the "one-shot" concept. This means that often the surgeon has only one attempt to place a screw in the correct position and that one misplaced screw can compromise the entire operation.[93,164,260,265,363]

Choice of Implant. Appropriate hardware must be selected, which usually means 1.5-mm screws in phalanges and 2- or 2.7-mm screws (with or without plates) in metacarpals. Plates are rarely indicated in the phalanges,[164,265] although there are several types of specialized implants such as Buchler's condylar plate,[58] which is specifically indicated for fractures close to the MP and PIP joints, and H plates for transverse fractures. Screw fixation alone is usually acceptable in long spiral oblique fractures in which the length of the fracture is greater than two[93,260,360] or two and a half times[193] the diameter of the bone. To avoid splintering of the bone, a fragment should exceed three times the thread diameter of the screw[164] or three to four times the diameter of the drill hole.[186] If interfragmental screws are used without a plate, it is important to employ the lag principle by overdrilling the proximal cortex.[110]

Drills and Taps. Use of the correct size drills and taps is imperative, and it is helpful to have the AO chart depicting such information posted in the operating room in clear view of the surgeon.

Technique of Tapping. When using the tap, care must be taken to avoid penetrating too deeply, especially when going from dorsal to palmar, where the flexor tendons are intimately contained in the fibro-osseous sheath and are at definite risk.[122] Because there is no calibration on the threads of the tap, the surgeon must first gauge the depth of penetration visually, although with experience, he or she comes to know instinctively when the opposite cortex has been penetrated.

Cortical Contact. Solid bone-to-bone contact must be achieved on the side opposite the plate.[164] If there is a cortical gap, it must be bone-grafted to prevent excessive tension on the plate and possible loss of purchase of the screws (Fig. 11-35).

Radiographic Control. X-rays should be taken in the operating room to confirm adequacy of reduction, hardware placement, and depth of screws.

Closure. Although not always possible, an attempt should be made to close the deep soft tissues, especially to restore the periosteum between the plate and the extensor tendon.

Tourniquet. The tourniquet should be released and good hemostasis established before closure.[265]

Goal of Surgical Intervention. One of the most important goals of the AO technique is to provide fracture stabilization secure enough to allow early active range of motion; if this goal is not achieved, the procedure must be considered to be at least a partial failure. The major cause of less than satisfactory stability is comminution of the fracture, which brings us back to the first principle: the surgeon must carefully assess the fracture preoperatively and honestly try to determine whether his or her AO skills are capable of providing stable internal fixation.

Hardware Removal. Screw removal is generally not necessary, and plate removal is probably not routinely required.[260] Stern and colleagues[363] reported removal of plates in only 25% of their cases, primarily for local tenderness. If the plates are removed, however, 4 to 6 months postoperatively is generally given as the appropriate time, followed by protection of the hand for 6 weeks to prevent refracture.[193,260]

The most common complication of the AO technique, especially in phalangeal fractures, is an active extensor lag in the PIP joint, and the postoperative exercise and splinting program must anticipate this

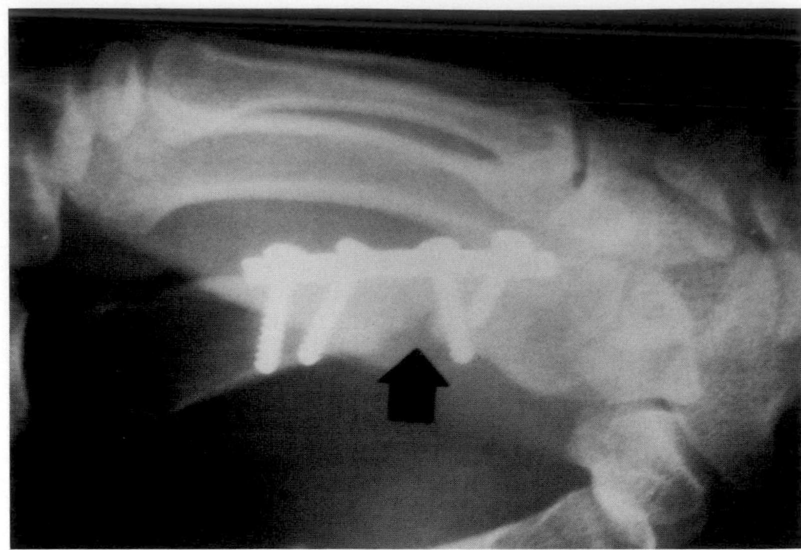

FIGURE 11-35. A fundamental principle of internal fixation is that there must be cortical contact on the side opposite the plate. This attempt at plate fixation of a comminuted metacarpal fracture failed because of lack of contact of the volar cortices. A bone graft should have been used to fill the gap (*arrow*).

potential problem.[129,186] That this is a recognized complication of the AO method is implied in the suggestion that plate removal may be combined with extensor tenolysis.[186]

Microplate Systems. Implants even smaller than those in the AO minifragment set, so-called microplates, have been used extensively in maxillofacial surgery, and a few reports of their application to hand fractures have begun to appear.[305,374] The largest such series is by Puckett and coworkers,[305] who are cautiously optimistic about their use but also describe several disadvantages with the available systems, including a maximum screw length of only 1 mm, allowing only unicortical fixation of the plates; the delicate 0.6-mm drill bits are easily bent; and questions regarding rigidity of stability (a longitudinal K-wire was "routinely" employed by one of the authors before allowing unprotected motion). In his discussion of this article, Jupiter[196] noted that this new class of plating systems raises several new questions (eg, the adequacy of unicortical versus bicortical fixation, the stability of tapped versus untapped screws, the effects of an enveloping plate on bone and soft tissues).

Comparison of Internal Fixation Methods

The relative strengths of different types of internal fixation modalities have been studied biomechanically in the laboratory by many investigators.# The results of these studies have frequently yielded conclusions that differ, and true comparisons among the various studies are virtually impossible because of the differing testing techniques used.[37,125] Barton[23] made the cogent observation that laboratory studies should reproduce the clinical situation (ie, the actual forces acting on the hand). Many of the previous studies tested implants in only one plane and therefore tended to favor the properties of a particular construct.

Most of these studies[36,37] have agreed that plates provide the most rigid fixation, with tension-band wiring[146] and intraosseous wiring[383] also being superior to K-wires. Even among plates, there are differences. Nunley and Kloen[286] tested the effect of several different proximal phalangeal plates on PIP motion. A straight or H plate was stronger than the minicondylar plate (palmar and dorsal stress testing) but they recommended the minicondylar for periarticular fractures because it restricted PIP flexion less.

More study must be done in this area because the optimum strength and rigidity for fracture healing are unknown.[241] The fundamental question that remains unanswered is, "How strong does internal fixation in the hand *have* to be?"

Open Reduction, Internal and External Fixation (ORIEF)

Although probably more commonly used in treatment of fractures of the distal radius, open reduction, internal and external fixation (ORIEF) is occasionally indicated in metacarpal and phalangeal fractures. In some of the more difficult comminuted intra-articular fractures, a combination of open reduction, external fixation, and internal fixation (often necessitating bone graft also) may the only way to restore some semblance of reasonably normal anatomy. Such cases should be undertaken only by surgeons who are expe-

References 36, 37, 146, 241, 244, 246, 248, 310, 383.

rienced with the use of both internal and external fixation techniques.

Amputation

An isolated fracture is virtually never an indication for amputation. However, when severe crush injuries have damaged tendons, nerves, and blood vessels in addition to bone, it may be the treatment of choice. Experienced trauma surgeons have suggested that primary amputation be considered only when there is irreparable damage to three tissue systems.[108] In the final analysis, however, the decision rests squarely on the judgment of the operating surgeon. Only the most obviously nonviable digits should be amputated as a primary procedure at the initial operation. If there is a reasonable possibility of viability, it is wise to reconstruct the digit as well as possible and allow the natural course of events to help determine the necessity for amputation.

Authors' Preferred Methods of Treatment

Extra-articular Fractures. A few extra-articular fractures of the proximal and middle phalanges do not require reduction; these include undisplaced fractures (Fig. 11-36) and impacted transverse fractures in satisfactory alignment. In the latter group, it is particularly important to be certain that neither rotation nor angulation has occurred at the fracture site. Rotation can be more readily appreciated by clinical examination than by x-ray. Angulation can occur in any plane but in proximal phalangeal fractures, it is almost always with apex volar (recurvatum). Angulation in this plane is easy to overlook unless true lateral radiographs of good quality are taken. Even a fracture that appears to be in excellent alignment in the posteroanterior view may have 25° to 30° or more recurvatum.[82] The base of the proximal phalanx is often not well seen in the lateral view, being obscured by superimposition of the other proximal phalanges. Careful interpretation of the x-rays is essential for accurate initial assessment of the degree of volar angulation in these fractures.

If one can be certain that the fracture is stable and neither angulated nor rotated, protection but not immobilization is required during the period of healing. We prefer buddy taping for these fractures, encouraging active range of motion exercises from the outset. Clinical and radiographic examinations are mandatory after about 1 week of such treatment, to be certain that position of the fracture has not changed.

For displaced extra-articular fractures that require reduction, our treatment plan generally follows the algorithm shown in Figure 11-37. Under suitable regional anesthesia (we generally prefer wrist blocks), a closed reduction maneuver is performed and x-rays are taken to evaluate the adequacy of reduction. If acceptable alignment and a stable position have been achieved, external immobilization (splint or cast) is applied. If the fracture can be reduced by closed methods but is unstable, we generally prefer percutaneous pin fixation (CRIF). If the fracture cannot be reduced by closed manipulation, then ORIF is indicated. With this general outline as a basis for discussion, the following are our preferred methods of treatment for the most common types of extra-articular fractures of the phalanges.

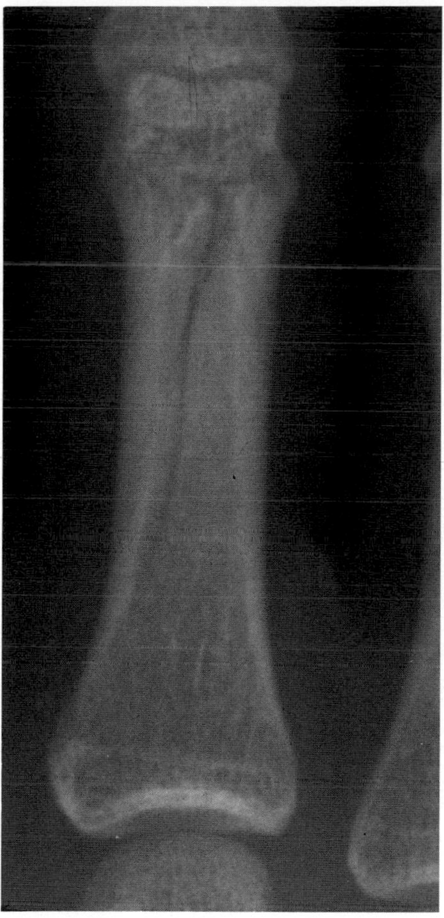

FIGURE 11-36. An example of a stable, undisplaced fracture of the proximal phalanx that can be treated by buddy taping to an adjacent normal digit.

Transverse Fracture at the Base of the Proximal Phalanx. As noted previously, the usual angulation in this fracture is recurvatum (apex volar), which we prefer to treat with Burkhalter's method of hyperflexion of the MP joint and active motion of the PIP joint (see Fig. 11-23). If the reduction cannot be held with

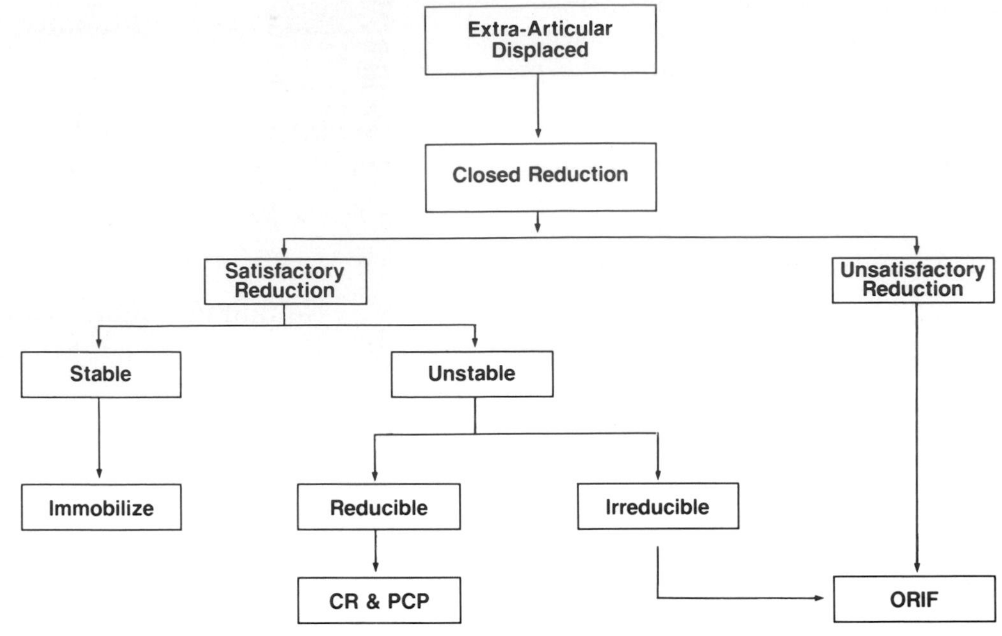

FIGURE 11-37. This algorithm is an overview of the authors' approach to the treatment of displaced extra-articular fractures of the phalanges. (CR & PCP – closed reduction and percutaneous pin fixation, or CRIF, ORIF – open reduction and internal fixation)

a splint, we use Eaton's closed intramedullary pinning technique (see Fig. 11-26C). These fractures rarely require open reduction.

Spiral Oblique Fracture of the Proximal Phalanx. This fracture (Fig. 11-38) is inherently unstable and usually requires internal fixation, although the choice must be made between CRIF and ORIF. If a satisfactory reduction can be obtained with closed manipulation (usually longitudinal traction combined with PIP flexion is sufficient, taking care to correct the rotational alignment), we prefer closed pinning of the fracture site directly, with two or three K-wires. This may be more difficult than it appears, and a fracture-reduction clamp (we prefer the Aesculap) and image intensifier control are of considerable help. Sometimes the fracture cannot be reduced satisfactorily by closed manipulation, in which case ORIF is mandatory.

Transverse Fracture at the Neck of the Proximal Phalanx. Although this fracture is more common in children, it can also occur in adults, and it is a classic "booby-trap" fracture.[155] Angulation is usually between 60° and 90° (apex volar); reduction is easy to obtain but difficult to maintain and almost impossible to monitor in a cast or splint because superimposition of the other fingers obscures satisfactory radiographic observation. For this reason, we generally prefer CRIF, flexing the PIP joint and passing a smooth K-wire either across or to the side of the PIP joint into the medullary canals of the distal and proximal fragments.

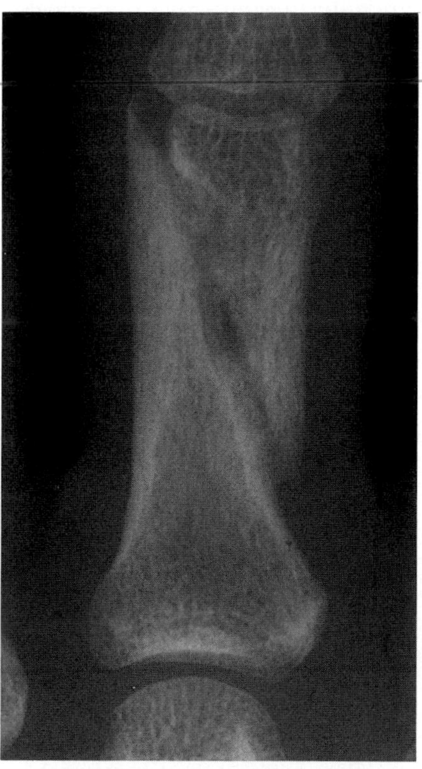

FIGURE 11-38. The extra-articular fracture most likely to be unstable after closed reduction is a long oblique fracture of the proximal phalanx. This fracture often requires internal fixation. The surgeon has a choice between closed reduction and percutaneous pinning or open reduction and internal fixation.

The pin can be removed at 2 to 3 weeks and motion at the PIP joint safely begun at that time. Occasionally, the distal fragment is rotated a full 180°, with the articular surface facing the proximal fracture surface, in which case ORIF is usually required.

Fractures of the Distal Phalanx. Extra-articular fractures of the distal phalanx rarely require internal fixation or even external immobilization. They are frequently associated with significant soft-tissue injury, including lacerations of the nail bed, and the most important primary care of these injuries should be directed at the soft-tissue damage. The one extra-articular fracture of the distal phalanx that requires operative treatment is a transverse fracture near the base in which the nail bed is trapped in the fracture site and must be extricated (see Fig. 11-4).

Comminuted Fractures of the Proximal and Middle Phalanges. These fractures are most commonly the result of crushing injuries or gunshot wounds and are usually open fractures. Concomitant soft-tissue injuries often complicate the treatment, and stable internal fixation is desirable to facilitate treatment of the soft tissues. Severely comminuted fractures are difficult—sometimes impossible—to restore satisfactorily by ORIF and are best treated with external fixation. Our preference for phalangeal fractures with significant loss of bone is delayed primary bone grafting, as described by Freeland and coworkers.[133]

Intra-articular Fractures. Truly undisplaced intra-articular fractures are uncommon but occasionally occur (Fig. 11-39). They are best treated by carefully guarded and protected early range of motion exercise, using the buddy taping system. Immobilization of such fractures often leads to prolonged or even permanent stiffness due to intra-articular adhesions. Again, careful and frequent clinical and radiographic examinations are necessary to check for displacement of the fragments during healing.

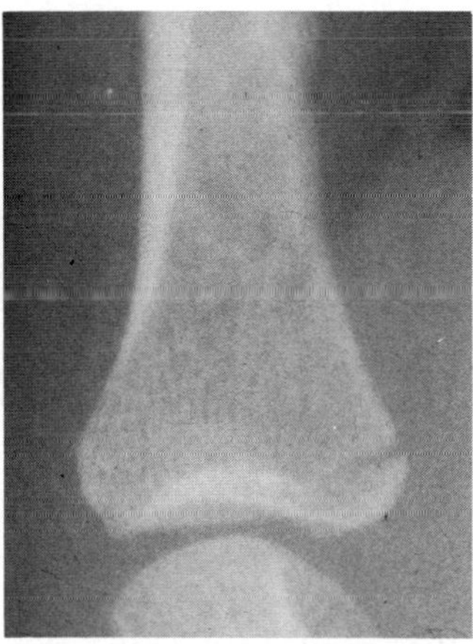

FIGURE 11-39. Truly undisplaced intra-articular fractures of the phalanges are uncommon. They can be treated by carefully guarded and protected early range of motion, using the buddy-taping system.

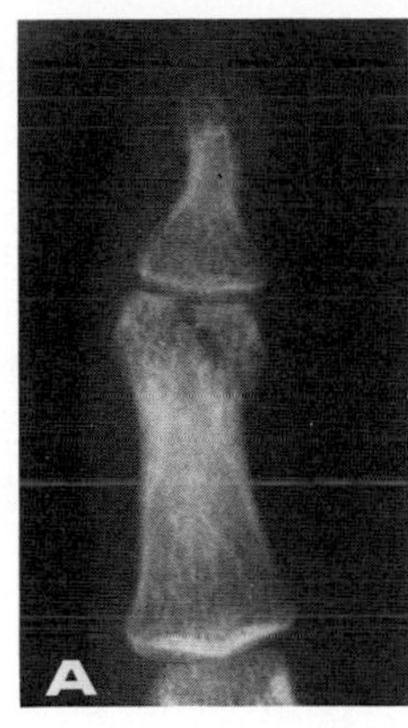

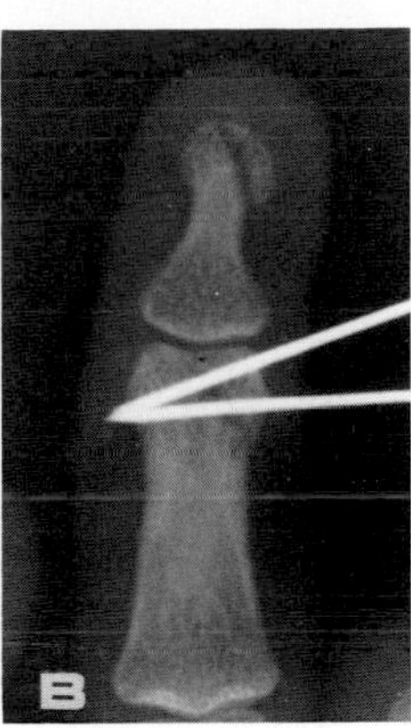

FIGURE 11-40. A fracture that virtually always demands internal fixation is a displaced fracture of one or both condyles of the proximal (or middle) phalanx. (**A**) This fracture most commonly splits off a single condyle, resulting in disruption of the joint and angular deformity of the finger. (**B**) This fracture should be treated with open reduction and exact anatomic restoration of the articular surface.

The goal of treatment in *most* displaced intra-articular fractures should be anatomic restoration of the joint surface by ORIF. This is particularly important in fractures involving the PIP joints and somewhat less so in the MP joints. Intra-articular fractures not requiring anatomic reduction include mallet fractures, which rarely require ORIF, and comminuted fracture-dislocations of the finger CMC joints.

Condylar Fractures. A fracture that virtually always demands internal fixation is a fracture of one or both condyles of the proximal phalanx (ie, at the level of the PIP joint).[209] A similar fracture occurs at the distal joint, involving the middle phalanx. This fracture most commonly splits off a single condyle (Fig. 11-40) but may have a Y configuration that displaces both condyles.

Weiss and Hastings[396] studied this fracture and emphasized the importance of clearly identifying the plane of the fracture line. They discovered that only 8 of their 38 fractures were in the purely sagittal plane; in 58%, the plane of the fracture was in neither the sagittal nor the coronal plane but what they termed an oblique palmar pattern. In such fractures, the distal fragment lies palmar to the proximal phalangeal shaft, and any form of internal fixation (whether by CRIF or ORIF) must be directed obliquely in a more palmar direction on the fracture side. They also advised against the use of a single K-wire for fixation, recommending instead multiple K-wires or an AO minifragment screw.

Failure to stabilize the condylar fracture usually

leads to significant displacement, resulting in angulation deformity and incongruity of the articular surface (Fig. 11-41). These fractures can often be treated with percutaneous pin fixation but only if anatomic alignment can be achieved by closed reduction. If this cannot be accomplished, ORIF is indicated. Adequate operative exposure is the key to success but it may be difficult to achieve. The surgeon must see the articular surface well enough to reduce the fracture anatomically but at the same time, the vital soft-tissue structures attached to the fragment must be preserved as carefully as possible to avoid devascularizing the bone. We prefer a dorsal approach, splitting the central slip in the midline down to its bony insertion, but extreme care must be taken not to weaken or detach the insertion itself. A mid-lateral incision avoids the dorsal structures of the extensor aponeurosis and is the preferred exposure when a screw or plate is to be used, but adequate exposure of the articular surface is often difficult with this approach, however. Freeland and Benoist[132] prefer to not open the joint unless it is essential to see, achieve, or confirm reduction (although in our experience it is often necessary to do this).

Some permanent stiffness of the PIP (or DIP) joint is not uncommon after any type of treatment of this injury, but internal fixation stable enough to allow early protected range of motion is the best method of minimizing this complication.

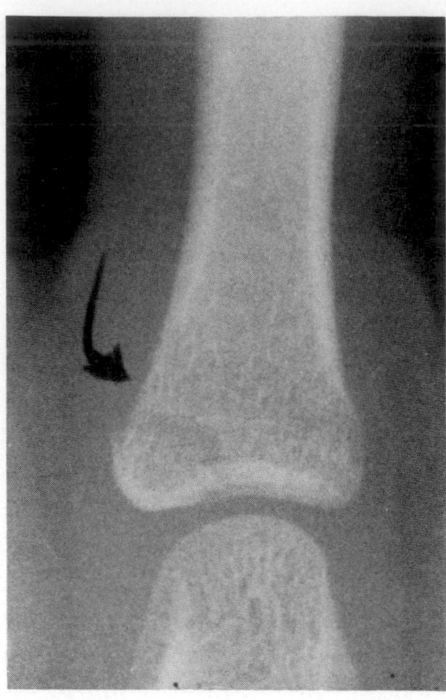

FIGURE 11-42. Nondisplaced marginal fractures of the base of the proximal phalanx can be adequately managed by buddy taping.

Avulsion Fractures at the Base of the Proximal Phalanx. Marginal fractures of the base of the proximal phalanx involving the MP joint usually represent avulsion fractures of the collateral ligament. Small or nondisplaced fragments (Fig. 11-42) can be adequately managed by buddy taping. Small fragments can either be fixed with tension-band wiring or excised and the collateral ligament reinserted into bone. Larger displaced fractures (Fig. 11-43) result in incongruity of the articular surface if they are not restored by ORIF. A dorsal approach that splits the extensor hood is generally used (preferably incising or excising the oblique portion on one side), but careful study of the preoperative x-rays is advised to choose the optimal approach. If the large avulsed fragment is seen to be more volar than dorsal, insertion of small K-wires or AO minifragment screws may be facilitated by a volar approach in which the flexor tendons are retracted and the volar plate reflected.

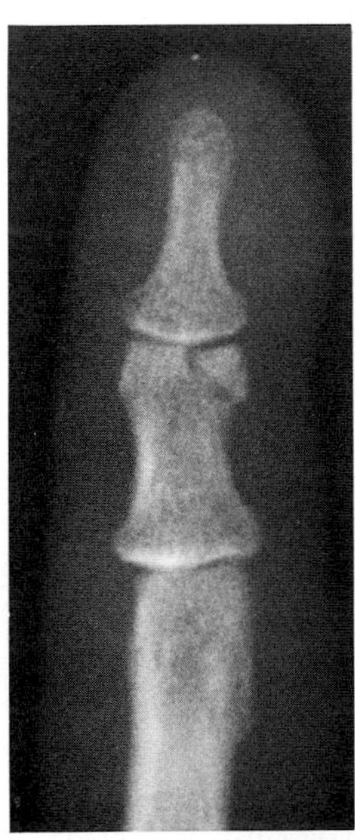

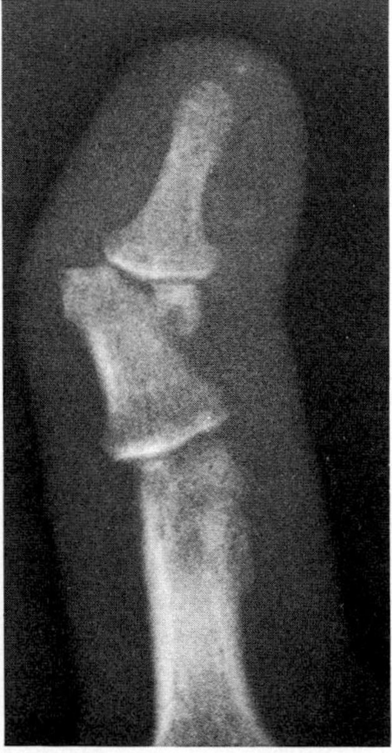

FIGURE 11-41. (*Left*) A condylar fracture of the middle or proximal phalanx should virtually always be pinned. (*Right*) Failure to do so will likely result in significant angular deformity and incongruity of the articular surface.

Avulsion Fractures at the Base of the Middle Phalanx. Intra-articular fractures that involve the base of the middle phalanx are usually one of three types: (1) a dorsal chip fracture, which represents an avulsion of bone by the central slip of the extensor tendon, creating a boutonniere deformity; (2) a volar lip fracture, usually combined with a dorsal dislocation or subluxation of the middle phalanx—the so-called fracture-dislocation of the PIP joint; and (3) a lateral chip fracture, representing avulsion of bone by the collateral ligament.

Boutonniere Injuries. Boutonniere or buttonhole deformity is caused by disruption of the central slip of

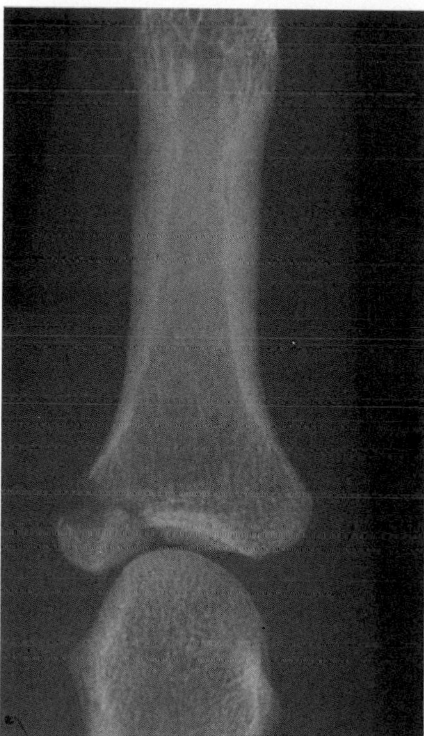

FIGURE 11-43. Displaced marginal fractures result in incongruity of the articular surface if they are not reduced. They usually require open reduction and internal fixation.

the extensor tendon combined with tearing of the triangular ligament on the dorsum of the middle phalanx, which allows the lateral bands to slip below the axis of the PIP joint. Rupture of the central slip causes loss of active extension of the middle phalanx, leading to a flexion deformity of the PIP joint. This is further aggravated by the pull of the lateral bands, which have become flexors of the joint. The PIP deformity is compounded by the limitation of flexion, both passive and active, that develops in the DIP joint. This results from the tenodesis effect of the displaced lateral bands and in time may lead to the fixed hyperextension deformity of the distal joint seen in the classic boutonniere lesion (Fig. 11-44).

Most boutonniere deformities are caused by rupture of the central slip directly from its bony insertion. No fracture is present radiographically, and the diagnosis must be made by clinical examination. The patient with acute injury usually presents not with a typical boutonniere deformity but simply with a swollen, painful PIP joint. Rupture of the central slip is differentiated from the more common injury to the collateral ligament by the location of the maximum area of tenderness on the dorsum rather than the sides of the joint and by the patient's inability to actively extend the PIP joint. If pain prevents active extension, it must be eliminated by digital or metacarpal nerve block, so that active motion can be tested. If a patient is suspected of having a ruptured central slip, x-rays of the involved finger should always be made; uncommonly, an avulsion fracture is seen at the dorsum of the base of the middle phalanx (Fig. 11-45). Patients with suspected central slip injuries should always be reexamined 7 to 10 days after the injury, when the boutonniere lesion may be more apparent.

A boutonniere lesion without a fracture should be treated closed, by splinting the PIP joint in full extension for 5 to 6 weeks (Fig. 11-46).[481,506] Souter[506] has shown that successful results can be achieved in closed boutonniere lesions in which treatment is delayed up to 6 weeks after injury. It is important that the distal joint not be immobilized; it must be actively and passively flexed during treatment. After the initial period of immobilization,

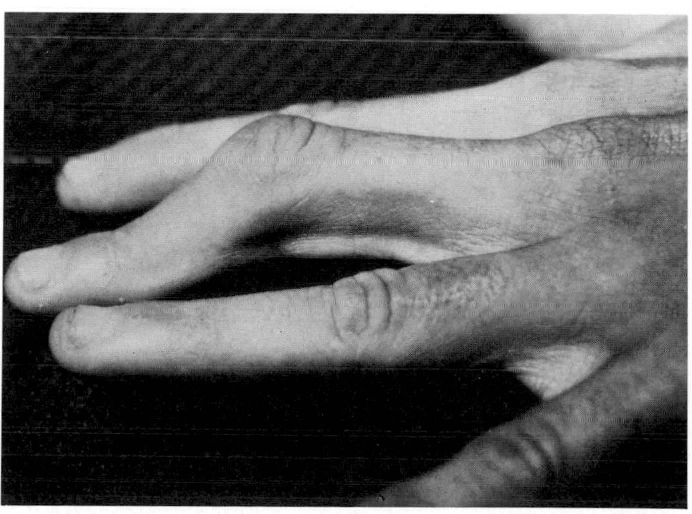

FIGURE 11-44. A typical boutonniere deformity with flexion of the proximal interphalangeal (PIP) joint and hyperextension of the distal interphalangeal joint. The acute boutonniere injury does not usually present with this typical deformity but with a swollen, painful PIP joint. Early diagnosis depends on careful clinical examination (see text).

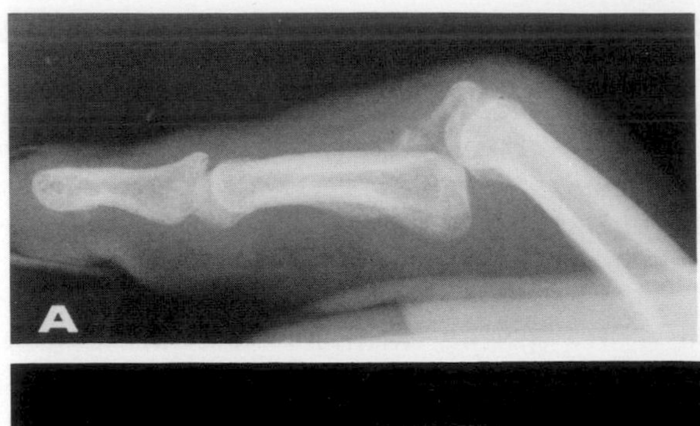

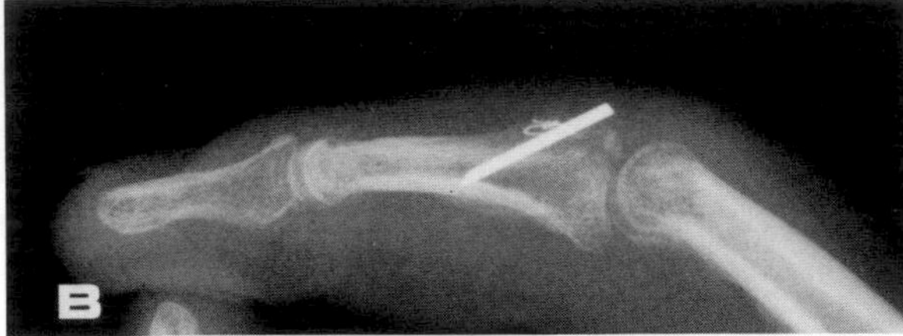

FIGURE 11-45. Most boutonniere injuries are purely soft-tissue lesions that can be treated by closed methods. (**A**) Occasionally, there is a sufficiently large fragment to result in a volar fracture-subluxation of the proximal interphalangeal joint. (**B**) Open reduction and internal fixation of this fracture is sometimes necessary.

a removable splint that holds the PIP joint should be worn at night for at least an additional 4 weeks. From the outset of treatment, the patient must be taught to actively and passively bend the distal joint while holding the PIP joint in full extension. Treatment should not be considered to be complete until active flexion of the distal joint is equal to that in the opposite normal finger.

A boutonniere injury with a large displaced avulsion fracture demands ORIF. At the time of operation, it is important also to repair the triangular ligament to correct the volar subluxation of the lateral bands, although care must be taken not to reef these tendons dorsally under excessive tension because this limits subsequent flexion of the joint. Postoperative immobilization should be limited to the PIP joint only (in full extension by using an external splint or with a smooth K-wire passed obliquely across the joint), and the patient should be carefully instructed in active assisted flexion of the distal joint.

Comminuted Intra-articular and "Pilon" Fractures. Severely comminuted intra-articular fractures that involve either the MP joint or the PIP joint are often not amenable to internal fixation, and attempts to fix such fractures by open reduction are fraught with difficulty and frustration. When these fractures involve the base of middle phalanx at the PIP joint, they are sometimes called "pilon" fractures.

Clearly the goal of treatment is restoration of joint congruity and motion. If that can be achieved by ORIF sufficiently stable to allow early motion, it is the best option. If open reduction is feasible, these difficult fractures often require a combination of internal fixation, external fixation, and bone grafting.

When the degree of comminution precludes a reasonable attempt at ORIF, two options are available: external fixation and dynamic traction. Before deciding how to treat one of these injuries, it is often helpful to obtain an x-ray, with the involved finger suspended in finger traps or distracted manually. If the x-ray shows improvement in the congruity of the articular surface, this gives some assurance that external fixation or traction may be advantageous. Conversely, if there is no significant improvement in the articular surface, nothing is to be gained from the use of skeletal traction alone. The surgeon must then decide whether he or she has the skills to fix the fracture with ORIF or ORIEF.

For comminuted intra-articular fractures with significant loss of bone, we prefer delayed primary bone grafting, as described by Freeland and associates.[133] In these situations, arthrodesis or reconstruction[263] of the involved joint generally is required.

Follow-Up Care and Healing Time of Phalangeal Fractures

There is a disturbing tendency to regard fractures of the phalanges as minor injuries and to neglect the important follow-up care they require. Complications

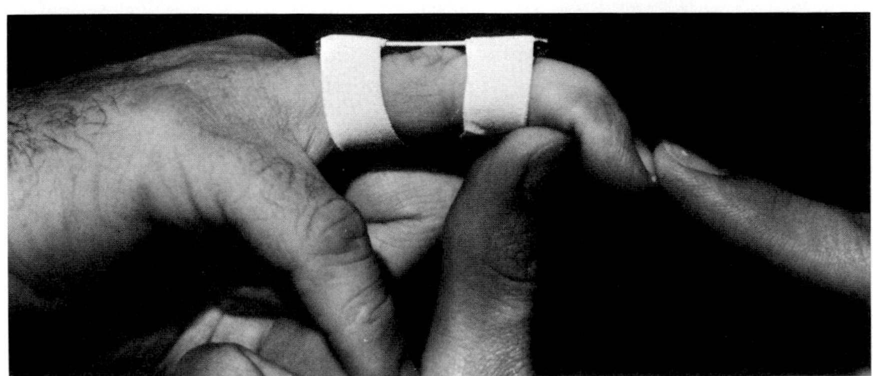

FIGURE 11-46. The treatment of closed boutonniere lesions entails two equally important elements: immobilization of the proximal interphalangeal joint in full extension and active and passive flexion of the distal interphalangeal joint.

often result from finger fractures when an inexperienced surgeon reduces a phalangeal fracture, immobilizes the injured digit, and then tells the patient to return in 3 weeks to have the splint removed. No matter how accurately the reduction is achieved and how carefully the splint is applied, it is imperative that the patient be examined clinically and radiographically from time to time during fracture healing. In particular, patients who are allowed early active motion should be seen periodically to be instructed and encouraged in the performance of specific exercises to minimize joint stiffness and to regain full active motion.

Immobilization of an injured digit should *not* be continued until consolidation at the fracture line is visible radiographically. Smith and Rider[353] demonstrated many years ago that the average "roentgenographic" healing time for fractures of the phalanges is 5 months, with the range being 1 to 17 months. The important point is that "clinical" healing is evident in 3 to 4 weeks. With the exception of mallet and boutonniere chip fractures, it is rarely necessary to immobilize a closed fracture of a phalanx for longer than 3 weeks and to do so is usually detrimental. Some protection should be afforded the digit for 3 more weeks; however, this is easily accomplished by the buddy taping system, which allows the patient to move the joints actively, even in unstable fractures, after the initial 3-week immobilization period.

A final point regarding the period of immobilization is that open fractures do not heal as rapidly as comparable closed fractures in the phalanges. Even in open fractures, however, external immobilization should rarely be continued for longer than 4 weeks.

Factors Influencing Results

Clearly, the skill of the surgeon is an important element in determining the outcome of fractures in the hand, but there are still many factors over which the surgeon has no control, including; violence of the original injury; associated soft-tissue damage[204,307]; contamination and devascularization of the wound; degree of comminution of the fracture; and age of the patient.[103] Strickland and colleagues[364] reviewed a large series of complicated fractures and concluded that age older than 50 years and associated tendon injuries (especially extensor) were two of the most important factors that compromised the result. A somewhat surprising finding in their study was that there was no meaningful difference in the ultimate performance of fractured digits after mobilization during each of the first 4 weeks after fracture, although immobilization for longer than 4 weeks was associated with poorer results.

In a similar study, Huffaker and coworkers[174] found that associated joint injury, more than one fracture in a finger, crush injury, tendon damage, and skin loss were the key factors causing limited range of motion in the injured finger. They further noted that crush injury, tendon damage, and skin loss in the fractured finger frequently caused loss of motion in the unaffected normal fingers. In a large prospective study from Hong Kong, patients with concomitant soft-tissue damage were three times as likely to have a poor result than those with simple, closed fractures.[76,306,347]

Complications of Phalangeal Fractures

Malunion

Undoubtedly the most common complication of phalangeal fractures is malunion; this may take several forms.

Malrotation. Correct rotational alignment is often difficult to maintain in the closed treatment of phalangeal fractures. Immobilizing an adjacent normal digit with the injured finger and carefully monitoring the planes of the fingernails helps to prevent this complication but when malrotation occurs, rotational osteotomy is frequently required. Royle[322] noted that rotational malalignment of less than 10° is usually well tolerated but deformity greater than this may impair hand function and require an osteotomy.

Some authors prefer to perform the osteotomy directly through the involved phalanx, using either a transverse[135,341] or a more complicated step-cut osteotomy.[225,240,298] In our opinion, however, this is more likely to result in stiffness of the MP or PIP joints and generally, we prefer Weckesser's technique[149,264,395,412] of performing the osteotomy through the cancellous base of the metacarpal, where rapid healing is ensured. Adequate fixation can usually be accomplished with K-wires[264] but an AO minifragment T-plate[236] provides a bit better stability and probably allows earlier active motion.

Weckesser[395] reported that it is possible to correct up to 25° of malrotation with this technique. Studies in cadaver hands by Gross and Gelberman[155] confirmed this for the small finger but suggested that only about 18° to 19° of correction is possible in the index, long, and ring fingers.

Pichora and coworkers[298] have described in detail the technique of step-cut osteotomy in the proximal phalanx or metacarpal. They believe that this method allows a wider range of correction, but it is considerably more difficult than a transverse osteotomy through the base of metacarpal.

In patients with a combined rotation and angulation deformity, the corrective osteotomy must be done at or near the malunion site.[381] Seitz and Froimson[341] have suggested the use of a mini external fixation device as an aid to correcting the rotational malalignment but we have not found this to be necessary.

Lateral Deviation. Radial or ulnar deviation after a healed fracture most commonly results from those situations in which there was actual bone loss at the time of injury (eg, in gunshot wounds, crush injuries). The simplest method of correcting lateral deviation is with a closing wedge osteotomy directly through the site of the malunion.[71] We prefer to do this by removing a small wedge that has been precisely measured on the preoperative x-rays, leaving the soft-tissue hinge intact at the apex of the wedge and using a single obliquely directed K-wire for fixation.[149] Froimson[135] has described another method for doing this with a series of progressively smaller burs, using the Hall drill (Fig. 11-47).

Volar Angulation. As noted, most fractures of the proximal phalanx tend to assume a position of volar (recurvatum) angulation at the fracture site. If this is not corrected at the time of reduction, severe residual angulation may occur, which frequently leads to a claw-like deformity of the finger (Fig. 11-48). Froimson[135,341] and Seitz recommend a dorsal opening wedge osteotomy at the malunion site but this requires a bone graft, and we generally prefer a volar closing wedge osteotomy.[149] The few millimeters of shortening caused by the closing wedge is compensated by correcting the angulation.

Fibrous Malunion. There is really not a word in our fracture lexicon that precisely defines this situation, although Fahmy and Harvey's[121] "maluniting fracture" comes close. These are fractures having a strong

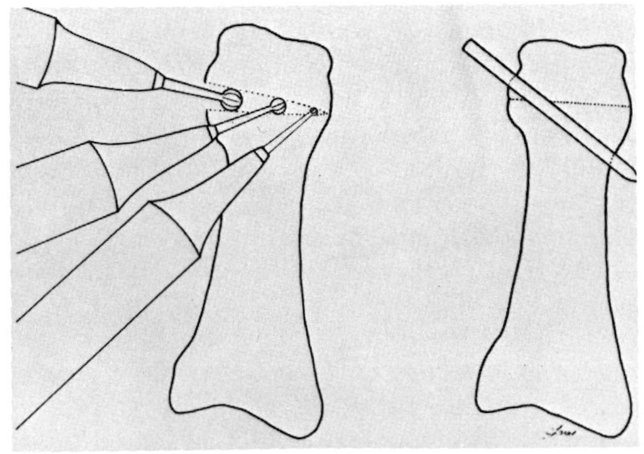

FIGURE 11-47. A relatively simple method of performing a closing wedge osteotomy to correct angular deformity of a phalanx by using progressively smaller burs with the Hall drill. (*Froimson, A.I.: Osteotomy for Digital Deformity. J. Hand Surg. 6:585, 1981.*)

fibrous union that appear to be an angulated malunion. The difference is that there is still some "give" or "spring" at the fracture site that permits correction by closed manipulation. Differentiation between a fibrous malunion and a solid (healed) malunion on plain x-rays may be difficult but the two are easily distinguished on stress x-rays. The fibrous malunion is correctable; the established malunion is not.

The implications for treatment are clear: an osteotomy is required for the solid malunion but the fibrous malunion, if manually correctable to satisfactory alignment, can be treated identical to a hypertrophic nonunion.

Displacement (Shortening). If a long spiral or short oblique fracture of the proximal phalanx is allowed to heal with shortening, a serious problem may develop. The distal spike of the proximal phalanx may impinge on the base of the middle phalanx, blocking PIP flexion (Fig. 11-49). If motion is significantly limited, surgical excision of the offending spike can restore good PIP motion (Fig. 11-50).[149]

Intra-articular Malunion. The most difficult malunion to correct is that which involves a joint surface, which reemphasizes the importance of anatomic reduction of intra-articular fractures. It is virtually impossible to restore a normal joint in these late situations but both Duncan and Jupiter[107] and Light and Bednar[227,228] have shown that some of these malunions can be improved with an intra-articular realignment osteotomy. These authors note several critical factors to achieve success with these difficult operations:

1. Precise preoperative planning using tomography.
2. Extensile exposure to see the entire joint surface clearly.
3. Minimal soft-tissue stripping.
4. Provisional K-wire fixation.
5. Intraoperative radiograph control.
6. Preferably miniplates to allow early postoperative motion.

Duncan and Jupiter[107] advised that better results were more likely if the operation were performed within 4 to 6 months of injury, and Light[227] observed that the quality of bone and size of fragment must be sufficient to allow firm fixation to permit early mobilization. The operation is most likely to be successful when there is a single segment of bone bearing a major portion of the articular surface that has healed in a malunited position.

Degenerative changes in the intact unfractured segment is a contraindication to realignment osteotomy. Joints having significant damage of the articular cartilage are often amenable only to arthrodesis, although

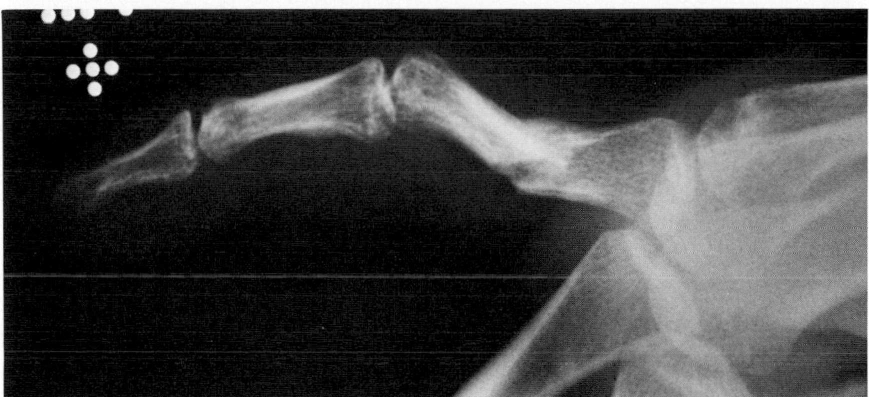

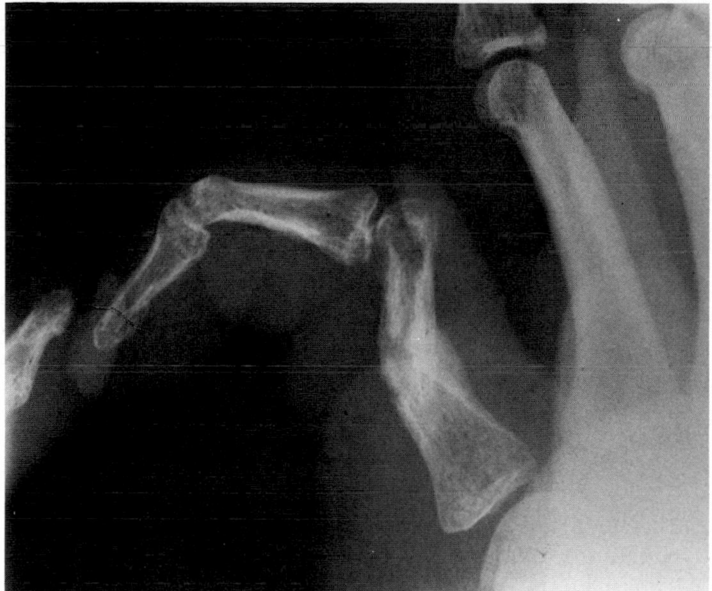

FIGURE 11-48. (*Top*) Recurvatum (volar angulation) deformity is a relatively common complication of fractures of the proximal phalanx. It generally results in a compensatory flexion deformity of the proximal interphalangeal (PIP) joint and limitation of motion in the PIP joint. (*Bottom*) Note that although the PIP joint is in maximum flexion radiographically, apparent (clinical) motion of the finger is limited to about 60°. Osteotomy is often required to correct this deformity.

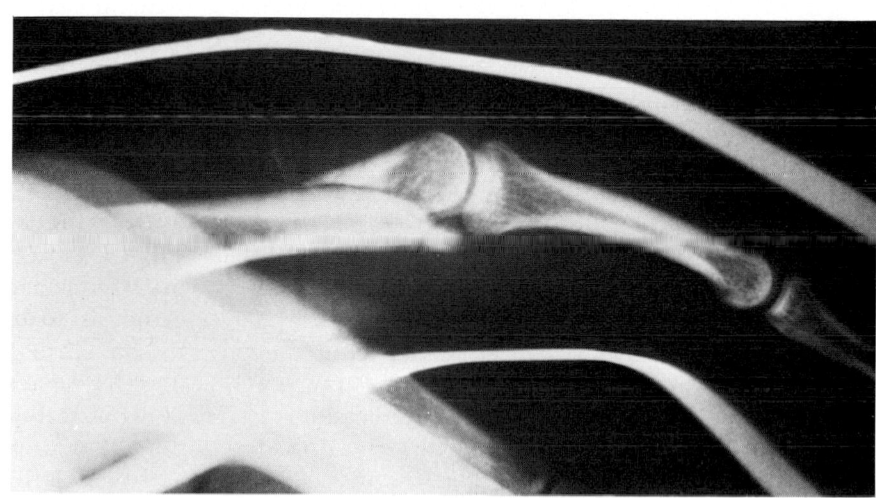

FIGURE 11-49. Oblique fractures of the proximal phalanx must be pulled out to length at the time of reduction. Failure to do so, as shown in this inadequate reduction, leaves a protruding volar spike that significantly limits PIP flexion.

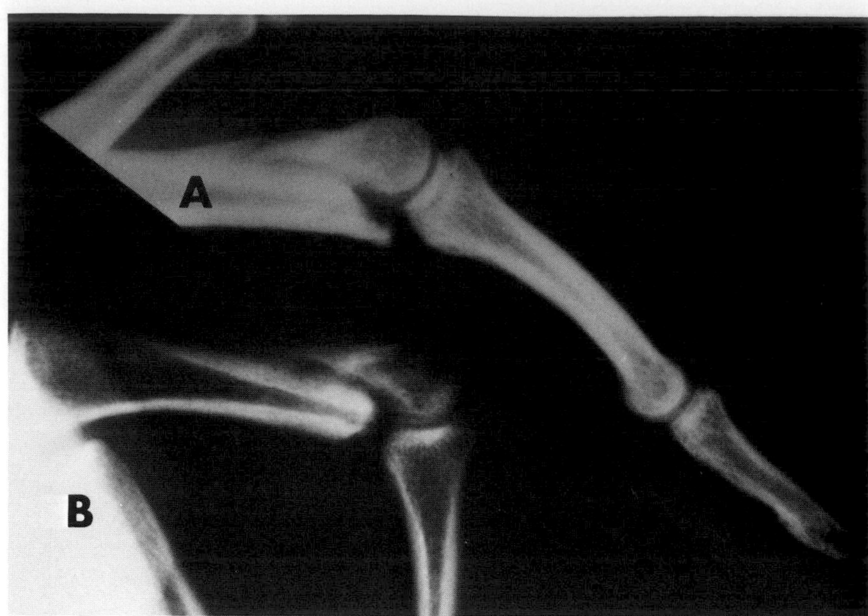

FIGURE 11-50. (**A**) Malunion of a proximal phalangeal fracture with a volar spike limiting flexion of the proximal interphalangeal joint. (**B**) Resection of the spike can improve flexion of the joint.

various forms of arthroplasty have been described, including partial articular homograft,[65] perichondral arthroplasty,[115] costal cartilage graft,[162] autogenous osteochondral graft from the ipsilateral second or third CMC joint,[183] metatarsophalangeal osteochondral autografts,[49] and Silastic implant arthroplasty.[180]

Nonunion. Nonunion of a phalangeal fracture is a relatively rare complication, and the diagnosis should not be made prematurely.[404] It must be remembered that radiographic union often requires 4 to 5 months to be complete and what appears to be delayed union may need only more time (Fig. 11-51).[353] Ohl and Smith[290] described the use of electrical stimulation in the treatment of delayed union of a phalanx but the efficacy of this modality in phalangeal fractures has not really been established.

Two distinctly different types of nonunion (hypertrophic and atrophic) have been described by the AO group,[275] and Segmüller and coworkers[340] have suggested that a ^{85}Sr bone scan may be helpful in differentiating the two. The atrophic type requires a bone graft; the hypertrophic nonunion does not.

Hypertrophic Nonunion. A true "elephant foot" hypertrophic type of nonunion as described by the AO group[394] is relatively uncommon in the hand. When it occurs, however, it should be treated by applying a basic AO principle; that is, that the application of a plate without taking down the fracture site provides sufficiently rigid fixation to allow the fibrous/cartilaginous tissue to undergo metaplasia to bone without the need for a bone graft.[55,275] The so-called "fibrous malunion" is amenable to this form of treatment if the angulation can be satisfactorily corrected with manipulation without taking down the fibrous union.

Atrophic Nonunion. Most nonunions in the hand are of the atrophic variety, and bone grafting is required in the treatment of this type.[394] Atrophic nonunion of the distal phalanx can be successfully stabilized and grafted through the volar midline approach described by Itoh and associates.[185] For infected nonunions, Jupiter and coworkers[197] have emphasized the importance of resecting back to normal bone, which creates a segmental defect. Although the treatment of each case must be individualized, for such segmental defects we generally prefer a corticocancellous graft, combined with internal fixation to achieve as much stability as possible.

Tendon Adherence. Especially in crush injuries and open fractures, scarring of the flexor or extensor tendons is common. Occasionally, prolonged immobilization may be the cause of tendon adherence. The first step in treatment is an intensive hand rehabilitation program, with appropriate exercise and splinting, and surgical treatment should be considered only after maximum passive joint motion has been regained. The diagnosis of flexor tendon adherence is made when the patient has a significant discrepancy between active and passive motion (Fig. 11-52). Treatment is tenolysis of the flexor tendons but such an operation is not to be entered into lightly. It is usually an extensive and technically difficult procedure, preferably done under some type of neurolept anesthesia that allows active motion on the table, to ensure complete correction of the problem. Stark and coworkers[359] have used

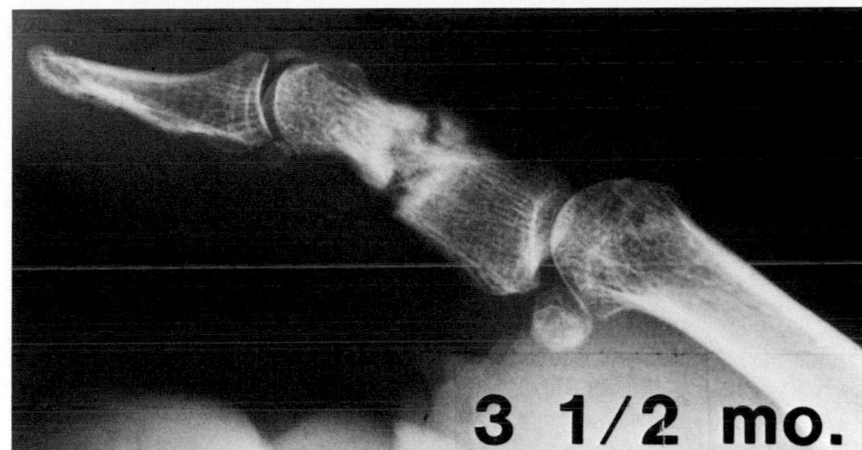

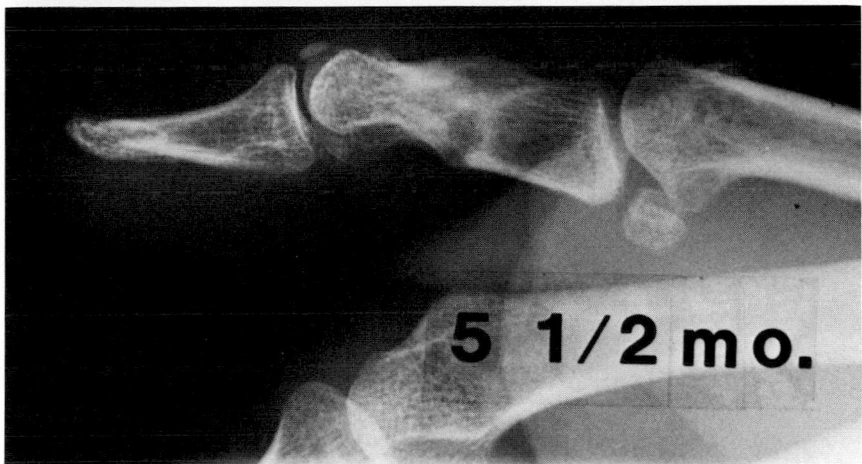

FIGURE 11-51. What may appear to be a nonunion of a phalangeal fracture (*top*) often requires only a bit more time (*bottom*). Phalangeal fractures can take up to 5 months to show radiographic healing.

Silastic sheeting as an interpositional material between tendon and bone in an effort to minimize recurrent adhesions. A highly motivated patient with a reasonably high pain threshold and an intensive postoperative rehabilitation program are also required to maintain the correction achieved at operation.

Because of the broad surface contact between the extensor aponeurosis and proximal phalanx, surgical tenolysis to correct an active extensor lag of the PIP joint is especially difficult; in our experience, extensor tenolysis has been less rewarding than tenolysis of the flexor tendons.

Soft-Tissue Interposition. Soft-tissue interposition within a fracture site is rarely a problem in the hand except in the distal phalanx, where the nail bed may become entrapped. The two major clues to this complication are avulsion of the root of the nail plate from beneath the proximal nail fold and widening of the fracture site in the lateral x-ray (see Fig. 11-4). Early recognition is essential because the nail bed must be surgically extricated from the fracture site and placed back in its normal anatomic position. It is preferred that the nail plate be replaced beneath the proximal nail fold rather than removed.[344]

An unusual case of soft-tissue interposition was reported by Sopher and coworkers,[356] in which closed reduction of an intra-articular fracture of the base of proximal phalanx was irreducible because the tendon of a dorsal interosseous muscle was caught in the fracture.

Joint Stiffness. Limitation of motion in the MP and IP joints after fracture treatment is not uncommon, but a well-supervised rehabilitation program of exercises and splinting restores good motion in most cases. Only after an adequate trial of such therapy should consideration be given to operative treatment.

Complications of Internal Fixation. Complications of internal fixation devices are discussed in the Internal Fixation section except for one rare complication, which is mentioned here.

Metal Allergy to Implants. Allergic reactions to metal implants is rare but has been documented in the literature.[157] The most common manifestations are

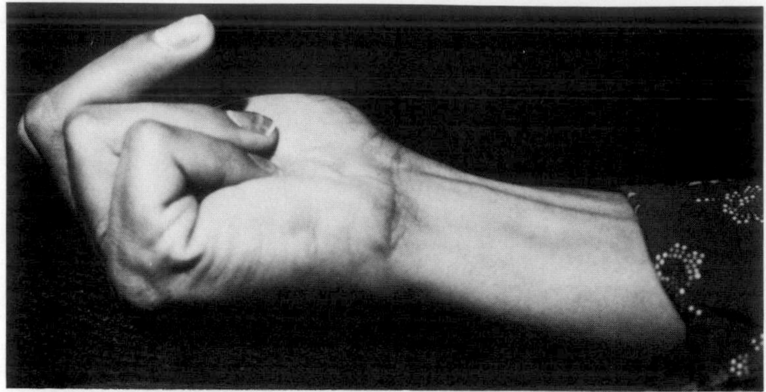

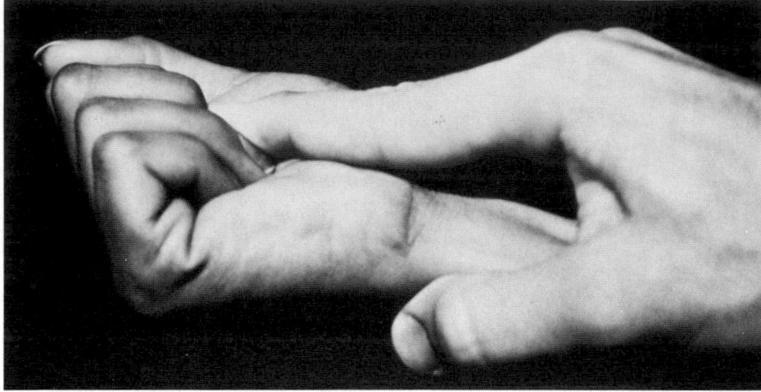

FIGURE 11-52. Adherence of the flexor tendons in a patient with a healed fracture of the proximal phalanx. Note the marked discrepancy between active (*top*) and passive (*bottom*) flexion and the absence of active flexion of the distal interphalangeal joint with simultaneous proximal interphalangeal flexion (*top*). Full active motion was restored in this finger with an extensive tenolysis of the flexor tendons.

dermatologic, including edema, eczema, urticaria, and bullous pemphigoid. The most commonly implicated ion is nickel, which is a major component of stainless steel, although cobalt and chromium have been suspected as causes. This is such a rare problem that it is anticipated infrequently and difficult to prove. Skin tests can be performed by a dermatologist or allergist if the diagnosis is suspected.

METACARPAL FRACTURES, EXCLUDING THE THUMB

Historical Perspective

Before 1932, according to Waugh and Ferrazzano,[393] practically all fractured metacarpals were treated by simple immobilization over a roller bandage, and there was little or no attempt to correct the displacement. Magnuson,[237] in 1928, and McNealy and Lichtenstein,[255] in 1932, advocated treating all metacarpal fractures with a straight dorsal splint, holding the wrist and fingers in extension. The extension method of treatment, with either a straight dorsal splint or a banjo splint, was recommended by Scudder,[338] Key and Conwell,[208] Cotton,[84] Owen,[291] and others. Neither method is currently considered acceptable for treating metacarpal fractures.

In 1935, Koch[212] wrote of the disabilities of the hand that resulted from stiffness when the MP joints were immobilized in extension; he advocated immobilizing the hand in the functional position.

Anatomy

The metacarpals are miniature long bones that are slightly arched in the long axis and concave on the palmar surface.[10,173] Their weakest point is just behind the head.[10]

The proximal ends of the index and long finger metacarpals articulate with the distal carpal row in practically immobile articulations, whereas those of the ring and little fingers have limited AP motion. The metacarpal shafts radiate like spokes of a wheel, terminating in the bulbous articular heads, which are weakly joined by transverse metacarpal ligaments. The collateral ligaments that join the metacarpal head to the proximal phalanx are relaxed in extension, permitting lateral motion, but become taut when the joint is fully flexed (Fig. 11-53, *left*). This occurs because of the unique shape of the metacarpal head, which acts as a cam. The distance in extension from the pivot point of the metacarpal to the phalanx is less than the distance in flexion, so that the collateral ligament is tightened on flexion of the MP joint (Fig. 11-53, *right*).

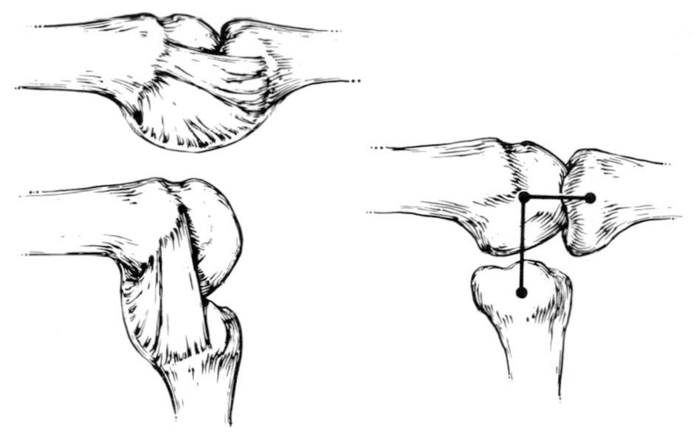

FIGURE 11-53. (*Left*) The collateral ligaments of the metacarpophalangeal joints are relaxed in extension, permitting lateral motion, but become taut when the joint is fully flexed. This occurs because of the unique shape of the metacarpal head, which acts as a cam. (*Right*) The distance from the pivot point of the metacarpal to the phalanx in extension is less than the distance in flexion, so that the collateral ligament is tight when the joint is flexed.

This anatomic point explains why the MP joints become stiff if the collateral ligaments are allowed to shorten, as they do when the MP joints are immobilized in extension.[190,317,318]

The dorsal and volar interosseous muscles arise from the shafts of the metacarpals and act as flexors at the MP joint. Their deforming force explains the dorsal angulation in metacarpal neck and shaft fractures.

Classification

Treatment of a metacarpal fracture is based on its anatomic location, whether it is stable or unstable, and the degree of comminution. Fractures of the metacarpals may be classified according their anatomic location: (1) metacarpal head (ie, distal to the insertion of the collateral ligaments), (2) metacarpal neck, (3) metacarpal shaft, and (4) base of the metacarpal.

Fractures of the Metacarpal Head

McElfresh and Dobyns[250] described a wide variety of fracture patterns in their series of metacarpal head fractures, noting that the second metacarpal was most commonly involved. If possible, these intra-articular fractures should be reduced anatomically and fixed with small K-wires (Fig. 11-54) or AO minifragment screws, although at times the degree of comminution may preclude satisfactory restoration of the articular surface. Small fragments are in jeopardy of developing avascular necrosis.[58]

Otherwise occult vertical articular fractures of the metacarpal head can be seen on the so-called "skyline" view of the metacarpal described by Eyres and Allen[117] (Fig. 11-55). These fractures are commonly the result of direct impact, especially the closed fist against a tooth, and as bite injuries, they should routinely be explored.

Severely comminuted intra- and periarticular fractures present a difficult challenge. Buchler[58] designed a minicondylar plate for such fractures but even this master AO surgeon admits that this implant has "unforgiving tolerances of application." The surgeon must make an honest preoperative assessment of whether he or she possesses the necessary technical skills to adequately fix the fracture. A distraction view taken with the finger in traction or with manual traction applied (under regional or general anesthesia) often gives a clearer picture of the degree of comminution. If this view reveals comminution that is too severe to allow restoration by open reduction but shows improvement in the articular surface with distraction, an external fixator or traction may be the appropriate treatment for that fracture. If the distraction view shows comminution that precludes open reduction and no improvement in articular alignment, nothing is to be gained from either fixation or prolonged immobilization. In such cases, a short period of splinting is indicated to alleviate pain, followed by early active motion to try to mold the fragments back into some sort of acceptable articular surface. The result, at best, will be limited motion without disabling pain.

Fractures of the Metacarpal Neck

Fractures of the fifth metacarpal neck are one of the most common yet most vexing fractures in the hand. The frequently used appellation "boxer's fracture" is really a misnomer because professional boxers rarely sustain this injury. It is common in brawlers and in those whose anger is taken out on a wall or other convenient but unyielding surface; thus, "fighter's fracture" is a more accurate description.

Virtually all fractures of the metacarpal neck have a typical angulation with apex dorsal and are inherently unstable because of the deforming muscle forces and frequent comminution of the volar cortex (Fig. 11-56). Because of this instability and the difficulties in maintaining reduction, many methods of treatment have been proposed.

It is important to distinguish the treatment of fractures involving the second and third metacarpal necks from that of the fourth and fifth metacarpal necks. As mentioned, there is considerably more mobility in the CMC joints of the ring and small fingers; for this reason, significantly less residual angulation can be tolerated in the second and third metacarpals.

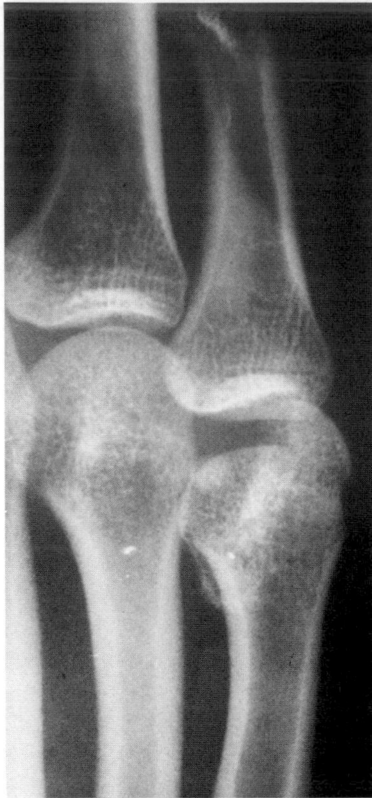
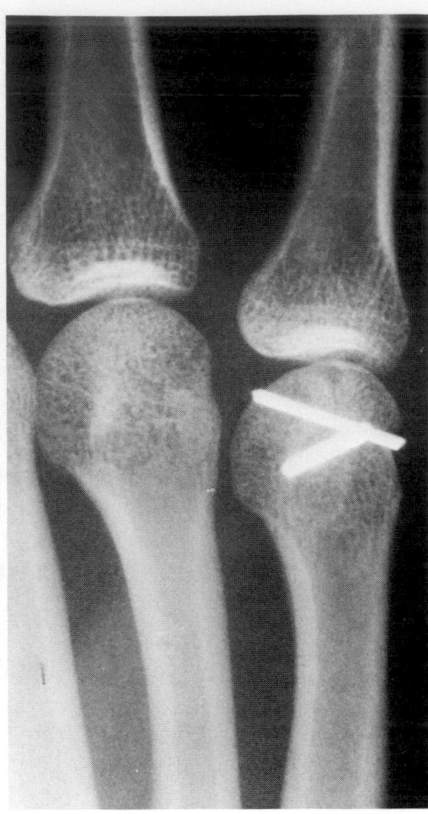

FIGURE 11-54. Displaced fractures of the metacarpal head that are not excessively comminuted (*left*) should be treated with anatomic open reduction and internal fixation (*right*).

Methods of Treatment

No Treatment or Minimal Immobilization. Substantial evidence in the literature from several countries suggests that good functional results can be achieved in patients with fractures of the fifth metacarpal without any attempt at reduction.[19,112,128,170,176,213,251] Excluding fractures with rotational deformity,[19] these authors recommend minimal splinting for pain relief only and gradual resumption of use of the hand. Some studies have shown satisfactory results with no splinting whatsoever[128] or with a so-called "functional cast" that covers only the hand and allows full wrist and finger mobility.[213] Another strong argument made in

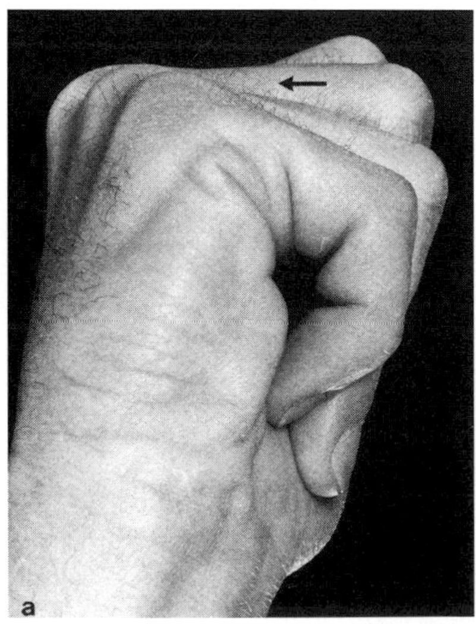
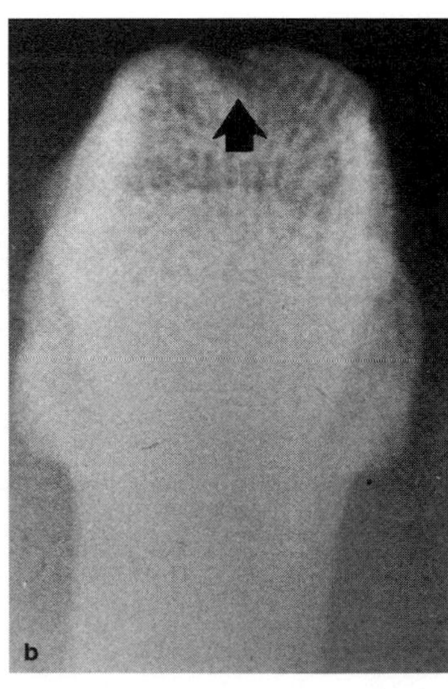

FIGURE 11-55. The "skyline" view of the metacarpophalangeal joint (**A**) may show a vertical impaction defect in the metacarpal head (**B,** *large arrow*), typically sustained in fistfight from tooth penetration through the extensor hood into the joint. (*Eyres, K.S., and Allen, T.R. Skyline View of the Metacarpal Head in the Assessment of Human Fight-Bite Injuries. J. Hand Surg. 18B:43–44, 1993.*)

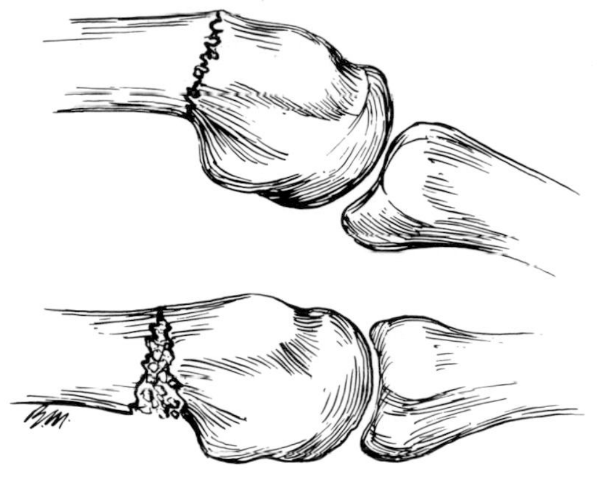

FIGURE 11-56. Fractures of the metacarpal neck are basically unstable because of comminution of the volar cortex. For this reason, the reduced fracture tends to settle back to its original angulated position.

defense of this method of treatment is by those who believe that a satisfactory reduction cannot be maintained with cast immobilization[251] and that recovery time is significantly shortened by not immobilizing the hand. The one drawback is that there is a cosmetic deformity (loss of prominence of the metacarpal head and a bump on the dorsum of the hand) directly proportional to the degree of angulation, although it is not certain that a similar deformity will not be present after an attempt at closed reduction and immobilization. Moreover, Theeuwen and coworkers[375] showed that there was no correlation between the degree of angulation and symptoms.

McKerrell and colleagues[251] reserved operative treatment for patients who demanded a better cosmetic result and were willing to accept a longer recovery time, but concluded that closed reduction was not indicated because cast or splint immobilization is ineffective in maintaining fracture reduction.

Closed Reduction and Immobilization With Plaster. One of the earlier and most popular methods of treatment was introduced by Jahss,[189] the so-called 90-90 method or the C-clamp treatment. This method takes advantage of the tightness of the collateral ligaments of the MP joint when the joint is flexed to 90°. With the tight collateral ligaments holding the loose metacarpal head, the PIP joint is flexed and the base of the proximal phalanx is used to push the metacarpal head back into position (Fig. 11-57). Because of the inherent instability of this fracture, Jahss maintained the reduction in plaster, with the finger flexed 90° at the MP joint and 90° at the PIP joint—the 90-90 position.

Jahss's method of *reducing* a metacarpal fracture is accepted by most authors but the use of the 90-90 position to *hold* the reduction has been widely condemned. Even though loss of reduction can be prevented with this position, we strongly advise that it not be used to immobilize a fracture. The possible complications of permanent stiffness of the PIP joint (Fig. 11-58) and skin sloughing over the dorsum of the PIP joint outweigh any loss of function secondary to a malaligned fracture.

Van Demark[379] used Jahss's method of immobilization but avoided the problem of pressure over the PIP joint by holding the finger acutely flexed in the palm with strips of $^{1}/_{2}$-inch adhesive. He reported good results but did not provide any cases with follow-up to support his method.

If the 90-90 position should not be used in immobilizing the fracture, how is the fracture to be held? Herein lies the difficulty, because it is difficult to hold a metacarpal fracture reduced with a cast or splint. Theoretically, the MP joint should be immobilized in 70° to 90° of flexion, and Ruby[323] has noted that the key is to avoid excessive cast material in the palm. This is difficult with an ulnar gutter splint and is best accommodated with anterior and posterior splints similar to the Burkhalter technique. The volar splint is cut off well proximal to the distal palmar crease, and the dorsal splint extends to but not beyond the PIP joint, holding the MP joint in flexion and allowing free movement of the PIP joint.

Closed Reduction and Functional Bracing. Several authors[123,141,142,386,389] have advocated that the reduction be maintained with various types of metal and plastic orthoses. One such device is the Galveston brace, a commercially available prefabricated splint that applies the basic concept of three-point fixation

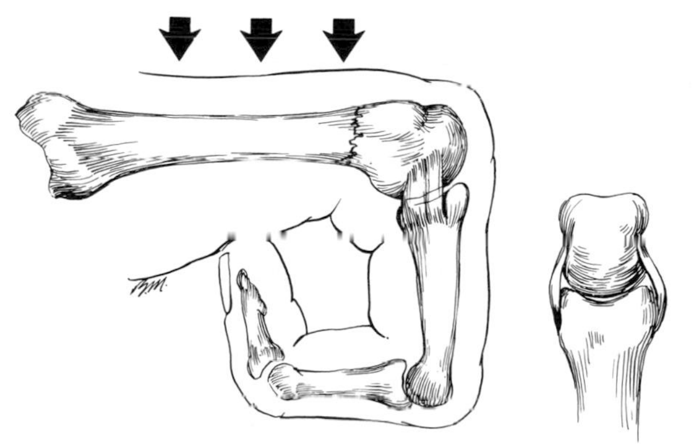

FIGURE 11-57. The so-called 90-90 method of reducing a fracture of the metacarpal neck. Although this is the accepted method of reducing fractures of the metacarpal neck, it should never be used to immobilize a fracture because of possible stiffness of the proximal interphalangeal joint (see Fig. 11-58) or skin slough over the dorsum of the joint.

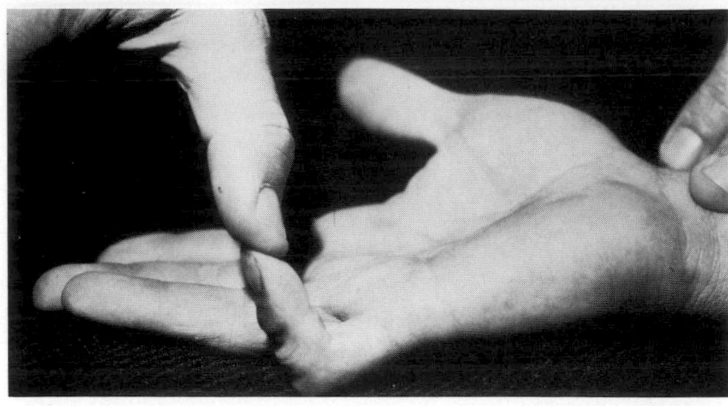

FIGURE 11-58. A 90° fixed flexion contracture of the proximal interphalangeal joint in a 26-year-old man after treatment of a metacarpal neck fracture in the 90-90 position.

of the fracture.[386,389] This method requires a compliant patient but even in cooperative patients, it is difficult to maintain precise positioning of the brace for the required 3 to 4 weeks. A study by Geiger and Karpman[137] showed that a even a snug but comfortably worn Galveston brace can exert more than 260 mm Hg pressure, exceeding the 100 mm Hg previously shown to cause skin necrosis. In response to their report of three patients with necrosis of the skin overlying the metacarpal, the manufacturer enlarged and altered the construction of the pads to minimize this potential complication.[292]

Closed Reduction and Internal Fixation (CRIF). There are two different methods of CRIF that can be used in the treatment of metacarpal fractures.

Closed Reduction and Intramedullary Fixation. Vom Saal,[390] Butt,[66] Clifford,[78] and Lord[233] popularized the use of intramedullary pin fixation, and Suman[366] used a combination of intramedullary and transverse pins. Intramedullary fixation has the disadvantage of requiring passage of the pins through the extensor mechanism at the level of the MP joint. Scarring of the extensor hood, with possible joint stiffness and loss of extension, is more likely to occur with this type of treatment if the pins are left in for more than 3 weeks.

Although most authors accept considerably more angulation in metacarpal neck fractures, Culver and Anderson[89] believe that no more than 20° angulation is acceptable in the fifth metacarpal and no more than 5° in the second and third metacarpals. In such patients, they prefer closed reduction and intramedullary pinning. A K-wire is introduced percutaneously, adjacent to the articular surface; the fracture is reduced; and the wire is advanced across the fracture into the metacarpal shaft. They note that one K-wire is often adequate but two provide more stable fixation. They cut off the wires beneath the skin and remove them at 4 weeks. The hand is protected in a splint for 2 weeks postoperatively.

Closed Reduction and Transverse Pinning. Another acceptable method of holding the reduction of a metacarpal fracture reduced is by transverse pinning of the fractured metacarpal to an adjacent intact metacarpal.[30,31,202,273,283,331,368,393] In 1936, Saypol and Slattery[331] introduced this method of transfixing the reduced metacarpal to the adjacent intact metacarpal(s) with smooth K-wires placed transversely proximal and distal to the fracture site (see Fig. 11-26*D*). They credited Lasher with originating the technique, and it was subsequently popularized in the late 1930s and early 1940s by Bosworth,[46] Waugh and Ferrazzano,[393] Berkman and Miles,[31] and others. Lamb and associates[216] reported excellent results with this method in a large series of patients.

The major advantage cited by most advocates of these percutaneous pin fixation techniques is that early motion can be started without the need for external splinting. The pins are generally left in place for 3 to 4 weeks, during which time the patient may be allowed to use the hand.

There is a difference of opinion regarding whether the pins should be cut off beneath the skin or left to protrude. The likelihood of pin-tract infection is minimized by burying the wires but many authors have reported leaving them out through the skin without serious problems from infection.[46,151,283,295,331,393]

External Fixation. Makeshift external fixation devices were developed as a logical extension of the transverse pinning method. Dickson[100] suggested that if the ulnar three metacarpals are all fractured, rigidity of fixation can be achieved by leaving the K-wires protruding through the skin and bonding them with methylmethacrylate (MMA) and a longitudinal interconnecting Kirschner-wire strut. Other authors have used similar homemade fixators with cement and rigid plastic tubes.[87,320,337] Shehadi[346] further refined this technique by forming the MMA rods inside clear plastic tubes slit open on one side and applied over the protruding K-wires. Bending the wires at right angles before applying the plastic tubes allows the fixator to be positioned out of the way. Eyres and coworkers[118] used a Charnley compression clamp attached to transverse 2-mm K-wires for treating various combinations of metacarpal fractures. Other authors have used commercially available fixators, including the Anderson,[34] AO,[31,355] and mini-Hoffman devices.[131,316,342] Czifer[91,92] of Hungary has designed a disposable mini external fixator that is both versatile and inexpensive but is not yet available in the United States. Stuchin and Kummer's[365] laboratory comparison of various methods showed that the commercial systems have a clearly superior pin but greater rigidity was achieved with certain configurations of reinforced bone cement.

For a discussion of the advantages of external fixation and specific points in technique, the reader is referred to the section on External Fixation.

The most appropriate indication for external fixation in the metacarpals is to maintain or restore length and alignment in severely comminuted fractures, especially those with segmental bone loss.[34,131,316] This is more likely to occur in fractures of the metacarpal shaft than in neck fractures, although external fixation may be the most appropriate form of treatment for severely comminuted intra-articular fractures of the metacarpal head, especially open fractures with bone loss.

Open Reduction and Internal Fixation. Open reduction and internal fixation is rarely indicated in acute metacarpal neck fractures and is reserved for those unusual cases in which the head has been displaced entirely off the metacarpal shaft (Fig. 11-59).[20,312,367] If open reduction is performed, a technique should be chosen that allows early active range of motion.

 *Authors' Preferred Method of Treatment*

As noted, reduction of a metacarpal neck fracture is usually easy, but maintenance of that reduction may be difficult. It actually may be impossible to hold an anatomic reduction with any type of external immobilization except perhaps Jahss's 90-90 method. At the same time, it must be reemphasized that the potential complications of the 90-90 method outweigh the advantages of an anatomic reduction, and we advise against the use of this technique.

Having tried virtually every type of splinting discussed in the preceding section, we have changed our ideas about fifth metacarpal neck fractures (fighter's fractures), and our indications for reduction are significantly different than they were in the first two editions of this book. We explain to the patient that even if the fracture is reduced and held in a splint or cast for 4 weeks, it is likely that he or she will have some residual angulation at the fracture site (a bump on the dorsum of the hand) and mild loss of prominence of the metacarpal head when making a fist. If the patient understands and accepts that the residual

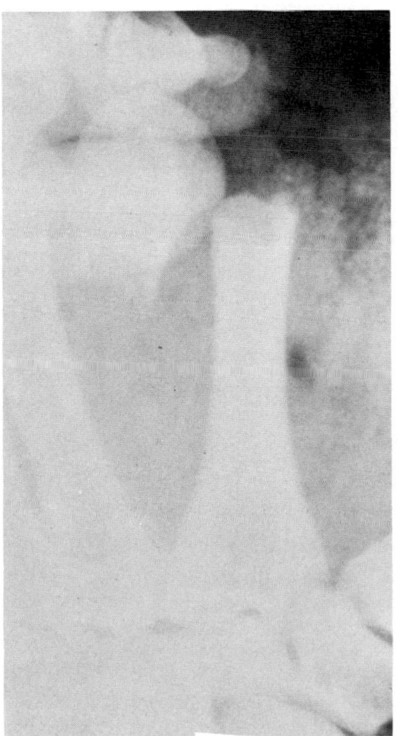
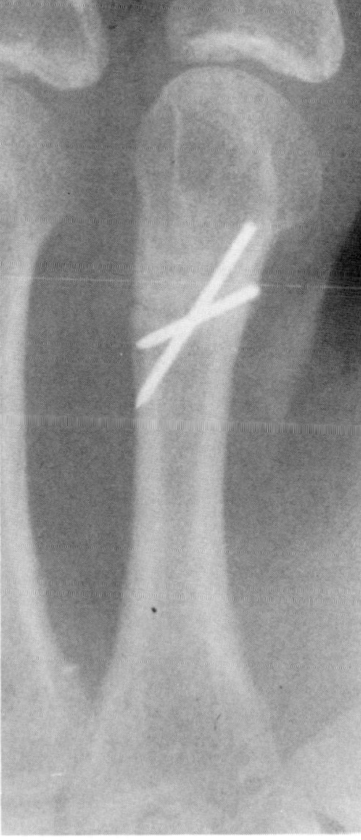

FIGURE 11-59. Open reduction and internal fixation is rarely indicated in acute neck fractures and is reserved for those unusual instances in which the metacarpal head and neck have been displaced entirely off the metacarpal shaft, as in this patient.

deformity probably will be purely cosmetic and that function probably will not be altered, treatment consists of a removable volar splint that is worn for comfort until the local pain and tenderness subside. Occasionally we use the Galveston brace, which may lesson the angulation deformity.

If the patient does not wish to accept any angulation, we recommend CRIF in the operating room. If open reduction is deemed appropriate, tension-band wiring with 24- or 26-gauge wire is a technique that generally provides sufficient stability to allow early active range of motion.

There is, however, a small group of patients with metacarpal neck fractures who fall into a middle ground between these two extremes. If the angulation is severe (ie, 40° or more), a functional deficit (pseudoclawing) may result (Fig. 11-60). In such patients, we sometimes perform a closed reduction under ulnar block anesthesia and immobilize the fracture for 4 weeks, using Burkhalter-type anterior and posterior splints. We explain to these patients that there will be some mild to moderate residual angulation, as noted previously, but the objective of the reduction is to minimize that angulation to eliminate any potential functional deficit.

In making this determination, it must be kept in mind that the normal metacarpal neck angle is about 15°, so that a measured angle of 30° on the injury films probably represents a true angle of only 15°.[16,128,375]

Because of the relative immobility of the second and third CMC joints, less angulation can be accepted in fractures of the metacarpal necks in the index and long fingers. Lane and coworkers[220] have noted that the true angulation of a second metacarpal neck fracture may be difficult to see in the routine three views of the hand; they recommend a reverse oblique view (Fig. 11-61) if such a fracture is suspected. Angulated fractures of these two metacarpal necks should probably be treated with either CRIF or ORIF.

Fractures of the Metacarpal Shaft

There are three important potential problems in the management of all metacarpal shaft fractures: shortening, dorsal angulation, and rotational malalignment. Several millimeters of shortening and varying degrees of dorsal angulation are compatible with normal function. Dorsal angulation rarely results in functional disability but some patients will be unhappy with the cosmetic appearance of a highly visible bump on the dorsum of the hand. The bump is usually more prominent in a metacarpal shaft fracture than it is in a neck fracture. Malrotation of a metacarpal is a serious complication because it usually interferes with normal flexion of the adjacent fingers.

Fractures of the metacarpal shaft are of three types: transverse, oblique, and comminuted.

Transverse Fractures

Transverse fractures are usually the result of a direct blow, and they generally angulate dorsally because of the interosseous muscles exerting a volar force (Fig. 11-62). After reduction, these fractures may be immobilized with Burkhalter-type volar and dorsal splints. Rotational alignment is more easily maintained by including an adjacent normal finger. The same principles that apply to angular deformity of neck fractures apply to shaft fractures. Minimal angulation can be accepted in the second and third metacarpals because there is no compensatory motion at the CMC joints. Some angulation of the fourth and fifth metacarpals may be accepted, although, as noted previously, some patients find the bump objectionable. The further the fracture

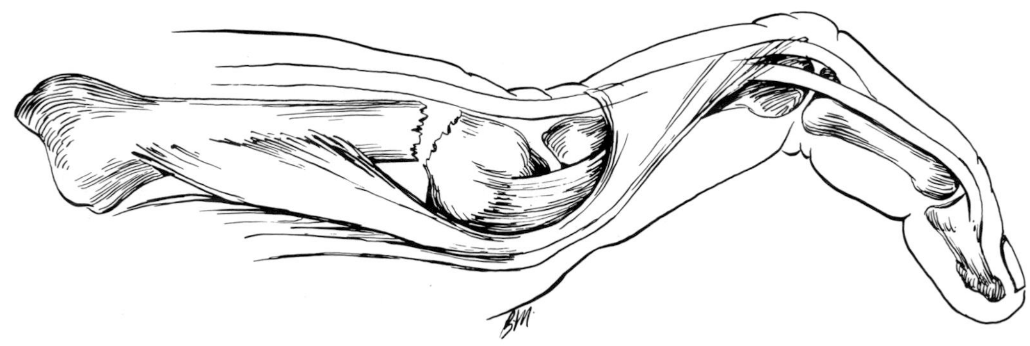

FIGURE 11-60. If the angulation in a metacarpal neck fracture is severe, pseudoclawing may result when the patient attempts to extend the finger. We have found this to be a good clinical test to supplement the evaluation of the severity of the angulation seen radiographically.

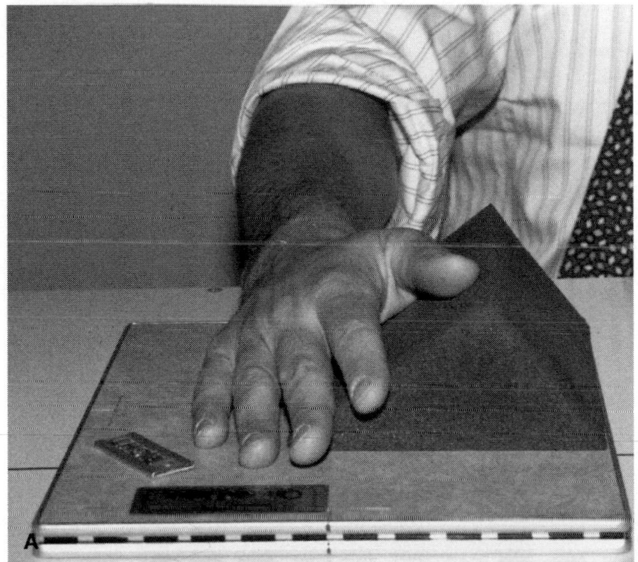

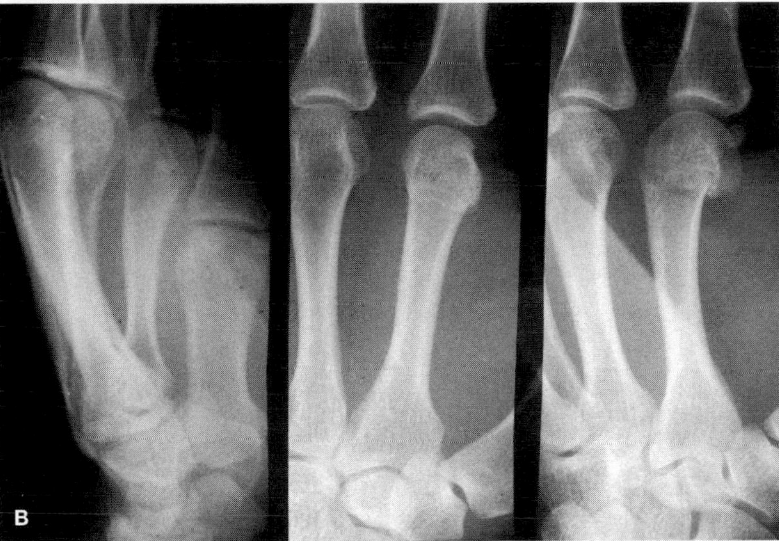

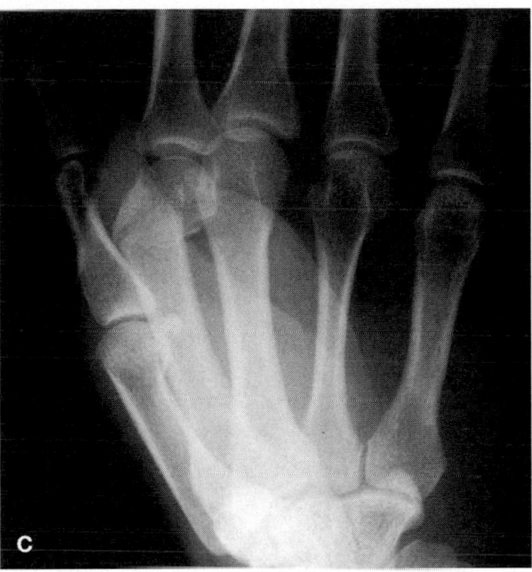

FIGURE 11-61. (**A**) Positioning for the reverse oblique view, which more accurately depicts angulation in fractures of the second metacarpal neck. Routine views of the hand (**B**) were interpreted as showing an impacted fracture of the second metacarpal neck but the reverse oblique view (**C**) demonstrated surprisingly marked angulation. *(Lane, C.S., Kennedy, J.F., and Kuschner, S.H.: The Reverse Oblique X-ray Film: Metacarpal Fractures Revealed. J. Hand Surg. 17A:504–506, 1992.)*

is from the MP joint, the more pronounced the dorsal angulation appears. Therefore, less angulation can be accepted in proximal or mid-shaft fractures than in fractures through the neck (Fig. 11-63).

If reduction is necessary, the same options are available as those discussed for metacarpal neck fractures. Most transverse metacarpal fractures have a significant amount of soft-tissue swelling, and maintenance of reduction may be difficult or impossible with external splinting or casting. If the swelling is not excessive, we prefer separate Burkhalter-type anterior and posterior plaster splints, although follow-up x-rays at 5 to 7 days are mandatory to detect loss of reduction.

CRIF is an acceptable method of treatment for some metacarpal shaft fractures, using either transverse or intramedullary pinning or a combination of the two.[366]

Saypol and Slattery's[331] transverse pinning to an adjacent metacarpal is more applicable to the border metacarpals (second and fifth) but may also be used for the inner metacarpals (third and fourth). Care must be taken to ensure proper rotational alignment and to avoid distraction at the fracture site.

If intramedullary fixation is used, we prefer to insert the pin into the side of the metacarpal head to avoid impaling the extensor hood. A longitudinal pin controls angulation but not rotation and must therefore

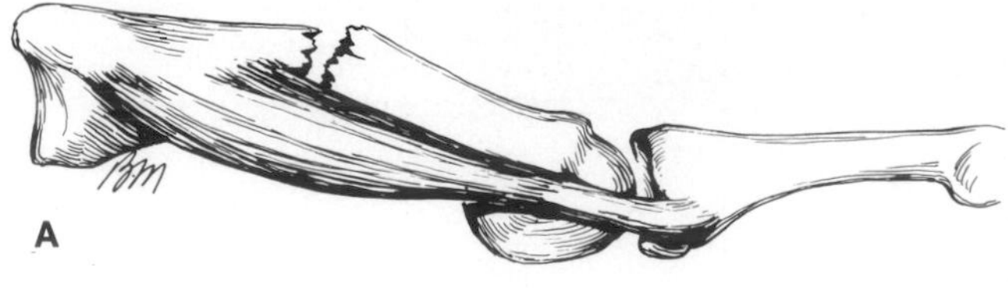

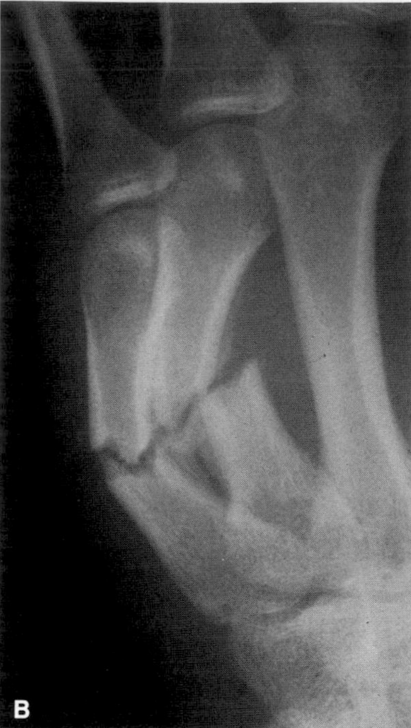

FIGURE 11-62. Transverse fractures of the metacarpal are usually the result of a direct blow. (**A**) They generally angulate dorsally because of the interosseous muscles exerting a volar force. (**B**) An x-ray showing the typical dorsal angulation of fractures of the metacarpal shafts.

be supplemented by either a transverse pin, external splinting, or buddy taping.

ORIF is indicated when the fracture cannot be reduced by closed manipulation. Other relative indications include multiple fractures and concomitant soft-tissue injury. As noted, skeletal stabilization is indicated either primarily or as delayed primary fixation (at 2 to 5 days) in patients who have complex open wounds with significant soft-tissue injury.

The relative advantages and disadvantages of the various types of internal fixation are discussed in Chapter 3. In addition to the standard forms of operative fixation discussed in that section under phalangeal fractures, Mennen[262] has described a "clamp-on" plate that can be used for ORIF of metacarpal shaft fractures.

Spiral Oblique Fractures

Spiral oblique fractures of the metacarpal shaft result from a torque force, with the finger acting as a long lever.[52] These fractures tend to shorten and rotate rather than angulate. The third and fourth metacarpals tend to shorten less because of the tethering effect of the deep transverse metacarpal ligaments (Figs. 11-64 and 11-65). At least 5 mm of shortening and probably up to 10 mm can be accepted without

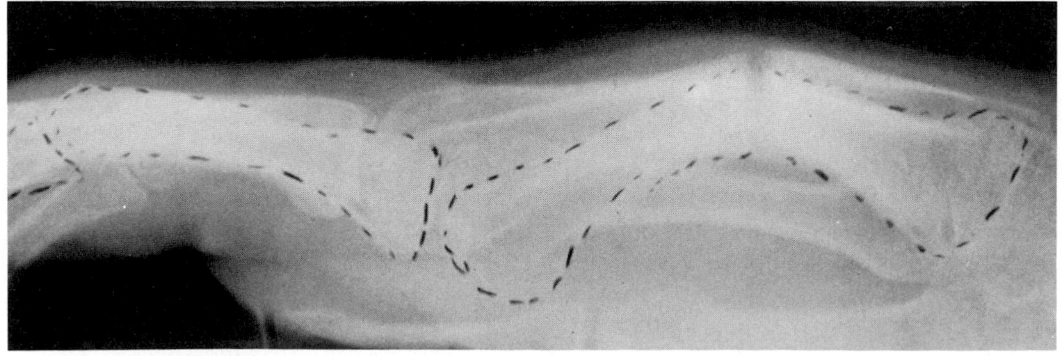

FIGURE 11-63. The farther the fracture is from the metacarpophalangeal joint, the more pronounced the dorsal angulation will appear and the greater the clawing will be. Therefore, less angulation can be accepted in mid-shaft fractures than in fractures through the neck of the metacarpal.

loss of function if there is no angulation or rotational malalignment.[39] Such fractures are easily treated with external immobilization (casts or splints). Greater amounts of shortening, rotational deformity, and fractures of multiple metacarpals are our indications for ORIF. For those few spiral fractures that require fixation, we prefer open reduction rather than closed manipulation because reduction may be difficult to accomplish without direct vison of the fracture site. Stable internal fixation can usually be achieved with K-wires,[111] AO lag screws,[164] or cerclage wiring.[154]

Another reasonable indication for internal fixation is the subcapital spiral oblique fracture, which if allowed to heal in the shortened position may result in impingement at the MP joint level (Fig. 11-66).

Comminuted Fractures

Comminuted fractures of the metacarpal shafts are caused by violent trauma (eg, crush injuries, gunshot wounds) and are frequently associated with a great deal of soft-tissue damage. If undisplaced and sufficiently stable to allow early finger motion, these fractures may be treated with external splinting. More commonly, however, they require a combination of internal and external fixation to facilitate the treatment of concomitant soft-tissue damage and to prevent skeletal collapse. Delayed primary bone grafting may be indicated if there is significant bone loss.[131]

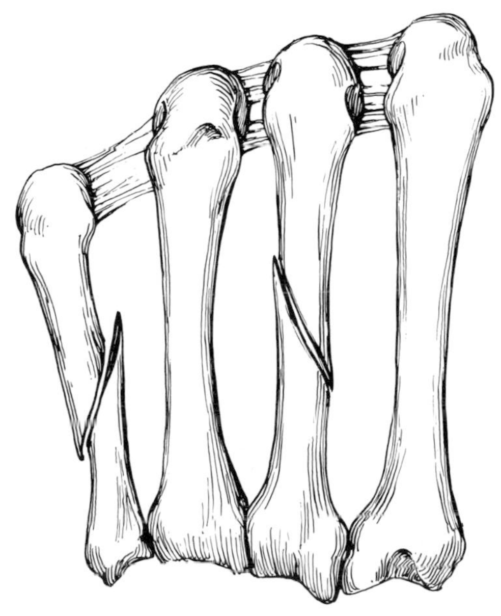

FIGURE 11-64. Oblique fractures of the metacarpals tend to shorten and rotate rather than angulate. The third and fourth metacarpals shorten less because of the tethering effect of the deep transverse metacarpal ligament. In the border second and fifth metacarpals, shortening and rotation are likely to be more pronounced.

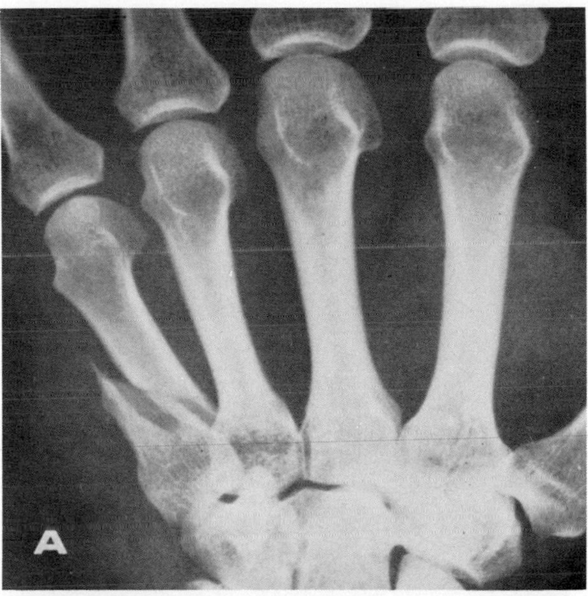

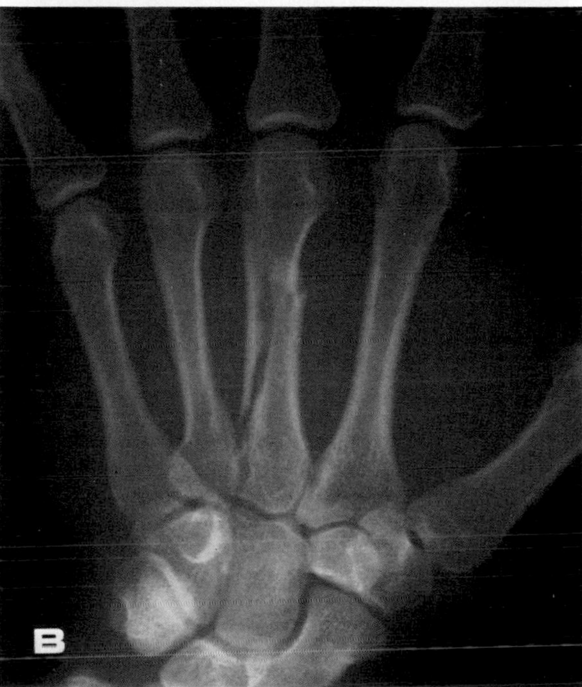

FIGURE 11-65. (**A**) An oblique fracture of the proximal shaft of the fifth metacarpal. Note the significant shortening (**B**) A long oblique fracture of the shaft of the third metacarpal. Note that only minimal shortening has occurred.

Fractures at the Base of the Metacarpal

Fractures at the base of the metacarpal are usually stable; however, the slightest rotational malalignment is greatly magnified at the fingertip. Figure 11-67 dem-

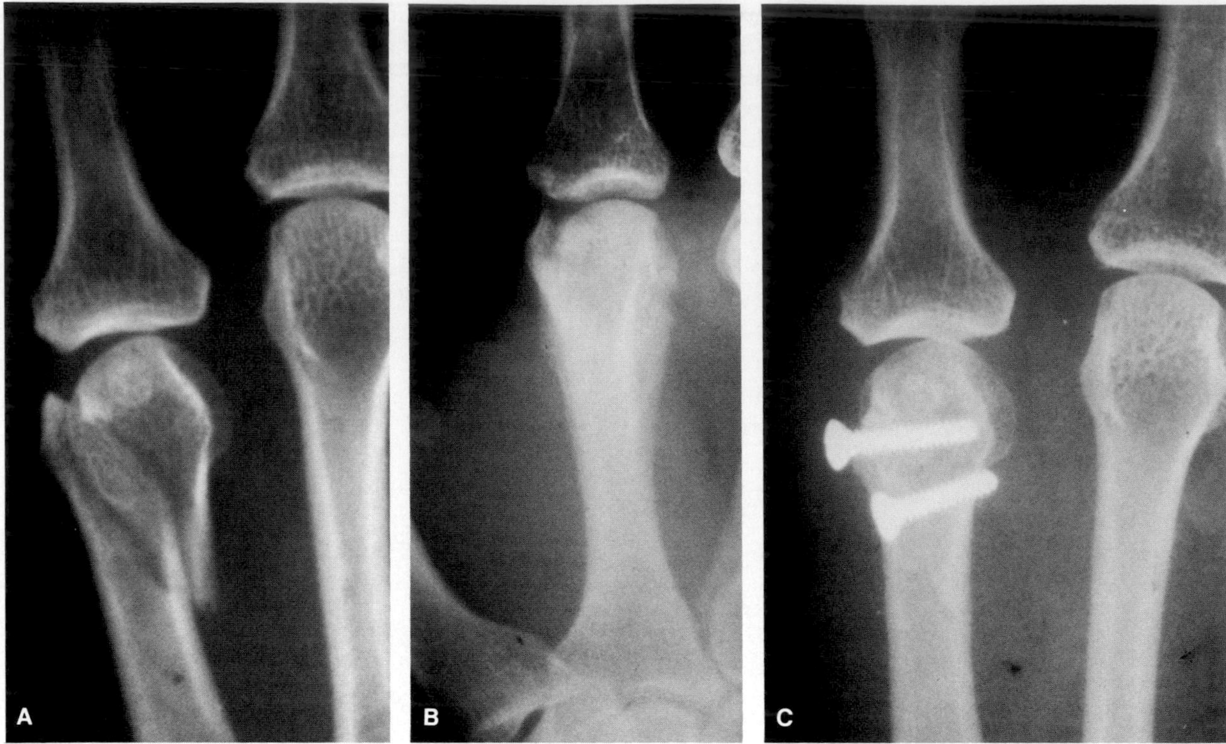

FIGURE 11-66. Most spiral oblique fractures of the metacarpals do not displace significantly and can be adequately treated with closed methods. However, if such a fracture involves the neck area (**A**), the fracture may heal such that the proximal spike may impinge on the metacarpophalangeal joint (**B**). This fracture is probably best treated with open reduction and internal fixation (**C**).

onstrates fractures at the base of the third, fourth, and fifth metacarpals, with rotation in all three fingers, leaving a wide gap between the index and long fingers.

Identification of occult fractures at the base of the metacarpal may be aided by the use of the Brewerton view[205] (see Fig. 11-113), polytomes, or a CT scan.[169] Intra-articular fractures at the base of the second metacarpal are particularly difficult to demonstrate radiographically, and the special view described by Mehara and Bhan[892] (see Fig. 11-111) may be useful when such a fracture is suspected. Unrecognized or untreated displaced intra-articular fractures at the bases of the metacarpals may result in subsequent arthrosis.

A relatively uncommon injury at the base of the metacarpal is an avulsion fracture attached to the insertion of the extensor carpi radialis longus (ECRL) or brevis. Most authors[98,321,377] reporting these unusual cases have recommended open reduction, but Crichlow and Hoskinson[86] concluded from their three cases that operative treatment is necessary only when the avulsed fragment causes a bothersome bony prominence. Sadr and Lalehzarian[329] treated a laborer who complained of weakness in his hand 1 year after injury; their case was surprising because the avulsed fragment could not be brought out to length and reattached anatomically only 12 days after the injury. We treated one patient who avulsed the ECRL insertion *without* a fragment of bone, in whom persistent symptoms required operative repair that was successful 6 weeks postinjury.

Complications of Metacarpal Fractures

The complications seen after metacarpal fractures are related to concomitant soft-tissue injury, malunion, overzealous treatment, or pin-tract problems.

Soft-Tissue Injury

Fractures involving the shafts and bases of the metacarpals are most commonly due to crushing injuries, and the fractures are often open, involving several metacarpals. Frequently, there is soft-tissue damage followed by massive edema. Concomitant extensor tendon damage is common, with adhesions being a likely sequela. Interosseous muscles may be damaged, and scarring may result in intrinsic contracture of the hand.

Stiffness of the MP and PIP joints is a not uncommon complication of multiple metacarpal fractures, espe-

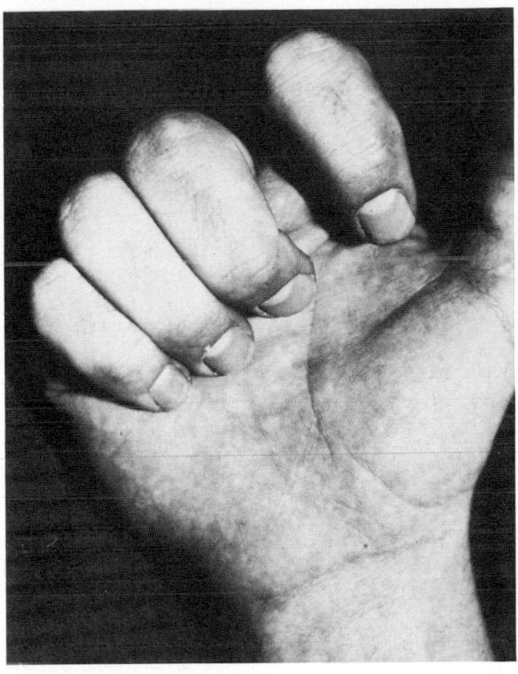

FIGURE 11-67. This patient had fractures at the bases of the third, fourth, and fifth metacarpals. All three healed with rotational deformity, leaving a wide gap between the index and long fingers. Correct rotational alignment is particularly difficult to achieve with multiple metacarpal fractures.

cially those associated with massive soft-tissue injury. The causes of joint stiffness are multiple, some of which are beyond the control of the surgeon, and may include any combination of the following:

1. Improper immobilization of the MP joints in extension.
2. Prolonged immobilization.
3. Intrinsic contracture.
4. Extrinsic contracture secondary to extensor tendon adherence.
5. Varying degrees of hand dysfunction syndrome. (reflex sympathetic dystrophy).

Prevention of stiffness is the best treatment but once it is present, prompt and careful evaluation of the patient is essential to determine the major cause or causes to initiate appropriate treatment.

Malunion—Angulation

Malunion of the metacarpal neck or shaft virtually always occurs with apex dorsal; the farther it is from the MP joint, the more noticeable the deformity and the more likely it is to disturb the intrinsic and extrinsic muscle balance and cause pseudoclawing or a painful grip. Thus, malunion of the shaft is more likely to be symptomatic than that involving the neck. Angulation up to about 30° is unlikely to cause problems but if symptoms warrant treatment, a corrective osteotomy is indicated. This can be done as an opening, closing,[149] or combination[376] wedge osteotomy. An opening wedge osteotomy requires a bone graft; therefore, we prefer a closing wedge osteotomy, which does not. Theoretically, a closing wedge osteotomy shortens the bone but this is probably compensated by straightening the angulation. The key to success with this procedure is precise preoperative planning of the osteotomy. Satisfactory fixation can be achieved with K-wires, tension-band wiring, or a dorsal miniplate.

Malunion—Rotational

Rotational malalignment is a serious complication of metacarpal fractures, and its prevention must be foremost in the mind of the physician managing these injuries. This problem is particularly likely to occur with fractures of the border metacarpals and is more difficult to control when more than one metacarpal is fractured (see Fig. 11-67). Malunion with rotational deformity may require a rotational osteotomy for correction.[79,299,395]

Pin-Tract Infections

Serious pin-tract infection from percutaneously placed K-wires is uncommon, even when the pins are left protruding through the skin. A slight amount of serous drainage is not unusual but this is rarely a problem if the pins are left in no longer than 4 weeks. Pin-tract problems can also be minimized by avoiding skin tension at the time of placement, bending the pins outside the skin to prevent migration, windowing the cast over the pins, and having the patient apply an antiseptic solution (eg, alcohol, hydrogen peroxide, Betadine) to the pin–skin interface several times a day.

Other general complications are discussed in the section on phalangeal fractures.

FRACTURES OF THE THUMB METACARPAL

The thumb is a unique digit, and fractures of the thumb metacarpal are distinctly different from those of other metacarpals. Most thumb metacarpal fractures occur at or near the base, and therefore a thorough knowledge of the anatomy of the CMC joint is essential to understand the mechanism of injury, the pathologic anatomy, and the treatment of these fractures (see section on Thumb CMC).

Classification

Four distinct fracture patterns may involve the base of the thumb metacarpal, as illustrated in Figure 11-68.[548,560,561] It is particularly important to differentiate intra-articular fractures from the extra-articular types because management of the two is different. Bennett's fracture-dislocation and Rolando's fracture are the intra-articular types, and the extra-articular fracture may have either a transverse or an oblique configuration. The epiphyseal fracture seen only in children is excluded from this discussion.

Bennett's Fracture

More properly called a fracture-dislocation, Bennett's fracture was first described by Bennett[528] in 1882 and has been discussed exhaustively in the world literature since. The mechanism of injury is an axial blow directed against the partially flexed metacarpal; not surprisingly, many of these injuries are sustained in fistfights. The fracture line characteristically separates the major part of the metacarpal from a small volar lip fragment, producing disruption of the CMC joint (Fig. 11-69). That an avulsion fracture occurs rather than a pure dislocation attests to the strength of the anterior oblique ligament (AOL), which anchors the volar lip of the metacarpal to the tubercle of the trapezium. Kuschner and coworkers[557] described an unusual variant of Bennett's fracture in which there was an avulsion fracture of the radial tubercle of the index metacarpal, with the ligament still attached to the ulnar beak of the thumb metacarpal base.

The two primary variables of a Bennett's fracture are the size of the volar lip fragment and the amount of displacement of the shaft. The base of the metacarpal is

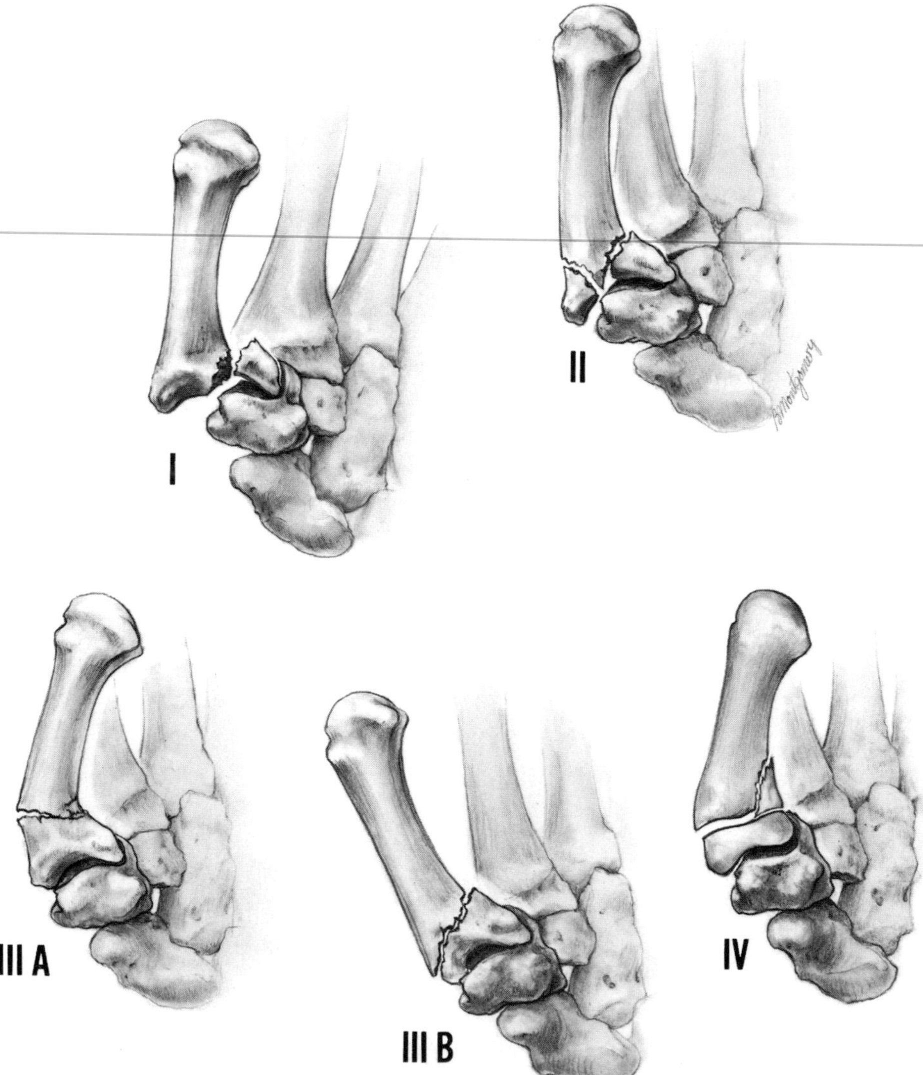

FIGURE 11-68. Four distinct fracture patterns may involve the base of the thumb metacarpal. Type I (Bennett's fracture-dislocation) and type II (Rolando's fracture) are intra-articular. These should be differentiated from type III extra-articular fractures, which may be either transverse or oblique. Type IV fractures are epiphyseal injuries seen in children. (*Green, D.P., and O'Brien, E.T.: Fractures of the Thumb Metacarpal. South. Med. J. 65:807, 1972.*)

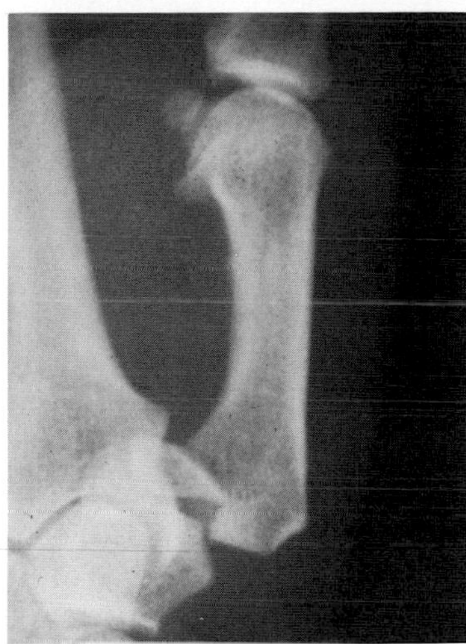

FIGURE 11-69. A typical Bennett's fracture-dislocation. The small volar lip fragment remains attached to the anterior oblique ligament that anchors the fragment to the tubercle of the trapezium.

pulled dorsally and radially by the abductor pollicis longus, while the distal attachment of the adductor levers the base further dorsally (Fig. 11-70).

Associated Injuries

Concomitant fractures of the trapezium seen with Bennett's fractures have been reported, for which ORIF is the recommended treatment.[542,566]

Rupture of the MP joint collateral ligaments (see Ulnar Collateral Ligament Injury) has been reported as a concomitant (and easily overlooked) injury with Bennett's fracture.[555]

Methods of Treatment

At least 20 methods of treatment have been advocated for Bennett's fracture since the first large clinical series with x-rays in 1904.[562] At one end of the therapeutic spectrum is Blum,[531] who proposed that reduction of the fracture was not necessary and that good results could be achieved with early active motion. Charnley,[535] Roberts and Kelly,[567] Böhler,[41] and Griffiths[549] separately advocated the use of a well-molded plaster cast. Griffiths[549] reported that even in unreduced Bennett's fractures, the results were not bad, noting that although these patients had some limitation of motion, they were generally free of pain. He concluded that the importance of the joint involvement in this fracture was generally overestimated. Cannon and coworkers[534] further supported this concept with a long-term follow-up study of patients treated nonoperatively, showing that 92% of these patients were asymptomatic at 10 years. They also found in a literature review that only 7 of 456 patients (1.5%) being treated surgically for painful CMC arthritis had a history of a Bennett's fracture. Other subsequent studies have shown that although many of these patients may develop varying degrees of arthritis, few have more than mild symptoms.[556,559,576]

James and Gibson[553] and Pollen[564] incorporated a felt pad into their casts to prevent the loss of reduction that frequently occurred with plaster alone. Robinson[568] and Watson-Jones[392] each advocated the use of continuous skin traction in addition to a cast, and Bunnell[59] described a method of skeletal traction that at one time was used rather extensively in the treatment of Bennett's fractures. Thoren[574,575] devised a unique method of applying oblique skeletal traction by using a hook inserted into the base of the first metacarpal. He believed that traction should be applied in the direction of *adduction and opposition* rather than abduction to bring the displaced shaft back into alignment with the volar lip fragment. Harvey and Bye[551] also suggested adduction as the preferred position of immobilization.

Numerous types of external splints have been advocated, including the Goldthwaite splint[536] and Goldberg's[546,547] felt pad attached to an outrigger. Ross and Sinclair[570] treated a series of patients with the Stader splint, a forerunner of the Roger Anderson device.

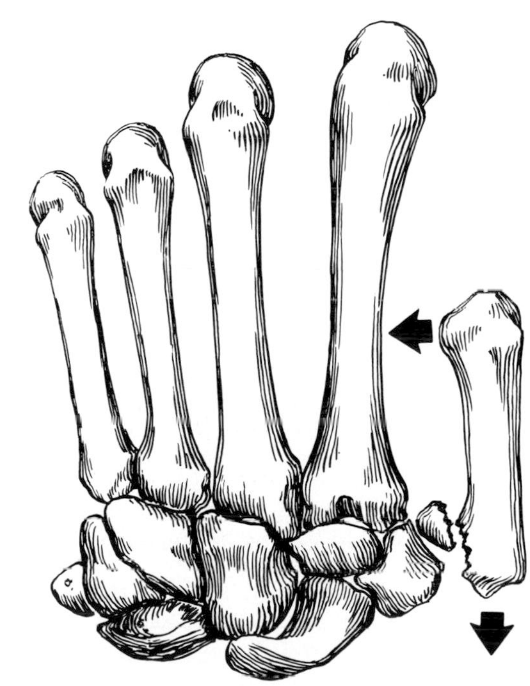

FIGURE 11-70. In a Bennett's fracture, the base of the metacarpal is pulled dorsally and radially by the abductor pollicis longus, and the adductor further levers the base into abduction.

Closed reduction and percutaneous pin fixation was originally described by Johnson,[554] using Waugh and Ferrazzano's[393] technique of transfixing a fractured metacarpal to an adjacent one. Wagner[578,579] later modified this method by passing a K-wire from the shaft of the first metacarpal into the trapezium rather than into the second metacarpal, and Salgeback and colleagues[571] used Wagner's technique but with two pins. Others[537,577] have gone back to percutaneous pin fixation from the thumb metacarpal into the second metacarpal instead of into the carpal bones. Wiggins and associates[580] used intramedullary wire fixation after closed reduction because of difficulty in positioning the wires in the manner described by Wagner.

In 1946, Ellis[539] was apparently the first to advocate open reduction, although in his technique the fracture site was not actually exposed. Instead, he reduced the base of the metacarpal and passed small pins into the trapezium, leaving them protruding as a buttress to hold the reduction of the metacarpal. Fisher[540] performed a limited open reduction by looping a No. 2 nylon or silk suture around the first metacarpal and passing this out as a pull-out suture in the palm. Badger[527] used a small screw for fixation, obviating plaster immobilization postoperatively.

Gedda and Moberg,[543,544] however, appear to have turned the tide in favor of open reduction with their conclusions that exact anatomic restoration of the articular surface is less likely to lead to posttraumatic arthritis. Subsequent studies[576] have shown a correlation between the quality of reduction and the likelihood of subsequent arthritis, but there does not appear to be good correlation between radiographic evidence of arthritis and significant symptoms.[532,556,559,563,571] Despite the absence of any good long-term studies supporting the concept that symptoms are directly related to joint incongruity, ORIF has become increasingly popular with surgeons as the treatment of choice. Recommended methods of fixation have included two 0.028-inch K-wires or a 2-mm AO screw for smaller fragments[541] and a 2.7-mm AO screw[541,573] or Herbert screw[552] for larger fragments. Foster and Hastings[541] noted that the screw diameter should not exceed 30% of the cortical surface of the volar lip fragment.

 *Authors' Preferred Method of Treatment*

Reports of good results from each of the preceding methods (many in articles with short-term follow-up) pose a perplexing dilemma for the surgeon choosing a plan of treatment for a patient having a Bennett's fracture. That so many types of splinting, traction, and other methods of immobilization have been described implies that it is often difficult to achieve and maintain reduction of the articular surface by nonoperative means. We therefore tend to prefer some type of internal fixation in an effort to hold the reduction. Our first choice is closed reduction and percutaneous pin fixation (CRIF).

Technique of CRIF for Bennett's Fracture. Under brachial block or general anesthesia, the surgeon applies longitudinal traction to the thumb while an assistant provides counter traction through the upper arm. The correct direction of pull is the most important element in achieving a satisfactory reduction. Successful reduction in acute cases does not require a strong traction force, but the direction of that gentle traction force is critical. The natural tendency is to abduct the thumb and lever the metacarpal into what is thought to be the reduced position. This does not reduce the fracture, but instead a gap is created at the fracture site. It must be remembered that the fundamental fracture axiom that the controllable distal fragment is to bring into alignment with the uncontrollable proximal fragment. In this case, the fragment over which we have no control is the small volar lip fragment that is still attached by the AOL to the trapezium. Recalling Thoren's premise regarding the direction of a traction force necessary to reduce this fracture, it is therefore imperative to bring the thumb metacarpal shaft into apposition with the volar lip fragment by *adducting the thumb and pushing the base of the thumb metacarpal toward the palm in an opposition movement.* Adequacy of reduction should then be verified with an image intensifier or smaller radiograph unit (Xi-scan or Fluoroscan). If joint congruity has been restored, the surgeon can hold the reduction with one hand and insert a 0.045-inch K-wire with the other hand. The pin enters the dorsal surface of the proximal third of the thumb metacarpal and is aimed toward either the second metacarpal, trapezoid, or trapezium (Fig. 11-71). No attempt is made to spear the small volar lip fragment with the K-wire, but the pin simply holds the metacarpal shaft in the reduced position. A second K-wire is usually used for added stability.

The pins are bent at a right angle outside the skin, any skin tension is relieved with a scalpel, the pins are cut off, and the tips covered with commercially available rubber caps. A thumb spica cast is applied, adding sufficient padding around the protruding wires to avoid pressure from the plaster. Within the first 7 to 10 days postoperatively, the patient is seen in the office to obtain x-rays to verify maintenance of reduction, and a fiberglass thumb spica cast is applied with a window for the patient to administer pin-tract care. The cast and pins are removed in the office at 4 weeks and a supervised therapy program is begun.

What constitutes an "acceptable" reduction is still

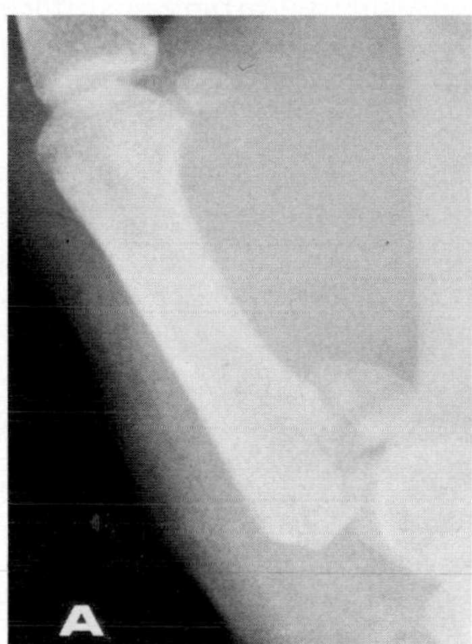

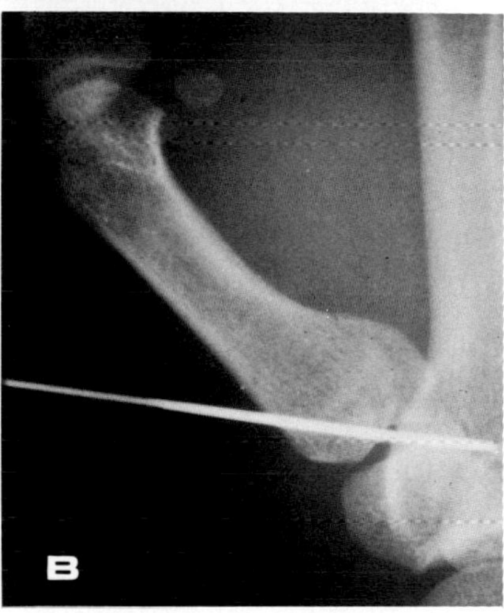

FIGURE 11-71. Our preferred method of treatment for Bennett's fracture is an initial attempt at closed reduction and percutaneous pin fixation. (**A**) A typical Bennett's fracture-dislocation. (**B**) Anatomic reduction was achieved by closed reduction and percutaneous pinning. Note that no attempt is made to transfix the small volar fragment; rather the purpose of the pin is to hold the shaft of the metacarpal in the reduced position after a reduction has been achieved by closed manipulation.

an unresolved issue. We formerly believed that it was imperative to accept nothing but a perfect anatomic reduction, but the results of Cannon and colleagues'[534] previously cited study and the lack of correlation between arthrosis and symptoms suggest that this may not be necessary, and we accept slight joint incongruity. Specifically, we try to correct the joint incongruity to less than 2 mm. Only if this cannot be accomplished with closed reduction (Fig. 11-72) do we resort to ORIF. A small AO cortical screw probably provides the best fixation but it should be used in this situation only by those familiar with AO principles and techniques. Small K-wires or a Herbert screw are acceptable alternatives.

After closed reduction and percutaneous pin fixation, a thumb spica cast is imperative until the K-wires are removed at 4 weeks. Unprotected motion is allowed sooner after open reduction if secure rigid fixation has been achieved.

Rolando's Fracture

In 1910, Rolando[569] described a fracture pattern that differed from the classic Bennett's fracture-dislocation. In the fracture that he reported, in addition to the volar lip fragment, a large dorsal fragment was present, resulting in a Y- or T-shaped intra-articular fracture. Although the classic Rolando's fracture is that pictured in Figure 11-68 (II), it should probably more properly be thought of as being a comminuted Bennett's fracture because in most cases, instead of having the simple Y or T configuration, there is severe comminution. Rolando observed that the prognosis was poor after this injury, despite treatment either in a cast or with skin traction. More than 75 years later, it remains a difficult fracture to treat but fortunately is the least common of the adult thumb metacarpal fractures.

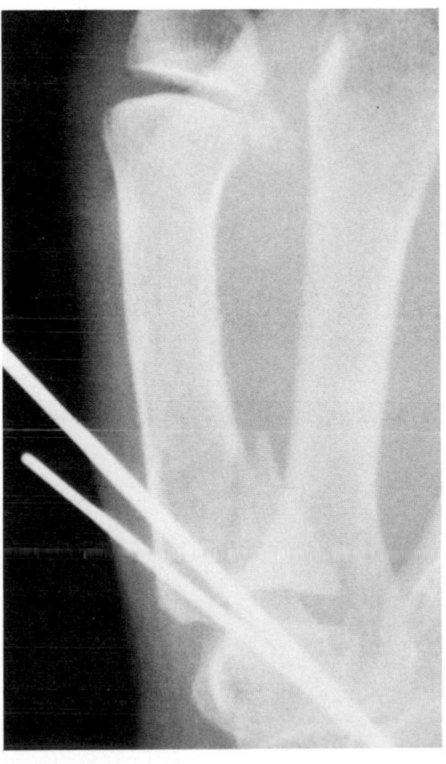

FIGURE 11-72. A Bennett's fracture in which a successful reduction was not achieved by the closed method. Although a perfect reduction is probably not necessary (see text), the amount of residual step-off in this joint is unacceptable. Either a second attempt at closed reduction or open reduction and internal fixation should be performed.

Methods of Treatment

The choice of treatment depends primarily on the severity of comminution of the fragments and to a lesser extent on the degree of displacement. ORIF should be attempted only if the volar and dorsal components are single large fragments.[541] More commonly, however, the base of the metacarpal is shattered into many fragments, and attempts at operative restoration are frustrating, if not impossible (Fig. 11-73). Operative fixation of comminuted fractures of the base of the thumb metacarpal should be attempted only by surgeons experienced in AO techniques in the hand because these are technically demanding procedures.[558] ORIF alone may not be sufficient, and one of the most experienced AO hand surgeons has reported good results with ORIEF, a combination of ORIF, external fixation, and bone grafting.[533]

For most surgeons who do not possess such technical skills, traction or external fixation may a reasonable alternative for the more comminuted varieties of these difficult injuries. Gelberman and associates[532,545] have reported good results in patients with Rolando's fracture using Thoren's method of oblique traction. Before skeletal traction is applied, however, it is advisable to take an x-ray while a longitudinal traction force is applied to see whether the articular surface has improved. If the joint surface has been reasonably restored, treatment with either traction or external fixation to maintain the reduction is justified; if it has not, little will be gained from the use of distraction.[552,565] Another method of holding the thumb metacarpal out to length is by percutaneous pin fixation to the second metacarpal.[577]

For severely comminuted fractures in which the joint surface is not significantly improved on the x-ray taken in traction, we prefer to immobilize the thumb for a minimal period to relieve pain and then begin early active motion in an attempt to remold the badly distorted articular surface. Because of the infrequency of Rolando's fracture, no one has reported a series comparing the results of different forms of treatment. In our experience, the tendency in the past has been to err on the side of overtreatment (ie, to attempt open reduction when it was virtually impossible to restore the articular surface). We repeat that significant comminution is a definite contraindication to operative treatment of this injury.

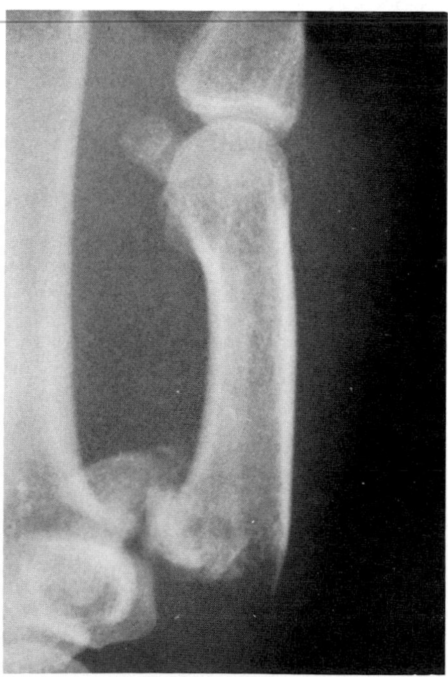

FIGURE 11-73. A Rolando's fracture rarely has only the large dorsal and volar fragments. More commonly, it is severely comminuted, as illustrated. In fractures such as this, open reduction and anatomic restoration of the articular surface are virtually impossible and should not be attempted by anyone except a most experienced AO surgeon. (*Green, D.P., and O'Brien, E.T.: Fractures of the Thumb Metacarpal. South. Med. J. 65:807, 1972.*)

Extra-articular Fractures

The extra-articular type is the most frequent fracture in the thumb metacarpal and the simplest to treat. Two basic patterns are seen (Fig. 11-74): a transverse fracture and a less common oblique one. It is particularly important to distinguish these extra-articular fractures from the more serious intra-articular Bennett's and Rolando's fractures because rarely is surgery indicated in the management of the extra-articular fractures. This differentiation is usually not difficult on careful study of the x-rays, although the oblique type may appear at first glance to be a Bennett's fracture. The distinguishing feature is that in the oblique extra-articular type, the fracture line does not enter the joint.

Treatment

One should resist the temptation to overtreat these extra-articular fractures. Anatomic reduction can usually be achieved readily by closed manipulation under regional or local anesthesia; the thumb is immobilized in a short-arm thumb spica cast for 4 weeks. Care must be taken to avoid hyperextension of the MP joint in plaster. Failure to achieve exact alignment of the fracture should not be considered an indication for open reduction. At the worst, the patient with an inadequately reduced transverse fracture is likely to have only a slight prominence at the base of the thumb and possibly some minimal limitation of thumb abduction. Even with 20° to 30° of residual angulation, however, there is usually no detectable limitation of motion.

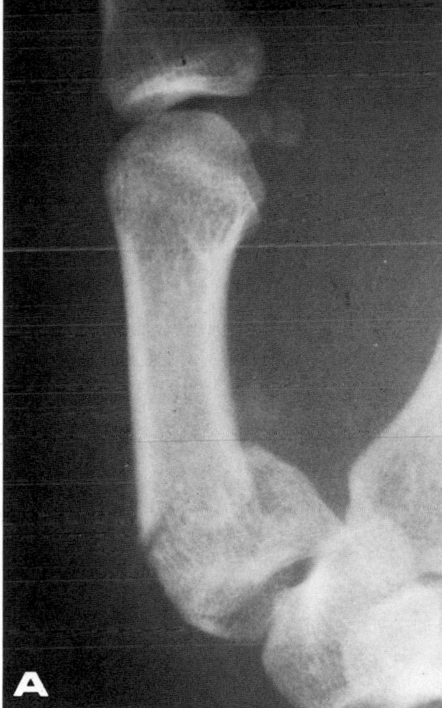
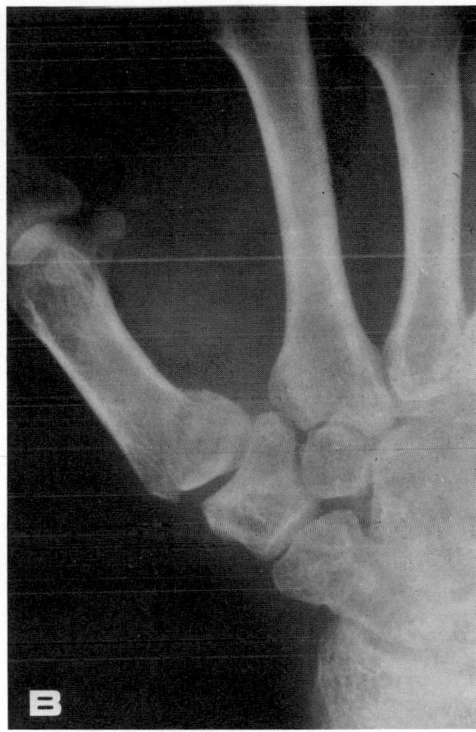

FIGURE 11-74. It is particularly important to distinguish these extra-articular thumb metacarpal fractures from the intra-articular varieties. (**A**) The most common fracture of the thumb metacarpal is a transverse extra-articular type. (**B**) Less commonly seen is an oblique extra-articular fracture. This is the fracture that is most frequently confused with a Bennett's fracture. Careful examination of the x-ray reveals that the fracture line does not enter the joint.

Occasionally, the oblique type of extra-articular fracture may prove to be somewhat unstable, particularly if there is marked vertical inclination of the fracture line. Even in this type of fracture, open reduction is not warranted. If plaster immobilization is unsuccessful in holding the reduction, percutaneous pinning provides a simple method of securing the reduction achieved by closed manipulation.

DISLOCATIONS OF THE DIP JOINT

Acute Injuries

Pure dislocations of the DIP joints of the fingers and the IP joint of the thumb are rare injuries. When they occur, they are almost always dorsal dislocations and are frequently associated with an open wound. A far more common injury occurring at the DIP joint is a mallet fracture-dislocation, in which the distal phalanx may subluxate volarly (see section on Mallet Fracture). Even the relatively uncommon avulsion of the FDP is more common than a pure dislocation of this joint. Bowers and Fajgenbaum[594] described volar plate avulsion of the DIP joint that mimics FDP avulsion, even to the point of causing inability to actively flex the DIP joint. They noted that this rare lesion may occur in the absence of actual dislocation of the joint. A similar case was reported by Lineaweaver and Mathes.[659]

Dorsal fracture-dislocations of the DIP joint are uncommon, and only two small series have been reported. Horiuchi and coworkers[630] found that acute cases were easy to reduce closed and could be held reduced with a K-wire either across the joint or as an internal extension block splint. Cases seen more than 3 weeks postinjury usually required open reduction, for which they preferred a mid-lateral or posterolateral approach.

Hamer and Quinton[625] successfully applied the closed reduction and dorsal extension block splint method to six patients having dorsal fracture-subluxation of the DIP joint.

Simultaneous DIP and PIP Dislocations

Simultaneous dislocation of the PIP and DIP joints in the same digit can occur in any finger but apparently these double dislocations are most common in the ring and small fingers. The best review article is by Andersen and Johannsen,[586] who collected 52 cases that were published between 1874, when the combination was first reported by Bartels, and 1992. Virtually all have appeared as case reports, and even the Hand Service of the Edinburgh Hospitals could find only eight cases in 10 years.[158]

If the swelling is mild, the finger may have a "stepladder" appearance, but Krishnan[650] noted that swelling may obscure the clinical diagnosis.[586] Radiographic examination is mandatory, especially a true lateral view of the individual digit. In most of the previously reported cases,** closed reduction was easily accomplished, usually under digital block[585,724] or without anesthesia. Postreduction immobilization has ranged from "brief"[158] to 3 weeks, although mild limitation of motion has been reported after 3 weeks of splinting.[586] The preferred position of immobilization is the intrinsic plus position (DIP and PIP joints in full extension). Delay in diagnosis or treatment may necessitate open reduction and compromise the result.[589,693] Good results were reported by most authors except Krebs and Gron,[649] whose patient ultimately required arthrodesis of the PIP joint for severe pain.

There has apparently been only one case report of triple dislocation (ie, simultaneous MP, PIP, and DIP in the same digit).[628] This patient was treated with closed reduction and 3 weeks immobilization. The result was good motion in the MP and PIP joints but limited motion in the DIP joint.

Irreducible DIP Dislocations

Irreducible dislocations have been reported in the DIP joint, and there appear to be at least four distinct mechanisms:

1. A pure dorsal dislocation in which the volar plate is avulsed from the neck of the middle phalanx and becomes entrapped in the joint, similar to a complex dislocation of the MP joint[642,683,688,700,704,705]
2. Entrapment of the long flexor tendon (FDP) in the joint, seen in a dislocation in which there is rupture of one collateral ligament.[360,676,689,694,704] (The radiographic key to diagnosis of FDP entrapment is marked lateral displacement of the distal phalanx)[360]
3. Entrapment of an osteochondral fragment[782] or a sesamoid (without attachment to the volar plate)[645] in the joint
4. Buttonholing of the condyles of middle phalanx volarly through a split in the FDP tendon[618]

Iftikhar[632] believed that the volar plate is more likely to be the obstructing element in closed injuries and FDP entrapment the obstructing element in open dislocations of the DIP joint.

Only one case of irreducible palmar dislocation of the DIP joint has been reported.[636]

Treatment

When seen early, DIP dislocations can almost always be easily reduced closed, and they are generally stable after reduction. Hyperextension and mediolateral stress examination should be performed after reduction; a short period (10 to 12 days) of immobilization of the DIP joint alone is usually adequate.[717]

The patient with an open DIP dislocation should be afforded all the standard acceptable treatment for any open joint injury (ie, thorough cleansing and irrigation) before open reduction.

If the dislocation is irreducible, open reduction is required.

Chronic (Unreduced) DIP Dislocations

Occasionally, a patient presents with an old, unreduced DIP (or thumb IP) dislocation. If the delay has been as long as 2 to 3 weeks, open reduction likely is required. This may be somewhat difficult technically because of contracture of the periarticular soft tissues, and the prognosis for joint motion is poor.

The joint can be exposed from dorsal, volar, or midlateral incisions. Having tried all of these, we believe that the dorsal approach provides the best exposure, although at least partial transection of the collateral ligament is usually required to see the joint fully and accomplish a reduction from any approach. The longer the joint has been unreduced, the more extensive is the soft-tissue dissection required and the more unstable the joint will be postoperatively.

The articular surfaces should be examined carefully at the time of operation. If there is extensive articular damage or erosion, primary arthrodesis is indicated.

DISLOCATIONS AND LIGAMENTOUS INJURIES OF THE PIP JOINT

The PIP joint occupies a position of unique importance in the hand. Loss of motion in this joint severely restricts function. Conversely, if flexion and extension can be maintained in the PIP joint when there is significant damage in the other small joints of the same finger, satisfactory hand function can be preserved. The propensity for stiffness in the PIP joint is great, not only after injury to the joint itself but even after prolonged immobilization of an otherwise normal joint. For this reason, the utmost care and concern should be given to injuries involving the PIP joint, and unnecessary immobilization of this joint should be avoided when other injuries in the hand are treated.

Anatomy

The PIP joint, although in some ways similar to the MP joint, has numerous important differences, which have been pointed out by Kuczynski.[11] The PIP joint has been described as a "sloppy hinge," designed

** References 585, 623, 626, 633, 635, 636, 648, 724, 726, 602, 623, 635.

mainly for flexion and extension but allowing 7° to 10° lateral deviation and slight rotation.[600,656] It is inherently more stable than the MP joint because of its bicondylar configuration, which gives it a modified tongue-in-groove appearance (Fig. 11-75). The shape of the head of the proximal phalanx is less eccentric than that of the metacarpal head, as seen in the lateral view, and therefore the cam effect is less significant (Fig. 11-76).

The collateral ligaments of the PIP joint are similar to those in the MP joint, with a cord-like collateral ligament proper and a lower accessory ligament (Fig. 11-77). The major difference is that tension in these ligaments is essentially the same in flexion as it is in extension. This is due primarily to two factors: the absence of the cam effect and the parallel alignment of the collateral ligaments, as compared with the divergence of the ligaments in the MP joint. The result of these anatomic peculiarities is that at least some part of the collateral ligament is taut in both flexion and extension.[3,672]

Normal range of motion in the PIP joints is usually at least 0° to 105° and in many fingers, flexion of 120° is easily obtained. As in the MP joint, the volar plate at this level has a firm distal attachment to the base of the middle phalanx and a more flexible proximal attachment to the neck of the proximal phalanx to allow folding with flexion of the joint. Kuczynski[11] has suggested that the volar plate is less mobile in the PIP joint than it is in the MP joint.

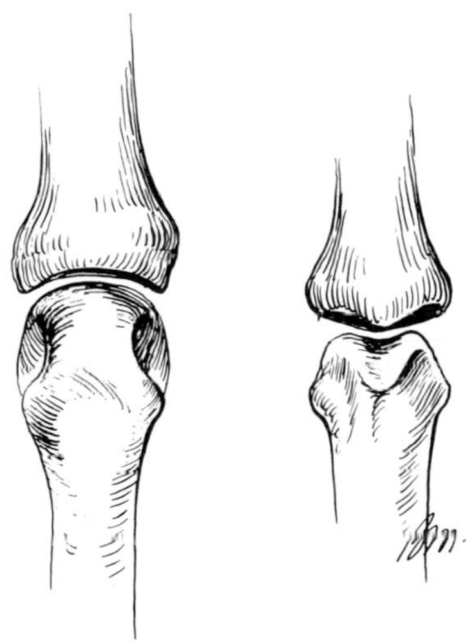

FIGURE 11-75. Comparison of the metacarpophalangeal (MP) and proximal interphalangeal (PIP) joints, as seen in the anteroposterior view. (*Left*) The MP joint is a condyloid joint in which the globular head of the metacarpal articulates with the reciprocally concave base of the proximal phalanx. It allows flexion, extension, abduction, adduction, and a limited amount of circumduction. (*Right*) The PIP joint is essentially a ginglymus or hinge joint, allowing only flexion and extension. It is inherently more stable than the MP joint because of its bicondylar configuration, which gives it a modified tongue-in-groove appearance.

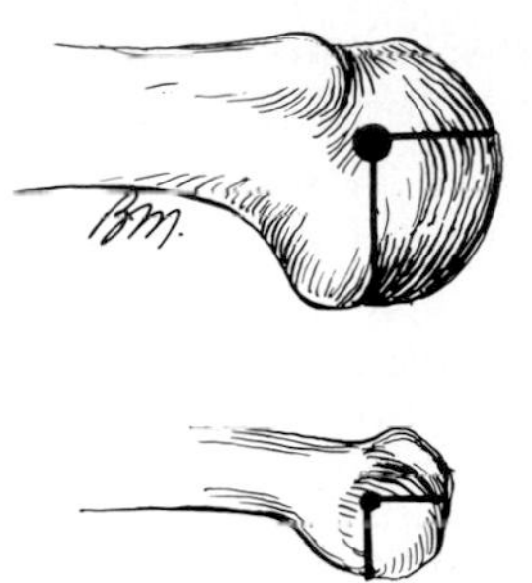

FIGURE 11-76. Comparison of the MP (*top*) and PIP (*bottom*) joints, as seen in the lateral view. The shape of the head of the proximal phalanx is less eccentric than that of the metacarpal head and therefore, the cam effect is less significant in the PIP joint.

Dorsally and dorsolaterally, the extensor hood mechanism envelops the joint, and Slattery[706] only recently described what he calls the dorsal plate of the PIP joint, which he believes is analogous to the patella in the knee.

On the volar aspect, the volar (palmar) plate separates the joint from the flexor tendons. (For more detailed descriptions of the anatomy of and around the PIP joint, the reader is referred to the monographs by Milford[13] and Bowers[596] and the articles by Haines,[9] Landsmeer,[12] and Tubiana and Valentin.[15]

Classification

Injuries of the PIP joints may be classified as collateral ligament injuries, volar plate injuries, dislocations, and fracture-dislocations. The most important clinical consideration in these injuries is to distinguish between those that are stable and those that are unstable. As a

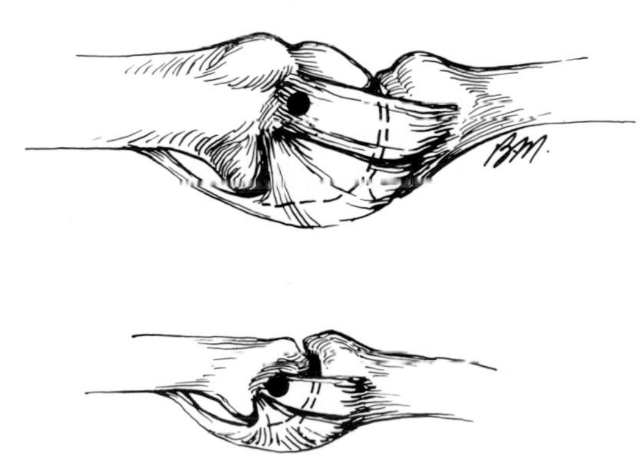

FIGURE 11-77. The collateral ligaments of the MP (*top*) and PIP (*bottom*) joints are similar. Both have a cord-like collateral ligament proper and a lower accessory ligament, which attaches directly into the volar plate.

general rule, those that are stable are easy to treat and have the best prognosis.

There is clearly a great deal of overlap among PIP joint injuries, especially those involving a combination of fractures and dislocation or subluxation. Several authors[596,627,662,702] have attempted to classify such injuries but no single system has yet received widespread acceptance.

Collateral Ligament Injuries

Collateral ligament injuries (lateral dislocations) are caused by abduction or adduction force applied to the finger, usually in the extended position.[665] Because of the long lever arm, the injury usually involves the PIP joint and is more frequently seen in sports such as football, wrestling, baseball, and basketball. The radial collateral ligament (RCL) is injured more often than the ulnar collateral ligament (UCL).

Collateral ligament injuries may be classified as acute or chronic and further subclassified as stable or unstable. McCue and colleagues[665] defined acute injuries in their series of patients as those diagnosed within 3 months of injury; most were seen within 3 weeks. We believe that any injury of the lateral ligament diagnosed after 6 weeks should be classified as being an old or chronic injury.

Diagnosis

Regardless of the apparent severity or suspected pathology, every injury of the PIP joint should be examined in a systematic and thorough fashion, which must include at least the following major points:

Tenderness
The examiner should attempt to ascertain whether the maximum tenderness is over the central slip (dorsal), the collateral ligaments (radial and ulnar), or the volar plate (volar).

Stability
The joint should be stressed radially and ulnarly to check the integrity of the collateral ligaments. This has traditionally been done with the PIP joint in full extension but researchers at the Mayo Clinic suggested that stability should also be tested with the joint flexed 20° to 30°.[672] They showed that, as in the knee, structures other than the collateral ligaments may provide stability of the PIP joint in full extension. They concluded that angulation greater than 20° in response to stress testing is abnormal and indicates loss of collateral ligament integrity.

Partial tears (sprains) of the collateral ligaments do not allow the joint to open up in excess of physiologic limits. In complete tears (ruptures), there is little or no resistance to lateral deviation stress, and the joint opens on the injured side. Complete tears that are suspected on clinical examination can be documented by stress radiographs, comparing these with stress films of the same digit in the uninjured hand.

Integrity of the volar plate is tested by passive hyperextension, comparing the range of hyperextension to the other fingers. Pain on testing the volar plate is probably a more important sign than the actual amount of hyperextension.

Range of Motion
Both active and passive range of motion should be observed, with specific emphasis on the patient's ability to actively extend the PIP joint completely. If he or she is unable to do so because of pain, the examination must be repeated under digital block anesthesia. Inability to actively extend the PIP joint against resistance is diagnostic of rupture of the central slip, and a boutonniere lesion results if the patient is not appropriately treated. In the early stages, there is no limitation of passive flexion of the DIP joint but within 1 to 2 weeks after injury, this test gains increasing significance. In the patient with a developing boutonniere lesion, passive flexion of the DIP joint will be limited if the PIP joint is held in maximum extension. We believe that passive DIP flexion with the PIP held in maximum extension is the best clinical test to differentiate an early developing boutonniere lesion from other injuries of the PIP joint.

Adequate X-rays
It is necessary to obtain at least two (PA and lateral) views of the involved finger. Of these, the most important is a true lateral view of the individual finger. More errors are made in the diagnosis of PIP joint injuries because of failure to obtain this x-ray than any other single reason. A lateral view of the hand is unacceptable because important details are obscured by superimposition of the other three fingers. An oblique view, although often helpful in delineating other injuries such as condylar fractures, often fails to demonstrate the presence or extent of a small intra-articular fracture at the base of the middle phalanx.

In patients who have chronic or old collateral ligament injuries, in whom treatment has been ineffective or no primary treatment was instituted, two signs are prominent: instability and swelling.[673] Instability may result from attenuation of the ligament or there may be total loss of continuity. Swelling at the site of collateral ligament injury is at times severe and painful, and it may be the patient's main complaint. This may be associated with limitation of joint motion. Swelling is due to excessive reparative connective tissue, which has been described by Moberg[673] as "ligamentous callus," at times possibly surrounding tiny avulsion fractures that are too small to be seen radiographically.[643]

Partial tears of the collateral ligament can be difficult to differentiate from complete ruptures on clinical examination alone; therefore, when instability is suspected, stress radiographs (Fig. 11-78) should be compared with those of a finger in the opposite hand. Kiefhaber and colleagues[643] performed extensive laboratory studies on collateral ligament instability and concluded that angulation of greater than 20° is diagnostic of complete rupture. Their studies showed that if the stress x-ray shows angulation of less than 20°, there is a 47% chance of complete rupture but in these patients, the connective tissue layer surrounding the collateral ligament is intact and this maintains the correct anatomic relation of the injured structures. In their study, 94% of PIP collateral ligament ruptures occurred at the proximal attachment, but Rhee and coworkers[696] demonstrated that in cadaveric experiments, the site of the disruption depended on the speed at which the ligaments were stressed.

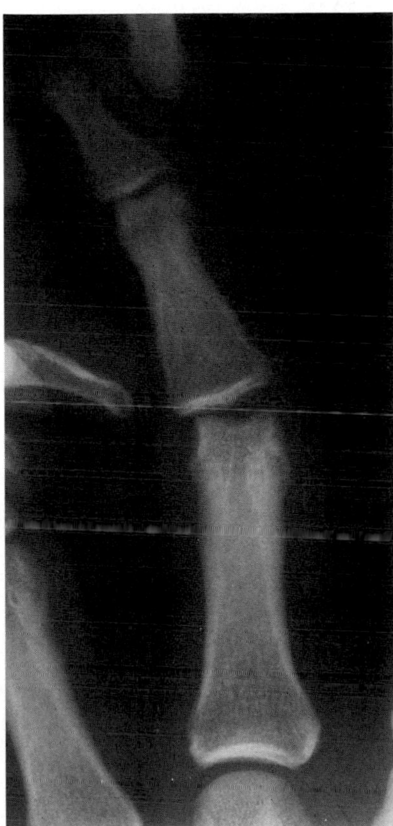

FIGURE 11-78. A stress x-ray of the proximal interphalangeal joint, showing apparent rupture of the radial collateral ligament.

Treatment

Acute Injuries With Partial Tears. Most authors agree that incomplete tears (sprains) of the collateral ligament should be treated with 2 to 5 weeks of buddy taping or immobilization, depending on the degree of severity.[666,673]

Authors' Preferred Method of Treatment

We prefer to treat all partial tears of the collateral ligaments with buddy taping. The injured finger is taped to a normal adjacent digit, and active motion is encouraged from the outset. The tape is worn continuously for 3 weeks and then only during periods of anticipated stress (eg, participation in sports) for an additional 3 weeks. Usually, an athlete is allowed to continue to play during the entire period of treatment.

Regardless of the method of treatment, however, two points must be made clear to the patient from the outset:

1. Full recovery (ie, reaching that point at which there is no residual soreness in the joint) is likely to take what seems to the patient an inordinately long time (usually several months, sometimes 12 to 18 months).
2. There almost certainly will be some permanent residual enlargement of the joint due to normal healing of the ligament with scar tissue.

Acute Injuries With Complete Tears. Treatment of complete tears (ruptures) of the collateral ligaments of the PIP joints is somewhat controversial. Some authors advocate simple immobilization of the finger, although the recommended position and duration of immobilization vary. Moberg[673] advocated immobilization of the PIP joint in the position of function for as long as 5 weeks. Eaton and Littler[611] advised immobilization of the joint in 25° to 30° flexion for 2 to 3 weeks, followed by buddy taping for further protection as active motion is begun. In discussing McCue's paper,[665] Coonrad suggested that the finger be immobilized for 3 to 4 weeks and that operative treatment be considered only if the joint is still unstable after that time. At one time, Milford[668] suggested splinting the PIP joint in 60° of flexion for 2 to 3 weeks for complete ruptures but he later advocated surgical repair in a young adult, especially for the RCL of the index finger.[669,671] Stern[711] reported a case in which the collateral ligament became entrapped between the central slip and the lateral band, preventing closed reduction and therefore requiring operative treatment.

In the only prospective comparison study published, Ali[584] presented a fairly convincing argument for repair of completely ruptured ligaments, demonstrating in his small series that morbidity was shorter in the patients treated surgically. A few other authors have advised surgical repair of all complete ruptures[639,665,695] but Bowers[593] suggested two specific indications for operative repair: (1) inability to achieve a perfectly congruent reduction, and (2) "unstressed instability." Wilson and Liechty[731] advised surgical repair for (1) instability demonstrated on active range of motion; (2) tissue interposition preventing joint motion; or (3) lack of joint congruity on radiographic evaluation.

Authors' Preferred Method of Treatment

We believe that most complete ruptures of the collateral ligaments of the PIP joints do not require operative treatment. Full-time buddy taping for 3 to 6 weeks is appropriate treatment for most of these injuries, especially in the long, ring, and small fingers. Figure 11-79 demonstrates normal stability of the joint 2 months after injury in a high school basketball player who had a complete rupture treated with buddy taping while he continued to play.

The major objection to advocating primary repair for all collateral ligament ruptures is that occasionally the additional operative trauma may result in some limitation of joint motion, which is likely to be more disabling than slight instability, if that should result from nonoperative treatment. As Flatt[615] has observed, surgical repair of the collateral ligament is delicate and difficult work. In our experience, it is unusual to obtain absolutely full range of motion after any type of operative procedure on the PIP joint. We agree with Milford[669,671] that operative repair probably should be considered for complete rupture of the RCL in the index finger of a young adult, where stability for pinch is more important than full range of motion.

Chronic or Old Complete Ruptures. Patients are occasionally seen with chronic laxity of a collateral ligament because the acute injury was treated either inadequately or not at all. As McCue and coworkers[665] have noted, the results of operative treatment in chronic injuries are less satisfactory than those of primary repair. For this reason, reconstruction of chronic ruptures should be considered only if the patient is significantly symptomatic. Moreover, if there is radiographic evidence of articular damage, reconstruction of the ligament is not likely to totally alleviate the patient's symptoms.

In our experience, late reconstruction of a PIP joint

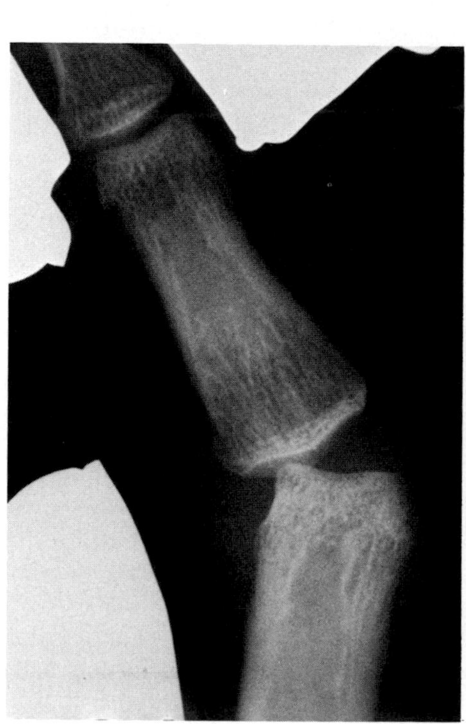

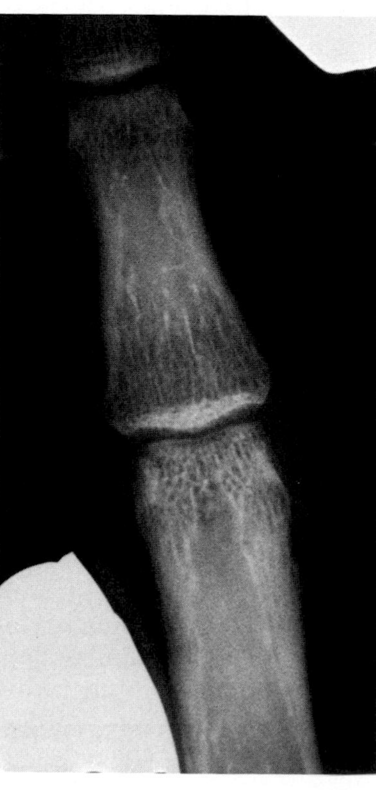

FIGURE 11-79. This high school athlete sustained a complete rupture of the collateral ligament of the proximal interphalangeal (PIP) joint, easily demonstrated clinically and by stress x-rays (*left*). Follow-up stress x-rays taken 2 months later, after 6 weeks of buddy taping, showed good stability of the joint (*right*). Most complete ruptures of the PIP joint collateral ligaments do not require operative repair.

collateral ligament is a difficult operation, and the results are somewhat unpredictable, which is attested to by the paucity of good clinical studies regarding this problem. Noting that the ligament may have healed with lengthening, Redler and Williams[695] merely shortened the ligament and sutured it "under proper tension," a surgical feat that may be somewhat difficult to gauge accurately at operation. In addition to shortening, McCue and associates[665] reinforced the late repair by transferring the radial slip of the superficialis insertion and reattaching it to the proximal end of the ligament with a Bunnell pull-out wire suture. Faithfull[614] reported good results after reconstruction of the lateral ligament with a narrow strip of volar plate detached proximally and sutured into the remnant of collateral ligament on the head of the proximal phalanx. Because chronic rupture of the collateral ligament is often accompanied by laxity of the volar plate, many of the repairs previously described in the literature employ combined techniques to reconstruct both structures.[653,682]

Dislocations of the PIP Joint

There are three types of dislocations of the PIP joint: dorsal, volar, and rotatory (Fig. 11-80).

Dorsal PIP Dislocations (Volar Plate Injury)

Dorsal dislocation is by far the most common type of dislocation in the PIP joint. The physician rarely has an opportunity to see the actual dislocation; reduction is usually accomplished by a coach, trainer, observer, or even the patient. The mechanism of injury is hyperextension of the joint but the patient frequently is unable to give a precise history of the mechanism. It is important, however, for the examiner to try to ascertain whether the initial displacement of the finger was dorsal or volar because the treatment implications of these two types of dislocations are radically different.

Although collateral ligament rupture is sometimes a concomitant feature of dorsal dislocation,[673] experi-

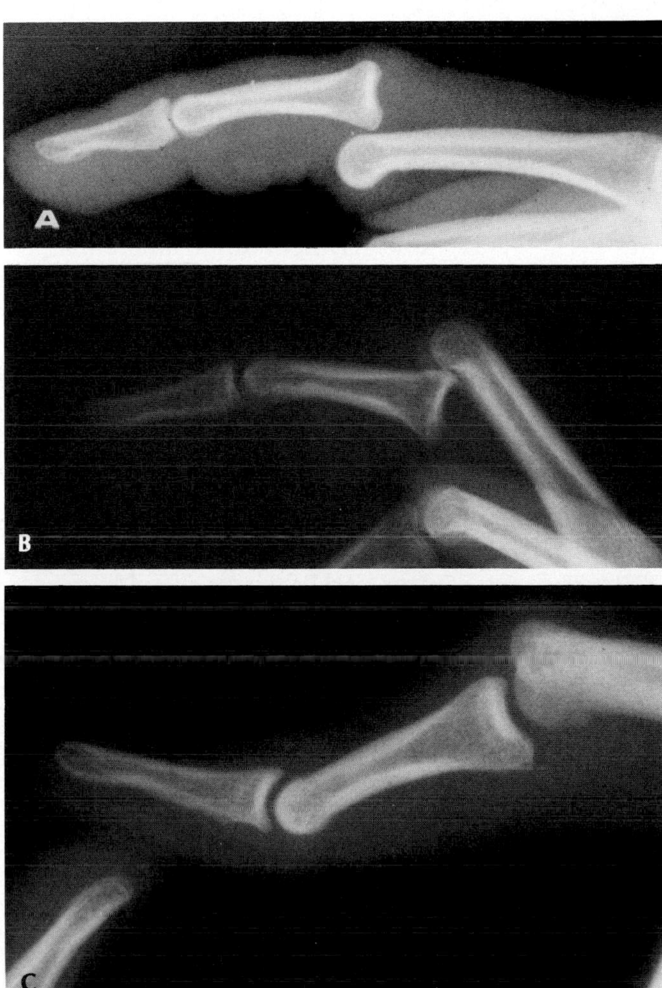

FIGURE 11-80. Dislocations of the proximal interphalangeal joints are of three types. Although the common dorsal dislocation (**A**) and the rare volar dislocation (**B**) are easy to reduce, the volar dislocation carries with it a greater likelihood for permanent impairment because of rupture of the central slip. (**C**) The most uncommon type of dislocation is rotatory subluxation. Note that the middle and distal phalanges are seen in true lateral profile and the proximal phalanx has an oblique orientation.

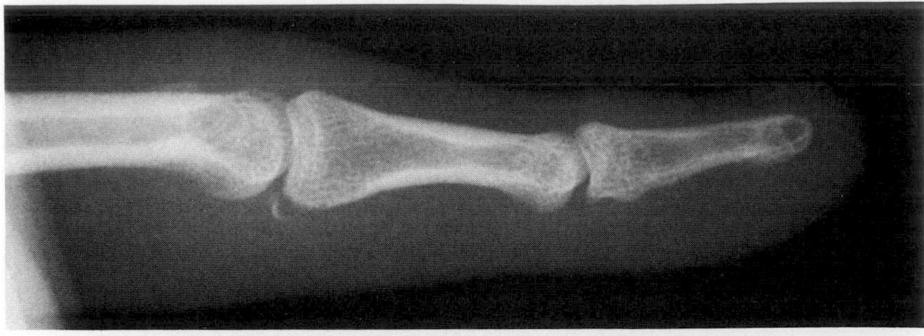

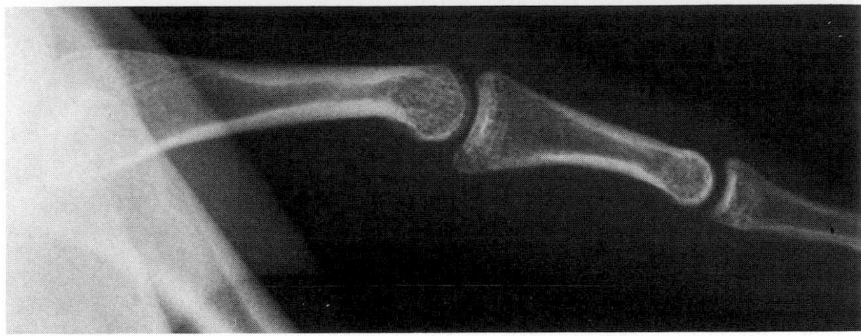

FIGURE 11-81. Two types of volar plate avulsion fractures: (*top*) a tiny chip with slight displacement and (*bottom*) a slightly larger fracture with no displacement. These are stable injuries and must be differentiated from the more serious unstable fracture-dislocation shown in Figure 11-82.

mental studies by Benke and Stableforth[590] demonstrated that this is not necessarily so in all cases. What must always occur with dorsal dislocation, however, is rupture of the volar plate. According to Bowers,[592] the plate is virtually always disrupted from its distal attachment into the base of the middle phalanx. This may occur with or without a small avulsion chip fracture[677] (Fig. 11-81), and it is important to differentiate this from the far more serious fracture-dislocation of the PIP joint, in which the volar lip fracture involves 20% to 70% of the articular surface and the joint is unstable after reduction (Fig. 11-82). The tiny avulsion fracture seen in simple volar plate injuries is rarely displaced and generally heals with only slight spurring of the volar beak of the middle phalanx. Moreover, the presence of the tiny chip provides the physician with clear radiographic evidence of the position of the avulsed volar plate.

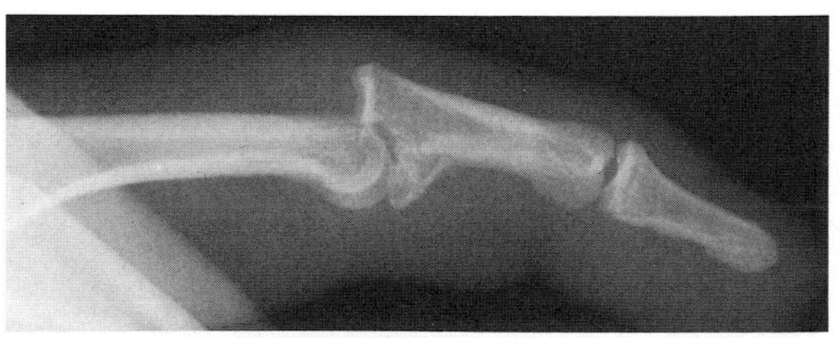

FIGURE 11-82. When the volar lip fracture of the middle phalanx involves 20% or more of the articular surface, the remainder of the middle phalanx subluxates dorsally. This unstable injury requires more sophisticated treatment than the small volar plate avulsion fractures shown in Figure 11-81. We generally prefer closed reduction and the dorsal extension block splint method of treatment for this PIP fracture-dislocation.

Rupture of the volar plate can occur with hyperextension injury of the PIP joint without actual dislocation. Zook and associates[736] pointed out that a transverse skin laceration over the volar aspect of the joint should alert the examiner that the volar plate has probably been torn. Even in the absence of such a laceration, a history of hyperextension injury of the PIP joint necessitates testing the stability of the volar plate by stressing the joint, under digital-block anesthesia if necessary.

Stern and Lee[713] studied *open* dislocations of the PIP joint and concluded that the severity of these injuries is generally underestimated. They emphasized the importance of volar plate repair in the operating room and advocated the use of parenteral antibiotics. Kjeldal[646] emphasized that debridement should precede reduction of the dislocation.

Complex (irreducible) dorsal dislocations of the PIP joint are relatively uncommon but have been reported. The structures blocking reduction have been noted to be the volar plate and the flexor tendons and in one case, the head of the proximal phalanx was entrapped between the superficialis and profundus tendons.[158,617,622,646,680]

Patel and associates[685] reported an unusual series of PIP injuries that they called bayonet dislocations because the x-rays showed displacement in both the AP and lateral projections. They postulated that *both* collateral ligaments were ruptured in these cases but seven of their eight cases were treated with closed reduction (the other case was seen late and treated operatively); therefore, no direct visual confirmation of this assumption was provided.

Diagnosis. If the patient is seen with an unreduced dislocation, x-rays should be taken before reduction. More commonly, however, he or she is seen after closed reduction has been done elsewhere, and the clinical appearance is a swollen, painful joint. The joint must be examined carefully.

Methods of Treatment

Acute Injuries. In the past, most authors advocated immobilization of the PIP joint after dorsal dislocation. Kuczynski's[11] extensive anatomic studies of the PIP joint led him to conclude that if immobilization of that joint cannot be avoided, it should be for as short a period as possible and in no more than 15° of flexion. Sprague[709] suggested 15° to 20° as the appropriate position and 3 weeks as the optimal duration of immobilization. Moller[674] recommended 2 weeks of immobilization for volar plate injuries with proximal tears and 3 to 4 weeks for those with distal avulsions, noting longer morbidity (soreness lasting up to several years) in the latter group. Zook's group[736] suggested that better results can be achieved with primary surgical repair of the plate.

The trend appears to be for less immobilization. Incavo and coworkers[634] showed no hyperextension laxity in their series of patients with volar plate avulsion injuries treated with immobilization of the PIP joint in full extension for 7 to 10 days, followed by buddy taping. Phair and coworkers[687] showed that patients with volar plate avulsion fractures 2 × 2 mm or smaller had less stiffness if treated by buddy taping. Soelberg and coworkers[707] advocated immediate active motion with an elastic double-finger bandage (a variant of buddy taping). If there is concern about hyperextension instability (which does not seem to be a common problem in the literature), protected motion can be achieved with a thermoplastic figure-of-eight splint that allows full flexion but provides a dorsal extension block.[655,712]

Authors' Preferred Method of Treatment

We prefer to treat all acute volar plate injuries or dorsal dislocations with 3 to 6 weeks of buddy taping. This allows early active motion and prevents hyperextension, which is to be avoided in these patients.

Most patients regain essentially full range of motion but as noted in the section on collateral ligament injuries, symptoms usually persist for 12 to 18 months, and some permanent swelling of the joint is to be expected, regardless of the method of treatment.[660]

The presence of a tiny avulsion chip fracture does not alter the plan of management but again, we emphasize that this must be differentiated radiographically from the far more serious fracture-dislocation of the PIP joint.

For open dislocations, we rarely repair the volar plate at the time of joint debridement. Postoperatively, we prefer to begin active motion about 3 to 4 days postoperatively. Generally, buddy taping is sufficient to prevent hyperextension of the joint but if added protection is desired, a dorsal extension block splint can be used for 3 weeks.

Chronic Injuries. Considering the frequency of dorsal dislocations and hyperextension injuries of the PIP joints, relatively few of these patients have chronic symptoms sufficiently troublesome to warrant operative treatment. Recurrent dorsal dislocations of the PIP joint are rare; symptomatic hyperextensibility of the joint secondary to laxity of the volar plate is only a bit more common. In some of these patients, a compensatory flexion deformity of the DIP joint may develop, resulting in a typical swan-neck appearance of the finger (Fig. 11-83). Bowers[592] reported satisfactory results in a small series of patients in whom he did late reattachment of the volar plate (4 months to 4 years after injury). Many other procedures have been described to correct this problem, all of which have as a common denominator shortening of the attenuated volar plate or creation of some type of check-rein tenodesis to prevent hyperextension of the joint.†† Other types of reconstructive procedures have been described for patients having combined chronic laxity of the collateral ligament and volar plate.[653,682]

A more common problem than symptomatic hyperextensibility or recurrent PIP dislocation is a flexion contracture of the PIP joint. This is generally believed to be due to scarring of the volar plate, with or without an associated chip fracture off the base of the middle phalanx, and has been called a pseudoboutonniere deformity by McCue and associates.[665] The problem can usually be corrected with dynamic splinting and exercise, although occasionally operative treatment may be necessary.[725]

Patients with stiff PIP joints (ie, with limited motion in both flexion and extension) should be treated initially with appropriate dynamic splinting. If supervised hand therapy fails to satisfactorily correct the limited motion, Eaton's[605,610] operation of excising the PIP collateral ligaments (usually both, occasionally one), can provide significantly improved motion. Although logic

†† References 581, 587, 603, 647, 690, 716, 728, 729.

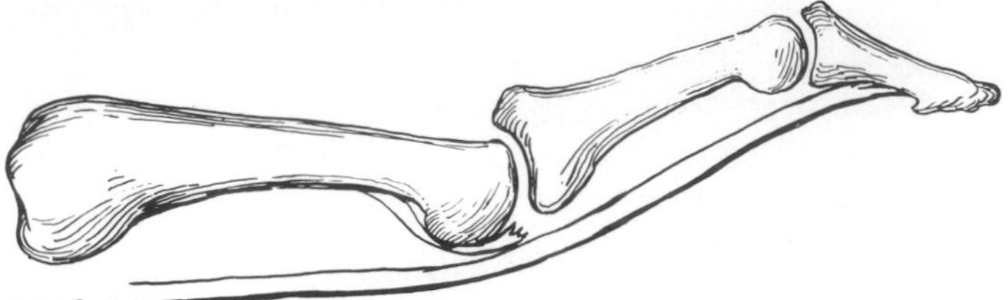

FIGURE 11-83. Volar plate injuries of the proximal interphalangeal joint may result in hyperextension deformity of the joint. Some patients may also have a compensatory flexion deformity of the distal interphalangeal joint, resulting in a swan-neck deformity.

suggests that this would make the joint unstable, Eaton's[605] clinical results and Minamikawa and coworkers'[672] biomechanical studies have shown that joints from which the collateral ligaments are excised usually remain stable. Moreover, under the stimulus of active motion, the postsurgical scar may remodel into a new collateral ligament capable of providing essentially normal stability.[605,610]

Volar PIP Dislocations

Acute Injuries. Volar dislocations of the PIP joint are relatively rare injuries. They may be pure dislocations (see Fig. 11-80*B*) or fracture-dislocations (fracture-sublaxations) (Fig. 11-84) but the implication of both types is the same: for this type of dislocation to occur, the central slip must be disrupted and the potential for boutonniere deformity is present. If the dislocation is reduced before the examiner sees the patient and no fracture is present to indicate that it was a volar dislocation, the pitfall is that it will be treated as though it were the more common dorsal dislocation. If the finger is treated with splinting in mild to moderate flexion or with buddy taping (both appropriate for a dorsal dislocation), a boutonniere deformity will develop.

Little is to be found in the literature regarding this uncommon injury. Spinner and Choi[708] reported the largest series (five cases), and their conclusion that open reduction and repair of the central slip is mandatory has been widely quoted. None of their cases had an adequate trial of primary nonoperative treatment, however. If the standard treatment for closed boutonniere lesions is nonoperative, it is not clear why operative repair of the central slip should be considered to be essential in the boutonniere lesion caused by a volar dislocation of the PIP joint. Indeed, Thompson and Eaton[718] advocated splinting of the joint in full extension for 3 weeks, followed by dynamic splinting. They advocated primary operative treatment only if the dislocations were irreducible, when the joint surfaces were incongruent after reduction, or when the active extensor lag was in excess of 30°.

Atypical volar dislocations can occur, such as the case reported by Crick and coworkers,[601] in which the fractured head of proximal phalanx was displaced through a rent in the central slip, thereby rendering it irreducible.

Authors' Preferred Method of Treatment

Unless the dislocation is irreducible by closed means, we prefer to treat this injury closed. After closed reduction of the dislocation, a true lateral x-ray of the finger

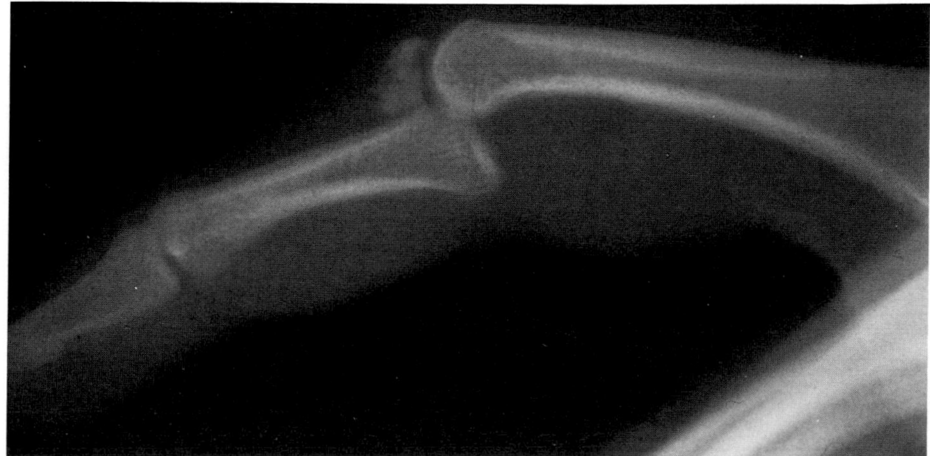

FIGURE 11-84. An unstable volar fracture-subluxation of the proximal interphalangeal joint.

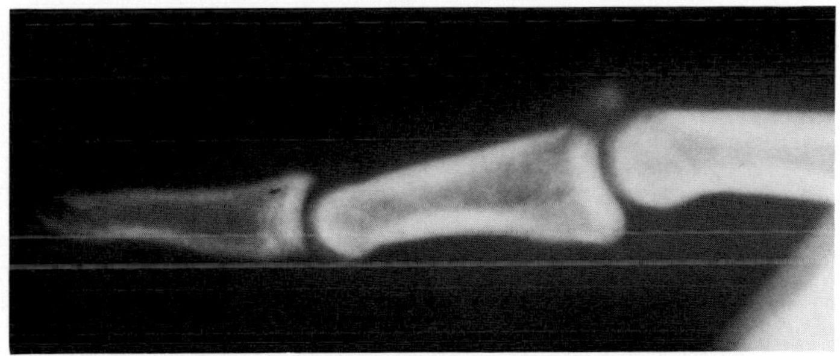

FIGURE 11-85. A stable dorsal fracture caused by avulsion by the central slip (analogous to a boutonniere lesion).

should be taken to ensure that there is normal congruity of the joint surfaces. The presence of an avulsion fracture at the dorsal base of the middle phalanx (Fig. 11-85) is not an indication for open reduction unless it is displaced and does not reduce adequately with the PIP joint in full extension. If these criteria are met, the treatment is the same as for a closed boutonniere lesion, that is immobilization of only the PIP joint in full extension with a dorsal splint or an obliquely placed 0.045-inch K-wire, combined with early active and passive flexion exercises of the DIP joint. Continuous splinting is maintained for 4 to 6 weeks, depending on the age of the patient (less time in older patients), followed by dynamic extension splinting during the day and static splinting at night (PIP joint in full extension) combined with active range of motion exercises.

If the dislocation cannot be reduced by closed manipulation or the joint surfaces are not congruent after an attempt at reduction, primary open reduction is indicated.

Chronic Injuries. Several authors[616,686,691] have discussed the problem of late recognition of volar PIP dislocations and the inevitably poor results in such cases. The key to recognition is a true lateral x-ray of the involved finger, both before and after reduction. Irreducible volar PIP dislocations have been reported but we believe that the literature on this subject has been unnecessarily confusing because of the failure to differentiate volar dislocation from rotatory subluxation. In our opinion, these are two distinctly different injuries based primarily on the status of the central slip. In volar dislocations, the central slip is ruptured but in rotatory subluxation, it is intact.

Inadequately treated or neglected old volar dislocations present either as a typical boutonniere deformity or as a flexion contracture of the PIP joint, with limited painful motion. A large series of such patients and the descriptions of operative techniques required to manage the unusual combination of injuries to the ruptured collateral ligament, volar plate, and extensor mechanism was reported by Peimer and associates.[686]

Rotatory PIP Subluxation

Rotatory subluxation of the PIP joint is uncommon but in our opinion, it is clearly a different injury from volar dislocation, even though previous reports in the literature have not always made this distinction.[637,640,644,675,678,692,704] The mechanism in most cases is a twisting injury,[681] and the resulting pathologic

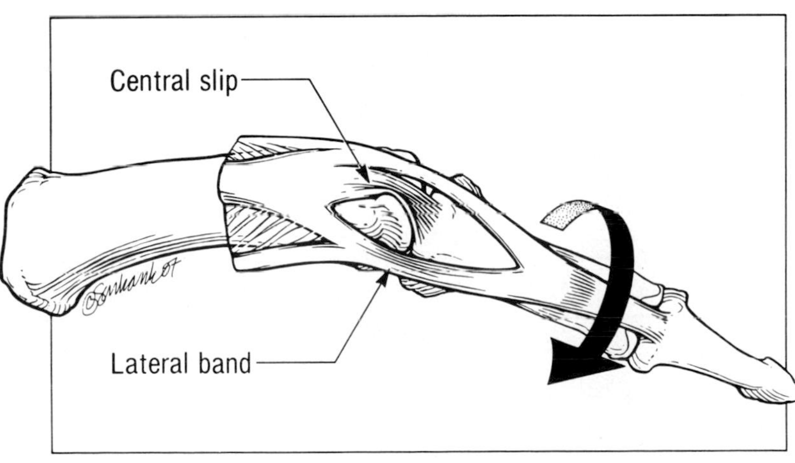

FIGURE 11-86. Rotatory subluxation of the proximal interphalangeal joint. The condyle of the head of the proximal phalanx is buttonholed between the lateral band and central slip, both of which remain intact.

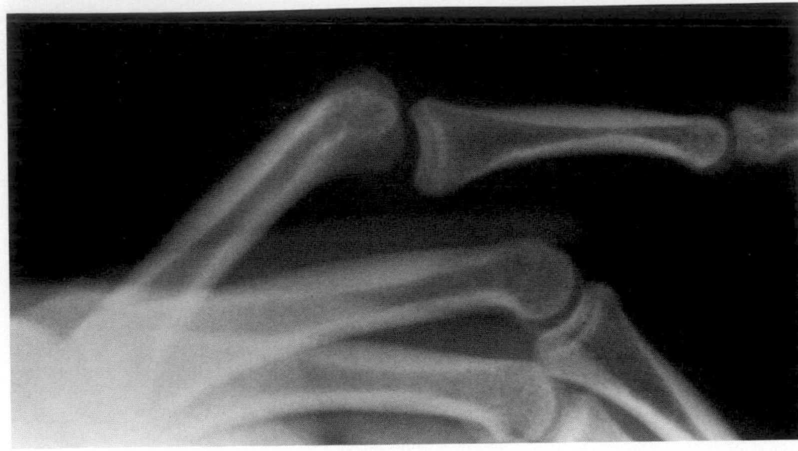

FIGURE 11-87. The radiographic key to diagnosis of rotatory subluxation of the proximal interphalangeal joint is a true lateral picture of the middle phalanx with a slightly obliqued configuration of the proximal phalanx or vice versa.

anatomy is buttonholing of one condyle of the head of the proximal phalanx through a longitudinal rent in the extensor hood between the central slip and lateral band, both of which remain intact (Fig. 11-86). The key radiographic feature of rotatory subluxation is seen in the lateral view, where there is a true lateral profile of the proximal phalanx and an oblique appearance of the middle phalanx (Fig. 11-87) or vice versa.

Treatment. In previous editions of this book, it was stated that this is always an irreducible dislocation but we have subsequently treated several patients successfully with the closed reduction maneuver described by Eaton and his colleagues.[609,718] Under digital-block anesthesia, gentle traction is applied to the finger with both the MP and PIP joints flexed to 90° (Fig. 11-88). This maneuver relaxes the volarly displaced lateral band and allows the band to be disengaged and to slip dorsally when a gentle rotational and traction force is applied. Further relaxation of the extensor mechanism can be achieved by extension of the wrist. A small pop may be felt as the lateral band reduces to its dorsal position. Successful reduction is followed by full active and passive motion of the PIP joint and must be confirmed by postreduction x-rays, especially a true lateral view of the involved digit. If the joint has been successfully reduced, no immobilization is required and early active motion can be started immediately, using buddy taping. Close follow-up is recommended to be certain that the patient does not develop a boutonniere deformity. Although the central slip is intact, it may be attenuated, and we have seen one patient who developed a mild boutonniere lesion after closed reduction of a rotatory subluxation.

Technique of Open Reduction of Rotatory PIP Sub-

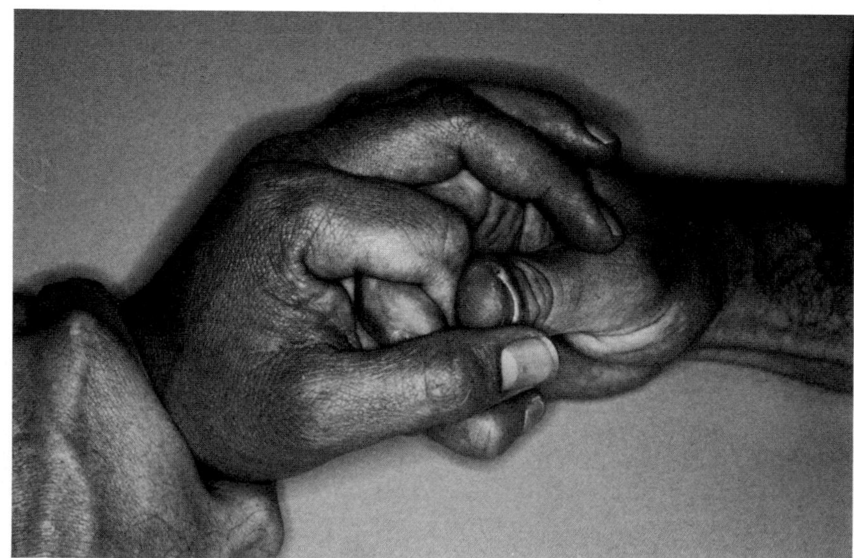

FIGURE 11-88. Eaton's[609,718] reduction maneuver for closed reduction of rotatory subluxation of the proximal interphalangeal (PIP) joint. The metacarpophalangeal and PIP joints are flexed to relax the lateral bands, and a gentle twisting motion is applied to the middle phalanx.

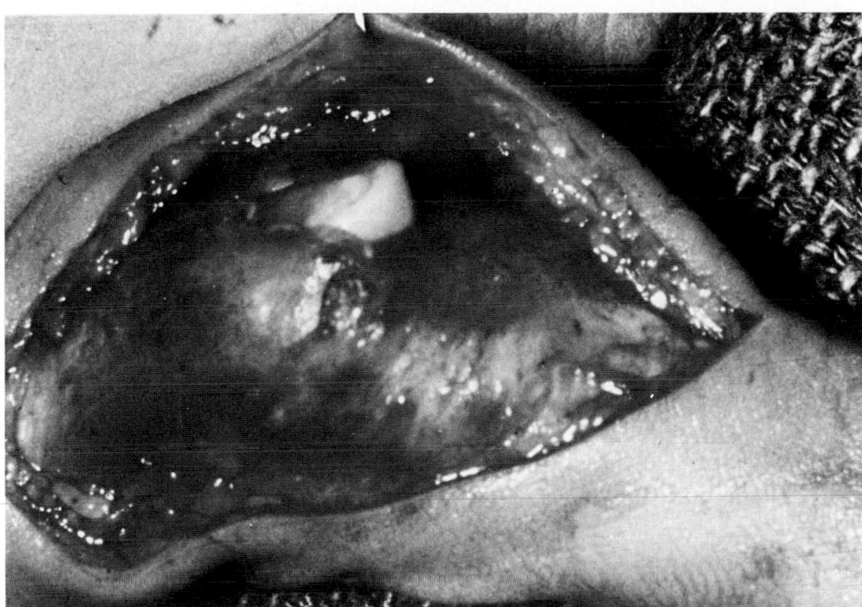

FIGURE 11-89. Rotatory subluxation of the proximal interphalangeal joint, as seen at operation. These uncommon injuries may be irreducible by closed methods because of buttonholing of the condyle of the proximal phalanx between the central slip and lateral band. The joint is usually stable after open reduction.

luxation. Failure of closed reduction is an indication for open reduction. The joint is exposed through a dorsal curved incision, which allows adequate visualization of the entire aponeurosis. A longitudinal rent is found between the intact central slip and one lateral band, with a condyle of the proximal phalanx protruding between these two structures (Fig. 11-89). It is relatively easy to reduce the condyle under direct vision by retracting the lateral band and lifting it from its volarly displaced position around to the side of the condyle. The collateral ligament should be inspected; if torn, it is repaired. Immediately after reduction, the joint should glide freely through a full range of passive motion. Because the central slip is intact, minimal postoperative immobilization is required, and we generally prefer to begin active range of motion at about 3 to 4 days postoperatively. If the collateral ligament is repaired, buddy taping for 3 to 4 additional weeks provides adequate protection.

Dorsal PIP Fracture-Dislocation

The most potentially disabling injury of the PIP joint is a dorsal fracture-dislocation. Usually, as the result of a jamming-type injury, the volar articular surface of the base of the middle phalanx is fractured (usually comminuted and involving up to 75% of the joint surface), and the remaining intact portion of the middle phalanx is subluxated dorsally above the head of the proximal phalanx. The middle phalanx remains partially in contact with the head of the proximal phalanx, and thus this injury is more properly called a fracture-subluxation, even though the term fracture-dislocation is more commonly used.

Diagnosis. The clinical picture is often not sufficiently dramatic to convey to an inexperienced physician the serious nature of the injury. The PIP joint is usually quite swollen, however, and both active and passive motion are severely limited and painful. *A true lateral x-ray is mandatory to confirm the diagnosis* (Fig. 11-90). Review of the x-ray reveals dorsal subluxation of the middle phalanx on the proximal phalanx, associated with the fracture of the volar lip of the middle phalanx. The fractured fragment involves at least one third of the volar articular surface of the middle phalanx and occasionally up to 75%.

In the lateral x-ray, the critical finding is the relative amount of the volar lip fragment that has been frac-

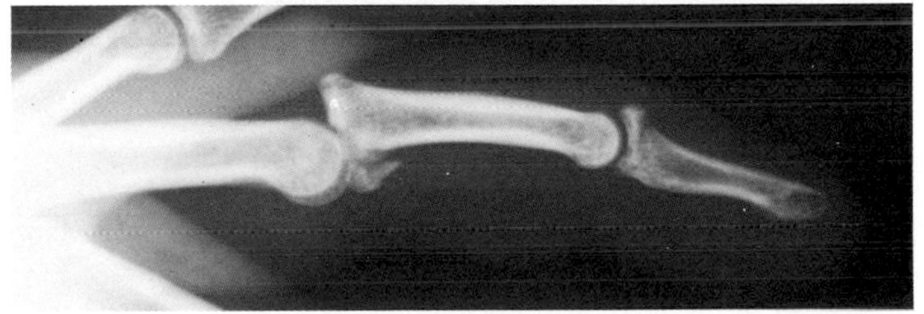

FIGURE 11-90. A classic fracture-dislocation of the proximal interphalangeal joint. There is a volar lip fracture, which is frequently comminuted, as in this patient, and the middle phalanx subluxates dorsally on the proximal phalanx. The injury is frequently missed initially because of the lack of gross clinical deformity and the failure to take an isolated true lateral x-ray of the involved digit.

tured or conversely stated, that percentage of the articular surface of base of middle phalanx that remains intact. The traditional method of determining this has been to calculate the size of the volar lip fragment or fragments as a percentage of the entire base of middle phalanx (Fig. 11-91*A*). Hamer and Quinton[624] noted, however, that this may give a spuriously high result because of the splaying of the base of middle phalanx. They recommended a second method, which is based on the constant relation between the diameter of the head of proximal phalanx and base of middle phalanx in the normal uninjured finger. They calculated this ratio to be 1 : 0.82, meaning that the head of proximal phalanx is normally 82% the diameter of base of middle phalanx. They thus concluded that a more accurate calculation of the relative size of the fracture fragment or fragments could be calculated from the formula shown in Figure 11-91*B*.

Regardless of the method of measuring the fracture size, it is important to recognize that x-rays fail to reveal the amount of cartilaginous damage. Therefore, the size of the fracture cannot be used as the sole criterion for predicting the future function of the joint.

Methods of Treatment

Acute Injuries. Treatment of the acute injury is controversial, and both closed and operative methods have been described. Shulze[703] advocated simple manipulative treatment by placing the joint into extreme flexion while applying traction on the finger. He held the finger in this position with adhesive tape strapping or a malleable aluminum splint, with gradual extension of the finger beginning at 7 to 10 days; all splinting was discontinued at 3 weeks. Unfortunately, he did not report any cases to demonstrate the effectiveness of his technique. Spray[710] reported two patients treated with taping of the finger in acute flexion with a slightly different technique for 2 and 5 weeks, respectively. Trojan[719] advocated closed reduction and percutaneous pin fixation of the joint with a K-wire for 4 to 6 weeks.

Robertson and coworkers[697] reported seven cases treated with a complicated tridirectional traction device designed to apply longitudinal and volar forces on the middle phalanx and a dorsal force on the proximal phalanx. Agee[582,583] subsequently described an ingenious force-couple device constructed with K-wires. Schenck[701] devised a technique that combines skeletal traction and passive motion, which he has used not only for fracture-dislocations but also for severely comminuted fractures of the base of the middle phalanx. There has been a flood of new devices and techniques for treating these more severely comminuted intra-articular fractures that are referred to as "pilon" fractures.

McElfresh and associates[666] first described the extension block splinting method, which is discussed in greater detail subsequently. Strong[715] devised a simpler technique that employs the dorsal extension block principle (Fig. 11-92), and a modification of this method was used by Lange and Engber[654] in three patients who had fracture-dislocations of the PIP joint combined with mallet finger injuries in the same digit.

At least two different authors[721,723] have described the use of a K-wire as an internal dorsal extension block splint, but the clinical results reported with this technique are a bit sparse.

Wilson and Rowland[730] reported the largest series of patients treated with ORIF. Only one of their patients obtained a full range of motion but only 4 of their 15 patients had acute injuries (less than 3 weeks postinjury). The major objections to primary open reduction are: 1) the volar lip fragment is almost invariably comminuted and the operation is therefore technically difficult; and 2) the 3-week period of postoperative immobilization recommended by the authors further enhances the likeli-

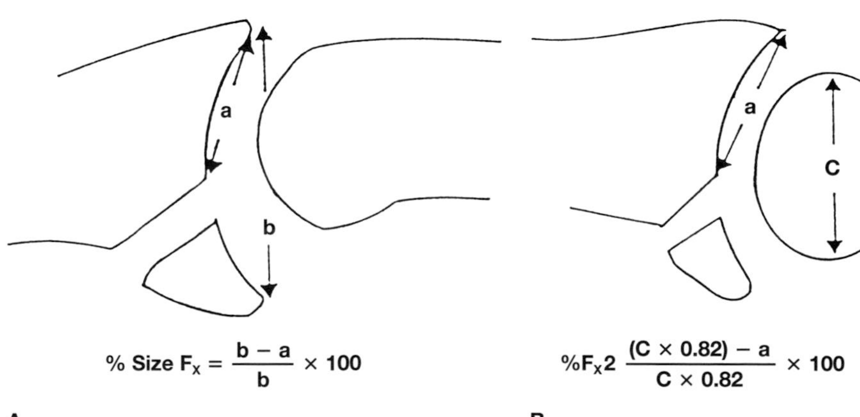

FIGURE 11-91. (**A**) The customary method of estimating the amount of involvement of the base of middle phalanx articular surface in proximal interphalangeal fracture-dislocations is to express it as a percentage of the base of middle phalanx. This may give a spuriously high percentage because of "splaying-out" of the comminuted volar fracture. Hamer and Quinton have suggested that a more accurate percentage can be obtained by using the formula shown in (**B**) which is based on measurements in normal hands that showed the diameter of the proximal phalanx to be 82% of the diameter of the base of the proximal phalanx. *(Hamer, D.W., and Quinton, D.N.: Dorsal Fracture Subluxation of the Proximal Interphalangeal Joints Treated by Extension Block Splintage. J Hand Surg. 17B:586–590, 1992.)*

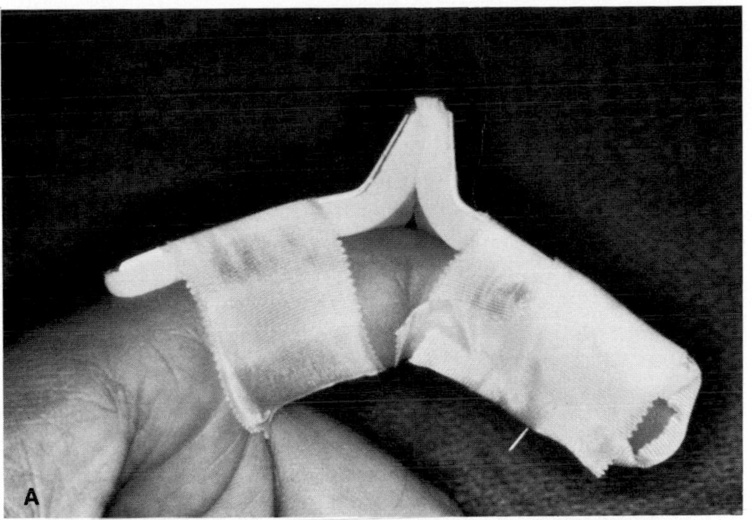

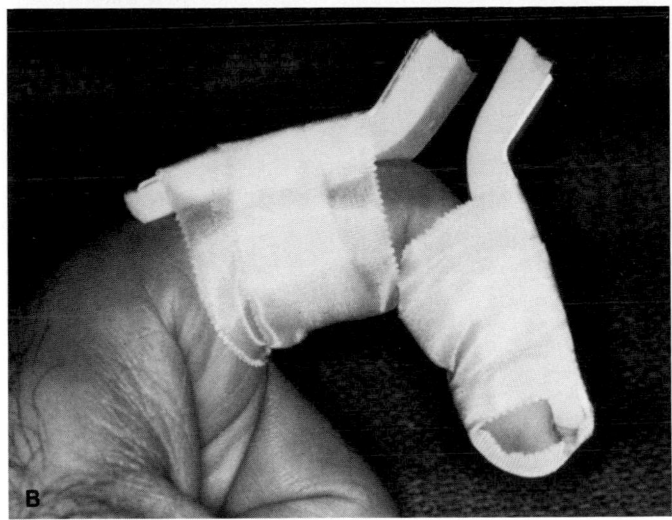

FIGURE 11-92. A simpler form of dorsal extension block splinting, made with two pieces of padded aluminum splint material bent to prevent extension at a predetermined level (**A**) and to allow flexion of the proximal interphalangeal (PIP) joint (**B**). This method should be used only in very reliable patients who understand the critical importance of not allowing the PIP joint to extend fully.

hood of stiffness in an already severely damaged joint. We therefore reserve primary open reduction for those rare cases in which the volar lip fragment is essentially a single large fragment comprising 30% or more of the articular surface.[619]

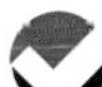 Authors' Preferred Method of Treatment

Our best results with this difficult injury have usually been obtained with the dorsal extension block splinting method described by McElfresh, Dobyns, and O'Brien.[606,666] The method requires careful attention to detail but can result in restoration of a full range of motion if properly applied.

This technique, however, should *not* be used if a satisfactory closed reduction cannot be achieved. Adequacy of reduction must be judged by congruity of the remaining intact articular surface of the middle phalanx with the head of the proximal phalanx (Fig. 11-93). The "V" sign described by Light[658] (Fig. 11-94) is indicative of an inadequately reduced joint. It is *not* necessary for the comminuted volar lip fragment to be anatomically reduced and usually it remains slightly depressed, but the subluxation of the joint must be reduced anatomically (Fig. 11-95).

If closed reduction cannot be accomplished in an acute injury, the dorsal extension block splinting method should not be used. In such cases, we prefer either ORIF, as described by Wilson and Rowland,[730] or Eaton's volar plate arthroplasty.[612] ORIF is a difficult operation, postoperative stiffness is common, and a long period of passive splinting is needed to restore maximum active range of motion. We consider ORIF only for those rare cases in which the volar lip fragment appears to be a single large fragment.

Technique of Dorsal Extension Block Splinting. Under digital or wrist block anesthesia, the PIP joint is reduced by longitudinal traction on the digit with

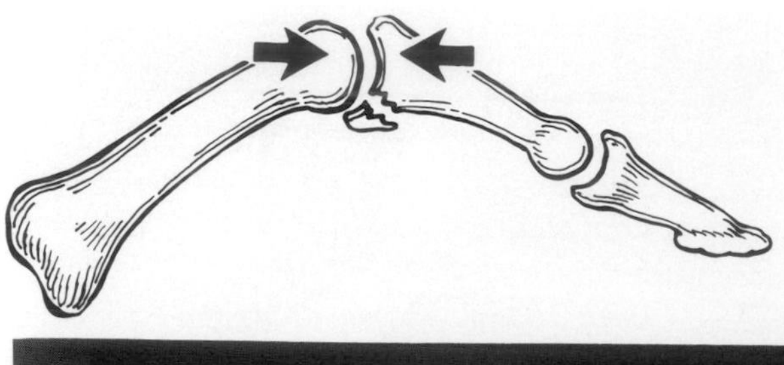

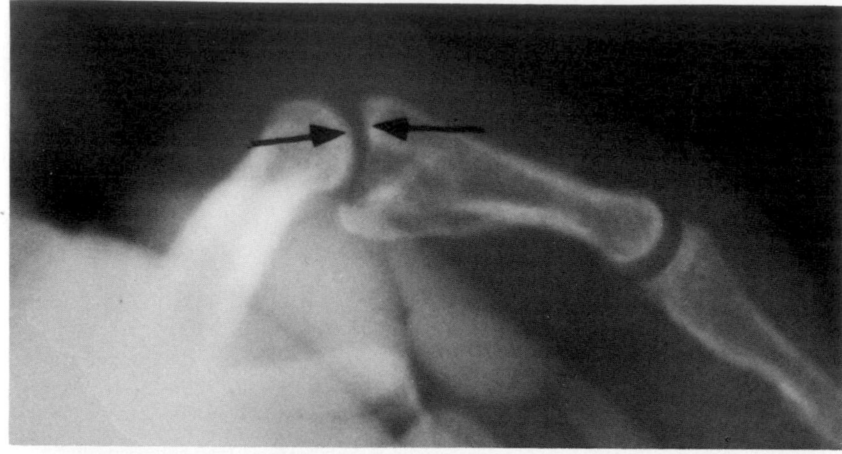

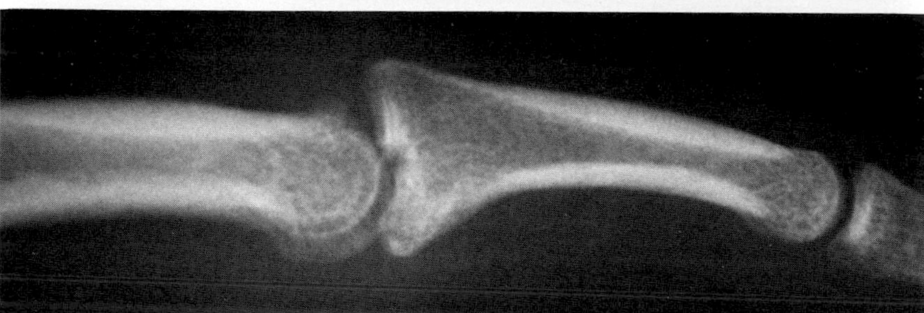

FIGURE 11-93. Adequacy of reduction in a proximal interphalangeal fracture-dislocation is judged by congruity between the remaining intact dorsal articular surface of the middle phalanx and the head of the proximal phalanx, as shown *top* and *center*. Compare this with the *bottom* figure, in which the joint is clearly *not* reduced. *(Strong, M.L.: A New Method of Entension-block Splinting for the Proximal Interphalangeal Joint—Preliminary Report. J. Hand Surg. 5:606–607, 1980.)*

simultaneous volarly directed pressure over the subluxated base of the middle phalanx. A lateral x-ray is taken to ensure that the joint can be reduced satisfactorily. Reduction is usually fairly easy to accomplish within a few days of injury but becomes increasingly difficult with time and may be impossible as early as 1 to 2 weeks after injury. If an adequate reduction cannot be documented radiographically, open reduction or volar plate arthroplasty is indicated. McElfresh and coworkers[730] reported success with this method in patients having 30% to 50% of the articular surface involved, and we have been able to use it effectively in some patients having up to 60% involvement.

If the initial test x-ray reveals satisfactory reduction (see Fig. 11-95), a short arm cast is applied, incorporating a 1-inch wide padded aluminum splint over the dorsum of the involved finger, extending about one-half inch beyond the tip of the digit (Fig. 11-96). The PIP joint is then reduced and the splint bent to conform to the amount of flexion required to maintain the reduction; usually this is about 60° but occasionally a bit more is necessary. A strip of adhesive tape is applied over the full extent of the aluminum splint and secured to the volar aspect of the cast to prevent inadvertent straightening of the splint (see Fig. 11-96*D*). An essential part of the technique is that the proximal segment of the finger must be held firmly to the splint with a strip of half-inch adhesive (see Fig. 7-96*A* through *C*); if this is not done, MP joint flexion causes the proximal phalanx to pull away from the splint, allowing extension of the PIP joint and loss of reduction. Immediately after application of the splint, another true lateral x-ray is taken to ensure that reduction has been maintained.

Active flexion of the involved finger is allowed and encouraged from the outset, with extension blocked by the splint. The patient is seen at weekly intervals and if a lateral x-ray shows continued maintenance of reduction, the adhesive tape holding the splint to the cast is cut, the splint is extended to reduce the amount of flexion in the PIP joint, and the tape is reapplied (Fig. 11-97). Usually, the flexion can be reduced about

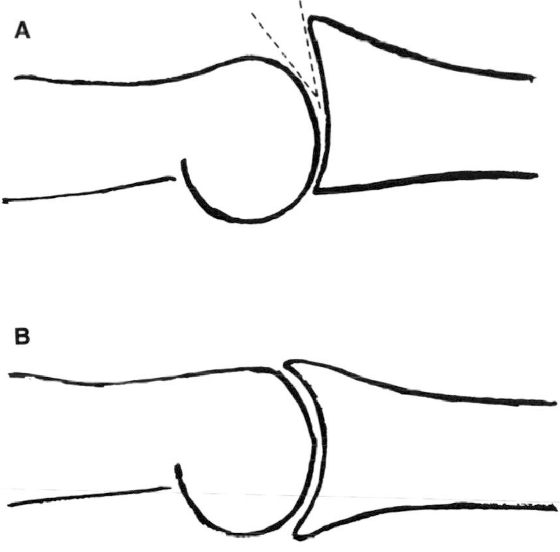

FIGURE 11-94. The "V" sign of incomplete reduction of a proximal interphalangeal fracture-dislocation. In a satisfactory reduction (**B**), there is parallel congruity between the dorsal base of the middle phalanx and head of the proximal phalanx. In an unsatisfactory reduction (**A**), these two surfaces are neither parallel nor congruent, and the two articular surfaces form a "V." (*Light, T.R.: Buttress Pinning Techniques. Orthop. Rev. 10:49, 1981.*)

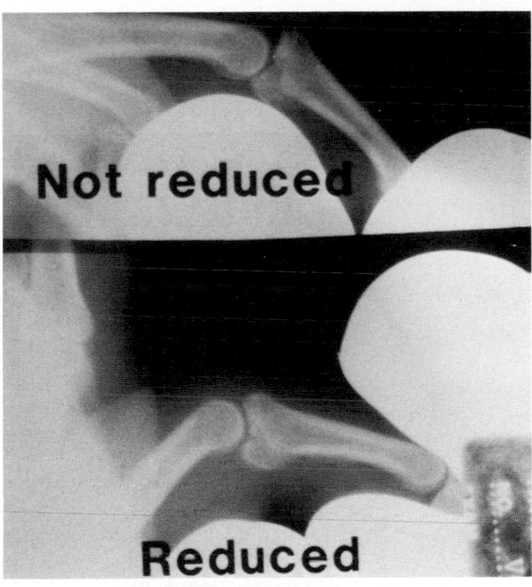

FIGURE 11-95. These two x-rays clearly show the difference between an unsatisfactory reduction of a proximal interphalangeal fracture-dislocation (**A**) and an acceptable reduction (**B**).

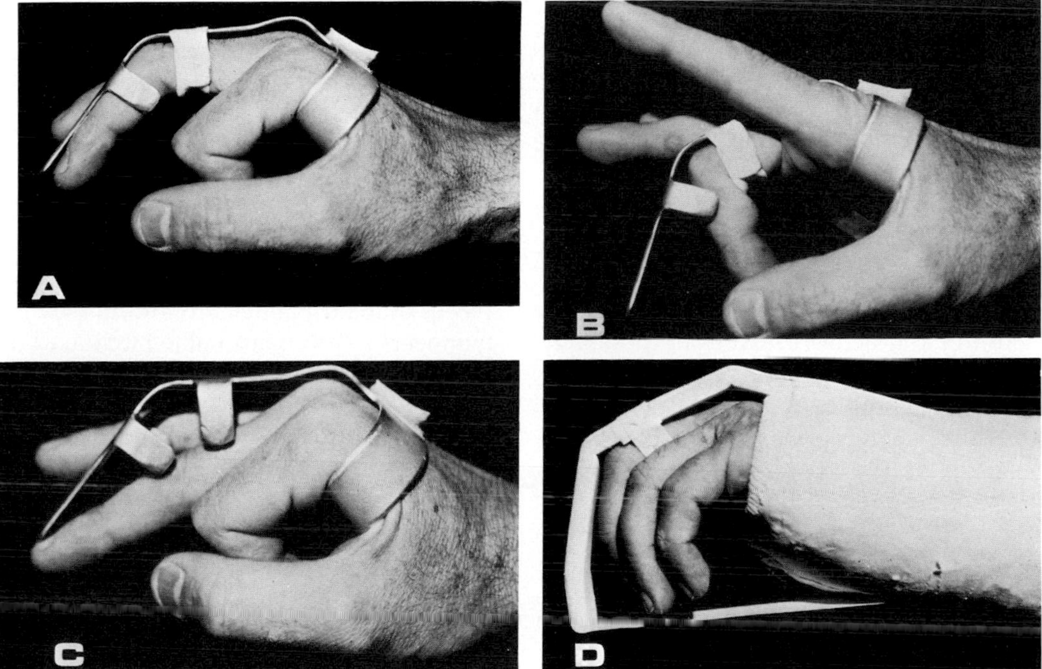

FIGURE 11-96. The dorsal extension block splint is useful in treating some unstable injuries of the proximal interphalangeal (PIP) joint. Extension of the PIP joint can be limited to a predetermined angle (**A**), while at the same time active flexion can be carried out by the patient (**B**). It is particularly important to secure the proximal phalanx to the splint because if this is not done, flexion of the metacarpophalangeal joint allows extension of the PIP joint, thereby negating the function of the splint (**C**). A custom-made orthosis is not necessary. The simplest way to construct the dorsal extension block splint is with a plaster (or fiberglass) gauntlet and a malleable outrigger that is firmly attached to the volar aspect of the cast to prevent bending in extension (**D**). The tip of the outrigger should extend about 1/2" beyond the tip of the finger to allow unrestricted active flexion.

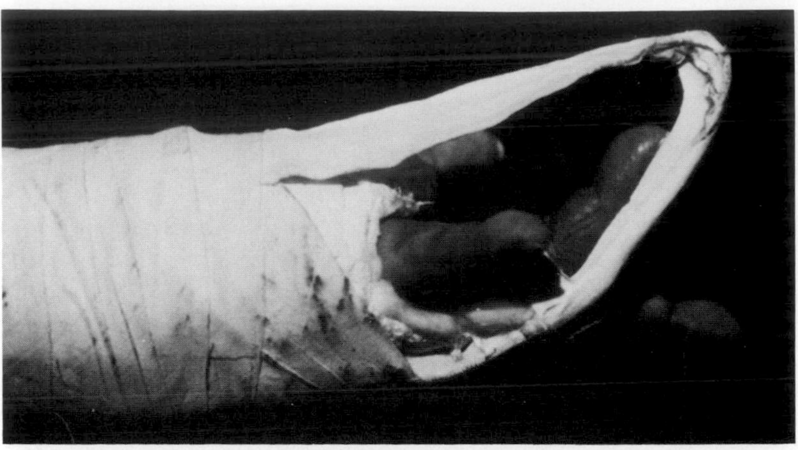

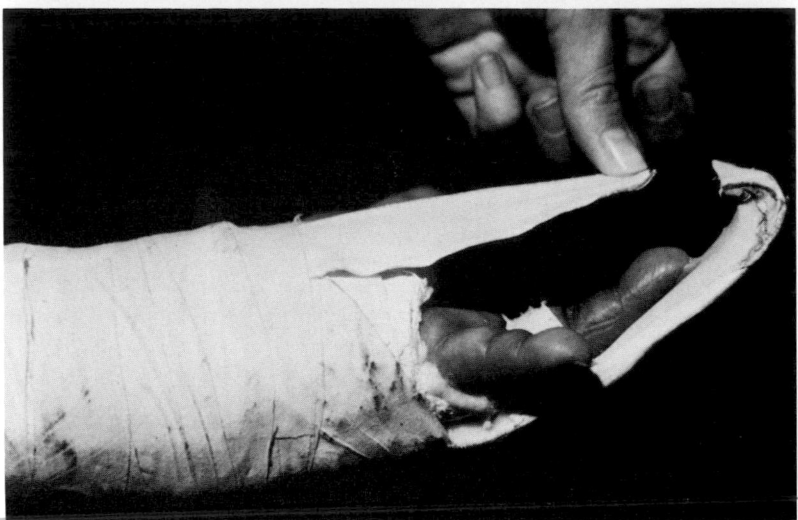

FIGURE 11-97. (*Top*) The outrigger in a dorsal extension block splint must be stabilized with tape to prevent its being inadvertently straightened. (*Bottom*) When the patient is seen at weekly intervals, the tape is cut to allow straightening of the splint and new tape is applied.

15° each week (Fig. 11-98). At 4 weeks, the splint is removed and buddy taping is worn for an additional 2 to 3 weeks. Most patients regain full active flexion from the beginning and achieve extension gradually over the 4-week period as the splint is extended. If the patient has not regained full extension of the PIP joint by 6 weeks, dynamic splinting may be used.

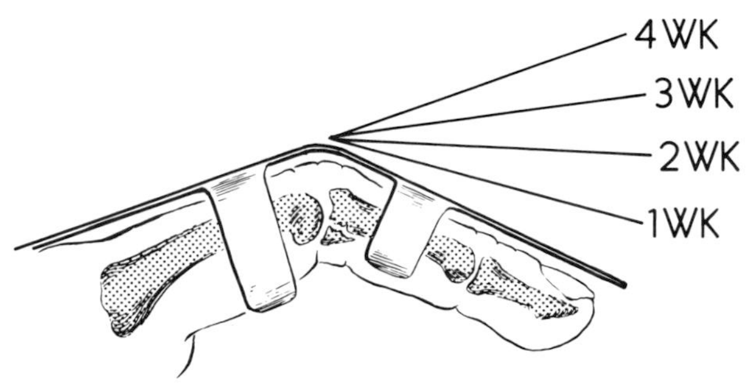

FIGURE 11-98. The amount of flexion in the dorsal extension block splint is gradually decreased over several weeks to minimize stiffness in the proximal interphalangeal joint.

We have limited experience with Strong's[715] simpler type of extension block splint fashioned from two pieces of foam-padded aluminum (see Fig. 11-92) but it appears to be a reasonable method to use in reliable, compliant patients.

Chronic Injuries. Despite the emphasis on the severity of this injury and repeated pleas for early recognition, fracture-dislocations of the PIP joint continue to be missed, and these patients present with stiff, painful PIP joints several weeks or even months after the initial injury. As noted, closed reduction is unlikely to be possible beyond 1 to 2 weeks, and other methods of treatment must be instituted.

Late open reduction using the technique described by Wilson and Rowland[730] may be used in some of these patients. They noted that stripping of the dorsal capsule and division of the collateral ligament and central slip are usually necessary in late cases. They also mentioned that an osteotomy of the united fragment is frequently necessary to improve alignment of the articular surface in old cases and they used a cortical bone graft from the adjacent proximal phalanx to support the reduced articular fragment. Zemel and associates[734] reported on the use of osteotomy and bone grafting for chronic PIP fracture dislocations, reporting good results for as long as 10 years postoperatively. McCue and coworkers[665] also used open reduction and osteotomy in late cases, although they did not find the addition of bone graft to be necessary.

Donaldson and Millender[607] were able to perform late open reduction without osteotomy by detaching the collateral ligament and performing a dorsal capsulotomy and "minimal freeing" of the extensor mechanism, which allowed reduction of the middle phalanx under direct vision. They pointed out the necessity of restoring the proximal volar pouch, which was consistently obliterated with scarring and adhesions.

Eaton[609] devised the volar plate arthroplasty for chronic irreducible fracture-dislocations of the PIP joint, which he has used up to 2 years after injury. Good long-term results have been reported from this salvage procedure.[612,664] Other authors have modified Eaton's technique slightly, primarily by using two separate sutures, one for either side of the volar plate instead of a single suture.[591,608]

Patel and Joshi[684] offered an alternative to volar plate arthroplasty. Using Schenck's[701] principle of simultaneous distraction and mobilization, they designed a mini phalangeal distractor, which first restores length and joint congruity and then allows active and passive motion. They reported results comparable to those in Eaton's series in their 11 patients treated with this method (see Dynamic Traction).

Authors' Preferred Method of Treatment

For chronic PIP fracture-dislocations, we prefer Eaton's volar plate arthroplasty.

The operation is technically difficult but good results can be achieved if the detailed operative technique described by Eaton and Malerich[612,664] is followed precisely.

Technique of Volar Plate Arthroplasty. The finger is exposed through a volar zigzag (Bruner) incision from the DIP crease to the MP crease, elevating a radial-based flap. The flexor sheath is excised from the A2 to the A4 pulley, and the flexor tendons are retracted to the side, taking care to protect the vincula. An essential feature of this operation is to "turn the joint inside out," so that the articular surface of the base of middle phalanx can be seen completely. This necessitates detaching the volar plate (which remains attached to the volar lip fragment) by incising along its lateral margins with the accessory collateral ligaments. Bone fragments are excised from the volar base of middle phalanx. The volar plate is detached as far distally as possible, leaving some volar periosteum if necessary, to create a proximally based pedicle of maximum length. To adequately see the joint in a chronic injury, it is necessary to *completely excise* both collateral ligaments, allowing the joint to be opened by hyperextension, as Eaton says, "like a shotgun." In acute injuries, the collateral ligaments do not need to be released because the joint exposure required is less and the ligaments have not shortened.

A transverse groove or trough is then created completely across the volar portion of the articular surface of the middle phalanx, and this must be done under direct vision. The trough can be made with an osteotome or small rongeur but it is important that it be at a right angle to the long axis of the finger to minimize subsequent angular deformity.

After the PIP joint has been reduced, passive range of motion must be tested. If the fingertip does not easily touch the distal palmar crease, incision of the dorsal capsule is necessary. This is done through a separate short incision on the dorsum of the joint, taking care to avoid detachment of the central slip.

The volar plate is then advanced distally into the trough, where it is securely approximated to bone with a pull-out suture passed through the extreme ends of the trough (Fig. 11-99). We prefer 2-0 or 3-0 Prolene. If the volar plate cannot be adequately advanced, the check-rein ligaments are transected or lengthened to allow further advancement, taking care to preserve the tiny vascular pedicle arising from the midline.

The volar plate is drawn into the articular defect, which effectively resurfaces the joint and should simultaneously reduce the phalanx. The joint need not be flexed more than 35° to maintain reduction. A 0.045-inch K-wire is passed obliquely across the joint, and the adequacy of reduction must be checked intraoperatively with a true lateral x-ray of the finger.

The K-wire is removed at 2 weeks, and active guarded motion with dorsal extension block splinting is begun. The pull-out suture is removed at 3 to 4 weeks and if full extension is not achieved by 6 weeks, dynamic splinting of the PIP joint is begun.

Dislocations and Ligamentous Injuries of the MP Joints (Excluding the Thumb)

Anatomy

The MP joint is a condyloid joint that allows flexion, extension, abduction, adduction, and a limited amount of circumduction.[7] The globular head of the metacarpal articulates with the reciprocally concave base of the proximal phalanx, although the surface

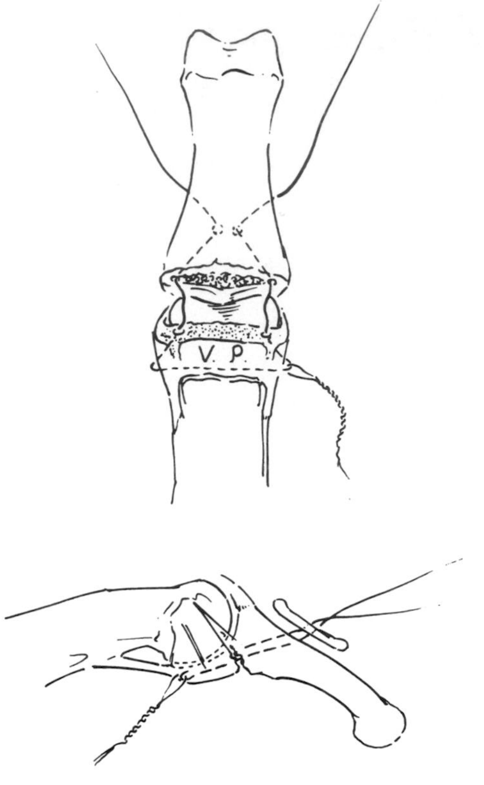

FIGURE 11-99. Eaton's volar plate arthroplasty is an operation that has withstood the test of time but his technique must be followed precisely to obtain good results (see text for details).

of the latter has a slightly less acute curve than the metacarpal head. The articular surface of the head is broader on its volar aspect than dorsally, allowing the recesses in the dorsolateral aspects of both sides of the head to accommodate the collateral ligaments. The stability of the joint depends on the collateral ligaments and volar plate, which together form a snug box-like configuration, as noted by Eaton[3] (Fig. 11-100).

Each collateral ligament has essentially two parts: an upper (dorsal) cord-like MP ligament and a lower accessory, or metacarpoglenoidal, ligament (see Fig. 11-77). The latter, which attaches directly into the volar plate, is less rigid, allowing it to fold on itself when the joint flexes. Lateral views show that the metacarpal head has an eccentric configuration: the distance from the center of rotation to the articular surface is greater in a volar direction than it is distally (see Fig. 11-76). This produces a cam-like effect on the collateral ligaments, making them tight in flexion and lax in extension. This can be readily demonstrated in a normal hand by noting that passive abduction and adduction are more restricted with the joint held in maximum flexion than in full extension. This eccentricity of the metacarpal head is the major reason that the MP joints are more likely to become stiff in extension than in flexion.

The volar plate of the MP joint is a relatively thick fibrocartilaginous condensation of the joint capsule forming the anterior wall of the joint. It is firmly attached distally to the base of the phalanx but its proximal attachment to the neck of the metacarpal is more areolar and flexible, allowing passive hyperextension of the joint and permitting the volar plate to fold on itself in flexion. The volar plates of the four palmar metacarpals are held together firmly by the deep transverse metacarpal ligament, which is actually continuous with the volar plate (Fig. 11-101).[739] Eaton[766] has called this the intervolar plate ligament.

Lateral MP Dislocations (Collateral Ligament Injuries)

Isolated injuries of the collateral ligaments of the finger MP joints are uncommon, presumably because of their relatively protected proximal position within the web space and the protection provided by the adjacent digits. For these reasons, the diagnosis may be missed early and the patient may present later with vague pain in the region of the MP joint. Most of these injuries appear to involve the RCL, and the mechanism of injury is usually an ulnarly directed force on the MP joint (James F. Murray, Toronto personal communication, 1982), usually combined with a hyperextension or flexion injury.

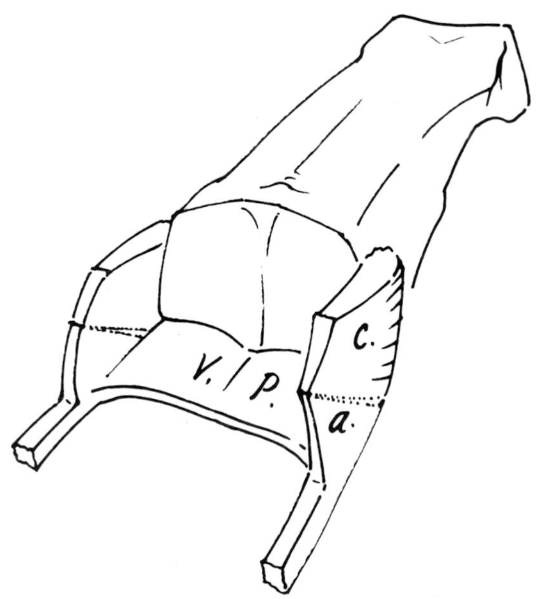

FIGURE 11-100. The stability of the metacarpophalangeal joint depends largely on the collateral ligaments and volar plate, which together form a snug box-like configuration. (*Eaton, R.G.: Joint Injuries of the Hand. Springfield, Ill., Charles C Thomas, 1970.*)

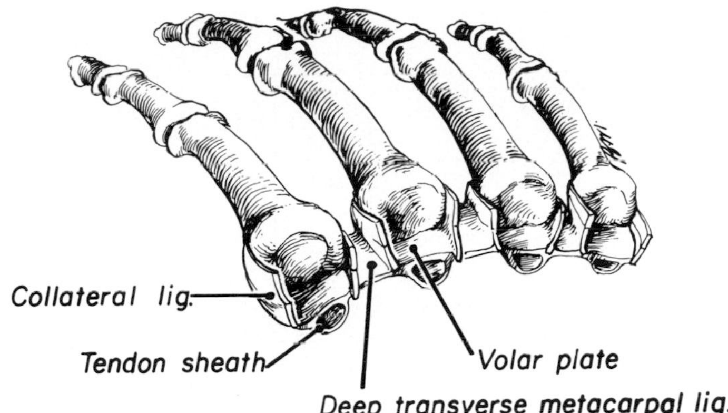

FIGURE 11-101. The volar plates of the four palmar metacarpals are held together firmly by the deep transverse metacarpal ligament, which is continuous with the volar plate. Eaton calls this the intervolar plate ligament.

Diagnosis. The diagnosis may be suggested by local tenderness and subtle swelling in the valley between the two metacarpal heads directly over the involved collateral ligament. The most specific and significant clinical sign is pain in response to lateral stress with the MP joint held in full flexion, with or without demonstrable instability. Because of the normal laxity of the collateral ligaments with the joint in full extension, stressing the normal MP joint in this position is usually not painful. Radiographs frequently demonstrate no abnormality but they may reveal a small avulsion fragment from the metacarpal head (Fig. 11-102). Even relatively large collateral ligament avulsion fractures may be difficult to see on routine x-rays,[773] and McElfresh and Dobyns[795] have suggested use of the Brewerton view (see Fig. 11-113). Other associated bony injuries include a significant intra-articular corner fracture at the base of the proximal phalanx (Fig. 11-103) in the acute injury or an area of cortical irregularity at the site of attachment of the collateral ligament in chronic injuries (Fig. 11-104).

Ishizuki[787] has reported the largest series of MP joint collateral ligament injuries. All of his 22 patients had arthrograms, which he thinks is the best method to

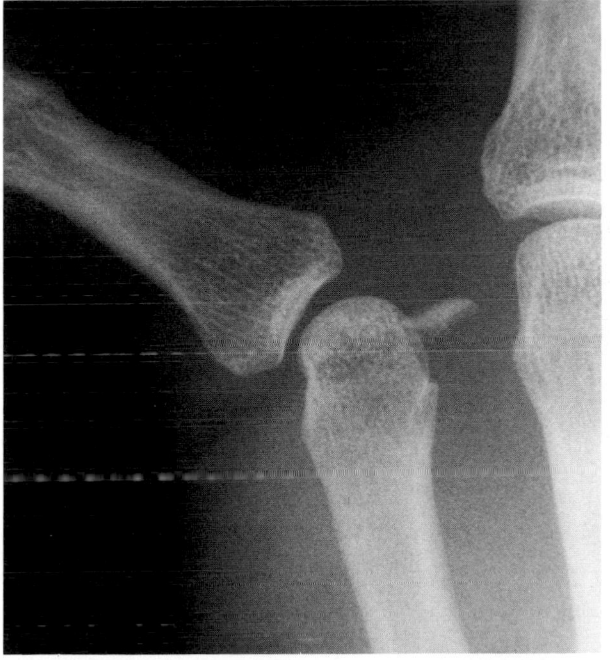

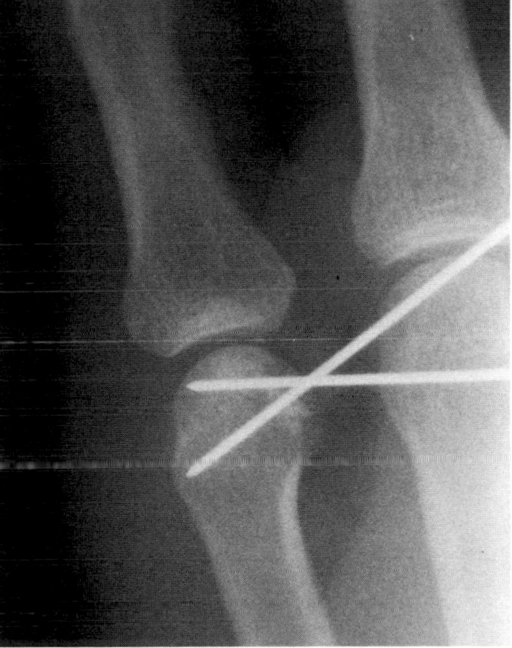

FIGURE 11-102. Occasionally, disruption of the collateral ligament of the metacarpophalangeal joint is associated with an avulsion fracture off the head of the metacarpal. If such a fracture is displaced (*left*), operative fixation is indicated (*right*).

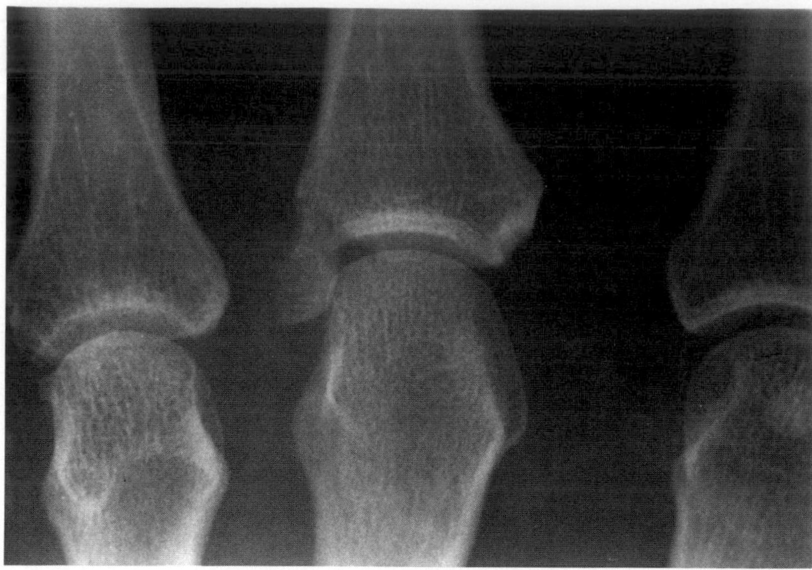

FIGURE 11-103. Another indication for open reduction of a metacarpophalangeal joint collateral ligament disruption is a large corner fracture of the base of the proximal phalanx.

determine whether surgical repair is necessary. The technique of MP joint arthrography is described in detail in his article.

Treatment

Acute Injuries. If the diagnosis is made early (within 10 to 14 days) and a significant avulsion fracture is not present radiographically, splinting of the joint in 50° flexion for 3 weeks is the recommended treatment,[766] although a few authors believe that grossly unstable joints should be repaired surgically.[763,787,814] A Stener-type lesion in which the sagittal band is interposed between the torn ends of the ligament has been reported by at least two separate authors.[787,814] If the x-rays show more than 2 to 3 mm displacement of a tiny avulsion chip or if the fragment involves more than 20% of the articular surface and is displaced or rotated, we believe that primary operative treatment is indicated. Our preferred methods are reinsertion of ligament avulsion (with or without a tiny chip fracture) using a pull-out suture or Mitek bone anchor, and internal fixation with small K-wires or tension-band wiring for corner fractures.

Chronic Injuries. As noted in the previous section, finger MP collateral ligament injuries are frequently missed early, and chronic symptoms may result, as suggested in the small series reported by Dray and

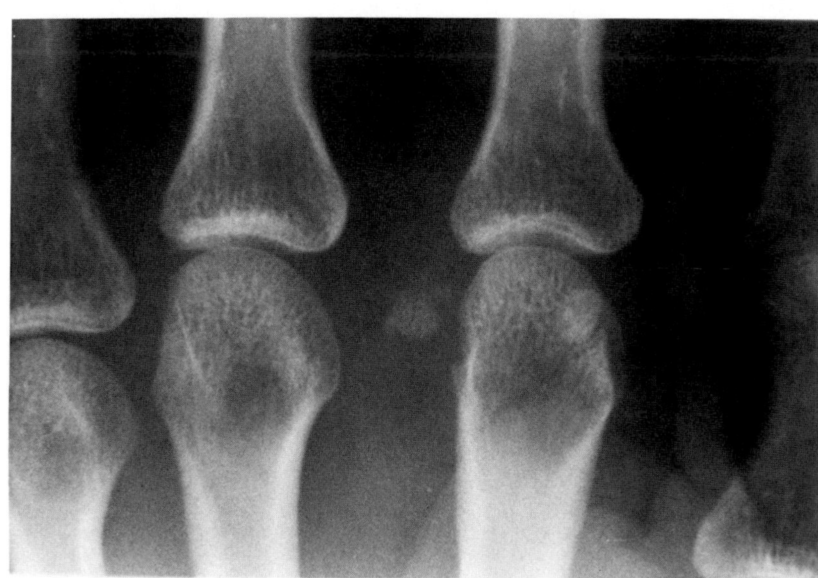

FIGURE 11-104. Late, untreated collateral ligament injuries of the metacarpophalangeal joint are occasionally associated with the appearance of heterotopic bone.

associates.[764] Although these authors advised against steroid injections, it has been our practice to treat patients presenting with chronic symptoms with an intra-articular steroid injection trial and 3 weeks of immobilization, followed by buddy taping to protect the ligament from further injury. Most of these patients continue to have symptoms for many months, sometimes taking up to 18 months to reach maximum improvement.[830]

If symptoms persist beyond this time, operative treatment is indicated but there is insufficient information in the literature to offer the surgeon clear guidance regarding the best method of surgical treatment. Our limited operative experience with this injury suggests that it may be difficult to identify reparable pathology in chronic cases, although several methods have been described for reconstruction of the ligament with a free tendon graft.[759,763,764]

Dorsal MP Dislocations

Two types of dorsal dislocation occur in the MP joint: simple and complex. It is important to differentiate between these two because simple dislocations can be reduced by closed manipulation, whereas complex dislocations are irreducible by closed methods and require open reduction. Both result from hyperextension injuries and in both, the volar plate is torn from its proximal insertion on the neck of the metacarpal. The two can usually be distinguished fairly easily by clinical and radiographic examination, and the surgeon should not have to resort to multiple unsuccessful attempts at closed reduction to conclude that he or she is contending with an irreducible dislocation.

Simple Dorsal Dislocation (Subluxation). Eaton[766] correctly refers to simple dorsal dislocation as subluxation of the joint because the articular surfaces are still in partial contact but with the proximal phalanx resting in 60° to 90° of hyperextension on the dorsum of the metacarpal head. These usually involve only a single finger but multiple simultaneous MP dislocations (including all four fingers) have been reported.[794,809] Closed reduction is relatively simple, although McLaughlin[796] cautioned that it is possible to convert a simple dislocation into a complex dislocation if the reduction is performed by traction alone.

Technique of Closed Reduction for Simple MP Dislocation. The proximal phalanx is first hyperextended 90° on the metacarpal and the base of the proximal phalanx is then *pushed* into flexion, maintaining contact at all times with the head of the metacarpal to prevent entrapment of the volar plate in the joint. The wrist and the IP joints are flexed during the maneuver to relax the flexor tendons, and the joint usually reduces easily with a palpable and audible "clunk."

Although the reduction can frequently be performed without anesthesia, we generally prefer to do it under wrist block because occasionally, pain may preclude a successful reduction and lead the surgeon to the erroneous conclusion that the patient has a complex dislocation.

Although a short (7- to 10-day) period of immobilization with the MP joint in 50° to 70° of flexion is acceptable treatment, we generally prefer to allow immediate active motion, preventing hyperextension by buddy taping alone. Recurrent dislocations or chronic symptoms after simple MP dislocations are rare.

Complex (Irreducible) MP Dislocation. Although Farabeuf[767] first coined the term complex dislocation in 1876, irreducible dislocation of the MP joints is said to have been described by Malgaigne in his 1855 text.[772,826] Isolated case reports appeared in the early English literature but it was not until 1957 that the pathologic anatomy became widely appreciated.[749,751,812] In that year, Kaplan[788] published his classic article in which he described the buttonholing of the metacarpal head into the palm and the anatomy of the constricting factors preventing reduction by closed methods. Although not all authors have agreed with Kaplan about the role of these various structures in preventing reduction, most agree that the most important element preventing reduction is interposition of the volar plate between the base of the proximal phalanx and the head of the metacarpal (Fig. 11-105).[750,760,776,778,798] In some open injuries, there may be other factors such as displacement of the flexor tendons that block reduction.[744]

Numerous case reports in the earlier literature inferred that this is a rare injury but larger series suggest that it is not as uncommon as formerly believed.‡‡

Recognition of a complex dislocation should be relatively simple because there are three clinical and radiographic clues to the diagnosis:

1. A complex dislocation does not present as dramatic an appearance as the simple dislocation (subluxation) described previously. The joint is only slightly hyperextended, with the proximal phalanx lying on the dorsum of the metacarpal head and the finger partially overlapping the adjacent digit. The IP joints are slightly flexed. Radiographically, the proximal phalanx and metacarpal are nearly parallel, with only slight angulation. Al-Qattan and Zuker[740] believe that

‡‡ References 742, 753, 776, 783, 796, 798, 802, 820.

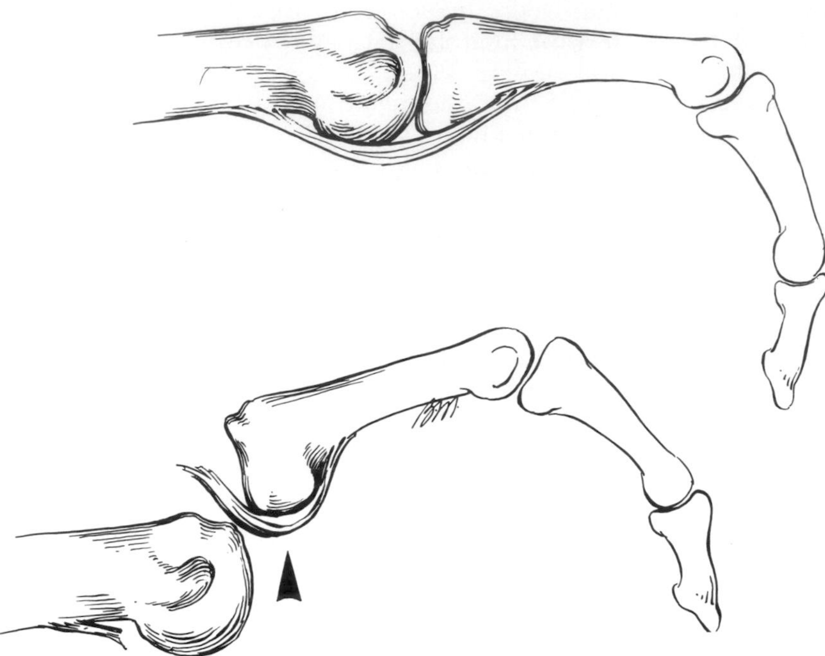

FIGURE 11-105. The single most important element preventing reduction in a complex metacarpophalangeal dislocation is interposition of the volar plate within the joint space, and it must be extricated surgically.

in some dorsal dislocations, a similar configuration of parallelism can exist in which the volar plate is not entrapped in the joint.

2. A consistent finding is puckering of the palmar skin. This is more difficult to see when the index finger is involved because the skin dimple lies within the proximal palmar crease (Fig. 11-106). When the central digits are involved, the skin pucker may have the appearance of a more longitudinally oriented groove.[738] It is more readily apparent when the dislocation occurs in the thumb and the dimple is present in the thenar eminence (see Fig. 11-125).
3. A pathognomonic radiographic sign of complex dislocation is the presence of a sesamoid within a widened joint space.[776,806,816,819] Because the sesamoids reside within the volar plate, the presence of a sesamoid within the joint space should be considered to be an unequivocal sign of a complex dislocation (Fig. 11-107). This finding should not be confused with a chip fracture of the metacarpal head, which may also occur but does not necessarily carry the same diagnostic significance. Tsuge and Watari[820] noted that this frequent concomitant injury represents an avulsion fracture of the ulnar tuberosity by the collateral ligament.

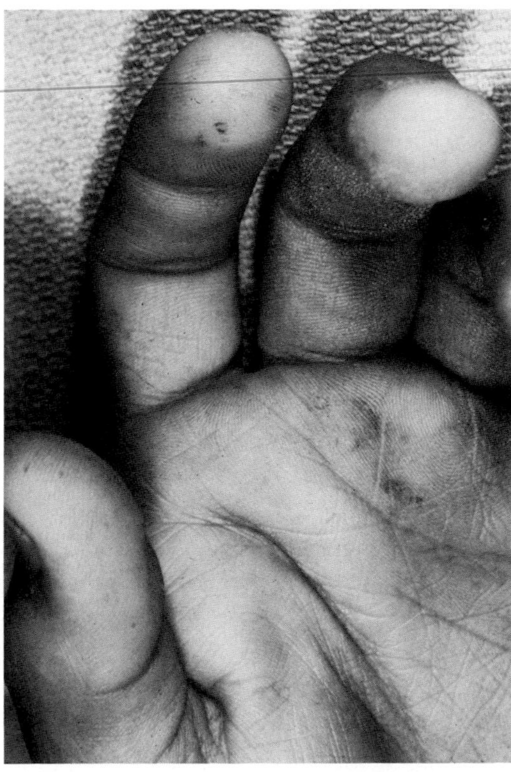

FIGURE 11-106. A particularly important clinical sign, which is virtually pathognomonic of a complex dislocation of the MP joint of index finger, is puckering of the skin in the proximal palmar crease.

Complex dislocations occur most commonly in the index finger, followed in incidence by the thumb and

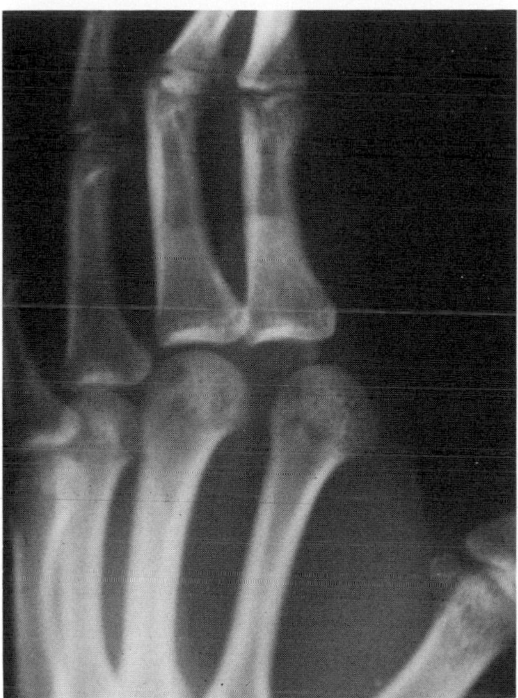

FIGURE 11-107. A pathognomonic radiographic sign of a complex dislocation is the presence of a sesamoid within the widened joint space. Since the sesamoids reside in the volar plate, the presence of the sesamoid within the joint space is indicative of interposition of the volar plate within the joint. (*Green, D.P., and Terry, G.C.: Complex Dislocation of the Metacarpophalangeal Joint. Correlative Pathological Anatomy. J. Bone Joint Surg. 55A:1482, 1973.*)

small finger and rarely, the long[805,825] and ring fingers.[738] Many other combinations have been described, including simultaneous dislocation of all four MP joints.§§ Multiple MP dislocations are not always complex, and in some cases may be reducible by closed manipulation.[768,809]

It is possible to have a concomitant fracture of the proximal phalanx in the same digit as a complex MP dislocation.[822]

Treatment. An attempt at closed reduction should be made in all dislocations of the MP joint. Even if the pathognomonic signs of a complex dislocation are present, the surgeon is justified in making a single attempt at gentle reduction under adequate anesthesia (preferably at least wrist block) but he or she should be prepared to follow this with an immediate open reduction if the manipulation is unsuccessful. The preferred method of closed reduction is that described by McLaughlin.[796] Malerich and associates[793] believe that relaxation of tension on the flexor tendons is critical, suggesting that the closed reduction maneuver should be performed with the wrist flexed.

Operative Treatment

The original operative approach to this injury was described by Farabeuf[767] as a dorsal releasing incision. Kaplan[788] presented the logical reasons that a volar approach offers the surgeon more direct visual access to the injury and facilitates the release.

Although most authors favor a volar approach for the open reduction of a complex MP dislocation, Becton and Carswell[752] advocated a dorsal approach, believing that it has the following advantages: (1) better exposure of the volar plate; (2) less likelihood of damage to the digital nerves; and (3) better access for accurate reduction and fixation of an osteochondral fracture of the metacarpal head, if present. Other authors[779,820] have also recommended the dorsal approach for similar reasons but it has been noted that the volar plate has to be split longitudinally from the dorsal approach to effect a reduction;[750,753] this is not necessary with the volar approach. It is easier to excise or fix a concomitant osteochondral fracture of the metacarpal head through the dorsal approach, which we use when the preoperative x-rays show such a fracture. Otherwise, we prefer the volar approach.

Technique of Open Reduction of Complex MP Dislocation. We believe that the volar approach provides the most direct access to the pathologic anatomy in a complex dislocation and unless there is a concomitant fracture of the metacarpal head, we use the incision suggested by McLaughlin,[796] which begins in the proximal palmar crease and turns distally along the midaxial line on the radial side of the index finger (Fig. 11-108). For dislocations in the small finger, an inci-

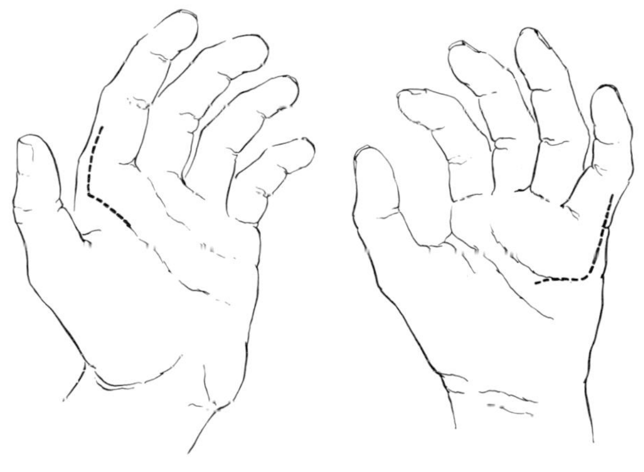

FIGURE 11-108. The authors' preferred incisions for open reduction of complex dislocations of the index finger (*left*) and small finger (*right*) metacarpophalangeal joints.

§§ References 737, 743, 779, 784, 785, 794, 824, 828, 1031.

sion in the proximal palmar crease is extended along the mid-ulnar aspect of the finger.

Of extreme importance in the surgical exposure is the vulnerable location of the neurovascular bundle, caused by displacement of the metacarpal head into the palm (Fig. 11-109). Invariably, the radial digital nerve and artery in the index finger (the ulnar bundle in the small finger) are tented tightly and superficially over the prominent metacarpal head, lying immediately beneath the skin. An overly aggressive skin incision can easily injure the neurovascular bundle.

Division of the superficial transverse metacarpal ligaments (transverse fibers of the palmar fascia) facilitates exposure. In the index finger, the metacarpal head is flanked on the radial side by the lumbrical muscle and on the ulnar side by the flexor tendons. In the small finger, the flexor tendons lie on the radial side, together with the lumbrical, and the tendon of the abductor digiti quinti lies on the ulnar side. These longitudinal structures must be retracted to provide better exposure of the joint but releasing them from around the metacarpal neck does not effect a reduction. The most important element preventing reduction is interposition of the volar plate between the base of the proximal phalanx and the head of the metacarpal. The plate has invariably been torn loose from its relatively loose membranous proximal attachment and is found to be wedged in tightly behind (dorsal to) the exposed metacarpal head. The volar plate must be removed manually from the joint before reduction can be accomplished. Avulsion of the volar plate from the neck of the metacarpal is necessarily accompanied by tearing of the plate on one or both sides from the adjacent deep transverse metacarpal (intervolar plate) ligament, but incompletely so. Extrication of the volar plate with a skin hook is facilitated if the partial tear between the volar plate and the deep transverse metacarpal ligament is completed by a short longitudinal incision (usually on both sides, occasionally on one side), as originally suggested by Flatt.[771]

If care has been taken in removing the volar plate from the joint, it is usually in good condition, with a firm insertion remaining into the base of the proximal phalanx.

It remains a moot and frequently argued point whether a true complex dislocation can be reduced by closed manipulation. Perhaps some so-called "complex" MP dislocations successfully reduced closed were actually the variant of simple dislocation described by Al-Qattan and Zuker,[740] in which the volar plate is not interposed in the joint. Our operative experience has led us to believe that successful closed reduction is not possible in a true complex MP dislocation but the issue is difficult to resolve because the mere fact of a successful reduction eliminates the opportunity to look and see whether the volar plate was actually entrapped.

Postoperative Care. The joint is invariably stable after reduction, easily confirmed at the operating table by passively moving the joint through a full range of motion. Thus, no immobilization is necessary postoperatively, and early active motion is encouraged, protecting the finger with buddy taping. If the surgeon is concerned about possible instability in hyperextension, a dorsal extension block splint can be used. Hubbard[782] has suggested the use of continuous passive motion postoperatively but we have not found this to be necessary.

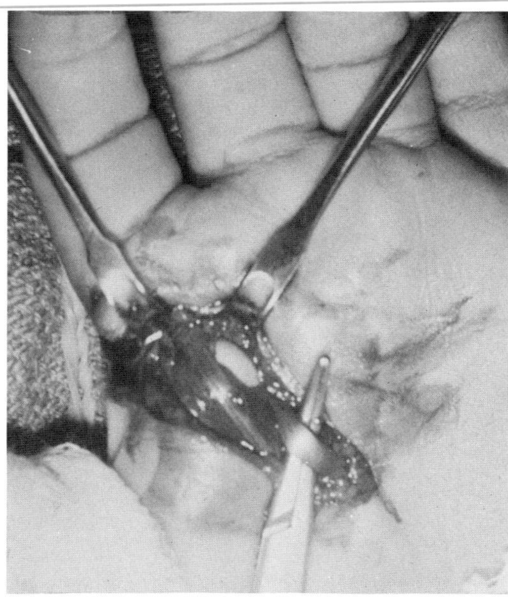

FIGURE 11-109. Of extreme importance in the open reduction of a complex metacarpophalangeal dislocation is the vulnerable location of the neurovascular bundle caused by displacement of the metacarpal head into the palm. Invariably, the digital nerve and artery are tented very tightly and superficially over the prominent metacarpal head and lie immediately beneath the skin.

Late Unreduced Complex MP Dislocation. The treatment of a late, untreated, or inadequately treated complex dislocation is considerably more complicated, and the end results are significantly compromised. Murphy and Stark[802] have reported their experience with these difficult injuries, and they note that a second, dorsal incision is necessary to excise the shortened UCL. None of their six patients with late complex dislocations regained normal range of motion in the finger.

Volar MP Dislocations

Volar dislocation of the MP joint is rare.[754,757,801,811,827] Perhaps because it is such an uncommon injury, the pathologic anatomy in volar MP dislocations is not as well understood as in the more common complex dorsal dislocation. The volar plate, collateral ligament, and dorsal capsule have all been implicated as a cause of irreducibility.[754,801,811,827] MRI in one patient with a 3-week-old volar MP dislocation was interpreted as showing interposition of the dorsal capsule but at operation, the origins of the collateral ligaments were also found to be invaginated into the joint.[800]

Because of our incomplete understanding of the actual pathologic anatomy in volar MP dislocations, some authors[754,801] have suggested that both dorsal and volar approaches may be necessary to achieve a reduction.

Locking of the MP Joint

Locking of the MP joint in flexion is a relatively uncommon problem. It must be differentiated clinically from the far more common trigger finger caused by stenosis of the flexor tendon sheath in the region of the A1 pulley. In a trigger finger, the "catching" characteristically occurs in the PIP joint, whereas in the condition being considered here, the locking is in the MP joint. The history may implicate a specific traumatic incident in which the finger locks after forcible active flexion of the digit or, more commonly, repeated episodes of catching of the finger after voluntary flexion. The patient may relate that he or she can passively extend the finger with pain, or the pain may have become so severe that the finger cannot be extended at all.

On examination, the flexor tendons are intact, and active flexion of the finger may be nearly normal. The key clinical finding is that the MP joint is typically flexed about 40° to 50° (Fig. 11-110), and attempts to straighten the digit are painful or even impossible.

The most frequently recognized cause appears to be the volar plate or collateral ligament catching on an osteophyte on either the side or the volar aspect of the metacarpal head.‖‖ The index finger is most commonly involved,[818] often in older patients with degenerative arthritis, and Goodfellow and Weaver[774] suggested that oblique x-rays of the hand frequently demonstrate these bony projections. Dibbell and Field[762] reported a similar mechanism in a patient having a malunited fracture of the metacarpal head. Other factors mentioned as causes include (1) loose bodies[792,806] or osteochondral fracture fragments;[815] (2) abnormal sesamoids;[769,770] (3) an abnormal fibrous band across the volar aspect of the joint (which may represent a chronic tear of the volar plate);[758,829] and (4) catching of the extensor hood on a dorsal osteophyte.[808]

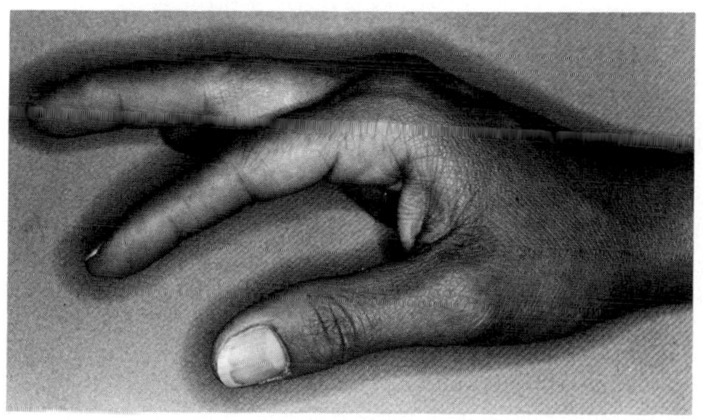

FIGURE 11-110. A patient with a "locked" metacarpophalangeal joint usually presents with the joint fixed in about 40° to 50° flexion.

Treatment. It has been suggested that these patients be observed[818] for at least a month[780] because spontaneous recovery has been reported in some patients.[745] Forceful manipulation is not recommended because this can cause fracture of the metacarpal head.[786,790] Newer reports, however, suggest that *gentle* manipulation may successfully "unlock" the finger, especially if the patient is seen soon after onset.[777,807] Guly and Azam[777] successfully treated three patients with longitudinal traction combined with alternate medial and lateral rotation under digital block anesthesia. Posner and coworkers[807] suggested distention of the joint with local anesthetic to aid in reduction. If closed reduction is unsuccessful, if spontaneous recovery does not occur, if the condition is painful, or if a fixed contracture of the joint is developing, operative treatment is indicated. The joint is explored through a volar approach,[818] with removal of any offending osteophytes from the metacarpal head or division of the abnormal fibrous bands.

CMC Dislocations (Excluding the Thumb)

Anatomy

The CMC joints of the fingers are arthrodial diarthroses (gliding joints), except the fifth, which is a modified saddle joint.[858] The bases of the metacarpals articulate with the distal row of the carpal bones and with each other in a complex interlocking configuration. This is especially true at the base of the second metacarpal, which is forked to receive the convex distal edge of the trapezoid and is also wedged tightly in between the base of the adjacent third metacarpal ulnarly and the trapezium radially.[876] This anatomic arrangement makes precise radiographic visualization of the second metacarpal-trapezoid joint somewhat difficult. Mehara and Bhan[892] described a special radiograph view (Fig.

‖‖ References 741, 745, 755, 762, 774, 780, 790, 813, 817.

11-111) that shows this area more clearly than is seen on routine views.

The joints are strengthened by tough intermetacarpal and CMC ligaments dorsally and volarly; the dorsal ligaments are stronger. Additional reinforcement is provided by the insertions of the wrist flexors and extensors into the bases of the second, third, and fifth metacarpals.

Essentially no movement is possible in the third metacarpal-capitate joint, which functions as the stable central post of the hand, as described by Flatt.[854] A limited amount of AP gliding is permitted at the base of the second metacarpotrapezoid joint but the articulations between the bases of the fourth and fifth metacarpals and the hamate are considerably more mobile. Most authors have assumed that up to 20° or 30° of motion is possible in these two joints, but Gunther's[861] cadaver studies revealed only 8° and 15° in the fourth and fifth CMC joints, respectively.

The fifth CMC joint is the most mobile because it is actually a saddle joint, similar to the articulation between the thumb metacarpal and the trapezium. A saddle joint is an articulation in which the opposing surfaces are reciprocally concavoconvex. Viewed from the dorsum, the distal surface of the hamate is convex; seen from the ulnar side, it is concave. The bases of both the fourth and fifth metacarpals articulate with the hamate; the distal surface of the hamate is divided into two facets by a faint ridge. The articular surface of the fourth metacarpal is generally transverse but Viegas and coworkers[915] have shown surprising anatomic variations of this joint in extensive cadaveric dissections. The obliquely oriented, sloping articular surface of the fifth CMC joint (Fig. 11-112) and the pull of the extensor carpi ulnaris inserting into the base of the fifth metacarpal are major factors that create instability in fracture-subluxations of this joint.

Two soft-tissue relations of the CMC joints are of extreme importance to the surgeon when operative intervention is required. The deep (motor) branch of the ulnar nerve lies immediately volar to the fifth CMC joint as it winds around the hook of the hamate, and the deep palmar arterial arch lies directly beneath the third metacarpal-capitate articulation.[857]

Mechanism of Injury

Despite attempts to reproduce CMC dislocations in the laboratory and many hypotheses based on clinical cases, the precise mechanism of these injuries remains somewhat speculative.[918] Generally, however, they tend to result either from extreme violence (eg, motor-

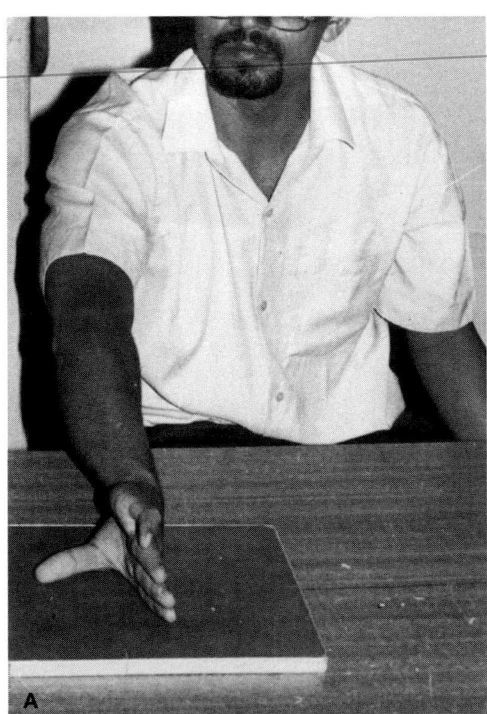

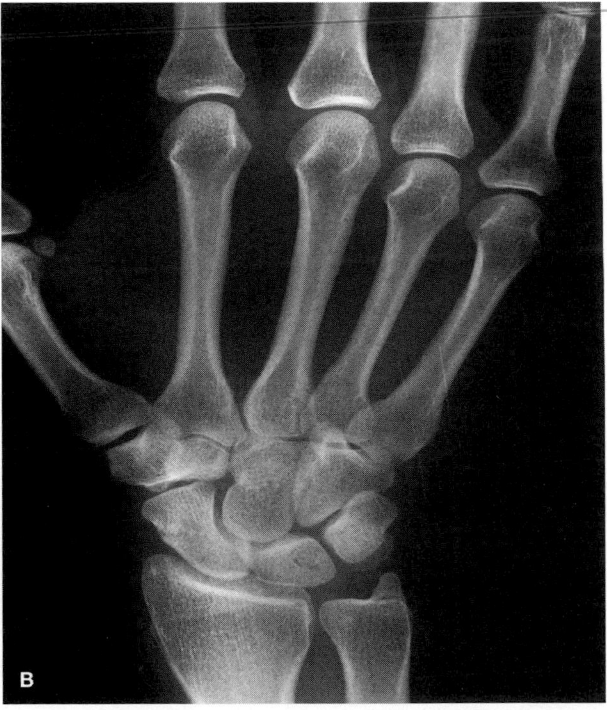

FIGURE 11-111. The area around the trapezoid is notoriously difficult to see clearly on routine radiographic examination. The view suggested by Mehara and Bhan (**A**) much more clearly shows the second metacarpal-trapezoid joint (**B**). *(Mehara, A.K., and Bhan, S.: Rotatory Dislocation of the Second Carpometacarpal Joint: Case Report. J Trauma 34:464–466, 1993.)*

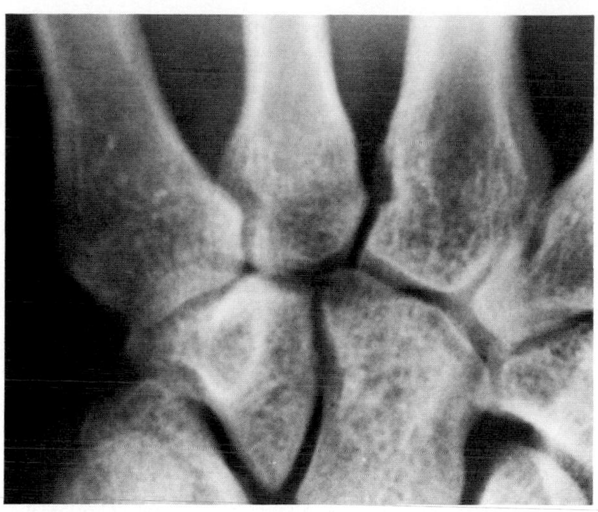

FIGURE 11-112. The bases of the fourth and fifth metacarpals both articulate with the hamate. The articular surface of the fourth metacarpal is transverse, and that of the fifth is oblique; the latter is partially responsible for instability of fracture-subluxations of this joint.

cycle accidents, crush injuries, blows from heavy falling objects)[864,885] or from hitting someone or something with the closed fist.[897] Dommisse and Lloyd[848] suggested that the type of fracture or dislocation of the fifth metacarpal is related to the mechanism of injury. They found that direct injury (a crushing blow) tends to produce angulated extra-articular fractures, which do not disrupt the CMC joint and are stable. In contrast, indirect injury is the cause of unstable intra-articular fracture-dislocations. They postulated that a lever type of strain in which the fifth metacarpal is forced into dorsiflexion causes a bipartite fracture-dislocation, and a direct blow to the metacarpal head produces a longitudinal force that results in a tripartite fracture-dislocation, with more proximal migration of the shaft. Their reason for differentiating these two types of fracture-dislocations was that in their experience, closed reduction and percutaneous pin fixation was more likely to be successful in the bipartite fracture than in the tripartite variety. Other authors have also postulated that the unstable fracture-dislocation is caused by a force acting along the longitudinal axis of the fifth metacarpal.[835,887,897]

In addition to isolated dislocations of each of the four individual joints, virtually every combination of CMC dislocations has been reported (even all five CMC joints, including the thumb).[832] Simultaneous dislocation of all four joints generally results from extreme trauma, such as having the hand run over by an automobile and is likely to be associated with multiple fractures and extensive soft-tissue damage.[882]

Most of these dislocations are dorsal but volar displacement of both the fifth and second CMC joints has been reported.[898,899,907,914] Thomas and coworkers[913] reported an unusual volar dislocation of the second CMC with a fragment of bone displaced into the palm. Proximal migration of the index metacarpal may occur when the trapezoid is dislocated into the palm.[849] Gunther and Bruno[862] described what they called a divergent dislocation (ie, dorsal displacement of the second and third and volar dislocation of the fourth and fifth CMC joints). Associated injuries have included dislocation of the fifth MP joint[911] and fractures of the hook of the hamate.[862,899]

Concomitant articular fractures of carpal bones in the distal row are not uncommon, especially the hamate.[856,873,879] Cain and coworkers[839] reported a series of such patients in whom the fourth metacarpal was fractured and the base of the fifth metacarpal was dislocated dorsally, associated with varying types of fractures of the hamate. Marck and Klasen[889] showed that lateral tomography is the best technique for clearly delineating the nature of these hamate fractures because the fracture line is usually in the coronal plane. Garcia-Elias[856] and his colleagues at the Mayo Clinic prefer polytomes (trispiral tomography).

Diagnosis

Clinical. The obvious clinical deformity that one may expect to see with this injury is often obscured by marked swelling of the hand. Even when the swelling is severe, however, maximum tenderness can generally be localized to the bases of the metacarpals. In dislocations of the fifth metacarpal-hamate joint, special attention should be directed to the integrity of the ulnar nerve[838,857,885,899] and in multiple dislocations, a careful assessment of all soft tissues, especially the circulation, must be made. Median nerve injury and avulsion of the wrist extensor tendons have been reported as associated injuries.[919]

Joseph and coworkers[875] have suggested that sprains of the CMC joints are considerably more common than generally believed, and chronic symptoms frequently result. Moreover, the literature still reflects that even frank dislocations are frequently missed when initially seen, and proper x-rays are mandatory.

Radiographic. Fisher and colleagues[852,853] have emphasized the principles of parallelism, symmetry, and overlapping articular surfaces in evaluating suspected injuries of the CMC joints. Initial radiographic examination should include the three standard views: PA, lateral, and oblique; the true lateral view is most likely to demonstrate the displacement of the base of the metacarpal.[847,867,912] Special views may be helpful, however, to determine the exact amount of displace-

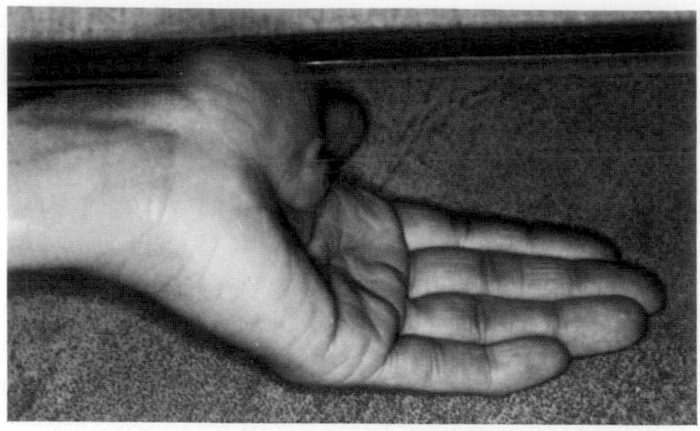

FIGURE 11-113. The Brewerton view has been suggested as a method of demonstrating occult fractures at the base of the metacarpals. The x-ray beam is angled 30° from the ulnar side of the hand.

ment and the extent of intra-articular comminution. Murless[895] demonstrated that an AP view (palm up with the forearm in supination) is more likely to show small detached fragments than is the standard PA (palm down) view. Bora and Didizian[835] stated that the most helpful view is with the forearm pronated 30° from a routine AP view (a 60° supination lateral), Niejchajev[897] showed that this position gives the best view of the fourth-fifth intermetacarpal space, and Kaye and Lister[877] suggested the Brewerton view[837] (Fig. 11-113) as a means of demonstrating occult fractures at the base of the metacarpal. Hindman and coworkers[169] pointed out the value of CT scans in identifying occult fractures at the base of the metacarpals, best seen in coronal and transaxial planes.

The second CMC joint is particularly difficult to see well on routine x-rays. Mehara and Bhan[892] described a special view that shows this metacarpal-trapezoid joint clearly (see Fig. 11-111).

An important point is to be aware of the possible coexistence of dislocation of one CMC joint associated with a displaced fracture of an adjacent metacarpal. Analogous to Monteggia and Galleazi fracture-dislocations in the forearm, the metacarpals are tethered proximally and distally, and if one metacarpal is shortened or significantly angulated, a careful look is necessary to rule out dislocation of the base of an adjacent metacarpal[872] (Fig. 11-114). A quick way to ascertain shortening of a metacarpal is with what Chmell and coworkers[842] called the oblique metacarpal line (ie, a straight line drawn on the x-ray connecting the heads of the ulnar three metacarpals). The amount of shortening of the involved metacarpal can be measured from this line, although comparison with the opposite uninjured hand is advised.

Our preference for evaluating CMC joint injuries, in addition to the standard PA and lateral views, includes oblique views with the hand pronated and supinated 30°, respectively, from the true lateral view. Additional oblique views with more or less forearm rotation may be indicated by what is seen in these initial films.

Treatment

Acute Injuries. Carpometacarpal dislocations are not rare injuries but they are sufficiently uncommon that most of the early literature regarding them was in the form of case reports or small series, with many recommendations for treatment based on limited clinical impressions and inadequate data. Reports have subsequently appeared of larger series from which reasonable guidelines for treatment can be gleaned.[846,856,881,885,897]

Methods of Treatment

Splinting Without Reduction. Good evidence suggests that intra-articular fractures of the base of the fifth metacarpal with minimal or no displacement can be adequately treated with a molded cast or splint for 3 to 4 weeks. Disagreement regarding treatment arises,

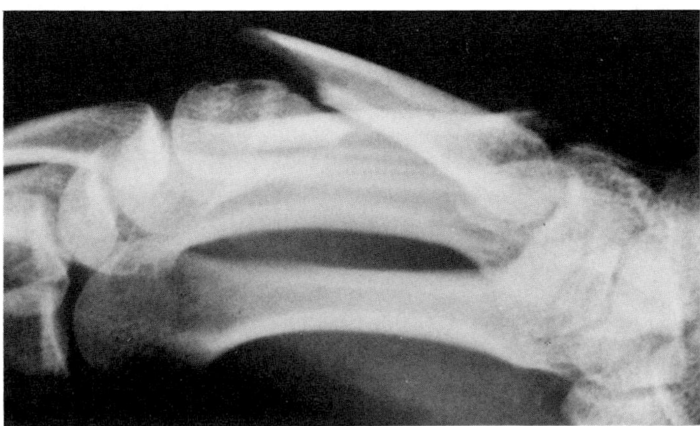

FIGURE 11-114. Whenever there is a displaced or angulated fracture of the base or the shaft of a metacarpal, particular care should be taken to look for dislocation of one or more adjacent carpometacarpal joints. In this patient, there is an angulated and shortened fracture of the fifth metacarpal and subluxation of the base of the fourth metacarpal.

however, in management of displaced intra-articular fracture-subluxations. Several authors,[880,905,909,920] especially in the older literature, have stated or implied that old, unreduced CMC dislocations ultimately become asymptomatic and produce no functional deficit. The validity of these conclusions is questionable because of the few cases and short follow-up periods reported. In 1974, however, Petrie and Lamb[902] published what is perhaps the only long-term (average, 4.5 years) follow-up study of numerous patients (23) having essentially untreated fracture-subluxations of the base of the fifth metacarpal. Their surprising results, which revealed only one patient with significant symptoms, may tend to dampen enthusiasm for open reduction of these injuries. Even considering this study, however, we cannot advocate total neglect for this fracture-dislocation because our experience agrees with that of the many authors who state that residual subluxation and incongruity of the CMC joints lead to pain and weakened grip in some patients.##

Closed Reduction and Cast Immobilization. Anatomic or at least acceptable closed reduction is usually not difficult to accomplish if the injury is recognized and treated early. The problem, however, is maintaining that reduction, especially in the presence of significant swelling.[872] If closed reduction and cast immobilization is selected as the method of treatment, careful radiographic monitoring must be done for the subsequent 3 to 4 weeks to detect resubluxation, which is likely. LaForgia and coworkers[884] reported successful treatment of a patient using only cast immobilization but their case was a rare pure fifth CMC dislocation with no associated fracture, which is probably a more stable injury.

Closed Reduction and Internal Fixation. Numerous authors[843,846,847,859,866,903,916] have demonstrated that the reduction can be maintained with percutaneously placed K-wires after reduction has been achieved by closed manipulation, including patients with concomitant carpal bone fractures.[856]

Technique of CRIF for CMC Fracture-Dislocations. With the patient under adequate anesthesia with complete muscle relaxation (general anesthesia or brachial block), a strong traction force is applied with finger traps and a counterweight across the upper arm. Uninterrupted traction for 5 to 10 minutes brings the metacarpals out to length but it does not necessarily reduce the dislocation, and direct pressure must be applied to the bases of the metacarpals to reduce them into their normal anatomic positions (Fig. 11-115). After full reduction has been verified by PA and lateral x-rays (or with the image intensifier) taken with the hand in traction, two or three 0.045-inch K-wires are passed percutaneously, stabilizing the involved metacarpal to an adjacent intact metacarpal or to the carpus itself or both. It is imperative to reduce the main shaft of the metacarpal (ie, the subluxation), and it is desirable to anatomically reduce the intra-articular fracture at the base of the metacarpal, although the latter is not always possible. We prefer to bend the pins at a right angle outside the skin to facilitate removal 4 weeks after reduction. The hand and wrist should be protected in a splint or cast for 4 to 6 weeks.

Open Reduction and Internal Fixation. Noting the similarity between the fracture-subluxation of the fifth CMC joint and Bennett's fracture in the thumb, numerous authors have advocated ORIF as the treatment of choice.[835,848,864,868,887,906] After discovering that their patients treated with open reduction did not fare as well as those treated with no reduction in the study previously cited, Petrie and Lamb[902] concluded that these two entities are anatomically but not functionally similar, and they argued that the case for open reduction is not strong.

Another problem with ORIF is whether the fracture is "fixable" or more precisely, whether the surgeon has the expertise to achieve anatomic reduction. Kjaer-Peterson and colleagues[881] found that in 7 of their 19 patients treated with ORIF, articular congruity was not improved, primarily because the actual comminution was greater than anticipated on the preoperative x-rays. It requires sound judgement to know which of these difficult fracture-dislocations are amenable to open reduction.

Certainly in some cases open reduction is indicated. Unsuccessful closed manipulation implies some impediment to reduction, including massive swelling,[865,908] interposed fracture fragments,[865,873,888] interposed soft-tissue structures such as the wrist extensor tendons,[865,886,892] or soft-tissue contracture secondary to delay in treatment.[846,891]

The literature suggests that open reduction is more likely to be necessary in multiple CMC dislocations.[865,882,893] In our opinion, open injuries should be treated with open reduction, debridement, appropriate wound care, and stabilization of the dislocations with multiple K-wires or minifragment T plates.

Open reduction also appears to be more frequently necessary in fracture-dislocations of the fifth CMC joint in which the base of the metacarpal is displaced radially across the bases of the other metacarpals than it is with the more common pattern of ulnar displacement.[896,905]

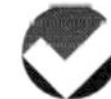

Authors' Preferred Method

For isolated fracture-subluxation of the CMC joints, including the fifth, we prefer CRIF. Mild to moderate incongruity of the articular surface is accepted (Fig.

References 840, 855, 864, 867, 868, 874, 878, 881.

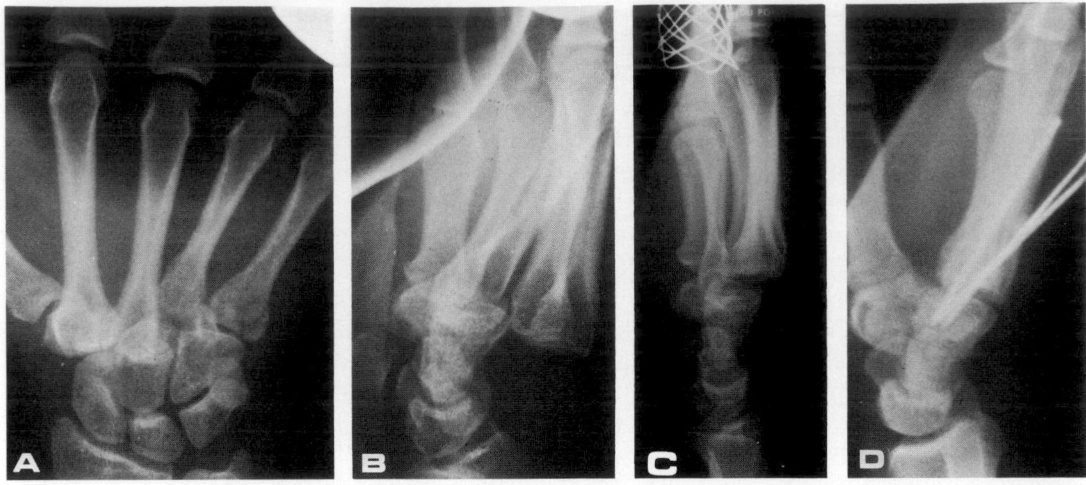

FIGURE 11-115. The steps in closed reduction of a carpometacarpal dislocation. (**A**) The anteroposterior view shows proximal displacement of the bases of the second and third metacarpals. Note also the fracture of the base of the fifth metacarpal. (**B**) The lateral view dramatically demonstrates dorsal dislocation of the bases of the second and third metacarpals. (**C**) The first step in reduction is to apply a strong traction force, best accomplished by finger traps, with countertraction across the upper arm. Traction brings the metacarpals out to length but it does not necessarily reduce the dislocation. Note that there is still dorsal subluxation of the bases of the metacarpals. Direct pressure must be applied to the bases of the metacarpals to restore their normal anatomic position. Because of the great propensity for recurrent subluxation after closed reduction alone, we believe that percutaneous pin fixation (**D**) should routinely be done at the time of closed reduction.

11-116), and the major emphasis is on reduction of the subluxation of the metacarpal shaft and restoration of length. This method works equally well when two adjacent joints are dislocated but we have never attempted to use it with three or four dislocations. Open reduction is more likely to be necessary in the patient having four CMC dislocations. In such situations, Hartwig and Louis[865] noted that reduction and stabilization of the base of the third metacarpal is the key to the reduction of the remaining metacarpals.

Operative treatment is necessary in all open dislocations, and despite the theoretic disadvantage of using internal fixation in an open wound, we believe that it is imperative to use as many K-wires as necessary to restore stability. The massive swelling so often a part of these injuries makes external splinting ineffectual in holding the reduction, and redislocation can be almost guaranteed if internal stabilization is not performed.

Chronic Injuries. Carpometacarpal dislocations are occasionally missed on initial examination and may present several weeks to months after injury. If the subluxation and joint incongruity are mild to moderate, we tend to favor no attempt at reduction for those injuries seen more than 3 weeks late. Using Petrie and Lamb's[902] series as the basis for this decision, we expect some of these patients to become relatively asymptomatic.

When the degree of displacement is marked or especially when multiple joints are involved, an attempt should probably be made to perform a late open reduction. Just how long after injury this can be successfully accomplished is not well documented in the literature, although Imbriglia[874] did so at 3.5 months and Fernyhough and Trumble[851] at 3 months. Bora and Didizian's[835] cases included open reductions performed as late as 6 months to 10 years after injury.

For the symptomatic patient with established posttraumatic arthritis, arthrodesis or arthroplasty is indicated.[835,864,865,875,910,917] Clendenin and Smith[845,910] suggested that the fifth CMC joint be fused in 20° to 30° of flexion and also that it is not necessary to fuse the adjacent fourth CMC joint if it is not involved. Surprisingly, none of their patients had any limitation of motion, presumably because of compensatory motion in the triquetro-hamate joint.[845] They used a corticocancellous graft carefully fitted into a slot across the joint, with or without Kirschner-wire fixation, similar to the technique described by Joseph and associates.[875]

Arthroplasty of the joint has been advocated by other authors. Black and colleagues[833] prefer simple resection of the impinging osteophytes without any attempt to reduce the subluxated dorsal fragment and shaft. Interposition arthroplasty is favored by others, using either a small Silastic great toe implant[860] or a rolled up tendon (anchovy).[842,855]

Most of the above articles refer to posttraumatic arthrosis in the more commonly injured fourth and fifth CMC joints. Carroll and Carlson[840] reported a series of

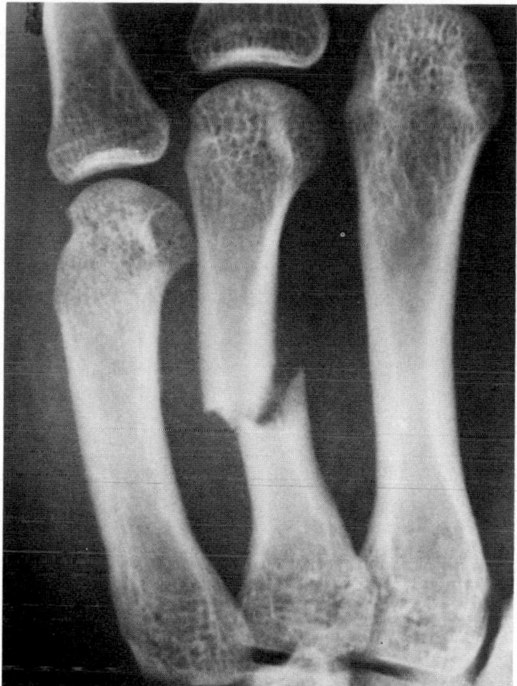

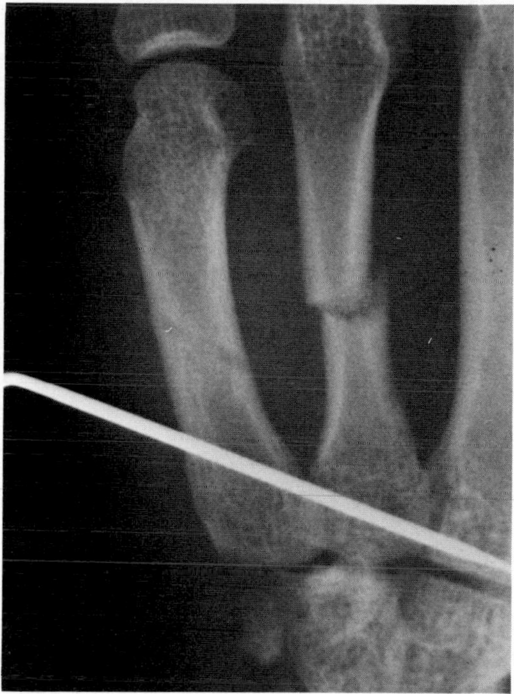

FIGURE 11-116. The major goal in closed reduction and percutaneous pin fixation of fracture-subluxations of the fifth carpometacarpal joint (*left*) is restoration of length; we accept mild incongruities of the articular surface, as shown on the *right*. Note also the angulated fracture of the shaft of the adjacent fourth metacarpal, a concomitant feature also illustrated in Figure 11-114.

patients with chronic injuries of the second and third CMC joints. This diagnosis, which is easy to overlook, was confirmed in their patients by intra-articular injection, and all were treated with arthrodesis of the involved joints. Konsens and Seitz[883] used the same technique in two patients.

THUMB MP JOINT

Anatomy

The MP joint of the thumb is basically a condyloid joint, allowing flexion, extension, abduction, adduction, and a limited amount of rotation.[954] The range of "normal" motion in the MP joint of the thumb varies widely (5° to 115°, according to Palmer and Louis[981]) and appears to be related to the contour of the metacarpal head.[963] Harris and Joseph[958] noted that motion in joints with flat or "flattish" metacarpal heads tends to be considerably limited. Shaw and Morris[998] postulated that MP joints with limited motion are more susceptible to ligament injury.

Coonrad and Goldner's[941] studies revealed that the normal range of abduction-adduction varies from 0° to 20°, with an average of 10° (measured with the joint in 15° of flexion). Mediolateral stability is provided mainly by the collateral ligaments.[1003]

On the ulnar aspect of the joint, the adductor pollicis muscle is inserted partly through the ulnar sesamoid bone into the volar plate and partly through a powerful tendon directly into the proximal phalanx, with additional fibers fusing with the ulnar expansion of the dorsal aponeurosis.[999,1003] This part of the dorsal aponeurosis is called the adductor aponeurosis, and it plays an important role in the pathomechanics of injuries of the UCL. The adductor aponeurosis directly overlies the ligament and must be divided to provide operative exposure of the ligament. Despite some contradictory studies by Kaplan,[964] most authors accept Stener's[1003] findings that passive (static) stability of the joint is provided by the collateral ligament, with the adductor aponeurosis providing active (dynamic) stabilization against violence tending to abduct the thumb.

Ulnar Collateral Ligament Injury or Gamekeeper's Thumb, Skier's Thumb

Mechanism of Injury

A sudden valgus (abduction) stress (probably combined with hyperextension) applied to the MP joint of the thumb results in partial or complete disruption of the UCL and volar plate.[1000] In 1955, Campbell[938] reported that chronic laxity of this ligament can develop without a specific incident of acute trauma, and he found this to be an occupational deformity in the hands of British gamekeepers. Their customary method of killing wounded rabbits was such that, over time, attenuation of the ligament resulted in chronic instability of the joint. Through common usage, the term *gamekeeper's thumb* has come to include any injury of the UCL, although most of these injuries seen are acute injuries rather than the chronic stretching of the ligament reported by Campbell.

Several authors[945,952,975] have suggested that acute injuries of the UCL of the thumb should more properly be called "skier's thumb" because this is probably the most common mechanism of injury and one of the most common ski injuries.[927,940,948,956,1010] Indeed, this injury was reported in the German literature in 1939 to 1940, and *skier's thumb* is the preferred appellation in Europe.[952,1005,1009] The ski pole has been implicated as the causative factor, and the incidence of injury appears to be essentially the same for all types of handles.[940,945,948,974,1010] The type of grip (ie, how or whether the strap is wrapped around the wrist) also does not appear to influence the chances of injury,[1010] although Primiano[984] suggested that if a strapless handle is used, injury is less likely to occur if the pole does not block full flexion of the IP joint. He reasoned that if the tip of the thumb extends beyond the guard on the handle, it may be the point of contact with the ground in a fall.

A special glove has been designed in an effort to protect the UCL.[949]

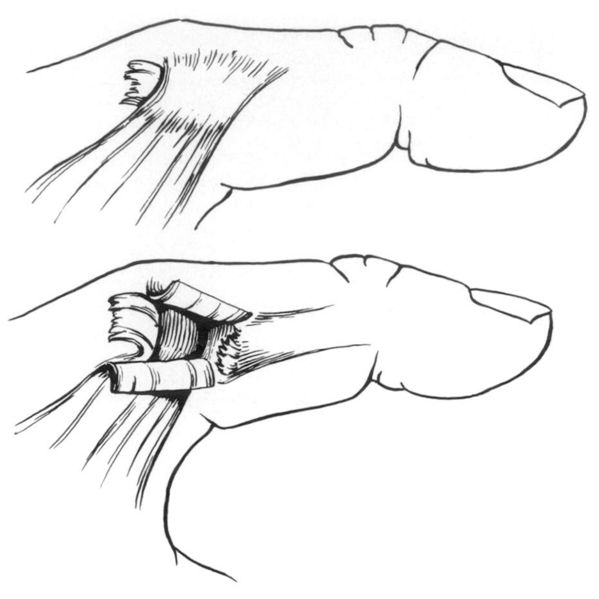

FIGURE 11-117. Stener has described how the ruptured end of the ulnar collateral ligament may become displaced and folded back on itself beneath the proximal edge of the adductor aponeurosis. Because of this frequent finding, most authors favor operative repair of complete rupture of the ulnar collateral ligament. (*Redrawn from Stener, B.: Displacement of the Ruptured Ulnar Collateral Ligament of the Metacarpo-phalangeal Joint of the Thumb. J. Bone Joint Surg. 44B:870, 1962.*)

Stener Lesion

Stener's[1003] important contribution to our understanding of this injury was the recognition that the adductor aponeurosis frequently becomes interposed between the two ends of the torn ligament, thereby preventing adequate healing (Fig. 11-117). The most frequent site of rupture is directly from the distal attachment of the ligament into the proximal phalanx, although interposition may occur even if the ligament is torn through its substance. Stener found this interposition in 25 of his 39 cases, and other authors have reported an incidence of the Stener lesion ranging from 14% to 83%.[967,976,982,1012,1018,1037] Our impression is that the Stener lesion is present in at least 50% of acute ruptures of the UCL.

Diagnosis

Clinical. The patient presents with a painful, swollen MP joint of the thumb. Usually, the point of maximum tenderness can be localized to the ulnar aspect of the joint. Abrahamsson and coworkers[922] suggested that the Stener lesion can be diagnosed on physical examination by palpation of a tender tumor at the level of the UCL just proximal to the MP joint, but Vihtonen and coworkers[1012] concluded that malposition of the end of the ligament could only be diagnosed with certainty at operation.

A particularly important point in the evaluation of these patients is to differentiate a sprain (partial tear) from a rupture (complete tear). The obvious way to do this is to determine the amount of radial deviation produced by abduction stress of the MP joint but this may be more difficult than it sounds. If the joint opens up easily (Fig. 11-118), the diagnosis of rupture is obvious, but pain and muscle spasm may limit passive abduction of the thumb and give a false-negative impression. Unless there is easily demonstrable gross instability, we believe that the abduction stress test should be performed under some type of anesthesia. Most authors‡‡‡ advocate local infiltration of the ligament; others prefer a block of the median and radial nerves at the wrist.[950,976,981] Testing should be done with the MP joint in both flexion and extension, and the opposite thumb should be used for comparison.

‡‡‡ References 931, 959, 965, 973, 981, 982, 995, 996.

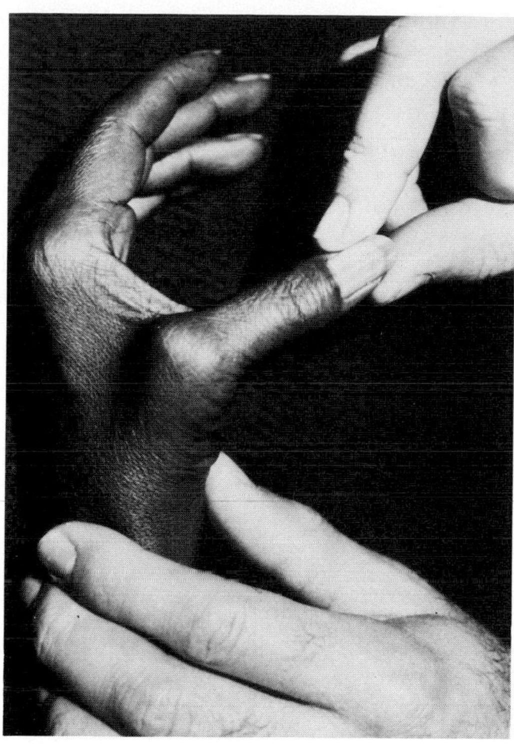

FIGURE 11-118. Valgus stress applied to the metacarpophalangeal joint of the thumb in a patient with complete rupture of the ulnar collateral ligament (so-called gamekeeper's or skier's thumb).

What constitutes an abnormal stress test remains somewhat controversial: Smith[1000] said 45°; Frank and Dobyns[950] and Bowers and Hurst[931] said more than 10° greater than the opposite side; and Palmer and Louis[981] said 35° (tested in full flexion). It may be difficult to measure the angle of abduction clinically, and Bowers and Hurst[931] noted that clinical estimates consistently were 5° to 15° greater than radiographic measurements in their studies. Therefore, if there is any question about the diagnosis, we believe that the stress test should be measured radiographically.

Rupture of the UCL can occur concomitantly with a fracture of the proximal phalanx, making the diagnosis difficult to suspect and even more difficult to confirm by stress examination.[955]

Radiographic. Some authors[950,1004] have suggested that routine x-rays should be made before stressing the joint, to prevent possible displacement of an undisplaced fracture. Three types of avulsion fractures may be seen in the initial films; the most common types are a small fragment pulled away from the base of the proximal phalanx (Fig. 11-119*A*) and a large intra-articular fracture involving one fourth or more of the articular surface of the base of the proximal phalanx (Fig. 11-119*B*). Louis and colleagues[972] have identified a third type of avulsion fracture that is attached not

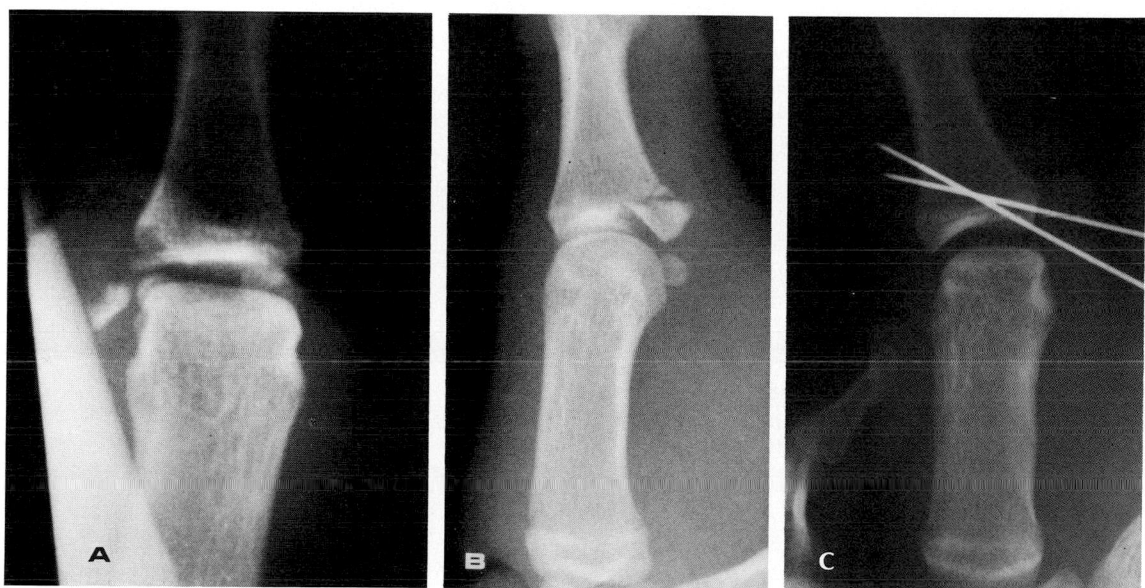

FIGURE 11-119. A gamekeeper's thumb may be associated with an avulsion fracture from the base of the proximal phalanx. This may be a very small fragment (**A**), or a large fragment involving one fourth or more of the articular surface (**B**). Either type, when displaced, requires open reduction. (**C**) A large, displaced fragment avulsed by the ulnar collateral ligament is best treated by open reduction and internal fixation with small, smooth K-wires or an AO minifragment screw. Smaller fragments are sometimes more readily fixed with a pull-out suture. (**A** *from Green, D.P.: Commonly Missed Injuries in the Hand. Am. Fam. Physician 7:118, 1973.*)

to the UCL but to the volar plate. Stothard and Caird's[1006] arthrographic studies showed two fractures that probably represented this type of injury, which is not unstable and can be treated with cast immobilization alone.

Studies of patients with skier's thumb injuries by surgeons in Davos, Switzerland, confirmed Louis and coworkers'[972] findings but identified yet another type of fracture, fragmentation of the volar ulnar portion of the proximal phalanx not attached to either the UCL or the volar plate, seen concomitantly with rupture of the UCL.[962] They concluded that stress x-rays should be taken in all patients having fractures at the base of the proximal phalanx, reasoning that even when the plain films show an undisplaced fracture, it cannot be assumed that the UCL is intact.

Stener and Stener[1004] have stressed the importance of differentiating avulsion and shear fractures (Fig. 11-120). The latter may originate from the *radial* side of the head of the metacarpal and are decidedly less common in our experience than the avulsion fractures, which arise from the ulnar aspect of the base of the proximal phalanx.

If no fracture is seen on the initial x-rays and a clear distinction cannot be made on clinical examination between sprain and rupture or if documentation of the rupture is desired, stress films are indicated. We believe that stress x-rays should be taken, even though Mogan and Davis[975] advised against their use. We agree with Engel and colleagues,[947] who stated that stress views without anesthesia are of questionable value. Bowers and Hurst[931] believe that the incomplete relief of pain provided by local infiltration anesthesia is a safeguard against further disruption of any of the torn structures but we prefer to perform the stress x-rays under median and radial nerve block at the wrist.

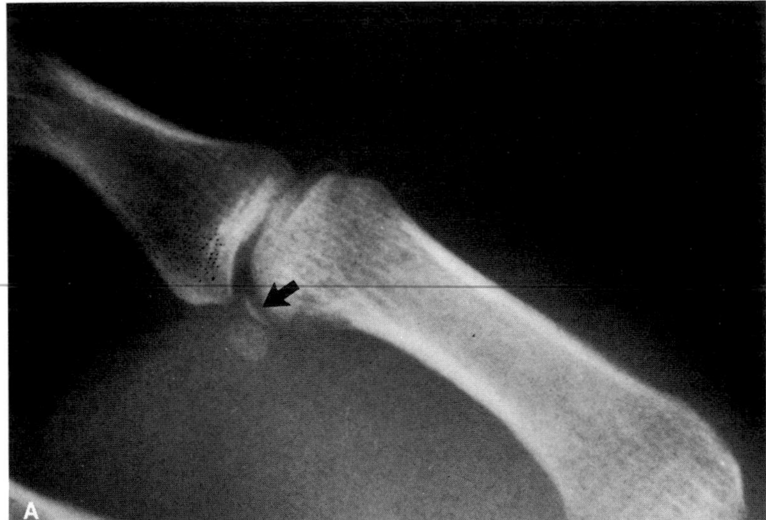

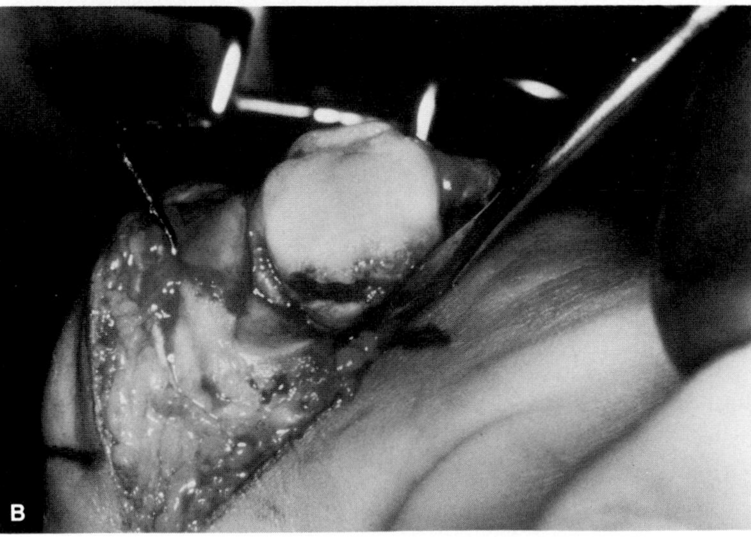

FIGURE 11-120. A shear fracture of the metacarpal head (**A** *arrow*) seen on the x-ray of a patient with a gamekeeper's thumb. These relatively uncommon fractures occur on the radial or volar (**B**) aspect of the metacarpal head and are different from the more typical fracture fragment that is avulsed by the ulnar collateral ligament (see Fig. 11-119).

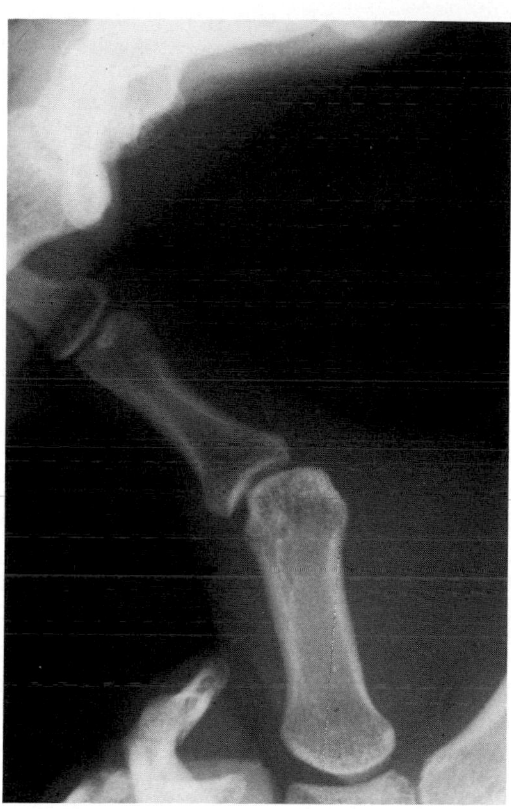

FIGURE 11-121. Routine x-rays of the thumb in a patient with a suspected gamekeeper's thumb may show no abnormality. If the instability is found on clinical examination, stress films should be taken to distinguish between a partial and a complete tear. This patient has a complete tear. Note also that the person stressing the thumb is not wearing leaded gloves, an important omission.

Films are taken with the MP joint in full extension, with radial abduction stress applied to the thumb by the surgeon wearing leaded gloves (Fig. 11-121). To our knowledge, no satisfactory method has yet been described to record radiographically the stress test performed with the MP joint in flexion.

Magnetic Resonance Imaging. With MRI becoming a standard method of identifying torn ligaments in the knee and other joints, it is logical to assume that it may have similar application in the thumb.[971] A cadaver study by Spaeth and coworkers[1002] showed that MRI was only 67% successful in differentiating a torn UCL from a normal ligament, but the technique was 100% sensitive in depicting displacement of a ruptured ligament (ie, the Stener lesion).

The cost of MRI technology is prohibitive for routine use at this time but if the use of more localized techniques can reduce the cost, MRI may become the standard method of identifying Stener lesions in the future.

Ultrasound. Bronstein and coworkers[934] demonstrated that ultrasound could be used to accurately identify artificially created ligament injuries in cadavers, including a simulated Stener lesion. Ultrasound examination cost is about 20% that of MRI and therefore may ultimately be a less expensive method of identifying the Stener lesion, although interpretation of ultrasound images entails skills that are not possessed by most orthopaedists and hand surgeons.

Arthrography. Several authors have attempted to evaluate ruptures of the MP collateral ligaments with arthrograms.[931,947,969,988,989,1014] This is done by injecting 1 to 2 mL of contrast material (1.2 mL 60% Renografin mixed with 0.8 mL 1% lidocaine) into the joint with a tuberculin syringe in the interval between the extensor pollicis brevis and RCL.[931,969] In our opinion, arthrography offers little additional information, unless it can be used to successfully identify the Stener lesion, which several authors have claimed is possible.[931,975,983] There is no question that this specific use of the arthrogram has great merit because it can aid the surgeon in deciding between operative and nonoperative treatment. We agree with other authors, however, who believe that it is difficult to identify the Stener lesion by arthrography with any degree of confidence.[974,1006]

Arthroscopy. Arthroscopy does not appear to have any value in the diagnosis or treatment of injuries of the MP joint collateral ligament but Vaupel and Andrews[1011] reported its use in one case to treat a chondral defect in the base of the proximal phalanx.

Treatment of Acute Injuries

Partial Tears. There is general agreement that partial tears (sprains) of the UCL should be treated nonoperatively. We prefer a well-molded thumb spica cast with the MP joint in slight flexion (hyperextension must be avoided) for 3 to 4 weeks. In a compliant patient, an Orthoplast splint is an acceptable alternative, and Sollerman and coworkers[1001] showed comparable results in patients treated with a cast versus a splint. Their functional splint actually allowed flexion-extension of the MP joint while preventing ulnar and radial deviation.

Rovere and associates[990] described a fiberglass "mini" thumb spica cast, which they used in hockey players, allowing continued participation in the sport. Primiano[985] advocated the use of a modified thumb spica cast that allows full flexion and extension of the wrist, and a similar "glove spica cast" was used for treatment of incomplete ruptures of skier's thumbs in Jackson Hole, Wyoming.[939]

Complete Tears. Since the publication of Stener's[1003] classic article in 1962, there has been increasingly strong support for the operative treatment of all acute ruptures of the UCL of the thumb[950,965,970,973,980,1000] even in the rare case of complete rupture in a child with an open epiphyseal plate.[1013,1015] A variety of techniques have been described for reinsertion of the ligament into bone, including pull-out sutures, direct suture to periosteum with Ethibond,[992] Mitek bone anchors,[930,961,986] and an absorbable polylactide tack.[1012]

Theoretically, a complete rupture without a Stener lesion can be treated satisfactorily nonoperatively, and Coonrad and Goldner[941] advocated cast immobilization for complete ruptures. Pichora and coworkers[983] reported satisfactory outcome in patients (including five thought to have a Stener lesion) treated with functional bracing, although their results are difficult to interpret because the data were reported only in mean values.

Authors' Preferred Method of Treatment

We prefer early operative repair of all acute UCL injuries for several reasons:

1. The Stener lesion is definitely present in numerous cases, and we are not confident that we can differentiate preoperatively the presence or absence of that lesion with any of the available modalities.
2. Operative repair of the acute tear is a relatively uncomplicated procedure having minimal morbidity.
3. As is true in ligamentous injuries in other joints, the results of primary repair are better than with any of the late reconstructive operations.[925,980]

Associated fractures that are also indications for operative treatment in our opinion are (1) a displaced intra-articular corner fracture involving 25% or more of the articular surface at the base of the proximal phalanx, and (2) a small avulsion fracture displaced more than 5 mm. Smith[1000] mentioned that volar subluxation of the proximal phalanx is also an indication for surgery.

Technique of Repair of Acute Rupture of the UCL MP Joint of the Thumb. The skin incision is centered over the dorsoulnar aspect of the MP joint. Gerber and associates[952] recommended a straight longitudinal incision 1 cm ulnar to the extensor pollicis longus tendon, although this can be gently curved. We prefer an elongated chevron incision but the apex of the incision should avoid the transverse skin web to prevent a subsequent scar contracture. Small sensory branches of the radial nerve must be identified and carefully protected throughout the procedure, because postoperative dysesthesia and even painful neuromas can result from scarring or damage of these cutaneous nerves.[945,960,980,993,997,1012] The key to the dissection is the adductor aponeurosis, which may be somewhat obscured by the displaced collateral ligament if a Stener lesion is present (see Fig. 11-117). The adductor aponeurosis is carefully divided a few millimeters from its insertion into the dorsal expansion, taking care to protect both ends for later repair. The joint capsule is exposed by retracting the dorsal and volar flaps of the hood, and the joint itself is inspected for articular damage; the volar plate and accessory collateral ligaments should be inspected also. If the major (cord) portion of the collateral ligament is torn in its substance, it is repaired with nonabsorbable sutures with the joint in 15° to 20° of flexion.

The most common type of pathology is separation of the ligament from the base of the proximal phalanx, with or without a small avulsion fracture. If this is found, the site of attachment of the ligament is roughened with a curet or a shallow groove is created with a rongeur just distal to the rim of articular cartilage at the base of proximal phalanx. The ligament is reattached with a pull-out suture over a button on the radial aspect of the thumb. Although monofilament wire was the traditional material used for pull-out sutures, we prefer 2-0 or 3-0 Prolene because its removal is far less painful for the patient. Also, we prefer to pull the suture out in the direction of its insertion (Fig. 11-122), obviating the need for the additional retrograde strand used with the classic Bunnell pull-out suture technique. The Mitek bone anchor is an acceptable alternative, although it does add extra cost to the operation ($375 charge to the patient in our hospital as of January 1995). If a good repair is achieved, and the joint is stable to gentle stress testing, no K-wire is needed across the joint.

We prefer to excise tiny avulsion fragments, advancing the ligament into the defect in the proximal phalanx, as described earlier for pure avulsion injuries. An alternative for small fragments is tension-band wiring, which avoids the potential problem of intra-operative fragmentation of the fragment (see Tension-Band Wiring).[928,966] Larger fragments should be anatomically reduced and held with 0.028-inch or 0.035-inch K-wires (two wires are usually necessary to prevent rotation) or an AO minifragment screw. The adductor tendon is carefully reattached to the dorsal expansion with 4-0 nonabsorbable sutures. The skin is closed with subcuticular sutures, and a plaster thumb spica splint is applied.

Postoperative Management. At 10 days, the splint and sutures are removed and a thumb spica cast is applied, leaving the IP joint free. The patient must be instructed in active and passive flexion exercises of the distal joint because some stiffness of this joint frequently results from dissection of the extensor hood. At 4 weeks, the cast is removed and flexion-extension exercises are

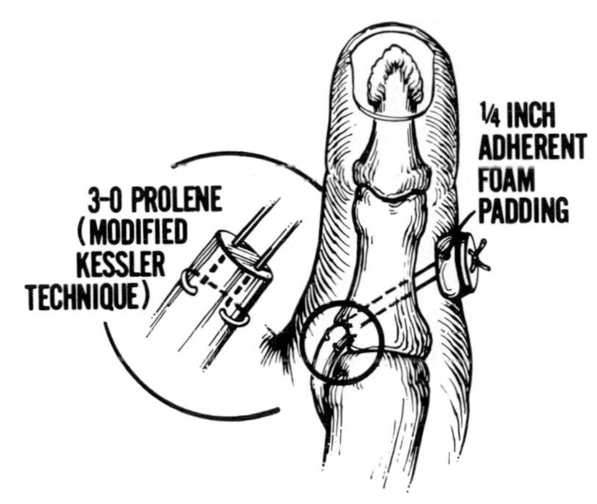

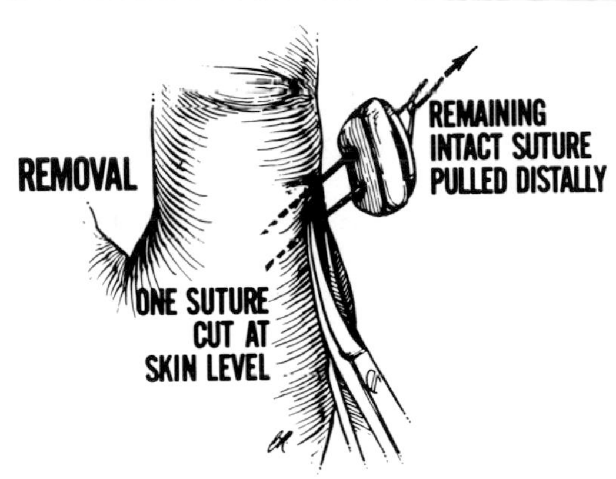

FIGURE 11-122. We prefer this type of pull-out suture over the standard Bunnell pull-out wire. No proximal loop is required because the suture is pulled distally at the time of removal. Removal of Prolene is considerably less painful for the patient than wire. This type of suture is applicable to any situation in which a pull-out suture is required.

instituted for the MP joint; a removable hand-based splint is worn to protect the thumb for an additional 2 to 3 weeks. Forceful stress and participation in strenuous athletic activities without splint protection are not allowed until 10 to 12 weeks after the operation, depending on the mobility of the MP joint and the strength of the thumb.

Bostock and Morris[929] reported no significant loss of MP motion postoperatively but they emphasized the importance of comparing motion with the opposite normal thumb. They did not mention IP motion but we have noted slightly limited IP motion in our patients, presumably due to some adherence of the extensor pollicis tendon.

Treatment of Chronic Injuries

If the patient is seen within 2 to 3 weeks of injury, operative repair can usually be accomplished with a reasonable chance of success. Unfortunately, chronic, untreated injuries of the UCL of the thumb are commonly seen for the first time weeks or months after injury.

Partial Tears. Untreated sprains of the MP collateral ligaments can produce long-term refractory symptoms, which may be difficult to fully alleviate. If there is no evidence of instability on stress examination, we generally treat these patients with cast or splint immobilization (with or without intra-articular steroid injection) for 3 weeks, followed by an intensive course of physical therapy. Perhaps the most important aspect of management of these patients is to make them aware of the chronicity of the problem, emphasizing that it is likely to take several months for their symptoms to subside.

Complete Tears. The patient with an untreated or inadequately treated rupture of the UCL with pain and demonstrable instability of the joint is a candidate for reconstruction because posttraumatic arthritis is likely to develop unless stability is restored. It must be emphasized, however, that no type of soft-tissue reconstruction relieves the patient's pain if posttraumatic arthritis is already established. If preoperative x-rays demonstrate significant arthritic changes or if significant articular damage is seen at operation, arthrodesis of the MP joint is the treatment of choice.[941,950,957,978]

Several operations have been described for late reconstruction of the UCL of the thumb. Alldred[924] used a free tendon graft from the fourth toe that was passed through drill holes in the base of the proximal phalanx and head of the metacarpal. Smith[1000] advocated a more sophisticated free tendon graft reconstruction, emphasizing the importance of correcting the volar subluxation of the proximal phalanx. He did this by making the transverse drill hole in the proximal phalanx volar to the axis of motion, so that the newly created reconstruction of the collateral ligament duplicates the normal ligament by passing distally and volarly from the metacarpal head to the base of the proximal phalanx. Littler's tendon graft technique has been described by Glickel and coworkers,[953] and Sennwald and coworkers[997] reported their results with a modification of Böhler's tendon graft technique. Breek and coworkers[932] used a modification of the palmaris longus graft technique, originally described by Strandell.[1007]

Although Strandell[1007] used a free graft in some cases, he also described a different technique using the extensor pollicis brevis tendon, leaving it attached to its normal insertion and passing the free end through a transverse drill hole in the head of the metacarpal to be reattached to the site of insertion of the original UCL. Frykman and Johansson[951] employed a slip of the abductor pollicis longus in a similar fashion. Sakellarides and DeWeese[993,995] also used the extensor pollicis brevis but with a bit more complicated type of reconstruction, and Ahmad and DePalma[923] reported a single case treated with yet another method of using the extensor pollicis brevis. Lamb and Angarita[968] used the palmaris longus tendon left attached at its distal insertion.

 Authors' Preferred Method

For the past 20 years, one of us has used a slight modification of the operation described by Neviaser and coworkers,[978] and this is our preference for late reconstruction of the UCL of the thumb. Our results[936] with this operation have been satisfactory but are not as predictable nor as uniformly successful as those of primary repair with acute ruptures. Osterman and colleagues[980] reported no functional difference between a free graft and Neviaser's operation but noted slightly less range of motion after the latter.

Modified Neviaser Technique for Late Reconstruction of the UCL MP Joint of the Thumb. The MP joint is exposed through a radially based chevron-type (dorsal zigzag) or gently curved longitudinal incision. The incision must extend far enough volarly to provide good exposure of the adductor tendon but care must be taken to avoid the transverse skin crease of the web to prevent subsequent scar contracture. Mogensen and Mattsson[976] have noted that the dorsal zigzag incision can be extended across the volar aspect of the joint if necessary. The dorsal sensory nerves are identified and carefully protected throughout the procedure. Tears in the capsule and ligaments are usually bridged by scar, and identification of these structures is more difficult than in the acute repair. Dissection is facilitated by identifying the adductor muscle and tracing its tendon distally to its insertion into the dorsal expansion. The adductor tendon is sharply divided a few millimeters from the extensor pollicis longus tendon (Figure 11-123*A*), and a plane is developed between the MP joint capsule and adductor tendon, preserving as much of the latter as possible. The location of the joint line must be identified before developing the capsular flap. This is most easily done by making the dorsal limb of the flap first, along an imaginary line corresponding to the dorsal border of the original UCL. A proximally based U-shaped casuloligamentous flap is then created by sharp dissection of the thickened, scarred remnant of UCL (Fig. 11-123*B*). The flap should conform generally to the original UCL (about 6 to 8 mm wide and 10 to 12 mm in length), based at the metacarpal origin of the ligament.

At this point, it is important to be sure that the flap has a secure attachment to the metacarpal head. Most UCL ligament injuries are avulsions from the base of proximal phalanx, and the metacarpal origin has not been disrupted. In those less common cases in which the injury was an avulsion of the proximal (metacarpal) attachment of the ligament (about 10% to 20% in our experience), the U-shaped capsular flap may have a relatively flimsy attachment to the metacarpal head. Using such a flap is likely to lead to failure, and when this situation is encountered, a free tendon graft operation should be considered instead of trying to reconstruct the UCL from the capsular flap.

The articular surface should also be inspected; if there is significant cartilage damage, an arthrodesis of the joint should be performed.

A narrow trough is created with a small rongeur, paralleling and immediately adjacent to the rim of articular cartilage along the ulnar base of proximal phalanx. If the trough is made slightly more volar than the normal ligament attachment, approximating the capsular flap to bone may help to correct the volar subluxation of proximal phalanx that is usually present in these chronic cases. The correct length of flap and placement of sutures can be determined by pulling the flap distally while the MP joint is held in full extension and maximum ulnar deviation. A modified Kessler-type suture, using 2-0 or 3-0 Prolene, secures a firm grasp of the flap, and the two suture ends are passed through the proximal phalanx. This is most easily done by passing two long Keith needles through the phalanx with a minidriver, entering the bone at the dorsal and volar margins of the trough (Fig. 11-123*C*). With the MP joint held by an assistant in slight flexion and maximum ulnar deviation, the sutures are tied over a foam pad and button (Fig. 11-123*D*). Additional reinforcement of the repair can be accomplished by suturing the flap to adjacent capsule and periosteum; ideally, the volar edge of the flap should be sutured to the volar plate.

The adductor tendon is then sutured directly into the repair site (capsular flap) or adjacent periosteum (Fig. 11-123*E*).

If appropriate tension has been restored in the capsular flap, the joint is stable to gentle stress-testing and a K-wire is neither needed nor recommended.

Postoperative management is identical to that for acute ligament repair.

Radial Collateral Ligament Injury

Injury of the RCL of the MP joint of the thumb is less common than that of the UCL. Perhaps partly for this reason, the injury is frequently not diagnosed early and in our experience, these patients

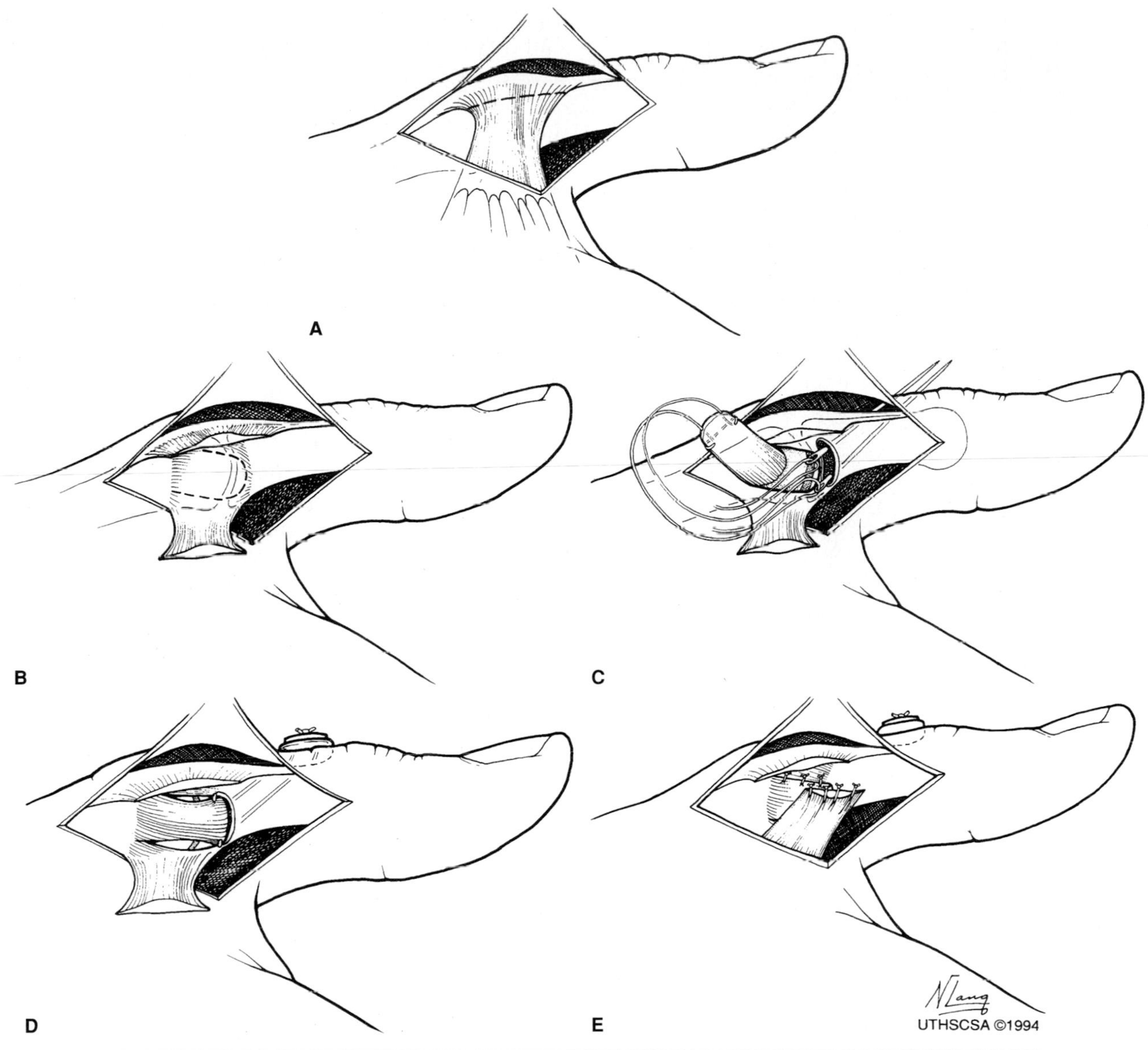

FIGURE 11-123. Modified Neviaser technique[936] for reconstruction of the ulnar collateral ligament. The two main components of the operation are creation of a proximal-based U-shaped flap of capsuloligamentous scar tissue for static support and reattachment of the adductor pollicis tendon for dynamic reinforcement (see text for details).

are almost always seen late. Such patients usually present with a tender prominence of the radial aspect of the metacarpal head (Fig 11-124) and often have pain with activities such as opening a large jar lid or a car door.[937]

Information in the literature is scanty regarding the acute management of such injuries but anatomically, a situation analogous to the Stener lesion cannot exist on the radial side of the thumb. Theoretically, nonoperative treatment (cast immobilization) of a complete rupture of the RCL is more likely to be successful than similar treatment of an UCL rupture. In one of the few collected series of such patients, Woods and coworkers[1017] advised primary repair for complete ruptures but Durham and coworkers[946] showed that the results were almost identical when they compared repair in acute RCL injuries with reconstruction in chronic injuries. Coyle[942] also showed highly successful results from late reconstruction of the RCL. Thus, the case for primary repair of ruptured RCL does not appear to be nearly as strong as the case for primary repair of ruptured UCL.

A capsular flap operation similar to that described

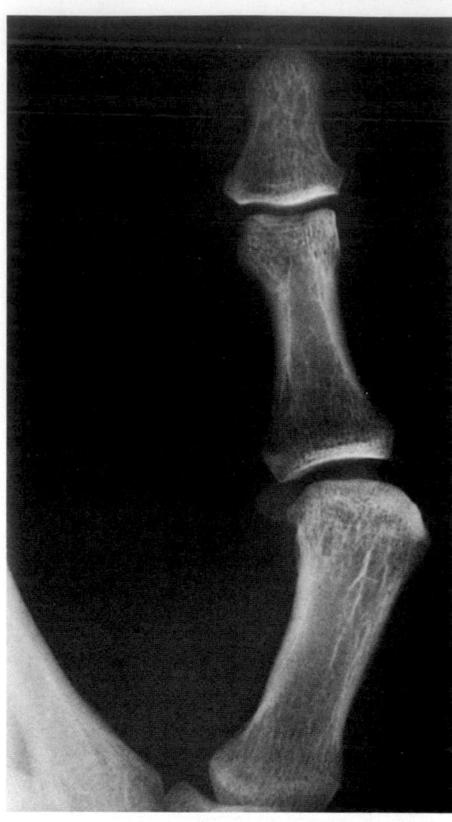

FIGURE 11-124. Patients with late, untreated injuries of the radial collateral ligament of the metacarpophalangeal joint of the thumb usually present with prominence of the radial condyle of the metacarpal.

for the UCL was apparently first suggested for reconstruction of the RCL by Sutro[1008] and advocated by Neviaser and Adams[977] and by Camp and associates.[937] Brewood and Menon[933] have described reconstruction using the extensor pollicis brevis tendon.

Authors' Preferred Method of Treatment

For patients who present acutely with rupture of the RCL, we prefer immobilization in a thumb spica cast for 3 to 4 weeks.

As noted, patients are more likely to present with chronic instability of the RCL. Unless there is gross instability, our initial management usually consists of splinting and often an intra-articular injection of the MP joint. We use a hand-based "mini" thumb spica Orthoplast splint that the patient wears initially full time for several weeks, followed by use during strenuous activity for several more months. Sometimes this results in reduction of symptoms to the point at which the thumb is not particularly bothersome to the patient but if symptoms persist, surgical treatment is advised.

In these patients, we prefer the Neviaser-type capsular flap reconstruction. The operation is performed in identical fashion except that for RCL reconstruction, the abductor pollicis brevis is used instead of the adductor.

Dislocations of the Thumb MP Joint

As in the fingers, dorsal dislocations are more common than volar dislocations in the thumb MP joint. These may be complex (irreducible), usually because of interposition of the volar plate,[1020] although entrapment of the flexor pollicis longus has also been reported.[1025,1033] Ostrowski[1034] reported an unusual irreducible dorsoulnar dislocation.

Volar dislocations seem to be almost always associated with collateral ligament ruptures and appear to be more commonly irreducible due to interposition of the dorsal capsule and one or both extensor tendons.[1024,1030,1032] Less severe dorsal capsular tears, with or without rupture of the extensor pollicis brevis, have also been reported.[1035]

Diagnosis

The most important initial step in management of the dorsal dislocation is to differentiate between a simple and a complex dislocation. As with MP dislocations in the fingers, it is usually possible to make this distinction based on clinical findings rather than to arrive at such a conclusion after repeated unsuccessful attempts at closed reduction. The resting position of the finger offers the first clue. In a simple dislocation (subluxation), the phalanx usually rests on the head of the metacarpal in nearly 90° of hyperextension. In a complex dislocation, the proximal phalanx is more nearly parallel to the metacarpal, with only slight hyperextension. The most important diagnostic clinical sign of a complex dislocation is a skin dimple found on the volar aspect of the thenar eminence (Fig. 11-125). Demonstration on x-ray of a sesamoid within the widened joint space is pathognomonic of a complex dislocation.

Methods of Treatment

Simple dislocations of the MP joint can be reduced easily by closed manipulation; complex dislocations cannot. Even in the presence of the pathognomonic skin dimple, however, we believe that a single attempt at closed reduction under adequate anesthesia should be made in all dorsal dislocations of this joint. McLaughlin[796] emphasized the point originally made

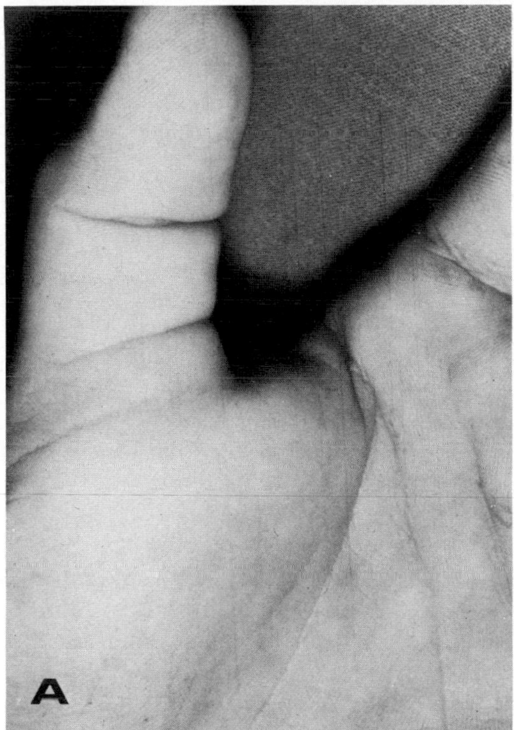

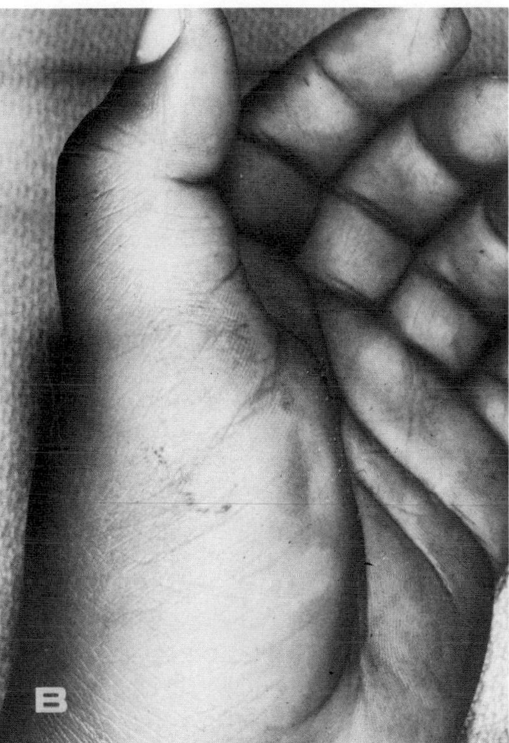

FIGURE 11-125. The most important diagnostic clinical sign of a complex dislocation in the thumb is a skin dimple found on the volar aspect of the thenar eminence. (**A**) This patient had a dislocation of the metacarpophalangeal (MP) joint of the thumb but no skin dimple was present. This was a simple dislocation that was easily reduced by closed manipulation. (**B**) This patient also had a dislocation of the MP joint of the thumb but the characteristic skin dimple was present over the thenar eminence. Closed reduction was unsuccessful and open reduction, which revealed interposition of the volar plate in the joint, confirmed the diagnosis of the complex dislocation.

by Farabeuf[767] that a simple dislocation can be converted into a complex dislocation by improper reduction. Closed reduction should be performed by first hyperextending the proximal phalanx as far as possible on the metacarpal and then *pushing* against the dorsal surface of the base of the phalanx with the IP joint in flexion. The wrist should be flexed to relax the tension on the flexor tendons. Attempting to reduce the deformity by traction and pulling the phalanx back into position may cause the volar plate to become interposed in the joint, thereby rendering it irreducible.

After a successful closed reduction, lateral stability of the joint should be carefully tested to check the integrity of both collateral ligaments. If there is evidence of complete rupture of one of the collateral ligaments, treatment should be directed toward management of this injury.

Usually, the joint is stable after closed reduction, and protected motion can be started almost immediately. Three to 6 weeks of protection with a removable thumb spica splint may minimize the prolonged MP joint soreness that these patients frequently experience. Few authors advocate immediate repair of the volar plate after a successful closed reduction because satisfactory healing usually occurs with adequate immobilization. In rare cases, improper healing of the plate may result in chronic pain, with either instability in hyperextension or flexion contracture from scarring, necessitating late reconstruction (see Volar Plate Injuries).

If closed manipulation of the dorsal dislocation fails, the surgeon should be prepared to follow this with an immediate open reduction. The joint is exposed through a volar or dorsal[765] approach, and the entrapped volar plate is extricated from the joint. The tendon of the flexor brevis may also be interposed, and the head of the metacarpal may be found to protrude through the bellies of the thenar intrinsic muscles. In two cases, we have found the tendon of the flexor pollicis longus wrapped around the neck of the metacarpal. Early protected motion should be instituted postoperatively because stiffness is more common after complex dislocation than it is after a simple dislocation.

Volar Plate Injuries

Relatively little has been written about hyperextension injuries of the MP joint of the thumb.[1031] A classic but somewhat difficult article to understand fully is that written by Stener[1050] in 1963, in which a distinction is made between the passive (volar plate and accessory collateral ligaments) and active (adductor pollicis and flexor pollicis brevis) restraints to hyperextension of the joint. Diagnosis is made by well-localized tenderness over the volar aspect of the joint and excessive hyperextension of the joint. Pain on passive hyperextension is a good diagnostic sign but if pain limits mobility in the joint, the examination must be performed under anesthesia (local infiltration or preferably, median and radial nerve block at the wrist) to obtain a reliable test. Hyperextension should be compared with the opposite uninjured thumb and tested with the IP joint flexed to relax the flexor pollicis longus.

Stener suggested that the position of the sesamoids may aid in differentiating between volar plate rupture and tear of the intrinsic muscles; if the sesamoids are displaced distally with the proximal phalanx on hyperextension stress, muscle tear should be suspected. He recommended that muscle rupture be treated operatively, and did so in three cases.

Yamanaka and colleagues[1040] reported a surprisingly large series of patients with "locking" of the MP joint of the thumb, which they identified as being a different entity from complex MP dislocation. In their 23 patients, the volar plate and radial sesamoid became "hung up" on the more prominent radial condyle of the metacarpal head. In seven patients, successful reduction was achieved by manipulation but 16 required open reduction; they advised a radial mid-lateral approach. Several other reports of locking of the MP joint have appeared, and it is curious that all but one[1019] of these studies have come from Japan.[1026,1028,1039,1046]

Treatment of Acute Injuries

Despite Stener's studies, there appears to be little support for his recommendation of primary repair of acute hyperextension injuries of the thumb. Most of these can probably be treated satisfactorily with thumb spica immobilization for 3 to 4 weeks, holding the MP joint in 15° to 20° flexion.

Treatment of Chronic Injuries

Chronic hyperextension instability of the MP joint of the thumb can cause pain with grasping and pinching. Posner and associates[1036,1037] have pointed out that it is important to differentiate a patient who has passive instability due to chronic volar plate injury from a patient who can actively hyperextend the MP joint voluntarily. The latter individual can stabilize the thumb in flexion when grasping or pinching but the patient with passive instability cannot.

Most patients with volar plate injuries of the MP joint of the thumb (often residual from a dorsal MP dislocation) do not have significant problems, although mild to moderate symptoms may persist for several months. Occasionally, a patient is seen who does have a painful or functional problem from chronic volar plate instability. Although this is a relatively uncommon entity, operative treatment may be required if the patient does not respond to nonoperative modalities (splinting, anti-inflammatory medications, and local injections).

Methods of Treatment. In some patients, it may be possible to simply reattach the volar plate (usually torn from its metacarpal neck origin), as suggested by Ishizuki and coworkers,[1046] although that which they referred to as reattachment is probably the same as that termed capsulodesis by other authors. Milch[1029] in 1929 was probably the first to suggest late repair of the volar plate for hyperextension instability but various techniques have been described for capsulodesis to correct MP joint hyperextension due to other causes (in the cerebral palsy patient by Filler and coworkers[1023] and in degenerative arthritis by Eaton and Floyd[1021]).

We have used Zancolli's[1041] procedure, although this is technically more difficult in the thumb than in the finger MP joints because of the large sesamoids in the thumb. To achieve maximum strength with the Zancolli technique, it is important to anchor the proximal end of the volar plate into bone with a pull-out suture but this may be difficult because of the larger sesamoids, which fill most of the volar plate, leaving little soft tissue with which to work. A modification of that technique is to denude the articular cartilage from the sesamoids and create a surgical synostosis between the sesamoids and the metacarpal neck. Schuurman and Bos[1038] reported satisfactory results with Filler's[1023] technique but they also commented that the operation was not easy.

Because of the technical difficulties in performing a volar capsulodesis, other authors have chosen to create a check-rein on the volar aspect of the MP joint by other means. Kessler[1027] constructed a criss-cross sling across the volar aspect of the MP joint, using the full length of the extensor pollicis brevis tendon (left attached at its insertion). Eiken[1022] used the palmaris longus tendon left attached at its insertion and passed along the volar aspect of the thumb to the base of the proximal phalanx. Posner and associates[1036] have treated this problem with a 1.5-cm advancement of the insertion of the conjoined tendon of the abductor pollicis brevis and flexor pollicis brevis, which may have the added advantage of providing dynamic resistance against hyperextension.

Arthrodesis is a reliable salvage procedure for the painful MP joint, especially if arthritic changes are present.

 Authors' Preferred Method of Treatment

Technique of Thumb MP Volar Capsulodesis. Indications for operative treatment in chronic MP joint instability are uncommon, and we have operated on only about a dozen such patients over a 25-year period. The joint is approached through a volar zigzag (Bruner) incision. The flexor sheath is incised longitudinally after first carefully identifying and gently retracting the neurovascular bundles, and the flexor pollicis longus tendon is retracted to expose the volar plate. Usually, the volar plate has been avulsed from its proximal (metacarpal neck) origin and if there is a secure attachment to the base of proximal phalanx, our first choice is to perform a capsulodesis. The volar plate is mobilized by incising along its lateral margins; if there is sufficient substance of the plate to advance it into a narrow trough in the neck of metacarpal, that is done with 2-0 or 3-0 Prolene, using a pull-out technique similar to that described for UCL reconstruction. If the soft-tissue portion of the volar plate is deficient, our next choice is to create a sesamoid-metacarpal synostosis by approximating the denuded sesamoids and the neck of metacarpal with K-wires or AO minifragment screws.

If good approximation of the volar plate (or sesamoids) to the metacarpal cannot be accomplished, we would abandon the capsulodesis and perform Posner and associates' advancement of the conjoined tendon.[1037]

Sesamoid Fractures

Fractures of the sesamoids are uncommon but need to be considered in the differential diagnosis of injuries of the MP joint of the thumb. Most people have five sesamoids in each hand: two at the thumb MP joint, one at the thumb IP joint, and one each at the MP joints of the index and little fingers.[1053] Although the latter three may occasionally be absent, the two thumb MP sesamoids are present in virtually 100% of the population and in this location they reside within the volar plate.[776,1053] The tendon of the adductor pollicis inserts into the ulnar sesamoid, and the tendon of the flexor pollicis brevis into the radial sesamoid.[1048] The flexor pollicis longus tendon passes between the two sesamoids, and the two bones may provide a static stabilizing force for the tendon.[1044] Bipartite sesamoids have been reported and should be differentiated from fractures.[1045,1049]

Sesamoids can apparently be fractured by direct trauma,[1044,1049] hyperextension,[1042,1046,1050] and possibly twisting injury.[1045] Separation of the fracture fragments implies disruption of the volar plate, as Stener[1050] noted, and has been demonstrated by arthrography.[1042]

The ulnar sesamoid is usually seen on the routine PA radiograph of the hand because the thumb is partially pronated in this view. A special view (Fig. 11-126) is required to profile the radial sesamoid.[1052]

Although Stener[1050] advocated surgical repair of sesamoid fractures, virtually all the case reports in the literature have been treated with simple immobilization for 3 to 5 weeks.### Most have had a satisfactory outcome but there is at least one report of a nonunion.[178]

Posttraumatic arthritis can occur between the sesamoids and the condyles of the metacarpal head (85% involving the radial sesamoid). In the only large series of such patients, there is no indication as to how many of these were preceded by a fracture of the sesamoid, although most of the patients had a history of either hyperextension or crush injuries of the thumb.[1052] In this series, Trumble and Watson[1052] treated symptomatic patients with excision of the involved sesamoid.

THUMB CMC JOINT

Anatomy

The CMC joint of the thumb is classically described as a saddle joint, although Eaton and Littler[1062] have noted that it is actually formed by two apposing saddles. The base of the first metacarpal is convex in the transverse (radioulnar) plane and concave in the vertical (dorsovolar) plate; the trapezium is concave in the transverse plane and convex in the vertical plane. The volar lip of the metacarpal is somewhat elongated, providing attachment for the volar (anterior oblique) ligament to the tubercle of the trapezium.

Littler[1074] reminded us that a remarkably accurate description of the ligaments at the base of the thumb was published in 1742 by Weitbrecht and subsequently translated into English by Kaplan.[1087] Most anatomists have accepted Pieron's[1080] description of four main ligaments supporting this joint: (1) anterior oblique ligament (AOL); (2) dorsoradial ligament (DRL); (3) posterior oblique ligament (POL); and (4) intermetacarpal ligament (IML) (Fig.11-127). Despite several scholarly studies, there is disagreement concerning which of these are most important, and the ligamentous anatomy of this joint remains somewhat

References 1042, 1043, 1045, 1047, 1049, 1051.

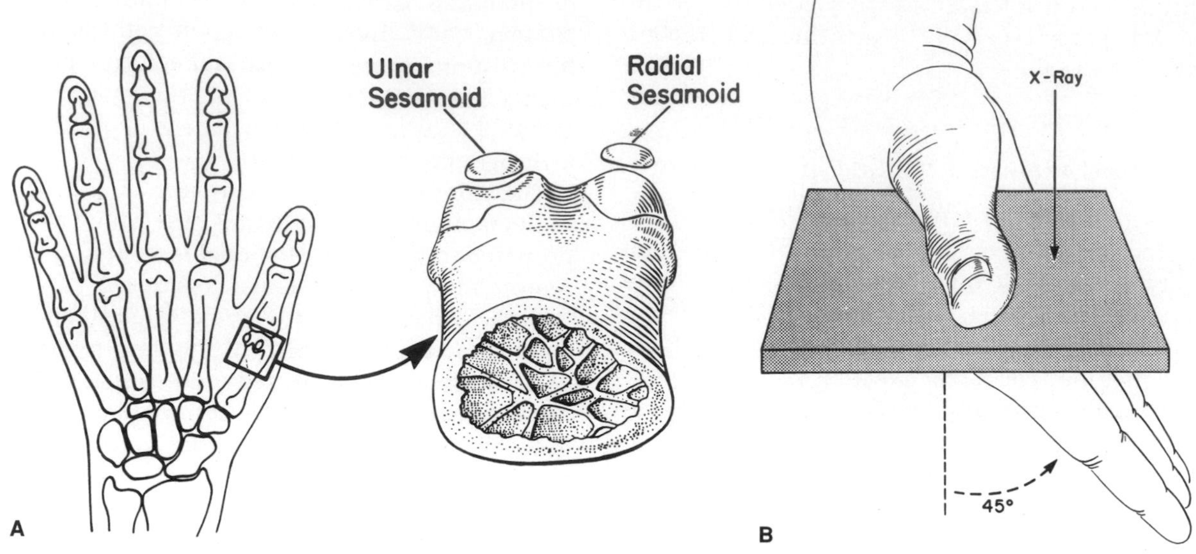

FIGURE 11-126. The radial sesamoid at the metacarpophalangeal level of the thumb (**A**) is not seen in routine x-rays but this view suggested by Trumble and Watson (**B**) profiles the joint between the radial sesamoid and metacarpal head. (*Trumble, T.E., and Watson, H.K. Posttraumatic Sesamoid Arthritis of the Metacarpophalangeal Joint of the Thumb. J. Hand Surg. 10A:94–100, 1985.*)

confusing, at least partly because of differences in terminology.**** Although most authors seem to consider the AOL to be the key structure maintaining thumb stability, others have concluded that the most important structure is the IML or the dorsoradial ligament.[1055,1062,1067,1079,1083]

The capsular and ligamentous attachments of the joint are relatively lax, allowing rotation of the thumb metacarpal on the trapezium. Rotation is blocked when the two saddles are tightly apposed to each other. The ligaments allow sufficient distraction of the two surfaces to permit rotation, while at the same time becoming taut enough in this elongated position to guide and limit axial rotation.[1071]

A true AP view (Robert view)[1073] is necessary to show the CMC joint adequately; it is taken with the hand in maximum pronation (Fig. 11-128).

**** References 1055, 1056, 1064, 1067, 1071, 1074, 1078, 1080, 1083.

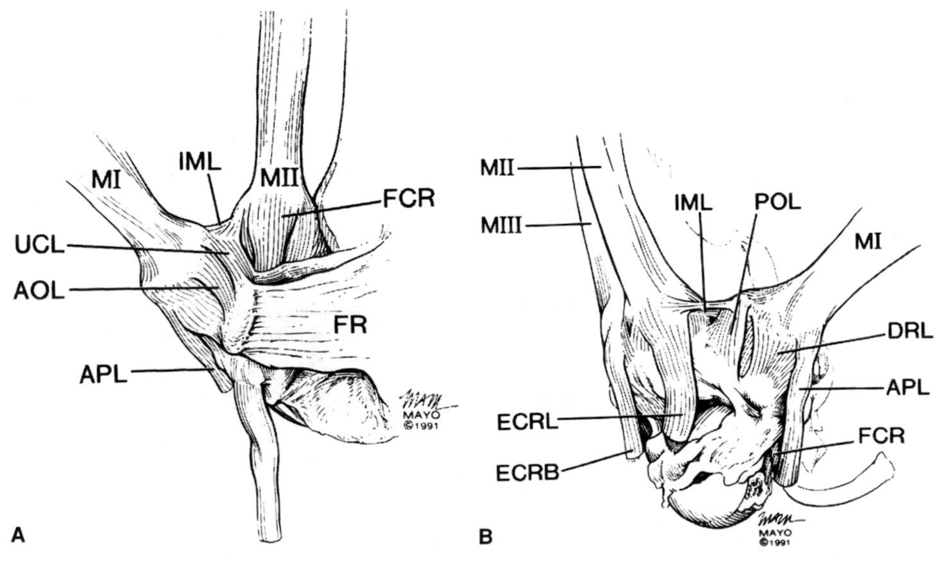

FIGURE 11-127. Palmar (**A**) and dorsal (**B**) line drawings of the basal joint of the thumb. The important ligaments include the anterior oblique ligament (*AOL*); dorsoradial ligament (*DRL*); posterior oblique ligament (*POL*); and first intermetacarpal ligament (*IML*). (*By permission of Mayo Clinic/Mayo Foundation. Imaeda, T., An, K., Cooney, W.P. III, and Linscheid, R. Anatomy of Trapeziometacarpal Ligaments J. Hand Surg. 18A:226–231, 1993.*)

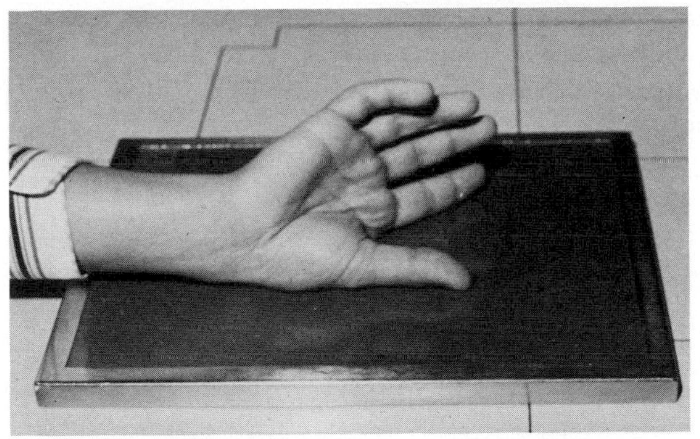

FIGURE 11-128. A true anteroposterior view (Robert view) is necessary to adequately show the carpometacarpal joint of the thumb. It is taken with the hand in extreme pronation.

Dislocation

Mechanism of Injury

Pure dislocations of the CMC joint of the thumb are uncommon. The mechanism appears to be a longitudinally directed force with the metacarpal in slight flexion, allowing the base of the metacarpal to be levered out in a dorsoradial direction. Johnson and coworkers[1069] suggested that motorcyclists are particularly prone to sustain this injury. Three of 12 individuals involved in motorcycle accidents in a single year were found to have dislocations of the CMC joint of the thumb, in all of whom the diagnosis was missed initially. They postulated the mechanism to be the handlebar driven into the first web space. The message here seems to be clear: signs of this injury should be sought in the motorcycle rider who is admitted with multiple trauma.

Because of the strong attachment of the AOL (and probably also the IML), an injury to this joint is most likely to fracture the volar beak of the metacarpal, resulting in a Bennett's fracture-subluxation of the joint. Other variants are dislocation of the joint in association with a fracture of the trapezium[1076,1084] and a concomitant fracture of the base of the second metacarpal (avulsed by the IML).[557] In the less common pure dislocation of the CMC joint, a tiny fragment of bone may be avulsed off the base of the metacarpal by the AOL.[1085,1086] These are usually isolated injuries but there have been case reports of simultaneous dislocation of the CMC and MP joints of the thumb.[1066,1077]

Treatment of Acute Injury

A pure dislocation of the CMC joint of the thumb without associated fracture (Fig. 11-129) is a deceptively difficult injury to treat. Closed reduction is simple but may be unstable. Even when the joint is temporarily stabilized after reduction with percutaneous pin fixation, the results are not entirely predictable, and residual subluxation or frank dislocation may recur after removal of the pins.

The unpredictable and often poor results with closed reduction led Burkhalter[1058] to explore surgically several of these injuries acutely in an effort to more clearly understand the pathologic anatomy. Similar to other authors who have operated on these injuries, he found that the volar ligament was intact.[1070,1081,1086] Burkhalter further noted that a sleeve of periosteum was present and that hyperpronation of the thumb metacarpal reduced the bone into this periosteal tube. These observations were later corroborated by Strauch and coworkers.[1083] Concluding that supination was an important element in the mechanism of injury, Burkhalter treated several subsequent patients with hyperpronation of the joint combined with percutaneous pin fixation for 6 weeks.

If Burkhalter's observations are correct and the volar ligament is intact, open reduction would not appear to offer any particular advantage, except perhaps in the rare situation of simultaneous MP and CMC dislocation, as reported by Moore and associates.[1077]

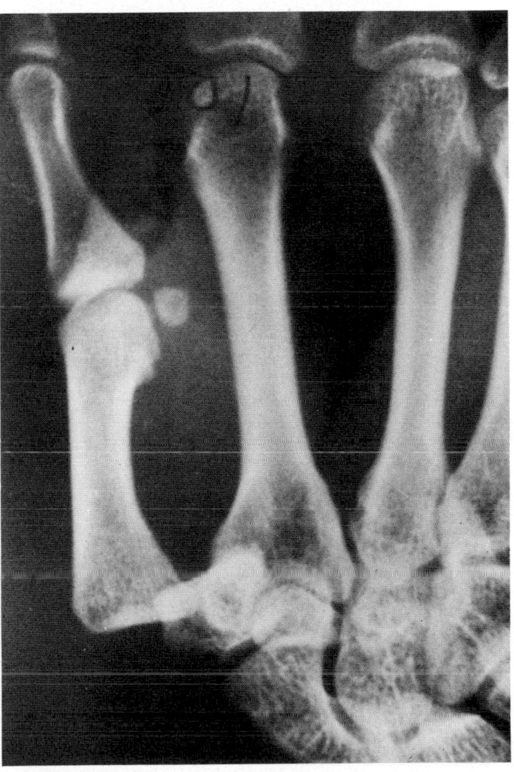

FIGURE 11-129. A pure dislocation of the carpometacarpal joint of the thumb without associated fracture is an uncommon injury. Closed reduction is easily achieved but extremely unstable.

In the largest series of these injuries reported (12 patients), Watt and Hooper[1085] found that closed reduction and cast immobilization were successful in some cases. They noted the importance of assessing stability of the joint immediately after reduction and of using a thumb spica cast alone only if the joint is stable. In their series, the best results were achieved in those patients treated on the day of injury.

Authors' Preferred Method of Treatment

Our experience with this uncommon injury is limited but based on Burkhalter's observations, our preference is closed reduction with the thumb hyperpronated, supplemented with percutaneously placed K-wires. A thumb spica cast is worn for 4 weeks, at which time the pins are removed but the joint is protected for 8 to 10 weeks.

Treatment of Chronic Injuries

In managing chronic subluxation of the CMC joint of the thumb, the surgeon should differentiate between posttraumatic and idiopathic subluxation. The latter, seen primarily in women and associated with degenerative arthritis, is far more common than instability of the joint resulting from a single traumatic episode, which is seen predominantly in men.

Chronic posttraumatic instability of the basilar joint of the thumb is so uncommon that virtually everything in the literature regarding treatment is in the form of single case reports. Attempts to stabilize the joint with various forms of free tendon grafts and tenodesis have been reported by Brunelli and associates,[1057] Slocum,[1082] Eggers,[1063] Kestler,[1070] Cho,[1060] and Jensen.[1068] The only technique that has been reported with any reasonably adequate number of patients and follow-up is that described by Eaton and Littler,[1062] although even in their series most of the patients had

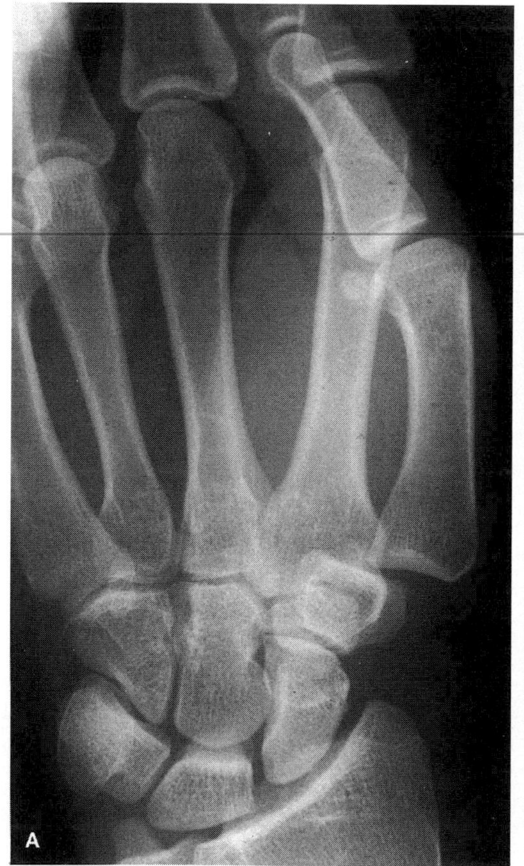

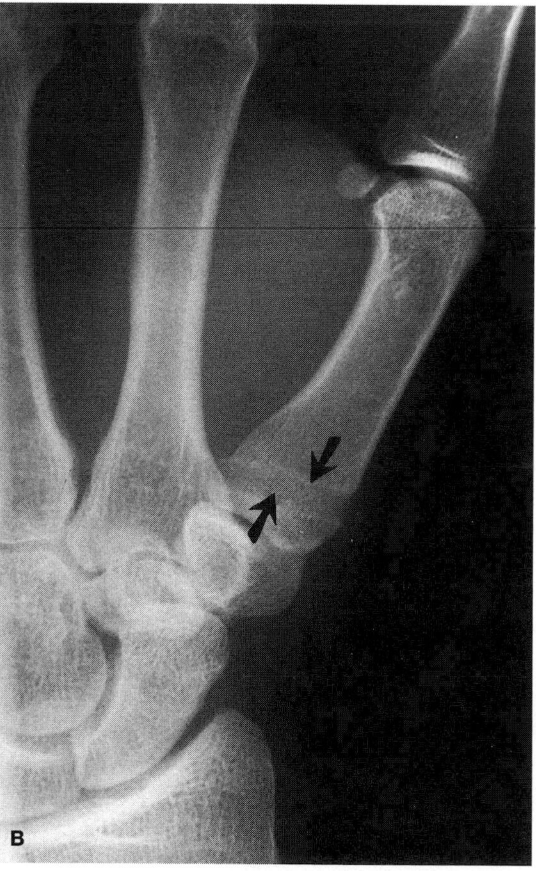

FIGURE 11-130. Residual instability of the basal joint of the thumb 1 week after a pure dislocation of the joint in an NBA basketball player (**A**). The joint could be subluxated easily (and painfully) in and out of place. After reconstruction using the Eaton-Littler technique, he returned to full competition with no protection needed for the thumb. In (**B**), *arrows* mark the path of the flexor carpi radialis tendon through the metacarpal.

the idiopathic degenerative type of subluxation. Other authors[1059,1085] have reported successful treatment of chronic CMC dislocations using this method of stabilizing the joint with a strip of flexor carpi radialis tendon, and Magnusson and associates[1075] have described a slight modification of the Eaton and Littler procedure.

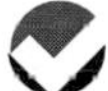

Authors' Preferred Method of Treatment

Because of the relatively rarity of this injury, we have minimal experience with late reconstruction of the CMC joint for chronic instability. Figure 11-130 shows the use of the Eaton-Littler type of reconstruction in a professional basketball player, suggesting that this operation can provide joint stability that appears to be both strong and durable.

It must be emphasized that if significant arthritis is present in the CMC joint, no type of tendon reconstruction procedure is likely to be successful, and arthroplasty or arthrodesis of the joint should be considered.

REFERENCES

ANATOMY

1. Allen, E.V.: Thromboangiitis Obliterans: Methods of Diagnosis of Chronic Occlusive Arterial Lesions Distal to the Wrist With Illustrative Cases. Am. J. Med. Sci. 178:237–244, 1929.
2. Cleland, J.: On the Cutaneous Ligaments of the Phalanges. J. Anat. Physiol. 12:526, 1878.
3. Eaton, R.G.: Joint Injuries of the Hand. Springfield, Ill., Charles C. Thomas, 1971.
4. Eyler, D.L., and Markee, J.F.: The Anatomy and Function of the Intrinsic Musculature of the Fingers. J. Bone Joint Surg. 36A:1–9,18–20, 1954.
5. Flatt, A.E.: The Care of Minor Hand Injuries, pp. 15–16. St. Louis, C.V. Mosby, 1959.
6. Gad, P.: The Anatomy of the Volar Part of the Capsules of the Finger Joints. J. Bone Joint Surg. 49B:362–367, 1967.
7. Goss, C.M.: Gray's Anatomy, 26th Ed, pp. 322–325,371–372. Philadelphia, Lea & Febiger, 1954.
8. Grayson, J.: The Cutaneous Ligaments of the Digits. J. Anat. 75:164–165, 1941.
9. Haines, R.W.: The Extensor Apparatus of the Finger. J. Anat. 85:251–259, 1951.
10. Kaplan, E.B.: Functional and Surgical Anatomy of the Hand, 2nd Ed, Philadelphia, J.B. Lippincott, 1965.
11. Kuczynski, K.: The Proximal Interphalangeal Joint: Anatomy and Causes of Stiffness in the Fingers. J. Bone Joint Surg. 50B:656–663, 1968.
12. Landsmeer, J.M.F.: Anatomical and Functional Investigations of the Human Finger, and Its Functional Significance. Acta Anat. [Suppl.] 24:1–69, 1955.
13. Milford, L.W.: Retaining Ligaments of the Digits of the Hand. Gross and Microscopic Anatomic Study. Philadelphia, W.B. Saunders, 1968.
14. Smith, R.J.: Non-ischemic Contractures of the Intrinsic Muscles of the Hand. J. Bone Joint Surg. 53A:1313–1331, 1971.
15. Tubiana, R.: and Valentin, P.: The Anatomy of the Extensor Apparatus of the Fingers. Surg. Clin. North Am. 44:897–918, 1964.

FRACTURES OF THE PHALANGES AND METACARPALS (EXCLUDING THE THUMB)

16. Abdon, P., Muhlow, A., Stigsson, L., Thorngren, K.G., and Werner, C.O.: Subcapital Fractures of the Fifth Metacarpal Bone. Arch. Orthop. Trauma Surg. 103:231–234, 1984.
17. Agee, J.: Treatment Principles for Proximal and Middle Phalangeal Fractures. Orthop. Clin. North Am. 23:35–40, 1992.
18. Alexander, H., Langrana, N., Massengill, J.B., and Weiss, A.B.: Development of New Methods for Phalangeal Fracture Fixation. J. Biomech. 14:377–387, 1981.
19. Arafa, M., Haines, J., Noble, J., and Carden, D.: Immediate Mobilization of Fractures of the Neck of the Fifth Metacarpal. Injury, 17:277–278, 1986.
20. Ashkenaze, D.M., and Ruby, L.K.: Metacarpal Fractures and Dislocations. Orthop. Clin. North Am. 23:19–33, 1992.
21. Ashmead, D. IV., Rothkopf, D.M., Walton, R.L., and Jupiter, J.B.: Treatment of Hand Injuries by External Fixation. J. Hand Surg. 17A:956–964, 1992.
22. Barton, N.: Conservative Treatment of Articular Fractures in the Hand. J. Hand Surg. 14A:386–390, 1989.
23. Barton, N.: Internal Fixation of Hand Fractures (Editorial). J. Hand Surg. 14B:139–141, 1989.
24. Barton, N.J.: Fractures of the Shafts of the Phalanges of the Hand. Hand 11:119–133, 1979.
25. Barton, N.J.: Fractures of the Hand (Review Article). J. Bone Joint Surg. 66B:159–167, 1984.
26. Bauer, A.R. Jr., and Yutani, D.: Computed Tomographic Localization of Wooden Foreign Bodies in Children's Extremities. Arch. Surg. 118:1084–1086, 1983.
27. Behrens, F.: General Theory and Principles of External Fixation. Clin. Orthop. 241:15–23, 1989.
28. Belpomme, C.: External Osteosynthesis of Distal Fractures of the Phalanges by Reposition-fixation of the Fingernail. Int. Surg. 60:219–222, 1975.
29. Belsky, M.R., Eaton, R.G., and Lane L.B.: Closed Reduction and Internal Fixation of Proximal Phalangeal Fractures. J. Hand Surg. 9A:725–729, 1984.
30. Belsole, R.: Physiological Fixation of Displaced and Unstable Fractures of the Hand. Orthop. Clin. North Am. 11:393–404, 1980.
31. Berkman, E.F., and Miles, G.H.: Internal Fixation of Metacarpal Fractures Exclusive of the Thumb. J. Bone Joint Surg. 25:816–821, 1943.
32. Billings, J.B., Zimmerman, M.C., Aurori, B., Parsons, J.R., and Swan, K.G.: Gunshot Wounds to the Extremities. Experience of a Level I Trauma Center. Orthop. Rev. 20:519–524, 1991.
33. Bilos, Z.J.: Compression Pin Fixation of Articular Phalangeal Fractures. Orthop. Rev. 12:125–127, 1983.
34. Bilos, Z.J., and Eskestrand, T.: External Fixator Use in Comminuted Gunshot Fractures of the Proximal Phalanx. J. Hand Surg. 4:357–359, 1979.
35. Bischoff, R., Buechler, U., De Roche, R., and Jupiter, J.: Clinical Results of Tension Band Fixation of Avulsion Fractures of the Hand. J. Hand Surg. 19A:1019–1026, 1994.
36. Black, D.M., Mann, R.J., Constine, R., and Daniels, A.U.: Comparison of Internal Fixation Techniques in Metacarpal Fractures. J. Hand Surg. 10A:466–472, 1985.
37. Black, D.M., Mann, R.J., Constine, R.M., and Daniels, A.U.: The Stability of Internal Fixation in the Proximal Phalanx. J. Hand Surg. 11A:672–677, 1986.
38. Blalock, H.S., Pearce, H.L., Kleinert, H., and Kutz, J.: An Instrument Designed to Help Reduce and Percutaneously Pin Fractured Phalanges. J. Bone Joint Surg. 57A:792–794, 1975.
39. Bloem, J.J.A.M.: The Treatment and Prognosis of Uncomplicated Dislocated Fractures of the Metacarpals and Phalanges. Arch. Chir. Neerlandicum 23:55–65, 1971.
40. Bohler, L.: The Treatment of Fractures, pp. 98–104. Vienna, Wilhelm Maudrich, 1929.
41. Bohler, L.: The Treatment of Fractures, 5th Ed, pp. 898–971. New York, Grune & Stratton, 1956.

42. Borden, J.: Complications of Fractures and Ligamentous Injuries of the Hand. Orthop. Rev. 1:29–38, 1972.
43. Borgeskov, S.: Conservative Therapy for Fractures of the Phalanges and Metacarpals. Acta Chir. Scand. 133:123–130, 1967.
44. Bosscha, K., and Snellen, J.P.: Internal Fixation of Metacarpal and Phalangeal Fractures With AO Minifragment Screws and Plates: A Prospective Study. Injury 24:166–168, 1993.
45. Bostman, O.M.: Absorbable Implants for the Fixation of Fractures. J. Bone Joint Surg. 73A:148–153, 1991.
46. Bosworth, D.M.: Internal Splinting of Fractures of the Fifth Metacarpal. J. Bone Joint Surg. 19:826–827, 1937.
47. Botelheiro, J.C.: Overlapping of Fingers due to a Malunion of a Phalanx Corrected by a Metacarpal Rotational Osteotomy—Report of Two Cases. J. Hand Surg. 10B:389–390, 1985.
48. Botte, M.J., Davis, J.L.W., Rose, B.A., et al.: Complications of Smooth Pin Fixation of Fractures and Dislocations in the Hand and Wrist. Clin. Orthop. 276:194–201, 1992.
49. Boulas, H.J., Herren, A., and Büchler, U.: Osteochondral Metatarsophalangeal Autografts for Traumatic Articular Metacarpophalangeal Defects: A Preliminary Report. J. Hand Surg. 18A:1086–1092, 1993.
50. Boyes, J.H.: Bunnell's Surgery of the Hand, 3rd Ed. Philadelphia, J.B. Lippincott, 1956.
51. Boyes, J.H.: Bunnell's Surgery of the Hand, 4th Ed. Philadelphia, J.B. Lippincott, 1964.
52. Boyes, J.H.: Bunnell's Surgery of the Hand, 5th Ed. Philadelphia, J.B. Lippincott, 1970.
53. Boyes, J.H., Wilson, J.N., and Smith, J.W.: Flexor Tendon Ruptures in the Forearm and Hand. J. Bone Joint Surg. 42A:637–646, 1960.
54. Brefort, G., Condamine, J.L., and Aubriot, J.H.: Functional Results of Seventy-Six Cases of Phalangeal and Metacarpal Fractures Studied Using a Hand Emergency Computer Card System. Ann. Chir. 5:25–35, 1986.
55. Brennwald, J.: Bone Healing in the Hand. Clin. Orthop. 214:7–10, 1987.
56. Brown, H.: Closed Crush Injuries of the Hand and Forearm. Orthop. Clin. North Am. 1:253–259, 1970.
57. Brunet, M.E., and Haddad, R.J.: Fractures and Dislocations of the Metacarpals and Phalanges. Clin. Sports Med. 5:773–781, 1986.
58. Buchler, U., and Fischer, T.: Use of a Minicondylar Plate for Metacarpal and Phalangeal Periarticular Injuries. Clin. Orthop. 214:53–58, 1987.
59. Bunnell, S.: Surgery of the Hand. Philadelphia, J.B. Lippincott, 1944.
60. Burkhalter, W.E.: Closed Treatment of Hand Fractures. J. Hand Surg. 14A:390–393, 1989.
61. Burkhalter, W.E., Butler, B., Metz, W., and Omer, G.: Experiences With Delayed Primary Closure of War Wounds of the Hand in Viet Nam. J. Bone Joint Surg. 50A:945–954, 1968.
62. Burkhalter, W.E., and Reyes, F.A.: Closed Treatment of Fractures of the Hand. Bull. Hosp. Jt. Dis. 44:145–162, 1984.
63. Burnham, P.J.: Physiological Treatment for Fractures of the Metacarpals and Phalanges. J.A.M.A. 169:663–666, 1959.
64. Burton, R.I., and Eaton, R.G.: Common Hand Injuries in the Athlete. Orthop. Clin. North Am. 4:809–838, 1973.
65. Bury, T.F., Stassen, L.P.S., and Van der Werken, C.: Repair of the Proximal Interphalangeal Joint With a Homograft. J. Hand Surg. 14A:657–658, 1989.
66. Butt, W.D.: Rigid Wire Fixation of Fractures of the Hand. Henry Ford Hosp. Bull. 4:134–143, 1956.
67. Butt, W.D.: Fractures of the Hand: I. Description. Can. Med. Assoc. J. 86:731–735, 1962.
68. Butt, W.D.: Fractures of the Hand: II. Statistical Review. Can. Med. Assoc. J. 86:775–779, 1962.
69. Butt, W.D.: Fractures of the Hand: III. Treatment and Results. Can. Med. Assoc. J. 86:815–822, 1962.
70. Caffee, H.H.: Atraumatic Placement of Kirschner Wires. Plast. Reconstr. Surg. 63:433–1979, 1994.
71. Campbell Reid, D.A.: Corrective Osteotomy in the Hand. Hand 6:50–57, 1974.
72. Carneiro, R.S., Okunski, W.J., and Heffernan, A.H.: Detection of a Relatively Radiolucent Foreign Body in the Hand by Xerography. Plast. Reconstr. Surg. 59:862–863, 1977.
73. Carr, R.W.: A Finger Caliper for Reduction of Phalangeal and Metacarpal Fractures by Skeletal Traction. South. Med. J. 32:543–546, 1939.
74. Caspi, I., Engel, J., and Lin, E.: Intra-articular Bone Formation in Hand Following Wire Fixation. Orthop. Rev. 13:91–92 1984, 1994.
75. Chasmar, L.R.: Metacarpal and Phalangeal Fractures. American Society for Surgery of the Hand Correspondence Newsletter, 1975.
76. Chow, S.P., Pun, W.K., So, Y.C., et al.: A Prospective Study of 245 Open Digital Fractures of the Hand. J. Hand Surg. 16B:137–140, 1991.
77. Chuinard, R.G., and D'Ambrosia, R.D.: Tooth Wounds and the Infected Fist. J. Bone Joint Surg. 59A:416–418, 1977.
78. Clifford, R.H.: Intramedullary Wire Fixation of Hand Fractures. Plast. Reconstr. Surg. 11:366–371, 1953.
79. Clinkscales, G.S. Jr.: Complications in the Management of Fractures in Hand Injuries. South. Med. J. 63:704–707, 1970.
80. Conolly, W.B.: The Spontaneous Healing of Hand Wounds. Aust. N.Z. J. Surg. 44:393–395, 1974.
81. Conwell, H.E., and Reynolds, F.C.: Key and Conwell's Management of Fractures, Dislocations, and Sprains, 7th Ed. St. Louis, C.V. Mosby, 1961.
82. Coonrad, R.W., and Pohlman, M.H.: Impacted Fractures in the Proximal Portion of the Proximal Phalanx of the Finger. J. Bone Joint Surg. 51A:1291–1296, 1969.
83. Cordrey, L.J.: Intramedullary "Pull-out" Wire Fixation in Surgery of the Hand. Arch. Surg. 8:51–64, 1981.
84. Cotton, F.J.: Dislocations and Joint Fractures, 2nd Ed.Philadelphia, W.B. Saunders, 1924.
85. Crawford, G.P.: Screw Fixation for Certain Fractures of the Phalanges and Metacarpals. J. Bone Joint Surg. 58A:487–492, 1976.
86. Crichlow, T.P.K.R., and Hoskinson, J.: Avulsion Fracture of the Index Metacarpal Base: Three Case Reports. J. Hand Surg. 13B:212–214, 1988.
87. Crockett, D.J.: Rigid Fixation of Bones of the Hand Using K-wires Bonded With Acrylic Resin. Hand 6:106–107, 1974.
88. Culver, J.E.: American Society for Surgery of the Hand Correspondence Newsletter, 1981.
89. Culver, J.E., and Anderson, T.E.: Fractures of the Hand and Wrist in the Athlete. Clin. Sports Med. 11:101–128, 1992.
90. Curry, G.J.: Treatment of Finger Fractures, Simple and Compound. Finger Amputations. Am. J. Surg. 71:80–83, 1946.
91. Cziffer, E.: The Use of the Manuflex Disposable Mini External Fixator. Orthopedics 12:163–166, 1989.
92. Cziffer, E.: Static Fixation of Finger Fractures. Hand Clin. 9:639–650, 1993.
93. Dabezies, E.J., and Schutte, J.P.: Fixation of Metacarpal and Phalangeal Fractures With Miniature Plates and Screws. J. Hand Surg. 11A:283–288, 1986.
94. DaCruz, D.J., Slade, R.J., and Malone, W.: Fractures of the Distal Phalanges. J. Hand Surg. 13B:350–352, 1988.
95. Davis, G.D.: A Ball Splint for Hand Fractures. Int. Clin. 1:182–183, 1928.
96. Davis, T.R.C., and Stothard, J.: Why All Finger Fractures Should be Referred to a Hand Surgery Service: A Prospective Study of Primary Management. J. Hand Surg. 15B:299–302, 1990.
97. De Jonge, J.J., Kingma, J., Van Der Lei, B., and Klasen, H.J.: Phalangeal Fractures of the Hand. An Analysis of Gender and Age-related Incidence and Aetiology. J. Hand Surg. 19B:168–170, 1994.
98. DeLee, J.C.: Avulsion Fracture of the Base of the Second Metacarpal by the Extensor Carpi Radialis Longus. J. Bone Joint Surg. 61A:445–446, 1979.
99. Dennys, L.J., Hurst, L.N., and Cox, J.: Management of Proximal Interphalangeal Joint Fractures Using a New Dynamic Traction Splint and Early Active Movement. J. Hand Therapy, Jan-Mar:16–24, 1992.

100. Dickson, R.A.: Rigid Fixation of Unstable Metacarpal Fractures Using Transverse K-wires Bonded With Acrylic Resin. Hand 7:284–286, 1975.
101. Diwaker, H.N., and Stothard, J.: The Role of Internal Fixation in Closed Fractures of the Proximal Phalanges and Metacarpals in Adults. J. Hand Surg. 11B:103–108, 1986.
102. Dobyns, J.H.: Articular Fractures of the Hand (Abstract). J. Bone Joint Surg. 48A:610, 1966.
103. Dobyns, J.H., Linscheid, R.L., and Cooney, W.P.: Fractures and Dislocations of the Wrist and Hand Then and Now. J. Hand Surg. 8:687–690, 1983.
104. Dove, A.F., Sloan, J.P., Moulder, T.J., and Barker, A.: Dressings of the Nailbed Following Nail Avulsion. J. Hand Surg. 13B:408–410, 1988.
105. Dugas, R., and D'Ambrosia, R.: Civilian Gunshot Wounds. Orthopedics 8:1121–1125, 1985.
106. Duncan, J., and Kettelkamp, D.B.: Low-velocity Gunshot Wounds of the Hand. Arch. Surg. 109:395–398, 1974.
107. Duncan, K.H., and Jupiter, J.B.: Intraarticular Osteotomy for Malunion of Metacarpal Head Fractures. J. Hand Surg. 14A:888–893, 1989.
108. Duncan, R.W., Freeland, A.E., Jabaley, M.E., and Meydrech, E.F.: Open Hand Fractures: An Analysis of the Recovery of Active Motion and of Complications. J. Hand Surg. 18A:387–394, 1993.
109. Eaton, R.G.: The Dangerous Chip Fracture in Athletes. Instr. Course Lect. 34:314–322, 1985.
110. Eaton, R.G.: Closed Reduction and Internal Fixation Versus Open Reduction and Internal Fixation for Displaced Oblique Proximal Phalangeal Fractures. Orthopedics 12:911–916, 1989.
111. Edwards, G.S., O'Brien, E.T., and Heckman, M.M.: Retrograde Cross-pinning of Transverse Metacarpal and Phalangeal Fractures. Hand 14:141–148, 1982.
112. Eichenholtz, S.N., and Rizzo, P.C.: Fracture of the Neck of the Fifth Metacarpal Bone—Is Overtreatment Justified? J.A.M.A. 178:151–152, 1961.
113. Elton, R.C., and Bouzard, W.C.: Gunshot and Fragment Wounds of the Metacarpus. South. Med. J. 68:833–843, 1975.
114. Emmett, J.E., and Breck, L.W.: A Review of Analysis of 11,000 Fractures Seen in a Private Practice of Orthopaedic Surgery, 1937–1957. J. Bone Joint Surg. 40A:1169–1175, 1958.
115. Engkvist, O., and Johansson, S.H.: Perichondrial Arthroplasty. A Clinical Study in Twenty-six Patients. Scand. J. Plast. Reconstr. Surg. 14:71–87, 1980.
116. Ersek, R.A., Gadaria, U., and Denton, D.R.: Nail Bed Avulsions Treated With Porcine Xenografts. J. Hand Surg. 10A:152–153, 1985.
117. Eyres, K.S., and Allen, T.R.: Skyline View of the Metacarpal Head in the Assessment of Human Fight-Bite Injuries. J. Hand Surg. 18B:43–44, 1993.
118. Eyres, K.S., Kreibich, N., and Allen, T.R.: Stabilization of Multiple Metacarpal Fractures: A New Use for the Charnley Toe-fusion Clamp. J. Hand Surg. 18B:192–194, 1993.
119. Fackler, M.L., and Burkhalter, W.E.: Hand and Forearm Injuries From Penetrating Projectiles. J. Hand Surg. 17A:971–975, 1992.
120. Fahmy, N.R.M.: The Stockport Serpentine Spring System for the Treatment of Displaced Comminuted Intra-articular Phalangeal Fractures. J. Hand Surg. 15B:303–311, 1990.
121. Fahmy, N.R.M., and Harvey, R.A.: The "S" Quattro in the Management of Fractures in the Hand. J. Hand Surg. 17B:321–331, 1992.
122. Fambrough, R.A., and Green, D.P.: Tendon Rupture as a Complication of Screw Fixation in Fractures in the Hand. A Case Report. J. Bone Joint Surg. 61A:781–782, 1979.
123. Ferraro, M.C., Coppola, A., Lippman, K., and Hurst, L.C.: Closed Functional Bracing of Metacarpal Fractures. Orthop. Rev. 12:49–56, 1983.
124. Field, L.D., Freeland, A.E., and Jabaley, M.E.: Midaxial Approach to the Proximal Phalanx for Fracture Fixation. Contemporary Orthop. 25:133–137, 1992.
125. Firoozbakhsh, K.K., Moneim, M.S., Howey, T., Castaneda, E., and Pirela-Cruz, M.A.: Comparative Fatigue Strengths and Stabilities of Metacarpal Internal Fixation Techniques. J. Hand Surg. 18A:1059–1068, 1993.
126. Fitzgerald, J.A.W., and Khan, M.A.: The Conservative Management of Fractures of the Shafts of the Phalanges of the Fingers by Combined Traction-Splintage. J. Hand Surg. 9B:303–306, 1984.
127. Flatt, A.E.: Closed and Open Fractures of the Hand. Postgrad. Med. J. 7:17–26, 1966.
128. Ford, D.J., Ali, M.S., and Steel, W.M.: Fractures of the Fifth Metacarpal Neck: Is Reduction or Immobilisation Necessary? J. Hand Surg. 14B:165–167, 1989.
129. Ford, D.J., El-Hadidi, S., Lunn, P.G., and Burke, F.D.: Fractures of the Phalanges: Results of Internal Fixation Using 1.5 mm and 2 mm A.O. Screws. J. Hand Surg. 12B:28–33, 1987.
130. Fornage, B.D., and Rifkin, M.D.: Ultrasound Examination of the Hand and Foot. Radiol. Clin. North Am. 26:109–129, 1988.
131. Freeland, A.E.: External Fixation for Skeletal Stabilization of Severe Open Fractures of the Hand. Clin. Orthop. 214:93–100, 1987.
132. Freeland, A.E., and Benoist, L.A.: Open Reduction and Internal Fixation Method for Fractures at the Proximal Interphalangeal Joint. Hand Clin. 10:239–250, 1994.
133. Freeland, A.E., Jabaley, M.E., Burkhalter, W.E., and Chaves, A.M.V.: Delayed Primary Bone Grafting in the Hand and Wrist After Traumatic Bone Loss. J. Hand Surg. 9A:22–28, 1984.
134. Freeland, A.E., and Roberts, T.S.: Percutaneous Screw Treatment of Spiral Oblique Finger Proximal Phalangeal Fractures. Orthopedics 14:384–388, 1991.
135. Froimson, A.I.: Osteotomy for Digital Deformity. J. Hand Surg. 6:585–589, 1981.
136. Fyfe, I.S., and Mason, S.: The Mechanical Stability of Internal Fixation of Fractured Phalanges. Hand 11:50–54, 1979.
137. Geiger, K.R., and Karpman, R.R.: Necrosis of the Skin Over the Metacarpal as a Result of Functional Fracture-Bracing. A Report of Three Cases. J. Bone Joint Surg. 71A:1199–1202, 1989.
138. Gilbert, F.J., Campbell, R.S.D., and Bayliss, A.P.: The Role of Ultrasound in the Detection of Non-Radiopaque Foreign Bodies. Clinical Radiol. 41:109–112, 1990.
139. Gingrass, R.P., Fehring, B., and Matloub, H.: Intraosseous Wiring of Complex Hand Fractures. Plast. Reconstr. Surg. 66:383—394, 1980.
140. Glasgow, M., and Lloyd, G.J.: The Use of Modified A.O. Reduction Forceps in Percutaneous Fracture Fixation. Hand 13:214–216, 1981.
141. Goldberg, D.: Metacarpal Fractures: A New Instrument for the Maintenance of Position After Reduction. Am. J. Surg. 72:758–766, 1945.
142. Goldberg, D.: Closed Functional Bracing of Metacarpal Fractures. Orthop. Rev. 13:139–141, 1984.
143. Gonzalez, M.H., McKay, W., and Hall, R.F. Jr.: Low-velocity Gunshot Wounds of the Metacarpal: Treatment by Early Stable Fixation and Bone Grafting. J. Hand Surg. 18A:267–270, 1993.
144. Gordon, L., and Monsanto, E.H.: Acute Vascular Compromise After Avulsion of the Distal Phalanx With the Flexor Digitorum Profundus Tendon. J. Hand Surg. 12A:259–261, 1987.
145. Gorosh, J., and Page, B.J. II: Treatment of Phalangeal Fractures of the Hand With Intraosseous Wire Fixation. Orthop. Rev. 18:800–806, 1989.
146. Gould, W.L., Belsole, R.J., and Skelton, W.H.: Tension-band Stabilization of Transverse Fractures: An Experimental Analysis. Plast. Reconstr. Surg. 73:111–115, 1984.
147. Granberry, W.M.: Gunshot Wounds of the Hand. Hand 5:220–228, 1973.

148. Green, D.P.: Commonly Missed Injuries in the Hand. Am. Fam. Physician 7:111–119, 1973.
149. Green, D.P.: Complications of Phalangeal and Metacarpal Fractures. Hand Clin. 2:307–328, 1986.
150. Green, D.P.: Non-articular Hand Fractures. The Case for Percutaneous Pinning. *In* Neviaser, R.J. (ed.): Controversies in Hand Surgery. New York, Churchill Livingstone, 1990.
151. Green, D.P., and Anderson: Closed Reduction and Percutaneous Pin Fixation of Fracture Phalanges. J. Bone Joint Surg. 55A:1651–1654, 1973.
152. Greene, T.L., Noellert, R.C., and Belsole, R.J.: Treatment of Unstable Metacarpal and Phalangeal Fractures With Tension Band Wiring Techniques. Clin. Orthop. 214:78–84, 1987.
153. Greene, T.L., Noellert, R.C., Belsole, R.J., and Simpson, L.A.: Composite Wiring of Metacarpal and Phalangeal Fractures. J. Hand Surg. 14A:665–669, 1989.
154. Gropper, P.T., and Bowen: Cerclage Wiring of Metacarpal Fractures. Clin. Orthop. 188:203–207, 1984.
155. Gross, M.S., and Gelberman, R.H.: Metacarpal Rotational Osteotomy. J. Hand Surg. 10A:105–108, 1985.
156. Grundberg, A.B.: Intramedullary Fixation for Fractures of the Hand. J. Hand Surg. 6:568–573, 1981.
157. Haas, S.B., and Savage, R.C.: Metacarpal Fracture Fixation With Interosseous Nylon Suture in a Patient With Metal Allergies. J. Hand Surg. 14A:107–110, 1989.
158. Hagan, H.J., and Hastings, H. II: Use of a Step-cut Osteotomy for Immediate Posttraumatic Proximal Interphalangeal Joint Fusion. J. Hand Surg. 15A:374–376, 1990.
159. Haggart, G.E.: Fractures of the Metacarpal, Metatarsal Bones, and Phalanges Treated by Skeletal Traction. Surg. Clin. North Am. 14:1203–1210, 1934.
160. Hall, R.F.: Closed Flexible Intramedullary Rodding of Metacarpal and Phalangeal Fractures. Orthop. Trans. 8:187–188, 1984.
161. Hall, R.F.: Treatment of Metacarpal and Phalangeal Fractures in Noncompliant Patients. Clin. Orthop. 214:31–36, 1987.
162. Hasegawa, T., and Yamano, Y.: Arthroplasty of the Proximal Interphalangeal Joint Using Costal Cartilage Grafts. J. Hand Surg. 17B:583–585, 1992.
163. Hasham, A.I.: Closed Flexor Profundus Injury. J. Trauma, 15:1067–1068, 1975.
164. Hastings, H.: Unstable Metacarpal and Phalangeal Fracture Treatment With Screws and Plates. Clin. Orthop. 214:37–52, 1994.
165. Hastings, H. II, and Ernst, J.M.J.: Dynamic External Fixation for Fractures of the Proximal Interphalangeal Joint. Hand Clin. 9:659–674, 1993.
166. Hawkins, L.G.: Splint Bracing for Unstable Proximal Diaphyseal and Metaphyseal Fractures of the Proximal Phalanx. Correspondence Newsletter, 1982.
167. Hedeboe, J.: Subcapital Fractures of the Fifth Metacarpal. A Classic Method of Treatment Is Abandoned. Ugeskr. Laeger 138:1766–1768, 1976.
168. Heim, U., and Pfeiffer, K.M.: Small Fragment Set Manual. Technique Recommended by the ASIF Group. New York, Springer-Verlag, 1982.
169. Hindman, B.W., Kulik, W.J., Lee, G., and Avolio, R.E.: Occult Fractures of the Carpals and Metacarpals: Demonstration by CT. A.J.R. 153:529–532, 1989.
170. Holst-Nielsen, F.: Subcapital Fractures of the Four Ulnar Metacarpal Bones. Hand 8:290–293, 1976.
171. Hotchkiss RN.: Compass Proximal Interphalangeal (PIP) Joint Hinge. Orthop Trans 1995. In Press.
172. Howard, L.D. Jr.: The Problem of Metacarpal Fractures of the Hand Due to War Wounds. Instr. Course Lect. 2:196–201, 1944.
173. Howard, L.D. Jr.: Fractures of the Small Bones of the Hand. Plast. Reconstr. Surg. 29:334, 1962.
174. Huffaker, W.H., Wray, R.C., and Weeks, P.M.: Factors Influencing Final Range of Motion in the Fingers After Fractures of the Hand. Plast. Reconstr. Surg. 63:82–87, 1979.
175. Hung, L.K., So, W.S., and Leung, P.C.: Combined Intramedullary Kirschner Wire and Intra-osseous Wire Loop for Fixation of Finger Fractures. J. Hand Surg. 14B:171–176, 1989.
176. Hunter, J.M., and Cowan, N.J.: Fifth Metacarpal Fractures in a Compensation Clinic Population. A Report on 133 Cases. J. Bone Joint Surg. 52A:1159–1165, 1970.
177. Ikuta, Y., and Tsuge, K.: Micro-bolts and Micro-screws for Fixation of Small Bones in the Hand. Hand 6:261–265, 1974.
178. Inada, Y., Tamai, S., Kawanishi, K., and Fukui, A.: Fifth Digit Sesamoid Fracture With Tenosynovitis. J. Hand Surg. 17A:915–917, 1992.
179. Inanami, H., Ninomiya, S., Okutsu, I., Tarui, T., and Fujiwara, N.: Dynamic External Finger Fixator for Fracture Dislocation of the Proximal Interphalangeal Joint. J. Hand Surg. 18A:160–164, 1993.
180. Iselin, F.: Arthroplasty of the Proximal Interphalangeal Joint After Trauma. Hand 7:41–42, 1975.
181. Iselin, F., and Thevenin, R.: Fixation of Fractures of the Digits With Intramedullary Flexible Screws. J. Bone Joint Surg. 56A:1096, 1974.
182. Iselin, M.: Avulsion Injuries of the Nail. Edinburgh, Churchill Livingstone, 1981.
183. Ishida, O., Ikuta, Y., and Kuroki, H.: Ipsilateral Osteochondral Grafting for Finger Joint Repair. J. Hand Surg. 19A:372–377, 1994.
184. Ishizuki, M., and Furuya, K.: Clinical Application of Sapphire Pins as an Internal Fixation Device for the Upper Extremity. J. Hand Surg. 16A:922–928, 1991.
185. Itoh, Y., Uchinishi, K., and Oka, Y.: Treatment of Pseudoarthrosis of the Distal Phalanx With the Palmar Midline Approach. J. Hand Surg. 8:80–84, 1983.
186. Jabaley, M.E., and Freeland, A.E.: Rigid Internal Fixation in the Hand: 104 Cases. Plast. Reconstr. Surg. 77:288–298, 1986.
187. Jablon, M.: Articular Fractures and Dislocations in the Hand. Orthop. Rev. 11:61–70, 1982.
188. Jahss, S.A.: Fractures of the Proximal Phalanges: Alignment and Immobilization. J. Bone Joint Surg. 18:726–731, 1936.
189. Jahss, S.A.: Fractures of the Metacarpals: A New Method of Reduction and Immobilization. J. Bone Joint Surg. 20:178–186, 1938.
190. James, J.I.P.: Fractures of the Proximal and Middle Phalanges of the Fingers. Acta Orthop. Scand. 32:401–412, 1962.
191. James, J.I.P.: Common, Single Errors in the Management of Hand Injuries. Proc. R. Soc. Med. 63:69–71, 1970.
192. James, J.I.P., and Wright, T.A.: Fractures of Metacarpals and Proximal and Middle Phalanges of the Finger. J. Bone Joint Surg. 48B:181–182, 1966.
193. Jones, W.W.: Biomechanics of Small Bone Fixation. Clin. Orthop. 214:11–18, 1987.
194. Jordan, S.E., and Greider, J.L.: The Angiocatheter in the Management of Hand Injuries. J. Hand Surg. 11A:446, 1986.
195. Joshi, B.B.: Percutaneous Internal Fixation of Fractures of the Proximal Phalanges. Hand 8:86–92, 1976.
196. Jupiter, J.B.: Discussion of Application of Maxillofacial Miniplating and Microplating Systems to the Hand. Plast. Reconstr. Surg. 92:708–709, 1993.
197. Jupiter, J.B., Koniuch, M.P., and Smith, R.J.: The Management of Delayed Union and Nonunion of the Metacarpals and Phalanges. J. Hand Surg. 10A:457–466, 1985.
198. Jupiter, J.B., and Lipton, H.A.: Open Reduction and Internal Fixation of Avulsion Fractures in the Hand: The Tension Hand Wiring Technique. Techniques Orthop. 6:10–18, 1991.
199. Jupiter, J.B., and Sheppard, J.E.: Tension Wire Fixation of Avulsion Fractures in the Hand. Clin. Orthop. 214:113–120, 1987.
200. Kaplan, I.B.: Carved Silastic Block Spacers. American Society for Surgery of the Hand Correspondence Newsletter, 1992:96.
201. Kaplan, L.: The Treatment of Fractures and Dislocations of the Hand and Fingers. Technic of Unpadded Casts for Carpal Metacarpal and Phalangeal Fractures. Surg. Clin. North Am. 20:1695–1720, 1940.

202. Karbelnig, M.J.: Fracture of the Metacarpal Shaft: A Method of Treatment. Calif. Med. 98:269–270, 1963.
203. Kasdan, M.L.: Fractures of the Hand and Wrist. Hand Clin. 9:359–367, 1993.
204. Kasdan, M.L., and June, L.A.: Returning to Work After a Unilateral Hand Fracture. J. Med. 35:132–135, 1993.
205. Kaye, J.J., and Lister, G.D.: Another Use for the Brewerton View (Letter). J. Hand Surg. 3:603, 1978.
206. Kelikian, H.: Osteotomy of the Finger. A Case Report. Bull. Northwestern Univ. Med. School 21:111–114, 1947.
207. Kessler, I., Hecht, O., and Baruch, A.: Distraction-lengthening of Digital Rays in the Management of the Injured Hand. J. Bone Joint Surg. 61A:83–87, 1979.
208. Key, J.A., and Conwell, H.E.: The Management of Fractures, Dislocations, and Sprains, 5th Ed. St. Louis, C.V. Mosby, 1951.
209. Kilbourne, B.C.: Management of Complicated Hand Fractures. Surg. Clin. North Am. 48:201–213, 1968.
210. Kilbourne, B.C., and Paul, E.G.: The Use of Small Bone Screws in the Treatment of Metacarpal, Metatarsal and Phalangeal Fractures. J. Bone Joint Surg. 40A:375–383, 1958.
211. King, T.: Principles in the Treatment of Hand Fractures as Shown in the Technique for a Closed Fracture of the Metacarpal Neck. Med. J. Aust. 1:570–573, 1962.
212. Koch, S.L.: Disabilities of Hand Resulting From Loss of Joint Function. J.A.M.A. 104:30–35, 1935.
213. Konradsen, L., Nielsen, P.T., and Albrecht-Beste, E.: Functional Treatment of Metacarpal Fractures. 100 Randomized Cases With or Without Fixation. Acta Orthop. Scand. 61:531–534, 1990.
214. Kumta, S.M., Spinner, R., and Leung, P.C.: Absorbable Intramedullary Implants for Hand Fractures. Animal Experiments and Clinical Trial. J. Bone Joint Surg. 74B:563–566, 1992.
215. Lamb, D.: Training in Hand Surgery. J. Hand Surg. 15B:148–150, 1990.
216. Lamb, D.W., Abernethy, P.A., and Raine, P.A.M.: Unstable Fractures of the Metacarpals: A Method of Treatment by Transverse Wire Fixation to Intact Metacarpals. Hand 5:43–48, 1973.
217. Lambotte, A.: Contribution to Conservative Surgery of the Injured Hand. Clin. Orthop. 214:4–6, 1987. (Reprinted from Arch. Franco-Belges. Chir. 31:759, 1928.)
218. Lamphier, T.A.: Improper Reduction of Fractures of the Proximal Phalanges of Fractures. Am. J. Surg. 94:926–930, 1957.
219. Lane, C.S.: Detecting Occult Fracture of the Metacarpal Head: The Brewerton View. J. Hand Surg. 2:131–133, 1977.
220. Lane, C.S., Kennedy, J.F., and Kuschner, S.H.: The Reverse Oblique X-ray Film: Metacarpal Fractures Revealed. J. Hand Surg. 17A:504 506, 1992.
221. Lee, M.L.H.: Intra-articular and Peri-articular Fractures of the Phalanges. J. Bone Joint Surg. 45B:103–109, 1963.
222. Lees, V.C., Wren, C., and Elliot, D.: Internal Splints for Prevention of First Web Contracture Following Severe Disruption of the First Web Space. J. Hand Surg. 19B:560–562, 1994.
223. Leonard, M.H.: The Solution of Lead by Synovial Fluid. Clin. Orthop. 64:255–261, 1969.
224. Levine, W.N., and Leslie, B.M.: The Use of Ultrasonography to Detect a Radiolucent Foreign Body in the Hand: A Case Report. J. Hand Surg. 18A.218–220, 1993.
225. Lewis, R.C., and Hartman, J.T.: Controlled Osteotomy for Correction of Rotation in Proximal Phalanx Fractures. Orthop. Rev. 11:11–15, 1973.
226. Lewis, R.C., Nordyke, M., and Duncan, K.: Expandable Intramedullary Device for Treatment of Fractures in the Hand. Clin. Orthop. 214:85–92, 1987.
227. Light, T.R.: Salvage of Intraarticular Malunions of the Hand and Wrist. The Role of Realignment Osteotomy. Clin. Orthop. 214:130–135, 1987.
228. Light, T.R., and Bednar, M.S.: Management of Intra-articular Fractures of the Metacarpophalangeal Joint. Hand Clin. 10:303–314, 1994.
229. Lipscomb, P.R.: Management of Fractures of the Hand. Am. Surg. 29:277–282, 1963.
230. Lister, G.: Intraosseous Wiring of the Digital Skeleton. J. Hand Surg. 3:427–435, 1978.
231. London, P.S.: Sprains and Fractures Involving the Interphalangeal Joints. Hand 3:155–158, 1971.
232. Loosli, A., and Garrick, J.G.: The Functional Treatment of a Third Proximal Phalanx Fracture. Am. J. Sports Med. 15:94–96, 1987.
233. Lord, R.D.: Intramedullary Fixation of Metacarpal Fractures. J.A.M.A. 164:1746–1749, 1957.
234. Lowdon, I.M.R.: Fractures of the Metacarpal Neck of the Little Finger. Injury, 17:189–192, 1986.
235. Lucas, G.L.: Internal Fixation in the Hand: A Review of Indications and Methods. Orthopedics 3:1083–1089, 1980.
236. Lucas, G.L., and Pfeiffer, C.M.: Osteotomy of the Metacarpals and Phalanges Stabilized by AO Plates and Screws. Ann. Chir. Main 8:30–38, 1989.
237. Magnuson, P.B.: Fractures of Metacarpals and Phalanges. J.A.M.A. 91:1339–1340, 1928.
238. Magnuson, P.B.: Fractures. Philadelphia, J.B. Lippincott, 1942.
239. Maitra, A., and Burdett-Smith, P.: The Conservative Management of Proximal Phalangeal Fractures of the Hand in an Accident and Emergency Department. J. Hand Surg. 17B:332–336, 1992.
240. Manktelow, R.T., and Mahoney, J.L.: Step Osteotomy: A Precise Rotation Osteotomy to Correct Scissoring Deformities of the Fingers. Plast. Reconstr. Surg. 68:571–576, 1981.
241. Mann, R.J., Black, D., Constine, R., and Daniels, A.U.: A Quantitative Comparison of Metacarpal Fracture Stability With Five Different Methods of Internal Fixation. J. Hand Surg. 10A:1024–1028, 1985.
242. Mansoor, I.A.: Fractures of the Proximal Phalanx of Fingers: A Method of Reduction. J. Bone Joint Surg. 51A:196–198, 1969.
243. Margles, S.W.: Intra-articular Fractures of the Metacarpophalangeal and Proximal Interphalangeal Joints. Hand Clin. 4:67–74, 1988.
244. Mason, S.M., and Fyfe, I.S.: Comparison of Rigidity of Whole Tubular Bones. J. Biomech. 12:367–372, 1979.
245. Massengill, J.B., Alexander, H., Langrana, N., and Mylod, A.: A Phlangeal Fracture Model—Quantitative Analysis of Rigidity and Failure. J. Hand Surg. 7:264–270, 1982.
246. Massengill, J.B., Alexander, H., Parson, J.R., and Schecter, M.J.: Mechanical Analysis of Kirschner Wire Fixation in a Phalangeal Model. J. Hand Surg. 4:351–356, 1979.
247. Match, R.M.: The Treatment of Fractures of the Hand and the Wrist. Orthop. Rev. 14:35–48, 1985.
248. Matloub, H.S., Jensen, P.L., Sanger, J.R., Grunert, B.K., and Yousif, N.J.: Spiral Fracture Fixation Techniques. A Biomechanical Study. J. Hand Surg. 18B:515–519, 1993.
249. Matloub, H.S., Prevel, C.D., Sanger, J.R., Yousif, N.J., Devine, C.A., and Romano, J.: Tire Explosion Injuries to the Upper Extremity. Ann. Plast. Surg. 29:559–563, 1992.
250. McElfresh, E.C., and Dobyns, J.H.: Intra-articular Metacarpal Head Fractures. J. Hand Surg. 8:383–393, 1983.
251. McKerrell, J., Bowen, V., Johnston, G., and Zondervan, J.: Boxer's Fractures—Conservative or Operative Management? J. Trauma, 27:486–490, 1987
252. McLain, R.F., Steyers, C., and Stoddard, M.: Infections in Open Fractures of the Hand. J. Hand Surg. 16A:108–112, 1991.
253. McMaster, P.E.: Tendon and Muscle Ruptures: Clinical and Experimental Studies on the Causes and Location of Subcutaneous Ruptures. J. Bone Joint Surg. 15:705–722, 1933.
254. McMaster, W.C.: Intraoperative Reduction of Phalangeal Fractures. Plast. Reconstr. Surg. 56:671–672, 1975.
255. McNealy, R.W., and Lichtenstein, M.E.: Fractures of the Metacarpals and the Phalanges. Surg. Gynecol. Obstet. 60:758–761, 1932.
256. McNealy, R.W., and Lichtenstein, M.E.: Fractures of the

Metacarpals and Phalanges. West. J. Surg. Obstet. Gynecol. 43:156–161, 1935.

257. McNealy, R.W., and Lichtenstein, M.E.: Fractures of the Bones of the Hand. Am. J. Surg. 50:563–570, 1940.
258. Meals, R.A.: American Society for Surgery of the Hand Correspondence Newsletter, 1986.
259. Meals, R.A., and Meuli, H.C.: Carpenter's Nails, Phonograph Needles, Piano Wires, and Safety Pins: The History of Operative Fixation of Metacarpal and Phalangeal Fractures. J. Hand Surg. 10A:144–150, 1985.
260. Melone, C.P.: Rigid Fixation of Phalangeal and Metacarpal Fractures. Orthop. Clin. North Am. 17:421–435, 1986.
261. Meltzer, H.: Wire Extension Treatment of Fractures of Fingers and Metacarpal Bones. Surg. Gynecol. Obstet. 55:87–89, 1932.
262. Mennen, U.: Metacarpal Fractures and the Clamp-on Plate. J. Hand Surg. 15B:295–298, 1990.
263. Menon, J.: Reconstruction of the Metacarpophalangeal Joint With Autogenous Metatarsal. J. Hand Surg. 8:443–446, 1983.
264. Menon, J.: Correction of Rotary Malunion of the Fingers by Metacarpal Rotational Osteotomy. Orthopedics 13:197–200, 1990.
265. Meyer, V.E., Chiu, D.T., and Beasley, R.W.: The Place of Internal Skeletal Fixation in Surgery of the Hand. Clin. Plast. Surg. 8:51–64, 1981.
266. Michon, J., and Delagoutte, J.P.: Crush Injuries of the Digital Extremities. *In* Pierre, M. (ed.): The Nail (G.E.M. Monograph). Edinburgh, Churchill Livingstone, 1981.
267. Milford, L.: The Hand. *In* Crenshaw A.H. (ed.): Campbell's Operative Orthopaedics, 5th Ed. St. Louis, C.V. Mosby, 1971.
268. Miller, W.R.: Fractures of the Metacarpals. Am. J. Orthop. 105–108, 1965.
269. Moberg, E.: The Use of Traction Treatment for Fractures of Phalanges and Metacarpals. Acta Chir. Scand. 99:341–352, 1950.
270. Moberg, E.: Emergency Surgery of the Hand. Edinburgh, E.S. Livingstone, 1968.
271. Mock, H.E., and Ellis, J.D.: The Treatment of Fractures of the Fingers and Metacarpals With a Description of the Author's Finger Caliper. Surg. Gynecol. Obstet. 45:551–556, 1927.
272. Moore, D.C.: Regional Block, 4th Ed. Springfield, Ill., Charles C. Thomas, 1967.
273. Morton, H.S.: Fractures of the Wrist and Hand. Can. Med. Assoc. J. 51:430–434, 1944.
274. Muller, M.E., Allgower, M., Schneider, R., and Willenegger, H.: Manual of Internal Fixation, 2nd Ed., pp. 42–43. New York, Springer-Verlag, 1979.
275. Muller, M.E., Allgwer, M., Schneider, R., and Willenegger, H.: Manual of Internal Fixation. Techniques Recommended by the AO Group, 2nd Ed., pp. 338. New York, Springer-Verlag, 1979.
276. Murray, C.R.: Fractures of the Bones of the Hand. N.Y. State J. Med. 36:1749–1761, 1936.
277. Nagle, D.J., af Ekenstam, F.W., and Lister, G.D.: Immediate Silastic Arthroplasty for Non-salvageable Intraarticular Phalangeal Fractures. Scand. J. Plast. Reconstr. Surg. 23:47–50, 1989.
278. Nagy, L.: Static External Fixation of Finger Fractures. Hand Clin. 9:651–657, 1993.
279. Namba, R.S., Kabo, J.M., and Meals, R.A.: Biomechanical Effects of Point Configuration in Kirschner-wire Fixation. Clin. Orthop. 214:19–22, 1987.
280. Nemethi, C.E.: Phalangeal Fractures. Treated by Open Reduction and Kirschner-wire Fixation. Indust. Med. Surg. 23:148–150, 1954.
281. Nichols, H.M.: Manual of Hand Injuries, 2nd Ed. Chicago, Year Book Medical Publishers, 1960.
282. Nordyke, M.D., Lewis, R.C., Janssen, H.F., and Duncan, K.H.: Biomechanical and Clinical Evaluation of Expandable Intramedullary Fixation Device. J. Hand Surg. 13A:129–134, 1988.
283. Norman, H.R.C.: Fractures of the Metacarpals Treated by a New Method. Can. Med. Assoc. J. 49:173–175, 1943.
284. Noyez, J., and Verstreken, J.: The Use of the Bilos Compression Pin in Hand Surgery. Acta Orthop. Belg. 53:75–79, 1987.
285. Nunley, J.A., Goldner, R.D., and Urbaniak, J.R.: Skeletal Fixation in Digital Replantation. Use of the "H" Plate. Clin. Orthop. 214:66–71, 1987.
286. Nunley, J.A., and Kloen, P.: Biomechanical and Functional Testing of Plate Fixation Devices for Proximal Phalangeal Fractures. J. Hand Surg. 16A:991–998, 1991.
287. O'Brien, E.T.: Fractures of the Metacarpals and Phalanges. *In* Green, D.P. (ed.): Operative Hand Surgery, 2nd Ed, pp. 709–775. New York, Churchill Livingstone, 1988.
288. O'Rourke, S.K., Gaur, S., and Barton, N.J.: Long-term Outcome of Articular Fractures of the Phalanges: An Eleven Year Follow Up. J. Hand Surg. 14B:183–193, 1989.
289. Ogunro, E.O.: External Fixation of Injured Nail Bed With the INRO Surgical Nail Splint. J. Hand Surg. 14A:236–241, 1989.
290. Ohl, M.D., and Smith, W.S.: The Treatment of a Phalangeal Delayed Union Using Electrical Stimulation. Orthopedics 11:585–588, 1988.
291. Owen, H.R.: Fractures of the Bones of the Hand. Surg. Gynecol. Obstet. 66:500–505, 1938.
292. Owens, C.: Necrosis of the Skin Over the Metacarpal as a Result of Functional Fracture-Bracing. A Report of Three Cases (Letter). J. Bone Joint Surg. 73A:789, 1991.
293. Packer, G.J., and Shaheen, M.A.: Patterns of Hand Fractures and Dislocations in a District General Hospital. J. Hand Surg. 18B:511–514, 1993.
294. Parsons, S.W., Fitzgerald, J.A.W., and Shearer, J.R.: External Fixation of Unstable Metacarpal and Phalangeal Fractures. J. Hand Surg. 17B:151–155, 1992.
295. Peacock, E.E.: Management of Conditions of the Hand Requiring Immobilization. Surg. Clin. North Am. 33:1297–1309, 1953.
296. Peacock, K.C., Hanna, D.P., Kirkpatrick, K., Breidenbach, W.C., Lister, G.D., and Firrell, J.: Efficacy of Perioperative Cefamandole With Postoperative Cephalexin in the Primary Outpatient Treatment of Open Wounds of the Hand. J. Hand Surg. 13A:960–964, 1988.
297. Pedersen, N.T., and Larsen, A.: Incidence of Flexion Contracture Following Fracture of the Fifth Metacarpal Treated by Jahss' Method. Ugeskr. Laeger 138:1765–1766, 1976.
298. Pichora, D.R., Meyer, R., and Masear, V.R.: Rotational Step-cut Osteotomy for Treatment of Metacarpal and Phalangeal Malunion. J. Hand Surg. 16A:551–555, 1991.
299. Pieron, A.P.: Correction of Rotational Malunion of a Phalanx by Metacarpal Osteotomy. J. Bone Joint Surg. 54B:516–519, 1972.
300. Pihlajamäki, H., Böstman, O., Hirvensalo, E., Törmälä, P., and Rokkanen, P.: Absorbable Pins of Self-reinforced Poly-L-Lactic Acid for Fixation of Fractures and Osteotomies. J. Bone Joint Surg. 74B:853–857, 1992.
301. Posner, M.A.: Injuries to the Hand and Wrist in Athletes. Orthop. Clin. North Am. 8:593–618, 1977.
302. Pratt, D.R.: Exposing Fractures of the Proximal Phalanx of the Finger Longitudinally Through the Dorsal Extensor Apparatus. Clin. Orthop. 15:22–26, 1959.
303. Pritsch, M., Engel, J., and Farin, I.: Manipulation and External Fixation of Metacarpal Fractures. J. Bone Joint Surg. 63A:1289–1291, 1981.
304. Pritsch, M., Engel, J., Tsur, H., and Farin, I.: The Fractured Metacarpal Neck: New Method of Manipulation and External Fixation. Orthop. Rev. 7:122–123, 1978.
305. Puckett, C.L., Welsh, C.F., Croll, G.H., and Concannon, M.J.: Application of Maxillofacial Miniplating and Microplating Systems to the Hand. Plast. Reconstr. Surg. 92:699–707, 1993.
306. Pun, W.K., Chow, S.P., So, Y.C., et al.: A Prospective Study on 284 Digital Fractures of the Hand. J. Hand Surg. 14A:474–481, 1989.
307. Pun, W.K., Chow, S.P., So, Y.C., et al.: Unstable Phalangeal

Fractures: Treatment by A.O. Screw and Plate Fixation. J. Hand Surg. 16A:113–117, 1991.

308. Putnam, M.D., and Walsh, T.M.: IV: External Fixation for Open Fractures of the Upper Extremity. Hand Clin. 9:613–623, 1993.
309. Quigley, T.B., and Urist, M.R.: Interphalangeal Joints: A Method of Digital Skeletal Traction Which Permits Active Motion. Am. J. Surg. 73:175–183, 1947.
310. Rayhack, J.M., Belsole, R.J., and Skelton, W.H.: A Strain Recording Model: Analysis of Transverse Osteotomy Fixation in Small Bones. J. Hand Surg. 9A:383–387, 1984.
311. Rayhack, J.M., and Bottke, C.A.: Intraosseous Compression Wiring of Displaced Articular Condylar Fractures. J. Hand Surg. 15A:370–373, 1990.
312. Rettig, A.C., Ryan, R., Shelbourne, K.D., McCarroll, J.R., Johnson, F. Jr., and Ahlfeld, S.K.: Metacarpal Fractures in the Athlete. Am. J. Sports Med. 17:567–572, 1989.
313. Reyes, F.A., and Latta, L.L.: Conservative Management of Difficult Phalangeal Fractures. Clin. Orthop. 214:23–30, 1987.
314. Rhoades, C.E., Soye, I., Levine, E., and Reckling, F.W.: Detection of a Wooden Foreign Body in the Hand Using Computed Tomography—Case Report. J. Hand Surg. 7:306–307, 1982.
315. Rider, D.L.: Fractures of the Metacarpals, Metatarsals, and Phalanges. Am. J. Surg. 38:549–559, 1937.
316. Riggs, S.A., and Cooney, W.P.: External Fixation of Complex Hand and Wrist Fractures. J. Trauma 23:332–336, 1983.
317. Riordan, D.C.: Fractures About the Hand. South. Med. J. 50:637–640, 1957.
318. Roberts, N.: Fractures of the Phalanges of the Hand and Metacarpals. Proc. R. Soc. Med. 31:793–798, 1938.
319. Robertson, D.C.: The Fusion of Interphalangeal Joints. Can. J. Surg. 7:433–437, 1964.
320. Rosenberg, L., and Kon, M.: An External Fixator in Finger Reconstruction. J. Hand Surg. 11B:147–148, 1986.
321. Rotman, M.B., and Pruitt, D.L.: Avulsion Fracture of the Extensor Carpi Radialis Brevis Insertion. J. Hand Surg. 18A:511–513, 1993.
322. Royle, S.G.: Rotational Deformity Following Metacarpal Fracture. J. Hand Surg. 15B:124–125, 1990.
323. Ruby, L.K.: American Society for Surgery of the Hand Correspondence Newsletter, 1982.
324. Ruedi, T.P., Burri, C., and Pfeiffer, K.M.: Stable Internal Fixation of Fractures of the Hand. J. Trauma 11:381–389, 1971.
325. Ruggeri, S., Osterman, A.L., and Bora, F.W.: Stabilization of Metacarpal and Phalangeal Fractures in the Hand. Orthop. Rev. 9:107–110, 1980.
326. Rush, L.V., and Rush, H.L.: Evolution of Medullary Fixation of Fractures by the Longitudinal Pin. Am. J. Surg. 78:324–333, 1949.
327. Russell, R.C., Williamson, D.A., Sullivan, J.W., Suchy, H., and Suliman, O.: Detection of Foreign Bodies in the Hand. J. Hand Surg. 16A:2–11, 1991.
328. Russotti, G.M., and Sim, F.H.: Missile Wounds of the Extremities: A Current Concepts Review. Orthopedics 8:1106–1116, 1985.
329. Sadr, B., and Lalehzarian, M.: Traumatic Avulsion of the tendon of Extensor Carpi Radialis Longus. J. Hand Surg. 12A:1035–1037, 1987.
330. Sanders, R.A., and Frederick, H.A.: Metacarpal and Phalangeal Osteotomy With Miniplate Fixation. Orthop. Rev. 20:449–456, 1991.
331. Saypol, G.M., and Slattery, L.R.: Observations on Displaced Fractures of the Hand. Surg. Gynecol. Obstet. 79:522–525, 1944.
332. Scheker, L.R.: Department of Technique: A Technique to Facilitate Drilling and Passing Intraosseous Wiring in the Hand. J. Hand Surg. 5:629–630, 1982.
333. Schenck, R.R.: The Dynamic Traction Method. Combining Movement and Traction for Intra-articular Fractures of the Phalanges. Hand Clin. 10:187–198, 1994.
334. Schlein, A.P., and Nathan, F.F.: A Dual Finger Fracture. Hand 4:171–172, 1972.
335. Schulze, H.A.: An Improved Skin-traction Technique for the Fingers. J. Bone Joint Surg. 29:222–224, 1947.
336. Scobie, W.H.: Crush Fracture of Sesamoid Bone of Thumb. Br. Med. J. 2:912, 1941.
337. Scott, M.M., and Mulligan, P.J.: Stabilizing Severe Phalangeal Fractures. Hand 12:44–50, 1980.
338. Scudder, C.L.: The Treatment of Fractures. Philadelphia, W.B. Saunders, 1926.
339. Segmuller, G.: Surgical Stabilization of the Skeleton of the Hand. Baltimore, Williams & Wilkins, 1977.
340. Segmüller, G., Cech, O., and Bekier, A.: Diagnostic Use of 85 Strontium in the Preoperative Evaluation of Non-union. Acta Orthop. Scand. 41:150–160, 1970.
341. Seitz, W.H., and Froimson, A.I.: Management of Malunited Fractures of the Metacarpal and Phalangeal Shafts. Hand Clin. 4:529–536, 1988.
342. Seitz, W.H., Gomez, W., Putnam, M.D., and Rosenwasser, M.P.: Management of Severe Hand Trauma With a Mini External Fixateur. Orthopedics 10:601–610, 1987.
343. Seitz, W.H. Jr., Froimson, A.I., Brooks, D.B., Postak, P., Polando, G., and Greenwald, A.S.: External Fixator Pin Insertion Techniques: Biomechanical Analysis and Clinical Relevance. J. Hand Surg. 16A:560–563, 1991.
344. Seymour, N.: Juxta-epiphysial Fracture of the Terminal Phalanx of the Finger. J. Bone Joint Surg. 48A:347–349, 1966.
345. Shapiro, J.S.: Power Staple Fixation in Hand and Wrist Surgery: New Applications of an Old Fixation Device. J. Hand Surg. 12A:218–227, 1987.
346. Shehadi, S.I.: External Fixation of Metacarpal and Phalangeal Fractures. J. Hand Surg. 16A:544–550, 1991.
347. Shibata, T., O'Flanagan, S.J., Ip, F.K., and Chow, S.P.: Articular Fractures of the Digits: A Prospective Study. J. Hand Surg. 18B:225–229, 1993.
348. Simon, R.R., and Wolgin, M.: Subungual Hematoma: Association With Occult Laceration Requiring Repair. Am. J. Emerg. Med. 5:302–304, 1987.
349. Simonetta, C.: The Use of "A.O." Plates in the Hand. Hand 2:43–45, 1970.
350. Slade JF, Chrostowski JH, Pomerance J, Wolfe SW.: Treatment of Unstable Fractures of the Proximal Interphalangeal Joint With Dynamic Traction and Immediate Active Motion. Presented at The American Society for Surgery of the Hand 49th Annual Meeting. Cincinnati, 1994.
351. Sloan, J.P., Dove, A.F., Maheson, M., Cope, A.N., and Welsh, K.R.: Antibiotics in Open Fractures of the Distal Phalanx? J. Hand Surg. 12B:123–124, 1987.
352. Smith, C.H.: Compound Fracture of the Fingers. Ann. Surg. 119:266–273, 1944.
353. Smith, F.L., and Rider, D.L.: A Study of The Healing of One Hundred Consecutive Phalangeal Fractures. J. Bone Joint Surg. 17:91–109, 1935.
354. Smith, R.J., and Peimer, C.A.: Injuries to the Metacarpal Bones and Joints. Adv. Surg. 2:341–374, 1977.
355. Smith, R.S., Alonso, J., and Horowitz, M.: External Fixation of Open Comminuted Fractures of the Proximal Phalanx. Orthop. Rev. 16:53–57, 1987.
356. Sopher, M., Gopalgi, B., and Spencer, J.D.: Interposition of the Dorsal Interosseous Tendon in a Fracture of the Base of the Proximal Phalanx of the Right Ring Finger. Injury 20:53–54, 1989.
357. Speed, K.: A Textbook of Fractures and Dislocations. Philadelphia, Lea & Febiger, 1942.
358. Stark, H.H.: Troublesome Fractures and Dislocations of the Hand. Instr. Course Lect. 19:130–149, 1970.
359. Stark, H.H., Boyes, J.H., Johnson, L., and Ashworth, C.R.: The Use of Paratenon, Polyethylene Film, or Silastic Sheeting to Prevent Restricting Adhesions to Tendons in the Hand. J. Bone Joint Surg. 59A:908–913, 1977.
360. Steel, W.M.: The A.O. Small Fragment Set in Hand Fractures. Hand 10:246–253, 1978.
361. Steel, W.M.: The Management of Fractures in the Hand (Editorial). J. Hand Surg. 15B:279–280, 1990.
362. Stern, P.J., Roman, R.J., Kiefhaber, T.R., and McDonough,

J.J.: Pilon Fractures of the Proximal Interphalangeal Joint. J. Hand Surg. 16A:844–850, 1991.
363. Stern, P.J., Wieser, M.J., and Reilly, D.G.: Complications of Plate Fixation in the Hand Skeleton. Clin. Orthop. 214:59–65, 1987.
364. Strickland, J.W., Steichen, J.B., Kleinman, W.B., Hastings, H., and Flynn, N.: Phalangeal Fractures. Factors Influencing Digital Performance. Orthop. Rev. 11:39–50, 1982.
365. Stuchin, S.A., and Kummer, F.J.: Stiffness of Small-bone External Fixation Methods: An Experimental Study. J. Hand Surg. 9A:718–724, 1984.
366. Suman, R.K.: Rigid Fixation of Metacarpal Fractures. J. R. Coll. Surg. Edinb. 28:51–52, 1983.
367. Suprock, M.D., Hood, J.M., and Lubahn, J.D.: Role of Antibiotics in Open Fractures of the Finger. J. Hand Surg. 15A:761–764, 1990.
368. Sutro, C.J.: Fracture of Metacarpal Bones and Proximal Manual Phalanges: Treatment With Emphasis on the Prevention of Rational Deformities. Am. J. Surg. 81:327–332, 1951.
369. Suzuki, Y., Matsunaga, T., Sato, S., and Yokoi, T.: The Pins and Rubbers Traction System for Treatment of Comminuted Intraarticular Fractures and Fracture-Dislocations in the Hand. J. Hand Surg. 19B:98–107, 1994.
370. Swanson, A.B.: Fractures Involving the Digits of the Hand. Orthop. Clin. North Am. 1:261–274, 1970.
371. Swanson, T.V., Szabo, R.M., and Anderson, D.D.: Open Hand Fractures: Prognosis and Classification. J. Hand Surg. 16A:101–107, 1991.
372. Teasdall, R.D., Aiken, M.A., Freeland, A.E., and Hughes, J.L.: Tire Explosion Injuries. Orthopedics 12:123–128, 1989.
373. Tennant, C.E.: Use of Steel Phonograph Needle as a Retaining Pin in Certain Irreducible Fractures of the Small Bones. J.A.M.A. 83:193, 1924.
374. Thaller, S.R., Powers, R., and Daniller, A.: Use of Maxillary Miniplates and Screw System in the Treatment of Hand Fractures: A Preliminary Report. Ann. Plast. Surg. 23:508–510, 1989.
375. Theeuwen, G.A.J.M., Lemmens, J.A.M., and van Niekerk, J.L.M.: Conservative Treatment of Boxer's Fracture: A Retrospective Analysis. Injury, 22:394–396, 1991.
376. Thurston, A.J.: Pivot Osteotomy for the Correction of Malunion of Metacarpal Neck Fractures. J. Hand Surg. 17B:580–582, 1992.
377. Treble, N., and Arif, S.: Avulsion Fracture of the Index Metacarpal. J. Hand Surg. 12B:38–39, 1987.
378. Vaccaro, A.R., Kupcha, P.C., and Salvo, J.P.: Accurate Reduction and Splinting of the Common Boxer's Fracture. Orthop. Rev. 19:994–995, 1990.
379. Van Demark, R.: A Simple Method of Treatment of Fractures of the Fifth Metacarpal Neck and Distal Shaft (Boxer's Fracture). South Dakota Medicine, 36:5–7, 1983.
380. van der Lei, B., Damen, A.L., Robinson, P.H., and Klasen, H.J.: Spiral Fracture of the Proximal Phalanx of the Index Finger by Finger Wrestling. Injury 23:560–566, 1992.
381. van der Lei, B., de Jonge, J., Robinson, P.H., and Klasen, H.J.: Correction Osteotomies of Phalanges and Metacarpals for Rotational and Angular Malunion: A Long-term Follow-up and a Review of the literature. J. Trauma 35:902–908, 1993.
382. van Egmond, D.B., Hovius, S.E.R., van der Meulen, J.C., and den Ouden, A.: Heat Recordings at Tips of Kirschner Wires During Drilling Through Human Phalanges. J. Hand Surg. 19A:648–652, 1994.
383. Vanik, R.K., Weber, R.C., Matloub, H.S., Sanger, J.R., and Gingrass, R.P.: The Comparative Strengths of Internal Fixation Techniques. J. Hand Surg. 9A:216–221, 1984.
384. Varela, C.D., and Carr, J.B.: Closed Intramedullary Pinning of Metacarpal and Phalanx Fractures. Orthopedics 13:213–215, 1990.
385. Vidal, J., Buscayret, C., and Connes, H.: Treatment of Articular Fractures by "Ligamentotaxis" With External Fixation. *In* Brooker, A.F. Jr., and Edwards, C.C. (eds.): External Fixation. The Current State of the Art, pp. 75–81. Baltimore, Williams & Wilkins, 1978.
386. Viegas, S.F.: New Method and Brace for Metacarpal Fractures. Surg. Rounds Orthop. 47–55, 1987.
387. Viegas, S.F., and Calhoun, J.H.: Lead Poisoning From a Gunshot Wound to the Hand. J. Hand Surg. 11A:729–732, 1986.
388. Viegas, S.F., Ferren, E.L., Self, J., and Tencer, A.F.: Comparative Mechanical Properties of Various Kirschner Wire Configurations in Transverse and Oblique Phalangeal Fractures. J. Hand Surg. 13A:246–253, 1988.
389. Viegas, S.F., Tencer, A., Woodard, P., and Williams, C.R.: Functional Bracing of Fractures of the Second Through Fifth Metacarpals. J. Hand Surg. 12A:139–143, 1987.
390. Vom Saal, F.H.: Intramedullary Fixation in Fractures of the Hand and Fingers. J. Bone Joint Surg. 35A:5–16, 1953.
391. Watson-Jones, R.: Fractures and Joint Injuries, 3rd Ed. Edinburgh, E.S. Livingstone, 1943.
392. Watson-Jones, R.: Fractures and Joint Injuries, 4th Ed. Edinburgh, E.S. Livingstone, 1956.
393. Waugh, R.L., and Ferrazzano, G.P.: Fractures of the Metacarpals Exclusive of the Thumb. A New Method of Treatment. Am. J. Surg. 59:186–194, 1943.
394. Weber, B.G., and Cech, O.: Pseudarthrosis. New York, Grune & Stratton, 1976.
395. Weckesser, E.C.: Rotational Osteotomy of the Metacarpal for Overlapping Fingers. J. Bone Joint Surg. 47A:751–756, 1965.
396. Weiss, A.C., and Hastings, H. II: Distal Unicondylar Fractures of the Proximal Phalanx. J. Hand Surg. 18A:594–599, 1993.
397. Widgerow, A.D., Edinburg, M., and Biddulph, S.L.: An Analysis of Proximal Phalangeal Fractures. J. Hand Surg. 12A:134–139, 1987.
398. Wise, R.A.: An Unusual Fracture of the Terminal Phalanx of the Finger. J. Bone Joint Surg. 21:467–469, 1939.
399. Woesner, M.E., and Sanders, I.: Xeroradiography: A Significant Modality in the Detection of Nonmetallic Foreign Bodies in Soft Tissues. J. Roentgenol. 115:636–640, 1972.
400. Wolfe, S.W., and Katz, L.D.: Intra-articular Impaction Fractures of the Phalanges. J. Hand Surg. 20A:1–7, 1995.
401. Woloszyn, J.T., Uitvlugt, G.M., and Castle, M.E.: Management of Civilian Gunshot Fractures of the Extremities. Clin. Orthop. 226:247–251, 1988.
402. Woods, G.L.: Troublesome Shaft Fractures of the Proximal Phalanx. Early Treatment to Avoid Late Problems at the Metacarpophalangeal and Proximal Phalangeal Joints. Hand Clin. 4:75–85, 1988.
403. Wray, R.C., and Weeks, P.M.: Management of Metacarpal Shaft Fractures. Mo. Med. 72:79–82, 1975.
404. Wray, R.C. Jr., and Glunk, R.: Treatment of Delayed Union, Nonunion, and Malunion of the Phalanges of the Hand. Ann. Plast. Surg. 22:14–18, 1989.
405. Wright, T.A.: Early Mobilization in Fractures of the Metacarpals and Phalanges. Can. J. Surg. 11:491–498, 1968.
406. Zacher, J.B.: Management of Injuries of the Distal Phalanx. Surg. Clin. North Am. 64:747–760, 1984.
407. Zimmerman, N.B., and Weiland, A.J.: Ninety-Ninety Intraosseous Wiring for Internal Fixation of the Digital Skeleton. Orthopedics 12:99–104, 1989.

FLEXOR DIGITORUM PROFUNDUS AVULSION

408. Zook, E.G.: Care of Nail Bed Injuries. Surg. Rounds 44–61, 1985.
409. Backe, H., and Posner, M.A.: Simultaneous Rupture of Both Flexor Tendons in a Finger. J. Hand Surg. 19A:246–248, 1994.
410. Blazina, M.E., and Lane, C.: Rupture of the Flexor Digitorum Profundus Tendon in Student Athletes. J. Am. Coll. Health 14:248–249, 1966.
411. Buscemi, M.J., and Page, B.J.: Flexor Digitorum Profundus Avulsions With Associated Distal Phalanx Fractures. Am. J. Sports Med. 15:366–370, 1987.
412. Bynum, D.K., and Gilbert, J.A.: Avulsion of the Flexor Digitorum Profundus: Anatomic and Biomechanical Considerations. J. Hand Surg. 13A:222–227, 1988.

413. Carroll, R.E., and Match, R.M.: Avulsion of the Flexor Profundus Tendon Insertion. J. Trauma 10:1109–1118, 1970.
414. Chang, W.H.J., Thomas, O.J., and White, W.L.: Avulsion Injury of the Long Flexor Tendons. Plast. Reconstr. Surg. 50:260–264, 1972.
415. Culver, J.E., Stanley, E.A., Amy, E.L., and Weiker, G.G.: Avulsion of the Profundus and Superficialis Tendons of the Ring Finger. Am. J. Sports Med. 9:184–186, 1981.
416. Eglseder, W.A., and Russell, J.M.: Type IV Flexor Digitorum Profundus Avulsion. J. Hand Surg. 15A:735–739, 1990.
417. Ehlert, K.J., Gould, J.S., and Black, K.P.: A Simultaneous Distal Phalanx Avulsion Fracture With Profundus Tendon Avulsion. A Case Report and Review of the Literature. Clin. Orthop. 283:265–269, 1992.
418. Gunter, G.S.: Traumatic Avulsion of the Insertion of Flexor Digitorum Profundus. Aust. N.Z. J. Surg. 30:1–8, 1960.
419. Langa, V., and Posner, M.A.: Unusual Rupture of a Flexor Profundus Tendon. J. Hand Surg. 11A:227–229, 1986.
420. Lanzetta, M., and Conolly, W.B.: Closed Rupture of Both Flexor Tendons in the Same Digit. J. Hand Surg. 17B:479–480, 1992.
421. Leddy, J.P.: Avulsions of the Flexor Digitorum Profundus. Hand Clin. 1:77–83, 1985.
422. Leddy, J.P., and Packer, J.W.: Avulsion of the Profundus Tendon Insertion in Athletes. J. Hand Surg. 2:66–69, 1977.
423. Manske, P.R., and Lesker, P.A.: Avulsion of the Ring Finger Flexor Digitorum Profundus Tendon: An Experimental Study. Hand 10:52–55, 1978.
424. McLaughlin, H.L.: Trauma.: Philadelphia, W.B. Saunders, 1960.
425. Ostrowski, D.M.: Avulsion of a Ring Finger Profundus Tendon With Separation of the Tendon From a Large Distal Phalanx Fracture Fragment. Orthopedics 14:1014–1017, 1991.
426. Posch, J.L., Walker, P.J., and Miller, H.: Treatment of Ruptured Tendons of the Hand and Wrist. Am. J. Surg. 91:669–681, 1956.
427. Reef, T.C.: Avulsion of the Flexor Digitorum Profundus: An Athletic Injury. Am. J. Sports Med. 5:281–285, 1977.
428. Robins, P.R., and Dobyns, J.H.: Avulsion of the Insertion of the Flexor Digitorum Profundus Tendon Associated With Fracture of the Distal Phalanx. A Brief Review. AAOS Symposium on Tendon Surgery in the Hand, pp. 151–156. St. Louis, C.V. Mosby, 1975.
429. Schwartz, G.B.: Flexor Digitorum Profundus Avulsion. A Unique Presentation. Orthop. Rev. 28:793–795, 1989.
430. Smith, J.H.: Avulsion of a Profundus Tendon With Simultaneous Intra-articular Fracture of the Distal Phalanx—Case Report. J. Hand Surg. 6:600–601, 1981.
431. Trumble, T.E., Vedder, N.B., and Benirschke, S.K.: Misleading Fractures after Profundus Tendon Avulsions: A Report of Six Cases. J. Hand Surg. 17A:902–906, 1992.
432. Wenger, D.R.: Avulsion of the Profundus Tendon Insertion in Football Players. Arch. Surg. 106:145–149, 1973.

MALLET FINGER AND BOUTONNIERE

433. Abouna, J.M., and Brown, H.: The Treatment of Mallet Finger. The Results in a Series of 148 Consecutive Cases and a Review of the Literature. Br. J. Surg. 55:653–667, 1968.
434. Auchincloss, J.M.: Mallet-finger Injuries: A Prospective, Controlled Trial of Internal and External Splintage. Hand 2:168–173, 1982.
435. Backdahl, M.: Ruptures of the Extensor Aponeurosis at the Distal Digital Joints. Acta Chir. Scand. 111:151–157, 1956.
436. Bischoff, R., Buechler, U., De Roche, R., and Jupiter, J.: Clinical Results of Tension Band Fixation of Avulsion Fractures of the Hand. J. Hand Surg. 19A:1019–1026, 1994.
437. Bowers, W.H., and Hurst, L.C.: Chronic Mallet Finger: The Use of Fowler's Central Slip Release. J. Hand Surg. 3:373–376, 1978.
438. Brooks, D.: Splint for Mallet Fingers. Br. Med. J. 1:1238, 1964.
439. Bunnell, S.: Surgery of the Hand, pp. 490–493. Philadelphia, J.B. Lippincott, 1944.
440. Burke, F.: Editorial: Mallet Finger. J. Hand Surg. 13B:115–117, 1988, 1994.
441. Casscells, S.W., and Strange, T.B.: Intramedullary Wire Fixation of Mallet Finger. J. Bone Joint Surg. 39A:521–526, 1957.
442. Casscells, S.W., and Strange, T.B.: Intramedullary Wire Fixation of Mallet Finger. J. Bone Joint Surg. 51A:1018–1019, 1969.
443. Cohn, B.T., and Froimson, A.I.: Case Report of a Rare Mallet Finger Injury. Orthopedics 9:529–531, 1986.
444. Crawford, G.P.: The Molded Polythene Splint for Mallet Finger Deformities. J. Hand Surg. 9A:231–237, 1984.
445. Damron, T.A., Engber, W.D., Lange, R.H., McCabe, R., Damron, L.A., Ulm, M., and Vanderby, R.: Biomechanical Analysis of Mallet Finger Fracture Fixation Techniques. J. Hand Surg. 18A:600–607, 1993.
446. Din, K.M., and Meggitt, B.F.: Mallet Thumb. J. Bone Joint Surg. 65B:606–607, 1983.
447. Elliott, R.A.: Injuries to the Extensor Mechanism of the Hand. Orthop. Clin. North Am. 1:335–354, 1970.
448. Elliott, R.A.: Splints for Mallet and Boutonniere Deformities. Plast. Reconstr. Surg. 52:282–285, 1973.
449. Evans, D., and Weightman, B.: The Pipflex Splint for Treatment of Mallet Finger. J. Hand Surg. 13B:156–158, 1988.
450. Flinchum, D.: Mallet Finger. J. Med. Assoc. Ga. 48:601–603, 1959.
451. Fowler, F.D.: New Splint for Treatment of Mallet Finger. J.A.M.A. 170:945, 1959.
452. Garberman, S.F., Diao, E., and Peimer, C.A.: Mallet Finger: Results of Early Versus Delayed Closed Treatment. J. Hand Surg. 19A:850–852, 1994.
453. Grundberg, A.B.: Anatomic Repair of Boutonniere Deformity. Clin. Orthop. 153:226–229, 1980.
454. Grundberg, A.B., and Reagan, D.S.: Central Slip Tenotomy for Chronic Mallet Finger Deformity. J. Hand Surg. 12A:545–547, 1987.
455. Hamas, R.S., Horrell, E.D., and Pierret, G.P.: Treatment of Mallet Finger Due to Intra-articular Fracture of the Distal Phalanx. J. Hand Surg. 3:361–363, 1978.
456. Harris, C., and Rutledge, G.L.: The Functional Anatomy of the Extensor Mechanism of the Finger. J. Bone Joint Surg. 54A:713–726, 1972.
457. Harris, C. Jr.: The Fowler Operation for Mallet Finger. J. Bone Joint Surg. 48A:613, 1966.
458. Hillman, F.E.: New Technique for Treatment of Mallet Fingers and Fractures of Distal Phalanx. J.A.M.A. 161:1135–1138, 1956.
459. Houpt, P., Dijkstra, R., and Storm Van Leeuwen, J.B.: Fowler's Tenotomy for Mallet Deformity. J. Hand Surg. 18B:499–500, 1993.
460. Hovgaard, C., and Klareskov, B.: Alternative Conservative Treatment of Mallet-finger Injuries by Elastic Double-finger Bandage. J. Hand Surg. 13B:154–155, 1988.
461. Howie, H.: The Treatment of Mallet Finger: A Modified Plaster Technique. N.Z. Med. J. 46:513, 1947.
462. Inoue, G.: Closed Reduction of Mallet Fractures Using Extension-block Kirschner Wire. J. Orthop. Trauma 6:413–415, 1992.
463. Isani, A.: Small Joint Injuries Requiring Surgical Treatment. Orthop. Clin. North Am. 17:407–419, 1986.
464. Iselin, F., Levame, J., and Godoy, J.: A Simplified Technique for Treating Mallet Fingers. Tenodermodesis. J. Hand Surg. 2:118–121, 1977.
465. Jones, N.F., and Peterson, J.: Epidemiologic Study of the Mallet Finger Deformity. J. Hand Surg. 13A:334–338, 1988.
466. Kaplan, E.B.: Mallet or Baseball Finger. Surgery, 7:784–791, 1940.
467. Kaplan, E.B.: Anatomy, Injuries and Treatment of the Extensor Apparatus of the Hand and the Digits. Clin. Orthop. 13:24–41, 1959.
468. Kinninmonth, A.W.G., and Holburn, F.: A Comparative Controlled Trial of a New Perforated Splint and a Traditional Splint in the Treatment of Mallet Finger. J. Hand Surg. 11B:261–262, 1986.

469. Kleinman, W.B., and Petersen, D.P.: Oblique Retinacular Ligament Reconstruction for Chronic Mallet Finger Deformity. J. Hand Surg. 9A:399–404, 1984.
470. Kon, M., and Bloem, J.J.A.M.: Treatment of Mallet Fingers by Tenodermodesis. Hand 14:174–176, 1982.
471. Lange, R.H., and Engber, W.D.: Hyperextension Mallet Finger. Orthopedics 6:1426–1431, 1983.
472. Lewin, P.: A Simple Splint for Baseball Finger. J.A.M.A. 85:1059, 1994.
473. Lind, J., and Hansen, L.B.: Abbrevatio: A New Operation for Chronic Mallet Finger. J. Hand Surg. 14B:347–349, 1989.
474. Littler, J.W.: The Voice of Polite Dissent. A New Method of Treatment for Mallet Finger. Plast. Reconstr. Surg. 58:499–500, 1976.
475. Littler, J.W., and Eaton, R.G.: Redistribution of Forces in the Correction of the Boutonniere Deformity. J. Bone Joint Surg. 49A:1267–1274, 1967.
476. Lubahn, J.D.: Mallet Finger Fractures: A Comparison of Open and Closed Technique. J. Hand Surg. 14A:394–396, 1989.
477. Mason, M.L.: Rupture of Tendons of the Hand. With a Study of the Extensor Tendon Insertions in the Fingers. Surg. Gynecol. Obstet. 50:611–624, 1930.
478. Mason, M.L.: Mallet Finger. Lancet, 266:1220, 1954.
479. Matev, I.: Transposition of the Lateral Slips of the Aponeurosis in Treatment of Long-standing "Boutonniere Deformity" of the Fingers. Br. J. Plast. Surg. 17:281–286, 1964.
480. Matev, I.: The Boutonniere Deformity. Hand 1:90–95, 1969.
481. McCue, F.C., and Abbott, J.L.: The Treatment of Mallet Finger and Boutonniere Deformities. Va. Med. 94:623–628, 1967.
482. McFarlane, R.M., and Hampole, M.K.: Treatment of Extensor Tendon Injuries of the Hand. Can. J. Surg. 16:366–375, 1973.
483. McMinn, D.J.W.: Mallet Finger and Fractures. Injury, 12:477–479, 1981.
484. Mikic, Z., and Helal, B.: The Treatment of the Mallet Finger by Oakley Splint. Hand 6:76–81, 1974.
485. Mirza, M.A., and Korber, K.E.: Inverted-U Incision for Exploration of the Distal Phalanx. Ideas and Innovations, 74:548–549, 1984.
486. Miura, T., Nakamura, R., and Torii, S.: Conservative Treatment for a Ruptured Extensor Tendon on the Dorsum of the Proximal Phalanges of the Thumb (Mallet Thumb). J. Hand Surg. 11A:229–233, 1986.
487. Mixa, T.M., Blair, S.J., and Dvonch, V.M.: Acute and Chronic Management of Mallet Finger. A Case Study. Orthopedics 8:1044–1046, 1985.
488. Moss, J.G., and Steingold, R.F.: The Long Term Results of Mallet Finger Injury: A Retrospective Study of One Hundred Cases. Hand 15:151–154, 1983.
489. Nichols, H.M.: Repair of Extensor Tendon Insertion in the Fingers. J. Bone Joint Surg. 33A:836–841, 1951.
490. Niechajev, I.A.: Conservative and Operative Treatment of Mallet Finger. Plast. Reconstr. Surg. 76:580–585, 1985.
491. Patel, M.R., Desai, S.S., and Lipson, L.B.: Conservative Management of Chronic Mallet Finger. J. Hand Surg. 11A:570–573, 1986.
492. Patel, M.R., Lipson, L.B., and Desai, S.S.: Conservative Treatment of Mallet Thumb. J. Hand Surg. 11A:45–47, 1986.
493. Pratt, D.R.: Internal Splint for Closed and Open Treatment of Injuries of the Extensor Tendon at the Distal Joint of the Finger. J. Bone Joint Surg. 34A:785–788, 1952.
494. Primiano, G.A.: Conservative Treatment of Two Cases of Mallet Thumb. J. Hand Surg. 11A:233–235, 1986.
495. Ramsay, R.A.: Mallet Finger. Lancet 2:1244, 1968.
496. Ratliff, A.H.C.: Mallet Finger: A Review of Forty-five Cases. Manch. Med. Gaz. 26:4, 1947.
497. Rayan, G.M., and Mullins, P.T.: Skin Necrosis Complicating Mallet Finger Splinting and Vascularity of the Distal Interphalangeal Joint Overlying Skin. J. Hand Surg. 12A:548–552, 1987.
498. Robb, W.A.T.: The Results of Treatment of Mallet Finger. J. Bone Joint Surg. 41B:546–549, 1959.
499. Roemer, F.J.: Hyperextension Injuries to the Finger Joints. Am. J. Surg. 80:295–302, 1950.
500. Rosenzweig, N.: Management of the Mallet Finger. S. Afr. Med. J. 24:831–832, 1950.
501. Schneider, L.H.: Fractures of the Distal Phalanx. Hand Clin. 4:537–547, 1988.
502. Schneider, L.H.: Commentary (On Mallet Finger Fracture Fixation Techniques—Damron et al-#445). J. Hand Surg. 18A:608, 1993.
503. Schneider, L.H.: Fractures of the Distal Interphalangeal Joint. Hand Clin. 10:277–285, 1994.
504. Shankar, N.S., and Goring, C.C.: Mallet Finger: Long-term Review of 100 Cases. J. R. Coll. Surg. Edinb. 37:196–198, 1992.
505. Smillie, I.S.: Mallet Finger. Br. J. Surg. 24:439–445, 1937.
506. Souter, W.A.: The Boutonniere Deformity. A Review of 101 Patients With Division of the Central Slip of the Extensor Expansion of the Fingers. J. Bone Joint Surg. 49B:710–721, 1967.
507. Souter, W.A.: The Problem of Boutonniere Deformity. Clin. Orthop. 104:116–133, 1974.
508. Spigelman, L.: New Splint for Management of Mallet Finger. J.A.M.A. 153:1362, 1953.
509. Stack, H.G.: Mallet Finger. Hand 1:83–89, 1969.
510. Stack, H.G.: A Modified Splint for Mallet Finger. J. Hand Surg. 11B:263, 1986.
511. Stark, H.H., Boyes, J.H., and Wilson, J.N.: Mallet Finger. J. Bone Joint Surg. 44A:1061–1068, 1962.
512. Stark, H.H., Gainor, B.J., Ashworth, C.R., Zemel, N.P., and Rickard, T.A.: Operative Treatment of Intra-articular Fractures of the Dorsal Aspect of the Distal Phalanx of Digits. J. Bone Joint Surg. 69A:892–896, 1987.
513. Stern, P.J., and Kastrup, J.J.: Complications and Prognosis of Treatment of Mallet Finger. J. Hand Surg. 13A:329–334, 1988.
514. Stewart, I.M.: Boutonniere Finger. Clin. Orthop. 23:220–226, 1962.
515. Thompson, J.S., Littler, J.W., and Upton, J.: The Spiral Oblique Retinacular Ligament (SORL). J. Hand Surg. 3:482–487, 1978.
516. Urbaniak, J.R., and Hayes, M.G.: Chronic Boutonniere Deformity: An Anatomic Reconstruction. J. Hand Surg. 6:379–383, 1981.
517. Van Demark, R.E.: A Simple Method of Treatment for Recent Mallet Finger. Mil. Surg. 107:385–386 1950, 1994.
518. Van Der Meulen, J.C.: The Treatment of Prolapse and Collapse of the Proximal Interphalangeal Joint. Hand 4:154–162, 1972.
519. Warren, R.A., Kay, N.R.M., and Ferguson, D.G.: Mallet Finger: Comparison Between Operative and Conservative Management in Those Cases Failing to Be Cured by Splintage. J. Hand Surg. 13B:159–160, 1988.
520. Warren, R.A., Kay, N.R.M., and Norris, S.H.: The Microvascular Anatomy of the Distal Digital Extensor Tendon. J. Hand Surg. 13B:161–163, 1988.
521. Warren, R.A., Norris, S.H., and Ferguson, D.G.: Mallet Finger: A Trial of Two Splints. J. Hand Surg. 13B:151–153, 1988.
522. Watson, F.M.: American Society for Surgery of the Hand Correspondence Newsletter, 1983.
523. Watson-Jones, R.: Fractures and Joint Injuries, 4th Ed., pp. 645–646. Edinburgh, E & S Livingstone, 1956.
524. Wehbe, M.A., and Schneider, L.H.: Mallet Fractures. J. Bone Joint Surg. 66A:658–669, 1984.
525. Weinberg, H., Stein, H.C., and Wexler, M.R.: A New Method of Treatment for Mallet Finger. A Preliminary Report. Plast. Reconstr. Surg. 58:347–349, 1976.
526. Williams, E.G.: Treatment of Mallet Finger. Can. Med. Assoc. J. 57:582, 1947.

FRACTURES OF THE THUMB METACARPAL

527. Badger, F.C.: Internal Fixation in the Treatment of Bennett's Fractures. J. Bone Joint Surg. 38B:771, 1956.
528. Bennett, E.H.: Fractures of the Metacarpal Bones. Dublin J. Med. Sci. 73:72–75, 1882.

529. Bennett, E.H.: On Fracture of the Metacarpal Bone of the Thumb. Br. Med. J. 2:12–13, 1886.
530. Billing, L., and Gedda, K.O.: Roentgen Examination of Bennett's Fracture. Acta Radiol. 38:471–476, 1952.
531. Blum, L.: The Treatment of Bennett's Fracture-Dislocation of the First Metacarpal Bone. J. Bone Joint Surg. 23:578–580, 1941.
532. Breen, T.F., Gelberman, R.H., and Jupiter, J.B.: Intra-articular Fractures of the Basilar Joint of the Thumb. Hand Clin. 4:491–501, 1988.
533. Buchler, U., McCollam, S.M., and Oppikofer, C.: Comminuted Fractures of the Basilar Joint of the Thumb: Combined Treatment by External Fixation, Limited Internal Fixation, and Bone Grafting. J. Hand Surg. 16A:556–560, 1991.
534. Cannon, S.R., Dowd, G.S.E., Williams, D.H., and Scott, J.M.: A Long-term Study Following Bennett's Fracture. J. Hand Surg. 11B:426–431, 1986.
535. Charnley, J.: The Closed Treatment of Common Fractures. Edinburgh, E & S Livingstone, 1961.
536. Cotton, F.J.: Dislocations and Joint Fractures. Philadelphia, W.B. Saunders, 1910.
537. Darte, D.A., Brink, P.R.G., and van Houtte, H.P.: Iselie's Operative Technique for Thumb Proximal Metacarpal Fractures. Injury 23:370–372, 1992.
538. Dial, W.B., and Berg, E.: Bennett's Fracture. Hand 4:229–235, 1972.
539. Ellis, V.H.: A Method of Treating Bennett's Fracture. Proc. R. Soc. Med. 39:21, 1946.
540. Fisher, E.: Bennett's Fracture in General Practice. Med. J. Aust. 1:434–438, 1976.
541. Foster, R.J., and Hastings, H.: Treatment of Bennett, Rolando, and Vertical Intraarticular Trapezial Fractures. Clin. Orthop. 214:121–129, 1987.
542. Garcia-Elias, M., Henríquez-Lluch, A., Rossignani, P., Fernandez De Retana, P., and Orovio De Elízaga, J.: Bennett's Fracture Combined With Fracture of the Trapezium. A Report of Three Cases. J. Hand Surg. 18B:523–526, 1993.
543. Gedda, K.O.: Studies on Bennett's Fracture: Anatomy, Roentgenology, and Therapy. Acta Chir. Scand. Suppl. 193, 1954.
544. Gedda, K.O., and Moberg, E.: Open Reduction and Osteosynthesis of the So-called Bennett's Fracture in the Carpometacarpal Joint of the Thumb. Acta Orthop. Scand. 22:249–256, 1953.
545. Gelberman, R.H., Vance, R.M., and Zakaib, G.S.: Fractures at the Base of the Thumb: Treatment With Oblique Traction. J. Bone Joint Surg. 61A:260–262, 1979.
546. Goldberg, D.: Thumb Fractures and Dislocations, A New Method of Treatment. Am. J. Surg. 81:227–231, 1951.
547. Goldberg, D.: Metacarpal and Thumb Fractures, A Dynamic Method of Treatment. Orthop. Rev. 7:37–42, 1978.
548. Green, D.P., and O'Brien, E.T.: Fractures of the Thumb Metacarpal. South. Med. J. 65:807–814, 1972.
549. Griffiths, J.C.: Fractures at the Base of the First Metacarpal Bone. J. Bone Joint Surg. 46B:712–719, 1964.
550. Griffiths, J.C.: Bennett's Fracture in Childhood. Br. J. Clin. Pract. 20:582–583, 1966.
551. Harvey, F.J., and Bye, W.D.: Bennett's Fracture. Hand 8:48–53, 1976.
552. Howard, F.M.: Fractures of the Basal Joint of the Thumb. Clin. Orthop. 220:46–51, 1987.
553. James, E.S., and Gibson, A.: Fractures of the First Metacarpal Bone. Can. Med. Assoc. J. 43:153–155, 1940.
554. Johnson, E.C.: Fracture of the Base of the Thumb: A New Method of Fixation. J.A.M.A. 126:27–28, 1944.
555. Kjaer-Petersen, K., Andersen, K., and Langhoff, O.: Combined Basal Metacarpal Fracture and Ligament Injury of the Metacarpophalangeal Joint of the Thumb. J. Bone Joint Surg. 73B:176–177, 1991.
556. Kjaer-Petersen, K., Langhoff, O., and Andersen, K.: Bennett's Fracture. J. Hand Surg. 15B:58–61, 1990.
557. Kuschner, S.H., Shepard, L., Stephens, S., and Gellman, H.: Fracture of the Index Metacarpal Base With Subluxation of the Trapeziometacarpal Joint. A Case Report. Clin. Orthop. 264:197–199, 1991.
558. Langhoff, O., Andersen, K., and Kjaer-Petersen, K.: Rolando's Fracture. J. Hand Surg. 16B:454–459, 1991.
559. Livesley, P.J.: The Conservative Management of Bennett's Fracture-Dislocation: A 26-Year Follow-up. J. Hand Surg. 15B:291–294, 1990.
560. Macey, H.B., and Murray, R.A.: Fractures About the Base of the First Metacarpal With Special Reference to Bennett's Fracture. South. Med. J. 42:931–935, 1949.
561. McNealy, R.W., and Lichtenstein, M.E.: Bennett's Fracture and Other Fractures of the First Metacarpal. Surg. Gynecol. Obstet. 56:197–201, 1933.
562. Miles, A., and Struthers, J.W.: Original Communications. Bennett's Fracture of the Base of the Metacarpal Bone of the Thumb. Edinburgh Med. J. 15:297–308, 1904.
563. Pellegrini, V.D.: Fractures at the Base of the Thumb. Hand Clin. 4:87–101, 1988.
564. Pollen, A.G.: The Conservative Treatment of Bennett's Fracture-subluxation of the Thumb Metacarpal. J. Bone Joint Surg. 50B:91–101, 1968.
565. Proubasta, I.R.: Rolando's Fracture of the First Metacarpal. Treatment by External Fixation. J. Bone Joint Surg. 74B:416–417, 1992.
566. Radford, P.J., Wilcox, D.T., and Holdsworth, B.J.: Simultaneous Trapezium and Bennett's Fractures. J. Hand Surg. 17A:621–623, 1992.
567. Roberts, J.B., and Kelly, N.A.: Treatise on Fractures. Philadelphia, J.B. Lippincott, 1916.
568. Robinson, S.: The Bennett Fracture of the First Metacarpal Bone: Diagnosis and Treatment. Boston Med. Surg. J. 158:275–276, 1908.
569. Rolando, S.: Fracture de la Base du Premier Metacarpien: Et Principalement sur une Variete non Encore Decrite. Presse Med. 18:303–304, 1910.
570. Ross, J.W., and Sinclair, A.B.: The Treatment of Bennett's Fracture With the Stader Splint. J. Can. Med. Serv. 3:507–511, 1946.
571. Salgeback, S., Eiken, O., Carstam, N., and Ohlsson, N.M.: A Study of Bennett's Fracture. Special Reference to Fixation by Percutaneous Pinning. Scand. J. Plast. Reconstr. Surg. 5:142–148, 1971.
572. Spangberg, O., and Thoren, L.: Bennett's Fracture: A Method of Treatment With Oblique Traction. J. Bone Joint Surg. 45B:732–739, 1963.
573. Stromberg, L.: Compression Fixation of Bennett's Fracture. Acta Orthop. Scand. 48:586–591, 1977.
574. Thoren, L.: A New Method of Extension Treatment in Bennett's Fracture. Acta Chir. Scand. 110:485–493, 1956.
575. Thoren, L.: Basal Fractures of the First Metacarpal Bone—A Method of Treatment by Excision. Acta Orthop. Scand. 27:40–48, 1957.
576. Timmenga, E.J.F., Blokhuis, T.J., Maas, M., and Raaijmakers, E.L.F.B.: Long-Term Evaluation of Bennett's Fracture. A Comparison Between Open and Closed Reduction. J. Hand Surg. 19B:373–377, 1994.
577. van Niekerk, J.L.M., and Ouwens, R.: Fractures of the Base of the First Metacarpal Bone: Results of Surgical Treatment. Injury 20:359–361, 1989.
578. Wagner, C.J.: Method of Treatment of Bennett's Fracture Dislocation. Am. J. Surg. 80:230–231, 1950.
579. Wagner, C.J.: Transarticular Fixation of Fracture-Dislocations of the First Metacarpal-carpal Joint. West. J. Surg. Obstet. Gynecol. 59:362–365, 1951.
580. Wiggins, H.E., Bundens, W.D. Jr., and Park, B.J.: A Method of Treatment of Fracture-Dislocations of the First Metacarpal Bone. J. Bone Joint Surg. 36A:810–819, 1954.

INTERPHALANGEAL JOINTS

581. Adams, J.P.: Correction of Chronic Dorsal Subluxation of the Proximal Interphalangeal Joint by Means of a Criss-cross Volar Graft. J. Bone Joint Surg. 41A:111–115, 1959.
582. Agee, J.M.: Unstable Fracture Dislocations of the Proximal

Interphalangeal Joint of the Fingers: A Preliminary Report of a New Treatment Technique. J. Hand Surg. 3:386–389, 1978.

583. Agee, J.M.: Unstable Fracture Dislocations of the Proximal Interphalangeal Joint. Treatment With the Force Couple Splint. Clin. Orthop. 214:101–112, 1987.
584. Ali, M.S.: Complete Disruption of Collateral Mechanism of Proximal Interphalangeal Joint of Fingers. J. Hand Surg. 9:191–193, 1984.
585. Ambrosia, J.M., and Linscheid, R.L.: Simultaneous Dorsal Dislocation of the Interphalangeal Joints in a Finger. Case Report and Review of the Literature. Orthopedics 11:1079–1080, 1988.
586. Andersen, M.B., and Johannsen, H.: Double Dislocation of the Interphalangeal Joints in the Finger. Case Report and Review of Publications. Scand. J. Plast. Reconstr. Hand Surg. 27:233–236, 1993.
587. Bate, J.T.: An Operation for the Correction of Locking of the Proximal Interphalangeal Joint of Finger in Hyperextension. J. Bone Joint Surg. 27:142–144, 1945.
588. Baugher, W.H., and McCue, F.C.: Anterior Fracture Dislocation of the Proximal Interphalangeal Joint. A Case Report. J. Bone Joint Surg. 61A:779–780, 1979.
589. Bayne, O., Chabot, J.M., Carr, J.P., and Evans, E.F.: Simultaneous Dorsal Dislocation of Interphalangeal Joints in a Finger. Clin. Orthop. 257:104–106, 1990.
590. Benke, G.J., and Stableforth, P.G.: Injuries of the Proximal Interphalangeal Joint of the Fingers. Hand 3:263–268, 1979.
591. Bilos, Z.J., Vender, M.I., Bonavolonta, M., and Knutson, K.: Fracture Subluxation of Proximal Interphalangeal Joint Treated by Palmar Plate Advancement. J. Hand Surg. 19A:189–196, 1994.
592. Bowers, W.H.: The Proximal Interphalangeal Joint Volar Plate. II: A Clinical study of Hyperextension Injury. J. Hand Surg. 6:77–81, 1981.
593. Bowers, W.H.: Management of Small Joint Injuries in the Hand. Orthop. Clin. North Am. 14:793–810, 1983.
594. Bowers, W.H., and Fajgenbaum, D.M.: Closed Rupture of the Volar Plate of the Distal Interphalangeal Joint. J. Bone Joint Surg. 61A:146, 1979.
595. Bowers, W.H., Wolf, J.W., Nehil, J.L., and Bittinger, S.: The Proximal Interphalangeal Joint Volar Plate: I. An Anatomical and Biomechanical Study. J. Hand Surg. 5:79–88, 1980.
596. Bowers, W.H.(.).: The Hand and Upper Limb. Volume 1. The Interphalangeal Joints. Edinburgh, Churchill Livingstone, 1987.
597. Buchanan, R.T.: Mechanical Requirements for Application and Modification of the Dynamic Force Couple Method. Hand Clin. 10:221–228, 1994.
598. Burton, R.I.: Small Joint Injuries of the Hand. Dynamic and Functional Implications. Hand Clin. 4:11–12, 1988.
599. Cole, I.C.: Principles and Guidelines in Hand Therapy and Rehabilitation During Recovery From Small Joint Injuries. Hand Clin. 4:123–131, 1988.
600. Craig, S.M.: Anatomy of the Joints of the Fingers. Hand Clin. 8:693–700, 1992.
601. Crick, J.C., Conners, J.J., and Franco, R.S.: Irreducible Palmar Dislocation of the Proximal Interphalangeal Joint With Bilateral Avulsion Fractures. J. Hand Surg. 15A:460–463, 1990.
602. Curran, A.J., McKiernan, M.V., and McCann, J.: Double Interphalangeal Joint Dislocation in a Little Finger. Injury, 23:138, 1992.
603. Curtis, R.M.: Treatment of Injuries of the Proximal Interphalangeal Joints of the Fingers. Curr. Pract. Orthop. Surg. 2:125–135, 1964.
604. De Smet, L., and Vercauteren, M.: Palmar Dislocation of the Proximal Interphalangeal Joint Requiring Open Reduction: A Case Report. J. Hand Surg. 9A:717–718, 1984.
605. Diao, E., and Eaton, R.G.: Total Collateral Ligament Excision for Contractures of the Proximal Interphalangeal Joint. J. Hand Surg. 18A:395–402, 1993.
606. Dobyns, J.H., and McElfresh, E.C.: Extension Block Splinting. Hand Clin. 10:229–237, 1994.
607. Donaldson, W.R., and Millender, L.H.: Chronic Fracture-subluxation of the Proximal Interphalangeal Joint. J. Hand Surg. 2:149–153, 1978.
608. Durham-Smith, G., and McCarten, G.M.: Volar Plate Arthroplasty for Closed Proximal Interphalangeal Joint Injuries. J. Hand Surg. 17B:422–428, 1992.
609. Eaton, R.G.: Joint Injuries of the Hand. Springfield, Ill., Charles C. Thomas, 1971.
610. Eaton, R.G.: The Founders Lecture: The Narrowest Hinge of My Hand. J. Hand Surg. 20A:149–154, 1995.
611. Eaton, R.G., and Littler, J.W.: Joint Injuries and Their Sequelae. Clin. Plast. Surg. 3:85–98, 1976.
612. Eaton, R.G., and Malerich, M.M.: Volar Plate Arthroplasty of the Proximal Interphalangeal Joint: A Review of Ten Years' Experience. J. Hand Surg. 5:260–268, 1980.
613. Espinosa, R.H., and Renart, I.P.: Simultaneous Dislocation of the Interphalangeal Joints in a Finger. Case Report. J. Hand Surg. 5:617–618, 1980.
614. Faithfull, D.K.: Treatment of Chronic Instability of the Digital Joints Using a Strip of Volar Plate. Hand 13:36–38, 1981.
615. Flatt, A.E.: The Care of Minor Hand Injuries, pp. 188–189. St. Louis, C.V. Mosby, 1959.
616. Freeman, B.H., Haskin, J.S. Jr., and Hay, E.L.: Chronic Anterior Dislocation of the Proximal Interphalangeal Joint. Orthopedics 8:385–388, 1985.
617. Garroway, R.Y., Hurst, L.C., Leppard, J. III; and Dick, H.M.: Complex Dislocations of the Proximal Interphalangeal Joint. A Pathoanatomic Classification of the Injury. Orthop. Rev. 13:21–28, 1984.
618. Ghobadi, F., and Anapolle, D.M.: Irreducible Distal Interphalangeal Joint Dislocation of the Finger: A New Cause. J. Hand Surg. 19A:196–198, 1994.
619. Green, A., Smith, J., Redding, M., and Akelman, E.: Acute Open Reduction and Rigid Internal Fixation of Proximal Interphalangeal Joint Fracture Dislocation. J. Hand Surg. 17A:512–517, 1992.
620. Green, D.P.: Dislocations and Ligamentous Injuries in the Hand and Wrist. *In* Evarts, C.M. (ed.): Surgery of the Musculoskeletal System. New York, Churchill Livingstone, 1983.
621. Green, D.P., and Rowland, S.A.: Fractures and Dislocations in the Hand. *In* Rockwood, C.A., and Green, D.P. (eds.): Fractures. Philadelphia, J.B. Lippincott, 1975.
622. Green, S.M., and Posner, M.A.: Irreducible Dorsal Dislocations of the Proximal Interphalangeal Joint. J. Hand Surg. 10A:85–87, 1985.
623. Hage, J.J., Reinders, J.F.M., and Schuwirth, L.: Simultaneous Dislocation of Both Interphalangeal Joints in a Finger. Arch. Orthop. Trauma Surg. 109:179–180, 1990.
624. Hamer, D.W., and Quinton, D.N.: Dorsal Fracture Subluxation of the Proximal Interphalangeal Joints Treated by Extension Block Splintage. J. Hand Surg. 17B:586–590, 1992.
625. Hamer, D.W., and Quinton, D.N.: Dorsal Fracture Subluxation of the Distal Interphalangeal Joint of the Finger and the Interphalangeal Joint of the Thumb Treated by Extension Block Splintage. J. Hand Surg. 17B:591–594, 1992.
626. Hardy, I., Russell, J., and McFarlane, I.: Simultaneous Dislocation of the Interphalangeal Joints in a Finger. J. Trauma 25:450–451, 1985.
627. Hastings, H., and Carroll, C.: Treatment of Closed Articular Fractures of the Metacarpophalangeal and Proximal Interphalangeal Joints. Hand Clin. 4:503–527, 1988.
628. Hindley, C.J.: Triple Dislocations in the Index Finger. J. Trauma 29:122–124, 1989.
629. Holtmann, B., Wray, R.C. Jr., and Weeks, P.M.: A Frequently Overlooked Injury in the Hand. Mo. Med. 73:477–481, 1976.
630. Horiuchi, Y., Itoh, Y., Sasaki, T., Tasaki, K., Iijima, K., and Uchinishi, K.: Dorsal Dislocation of the D.I.P. Joint With Fracture of the Volar Base of the Distal Phalanx. J. Hand Surg. 14B:177–182, 1989.
631. Hutchison, J.D., Hooper, G., and Robb, J.E.: Double Dislocations of Digits. J. Hand Surg. 16B:114–115, 1991.
632. Iftikhar, T.B.: Long Flexor Tendon Entrapment Causing Open Irreducible Dorsoradial Dislocation of Distal Interphalangeal

Joint of the Finger. A Case Report. Orthop. Rev. 11:117–119, 1982.
633. Ikpeme, J.O.: Dislocation of Both Interphalangeal Joints of One Finger. Injury, 9:68–70, 1977.
634. Incavo, S.J., Mogan, J.V., and Hilfrank, B.C.: Extension Splinting of Palmar Plate Avulsion Injuries of the Proximal Interphalangeal Joint. J. Hand Surg. 14A:659–661, 1989.
635. Inoue, G., Kino, Y., and Kondo, K.: Simultaneous Dorsal Dislocation of Both Interphalangeal Joints in a Finger. Am. J. Sports Med. 21:323–325, 1993.
636. Inoue, G., and Maeda, N.: Irreducible Palmar Dislocation of the Distal Interphalangeal Joint of the Finger. J. Hand Surg. 12A:1077–1079, 1987.
637. Inoue, G., and Maeda, N.: Irreducible Palmar Dislocation of the Proximal Interphalangeal Joint of the Finger. J. Hand Surg. 15A:301–304, 1990.
638. Isani, A.: Small Joint Injuries Requiring Surgical Treatment. Orthop. Clin. North Am. 17:407–419, 1986.
639. Isani, A., and Melone, C.P. Jr.: Ligamentous Injuries of the Hand in Athletes. Clin. Sports Med. 5:757–772, 1986.
640. Johnson, F.G., and Greene, M.H.: Another Cause of Irreducible Dislocation of the Proximal Interphalangeal Joint of a Finger. A Case Report. J. Bone Joint Surg. 48A:542–544, 1966.
641. Jones, N.F., and Jupiter, J.B.: Irreducible Palmar Dislocation of the Proximal Interphalangeal Joint Associated With an Epiphyseal Fracture of the Middle Phalanx. J. Hand Surg. 10A:261–264, 1985.
642. Khuri, S.M.: Irreducible Dorsal Dislocation of the Distal Interphalangeal Joint of the Finger. J. Trauma. 24:456–457, 1984.
643. Kiefhaber, T.R., Stern, P.J., and Grood, E.S.: Lateral Stability of the Proximal Interphalangeal Joint. J. Hand Surg. 11A:661–669, 1986.
644. Kilgore, E.S., Newmeyer, W.L., and Brown, L.G.: Post-traumatic Trapped Dislocations of the Proximal Interphalangeal Joint. J. Trauma 16:481–487, 1976.
645. Kitagawa, H., and Kashimoto, T.: Locking of the Thumb at the Interphalangeal Joint by One of the Sesamoid Bones. A Case Report. J. Bone Joint Surg. 66A:1300–1301, 1984.
646. Kjeldal, I.: Irreducible Compound Dorsal Dislocations of the Proximal Interphalangeal Joint of the Finger. J. Hand Surg. 11B:49–50, 1986.
647. Kleinert, H.E., and Kasdan, M.L.: Reconstruction of Chronically Subluxated Proximal Interphalangeal Finger Joint. J. Bone Joint Surg. 47A:958–964, 1965.
648. Konsens, R.M., Cohn, B.T., and Froimson, A.I.: Double Dislocation of the Fifth Finger. Orthopedics 10:1061–1062, 1987.
649. Krebs, B., and Gron, L.K.: Simultaneous Dorsal Dislocation of Both Interphalangeal Joints in a Finger. Br. J. Sports Med. 18:217–219, 1984.
650. Krishnan, S.G.: Double Dislocation of a Finger. A Case Report. Am. J. Sports Med. 7:204–205, 1979.
651. Kuczynski, K.: The Proximal Interphalangeal Joint. Anatomy and Causes of Stiffness in the Fingers. J. Bone Joint Surg. 50B:656–663, 1968.
652. Kuczynski, K.: Less-known Aspects of the Proximal Interphalangeal Joints of the Human Hand. Hand 7:31–33, 1975.
653. Lane, C.S.: Reconstruction of the Unstable Proximal Interphalangeal Joint: The Double Superficialis Tenodesis. J. Hand Surg. 3:368–369, 1978.
654. Lange, R.H., and Engber, W.D.: Proximal Interphalangeal Joint Fracture-Dislocation Associated With Mallet Finger. Orthopedics 6:571–575, 1983.
655. Laporte, J.M., Berrettoni, B.A., Seitz, W.H. Jr., Winsberg, D., and Froimson, A.I.: The Figure-of-Eight Splint for Proximal Interphalangeal Joint Volar Plate Injuries. Orthop. Rev. 21:457–461, 1992.
656. Leibovic, S.J., and Bowers, W.H.: Anatomy of the Proximal Interphalangeal Joint. Hand Clin. 10:169–178, 1994.
657. Levy, I.M., and Liberty, S.: Simultaneous Dislocation of the Interphalangeal and Metacarpophalangeal Joints of the Thumb: A Case Report. J. Hand Surg. 4:489–490, 1979.
658. Light, T.R.: Buttress Pinning Techniques. Orthop. Rev. 10:49–55, 1981.
659. Lineaweaver, W., and Mathes, S.J.: Distal Avulsion of the Palmar Plate of the Interphalangeal Joint of the Thumb. J. Hand Surg. 13A:465–467, 1988.
660. Liss, F.E., and Green, S.M.: Capsular Injuries of the Proximal Interphalangeal Joint. Hand Clin. 8:755–768, 1992.
661. London, P.S.: Sprains and Fractures Involving the Interphalangeal Joints. Hand 3:155–158, 1971.
662. Lubahn, J.D.: Dorsal Fracture Dislocations of the Proximal Interphalangeal Joint. Hand Clin. 4:15–24, 1988.
663. Lucas, G.L.: Volar Plate Advancement. Orthop. Rev. 4:13–16, 1975.
664. Malerich, M.M., and Eaton, R.G.: The Volar Plate Reconstruction for Fracture-Dislocation of the Proximal Interphalangeal Joint. Hand Clin. 10:251–260, 1994.
665. McCue, F.C., Honner, R., Johnson, M.C., and Gieck, J.H.: Athletic Injuries of the Proximal Interphalangeal Joint Requiring Surgical Treatment. J. Bone Joint Surg. 52A:937–956, 1970.
666. McElfresh, E.C., Dobyns, J.H., and O'Brien, E.T.: Management of Fracture-Dislocation of the Proximal Interphalangeal Joints by Extension-block Splinting. J. Bone Joint Surg. 54A:1705–1711, 1972.
667. Meyn, M.A. Jr.: Irreducible Volar Dislocation of the Proximointerphalangeal Joint. Clin. Orthop. 158:215–218, 1981.
668. Milford, L.: The Hand. *In* Crenshaw, A.H. (ed.): Campbell's Operative Orthopaedics, 4th Ed., p. 166. St. Louis, C.V. Mosby, 1963.
669. Milford, L.: The Hand. *In* Crenshaw, A.H. (ed.): Campbell's Operative Orthopaedics. 5th Ed., pp. 188–189. St. Louis, C.V. Mosby, 1971.
670. Milford, L.: The Hand. *In* Edmonson, A.S., and Crenshaw, A.H. (eds.): Campbell's Operative Orthopaedics, 6th Ed., pp. 160. St. Louis, C.V. Mosby, 1980.
671. Milford, L.: Interphalangeal Dislocations. *In* Crenshaw, A.H. (ed.): Campbell's Operative Orthopaedics, pp. 249–253. St. Louis, C.V. Mosby, 1987.
672. Minamikawa, Y., Horii, E., Amadio, P.C., Cooney, W.P., Linscheid, R.L., and An, K.: Stability and Constraint of the Proximal Interphalangeal Joint. J. Hand Surg. 18A:198–204, 1993.
673. Moberg, E.: Fractures and Ligamentous Injuries of the Thumb and Fingers. Surg. Clin. North Am. 40:297–309, 1960.
674. Moller, J.T.: Lesions of the Volar Fibrocartilage in Finger Joints. A 2-year Material. Acta Orthop. Scand. 45:673–682, 1974.
675. Murakami, Y.: Irreducible Volar Dislocation of the Proximal Interphalangeal Joint of the Finger. Hand 6:87–90, 1974.
676. Murakami, Y.: Irreducible Dislocation of the Distal Interphalangeal Joint. J. Hand Surg. 10B:231–232, 1985.
677. Nance, E.P., Kaye, J.J., and Milek, M.A.: Volar Plate Fractures. Radiology, 133:61–64, 1979.
678. Neviaser, R.J., and Wilson, J.N.: Interposition of the Extensor Tendon Resulting in Persistent Subluxation of the Proximal Interphalangeal Joint of the Finger. Clin. Orthop. 83:118–120, 1972.
679. Nichols, H.M.: Manual of Hand Injuries, 2nd Ed., p. 310. Chicago, Year Book Medical Publishers, 1960.
680. Oni, O.O.A.: Irreducible Buttonhole Dislocation of the Proximal Interphalangeal Joint of the Finger (A Case Report). J. Hand Surg. 10B:100, 1985.
681. Ostrowski, D.M., and Neimkin, R.J.: Irreducible Palmar Dislocation of the Proximal Interphalangeal Joint. A Case Report. Orthopedics 8:84–86, 1985.
682. Palmer, A.K., and Linscheid, R.L.: Irreducible Dorsal Dislocation of the Distal Interphalangeal Joint of the Finger. J. Hand Surg. 2:406–408, 1977.
683. Palmer, A.K., and Linscheid, R.L.: Chronic Recurrent Dislocation of the Proximal Interphalangeal Joint of the Finger. J. Hand Surg. 3:95–97, 1978.
684. Patel, M.R., and Joshi, B.B.: Distraction Method for Chronic

Dorsal Fracture Dislocation of the Proximal Interphalangeal Joint. Hand Clin. 10:327–337, 1994.
685. Patel, M.R., Pearlman, H.S., Engler, J., and Lavine, L.S.: Transverse Bayonet Dislocation of the Proximal Interphalangeal Joint. Clin. Orthop. 133:219–226, 1978.
686. Peimer, C.A., Sullivan, D.J., and Wild, D.R.: Palmar Dislocation of the Proximal Interphalangeal Joint. J. Hand Surg. 9A:39–48, 1984.
687. Phair, I.C., Quinton, D.N., and Allen, M.J.: The Conservative Management of Volar Avulsion Fractures of the P.I.P. Joint. J. Hand Surg. 14B:168–170, 1989.
688. Phillips, J.H.: Irreducible Dislocation of a Distal Interphalangeal Joint: Case Report and Review of Literature. Clin. Orthop. 154:188–190, 1981.
689. Pohl, A.L.: Irreducible Dislocation of a Distal Interphalangeal Joint. Br. J. Plast. Surg. 29:227–229, 1976.
690. Portis, R.B.: Hyperextensibility of the Proximal Interphalangeal Joint of the Finger Following Trauma. J. Bone Joint Surg. 36A:1141–1146, 1954.
691. Posner, M.A., and Kapila, D.: Chronic Palmar Dislocation of Proximal Interphalangeal Joints. J. Hand Surg. 11A:253–258, 1986.
692. Posner, M.A., and Wilenski, M.: Irreducible Volar Dislocation of the Proximal Interphalangeal Joint of a Finger Caused by Interposition of an Intact Central Slip. A Case Report. J. Bone Joint Surg. 60A:133–134, 1978.
693. Rajoo, R.D., Govender, S., and Goga, I.E.: Simultaneous Dislocation of the Interphalangeal Joints. S. Afr. Med. J. 77:45–46, 1990.
694. Rayan, G.M., and Elias, L.S.: Irreducible Dislocation of the Distal Interphalangeal Joint Caused by Long Flexor Tendon Entrapment. Orthopedics 4:35–37, 1981.
695. Redler, I., and Williams, J.T.: Rupture of a Collateral Ligament of the Proximal Interphalangeal Joint of the Fingers. Analysis of Eighteen Cases. J. Bone Joint Surg. 49A:322–326, 1967.
696. Rhee, R.Y., Reading, G., and Wray, R.C.: A Biomechanical Study of the Collateral Ligaments of the Proximal Interphalangeal Joint. J. Hand Surg. 17A:157–163, 1992.
697. Robertson, R.C., Cawley, J.J. Jr., and Faris, A.M.: Treatment of Fracture-Dislocation of the Interphalangeal Joints of the Hand. J. Bone Joint Surg. 28:68–70, 1946.
698. Rodriguez, A.L.: Injuries to the Collateral Ligaments of the Proximal Interphalangeal Joints. Hand 5:55–57, 1973.
699. Ron, D., Alkalay, D., and Torok, G.: Simultaneous Closed Dislocation of Both Interphalangeal Joints in One Finger. J. Trauma 23:66–67, 1982.
700. Salamon, P.B., and Gelberman, R.H.: Irreducible Dislocation of the Interphalangeal Joint of the Thumb. Report of Three Cases. J. Bone Joint Surg. 60A:400–401, 1978.
701. Schenck, R.R.: Dynamic Traction and Early Passive Movement for Fractures of the Proximal Interphalangeal Joint. J. Hand Surg. 11A:850–858, 1986.
702. Schenck, R.R.: Classification of Fractures and Dislocations of the Proximal Interphalangeal Joint. Hand Clin. 10:179–185, 1994.
703. Schulze, H.A.: Treatment of Fracture-Dislocations of the Proximal Interphalangeal Joints of the Fingers. Mil. Surg. 99:190–191, 1946.
704. Selig, S., and Schein, A.: Irreducible Buttonhole Dislocation of the Fingers. J. Bone Joint Surg. 22:436–441, 1940.
705. Simpson, M.B., and Greenfield, G.Q.: Irreducible Dorsal Dislocation of the Small Finger Distal Interphalangeal Joint: The Importance of Roentgenograms—Case Report. J. Trauma 31:1450–1454, 1991.
706. Slattery, P.G.: The Dorsal Plate of the Proximal Interphalangeal Joint. J. Hand Surg. 15B:68–73, 1990.
707. Soelberg, M., Gebuhr, P., and Klareskov, B.: Interphalangeal Dislocations of the Fingers Treated by an Elastic Double-Finger Bandage. J. Hand Surg. 15B:66–67, 1990.
708. Spinner, M., and Choi, B.Y.: Anterior Dislocation of the Proximal Interphalangeal Joint. A Cause of Rupture of the Central Slip of the Extensor Mechanism. J. Bone Joint Surg. 52A:1329–1336, 1970.
709. Sprague, B.L.: Proximal Interphalangeal Joint Injuries and Their Initial Treatment. J. Trauma 15:380–385, 1975.
710. Spray, P.: Finger Fracture-Dislocation Proximal at the Interphalangeal Joint. J. Tenn. Med. Assoc. 59:765–766, 1966.
711. Stern, P.J.: Stener Lesion After Lateral Dislocation of the Proximal Interphalangeal Joint—Indication for Open Reduction. J. Hand Surg. 6:602–603, 1981.
712. Stern, P.J.: The Figure of 8 Splint. American Society for Surgery of the Hand Correspondence Newsletter, 1990:61.
713. Stern, P.J., and Lee, A.F.: Open Dorsal Dislocations of the Proximal Interphalangeal Joint. J. Hand Surg. 10A:364–370, 1985.
714. Stripling, W.D.: Displaced Intra-articular Osteochondral Fracture—Cause for Irreducible Dislocation of the Distal Interphalangeal Joint. J. Hand Surg. 7:77–78, 1982.
715. Strong, M.L.: A New Method of Extension-block Splinting for the Proximal Interphalangeal Joint—Preliminary Report. J. Hand Surg. 5:606–607, 1980.
716. Swanson, A.B.: Surgery of the Hand in Cerebral Palsy and Muscle Origin Release Procedures. Surg. Clin. North Am. 48:1129–1137, 1968.
717. Thayer, D.T.: Distal Interphalangeal Joint Injuries. Hand Clin. 4:1–4, 1988.
718. Thompson, J.S., and Eaton, R.G.: Volar Dislocation of the Proximal Interphalangeal Joint (Abstract). J. Hand Surg. 2:232, 1977.
719. Trojan, E.: Fracture Dislocation of the Bases of the Proximal and Middle Phalanges of the Fingers. Hand 4:60–61, 1972.
720. Tully, J.G. Jr., Kaphan, M.L., and Burack, N.D.: Compound Complex Dislocation of Proximal Interphalangeal Joint. Orthop. Rev. 14:81–84, 1985.
721. Twyman, R.S., and David, H.G.: The Doorstop Procedure. A Technique for Treating Unstable Fracture Dislocations of the Proximal Interphalangeal Joint. J. Hand Surg. 18B:714–715, 1993.
722. Vicar, A.J.: Proximal Interphalangeal Joint Dislocations Without Fractures. Hand Clin. 4:5–13, 1988.
723. Viegas, S.F.: Extension Block Pinning for Proximal Interphalangeal Joint Fracture Dislocations: Preliminary Report of a New Technique. J. Hand Surg. 17A:896–901, 1992.
724. Watson, F.M. Jr.: Simultaneous Interphalangeal Dislocation in One Finger. J. Trauma 23:65, 1982.
725. Watson, H.K., Light, T.R., and Johnson, T.R.: Checkrein Resection for Flexion Contractures of the Middle Joint. J. Hand Surg. 4:67–71, 1979.
726. Weseley, M.S., Barenfeld, P.A., and Eisenstein, A.L.: Simultaneous Dorsal Dislocation of Both Interphalangeal Joints in a Finger. A Case Report. J. Bone Joint Surg. 60A:1142, 1978.
727. Whipple, T.L., Evans, J.P., and Urbaniak, J.R.: Irreducible Dislocation of a Finger Joint in a Child. A Case Report. J. Bone Joint Surg. 62A:832–833, 1980.
728. Wiley, A.M.: Chronic Dislocation of the Proximal Interphalangeal Joint: A Method of Surgical Repair. Can. J. Surg. 8:435–439, 1965.
729. Wiley, A.M.: Instability of the Proximal Interphalangeal Joint Following Dislocation and Fracture Dislocation: Surgical Repair. Hand 2:185–190, 1970.
730. Wilson, J.N., and Rowland, S.A.: Fracture-Dislocation of the Proximal Interphalangeal Joint of the Finger. Treatment by Open Reduction and Internal Fixation. J. Bone Joint Surg. 48A:493–502, 1966.
731. Wilson, R.L., and Liechty, B.W.: Complications Following Small Joint Injuries. Hand Clin. 2:329–345, 1986.
732. Wong, J.T.M.: Extensor Mechanism Preventing Reduction of Finger (Abstract). Med. J. Aust. 1:101, 1978.
733. Woods, G.L., and Burton, R.I.: Avoiding Pitfalls in the Diagnosis of Acutely Injured Proximal Interphalangeal Joint. Clin. Plast. Surg. 8:95–105, 1981.
734. Zemel, N.P., Stark, H.H., Ashworth, C.R., and Boyes, J.H.: Chronic Fracture Dislocation of the Proximal Interphalangeal

Joint—Treatment by Osteotomy and Bone Graft. Orthop. Trans. 4:5–6, 1980.
735. Zielinski, C.J.: Irreducible Fracture-Dislocation of the Distal Interphalangeal Joint. J. Bone Joint Surg. 65A:109–110, 1983.
736. Zook, E.G., Van Beek, A.L., and Wavak, P.: Transverse Volar Skin Laceration of the Finger: A Sign of Volar Plate Injury. Hand 11:213–216, 1979.

METACARPOPHALANGEAL JOINTS

737. Adler, G.A., and Light, T.R.: Simultaneous Complex Dislocation of the Metacarpophalangeal Joints of the Long and Index Fingers. J. Bone Joint Surg. 63A:1007–1009, 1981.
738. Al-Qattan, M.M., and Murray, K.A.: An Isolated Complex Dorsal Dislocation of the MP Joint of the Ring Finger. J. Hand Surg. 19B:171–173, 1994.
739. Al-Qattan, M.M., and Robertson, G.A.: An Anatomical Study of the Deep Transverse Metacarpal Ligament. J. Anat. 182:443–446, 1993.
740. Al-Qattan, M.M., and Zuker, R.M.: Scissoring Deformity After Closed Reduction of a Dorsal Subluxation of the MP Joint of the Middle Finger. J. Hand Surg. 19B:368–370, 1994.
741. Alldred, A.: A Locked Index Finger. J. Bone Joint Surg. 36B:102–103, 1954.
742. Andersen, J.A., and Gjerloff, C.C.: Complex Dislocation of the Metacarpophalangeal Joint of the Little Finger. J. Hand Surg. 12B:264–266, 1987.
743. Araki, S., Ohtani, T., and Tanaka, T.: Open Dorsal Metacarpophalangeal Dislocations of the Index, Long, and Ring Fingers. J. Hand Surg. 12A:458–460, 1987.
744. Araki, S., Uchiyama, M., Nishimura, T., and Mishima, S.: Irreducible Open Dislocation of the Metacarpophalangeal Joint of the Small Finger. J. Hand Surg. 17A:1146–1147, 1992.
745. Aston, J.N.: Locked Middle Finger. J. Bone Joint Surg. 42B:75–79, 1960.
746. Baldwin, L.W., Miller, D.L., Lockhart, L.D., and Evans, E.B.: Metacarpophalangeal-joint Dislocations of the Fingers. A Comparison of the Pathological Anatomy of Index and Little Finger Dislocations. J. Bone Joint Surg. 49A:1587–1590, 1967.
747. Barash, H.L.: An Unusual Case of Dorsal Dislocation of the Metacarpophalangeal Joint of the Index Finger. Clin. Orthop. 83:121–122, 1972.
748. Barenfeld, P.A., and Weseley, M.S.: Dorsal Dislocation of the Metacarpophalangeal Joint of the Index Finger Treated by Late Open Reduction. J. Bone Joint Surg. 54A:1311–1313, 1972.
749. Barnard, H.L.: Dorsal Dislocation of the First Phalanx of the Little Finger. Reduction by Farabeuf's Dorsal Incision. Lancet 1:88–90, 1901.
750. Barry, K., McGee, H., and Curtin, J.: Complex Dislocation of the Metacarpo-phalangeal Joint of the Index Finger: A Comparison of the Surgical Approaches. J. Hand Surg. 13B:466–468, 1988.
751. Battle, W.H.: Backward Dislocation of the Fingers Upon the Metacarpus. Lancet 1:1223–1224, 1888.
752. Becton, J.L., and Carswell, A.S.: The Natural History of an Unreduced Dislocated Index Finger Metacarpophalangeal Joint in a Child. J. Med. Assoc. Ga. 64:413–415, 1975.
753. Becton, J.L., Christian J.D.J., Goodwin, H.N., and Jackson, J.G. III: A Simplified Technique for Treating the Complex Dislocation of the Index Metacarpophalangeal Joint. J. Bone Joint Surg. 57A:698–700, 1975.
754. Betz, R.R., Browne, E.Z., Perry, G.B., and Resnick, E.J.: The Complex Volar Metacarpophalangeal-joint Dislocation. A Case Report and Review of the Literature. J. Bone Joint Surg. 64A:1374–1375, 1982.
755. Bloom, M.H., and Bryan, R.S.: Locked Index Finger Caused by Hyperflexion and Entrapment of Sesamoid Bone. J. Bone Joint Surg. 47A:1383–1385, 1965.
756. Bohart, P.G., Gelberman, R.H., Vandell, R.F., and Salamon, P.B.: Complex Dislocations of the Metacarpophalangeal Joint. Operative Reduction by Farabeuf's Dorsal Incision. Clin. Orthop. 164:208–210, 1982.
757. Boland, D.: Volar Dislocation of the Ring Finger Metacarpophalangeal Joint. Orthop. Rev. 13:69–72, 1984.
758. Bruner, J.M.: Recurrent Locking of the Index Finger Due to Internal Derangement of the Metacarpophalangeal Joint. J. Bone Joint Surg. 43A:450–453, 1961.
759. Buchler, U.: American Society for Surgery of the Hand Correspondence Newsletter, 1987.
760. Burman, M.: Irreducible Hyperextension Dislocation of the Metacarpophalangeal Joint of a Finger. Bull. Hosp. Jt. Dis. 14:290–291, 1953.
761. Cunningham, D.M., and Schwarz, G.: Dorsal Dislocation of the Index Metacarpophalangeal Joint. Plast. Reconstr. Surg. 56:654–659, 1975.
762. Dibbell, D.G., and Field, J.H.: Locking Metacarpal Phalangeal Joint. Plast. Reconstr. Surg. 40:562–564, 1967.
763. Doyle, J.R., and Atkinson, R.E.: Rupture of the Radial Collateral Ligament of the Metacarpo-phalangeal Joint of the Index Finger: A Report of Three Cases. J. Hand Surg. 14B:248–250, 1989.
764. Dray, G., Millender, L.H., and Nalebuff, E.A.: Rupture of the Radial Collateral Ligament of a Metacarpophalangeal Joint to One of the Ulnar Three Fingers. J. Hand Surg. 4:346–350, 1979.
765. Dutton, R.O., and Meals, R.A.: Complex Dorsal Dislocation of the Thumb Metacarpophalangeal Joint. Clin. Orthop. 164:160–164, 1982.
766. Eaton, R.G.: Joint Injuries of the Hand. Springfield, Ill., Charles C. Thomas, 1971.
767. Farabeuf, L.H.F.: De la luxation du ponce en arriere. Bull. Soc. Chir. 11:21–62, 1876.
768. Ferguson, D.B., Moore, G.P., and Hieke, K.A.: Dorsal Dislocation of Four Metacarpophalangeal Joints. Ann. Emerg. Med. 18:204–206, 1989.
769. Flatt, A.E.: Recurrent Locking of an Index Finger. J. Bone Joint Surg. 40A:1128–1129, 1958.
770. Flatt, A.E.: A Locking Little Finger. J. Bone Joint Surg. 43A:240–242, 1961.
771. Flatt, A.E.: Fracture-Dislocation of an Index Metacarpophalangeal Joint and an Ulnar Deviating Force in the Flexor Tendons. J. Bone Joint Surg. 48A:100–104, 1966.
772. Fultz, C.W., and Buchanan, J.R.: Complex Fracture-Dislocation of the Metacarpophalangeal Joint. Case Report. Clin. Orthop. 227:255–260, 1988.
773. Gee, T.C., and Pho, R.W.H.: Avulsion-fracture at the Proximal Attachment of the Radial Collateral Ligament of the Fifth Metacarpophalangeal Joint—A Case Report. J. Hand Surg. 7:526–527, 1982.
774. Goodfellow, J.W., and Weaver, J.P.A.: Locking of the Metacarpophalangeal Joints. J. Bone Joint Surg. 43B:772–777, 1961.
775. Gordon, M.H.: Irreduceable Metacarpophalangeal Dislocations. Bull. Hosp. Jt. Dis. 37:164–171, 1976.
776. Green, D.P., and Terry, G.C.: Complex Dislocation of the Metacarpophalangeal Joint. Correlative Pathological Anatomy. J. Bone Joint Surg. 55A:1480–1486, 1973.
777. Guly, H.R., and Azam, M.A.: Locked Finger Treated by Manipulation. A Report of Three Cases. J. Bone Joint Surg. 64A:73–75, 1982.
778. Gustilo, R.B.: Dislocation of the Metacarpophalangeal Joint of the Index Finger. Minn. Med. 1119–1121, 1966.
779. Hall, R.F. Jr., Gleason, T.F., and Kasa, R.F.: Simultaneous Closed Dislocations of the Metacarpophalangeal Joints of the Index, Long, and Ring Fingers: A Case Report. J. Hand Surg. 10A:81–85, 1985.
780. Harvey, F.J.: Locking of the Metacarpophalangeal Joints. J. Bone Joint Surg. 56B:156–159, 1974.
781. Honner, R.: Locking of the Metacarpophalangeal Joint From a Loose Body. Report of a Case. J. Bone Joint Surg. 51B:479–481, 1969.
782. Hubbard, L.F.: Metacarpophalangeal Dislocations. Hand Clin. 4:39–44, 1988.

783. Hunt, J.C., Watts, H.B., and Glasgow, J.D.: Dorsal Dislocation of the Metacarpophalangeal Joint of the Index Finger With Particular Reference to Open Dislocation. J. Bone Joint Surg. 49A:1572–1578, 1967.
784. Iftikhar, T.B., and Kaminski, R.S.: Simultaneous Dorsal Dislocation of MP Joints of Long and Ring Fingers. A Case Report. Orthop. Rev. 10:71–72, 1981.
785. Imbriglia, J.E., and Sciulli, R.: Open Complex Metacarpophalangeal Joint Dislocation. Two Cases: Index Finger and Long Finger. J. Hand Surg. 4:72–75, 1979.
786. Inoue, G., Nakamura, R., and Miura, T.: Intra-articular Fracture of the Metacarpal Head of the Locked Index Finger Due to Forced Passive Extension. J. Hand Surg. 13B:320–322, 1988.
787. Ishizuki, M.: Injury to Collateral Ligament of Metacarpophalangeal Joint of a Finger. J. Hand Surg. 13A:456–460, 1988.
788. Kaplan, E.B.: Dorsal Dislocation of the Metacarpophalangeal Joint of the Index Finger. J. Bone Joint Surg. 39A:1081–1086, 1957.
789. Koniuch, M.P., Peimer, C.A., VanGorder, T., and Moncada, A.: Closed Crush Injury of the Metacarpophalangeal Joint. J. Hand Surg. 12A:750–757, 1987.
790. Langenskiold, A.: Habitual Locking of a Metacarpophalangeal Joint by a Collateral Ligament, a Rare Cause of Trigger Finger. Acta Chir. Scand. 99:72–78, 1949.
791. Le Clerc, R.: Luxations de lindex sur son metacarpien. Rev. D'Orthop. 2:227–242, 1911.
792. Lutter, L.D.: A New Cause of Locking Fingers. Clin. Orthop. 83:131–134, 1972.
793. Malerich, M.M., Eaton, R.G., and Upton, J.: Complete Dislocation of a Little Finger Metacarpal Phalangeal Joint Treated by Closed Technique. J. Trauma 20:424–425, 1980.
794. McCarthy, L.J.: Open Metacarpophalangeal Dislocations of the Index, Middle, Ring, and Little Fingers. J. Trauma 20:183–185, 1980.
795. McElfresh, E.C., and Dobyns, J.H.: Intra-articular Metacarpal Head Fractures. J. Hand Surg. 8:383–393, 1983.
796. McLaughlin, H.L.: Complex "Locked" Dislocation of the Metacarpophalangeal Joints. J. Trauma 5:683–688, 1965.
797. Milch, H.: Subluxation of the Index Metacarpophalangeal Joint. Case Report. J. Bone Joint Surg. 47A:522–523, 1965.
798. Miller, P.R., Evans, B.W., and Glazer, D.A.: Locked Dislocation of the Metacarpophalangeal Joint of the Index Finger. J.A.M.A. 203:138–139, 1968.
799. Minami, A., An, K., Cooney, W.P., Linscheid, R.L., and Chao, E.Y.S.: Ligament Stability of the Metacarpophalangeal Joint: A Biomechanical Study. J. Hand Surg. 10A:255–260, 1985.
800. Mlsna, J., Hanel, D.P., and Kneeland, B.: Complex Volar Metacarpophalangeal Joint Dislocations: Pathologic Anatomy as Viewed by MRI. Orthopedics 16:1350–1352, 1993.
801. Moneim, M.S.: Volar Dislocation of the Metacarpophalangeal Joint. Pathologic Anatomy and Report of Two Cases. Clin. Orthop. 176:186–189, 1983.
802. Murphy, A.F., and Stark, H.H.: Closed Dislocation of the Metacarpophalangeal Joint of the Index Finger. J. Bone Joint Surg. 49A:1579–1586, 1967.
803. Murray, J.F. Personal communication, 1982.
804. Myers, W.J.: Isolated Middle Finger Complex Dorsal Dislocation of the Metacarpophalangeal Joint. Orthopedics 17:952–954, 1994.
805. Nussbaum, R., and Sadler, A.H.: An Isolated, Closed, Complex Dislocation of the Metacarpophalangeal Joint of the Long Finger: A Unique Case. J. Hand Surg. 11A:558–561, 1986.
806. Nutter, P.D.: Interposition of Sesamoids in Metacarpophalangeal Dislocations. J. Bone Joint Surg. 22:730–734, 1940.
807. Posner, M.A., Langa, V., and Green, S.M.: The Locked Metacarpophalangeal Joint: Diagnosis and Treatment. J. Hand Surg. 11A:249–253, 1986.
808. Quinton, D.N.: Dorsal Locking of the Metacarpophalangeal Joint. J. Hand Surg. 12B:62–63, 1987.
809. Ramirez Ruíz, G., Combalía Aleu, A., Valer Tito, A., Bordas Sales, J.L., and Rofes Capo, S.: Simultaneous Subluxation of the Metacarpophalangeal Joints of All Four Fingers: A Case Report. J. Hand Surg. 10A:78–80, 1985.
810. Rankin, E.A., and Uwagie-Ero, S.: Locking of the Metacarpophalangeal Joint. J. Hand Surg. 11A:868–871, 1986.
811. Renshaw, T.S., and Louis, D.S.: Complex Volar Dislocation of the Metacarpophalangeal Joint: A Case Report. J. Trauma 13:1086–1088, 1971.
812. Ridge, E.M.: Dorsal Dislocation of the First Phalanx of the Little Finger. Lancet 1:781, 1901.
813. Robins, R.H.C.: Injuries of the Metacarpophalangeal Joints. Hand 3:159–163, 1971.
814. Schubiner, J.M., and Mass, D.P.: Operation for Collateral Ligament Ruptures of the Metacarpophalangeal Joints of the Fingers. J. Bone Joint Surg. 71B:388–389, 1989.
815. Schuind, F.: Locked Metacarpo-phalangeal Joint Due to an Intra-articular Fracture of the Metacarpal Head. A Case Report. J. Hand Surg. 17B:148–150, 1992.
816. Silberman, W.W.: Clear View of the Index Sesamoid: A Sign of Irreducible Metacarpophalangeal Joint Dislocation. J. Am. Coll. Emerg. Physicians 8:371–373, 1979.
817. Smith, R.J., and Sturchio, E.A.: The Locked Metacarpophalangeal Joint. Bull. Hosp. Jt. Dis. 29:205–211, 1968.
818. Stewart, G.J., and Williams, E.A.: Locking of the Metacarpophalangeal Joints in Degenerative Disease. Hand 13:147–151, 1981.
819. Sweterlitsch, P.R., Torg, J.S., and Pollack, H.: Entrapment of a Sesamoid in the Index Metacarpophalangeal Joint. J. Bone Joint Surg. 51A:995–998, 1969.
820. Tsuge, K., and Watari, S.: Dorsal Dislocation of the Metacarpophalangeal Joint of the Index Finger. Hiroshima J. Med. Sci. 22:65–81, 1973.
821. Umansky, A.L.: The Dislocated Index Metacarpophalangeal Joint (Abstract). J. Bone Joint Surg. 45A:216, 1963.
822. Viegas, S.F., Heare, T.C., and Calhoun, J.H.: Complex Fracture-Dislocation of a Fifth Metacarpophalangeal Joint: Case Report and Literature Review. J. Trauma 29:521–524, 1989.
823. von Raffler, W.: Irreducible Dislocation of the Metacarpophalangeal Joint of the Finger. Clin. Orthop. 35:171–173, 1964.
824. Wilhelmy, J., and Hay, R.L.: Dual Dislocation of Metacarpophalangeal Joints. Hand 4:168–170, 1972.
825. Williams, J.S. Jr., Kamionek, S., Weiss, A.C., and Akelman, E.: The Surgical Approach in Non-Border Digit Complex Dislocations of the Metacarpophalangeal Joint. Orthop. Rev. 23:601–605, 1994.
826. Wolov, R.B.: Complex Dislocations of the Metacarpophalangeal Joints. Orthop. Rev. 17:770–775, 1988.
827. Wood, M.B., and Dobyns, J.H.: Chronic, Complex Volar Dislocation of the Metacarpophalangeal Joint. Report of Three Cases. J. Hand Surg. 6:73–76, 1981.
828. Wright, C.S.: Compound Dislocations of Four Metacarpophalangeal Joints. J. Hand Surg. 10B:233–235, 1985.
829. Yancey, H.A. Jr., and Howard, L.D. Jr.: Locking of the Metacarpophalangeal Joint. J. Bone Joint Surg. 44A:380–382, 1962.
830. Zemel, N.P.: Metacarpophalangeal Joint Injuries in Fingers. Hand Clin. 8:745–753, 1992.

CMC JOINTS (EXCLUDING THE THUMB)

831. Berg, E.E., and Murphy, D.F.: Ulnopalmar Dislocation of the Fifth Carpometacarpal Joint—Successful Closed Reduction: Review of the Literature and Anatomic Reevaluation. J. Hand Surg. 11A:521–525, 1986.
832. Bergfield, T.G., Dupuy, T.E., and Aulicino, P.L.: Fracture-Dislocations of all Five Carpometacarpal Joints: A Case Report. J. Hand Surg. 10A:76–78, 1985.
833. Black, D.M., Watson, H.K., and Vender, M.I.: Arthroplasty of the Ulnar Carpometacarpal Joints. J. Hand Surg. 12A:1071–1074, 1987.
834. Bloom, M.L., and Stern, P.J.: Carpometacarpal Joints of Fingers. Their Dislocation and Fracture-Dislocation. Orthop. Rev. 12:77–82, 1983.
835. Bora, F.W. Jr., and Didizian, N.H.: The Treatment of Injuries

to the Carpometacarpal Joint of the Little Finger. J. Bone Joint Surg. 56A:1459–1463, 1974.
836. Breiting, V.: Simultaneous Dislocation of the Bases of the Four Ulnar Metacarpals Upon the Last Row of Carpals. Hand 15:287–289, 1983.
837. Brewerton, D.A.: A Tangential Radiographic Projection for Demonstrating Involvement of the Metacarpal Head in Rheumatoid Arthritis. Br. J. Radiol. 40:233, 1967.
838. Buzby, B.F.: Palmar Carpo-metacarpal Dislocation of the Fifth Metacarpal. Ann. Surg. 100:555–557, 1934.
839. Cain, J.E., Shepler, T.R., and Wilson, M.R.: Hamatometacarpal Fracture-Dislocation: Classification and Treatment. J. Hand Surg. 12A:762–767, 1987.
840. Carroll, R.E., and Carlson, E.: Diagnosis and Treatment of Injury to the Second and Third Carpometacarpal Joints. J. Hand Surg. 14A:102–107, 1989.
841. Chen, V.T.: Dislocation of Carpometacarpal Joint of the Little Finger. J. Hand Surg. 12B:260–263, 1987.
842. Chmell, S., Light, T.R., and Blair, S.J.: Fracture and Fracture Dislocation of Ulnar Carpometacarpal Joint. Orthop. Rev. 11:73–80, 1982.
843. Clement, B.L.: Fracture-Dislocation of the Base of the Fifth Metacarpal. A Case Report. J. Bone Joint Surg. 17:498–499, 1945.
844. Clendenin, M.B., and Smith, R.J.: Metacarpo-hamate Arthrodesis for Post-traumatic Arthritis. Orthop. Trans. 6:168, 1982.
845. Clendenin, M.B., and Smith, R.J.: Fifth Metacarpal/Hamate Arthrodesis for Posttraumatic Osteoarthritis. J. Hand Surg. 9A:374–378, 1984.
846. De Beer, J.D., Maloon, S., Anderson, P., Jones, G., and Singer, M.: Multiple Carpo-Metacarpal Dislocations. J. Hand Surg. 14B:105–108, 1989.
847. Dennyson, W.G., and Stother, I.G.: Carpometacarpal Dislocation of the Little Finger. Hand 8:161–164, 1976.
848. Dommisse, I.G., and Lloyd, G.J.: Injuries to the Fifth Carpometacarpal Region. Can. J. Surg. 22:240–244, 1979.
849. Dunkerton, M., and Singer, M.: Dislocation of the Index Metacarpal and Trapezoid Bones. J. Hand Surg. 10B:377–378, 1985.
850. Fayman, M., Hugo, B., and de Wet, H.: Case Report. Simultaneous Dislocation of All Five Carpometacarpal Joints. Plast. Reconstr. Surg. 82:151–154, 1988.
851. Fernyhough, J., and Trumble, T.: Case Report. Late Posttraumatic Carpometacarpal Dislocation of the Ring and Little Finger. J. Orthop. Trauma 4:200–203, 1990.
852. Fisher, M.R., Rogers, L.F., and Hendrix, R.W.: Systematic Approach to Identifying Fourth and Fifth Carpometacarpal Joint Dislocations. A.J.R. 140:319–324, 1983.
853. Fisher, M.R., Rogers, L.F., and Hendrix, R.W.: Carpometacarpal Dislocations. CRC Crit. Rev. Diagn. Imaging 22:95–126, 1994.
854. Flatt, A.E.: The Care of Minor Hand Injuries. St. Louis, C.V. Mosby, 1959.
855. Gainor, B.J., Stark, H.H., Ashworth, C.R., Zemel, N.P., and Rickard, T.A.: Tendon Arthroplasty of the Fifth Carpometacarpal Joint for Treatment of Posttraumatic Arthritis. J. Hand Surg. 16A:520–524, 1991.
856. Garcia-Elias, M., Bishop, A.T., Dobyns, J.H., Cooney, W.P., and Linscheid, R.L.: Transcarpal Carpometacarpal Dislocations, Excluding the Thumb. J. Hand Surg. 15A:531–540, 1990.
857. Gore, D.R.: Carpometacarpal Dislocation Producing Compression of the Deep Branch of the Ulnar Nerve. J. Bone Joint Surg. 53A:1387–1390, 1971.
858. Goss, C.M.: Gray's Anatomy, 26th Ed., pp. 371–372. Philadelphia, Lea & Febiger, 1954.
859. Green, D.P., and Rowland, S.A.: Carpometacarpal Dislocations (Excluding the Thumb). *In* Rockwood, C.A., and Green, D.P. (eds.): Fractures, pp. 323–327. Philadelphia, J.B. Lippincott, 1975.
860. Green, W.L., and Kilgore, E.S.: Treatment of Fifth Digit Carpometacarpal Arthritis With Silastic Prosthesis. J. Hand Surg. 6:510–514, 1981.
861. Gunther, S.F.: The Carpometacarpal Joints. Orthop. Clin. North Am. 15:259–277, 1984.
862. Gunther, S.F., and Bruno, P.D.: Divergent Dislocation of the Carpometacarpal Joints: A Case Report. J. Hand Surg. 10A:197–201, 1985.
863. Gurland, M.: Carpometacarpal Joint Injuries of the Fingers. Hand Clin. 8:733–744, 1992.
864. Hagstrom, P.: Fracture Dislocation in the Ulnar Carpometacarpal Joints. Open Reduction and Pinning—A Case Report. Scand. J. Plast. Reconstr. Surg. 9:249–251, 1975.
865. Hartwig, R.H., and Louis, D.S.: Multiple Carpometacarpal Dislocations. J. Bone Joint Surg. 61A:906–908, 1979.
866. Harwin, S.F., Fox, J.M., and Sedlin, E.D.: Volar Dislocation of the Bases of the Second and Third Metacarpals. J. Bone Joint Surg. 57A:849–851, 1975.
867. Hazlett, J.W.: Carpometacarpal Dislocations Other Than the Thumb. A Report of 11 Cases. Can. J. Surg. 11:315–322, 1968.
868. Helal, B., and Kavanagh, T.G.: Unstable Dorsal Fracture-Dislocation of the Fifth Carpometacarpal Joint. Injury, 9:138–142, 1977.
869. Henderson, J.J., and Arafa, M.A.M.: Carpometacarpal Dislocation. An Easily Missed Diagnosis. J. Bone Joint Surg. 69B:212–214, 1987.
870. Hindman, B.W., Kulik, W.J., Lee, G., and Avolio, R.E.: Occult Fractures of the Carpals and Metacarpals: Demonstration by CT. A.J.R. 153:529–532, 1989.
871. Ho, P.K., Choban, S.J., Eshman, S.J., and Dupuy, T.E.: Complex Dorsal Dislocation of the Second Carpometacarpal Joint. J. Hand Surg. 12A:1074–1076, 1987.
872. Hsu, J.D., and Curtis, R.M.: Carpometacarpal Dislocations on the Ulnar Side of the Hand. J. Bone Joint Surg. 52A:927–930, 1970, 1994.
873. Hutchinson, M.R., Smith, J., and Hodgman, C.G.: Isolated Fracture-Dislocation of the Fourth Carpometacarpal Joint. A Report of Two Cases. Orthop. Rev. 22:1038–1045, 1993.
874. Imbriglia, J.E.: Chronic Dorsal Carpometacarpal Dislocations of the Index, Middle, Ring, and Little Fingers: A Case Report. J. Hand Surg. 4:343–345, 1979.
875. Joseph, R.B., Linscheid, R.L., Dobyns, J.H., and Bryan, R.S.: Chronic Sprains of the Carpometacarpal Joints. J. Hand Surg. 6:172–180, 1981.
876. Kaplan, E.B.: Functional and Surgical Anatomy of the Hand. 2nd Ed., pp. 28–35, 134. Philadelphia, J.B. Lippincott, 1965.
877. Kaye, J.J., and Lister, G.D.: Another Use for the Brewerton View (Letter). J. Hand Surg. 3:603, 1978.
878. Ker, H.R.: Dislocation of the Fifth Carpo-metacarpal Joint. J. Bone Joint Surg. 37B:254–256, 1955.
879. Kerr, H.D.: Hamate-Metacarpal Fracture Dislocation. J. Emerg. Med. 10:565–568, 1992.
880. Kinnett, J.G., and Lyden, J.P.: Posterior Fracture-Dislocation of the IV Metacarpal Hamate Articulation Case Report. J. Trauma 19:290–291, 1979.
881. Kjaer-Petersen, K., Jurik, A.G., and Petersen, L.K.: Intra-Articular Fractures at the Base of the Fifth Metacarpal. A Clinical and Radiographical Study of 64 Cases. J. Hand Surg. 17B:144–147, 1992.
882. Kleinman, W.B., and Grantham, S.A.: Multiple Volar Carpometacarpal Joint Dislocation. J. Hand Surg. 3:377–382, 1978.
883. Konsens, R.M., and Seitz, W.H. Jr.: Post-traumatic Arthrosis of the Index Carpometacarpal Joint. A Rationale for Treatment and Report of Two Cases. Orthopedics 10:1429–1433, 1987.
884. Laforgia, R., Specchiulli, F., and Mariana, A.: Dorsal Dislocation of the Fifth Carpometacarpal Joint. J. Hand Surg. 15A:463–465, 1990.
885. Lawlis, J.F. III, and Gunther, S.F.: Carpometacarpal Dislocations. Long-term Follow-up. J. Bone Joint Surg. 73A:52–59, 1991.
886. Lewis, H.H.: Dislocation of the Second Metacarpal Report of a Case. Clin. Orthop. 93:253–255, 1973.

887. Lilling, M., and Weinberg, H.: The Mechanism of Dorsal Fracture Dislocation of the Fifth Carpometacarpal Joint. J. Hand Surg. 4:340–342, 1979.
888. Lyman, C.B.: Backward Dislocation of the Second Carpometacarpal Articulation. Ann. Surg. 43:905–906, 1906.
889. Marck, K.W., and Klasen, H.J.: Fracture-Dislocation of the Hamatometacarpal Joint: A Case Report. J. Hand Surg. 11A:128–130, 1986.
890. McLean, E.H.: Carpometacarpal Dislocation. J.A.M.A. 79:299–300, 1922, 1994.
891. McWhorter, G.I.: Isolated and Complete Dislocation of the Fifth Carpometacarpal Joint Open Operation. Surg. Clin. North Am. 2:793–796, 1918.
892. Mehara, A.K., and Bhan, S.: Rotatory Dislocation of the Second Carpometacarpal Joint: Case Report. J. Trauma 34:464–466, 1993.
893. Metz, W.R.: Multiple Carpo-metacarpal Dislocations. With the Report of a Case. New Orleans Med. Surg. J. 79:327–330, 1927.
894. Mueller, J.J.: Carpometacarpal Dislocations Report of Five Cases and Review of the Literature. J. Hand Surg. 11A:184–188, 1986.
895. Murless, B.C.: Fracture-Dislocation of the Base of the Fifth Metacarpal Bone. Br. J. Surg. 31:402–404, 1943.
896. Nalebuff, E.A.: Isolated Anterior Carpometacarpal Dislocation of the Fifth Finger: Classification and Case Report. J. Trauma 8:1119–1123, 1968.
897. Niechajev, I.: Dislocated Intra-articular Fracture of the Base of the Fifth Metacarpal: A Clinical Study of 23 Patients. Plast. Reconstr. Surg. 75:406–410, 1985.
898. North, E.R., and Eaton, R.G.: Volar Dislocation of the Fifth Metacarpal. Report of Two Cases. J. Bone Joint Surg. 62A:657–659, 1980.
899. O'Rourke, P.J., and Quinlan, W.: Fracture Dislocation of the Fifth Metacarpal Resulting in Compression of the Deep Branch of the Ulnar Nerve. J. Hand Surg. 18B:190–191, 1993.
900. Oni, O.O.A., and Mackenny, R.P.: Multiple Dislocations of the Carpometacarpal Joints. J. Hand Surg. 11B:47–48, 1986.
901. Peterson, P., and Sacks, S.: Fracture-Dislocation of the Base of the Fifth Metacarpal Associated With Injury to the Deep Motor Branch of the Ulnar Nerve A Case Report. J. Hand Surg. 11A:525–528, 1986.
902. Petrie, P.W.R., and Lamb, D.W.: Fracture-Subluxation of Base of Fifth Metacarpal. Hand 6:82–86, 1974.
903. Rawles, J.G.: Dislocations and Fracture-Dislocations at the Carpometacarpal Joints of the Fingers. Hand Clin. 4:103–112, 1988.
904. Resnick, S.M., Greene, T.L., and Roeser, W.: Simultaneous Dislocation of the Five Carpometacarpal Joints. Clin. Orthop. 192:210–214, 1985.
905. Roberts, N., and Holland, C.T.: Isolated Dislocation of the Base of the Fifth Metacarpal. Br. J. Surg. 23:567–571, 1936.
906. Sandzen, S.C.: Fracture of the Fifth Metacarpal Resembling Bennett's Fracture. Hand 5:49–51, 1973.
907. Schutt, R.C., Boswick, J.A., and Scott, F.A.: Volar Fracture-Dislocation of the Carpometacarpal Joint of the Index Finger Treated by Delayed Open Reduction. J. Trauma 21:986–987, 1981.
908. Shephard, E., and Solomon, D.J.: Carpo-metacarpal Dislocation. A Report of Four Cases. J. Bone Joint Surg. 42B:772–777, 1960.
909. Shorbe, H.B.: Carpometacarpal Dislocations. A Report of a Case. J. Bone Joint Surg. 20:454–457, 1938.
910. Smith, R.J.: Malunion of the Base of the Fifth Metacarpal Fracture and Dislocation. American Society for Surgery of the Hand Correspondence Newsletter, 1980.
911. Stevanovic, M.V., and Stark, H.H.: Dorsal Dislocation of the Fourth and Fifth Carpometacarpal Joints and Simultaneous Dislocation of the Metacarpophalangeal Joint of the Small Finger A Case Report. J. Hand Surg. 9A:714–716, 1984.
912. Storm, J.O.: Traumatic Dislocation of the Fourth and Fifth Carpo-metacarpal Joints: A Case Report. J. Hand Surg. 13B:210–211, 1988.
913. Thomas, W.O., Gottliebson, W.M., D'Amore, T.F., Harris, C.N., and Parry, S.W.: Isolated Palmar Displaced Fracture of the Base of the Index Metacarpal: A Case Report. J. Hand Surg. 19A:455–456, 1994.
914. Tountas, A.A., and Kwok, J.M.K.: Isolated Volar Dislocation of the Fifth Carpometacarpal Joint. Case Report. Clin. Orthop. 187:172–175, 1984.
915. Viegas, S.F., Crossley, M., Marzke, M., and Wullstein, K.: The Fourth Carpometacarpal Joint. J. Hand Surg. 16A:525–533, 1991.
916. Wainwright, D.: Fractures of the Metacarpals and Phalanges. Proc. R. Soc. Med. 57:598–599, 1964.
917. Watson-Jones, R.: Fractures and Joint Injuries, 4th Ed., p. 635. Edinburgh, E & S Livingstone, 1956.
918. Waugh, R.L., and Yancey, A.G.: Carpometacarpal Dislocation. With Particular Reference to Simultaneous Dislocation of the Bases of the Fourth and Fifth Metacarpals. J. Bone Joint Surg. 30A:397–404, 1948.
919. Weiland, A.J., Lister, G.D., and Villarreal-Rios, A.: Volar Fracture Dislocations of the Second and Third Carpometacarpal Joints Associated With Acute Carpal Tunnel Syndrome. J. Trauma 16:672–675, 1976.
920. Whitson, R.O.: Carpometacarpal Dislocation. A Case Report. Clin. Orthop. 6:189–195, 1955.
921. Wiley, A.M., and Dommisse, I.: Disabilities Following Basal Fractures and Dislocations of the Ulnar Border of the Hand. Orthop. Rev. 5:43–47, 1976.

MP JOINT OF THE THUMB—COLLATERAL LIGAMENT INJURIES

922. Abrahamsson, S., Sollerman, C., Lundborg, G., Larsson, J., and Egund, N.: Diagnosis of Displaced Ulnar Collateral Ligament of the Metacarpophlanageal Joint of the Thumb. J. Hand Surg. 15A:457–460, 1990.
923. Ahmad, I., and DePalma, A.F.: Treatment of Gamekeeper's Thumb by a New Operation. Clin. Orthop. 103:167–169, 1974.
924. Alldred, A.J.: Rupture of the Collateral Ligament of the Metacarpo-phalangeal Joint of the Thumb. J. Bone Joint Surg. 37B:443–445, 1955.
925. Arnold, D.M., Cooney, W.P., and Wood, M.B.: Surgical Management of Chronic Ulnar Collateral Ligament Insufficiency of the Thumb Metacarpophalangeal Joint. Orthop. Rev. 21:583–588, 1992.
926. Baily, R.A.J.: Some Closed Injuries of the Metacarpophalangeal Joint of the Thumb. J. Bone Joint Surg. 45B:428–429, 1963.
927. Bezes, P.M.H.: Severe Metacarpophalangeal Sprain of the Thumb in Ski Accidents. Ann. Chir. Main 3:101–112, 1984.
928. Bischoff, R., Buechler, U., De Roche, R., and Jupiter, J.: Clinical Results of Tension Band Fixation of Avulsion Fractures of the Hand. J. Hand Surg. 19A:1019–1026, 1994.
929. Bostock, S., and Morris, M.A.: The Range of Motion of the MP Joint of the Thumb Following Operative Repair of the Ulnar Collateral Ligament. J. Hand Surg. 18B:710–711, 1993.
930. Bovard, R.S., Derkash, R.S., and Freeman, J.R.: Grade III Avulsion Fracture Repair on the UCL of the Proximal Joint of the Thumb. Orthop. Rev. 23:167–169, 1994.
931. Bowers, W.H., and Hurst, L.C.: Gamekeeper's Thumb. Evaluation by Arthrography and Stress Roentgenography. J. Bone Joint Surg. 59A:519–524, 1977.
932. Breek, J.C., Tan, A.M., Van Thiel, T.P.H., and Daantje, C.R.E.: Free Tendon Grafting to Repair the Metacarpophalangeal Joint of the Thumb. Surgical Techniques and a Review of 70 Patients. J. Bone Joint Surg. 71B:383–387, 1989.
933. Brewood, A.F.M., and Menon, T.J.: Combined Reconstruction of Volar and Radial Instability of a Thumb Metacarpophalangeal Joint. J. Hand Surg. 9B:333–334, 1984.
934. Bronstein, A.J., Koniuch, M.P., and van Holsbeeck, M.: Ultrasonographic Detection of Thumb Ulnar Collateral Ligament

Injuries: A Cadaveric Study. J. Hand Surg. 19A:304–312, 1994.

935. Browne, E.Z., Dunn, H.K., and Snyder, C.C.: Ski Pole Thumb Injury. Plast. Reconstr. Surg. 58:19–23, 1976.

936. Butler, T.E. Jr., and Green, D.P.: Reconstruction of Chronic Ulnar Collateral Ligament Instability of the Thumb Metacarpophalangeal Joint With a Modified Neviaser Technique. Accepted for Publication, J. Hand Surg., 1995.

937. Camp, R.A., Weatherwax, R.J., and Miller, E.B.: Chronic Posttraumatic Radial Instability of the Thumb Metacarpophalangeal Joint. J. Hand Surg. 5:221–225, 1980.

938. Campbell, C.S.: Gamekeeper's Thumb. J. Bone Joint Surg. 37B:148–149, 1955.

939. Campbell, J.D., Feagin, J.A., King, P., Lambert, K.L., and Cunningham, R.: Ulnar Collateral Ligament Injury of the Thumb. Treatment With Glove Spica Cast. Am. J. Sports Med. 20:29–30, 1992.

940. Carr, D., Johnson, R.J., and Pope, M.H.: Upper Extremity Injuries in Skiing. Am. J. Sports Med. 9:378–383, 1981.

941. Coonrad, R.W., and Goldner, J.L.: A Study of the Pathological Findings and Treatment in Soft-tissue Injury of the Thumb Metacarpophalangeal Joint. J. Bone Joint Surg. 50A:439–451, 1968.

942. Coyle, M.P. Jr.: Radial Collateral Ligament Injuries of Thumb MPJ: Treatment by Soft-tissue Advancement and Bony Reattachment. Presented at the 49th Annual Meeting, American Society for Surgery of the Hand, Cincinnati, 1994.

943. Curtis, D.J., and Downey, E.F. Jr.: A Simple First Metacarpophalangeal Stress Test. Radiology, 148:855–856, 1983.

944. Davis, P.H.: Arthrography of the Thumb Metacarpo-phalangeal Joint. American Society for Surgery of the Hand Correspondence Newsletter, 1975.

945. Derkash, R.S., Matyas, J.R., Weaver, J.K., et al.: Acute Surgical Repair of the Skier's Thumb. Clin. Orthop. 216:29–33, 1987.

946. Durham, J.W., Khuri, S., and Kim, M.H.: Acute and Late Radial Collateral Ligament Injuries of the Thumb Metacarpophalangeal Joint. J. Hand Surg. 18A:232–237, 1993.

947. Engel, J., Ganel, A., Ditzian, R., and Militeanu, J.: Arthrography as a Method of Diagnosing Tear of the Ulnar Collateral Ligament of the Metacarpophalangeal Joint of the Thumb ("Gamekeeper's Thumb"). J. Trauma 19:106–109, 1979.

948. Engkvist, O., Balkfors, B., and Lindsj, U.: Thumb Injuries in Downhill Skiing. Int. J. Sports Med. 3:50–55, 1982.

949. Fairclough, J.A., and Mintowt-Czyz, W.J.: Skier's Thumb—A Method of Prevention. Injury, 17:203–204, 1986.

950. Frank, W.E., and Dobyns, J.: Surgical Pathology of Collateral Ligamentous Injuries of the Thumb. Clin. Orthop. 83:102–114, 1972.

951. Frykman, G., and Johansson, O.: Surgical Repair of Rupture of the Ulnar Collateral Ligament of the Metacarpophalangeal Joint of the Thumb. Acta Chir. Scand. 112:58–64, 1956.

952. Gerber, C., Senn, E., and Matter, P.: Skier's Thumb. Surgical Treatment of Recent Injuries to the Ulnar Collateral Ligament of the Thumb's Metacarpophalangeal Joint. Am. J. Sports Med. 9:171–177, 1981.

953. Glickel, S.Z., Malerich, M., Pearce, S.M., and Littler, J.W.: Ligament Replacement for Chronic Instability of the Ulnar Collateral Ligament of the Metacarpophalangeal Joint of the Thumb. J. Hand Surg. 18A:930–941, 1993.

954. Goss, C.M.: Gray's Anatomy of the Human Body, 26th Ed., pp. 324,372–373. Philadelphia, Lea & Febiger, 1954.

955. Gottlieb, J.O., and Boe, S.: Combination of Rupture of the Ulnar Collateral Ligament and Spiroid Fracture of the Thumb. Case Report. Scand. J. Plast. Reconstr. Surg. 23:75–76, 1989.

956. Gutman, J., Weisbuch, J., and Wolf, M.: Ski Injuries in 1972–1973. A Repeat Analysis of a Major Health Problem. J.A.M.A. 230:1423–1425, 1974.

957. Hagan, H.J., and Hastings, H.: Fusion of the Thumb Metacarpophalangeal Joint to Treat Posttraumatic Arthritis. J. Hand Surg. 13A:750–753, 1988.

958. Harris, H., and Joseph, J.: Variation in Extension of the Metacarpo-phalangeal and Interphalangeal Joints of the Thumb. J. Bone Joint Surg. 31B:547–559, 1949.

959. Heller, J.: Complete Avulsion of the Ligamentous Apparatus of the Metacarpophalangeal Joint of the Thumb. Surg. Gynecol. Obstet. 116:95–98, 1963.

960. Helm, R.H.: Hand Function After Injuries to the Collateral Ligaments of the Metacarpophalangeal Joint of the Thumb. J. Hand Surg. 12B:252–255, 1987.

961. Hildreth, D.H., and Oxford, K.: Use of the Mitek Ligament Anchor System for Repair of Collateral Ligament Injuries of the Thumb. Submitted for Publication, 1994.

962. Hintermann, B., Holzach, P.J., Schütz, M., and Matter, P.: Skier's Thumb—The Significance of Bony Injuries. Am. J. Sports Med. 21:800–804, 1993.

963. Joseph, J.: Further Studies of the Metacarpophalangeal and Interphalangeal Joints of the Thumb. J. Anat. 85:221–229, 1951.

964. Kaplan, E.B.: The Pathology and Treatment of Radial Subluxation of the Thumb With Ulnar Displacement of the Head of the First Metacarpal. J. Bone Joint Surg. 43A:541–546, 1961.

965. Kessler, I.: Complex Avulsion of the Ulnar Collateral Ligament of the Metacarpophalangeal Joint of the Thumb. Clin. Orthop. 29:196–200, 1961.

966. Kozin, S.H., and Bishop, A.T.: Tension Wire Fixation of Avulsion Fractures at the Thumb Metacarpophalangeal Joint. J. Hand Surg. 19A:1027–1031, 1994.

967. Lamb, D.W., Abernethy, P.J., and Fragiadakis, E.: Injuries of the Metacarpophalangeal Joint of the Thumb. Hand 3:164–168, 1971.

968. Lamb, D.W., and Angarita, G.: Ulnar Instability of the Metacarpophalangeal Joint of Thumb. J. Hand Surg. 10B:113–114, 1985.

969. Linscheid, R.L.: Arthrography of the Metacarpophalangeal Joint. Clin. Orthop. 103:91, 1974.

970. Linscheid, R.L., Grainger, R.W., and Johnson, E.W.: The Thumb Metacarpophalangeal Joint. Injuries. Minn. Med. 55:1037–1040, 1972.

971. Louis, D.S., and Buckwalter, K.A.: Magnetic Resonance Imaging of the Collateral Ligaments of the Thumb. J. Hand Surg. 14A:739–741, 1989.

972. Louis, D.S., Huebner, J.J. Jr., and Hankin, F.M.: Rupture and Displacement of the Ulnar Collateral Ligament of the Metacarpophalangeal Joint of the Thumb. Preoperative Diagnosis. J. Bone Joint Surg. 68A:1320–1326, 1986.

973. McCue, F.C., Hakala, M.W., Andrews, J.R., and Gieck, J.H.: Ulnar Collateral Ligament Injuries of the Thumb in Athletes. J. Sports Med. 2:70–80, 1974.

974. Miller, R.J.: Dislocations and Fracture Dislocations of the Metacarpophalangeal Joint of the Thumb. Hand Clin. 4:45–65, 1988.

975. Mogan, J.V., and Davis, P.H.: Upper Extremity Injuries in Skiing. Clin. Sports Med. 1:295–308, 1982.

976. Mogensen, B.A., and Mattsson, H.S.: Post-traumatic Instability of the Metacarpophalangeal Joint of the Thumb. Hand 12:85–90, 1980.

977. Neviaser, R.J., and Adams, J.P.: Complications of Treatment of Injuries to the Hand. *In* Epps, C.H. (ed.): Complications in Orthopaedic Surgery. Philadelphia, J.B. Lippincott, 1978.

978. Neviaser, R.J., Wilson, J.N., and Lievano, A.: Rupture of the Ulnar Collateral Ligament of the Thumb (Gamekeeper's Thumb). J. Bone Joint Surg. 53A:1357–1364, 1971.

979. Newland, C.C.: Gamekeeper's Thumb. Orthop. Clin. North Am. 23:41–48, 1992.

980. Osterman, A.L., Hayken, G.D., and Bora, F.W.: A Quantitative Evaluation of Thumb Function After Ulnar Collateral Repair and Reconstruction. J. Trauma 21:854–861, 1981.

981. Palmer, A.K., and Louis, D.S.: Assessing Ulnar Instability of the Metacarpophalangeal Joint of the Thumb. J. Hand Surg. 3:542—546, 1978.

982. Parikh, M., Nahigian, S., and Froimson, A.: Gamekeeper's Thumb. Plast. Reconstr. Surg. 58:24–31, 1976.

983. Pichora, D.R., McMurtry, R.Y., and Bell, M.J.: Gamekeepers

Thumb: A Prospective Study of Functional Bracing. J. Hand Surg. 14A:567–573, 1989.

984. Primiano, G.A.: Skiers' Thumb Injuries Associated With Flared Ski Pole Handles. Am. J. Sports Med. 13:425–427, 1985.
985. Primiano, G.A.: Functional Cast Immobilization of Thumb Metacarpophalangeal Joint Injuries. Am. J. Sports Med. 14:335–339, 1986.
986. Rehak, D.C., Sotereanos, D.G., Bowman, M.W., and Herndon, J.H.: The Mitek Bone Anchor: Application to the Hand Wrist and Elbow. J. Hand Surg. 19A:853–860, 1994.
987. Reikeras, O., and Kvarnes, L.: Rupture of the Ulnar Ligament of the Metacarpophalangeal Joint of the Thumb. Arch. Orthop. Trauma Surg. 100:175–177, 1982.
988. Resnick, D., and Danzig, L.A.: Arthrographic Evaluation of Injuries of the First Metacarpophalangeal Joint Gamekeeper's Thumb. A.J.R. 126:1046–1052, 1976.
989. Rosenthal, D.I., Murray, W.T., and Smith, R.J.: Finger Arthrography. Radiology, 137:647–651, 1980.
990. Rovere, G.D., Gristina, A.G., Stolzer, W.A., and Garver, E.M.: Treatment of "Gamekeeper's Thumb" in Hockey Players. J. Sports Med. 3:147–151, 1975.
991. Ruby, L.K.: Common Hand Injuries in the Athlete. Orthop. Clin. North Am. 11:819–839, 1980.
992. Saetta, J.P., Phair, I.C., and Quinton, D.N.: Ulnar Collateral Ligament Repair of the Metacarpo-phalangeal Joint of the Thumb: A Study Comparing Two Methods of Repair. J. Hand Surg. 17B:160–163, 1992.
993. Sakellarides, H.T.: Treatment of Recent and Old Injuries of the Ulnar Collateral Ligament of the MP Joint of the Thumb. Am. J. Sports Med. 6:255–262, 1978.
994. Sakellarides, H.T.: The Surgical Treatment of Old Injuries of the Collateral Ligaments of the MP Joint of the Thumb Using the Extensor Pollicis Brevis Tendon (A Long-term Follow-up of 100 Cases). Bull. Hosp. Jt. Dis. 44:449–458, 1984.
995. Sakellarides, H.T., and DeWeese, J.W.: Instability of the Metacarpophalangeal Joint of the Thumb. Reconstruction of the Collateral Ligaments Using the Extensor Pollicis Brevis Tendon. J. Bone Joint Surg. 58A:106–112, 1976.
996. Schultz, R.J., and Fox, J.M.: Gamekeeper's Thumb. N.Y. State J. Med. 73:2329–2331, 1973.
997. Sennwald, G., Segmüller, G., and Egli, A.: The Late Reconstruction of the Ligament of the Metacarpo-phalangeal Joint of the Thumb. Ann. Chir. Main 6:15–24, 1987.
998. Shaw, S.J., and Morris, M.A.: The Range of Motion of the Metacarpo-phalangeal Joint of the Thumb and Its Relationship to Injury. J. Hand Surg. 17B:164–166, 1992.
999. Smith, M.A.: The Mechanism of Acute Ulnar Instability of the Metacarpophalangeal Joint of the Thumb. Hand 12:225–230, 1980.
1000. Smith, R.J.: Post-traumatic Instability of the Metacarpophalangeal Joint of the Thumb. J. Bone Joint Surg. 59A:14—21, 1977.
1001. Sollerman, C., Abrahamsson, S., Lundborg, G., and Adalbert, K.: Functional Splinting Versus Plaster Cast for Ruptures of the Ulnar Collateral Ligament of the Thumb. A Prospective Randomized Study of 63 Cases. Acta Orthop. Scand. 62:524–526, 1991.
1002. Spaeth, H.J., Abrams, R.A., Bock, G.W., et al.: Gamekeeper Thumb: Differentiation of Nondisplaced and Displaced Tears of the Ulnar Collateal Ligament With MR Imaging. Radiology 188:553–556, 1993.
1003. Stener, B.: Displacement of the Ruptured Ulnar Collateral Ligament of the Metacarpophalangeal Joint of the Thumb. A Clinical and Anatomical Study. J. Bone Joint Surg. 44B:869–879, 1962.
1004. Stener, B., and Stener, I.: Shearing Fractures Associated With Rupture of Ulnar Collateral Ligament of Metacarpophalangeal Joint of Thumb. Injury, 1:12–16, 1969.
1005. Sternbach, G., C.S. Campbell: Gamekeeper's Thumb. J. Emerg. Med. 1:345–347, 1984.
1006. Stothard, J., and Caird, D.M.: Experience With Arthrography of the First Metacarpophalangeal Joint. Hand 13:257–266, 1981.
1007. Strandell, G.: Total Rupture of the Ulnar Collateral Ligament of the Metacarpophalangeal Joint of the Thumb. Results of Surgery in 35 Cases. Acta Chir. Scand. 118:72–80, 1959.
1008. Sutro, C.J.: Pollex Valgus (A Bunion-like Deformity of the Thumb Corrected by Surgical Intervention). Bull. Hosp. Jt. Dis. 18:135–139, 1957.
1009. Van Der Kloot, J.F.V.: Injury to the Ulnar Ligament of the Thumb. Arch. Chir. Neerl. 17:179–185, 1965.
1010. Van Dommelen, B.A., and Zvirbulis, R.A.: Upper Extremity Injuries in Snow Skiers. Am. J. Sports Med. 17:751–753, 1989.
1011. Vaupel, G.L., and Andrews, J.R.: Diagnostic and Operative Arthroscopy of the Thumb Metacarpophalangeal Joint. A Case Report. Am. J. Sports Med. 13:139–141, 1985.
1012. Vihtonen, K., Juutilainen, T., Pätiälä, H., Rokkanen, P., and Trmälä, P.: Reinsertion of the Ruptured Ulnar Collateral Ligament of the Metacarpophalangeal Joint With an Absorbable Self-reinforced Polylactide Tack. J. Hand Surg. 18B:200–203, 1993.
1013. Wallace, D.A., and Carr, A.J.: Rupture of the Ulnar Collateral Ligament of the Thumb in a 5-Year-Old Girl. J. Hand Surg. 18B:501, 1993.
1014. Weston, W.J.: The Normal Arthrograms of the Metacarpophalangeal, Metatarso-phalangeal and Inter-phalangeal Joints. Aust. Radiol. 13:211–218, 1969.
1015. White, G.M.: Ligamentous Avulsion of the Ulnar Collateral Ligament of the Thumb of a Child. J. Hand Surg. 11A:669–672, 1986.
1016. Wilppula, E., and Nummi, J.: Surgical Treatment of Ruptured Ulnar Collateral Ligament of the Metacarpophalangeal Joint of the Thumb. Injury, 2:69–72, 1970.
1017. Woods, D.W., Mudge, M.K., and Wood, V.E.: Radial Instability of the Thumb Metacarpophalangeal Joint: A Clinical and Cadaveric Study. Presented at the Scientific Exhibit, AAOS Annual Meeting, San Francisco, 1987.
1018. Zilberman, Z., Rotschild, E., and Krauss, L.: Rupture of the Ulnar Collateral Ligament of the Thumb. J. Trauma 5:447–481, 1965.

MP JOINT OF THE THUMB—DISLOCATIONS AND VOLAR PLATE INJURIES

1019. Desai, S.S., and Morgan, W.J.: Locked Thumb Metacarpophalangeal Joint Caused by Sesamoid Entrapment. J. Hand Surg. 16A:1052–1055, 1991.
1020. Dutton, R.O., and Meals, R.A.: Complex Dorsal Dislocation of the Thumb Metacarpophalangeal Joint. Clin. Orthop. 164:160–164, 1982.
1021. Eaton, R.G., and Floyd, W.E. III: Thumb Metacarpophalangeal Capsulodesis: An Adjunct Procedure to Basal Joint Arthroplasty for Collapse Deformity of the First Ray. J. Hand Surg. 13A:449–453, 1988.
1022. Eiken, O.: Palmaris Longus-tenodesis for Hyperextension of the Thumb Metacarpophalangeal Joint. Scand. J. Plast. Reconstr. Surg. 15:149–152, 1981.
1023. Filler, B.C., Stark, H.H., and Boyes, J.H.: Capsulodesis of the Metacarpophalangeal Joint of the Thumb in Children With Cerebral Palsy. J. Bone Joint Surg. 58A:667–670, 1976.
1024. Gunther, S.F., and Zielinski, C.J.: Irreducible Palmar Dislocation of the Proximal Phalanx of the Thumb—Case Report. J. Hand Surg. 7:515–517, 1982.
1025. Hughes, L.A., and Freiberg, A.: Irreducible MP Joint Dislocation Due to Entrapment of FPL. J. Hand Surg. 18B:708–709, 1993.
1026. Inoue, G., and Miura, T.: Locked Metacarpo-phalangeal Joint of the Thumb. J. Hand Surg. 13B:469–473, 1988.
1027. Kessler, I.: A Simplified Technique to Correct Hyperextension Deformity of the Metacarpophalangeal Joint of the Thumb. J. Bone Joint Surg. 61A:903–905, 1979.
1028. Kojima, T., Nagano, T., and Kohno, T.: Causes of Locking Metacarpophalangeal Joint of the Thumb and Its Non-operative Treatment. Hand 11:256–262, 1979.

1029. Milch, H.: Recurrent Dislocation of Thumb. Capsulorrhaphy. Am. J. Surg. 6:237–239, 1929.
1030. Miyamoto, M., Hirayama, T., and Uchida, M.: Volar Dislocation of the Metacarpophalangeal Joint of the Thumb—A Case Report. J. Hand Surg. 11B:51–54, 1986.
1031. Moberg, E., and Stener, B.: Injuries to the Ligaments of the Thumb and Fingers. Diagnosis, Treatment and Prognosis. Acta Chir. Scand. 106:166–186, 1953.
1032. Moneim, M.S.: Volar Dislocation of the Metacarpophalangeal Joint. Pathological Anatomy and Report of Two Cases. Clin. Orthop. 176:186–189, 1983.
1033. Onuba, O., and Essiet, A.: Irreducible Dislocation of the Metacarpophalangeal Joint of the Thumb Due to Tendon Interposition. J. Hand Surg. 12B:60–61, 1987.
1034. Ostrowski, D.M.: Irreducible Dorsoulnar Dislocation of the Proximal Phalanx of the Thumb. J. Hand Surg. 16A:121–124, 1991.
1035. Palmer, R.E.: Injury to Dorsal MCP Joint of the Thumb. Orthop. Rev. 11:127–129, 1982.
1036. Posner, M.A., Langa, V., and Ambrose, L.: Intrinsic Muscle Advancement to Treat Chronic Palmar Instability of the Metacarpophalangeal Joint of the Thumb. J. Hand Surg. 13A:110–115, 1988.
1037. Posner, M.A., and Retaillaud, J.: Metacarpophalangeal Joint Injuries of the Thumb. Hand Clin. 8:713–732, 1992.
1038. Schuurman, A.H., and Bos, K.E.: Treatment of Volar Instability of the Metacarpophalangeal Joint of the Thumb by Volar Capsulodesis. J. Hand Surg. 18B:346–349, 1993.
1039. Tsuge, K., and Watari, S.: Locking Metacarpophalangeal Joint of the Thumb. Hand 6:255–260, 1974.
1040. Yamanaka, K., Yoshida, K., Inoue, H., Inoue, A., and Miyagi, T.: Locking of the Metacarpophalangeal Joint of the Thumb. J. Bone Joint Surg. 67A:782–787, 1985.
1041. Zancolli, E.: Structural and Dynamic Bases of Hand Surgery, 2nd Ed., pp. 212–213. Philadelphia, J.B. Lippincott, 1979.

MP JOINT OF THE THUMB—SESAMOID FRACTURES

1042. Bell, M.J., McMurtry, R.Y., and Rubenstein, J.: Fracture of the Ulnar Sesamoid of the Metacarpophalangeal Joint of the Thumb—An Arthrographic Study. J. Hand Surg. 10B:379–381, 1985.
1043. Clarke, P., Braunstein, E.M., Weissman, B.N., and Sosman, J.L.: Case Reports. Sesamoid Fracture of the Thumb. Br. J. Radiol. 56:485, 1983.
1044. Gibeault, J.D., Saba, P., Hoenecke, H., and Graham, A.: The Sesamoids of the Metacarpo-phalangeal Joint of the Thumb: An Anatomical and Clinical Study. J. Hand Surg. 14B:244–247, 1989.
1045. Hansen, C.A., and Peterson, T.H.: Fracture of the Thumb Sesamoid Bones. J. Hand Surg. 12A:269–270, 1987.
1046. Ishizuki, M., Nakagawa, T., and Ito, S.: Hyperextension Injuries of the MP Joint of the Thumb. J. Hand Surg. 19B:361–367, 1994.
1047. Jones, R.P., and Leach, R.E.: Fracture of the Ulnar Sesamoid Bone of the Thumb. Am. J. Sports Med. 8:446–447, 1980.
1048. Patel, M.R., Pearlman, H.S., Bassini, L., and Ravich, S.: Fractures of the Sesamoid Bones of the Thumb. J. Hand Surg. 15A:776–781, 1990.
1049. Sinberg, S.E.: Fracture of a Sesamoid of the Thumb. J. Bone Joint Surg. 22:444–445, 1940.
1050. Stener, B.: Hyperextension Injuries to the Metacarpophalangeal Joint of the Thumb—Rupture of Ligaments, Fracture of Sesamoid Bones, Rupture of Flexor Pollicis Brevis. An Anatomical and Clinical Study. Acta Chir. Scand. 125:275–293, 1963.
1051. Streatfeild, T., and Griffiths, H.F.: Fracture of a Sesamoid Bone. Lancet 1:1117, 1934.
1052. Trumble, T.E., and Watson, H.K.: Posttraumatic Sesamoid Arthritis of the Metacarpophalangeal Joint of the Thumb. J. Hand Surg. 10A:94–100, 1985.
1053. Wood, V.E.: The Sesamoid Bones of the Hand and Their Pathology. J. Hand Surg. 9B:261–264, 1984.

CMC JOINT OF THE THUMB

1054. Barmakian, J.T.: Anatomy of the Joints of the Thumb. Hand Clin. 8:683–691, 1992.
1055. Bojsen-Moller, F.: Osteoligamentous Guidance of the Movements of the Human Thumb. Am. J. Anat. 147:71–80, 1976.
1056. Bojsen-Moller, F.B.: Osteoligamentous Guidance of the Movements of the Human Thumb. Am. J. Anat. 147:71–80, 1976.
1057. Brunelli, G., Monini, L., and Brunelli, F.: Stabilisation of the Trapezio-metacarpal Joint. J. Hand Surg. 14B:209–212, 1989.
1058. Burkhalter, W.E.: American Society for Surgery of the Hand Correspondence Newsletter, 1981.
1059. Chen, V.T.: Dislocation of the Carpometacarpal Joint of the Thumb. J. Hand Surg. 12B:246–251, 1987.
1060. Cho, K.O.: Translocation of the Abductor Pollicis Longus Tendon. A Treatment for Chronic Subluxation of the Thumb Carpometacarpal Joint. J. Bone Joint Surg. 52A:1166–1170, 1970.
1061. Eaton, R.G.: Joint Injuries of the Hand, pp. 66–70. Springfield, Ill., Charles C. Thomas, 1971.
1062. Eaton, R.G., and Littler, J.W.: Ligament Reconstruction for the Painful Thumb Carpometacarpal Joint. J. Bone Joint Surg. 55A:1655 1666, 1973.
1063. Eggers, G.W.N.: Chronic Dislocation of the Base of the Metacarpal of the Thumb. J. Bone Joint Surg. 27:500–501, 1945.
1064. Haines, R.W.: The Mechanism of Rotation at the First Carpometacarpal Joint. J. Anat. 78:44–46, 1944.
1065. Hooper, G.J.: An Unusual Variety of Skier's Thumb. J. Hand Surg. 12A:627–629, 1987.
1066. Ibrahim, S., and Noor, M.A.: Simultaneous Dislocations of the Carpometacarpal and Metacarpophalangeal Joints of the Thumb. Injury, 24:343–344, 1993.
1067. Imaeda, T., An, K., Cooney, W.P. III, and Linscheid, R. Anatomy of Trapeziometacarpal Ligaments. J. Hand Surg. 18A:226–231, 1993.
1068. Jensen, J.S.: Operative Treatment of Chronic Subluxation of the First Carpometacarpal Joint. Hand 7:269–271, 1975.
1069. Johnson, S.R., Jones, D.G., and Hoddinott, H.C.: Missed Carpometacarpal Dislocation of the Thumb in Motorcyclists. Injury 18:415–416, 1987.
1070. Kestler, O.C.: Recurrent Dislocation of the First Carpometacarpal Joint. Repaired by Functional Tenodesis. J. Bone Joint Surg. 28A:858–861, 1946.
1071. Kuczynski, K.: Carpometacarpal Joint of the Human Thumb. J. Anat. 118:119–126, 1974.
1072. Kuschner, S.H., Shepard, L., Stephens, S., and Gellman, H.: Fracture of the Index Metacarpal Base With Subluxation of the Trapeziometacarpal Joint. A Case Report. Clin. Orthop. 264:197–199, 1991.
1073. Lasserre, C., Pauzat, D., and Derennes, R.: Osteoarthritis of the Trapezio-metacarpal Joint. J. Bone Joint Surg. 31B:534–536, 1949.
1074. Littler, J.W.: Trapeziometacarpal Joint Injuries. Hand Clin. 8:701–711, 1992.
1075. Magnusson, A., Bertheussen, K., and Weilby, A.: Ligament Reconstruction of the Thumb Carpometacarpal Joint Using a Modified Eaton and Littler Technique. J. Hand Surg. 10B:115–116, 1985.
1076. Mody, B.S., and Dias, J.J.: Carpometacarpal Dislocation of the Thumb Associated With Fracture of the Trapezium. J. Hand Surg. 18B:197–199, 1993.
1077. Moore, J.R., Webb, C.A., and Thompson, R.C.: A Complete Dislocation of the Thumb Metacarpal. J. Hand Surg. 3:547–549, 1978.
1078. Napier, J.R.: The Form and Function of the Carpometacarpal Joint of the Thumb. J. Anat. 89:362–369, 1955.
1079. Pagalidis, T., Kuczynski, K., and Lamb, D.W.: Ligmentous Stability of the Base of the Thumb. Hand 13:29–35, 1981.
1080. Pieron, A.P.: The Mechanism of the First Carpometacarpal (CMC) Joint. An Anatomical and Mechanical Analysis. Acta Orthop. Scand. 148:7–104, 1973.
1081. Shah, J., and Patel, M.: Dislocation of the Carpometacarpal

Joint of the Thumb. A Report of Four Cases. Clin. Orthop. 175:166–169, 1983.
1082. Slocum, D.B.: Stabilization of the Articulation of the Greater Multangular and the First Metacarpal. J. Bone Joint Surg. 25A:626–630, 1943.
1083. Strauch, R.J., Behrman, M.J., and Rosenwasser, M.P.: Acute Dislocation of the Carpometacarpal Joint of the Thumb: An Anatomic and Cadaver Study. J. Hand Surg. 19A:93–98, 1994.
1084. Tolat, A.R., and Jones, M.W.: Carpometacarpal Dislocation of the Thumb Associated With Fracture of the Trapezium. Injury 21:411–412, 1990.
1085. Watt, N., and Hooper, G.: Dislocation of the Trapezio-metacarpal Joint. J. Hand Surg. 12B:242–245, 1987.
1086. Wee, J.T.K., Chandra, D., and Satku, K.: Simultaneous Dislocations of the Interphalangeal and Carpometacarpal Joints of the Thumb: A Case Report. J. Hand Surg. 13B:224–226, 1988.
1087. Weitbrecht, J.: Syndesmology Or A Description of the Ligaments of the Human Body, pp. VII–X,48,150–152. Philadelphia, W.B. Saunders Company, 1969.

Rockwood and Green's Fractures in Adults, Fourth Edition,
edited by Charles A. Rockwood, David P. Green, Robert W. Bucholz and James D. Heckman.
Lippincott-Raven Publishers, Philadelphia © 1996.

CHAPTER 12

Fractures and Dislocations of the Wrist

William P. Cooney, III, Ronald L. Linscheid,
and James H. Dobyns

The wrist is a specialized region of the upper extremity that extends from the carpometacarpal joints to the proximal border of the pronator quadratus. The dictionary definitions of the wrist and carpus may be considered identical, but the wrist (from the Middle English *wraeston,* to "twist") generally covers a larger area of interest than the carpus, which is intended to refer only to the two rows of bones between the distal radius and metacarpals. The wrist is the interconnecting group of joints between the hand and forearm and, in common parlance, includes the midcarpal and radiocarpal joints and the distal radioulnar joint (DRUJ). The orientation of the wrist is based on skeletal landmarks of the distal radius.[282] Motion is described in terms of radiocarpal flexion–extension and radioulnar deviation, as well as DRUJ pronation and supination (Fig. 12-1).

The carpus is a complex unit of bony articulations that transfers the force and motion of the hand to the supportive forearm and upper extremity.[171,284,323] Rather than a simple hinge joint such as the elbow, or a ball-socket joint such as the hip, the wrist involves a delicate interaction between eight carpal bones that are divided into two carpal rows, the mechanical equivalent of which is not easily simulated.[118,208,284,462] Whereas the primary motions are flexion–extension and radioulnar deviation, the actual motion of carpal bones is much more complex (Fig. 12-2).[118,282] The primary axis of motion resides within the head of the capitate,[361] which is not a singular point but rather an oblique screw axis for combined motions of wrist extension–radial deviation and wrist flexion–ulnar deviation that are quite normal planes of daily movement (see Fig. 12-2). To produce this natural movement, individual carpal bones not only turn up and down and back and forth but also spin and roll about their own axes. To understand the pathophysiology of wrist fractures and dislocations, these functional components need to be understood (see Kinematics).

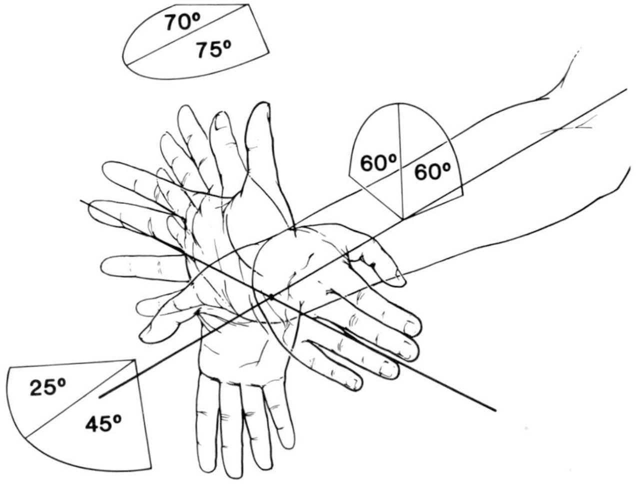

FIGURE 12-1. Global motion of the wrist and forearm. The wrist has three degrees of freedom through a complex mechanical arrangement that allows approximately 145° of flexion—extension movement (FEM), 70° of radioulnar deviation (RUD), and 120° of pronosupination through the forearm radioulnar joints. The last provides the torque to accomplish twisting motions.

Equally important are the muscles and tendons that move the wrist. Their actions are tightly constrained so that their effect on motion and transmission of force can be carefully controlled.

HISTORICAL REVIEW

Undoubtedly the ancients were aware of wrist problems, but not much was written until the beginning of the 19th century. A theme, reflected in the writings of the continental physicians, was that most injuries of this area were dislocations of the wrist. Jeanne and Mouchet,[268] Malgaigne,[344] Desault,[144] and others[145,157] diagnosed by clinical examination or confirmed by autopsy dislocations and luxations of the carpus. Sir Astley Cooper produced the first book on wrist injuries, *A Treatise on Dislocations and Fractures of Joints,* in 1822. It remained for Colles of Dublin[110] and Pouteau of France[439] to differentiate between fractures of the distal radius and wrist dislocations. In the United States, Barton[34] described the volar and dorsal fracture–dislocations of the radiocarpal joint, and Pilcher[436] identified the difference between intra-articular and extra-articular distal radius fractures by description and illustration. The discovery of the x-ray by Roentgen allowed swift progression in understanding and classifying traumatic injuries of the wrist. Destot[145] produced a remarkable discussion of a variety of wrist injuries in 1926.

Twenty years ago, when the first version of this chapter on wrist fracture and dislocations was written,[152] the concept of wrist instability had changed only modestly from these earlier writings. It was the work of Lambrinudi,[221,308] Bolton,[221] and later Fisk[183] that recognized that both fracture of the scaphoid and carpal ligament injuries would produce carpal instability. Fisk, in a landmark Hunterian Lecture presentation in 1968,[182] detailed the role of scaphoid fracture producing carpal instability and ultimately carpal collapse. In 1972, Linscheid and coworkers[329] defined traumatic instability of the wrist, bringing forth concepts of dorsal and volar intercalated carpal instability based on the ideas of Landsmeer[309] (DISI and VISI). The term "sprain" of the wrist took on new meaning, and the real importance of ligament injuries in producing wrist instability equal to that of wrist fractures became appreciated. The concept of carpal instability has been expanded widely as a result of careful clinical studies

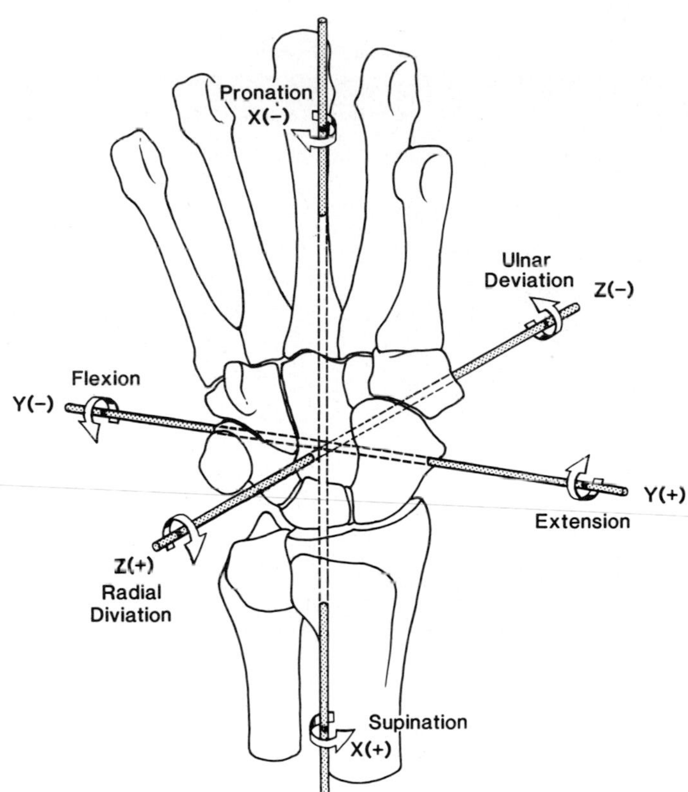

FIGURE 12-2. A coordinate system to describe the screw axis of the wrist, which passes through the head of the capitate for flexion $Y(-)$ and extension $Y(+)$; radial deviation $Z(+)$ and ulnar deviation $Z(-)$; and pronation $X(-)$ and supination $X(+)$.

and anatomical and biomechanical analyses of the specific pathology involved.[153,327,514] As a result, clear concepts and classifications of the different types of carpal instability have evolved (Table 12-1).

Carpal instability may occur from a variety of different fractures or dislocations with a combination of ligament, bone, capsule, and tendon injury.[118,119,153,356,414] Ligament repair and proper reconstruction of fractured carpal components serve to preserve these support structures for maintenance of normal joint alignment and transmission of forces within this highly tuned and mechanically complex unit.

New information on muscle and tendon physiology,[77] vascularity of the carpal bones,[213,519] the location and function of intrinsic and extrinsic wrist ligaments,[50,210,357] and the three-dimensional motion of individual carpal bones[130,461,490,561] has increased immeasurably our understanding of the surgical anatomy of the wrist. This will assist our efforts toward timely and anatomically accurate reconstruction after acute or delayed trauma.

SURGICAL ANATOMY

General Anatomy

From the carpometacarpal joints to the distal border of the pronator quadratus, most of the soft tissues that pass the wrist are bound within rigid compartments.[317,318] On the dorsal side the extensor tendons pass under an extensor retinaculum that holds them close to bone and maintains their uniform mechanical relationship to the carpus.[518] The six extensor compartments (Fig. 12-3) separate the following tendons: radial wrist abductor (abductor pollicis longus) and short thumb extensor (extensor pollicis brevis) from the radial wrist extensors (extensor carpi radialis longus and extensor carpi radialis brevis); the long thumb extensor (extensor pollicis longus) in a separate tunnel as it wraps ulnarly around Lister's tubercle; the common finger extensors (extensor digitorum communis) in the fourth or central compartment; the single extensor digiti minimi tendon (extensor digiti minimi) to the fifth digit; and the last or sixth compartment, residing in a groove adjacent to the ulnar styloid, holds the ulnar wrist extensor (extensor carpi ulnaris).[543]

The volar wrist tendons are tightly constrained within a special compartment, the carpal tunnel (thumb and finger long flexor tendons), except for the flexor carpi radialis in a separate compartment, the flexor carpi ulnaris, and palmaris longus (see Fig. 12-3). The flexor carpi radialis and flexor carpi ulnaris control wrist flexion and are uniquely placed to enhance their mechanical advantage through the mechanical effect of scaphoid and pisiform bones on the tendon moment arm. The flexor carpi ulnaris is the most powerful wrist muscle be-

TABLE 12-1
*Carpal Instability (Mayo Classification)**

Instability (Subluxation)	Dislocation (Luxation)	Fracture–Dislocation
PERILUNATE		
Partial or residual	Various stage†	Transosseous
CID type		Transscaphoid perilunate†
Scapholunate dissociation with DISI†		Transradiostyloid perilunate
Lunatotriquertral dissociation with VISI		Other combinations
RADIOCARPAL		
CIND type	Dorsal†	Dorsal Barton's
VISI	Volar	Volar Barton's†
DISI	Ulnar	Radial styloid with carpal translation (ulnar, dorsal, radial, volar)
Ulnar translation†		Lunate fossa with carpal translation
CIC	Various	
MIDCARPAL		
CIND type	Potential (but so rare as to be unique)	Malunited Colles' fracture (potential, but so rare as to be unique)
Triquetrohamate (VISI > DISI)†		With primary MC instability
Scaphotrapeziotrapezoidal (VISI > DISI)		With secondary MC instability
Capitolunate (DISI > VISI)		
Diffuse laxity (DISI > VISI)		

CID, Carpal instability dissociative; CIND, carpal instability nondissociative; CIC, carpal instability combined.
* Instability, dislocations, and fracture–dislocation combined are the most common wrist destabilization pattern.
† The most common instability pattern of the group.

cause of its multiple short muscle fibers.[77] The extrinsic tendons of the digits, with the exception of the thumb, are grouped centrally in the frontal plane to afford minimal angulation to the wrist during use, while the wrist motors are grouped peripherally to exert optimum control of the position of the wrist. It is unusual and often pathologic for a muscle belly to cross the wrist, because tendons transmit muscle force efficiently with minimal utilization of space. As a consequence, there is little soft-tissue protection for the accompanying median and ulnar nerves and ulnar and radial arteries.

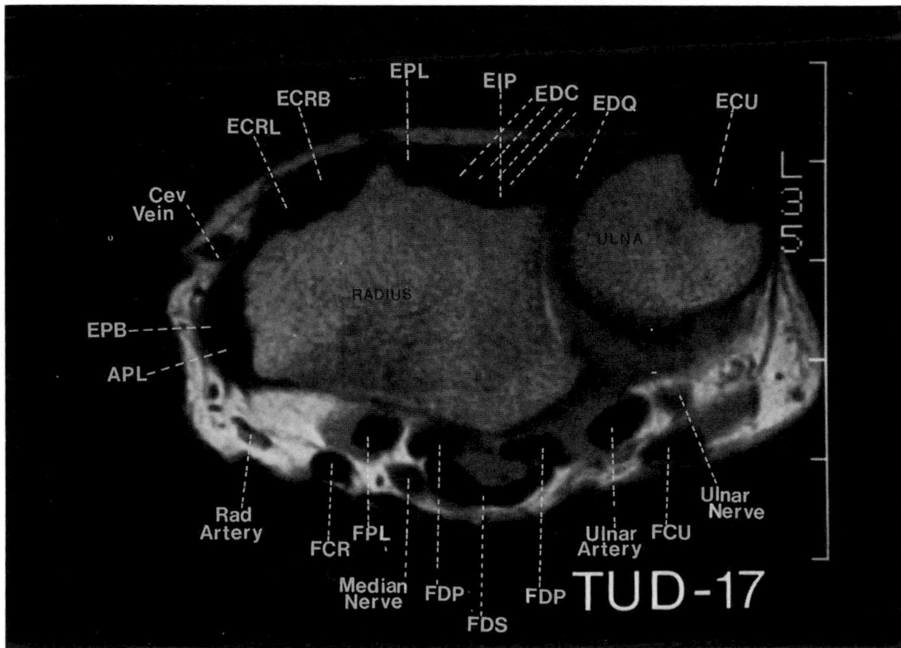

FIGURE 12-3. Cross-sectional anatomy of the wrist shown on an MRI through the distal radioulnar joint. Flexor and extensor tendons of the fingers are grouped over the center of rotation so as to impart minimal deviation radially or ulnarly, except for the thumb extrinsic tendons. The wrist motors are distributed peripherally to provide maximum moment arms or establish a wrist position. Dorsal structures, left to right: cephalic vein (Cev Vein); extensor carpi radialis longus (ECRL); extensor carpi radialis brevis (ECRB); extensor pollicis longus (EPL); extensor indicis proprius (EIP); extensor digitorum communis (EDC); extensor digiti quinti (EDQ); extensor carpi ulnaris (ECU). Palmar structures, left to right: extensor pollicis brevis (EPB); abductor pollicis longus (APL); radial artery (Rad Artery); flexor carpi radialis (FCR); flexor pollicis longus (FPL); flexor digitorum profundus (FDP); flexor digitorum superficialis (FDS); flexor carpi ulnaris (FCU).

These structures are in close proximity to the wrist dorsal and volar ligaments and underlying bones, rendering them susceptible to injury with wrist trauma.

Topographic Anatomy and Clinical Examination

Clinical examination of the wrist begins with an appreciation of the topographic anatomy of the wrist (Fig. 12-4).[75,325,349] Dorsally, the wrist extensor tendons can be seen and palpated within each of the six extensor compartments. On the radial side of the wrist, the tendons of the first compartment (extensor pollicis brevis and abductor pollicis longus) and third compartment (extensor pollicis longus) border the radial and ulnar sides of the anatomical snuff box. One can palpate proximally in the snuff box the radial styloid and, in the mid-third, the waist and distal third of the scaphoid. At the distal end of the snuff box the scapho-trapeziotrapezoidal joint is identified. Moving ulnarly to the extensor pollicis longus is an important landmark, Lister's tubercle, which is the key to identifying both dorsal wrist ganglia, the junction of the scapholunate joint and dorsal scapholunate interosseous ligament. Beneath the extensor tendons the lunate is not easily identified, but the capitate can be felt proximal to the carpometacarpal joint. A prominence in this region is consistent with a *carpe bossu* (carpal boss) or carpometacarpal joint arthrosis.[278] On the ulnar side of the wrist, the ulnar head and styloid are identified. Just distal are the ulnar side of the lunate, the triquetrum, and the lunatotriquetral joint. The ulnar styloid can be noted to change position volarly with pronation and dorsally with supination. The extensor carpi ulnaris maintains a constant relationship adjacent to the styloid within its own extensor compartment.

On the volar side of the wrist, an elliptical bony prominence at the base of the thenar muscles, consisting of the trapezial ridge and scaphoid tuberosity, is the most obvious radial bony landmark. The radial artery is lateral and the flexor carpi radialis is medial to these structures. As one follows the wrist flexion crease ulnarly, the tendon of the palmaris longus is evident. The position of the median nerve just radial to the palmaris longus may be detected by eliciting Tinel's sign. The finger flexor tendons surround the nerve. The lunate, capitate, and body of the triquetrum are deep to these. The ulnar border of the carpal tunnel is formed by palmar fascia, the volar carpal ligament, and the distal edge of the hook of the hamate. The palmar arch pulsates beyond the hook and can be traced proximally as the ulnar artery. There is considerable variability in the location of the palmar arch with respect to the boundaries of Guyon's canal. The pisiform is prominent at the base of the hypothenar muscles, articulating dorsally with the triquetrum and held within the flexor carpi ulnaris. It protects the ulnar side of Guyon's canal.

In the diagnosis of specific wrist injuries, these topographic landmarks are of great value.[325] For example, a scaphoid waist fracture will produce pain and elicit tenderness within the radial snuffbox (see Fig. 12-4). Over the dorsal radius, fractures of the radial styloid, radial metaphysis, or lunate fossa of the distal radius can be determined. Scapholunate ligament injuries will demonstrate tenderness just distal to Lister's tubercle, and pain or crepitus produced by ballottement of the scaphoid against the dorsal rim of the distal radius may suggest interosseous ligament damage (see

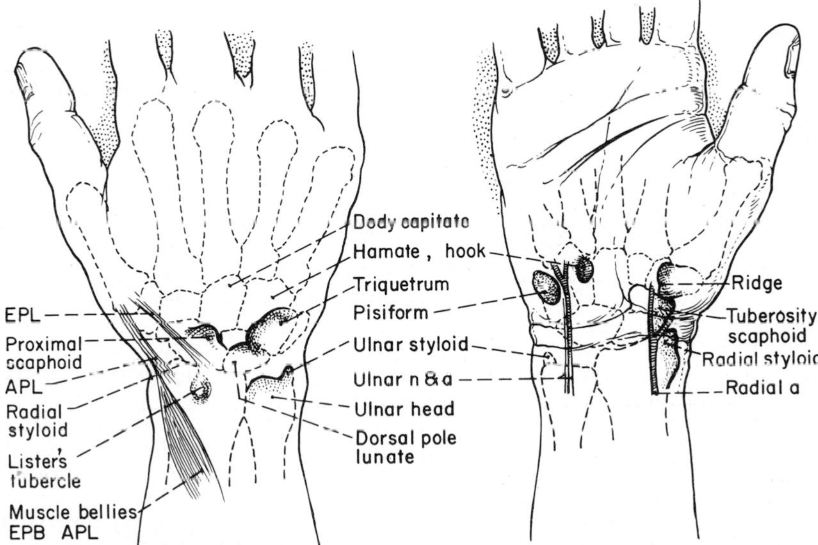

FIGURE 12-4. Topographical anatomy of the right hand. Bony prominences, readily palpated at the wrist, may be used to locate most major structures, by either palpation or stereotactic approximation. Various movements of the wrist increase the accessibility of certain bony prominences (eg, the dorsal poles of the scaphoid and lunate, the tuberosity of the scaphoid, the body of the scaphoid in the snuffbox, the hamate, the triquetrum, and the pisiform). The ulnar styloid presents in various positions, depending on rotation of the wrist. It is at the ulnar-palmar position in full pronation and the dorso-radial position in full supination.

Fig. 12-4). Pain, tenderness, and restricted radial deviation of the wrist may be caused by radial styloid-scaphoid arthritis proximally in the anatomical snuffbox or from scaphotrapeziotrapezoidal arthritis distally. Tenderness of the dorsal lunate may suggest Kienböck's disease, while more ulnar tenderness suggests tears of the triangular fibrocartilage (TFC) or lunatotriquetral ligament (see Fig. 12-4). Knowing the normal position of the extensor carpi ulnaris tendon and ulnar styloid helps to differentiate extensor carpi ulnaris tendinitis from distal radioulnar problems.[91]

A number of provocative tests based on the underlying topographic anatomy (see Carpal Instabilities) can be performed to confirm or eliminate fracture or ligament injuries. Similar stress testing can assess flexor or extensor tendon damage. Accurate palpation of the cutaneous or deep peripheral nerves and testing the vascular supply through the radial and ulnar and arteries and palmar arch can elicit a site of injury. If there are significant fractures or dislocations of the wrist, the normal alignment of the carpal bones will be displaced, and clinical examination will provide a correct diagnosis before the confirmatory radiologic examinations are completed.

Bones and Joints

The wrist is composed of the distal radius and ulna, the proximal and distal carpal rows, and the base of the metacarpals (Fig. 12-5). The distal carpal row (trapezium, trapezoid, capitate, hamate) forms a rigid, supportive transverse arch upon which the five metacarpals of the hand are firmly supported. The trapezium, cantilevered radiovolarly from the trapezoid, interfaces the thumb with the proximal row. There is motion of 10° to 20° at the scaphotrapezial joint and 30° to 42° of rotation and flexion–extension at the metacarpotrapezial joint. Under repetitive stress, the trapezium may shift radially and volarly, increasing compressive stress on the distal scaphoid. The capitate and trapezoid, which shift minimally on each other, are tightly articulated with the second and third meta-

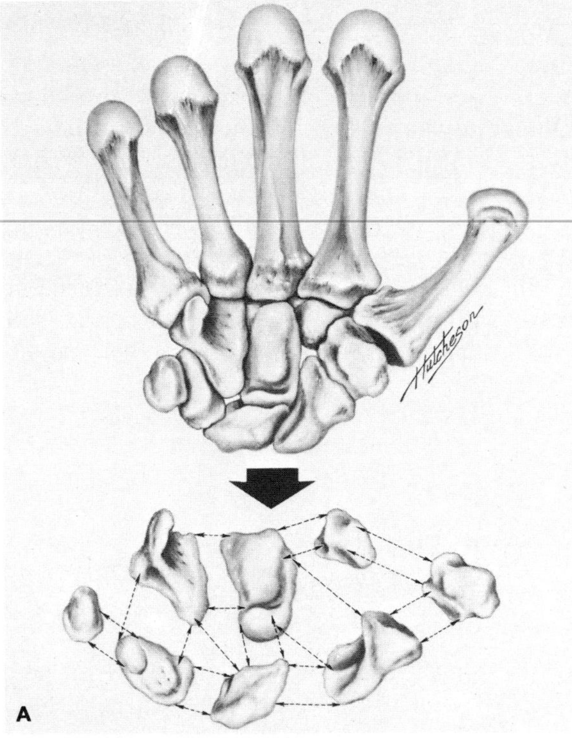

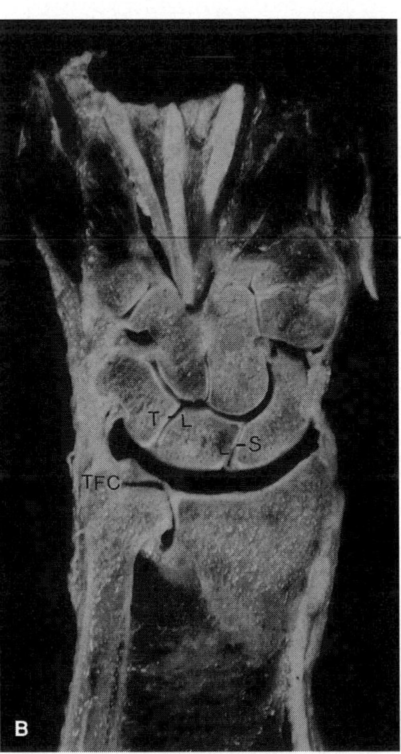

FIGURE 12-5. (**A**) Exploded view of the carpal bones. The wrist is composed of two rows of bones that provide motion and transfer of forces. The distal row (trapezium, trapezoid, capitate, and hamate) is quite stable and moves as a unit. The proximal row (scaphoid, lunate, and triquetrum) is potentially unstable. The carpal bones are supported by extrinsic ligaments attached to roughened areas on the dorsal and volar surfaces, and by intrinsic ligaments attaching intra-articular components, particularly between the scaphoid, lunate, and triquetrum. The radial side of the wrist, exemplified by the scaphoid, provides flexion-extension control over the lunate and distal carpal row. The ulnar side of the wrist exerts rotational control and stability. (**B**) Cross-sectional anatomy of the wrist demonstrating the intrinsic scapholunate (SL) and lunatotriquetral (LT) ligaments and the triangular fibrocartilage (TFC). Full visualization of these structures can be achieved by arthroscopic examination of the wrist. *(A modified from Taleisnik, J. and Kelly, P.J.: The Extraosseous and Intraosseous Blood Supply of the Scaphoid Bone. J. Bone Joint Surg. 48A:1125–1137, 1966.)*

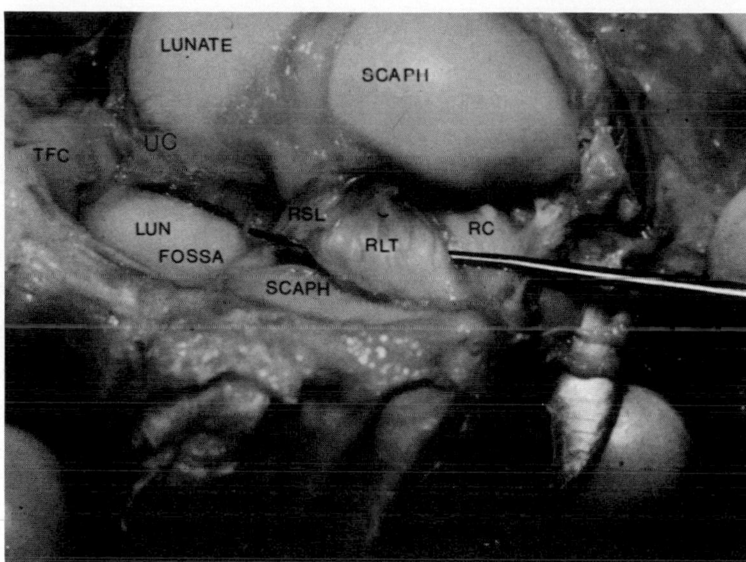

FIGURE 12-6. Intra-articular proximal-to-distal view. Intracapsular ligaments of the wrist include the radiocapitate (RC), radiolunatotriquetral (RLT), radioscapholunate (RSL), and ulnocarpal (UC) ligaments. These ligaments originate from the volar flare of the distal radius (scaphoid and lunate fossae), and insert on the volar aspects of the proximal carpal row. The triangular fibrocartilage (TFC) extends from ulnar aspect of the distal radius and inserts at the base of the ulnar styloid.

carpals. The double chevron shape of the second metacarpal on the trapezoid and the third metacarpal styloid on the capitate provide a rigid central strut for the hand. The capitate and hamate slide slightly on each other with wrist motions. Distally they allow moderate motion for the ulnar two metacarpals to enhance the gripping adaptation for the hand. The interlocking of the fifth metacarpal on the ulnar half of the hamate, along with strong volar carpometacarpal ligaments, provides stability.

The proximal carpal row consists of the lunate and triquetrum and, in an anatomical sense, the entire scaphoid. The scaphoid is, however, uniquely positioned to function mechanically as part of both the distal and carpal rows (see Fig. 12-5**B**).[341] The short intrinsic ligaments that bind these three bones together around their convex proximal surfaces coordinate their mechanical behavior (Fig. 12-6).

Articular Surfaces

The articular surfaces of each of the joints that make up the wrist have important roles in subsequent integrated movements of the wrist.[90,317]The eight carpal bones are influenced by the shape of the distal radius, the distal ulna, and triangular fibrocartilage complex (TFCC). The distal articular surface of the radius is concave and tilted in two planes. In the sagittal plane, there is an average of 14° volar tilt; in the frontal plane, there is an average ulnar inclination of 22°. The TFC is the ulnar continuation of the distal radius and presents a concave surface for articulation with the lunate and triquetrum distally and the head of the ulna proximally. In certain conditions, such as Madelung's deformity or rheumatoid arthritis, the ulnar slope of the radius is accentuated, producing an ulnar shift of the carpus. The variable length of the ulna as a positive or

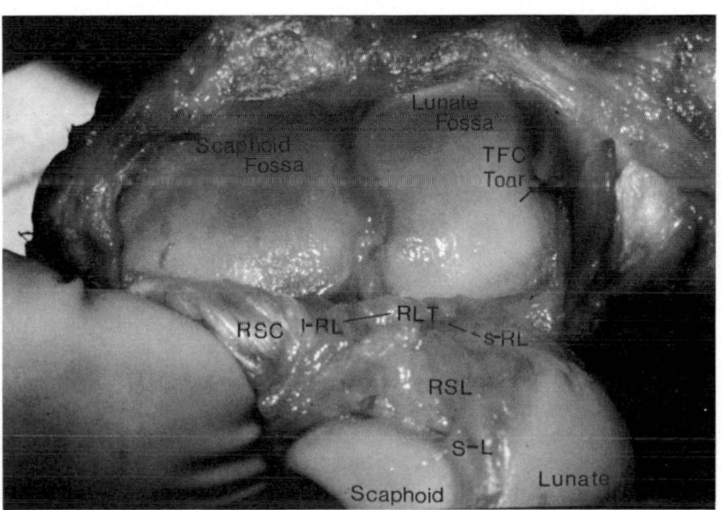

FIGURE 12-7. Intra-articular distal-to-proximal view. The volar radioscapholunate (RSL) and radiolunatotriquetral (RLT) ligaments blend with the volar aspect of the scapholunate (SL) interosseous ligaments (s-RL, short radiolunate and l-RL long radiolunate are subdivisions of the radiolunatotriquetral ligament, RLT).

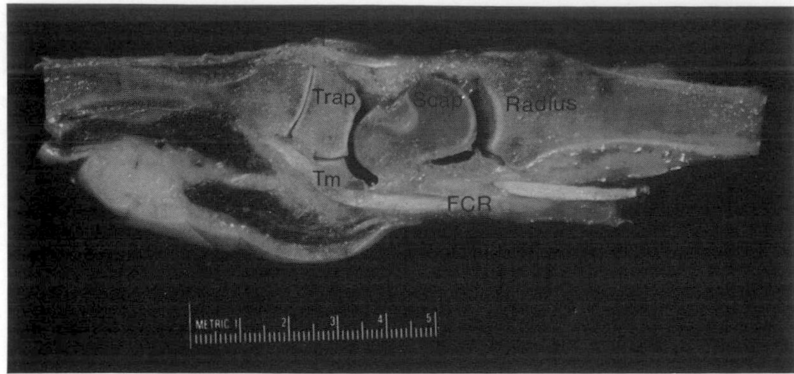

FIGURE 12-8. Sagittal view through the radius, scaphoid, and trapeziotrapezoidal joints. Note joint configuration, the volar ligaments, the bow-stringing of the FCR tendon around the scaphoid tuberosity (Trap, trapezoid; Tz, trapezium; Scap, scaphoid; FCR, flexor carpi radialis).

negative variance may influence the carpal position.[130] When it comes into contact with the proximal carpal row it can force a volar tilt to the lunate and triquetrum (ie, volar intercalated segment instability [VISI] deformity).

The distal radius presents three articular surfaces (scaphoid, lunate fossa and sigmoid notch) for the scaphoid, lunate, and distal ulna, respectively. These joint surfaces are important in judging congruent alignment of the wrist after fractures (Colles' type)[76] and in suggesting ligament injuries (dissociation) (Fig. 12-7).[153] A malalignment of the distal radius with loss of volar tilt can also produce a secondary carpal instability.[19,320,521]

The midcarpal joint has a unique articular surface shape, which, as a whole, resembles an acetabulum centered on the scaphoid and lunate distal articular surfaces. In fact, the midcarpal joint is a combination of three different types of articulation.[118] Laterally, there is a convex distal scaphoid surface articulating with the trapezium and trapezoid (Fig. 12-8). The central part of the midcarpal joint is a concavity of the scaphoid and lunate receiving a convex proximal head of the capitate (Fig. 12-9). Finally, the medial joint of hamate and triquetrum is helicoid, providing for a sliding movement of the hamate on the triquetrum that influences angulation of the proximal row with wrist movements[552] (see Kinematics).

The TFC is the main stabilizer of the DRUJ.[73,290,427,428] It originates from firm attachments on the medial border of the distal radius and inserts into the base and around the tip of the ulnar styloid, separating the ulnar styloid from the radiocarpal joint of the ulnar styloid.[317] It gives origin to the volar ulnocarpal ligaments and blends imperceptibly into the volar and dorsal radioulnar ligaments,[516] giving the appearance of one discrete structure. The cartilage component is thinnest in the central or middle third of the TFC and thickens at the peripheral margins. The TFC blends distally into the ulnar collateral ligament complex (see Fig. 12-9).[424,428] The space between the distal ulna and the TFC is the recessus sacciformis. As a result of phylogenic adaptation of the wrist, a vestigial meniscus of the ulnotriquetral joint merges imperceptibly with the TFC distally.

The wrist is a very congruent structure, with close contact of the articular surfaces during the global motion, combining wrist flexion–extension and radioulnar deviation.[341] Each carpal bone can move three-dimensionally in space, rotating, flexing, or extending as well as deviating in response to various wrist positions.[139,461] Conceptually, it resembles a Rubik cube, in which motion of each component bone will have an effect on adjacent carpal bones.

The wrist must be considered in terms of three-dimensional motion and structure.[171,561] Fractures and dislocations rarely involve only one carpal bone or joint, and radiographic imaging that assists evaluation in three dimensions is needed to understand the pathology that may exist.[394,403]

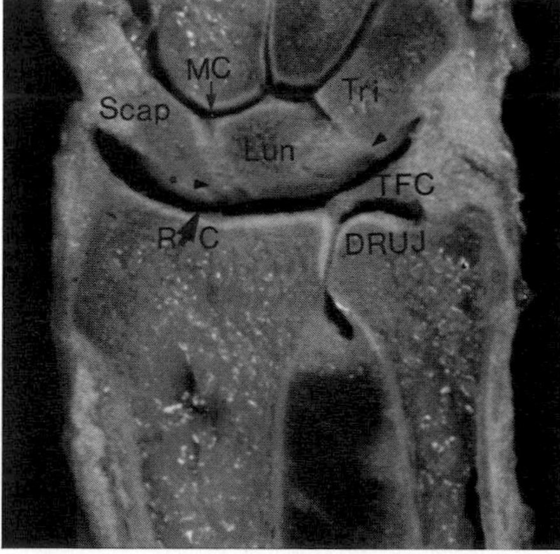

FIGURE 12-9. Cross-section anatomy (coronal view) demonstrates the intra-osseous ligaments (*small arrows*) that imperceptibly blend the scaphoid (SCAP), lunate (LUN) and triquetrum (TRIQ) to each other and separate the radiocarpal joint (RC) from the midcarpal joint (MC). The triangular fibrocartilage (TFC) is an ulnar extension of the articular surface of the distal radius, and separates the radiocarpal from the distal radioulnar joint (DRUJ). It is the main stabilizer of the distal radioulnar joint.

Ligaments of the Wrist

There are two major groups of ligaments of the wrist (Fig. 12-10): extrinsic and intrinsic.[48,357,516] The extrinsic ligaments are those that link the carpal bones to the radius, ulna, and metacarpals. The intrinsic ligaments interconnect individual carpal bones.[48,118,133] The transverse carpal ligament (transverse retinaculum) is an extrinsic ligament of the wrist that connects the scaphoid tuberosity and trapezial ridge with the hamulus and pisiform to provide structural integrity to the proximal carpal arch, as well as to constrain the flexor tendons. It connects medially through the pisiform and hypothenar deep fascia with the dorsal retinaculum,

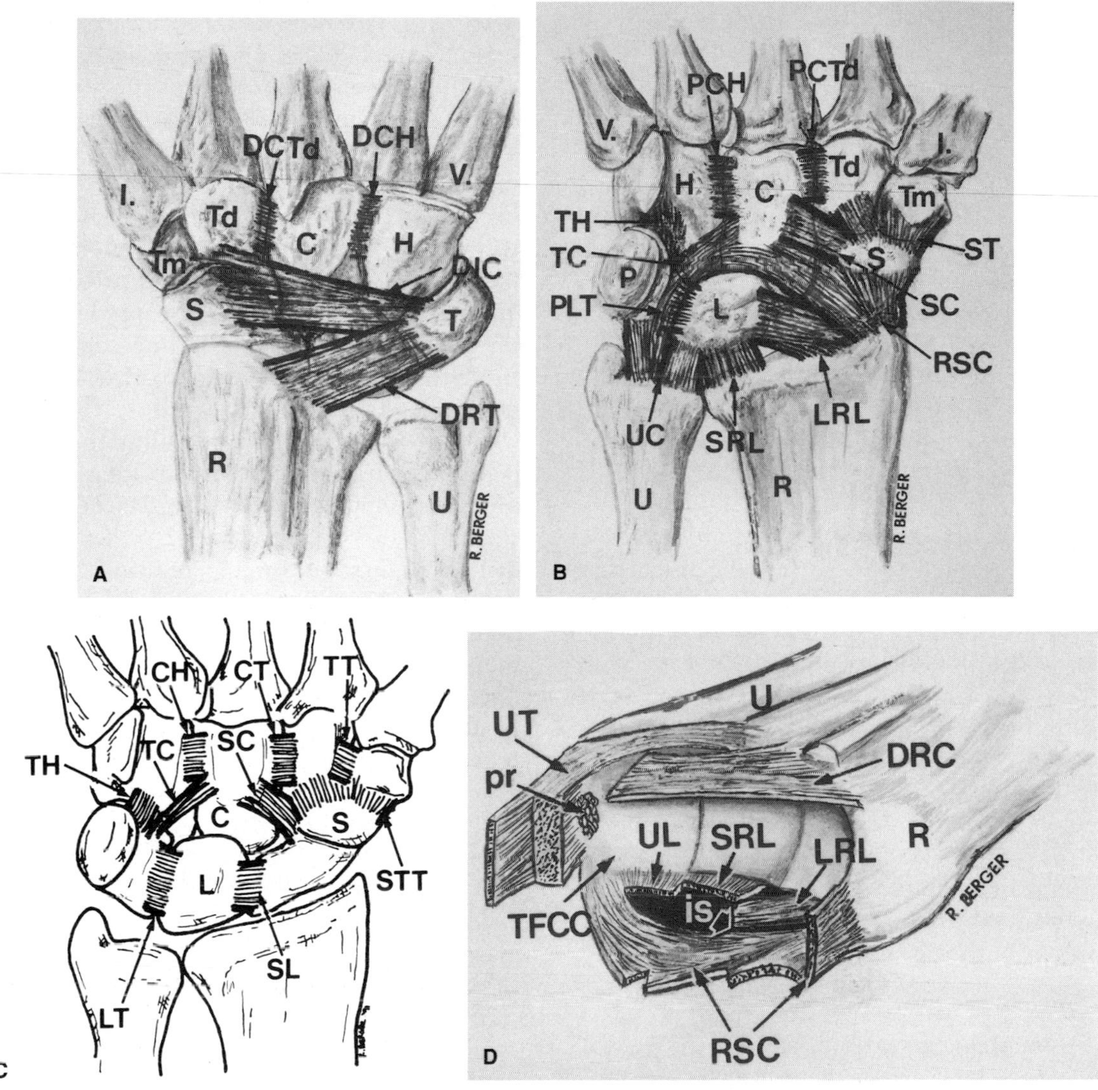

FIGURE 12-10. (**A**) Dorsal extrinsic ligaments of the wrist. dorsal intercarpal ligament (DIC); dorsal radiotriquetral ligament (DRT); trapezium (Tm); trapezoid (Td); capitate (C); hamate (H); scaphoid (S); triquetrum (T). (**B**) Volar extrinsic ligaments of the wrist: scaphotrapezial (ST); radioscaphocapitate (RSC); scaphocapitate (SC); long radiolunate (LRL); short radiolunate (SRL); ulnocarpal (UC); palmar lunatotriquetral (PLT); triquetral-capitate (TC); triquetral-hamate (TH); lunate (L); scaphoid (S); pisiform (P). (**C**) Intrinsic ligaments of the wrist: scapholunate (SL); lunatotriquetral (LT); scaphotrapeziotrapezoidal (STT); scaphocapitate (SC); triquetral capitate (TC); triquetral-hamate (TH); capitohamate (CH); capito-trapezoidal (CT); trapezio-trapezoidal (TT). *C,* capitate; *S,* scaphoid; *L,* lunate. (**D**) Axial view of the wrist with the carpal bones removed (after Berger). *R,* radius; *DRC,* dorsal radiocarpal ligament; *U,* ulna; *UT,* ulnotriquetral ligament; Pr, prestyloid recess; *UL,* ulnolunate ligament; *SRL,* short radiolunate ligament; *IS,* isthmus between palmar carpal ligaments; *LRL,* long radiolunate ligament; *RSR,* radioscaphocapitate ligament. (**E**) Axial view of the wrist with the proximal carpal row reflected palmarly, showing the palmar carpal ligaments: *RSC,* radioscaphocapitate, *LRL,* long radiolunate; *SRL,* short radiolunate ligament; *SF,* scaphoid fossa; *LF,* lunate fossa; *IP,* interfossa prominence; *IS,* isthmus between palmar carpal ligaments; *S,* scaphoid; *L,* lunate; *U,* ulna; *R,* radius.

continues

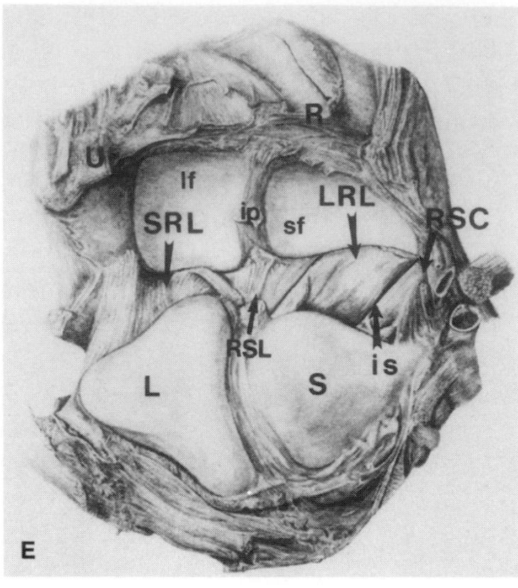

FIGURE 12-10. (continued)

completing a circumferential superficial ligament complex.[518]

Extrinsic Ligaments

The deeper extrinsic ligaments[48,50] are intracapsular ligaments best observed from within the radiocarpal and midcarpal joints. From an external view, the ligaments appear as condensations of fibrous capsule and are difficult to distinguish through the superficial adventitia. They are quite prominent from the intra-articular aspect of the joint (see Fig. 12-7). The volar wrist ligaments originate laterally from a radial-volar facet of the radial styloid and are directed in a distal-ulnar direction, where they meet ligaments originating medially from the TFC and the distal ulna. The stronger and more oblique radial ligaments prevent the carpus from translating ulnarly on the medially angulated slope of the distal radius. The volar extrinsic ligaments consist of two V-shaped ligamentous bands: one is proximal and connects the forearm to the proximal carpal row; one is distal and connects the forearm to the distal carpal row. The distal limb of the volar extrinsic ligaments (the arcuate ligaments) consists of the radioscaphocapitate ligament laterally and the ulnocapitate ligament medially (see Fig. 12-10**B**). The proximal limb consists of the radiolunatotriquetral and radioscaphoid ligaments laterally and the ulnolunate and ulnotriquetral ligaments medially. The radioscaphoid ligament that inserts onto the tuberosity of the scaphoid is the radial expansion of the radiocapitate ligament, which courses over the palmar concavity of the scaphoid proximal to the tuberosity before inserting on the palmar aspect of the keel and neck of the capitate. It forms a fulcrum over which the scaphoid rotates (see Fig. 12-8) and usually does not have ligamentous insertion into the scaphoid itself. The distal portion of the radiocapitate and ulnocapitate ligaments (distal V) do not attach to the head of the capitate but forms a support sling commonly referred to as the arcuate ligament. Between these two rows of ligaments is a thinned area termed the *space of Poirier*.[437] This area expands when the wrist is dorsiflexed and disappears in palmar flexion. A rent develops during dorsal dislocations, and it is through this interval that the lunate displaces into the carpal canal.[355] The radiocapitate ligament is superficial to the radiolunate, and the former slips over the latter in flexion.

The dorsal ligaments of importance are the radiotriquetral and scaphotriquetral (dorsal intercarpal) ligaments, which describe a V-shape from the dorsal aspect of the distal radius near Lister's tubercle to the triquetrum and then back to the dorsal scaphoid rim (see Fig. 12-10**A**).[323,538] The radial capsule is thickened, melding into the radioscaphoid ligament, while the ulnodorsal capsule is augmented by the floors of the fifth and sixth dorsal compartments. There are no true collateral ligaments.

The extrinsic palmar radiolunate ligaments have been subdivided into short and long radiolunate ligaments (see Fig. 12-10**B**). The radioscapholunate ligament of Testut[523] and Kuenz,[304] seen well from the inside of the joint, originates from the palmar aspect of the ridge between the scaphoid and lunate fossae and inserts into the scapholunate interosseous ligament; it acts as a neurovascular supply to the scapholunate interosseous membrane (see Figs. 12-6 and 12-7). Anatomical studies,[50], arthroscopic observation, and mechanical testing demonstrate low tensile force and suggest that the radioscapholunate is not a true extrinsic ligament of the wrist.[68]

The final group of extrinsic ligaments support the midcarpal joint and couple the distal carpal bones to each other. On the radial side of the wrist, a V-shaped scaphotrapezial ligament extends from the scaphoid tuberosity to the volar tubercle of the trapezium. Adjacent to it medially are the scaphocapitate and palmar capitotrapezial ligaments and the capitotrapezoidal ligament. On the ulnar side of the wrist, the triquetrocapitate and triquetrohamate ligaments are a continuation of the ulnotriquetral ligament.[10]

Intrinsic Ligaments

The intra-articular intrinsic ligaments of the wrist connect adjacent carpal bones.[329,357,516] They are collections of relatively short fibers that bind the bones of either the proximal or distal carpal rows to each other (see Figs. 12-7 and 12-9).

In the proximal carpal row, the ligaments are intra-articular, connecting the scaphoid to the lunate and the lunate to the triquetrum. There is a contiguous blending of the interosseous ligaments with the joint articular cartilage. Laterally, the strong scapholunate interosseous ligament has been shown to consist of three components: volar, central, and dorsal. The scapholunate ligament follows the proximal edge of the two bones to the dorsal surface, where there is a thickened collection of fibers that describe a scapholunate ligament.[333,357,460] This has an important role in carpal stability.[460] The longer fibers of the palmar portion of the scapholunate interosseous membrane allow the scaphoid flexibility as it rotates on the lunate. The dorsal third of the ligament is the strongest, while the volar ligament has more laxity. The central third appears to be cartilaginous, blending with the adjacent cartilage of scaphoid and lunate.

The lunatotriquetral interosseous membrane[449,539,540] is similarly formed by stout transverse fibers connecting the proximal edges of triquetrum and lunate. It interdigitates with the dorsal radiotriquetral ligament and palmar ulnotriquetral, ulnolunate, and radiolunatotriquetral insertions. The volar third of the lunatotriquetral ligament is stronger than the dorsal third, supported by strong volar ulnocarpal ligaments. Its fibers are more taut, making for a closer lunatotriquetral than scapholunate kinematic relationship. The disposition of these ligaments and their strengths are of considerable importance in the kinematics of the joint and the mechanisms of injury.[333,356]

Neurovascular Supply

The innervation and blood supply of the wrist come from the regional nerves and vessels.[429] The nerves include the main trunk of the ulnar nerve, running deep to the flexor carpi ulnaris tendon and into Guyon's canal; the main trunk of the median nerve, running between and deep to the flexor carpi radialis and the palmaris longus into the carpal tunnel; the anterior interosseous branch of the median nerve, lying on the interosseous membrane between the ulna and the radius; the posterior interosseous branch of the radial nerve, lying on the posterior surface of the radioulnar interosseous membrane; the superficial sensory branch of the radial nerve, emerging dorsally from beneath the brachioradialis tendon about 5 cm proximal to the radial styloid; and the dorsal cutaneous branch of the ulnar nerve, which branches from the main ulnar trunk and lies subcutaneously across the ulnocarpal sulcus. The palmar cutaneous branch of the median nerve arises from its main trunk, about 4 cm proximal to the wrist crease. These subsidiary branches to the median, ulnar, and radial nerves are readily damaged by lacerations, incisions, and contusions. They are easily visualized just deep to the superficial veins and should be protected. The potential for a neuralgic pain syndrome is common to all of them.

Circulation of the wrist is obtained through the radial, ulnar, and anterior interosseous arteries and the deep palmar arch (Fig. 12-11). The extraosseous arterial pattern is formed by an anastomotic network of three dorsal and three palmar arches connected longitudinally at their medial and lateral borders by the radial and ulnar arteries.[216,217] The dorsal interosseous does not make a substantial contribution (see Fig. 12-11**A**). In addition to transverse and longitudinal anastomoses, there are dorsal to volar interconnections between the dorsal and volar branches of the anterior interosseous artery (Fig. 12-11**B**).

The palmar transverse arches are the radiocarpal, intercarpal, and deep palmar arch (Fig. 12-11**C**). Two recurrent vessels, one radial and one ulnar, traverse proximally to frequently anastomose with the terminal branches of the anterior division of the anterior interosseous artery. The radiocarpal arch provides the predominant blood supply to the palmar surface of the lunate and triquetrum. The radial and ulnar recurrent arteries supply the distal carpal row. With such a broad collateral circulation present at the wrist, it is rare that damage to one aspect of this extrinsic circulation has a significant effect on the blood supply of the wrist.

The intrinsic blood supply to the carpal bones is an important factor in the incidence of avascular necrosis after trauma.[214,519] Latex injection techniques demonstrate three patterns of intraosseous vascularization. The bones in the first group, scaphoid,[440] capitate (see Fig. 12-11**D** and **E**),[410] and about 20% of lunate (see Fig. 12-11**C**), are supplied by a single vessel and thus are at risk for avascular necrosis. The trapezium, triquetrum, pisiform, and 80% of the lunate receive nutrient arteries through two nonarticular surfaces and have consistent intraosseous anastomoses with a resultant rare occurrence of avascular necrosis. The trapezoid and hamate lack an intraosseous anastomosis and, after fracture, can have avascular fragments.[216] These observations extend previous work, which showed that the blood supply to most carpal bones enters the distal half, leaving the proximal half at risk. There is no interval, for example, by which the scaphoid can be approached without endangering some of the branches that supply its circulation.[71] With proximal scaphoid fracture the danger of devascularizing the proximal fragment exists. It is important to identify and protect the dorsal and volar radial artery branches to the scaphoid. The lunate blood supply[213] is constantly endangered by common dorsal approaches to the wrist, but the blood supply from the palmar radiocarpal arch is usually sufficient. With fracture–dislocations of the wrist the palmar radiolunate ligament usu-

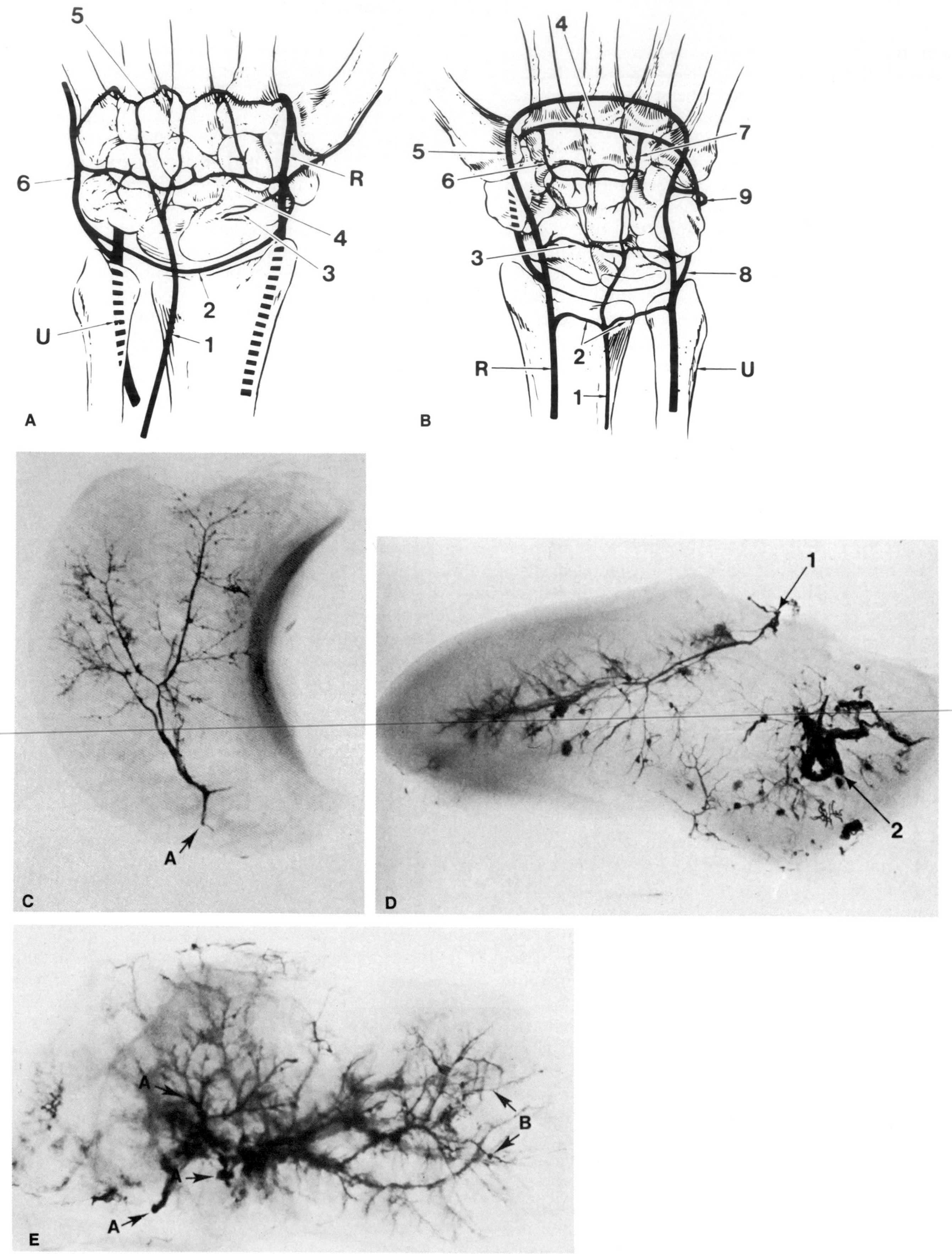

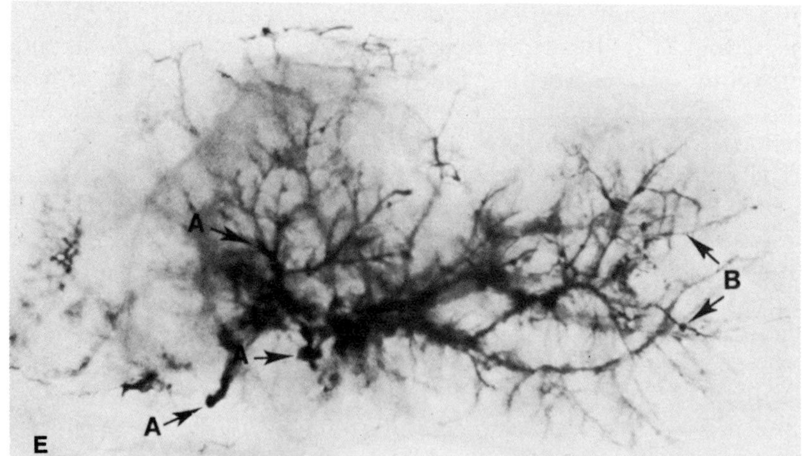

FIGURE 12-11.

ally remains intact, because the dislocation is distal through the space of Poirier.

MECHANISMS OF INJURY

The most common mechanism of injury (Fig. 12-12) to the wrist is an axial compressive force applied with the wrist in hyperextension, in which the palmar ligaments are placed under tension and the dorsal joint surfaces are compressed and subject to shear stresses, especially if the wrist is extended beyond its physiologic limits.[327,328,356,487,542] Depending on the degree of radial or ulnar deviation, a ligament or bone injury or a combination of both will result. The amount of energy absorbed, the direction of the applied force, its point of application, and the strength of the bone and ligaments all have a distinct bearing on the pathology and severity of injury (Fig. 12-13).[165,186,367] For example, a scaphoid fracture appears to occur when the wrist is dorsiflexed past 97° and radially deviated 10°.[553] In this position, the proximal pole of the scaphoid is held viselike by the radius and the proximal radioscaphocapitate ligament, while the distal pole of the bone is carried dorsally by the trapeziocapitate complex. The lunate is unloaded. The radioscaphoid ligament is relaxed by the radial deviation and cannot alleviate the tensile stresses accumulating on the radiopalmar aspect of the scaphoid. The tensile fracture then propagates dorsally. The fracture can be transverse, oblique, or comminuted depending on the direction of the applied loads (Fig. 12-14).[553]

Common injuries include a fall from a height, a sports-related collision, or a motor vehicle accident. The injured individual straightens the arm for protection, and the body weight and exterior force are concentrated across the wrist. Other mechanisms include palmar flexion, as occurs in an over-the-handlebars motorcycle accident or twisting injuries in sports where the hand is forcefully rotated against the stationary body. With similar loads, an athlete may suffer no significant injury, while the immature individual sustains a physeal separation and the elderly person suffers a comminuted and displaced distal radius fracture.

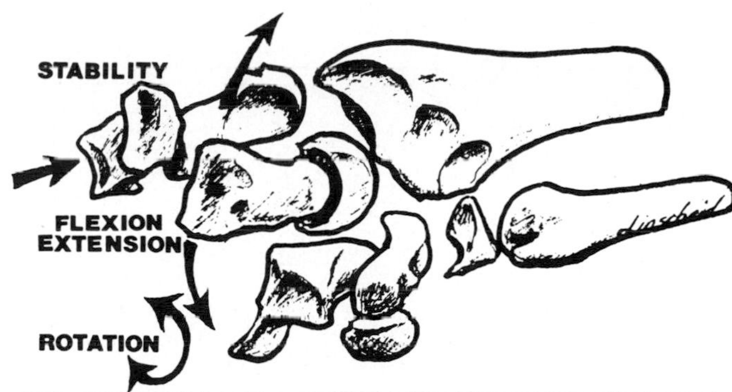

FIGURE 12-12. Perilunar dislocation of the wrist occurs in hyperextension. Disruption occurs at the scapholunate area and progresses into the space of Poirier and then through the lunatotriquetral space. At times, the sequence of injury may be reversed, depending on the orientation at impact. *Forme frustes* are responsible for scapholunate or lunatotriquetral dissociations and a variety of wrist sprains.

Mayfield, Kilcoyne, and Johnson[355,356,272] independently have pointed out that many injuries of the wrist appear to be sequential variants of perilunate dislocations (Fig. 12-15). Minor injuries such as sprains (stretch or partial tears of carpal ligaments) result from low-energy forces. Ligament tears involve more substantial force to the hand, as when the capitate forcibly separates the scaphoid and lunate interval, tearing the interosseous ligament. Higher energy forces result in carpal bone fractures or ligamentous disruptions of both intrinsic and extrinsic ligaments or, in the most severe injury, fracture–dislocations or perilunate dislocations of the wrist. The majority of these injuries occur around the lunate, which as the "carpal keystone" is held most securely to the distal radius. As such, perilunate and lunate dislocations involve the greatest expenditure of force during wrist injuries.

FIGURE 12-11. (**A**) Schematic drawing of the arterial supply of the dorsum of the wrist. *R*, radial artery; *U*, ulnar artery; *1*, dorsal branch, anterior interosseous artery; *2*, dorsal radiocarpal arch; *3*, branch to the dorsal ridge of the scaphoid; *4*, dorsal intercarpal arch; *5*, basal metacarpal arch; *6*, medial branch of the ulnar artery. (**B**) Schematic drawing of the arterial supply of the palmar aspect of the wrist. *R*, radial artery; *U*, ulnar artery; *1*, palmar branch, anterior interosseous artery; *2*, palmar radiocarpal arch; *3*, palmar intercarpal arch; *4*, deep palmar arch; *5*, superficial palmar arch; *6*, radial recurrent artery; *7*, ulnar recurrent artery; *8*, medial branch, ulnar artery; *9*, branch off ulnar artery contributing to the dorsal intercarpal arch. (**C**) Lunate. Lateral view, showing a single large vessel entering the palmar surface and branching within the bone to provide the sole blood supply. This pattern was seen in 20% of the specimens. (**D**) Photograph of a specimen showing the internal vascularity of the scaphoid (*1*, dorsal branch of the radial artery; *2*, volar scaphoid branch.) (**E**) Capitate. Dorsal view, following clearing by Spalteholz technique. Nutrient vessels enter the distal third (A), with retrograde course towards the proximal articular surface and (B), terminal vessels enter into the head of the capitate. (***A,B:*** *Gelberman, R.H.; Panagis, J.S.; Taleisnik, J.; Baumgaertner, M.: The Arterial Anatomy of the Human Carpus. I: The Extraosseous Vascularity. J. Hand Surg., 8(4):367–375, 1983.* ***C,E:*** *Gelberman, R.H.; Panagis, J.S.; Taleisnik, J.; Baumgaertner, M.: The Arterial Anatomy of the Human Carpus. II: The Intraosseous Vascularity. J. Hand Surg., 8(4):375–382, 1983.* ***D:*** *Gelberman, R.H.; Menon, J.: The Vascularity of the Scaphoid Bone. J. Hand Surg., 5(5):508–513, 1980.)*

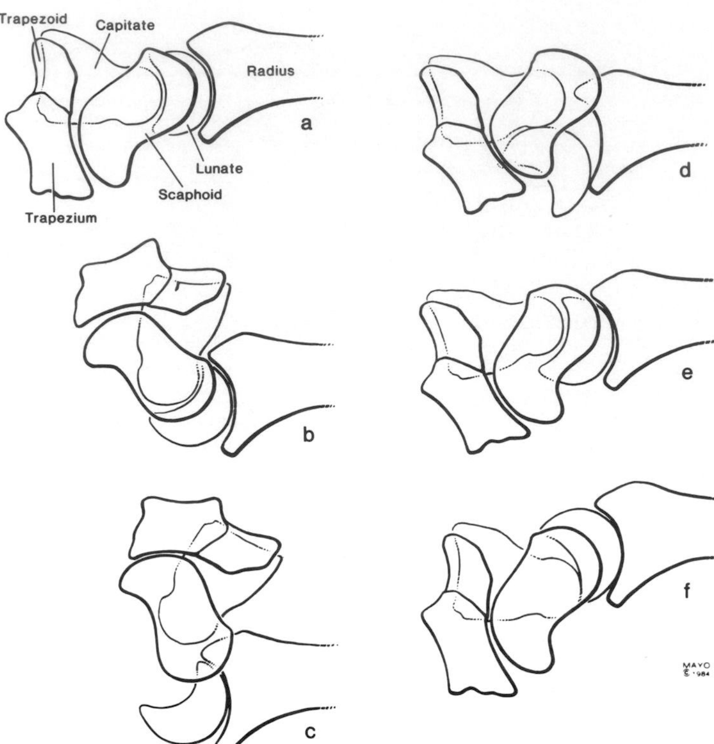

FIGURE 12-13. Perilunar dislocation progresses from the neutral position *a,* to extension *b,* to displacement dorsally *c.* As the dislocation rebounds, the carpus may partially displace and flex the lunate. Scapholunate dissociation may develop, or with more extensive ligamentous damage, the carpus may settle into a volar dislocation (*d*). This implies more disruption of the ulnar aspect of the proximal row.

After ligamentous injury, use of the hand potentiates carpal instability, because normal activities generate joint compressive forces that are transmitted across the carpus to the distal radius and to the restraining ligaments.

From the proximal carpal row, the compression loads are transmitted across the radiocarpal joint and, to a lesser degree, across the TFC to the distal ulna.[165] In the normal setting the force distribution is 80/20, with the distal radius accepting the larger load. With the wrist in a neutral position, the loaded carpus will tend to slide down the palmar and ulnarly inclined articular surface of the distal radius. The extrinsic radiocarpal ligaments resist this ulnar translation to maintain carpal alignment and stability.

Compressive loads across the TFC are accepted by the head of the distal ulna, depending on the relative length of the ulna with respect to the articular surface of the distal radius (positive or negative ulnar variance).[544] Redistribution of forces in the forearm are influenced by rotation, ulnar variance, and integrity of the muscles and interosseous membrane.

KINEMATICS

The global motion of the wrist is composed of flexion, extension, and radioulnar deviation (see Fig. 12-1) at the radiocarpal joint, and axial rotation around the DRUJ.[323,341,471] The radiocarpal articulation acts as a universal joint, allowing a small degree of intercarpal motion around the longitudinal axis related to the rotation of individual carpal bones.[307] The forearm accounts for the most rotation (about 140°) and supplies the hand with the strength necessary to apply vigorous torque. Radiocarpal joint motion is primarily flexion–extension of nearly equal proportions (70° each), and radial and ulnar deviation of 20° and 40°, respectively.[86] This amount of motion is possible as a result of complex arrangements between the two carpal rows.[25,171] The wrist motors are attached to the metacarpal bases, but because the carpometacarpal joints are rather rigid, angular deflection is readily transmitted to the distal carpal row and then to the proximal carpal row. The latter, an intercalated segment of connected bones without tendon or muscle attachments,[309,484] is pushed back and forth in response to forces applied distally from the hand. Its stability is dependent on the complex ligament structure described previously and the contours of the articular surfaces. During flexion and extension, each carpal row angulates in the same direction with nearly equal amplitude and in a synchronous fashion (Fig. 12-16).[139,171,560,561] During radioulnar deviation, however, the proximal row exhibits a secondary angulation in the sagittal plane to the synchronous motion occurring in the coronal plane. Radial deviation induces flexion of the obliquely situated scaphoid as the

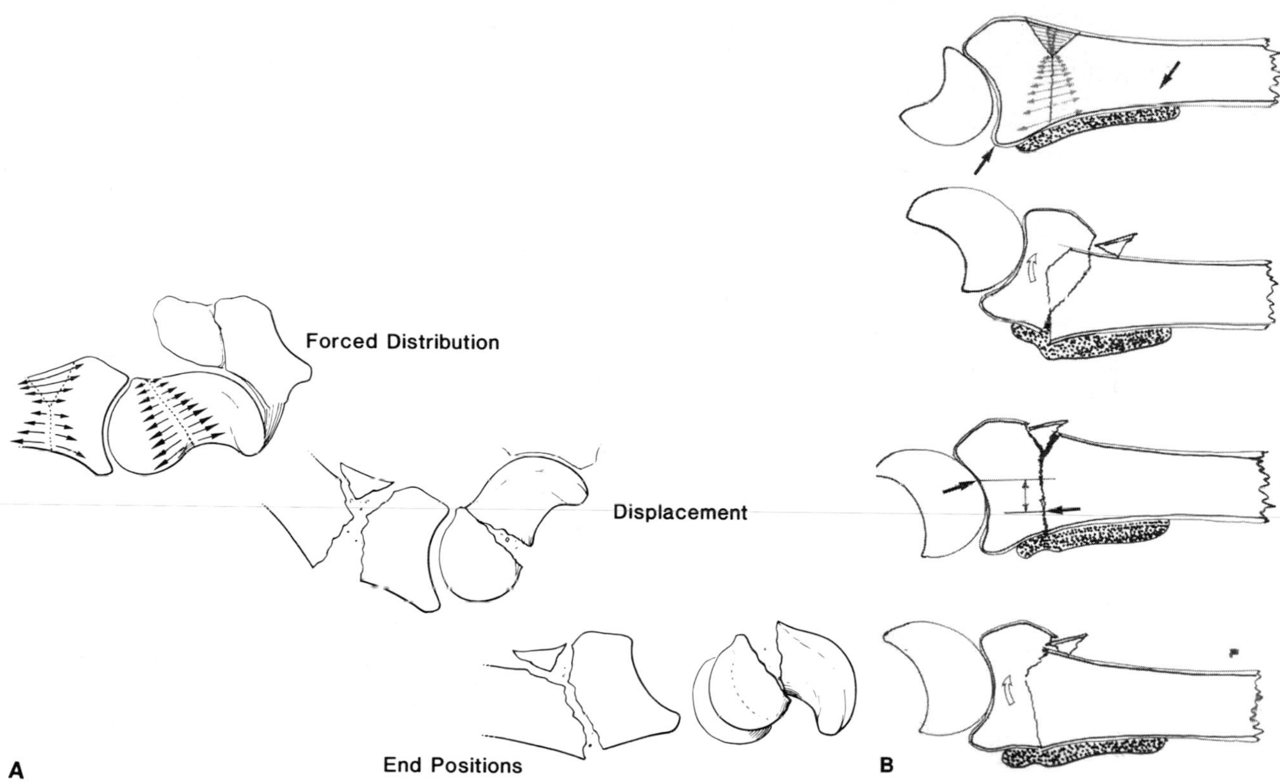

FIGURE 12-14. (**A**) Pathomechanics of scaphoid and distal radius fractures. A radial fracture occurs because of excessive tensile forces on the palmar cortex. Near the dorsal cortex these forces become compressive, and the fracture propagates through shear stresses at 45° angles to produce dorsal comminution. The scaphoid fracture also occurs in tension volarly, but propagation continues in tension through the dorsal cortex, in most instances due to the decompressing effect of the midcarpal joint. (**B**) Fractures of the distal radius. A forced directed 40°–90° to the horizontal produces tension palmarly and compression dorsally (*top*). The fracture occurs with dorsal displacement, dorsal angulation and loss of radial length; comminution and butterfly fragments occur dorsally (*second from top*). Reduction occurs around the stable palmar cortex, which must compensate against the lunate force (large arrow) that will tend to cause recurrence of dorsal angulation about a palmar fulcrum (large arrow at right; moment arm between lighter double arrow) (*second from bottom*). Loss of reduction with dorsal angulation and shortening if lunate compressive forces (forces from hand and forearm muscles) are not counter-acted by a cast or external fixation neutralization (*bottom*).

trapezium approaches the radius. Through the dorsal aspect of the scapholunate ligament, this motion is transmitted sequentially to the lunate and triquetrum, which flex approximately 25°.[323,333,341,461] As the carpus moves back to neutral and onto full ulnar deviation, the proximal row extends and supinates with respect to the radius. The scaphoid can be observed to extend with ulnar deviation, but it is the proximal migration of the hamate that forces the triquetrum to displace volarly and extend, bringing the lunate with it. This conjunct rotation by varying the length and contour of the proximal carpal row allows for extensive excursion of the wrist while maintaining stability around a longitudinal axis.[323,407] This facility has been described as the "variable geometry" of the proximal carpal row.[281]

When this mechanism is disrupted by fracture or ligamentous injury, the wrist becomes destabilized.[89,329] The usual arcs of motion are no longer synchronous, and the intercarpal contact patterns change. A snap, catch, or clunk can be appreciated with motion of the wrist, particularly when under a compressive load. Instability leads, in time, to degenerative changes as a consequence of increased local shear forces and abnormal contact across radiocarpal and midcarpal joints. The concept of advancing arthritic collapse particularly after scapholunate dissociation (SLD) and scaphoid fracture has now been clearly delineated. Similar degenerative changes occur on the ulnar side of the wrist between the lunate, triquetrum, and distal ulna—the so-called ulnocarpal impaction syndrome.

Normally, in the coronal plane, the center of rotation of the wrist is located within a small area in the capitate neck (see Fig. 12-2). A line drawn through the axis of rotation parallel with the anatomical axis of the forearm will, with the hand in a neutral position, pass through the head and base of the third metacarpal, the capitate, the radial aspect of the lunate, and

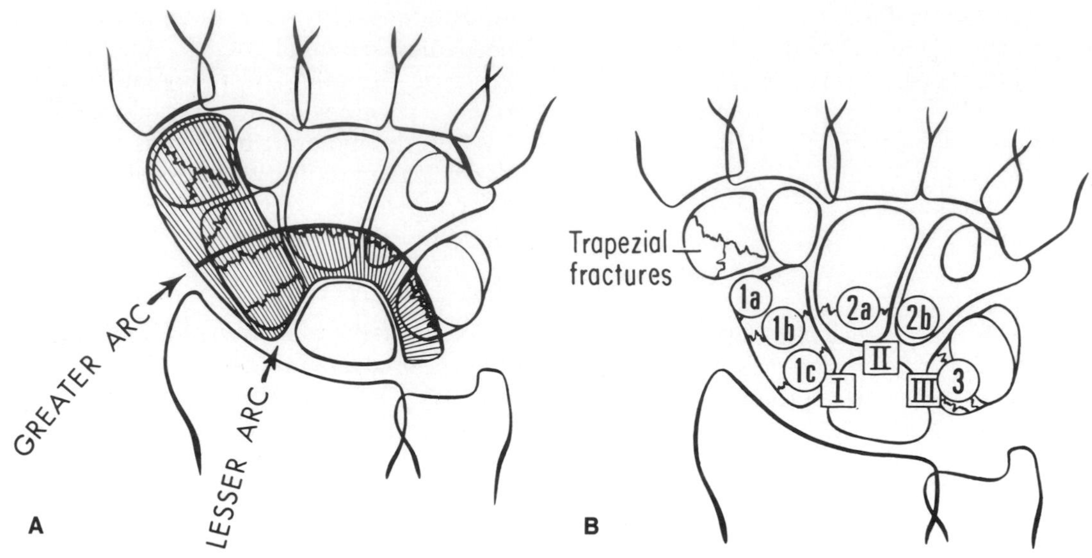

FIGURE 12-15. Vulnerable zones of the carpus. (**A**) A *lesser arc injury* follows a curved path through the radial styloid, midcarpal joint, and lunatotriquetral space. A *greater arc injury* passes through the scaphoid, capitate, and triquetrum. (**B**) Lesser and greater arc injuries can be considered as three stages of perilunate fracture or ligament instabilities. (*Johnson, R.P.: The Acutely Injured Wrist and Its Residuals. Clin. Orthop., 149:33–44, 1980.*[272])

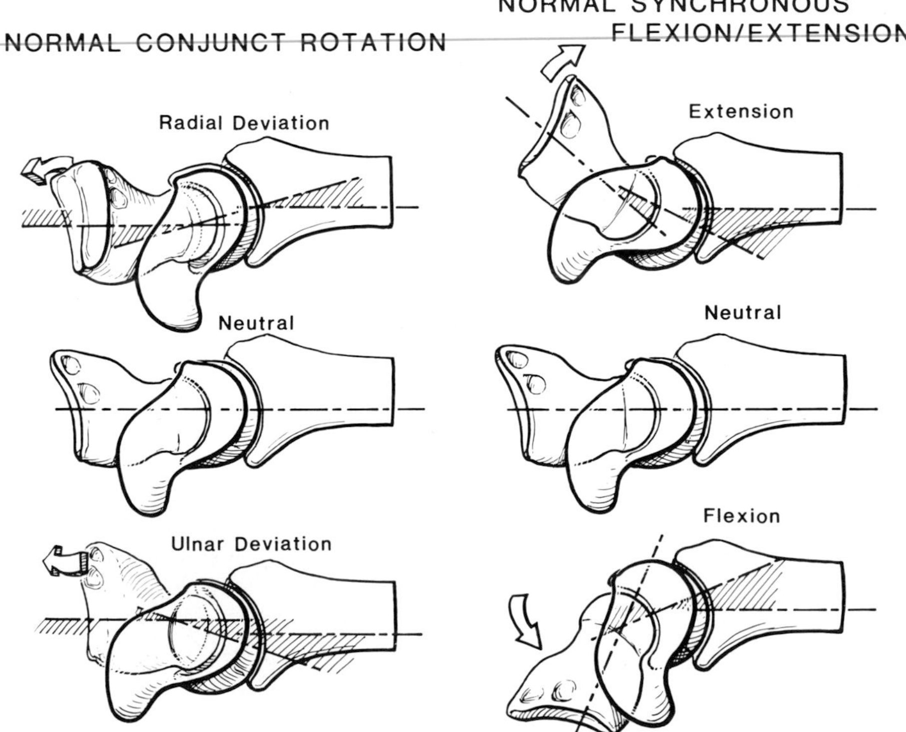

FIGURE 12-16. Conjunct rotation of the entire proximal carpal row occurs in flexion during radial deviation (*upper left*). The axes of the radius and carpal rows are colinear in neutral (*middle left*), and the proximal row extends with ulnar deviation (*lower left*). Angulatory excursions of the proximal and distal rows are essentially equal in amplitude and direction during flexion (*lower right*) and extension (*upper right*). This may be described as synchronous angulation.

the center of the lunate fossa of the radius.[361] The muscle forces in this plane are nearly equally distributed to either side (see Fig. 12-3).

In the sagittal plane with the wrist in neutral flexion–extension, a line passing through the longitudinal axis of the capitate, lunate, and radius will show these to be nearly superimposed or co-linear (Fig. 12-17). The scaphoid axis lies 45° to the above line and passes between the lunate and capitate in a fashion that provides optimal stability to the midcarpal joint. The scaphoid acts as a stabilizing strut or column to support the inherently unstable central column.[329,402] By virtue of its obliquity, the scaphoid will flex when under compressive load and exerts a similar force on the lunate. The lunate, however, is also under the influence of the triquetrum, which inherently prefers to extend. For this reason, the lunate may be thought of as being in a state of dynamic balance between two antagonists when allowed to do so, for example, after ligament injury or fracture of the scaphoid and triquetrum. It tends to lie in the position of least mechanical potential energy (Fig. 12-18**A**). What we recognize clinically and radiographically as DISI and VISI are positions of carpal instability.

When the dynamic balance is interrupted, the lunate will tend to flex with loss of ulnar support from the triquetrum (see Fig. 12-18**C**). It will extend when the situation is reversed by loss of radial stability (see Fig. 12-18**B**).[460] When the lunate slips into a statically fixed position, arbitrarily considered as greater than 15° of flexion or 10° of extension, conditions defined as volar intercalated segment instability (VISI) or dorsal intercalated segment instability (DISI), respectively, are present (Fig. 12-19).[309] The relative alignment of the scaphoid to the lunate, which approximates 45°, is also important. When this exceeds 70°, the ligamentous linkage between the scaphoid and lunate is usually inoperative. The lunate then generally adopts an extended position (ie, DISI) and maintains this position even during

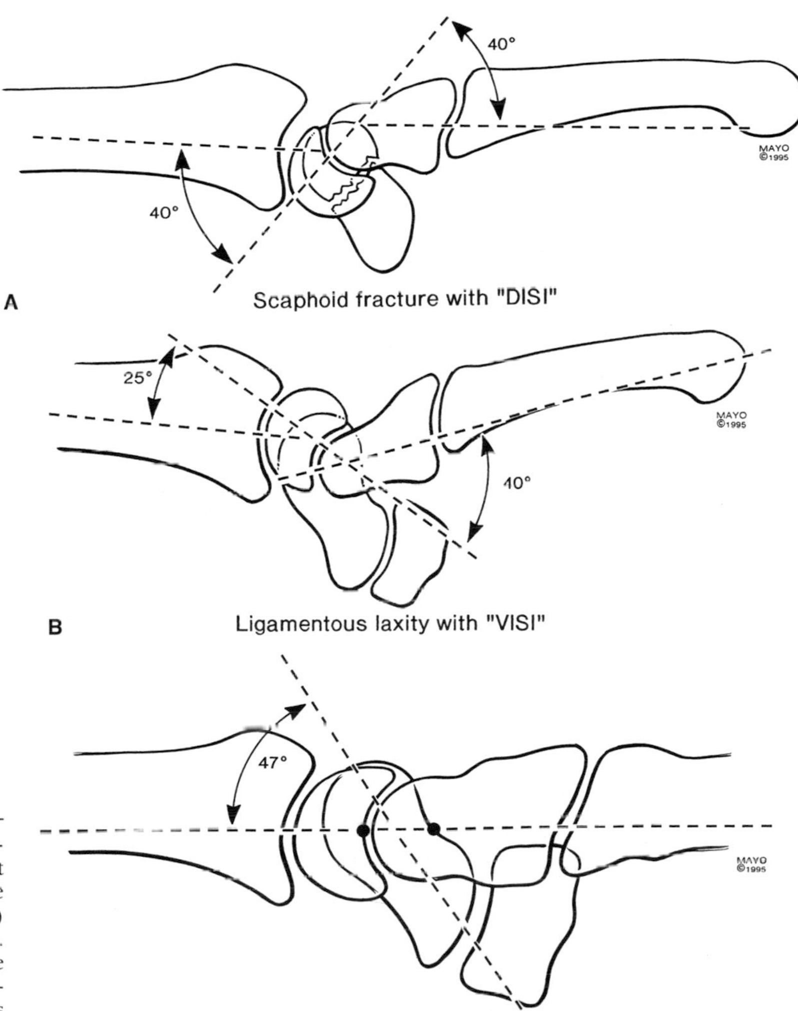

FIGURE 12-17. Diagramatic representation of carpal instability. (**A**) DISI deformity—dorsal intercalated segment instability. DISI deformity is associated with scapholunate ligament disruption or a displaced scaphoid fracture. (**B**) VISI deformity—volar intercalated segment instability. VISI deformity is usually associated with disruption of the lunatotriquetral ligament complex. (**C**) Normal longitudinal alignment of the carpal bones with the scaphoid axis at a 47° angle to the axes of the capitate, lunate, and radius.

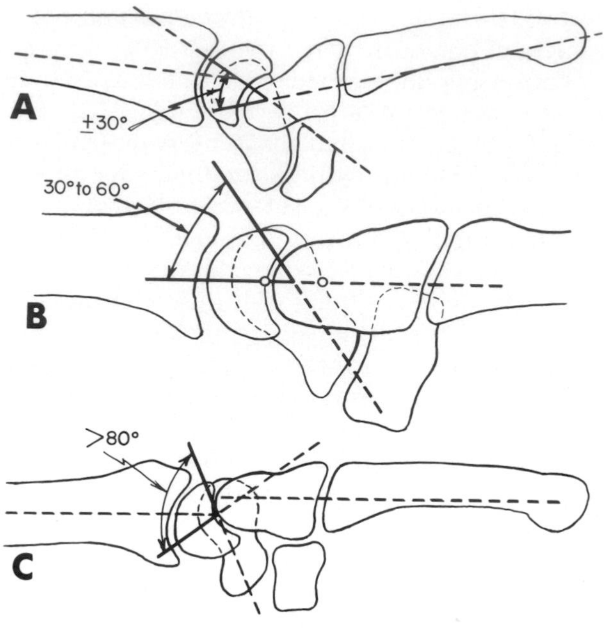

FIGURE 12-18. (**A**) Abnormal palmar flexion of the lunate and scaphoid with ± 30° volar tilt, diagnostic of a VISI deformity. (**B**) Normal carpal alignment with lunate and capitate colinear and scaphoid angled 45° (normal, 30°–60°), ± 15° to the sagittal plane of forearm. (**C**) Abnormal dorsiflexion of the lunate with a vertical scaphoid; scapholunate angle >80° (normal, 45°–60°), typical DISI deformity.

radial deviation, thus interrupting the normal conjunct rotation and the spatial adaptability of the proximal row. The same is true when the lunate is fixed in flexion whereas the lunate and triquetrum are no longer linked and a VISI deformity results such that the wrist will not extend even during ulnar deviation (see Radiographic Examination).

The proximal carpal row is also variably unstable in the coronal plane owing to the obliquity of the radial articular surface to the plane perpendicular to the longitudinal axis. Joint compressive forces lead the proximal row to slide ulnarly down this inclined plane (Fig. 12-20). This is resisted primarily by the extrinsic palmar radiocarpal ligaments, which run from the radial styloid to the capitate and lunate, and, to a lesser extent, by the concavity produced by the TFC and underlying ulnar head. Injuries to these structures may allow a partial or complete ulnar translation of the proximal row (see Carpal Instabilities).[323]

Architecturally, the carpus consists of transverse and longitudinal arches of the hand that provide structural integrity to withstand extrinsically applied stresses. The faceted, interlocking, rigid second and third carpometacarpal joints provide the primary support for the longitudinal arch, while the flattened surfaces of the distal carpal bones supported by short stout intercarpal

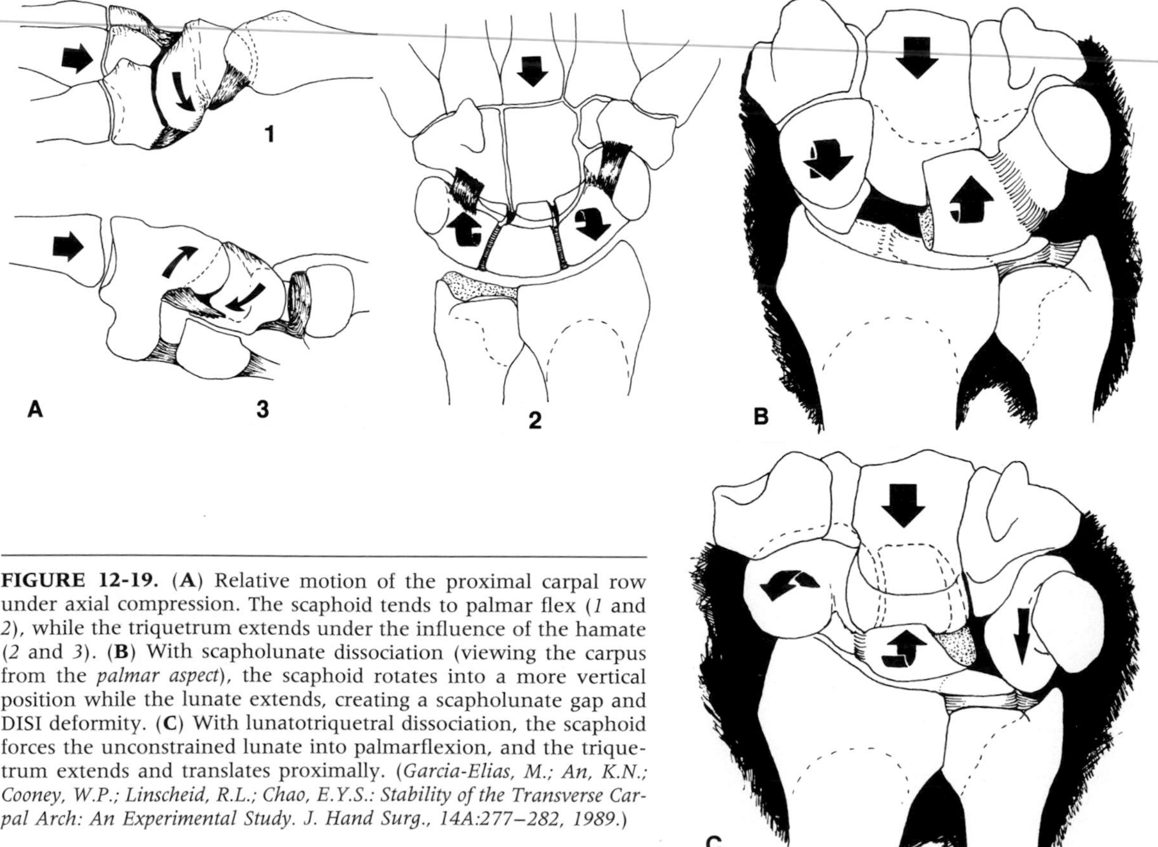

FIGURE 12-19. (**A**) Relative motion of the proximal carpal row under axial compression. The scaphoid tends to palmar flex (*1* and *2*), while the triquetrum extends under the influence of the hamate (*2* and *3*). (**B**) With scapholunate dissociation (viewing the carpus from the *palmar aspect*), the scaphoid rotates into a more vertical position while the lunate extends, creating a scapholunate gap and DISI deformity. (**C**) With lunatotriquetral dissociation, the scaphoid forces the unconstrained lunate into palmarflexion, and the triquetrum extends and translates proximally. (*Garcia-Elias, M.; An, K.N.; Cooney, W.P.; Linscheid, R.L.; Chao, E.Y.S.: Stability of the Transverse Carpal Arch: An Experimental Study. J. Hand Surg., 14A:277–282, 1989.*)

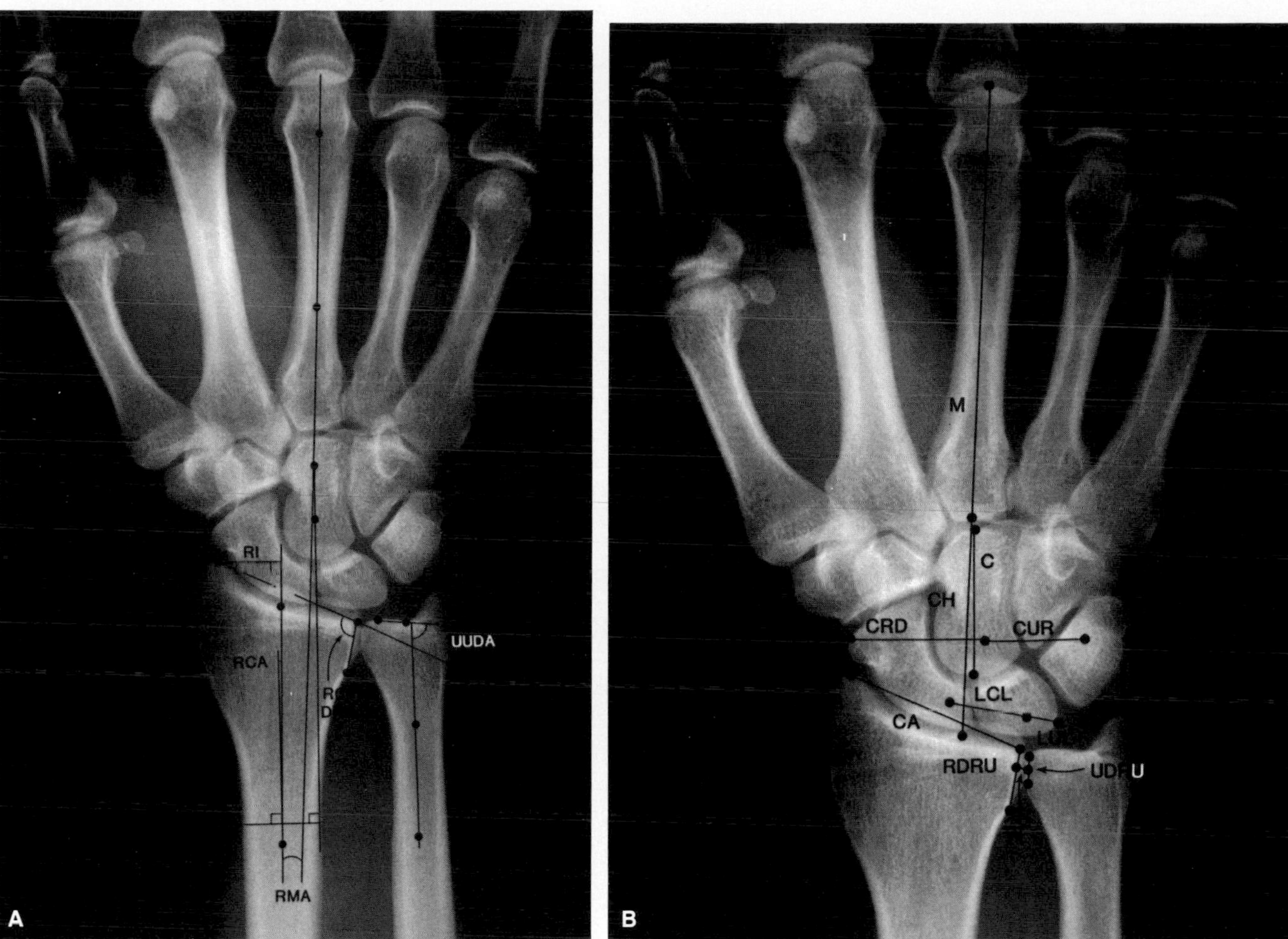

FIGURE 12-20. X-ray mapping of the distal radius and ulna. (**A**) Angular measurements of the distal radius and ulna. *RCA,* radiocapitate angle (N = 1° ± 8°); *RI,* radial inclination (N = 24° ± 2.5°); *RCJ-DRUJ,* angle of the radiocarpal joint to the radial margin of the distal radioulnar joint (N = 108 ± 6°); *UUDA,* angle of main axis of ulna to the dome of the ulna (N = 90° ± 8.1°). (**B**) Mean length of the articular surface of distal radius and ulna. *CRD,* carpal radial distance (N = 20.1 mm ± 1.4) (center of capitate to radial styloid); *CUR,* carpal ulnar distance (N = 18.5 mm ± 3.5) (center of capitate to center of ulnar shaft and base of ulnar styloid), N = 17.1 ± 3.3; *CH,* carpal height (distal capitate to distal radius articular surface) N = 35.6 mm ± 12.4, carpal height ratio (%) 54.3 ± 3.9; *CA,* cord of the arc of the radiocarpal joint, N = 30.9 mm ± 1.7; *RDRU,* length of the radial part of the distal radioulnar joint (sigmoid notch), N = 8.0 mm ± 1.5; *UDRU,* length of the ulnar part of the distal radioulnar joint, N = 6.7 mm ± 1.0; *CUR,* length capitate to axis ulna (carpal-ulnar ratio index CUR/M % = 27.1 ± 15); *LCL,* covered length of the lunate (by the radius); *LUL,* uncovered length of lunate (contact with triangular fibrocartilage), N = 6.1 mm ± 2.5; *W,* width distal radioulnar joint (N = 1.7 mm ± 0.5).

ligaments do the same for the proximal transverse arch.[278] Even these structures can relent to applied forces, which may weaken or disrupt the support arches of the hand and wrist (see section on axial collapse patterns).

IMAGING OF THE WRIST

Radiographic Examination

With rare exceptions such as isolated soft-tissue injury or tenosynovitis, imaging is an absolute requirement in the diagnosis of injury or disease involving the wrist.[153,222,223,299,325,329,474,514] The two most important views are the posteroanterior (PA) and the lateral, each taken in an exact neutral position (Fig. 12-21). To these two views, we often add so-called motion views of maximal radial deviation and maximal ulnar deviation and lateral views in maximal flexion and maximal extension. These six views are adequate in more than 90% of cases in diagnosing fractures and dislocations in this area. The shifting of the carpal bones in the various positions changes the overlap pattern sufficiently so that most fracture lines can be seen readily on one or more of the views. When there is still suspicion of an occult fracture,

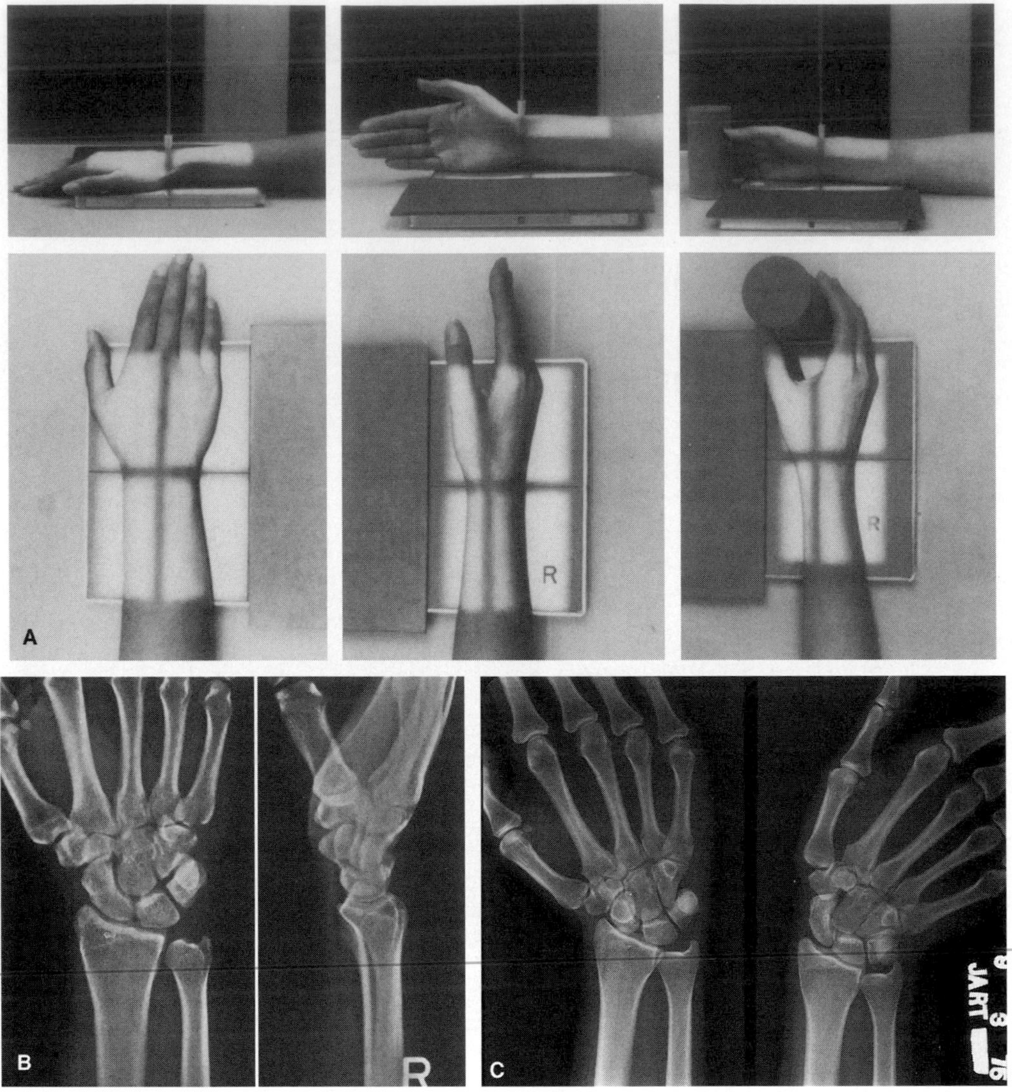

FIGURE 12-21. PA and lateral views of the wrist. The patient sits next to the table with the hand and wrist palm down on the cassette. In a true PA, there should be no overlap of the distal radioulnar articulation. On a true lateral, the radius and ulna should be superimposed as should all of the metacarpals. (**A**) Correct positioning for PA and lateral views of the wrist. (**B**) PA and lateral x-rays of the right wrist. (**C**) Radial and ulnar deviation of the right wrist. *(Bernauer, A., and Berquist, T.: Orthopaedic Positioning in Diagnostic Radiology. In Urban, et al. Baltimore, Munich, 1983.)*

proximal and distal oblique views of the wrist can be diagnostic (see Fig. 12-22).[155A]

Carpal Bone Angles

In addition, the more subtle changes in the normal relationships of the carpal bones can usually be visualized and measured in one or more of the views. The important angular relationships are probably best visualized in the lateral views and an attempt should be made to outline the carpal bones on the lateral x-rays (see Figs. 12-17, 12-53, 12-65, and 12-92) and to determine the (intercarpal) angles between the carpal bones. With the wrist in neutral position, the longitudinal axes of the long finger metacarpal, the capitate, the lunate, and the radius in the normal wrist all fall on the same line—a line drawn through the center of the head of the third metacarpal, the center of the head of the capitate, the midpoints of the convex proximal and the concave distal joint surfaces of the lunate, and the midpoint of the distal articular surface of the radius (see Fig. 12-17**C**). The longitudinal axis of the scaphoid is drawn through the midpoints of its proximal and distal poles. Using these axes, it is possible to measure angles that define the positions of the carpal bones. For example, the scapholunate angle formed by the intersection of the longitudinal axes of the scaphoid and the lunate averages 47° and

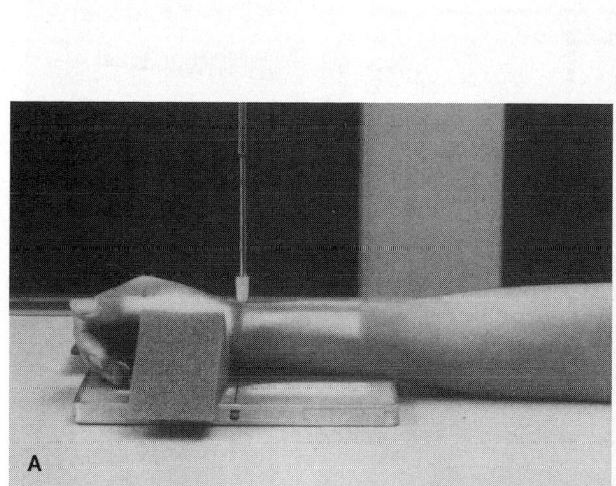

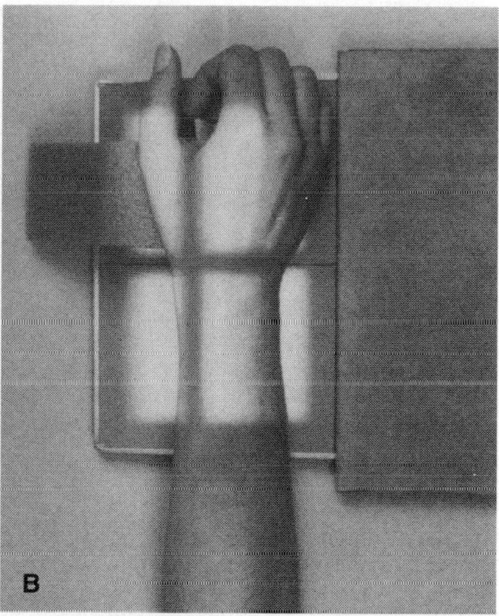

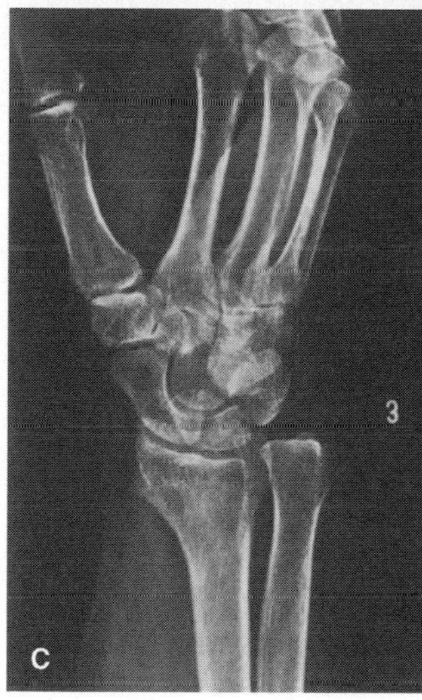

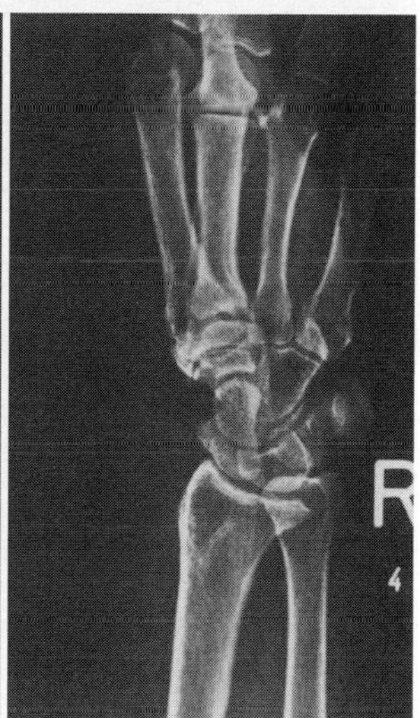

FIGURE 12-22. Scaphoid-radial oblique (supinated PA) view. (**A**) The forearm is positioned on the x-ray table with the wrist centered on the cassette. (**B**) The forearm is pronated 45° from neutral and supported with a wedge support. (**C**) This positioning portrays a full length profile view of the scaphoid particularly useful in detecting scaphoid fractures (*left*). By comparison, the ulnar oblique view (*right*) shows overlap of the scaphoid by the capitate and lunate, and only the radioscaphoid joint is well demonstrated. (*From Bernaeu, A. and Berquist, T.H.: Orthopaedic Positioning in Diagnostic Radiology. Urban and Schwazenberg, Baltimore, Munich, 1983.*)

ranges from 30° to 60° in normal wrists (see Fig. 12-17). An angle greater than 70° suggests instability, and one greater than 80° is almost certain proof of carpal instability. A capitolunate angle of more than 20° is also strongly suggestive of carpal instability.

When the lunate lies palmar to the capitate but faces dorsally, the collapse pattern is one of dorsal flexion instability (ie, DISI); this pattern is much more common in post-traumatic situations. If the lunate lies dorsal to the capitate and is flexed palmarward, the collapse pattern is one of volar flexion instability (ie, VISI) (see Figs. 12-18 and 12-19). The DISI pattern is most commonly observed with displaced scaphoid fractures and SLD while the VISI pattern is more likely to be associated with lunatotriquetral dissociation.

Whereas the lateral x-ray defines the degree and type of carpal instability, both SLD and, to a lesser degree, lunatotriquetral dissociation (LTD) may be marked by more dramatic changes on the posteroanterior view (Fig. 12-23). The normal x-ray should show a fairly constant space between the scaphoid and lunate, lunate and triquetrum, which is maintained throughout the range of motion. For instance, the joint width between the scaphoid and the lunate is normally 1 to 2 mm, although it is wider in ulnar deviation than in radial deviation. However, with SLD, an increasing gap appears, which may in time be wide enough to accept proximal migration of the entire capitate head. A spread of more than 3 mm is considered abnormal. In addition, the scaphoid flexes palmarward; this gives the scaphoid less of an elongated profile on the posteroanterior view and projects the cortical waist of the scaphoid as an overlapping ring of bone inside the scaphoid projection (the "cortical ring sign"). The lunate also moves into DISI collapse position, and this can also be noted on the posteroanterior view by the increasing overlap of the capitate silhouette by a lunate horn (wedge shape with volar horn underlap).

With LTD, a gap between the two bones is not usually evident but a break in the normal carpal arc of the

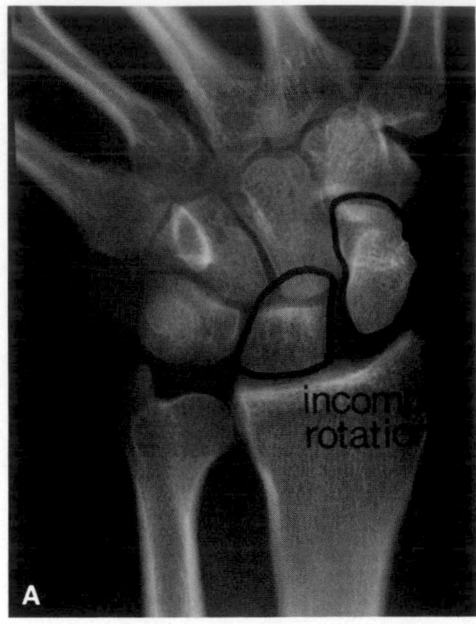

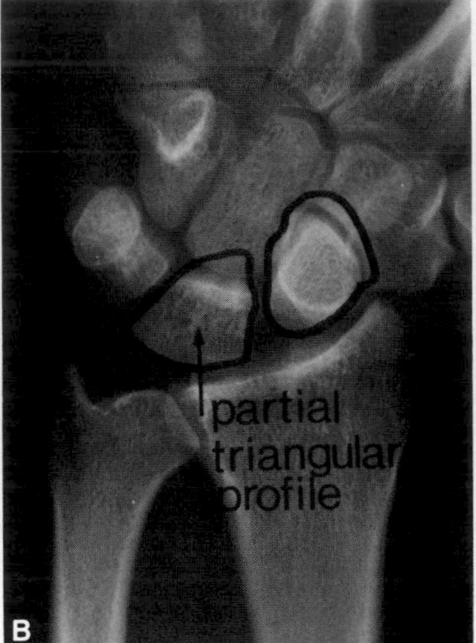

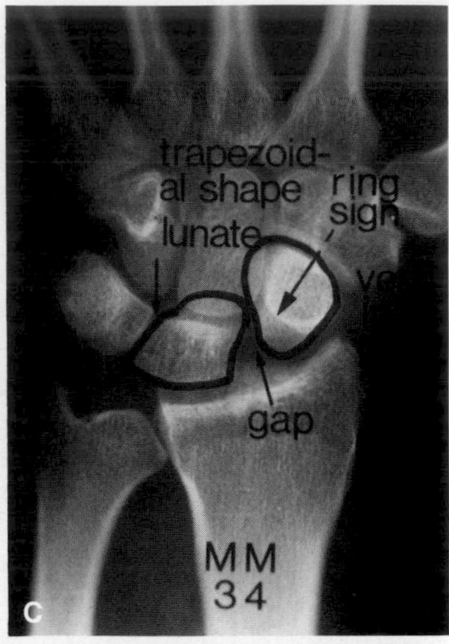

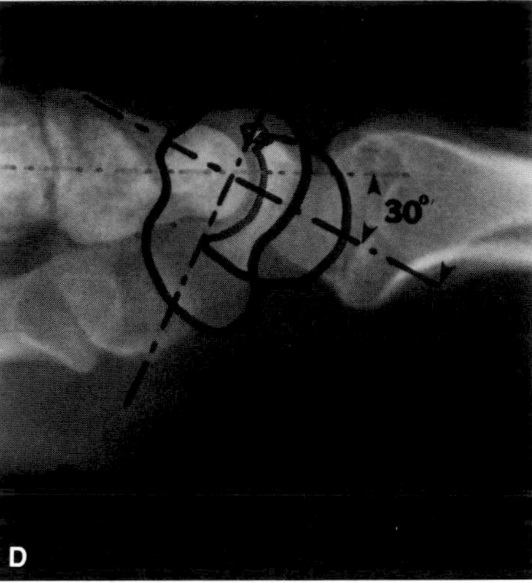

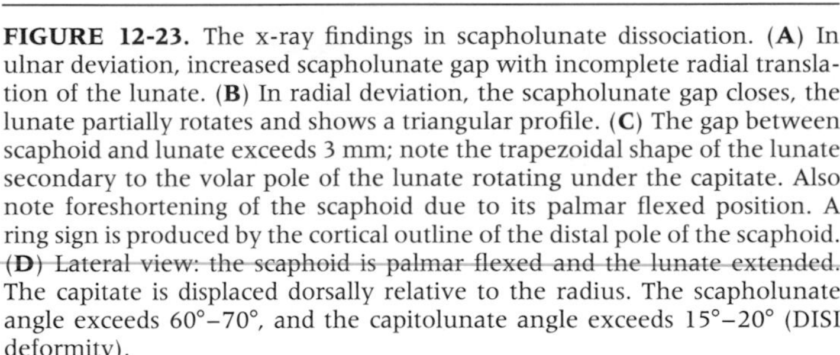

FIGURE 12-23. The x-ray findings in scapholunate dissociation. (**A**) In ulnar deviation, increased scapholunate gap with incomplete radial translation of the lunate. (**B**) In radial deviation, the scapholunate gap closes, the lunate partially rotates and shows a triangular profile. (**C**) The gap between scaphoid and lunate exceeds 3 mm; note the trapezoidal shape of the lunate secondary to the volar pole of the lunate rotating under the capitate. Also note foreshortening of the scaphoid due to its palmar flexed position. A ring sign is produced by the cortical outline of the distal pole of the scaphoid. (**D**) Lateral view: the scaphoid is palmar flexed and the lunate extended. The capitate is displaced dorsally relative to the radius. The scapholunate angle exceeds 60°–70°, and the capitolunate angle exceeds 15°–20° (DISI deformity).

proximal carpal row can be seen. Another associated deformity that may be seen with either dorsiflexion or palmar flexion instability is that of ulnar translocation of the carpus (Fig. 12-24) in which the lunate alone (type II) or scaphoid and lunate together (type I) slide ulnarly with respect to the distal radius, translating in effect the entire carpus in an ulnar direction.[329,447]

Carpal height is another way of evaluating carpal alignment (see Fig. 12-20).

Special Imaging Techniques

Special imaging studies that we have found helpful in the diagnosis of wrist injury and, particularly, carpal instability include polyspiral and trispiral tomography, computed tomographic (CT) scanning, and magnetic resonance imaging (MRI).[51,57,222,430,438] Polytomography should ideally be taken in two planes.[58] CT with cross-sectional scanning of the carpus[169,468] can be diagnostic for scaphoid malunion and displaced nonunion, capitate fractures, carpal tunnel impingement, and transosseous fracture–dislocations. CT scans are impressive in depicting displacement of distal radius fractures, including displacement of articular fragments and subluxation or dislocation of the DRUJ. MRI[20,57] (Fig. 12-25) and ultrasound[188] may provide specific information on stress fractures (scaphoid, capitate, lunate) and avascular necrosis. Bone scans,[40,45,202] while not diagnostic, can assist in confirming a suspected fracture or ligament avulsion injury (Fig. 12-26). Stress x-rays[244] (including traction views) may reveal unsuspected pathology, particularly in fracture–dislocations of the wrist. Arthrography,[49,224,286,315,451] videoradiography,[299,367,474,476] and arthroscopy[68,458] are techniques that can greatly assist in the diagnosis of carpal ligament injuries, as well as both static and dynamic carpal instabilities.

Advanced imaging techniques now include selected use of three-dimensional imaging[45a,394,403,555] in plan-

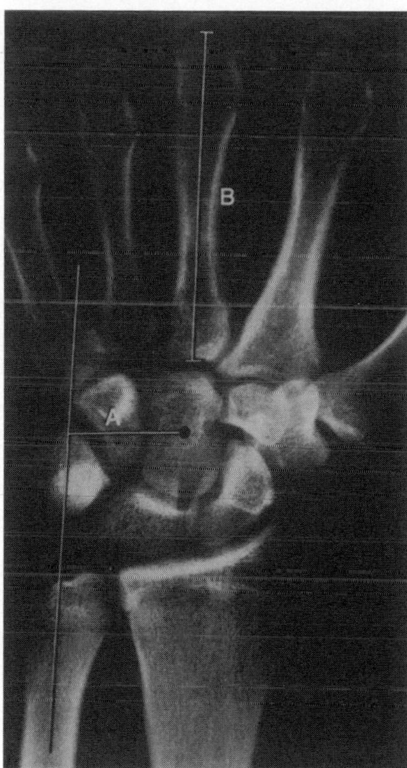

FIGURE 12-24. Ulnar carpal alignment of the wrist. This distance is measured on an AP x-ray. Normally the ratio is 0.30 (A/B = 0.30, ±0.3) where *B* is the length of the third metacarpal and *A* is the midline of the ulnar shaft to the midpoint of the capitate.

ning reconstructive procedures for malunions and nonunions associated with scaphoid fractures, distal radius fractures, and carpal fracture–dislocations.

At the present time, the ancillary radiographic methods that we use most commonly are the carpal tunnel view,[313,340,345,559] arthrography, videoradiography[567] with stress loading, polytomography, and cross-sectional CT scanning. MRI has frequent application in detecting occult fractures, avascular necrosis of scaphoid and lunate, and soft-tissue lesions, including TFC tears. Studies suggest that MRI may, in fact, assist in assessing extrinsic ligaments such as palmar radiocarpal ligaments.[50a] Wrist arthroscopy is an important adjuvant to arthrography, and the current techniques are complementary to each other.[458]

CLASSIFICATION OF WRIST INJURIES AND CARPAL INSTABILITY

The role of instability in carpal injuries has assumed increasing importance since the concept was introduced in the first edition of this book and subsequently substantially expanded.[324] For a number of years we have been content with a classification system that uses a combination of the basic diagnostic terms: instability (subluxation), dislocation (luxation), fracture–dislocation, and the direction (or type) of the instability (see Table 12-1). Dislocations and fracture–dislocations are always unstable injuries. Fractures and sprains may be stable or unstable, and treatment algorithms are frequently based on this classification. Carpal instabilities may be obvious on standard x-rays or may require special imaging techniques or special maneuvers for demonstration.[205,329,332] The most common types of carpal instability are associated with perilunate dislocations. In identifying perilunate instability, one emphasizes the central alignment in a three-link system of rows (radius, proximal carpal row, distal carpal row). Normal balance, as visualized on a lateral x-ray of the carpus, is usually assessed by the co-linear alignment of the central column of those rows (radius, lunate, capitate–third metacarpal). Although there is a spectrum of normal on either side of this co-linear alignment, a deviation of more than about 15° either way between the links of this chain should be considered abnormal and viewed as a lax, diseased, or damaged joint system. The terms for the principal collapse positions remain *DISI* and *VISI*.[13,329,330]

Although other types of carpal instability are common and create confusion, one must begin with an understanding of the concepts of perilunate instability.[119,153,355,483,514] Perilunate instability is based on the premise that the lunate is the "carpal keystone" and that its relationship with the distal radius is critical. All of the carpal bones of the proximal carpal row are linked together by strong interosseous ligaments. Reduction of the triquetrum, capitate, and scaphoid back

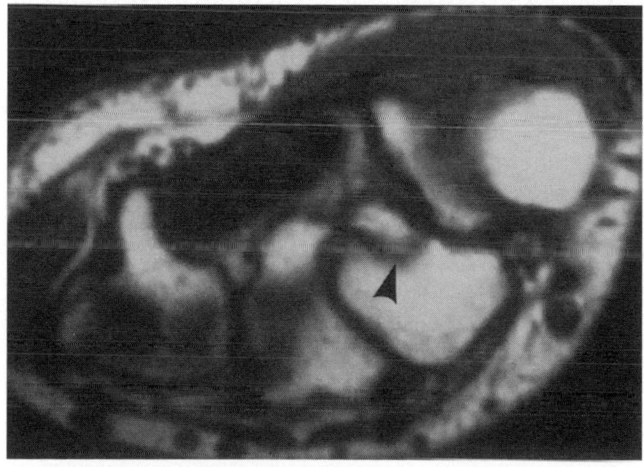

FIGURE 12-25. MRI of the wrist. Axial SE500/20 image of the wrist in a patient with post-traumatic pain. A fracture of the trapezoid (*arrow*) is detected. (*From Berquist, T.H.: The Hand and Wrist. In Imaging of Orthopedic Trauma, 2nd ed., Raven Press, New York, 1992.*)

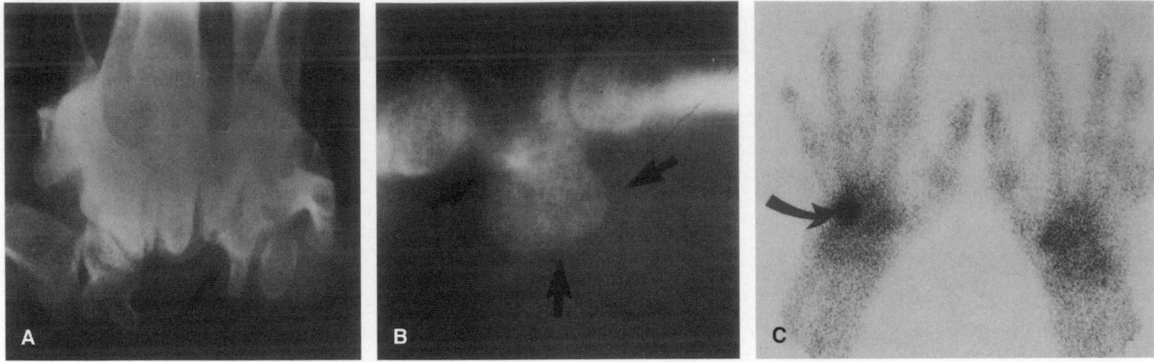

FIGURE 12-26. The bone scan is a useful tool for identifying the site of occult pathology. (**A**) A carpal tunnel view demonstrating the hook of the hamate (*arrow*). A fracture is not clearly seen. (**B**) Trispiral tomogram clearly demonstrates the fracture (*arrows*) with a Y configuration. (**C**) A bone scan with 99mTc demonstrates increased uptake in the region of the hamate. (*From Wood, M.B. and Berquist, T.H.: The Hand and Wrist. In Imaging of Orthopedic Trauma, 2nd ed. Raven Press, New York, 1992.*

to the lunate is essential to restore the integrity of the proximal carpal row and its alignment with the distal carpal bones. The theory of carpal kinematics therefore takes precedence over other theories because it is based on mechanism of injury (ie, perilunate dislocations) and the necessity of restoring carpal bone alignment to maintain normal carpal kinematics. Concepts of radial-sided, central, and ulnar-side instabilities of the wrist are also helpful in understanding the different types of wrist injuries, although these arbitrary designations may not be, strictly speaking, physiologic.[327,355,538] The lateral or radial side of the wrist provides longitudinal stability; the central segment, flexion–extension capability; and the medial or ulnar side, rotational stability (see Fig. 12-5). Carpal instability can result from fractures and dislocations of the wrist that affect one or more of these carpal columns.[151] On the lateral side of the wrist, for example, fractures can involve either the trapezium, scaphoid, and radial styloid (area of ligament origins), or ligament injuries can occur between the scaphoid and lunate or scaphoid and trapezium. Combinations of injuries produce wrist fracture–dislocations with variations on the theme of perilunate instability (eg, transscaphoid or transradiostyloid perilunate dislocations).[114] As lateral-sided disruption propagates centrally, perilunate ligament tears present as dorsal and volar perilunate dislocations and may culminate in complete lunate dislocation. Eventually, destabilizing injury reaches the medial (rotational) side of the wrist, and triquetrohamate and lunatotriquetral injuries are seen, occasionally with avulsion or chip fractures from either the dorsal or volar surface of the triquetrum. Injury patterns can vary between the radial and ulnar sides of the wrist as well as between radiocarpal and midcarpal joints depending on the direction and magnitude of the force.

Instability that involves the proximal wrist presents as radiocarpal subluxations or dislocations (ulnar, dorsal, or volar translations). Secondary instability at the radiocarpal or midcarpal joint results from attenuated volar radiocarpal ligament injuries or from malaligned distal radius fractures (excessive dorsal angulation of the distal radius).

In an attempt to further classify wrist instability, Dobyns and Linscheid divided them into two broad categories[118]: carpal instability dissociative (CID)[154] and carpal instability nondissociative (CIND).[155] The original concepts of carpal instability described by Fisk[182] and Linscheid and associates[329] considered CID to involve scaphoid fracture, SLD, or LTD. The more recent concept has included nondissociative injuries,[155] in which collapse patterns occur in which the bones of each carpal row are still strongly attached to each other (ie, the interosseous ligaments are intact) but extensor wrist ligaments are injured (torn or attenuated). Unfortunately, carpal injuries are not always so clear-cut. Dissociative patterns of instability may occur with nondissociative patterns, leading to complexities of both diagnosis and management. We use the acronym CIC to describe this combination as "combined or complex instability of the carpus."

Carpal instabilities lead to abnormal positioning or alignment of the carpal bones by fracture, ligament injury, or both.[13] The most common patterns of carpal malalignment as described earlier are (1) DISI, in which the lunate is dorsiflexed abnormally for any given wrist position; (2) VISI, in which the lunate appears abnormally volar flexed; and (3) ulnar translocation, in which the lunate is abnormally displaced ulnarly from the lunate fossa of the distal radius.

In one study, researchers identified a separate group of *axial carpal instabilities,*[209] which are characterized by bone and ligament disruptions between the bones of the distal carpal row, adjacent metacarpals, and proximal carpal elements. Because they involve intrinsic ligament injuries, they are classified as CID injuries.

In applying this classification to acute wrist injuries, the most common types of CID occur between bones of the proximal carpal row (eg, scaphoid fracture or tear of the scapholunate or lunatotriquetral ligaments). The transscaphoid perilunate or pure perilunate dislocations provide the highest degree of dissociative carpal instabilities.

Unstable scaphoid fractures[184,252] frequently result in a dissociative type of carpal instability. The radial side or column of the wrist becomes unstable. The distal scaphoid continues to follow the palmar flexion tendency, while the proximal fragment follows the lunate into extension. This results in a DISI type of carpal malalignment. As the distal carpal row migrates proximally, compressive force from the trapezium results in greater mid scaphoid angulation and additional carpal collapse.

Scapholunate dissociation, also a radial-side carpal instability, involves a substantial disruption of the ligament between the scaphoid and lunate.[329] Lesser degrees of ligament attenuation or partial tear can occur. The scaphoid, devoid of proximal ligament attachments, rotates around the palmar radiocapitate ligament, resulting in a dorsal rotary subluxation of the proximal pole. The lunate follows the triquetrum into extension, and a dorsally angulated lunate results (DISI). The primary constraint to SLD is the dorsal half of the scapholunate interosseous membrane, followed by the palmar third to half of the ligament with secondary constraints being the palmar radiocapitate and distal scaphotrapezial ligaments.

Lunatotriquetral dissociation, an ulnar-side carpal instability, involves a substantial disruption of the lunatotriquetral and volar radiolunatotriquetral ligaments and attenuation or rupture of dorsal radiotriquetral attachments. LTD has been divided into three stages, depending on involvement of these three ligaments. In stage III, in which lunatotriquetral, volar radiolunatotriquetral, and dorsal radiolunatotriquetral ligaments are torn, a VISI collapse deformity occurs as the scaphoid induces the lunate into a further flexion stance while the triquetrum extends.[530,538]

CIND can be classified into three groups based on the level of involvement: radiocarpal, midcarpal, and combined radiomidcarpal.[118] The radiocarpal instabilities are commonly associated with complete or partial radiocarpal dislocation or Barton's volar-dorsal fracture–dislocations of the distal radius. The midcarpal instabilities relate to loss of ligament support from the extrinsic scaphotrapezial, scaphocapitate, and triquetrocapitate ligaments. These problems are rarely noted acutely and represent chronic or late presentations of unrecognized sprains of the wrist, often superimposed on a lax ligamentous habitus. Secondary CIND-type midcarpal instabilities that lead to a VISI-type deformity can be seen after malunited distal radius fractures. Combined CID/CIND/CIC are frequent sequelae of the various carpal dislocations (radiocarpal, perilunate, midcarpal), implying severe damage to both the intrinsic and extrinsic radiocarpal ligaments.

The easiest way to differentiate between dissociative and nondissociative instabilities is to perform an arthrogram and note the presence or absence of dye flow between midcarpal and radiocarpal joints. If there is dye flow between compartments, one is probably dealing with a dissociative instability (CID). A lack of communication between the radiocarpal and midcarpal joint favors a nondissociative collapse (CIND). There are multiple reasons for nondissociative proximal carpal row collapse. In the normal wrist, the proximal carpal row is stabilized both proximally and distally by a complex of capsuloligamentous restraints. Damage to these restraints on *either* side of the proximal carpal row may lead to collapse. The imaging and clinical appearance of the proximal carpal row may be the same whether the destabilization is radiocarpal or midcarpal.

FRACTURES OF THE DISTAL RADIUS

Eponyms

Modern treatment of fractures of the distal radius requires a clearer definition of the different types of fracture and clarification of the various eponyms associated with this injury. Of all of the fractures that affect the upper extremity, the distal radius fracture is among the most common. Historically, the accurate descriptions of this fracture are ascribed to Pouteau (1783)[439] and Colles (1814),[110] for whom it is classically named. In time, other descriptions of distal radius fractures were credited to Barton (1838),[35] Smith (1854),[494] and Dupuytren (1847).[157] It is more important today to determine the nature of the fracture and to describe the pathology involved than to link diagnosis and treatment to a single name. The type, direction, and amount of displacement are the most important factors[234] relating to treatment and, in this chapter, discussion is directed to the features emphasized as we sort through the preferred methods of treatment for fractures of the distal radius.

Anatomy

The distal radius joint and DRUJ support the carpus with three separate articulations that are of concern in treatment of fractures of the distal radius. The scaphoid fossa and lunate fossa are two concave articular surfaces separated by a dorsal-volar ridge, which define clear articulations for the lunate and scaphoid (see Figs. 12-6 and 12-7). A separate articulation, the sigmoid notch, is present for the head of the ulna. This notch is also concave for contribution to the stability of the distal ulna. The distal articular surface of the radius is aligned to the longitudinal axis of the radius at 14° of volar tilt and 22° of ulnar inclination (see Fig. 12-20). The ulnar side of the wrist is supported in addition by the TFC, which articulates with both the lunate and triquetrum. In various degrees of radioulnar deviation, there is greater or lesser contact with the TFC. The length of the ulna varies with pronation and supination, and there are varying degrees of positive or ulnar variance that affect the amount of force transmitted between the radius and the TFC.

The dorsal and palmar ligaments of the wrist attached to the distal radius, previously described in the section on ligaments of the wrist, are important in the mechanism of fracture and subsequent fragment displacement. These areas include the radial styloid, palmar scaphoid, and palmar lunate facet, where the long and short radiolunate and radiocapitate ligaments originate. The dorsal radiotriquetral ligament and the attachments of the dorsal retinaculum are at the first compartment, Lister's tubercle, and the ulnar rim.

The attachments of the dorsal and palmar radioulnar ligaments of the TFC originate on the ulnar aspect of the distal radius (ulnar edge of lunate fossa) and have importance in lunate fossa fractures (die-punch fractures), disruptions of the TFC, and DRUJ injuries. The radial border of the TFC is attached along the entire margin of the lunate fossa at its border with the sigmoid notch while the ulnar attachment of the TFC begins at the base of the ulnar styloid and extends ulnarly and distally around the ulnar styloid to insert on the triquetrum and proximal hamate.

Mechanisms of Injury

Fractures of the distal radius occur most often from falls on the outstretched hand. The amount of force necessary experimentally to produce these fractures varies in the dorsiflexed wrist from 105 to 440 kg, with a mean of 195 kg for women and 282 kg for men.[198] Fractures of the distal radius are produced when the dorsiflexion of the wrist varies from 40° to 90°,[553] with lesser amounts of force being required at smaller angles. Although the exact mechanism of fracture is not clear, the generally sharp fracture on the palmar aspect of the radial metaphyseal area, compared with the dorsally comminuted fragments, suggests that the radius may first fracture in tension on its palmar surface, with the fracture propagating dorsally where bending moment forces induce compression stresses (see Fig. 12-14). This results in the dorsal cortex comminuting as the fracture proceeds along 45° shear stress lines. Cancellous bone is compacted, further reducing dorsal stability. A high-tensile loading of the palmar radiocarpal ligaments is necessary to transmit the tensile loading to the palmar cortex. Distal radius fractures that have a shear or compression component produce intra-articular fractures that are considerably more unstable than the bending metaphyseal extra-articular fractures. Concomitant ligamentous injuries are therefore to be expected.

Classification

The presentation of a classification of fractures of the distal radius must begin with an initial recognition of the different common types of fracture. Colles' fracture is the most common. It involves the distal metaphysis of the radius, which is dorsally displaced and angulated. It occurs within 2 cm of the articular surface and may extend into the distal radiocarpal joint or DRUJ.[321] Dorsal angulation (silver fork deformity), dorsal displacement, radial angulation, and radial shortening are present. There is often an accompanying fracture of the ulnar styloid, which may signify avulsion of the TFC insertion.

Smith's fracture,[494] or reverse Colles' fracture, is a volar angulated fracture of the distal radius with a "garden spade" deformity.[336] The hand and wrist are displaced forward or volarly with respect to the forearm. The fracture may be extra-articular, intra-articular, or part of a fracture–dislocation of the wrist (Fig. 12-27).

Barton's fracture is actually a fracture–dislocation or subluxation in which the rim of the distal radius,

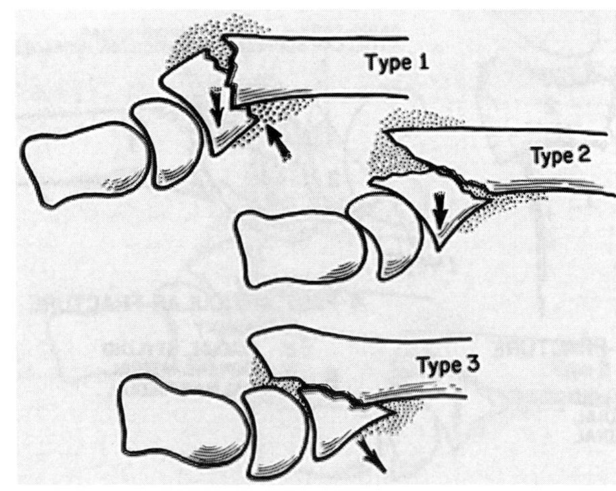

FIGURE 12-27. Modified Thomas classification of Smith's fractures. *Type I* is extra-articular, *type II* crosses into the dorsal articular surface, and *type III* enters the radiocarpal joint (and is equivalent to a volar Barton's fracture-dislocation).

dorsally or volarly, is displaced with the hand and carpus.[336,432] It is different from a Colles or Smith fracture in that the dislocation is the most clinically and radiographically obvious abnormality, with the radial fracture noted secondarily. Some Colles' fractures resemble some Barton fractures when there is significant comminution of the dorsal surface and the fracture location is quite distal on the radius. The volar Barton fracture is equivalent to a Smith type III fracture, because both involve palmar dislocation of the carpus associated with an intra-articular distal radius component. Based on mechanism of injury, Fernandez has classified distal radius fractures as compression, bending, shear, with intra-articular three-part and four-part components.

Although a number of different classifications have been advanced for fractures of the distal radius, a recent classification that is treatment based and easy to remember is presented. The Frykman classification[198] was used in the previous edition and has served as a reasonable, although somewhat cumbersome, method of recognition of different fracture types (Table 12-2; Fig. 12-28). The present "universal" classification is modified from Gartland and Werley[211] and Sarmiento (Fig. 12-29) and emphasizes the increasing awareness that different treatment modalities are indicated for the variations that exist in distal radius fractures.

Fractures of the distal radius can be broadly classified as extra-articular or intra-articular.[211] The extra-articular fractures are generally referred to as Colles' fractures. Extra-articular fractures are either type I, nondisplaced and stable, or type II, displaced and unstable. Intra-articular fractures, conversely, are either nondisplaced, type III, or displaced, type IV.

TABLE 12-2
Frykman Classification of Colles' Fractures

	Distal Ulnar Fracture	
Fractures	***Absent***	***Present***
Extra-articular	I	II
Intra-articular involving radiocarpal joint	III	IV
Intra-articular involving distal radioulnar joint	V	VI
Intra-articular involving both radiocarpal and distal radioulnar joint	VII	VIII

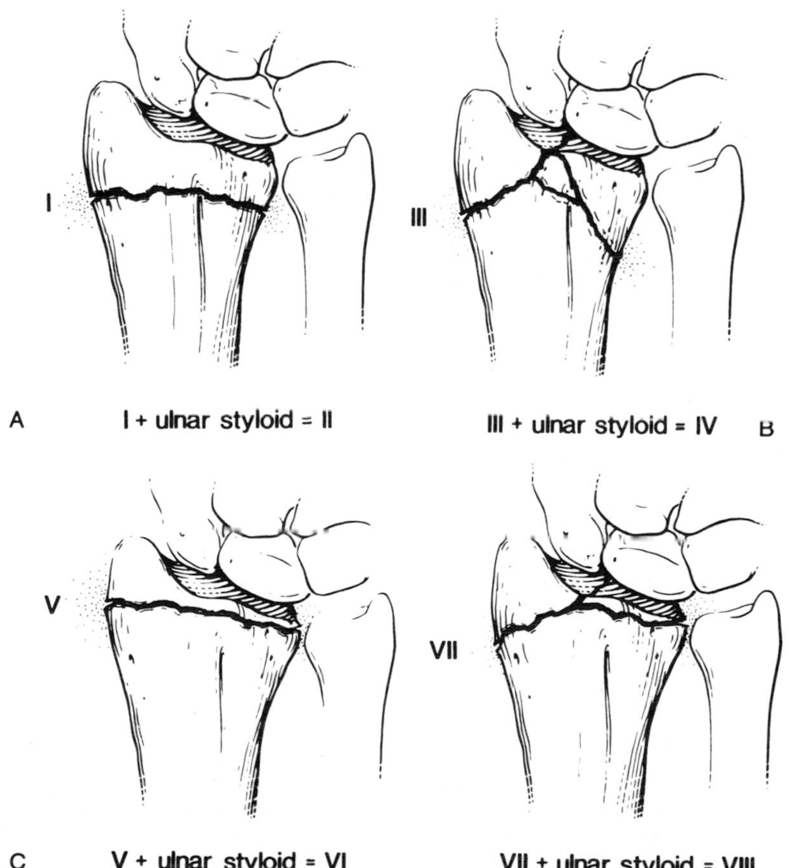

FIGURE 12-28. Frykman classification of distal radius fractures. (**A**) Frykman Type I/II-extra-articular. (**B**) Frykman Type III/IV-intra-articular radiocarpal joint. (**C**) Frykman Type V/VI-intra-articular distal radioulnar joint. (**D**) Frykman Type VII/VIII-intra-articular radiocarpal *and* distal radioulnar joints.

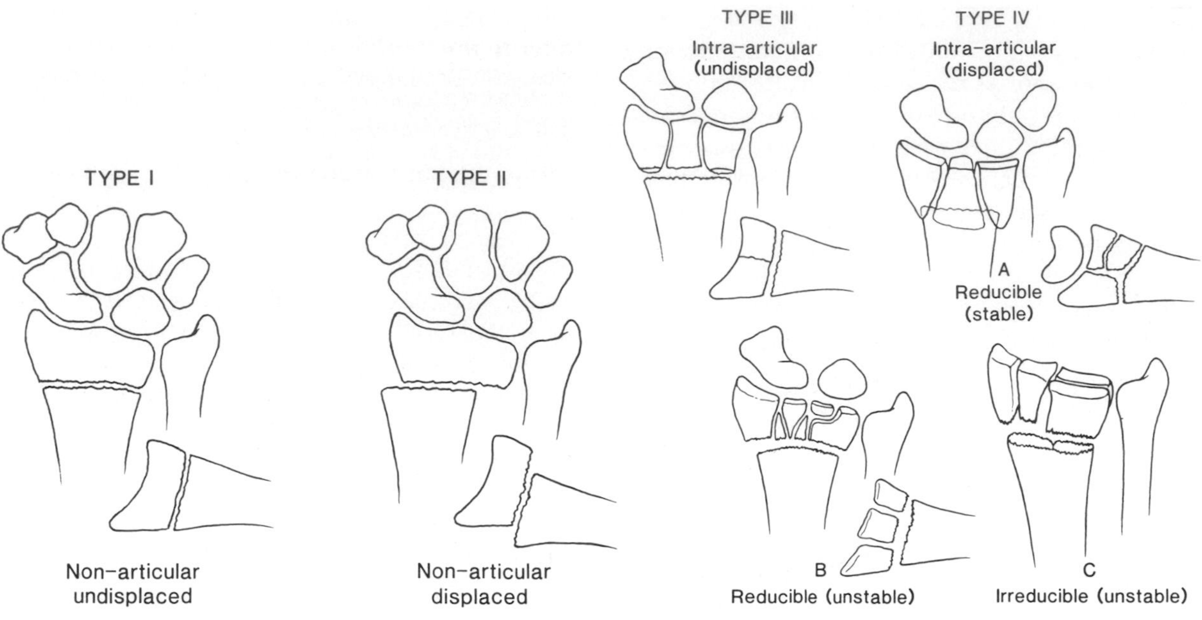

FIGURE 12-29. Universal classification of dorsally displaced distal radius fractures. *Type I:* extra-articular, undisplaced; *type II:* extra-articular, displaced; *type III:* intra-articular, undisplaced; *type IV:* intra-articular, displaced: (*A*) reducible, stable; (*B*) reducible, unstable; (*C*) irreducible, unstable. (*Modified from Gartland, J.J., Jr. and Werley, C.W.: Evaluation of Healed Colles' Fractures. J. Bone Joint Surg. 33A:895–907, 1951; and from Sarmentio, A.; Pratt, G.W.; Berry, N.C.; Sinclair, W.F.: Colles' Fractures: Functional Bracing in Supination. J. Bone Joint Surg. 57A:311–317, 1975.*)

The displaced type IV has three subcategories: (A) reducible, stable; (B) reducible, unstable; and (C) complex irreducible (see Fig. 12-29). The treatment decisions are based on the extent of potential instability. The degree of initial displacement provides some criteria for determining instability. In our experience,[120] an unstable fracture is one that presents with greater than 20° of dorsal angulation, has marked dorsal comminution, and has radial shortening of 10 mm or more. Secondary instability is present when closed reduction and cast immobilization fails to maintain the initial reduction, and there is residual dorsal angulation of 10° or more and greater than 5 mm of radial shortening. Stable fractures are usually extra-articular with mild to moderate displacement and when reduced do not redisplace to the original deformity. Unstable fractures are more commonly comminuted and shortened and have articular fractures that involve not only the radiocarpal joint but also the DRUJ. These fractures are associated with a higher rate of complications, including loss of reduction, median nerve injury, and instability of the DRUJ.[115]

Intra-articular fractures of the distal radius have been recognized as having different requirements for treatment than the extra-articular fractures. In addition to the modified Gartland universal classification, several other classifications of intra-articular fractures have been proposed. The Melone[362] classification (Fig. 12-30) recognizes articular fractures as comprising four basic components: the shaft, radial styloid, and dorsal medial and palmar medial components. Variations on the involvement of these fracture fragments results in four different types of intra-articular fractures. Type I is nondisplaced and minimally comminuted; type II fractures (die-punch fractures) are unstable with moderate to severe displacement. Comminution of the anterior cortex suggest instability. Type III fractures involve an additional fracture component from the shaft of the radius that can project into the flexor compartment. Type IV fractures involve a transverse split of the articular surfaces with rotational displacement. Unsuccessful dorsal reductions are common with Melone types II, III, and IV.

To clearly separate the articular surfaces that may individually be involved with distal radius fractures, we have proposed a modified (Mayo Clinic) classification (Fig. 12-31) *in which the scaphoid, lunate, and sigmoid notch fossae of the distal radius are considered as separate articulations.*[368A] Type I fractures are intra-articular but nondisplaced. Type II fractures are displaced involving the radioscaphoid joint (Fig. 12-32**A**). Type III fractures are displaced involving the radiolunate joint. Type IV fractures are displaced involving both the radioscaphoid and lunate joints and

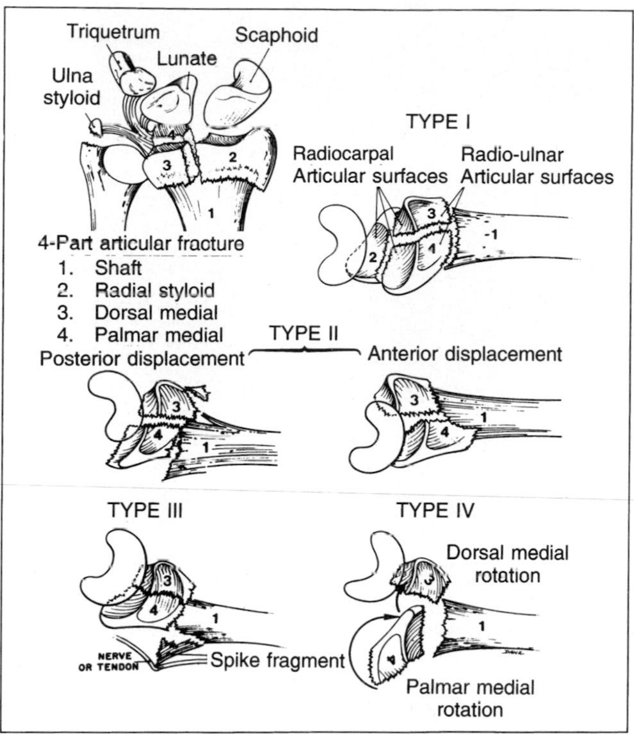

FIGURE 12-30. Melone's intra-articular fracture classification. This classification of articular fractures is based on consistent fracture patterns resulting from the characteristic die-punch mechanism of injury. The fractures generally comprise four basic components. The key medial fragments, owing to their pivotal position, are the cornerstones of both the radiocarpal and distal radioulnar joints, and have been termed the medial complex. Displacement of this complex is the basis for categorization of the articular fracture into specific types. (*Melone, C.P., Jr.: Unstable Fractures of the Distal Radius. In Lichtman, D.M. (ed)): The Wrist and Its Disorders. Philadelphia, W.B. Saunders, 1987.*)

the sigmoid fossa of the distal radius. The radioscaphoid joint fracture (type II) involves the radial styloid (chauffeur's fracture), is associated with scapholunate ligament tears, and has significant dorsal angulation and radial shortening. The radiolunate fracture (type III) (see Fig. 12-32**B**) is the die-punch or lunate load fracture and is often irreducible by traction alone. The combined radioscaphoid and lunate fracture (type IV) (see Fig. 12-32**C**) is often a more comminuted fracture involving all of the major joint articular surfaces and almost always includes a fracture component into the DRUJ.

The purpose of both the Melone[362] and the Mayo Clinic classifications of distal radius fractures is to call attention to the intra-articular fracture, which must be identified as distinct variants of Colles' fracture and which demands more aggressive treatment. Either of these classifications fit well as further subdivisions of the universal classification of distal radius fractures: type IV—intra-articular (see Fig. 12-29).

Throughout the remainder of this chapter, the various types of fracture designations (I, II, III, and IV) refer to the "universal" classification (see Fig. 12-29).

Clinical Findings

Within the thin osteoporotic cortices in the elderly, an extra-articular metaphyseal fracture generally occurs. In younger patients, an intra-articular fracture with displacement of the joint surfaces is more likely. The mechanism of injury, however, may cause compression, shear, or displaced three-part or four-part intra-articular fractures in all ages of patients.

On clinical examination, there is obvious deformity of the wrist with dorsal displacement of the hand in the Colles-type fracture (or dorsal Barton's fracture) or palmar displacement of the hand and wrist in the Smith-type fracture (palmar Barton's fracture).[321] The dorsal aspect of the hand and wrist are usually quite swollen, and ecchymosis may be present, especially in the elderly. The wrist should be examined for tenderness not only about the radial fracture site but also at the distal ulna, elbow, and shoulder. Median nerve function and flexor and extensor tendon action should be tested.[82,104,492,527] Instability of the distal ulna should be assessed, usually after local or regional anesthesia

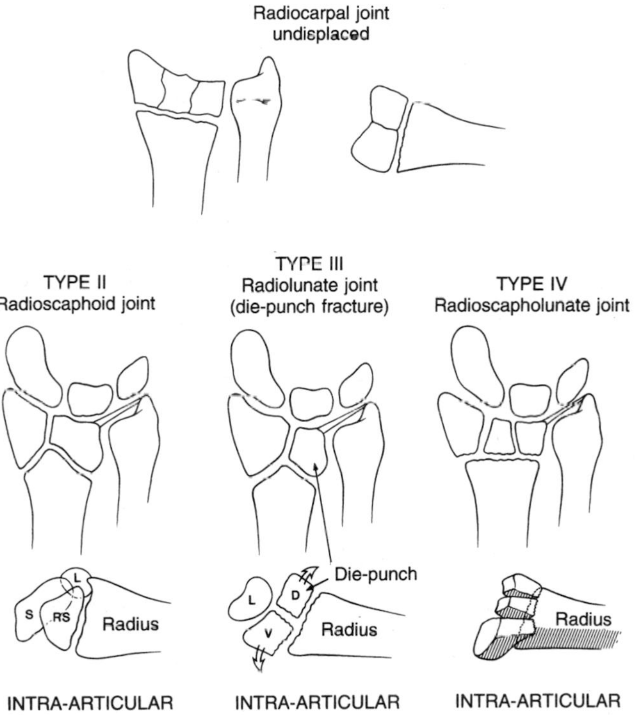

FIGURE 12-31. Mayo Classification for intra-articular fractures of the distal radius. Type I–undisplaced, extra-articular to radiocarpal joint. Type II–intra-articular radioscaphoid joint. Type III–intra-articular radiolunate joint. Type IV–intra-articular radioscaphoid and radiolunate joint.

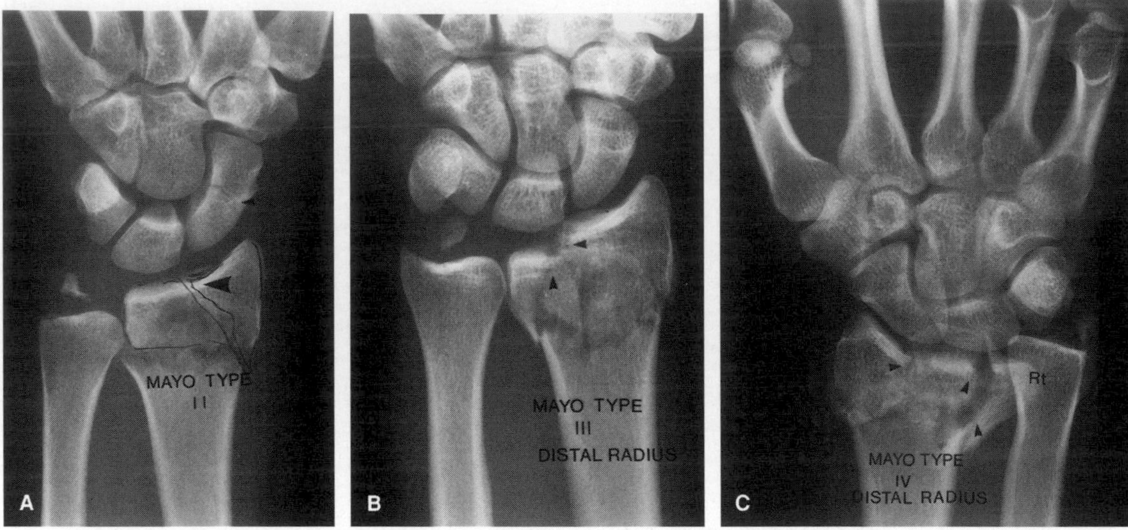

FIGURE 12-32. (**A**) A Mayo Type II distal radius fracture that is displaced into the radioscaphoid joint (*large arrow*). Note the associated scaphoid waist fracture (*small arrow*) and a displaced ulnar styloid fracture. (**B**) A Mayo Type III intra-articular fracture into the radiolunate joint, a displaced "die-punch fracture" of the lunate fossa of distal radius. (**C**) A Mayo Type IV complex intra-articular fracture involving the radioscaphoid, radiolunate and distal radioulnar joints.

has been obtained and again after reduction and fixation of the distal radius fracture.

Associated Injuries and Complications

Median Nerve Injury

As a result of the original trauma, distal radius fractures are associated with a number of soft-tissue injuries and a variety of potential complications (Table 12-3). The most common associated problem is damage to the median nerve.[115,297,340] In our own Mayo Clinic experience, chronic median neuropathy occurred in 23% of 536 distal radius fractures and acute median neuropathy occurred in 13%.[115] With forceful hyperextension, the median nerve is placed under considerable tension. Displacement of fracture fragments can cause direct nerve injury. Inadequate or delayed reduction, hematoma formation, and increased compartment pressure may produce additional pressure on the nerve. In this review of complications of distal radius fractures, median nerve injury had the most serious sequelae.[115]

Prompt reduction of the fracture in the emergency department can help reduce the extent of compression and compromised vascularity. Ade-

TABLE 12-3
Complications of Colles' Fracture

EARLY
Difficult reduction; unstable reduction maintained only by extreme position
Depressed major articular components
Distal radioulnar subluxation, dislocation
Median or ulnar nerve stretch, contusion, or compression[532]
Acute carpal tunnel syndrome
Post-reduction swelling; compartment syndromes[532]
Errors in external fixation (peripheral nerve injuries)
Tendon damage
Pain dysfunction syndromes (early)
Associated carpal injury
INTERMEDIATE AND LATE
Loss of reduction and secondary deformity
Malunion and secondary intercarpal collapse deformity
Radiocarpal arthrosis—inadequate articular surface reduction
Distal radioulnar dissociation and arthrosis
Stiff hand; shoulder-hand syndrome; arthritic flare
Pain dysfunction syndrome
Median nerve compression; carpal tunnel syndrome; occasionally ulnar or radial nerve compression
Tendinous adhesion in the flexor compartment
Extensor pollicis longus tendon rupture[308,399,492,527]
Nonunion

quate anesthesia, axillary block, Bier block, or general anesthesia are preferable to hematoma block or intravenous analgesics, except for expedient decompression of the median nerve. Adequate reduction will often relieve paresthesias within a few days. If the symptoms are severe or increasing, carpal tunnel decompression is warranted.[41,352] Open reduction of the fracture or application of external fixation may be applied simultaneously. For mild, chronic median neuropathy, observation may be employed for 3 or 4 months, but the neuropathy should not be ignored. Pain dysfunction, including severe reflex sympathetic dystrophy, is the most devastating sequela that can follow acute median neuropathy.

Loss of Reduction

In most displaced fractures of the radius, loss of reduction is likely to occur unless measures are initiated acutely to prevent redisplacement (Fig. 12-33). Primary percutaneous pin fixation or external fixation should be considered if the original fracture reduction is considered unstable. Fracture stability may be judged at the time of reduction. If there is immediate redisplacement of fracture fragments despite sugar-tong splint or cast support, the fracture is presumed unstable. If the fracture fragments cannot be easily reduced with longitudinal traction, the fracture is probably unstable. Our treatment plan is to obtain as good a closed reduction as possible acutely in the emergency department. If the fracture is unstable, then the patient is scheduled for operating room treatment either the same day or within 48 hours of injury. Even with excellent reduction and adequate casting, there is often gradual shortening at the fracture site as healing occurs. Ideally this should be prevented by adding pin fixation to cast support or by proceeding to external fixation alone or combined with open fracture reduction and internal fixation (Fig. 12-34).

Late, unrecognized loss of reduction is associated with arthritis of the radiocarpal joint and DRUJ[192] and was the second most common cause of late complications from distal radius fractures in our series. Rereduction is possible up to 3 weeks from the time of injury, and radiographic reevaluation of fracture alignment is recommended weekly to prevent loss of reduction, malunion,[270,278a] or the rare nonunion.[246]

Distal Radioulnar Joint

Injury to the TFC is an often unrecognized element of distal radius fractures.[164,261] Although the exact incidence is unknown, we would estimate that approximately 50% of fractures have clinically significant injury to the TFC. These injuries include avulsion of the TFC from the ulnar styloid, in-substance tears of the peripheral rim, and displacement of the lunate fossa with the TFC.[164] It is difficult to test the stability of the distal ulna acutely without incurring redisplacement of the reduced radial fracture. If the ulnar styloid is displaced, it is likely that the TFC will provide diminished support. Placing the forearm in neutral rotation in a long-arm cast situates the TFC in the best alignment for healing. Marked pronation is to be avoided, because this inclines the ulnar head to displace dorsally. By the same token, supination with imperfect radial fragment reduction may result in palmar subluxation of the ulnar head. We would continue long-arm casting for at least 3 weeks, or until forearm rotation is not symptomatic.

To date there have been few advocates for reattachment of the TFC to the ulnar styloid or styloid fixation, but it should be considered when there is gross instability and the ulnar styloid is displaced more than 3 mm and the ulnar styloid fragment is large, implying total detachment.

Open Fractures

It is unusual to have an open fracture of the distal radius, but when this occurs it is an indication for emergency operative treatment. Any open injury, even an inside-out puncture wound, should be debrided and the fracture site irrigated using pulsed lavage. If the wound is a result of low-energy trauma, primary closure is acceptable, but if the wound is contaminated, contused, or greater than 2 cm as the result of high-energy trauma, then debridement and delayed wound closure are recommended. External fixation to maintain fracture reduction and allow wound access for dressing changes is preferred. Open reduction and internal fixation with plates or multiple pins is usually contraindicated. The exception would be the small inside-out wound that is primarily closed. Operative quantitative cultures are advisable before starting a broad-spectrum antibiotic. Wound closure is performed at 48 to 72 hours.

Treatment

Nondisplaced Fractures

Some distal radius fractures in the elderly are nondisplaced or minimally displaced stable fractures. The goals of treatment in these cases are to protect the area of fracture from further injury and to mobilize the hand and wrist as soon as symptoms allow. Many forms of cast and splints have been described, and the selection can be left to the surgeon's preference.[469,545] Some form of three-point fixation is needed, with a dorsal splint holding the wrist in slight flexion and ulnar deviation. The length of immobilization varies from 3 to 6 weeks. Pain-free motion of the fingers, forearm, and elbow are prerequisites for choosing short-arm cast or splint immobilization.

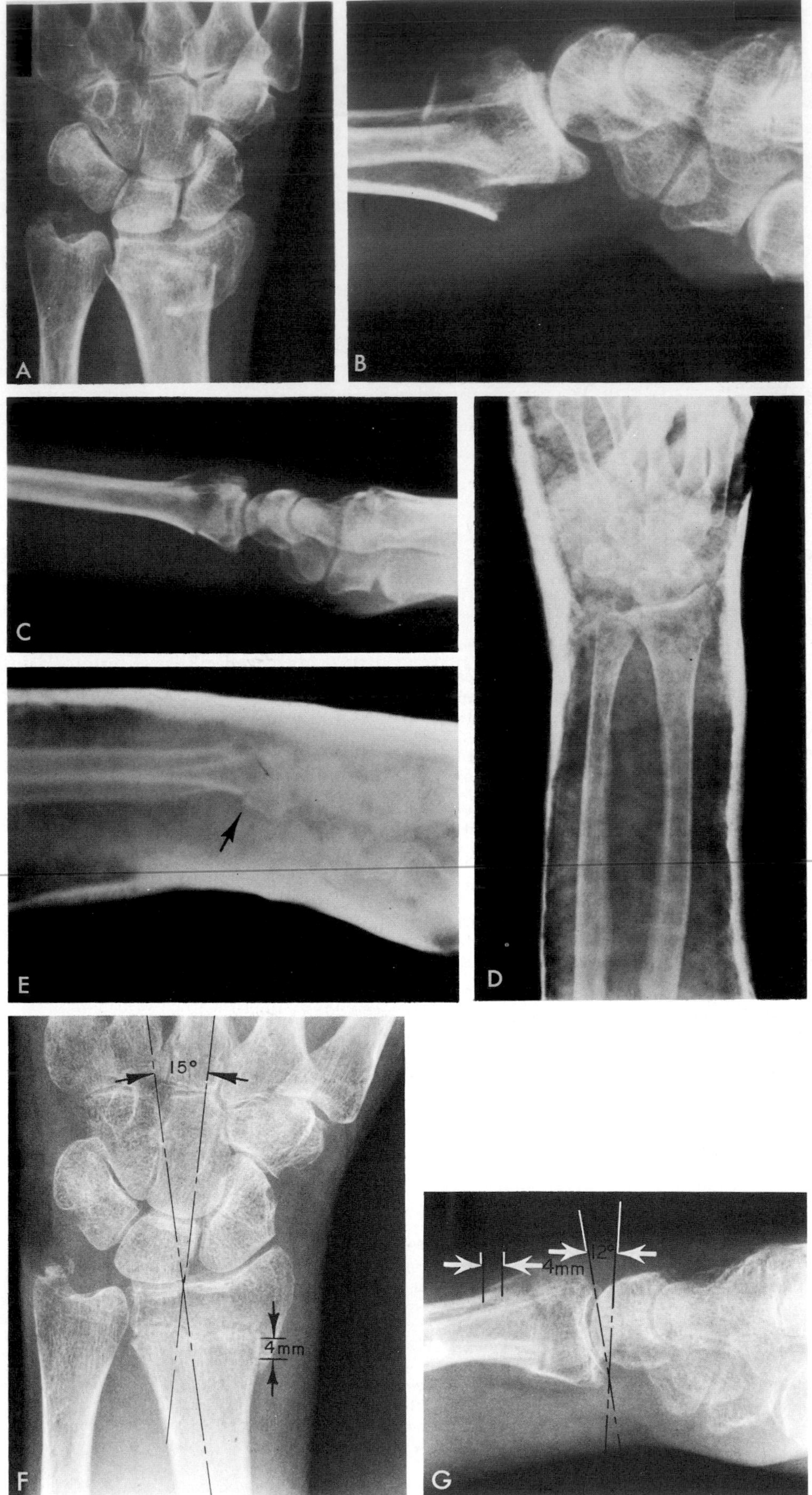

FIGURE 12-33.

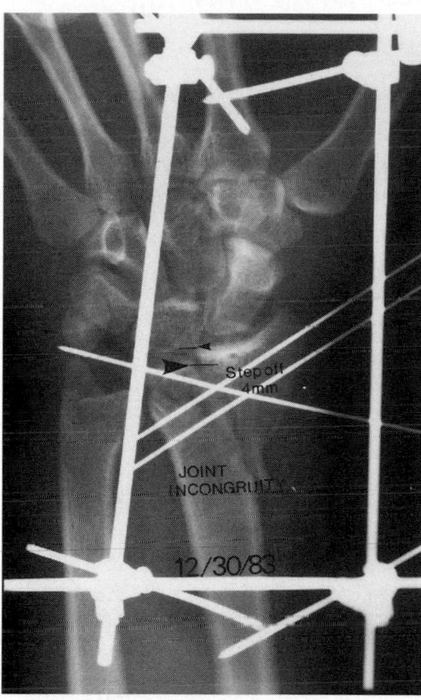

FIGURE 12-34. A comminuted fracture of the distal radius treated by external fixation and closed percutaneous pinning. Note failure to reduce the articular surface, with a residual 4 mm step-off and joint incongruity. Open reduction and internal fixation rather than percutaneous closed pinning would have been preferred in this situation.

Authors' Preferred Method of Treatment

For stable nondisplaced or minimally displaced extra-articular fractures (universal classification type I; see Fig. 12-29), we prefer treatment with a light, short-arm fiberglass or plaster cast, either at the time of presentation or within 48 hours if a sugar-tong splint was applied in the presence of initial swelling. The cast is applied with the fingers in light traction to help prevent settling (Fig. 12-35).[431] For type II displaced fractures, a closed reduction and long-arm cast is applied with the wrist and hand in traction to help maintain the reduction. At the time of cast change, we replace the limb in traction, provide 8 to 10 pounds (4 to 5 kg) of countertraction and reapply the long-arm cast. A neutral position of the wrist is desirable. If the fracture was originally slightly displaced, the wrist is placed in no more than slight flexion and ulnar deviation for 3 weeks. Alternative treatment for extra-articular fractures include percutaneous pins (see Fig. 12-34), Rayhack radius to ulna pins (Fig. 12-36), or the Kapandji percutaneous pinning technique (Fig. 12-37). We recommend supportive cast or splints with any of the percutaneous fixation techniques.

For nondisplaced or minimally displaced fractures that are stable but have intra-articular extensions (type III), percutaneous pin fixation may be added where a potential for fracture settling or displacement of the articular fragments is a concern. A short-arm cast is used with percutaneous pins, and the pins are usually removed after 3 to 4 weeks.

Usually by 6 weeks, clinical and radiographic examination demonstrate progression of fracture healing. A custom-designed splint or commercial protective splint is applied. The splint is removed for bathing and exercises and gradually removed over 2 to 3 weeks when the fracture is solidly healed. Most patients favor the splint for protection, particularly in icy climates. Instructions in active-assisted wrist motion are demonstrated to the patient. These exercises, known as "the six pack" of hand exercises and first described by the senior author (JHD), emphasize complete finger and wrist excursion (see p. 854). Most patients are able to perform these exercises and rehabilitation on their own, but their progress is checked periodically.

Displaced Fractures

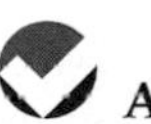

Authors' Preferred Method of Treatment

In the treatment of displaced fractures of the radius, determining the specific fracture type within the Universal Classification provides an excellent guide to

FIGURE 12-33. A 54-year-old housewife fell on the palm of her left hand after slipping on ice and sustained a Frykman type VI Colles' fracture. (**A,B**) The fracture line enters the distal radioulnar joint. There is a small avulsion fracture of the ulnar styloid, dorsal angulation of 25°, radial shortening, and dorsal displacement. (**C**) Dorsal angulation was corrected with traction in Chinese finger traps. There is a sharp fracture line on the palmar aspect. The distal fragment lacks approximately 1 mm of complete reduction. There is a comminuted fracture surface dorsally, with evidence of compaction of cancellous bone. (**D**) Postreduction x-rays taken after a circular above elbow plaster cast was applied with the forearm in slight supination, showing correction of radial length and radial angulation. (**E**) The lateral view shows that the volar cortex was overcorrected slightly (*arrow*), thus locking its position. Angulation of the articular surface approaches normal palmar flexion of 10° to 15°. The cast is well-molded about the forearm, and three-point fixation has been achieved. The cast was split along its ulnar margin to accommodate swelling. (**F,G**) Six weeks later, the fracture shows settling. Radial angulation of 15°, radial shortening of 4 mm, and loss of normal palmar-flexed position of the articular surface to 12° dorsiflexion have occurred in cast. The ulnar styloid appears to be uniting. Clinically, this was an acceptable result. Six months after fracture, there was full range of motion of the fingers, but wrist extension was limited to 50°. The woman had slight residual discomfort on supination with active use of the hand.

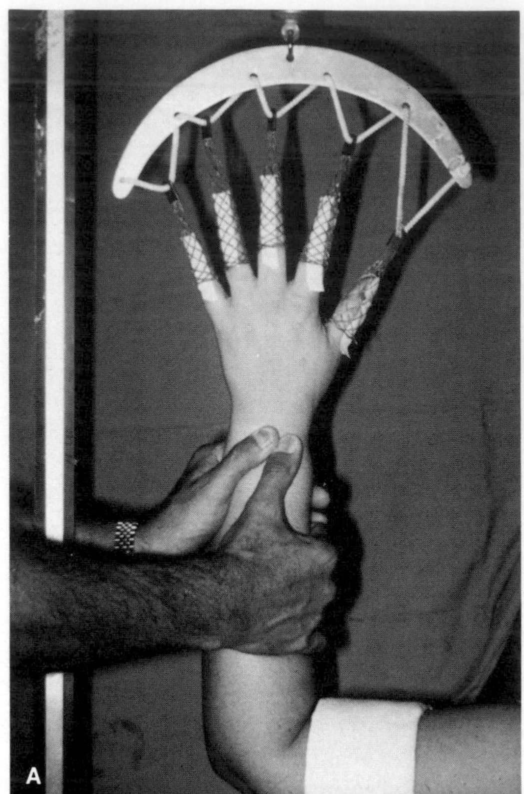

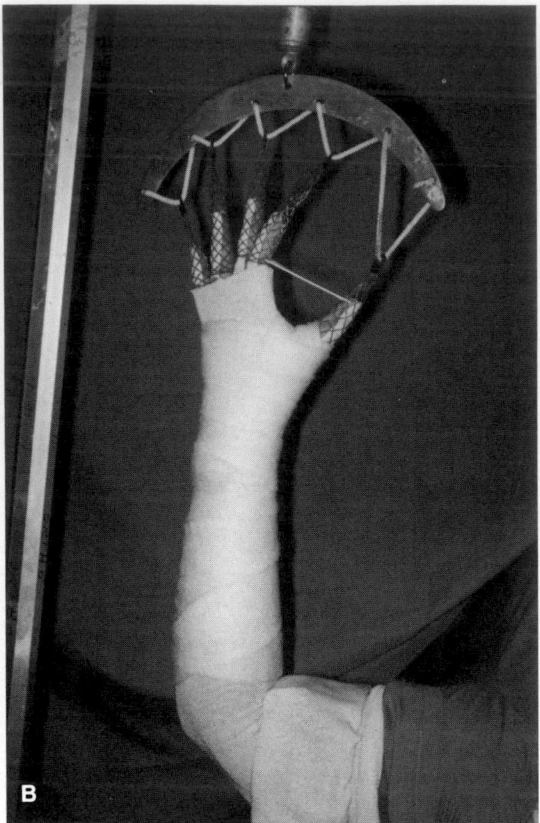

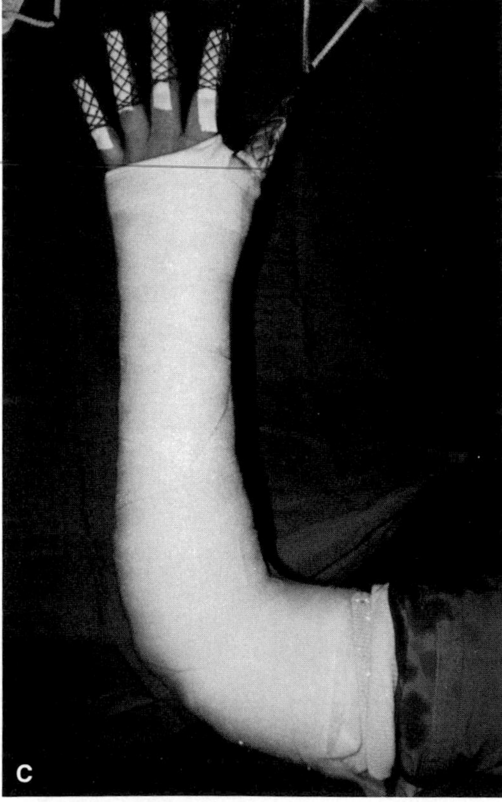

FIGURE 12-35. Our preferred technique of closed reduction for fractures of the distal radius. Undisplaced fractures are treated in a short-arm cast, while displaced fractures are treated in a long-arm cast. Displaced fractures require (**A**) gentle manipulation and sustained traction, and (**B,C**) application of the long-arm cast while maintaining traction. The finger traps are removed and the cast trimmed to allow for full finger and thumb motion.

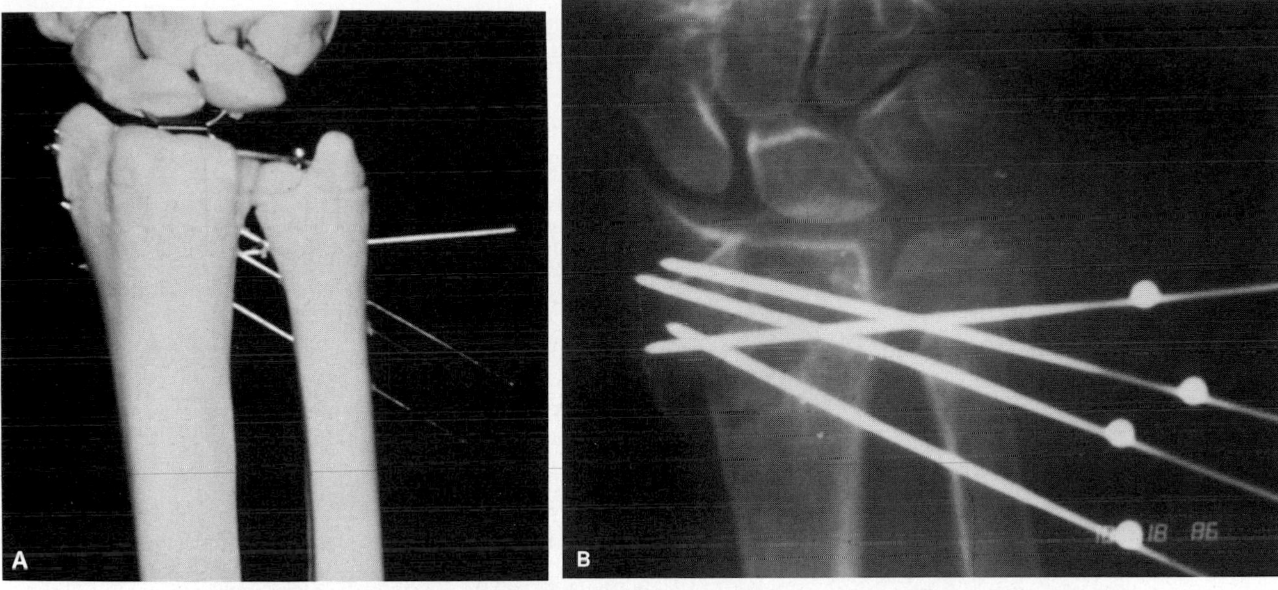

FIGURE 12-36. Rayhack technique of percutaneous pin fixation of the distal radius with K-wires (0.45″ to 0.625″) inserted from the subarticular region of the distal radius into the stable distal ulna. (**A**) Bone model showing the percutaneous pin technique. (**B**) Pin fixation of a type II, extra-articular displaced distal radius fracture. (Courtesy of John Rayhack, M.D.)

selecting the preferred form of treatment (see Fig. 12-29). The principles involve first obtaining an anatomical reduction and then maintaining that reduction with appropriate methods of immobilization.[63] The importance of anatomical reduction has been demonstrated by clinical studies of the natural history of incompletely reduced fractures,[530b] as well as by laboratory assessment of forces and stress loading across the radiocarpal joint. Knirk and Jupiter,[298] Bradway and associates,[76] and others[38,219,362] have correlated the outcome after distal radius fractures with the initial and final fracture displacement. When part of the joint articular surface was displaced more than 2 mm, radial shortening was greater than 5 mm, or dorsal angulation exceeded 20°, less than optimal results were seen. Post-traumatic arthritis was present at the radiocarpal and radioulnar joints in such patients. Wrist motion was decreased, grip strength was less than 50% of normal, and carpal subluxation with wrist instability was evident[19,360] (see Carpal Instabilities). These clinical observations have been confirmed by laboratory studies, which show that the effect of loss of radial length creates increased loads across the ulnocarpal joint and decreased force concentration across the radiocarpal joint. Every effort should be made to restore normal length, alignment, and articular surface congruency of the distal radius.[300,431,443a]

Closed Reduction

An accurate reduction of the fracture is the first step in treatment. Böhler[63] recommended in 1922 that this be performed by longitudinal traction to the hand with countertraction through the forearm. Today, the use of finger-trap traction with proximal brachial countertraction is preferred (see Fig. 12-35). The application of hyperextension and flexion maneuvers to break up the impaction is not recommended. Traction is placed through the thumb, index, and long fingers, and a self-sustained traction holder applies 6 to 12 pounds of countertraction. An axillary block or Bier block is recommended in displaced fractures, because a hematoma block may not provide sufficient anesthesia for distraction reduction. With a dorsally displaced fracture, the reduction is then performed by pushing the distal fragment distally and palmarly while holding the proximal fragment with the fingers around the forearm (see Fig. 12-35). When pressure is released, the distal fragment frequently springs back dorsally. Pronation and ulnar deviation of the distal component may also be necessary. Anteroposterior and lateral x-rays are taken to assess the accuracy of the reduction. The goal is to convert the dorsal angulation to neutral or to a slight volar tilt, as well as to regain radial length. Alignment or slight overreduction of the palmar cortices is essential to prevent redisplacement, because there is little dorsal cortical support in most of these fractures. It should not be necessary to manipulate the wrist in pronation or wrist flexion to obtain or hold the reduction. The Cotton-Loder position of forced wrist flexion should be avoided in holding fracture reduction.

For a dorsal Barton fracture, the reduction is performed in the same manner as a Colles' fracture, but

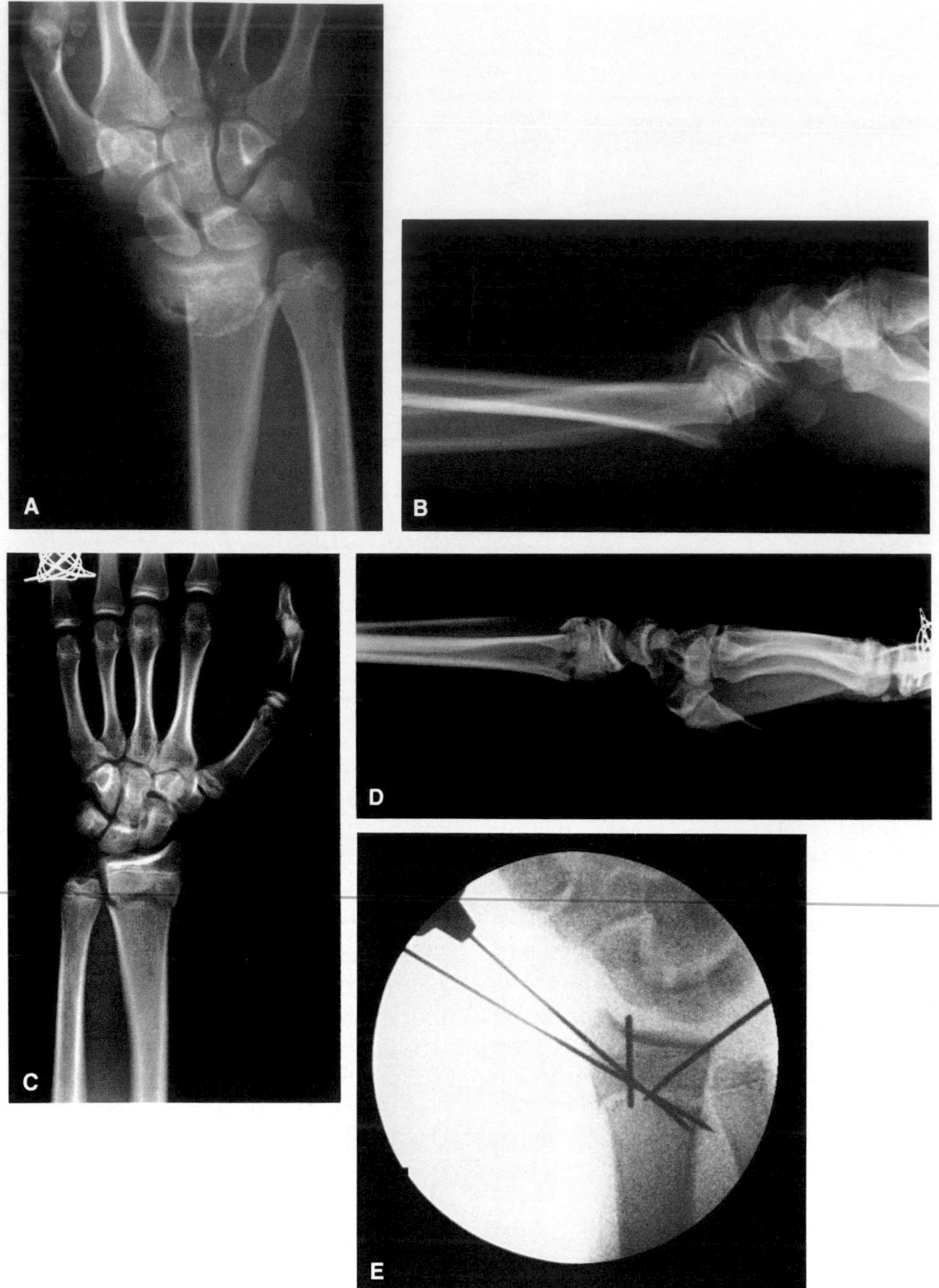

FIGURE 12-37. Kapandji technique of intra-focal percutaneous pin fixation. An extra-articular, type II, displaced fracture of the distal radius in a 17-year-old basketball player injured during practice. (**A**) Radial angulation of the fracture. (**B**) Dorsal angulation of 50°. (**C**) Traction restored to radial length. (**D**) The lateral reduction was incomplete, with residual dorsal displacement of the distal fracture component. (**E**) Intra-focal pinning, image view, PA.

continues

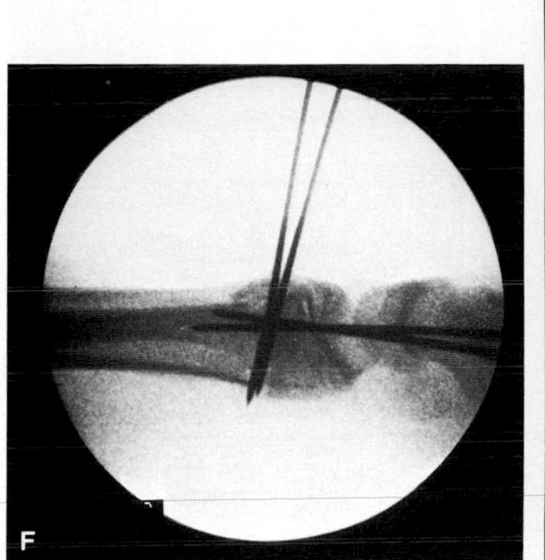

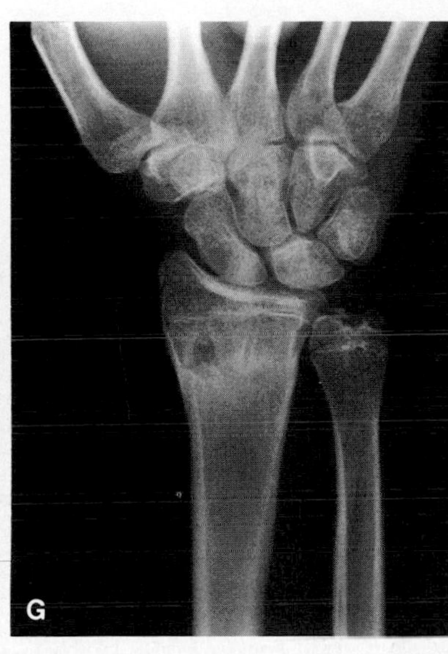

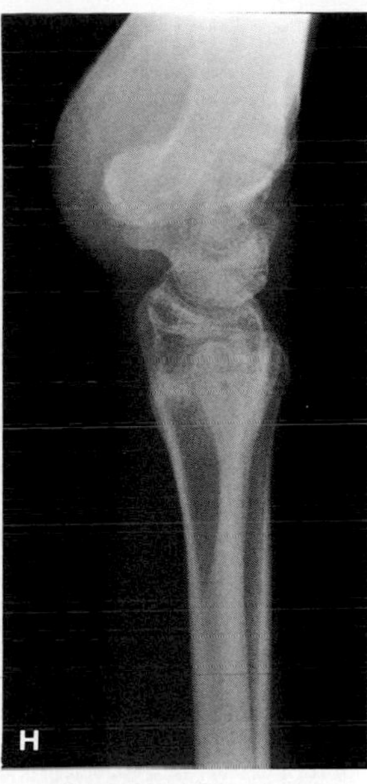

FIGURE 12-37. (continued) (**F**) Intra-focal pinning, lateral view. Note improved reduction from the wedging effect of the intra-focal (intra-fracture site) K-wires (0.045″). (**G,H**) Healed and anatomically aligned distal radius.

most of these are unstable and pin fixation or open reduction may be needed to maintain reduction. For a Smith's fracture with palmar displacement and palmar angulation of the distal fracture component, traction is used to disimpact the bone surfaces, and dorsal displacement and supination are applied to the distal fragment. Smith's fracture types II and III (see Fig. 12-27) may be unstable, and closed reduction may be insufficient (Fig. 12-38). Image intensification is of immeasurable value in assisting fracture reduction, especially if percutaneous pin fixation is performed. Plain films, however, are essential to assess the final accuracy of the reduction, because fluoroscopic imaging often lacks the clarity required.[399]

Five to 10 pounds is used for initial distraction. Occasionally, 15 to 20 pounds (8 to 10 kg) is needed for disimpaction. The wrist should not be maintained with this much distraction during external fixation or pin fixation because the weight of the extremity or 5 pounds countertraction should be sufficient.

If closed reduction of a fracture is unsuccessful, open reduction of the radius may be required (including bone grafting), especially to restore joint articular surfaces to normal contour and length, because functional results mirror the radiographic results (Fig. 12-39). Failure to restore articular alignment and congruity may lead to late collapse and quite unsatisfactory results (Fig. 12-40).

Cast Immobilization

After reduction of the fracture is achieved, many methods are available to maintain alignment and prevent redisplacement. The method of immobilization selected depends on the classification status of the fracture (see Fig. 12-29): Is the fracture extra-articular or intra-articular? Is the reduction stable or unstable? How significant is the displacement and amount of comminution present? For most fractures, closed reduction and cast immobilization is preferred. Traction maintained during application allows molding three-point pressure into a long-arm cast. The palmar cortices must be aligned and the distal fragment slightly overreduced to hold length. Three-point pressure is then applied by molding dorsally over the distal fragment and proximal forearm and palmarly over the distal forearm. Excessive flexion and ulnar deviation may actually increase the tendency to redisplacement by displacing the contact area at the radiocarpal joint dorsally; therefore, the wrist is placed in neutral or very slight flexion. The dorsal capsule has less ability to maintain reduction by ligamentotaxis, and fracture stability itself is necessary. Shortening and redisplacement can be minimized when the cast is applied in this fashion, but some subsequent settling is unavoidable.

Excessive wrist flexion also compromises the carpal tunnel and normal flexor tendon function. The forearm should be in neutral rotation in a long-arm cast, so that the ulnar head is fully seated in the sigmoid notch. Restoration of both pronation and supination is more easily achieved from this position.

External Fixation

In many comminuted and displaced fractures of the distal radius, cast immobilization will not be effective in maintaining the fracture reduction.[26,107,113,120,392,477] Despite skillful cast application, there are fractures that

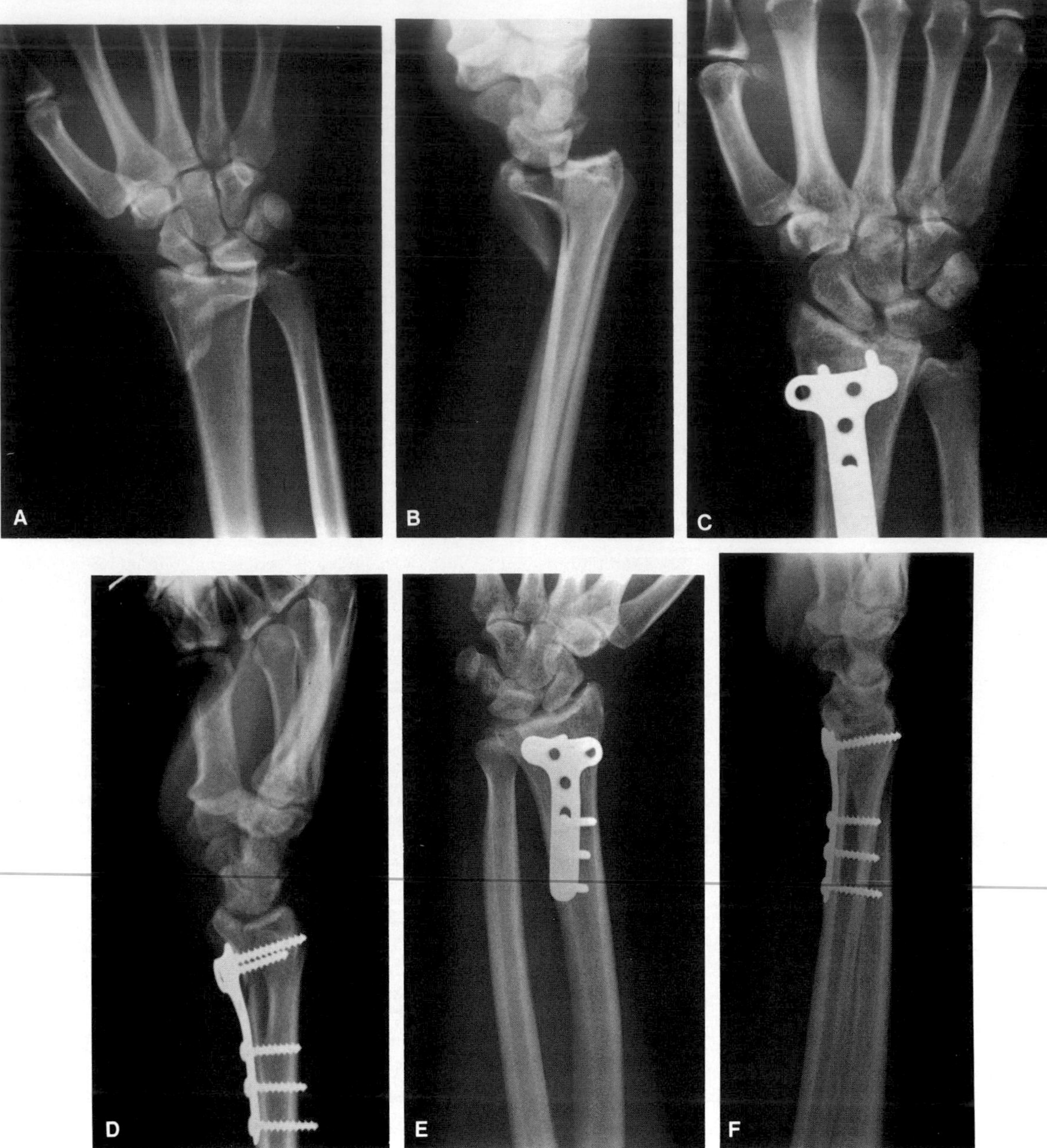

FIGURE 12-38. Smith's fracture. Palmar displacement of the carpus with a distal radius fracture in a 26-year-old plumber who fell forward from his motorcycle. (**A**) In the PA view there is an oblique fracture through the radius. Note the double shadow over the lunate, indicating volar displacement. (**B**) The lateral view shows a fracture of the distal radial articular surface with volar displacement of the carpus; a comminuted intra-articular fracture (Thomas type III). (**C,D**) Open reduction and volar buttress plate fixation. Distal screws were used to hold reduction of the intra-articular fracture components. (**E,F**) Reduction well-maintained (1 year later), with excellent alignment of the joint articular surface and a well-united fracture.

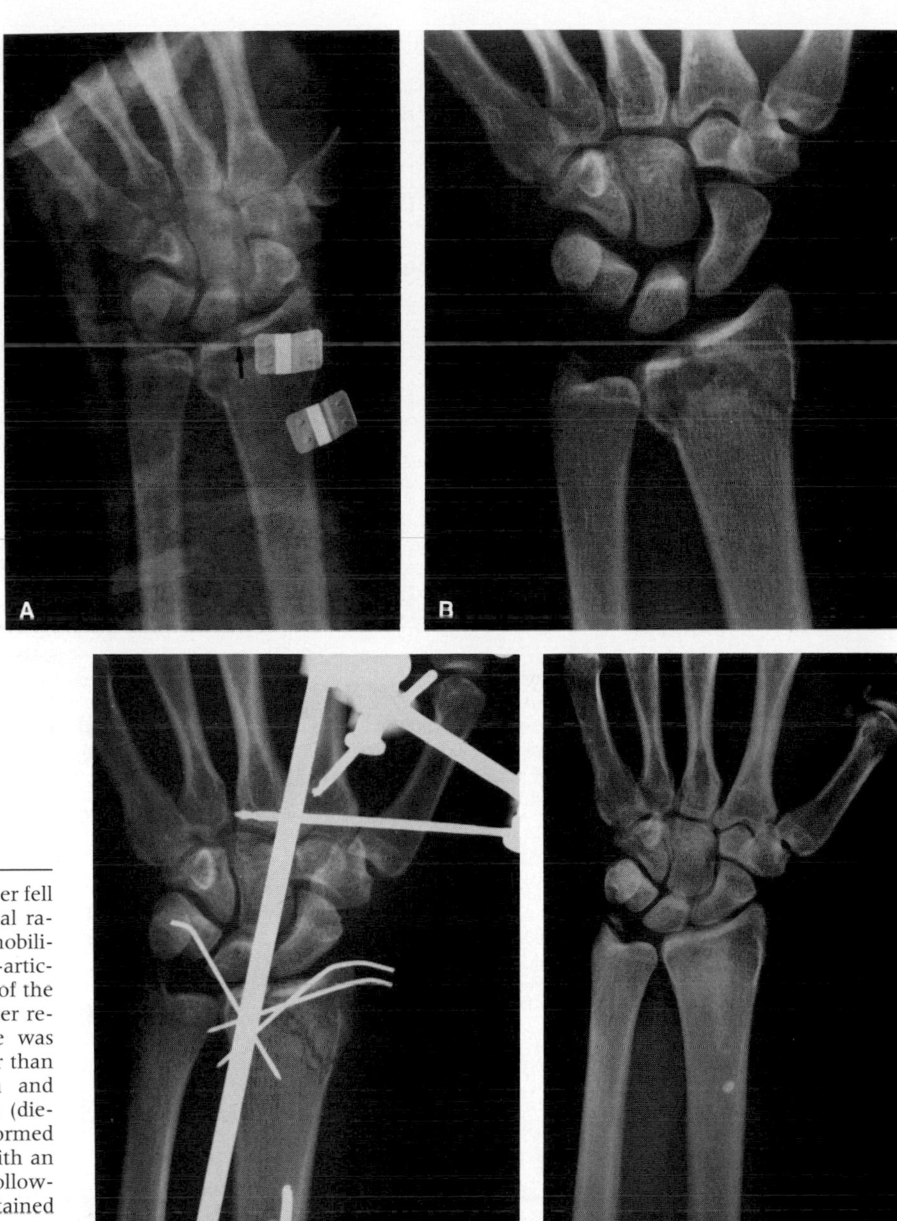

FIGURE 12-39. A 32-year-old carpenter fell from a building, fracturing his left distal radius. (**A**) Closed reduction and cast immobilization was performed. A persistent intra-articular step-off involving the lunate fossa of the distal radius was noted (*arrow*). (**B**) After rereduction with further traction, there was still an intra-articular step-off of greater than 3 mm. (**C**) Limited open reduction and K-wire fixation across the lunate fossa (die-punch) fracture component was performed under sustained traction maintained with an external fixation frame. (**D**) At 4 years follow-up, an anatomic reduction was maintained without evidence of radiocarpal arthrosis. Note the minor complication of a retained fixation pin tip.

are inherently unstable and therefore require immobilization by fixed traction. In the Frykman classification,[198] these fracture types are usually types VII and VIII, in which comminution and displacement are present in addition to intra-articular involvement. Melone has called attention to intra-articular fractures as four-part fractures of increasing severity through four types. Primary external fixation[314,477] should be considered for Universal Classification fracture types II, IVA, and IVB (see Fig. 12-29). Secondary external fixation is indicated when there is loss of reduction after cast immobilization.[113]

Factors that mitigate against adequate reduction include dorsal comminution, interposition of soft tissues palmarly, a tendency for dorsal displacement and dorsal angulation of the distal fragment to occur dynamically from soft-tissue tension, and greater radial than ulnar instability. To overcome these problems, palmar stability must be obtained by adequate locking of the palmar cortices and counterforce application to the dorsoradial compressive force. For the latter, the concept of using an external distraction apparatus is appealing. It must be remembered, however, that traction applied in this manner is not well transmitted to the dorsal rim of the radius by ligamentotaxis, because the dorsal ligaments run obliquely and tend to stretch apart rather than exert equivalent force to the distal fragment from the external fixator.[37]

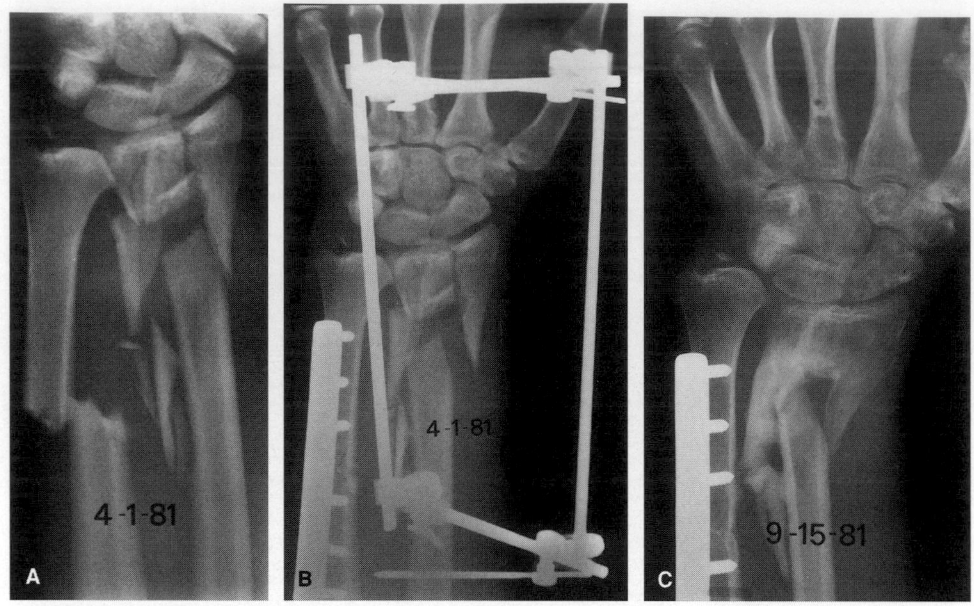

FIGURE 12-40. A comminuted open fracture of the distal radius including the radiocarpal joint and radial shaft, with displacement of the distal shaft of the ulna. (**A**) An AP x-ray prior to definitive reduction but with an air splint applied. (**B**) Treatment by closed reduction of the radius and application of an external fixator frame, compression plate fixation of the ulna, and no bone grafting. (**C**) Late collapse of the radius resulting in malunion. Prevention of deformity by early bone grafting, combined with open reduction and internal fixation of the radius, would have been indicated.

Our current preference is to accurately reduce the fracture of the distal radius acutely in the emergency department, using traction and adequate anesthesia. If the fracture is considered unstable, we schedule the patient for immediate definitive treatment in the operating room or within 48 hours, as scheduling permits. The specific method of external fixation is less important in treatment of these fractures than adhering to the principle of maintaining reduction with fixed traction (Fig. 12-41).[200,269,405,453,454,458,485] In selecting an external fixator, we prefer a half frame on the radial side of the wrist and forearm for comminuted fractures, combining Kirschner-wire fixation and bone grafting with the external fixation as necessary. Our experience has included the Hoffman C-series, Orthofix, and ASIF half-frame devices; the Roger Anderson, Mini-Hoffman (Judet), and Ace Colles quadrilateral frame devices; and the Orthologic frame.[120]

The fixation frame is assembled and tightened only after the fracture has been completely reduced. With the exception of devices designed to aid in fracture reduction (eg, Wrist Jack, Hand Biomechanics Laboratory, Sacramento, CA), we believe that the frame and pins should not be used to obtain the reduction but only provide minor adjustment in length, angulation, and rotation. The preferred sequence is longitudinal traction, insertion of half pins, fracture reduction, and assemblage of the external fixator while the wrist is maintained in traction. Newer models of lightweight radiolucent carbon frames aid in the process and allow for improved imaging of the fracture reduction. With all frames, the external fixation can be supplemented with percutaneous pins through the radial styloid for certain intra-articular fractures. A limited open reduction with the external fixation frame in position can also be performed (see p. 789). We have not had experience with external fixation frames that allow early motion through a lateral hinged joint.[106] External fixation with a mini-Hoffman frame in which the pins are placed only into the distal radius and not across the carpus has had limited application in extra-articular distal radius fractures in patients with excellent bone stock and is an acceptable alternative. Manipulation of intra-articular fragments with percutaneous pins may also be accomplished after the frame is applied. Care must be taken to avoid excessive distraction. The pins-and-plaster technique of external fixation,[107] although appealing in concept,[94] is often difficult in practice.[101,230] Application of the plaster around the pins may prolong the procedure sufficiently to prevent adequate molding of the cast.[101] Subsequent dorsal redisplacement and angulation of the distal fragment has been one factor in our dissatisfaction with the pins-and-plaster technique.

External fixation is maintained for a minimal period of 6 to 8 weeks. After removal of the external fixation

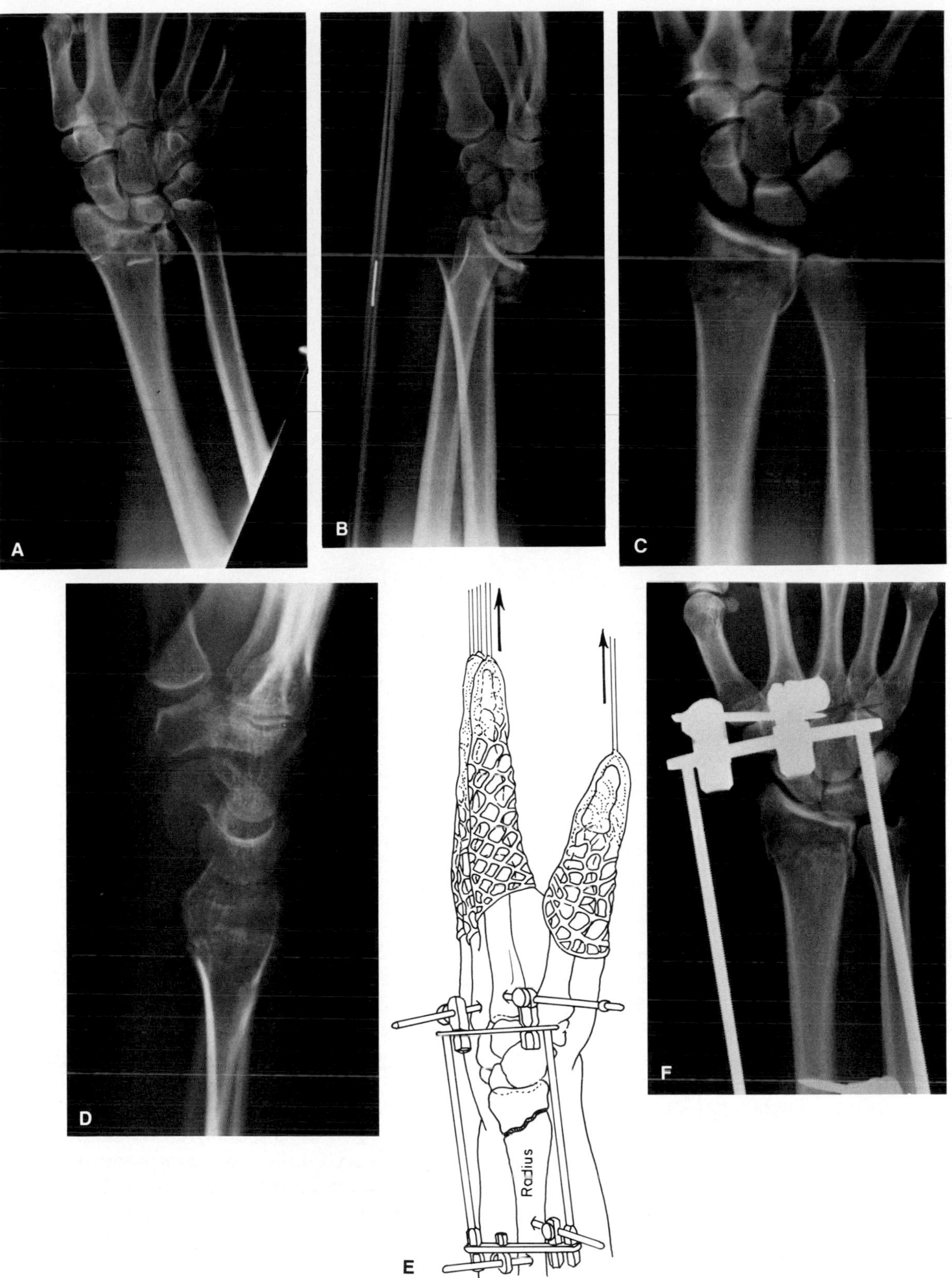

FIGURE 12-41. A 32-year-old teacher fell on ice and sustained this intra-articular distal radius fracture (type IV). (**A**) Her intra-articular fracture involved the lunate fossa of the distal radius. (**B**) Lateral view showing dorsal angulation of 65° with dorsal comminution. (**C**) Traction view, with anatomic reduction achieved. (**D**) Anatomic alignment of the palmar cortex (buttress effect). (**E**) External fixation with a quadrilateral frame was used to maintain the reduction. (**F,G**) Radiographic appearance (PA and lateral) at 4 weeks; reduction maintained. (**H,I**) End result with nearly normal anatomic alignment of the distal radius 7 months postinjury.

continues

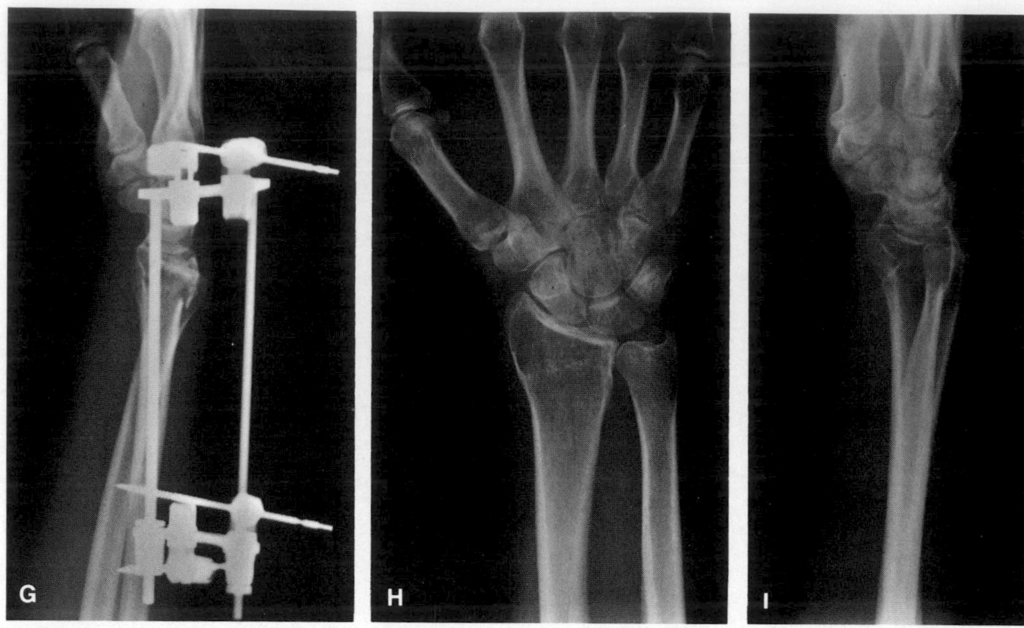

FIGURE 12-41. (continued)

frame and pins, removable splint protection is used for 2 to 3 weeks, because gentle motion is encouraged. Pins can be removed on an outpatient basis with the use of local anesthesia. Physical therapy should be considered, because distraction across the wrist may delay the return of motion and strength. Pin-tract infection and pin loosening are the major problems with this technique.[554]

Percutaneous Pin Fixation

For displaced fractures of the radius, the use of percutaneous pins[105,142,279] has been an accepted practice either alone or to supplement external fixation. Most commonly it is used with a cast or splint. Braun suggested the use of percutaneous pins to assist in obtaining palmar tilt to the distal radius and then using dorsal pin and external fixation to maintain fracture alignment.[77a] Percutaneous pins are considered for Universal Classification type II, type III, and type IVA fractures. Some surgeons use pins when slippage in the cast is a concern or when the patient is considered unreliable.

A number of techniques have been described. Steinmann pins can be placed down the radial shaft, so that one is inserted through the styloid and the other through the dorsoulnar corner of the distal fragment as intramedullary fixation. The tension produced in the pins as they deflect against the proximal cortices effectively maintains reduction. The ends of the pins are bent at a right angle and are connected with a small metal clamp to prevent rotation.

A second technique involves passing Kirschner wires through the radial styloid with the wrist in traction. The pins are drilled proximally through the radial styloid until they penetrate the intact cortex of the shaft.[105] Kirschner wires of 0.045- to 0.0625-inch diameter are selected, with smaller pins for women and larger pins for men. The pin insertion is performed with a power Kirschner-wire driver to allow the surgeon to hold part of the reduction with one hand during the Kirschner-wire insertion. Variations include drilling first through the ulna until the pin reaches the inner cortex of the radial styloid[142] or drilling through the radial styloid until it is completely through the ulna (Rayhack technique) (see Fig. 12-36**A**). Above-elbow cast or splint immobilization must be used if the pins pass between the radius and ulna.

Another method of percutaneous pin fixation is the intrafocal pin technique of Kapandji (see Fig. 12-37).[279] In this technique, the Kirschner wires are introduced into the fracture site itself, rather than through the distal fracture fragment. The Kirschner wire can be used to wedge open the fracture reduction and then to prevent the distal fragments from redisplacement. A total of four Kirschner wires are used with this technique (two dorsal and two volar). Kapandji's original technique involved "feeling for the fracture site" with the tip of the K-wire, followed by manual insertion; however, we prefer image intensification fluoroscopy to assist the insertion. X-rays confirm pin placement. All such procedures are carried out under full sterile preparation and draping. Either overhead traction or a lateral traction arm board can be used. After insertion, the Kirschner wires are cut short outside the skin and capped. A sponge padding with an occlusive dressing prevents skin irritation. A short-arm cast is worn for 3 to 6 weeks, depending on the degree of fracture stability. In some cases the cast can be removed at 3 weeks, a splint applied, and radiocarpal motion started with the pins in place. Some authors recommend windowing the cast and making stress-relieving skin incisions if swelling results in pin-site irritation. Careful patient follow-up is needed with all three of these techniques.

Percutaneous pin fixation is an excellent technique, provided the distal radius is not severely comminuted or osteoporotic, because the trabecular bone of the metaphysis provides little inherent stability. It is especially useful for unstable fractures, both extra-articular and intra-articular, in combination with external fixation.

Open Reduction

One of the recent advances in the treatment of distal radius fractures is the more frequent application of open reduction and internal fixation, especially for intra-articular fractures (Fig. 12-42).[29,32,38,303,362,368a,480]

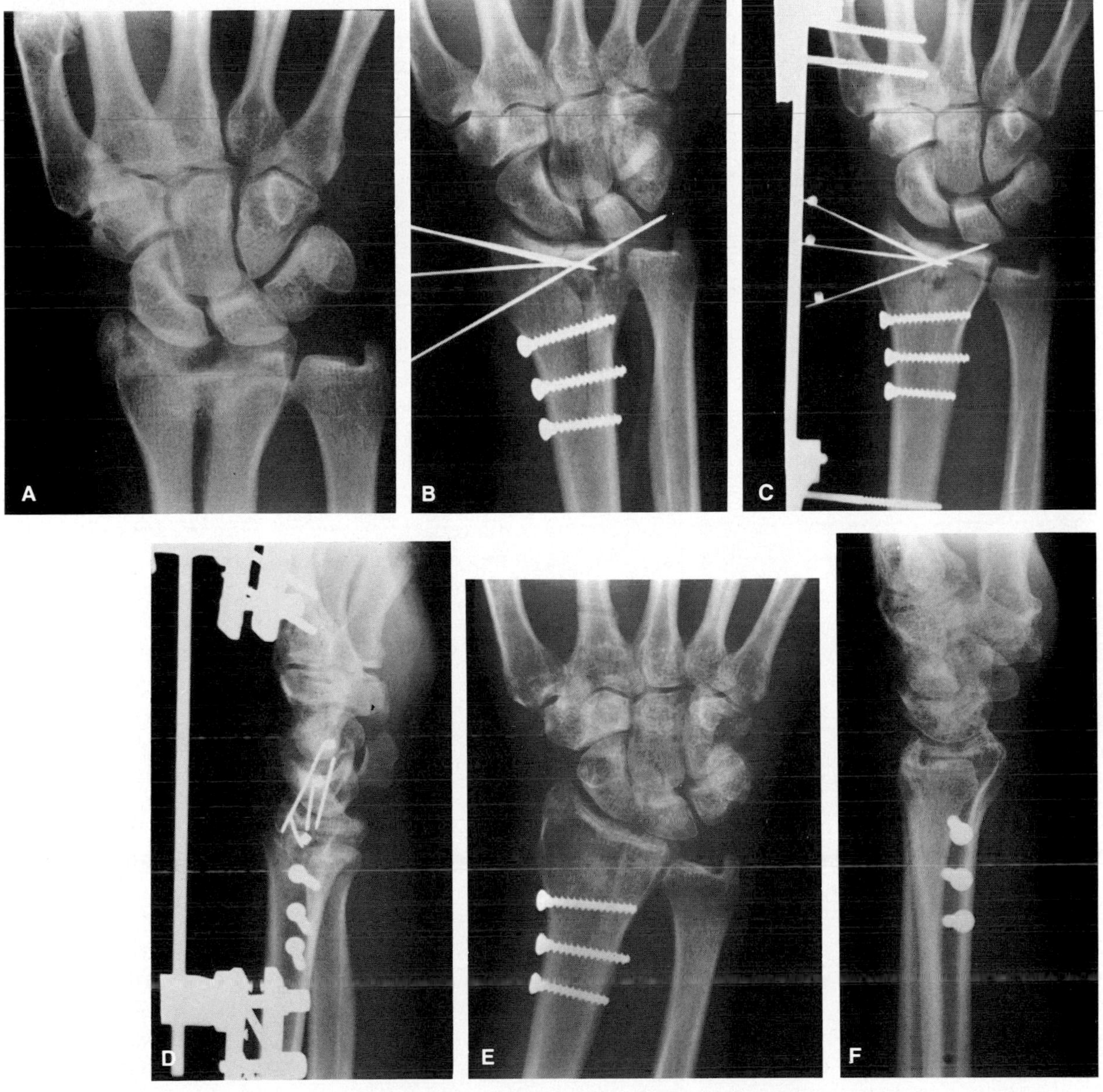

FIGURE 12-42. A displaced intra-articular fracture in a 43-year-old motorcyclist was treated with open reduction and internal and external fixation. (**A**) Extensive intra-articular involvement of the scaphoid and lunate fossae with a longitudinal split component. (**B**) After open reduction, the articular fracture component was fixed with K-wires, and the shaft fracture component was transfixed with cortical bone screws. (**C,D**) An external fixation frame was used for 3 weeks to maintain distraction across the carpus and to prevent compression of the articular surface of the distal radius. Motion of the radiocarpal joint was started at 6 weeks. (**E,F**) At follow-up, the articular surface reduction was maintained without evidence of radiocarpal joint abnormality.

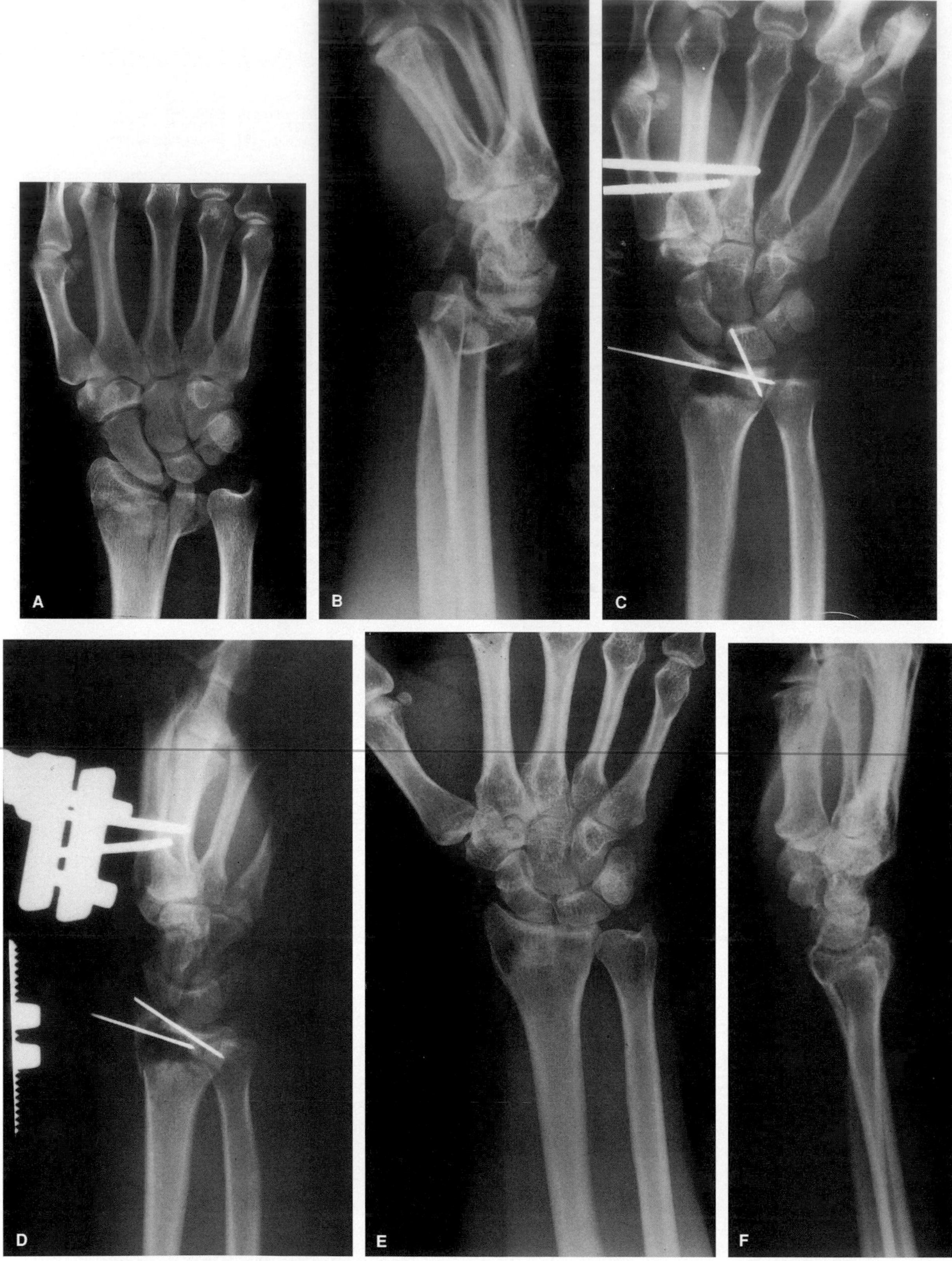

FIGURE 12-43. A comminuted intra-articular fracture of the distal radius. (**A,B**) Melone Type III split fracture of the lunate fossa of the distal radius with severe comminution, dorsal angulation and radial shortening. (**C,D**) After traction, external fixation and open reduction of the joint articular surface and restoration of the lunate fossa held with K-wires (note bone loss). (**E,F**) Fifteen months after treatment. Normal alignment of the articular surface of the distal radius; restoration of radial length and dorsal-palmar tilt. *(From Bradway, J.; Arnadio, P.C.; Cooney, W.P.: J Bone Joint Surg. 71:839–847, 1989.)*

The primary indication is articular fragment displacement,[219] which, if left unreduced, leads to radiocarpal or radioulnar arthritis. Although the magnitude of forces across the wrist joint is not known, some investigators have estimated these at 10 to 12 times the grip force. Strenuous activity may require withstanding over 500 pounds of compressive force. Thus, accurate reduction of the intra-articular joint surfaces should be considered along with factors of age, occupation, and activity level during the decision as to whether fracture alignment can best be obtained with closed or open reduction.

The options for open reduction include a longitudinal dorsal approach, a volar approach, a limited transverse dorsal approach, or reduction under arthroscopic control.

Open reduction is preferred when joint incongruity is evident by articular surface displacement of more than 2 mm (see Fig. 12-42).[38,76] For a dorsally displaced fracture, a limited dorsal transverse incision is used, distracting the wrist either in traction or with an external fixator. The extensor retinaculum between the third and fourth extensor compartments is reflected, and the wrist capsule is divided in line with the skin incision. A nerve hook, Freer elevator, or percutaneously placed pins can be used to elevate the joint fracture fragments. If there is more than 4 to 5 mm of impaction, a bone graft from the iliac crest or an allograft is recommended to fill the metaphyseal defect (Fig. 12-43). Early return of wrist motion with removal of external fixation at 3 to 4 weeks has been reported after bone grafting of acute distal radius fractures.

The choice of fixation depends on the fracture configuration.[314] External fixation supplemented with Kirschner wires that hold the intra-articular fracture components is preferred (see Fig. 12-40). A mini-plate (AO/ASIF) is chosen when more proximal comminution is present or for depressed fractures involving primarily the lunate fossa of the distal radius (Melone type IV) (Fig. 12-44).[219,265] The dorsal approach for plate fixation involves a longitudinal incision, reflection of the extensor retinaculum, removal of Lister's tubercle, and subperiosteal exposure of the fracture (Fig. 12-45). Temporary Kirschner-wire fixation while the defect is packed with a bone graft is usually necessary before application of a mini T-plate. Distal comminution precludes the use of screws in the distal fragment. For the lunate fossa fracture (die-punch fracture) both Kirschner wires and small AO plates have been used to maintain the reduction. Bone graft is often required when internal fixation is performed because a loss of cancellous bone is generally present.

A palmarly displaced fracture of Smith's or palmar Barton's type is better approached through a palmar incision, with application of a buttress plate as described by Ellis (see Fig. 12-38).[166] The incision is made through a proximally extended carpal tunnel incision, with reflection of the pronator quadratus from the radius. The plate is contoured to fit the metaphyseal curvature, and distal fragment screws are rarely indicated. This approach may also be necessary to retrieve muscle, tendon,[399] or periosteum that is entrapped and preventing reduction of a dorsally angulated fracture. A displaced volar spike (Melone type III) fracture may also require a volar approach with internal fixation with a mini fragment condylar plate (Fernandez).

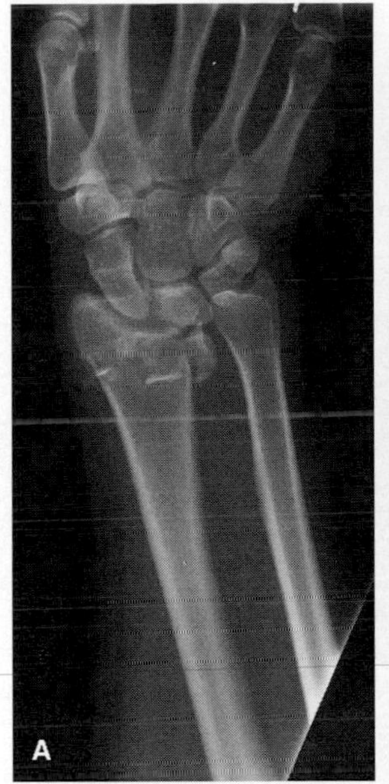

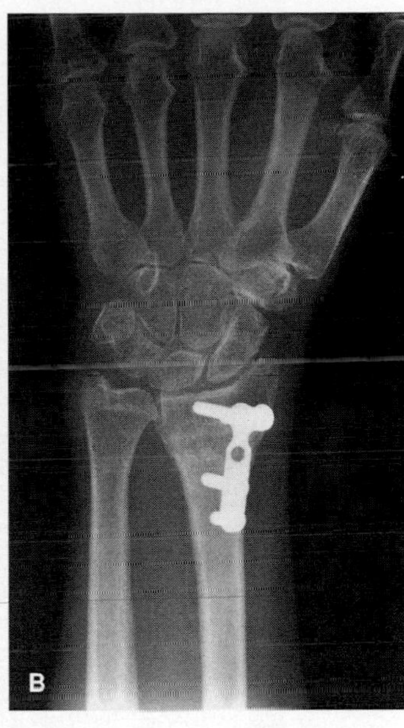

FIGURE 12-44. (**A**) An intra-articular fracture of the distal radius involving the lunate fossa (Melone Type IV). Note displacement of the articular surface ulnarly including the sigmoid notch of the distal radioulnar joint. (**B**) Open reduction and internal fixation was performed through a dorsal approach. A mini-ASIF plate was applied to hold reduction of the lunate fossa.

During open reduction of the distal radius, the surgeon needs to examine the articular surface reduction of the radioscaphoid and radiolunate joints and the DRUJ and treat each appropriately. There is little indication for primary excision of the distal ulna.[148]

Barton's Fracture. A palmar Barton (Smith III) is ideally treated by a palmar buttress plate.[29,30] A dorsal Barton (intra articular Colles) is best treated by closed reduction and external fixation if an adequate reduction can be maintained.[141] Otherwise, open reduction and percutaneous pins, compressive screws, or a dorsal buttress plate can be used.[432,534] Arthroscopic reduction of dorsal Barton's fracture offers an alternative that limits exposure of the dorsal carpus and that may help to maintain blood supply to the dorsal fracture components. Skill in wrist arthroscopy is required for this type of procedure.

Chauffeur's Fracture. The radial styloid fracture can

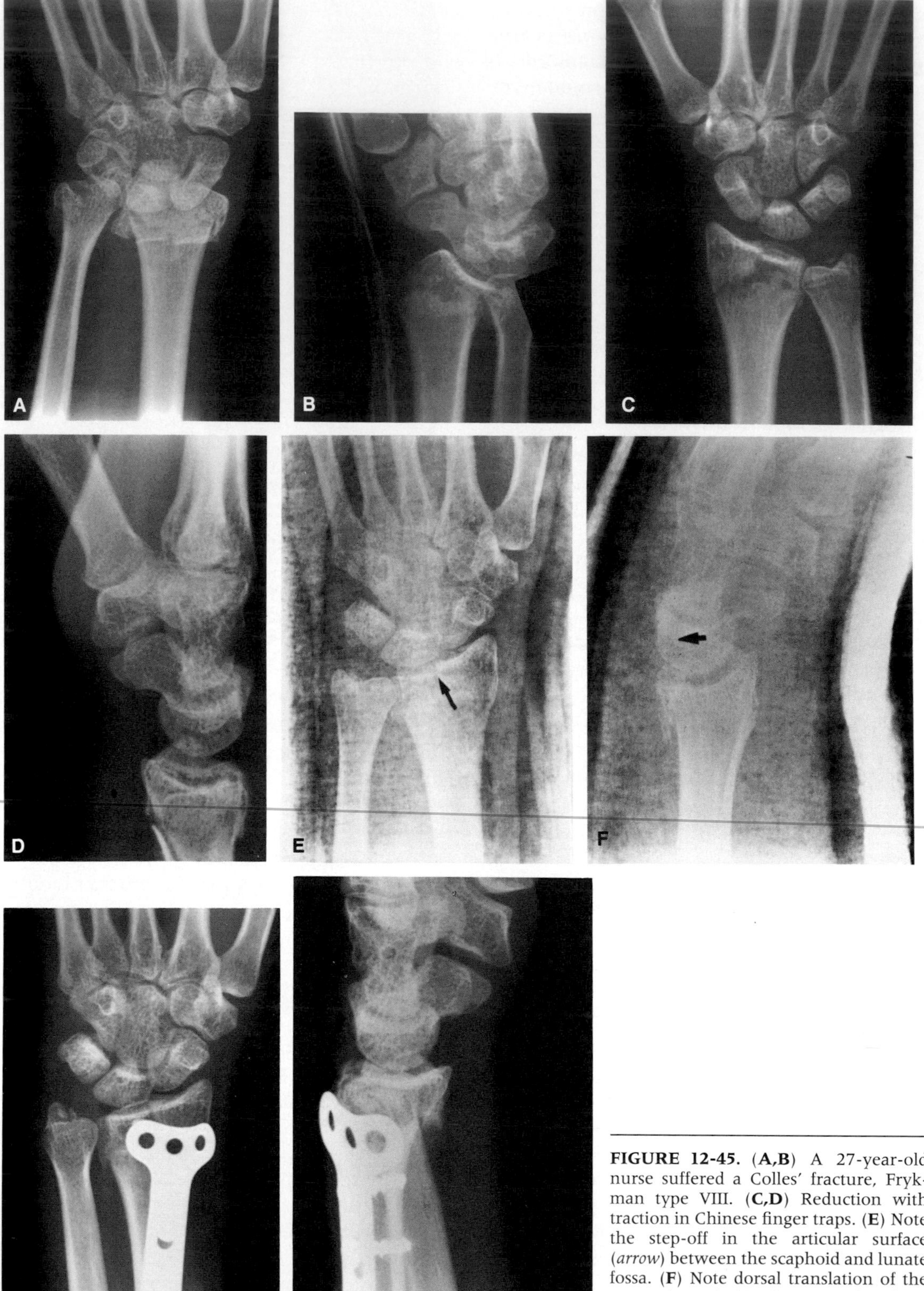

FIGURE 12-45. (**A,B**) A 27-year-old nurse suffered a Colles' fracture, Frykman type VIII. (**C,D**) Reduction with traction in Chinese finger traps. (**E**) Note the step-off in the articular surface (*arrow*) between the scaphoid and lunate fossa. (**F**) Note dorsal translation of the carpus (*arrow*). (**G,H**) Improved realignment of the articular surface following open reduction.

usually be treated with closed reduction and percutaneous pin fixation. If, however, the fracture is displaced more than 3 mm, there may be an associated scapholunate[39] dissociation for which we would favor open reduction, repair of the ligament, and anatomical reduction of the radial styloid. Percutaneous pins that, at most, penetrate only two cortices are subject to erosive loosening within the trabecular bone of the metaphysis; therefore, trabecular screws may offer greater security for fixation. Very accurate anatomical alignment is essential to prevent secondary post-traumatic arthrosis.

Smith's Fracture. Open reduction and internal fixation (or external fixation) is the treatment of choice for palmar displaced fractures, especially the intra-articular types II and III.[336,524] External fixation for open Smith's fractures is acceptable for wound considerations.[113] Careful reduction with radiographic control and supplemental Kirschner wires may be needed for Smith's type II fractures, to ensure anatomical alignment of the radiocarpal joint.[166] It is rarely necessary to have distal screws in using the buttress plate for most Smith fractures, and there is a risk of screws penetrating either the radiocarpal joint or extruding dorsally to affect the wrist and finger extensor tendons. A mini fragment plate is the exception to the general rule.

CARPAL INSTABILITIES

Severe wrist injuries with dislocation or fracture–dislocation often develop a wrist instability pattern after spontaneous or manipulative relocation.[272,481] The perilunate dislocation pattern provides a whole spectrum of wrist sprains, fractures, dislocations, and instabilities (Fig. 12-46).[229,272,330,514,478,525] This injury pattern usually begins radially and destabilizes through the body of the scaphoid (scaphoid fracture) or through the scapholunate interval (ie, SLD).[354] Further destabilization passes distal between the capitate and lunate, either through the space of Poirier between the proximal and distal palmar V-ligaments or through the capitate (transcapitate fracture), and then ulnar to the lunate, either through hamate and triquetrum or through the lunatotriquetral interval.[354–356] This type of perilunate dislocation usually results in a DISI collapse pattern, because the stabilizing influence of the scaphoid is lost first and foremost.

A similar pattern of destabilization can begin ulnarly and propagate radialward around the lunate, such that the lunate is first dissociated from the triquetrum.[449,530,538] The lunate may retain sufficient bonding to the scaphoid that the residual collapse pattern is VISI. Both of these collapse patterns are dissociative (ie, CID) because there is disruption of the ligament bond or the bone structure between the lunate and one or both of the adjacent carpal bones (ie, SLD, LTD, or lunatocapitate dissociation).[118]

Radiocarpal dislocation is a less common injury, sometimes ligamentous only, but more commonly includes a fragment of the radius. It is recognized and traditionally called either a palmar or dorsal Barton fracture–dislocation or as radiocarpal subluxation or dislocation. Either a VISI or DISI instability is possible, and it may be either dissociative or nondissociative, depending on the degree of damage

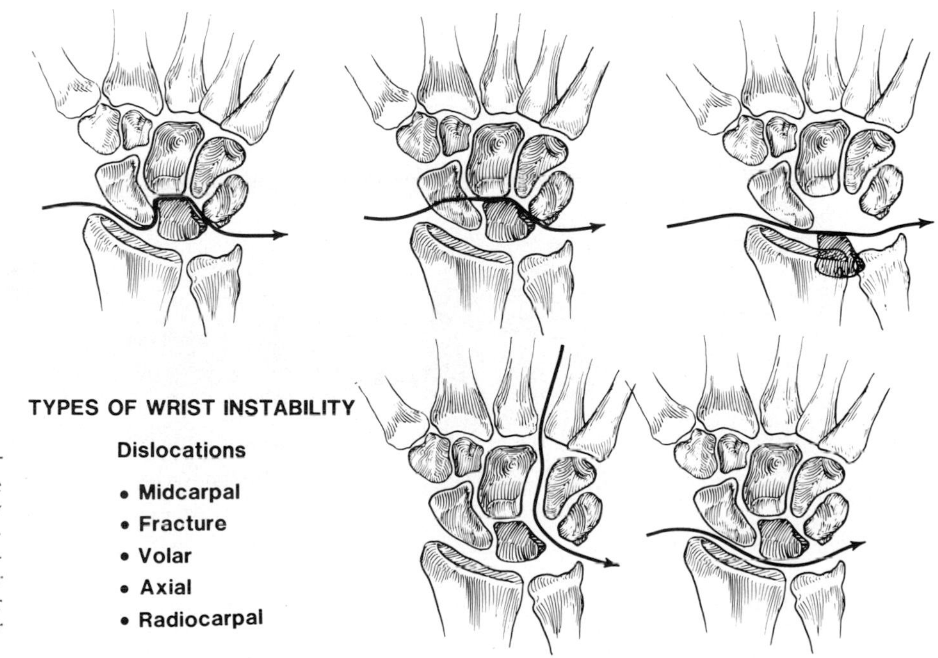

FIGURE 12-46. Types of perilunate dislocations. Perilunate dislocations may be purely ligamentous dislocations (*upper left*); fracture-dislocations (*upper center*); volar lunate dislocations (*upper right*); axial dislocations (*lower left*); or pure radiocarpal dislocations (*lower right*).

done to the ligamentous bonds of the proximal carpal row.

There are three other radiocarpal instabilities: ulnar translation of the entire carpus, dorsal translation instabilities, and occasionally volar translation instabilities.[447,470,472] Combinations of these instabilities may occur, although one deformity pattern is usually predominant. The basic patterns are similar in instability, dislocation, and fracture–dislocation, suggesting a spectrum of problems that arise as variations occur in the linkage system within the carpus (see Table 12-1). Using these concepts, it is possible to group all known injuries that result in carpal instability into interrelated categories.

TABLE 12-4
Carpal Instability Evaluation Plan

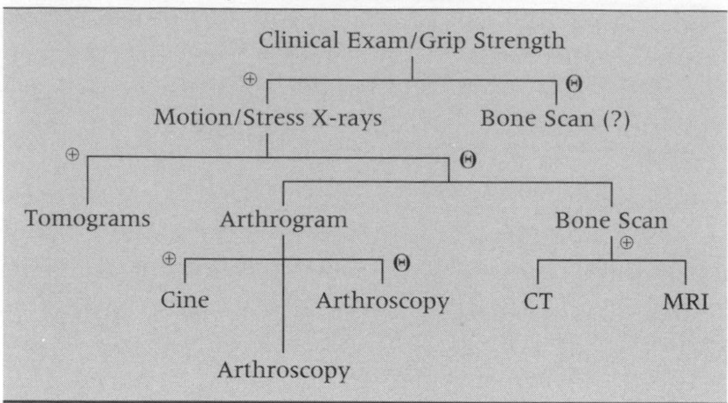

Signs and Symptoms

A general evaluation plan is needed to assess carpal instability (Table 12-4). The most constant and dependable sign of carpal injury is well-localized tenderness. Fractures of the scaphoid, for example, are most tender to pressure in the anatomical snuffbox. Scapholunate and lunate injuries cause tenderness just distal to Lister's tubercle (Fig. 12-47**A**).[238] Triquetral, lunatotriquetral, and triquetrohamate ligament injuries result in tenderness over the dorsal margin of the appropriate bone, usually a fingerbreadth distal to the ulnar head. Other clinical findings are highly variable and depend on the extent of carpal disruption, with more traumatic carpal disruption seen in perilunate dislocations. Tenderness and swelling are general rather than localized. There may be swelling that is severe and generalized or discrete and barely detectable. Changes in alignment of the hand, wrist, and forearm may be clinically evident on inspection of the extremity. Swelling over the proximal carpal row is suggestive of a ligament avulsion with or without a chip fracture. Marked prominence of the entire carpus dorsally is suggestive of a perilunate dislocation. Compressive stresses applied actively or passively may produce pain at the site of damage (see Fig. 12-47**B**) and result in snaps, clicks, shifts, and thuds, which are palpable and audible.[102,229]

Provocative Stress Tests

There are several clinical stress tests that assist in the diagnosis of carpal instability diagnosis.[102,222,474] For scapholunate instability, these include (1) the scaphoid lift test, which is a reproduction of pain with dorsal-palmar shifting of the scaphoid; (2) the Watson test,[550] which is painful dorsal scaphoid displacement instability as the wrist is moved from ulnar to radial deviation with the tuberosity compressed; and (3) the bone

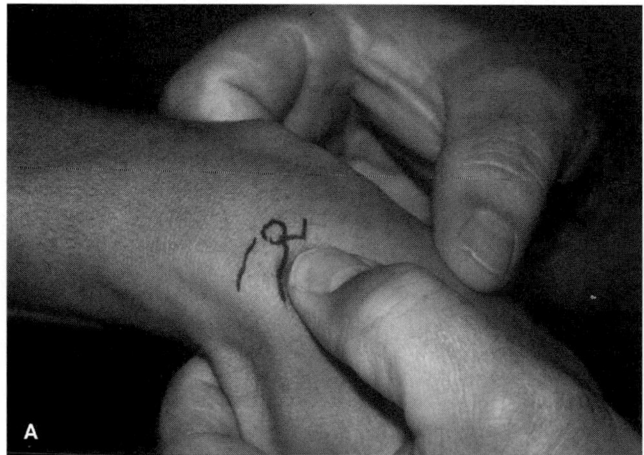

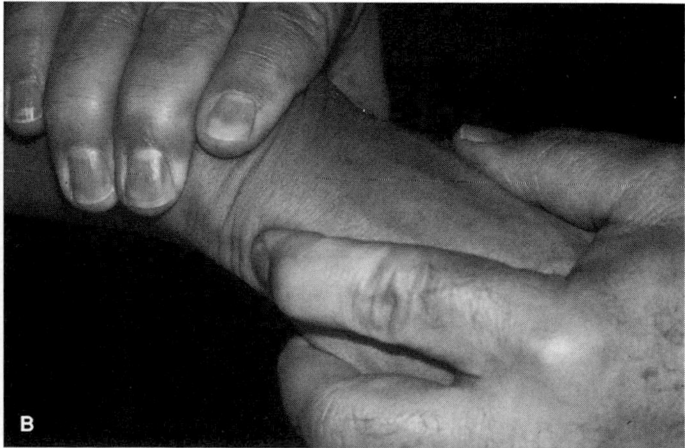

FIGURE 12-47. Clinical examination of the wrist. (**A**) Palpation over the scaphoid and lunate just distal to Lister's tubercle that produces pain in patients with a ganglion cyst or scapholunate dissociation. (**B**) Tenderness in the snuffbox just distal to the radial styloid is suggestive of a scaphoid fracture.

scaphoid shift test,[309a] which leads the distal scaphoid to subluxate the proximal scaphoid.

For lunatotriquetral instability, there is the ballottement test (also called shear or shuck test), in which the triquetrum is displaced dorsally and palmarly on the lunate, demonstrating increased excursion over the normal side and often a painful crepitus. The compression test is a similar displacement of the triquetrum ulnarly during radioulnar deviation, which is also painful. A lax ligamentous habitus is often associated with the ability to subluxate the midcarpal joint by displacing the carpometacarpal unit on the radiocarpal.[509,510] Tendon displacements with audible snaps are easily produced by some persons but are seldom symptomatic.

Distraction can be a good clue to a "lax wrist" or a damaged area, particularly when viewed under fluoroscopic imaging with static traction (approximately 25 pounds) applied. Stress loading the wrist with compression and motion from radial to ulnar deviation may simulate midcarpal instability and produce a "catch-up clunk" as the proximal row of carpal bones snap from a flexion to an extension stance. These and the other movement abnormalities must be correlated with history, clinical findings, and radiologic findings to provide a proper diagnosis.[345]

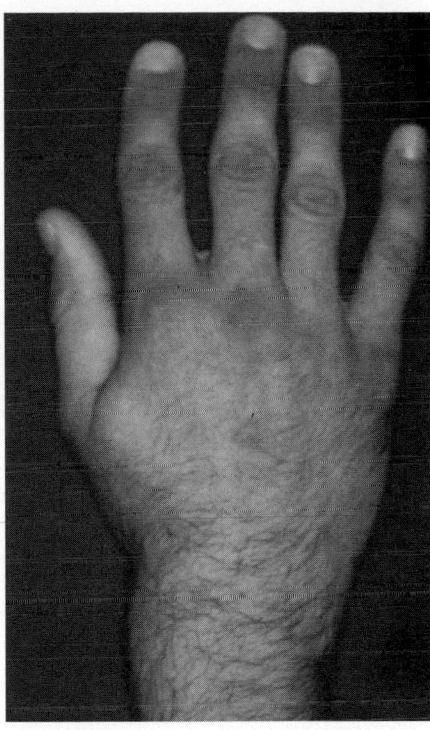

FIGURE 12-49. Clinical appearance of ulnar translocation of the carpus. Note prominence of the radial styloid and ulnar displacement of the carpus.

Post-Traumatic Carpal Instability

Carpal instability was introduced as a category of injury to the wrist in the first edition of this text (1975), emphasizing the traumatic causes. Subsequent experience has expanded its utility and applicability to the point that most wrist injuries can now be appreciated as having an element of carpal instability. First-degree sprains and fractures are usually not associated with instability,[328] but prior trauma, congenital laxity, inflammation, or disease may elevate even these injuries into the instability category. Second- and third-degree sprains, dislocations, and fracture–dislocations are likely to develop carpal instability.[540a] The clinical groups to be discussed that we consider post-traumatic carpal instability are radiocarpal, perilunate, midcarpal, and axial injuries. DRUJ injuries are discussed separately.

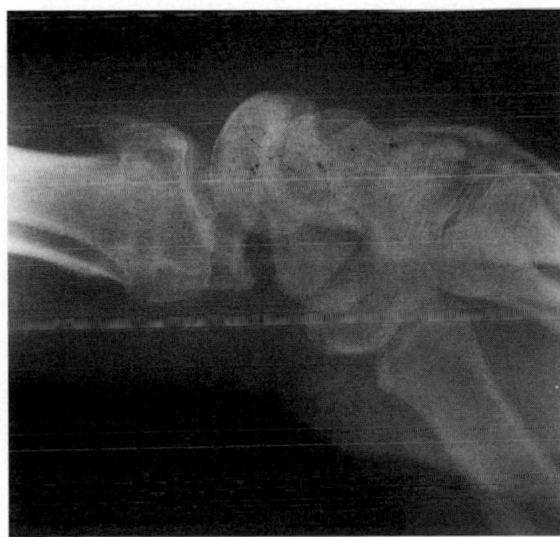

FIGURE 12-48. Dorsal radiocarpal instability following a dorsally angulated fracture of the distal radius. The lunate has displaced (subluxated) dorsally with secondary palmar flexion of the capitate to maintain the wrist and hand in alignment.

Radiocarpal Instability

Radiocarpal instability is an injury that results in loss of alignment of the proximal carpal row with the distal radius (Fig. 12-48). Diagnosis of these injuries is made from a history of appropriate trauma followed by the usual initial findings of swelling, deformity, tenderness, and pain. Swelling and tenderness are most noticeable dorsally at the radiocarpal level and aggravated by wrist motions. Deformity may be an ulnar, dorsal, or palmar shift of the carpus. For definitive diagnosis, some deformity should be visible on standard x-rays, although provocative stress may be required to demonstrate dynamic (rather than static) radiocarpal instability.

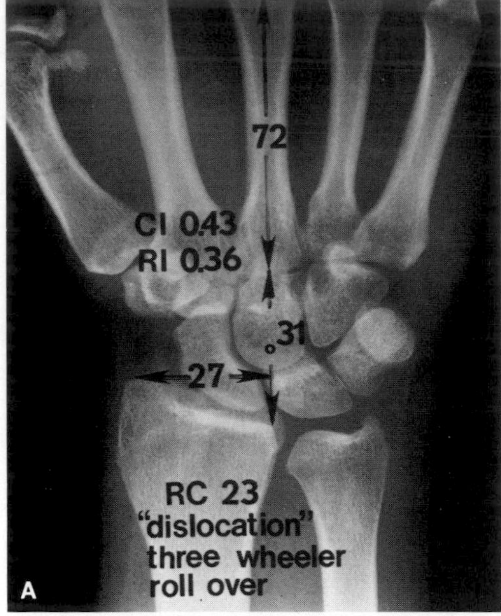

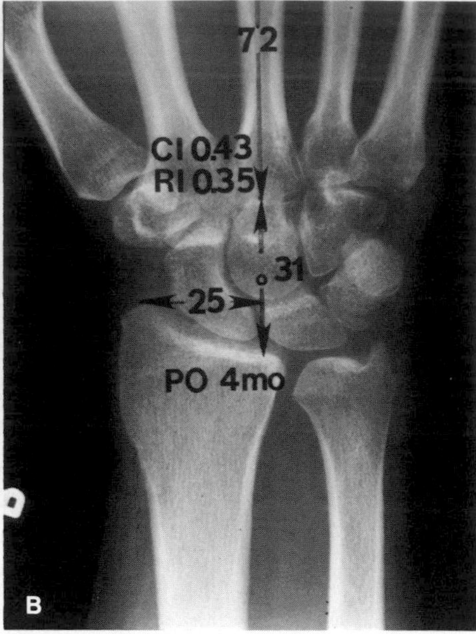

FIGURE 12-50. Ulnar translation. (**A**) A 23-year-old man who was injured in an all-terrain vehicle rollover. Note lunate displacement and increased radioscaphoid gap. Increased ulnar translation index (radiostyloid capitate head distance/length third metacarpal, Chamay). (**B**) Four months postoperatively there is partial recurrence of the ulnar translation after repair of the radiolunate and radiocapitate ligaments to the radial styloid.

The most common injuries at the radiocarpal joint are the well-known fracture–dislocations of the distal radius and carpus[475]; these are commonly known as palmar and dorsal Barton's fracture-dislocations, radial styloid fracture–dislocations (chauffeur's) (see Fractures of the Distal Radius), and die-punch fracture–dislocations. Less common are the pure ligamentous radiocarpal injuries,[56] which may destabilize the wrist in one of three directions—ulnarly, as ulnar translation; dorsally, as dorsal translation; or palmarly, as palmar translation.[118,228] True dislocations without fracture of the bony margins are rare, and they may sometimes spontaneously reduce, making it even more difficult to demonstrate them. However, they are occasionally seen in unreduced, dramatic fashion with the carpus dorsal to the radius, palmar to the radius, or ulnar to the radius.

Ulnar translation is the most frequent radiocarpal instability (Fig. 12-49). It may occur acutely, develop gradually, or be observed as a late residua or sequela of a perilunate dislocation.[447] It may occur after radiocarpal level injury, where the radiocarpal ligaments are avulsed from their styloidal origins, or after perilunate injury. Clinically, the carpus and hand are offset ulnarly (see Fig. 12-49). The radiographic appearance is often dramatic, with the lunate positioned just distal to the ulna and a large space between the radial styloid and the scaphoid (Fig. 12-50). If the perilunate destabilization is also involved, the lunate and triquetrum slide ulnarly, opening a gap between scaphoid and lunate. In some cases the ulnar shift is subtle, and a decrease in the ulnocarpal index (Chamay[100]) may provide the only clue to diagnosis (see Fig. 12-20). Ulnar translation is also commonly seen in diseases

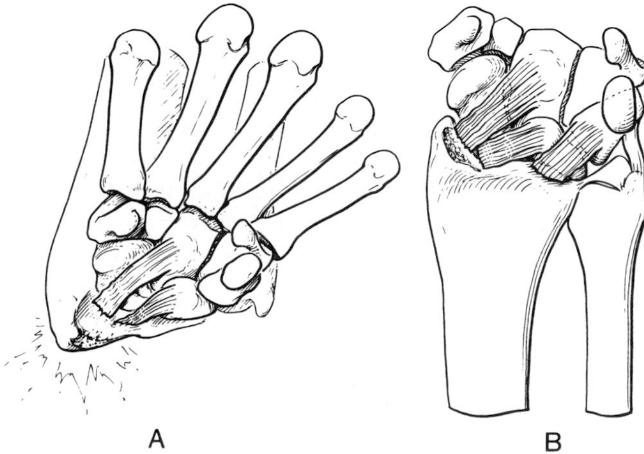

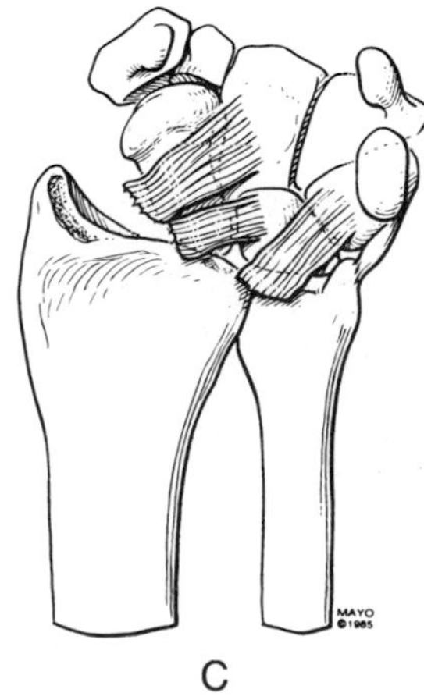

FIGURE 12-51. Ligament damage associated with carpal dislocations. Radiocarpal ligaments are torn or avulsed from the palmar radial aspect of the distal radius, leading to dorsal or ulnar (or both) displacement of the carpus.

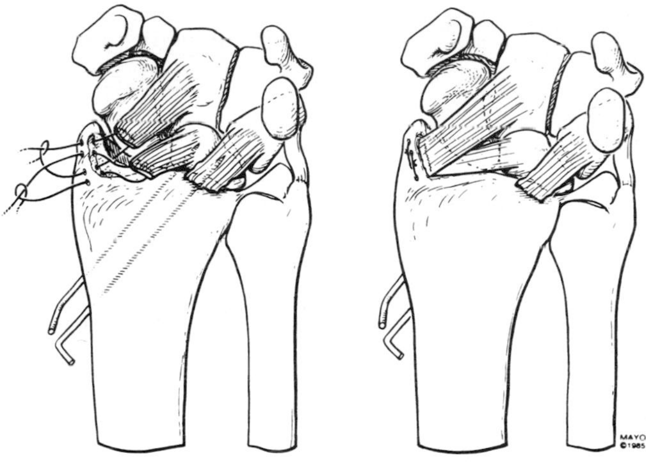

FIGURE 12-52. Method of repair of the radiocarpal ligaments to the radial styloid following reduction and K-wire stabilization to the lunate (for ulnar translation).

such as rheumatoid arthritis and in developmental deformities such as Madelung's deformity.

Dorsal translation of the carpus and ulnar translation can be seen in two modes: one a true instability secondary to ligament damage (Fig. 12-51), the other an apparent instability due to a carpal shift in response to a change in position of the distal radial articular surface (see Fig. 12-48). Ulnar translation may occur with an increase in the radial to ulnar slope of the distal radius. Dorsal translation usually occurs after a loss of the normal palmar slope of the distal radius from a flexion angle to an extension angle. The latter is a common problem after collapse of a distal radius fracture. The degree of shift of the carpus in response to the new extension slope of the distal radial surface depends to some extent on laxity of the carpal support ligaments or injury to those ligaments, but even a normal carpus will reposition itself on the changed slope of the distal radius in such a fashion as to maintain the hand parallel to the forearm.

Treatment of Radiocarpal Instability

Unusual dislocations of the radiocarpal joint require immediate reduction, because the deformity of such a dislocation threatens neurovascular structures in the area. Whereas reduction is possible,[556] maintaining or holding the reduction is difficult. We believe that open treatment, both dorsal and palmar, should be considered in most carpal dislocations, because residual deformity after these injuries is almost universal. In the acute situation, repair of the damaged extrinsic ligament systems both palmarly and dorsally, along with temporary percutaneous wires for 6 to 8 weeks, is nec-

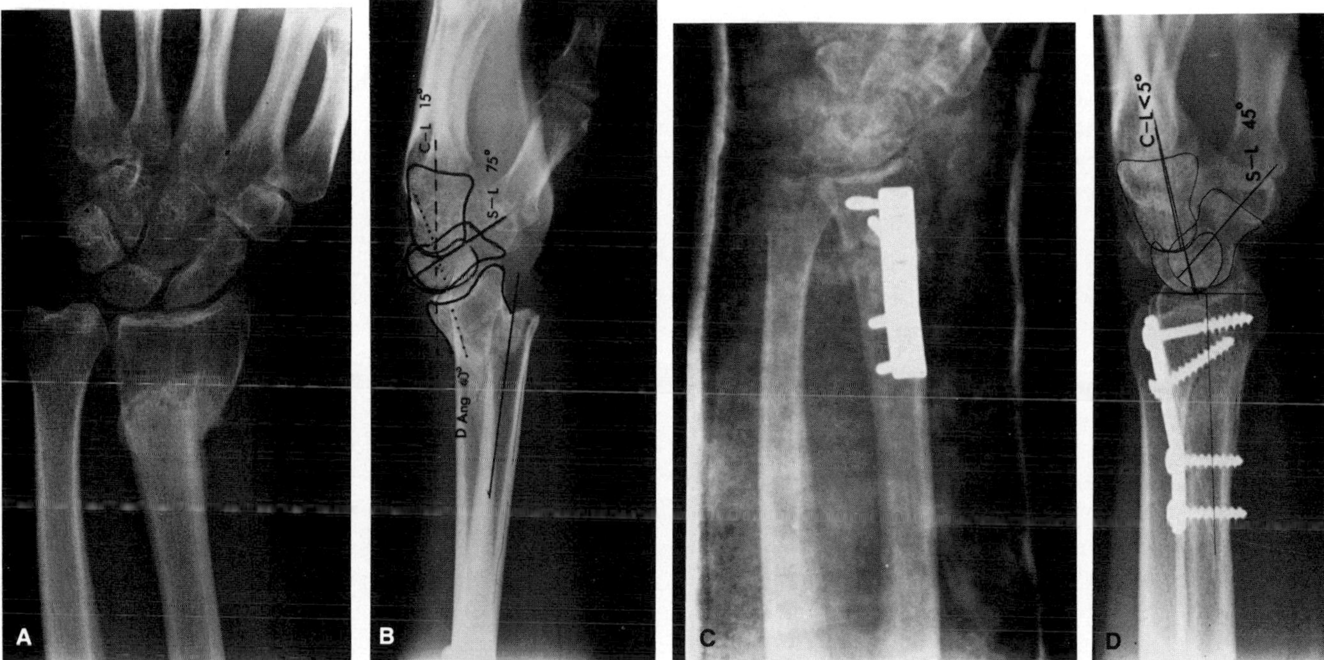

FIGURE 12-53. Corrective osteotomy for malunion of the distal radius. (**A**) Shortening and radial deviation of the distal radius (PA view) and (**B**) dorsal angulation and DRUJ subluxation (lateral view) associated with wrist pain and weakness of grasp. Radiocarpal and midcarpal angulation measurements show a radiocarpal (*RC*) angle of 40° from neutral, and scapholunate (*SL*) angle of 75°. (**C**) Corrective osteotomy and interposition iliac crest graft restored radial length. (**D**) Lateral x-ray shows slight carpal instability. Note improvement in the radiocarpal and scapholunate angles. The patient's symptoms were significantly improved.

essary to avoid late displacement and loss of carpal reduction. We also prefer operative ligament repair (Fig. 12-52) for those conditions that do not initially manifest as a complete dislocation but are diagnosed sometime afterward by an ulnar shift of the carpus.

If the carpal shift is the result of the dorsal radial articular surface, the best management is complete reduction and immobilization of the distal radial fracture by Kirschner wires or appropriate condylar or T-plates. One should be certain that the reduction also results in realignment of the carpus, because additional carpal ligament injury is possible.

Late cases of distal radius fracture deformity may require corrective osteotomy and bone graft to restore the position of the radial articular surface (Fig. 12-53). Late identification of ulnar translation deformity or dorsal or palmar translation deformity has responded poorly to ligament repairs.[447] The most certain method of controlling possible recurrence of deformity is to carry out a partial or total radiocarpal arthrodesis. Radiolunate fusion has been our preferred technique for this situation, although the variabilities of joint surface damage may suggest radioscaphoid fusion in some cases and radioscapholunate fusion in others.[326] The latter is usually indicated in the combinations of radiocarpal and perilunate destabilization.

Perilunate Instability

Perilunate instability is an injury (ligament or fracture) that occurs around the lunate bone that usually remains aligned with the distal radius (see Fig. 12-13). Perilunate injuries are the most common of the carpal instability patterns.[2,114] These injuries present as pure ligament injuries (ie, SLD and LTD)[64,66]; as perilunate dislocations[6,21,30,55]; and as transosseous, perilunate fracture–dislocations (transscaphoid, perilunate dislocations; transradiostyloid, perilunate dislocations; and transscaphoid, transcapitate, perilunate dislocations).[60,114,176] The two pure ligament injuries SLD[338] and LTD[449] usually occur alone; they may follow, however, incomplete treatment of perilunate SLD[338] and LTD,[449] dislocations or fracture–dislocations. They may also occur in conjunction with other regional injuries such as SLD with fractures of the distal radius, with Kienböck's disease, with scaphoid fractures, or as LTD with ulnocarpal impingement or TFCC tears. Such combinations modify treatment priorities. Here we consider each entity alone, as if no associations are present.

Scapholunate Dissociation

Representing a ligament analogue of the scaphoid fracture, this injury is the most common and most significant ligament injury of the wrist. It is a spectrum of injury ranging from grade I sprains through all gradations of ligament destabilization to scaphoid disloca-

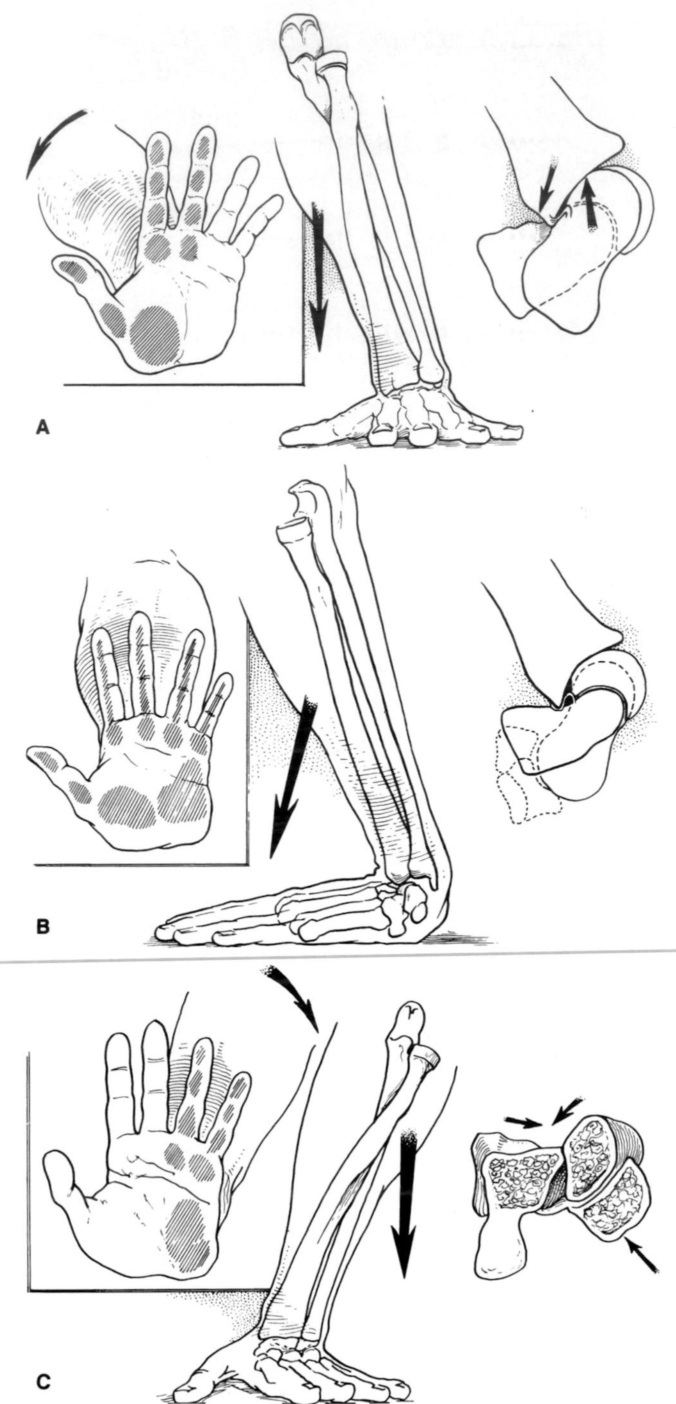

FIGURE 12-54. Mechanism of perilunate ligament injuries. (**A**) Dorsiflexion, pronation, and radial deviation load across the radioscaphoid fossa. Torque continues to the ulnar side of wrist. Scaphoid fracture, lunatotriquetral ligament tear, or transscaphoid perilunate dislocation may result. (**B**) Dorsiflexion in neutral stresses the midcarpal space. A capitate or lunate fracture may result, or the distal radius will fracture. (**C**) Dorsiflexion in ulnar deviation and supination loads the ulnar side of the wrist and DRUJ. Scapholunate dissociation, triquetrohamate sprain, or perilunate dislocation may result. Tensile stresses of the palmar ligaments may initiate failure at varying locations, depending on the position of the wrist at impact.

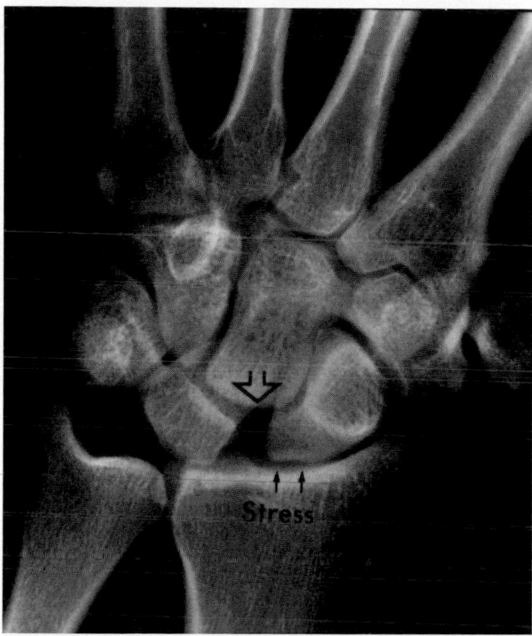

FIGURE 12-55. Grip view of the wrist (PA) demonstrates scapholunate dissociation by forcing the capitate to spread and rotate the scaphoid and lunate apart. Note the increased scapholunate gap, the foreshortened scaphoid, and the ring sign projection of the vertically oriented scaphoid.

tion.[274,328,412,460] The clinical consequences of the injury depend on the tightness or laxity of the associated and generalized capsuloligamentous system of the wrist and an associated palmar radiocarpal or midcarpal ligament damage. Developmental factors of consequence include an ulna-minus configuration of the wrist,[130] the slope of the radial articular surface, and lunatotriquetral coalition. All are probable risk factors.

The mechanism of injury[118] is similar to that of the scaphoid fracture with stress loading of the extended carpus, except it is usually in ulnar (Fig. 12-54) rather than radial deviation. Prior injury, repetitive injury, or the presence of acute or chronic synovitis modifies the degree of stress required to the point that the index event may be fairly trivial, such as slamming a car door or catching a basketball.

The diagnosis is made by the appropriate history, complaint localized to the scapholunate area (see Fig. 12-47), and physical findings of tenderness, swelling, or deformity in the scapholunate area. The degree of associated stability may be sufficient that only provocative stress[102] will reveal the classic findings. An easy provocative maneuver is a vigorous grasp that induces pain; another indication is decreasing repetitive grip strength.[131] The patient may also demonstrate pain during flexion–extension or radioulnar deviation. Provocative stress is often accompanied by a click in the region of the proximal scaphoid and sometimes by a visible deformity dorsally.[264] The Watson test (scaphoid shift test), which can produce a painful dorsal protuberance of the proximal pole of the scaphoid, is highly suggestive of SLD (see Signs and Symptoms).[309a,546b] As the scaphoid flexes to a more vertical orientation with radial deviation, tuberosity compression forces proximal pole subluxation dorsal to the lip of the radius. This test is not absolutely specific for SLD, because it may reposition the entire proximal carpal row if the row, rather than the individual scaphoid, is unstable. In addition, in individuals with lax ligaments there may be false-positive signs of dorsal subluxation of the scaphoid that are not pathologic.

Scapholunate dissociations may be severe enough or old enough to be fixed in malposition with scaphoid flexion and a fixed excessive space between scaphoid and lunate (see Fig. 12-23). A scapholunate gap greater than 3 mm is suspect, and a gap greater than

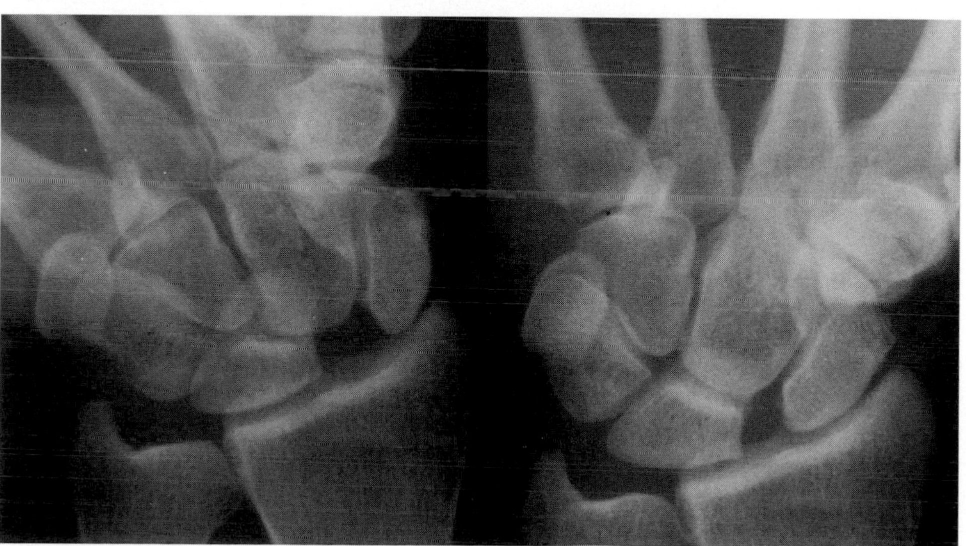

FIGURE 12-56. Scapholunate dissociation. Scapholunate diastasis (increased gap) is noted with radial (*right*) and ulnar (*left*) deviation stress views of the wrist.

5 mm is confirmatory.[386] The lateral radiographic appearance of a scapholunate angle greater than 60° is suspect; if the angle is greater than 80°, the x-ray appearance is confirmatory. A capitolunate or radiolunate angle greater than 15° is suspect but if greater than 20° it is confirmatory.[311b] If these findings are not present, the provocative maneuvers discussed earlier may cause them to appear. If scapholunate instability cannot be seen with grip x-rays or radioulnar stress x-rays (Fig. 12-55 and 12-56), then video fluoroscopy using standard and provocative stress motions is observed and recorded. Arthrography[132,315] is then performed to demonstrate dye flow from radiocarpal to midcarpal joint between the scaphoid and lunate (Fig. 12-57). It is possible, however, to have an attenuated but still intact scapholunate membrane or a ligament flap that acts as a valve, so that a negative arthrogram does not necessarily rule out the diagnosis. Conversely, a positive arthrogram does not necessarily imply the cause for clinical symptoms.[98a] It is the combination of clinical symptoms and radiographic findings that is essential. A midcarpal arthrogram may be more diagnostic than a radiocarpal arthrogram, and triple injection arthrograms (radiocarpal, midcarpal, and dis-

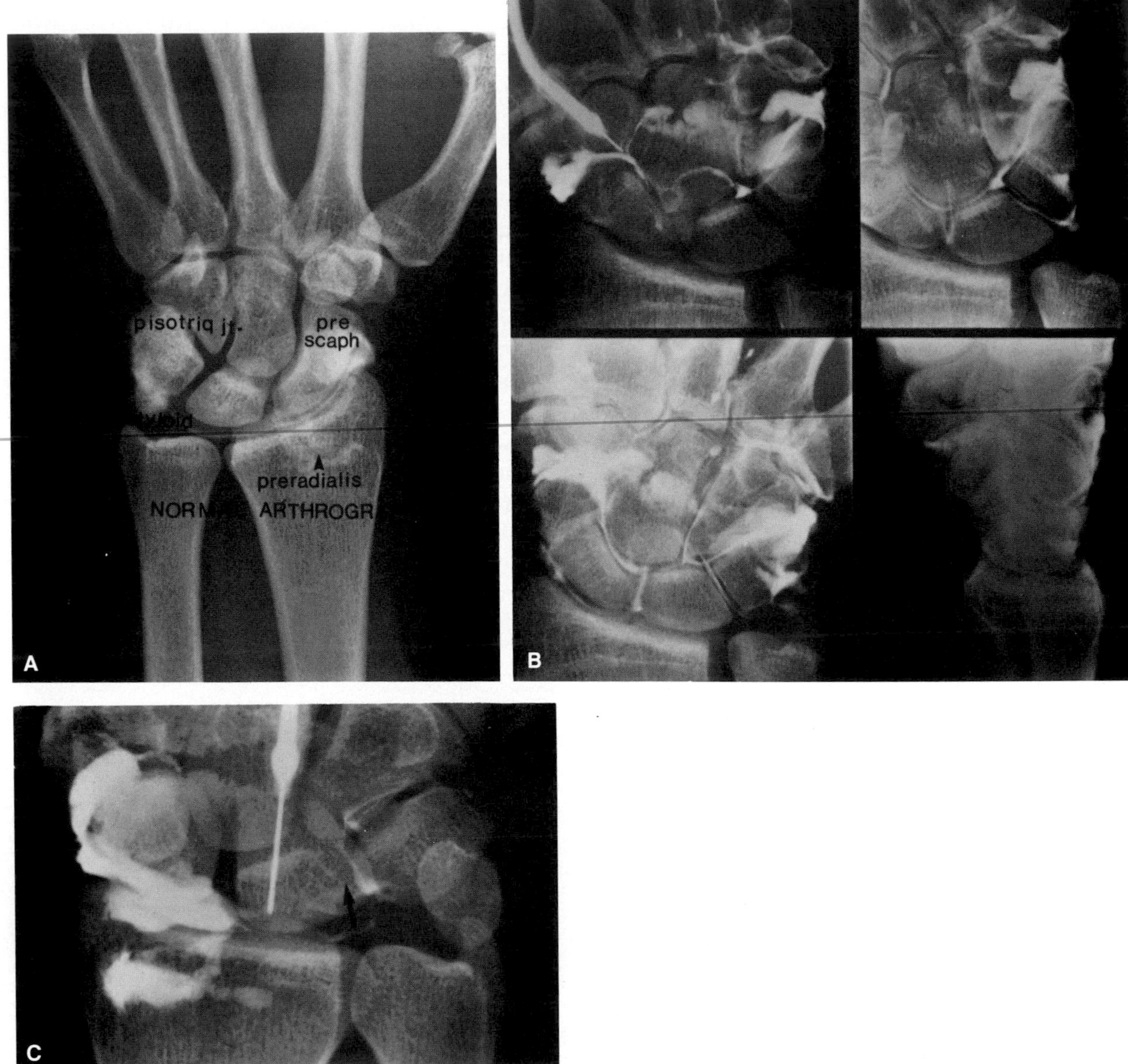

FIGURE 12-57. Wrist arthrography. (**A**) Normal radiocarpal arthrogram. Recesses of the prescaphoid, preradialis, prestyloid (ulnar), and pisotriquetral joints have filled. (**B**) Midcarpal arthrogram (serial x-rays) shows gradual presence of dye in the scapholunate and lunotriquetral intervals (*top right*), suggesting a lunatotriquetral ligament tear. The radiocarpal joint (*left bottom*) fills, confirming an interosseous ligament tear. (**C**) Abnormal radiocarpal arthrogram with contrast across the lunatotriquetral interval (*arrow*).

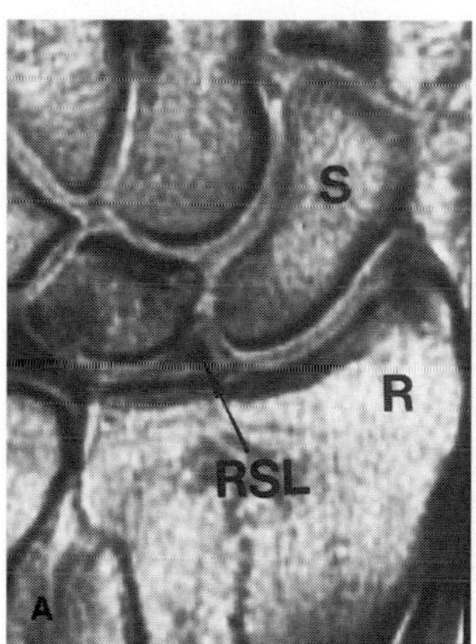

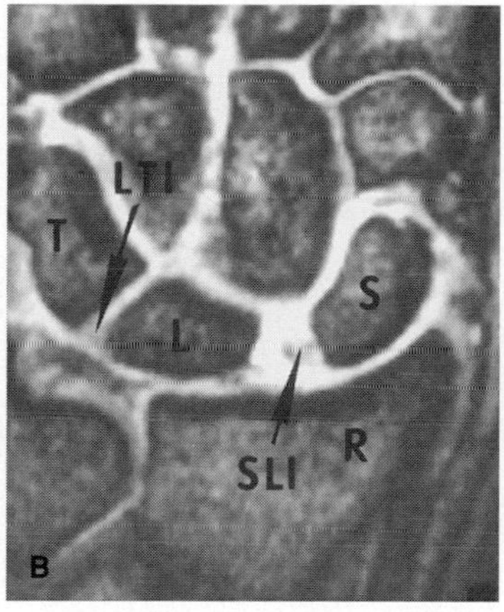

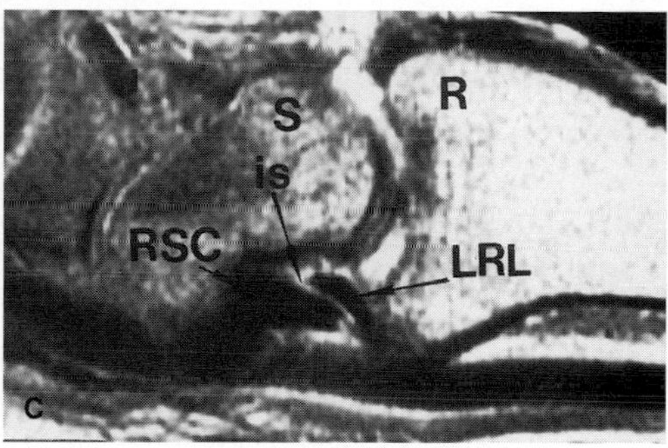

FIGURE 12-58. Magnetic resonant imaging to evaluate scapholunate (SL) ligament injury. (**A**) MRI showing increased signal along the radioscapholunate ligament (RSL) with normal scapholunate interspace. (**B**) MRI showing widened SL gap and presumed tear of scapholunate interosseous ligament (SLI). (**C**) Lateral MRI view showing intact radioscaphocapitate (RSC) and long radiolunate ligaments (LRL). *S*, scaphoid; *R*, radius; *IS*, isthmus between palmar carpal ligaments.

tal radioulnar) are preferred by some.[315] MRI may be helpful in discriminating a partial ligament tear or attenuation from an intact ligament (Fig. 12-58).

Arthroscopy can be used to determine the extent of ligament disruption and presence of radioscaphoid arthritis.[68,458] We view arthrography and arthroscopy as complementary procedures, noting the studies that suggest that bilateral arthrograms can demonstrate similar lesions in the asymptomatic wrist.[121a]

Treatment. The treatment of SLD has changed significantly over the past 10 years.[329] It is best to consider different options for treatment based in part on the duration of injury, extent of ligament involvement, and associated carpal instabilities.[118,119,324,423] We recommend different treatment plans depending on whether the injury is acute, subacute, or late carpal instability. A list of treatment alternatives is presented, followed by specific recommendations for acute, subacute, and chronic scapholunate instability. For confirmed cases of scapholunate instability, the list of treatment options includes at least the following:

1. Protection only in a supportive cast or splint until the natural healing process has concluded. In an acute injury, three-point pressure on the volar scaphoid, dorsal capitate, and dorsal aspect of the distal radius can occasionally support and maintain the reduction.[153]
2. Closed reduction and percutaneous pin fixation under image control; a support cast is worn for 8 weeks followed by splint immobilization.[149]
3. Arthroscopic controlled reduction and percutaneous pin fixation.
4. Open reduction and internal fixation plus ligament repair.[119,329]
5. Open reduction, ligament repair with soft-tissue augmentation, with internal fixation.[61]
6. Intercarpal fusion.[296,548]
7. Proximal row carpectomy[81,277] or wrist fusion.[240,408]

Twenty years ago, reconstruction of the scapholunate ligament was recommended by a technique of tendon graft woven through the scaphoid, lunate, and the volar lip of the distal radius.[153,328,329,423] Although clinical results were often satisfactory (about 75% good or excellent),[225] radiographic correlation was less evident, and these procedures were very difficult to perform.[423] Ligament repair was superseded in many instances by fusion of the distal scaphoid to the trapezium or capitate.[294,295,296] These techniques address only one part of the problem, the unstable scaphoid, and ignore the instability present in the rest of the carpus (ie, lunate and capitate). Difficulty in obtaining congruency of the proximal radioscaphoid articulation at surgery,[62] a significant incidence of nonunion, and late degenerative changes have been noted. The long-term efficacy of intercarpal fusion[294] is under increasing scrutiny, and the trend is to look for more reliable ligament and soft-tissue repairs for SLD,[227,514] particularly those presenting early. The controversy between repair and intercarpal fusions will not be resolved soon, but the latter are indicated for late or chronic instability.[550] In the methods of treatment to follow, new concepts in repair or reconstruction of these ligaments are presented, as well as a review of current techniques for limited intercarpal fusions.

Acute and Subacute Scapholunate Dissociation. *Authors' Preferred Method of Treatment.* Anatomical res-

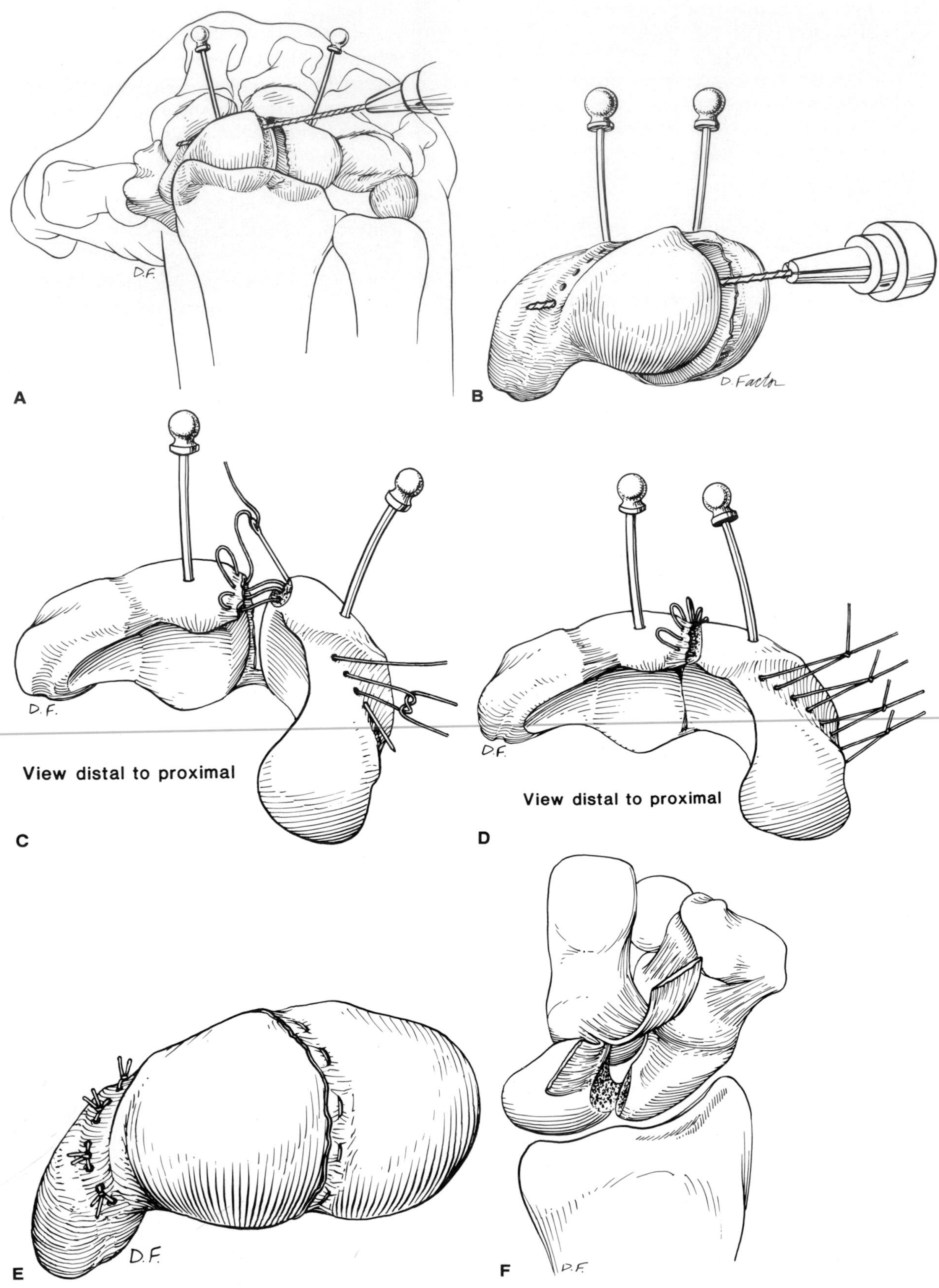
D.F.
D.Factor
A
B
D.F.
View distal to proximal
C
D.F.
View distal to proximal
D
D.F.
E
D.F.
F

FIGURE 12-59.

toration of the scapholunate complex by ligament repair is a realistic goal when the patient presents early (Fig. 12-59).[149,227] Early confirmation of the diagnosis is done by clinical examination, stress x-ray studies, or arthrography. Arthroscopy of the wrist[68] can assist in confirming the diagnosis and determining the location and extent of ligamentous damage. The patient who has a mild partial ligament tear may be treated more conservatively than those with significant carpal instability. The patient with an injury less than 4 weeks old is considered to have an acute tear; if more than 4 but less than 24 weeks, it is a subacute tear. If the time is greater than 6 months from injury, the tear is chronic and may be reducible or irreducible. Depending on the mechanism of injury and amount of force across the wrist, the scapholunate ligament may be accompanied by injuries to the palmar radiocarpal and lunatotriquetral ligament or the TFC.

We believe that ligament repair should be considered in all acute scapholunate injuries, unless the carpus is easily reduced anatomically by closed techniques and remains reduced in sequential x-rays without carpal malalignment by the criteria mentioned previously. An increasing scapholunate angle exceeding 60°, a lunatocapitate angle exceeding 15°, or an increasing scapholunate gap greater than 3 mm is an indication for operative intervention. There are a number of different reconstruction alternatives, but the most common and direct ones are presented here.

Acute Ligament Tear—Repair Technique. The principles for ligament repair (see Fig. 12-59) are similar for acute and subacute injuries. The type of repair depends on the quality of the local tissues. Usually, there is sufficient local tissue to perform a direct repair for acute and subacute injuries using the techniques described by Linscheid and Dobyns[332a] and Taleisnik.[311c] The usual technique involves the following:

1. A dorsal incision is centered over Lister's tubercle, reflecting the dorsal wrist capsule to preserve the dorsal intercarpal and dorsal radiotriquetral ligaments using a radial based capsular flap. The radial capsule is reflected from the scaphoid to its waist.
2. Reduction of the lunate and scaphoid is performed with Kirschner-wire "joysticks" inserted in a dorsal to palmar direction.
3. The rim of the proximal scaphoid is freshened to subcortical bone with a small, high-speed bur.
4. When the ligament is attached to the lunate (the usual case), holes are drilled from the waist of the scaphoid in a proximal and medial direction to exit at the scapholunate articulation.
5. Nonabsorbable sutures (2-0 or 3-0 Mersilene) are placed in the scapholunate ligament, palmar to dorsal. The suture is pulled back through the scaphoid with a second suture on a straight needle.
6. When the sutures for repair are in place, the scaphoid and lunate are reduced with joysticks held in the reduced or slightly overreduced position with pins across the scapholunate and, if needed, radiolunate articulations.
7. The sutures are tied and the capsule repaired.
8. Reinforcing this repair with the radioscaphoid tether (see next section) is suggested.

Alternatives for repair include intraosseous suture-retaining plugs (eg, Mitek, Statac) placed along the ulnar rim of the scaphoid (or lunate), depending on the site of ligament detachment. The principle involved is to repair the scapholunate ligament tightly down to a fresh bone edge to provide a source for ligament healing.

Subacute Ligament Tear—Repair Technique. For subacute scapholunate ligament tears, the addition of local tissue (alone or additionally) may be necessary if the scapholunate ligament has retracted or is deficient. Blatt's technique[67] reflects a proximally based dorsal capsule flap onto the scapholunate interspace, and this is sutured tautly to the dorsal scaphoid to act as a tether to the proximal pole (Fig. 12-60). This flap can be added to the ligament repair process described earlier by placing nonabsorbable sutures from the lunate ligament remnant into the capsular tissue and then out through the scaphoid.

An alternative method is to use a strip of tendon from the radial wrist extensors (extensor carpi radialis longus or extensor carpi radialis brevis), but tendon tissue is not an ideal ligament replacement, and capsular tissue is preferred (Fig. 12-61). Capsular tethers can also be created from the dorsal intercarpal ligament, which is left attached to the distal scaphoid, pulled

FIGURE 12-59. Ligament repairs for scapholunate dissociation. (**A**) The scapholunate interosseous membrane (SLIOM) is retained on the lunate. K-wires are introduced into the scaphoid and lunate as toggle arms ("joysticks"). Both bones are decorticated to the SLIOM attachment. (**B**) Drill holes are made from the proximal scaphoid to the lateral scaphoid sulcus distally (Taleisnik technique). (**C**) Sutures are passed through the SLIOM and are retrieved internally with retrograde straight needles or looped wires. (**D**) Reduction of the lunate by flexion and the scaphoid by extension using joy sticks. (**E**) The sutures are tied after pulling the remnant of the SLIOM tautly against the scaphoid rim. (**F**) SLURPIE procedure. Volar approach with decortication of the contiguous surfaces of the scaphoid and lunate. Fixation is with threaded K-wires after reduction, and the palmar ligaments are repaired.

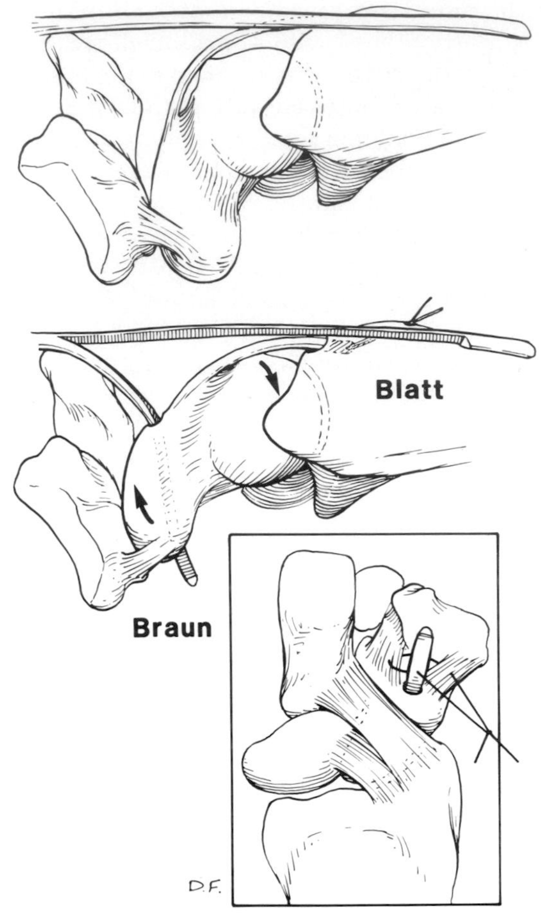

FIGURE 12-60. Capsulodesis for carpal instability. (*Top*) The scaphoid is flexed and subluxated at the STT joint. (*Middle*) Dorsal capsulodesis as described by Blatt. (*Bottom*) Palmar capsulodesis with a slip of ECRB passed through the scaphoid (Braun).

taut (extending the flexed scaphoid), and attached proximally to the distal radius.

In both subacute and severe acute scapholunate tears, palmar extrinsic ligament attenuation may be found. Use of the arthroscope intraoperatively helps to identify these conditions and plan appropriate incisions. A palmar approach with direct ligament repair by nonabsorbable sutures can be performed. If there is deficient tissue in the subacute case, part of the flexor carpi radialis can be used to augment the repair process by placing drill holes through the proximal scaphoid and radial half of the lunate and passing one half of the flexor carpi radialis tendon in a circular fashion to reinforce dorsal and palmar ligaments (Fig. 12-62). Palmarly, the radioscaphocapitate and radiolunate ligaments may be advanced into the gap as described by Conyers. With a large, complete scapholunate ligament tear, that is, a wide scapholunate gap of 5 mm or more, palmar ligament repair is usually needed. A carpal tunnel incision extended slightly radially is performed, and the damaged area is identified with a probe inserted from a separate dorsal incision. The interval between the radioscaphocapitate ligament and long radiolunate ligament is developed. Sutures may then be placed through the scaphoid proximal pole or remnants of the interosseous membrane, which are then used to pull the radiolunate ligament against the proximal pole to hold the overreduction of the proximal scaphoid, which is stabilized by Kirschner wires. The purpose of this palmar repair is to bring the dorsal subluxated and rotated proximal scaphoid in apposition with the palmar intracapsular ligaments.

Whether the approach is dorsal or palmar or combined, tight repair of the capsular structures is required for acute or subacute dissociation. Internal fixation for a minimal period of 8 weeks is preferred, supplemented with a supportive thumb spica cast. After cast removal, an orthoplast splint is worn as muscle strength and joint motion are restored. Return to work or athletic competition is best delayed for a minimum of 6 months, with continued protection during athletic competition.

Chronic Scapholunate Instability—Repair Technique. *Author's Preferred Method of Treatment.* In cases that present more than 6 months from the time of

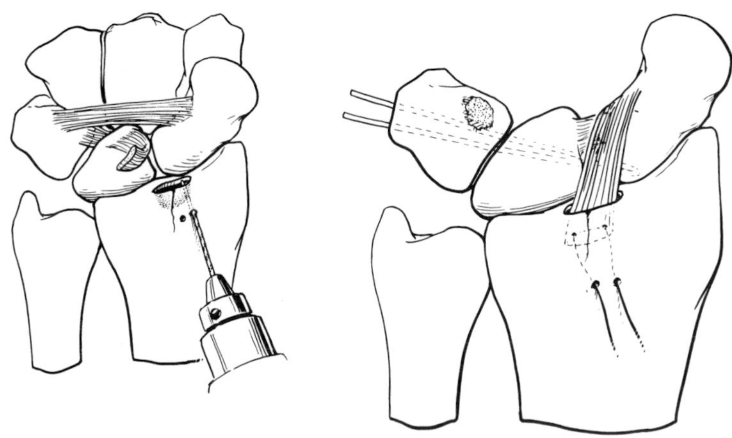

FIGURE 12-61. Dorsal intercarpal ligament capsulodesis. This capsulodesis uses the dorsal intercarpal ligament left attached to the distal scaphoid and brought proximal to be tethered to the distal radius.

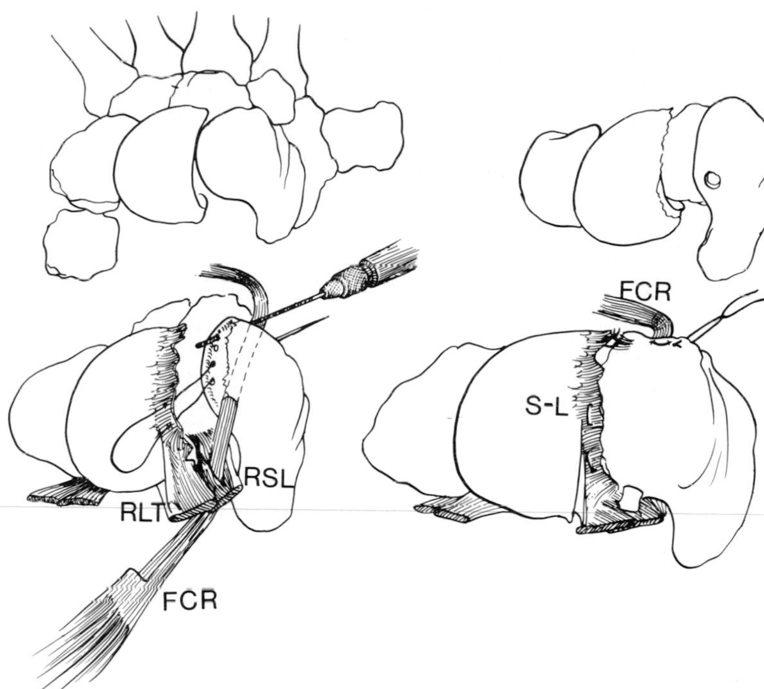

FIGURE 12-62. Augmentation of scapholunate ligament repair using half of the flexor carpi radialis (*FCR*) tendon. The scapholunate ligament repair is similar to techniques described in Figure 12-59, with drill holes placed through the scaphoid to the lunate ligament remnant. The dorsal scapholunate ligament is repaired and augmented with a portion of the tendon graft. *RLT*, radiolunotriquetral; *S-L*, scapholunate ligament; *RSL*, radioscapholunate.

injury, alternatives for treatment are based on the ability to reduce the carpal instability, the stress demands on the patient's wrist, and the absence of degenerative changes within the carpus. When feasible, restoration of normal carpal anatomy by repair and reconstruction of the support ligaments of the wrist remain, in our opinion, the preferred treatment. This requires sufficient local tissue for repair and a correctable carpal instability. When the patient presents with a fixed carpal deformity, that is, if the rotational subluxation of the scaphoid or dorsal angulated lunate (DISI) cannot be reduced, or when local degenerative changes or work demands that require heavy lifting or repetitive stress loading are present, the alternative of partial or complete fusion of the wrist may be preferred.[294,295,296,546,550]

Current techniques for ligament reconstruction include the dorsal capsular flap procedure,[61] a palmar ligament reefing procedure,[111] and combined dorsal and volar procedures that add flexor or extensor tendon tissue to the repair site. The goal of each of these repair techniques involves the addition of local tissue to provide a collagen framework for future stability. Our preferred approach is to start with a dorsal midline incision with access to the wrist between the extensor pollicis longus and the radial wrist extensors laterally and the extensor digitorum communis medially. Because capsular flaps are needed for the reconstruction, they should be anticipated and created during the exposure, preserving for future use, as necessary, the dorsal radiotriquetral and dorsal intercarpal ligaments.

For the Blatt type of capsule reconstruction (see Fig. 12-60),[61] a long, rectangular flap is made, about 1.5 cm wide, based on the dorsal aspect of the distal radius. For a distal-based flap, one can release the dorsal scaphotriquetral ligament (dorsal intercarpal ligament) from the triquetrum, leaving it attached to the scaphoid rim distally (see Fig. 12-61). The triquetral insertion is brought proximally and sutured to the distal radius. Some surgeons prefer to use part of the extensor carpi radialis brevis left attached distally and reflect it proximally into the scapholunate interval, where it is interwoven into the repair. In the Blatt procedure, the dorsal flap of wrist capsule is sutured under tension distal to the scaphoid center of rotation, so that it tethers the proximal pole in the scaphoid fossa. The flap is sutured to reinforce the local tissue of the scapholunate interval.

Wrist extensor or flexor tendon augmentation procedures require placement of drill holes in bone. This requires precision and technical skill from the surgeon. In this procedure, drill holes are carefully placed in a dorsal-to-volar direction through the scaphoid and enlarged with an awl. Half of the tendon is placed through the scaphoid drill hole dorsal to palmar and then back through the lunate, palmar to dorsal. The scapholunate joint is reduced with joysticks and the ligament repair tightened and sutured. Kirschner wires are inserted to help maintain reduction. An alternative technique is to take part of an extensor or flexor tendon after passing it to or through the long radiolunate ligament and then pull it through the scapholunate interval, where it augments the local ligament repair. A combined dorsal-volar approach is needed to perform these procedures effectively. There is increased risk from placing holes in bone, but they do provide a strong static control of the scaphoid as well as adding local tissue for ligament repair.

The palmar approach for scapholunate ligament repair (Conyers' technique)[111] is performed through a carpal tunnel incision. A probe or needle passed dorsal to palmar is helpful in locating the ligament tear and palmar ligament intervals. Flaps of radioscaphocapitate and long radiolunate ligaments are reflected laterally and medially. The cartilage surfaces that are contiguous to scaphoid and lunate are denuded to subchondral bone to encourage a strong syndesmosis. The scaphoid and lunate are then reduced and pinned with threaded wires that are left in place 8 weeks or more. The palmar ligaments are snugly repaired. Motion is delayed 10 to 12 weeks to encourage adequate strength of the syndesmosis.

To correct the malalignment of the carpus, we recommend the following steps in each of these techniques:

1. It is necessary to reduce and pin the lunate to the distal radius or to the distal carpal row to correct lunate dorsal angulation.
2. The scaphoid is reduced to the lunate and the scapholunate interval is pinned. Overreduction of the lunate and scaphoid is preferable.
3. Supplemental fixation of the scaphoid to the capitate or trapezium may be considered (Fig. 12-63).

The greater the difficulty in obtaining the reduction or holding the reduction, the more critical strong internal fixation is and the more likely it is that the soft-tissue repair will not be successful. For reduction of the scaphoid and lunate, the use of Kirschner-wire joysticks is helpful. Manual assistance by direct pressure palmarly over the tuberosity of the distal (vertical) scaphoid along with downward pressure on the capitate may be needed. Lateral and posteroanterior x-rays are necessary to confirm that the reduction or overreduction has been obtained before final capsule closer.

After scapholunate ligament reconstruction, immobilization in a thumb spica cast is recommended for 8 to 10 weeks. Splint immobilization for an additional 4 weeks is suggested to allow for collagen tissue healing with gradual stress loading. Supporting splints are best worn intermittently for 6 months to prevent sudden stress to the wrist and allow further collagen maturation.

Scaphotrapeziotrapezoidal (STT) Fusion The decision regarding intercarpal fusion for SLD is based on the length of time from the original injury, the degree of ligament disruption, and the ability to reduce the carpal instability. Additional important factors are work and strength expectations of the patient.[435] Findings of radio-

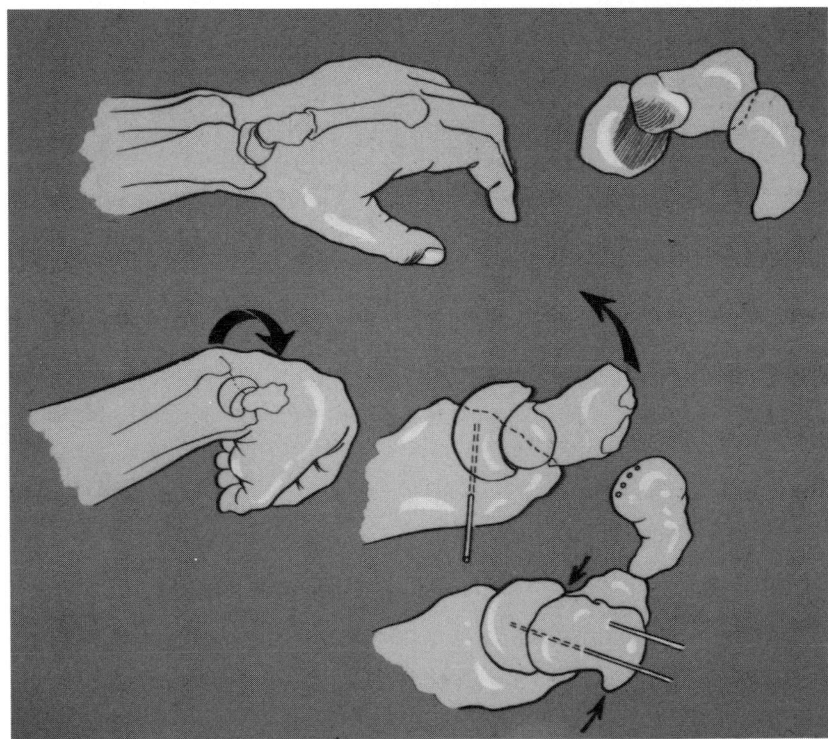

FIGURE 12-63. Principles of correcting carpal malalignment. (*Top*) Typical instability pattern with the lunate extended and scaphoid and capitate flexed with respect to the distal radius. (*Middle*) The lunate is reduced by flexion of the wrist, and the lunate is pinned in the reduced position (radiolunate Kirschner wire). Extending the wrist then reduces or aligns the scaphoid and lunate. (*Bottom*) Following scapholunate ligament repair (or reconstruction), the scaphoid and lunate are pinned in the reduced position.

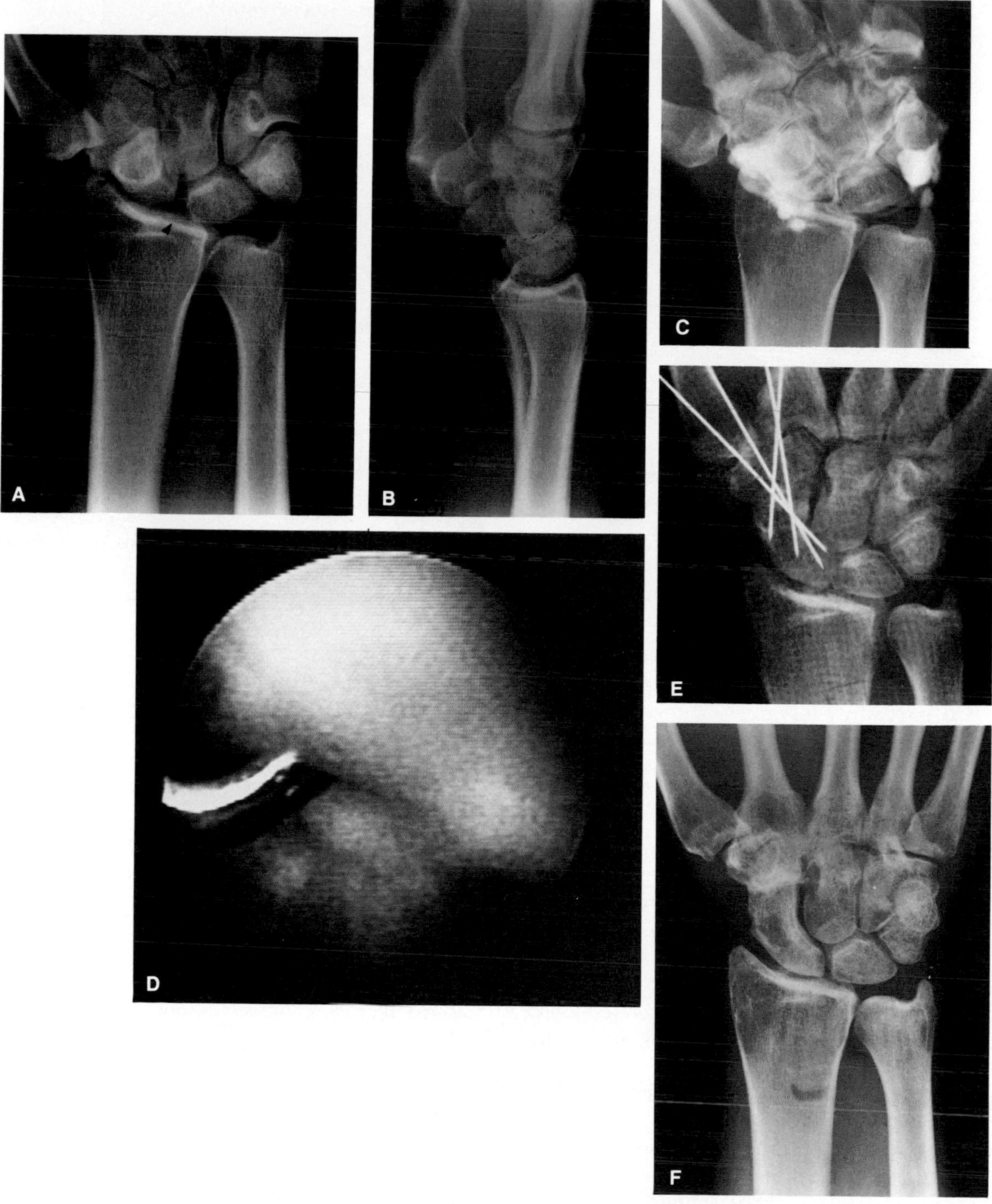

FIGURE 12-64. A 36-year-old attorney and riding-enthusiast fell from his bicycle 18 months prior to presentation. He complained of persistent wrist pain, loss of strength, and swelling with use. (**A,B**) PA and lateral x-rays demonstrate a scapholunate gap of 4 mm and rotatory subluxation of the scaphoid. Palmar flexion of the lunate is unusual and suggests additional extrinsic wrist ligament damage. (**C**) A wrist arthrogram showed evidence of an intercarpal ligament tear with contrast passing through the scapholunate interval. (**D**) Arthroscopy was performed to confirm the suspected pathology and to determine the degree of instability. Gross instability between the scaphoid and lunate was noted. (**E**) Fusion of the scaphotrapeziotrapezoidal (STT) joint was performed with a distal radius bone graft and crossed K-wires. (**F**) At 2 years, the fusion was solid with no evidence of radioscaphoid impingement.

continues

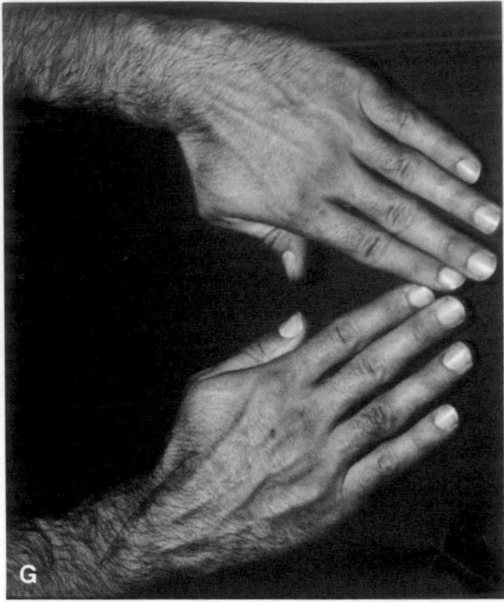

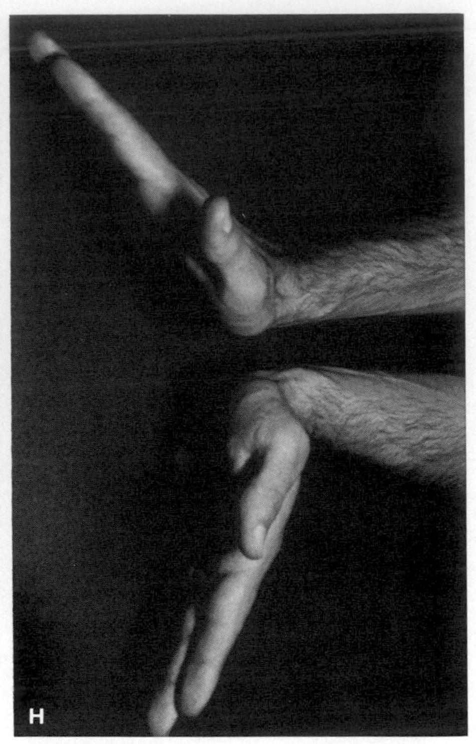

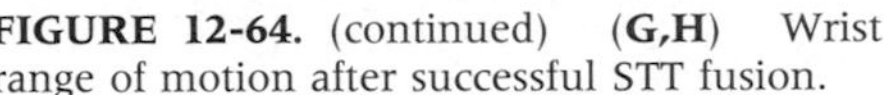

FIGURE 12-64. (continued) (**G,H**) Wrist range of motion after successful STT fusion.

carpal and midcarpal arthritis should influence the decision toward intercarpal fusion.[547] Of the partial wrist fusions performed for wrist instability, the scaphotrapeziotrapezoidal (triscaphe) fusion has had the widest clinical application (Fig. 12-64).[128,159,296,546,548] As described by Watson,[550] the purpose of this procedure is to stabilize the distal scaphoid and thereby hold the proximal pole more securely within the scaphoid fossa of the distal radius. This operation can be performed through a transverse incision centered over the scaphotrapeziotrapezoidal joint or with the universal longitudinal incision.[159] Arthroscopic examination of both midcarpal and radiocarpal joints may determine the extent of scapholunate ligament and articular cartilage damage, aiding in the choice of preferred treatment.

With either scaphotrapeziotrapezoidal fusion[294,295] or the equivalent scaphocapitate fusion,[208,366] an important component of the procedure is to reduce the vertical (palmar-flexed) scaphoid, close the scapholunate interval, and maintain carpal height.[366,456] Radiographic control is recommended. The ideal flexion angle of the scaphoid is 45°. Fixation of the scaphotrapeziotrapezoidal or scaphocapitate joints is performed with Kirschner wires, screws, or staples. A bone graft from the distal radius or iliac crest is placed between the decorticated distal scaphoid and proximal surface of the trapezium and trapezoid (scaphotrapeziotrapezoidal fusion) or between the medial articular surface of the scaphoid and the lateral surface of the capitate (scaphocapitate fusion). Once scaphoid alignment is achieved, cancellous bone graft is inserted and Kirschner wires are placed to support the fusion area. Pre-reduction placement of Kirschner wires into the scaphoid facilitates correct orientation after reduction.[546]

Immobilization for intercarpal fusion is usually 8 weeks in a thumb spica cast, followed by a support splint for 4 to 6 weeks. Tomography of the wrist can help determine the degree of consolidation at the fusion site. In our experience, 6 weeks is usually a sufficient time to allow for unprotected wrist motion after an intercarpal fusion. Radiocarpal impingement[197,294] as a complication of scaphotrapeziotrapezoidal fusion has led to the recommendation that a concomitant radial styloidectomy be included.[455]

Intercarpal Fusion

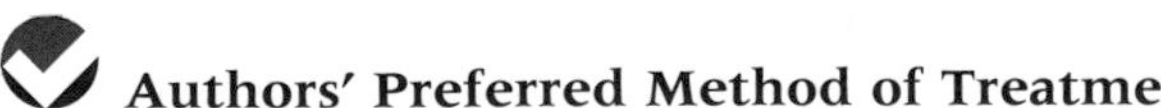

Authors' Preferred Method of Treatment

We consider localized fusion to be preferable in certain conditions of wrist instability. One of these is the fixed deformity that is difficult or impossible to reduce and tends to re-deform unless strong reduction force is maintained. Some carpal deformities are irreducible without extensive soft-tissue release, which may cause damage to circulation and joint surfaces; these are better treated with a salvage procedure. This intermediate group between the reducible and salvage groups are probably better treated with intercarpal fusion (eg, scaphotrapeziotrapezoidal or scaphocapitate). Where there is scaphotrapeziotrapezoidal joint damage as well as SLD,[243] scaphotrapeziotrapezoidal fusion with the scaphoid properly reduced is preferable. In the special situation of SLD and Kienböck's disease, either scaphotrapeziotrapezoidal or scaphocapitate fusion is preferable, plus whatever direct intervention may be desired for the lunate.

SLD and LTD may be present together. The SLD is usually the most unstable of the two, and control of both may be indicated. Lunatotriquetral fusion increases the force on the scapholunate ligament repair and should be avoided. Joint surface damage of the proximal scaphoid may require other types of localized fusion, such as radioscaphoid or capitolunate fusion, the former retaining and the latter discarding the scaphoid.

There may be an associated instability of the proximal carpal row as well as the dissociative instability between scaphoid and lunate. The ligament-tether augmentations described subsequently often control such instability. If the tendency for either severe DISI or VISI is marked and it is thought that soft-tissue restraint will not control it, a localized fusion may be preferable. If the instability seems to be primarily at the radiocarpal level, radiolunate or radioscapholunate fusion is preferable; if it is primarily at the midcarpal level, scaphocapitate or scapholunatocapitate fusion should be satisfactory.

Lunatotriquetral Dissociation

Lunatotriquetral dissociation involves a partial or complete tear of interosseous ligaments between the lunate and triquetrum.[449,538] It may present as an isolated injury, as part of the spectrum of perilunate dislocation, or in association with ulnocarpal impingement and TFC injuries.[350,449] The pathomechanics of lunatotriquetral injury that accompany perilunate dislocation are well known,[355,540] but the mechanism of isolated injury requires further study.[530] Because the lunatotriquetral joint is more stable than the scapholunate joint, it seems apparent that associated ligament damage, particularly to the dorsal radiotriquetral ligament or palmar ulnocarpal ligaments, must be present before severe, fixed deformities can occur. Diagnosis of lunatotriquetral instability involves a history of specific injury with residua of pain and weakness. Tenderness is present dorsally over the lunatotriquetral joint, and ballottement of the unstable triquetrum may be possible.[449] Stress loading of the lunatotriquetral joint (compression, ballottement, or shear) helps to confirm the diagnosis.

Radiographic diagnosis is more difficult than the diagnosis of SLD because the subtle findings are less pronounced and the provocative, stress-induced deformity is less frequent (Fig. 12-65). Subtle angle changes may be demonstrated with special imaging of the wrists,[223] but usually wrist arthrography or arthroscopy is needed to demonstrate the loss of membrane continuity between lunate and triquetrum with direct communication between the radiocarpal and midcarpal joints. Occasionally, alteration of the proximal or distal carpal arcs may be present. Fixed deformities are usually VISI,[465,530] because there is dissociation between lunate and triquetrum, and the usual pattern is for the lunate to follow the scaphoid into flexion while the triquetrum extends and supinates by sliding distally and palmarly on the hamate. Studies[538] demonstrate that a tear of the palmar lunatotriquetral ligament, dorsal radiotriquetral ligament, or palmar ulnocarpal ligaments is necessary in addition to lunatotriquetral ligament tear for the VISI deformity to develop. Isolated interosseous lunatotriquetral ligament tears usually will not produce a VISI collapse

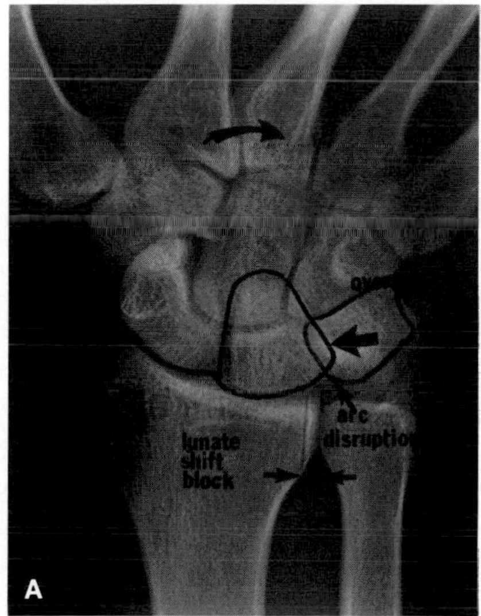

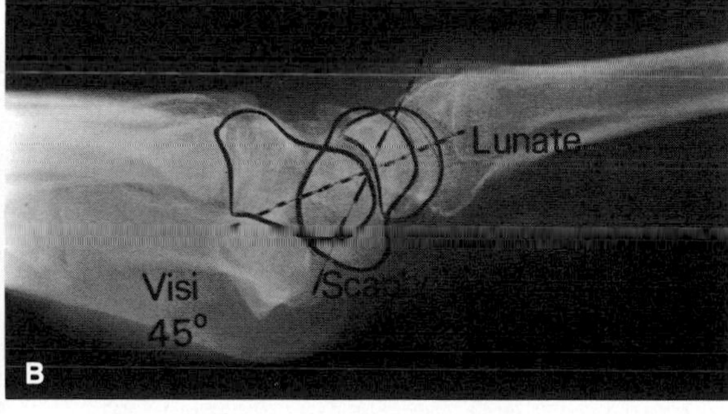

FIGURE 12-65. Lunatotriquetral dissociation. (**A**) The PA view demonstrates irregularity of the lunatotriquetral arc and a triangular appearance of the lunate. (**B**) The lunate together with the scaphoid is flexed relative to the dissociated triquetrum. (*Reagan, D.S.; Linscheid, R.L.; Dobyns, J.H.: Lunotriquetral Sprains. J. Hand Surg. 9A(4):502–514, 1984.*)

deformity, unless there is secondary extrinsic carpal ligament attenuation or injury. Lunatotriquetral ligament defects are common with ulnocarpal impingement and may represent the end stage of ulnar wrist instability.

Treatment. Acute LTD with minimal deformity is ideally treated with a support cast, adding closed reduction and internal fixation of lunate to triquetrum if there is displacement.

A special splint that supports the lunatotriquetral joint by maintaining mild, support pressure underneath the pisiform, over the dorsal aspect of the distal ulna, and under the tuberosity of the distal scaphoid with the wrist in extension and ulnar deviation helps to reduce the dissociating stresses.

LTD with angular deformity or with unsatisfactory results from previous treatment may need open treatment, particularly in the subacute or acute phase. Open reduction, repair of lax or damaged ligaments, and temporary internal fixation with percutaneous wires across the triquetrum and lunate left in place for 6 to 8 weeks is recommended for isolated lunatotriquetral ligament tears (Fig. 12-66). All ligaments that seem to be concerned with lunatotriquetral stability should be tightened as necessary, although this is by no means easy to accomplish. The interosseous ligament repair is usually done in a fashion similar to that described for the scapholunate repair, through a dorsal approach in the floor of the fifth dorsal compartment (Fig. 12-67). The ligament is more likely to be stripped from the triquetrum. Capsular flaps are useful for reinforcing the dorsal portion of such a repair or augmenting the dorsal radiotriquetral and dorsal scaphotriquetral ligament system. For late presentations with

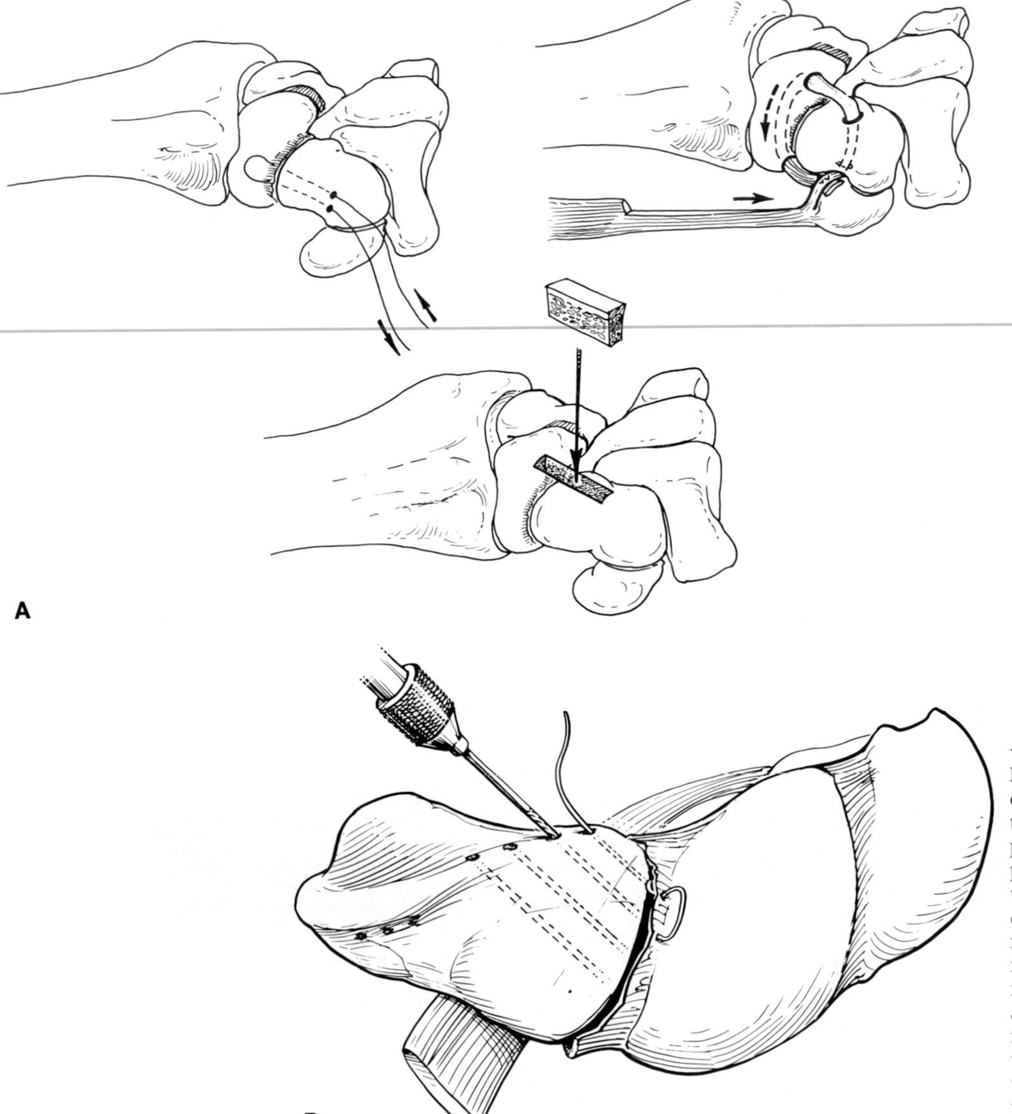

FIGURE 12-66. Lunatotriquetral dissociation. (**A**) Treatment options include direct ligament repair (*top left*), augmentation of repair with half of the flexor carpi ulnaris (*top right*), and lunatotriquetral fusion (*bottom*). (**B**) Schematic diagram of the technique to repair the lunatotriquetral ligament involves drill holes placed across the waist of the triquetrum into the lunatotriquetral interval with a nonabsorbable suture of the lunate remnant. The repair is protected with K-wire fixation for 6 weeks.

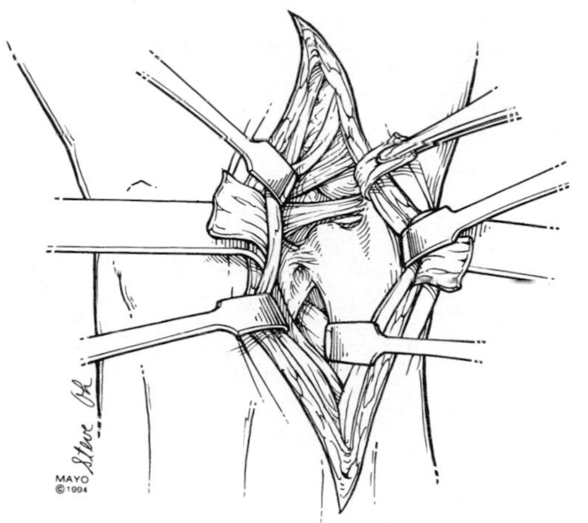

FIGURE 12-67. Dorsal approach for lunatotriquetral ligament injuries. A dorsal curvilinear incision is centered along the fourth metacarpal distally and distal radioulnar joint proximally. The extensor retinaculum is reflected between the fifth and sixth compartments. The ulnar radiocarpal joint is opened with an ulnar-based flap, and the dorsal radiotriquetral ligament may be attached distally as a radial-based flap.

complete ligament disruption and no tissue for repair, ligament reconstruction using part of the extensor carpi ulnaris tendon is recommended (Fig. 12-68). The technique involves drill holes through the triquetrum (dorsal to palmar) and lunate similar to late scapholunate ligament reconstruction. It is important to advance or repair the dorsal radiotriquetral ligament, which effectively pulls the lunate and triquetrum dorsally and proximally reducing the VISI deformity.

If it appears that soft-tissue repairs cannot control the tendency to recurrent deformity, lunatotriquetral fusion may be indicated (Fig. 12-69). Repair of the dorsal radiotriquetral ligament should also be performed so that a CID-type VISI deformity is not converted to a CIND-type VISI deformity after fusion. In most cases, we prefer ligament augmentation procedures that provide satisfactory stabilization; these are preferred over lunatotriquetral, radiolunate, or radiolunatotriquetral fusion.[528] Concomitant ulnar shortening procedures should be considered (especially with ulnar plus variance) to tighten the palmar ulnocarpal ligaments in addition to lunatotriquetral fusion or ligament reconstruction.

Perilunate Dislocations and Fracture–Dislocations

The concept of perilunate instability of the wrist has been developed based on a common mechanism of ligament disruption that begins radially and propagates around or through the lunate to the ulnar side of the carpus.[232,355,356,412,414,539,540] A similar pattern that begins ulnarly and propagates radially also occurs but is not as well documented experimentally. SLD and LTD often remain as the residual problems, even after relocation of the perilunate injury. Recurrence of carpal instability is common whether the injury involves the "lesser arc" injury through ligamentous tissue or the "greater arc" injury through bone, or some combination of the two (see Figs. 12-15 and 12-54).[272,356,374] The most common pattern of perilunate instability is the transscaphoid perilunate dislocation,[31,114] sometimes given the eponym of de Quervain's injury.[143]

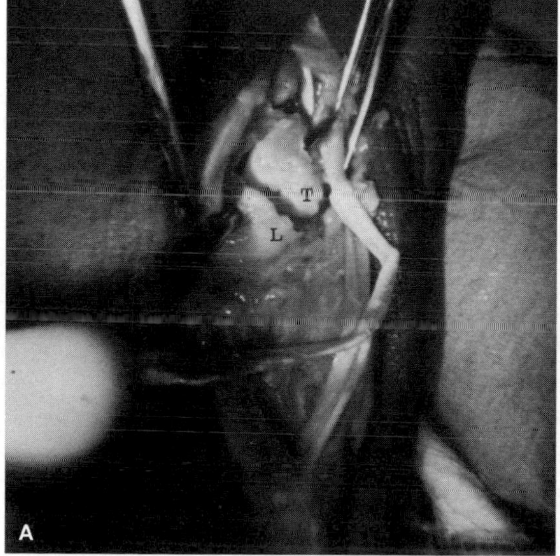

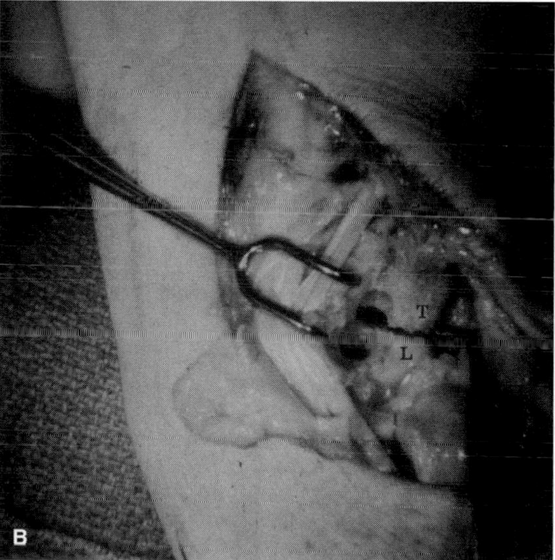

FIGURE 12-68. (**A**) Surgical exposures for a ligament reconstruction using half of the extensor carpi ulnaris tendon (forceps at upper left), which is passed through drill holes in the dorsal lunate and triquetrum. *L*, lunate; *T*, triquetrum. (**B**) Fusion of the lunatotriquetral joint. Dorsal exposure of the lunate (L) and triquetrum (T) with the dorsal surface prepared for an inlay bone graft.

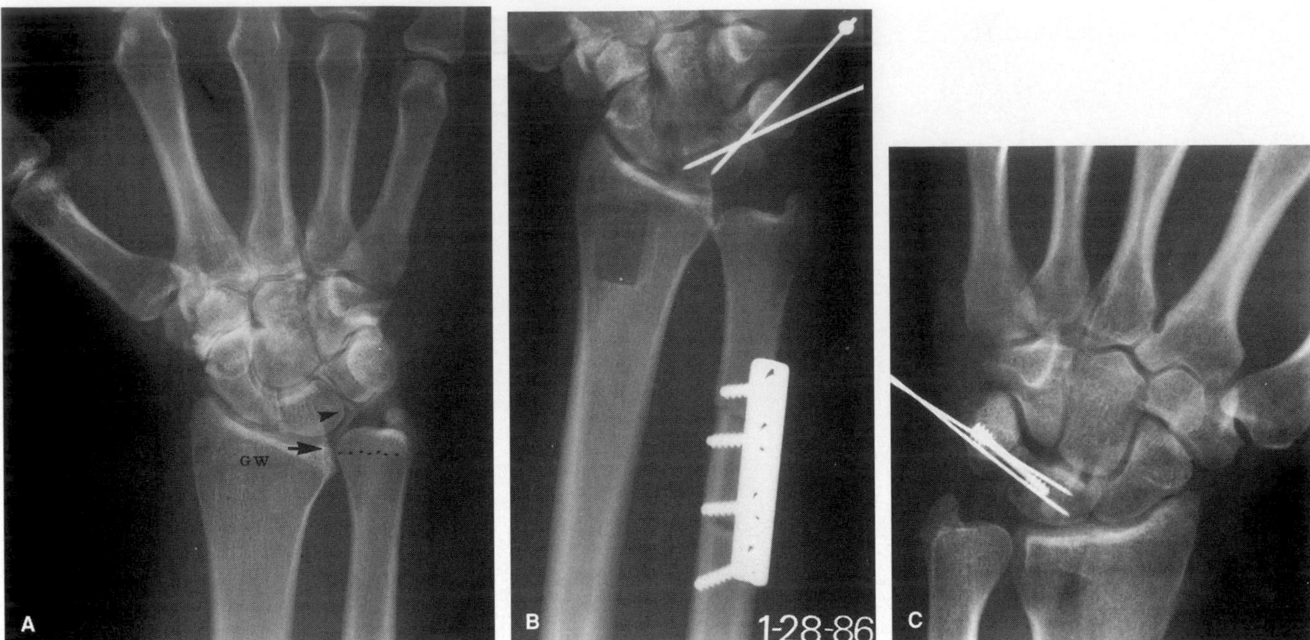

FIGURE 12-69. Lunatotriquetral (LT) dissociation. This 56-year-old carpenter presented with persistent ulnar wrist pain. (**A**) PA x-ray shows positive ulnar variance (*large arrow*) and arthrographic evidence of an LT tear (*small arrow*). (**B**) A lunatotriquetral fusion was done with interposition graft from the distal radius, combined with shortening of the ulna using a 4-hole compression plate (a 6 hole plate is now recommended). (**C**) Alternative lunatotriquetral fusion technique using a Herbert screw and Kirschner wires with an interposition bone graft.

Signs and Symptoms. Diagnosis is established by history of a hyperextension injury and persistent pain, swelling, and deformity.[253b,533] These high-energy injuries produce great deformity and soft-tissue damage. A common clinical presentation includes median nerve injury, but ulnar neuropathy, arterial injury, and tendon damage may also be seen.[504] The pattern of skeletal deformity is variable.[232,398] The hand and distal carpal row usually remain intact, but the disruption pattern between distal and proximal carpal rows is quite variable with the transscaphoid fracture dislocation.[464] The distal scaphoid dislocates with the distal row, leaving the proximal scaphoid and lunate in near-normal relationship to the forearm. When the perilunate ligament ruptures, typically the lunate remains bonded to some degree with the radius and the remainder of the carpus dislocates, usually dorsally.[112] Occasionally, the lunate is displaced and rotated palmarly and the remainder of the carpus settles into a semi-normal alignment with the distal radius. In some instances, the initial dislocation of the majority of the carpus may be volar.[6,228] In the usual situation, the dorsally displaced carpus rebounds to come to rest upon the dorsum of the lunate.[233,218,367] Occasionally, even the volar attachment of lunate is torn, allowing extrusion into the forearm or through the skin.

Radiographic Examination. Diagnosis can be made without x-rays, but the specifics of damage to soft tissue and bone are better appreciated with improved imaging techniques. The basic pattern can be discerned on standard posteroanterior and lateral x-rays (Fig. 12-70), but details of instability, fracture, and fragmentation are much better appreciated with traction views obtained with 5 to 10 pounds of finger-trap traction (Fig. 12-71). Approximately 20% of these dislocations are misinterpreted on the initial x-rays. Additional studies of particular value include polytomography, CT scanning, and MRI. Arthrography and arthroscopy may have a useful role in determining the details of injury, if open reduction of the fracture–dislocation is questioned.

Treatment. Acute injuries may be divided into two groups: those that spontaneously reduce or are easily reduced by closed reduction methods and those that are either open, irreducible, or unstable, once reduced.[2,267] Many of those from the first group will become unstable, making distinction between the two groups hazardous. This feature has led some surgeons to recommend open treatment of all perilunate dislocations and fracture–dislocations.[262a] Nevertheless, there are some spontaneous reductions that are so stable that it is difficult to determine whether a full, perilunate-type dislocation took place; and there are others that reduce and can be maintained in near-normal alignment in casts and splints. The trend, however, is to suggest that all perilunate injuries require open

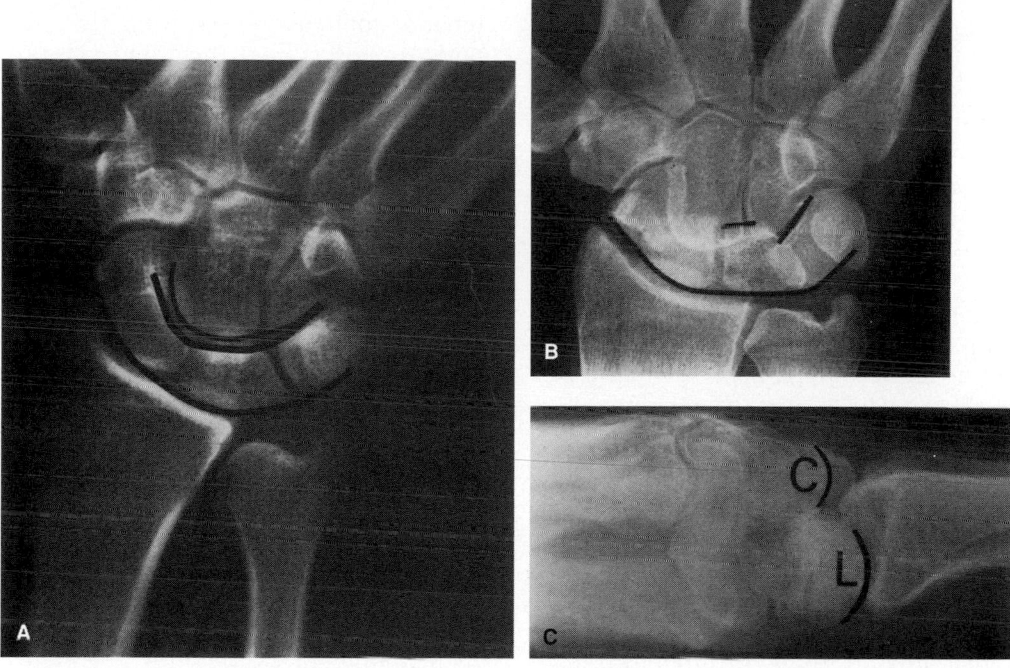

FIGURE 12-70. Fracture-dislocation of wrist. (**A**) Normal carpal arcs in the proximal row, midcarpal joint, and distal row arc are smooth and concentric. (**B**) Disruption of carpal arcs in a perilunate dislocation. (**C**) Lateral x-ray of a dorsal perilunate dislocation (*C*, capitate; *L*, lunate.)

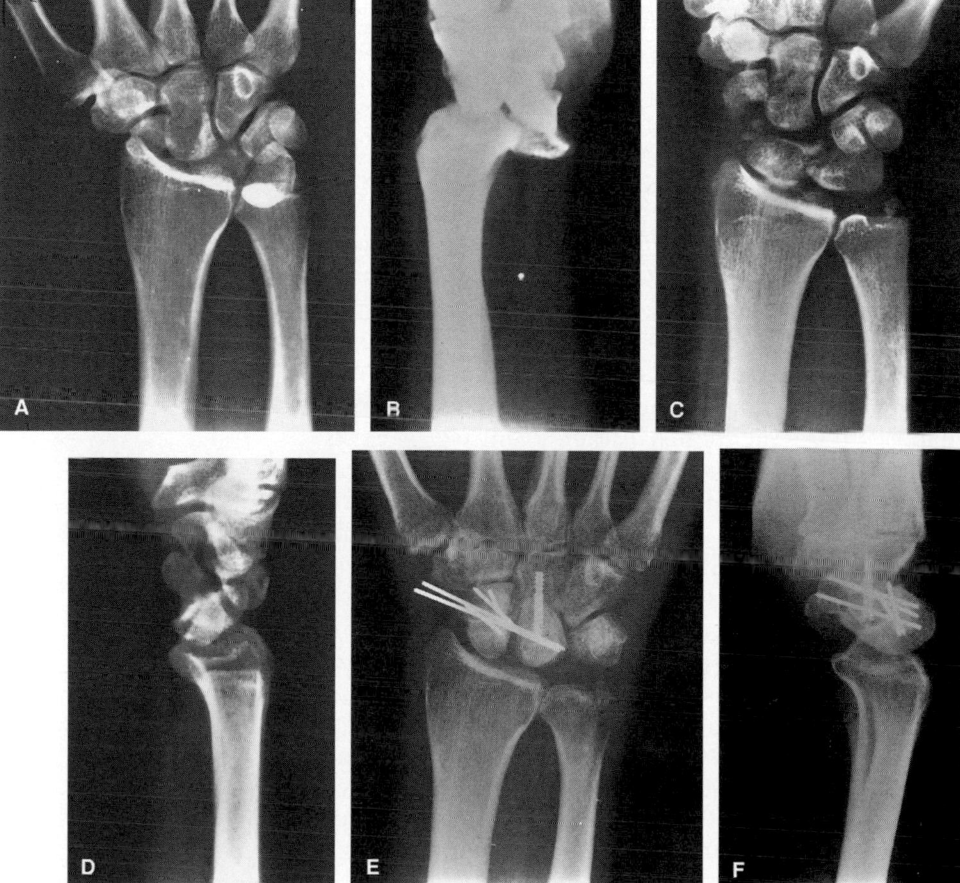

FIGURE 12-71. Trans-scaphoid transcapitate, perilunate dislocation. (**A**) PA view of the wrist shows proximal migration of the capitate, displaced proximal carpal row, and disrupted carpal arcs. (**B**) Lateral view demonstrates a lunate dislocation (type IV perilunate instability) with "spilled tea-cup sign" of the lunate articular surface facing palmarly. (**C**) Distraction view (in traction) helps to more clearly establish the diagnosis of a trans-scaphoid (displaced) transcapitate (undisplaced) fracture dislocation, with the lunate and proximal scaphoid partially reduced to the distal radius. (**D**) Lateral traction view shows the lunate to be reduced but the distal scaphoid and capitate are still displaced. (**E**) PA view following open reduction and retrograde Herbert screw fixation of the capitate and multiple Kirschner wires to fix the comminuted scaphoid fracture. The lunate is reduced in the lunate fossa of the distal radius and the scaphoid is cross-pinned. (**F**) Lateral view showing dorsal displacement of the lunate secondary to loss of palmar radiolunate ligament and failure to fully reduce and hold the radiolunate reduction. We consider this a secondary loss of reduction from unrecognized injury to the palmar radiocarpal ligaments.

reduction because open assessment almost always discloses more damage than anticipated.[114,232] Those injuries that reduce to normal alignment and that are treated by closed reduction and cast require monitoring on a daily basis for the first week and on a weekly basis thereafter because studies have demonstrated improved results with open treatment.

The majority of perilunate injuries fall into the open, irreducible, or unstable group, often with neurovascular problems.[112,114,233,414] This group is best treated by open investigation and repair.[2,114,374,387] If there are neurovascular problems, a palmar approach allows access for median nerve decompression, vascular repair if needed, as well as repair of torn palmar carpal ligaments. Combined with a dorsal approach, this allows both intra-articular and extra-articular damage to be assessed and treated adequately. The surgical access planes are similar to those for treatment of scapholunate and lunatotriquetral dissociation, except that it is necessary to release the carpal tunnel.[233] The palmar capsule should be examined either along its attachments to the radial rim or through the often torn space of Poirier; the dorsal capsule is usually opened along its origins from the dorsal radial rim, as well as longitudinally in the space between the second and fourth extensor compartments.

For discussion purposes, the perilunate-type injuries are divided into acute (less than) and chronic (more than) 3 months old. Acute injury are further subdivided into those that are easily reducible and those that are open, irreducible, and unstable. The chronic injuries are divided into those previously untreated and those for which previous treatment has failed. Severity of injury must be assessed for both the bone and soft tissues carefully.

Acute (Reduced or Reducible) Perilunate Injury. Some injuries are seen that have probably been dislocated but appear to be reduced at initial assessment. Ways of confirming this suspicion include stress-test imaging, arthroscopy, and open exploration. Dislocations can reduce with traction or manipulation to a near-normal alignment. As mentioned earlier, controversy exists as to whether all such injuries should be explored, repaired, and internally fixed, even though some perilunatc injuries heal satisfactorily and remain stable with closed management.[114,387,414] Similarly, we recommend open reduction and internal fixation of perilunate injuries unless other life-threatening problems take precedence or if the surgeon is not totally familiar with the operative techniques. Closed reduction with appropriate cast application and cast changes can produce satisfactory results, although it is difficult and unpredictable.[114] Open treatment does not guarantee stability, a good result, or avoidance of complications. Loss of reduction with cast loosening is common. Cast changes with careful maintenance maneuvers may be required during the first 3 to 4 weeks. The basic maintenance maneuver used from the outset is a three-point support system, including pads under the palmar aspect of the scaphoid tuberosity and pisiform, plus dorsal pads over the neck of the capitate and over the proximal pole of the scaphoid. The pad under the tuberosity helps to lift and elongate the scaphoid, while the dorsal pad helps control the proximal scaphoid. The pisiform pad transmits a support to the triquetrum, diminishing its tendency to extend (Fig. 12-72). The dorsal pad over the capitate neck depresses the distal row on the proximal row, which derotates the extension of the proximal carpal row. Anatomical reduction is so difficult to maintain that some surgeons prefer percutaneous fixation over external support (cast immobilization alone) in most cases. The stability characteristics of the specific wrist reveal themselves by the difficulty noted in maintaining reduction with external support alone. If reduction is too difficult to either achieve or hold, that becomes the indication for open reduction and repair. The success of closed reduction methods requires adequate imaging with good, standardized posteroanterior and lateral views of the wrist or special imaging techniques.

Acute (Irreducible or Unstable) Perilunate Injury. If treatment is unsuccessful or if the injury is open, irreducible, unstable, or compromised neurovascularly, then open reduction, repair, and external or internal fixation is indicated.[174,180,233] There is value in both palmar and dorsal approaches. It is easier to examine the cartilage surfaces and intra-articular fragments

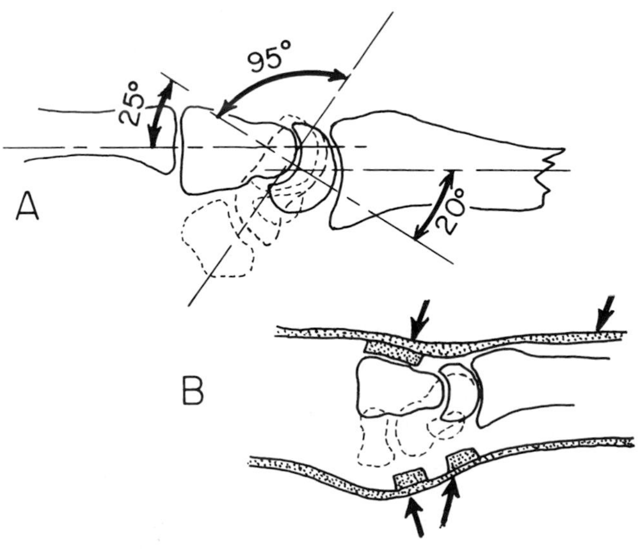

FIGURE 12-72. The authors' preferred technique of cast application for fracture-dislocations of the wrist using three-point fixation. (**A**) Dorsal instability pattern: capitolunate angle 25°; scapholunate angle 95°; radiolunate angle 20°. (**B**) Reduction is accomplished by pressure applied dorsally over the capitate and distal radius and palmarly over the distal pole of the scaphoid and the pisiform.

through the dorsal approach. It is easier to observe and repair palmar ligamentous damage through the palmar approach, and a palmar approach is essential if neurovascular injuries or flexor tendons are to be assessed. Transscaphoid fractures are often approached from the volar aspect if internal fixation is desired. However, the use of a volar approach only to place a Herbert screw or similar device, ignoring the other widespread requirements of this extensive injury, is inappropriate. It is more important to assess all elements of the injury, restore normal configuration of bony elements, and repair soft-tissue damage than to be concerned with the type of fixation device. The reduction and internal fixation should be centered around the lunate. The lunate must be aligned and pinned first to the distal radius. The lunatotriquetral joint is next reduced and pinned, and ligaments are repaired as needed. The capitolunate joint alignment is then evaluated and correct co-linear alignment is assessed. Lastly, the scapholunate joint (or transscaphoid fracture) is reduced and held with internal fixation. Compression screws are also quite helpful but must be used in concert with other forms of carpal reduction and fixation and not be relied on alone. Kirschner wires that can be inserted swiftly and repetitively are adequate for stabilization. External fixation is a reasonable alternative for complex perilunate dislocation and fracture–dislocations in our experience and that of others[180a] to provide a method of stabilization that allows for more secure ligament repair and fracture fixation.

Special Problems. The two types of perilunate dislocation and fracture–dislocation are the lesser arc or transligamentous injury and the greater arc or transosseous pattern (see Fig. 12-15). Within these major patterns there are many variant patterns.[220] For instance, the scaphoid and lunate may remain partly or totally bonded by ligamentous connections,[21,109,420] and the remainder of the carpus may disrupt around these two bones. In transosseous perilunate fracture–dislocations, a wide spectrum of fracture types is seen, such as transradiostyloid, transscaphoid (Fig. 12-73), transcapitate, and transtriquetral in various combinations (see Fig. 12-73).[22] Probably the most common distortions are those of the proximal capitate and the proximal scaphoid fragment.[348] The capitate fragment is frequently turned 180°, so that its articular surface faces the raw cancellous surface of the major capitate fragment.[281a,348,385,410,503,533] Both capitate and scaphoid fragments (see Figs. 12-73 and 12-74) are devascularized by displacement. Any such bony fragment displacement is best anatomically reduced and fixed. Multiple Kirschner wires inserted proximal to distal and left buried within the proximal capitate or scaphoid or retrograde insertion of a Herbert screw is recommended. Healing is surprisingly good, and restoration of bony architecture is the norm. Autogenous bone graft to restore scaphoid length may be required. Restoration of bony architecture, joint congruency, alignment, and capsular attenuation is probably sufficient in the majority of acute cases of perilunate disruption.

Soft-tissue damage is common in these high-energy lesions, and it may be obvious that a severe neuropathy or vascular deficiency has occurred. When these are present, open treatment and evaluation of the structures at risk is essential. Treatment of vascular and nerve injuries should proceed once the fractures are stabilized. Median or ulnar neuropathy, if severe or increasing, is an indication for surgical exploration.

Chronic, Perilunate-Type Injuries. Untreated injuries of this type may be seen months or years after the initial injury.[152,489] The patient is more likely to present because of increasing nerve symptoms or tendon rupture than because of wrist deformity, to which the patient has often become accustomed. These very late problems nearly always require some type of salvage operation, and this is discussed elsewhere. However, those injuries seen within 3 to 6 months are still potentially treatable by open reduction, although this will be more difficult because of articular changes and capsular contracture (Fig. 12-75).[489] A good clue to the potential for reduction is distraction of the carpal elements on x-rays obtained with 25 to 30 pounds of traction. An attempt at reduction, repair, and internal fixation should be offered if carpal bone realignment is feasible, because even in late cases results can be surprisingly good. Extensive dissection may be required.[218]

Another group of chronic, perilunate-type injuries includes those where prior treatment has not been completely successful. Depending on the time of presentation from injury and extent of prior surgery, options for treatment are identical to those of acute treatment. When a bone or bone fragment has been removed (eg, proximal scaphoid or capitate fragment), the alternatives are to rehabilitate the limb and assess the functional level or to consider a salvage procedure such as radiocarpal fusion[147,240] or proximal row carpectomy.[21,126,185,262,408]

Midcarpal Instabilities

Midcarpal instabilities are associated with or result directly from extrinsic ligament injuries of the wrist. The difficulties of diagnosing carpal instability of the nondissociative type (CIND) have already been discussed with regard to the radiocarpal instabilities (see Table 12-1).[154,473] The history and the physical findings differ little between radiocarpal and midcarpal types of CIND, unless a history of recent injury and a localized area of tenderness are both present.[85,155,273,320,335,517] Imaging findings are also almost identical for radiocar-

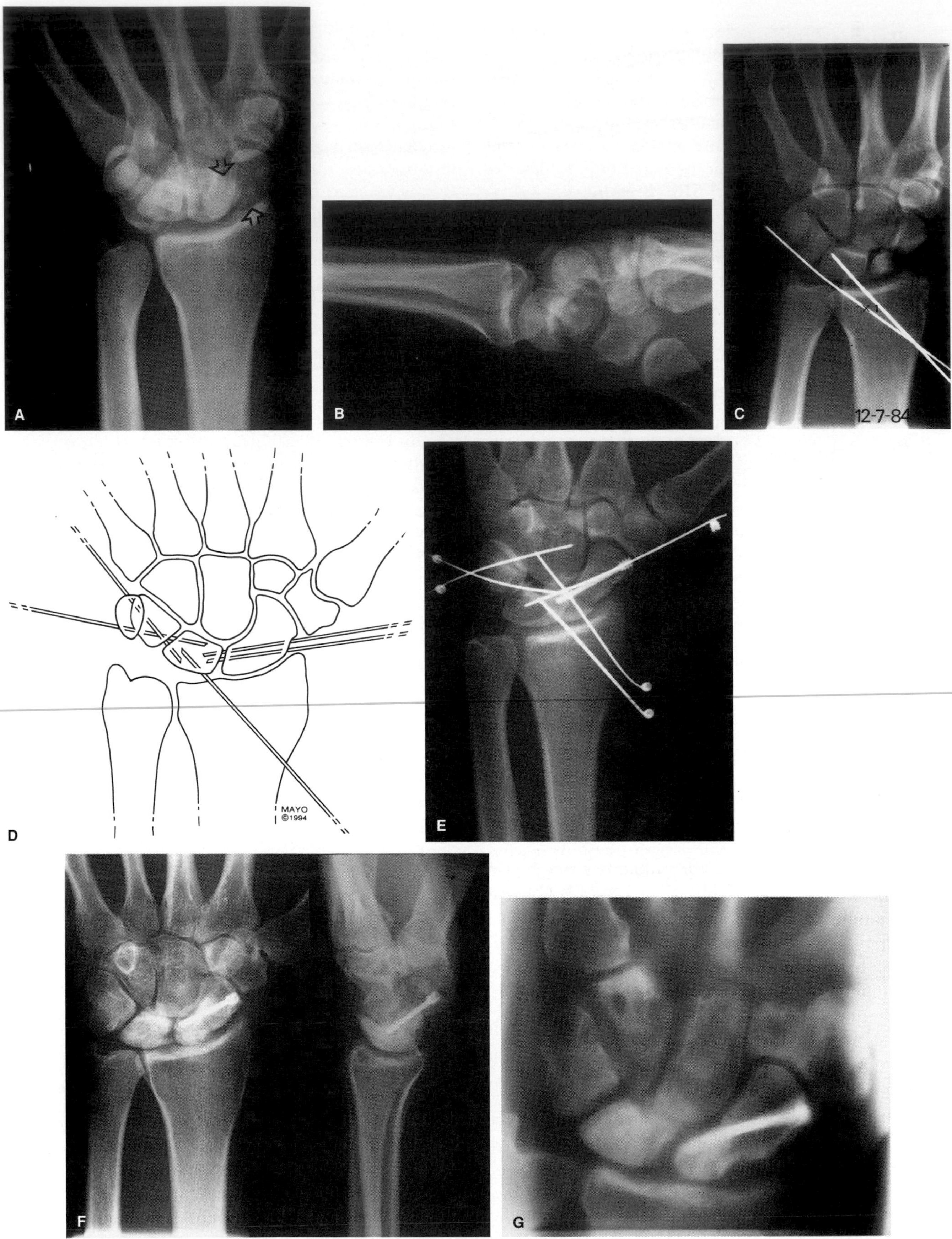

FIGURE 12-73.

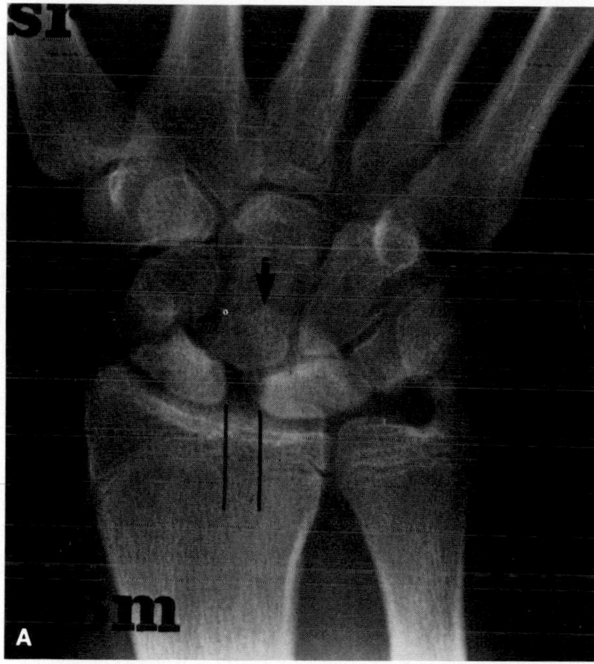

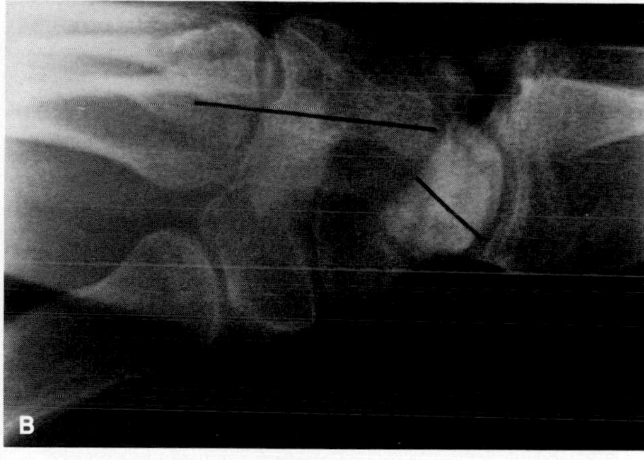

FIGURE 12-74. Transscaphoid, transcapitate perilunate dislocation. (**A**) A displaced scaphoid fracture (*small arrows*), increased scapholunate interval, and undisplaced capitate fracture (*large arrow*). Note increased density and bone cysts in the proximal scaphoid and lunate. (**B**) Persistent dorsal subluxation of the capitate and capitolunate instability is present.

pal or midcarpal CIND, and drawing a careful distinction between these uncommon and unusual injuries is difficult. Either VISI or DISI deformity or alternating patterns may occur at either level (Fig. 12-76).[154,320,335] In the early stages, these patterns of deformity may be so subtle that they are difficult to detect. Comparison of video motion patterns of the symptomatic wrist to the normal contralateral wrist is often useful. These difficulties are compounded by the fact that ligament insufficiency, which is usually post-traumatic but occasionally congenital, may be present at both radiocarpal and midcarpal levels. Visualizing both joints and the intervening proximal carpal row by arthroscopy or surgery gives the final opportunity to decide where the instability is most noticeable. Inflammatory synovitis and clear ligament laxity are the diagnostic signs. Even then, one may have to judge from subtle deviations from the norm, because the attenuation may not be obvious.

Several studies have added to our ability to diagnose midcarpal instability. Johnson and Carrera[273] described 12 cases in which laxity or attenuation of the radioscaphocapitate ligament was present. The diagnosis was made by midcarpal stress test in which a pathologic clunk could be reproduced by dorsal-palmar subluxation of the midcarpal joint. A painful snap could be produced with a sudden dorsal subluxation and ulnar shift of the lunate. With good cineradiography, moving the compressed carpus through the normal range of motion and with subluxation stresses applied during movement, one can produce the same catch or clunk that presented clinically. Differentially testing the midcarpal row and radiocarpal level may help one decide which is the more unstable.

A second clinical test[343] involves dynamic instability through the midcarpal joint produced by extension with radioulnar deviation, producing a "catch-up" clunk as the proximal row snaps from flexion into extension (Fig. 12-77).[558] The clinical literature suggests that triquetrohamate instability, presumed due to damage to the ulnar arm of the palmar arcuate ligament, is the most common cause for midcarpal instability, but dorsal ligament laxity (dorsal radiotrique-

FIGURE 12-73. Principles of reduction of a transscaphoid perilunate dislocation. (**A**) PA view of the carpus showing the distal scaphoid (*up arrow*) and proximal scaphoid (*down arrow*), with the proximal displaced capitate aligned to the articular surface of distal radius. (**B**) In the lateral view, the lunate is aligned with the distal radius but not the capitate (which is dorsally displaced), nor the scaphoid. (**C**) Reduction of the lunate to the distal radius (aligned and held with Kirschner wires). (**D**) Schematic diagram showing reduction and K-wire fixation of the lunate to distal radius; triquetrum to lunate; and fixation of either a scaphoid fracture or scapholunate dissociation with Kirschner wires. (**E**) Internal fixation of a carpal dislocation with K-wires (0.035–0.045 inch) and Herbert screw (antegrade inserted). (**F**) After K-wire removal and fracture healing showing maintenance of carpal alignment. (**G**) PA tomogram demonstrates residual ischemic changes in the proximal scaphoid and lunate. This ischemia usually resolves with fracture and ligament healing as revascularization occurs.

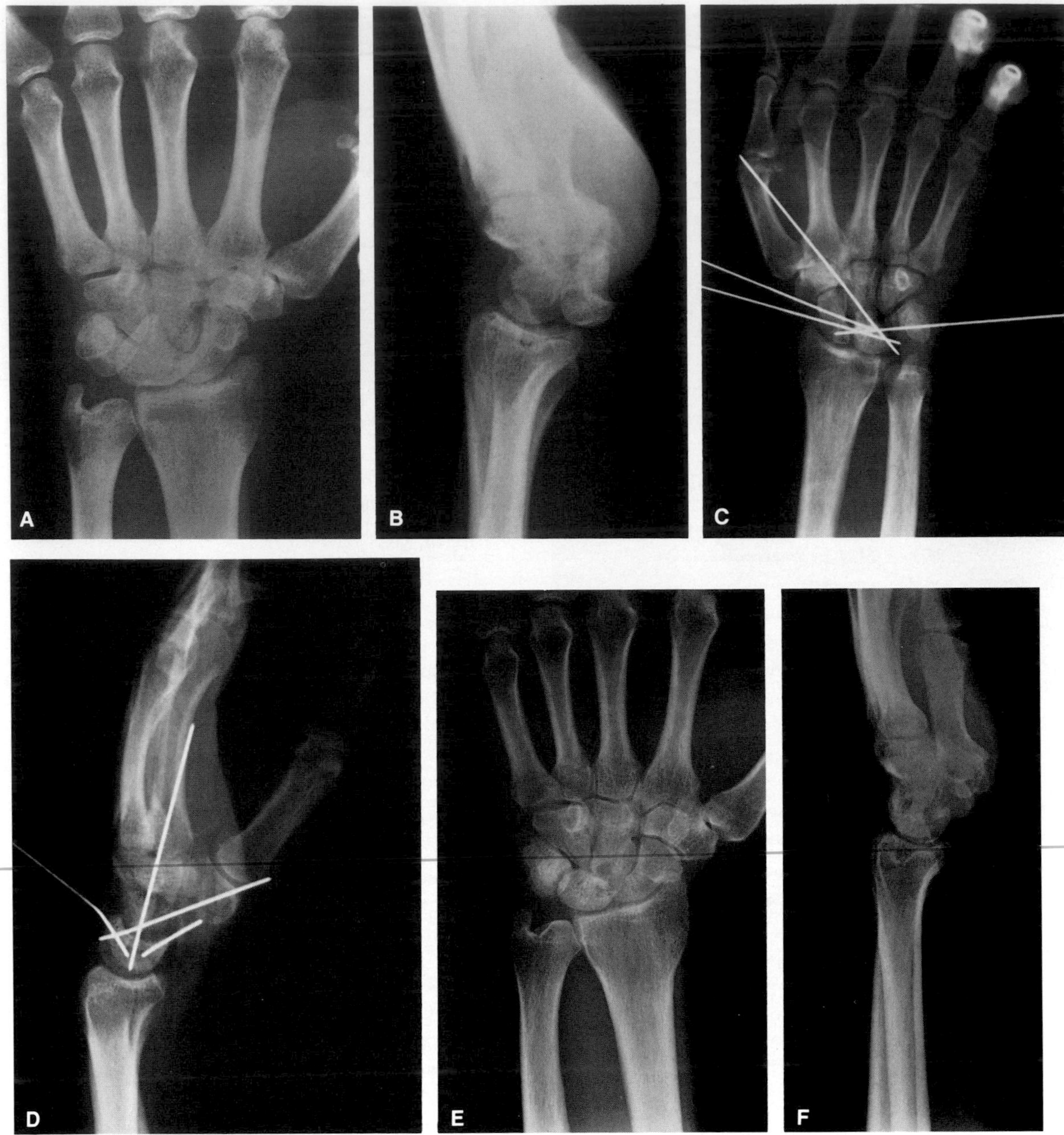

FIGURE 12-75. Chronic perilunate dislocation treated by open reduction. (**A**) PA and (**B**) lateral x-rays of the nondominant hand of a patient who was seen at our institution 17 weeks after a forced extension injury resulted in perilunate dislocation. The patient was unable to work because of severe, intolerable pain. Grip strength measured 12% of the opposite hand. (**C**) PA and (**D**) lateral x-rays at the time of open reduction and temporary K-wire fixation. The scapholunate and lunotriquetral ligaments were also repaired at this time. (**E**) PA and (**F**) lateral films 12 months postoperation demonstrate maintenance of reduction. The patient had returned to heavy farm work and reported occasional mild pain after heavy lifting. Grip strength measured 73% of the opposite dominant hand. (*Siegert, J.J., Frassica, F.J., Amadio, P.C.: Treatment of Chronic Perilunate Dislocations. J. Hand Surg. 13A(2):206–012, 1988.*)

tral and dorsal intercarpal) may also be important.[10,320] Our clinical experience suggests that radiocarpal causes of proximal carpal row instability are as common as midcarpal causes. Midcarpal instability may be associated with radioscaphocapitate ligament attenuation,[335] leading to loss of radiocarpal wrist stability as well as midcarpal instability.[530] Experience is not yet sufficient to judge how the incidence of midcarpal instability compares with other forms of carpal instability, and therefore treatment alternatives remain limited. Localized fusion placed at the wrong level will not correct the problem, and we have seen instances of satisfactory midcarpal fusion followed by symptomatic radiocarpal instability.

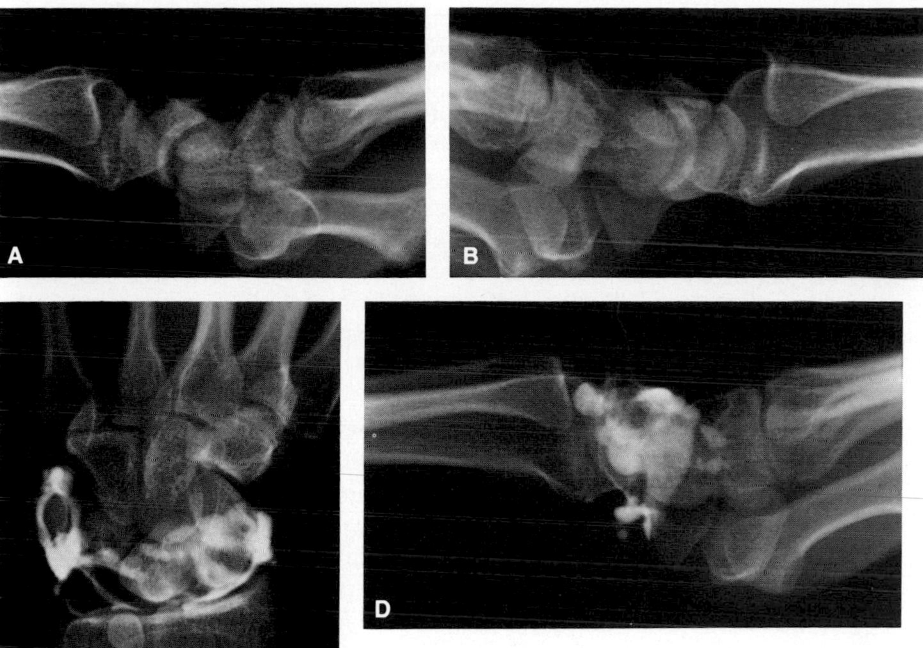

FIGURE 12-76. Carpal instability nondissociative (CIND). (**A**) The left wrist shows a VISI deformity secondary to catching a thrown 20-pound weight. The wrist was weak and painful, and a snapping motion could be elicited. (**B**) The right wrist shows normal alignment of the midcarpal joint. (**C,D**) Normal PA and lateral radiocarpal arthrogram views confirm that the VISI deformity is related to extrinsic and not intrinsic carpal ligament injury.

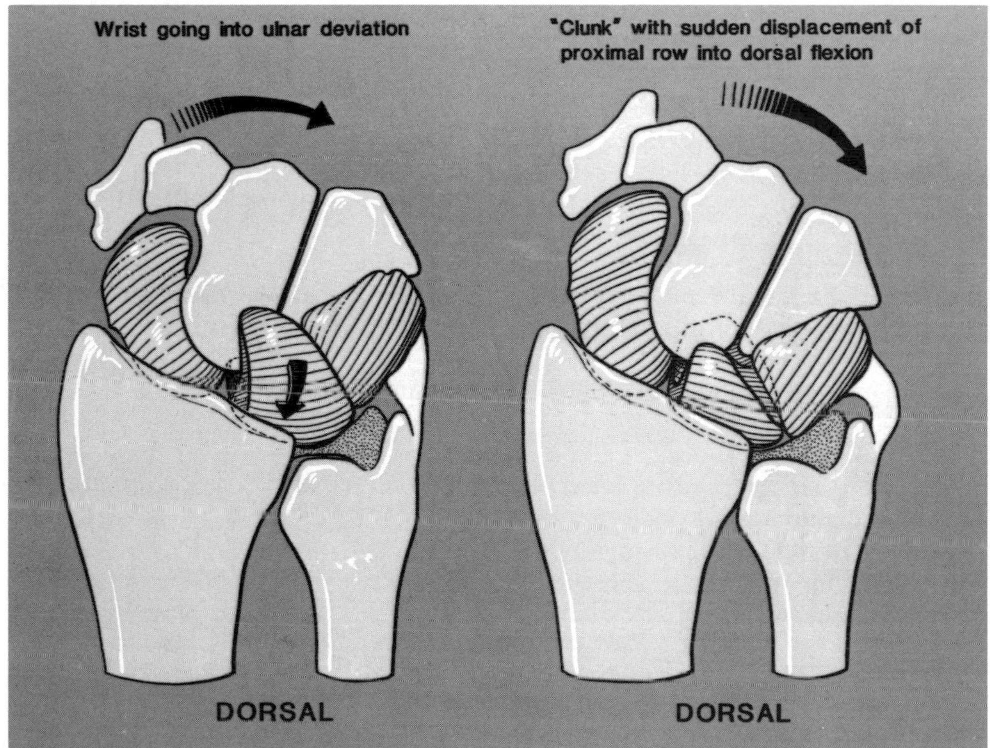

FIGURE 12-77. Catch-up clunk. Carpal instability nondissociative (CIND) is often characterized by sudden displacement of the lunate during radial to ulnar deviation. The palmar-flexed lunate catches as it slides up the radial inclination, then suddenly displaces radially and dorsiflexes with an audible and palpable "clunk." The end positions are normal, but occur as an interrupted rather than a smooth motion transition.

Treatment

There is no preferred procedure that can be universally applied for midcarpal instability.[343] A careful review of our experience in treating this problem indicates about equally satisfactory results with both nonoperative and surgical treatment. A solid radius-to-metacarpal (wrist) fusion should solve any instability problem, but the penalties of that treatment are so severe that it should not be applied, unless one is dealing with a fixed deformity and significant arthritis. Many of these wrist problems occur in individuals with congenitally or post-traumatically lax wrists,[509,510] who can control the subluxation tendency to some degree by the sequence of muscle contraction. In such instances, external support, limiting the provocative wrist motion, plus musculotendinous training may suffice.

For those with relatively normal joint surfaces but uncontrollable symptoms, the treatment plan is similar to that outlined for radiocarpal instability. If a specific lesion can be identified, such as damage to radial arcuate (radioscaphocapitate) ligament, the ulnar palmar arcuate (triquetrocapitate) ligament, or the scaphotrapeziotrapezoidal capsule, direct repairs are indicated with temporary percutaneous fixation in the corrected alignment. A reasonable repair for a midcarpal VISI instability (VISI-CIND) is to close the space of Poirier palmarly[273] or to construct a dorsal radiocarpal tether between radius and proximal carpal row that limits proximal row excursion. Conversely, for a midcarpal CIND-DISI pattern, one could augment dorsally between proximal carpal row and mid-metacarpal base. If manual reduction is incomplete or recurrence after reduction is rapid at the midcarpal joint, localized fusion across the midcarpal joint is preferable.[85,248,482,528] Radiocarpal fusion is more likely to control the unstable proximal carpal row.[326] Soft-tissue augmentation or repair should be protected for 8 weeks with percutaneous pins and external support part time for another 8 weeks. Proximal row carpectomy is a satisfactory salvage procedure.[408,500]

Midcarpal Instability Secondary to Malangulation of the Distal Radius

There are two conditions that can produce proximal carpal row malalignment secondary to deformity of the distal radius. The less common is ulnar translation of the carpus from Madelung's deformity. This condition is due to increased radial-to-ulnar slope of the distal radial articular surface. It is developmental (but occasionally post-traumatic).[536] A much more common problem is post-traumatic deformity of the distal radius related to the attempt of the hand to realign itself with the forearm in the presence of an extension malunion of the distal radius (see Fig. 12-53). In such circumstances, the carpus has two alternatives, one of which is to translate dorsally on the radial articular surface and articulate with only the dorsal half of that radial surface.[52,521] The carpus remains aligned, as does the hand, so that function and appearance remain reasonably good. The carpus is more prominent dorsally and motion is somewhat restricted, particularly flexion, but patients with this realignment pattern infrequently seek additional treatment. More commonly, the proximal carpal row stays aligned normally with the distal radius, but a flexion angulation, DISI, develops at the midcarpal level. Furthermore, the proximal carpal row cannot slide normally in either the radioulnar plane or the dorsopalmar plane to permit a normal pattern of wrist motion. Over time, this may be accompanied by wrist discomfort, grip weakness, and eventually abnormal wear patterns at both the radiocarpal and midcarpal levels.

Appropriate treatment for midcarpal instability secondary to a distal radius fracture is corrective radial osteotomy with restoration of length and angulation (see Fig. 12-53).[19,179,497] If there are no associated problems, the carpal malalignment should improve as the distal radius is corrected. Open-wedge osteotomy of the distal radius, bone graft, and plate fixation is the current preference. If there are associated instabilities of the distal ulna, DRUJ problems, or fixed deformity of the carpus, then further surgical alternatives, such as ulnar shortening, DRUJ stabilization, or midcarpal joint fusion, may need to be addressed at the same time.

Axial Instabilities

Axial (longitudinal) instabilities are a type of carpal instability in which the injury affects longitudinal support or alignment of the wrist rather than transverse alignment of the proximal and distal carpal rows. Crush injuries that flatten the hand cause this "axial" instability. Axial instabilities have been separately categorized from other carpal injuries (Fig. 12-78).[93,204,209,396,413,441] These represent longitudinal fracture–dislocations of the wrist and, for the most part, are caused by high-energy injuries. Traumatic causes have included an exploding truck tire, crushing under heavy objects, and high-pressure machine compression.[204] The basic pathophysiology is collapse of the carpal arch, often with tearing or avulsion of the bony origins of the transverse carpal ligament.[206,207] The focus of this injury is usually in the distal carpus and adjacent metacarpals, occasionally extending either distally into the intermetacarpal area or proximally through the proximal carpal row (Fig. 12-79).[239] The most common pattern is separation of either radial or ulnar "columns" of the carpus with their metacarpal rays from the central carpus.[209] From our review of the more common patterns, a proposed nomenclature is axial-radial,

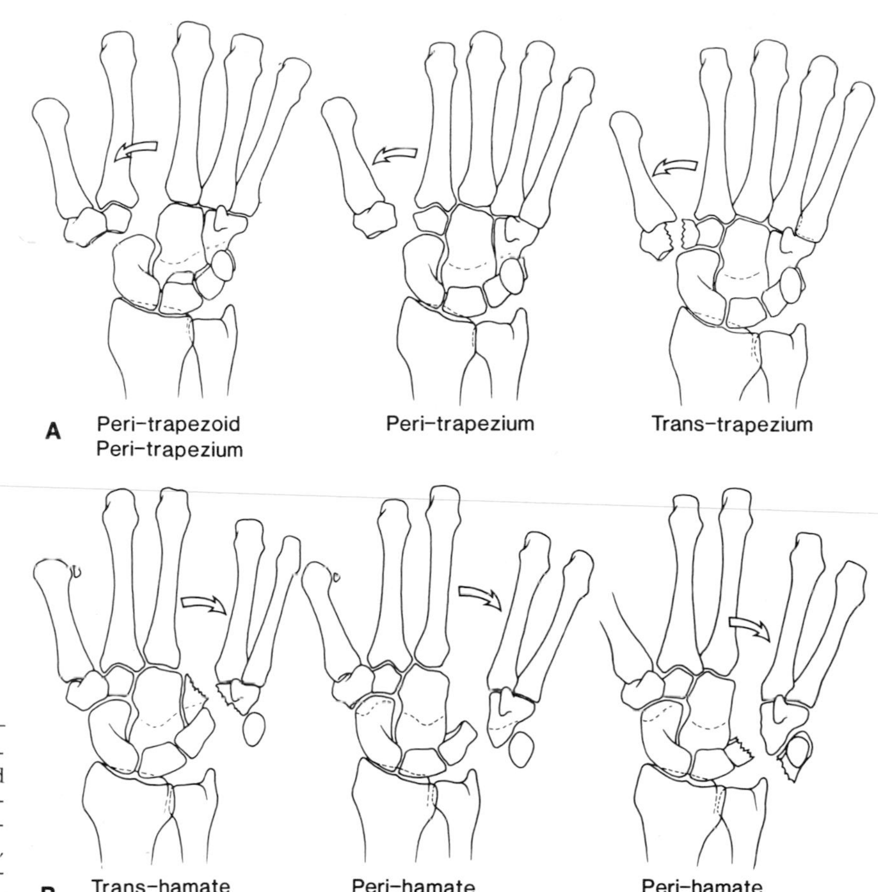

FIGURE 12-78. Axial disruptions of the carpus. (**A**) Axial-radial disruption, peritrapezoid and peritrapezial types. (**B**) Axial-ulnar disruptions, transhamate, perihamate, and transtriquetral types. (*Garcia-Elias, M., Dobyns, J.H., Cooney, W.P., Linscheid, R.L.: Traumatic Axial Dislocation of the Carpus. J. Hand Surg. 14A(3):446–457, 1989.*)

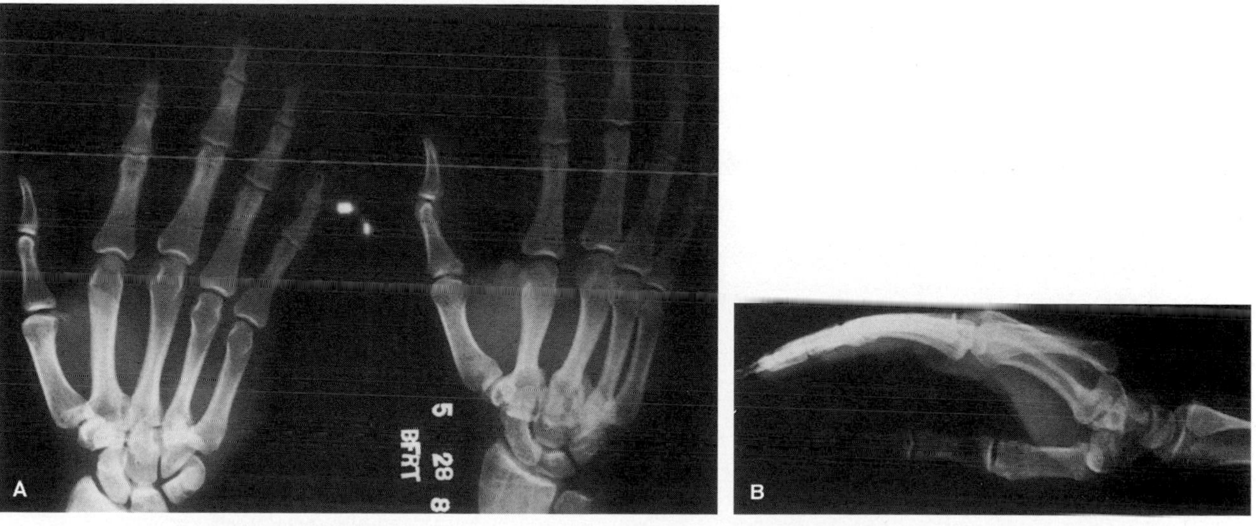

FIGURE 12-79. (**A**) Complete fracture-dislocation of the second through fifth carpometacarpal joints. Note overlapping of the metacarpal and distal carpal bones (*right*). (**B**) A lateral view shows the displacement even more clearly.

axial-ulnar, or a combination of the two fracture–dislocations (see Fig. 12-78). The carpal elements involved are usually indicated by the term *peri,* if the discontinuity is primarily ligamentous, as in peritrapezial or peritrapezoidal-trapezial. If the discontinuity is through bone, the term *trans* is employed, as in transtrapezial or transtrapeziotrapezoidal. The accompanying soft-tissue disruption is often of more importance than the bone and joint disruption. Neurovascular injury is frequent, sometimes to the point of nonviability of digits.

Diagnosis is established by the history of a force propagating in a sagittal plane (ie, dorsal to palmar crush), often with evidence of severe soft-tissue damage, swelling, and open wounds. Standard x-rays should confirm the diagnosis, although the carpal malalignment may be subtle and escape notice. A high index of suspicion is needed. Provocative stress x-rays, tomography, CT scanning, or MRI should be obtained preoperatively. Evidence of nerve, vascular, musculotendinous, and ligamentous damage is usually present, often to a severe degree. Instances of median neuropathy are less than expected, probably because the carpal tunnel is usually decompressed by the injury.

Treatment

A complete assessment is needed in these injuries for planning of both soft-tissue and joint repair. Urgent surgical intervention is often indicated to salvage neurovascular function and restore skeletal alignment (Fig. 12-80).[93] Massive swelling may necessitate decompression of compartments not already decompressed by the injury. Traction can help reduce the axial displacement. Fractures and dislocations, once reduced, can be maintained by Kirschner wires and lag screws. Transcarpal or metacarpal K-wire fixation is usually necessary to prevent redisplacement. Early *active* motion of the hand helps prevent adhesions of the flexor and extensor tendons. Rehabilitation is often prolonged, and prognosis depends on the severity of soft-tissue damage.

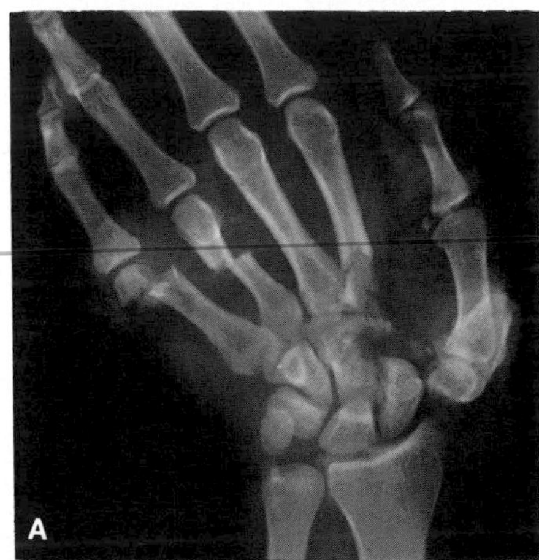

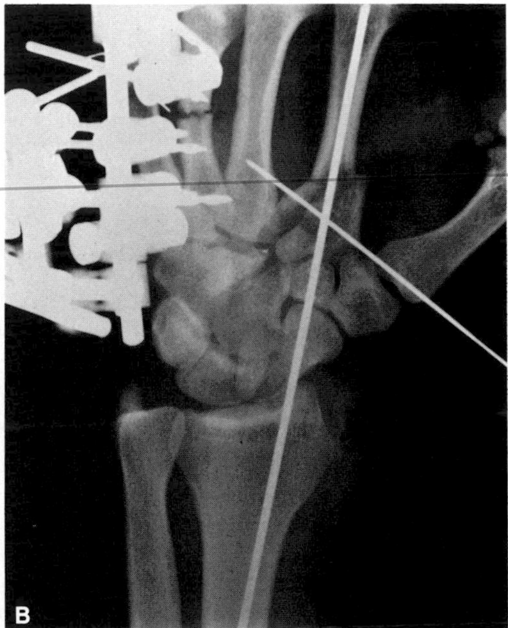

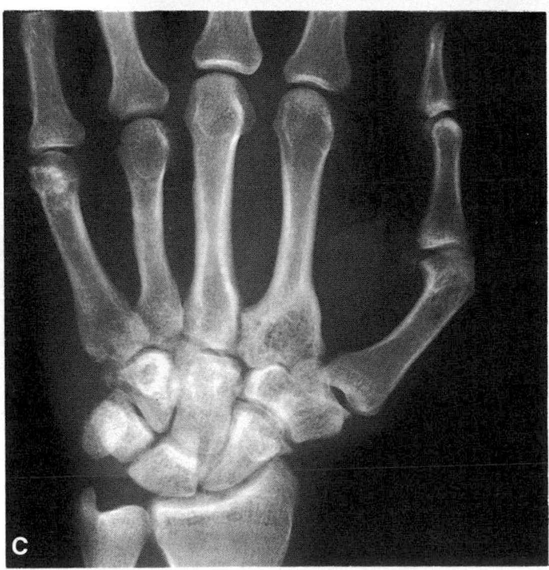

FIGURE 12-80. A peritrapezial-trapezoidal axial dissociation in a 19-year-old man who sustained a crush injury of his left wrist. He had associated injuries of intrinsic muscles and extensor tendons, along with fractures of the index, ring, and little metacarpal fractures. (**A**) Radial axial dislocation of the thumb ray through the trapezium and trapezoid articulation with the scaphoid and capitate. Note transverse fractures of the fourth and fifth metacarpals. (**B**) Transverse and axial K-wire fixation of the radial axial fracture-dislocation, and external fixation of the open metacarpal fractures. (**C**) Six years following injury, the skeleton is well aligned. There were residual intrinsic contractures.

FRACTURES OF THE OTHER CARPAL BONES (Excluding the Scaphoid and Lunate)

Mechanisms of Injury

Triquetrum

Fractures of the triquetrum result from a direct blow or from an avulsion injury that may include ligament damage.[36,137,150,203] The triquetrum may be fractured transversely during a perilunate dislocation, but it usually displaces dorsally with the distal carpal row away from the lunate (Fig. 12-81).[87,203] The most common triquetral fracture is probably the impingement shear fracture[69,316] of ulnar styloid against dorsal triquetrum, occurring with the wrist in extension and ulnar deviation, particularly when a long ulnar styloid is present.[203,316] Shear impingement by the hamate against the posteroradial projection of the triquetrum can occur with the wrist in extension and ulnar deviation. A bone avulsion with either dorsal or palmar ligaments stripped from their triquetral insertions can also occur. The triquetrum is rarely dislocated alone because of the strong ligamentous support dorsally, palmarly, and ulnarly. Isolated case reports have been described.[54,196]

Trapezium

Fracture through the articular surface of the trapezium is produced by the base of the first metacarpal being driven into the articular surface of the trapezium by the adducted thumb (Fig. 12-82).[17,123,172,275,359] Avulsion fractures caused by the capsular ligaments can occur during forceful deviation, traction, or rotation.[87,271,416] Direct blows to the palmar arch area or forceful distraction of the proximal palmar arch may result in avulsion of the ridge of the trapezium by the

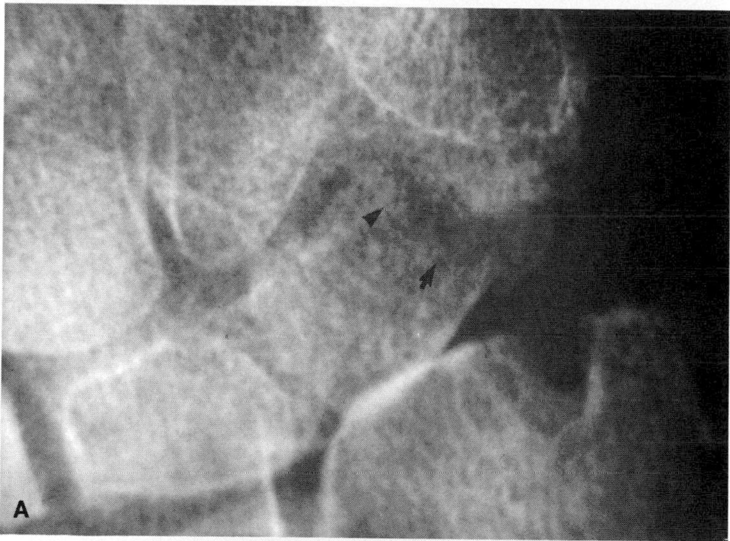

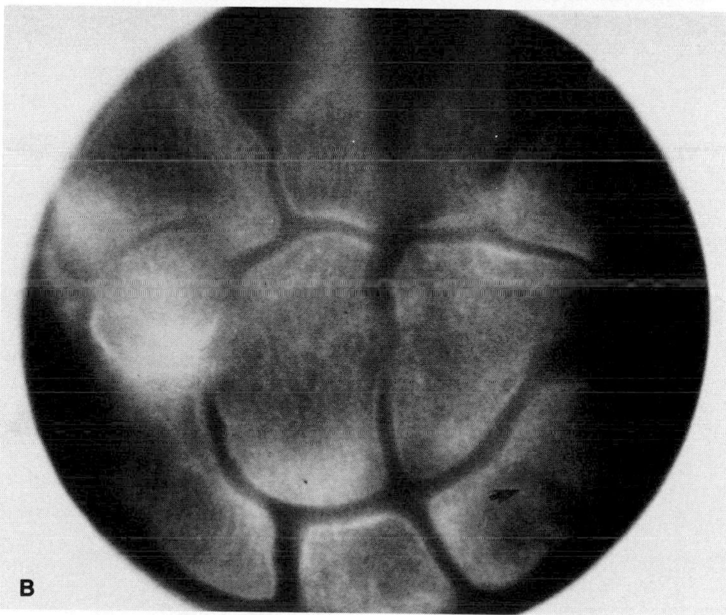

FIGURE 12-81. Triquetral fractures. (**A**) An isolated fracture through the body of the triquetrum from an apparent impaction load from the distal ulna. This fracture may also occur from a greater arc injury of the carpus (see Fig. 12-15). (**B**) A tomogram confirms an undisplaced fracture in the body of the triquetrum.

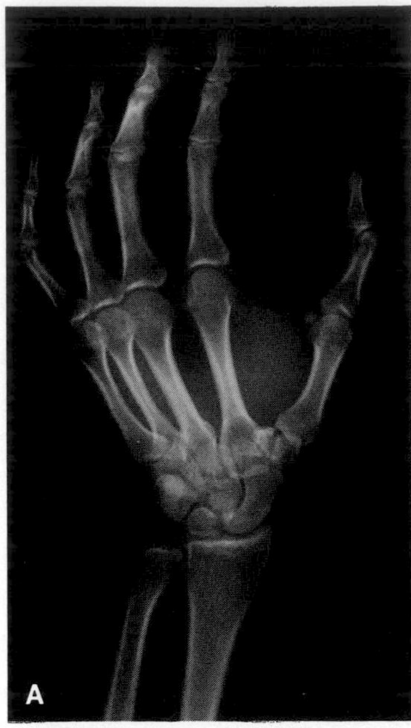

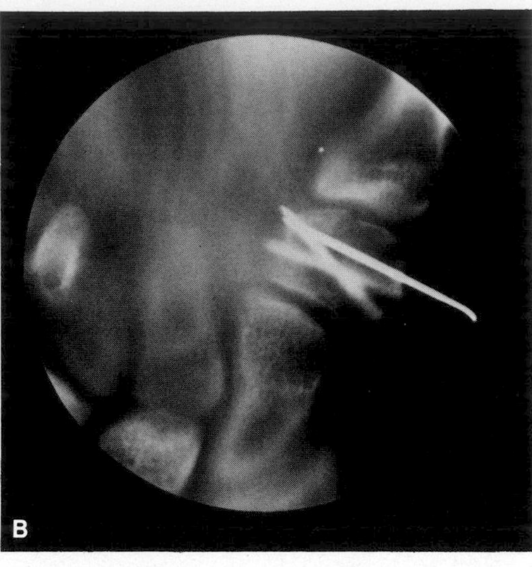

FIGURE 12-82. Fracture of the trapezium. (**A**) A comminuted fracture on the radial side of the trapezium with displacement of the first metacarpal base. (**B**) Open reduction and internal fixation with K-wires was performed to realign the joint articular surface.

transverse carpal ligament.[123,150,421] Dislocations are occasionally seen.[254,479,486,488,505,512]

Pisiform

The pisiform is generally injured during a fall on the dorsiflexed, outstretched hand.[69,150] A direct blow while the pisiform is held firmly against the triquetrum under tension from the flexor carpi ulnaris leads to either avulsion of its distal portion with a vertical fracture or an osteochondral compression fracture at the pisotriquetral joint (Fig. 12-83). Subluxation or dislocation may occur, usually with a combination of wrist extension and flexor carpi ulnaris contraction.[376,535]

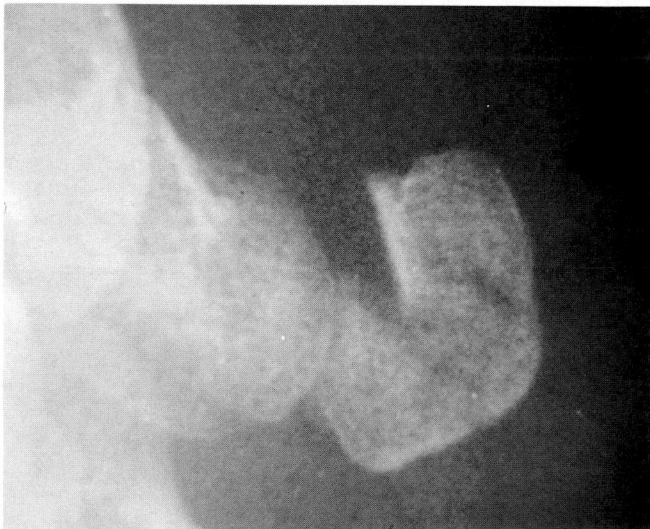

FIGURE 12-83. Pisiform fracture. A rather unusual displaced fracture through the body of the pisiform, from a direct blow to the palmar surface of the hand. Treatment was excision of the pisiform.

Hamate

The hamate may be fractured through its distal articular surface,[347] through the other articular surfaces, or through the hook (hamulus) of the hamate,[23,59,271] the proximal pole, or the body.[11,69,87,334,373,415,493,502] The hamate may also be dislocated by direct violence.[416] A dorsally displaced articular fracture, the distal portion of the hamate with fifth metacarpal subluxation, occurs when force is applied along the shaft as from a fall or a blow from a fist. Fracture of the hook of the hamate may occur from a fall on the dorsiflexed wrist, with tension exerted through the transverse carpal ligament and pisohamate ligament (Fig. 12-84).[59,78,97,381] More commonly, sports-related fracture of the hook occurs from the use of clubs, bats, or racquets.[502] Direct force exerted by these objects against the hypothenar eminence or transverse carpal ligament has been implicated. The fracture generally occurs at the base of the hamulus, although avulsion fracture of the tip also may be seen. Osteochondral fracture of the proximal pole probably occurs from impaction injuries against the articular surface of the lunate during dorsiflexion and ulnar deviation. Osteochondral fractures of the triquetral and hamate articular surface may occur in a similar fashion or from a shearing injury, such as that which occurs when a trapped hand is wrenched violently against a steering wheel. Fractures of the body of the hamate[193] and dislocation of the hamate[237] are generally caused by blast injuries or by direct crushing injuries, such as punch-press accidents.

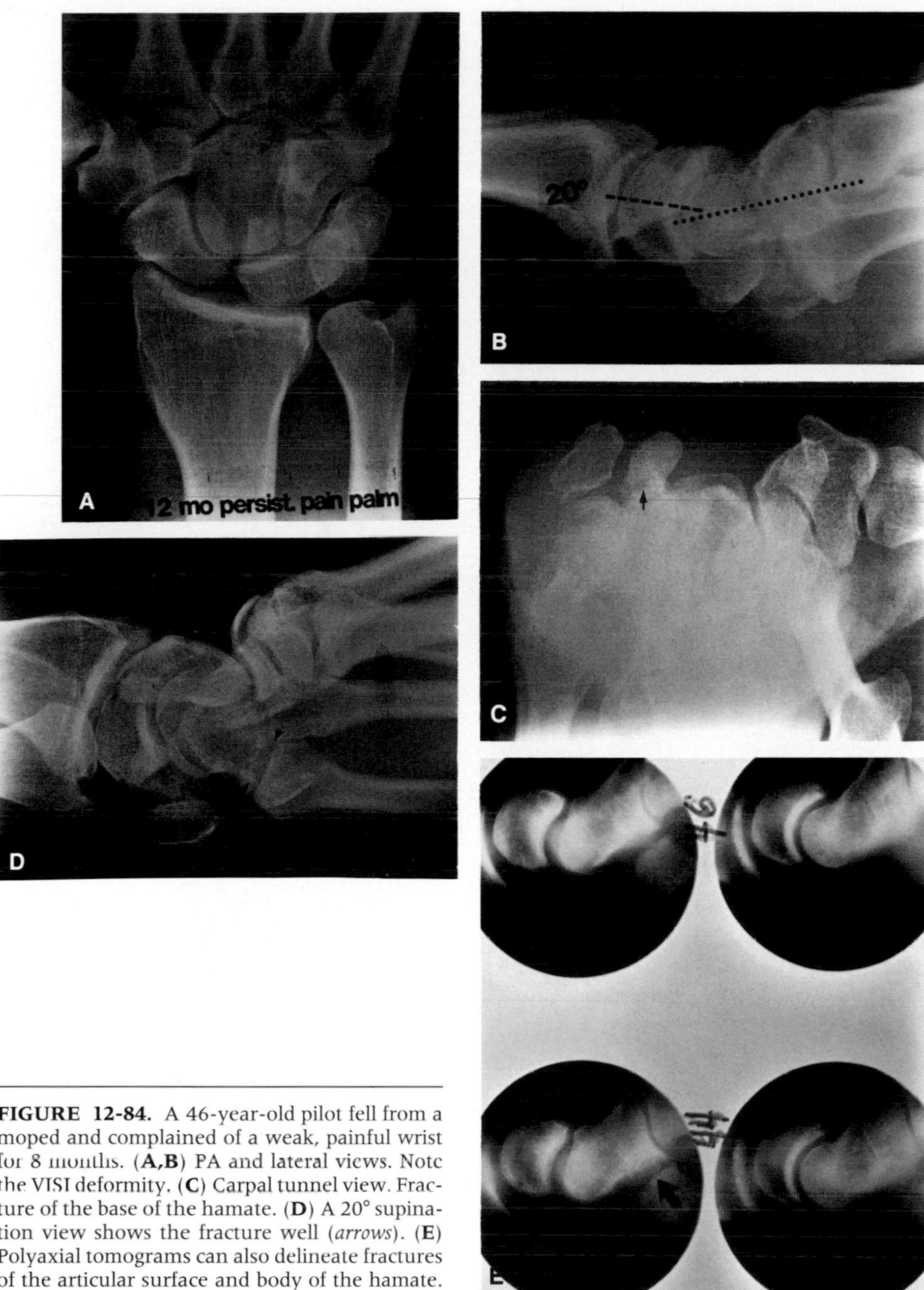

FIGURE 12-84. A 46-year-old pilot fell from a moped and complained of a weak, painful wrist for 8 months. (**A,B**) PA and lateral views. Note the VISI deformity. (**C**) Carpal tunnel view. Fracture of the base of the hamate. (**D**) A 20° supination view shows the fracture well (*arrows*). (**E**) Polyaxial tomograms can also delineate fractures of the articular surface and body of the hamate.

Capitate

Because of its protected position, the body of the capitate is seldom fractured (Fig. 12-85).[3,150,337,338,446,450] Nonunions of the capitate with fracture site erosion and secondary DISI deformity have been recorded.[375] Direct force or crushing blows usually occur with associated injury to the metacarpals and other carpal bones. The capitate, in association with perilunate fracture–dislocation, is more susceptible to fracture through the neck of the bone.[446] A variation of this is the "naviculocapitate syndrome,"[174] in which the capitate and scaphoid are fractured but no dislocation is observed. Because fractures of the scaphoid and the capitate are only stage 1 or stage 2 of the spectrum of injury that culminates in a transscaphoid, transcapitate, perilunate dislocation of the carpus, it is not surprising that the capitate fragment can be frequently rotated 90° to 180° with the articular surface displaced anteriorly or facing the fracture surface of the capitate neck. Without reduction, avascular necrosis will result. In wrist fracture–dislocations, subtle osteochrondral injuries can be easily overlooked. The mechanism of injury is impingement of the capitate against the dorsal lip of the radius during hyperdorsiflexion, although an opposite mechanism—that of a fall on the hyperflexed

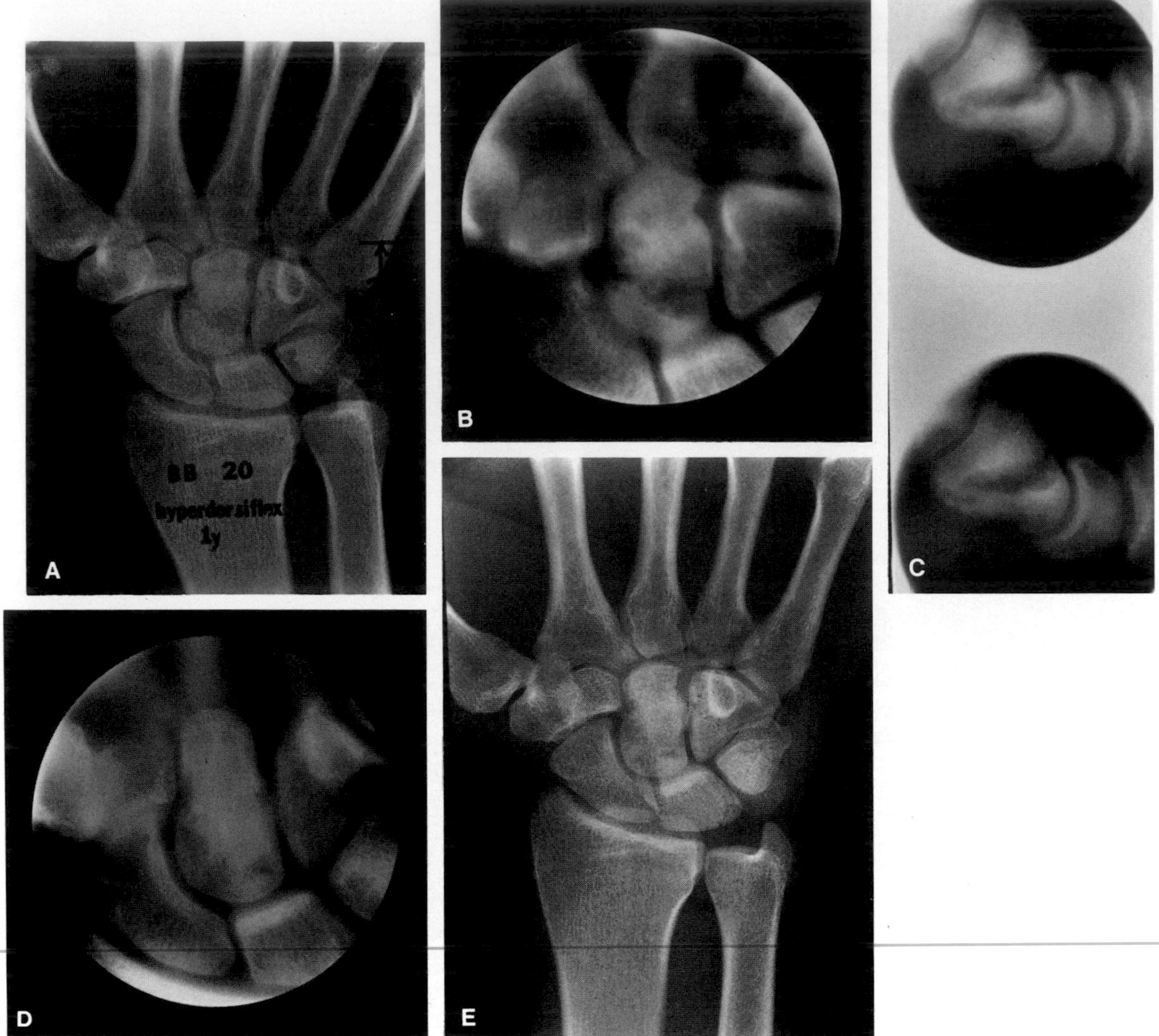

FIGURE 12-85. A 20-year-old softball player hyperextended his wrist 1 year prior to examination. He had persistent pain in the mid carpus. (**A**) An AP x-ray was apparently normal except for a suspicious capitate fracture. (**B**) AP polyaxial tomograms demonstrated a fracture nonunion through the body of the capitate, with foreshortening. (**C**) The lateral view showed dorsal displacement of the distal fragment. (**D**) The capitate healed 5 months after open reduction, distraction, and fixation with a keyed corticocancellous graft. Note sclerosis and mild avascular changes. (**E**) Final radiographic appearance, showing the united capitate.

wrist—has also been suggested. Nonunion and ischemia after injury[338,375,444] are rare in the capitate, but they do occur.[445]

Trapezoid

Injury to the trapezoid is generally associated with forces applied through the second metacarpal (see Fig. 12-80).[305] Because of its shape and position, the trapezoid is rarely fractured, although axial loading of the second metacarpal can cause dorsal dislocation with rupture of the capsular ligaments.[305,365,452] Palmar dislocation has also been reported. Ligamentous instability produced by similar injury or osteochondral injuries to the trapezoid–second metacarpal, capitate–third metacarpal, or metacarpohamate joints often escapes detection. Blast or crush forces can also disrupt the trapezoid sufficient to dislocate or fracture it.

Signs and Symptoms

The signs and symptoms of injuries to the individual carpal bones are pain and tenderness appropriately situated for the injury. Localized swelling, prominence, and limited motion may be present. Stress of muscle–tendon units inserted on or supported by the injured structure may localize symptoms. A knowledge of the deep and topographic anatomy should locate the injury specifically. Neurovascular signs are unusual with these isolated carpal injuries, except for injury of the pisiform and the hook of the hamate, which may affect the ulnar nerve and artery. Tendons on both the flexor and extensor surfaces pass near carpal bone surfaces.[66a] Either the fresh raw surface of recent fracture or the roughened exostosis of an old nonunion or malunion may damage any of the flexor or extensor tendons that pass over the carpus.[127]

Radiographic Examination

Triquetrum

Dorsal chip fractures of the triquetrum are easily overlooked on the anteroposterior view because of the normal superimposition of the dorsal lip on the lunate.[313] Such fractures are usually seen in one of the three lateral views of the recommended motion studies of the wrist; if not, a slightly oblique, pronated lateral view will project the triquetrum even more dorsal to the lunate. Transverse fractures of the triquetral body are usually easily identified on the anteroposterior view.

Trapezium

If fractures of the body of the trapezium cannot be seen on standard views, a true anteroposterior x-ray such as the Robert view to outline the trapezium and first metacarpal base without superimposition may be useful.

Fracture of the trapezial ridge is difficult to identify without carpal tunnel views that silhouette the ridge.

Pisiform

Special views are required to see pisiform injuries. A lateral view of the wrist with the forearm in 20° to 45° supination (see Fig. 12-84) and carpal tunnel views (see Fig. 12-26) are useful. If subluxation of the pisotriquetral joint is suspected, the diagnosis is made when one or more of the following are present: (1) a joint space more than 4 mm in width, (2) loss of parallelism of the joint surfaces greater than 20°, and (3) proximal or distal overriding of the pisiform amounting to more than 15% of the width of the joint surfaces. The wrist must be in a neutral position during these observations.

Hamate

Fractures and dislocations of the hamate are usually identified on posteroanterior or anteroposterior views.[161,334] A dislocation usually results in some rotation that alters the contour of the bone and the normal oval appearance of the hamulus. Fracture of the hook of the hamate is best visualized on the carpal tunnel or 20° supination oblique view.[97,191,430] When there is still doubt, polytomography or CT scanning can confirm the fracture.[161,273a] The hook of the hamate is said to ossify independently and occasionally may fail to fuse with the body of the hamate. This separate bone, known as the os hamulus proprium, can be mistaken for a fracture. Chondral articular injuries are seldom visualized on x-rays.

Capitate

Fractures of the capitate can usually be identified on standard posteroanterior x-rays, although motion studies are recommended to look for displacement. A lucent line through the neck of the capitate may be isolated or may be combined with other fractures or fracture–dislocations.[337,338,533] In such instances, the head of the capitate should be identified on the lateral view to determine if it has been rotated or displaced. Tomography and MRI may be necessary to detect occult capitate fractures. MRI provides information regarding vascularity of the proximal capitate.

Trapezoid

A trapezoid dislocation or fracture–dislocation is seen on the anteroposterior view as a loss of the normal relationship between the second metacarpal base and the trapezoid. The trapezoid may be superimposed over the trapezium, or the capitate and the second metacarpal may be proximally displaced. Oblique views and tomography may be helpful because the trapezoid is difficult to visualize on routine posteroanterior, anteroposterior, or lateral views of the wrist.

Treatment

Isolated injuries of the carpal bones are treated similarly if nondisplaced. Most respond to 6 weeks of support in a short-arm plaster cast or splint (even fractures of the hamate[557a]). In a few instances, such as the fracture of the neck of the capitate, in which there is instability or vascular deprivation, more complete rest of the upper limb muscles is gained by using a long-arm, full-digit cast, plus internal fixation by Kirschner wires or screws if displacement is evident.

Dislocations or displaced fractures should be treated in the same fashion. Satisfactory reduction can be accomplished in a finger-trap apparatus with countertraction on the arm and good muscle relaxation. Direct manipulative pressure may be required. If the reduction is unsatisfactory, open reduction and internal fixation[191,193,194] (Kirschner wires, screws, staples) should be used. A fracture of the hook of the hamate may be the sole exception when excision[59,93A,201a,502] is preferred to open reduction and internal fixation.[549] Even some fractures that are satisfactorily reduced by closed methods may be unstable enough to require percutaneous pin fixation or compression screw fixation (capitate,[452a] hamate). Fractures at the carpometacarpal joint frequently need such fixation. Other indications for open reduction include gross comminution involving an important joint (eg, the trapezium at the thumb carpometacarpal joint will require bone graft to replace bone loss), fusion for irreparable joint damage, or excisional arthroplasty. Revascularization procedures may see increasing use. In a few circumstances in which there is persistent instability, external fixation with slight distraction may be useful.

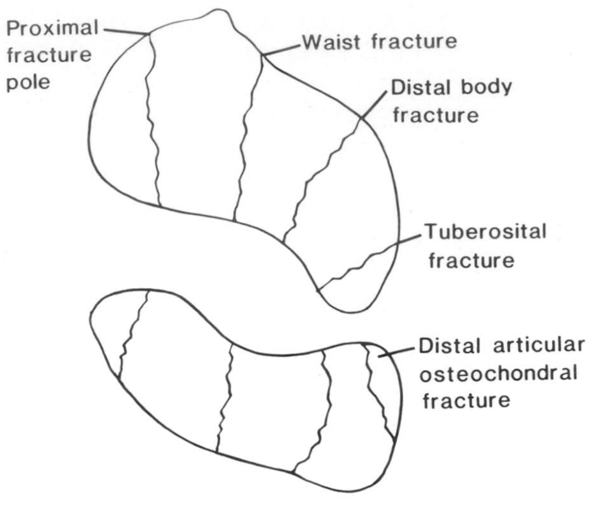

FIGURE 12-86. Types of scaphoid fractures. The scaphoid is susceptible to fractures at any level. Approximately 65% occur at the waist, 15% through the proximal pole, 10% through the distal body, 8% through the tuberosity, and 2% in the distal articular surface.

FRACTURES OF THE SCAPHOID

Fractures of the scaphoid are among the most common fractures of the wrist after fractures of the distal radius and represent the most common fracture of a carpal bone.[150,393,537] The position of the scaphoid on the radial side of the wrist, as a proximal extension of the thumb ray, makes it vulnerable to injury. Not only does the scaphoid mechanically link the proximal and distal carpal rows, but it is also firmly attached at both ends to strong ligament systems that limit and control its motion.[47,357,505,516] It is self-evident that the scaphoid flexes with wrist flexion and extends with wrist extension, but it also flexes during radial deviation and extends with ulnar deviation. These factors make immobilization of scaphoid fractures difficult, especially when there is displacement. This change in position of the scaphoid during different planes of wrist motion confirms the scaphoid's role as the mechanistic key that controls wrist stability and serves as the principal bony support between the proximal and distal carpal rows and for carrying compressive loads from the hand across the wrist to the distal forearm. There are two different mechanisms of scaphoid fracture that may explain the differences in clinical presentation—compression injury and hyperextension, bending injury (Fig. 12-86). The compression fracture from a more longitudinal load or impaction of the wrist leads to intraction of the scaphoid without displacement. Tensile stresses generated palmarly when excessive hyperextension is applied to the wrist and when tensile forces exceed bone strength produce a fracture through the scaphoid that commonly results in fracture displacement. As a result of these two different mechanisms, scaphoid fractures can present as nondisplaced, stable fractures or as displaced, unstable fractures.[138,245]

The scaphoid is an irregularly shaped bone, more resembling a deformed peanut than the boat for which it is named. It rests in a plane at 45° to the longitudinal axis of the wrist. Articular cartilage covers 80% of the surface. The proximal pole is constrained to the lunate by an interosseous ligament. The distal pole has a V-shaped scaphotrapezial ligament, a scaphocapitate ligament, and a dorsal capsule. It rests on and can be attached along the ulnar aspect of the waist to the radioscaphocapitate ligament. The only other capsular influence is where the dorsal intercarpal ligament inserts obliquely on a roughened ridge and brings the primary blood supply that enters the scaphoid. Otherwise, the scaphoid has no ligamentous or tendinous attachments and acts with the rest of the proximal carpal row as "intercalated segments" subjected to the forces acting on them.[89,309] Compressive forces, acting across a three-link structure, cause a zig-zag collapse deformity. With a scaphoid fracture, the distal scaphoid tends to flex and the proximal scaphoid extends with the proximal carpal row. As a consequence, angulation occurs at the fracture site, which gaps open dorsally and gradually assumes the so-called humpback deformity.[18,331,388,491] Studies have shown that this deformity may occur at the time of fracture and result in immediate malposition of the scaphoid fragments into radial as well as dorsal angulation.[490] Failure to correct such deformity leads to fracture malalignment, nonunion, or malunion.[322,342]

Despite the lack of direct tendon attachment, joint compressive forces, trapezial–scaphoid shear stress, and capitolunate rotation moments exert control on the scaphoid. As a consequence of these biologic and mechanical factors, scaphoid fractures have a high incidence of nonunion (8% to 10%), frequent mal-

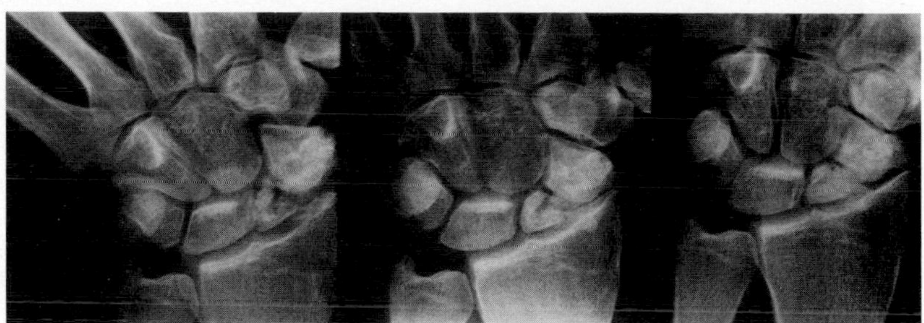

FIGURE 12-87. Scaphoid fracture (motion views). (*Left*) With ulnar deviation, a radial gap develops. Neutral deviation (*center*); the fracture line is still obvious. (*Right*) Radial deviation closes the gap. Note the radioscaphoid arthrosis involving the distal pole of scaphoid.

union, and late sequelae of carpal instability and posttraumatic arthritis. Next we examine the diagnosis and treatment of acute scaphoid fractures and address the treatment options available when scaphoid union is either delayed or absent.

Acute Scaphoid Fractures

Acute fractures of the scaphoid were first recognized in 1889 by Cousin and Destot[145] before the discovery of x-ray. A clear description was made later, in 1919, by Mouchet and Jeanne.[268] Scaphoid fractures are usually an injury of young men occurring after a fall, athletic injury, or motor vehicle accident. The mechanism of fracture is usually considered a bending fracture with compression dorsal and tension palmar. However, axial loading compression injuries have been suggested as another mechanism, particularly in the nondisplaced, stable fracture.[256a] Scaphoid fractures in children are uncommon, because the physis of the distal radius usually fails first.[7,103,173,235,311,531] Concomitant fractures of the distal radius and scaphoid have been reported.[256b,530a,531] Similarly, in the elderly, the distal radial metaphysis usually fails with fracture before the scaphoid fractures.

The patient often presents to the emergency department complaining of wrist pain and may be diagnosed as having a "sprain" of the wrist. In sports injuries it is not uncommon for the wrist injury to go unnoticed, with the request for evaluation and treatment delayed.[342] Fractures of the scaphoid in adolescents, previously believed uncommon, are now being reported more frequently and with different clinical appearance.[377a,500a]

Signs and Symptoms

The diagnosis of a scaphoid fracture is made on clinical examination where the index of suspicion is raised and by proper radiographic examination, by which the diagnosis is confirmed (see Fig. 12-47**B**).[146] Clinical examination should demonstrate tenderness in the snuffbox region of the wrist, over the tuberosity, or on the proximal pole of the scaphoid just distal to Lister's tubercle. Range of motion is reduced but not dramatically. There is usually pain at the extremes of motion. Swelling or ecchymosis is not present except in fracture–dislocations. Clearly, these same physical findings may be present with ligamentous injuries of the wrist, and thus whenever there are any findings suggestive of a scaphoid fracture,[124,146] the patient should be treated for a suspected scaphoid fracture.[103]

Radiographic Examination

Radiographic diagnosis of a scaphoid fracture often requires special views and occasionally special tests.[160,173,468] The emergency posteroanterior and lateral x-rays[146] should also include a scaphoid view (see Fig. 12-22), which puts the scaphoid in profile. Motion views of the wrist (Fig. 12-87) (flexion–extension and radial and ulnar deviation) may demonstrate fracture displacement, which is an indication of an unstable scaphoid fracture. These same x-rays should be repeated at 2 to 3 weeks if the initial films were negative. It is imperative for the treating physician to make the diagnosis at this time, because a

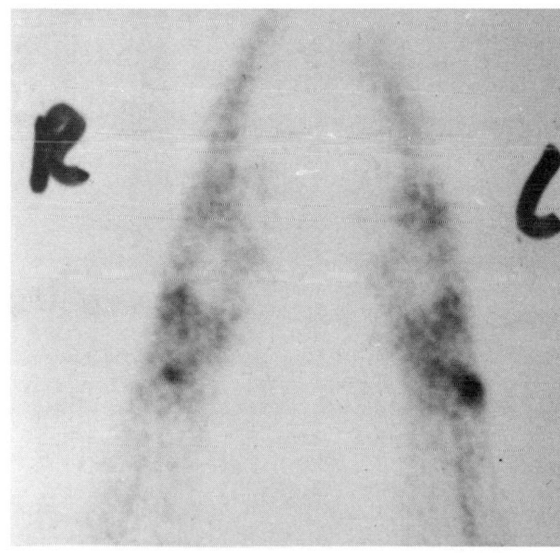

FIGURE 12-88. Scaphoid fracture with delayed early diagnosis strongly suggested by positive technetium 99m bone scan.

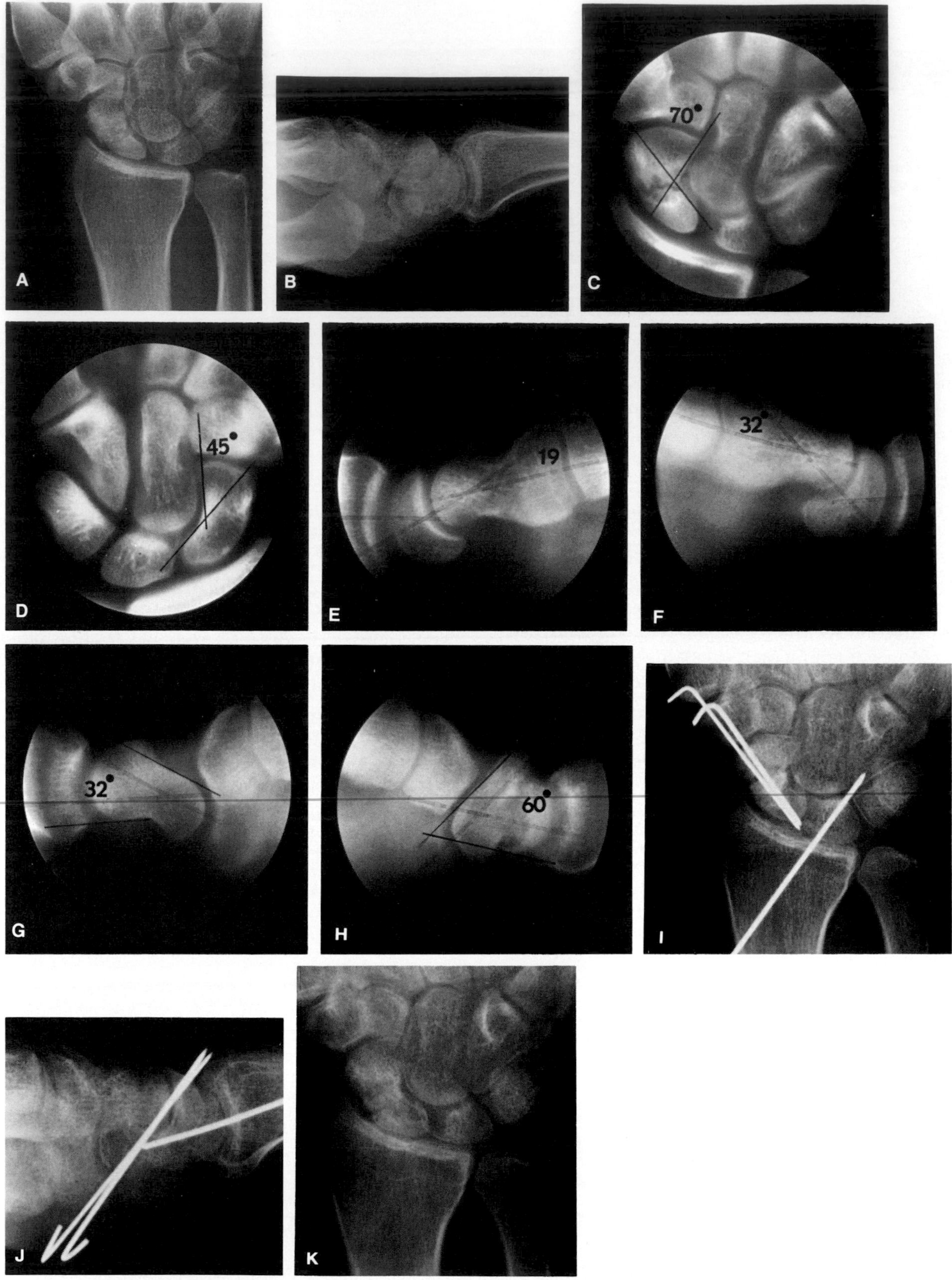

FIGURE 12-89. A 19-year-old man sustained a scaphoid fracture 1 year ago. (**A**) AP view: radial displacement and resorption. Note the elongated volar pole of lunate. (**B**) Lateral view showing DISI deformity. (**C,D**) Tomograms. The AP intrascaphoid angle is 70° on the fracture side, (**C**), 45° on the normal side (**D**). (**E,F**) The capitolunate angles are 19° on the normal side (**E**) 32° on the fracture side (**F**) with dorsal displacement of the capitate. (**G,H**) The intrascaphoid sagittal angles are 32° on the normal side (**G**), 60° on the fracture side (**H**), with dorsal displacement of the capitate. (**I,J**) Six weeks postoperation, interpositional bone graft with K-wire fixation of the fracture combined with derotation and pinning of the lunate. (**K**) Three months postoperation, showing healed scaphoid.

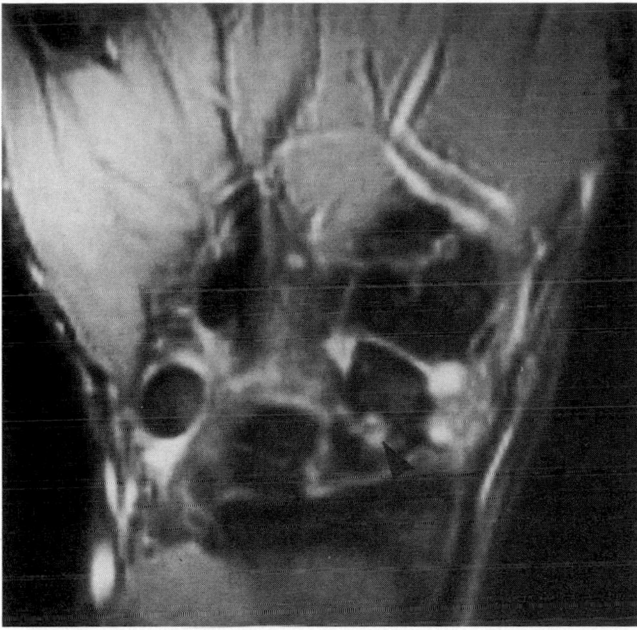

FIGURE 12-90. Magnetic resonance imaging. T-1 weighted image of the wrist demonstrating an acute scaphoid fracture (*arrow*) between the proximal and distal poles. Vascularity of the scaphoid is normal.

delay in diagnosis increases the incidence of scaphoid nonunion.[160] If a diagnosis still cannot be confirmed with confidence on routine films, a technetium bone scan (Fig. 12-88),[45,202,411,417] polytomography (Fig. 12-89),[58,223,403] or MRI (Figs. 12-90 and 12-91)[51,261a] of the wrist is recommended, in that order of preference.[222,411,417,438,525a] Ultrasonography and intrasound vibration examination have also been used to detect the occult, undiagnosed scaphoid fracture.[102a,181a] We have been impressed with the ability of both CT scanning[276a] and MRI to clearly show a scaphoid fracture when both plain films and even polytomography were not diagnostic of a fracture.[57,261a] Most authorities recommend bone scintigraphy as the procedure of choice for a suspected but unconfirmed fracture.[45,202,444a,525a,525b]

When instability of the scaphoid is suspected, careful analysis of the lateral x-ray for intrascaphoid angulation or a dorsally tilted lunate is recommended (Fig. 12-92). Motion views comparing scaphoid position during radial and ulnar deviation may also demonstrate motion at the fracture site (see Fig. 12-87). Polytomography, however, is a good method to determine scaphoid displacement.[51] Lateral tomography or lateral CT (and axial) scanning can be used to measure the exact degree of intrascaphoid angulation or displacement (see Fig. 12-92).[332,468] Three-dimensional imaging of scaphoid fractures and fracture nonunions has been reported both to assess displacement mechanisms as well as to plan treatment.[45a] From biplanar trispiral tomography, we have studied the range of normal angulation of the scaphoid to detect displacement and instability.[490,491] Measurements appear to be reproducible to within 5° and, when compared with the uninvolved scaphoid, provide information to assess not only the presence of displacement but the accuracy of reduction. Three-dimensional representation of the scaphoid using CT scanning and three-dimensional imaging provides the ability to describe displacement in all three planes and has promising clinical application.[45,394,403]

Differentiation between an acute scaphoid fracture and a scaphoid nonunion is important for planning treatment, and only proper x-rays can make the difference evident. Not uncommonly, a second injury will draw attention to a minimally symptomatic nonunion aggravated by the recent event. The

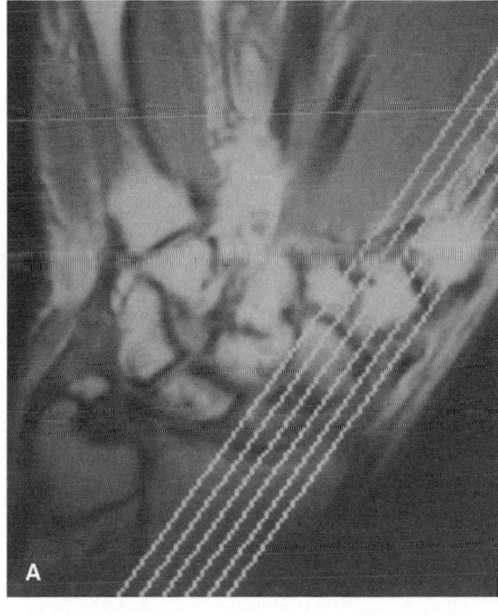

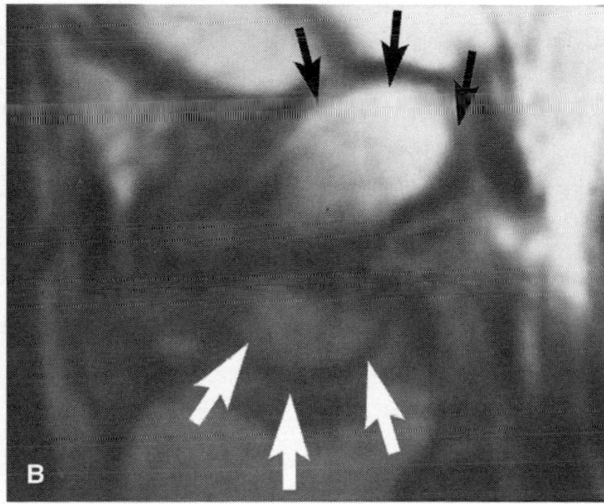

FIGURE 12-91. MRI in the scaphoid-sagittal parallel format (*left*) provides a clear view of the proximal (*white arrows*) and distal poles of the scaphoid (*dark arrows*), showing scaphoid angulation.

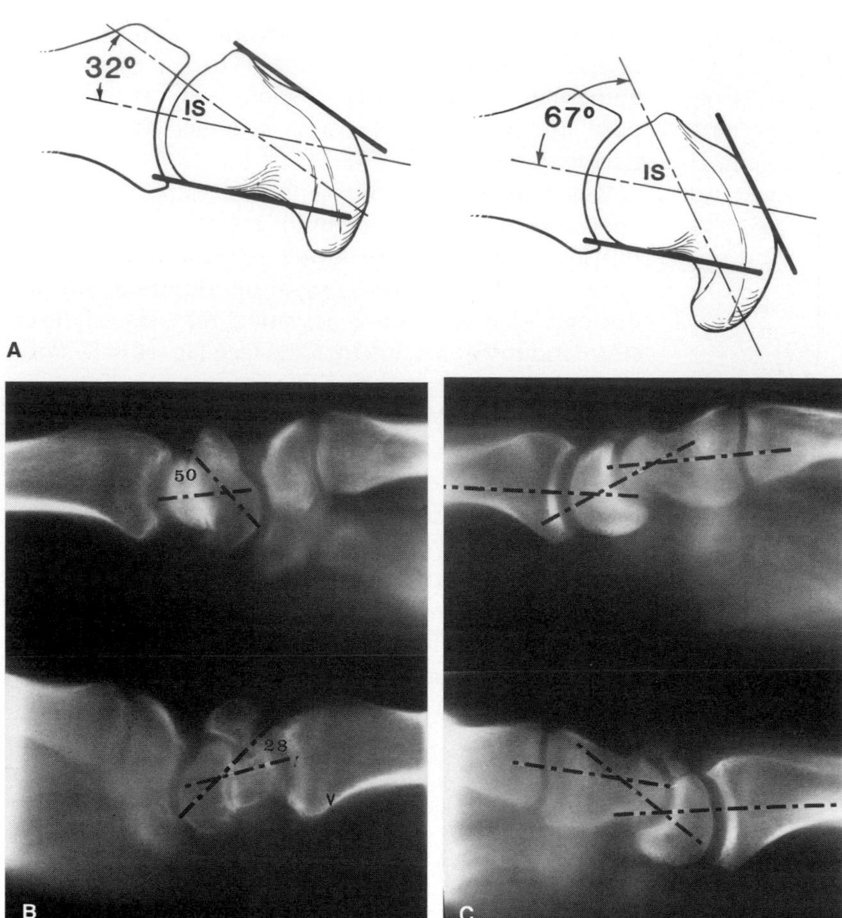

FIGURE 12-92. Scaphoid angulation. (**A**) Normal scaphoid and humpback scaphoid deformity. The normal lateral intrascaphoid (IS) angle is 30° ± 5°. The humpback deformity IS angle measures 67° and the normal scaphoid 32°. (**B**) Bilateral displaced scaphoid fractures with malunion showing an abnormal intrascaphoid angle of 50° (*top*) and a normal angle 28° (*bottom*), despite dorsal comminution. (**C**) Capitolunate angles are helpful in assessing carpal instability. At the top, the capitolunate angle measures 35° and on the bottom, 25°. Both angles confirm carpal instability associated with displaced scaphoid fractures.

acute scaphoid fracture is represented by a single line through the bone, occasionally with dorsal-radial comminution and dorsal angulation. Late presentation of a fracture or established nonunion, conversely, will demonstrate resorption at the fracture site (evident as a space between the fragments), subchondral sclerosis, and displacement on both the posteroanterior and lateral x-rays.[12] A true pseudarthrosis separates delayed acute fracture from established nonunions. The longer the period of time since injury, the greater the cystic resorption, the denser the sclerosis, the more prominent the shortening of the scaphoid, and the greater the loss of carpal height. Secondary degenerative changes are usually present by 10 to 15 years.[322]

Classification

Fractures of the scaphoid may be classified either by the location of the fracture within the bone or by the amount of fracture displacement (stability).

Location

Classification by anatomical location has many proponents, some of whom attempt to correlate fracture union rate with the site of injury (see Fig. 12-86). Five different fracture sites have been described: tuberosity, distal third, waist, proximal third, and distal osteochondral fractures.[116,537] All but the tuberosity fractures are intra-articular to a greater or lesser degree.[122,252,443] From a series of scaphoid fractures carefully studied, waist fractures accounted for 80%, proximal pole, 15%; tuberosity, 4%; and distal articular, 1%. Nonunion of the distal scaphoid has only recently been recognized and reported.[384a] The other anatomical classification is based on the direction of the fracture, with horizontal, oblique, avulsion, and comminuted types described.

The healing time for these different fracture types ranges from 4 to 6 weeks for tuberosity fractures, 10 to 12 weeks for distal third and waist fractures, and 12 to 20 weeks for proximal pole fractures.

The blood supply of the scaphoid is critical in regard to fracture location. Gelberman's work[214] confirmed earlier studies,[519] demonstrating that the major blood supply comes from the scaphoid branches of the radial artery, entering the dorsal ridge and supplying 70% to 80% of the bone, including the proximal pole. The second major group of vessels enters the scaphoid tubercle, perfusing only the distal 30% of the bone. With fractures through the waist and proximal third, revascularization will occur only with fracture healing. One can assume that with proper treatment nearly 100% of tuberosity and distal third scaphoid will heal; 80% to 90% of fractures at the waist will heal; and only 60% to 70% of proximal pole fractures will heal. Similarly, oblique or shear fractures have been shown to have delayed healing in comparison to horizontal fractures. Comminuted or distracted osteochrondral fractures will have the poorest rate of union.

Stability

The second major classification of scaphoid fractures subdivides them into either stable or unstable fractures.[116,252] A stable fracture is one that is nondisplaced, and it may have an intact cartilage envelope. That is, the fracture may occur within the bony substance of the scaphoid, usually from an impaction rather than a bending mechanism, incompletely separating the two fracture components. X-rays in two planes, as well as motion views, do not show any step-off or displacement of these fractures. The unstable scaphoid fracture, conversely, is by definition displaced with a step-off of 1 mm or more of angulation of the scaphoid in a lateral x-ray (Fig. 12-93). Rotational displacement can also be detected. The rate of fracture union and options for treatment change dramatically when one compares unstable and stable scaphoid fractures. Unstable fractures can be simply displacement from bending fracture mechanisms or from high energy, leading to fracture–dislocations of the wrist.

Treatment

Nondisplaced Fractures

The primary treatment for acute fractures of the scaphoid is cast or splint immobilization.[506,559b] As mentioned earlier, when there is any question regarding the presence of a scaphoid fracture, cast immobilization is recommended for 2 to 3 weeks until the diagnosis can be reassessed. The debate between long- and short-arm casts, as well as the position of immobilization, has not been definitely answered, but findings of recent studies should influence our decision.[35a,395] In one prospective study, Gellman and coauthors compared short- and long-thumb spica casts and noted decreased time to union and reduced rates of delayed union and nonunion with a long-arm thumb spica cast.[217] The findings in this study agree with those of earlier reports[84,183,226,537] that noted higher rates of healing with a long-arm cast for 4 to 6 weeks. Conversely, those surgeons who prefer a short-arm thumb spica cast point to 95% union rates in their personal series. Furthermore, a study from Nottingham, England, suggests that the thumb does not need to be included, provided the wrist is immobilized in the treatment of the acute, nondisplaced fracture.[105a] Tuberosity fractures are undoubtedly suitable for a short-arm cast, while patients with proximal pole fractures are candidates for a long-arm cast (if not open fracture treatment).

The recommended position of immobilization for scaphoid fractures varies from full extension to slight flexion, with varying degrees of radial or ulnar deviation. The amount of fracture displacement, alignment in both the posteroanterior and lateral planes, and associated injuries have been analyzed by several biomechanical studies, suggesting that a position of neutral flexion–extension and slight ulnar deviation is the preferred position of nondisplaced and minimally displaced scaphoid fractures. To reduce the stress produced by the volar and radiocapitate ligament, Weber and Chao[553] recommended radial deviation and palmar flexion. This position makes radiographic assess-

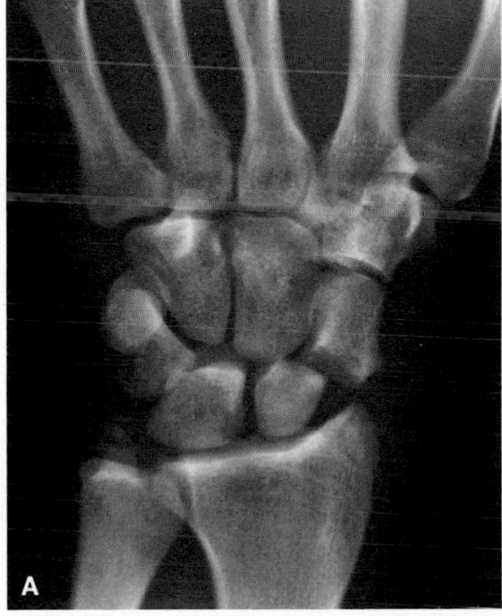

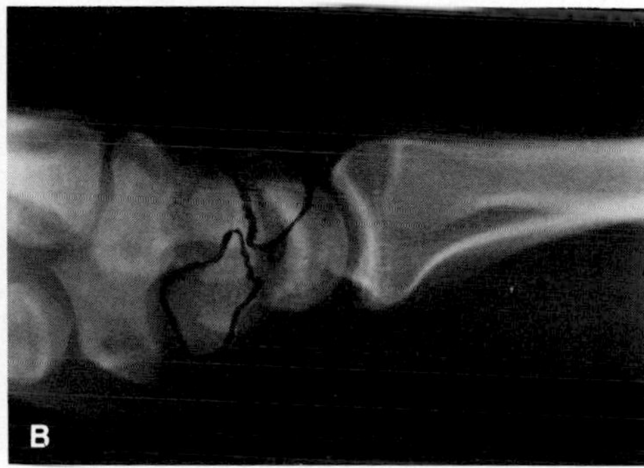

FIGURE 12-93. Unstable scaphoid fracture. Displacement greater than 1 mm is defined as an unstable scaphoid fracture. A displaced scaphoid fracture of this degree is inherently unstable and usually requires open reduction and internal fixation.

ment difficult. From an analysis of simulated displaced fractures,[491] it would appear that slight radial or ulnar deviation is acceptable, along with neutral flexion–extension. If the effect of lunate extension on dorsal gapping of the fracture site is important, then an attempt at flexing the lunate should help control the scaphoid reduction. This can be accomplished by careful molding of the cast. A depression is created over the capitate neck while displacing the carpometacarpal area relative to the forearm. The capitate tends to derotate the lunate and proximal pole, providing better coaptation of the fracture fragments (Fig. 12-94).

For nondisplaced stable scaphoid fractures (Fig. 12-95), we recommend a long-arm thumb spica cast, with the wrist in neutral deviation and neutral flexion–extension for 6 weeks, followed by a short-arm thumb spica cast until there is radiographic union confirmed by polytomography.[116] The union rate should exceed 95%. Delay in recognition, delay in initial treatment, and proximal third location of the fracture all negatively influence fracture healing.

Displaced Fractures

Author's Preferred Method of Treatment. Displaced fractures of the scaphoid require treatment different from that for nondisplaced fractures. A displaced fracture, by definition, is one with greater than 1 mm of step-off or more than 60° of scapholunate or 15° of lunatocapitate angulation as observed on either plain x-rays or tomography.[117] The degree of instability may vary, and thus there are different choices for fracture treatment. We believe that there is still a role for a

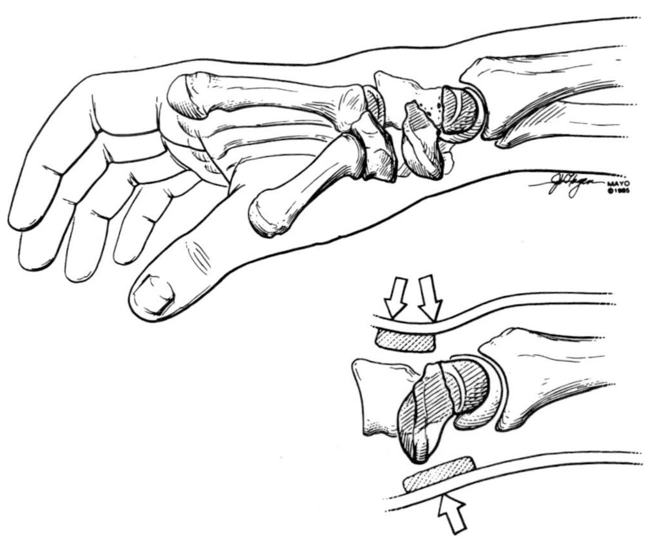

FIGURE 12-94. Closed reduction of a displaced scaphoid fracture by three-point pressure. Upward pressure is applied from the palmar side on the distal pole of the scaphoid, and downward pressure is applied dorsally on the capitate and lunate. Displacement of the capitate palmarly rotates the lunate and proximal pole into flexion and closes the dorsal scaphoid gap.

carefully applied long-arm thumb spica cast in the treatment of displaced scaphoid fractures, provided that the fracture can be acceptably reduced and the reduction maintained. To effect the reduction, three-point pressure on the tubercle of the distal scaphoid palmarly is combined with dorsal pressure over the capitate and dorsal support at the distal radius, which helps reduce and maintain the dorsal lunate angulation (see Fig. 12-94). An acceptable reduction includes alignment with less than 1 mm of displacement and a scapholunate angle of not more than 60°. With lateral tomography (or CT scanning), lateral intrascaphoid angulation should not exceed 25° ± 5°, and the posteroanterior angulation should be not more than 35° ± 5°.

If an accurate fracture reduction cannot be obtained, then other methods of treatment should be considered. These include closed reduction and percutaneous pin fixation, open reduction and pin fixation,[167] and open reduction and compression screw fixation (Figs. 12-96 and 12-97).[88,140,251,253,310] For acute displaced fractures that cannot be easily reduced, we recommend open reduction and Kirschner-wire or compression screw fixation of the scaphoid. The technique we prefer is to realign the proximal scaphoid and lunate to the distal radius and secure them with Kirschner wires. The proximal fracture components are stabilized by this procedure. The distal scaphoid can then be reduced onto the proximal fragments and fixed in that position. In addition to Kirschner-wire fixation or compression screw (AO, Herbert), a long-arm thumb spica cast is maintained for 6 weeks. After Kischner-wire removal, a short-arm cast is applied until fracture healing is confirmed radiographically (preferably with polytomography or CT scan).

With the advent of new compression screws and staples for the scaphoid, internal fixation has become more popular.[88,253,301,301a,310,346,442,443a,492a,559a] These procedures provide more rigid fixation for the scaphoid and allow earlier wrist motion.[446a] A number of authors have reported their experience with such techniques, but consensus on the role of screw fixation appears to suggest a definite role for early internal fixation of the scaphoid.[1,110A,121,187,253a,310,389,397,442] Several authors have reported significant problems with screw fixation of acute scaphoid fractures.[1,212,353,389] We reviewed 20 patients with displaced scaphoid fractures in which open reduction and internal fixation was performed early, less than 6 weeks. Nineteen of 20 healed. A comminuted fracture had delayed healing and required a Russe bone graft. Motion and strength were improved over cast immobilization, and patients returned to work and other activities by an average of 3 months. Although strong fixation is provided initially, should fracture union not occur, loosening of the screw and loss of fixation has been reported. A biomechanical analysis compared the fixation strength

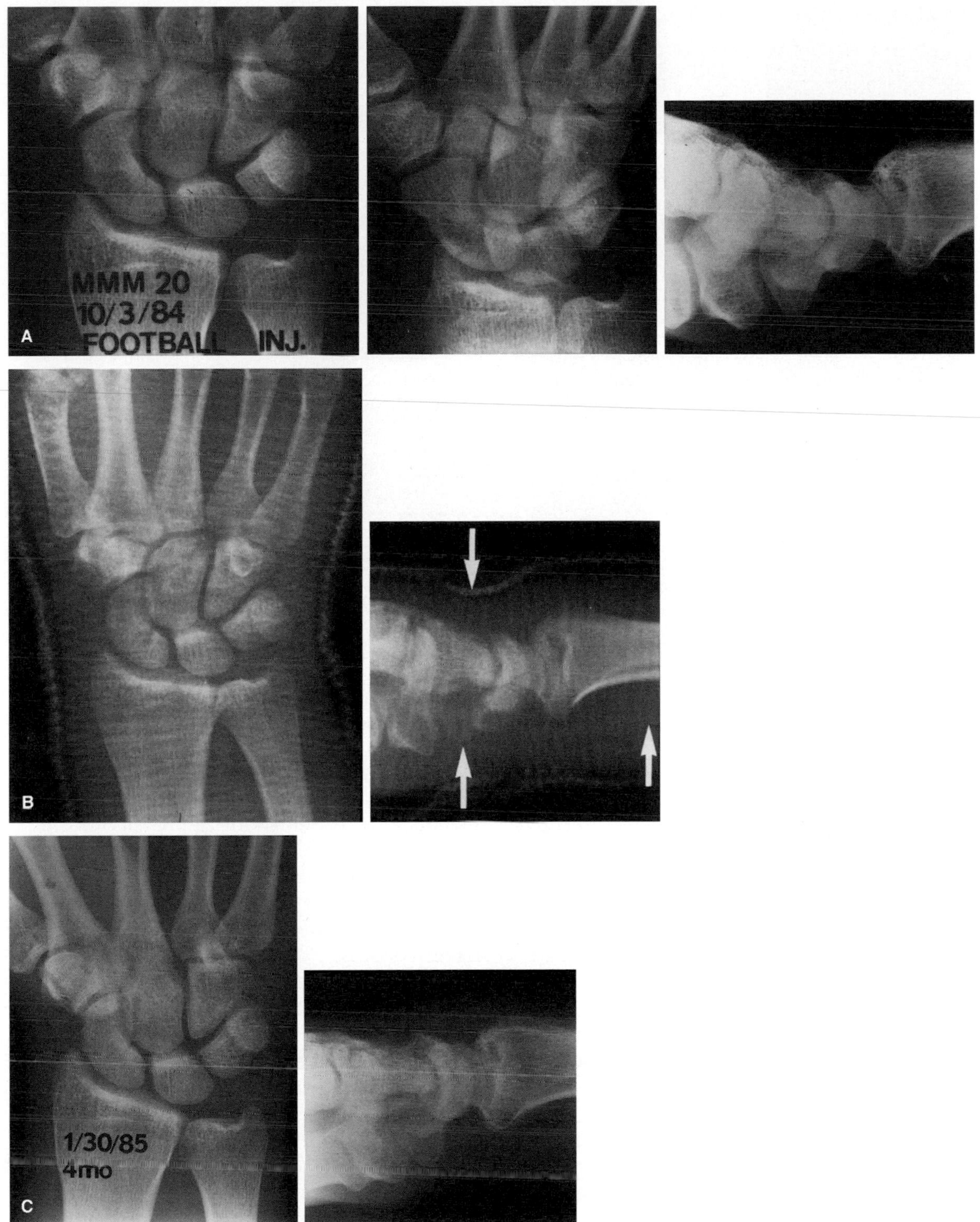

FIGURE 12-95. An acute, undisplaced scaphoid fracture in a 20-year-old football player. (**A**) An undisplaced fracture in the proximal third of the scaphoid. (**B**) Treatment was immobilization in a thumb spica cast with the wrist in neutral flexion-extension with slight radial deviation to relax the radioscaphocapitate ligament. Note careful molding of the plaster palmar distal scaphoid (*left bottom arrow*), dorsal capitate (*top arrow*), and proximal radius (*right bottom arrow*). (**C**) The fracture was thought by the radiologist to be healed at 4 months. Normal carpal alignment. (**D**) Tomography suggested delayed union (*left*) and showed slight lateral angulation of the scaphoid (*right*). Further protective splinting was recommended.

continues

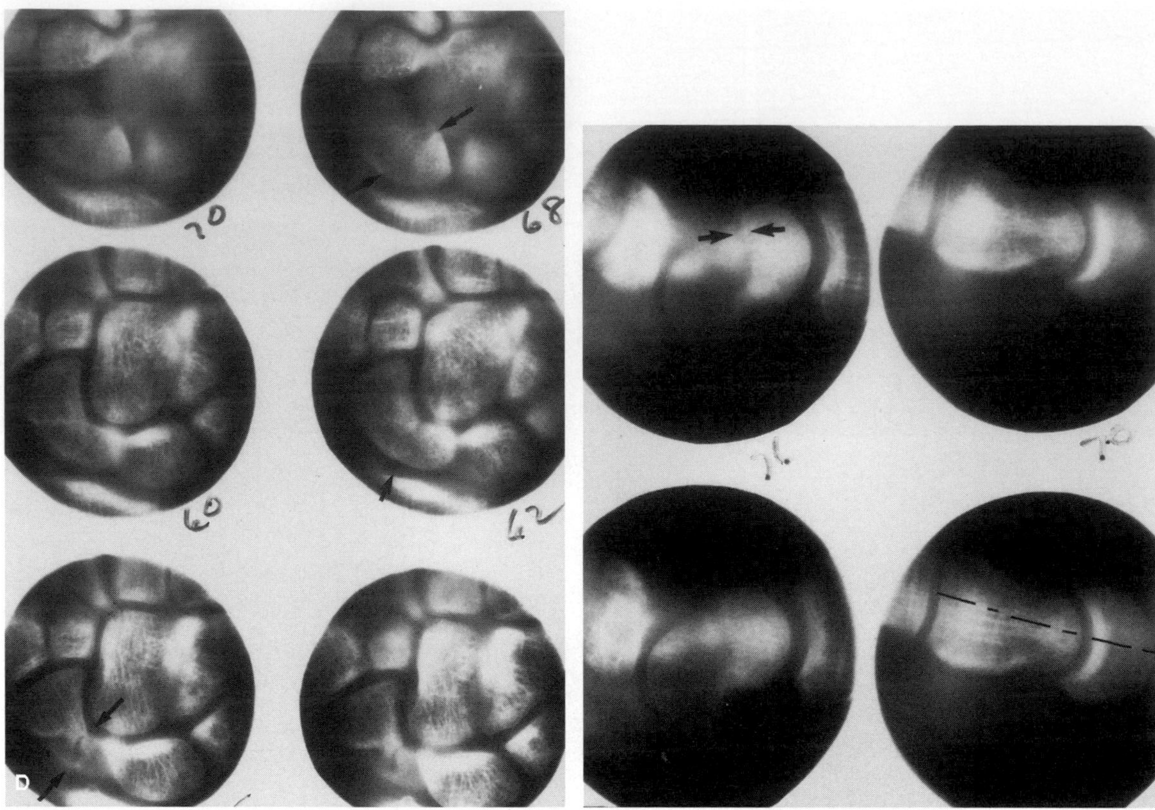

FIGURE 12-95. (continued)

of different bone screws and noted less interfragmentary compression with the Herbert screw than was anticipated from its unique design of differential thread-pitch between the distal and proximal screw ends. The correct application of fracture reduction and alignment devices is essential for anatomical screw placement.[110a] The development of cannulated screws placed over a Kirschner wire or use of intraoperative imaging has improved the technical factors associated with fracture fixation.[70,187]

The current role for compression screw fixation of scaphoid fractures is limited to displaced fractures, displaced proximal pole fractures,[140] and fracture–dislocations.[150] Postfixation cast immobilization is recommended despite proposals for early motion at 2 to 3 weeks.[251] Conclusive studies comparing compression screws with Kirschner wires or cast immobilization of displaced scaphoid fractures are needed. However, the role of open reduction and screw fixation is more commonly recommended and being used.

Scaphoid Nonunion

Treatment

Stable Nonunions

In the treatment of nonunion of the scaphoid it is essential to maintain the important principles of fracture healing and at the same time secure correct scaphoid alignment. Should an asymptomatic patient with scaphoid nonunion have surgical treatment recommended? Today, more longitudinal or outcome studies do favor operative intervention to prevent the late sequelae of traumatic arthritis.[157a,342,462] Four principles to follow include (1) preservation of blood supply, (2) bone apposition by inlay graft, (3) internal fixation for fracture stability, and (4) correction of carpal instability.[117,358,400] Failure of scaphoid bone grafting appears to be associated with inadequate vascularization, unsatisfactory fracture immobilization, insufficient length of immobilization, and instability or displacement. A number of questions are currently being asked regarding the treatment of choice for a nondisplaced scaphoid nonunion. What is the effect of operative approach on the blood supply? How should avascular necrosis of the scaphoid be confirmed? Is there a role for electrical stimulation of nondisplaced scaphoid nonunions? Is internal fixation of the scaphoid nonunion necessary when the nonunion is not displaced?

Russe Bone Graft. From a survey of the literature[24,156,395] and our experience, it appears that a Rüsse-type inlay bone graft of the scaphoid is the treatment of choice to which other procedures should be compared (Fig. 12-98).[463,501,506] From a review of four different treatment options, the volar Russe[463] type or dorsal-radial Matti[34,351] type had union rates of 86%

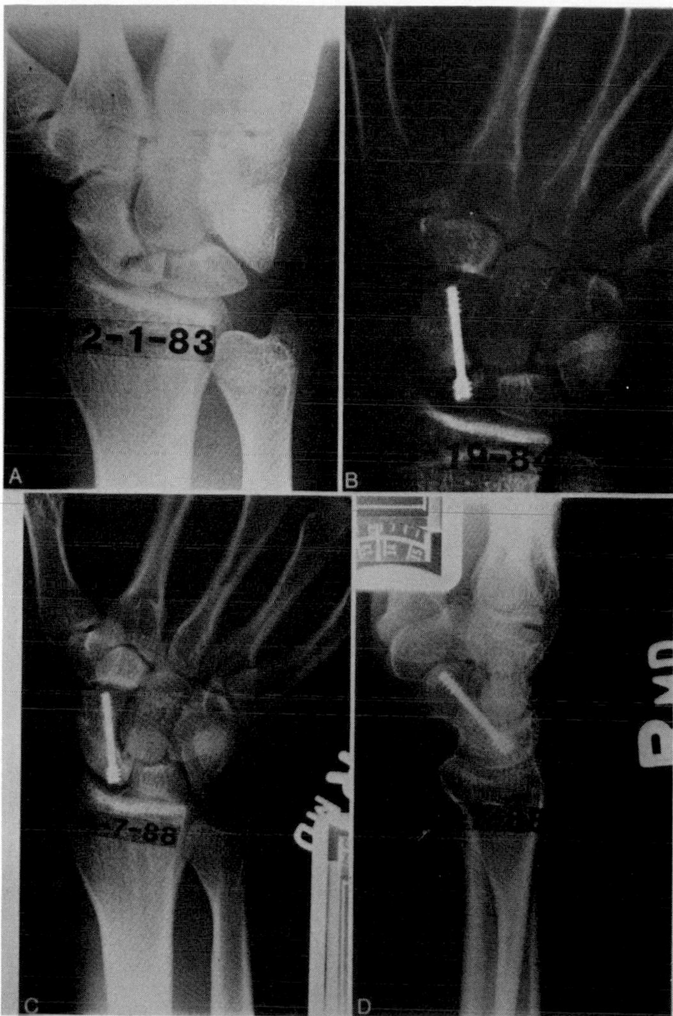

FIGURE 12-96. A small proximal pole scaphoid fracture treated with a Herbert screw inserted from the proximal pole. The fracture is reduced from a dorsal approach and the screw inserted through articular cartilage and countersunk. (**A**) Preoperative appearance. (**B**) Immediate postoperative Herbert screw insertion. (**C,D**) Six-year follow-up PA and lateral x-rays. No degenerative changes from proximal screw insertion into the scaphoid articular cartilage. (*DeMaagd, R.L., Engber, W.D.: Retrograde Herbert Screw Fixation for Treatment of Proximal Pole Scaphoid Nonunions. J. Hand Surg. 14A:996–1003, 1989.*)

and 92%, respectively.[117] Studies by others confirm the excellent results associated with the Russe procedure and report union rates of 85% to 97% for Russe grafting of stable scaphoid nonunions.[24,34,155,395] The need for internal fixation of nondisplaced fractures has been questioned by some, but one study demonstrated a 97% healing rate after combining a Russe procedure with internal fixation.

Author's Preferred Method of Treatment. Our preference and treatment of choice for scaphoid nonunion is palmar grafting similar to the approach modified by Russe.[112] The bone graft is a combination corticocancellous graft. Russe (as reported by Green)[231] has recommended using a double cortical graft placed side by side (see Fig. 12-98). His technique emphasized the need to remove the avascular bone and fibrous tissue through a palmar bone window, thoroughly excavating both the proximal and distal poles with a curette. We prefer a corticocancellous graft from the iliac crest, which is inset palmarly and serves to bridge the fracture gap and correct any displacement or angulation of the scaphoid that has occurred (Fig. 12-99). Supplemental fixation with a Kirschner wire or wires is preferred. Postoperative immobilization in a long-arm thumb spica cast is maintained for 6 weeks. The Kirschner wires are removed and a short-arm thumb spica cast is worn until fracture union is demonstrated on tomography. A radial styloid or radial metaphysis bone graft can be selected, but the ilium offers a stronger, more compact, trabecular graft that is easier to sculpt for proper fill. Vascularized bone grafts from the distal radius (radial artery)[255,306] or distal ulna (ulnar artery)[236] have also been described.

The presence of *diminished* vascularity of the proximal scaphoid[79] is not a contraindication to a palmar inlay bone graft. If fracture union can be achieved, the relative avascularity will improve. The time to union is, however, slower, and the rate of nonunion is increased. Therefore, it is advantageous to confirm avascular necrosis to determine length and prognosis for successful treatment. Methods of assessing avascular necrosis include bone scan, tomography, and MRI.[175]

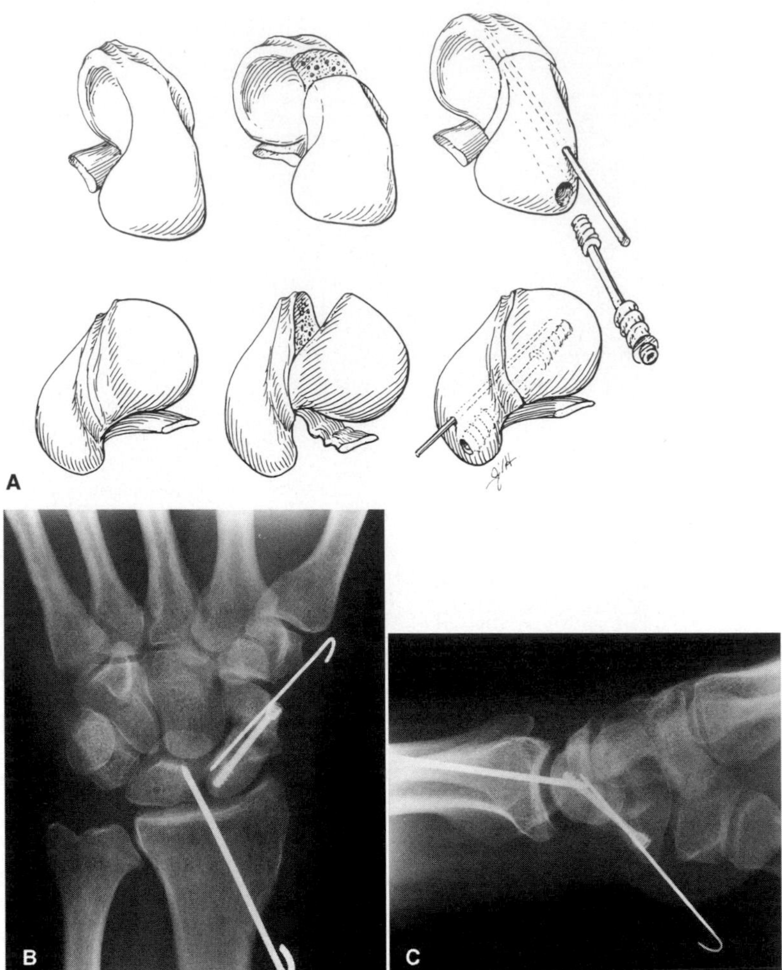

FIGURE 12-97. (**A**) Schematic illustration of compression screw insertion of a displaced scaphoid fracture. Reduction with K-wire fixation is performed prior to screw insertion. (Viewed distal to proximal at the *top* and lateral-radial at the *bottom*). (**B**) An acute, comminuted fracture of the distal third of scaphoid reduced with internal fixation with a Kirschner wire and Herbert screw. Correction of dorsal tilt of lunate is performed prior to scaphoid reduction; the lunate is held with a K-wire. (**C**) Lateral view of re-aligned proximal scaphoid and lunate with internal fixation to the distal scaphoid.

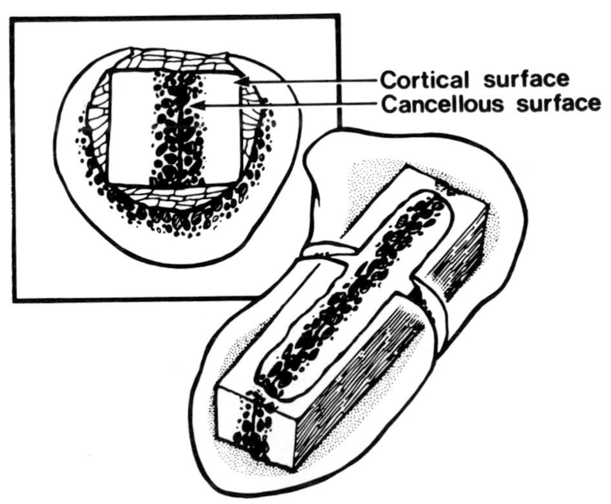

FIGURE 12-98. Russe bone graft. Two corticocancellous struts are placed in the excavated scaphoid through a volar approach. The remainder of the cavity is packed with cancellous chips. No power equipment is used, to avoid overheating the bone. The curetted interior surfaces of the scaphoid are closely inspected for evidence of vascularity. (*Green, D.P.: The Effect of Avascular Necrosis on Russe Bone Grafting for Scaphoid Nonunion. J. Hand Surg. 10A:597–605, 1985.*)

The latter technique is undoubtedly the most sensitive and specific. It can provide sequential information on revascularization of the scaphoid.[433a] Tomography is a better method of assessing fracture union and may be just as sensitive and specific in determining avascular changes. The only definitive test for confirming avascular necrosis, however, is the observation at surgery of the presence or absence of bleeding from bone. Green[231] reported that when the proximal pole was *completely* avascular (total lack of bone bleeding), the likelihood of successful healing with a graft was virtually nil. If the proximal scaphoid is *completely* avascular (Preiser's disease[537a]), an alternative procedure such as intercarpal fusion,[548] excision of the proximal scaphoid,[158] interposition arthroplasty,[46] proximal row carpectomy,[144a] or scaphoid allograft[98] should be considered. Another alternative is some type of vascularized bone graft.[562]

Electrical Stimulation. Electrical stimulation (pulsed electromagnetic stimulation [PEMS]) has been proposed for nondisplaced scaphoid nonunion.[5,43,67,199] Studies suggest that it has a role for fractures 3 to 6

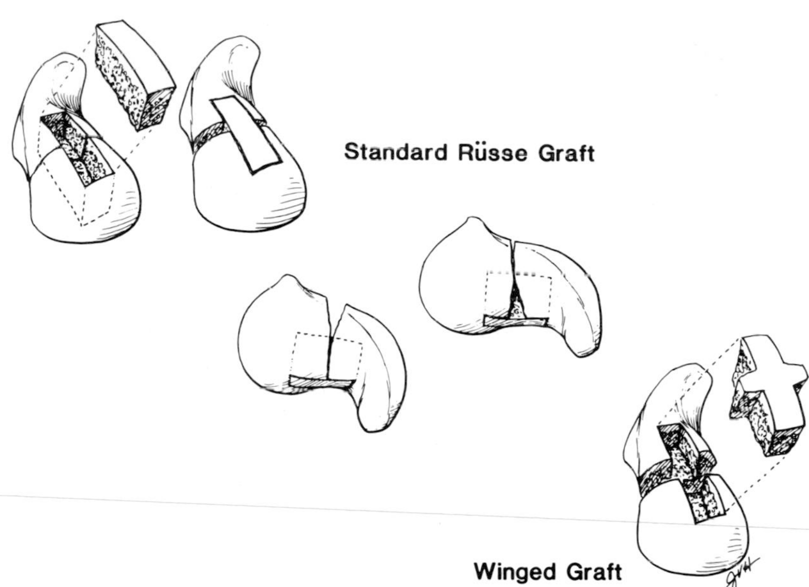

FIGURE 12-99. Standard Russe and Mayo "winged" Russe bone graft. The original Russe technique relied on packing a corticocancellous bone graft into a trough curetted through the volar cortex of both the proximal and distal fragments (although Russe placed the graft *inside* the cavity rather than in the cortical trough as shown here, *left*). Because the volar cortex is often foreshortened by erosion of the fragments, loss of length is difficult to correct without introducing a cortical graft (*center*). Our modification of the Russe technique involves using a "winged" corticocancellous iliac graft that is impacted into a volar trough to lengthen the scaphoid (*right*).

months old. In a study of 44 nonunited fractures that were at least 6 months old, union was achieved in 35, combining electrical stimulation and a thumb spica cast.[199] This study and an unpublished report[43] demonstrated better union with a long-arm cast than a short-arm thumb spica cast. Union rates from these series were 80% and 92%, respectively. The length of stimulation varied from 8 to 10 hours per day.

The controversy regarding the use of electrical stimulation in the treatment of scaphoid nonunions, however, remains unsettled, because there have been no controlled patient series comparing cast immobilization alone with electrical stimulation in these studies. Its use in unstable, angulated, displaced nonunions is not indicated. Newer types of pulsed electromagnetic fields with a shorter stimulation period are now available (Orthologic Co., Phoenix, AZ), but there have been no published reports on their use in treatment of scaphoid nonunions.

Unstable Nonunions

From the work of Fisk[182,183] and later from that of Linscheid and colleagues,[329] instability of the carpus as a result of scaphoid nonunion has had increased recognition. Displaced scaphoid fractures are more difficult to diagnose[168] and treat, and nonunions of the scaphoid with displacement have a lower rate of union with an increased potential for radioscaphoid arthritis.[95,117,307,342,462] Techniques to improve scaphoid alignment by palmar and radiopalmar bone grafting have been developed to correct scaphoid malalignment[18,184] and to restore normal scaphoid length.[177,178] A number of authors have reported their experience with interposition bone grafting for displaced scaphoid nonunions with internal fixation such as the Herbert screw,[70,121,346] conventional lag screw,[178] Enders plate,[258a] and multiple Kirschner wires,[177] reporting results equal to or superior to the Rüsse graft.[452b] Comparative studies on this issue, however, are only a few.[405a]

Authors' Preferred Method of Treatment

The indications for interposition grafting include gross motion at the nonunion site, scaphoid resorption, and loss of carpal height.[184,331] A dorsal-radial operative approach (Fig. 12-100) can be utilized with Kirschner wire internal fixation. More commonly, the operative procedure involves an anterior interposition bone graft, with size based on comparative scaphoid views of the opposite wrist and intraoperative measurements. An extended palmar Russe approach between the radial artery and flexor carpi radialis is used to expose the scaphoid. A gap is noted as the nonunion is debrided. With the two fragments gently distracted and aligned, reduction is held with a Kirschner wire. The size of the defect is measured in width and depth, and with an oscillating saw the exact dimensions of the graft are removed from the iliac crest. With the graft in place and the scaphoid reduced and held with a Kirschner wire, a Herbert screw is inserted by the technique described by its originator (Fig. 12-101). If there is marked DISI angulation of the lunate, it is best to reduce the lunate and proximal scaphoid by flexing the wrist and pinning the lunate in a reduced position through the radial styloid first.[331,401] An alternative procedure is to use multiple Kirschner wires as described by Fernandez (see Fig. 12-89) or dorsal-radial operative approach (see Fig. 12-100).[177] Displaced, small proximal pole fractures are best approached dorsally.[156a,546a]

The results of treatment in our series demonstrated

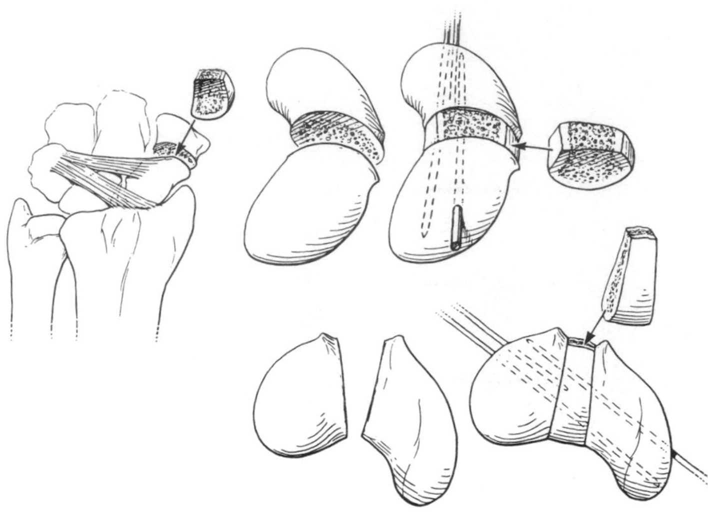

FIGURE 12-100. Interposition bone graft for scaphoid nonunion. Schematic illustration of a trapezoidal wedge graft (usually from the iliac crest). The graft is interposed between the proximal and distal scaphoid fragments and held with Kirschner wires. Exposure is from a dorsal-radial approach.

a union rate of 81%, although two cases required a secondary interposition graft.[121] Carpal instability as measured by the scapholunate angle was corrected from a preoperative mean of 65° to a postoperative mean of 54°. The capitolunate angle improved from 15° to 3.5°, and the carpal height ratio improved from 0.51 to postoperative 0.54. Complications were related to incorrect placement of the Herbert screw and to resorption of the bone graft. This was usually associated with failure of healing to the proximal pole. Interposition grafting is preferred when the palmar gap exceeds 3 mm or more. A modification of the Russe procedure using a cross-shaped corticocancellous graft or an extended Russe bicortical graft inserted into the troughs in either pole to prop the scaphoid open for restoration of length may also be used (see Fig. 12-99). Improved imaging may provide the technical basis for more accurate bone graft configuration, scaphoid reconstruction, and internal fixation, making interposition grafting more practical and easier for the surgeon.[45a,405b]

A radial approach with partial radial styloidectomy may be indicated in patients with a severe humpback scaphoid deformity, to judge the necessary degree of corrective realignment. The dorsal osteophyte of the humpback should be excised to assist in the reduction. This procedure should be chosen with caution, because the traditional Matti-Russe graft has a superior union rate and is capable of correcting mild carpal instability. The Russe technique remains the gold standard to which other scaphoid grafting procedures must be compared.

It may be difficult to completely correct carpal instability in long-standing cases, and these patients may be better served by various salvage procedures.

Vascularized Bone Graft. A vascularized bone graft to the scaphoid[562] for established nonunion is recommended for (1) avascular necrosis, (2) failed bone grafting procedure (eg, failed Russe or interposition graft), and (3) Preiser's disease. The vascular bone graft can be harvested from the distal radius (second dorsal compartment) or from the second metacarpal. A dorsal-radial approach is required (Fig. 12-102). We recommend harvesting the vascular graft first from the radius, using loop magnification. The radial artery branches are then dissected and followed to the radius. The rectangular bone graft is then harvested with great care taken to protect the vascular pedicle. The scaphoid is approached dorsoradially, and the nonunion site is excavated. Kirschner wires are positioned by retrograde insertion and then the vascularized bone graft is inserted. With the graft in place, the Kirschner wires are drilled across the nonunion site. A radial styloidectomy may be required because the breadth (width) of the scaphoid is usually increased.

For avascular necrosis of the scaphoid, one must remove all of the avascular bone (usually proximal third). The vascular graft is inlaid with care taken to protect the pedicle, and additional cancellous bone may be packed around the vascular graft. Kirschner wire fixation is used if the scaphoid appears unstable. For a failed primary bone graft, the previous graft fragments must be removed and a fresh surface created between the ends of each fragment. The vascular graft is inserted usually as an inlay graft or alternatively as an interposition graft. Kirschner wire or compression screw fixation is usually recommended. Cast immobilization is continued until tomograms show solid healing.

For Preiser's disease[537a] (avascular necrosis of the entire scaphoid), a vascularized bone graft is the procedure of choice if nonoperative methods (splint, rest, electrical stimulation) fail to resolve the problem. If the scaphoid begins to show collapse similar to that seen in a nonunion, bone grafting (preferably a vascularized graft from the distal radius) is recommended. The technique is similar to that described in the preceding paragraph except

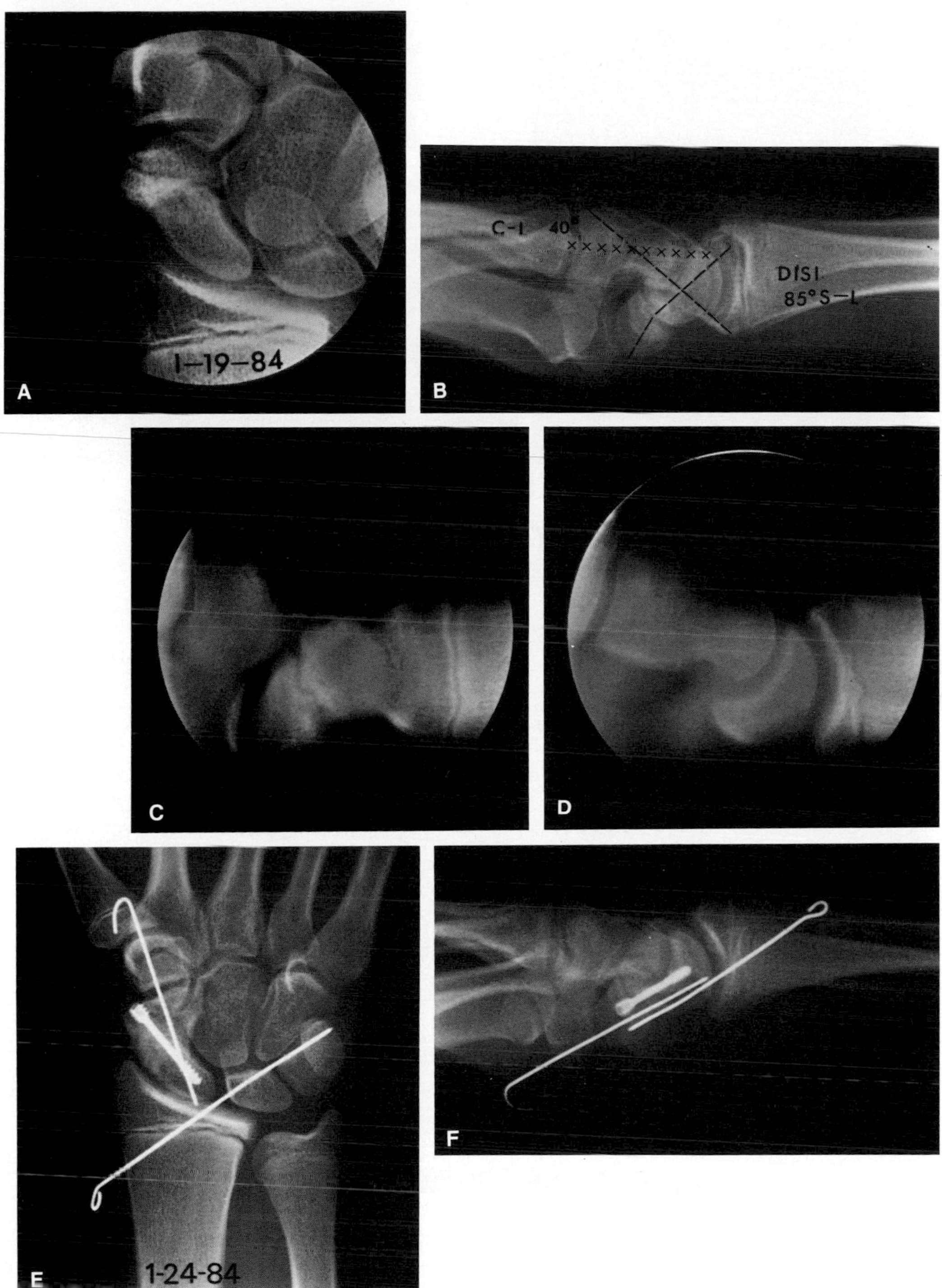

FIGURE 12-101. A 17-year-old high school athlete presented with a painful wrist 9 months following a "sprained wrist" sustained in senior-year football. (**A**) X-rays revealed a distal scaphoid fracture with radial angulation. (**B**) Capitolunate (40°) and scapholunate (85°) malalignment were present. (**C**) A lateral tomogram demonstrated volar resorption and angulation through the nonunion site, the so-called humpback scaphoid. (**D**) Dorsiflexion of the lunate and capitolunate subluxation. (**E,F**) Open reduction, interposition volar wedge bone graft with internal fixation was performed. The proximal scaphoid and lunate were reduced first and pinned; the distal scaphoid was reduced with the interposition bone graft in place and pinned; the Herbert screw was inserted. (**G,H**) Scaphoid union and correction of carpal instability was obtained. (**I**) Operative approach for anterior wedge graft using an extended Russe incision to the scaphotrapezial joint (*A*); interposition iliac crest bone graft (*B*) and internal fixation with Herbert screw (*C*). (**I,** *Cooney, W.P.; Linscheid, R.L.; Dobyns, J.H.; and Wood, M.B.: Scaphoid Non-union: Role of Interposition Bone Grafts. J. Hand Surg. 13A:635–650, 1988.*)

continues

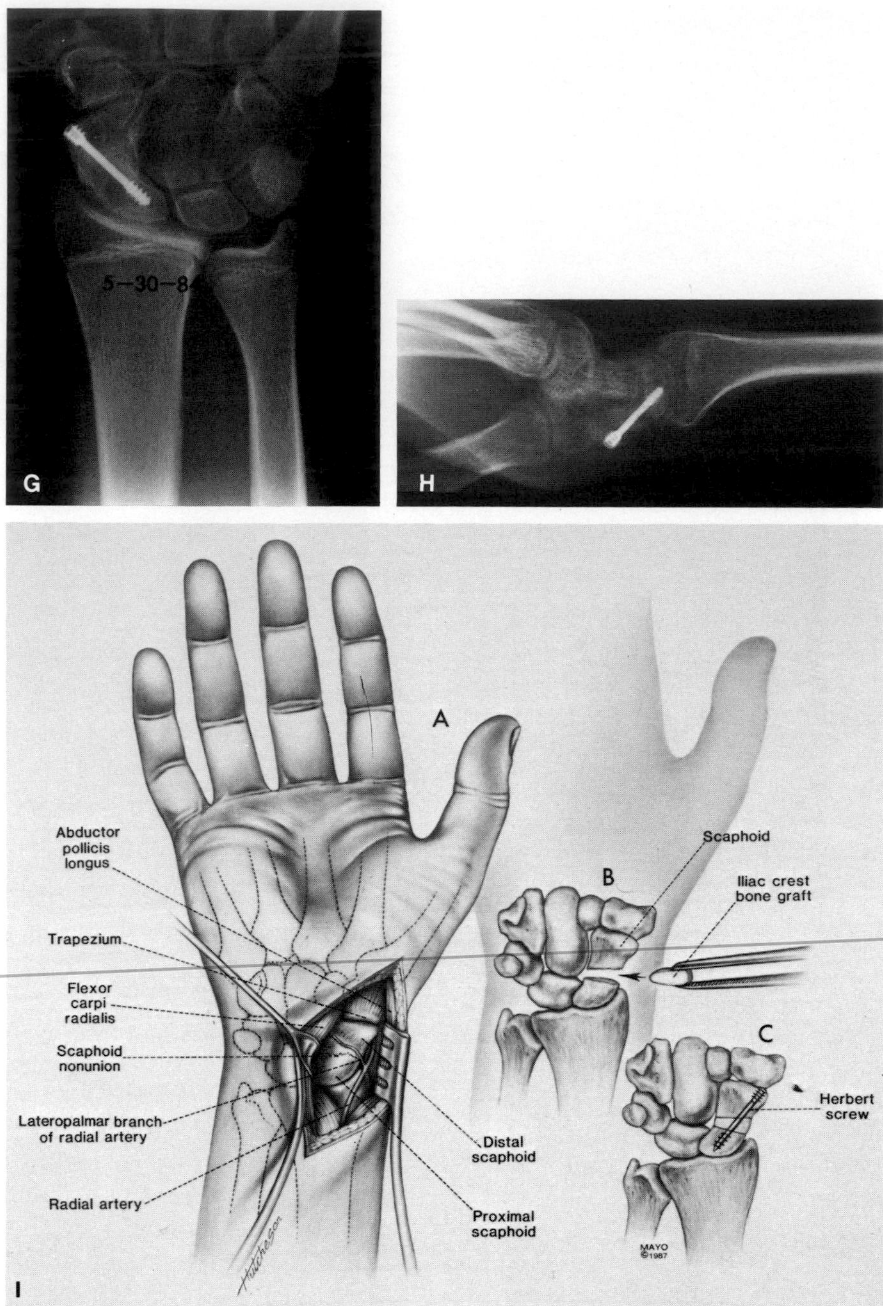

FIGURE 12-101. (continued)

that the entire scaphoid is excavated of avascular bone. Cast immobilization is recommended as with a fracture nonunion. Long-term splint protection may be needed for up to 6 months because revascularization is a slow process in Preiser's disease.

LUNATE FRACTURES (KIENBÖCK'S DISEASE)

Fractures of the lunate are relatively uncommon[44,99,260,384,522] and often unrecognized, at least until they progress to osteochondrosis of the lunate, at which time they become symptomatic and are diagnosed as Kienböck's disease.[83,287,522] The latter is a condition for which no consistently reliable treatment has been found, and it produces significant disability in a generally young and productive segment of society.[44,368,467] The problem encompasses several aspects of wrist injuries that result in early neglect. First, the injury may be considered a sprain and ignored by the patient. Second, initial x-rays may be negative, because the fracture line remains occult for several weeks, as sometimes seen in the scaphoid. Third, be-

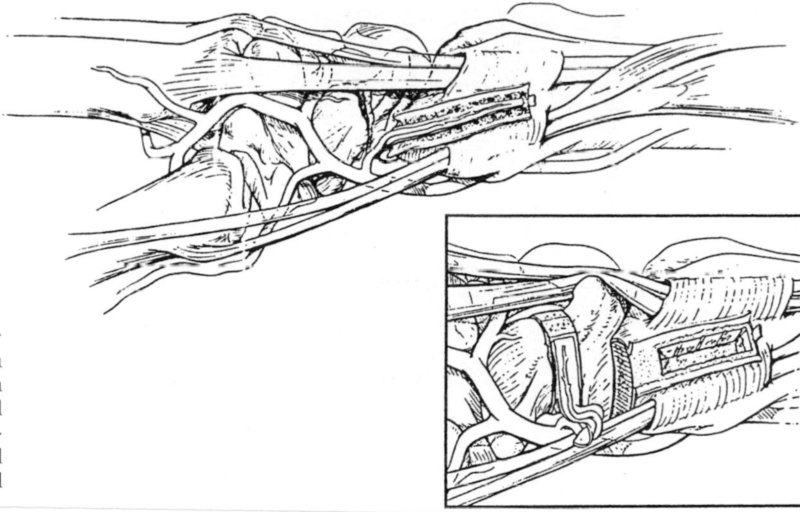

FIGURE 12-102. Vascularized bone graft from the distal radius. Supra-retinacular branches from the radial artery are dissected to the metaphyseal area of the distal radius between the first and second dorsal extensor compartments. A vascularized cortico-cancellous graft can then be harvested and reflected distally (*inset*) into the scaphoid.

cause the lunate is covered by superimposed images of the radius, ulna, and other carpal bones, even lateral x-rays may be read as normal (Fig. 12-103). Fourth, osteonecrosis may be the result of interruption of the vascular supply to the lunate,[216,260,287] which shows no radiographic evidence of injury until sclerosis and osteochondral collapse are seen. Finally, reconstitution of the lunate to its former condition has so far evaded our surgical abilities.[466] There is the observation that this entity is more prevalent in patients with an ulnar minus variant. Much of the current treatment methods are based on trying to redistribute the compressive forces across the joint to unload the collapsing part of the lunate. New techniques combining distraction (external fixation) to unload the wrist revascularization and limited internal fixation may provide resolution to Kienböck's disease, but thus far their effectiveness has not been proven in controlled series.

Anatomy

The lunate sits like a keystone in the proximal carpal row in the well-protected concavity of the lunate fossa of the radius, anchored on either side by the interosseous ligaments to the scaphoid and triquetrum with which it articulates. Distally, the convex capitate head fits congruently into the concavity of the lunate. The joint reaction force from the capitate and radius squeezes the lunate ulnarly. The proximal horn of the hamate has a variable articular facet on the distal ulnar surface of the lunate, and ulnar deviation increases the degree of contact of these two bones. The vascular supply of the lunate is primarily through the proximal carpal arcade both dorsally and palmarly.[364] Both Lee[312] and Gelberman and associates[213] have shown the intralunate anastomoses to be of three main types, which can be characterized as I, Y, and X. The degree of cross flow between the two systems is probably subject to considerable variation, and the redundancy available for adequate perfusion of the bone is unknown.

Mechanisms of Injury

Most patients with fractures of the lunate have a history of a hyperextension injury, such as a fall on the outstretched hand.[14] Occasionally, repetitive use of the hand or a strenuous push will give rise to a "snap" in the wrist. In extension, the lunate is displaced onto the palmar aspect of the lunate fossa and rotated dorsally. The capitate drives against the palmar horn and at the same time pushes the lunate ulnarly. This is resisted by the radiolunate ligament, which exerts tension at its lunate insertion. If there is an ulnar minus variant,[406] the support offered by the TFC and ulnar head will be minimal, and even less when the hand is pronated. The compressive stresses over the proximal convexity of the lunate shift dramatically at the interface between the TFC and radial articular surface. The lack of ulnar support may also allow proximal displacement of the triquetrum, placing further tensile stress on the lunate surface through the lunatotriquetral ligament. This appears to provide a reasonable scenario for the transverse fractures that occur in the sagittal plane (see Fig. 12-103). Avulsions of the dorsal pole are more likely due to tension that develops in the scapholunate ligament, because these are frequently seen with SLD. Avulsion fractures of the ulnar aspect of the palmar pole are usually associated with a perilunar dislocation variant. It is also possible that sufficient stress develops where the arteries penetrate the bone to induce devascularization. In this situation, avascularity would precede fracture, rather than vice versa. Indeed, there is considerable evidence that

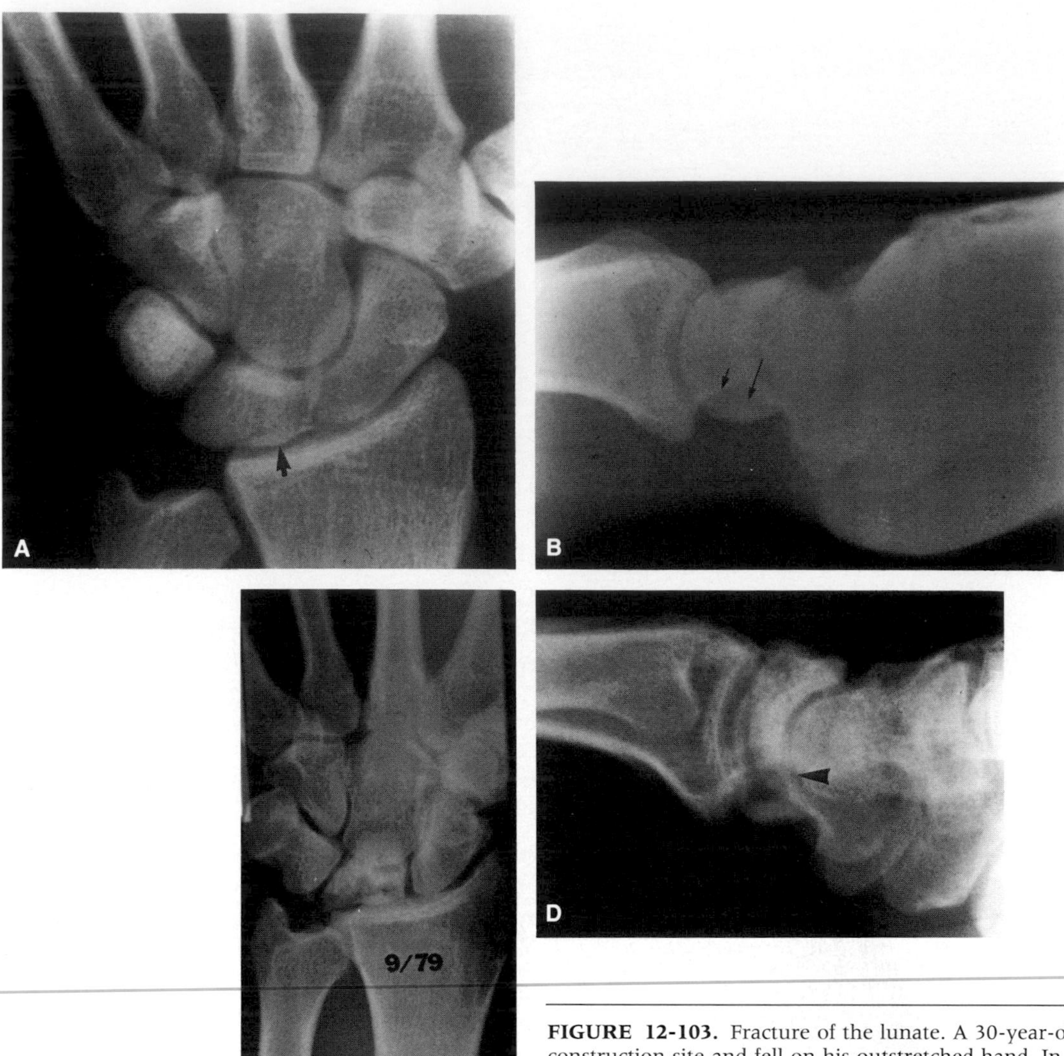

FIGURE 12-103. Fracture of the lunate. A 30-year-old man slipped on a muddy construction site and fell on his outstretched hand. In retrospect, both the AP (**A**) and lateral (**B**) views were questionable. The fracture line parallel with volar line of the radial styloid was missed at the time of the initial examination. (**C**) The AP view shows development of stage III Kienböck's disease over the ensuing 22 months. (**D**) Lateral view shows displacement of the volar pole below the rim of the radius.

both mechanisms can be responsible for Kienböck's disease and that several contributing factors (trauma, ulnar variance, vascularity) interact to result in the radiographic and clinical entity called Kienböck's disease.[20,448]

Classification

Fresh fractures of the lunate include dorsal and palmar horn avulsion fractures, usually more often from the radial corner than from the ulnar corner.[201] Fractures in the body are most often transverse in the coronal plane. The more common of these is between the mid and palmar thirds of the body. A fracture in the sagittal plane suggests that the differential stress across the radioulnar step-off is causative. Collapse of the radial aspect of the lunate is more apparent than on the ulnar side.

Part of the difficulty in describing fractures of the lunate is that the fragmentation that occurs in Kienböck's disease presents confusion between an initiating fracture and the fragmentation due to secondary subcortical collapse patterns.[9] Kienböck's disease is often classified in four or five stages according to the Stahl,[499] DeCoulx,[138] or Lichtman[319] classifications (Table 12-5; Fig. 12-104). Staging is based on the posteroanterior radiographic appearance, which gives only a partial picture of the condition of the lunate. Ideally, polyaxial tomography or CT scanning should be used for classification purposes.[9,51] Palmer has a further subdivision that may assist in determining treatment. Radiodensity changes alone are unreliable criteria for

TABLE 12-5
Kienböck's Disease: Classification of Radiographic Stages (Stahl/Lichtman)

Stage	Description
I	Normal appearance or linear or compression fracture (on tomogram)
II	Bone density change (sclerosis); slight collapse of radial border
III	Fragmentation, collapse, cystic degeneration; loss of carpal height; capitate proximal migration; scaphoid rotation (S-L dissociation)
IV	Advanced collapse; scaphoid rotation; sclerosis; osteophytes of the radiocarpal joint

(After Lichtman, D.M., Alexander, A.H., Mack, G.R., and Gunther, S.F.: Kienböck's Disease: Update on Silicone Replacement Arthroplasty. J. Hand Surg., 7A:343, 1982.)

Kienböck's disease, for which the characteristic change is deformity. Not all radiodense lunates deform; if they do not do so, the unique problems associated with Kienböck's disease do not develop.

Radiographic Findings

After the scaphoid, the lunate is the next most fractured carpal bone. As already emphasized, the fracture may be difficult to visualize early, because a nondisplaced crack is often hidden by the superimposed structures (see Fig. 12-103**A**). The best example of this problem is the palmar cortical line of the radial styloid, which is aligned with the division between the dorsal and palmar thirds of the lunate, where a transverse fracture often occurs. The anteroposterior view of this is in a plane almost perpendicular to the fracture, which is overlapped by the radial rims and, therefore, is not apparent. The palmar horn of the lunate is hidden by the pisiform and scaphoid shadows (see Fig. 12-103**B** and **D**). For these reasons, clinical suspicion must take precedence over the findings on plain films.[378] A technetium-99m bone scan will be positive within 24 hours of injury. Oblique films help to throw minute fracture lines into focus on some occasions, but CT scans or polyaxial tomograms, preferably of the trispiral type, provide more precise detail (Fig. 12-105). Distraction of a transverse fracture by the intrusion of the capitate, for instance, is easily recognized on tomography but seldom on plain films. Palmar subluxation of the capitate with a palmar horn fracture of the lunate is unlikely to be missed on tomography. When osteonecrotic changes have supervened, they are often apparent in some detail by tomography before there is more than a suspicion on regular films. The stage of osteonecrosis is frequently noted to be more advanced than was apparent on standard x-rays. In fact, classification is best made from tomograms as well as decision regarding treatment alternatives and prognosis. It is also possible to differentiate the primary fracture from the secondary fractures associated with fragmentation. Fragmentation and collapse generally affect the lunate overlying the radial contact area, especially in those wrists with an ulna minus variant.[170,215,302,406] Additional findings that may be of importance in treatment are the carpal height ratio[361] and the radioscaphoid angle, as a measure of carpal collapse.

MRI has increased our appreciation of the vascular changes that occur within a few days of injury.[20,496] Nakamura has demonstrated that MRI is an excellent tool to assess vascularity and to demonstrate revascularization as well as healing. MRI will show evidence

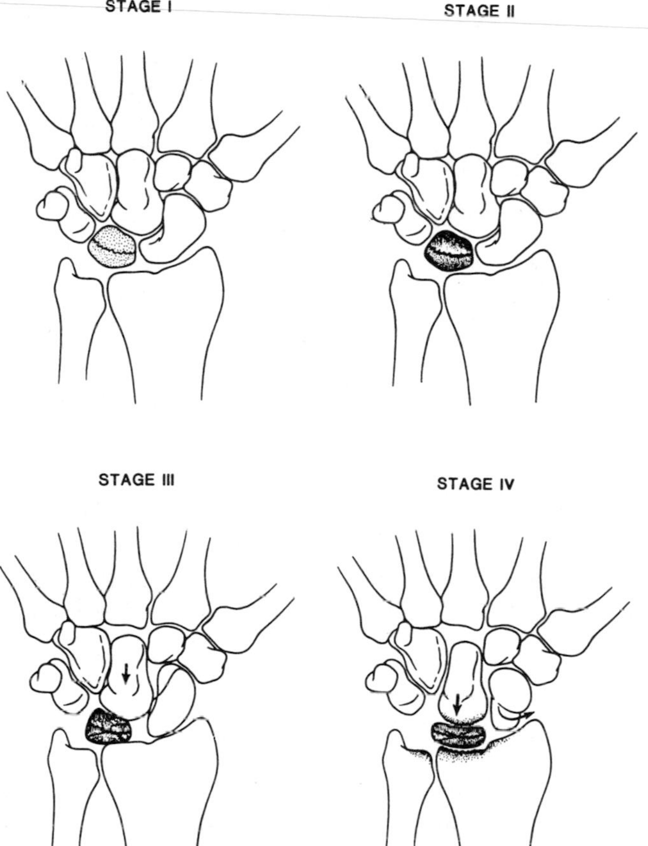

FIGURE 12-104. Staging of Kienböck's disease (after Lichtman). *Stage I:* Routine x-rays (PA, lateral) are normal but tomography may show a linear fracture; usually transverse through the body of the lunate. MRI will confirm avascular changes. *Stage II:* Bone density increase (sclerosis) and a fracture line are usually evident on the PA x-ray. PA and lateral tomograms demonstrate sclerosis, cystic changes, and often a clear fracture. There is no collapse deformity. *Stage III:* Advanced bone density changes are present with fragmentation, cystic resorption, and collapse. The diagnosis is evident from the PA x-ray. Tomograms (PA, lateral) demonstrate the degree of lunate infraction and amount of fracture displacement. Proximal migration of the capitate is present and there is mild to moderate rotary alignment of the scaphoid. *Stage IV:* Perilunate arthritic changes are present with complete collapse and fragmentation of the lunate. Carpal instability is evident with scaphoid malalignment and capitate displacement into the lunate space.

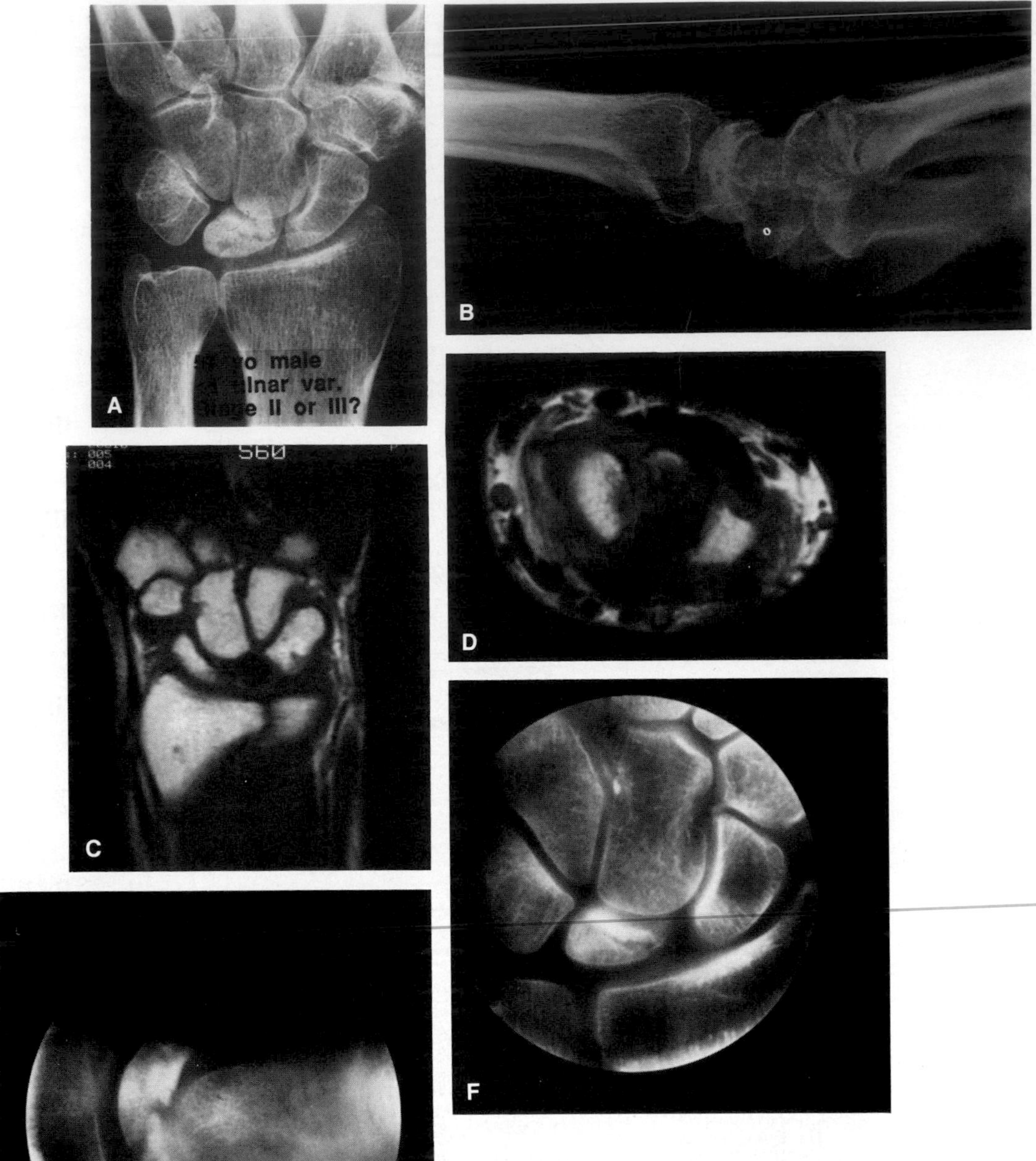

FIGURE 12-105. A 57-year-old man with pain in the left wrist after a fall. (**A**) PA view shows sclerosis of the lunate, with a +1 ulnar variance. (**B**) Displacement of the volar pole of the lunate. (**C,D**) MRI, showing avascularity of the entire lunate. (**E,F**) Trispiral tomograms. Lateral view shows displacement of the volar pole, extrusion of fragments by the capitate, and collapse of the proximal cortical area (**E**). Sclerosis of the lunate, increased scapholunate space, and intra-trabecular collapse (**F**).

of diminished vascularity before changes are apparent on x-ray, and this modality is now the imaging procedure of choice for early evaluation of Kienböck's disease.

Eponyms

Kienböck's disease is the well-known eponym for avascular necrosis with deformity of the carpal lunate. It is also described as lunatomalacia, osteonecrosis, and osteochondritis of the lunate.

Treatment

Acute Lunate Fractures

The most important factor in treating a fractured lunate is recognition that the fracture may progress to carpal instability, nonunion, or avascular necrosis. Under no circumstances should even a simple fracture of the lunate be treated expectantly in a cast or splint without provision for follow-up studies at close intervals for the first several weeks. Ideally, this should include tomography and, in some instances, MRI. If there is evidence of separation of the lunate fragments by the intrusion of the capitate, union will not be possible and the risk of avascular necrosis is sharply increased. The concentration of compressive stresses at the acute angulation of the fracture site prevents the establishment of intraosseous anastomoses.[256] Although the efficacy of internal fixation of the lunate is unproven and the obstacles to successful reduction and fixation are substantial, the consequences of inaction are quite certain. Distraction with an external fixator may allow the lunate fragments to coapt. If there is an ulnar minus variant, a leveling procedure, such as radial recession[15,291] or ulnar lengthening,[27,459,526] can reduce the joint compressive stresses (Fig. 12-106).[15,291,383,404,419,434,508,513,526,529] Immobilization during the expectant period should include a long-arm or Munster-type cast, well molded over the wrist to compress the lunate area.

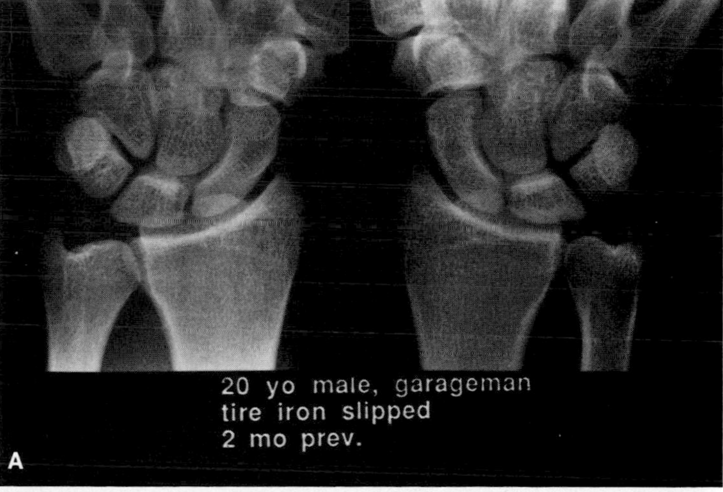

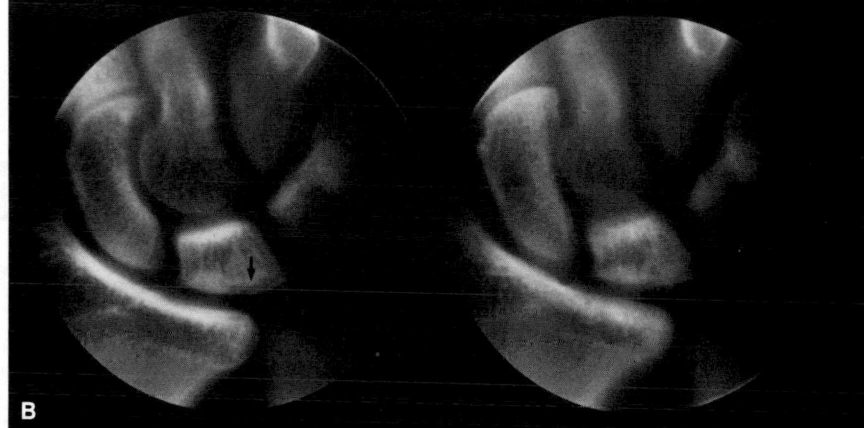

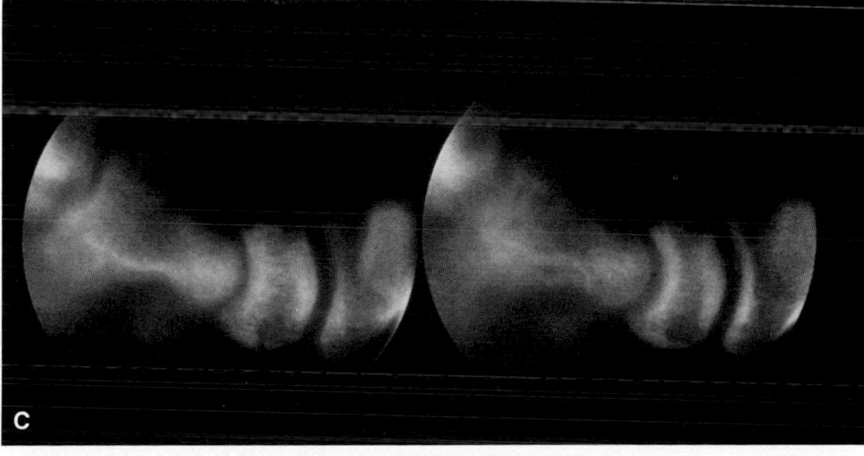

FIGURE 12-106. A 20-year-old garageman injured his wrist when a tire iron slipped. (**A**) Normal left wrist; infraction and early collapse of the right lunate; ulnar variance −2 mm. (**B,C**) AP and lateral variance tomograms demonstrate a fracture through the volar pole of the lunate. (**D,E**) Radial recession to create +1 mm ulnar variance; at 6 weeks (**D**) healing is apparent on the 12-week tomograms (**E**).

continues

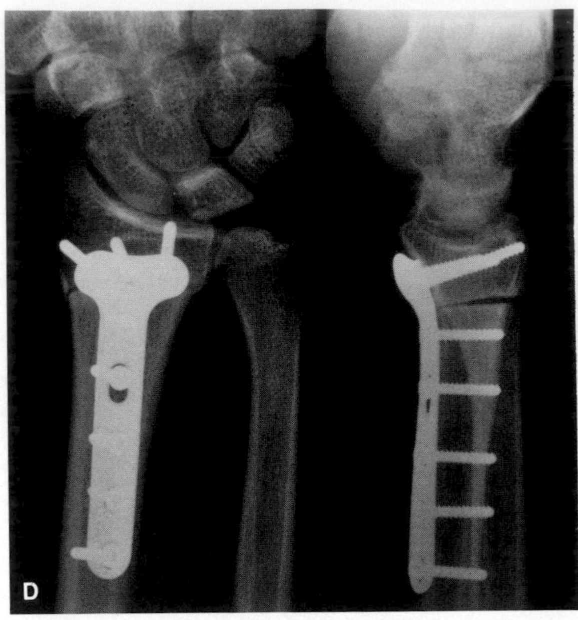

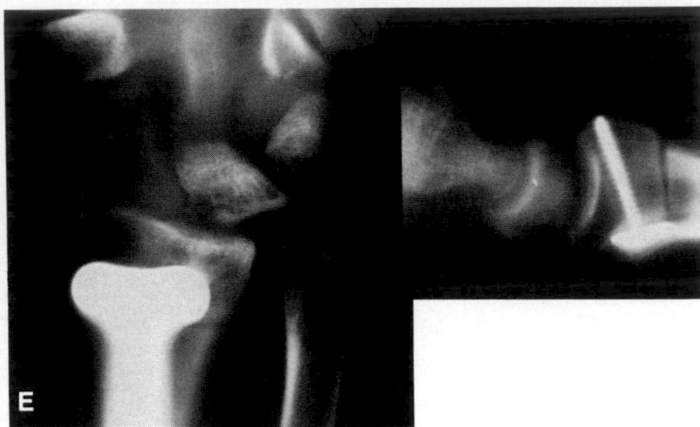

FIGURE 12-106. (continued)

Established Kienböck's Disease

When Kienböck's disease is established, leveling procedures seem to be the most efficacious approaches to treatment.[467] They do not violate the proximal row, as do the excision replacement procedures,[96,256,285,434,457,511,551,557] and they do relieve forces on the lunate.[433,457,511] Several long-term studies show adequate symptomatic relief and return to work after radial shortening,[15,404] radial wedge osteotomy,[405c] or ulnar lengthening.[27] The revascularization procedures[190] have not yet fulfilled their expectations,[16,190] especially without long-term simultaneous decompressive procedures.[380,390] Salvage procedures include proximal row carpectomy, wrist denervation,[87a] and arthrodesis. Excision and prosthetic replacements are rarely indicated for acute fractures[319] and are now seriously questioned for late cases because of silicone synovitis.[96,293,433]

Prognosis

Healing of nondisplaced lunate fractures, especially of avulsion injuries at the dorsal or volar horns, is relatively good. A transverse fracture of the body will heal if it remains nondisplaced, particularly in adolescents. Nonunion of a lunate body fracture is rare, because most progress to Kienböck's disease. Carpal collapse may occur in advanced Kienböck's disease (stages III, IV). The progressive disintegration of the lunate leads to degenerative changes. Over some years, some of these tend to stabilize and the symptoms may become tolerable at a decreased functional level. Others progress to radiolunate and capitolunate arthritis. Prompt treatment of lunate fractures and early operative intervention, therefore, seems warranted.

COMPLICATIONS OF CARPAL BONE INJURIES

Refracture

The incidence of refracture in the carpal bones is unknown. However, the frequent reinjury of the wrist associated with scaphoid fractures that appear to be healing at 8 or even 12 weeks but are found a few years later to have nonunion suggest that refracture is not infrequent. On the other hand, it is possible that some of these fractures never healed completely. The use of a protective splint for a considerable time, even after the fracture is thought to be healed, is recommended. Follow-up should be more carefully monitored longer than for other fractures. If clinical findings or routine x-rays are questionable, the status of union should be checked by polytomography, CT scan, or special x-rays, such as giant views.[367] If avascular necrosis is suspected, MRI is recommended.

Nerve Injury

Nerve injury is relatively common with carpal injuries.[41,297,532] Almost all dislocations and fracture–dislocations of the carpus have at least transient median nerve symptoms, and many have a sufficient neuropathy to suggest axonotmesis. Those with immediate significant signs of neuropathy are more likely due to direct contusion, hematoma, or stretching of the nerve. Those with slowly increasing signs during the first week are more likely due to an incipient carpal tunnel syndrome aggravated by the injury.

Other carpal injuries associated with neuropathy are fractures of the hamate hook[257] and the pisiform, both of which render the juxtaposed ulnar nerve susceptible to injury.[11] Damage to the articular nerve branches may be responsible for chronic wrist sprain pain (eg, the dorsal interosseous nerve at the radiocarpal interval). Damage to the dorsal sensory branches of the radial or ulnar nerves is probably due most often to the pressure of the support apparatus (splint or cast), rather than to direct injury. Vascular injury of significant degree associated with carpal injuries is uncommon.

Nonunion

Nonunion occurs in several of the carpal bones, probably because of intermittent forceful compressive stresses, the difficulty of maintaining immobility, and frequent lack of early diagnosis. Scaphoid nonunion[117] is the most common, but similar problems have been observed in the capitate,[195,276,288,375] lunate, pisiform, and hook of hamate.[59,502] Malunion and delayed union also occur for the same reasons.[18] Treatment of nonunion by closed methods is usually unsuccessful. Open reduction and internal fixation are usually necessary. Open reduction with bone graft to restore carpal bone configuration and carpal height is often preferable.

Pain Dysfunction Syndrome

Dysfunction and dystrophy,[17,28,65,292,418] which combine to be a common serious complication of wrist injuries, can be best introduced by a quotation from John Rhea Barton.

> I do not know of any subject on which I have been more frequently consulted than on deformities, rigid joints, inflexible fingers, loss of the pronating and supinating motions and on neuralgic complaints resulting from injuries of the wrist, and of the carpal extremity of the forearm—one or more of these evils have been left, not merely as a temporary inconvenience, but as a permanent consequence.[35]

The many disabilities that lead to upper limb dysfunction, often referred to as the shoulder-hand syndrome, are common complications of wrist injuries, particularly those that occur in the older age group. The dramatic presentation of the causalgia type[379] has drawn particular attention to the effect of reflex sympathetic dystrophy in such conditions.[379] Nevertheless, the number of cases in which this is the principal factor is relatively small. Shoulder-hand syndrome is a better choice, because the shoulder and hand are the most commonly involved, and hand and wrist involvement more than shoulder involvement.[382] The forearm, elbow, shoulder girdle, and neck are less commonly involved with pain and limitation of motion.

To cover this spectrum of disabilities, we use the term *pain dysfunction syndrome*.[17] The common denominator of all forms is that of dysfunction, usually precipitated by pain that may be focal, multiple sited, or even referred.[418] We further try to identify the pain that is sympathetic mediated from somatic mediated pain, noting differences in presentation, treatment alternatives, and prognosis. Sympathetic pain typical of sympathetic dystrophy is that of dysesthetic pain that is associated with hyperhidrosis, erythematous inflammatory response about finger joints, and general reflex response to most stimuli; thus it is generally recognized early. Positive bone scan, osteoporosis, and Q-SAART testing help to confirm the diagnosis.[297a] Response to sympathetic blocks is usually noticeable and effective in the case of true sympathetic dystrophy.

Somatic nerve pain, on the other hand, relates to a single peripheral nerve autonomous zone, consists of more burning, laminating pain, and is not associated with sympathetic overflow. Isolated radial sensory nerve injury or persistent median neuropathy from carpal injury left untreated are examples of somatic dystrophy. Isolated peripheral nerve blocks will relieve pain and help confirm the diagnosis. Sympathetic blocks are not helpful other than to demonstrate that the pain dysfunction is not a sympathetic dystrophy.

Sudeck's atrophy or osteoporosis associated with pain and dysfunction is one portion of the spectrum that occurs after carpal injuries and particularly after median nerve irritation that is generally more sympathetic than somatic; however, both aspects of peripheral neuropathy can coexist after peripheral nerve damage.[507] The osteoporosis commonly seen after carpal injury is usually a disuse phenomenon, not the Sudeck type. Treatment consists in identifying and coping with as many of the causes as possible. The most common physiologic pain sources are (1) the injury area generally, (2) autonomic dysfunction, (3) peripheral nerve elements, (4) synovial lined structures, and (5) musculoskeletal trigger areas.[17] Successful treatment of one source alone may allow resolution. Generally, however, combined efforts are needed by (1) controlling pain (peripheral or sympathetic nerve blocks); (2) physical therapy (mainly active assisted); (3) occupational re-education, making the patients help themselves; and (4) psychologic support, which includes reassurance that the condition will improve given time and appropriate treatment. "No pain, no gain" is the biggest detriment to resolution of most pain dysfunctions.

Active psychiatric support may be needed. More often evaluation and recommendations are useful with regard to (1) estimates of the degree of neurotic, psychotic, or motivational enhancement of the problem; (2) drug dependency or utility of drugs in management; and (3) suitability of the patient for surgery, for a pain-management center, and so forth. The number of patients with some degree of pain dysfunction syndrome argues for a prophylactic plan that includes (1) control of pain, first by ensuring that treatment methods, such as cast or external fixation frames, are not causative; (2) control of dysfunction, beginning with relaxation and rehabilitation techniques for the injured part; and (3) monitoring and graduated retraining to work-level function. One should assume that this process will take a year and be happy when it does not.

Ischemic Contractures

Closed compartment syndromes, both of the forearm or Volkmann type and of the intrinsic compartments of the hand, are not uncommon, particularly if associated with a crush injury.[541] Thus, rigid casts or dressings must be avoided, and careful attention must be paid to all severe and increasing pains that are referred to muscle, nerve, or vascular compartments. Immediate measurement of hand, carpal tunnel, and forearm compartments is essential. If rest, elevation, and resilient bulky dressings are unavailing, remeasurement of compartment pressures followed by surgical decompression is indicated. A wait and watch approach may lead to disastrous consequences. Clinical signs may mislead, and a palpable pulse means nothing in the presence of persistent pain. Similarly, narcotics to control pain after fractures or dislocations are rarely indicated and should be a sign of potential ischemic muscle and nerve damage. It is better to err on acting too soon than not soon enough. Impending contractures (ischemia) must be promptly treated.

Post-Traumatic Changes

Part of the differential diagnosis includes excluding stress fracture and impingement problems. Stress fractures have been noted in the carpus.[202,266] Osteolytic and cystic changes, secondary to episodes of single or repetitive stress, have been reported, especially in certain athletes. In boxers, a condition similar to carpal bossu or os styloideum has been noted, with ridging and exostosis formation, secondary to chondral changes at the carpometacarpal, intercarpal, or intermetacarpal joints of the index and mid finger.[87] Similar chondral defects, eburnation, and ridging have been noted at areas of joint impingement where contact occurs during extreme dorsiflexion at the radioscaphoid joint, as in gymnastics, between distal ulna and lunate. Similar impingement syndromes, usually with considerably more exostosis formation, are seen after dorsal chip fractures of the carpus or Colles' fractures. Associated with these or presenting alone are other post-traumatic residua that include intra-articular ligament or TFC tears; osteochondral injury; bone osteophytes on scaphoid, lunate, triquetrum and radial styloid; as well as localized areas of synovitis and ganglion formation. It is important in the differential diagnosis of wrist injuries to look for response to repetitive load that cause these stress reactions and formations. The advent of wrist arthroscopy has helped significantly to discover this unsuspected intra-articular problem.

U Other Complications

Skin loss, infection, and pathologic fractures are also complications in wrist injuries. All associated injuries to neighboring muscles and joints are common with acute carpal injuries. Secondary arthrosis may, much later, lead to damage of the deep flexors or the extensors because traumatic arthritis is present to some degree in almost all carpal injuries and may be severe, depending on the degree of chondral-surface damage. Fibrous ankylosis of the carpal joints is associated with the extent of traumatic arthrosis, the degree and persistence of hemorrhage and edema, the length of immobility, and the position during immobilization. The wrist ankylosed in flexion makes satisfactory hand function impossible.

INJURIES OF THE DISTAL RADIOULNAR JOINT

Injuries of the DRUJ are recognized as integral parts of other fractures that involve the wrist. Colles', Smith's, Essex-Lopresti's, and Galeazzi's fractures are the most common, yet isolated fracture or fracture–dislocation of the DRUJ is equally important.[92,108,164,371] Despite this, they are often relegated to secondary consideration. Until recently, excision of the ulnar head was considered an easy and safe way of dealing with symptoms related to the DRUJ. An increasing awareness of secondary problems after distal ulna excision has diminished this popularity, and a number of alternatives are now considered preferable. There are a significant number of localized injuries to the DRUJ and ulnar aspect of the wrist.[133,241,250] The diagnosis of many of these problems is difficult because physical and radiographic findings are often subtle or confusing. Interest in the problems of the DRUJ has increased considerably since the previous editions of this book.

Surgical Anatomy

The DRUJ provides the distal joint for forearm rotation, the axis of which runs from the center of the radial head proximally to the foveal area of the ulnar head distally (Fig. 12-107).[73,162,280,310,457] The ulnar head has two articular surfaces: the pole, which supports the carpal articulation and is covered by the TFC; and the seat, which articulates with the sigmoid notch of the radius. The TFC is a complex homogeneous structure, composed of the dorsal and palmar radioulnar ligaments, the articular disk,[108] "meniscus homologue," ulnar collateral ligament, and floor of the sixth dorsal compartment.[317,318,370] The TFC transfers force from the carpus to the ulna, extends the radiocarpal articulation, constrains the ulnocarpal joint, and stabilizes the DRUJ.[290] The radioulnar ligaments arise along the margins of the sigmoid notch of the radius and follow a helical course to converge to an insertion on the base of the ulnar styloid and the fovea of the ulnar pole.[280] On cross section,[289] the ulnar head is slightly elliptical and presents its major axis to the shallow sigmoid notch when in the neutral position. The seat of the ulnar head slides dorsally on the shallow articular crescent of the sigmoid notch during pronation and palmarly with supination.[162] This accounts for the greater prominence of the ulnar head clinically with pronation. The dorsal and palmar radioulnar ligaments that provide the boundaries of the TFC aid in guiding this motion.[427] The dorsal radioulnar ligament is taut in pronation, but it is the palmar ligament that actually prevents dorsal dislocation of the ulna on the radius. The palmar ligament is taut in supination, but it is the dorsal radioulnar ligament that is the key support preventing palmar dislocation. Only in the neutral position can the ulnar head be balloted dorsovolarly to test stability, a finding more apparent in lax-jointed individuals. There is also a variable amount of longitudinal play in the joint with pronosupination, radioulnar deviation, and forceful grasp. The TFC also acts as a shock absorber between the carpus and the ulnar head.[428]

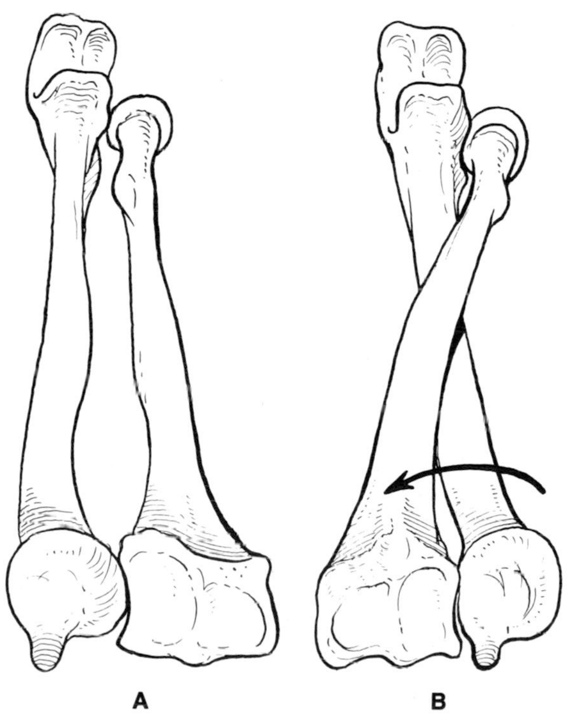

FIGURE 12-107. (**A**) In supination, the ulnar head rests against the volar rim of the sigmoid notch. (**B**) In pronation, the ulnar head rests against dorsal lip of the sigmoid notch.

The relative length of the ulna to the radius is described as ulnar variance, which is measured when the forearm is at rest with the elbow and shoulder flexed 90° and the wrist is in neutral flexion–extension and radial-ulnar deviation.[425] Neutral variance is present if the ulnar head is level with the articular concavity of the lunate fossa in a line perpendicular to the anatomical axis of the forearm. In pronation, the radius migrates proximally, creating a relative positive ulnar variance; and in supination, the radius is more distal, portraying a negative ulnar variance. Midportion x-rays are therefore important in assessing this variance. Statically in the ulnar neutral wrist, the relative load across the radioulnar complex is 80% radial and 20% ulnar. With 4 mm of ulna plus, the load changes to approximately 60% radial and 40% ulnar, whereas with an ulna minus the entire load is assumed by the radius.[427] There is increasing evidence to suggest that ulna variance plays a part in a number of symptomatic responses to injury and sustained use.

The final important stabilizer of the DRUJ is provided by the extensor carpi ulnaris and its related tendon sheath. The tendon sheath lies in a groove on the ulnar head radial to the styloid process.[498] It has been suggested that the floor of the sheath and the tendon act as a static and dynamic collateral ligament, respectively.[427] As it is fixed to the ulna, its relative position changes from dorsoulnar to ulnovolar as the radius moves from full supination to pronation. The dorsal and palmar capsules of the DRUJ are lax and provide minimal support.

Mechanisms of Injury

The DRUJ is subjected to a variety of stresses during everyday activity as well as from falls, twisting injuries, and overloads.[369] The joint is particularly vulnerable when in pronation.[92,457,495] The ulnar head lies on the dorsal rim of the sigmoid notch and is also dorsal to the carpus. With ulnar deviation, the triquetrum compresses the TFC into the palmar aspect of the ulnar head. With hyperpronation the ulnar ligament com-

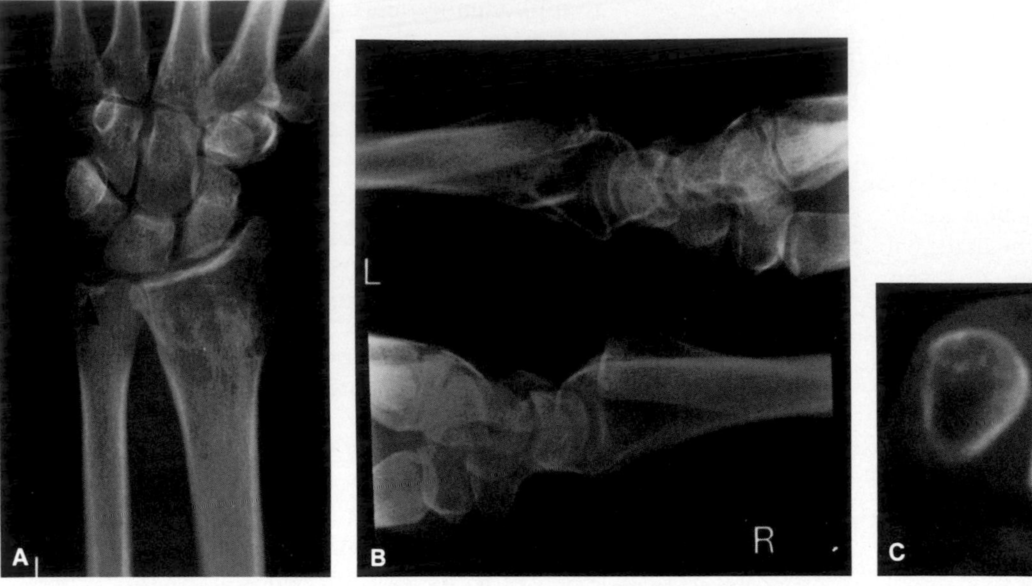

FIGURE 12-108. (**A**) AP—an ulnar styloid fracture and narrowed distal radioulnar joint of the left wrist. (**B**) Lateral–dorsal subluxation of the right ulnar head (*bottom*) in comparison to normal left wrist (*top*). Note that the ulnar head lies well above the triquetral silhouette. (**C**) CT scan showing dorsal subluxation of the ulnar head.

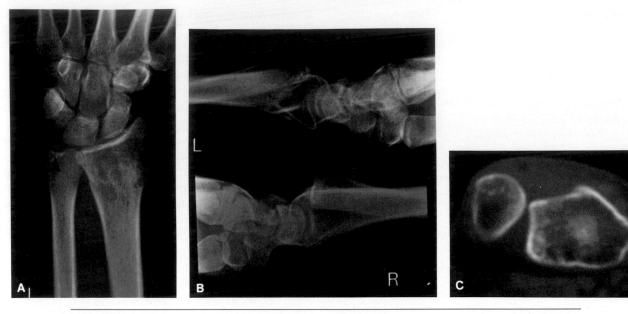

plex is twisted tautly about the palmarly displaced ulnar styloid, forcing the ulnar head dorsally.[259,495] Both of these mechanisms will force further dorsal subluxation of the ulnar head and disrupt the dorsal capsule, tearing the TFC from the bone of the ulnar styloid, or a palmar radioulnar ligament tear will occur.[242] Palmar dislocation of the ulnar head invariably occurs with the forearm loaded in supination, where the stretched palmar capsule provides little support to resist a pronatory torque applied to the heel of the palm.[125,134,457] The injured dorsal radioulnar ligament is not capable of preventing the dislocating force. Each of these mechanisms may induce chondromalacia of the seat of the ulnar head by shear stress to the cartilage surfaces as they override the rims of the sigmoid notch (Fig. 12-108). The tip of the ulnar styloid may be avulsed or sheared off. A fracture through the base of the ulnar styloid suggests an avulsion of the TFC insertions. The TFC may also be injured by direct compression or shearing stresses between the ulnar head and carpus. An ulna plus variant is often associated with these injuries. Likewise, the radial origins or ulnar insertions may be avulsed by the aforementioned mechanisms and can be associated with injury to the tendon sheaths, carpal ligaments, and joints in close proximity.[73,186]

Classification of Injuries of the DRUJ and Associated Conditions

By convention we speak of dorsal and palmar dislocations of the ulnar head. Chondromalacia or osteochondral defects of the ulnar seat may be associated with these injuries or with a lax ligamentous habitus. TFC injuries and ulnolunate impactions are often related to a positive ulna variance. The three worst injuries appear to be (1) dislocation of ulna with (a) soft-tissue tear or (b) bone avulsion injury of the ulnocarpal complex; (2) fracture–dislocation of the DRUJ (ie, Galeazzi, Essex-Lopresti); and (3) intra-articular fractures of the distal radius that involve the DRUJ. A broad classification follows, recognizing there are often subtleties and interrelations that may occur.[515]

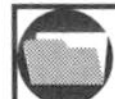

Classification

Dislocations/subluxations:[189,377,391,420]
- Ulna dorsal—with or without chondromalacia or osteochondral fracture
- Ulna volar—with or without accompanying radial fracture

Posttraumatic arthrosis:
- Ulnar pole
- Sigmoid notch of radius, with or without intraarticular radial fracture
- Ulnar seat

TFC injuries:[371,409,422]
- Acute tears
  - central, radial rim, palmar, ulnar styloidal
- Chronic tears
  - stellate central, ragged radial rim, ulnar styloidal

Styloid fractures:
- Tip, osteochondral
- Mid-styloid

Base—with or without TFC disruption; radioulnar instability
Ulnar head—with or without avulsion, floor of sixth compartment, with or a without displacement
Impaction injuries:
Ulnocarpal—functional, ulna plus variance, with or without TFC perforation
Ulnolunate—chronic, ulnar or lunate cortical sclerosis, cyst formation
Triquetrostyloid—elongated styloid process, triquetral rim avulsion?
ECU subluxation:[91]
Lax ligamentous habitus
Associated ulnocarpal injuries or conditions
Lunatotriquetral tears—with or without ulnocarpal impingement
Triquetrohamate impaction
Triquetropisiform chondromalacia
Osteochondral loose bodies
Occult carpal fractures
Carpal instabilities

Signs and Symptoms

Pain on the ulnar aspect of the wrist, usually accentuated with certain movements, and weakness are common complaints.[391,515] Rotation stress of the forearm and pain at the extremes of forearm rotation are different than pain associated with carpal rotation. In examining the forearm and DRUJ, the hand and carpus should be left free. In such testing, limitation of some motions, snapping, and "giving way" may be included. Dorsal subluxation of the ulna is suggested by ulnar head prominence when the forearm is pronated and by marked limitation of supination.[420] A positive "piano key" sign is a classic sign of instability. It can be positive dorsal, ballotting the distal ulna from dorsal to palmar, or it can be positive palmar, by lifting the pisiform and associated carpus dorsal to radial, that is, the palmar displaced distal radius and carpus. Palmar dislocation is evident by apparent narrowing of the forearm, a dimple where the ulnar head should be, and limited pronation. Chondromalacic pain may be elicited with ballottement of the distal ulna in various positions of forearm rotation. TFC tear and ulnocarpal impingement symptoms may be exaggerated by compressing the ulnar head and pisiform between index finger and thumb, followed by ulnar deviation.[409] Tenderness is elicited by pressure at the sulcus below the ulnar styloid, the "ulnar snuffbox." Crepitus is occasionally found during forearm rotation and radioulnar deviation. Disruption of the TFC insertions on the ulna allows an increased passive mobility of the ulnar head on the radius, especially as compared with the opposite wrist. Styloid fractures and loose bodies present with localized tenderness directly over the styloid. Extensor carpi ulnaris subluxation is demonstrated by turning both supinated forearms toward the examiner and forcibly resisting ulnar deviation. This causes the affected tendon to slip out of its groove and bowstring ulnarly. Lunatotriquetral tears are tender directly over the joint, and the symptoms are exaggerated by ballottement dorsovolarly, by radioulnar or ulnoradial triquetral displacement or by pisotriquetral lifting against the stable lunate. Triquetrohamate pain is differentiated by accentuating in extension and ulnar deviation triquetral hamate stress while pisotriquetral degenerative changes are reproduced by grinding the bones together.

Radiographic Findings

Confirmation of a dorsal ulnar dislocation is often difficult on plain films but usually evident on a cross-sectional CT scan (see Fig. 12-108**C**).[289,377,420] This will also show fractures and deformity of the sigmoid notch and osteochondral defects. A palmar dislocation is easily recognized on a CT scan but is often apparent on plain films, when carefully examined, because the ulnar head is superimposed beneath the edge of the sigmoid notch on the anteroposterior (coronal) view and displaced volar to the radius on the sagittal (lateral) view (Fig. 12-109). An ulna plus variant is often seen on the x-rays of patients with TFC tears, ulnocarpal impingements, and lunatotriquetral tears.[425]

Arthrograms can be helpful (Fig. 12-110**B**),[49] but some specifics of technique may be necessary to prevent a false-negative result.[451] The prestyloid recess and the pisotriquetral spaces are normal and must not

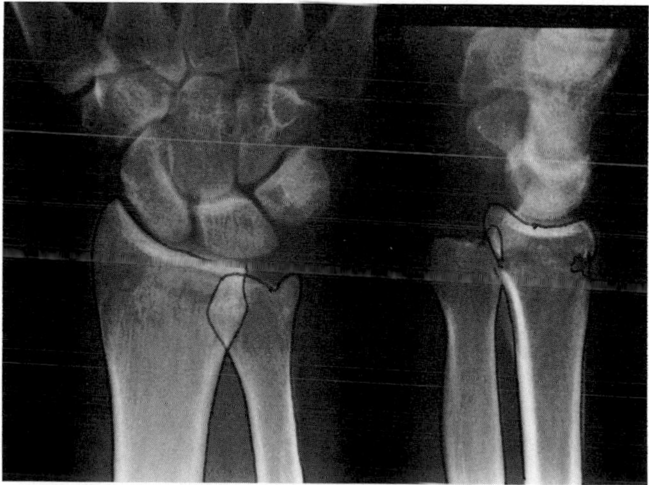

FIGURE 12-109. Palmar dislocation of the ulnar head associated with a minimally displaced distal radial fracture. There is narrowing of the anteroposterior silhouette and widening of the lateral silhouette, both clinically and on x-ray.

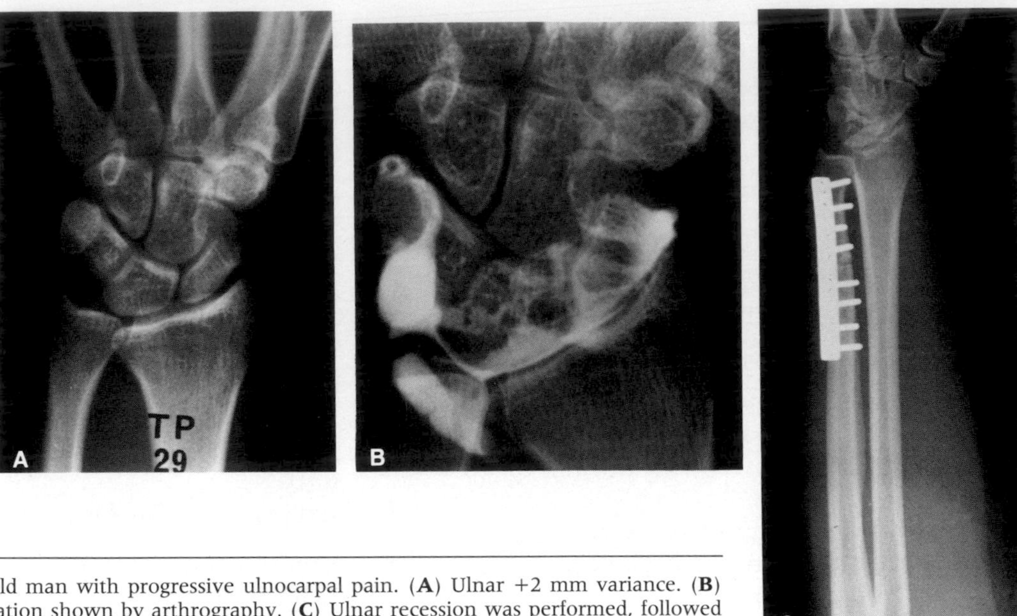

FIGURE 12-110. A 29-year-old man with progressive ulnocarpal pain. (**A**) Ulnar +2 mm variance. (**B**) Triangular fibrocartilage perforation shown by arthrography. (**C**) Ulnar recession was performed, followed by 8 weeks cast immobilization. The patient was allowed to return to full activities, and he had no pain.

be considered evidence of injury. A two- or three-phase study sequentially injecting the midcarpal and radiocarpal joints and the DRUJ is sometimes indicated to be sure that a torn flap of the TFC or lunatotriquetral ligament is not blocking the flow of dye. These studies should be done under the image intensifier and recorded on videotape during wrist motions. Extra-articular disruption of the TFC at the ulnar styloid, for instance, will not be seen on most radiocarpal studies but would be revealed on a DRUJ study. Fractures may require special views on occasion. Ulnolunate impaction sclerosis and cystic changes are readily identified on tomography. MRI studies will be increasingly valuable, because they show effusions in the DRUJ, chondral lesions, and often the TFC and ligament tears.

Treatment

Dorsal subluxation, recognized early, will respond to reduction with the forearm in *supination* and held in a long-arm cast for 6 weeks.[8] A variety of operations for chronic dislocations have been suggested. These usually employ an augmentation of the ligamentous structures with a strip of tendon.[258] Repair of a peripherally torn TFC should be included. We prefer to include tightening of the ulnocarpal capsule to this repair, because there is often a concomitant carpal supination.

A fresh palmar dislocation[133] may reduce with manipulation and pronation, but open reduction is often necessary because the ulnar head is sometimes locked on the undersurface of the radius (see Fig. 12-109). Access between the ulnar neurovascular bundle and the flexor profundi tendons will allow the ulna to be pried back into position. An osteochondral indentation may be noted. Immobilization in pronation is usually sufficient to prevent redislocation.

Repair of a torn TFC or ulnar styloid fracture is justified.[121b,409] The same is true when a peripheral injury destabilizes the ulnar TFC by fracturing the styloid or tears the styloid insertion, especially in the athlete or active younger adult. Such repairs can prevent chronic radioulnar instability. A more extensive tearing of the floor of the sixth compartment and ulnocarpal ligaments may be seen. Small ulnar styloid fractures are seldom of significance, but fractures through the base usually imply that the integrity of the TFC is compromised. Immobilization is preferred for 6 weeks, but if there is marked displacement of more than 3 mm, open reduction with internal fixation should be performed.

Central and radial tears of the TFC may be treated by several methods.[363,426] Arthroscopy enthusiasts have popularized arthroscopic debridement of the central portion of the TFC as the treatment of choice because of the rapid rehabilitation. A "wafer" excision of a few millimeters of the distal ulna, preserving the radioulnar joint, has been reported as showing good results. Others recommend an open resection of the distal ulna articular surface for chronic TFC tears and ulna impaction syndrome.[173a] In our hands, there have also been satisfactory results with ulnar recession (shortening) (see Fig. 12-110).[136] This preserves the ulnar head intact, corrects the ulnar plus variance, allows the TFC to heal or be repaired, and provides exposure for concomitant repair of the lunatotriquetral ligament, if indicated. The obvious disadvantage is the presence of an ulnar plate and a longer healing period. Acute repair of radial rim tears (tears at the edge of the lunate fossa of the distal radius) and volar ulnocarpal ligaments should also be performed.[121b] Other occasional procedures are pisiformectomy, ulnar styloid excision, triquetral cheilotomy, and loose body removal.

Excision of the ulnar head, the Darrach procedure,[135,148,163] is occasionally indicated when there is irreparable damage in the DRUJ itself. In some patients the results appear to be quite good,[247] while in others ulnar head excision is disastrous (Fig. 12-111).[53,339,372] Those patients most likely to have a poor result are young women with a loose-jointed habitus. Complications of distal ulnar excision include narrowing of the interosseous space, instability of the ulnar stump, impaction of the stump against the radius, and snapping with rotatory motions. Later the radius shows scalloping, the ulnar stump remodels into a penciled appearance, and there is persistent weakness.[53] Reconstructive procedures at this stage are unpredictable and often lead to multiple operations.

An alternative procedure, the Sauve-Kapandji, involves fusion of the DRUJ with a proximal pseudarthrosis, which has the purpose of stabilizing the ulna side of the wrist yet preserving forearm rotation. Partial ulnar head excisions with preservation of the styloid and its attachments, with or without soft-tissue interposition, may provide better stability but are not free of complications.[74] Preservation of the DRUJ by recession,[72] corrective angulatory osteotomy,[179] or ligamentous stabilizing procedures[80,259] should take precedence, if at all possible. In malunited Colles' fractures, radial corrective osteotomies should be considered.

Dislocation of the extensor carpi ulnaris has been treated by augmenting the dorsal fascial roof of the sixth compartment with a leaf of the overlying dorsal retinaculum or reflecting the extensor retinacular proper with a radial-based flap. A stronger repair results when adjacent retinacular tissue is reflected over for support.[91]

Prognosis

Dorsal subluxations of the ulna may recur or worsen without adequate treatment but are generally responsive to treatment as outlined. Palmar dislocations become firmly locked and difficult to reduce after 2 or 3 weeks. An osteochondral lesion worsens with time, as will instabilities of the DRUJ. Symptoms of TFC tears may fluctuate but do not repair themselves spontaneously in most instances. The same is true of ulnar impaction syndromes and lunatotriquetral tears.

Complications

Transient sensory symptoms may be the result of irritation of the ulnar nerve in Guyon's canal or at its dorsal sensory branch with the previously discussed conditions, although permanent damage is rare. The development of progressive instability is possible with the injuries that affect the TFC. Osteochondral lesions lead to degenerative arthritis, as do the impaction syndromes. Surgical procedures also occasionally develop complications, such as already discussed under the Darrach procedure. Failure of TFC and ligament repairs as well as nonunion of ulnar osteotomies occur at times.

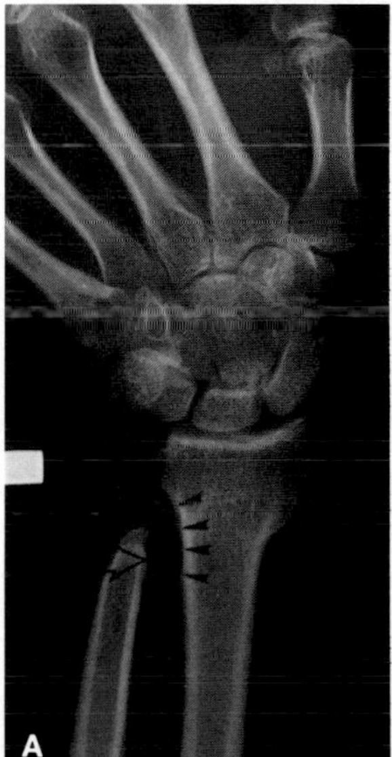

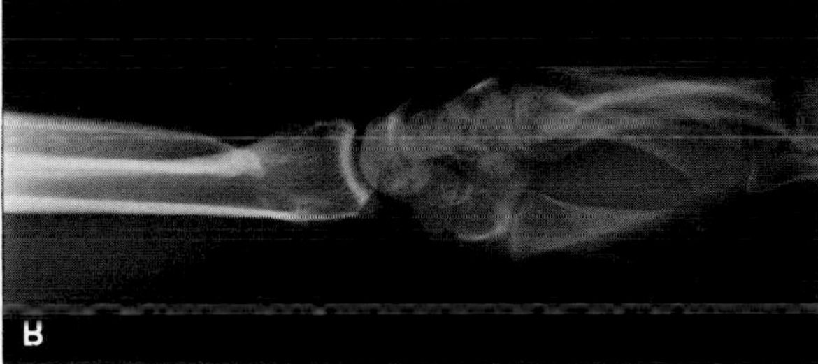

FIGURE 12-111. A 20-year-old laborer had a distal radius fracture with moderate dorsal angulation and distal radioulnar joint discomfort. Excision of ulnar head resulted in increased weakness, snapping, and loss of rotation. PA (**A**) and lateral (**B**) x-rays show scalloping of radial metaphysis secondary to lunate stump impingement (*arrows*). A radial corrective osteotomy might have been a better alternative than resection of the distal ulna in this working man.

PROGNOSIS IN CARPAL INJURIES

In general, the prognosis for recovery from many of these injuries is good, provided diagnosis is made early and appropriate management is carried out swiftly. The time for recovery varies, depending on the type of injury and the treatment requirements, particularly the length of time required for support and healing of damaged tissues. Recovery is practically never complete, if residual deformity involves a joint surface. Severe deformity, such as recurrent or persistent dislocation, collapse deformity, or chondral damage, nearly always results in disability sufficient to warrant a reconstructive procedure such as excisional or fibrous arthroplasties to partial carpal arthrodesis. These procedures, when properly selected, are adequate, but significant disability always results.

POST-TREATMENT CARE AND REHABILITATION OF CARPAL INJURIES

Post-injury splinting and rehabilitation are an essential component of nearly every wrist injury. The type of support apparatus used for each condition has been included under the individual topics. Generally, palmar surface splints, combined with resilient dressings, are used during the immediate post-trauma period of reaction and swelling. After this, the minimal support used should be a short-arm wrist support splint. The maximal support can be a long-arm cast for certain scaphoid fractures and other precarious carpal body fractures. Some external fixators or internal fixation may be secure enough to minimize external support and allow earlier return to function. Dislocations and fracture–dislocations are treated with supports similar to those used in carpal body fractures, unless there has been associated internal fixation. Kirschner wires, when used percutaneously or for open reduction, are usually left protruding, with the external portion bent at right angles to avoid migration. Antibiotic ointment is applied around the pin site. These cause little trouble (less so in our experience than do buried pins) but must be monitored closely for evidence of looseness or inflammation or both.

Generally, inflammation is preceded by loosening of a pin. A loose pin should be removed immediately. The first sign of loosening is that the pin can be rotated with manual force alone. In most instances, even snug Kirschner wires are removed in 6 to 8 weeks. The return of a complete range of motion, even in normal joints, can be expected *to take about as long as the joint was totally immobilized*. The return of comfort and full strength, as judged by the return of grip power and repetitive grip endurance, takes about *four times* as long as the time that the part was rigidly supported. Nevertheless, the permanently disabling residua associated with pain dysfunction syndrome[17] almost always can be avoided by careful attention to (1) instituting and maintaining shoulder elevation exercises throughout the course of treatment, (2) observing and halting the progression of any neurologic or circulatory deficits, (3) observing and remedying all pain and swelling, (4) avoiding extreme positioning of any joint or part, (5) initiating digit exercises as soon as feasible, and (6) bringing the wrist to a neutral or slightly extended position as soon as this is safe.

Shoulder exercises of the Codman type should be undertaken in all wrist injuries. This motion and use of the hand and shoulder serve as pump for the extremity to reduce swelling when some disability of the shoulder restricts elevation. Even greater attention is paid to the shoulder. The key shoulder exercise to avoid shoulder-hand syndrome is active elevation and rotation. This should be carried out a minimum of 50 times each day if possible. Almost any digit exercise is useful, provided a full range of possible motion is carried out, with the maximal force that is comfortable. Wiggling exercises are inadequate. To ensure that each joint has the maximal chance of being carried through its particular range of motion, we use a set of six exercises (the "six pack hand exercises"): (1) maximal extension of all digits, (2) thumb to each fingertip, (3) the grasp or fist exercise with all fingers flexing to the palmar crease or as near as possible to it, (4) the "claw" exercise with the metacarpophalangeal joints of the fingers kept extended but the interphalangeal joints maximally flexed, (5) the "tabletop" exercise with the metacarpophalangeal joints maximally flexed but the interphalangeal joints extended, and (6) abduction–adduction of all digits in the radioulnar plane.

With these precautions and a gradual increase of function with both duration and force carefully controlled, rehabilitation is seldom a problem, yet not an area to ignore. Occasionally, physical therapy modalities, manipulation under anesthesia, articular corticosteroid injection, splinting, and particularly re-education may be required. Re-education with normal patterns of relaxation and integrated contraction are difficult and almost impossible if pain, apprehension, or distraction interferes. The principal resource here is a good, patient therapist, but chemical assistance (eg, blocks) may be needed. Inhibition of some or all of the motors that control the wrist and digits may be so ingrained a pattern that special training may be necessary. The most common instance of this is inhibition of the wrist extensors when pain is associated with wrist extension or when deformity decreases the moment arm distance between the center of wrist motion and the wrist extensor tendon. The patient attempts to extend the wrist with the finger extensors, making it impossible to extend the wrist and make a fist at the same time. The sooner this and other abnormal co-contractions can be identified and corrected, the smoother rehabilitation will be. Recovery from wrist injury is a challenging endeavor, but it must be understood and successfully managed because the injury is frequent; loss of time, productivity, and important skills is common.

REFERENCES

1. Adams, B.D., Blair, W.F., Reagan, D.S., and Grundberg, A.B.: Technical Factors Related to Herbert Screw Fixation. J. Hand Surg., 13A:893–899, 1988.

1a. Adams, B.D., Frykman, G.K., and Taleisnik, J.: Treatment of Scaphoid Nonunion With Casting and Pulsed Electromagnetic Fields. J. Hand Surg. 17A:910–913, 1992.

2. Adkinson, J.W., and Chapman, M.W.: Treatment of Acute Lunate and Perilunate Dislocations. Clin. Orthop., 164:199–207, 1982.

3. Adler, J.M., and Shaftan, G.W.: Fractures of the Capitate. J. Bone Joint Surg., 44A:1537–1547, 1962.

4. Agerholm, J.C., and Goodfellow, J.W.: Avascular Necrosis of the Lunate Bone Treated by Excision and Prosthetic Replacement. J. Bone Joint Surg., 45B:110–116, 1963.

5. Ahl, T., Andersson, G., Herberts, P., and Kalen, R.: Electrical Treatment of Non-United Fractures. Acta Orthop. Scand., 55:585–588, 1984.

6. Aitken, A.P., and Nalebuff, E.A.: Volar Transnavicular Perilunar Dislocation of the Carpus. J. Bone Joint Surg., 42A:1051–1057, 1960.

7. Albert, M.C., and Barre, P.S.: A Scaphoid Fracture Associated With a Displaced Distal Radial Fracture in a Child. Clin. Orthop., 240:232–235, 1989.

8. Albert, S.M., Wohl, M.A., and Rechtman, A.M.: Treatment of the Disrupted Radioulnar Joint. J. Bone Joint Surg., 45A:1373–1381, 1963.

9. Alexander, A.H., and Lichtman, D.M.: Kienböck's Disease. Orthop. Clin. North Am., 17:461–472, 1986.

10. Alexander, C.E., and Lichtman, D.M.: Ulnar Carpal Instabilities. Orthop. Clin. North Am., 15:307–320, 1984.

11. Ali, M.A.: Fracture of the Body of the Hamate Bone Associated With Compartment Syndrome and Dorsal Decompression of the Carpal Tunnel. J. Hand Surg., 11B:207–210, 1986.

12. Allen, P.R.: Idiopathic Avascular Necrosis of the Scaphoid: Report of Two Cases. J. Bone Joint Surg., 65B:333–335, 1983.

13. Allieu, Y.: Carpal Instability Revisited: Ligamentous Instabilities and Intracarpal Malalignments. Ann. Chir. Main Memb. Super., 3:317–321, 1984.

14. Almquist, E.E.: Kienböck's Disease. Clin. Orthop., 202:68–78, 1986.

15. Almquist, E.E., and Burns, J.F.: Radial Shortening for the Treatment of Kienböck's Disease—A Five to Ten Year Follow-Up. J. Hand Surg., 7:348–352, 1982.

16. Alnot, J.Y., Badelon, O., Sommariva, L., Bocquet, L., and Grossin, M.: Necrotic Bone Segment Revascularization by the Transfer of a Vascular Bundle: Experimental Study in the Rat. Ann. Chir. Main Memb. Super., 1:274–276, 1982.

17. Amadio, P.C.: Current Concepts Review: Pain Dysfunction Syndromes. J. Bone Joint Surg., 70A:944–949, 1988.

18. Amadio, P.C., Berquist, T.H., Smith, D.K., Ilstrup, D.M., Cooney, W.P., and Linscheid, R.L.: Scaphoid Malunion. J. Hand Surg., 14A:679–687, 1989.

19. Amadio, P.C., and Botte, M.J.: Treatment of Malunion of the Distal Radius. Hand Clin., 3:541–559, 1987.

20. Amadio, P.C., Hanssen, A.D., and Berquist, T.H.: The Genesis of Kienböck's Disease: Evaluation of a Case by Magnetic Resonance Imaging. J. Hand Surg., 12A:1044–1049, 1987.

21. Amamilo, S.C., Uppal, R., and Samuel, A.W.: Isolated Dislocation of Carpal Scaphoid. J. Hand Surg., 10B:385–388, 1985.

22. Anderson, W.J.: Simultaneous Fracture of the Scaphoid and Capitate in a Child. J. Hand Surg., 12A:271–273, 1987.

23. Andress, M.R., and Peckar, V.G.: Fracture of the Hook of the Hamate. Br. J. Radiol., 43:141–143, 1970.

24. Andrews, J., Miller, G., and Haddad, R.: Treatment of Scaphoid Nonunion by Volar Inlay Distal Radius Bone Graft. J. Hand Surg., 10B:214–216, 1985.

25. Andrews, J.G., and Youm, Y.: A Biomechanical Investigation of Wrist Kinematics. J. Biomech., 12:83–83, 1979.

26. Andrianne, Y., Donkerwolcke, M., Hinsenkamp, M., Quintin, J., Rasquin, C., El Banna, S., and Burny, F.: Hoffman External Fixation of Fractures of the Radius and Ulna: A Prospective Study of Fifty-Three Patients. Orthopedics, 7:845–850, 1984.

27. Armistead, R.B., Linscheid, R.L., Dobyns, J.H., and Beckenbaugh, R.D.: Ulnar Lengthening in the Treatment of Kienböck's Disease. J. Bone Joint Surg., 64A:170–178, 1982.

28. Atkins, R.M., Duckworth, T., and Kanis, J.A.: Algodystrophy Following Colles' Fracture. J. Hand Surg., 14B:161–164, 1989.

29. Auffray, Y., and Comtet, J.J.: The Role of Osteosynthesis of the Anterior Surface in Fractures of the Distal End of the Radius (in French). Lyon Med., 219:193–198, 1968.

30. Aufranc, O.E., Jones, W.N., and Turner, R.H.: Anterior Marginal Articular Fracture of Distal Radius. J.A.M.A., 196:788–791, 1966.

31. Aufranc, O.E., Jones, W.N., and Turner, R.N.: Transnavicular Perilunar Carpal Dislocation. J.A.M.A., 181:130–133, 1962.

32. Axelrod, T., Paley, D., Green, J., and McMurtry, R.Y.: Limited Open Reduction of the Lunate Facet in Comminuted Intra-Articular Fractures of the Distal Radius. J. Hand Surg., 13A:372–377, 1988.

33. Balfour, G.W.: Diagnosis of Oblique Fractures of the Distal Ulna Using an Extended Pronated View of the Wrist: Case Report. Orthopedics, 13:247–250, 1990.

34. Barnard, L., and Stubbins, S.G.: Styloidectomy of the Radius in the Surgical Treatment of Non-Union of the Carpal Navicular: A Preliminary Report. J. Bone Joint Surg., 30A:98–102, 1948.

35. Barton, J.R.: Views and Treatment of an Important Injury to the Wrist. Med. Examiner, 1:365, 1838.

35a. Barton, N.J.: Twenty Questions About Scaphoid Fractures. J. Hand Surg., 17B:289-310, 1992.

36. Bartone, N.F., and Grieco, R.V.: Fractures of the Triquetrum. J. Bone Joint Surg., 38A:353–356, 1956.

37. Bartosh, R.A., and Saldana, M.J.: Intraarticular Fractures of the Distal Radius: A Cadaveric Study to Determine if Ligamentotaxis Restores Radiopalmar Tilt. J. Hand Surg., 15A:18–21, 1990.

38. Bassett, R.L.: Displaced Intraarticular Fractures of the Distal Radius. Clin. Orthop., 214:148–152, 1987.

39. Bassett, R.L., and Ray, M.J.: Carpal Instability Associated With Radial Styloid Fracture. Orthopedics, 7:1356–1361, 1984.

40. Bastillas, J., Vasilas, A., Pizzi, W.F., and Gokcebay, T.: Bone Scanning in the Detection of Occult Fractures. J. Trauma, 21:564, 1981.

41. Bauman, T.D., Gelberman, R.H., Mubarak, S.J., and Garfin, S.R.: The Acute Carpal Tunnel Syndrome. Clin. Orthop., 156:151–156, 1981.

42. Baumann, J.U., and Campbell, R.D. Jr.: Significance of Architectural Types of Fractures of the Carpal Scaphoid and Relation to Timing of Treatment. J. Trauma, 2:431–438, 1962.

43. Beckenbaugh, R.D.: Diagnosis and Treatment of Scaphoid Fracture Nonunion. Adv. Orthop., 1(3):1-24, 1985.

44. Beckenbaugh, R.D., Shives, T.C., Dobyns, J.H., and Linscheid, R.L.: Kienböck's Disease: The Natural History of Kienböck's Disease and Consideration of Lunate Fractures. Clin. Orthop., 149:98–106, 1980.

45. Belsole, R.J., Eikman, E.A., and Muroff, L.R.: Bone Scintigraphy in Trauma of the Hand and Wrist. J. Trauma, 21:163–166, 1981.

45a. Belsole, R.J., Hilbelink, D.R., Llewallyn, J.A., Dale, M., Greene, T.L., and Rayhack, J.M.: Computed Analysis of the

Pathomechanics of Scaphoid Waist Fracture. J. Hand Surg. 16A:899–906, 1991.
46. Bentzon, P.G.K., and Madsen, A.R.: On Fracture of Carpal Scaphoid Bone: Method for Operative Treatment of Inveterate Fractures. Acta Orthop. Scand., 16:30–39, 1945.
47. Berger, R.A., Blair, W.F., Crowninshield, R.D., and Flatt, A.E.: The Scapholunate Ligament. J. Hand Surg. 7:87–91, 1982.
48. Berger, R.A., and Blair, W.F.: The Radioscapholunate Ligament: A Gross and Histologic Description. Anat. Rec., 210:393–404, 1984.
49. Berger, R.A., Blair, W.F., and El-Khoury, G.Y.: Arthrotomography of the Wrist: The Triangular Fibrocartilage Complex. Clin. Orthop., 172:257–264, 1983.
50. Berger, R.A., and Landsmeer, J.M.F.: The Palmar Radiocarpal Ligaments: A Study of Adult and Fetal Human Wrist Joints. Iowa Orthop. J., 5:32–41, 1985.
51. Berquist, T.H. (ed.): Imaging of Orthopedic Trauma and Surgery. Philadelphia, W.B. Saunders, 1986.
52. Bickerstaff, D.R., and Bell, M.J.: Carpal Malalignment in Colles' Fractures. J. Hand Surg., 14B:155–160, 1989.
53. Bieber, E.J., Linscheid, R.L., Dobyns, J.H., and Beckenbaugh, R.D.: Failed Distal Ulna Resections. J. Hand Surg., 13A:193–200, 1988.
54. Bieber, E.J., and Weiland, A.J.: Traumatic Dorsal Dislocation of the Triquetrum: A Case Report. J. Hand Surg., 9A:840–842, 1984.
55. Bilos, J., and Hui, P.W.: Dorsal Dislocation of the Lunate With Carpal Collapse. J. Bone Joint Surg., 63A:1484–1486, 1981.
56. Bilos, Z.J., Pankovich, A.M., and Yelda, S.: Fracture–Dislocation of the Radiocarpal Joint. J. Bone Joint Surg., 59A:198–203, 1977.
57. Binkovitz, L.A., Ehman, R.L., Cahill, D.R., and Berquist, T.H.: Magnetic Resonance Imaging of the Wrist. Radiographics, 8(6):1171–1202, 1988.
58. Biondelle, P.R., Vannier, M.W., Gilula, L.A., and Knapp, R.: Wrist: Coronal and Transaxial Scanners. Radiology, 163:149–151, 1989.
59. Bishop, A.T., and Beckenbaugh, R.D.: Fracture of the Hamate Hook. J. Hand Surg., 13A:135–139, 1988.
60. Black, D.M., Watson, H.K., and Vender, M.I.: Scapholunate Gap With Scaphoid Nonunion. Clin. Orthop., 224:205–209, 1987.
61. Blatt, G.: Capsulodesis in Reconstructive Hand Surgery: Dorsal Capsulodesis for the Unstable Scaphoid and Volar Capsulodesis Following Excision of the Distal Ulna. Hand Clin., 3:81–102, 1987.
62. Blevens, A.D., Light, T.R., Jablonsky, W.S., Smith, D.G., Patwardhan, A.G., Guay, M.E., and Woo, T.S.: Radiocarpal Articular Contact Characteristics With Scaphoid Instability. J. Hand Surg., 14A:781–790, 1989.
63. Böhler, L.: The Treatment of Fractures. Translated by Tretter, H., Luchini, H.B., Kreuz, K., Rüsse, O.A., and Bjornson, R.G.B., from the 13th German ed. New York, Grune & Stratton, 1956.
64. Bollen, S.R.: Peri-Triquetral-Lunate Dislocation Associated With Ulnar Nerve Palsy. J. Hand Surg., 13B:456–457, 1988.
65. Bonica, J.J.: Causalgia and Other Reflex Sympathetic Dystrophies. Postgrad. Med. 53:143, 1973.
66. Bonnel, F., and Allieu, Y.: The Radioulnocarpal and Midcarpal Joints: Anatomical Organisation and Biomechanical Basis. Ann. Chir. Main Memb. Super., 3:287–296, 1984.
67. Bora, F.W., Osterman, A.L., and Brighton, C.T.: The Electrical Treatment of Scaphoid Non-Union. Clin. Orthop., 161:33–38, 1981.
68. Botte, M.J., Cooney, W.P., and Linscheid, R.L.: Arthroscopy of the Wrist: Anatomy and Technique. J. Hand Surg., 14A:313–316, 1989.
69. Botte, M.J., and Gelberman, R.H.: Fractures of the Carpus, Excluding the Scaphoid. Hand Clin., 3:149–161, 1987.
70. Botte, M.J., and Gelberman, R.H.: Modified Technique for Herbert Screw Insertion in Fractures of the Scaphoid. J. Hand Surg., 12A:149–150, 1987.
71. Botte, M.J., Mortensen, W.W., Gelberman, R.H., Rhoades, C.E., and Gellman, H.: Internal Vascularity of the Scaphoid in Cadavers After Insertion of the Herbert Screw. J. Hand Surg., 13A:216–222, 1988.
72. Boulas, H.J., and Milek, M.A.: Ulnar Shortening for Tears of the Triangular Fibrocartilaginous Complex. J. Hand Surg., 15A:415–420, 1990.
72a. Boulas, H.J., and Miler, M.A.: Hook of Hamate Fractures: Diagnosis, Treatment, and Complications. Orthop. Rev., 19:518–529, 1990.
73. Bowers, W.H.: Distal Radioulnar Joint. *In* Green, D.P. (ed.): Operative Hand Surgery, pp. 743–769. Philadelphia, J.B. Lippincott, 1982.
74. Bowers, W.H.: Distal Radioulnar Joint Arthroplasty: The Hemiresection–Interposition Technique. J. Hand Surg., 10A:169–178, 1985.
75. Boyes, J.H.: Bunnell's Surgery of the Hand, 4th ed., pp. 292–293. Philadelphia, J.B. Lippincott, 1964.
76. Bradway, J.K., Amadio, P.C., and Cooney, W.P.: Open Reduction and Internal Fixation of Displaced, Comminuted Intra-Articular Fractures of the Distal End of the Radius. J. Bone Joint Surg., 71A:839–847, 1989.
77. Brand, P., Beach, R.B., and Thompson, D.E.: Relative Tension and Potential Excursion of Muscles in the Forearm and Hand. J. Hand Surg., 6A:209–219, 1981.
78. Bray, R.J., Swafford, A. R., and Brown, R.L.: Bilateral Fractures of the Hook of the Hamate. J. Trauma, 25:174–175, 1985.
79. Bray, T.J., and McCarroll, H.R. Jr.: Preiser's Disease: A Case Report. J. Hand Surg., 9A:730–732, 1984.
80. Breen, T.F., and Jupiter, J.B.: Extensor Carpi Ulnaris and Flexor Carpi Ulnaris Tenodesis of the Unstable Distal Ulna. J. Hand Surg., 14A:612–617, 1989.
81. Briggs, B.T., Cooney, W.P., and Linscheid, R.L.: Proximal Row Carpectomy (Abstract). Orthop. Trans., 2:216, 1978.
82. Broder, H.: Rupture of Flexor Tendons, Associated With a Malunited Colles Fracture. J. Bone Joint Surg., 36A:404–405, 1954.
83. Brolin, I.: Post-Traumatic Lesions of the Lunate Bone. Acta Orthop. Scand., 34:167–182, 1964.
84. Broome, A., Cedell, C.A., and Colleen, S.: High Plaster Immobilization for Fracture of the Carpal Scaphoid Bone. Acta Chir. Scand., 128:42–44, 1964.
85. Brown, D.E., and Lichtman, D.M.: Midcarpal Instability. Hand Clin., 3:135–140, 1987.
86. Brumbaugh, R.B., Crowninschield, R.D., Blair, W.F., and Andrews, J.G.: An In-Vivo Study of Normal Wrist Kinematics. J. Biomech. Eng., 104:176–181, 1982.
87. Bryan, R.S., and Dobyns, J.H.: Fractures of the Carpal Bones Other Than Lunate or Navicular. Clin. Orthop., 149:107–111, 1980.
88. Bunker, T.D., McNamee, P.B., and Scott, T.D.: The Herbert Screw for Scaphoid Fractures. J. Bone Joint Surg., 69B:631–634, 1987.
89. Burgess, R.C.: The Effect of a Simulated Scaphoid Malunion on Wrist Motion. J. Hand Surg., 12A:774–776, 1987.
90. Burgess, R.C.: The Effect of Rotatory Subluxation of the Scaphoid on Radio-Scaphoid Contact. J. Hand Surg., 12A:771–774, 1987.
91. Burkhart, S.S., Wood, M.B., and Linscheid, R.L.: Posttraumatic Recurrent Subluxation of the Extensor Carpi Ulnaris Tendon. J. Hand Surg., 7:1–3, 1982.
92. Buterbaugh, G.A., and Palmer, A.K.: Fractures and Dislocations of the Distal Radioulnar Joint. Hand Clin., 4:361–375, 1988.
93. Cain, J.E. Jr., Shepler, T.R., and Wilson, M.R.: Hamatometacarpal Fracture–Dislocation: Classification and Treatment. J. Hand Surg., 12A:762–767, 1987.
93a. Carroll, R.E., and Lakin, J.F.: Fracture of the Hook of the Hamate: Acute Treatment. J. Trauma, 34:803–805, 1993.
94. Carrozzella, J., and Stern, P.J.: Treatment of Comminuted Distal Radius Fractures With Pins and Plaster. Hand Clin., 4:391–397, 1988.
95. Carrozzella, J.C., Stern, P.J., and Murdock, P.A.: The Fate of Failed Bone Graft Surgery for Scaphoid Nonunions. J. Hand Surg., 14A:800–806, 1989.

96. Carter, P.R., Benton, L.J., and Dysert, P.A.: Silicone Rubber Carpal Implants: A Study of the Incidence of Late Osseous Complications. J. Hand Surg., 11A:639–644, 1986.
97. Carter, P.R., Eaton, R.G., and Littler, J.W.: Ununited Fracture of the Hook of the Hamate. J. Bone Joint Surg., 59A:583–588, 1977.
98. Carter, P.R., Malinin, T.I., Abbey, P.A., and Sommerkamp, T.G.: The Scaphoid Allograft: A New Operation for Treatment of the Very Proximal Scaphoid Nonunion or for the Necrotic, Fragmented Scaphoid Proximal Pole. J. Hand Surg., 14A:1–12, 1989.
99. Cetti, R., Christensen, S-E., and Reuther, K.: Fracture of the Lunate Bone. Hand, 14:80–84, 1982.
100. Chamay, A., and Della Santa, D.: Cinematique du Poignet Rheumatoids Après Resection de la Tête du Culitus: A Propos de 35 Cas. Ann. Chim., 34:711–718,1980.
101. Chapman, D.R., Bennett, J.B., Bryan, W.J., and Tullos, H.S.: Complications of Distal Radial Fractures: Pins and Plaster Treatment. J. Hand Surg., 7:509–512, 1982.
102. Chen, S.C.: The Scaphoid Compression Test. J. Hand Surg., 14B:323–325, 1989.
103. Christodoulou, A.G., and Colton, C.L.: Scaphoid Fractures in Children. J. Pediatr. Orthop., 6:37–39, 1986.
104. Christophe, K.: Rupture of the Extensor Pollicis Longus Tendon Following Colles' Fracture. J. Bone Joint Surg., 35A:1003–1005, 1953.
104a. Chun, S., Wicks, B.P., Meyerdierks, E., Werner, F., and Mosher, J.F. Jr.: Two Modifications for Insertion of the Herbert Screw in the Fractured Scaphoid. J. Hand Surg., 15A:669–671, 1990.
105. Clancy, G.J.: Percutaneous Kirschner Wire Fixation of Colles Fractures. J. Bone Joint Surg., 66A:1008–1014, 1984.
105a. Clay, N.R., Dias, J.J., Costigan, P.S., Gregg, P.J., and Barton, N.J.: Need the Thumb be Immobilized in Scaphoid Fractures. J. Hand Surg., 73B:828–832, 1991.
106. Clyburn, T.A.: Dynamic External Fixation for Comminuted Intra-Articular Fractures of the Distal End of the Radius. J. Bone Joint Surg., 69A:248–254, 1987.
107. Cole, J.M., and Obletz, B.E.: Comminuted Fractures of the Distal End of the Radius Treated by Skeletal Transfixion in Plaster Cast: An End-Result Study of Thirty-Three Cases. J. Bone Joint Surg., 48:931–945, 1966.
108. Coleman, H.M.: Injuries of the Articular Disc at the Wrist. J. Bone Joint Surg., 42B:522–529, 1960.
109. Coll, G.A.: Palmar Dislocation of the Scaphoid and Lunate. J. Hand Surg., 12A:476–480, 1987.
110. Colles, A.: On the Fracture of the Carpal Extremity of the Radius. Edinb. Med. Surg. J., 10:182–186, 1814.
110a. Compson, J.P., and Heatly, F.W.: Imaging the Position of a Screw Within the Scaphoid: A Clinical, Anatomical and Radiological Study. J. Hand Surg., 18B:716–724, 1993.
111. Conyers, D.J.: Scapholunate Intraosseous Reconstruction and Imbrication of the Palmar Carpal Ligaments. J. Hand Surg., 15A:690–700, 1990.
112. Conway, W.F., Gilula, L.A., Manske, P.R., Kriegshauser, L.A., Rholl, K.S., Resnik, C.: Translunate, Palmar Perilunate Fracture–Subluxation of the Wrist. J. Hand Surg., 14A:635–639, 1989.
113. Cooney, W.P.: External Fixation of Distal Radius Fractures. Clin. Orthop., 180A:44–49, 1983.
114. Cooney, W.P., Bussey, R., Dobyns, J.H., and Linscheid, R.L.: Difficult Wrist Fractures: Perilunate Fracture–Dislocations of the Wrist. Clin. Orthop., 214:136–147, 1987.
115. Cooney, W.P., Dobyns, J.H., and Linscheid, R.L.: Complications of Colles' Fractures. J. Bone Joint Surg., 62A:613–619, 1980.
116. Cooney, W.P., Dobyns, J.H., and Linscheid, R.L.: Fractures of the Scaphoid: A Rational Approach to Management. Clin. Orthop., 149:90–97, 1980.
117. Cooney, W.P., Dobyns, J.H., and Linscheid, R.L.: Nonunion of the Scaphoid: Analysis of the Results from Bone Grafting. J. Hand Surg., 5:343–354, 1980.
118. Cooney, W.P., Garcia-Elias, M., Dobyns, J.H., and Linscheid, R.L.: Anatomy and Mechanics of Carpal Instability. Surg. Rounds Orthop., 1:15–24, 1989.
119. Cooney, W.P., Linscheid, R.L., and Dobyns, J.H.: Carpal Instability: Ligament Repair and Reconstruction. *In* Neviaser, R.J. (ed.): Controversies in Hand Surgery, pp. 125–145. New York, Churchill Livingstone, 1990.
120. Cooney, W.P., Linscheid, R.L., and Dobyns, J.H.: External Pin Fixation for Unstable Colles' Fractures. J. Bone Joint Surg., 61A:840–845, 1979.
121. Cooney, W.P., Linscheid, R.L., Dobyns, J.H., and Wood, M.B.: Scaphoid Nonunion: Role of Anterior Interpositional Bone Grafts. J. Hand Surg., 13A:635–650, 1988.
121a. Cooney, W.P.: Evaluation of Chronic Wrist Pain by Arthrography, Arthroscopy and Arthrotomy. J. Hand Surg. 18A:41–66, 1993.
121b. Cooney, W.P., Linscheid, R.L., and Dobyns, J.H.: Triangular Fibrocartilage Tears. J. Hand Surg., 19A:143–154, 1994.
122. Cooney, W.P., Ripperger, R.R., and Linscheid, R.L.: Distal Pole Scaphoid Fractures. Orthop. Trans., 4:18, 1980.
123. Cordrey, L.J., and Ferrer-Torells, M.: Management of Fractures of the Greater Multangular: Report of Five Cases. J. Bone Joint Surg., 42A:1321–1322, 1963.
124. Corfitsen, M., Christensen, S.E., and Cetti, R.: The Anatomical Fat Pad and the Radiological "Scaphoid Fat Stripe." J. Hand Surg., 14B:326–328, 1989.
125. Cox, F.J.: Anterior Dislocation of the Distal Extremity of the Ulna. Surgery, 12:41–45, 1942.
126. Crabbe, W.A.: Excision of the Proximal Row of the Carpus. J. Bone Joint Surg., 46B:708–711, 1964.
127. Crosby, E.B., and Linscheid, R.L.: Rupture of the Flexor Profundus Tendon of the Ring Finger Secondary to Ancient Fracture of the Hook of the Hamate: Review of the Literature and Report of Two Cases. J. Bone Joint Surg., 56A:1076, 1974.
128. Crosby, E.B., Linscheid, R.L., and Dobyns, J.H.: Scaphotrapezial Trapezoidal Arthrosis. J. Hand Surg., 3:223–234, 1978.
129. Curtiss, P.H. Jr.: The Hunchback Carpal Bone. J. Bone Joint Surg., 43A:392–394, 1961.
130. Czitrom, A.A., Dobyns, J.H., and Linscheid, R.L.: Ulnar Variance in Carpal Instability. J. Hand Surg., 12A:205–208, 1987.
131. Czitrom, A.A., and Lister, G.D.: Measurement of Grip Strength in the Diagnosis of Wrist Pain. J. Hand Surg., 13A:16–19, 1988.
132. Dalinka, M.K., Turner, M.L., Osterman, A.L., and Batra, P.: Wrist Arthrography. Radiol. Clin. North Am., 19:217, 1981.
133. Dameron, T.B. Jr.: Traumatic Dislocation of the Distal Radioulnar Joint. Clin. Orthop., 83:55–63, 1972.
134. Darrach, W.: Anterior Dislocation of the Head of the Ulna. Ann. Surg., 56:802–803, 1912.
135. Darrach, W.: Partial Excision of Lower Shaft of Ulna for Deformity Following Colles' Fracture. Ann. Surg., 57:764–765, 1913.
136. Darrow, J.C., Linscheid, R.L., Dobyns, J.H., Mann, J.M., Wood, M.B., and Beckenbaugh, R.D.: Distal Ulnar Recession for Disorders of the Distal Radioulnar Joint. J. Hand Surg., 10A:482–491, 1985.
137. De Beer, J.DeV., and Hudson, D.A.: Fractures of the Triquetrum. J. Hand Surg., 12B:52–53, 1987.
138. Decoulx, P., Duquency, A., and Ammau-Stein, J.: Maladie da Kienboch: Traitment Chirurgical. Lille Chir., 231–250, 1965.
139. Dehne, E., Deffer, P.A., and Feighney, R.E.: Pathomechanics of the Fracture of the Carpal Navicular. J. Trauma, 4:96–113, 1964.
139. de Lange, A., Kauer, J.M.G., and Huiskes, R.: Kinematic Behavior of the Human Wrist Joint: A Roentgen-Stereophotogrammetric Analysis. J. Orthop. Res., 3:56–64, 1985.
140. DeMaagd, R.L., and Engber, W.D.: Retrograde Herbert Screw Fixation for Treatment of Proximal Pole Scaphoid Nonunions. J. Hand Surg., 14A:996–1003, 1989.
141. De Oliveira, J.C.: Barton's Fractures. J. Bone Joint Surg., 55A:586–594, 1973.
142. DePalma, A.F.: Comminuted Fractures of the Distal End of the Radius Treated by Ulnar Pinning. J. Bone Joint Surg., 34A:651–662, 1952.
143. deQuervain, F.: Clinical Surgical Diagnosis for Students and

Practitioners. (Translated by J. Snowman from 4th ed.) New York, William Wood & Co., 1913.
144. Desault, P.J.: A Treatise on Fractures, Luxations and Other Affections of the Bones (Bichat X.] and Caldwell C. [trans.]). Philadelphia, Fry & Kammerer, 1805.
144a. DeSmet, L., Aerts, P., and Fabry, M.S.: Avascular Necrosis of the Scaphoid (Preiser): Report of 3 Cases Treated With Proximal Row Carpectomy. J. Hand Surg., 17A:907-910, 1992.
145. Destot, E.A.J.: Injuries of the Wrist: A Radiological Study (Atkinson, F.R.B. [trans.]). New York, Paul B. Hoeber, 1926.
146. Dias, J.J., Thompson, J., Barton, N.J., and Gregg, P.J.: Suspected Scaphoid Fractures: The Value of Radiographs. J. Bone Joint Surg., 72B:98–101, 1990.
147. Dick, H.M.: Wrist Arthrodesis. *In* Green, D.P. (ed.): Operative Hand Surgery, 2nd ed., vol. 1, pp. 155–166. New York, Churchill Livingstone, 1988.
148. Dingman, P.V.C.: Resection of the Distal End of the Ulna (Darrach Operation): An End-Result Study of Twenty-Four Cases. J. Bone Joint Surg., 34A:893–900, 1952.
149. Dobyns, J.H.: Invited Comment: Ligamentous Reconstruction for Chronic Intercarpal Instability (article by Glickel, S.Z., and Millender, L.H.). J. Hand Surg., 9A:526–527, 1984.
150. Dobyns, J.H., Beckenbaugh, R.D., Bryan, R.S., Cooney, W.P., Linscheid, R.L., and Wood, M.B.: Fractures of the Hand and Wrist. *In* Flynn, J.E. (ed.): Hand Surgery, 3rd ed., pp. 111–180. Baltimore, Williams & Wilkins, 1982.
151. Dobyns, J.H., and Linscheid, R.L.: Complications of Fractures and Dislocations of the Wrist. *In* Epps, C.H. Jr. (ed.): Complications in Orthopaedic Surgery, vol. 1, pp. 271–352. Philadelphia, J.B. Lippincott, 1978.
152. Dobyns, J.H., and Linscheid, R.L.: Fractures and Dislocations of the Wrist. *In* Rockwood, C.A. Jr., and Green, D.P. (eds.): Fractures, pp. 345–440. Philadelphia, J.B. Lippincott, 1975.
153. Dobyns, J.H., Linscheid, R.L., Chao, E.Y.S., Weber, E.R., and Swanson, G.E.: Traumatic Instability of the Wrist. A.A.O.S. Instr. Course Lect., 24:182–199, 1975.
154. Dobyns, J.H., Linscheid, R.L., and Cooney, W.P.: Fractures and Dislocations of the Wrist and Hand, Then and Now. J. Hand Surg., 8:687–691, 1983.
155. Dobyns, J.H., Linscheid, R.L., and Macksoud, W.S.: Proximal Row Instability Nondissociative. Orthop. Trans., 9:574, 1985.
155a. Doffner, R.N., Emmerlung, E.W., and Buterbaugh, G.A.: Proximal and Distal Oblique Radiography of the Wrist: Value in Occult Injuries. J. Hand Surg., 17A:499–503, 1992.
156. Dooley, B.J.: Inlay Bone Grafting for Non-Union of the Scaphoid Bone by the Anterior Approach. J. Bone Joint Surg., 50B:102–109, 1968.
156a. DosReis, F.B., Koeberle, G., Leite, N.M., Katchburian, M.V.: Internal Fixation of Scaphoid Injuries Using the Herbert Screw Through a Dorsal Approach. J. Hand Surg., 18A:792–797, 1993.
157. Dupuytren, B.: On the Injuries and Diseases of Bones (Le Gros Clark, F. ed., trans.]). London, Sydenham Society, 1847.
157a. Duppe, H., Johnell, O., Lundborg, G., Karlsson, M., and Redlund-Johnell, I.: Long Term Results of Fracture of the Scaphoid: A Follow-up Study of More than 30 Years. J. Bone Joint Surg., 76A:249-252, 1994.
158. Dwyer, R.C.: Excision of the Carpal Scaphoid for Ununited Fractures. J. Bone Joint Surg., 31B:572–577, 1949.
159. Eckenrode, J.F., Louis, D.S., and Greene, T.L.: Scaphoid-Trapezium-Trapezoid Fusion in the Treatment of Chronic Scapholunate Instability. J. Hand Surg., 11A:497–502, 1986.
160. Eddeland, A., Eiken, O., Hellgren, E., and Ohlsson, N.M.: Fractures of the Scaphoid. Scand. J. Plast. Reconstr. Surg., 9:234–239, 1975.
161. Egawa, M., and Asai, T.: Fracture of the Hook of the Hamate: Report of Six Cases and the Suitability of Computerized Tomography. J. Hand Surg., 8:393–398, 1983.
162. Ekenstam, F.W.: The Distal Radio Ulnar Joint: An Anatomical, Experimental and Clinical Study With Special Reference to Malunited Fractures of the Distal Radius (thesis). Uppsala Universitet, 1984, pp. 1–55.
163. Ekenstam, F.W., Engkvist, O., and Wadin, K.: Results From Resection of the Distal End of the Ulna After Fractures of the Lower End of the Radius. Scand. J. Plast. Reconstr. Surg., 16:177–181, 1982.
164. Ekenstam, F.W., Jakobsson, O.P., and Wadin, K.: Repair of the Triangular Ligament in Colles' Fracture: No Effect in a Prospective Randomized Study. Acta Orthop. Scand., 60:393–396, 1989.
165. Ekenstam, F.W., Palmer, A.K., and Glisson, R.R.: The Load on the Radius and Ulna in Different Positions of the Wrist and Forearm. Acta Orthop. Scand. 55:363–365, 1984.
166. Ellis, J.: Smith's and Barton's Fractures: A Method of Treatment. J. Bone Joint Surg., 47B:724–727, 1965.
167. Ender, H.G., and Herbert, T.J.: Treatment of Problem Fractures and Nonunions of the Scaphoid. Orthopedics, 12:195–202, 1989.
168. Engdahl, D.E., and Schacherer, T.G.: A New Method of Evaluating Angulation of Scaphoid Nonunions. J. Hand Surg., 14A:1033–1034, 1989.
169. Engel, J., Salai, M., Yaffe, B., and Tadmor, R.: The Role of Three Dimension Computerized Imaging in Hand Surgery. J. Hand Surg., 12B:349–352, 1987.
170. Epner, R.A., and Bowers, W.H.: Ulnar Variance—The Effect of Wrist Positioning and Roentgen Filming Technique. J. Hand Surg., 7:298–305, 1982.
171. Erdman, A.G., Mayfield, J.K., Dorman, F., Wallrich, M., and Dahlof, W.: Kinematic and Kinetic Analysis of the Human Wrist By Steroscopic Instrumentation. J. Biomech. Eng., 101:124–133, 1979.
172. Failla, J.M., and Amadio, P.C.: Recognition and Treatment of Uncommon Carpal Fractures. Hand Clin., 4:469–476, 1988.
173. Faulkner, D.M.: Bipartite Carpal Scaphoid. J. Bone Joint Surg., 10:284–289, 1928.
173a. Feldon, P., Terrano, A.L., and Belsky, M.R.: Wafer Distal Ulna Resection for TFC Tears and/or Ulna Impaction Syndrome. J. Hand Surg., 17A:731–737, 1992.
174. Fenton, R.L.: The Naviculo-Capitate Fracture Syndrome. J. Bone Joint Surg., 38A:681–684, 1956.
175. Ferlic, D.C., and Morin, P.: Idiopathic Avascular Necrosis of the Scaphoid: Preiser's Disease? J. Hand Surg., 14A:13–16, 1989.
176. Fernandes, H.J.A., Koberle, G., Ferreira, G.H.S., and Camargo, J.N. Jr.: Volar Transscaphoid Perilunar Dislocation. Hand 15:276–280, 1983.
177. Fernandez, D.L.: A Technique for Anterior Wedge-Shaped Grafts for Scaphoid Nonunions With Carpal Instability. J. Hand Surg., 9A:733–737, 1984.
178. Fernandez, D.L.: Anterior Bone Grafting and Conventional Lag Screw Fixation to Treat Scaphoid Nonunions. J. Hand Surg., 15A:140–147, 1990.
179. Fernandez, D.L.: Correction of Post-Traumatic Wrist Deformity in Adults by Osteotomy, Bone Grafting, and Internal Fixation. J. Bone Joint Surg., 64A:1164, 1982.
180. Fernandez, D.L., and Ghillani, R.: External Fixation of Complex Carpal Dislocations: A Preliminary Report. J. Hand Surg., 12A:335–347, 1987.
180a. Fernandez, D.L.: Technique and Results of External Fixation of Complex Carpal Injuries. Hand Clin., 9:625–637, 1993.
181. Fick, R.: Handbuch der Anatomie und Mechanik der Gelenke: Unter Berucksichtigung der Bewegenden Muskeln: I. Anatomie der Gelenke: II. Allgemeine Gelenk und Muskelmechanik: III. Spezielle Gelenk und Muskelmechanik. Jena, Gustav Fischer Verlag, 1904–1911.
181a. Finkenberg, J.G., Hotter, E., Kelly, C., Zinar, D.M.: Diagnosis of Occult Scaphoid Fractures by Intrasound Vibration. J. Hand Surg. 18A:4–7, 1993.
182. Fisk, G.R.: Carpal Instability and the Fractured Scaphoid. Ann. R. Coll Surg. Edinb., 46:63–76, 1970.
183. Fisk, G.R.: An Overview of Injuries of the Wrist. Clin. Orthop., 149:137–144, 1980.
184. Fisk, G.R.: The Wrist: Review Article. J. Bone Joint Surg., 66B:396–407, 1984.
185. Fitzgerald, J.P., Peimer, C.A., and Smith, R.J.: Distraction Resection Arthroplasty of the Wrist. J. Hand Surg., 14A:774–781, 1989.
186. Flatt, A.E.: Biomechanics of the Hand and Wrist. *In* Evarts,

C.M. (ed.): Surgery of the Musculoskeletal System, 2nd ed., vol. I, pp. 311–329. New York, Churchill Livingstone, 1990.

187. Ford, D.J., Khoury, G., El-Hadidi, S., Lunn, P.G., and Burke, F.D.: The Herbert Screw for Fractures of the Scaphoid: A Review of Results and Technical Difficulties. J. Bone Joint Surg., 69B:124–127, 1987.
188. Fornage, B.D., Schernberg, R.L., and Rifkin, M.D.: Ultrasound Examination of the Hand. Radiology, 155:785–788, 1985.
189. Foster, R.J., and Hansen, S.T.: Management of Acute Distal Radioulnar Dislocations Associated With Radial Shaft Substance Loss. J. Hand Surg., 10A:72–75, 1985.
190. Foucher, G., and Saffar, P.L.: Revascularization of the Necrosed Lunate, Stages I and II, With a Dorsal Intermetacarpal Arteriovenous Pedicle. J. Chir. Main., 1:259, 1982.
191. Foucher, G., Schuind, F., Merle, M., and Brunelli, F.: Fractures of the Hook of the Hamate. J. Hand Surg., 10B:205–210, 1985.
192. Fourrier, P., Bardy, A., Roche, G., Cisterne, J.P., and Chambon, A.: Approach to a Definition of Mal-Union Callus After Pouteau–Colles Fractures. Int. Orthop. 4:299–305, 1981.
193. Freeland, A.E., and Finley, J.S.: Displaced Dorsal Oblique Fracture of the Hamate Treated With a Cortical Mini Lag Screw. J. Hand Surg., 11A:656–658, 1986.
194. Freeland, A.E., and Finley, J.S.: Displaced Vertical Fracture of the Trapezium Treated With a Small Cancellous Lag Screw. J. Hand Surg., 9A:843–845, 1984.
195. Freeman, B.H., and Hay, E.L.: Nonunion of the Capitate: A Case Report. J. Hand Surg., 10A:187–190, 1985.
196. Frykman, E.: Dislocation of the Triquetrum: Case Report. Scand. J. Plast. Reconstr. Surg., 14:205, 1980.
197. Frykman, E.B., Ekenstam, F., and Wadin, K.: Triscaphoid Arthrodesis and Its Complications. J. Hand Surg., 13A:844–849, 1988.
198. Frykman, G.: Fracture of the Distal Radius Including Sequelae—Shoulder-Hand-Finger Syndrome, Disturbance in the Distal Radio-Ulnar Joint, and Impairment of Nerve Function: A Clinical and Experimental Study. Acta Orthop. Scand., 108(Suppl.):1–153, 1967.
199. Frykman, G.K., Taleisnik, J., Peters, G., et al.: Treatment of Nonunited Scaphoid Fractures by Pulsed Electromagnetic Field and Cast. J. Hand Surg., 11A:344–349, 1986.
200. Frykman, G.K., Tooma, G.S., Boyko, K., and Henderson, R.: Comparison of Eleven External Fixators for Treatment of Unstable Wrist Fractures. J. Hand Surg., 14A:247–254, 1989.
201. Fu, F.H., and Imbriglia, J.F.: An Anatomical Study of the Lunate Bone in Kienböck's Disease. Orthopedics, 8:483–487, 1985.
201a. Futami, T., Aoki, H., Tsukamoto, Y.: Fractures of the Hook of the Hamate in Athletes. Acta Orthop. Scand. 64:469–471, 1993.
202. Ganel, A., Engel, J., Oster, Z., and Farine, I.: Bone Scanning in the Assessment of Fractures of the Scaphoid. J. Hand Surg., 4:541, 1979.
203. Garcia-Elias, M.: Dorsal Fractures of the Triquetrum: Avulsion or Compression Fractures? J. Hand Surg., 12A:266–268, 1987.
204. Garcia-Elias, M., Abanco, J., Salvador, E., and Sanchez, R.: Crush Injury of the Carpus. J. Bone Joint Surg., 67B:286–289, 1985.
205. Garcia-Elias, M., An, K.N., Amadio, P.C., Cooney, W.P., and Linscheid, R.L.: Reliability of Carpal Angle Determinations. J. Hand Surg., 14A:1017–1021, 1989.
206. Garcia-Elias, M., An, K.N., Cooney, W.P., Linscheid, R.L., and Chao, E.Y.S.: Stability of the Transverse Carpal Arch: An Experimental Study. J. Hand Surg., 14A:277–282, 1989.
207. Garcia-Elias, M., An, K.N., Cooney, W.P., Linscheid, R.L., and Chao, E.Y.S.: Transverse Stability of the Carpus: An Analytical Study. J. Orthop. Res., 7:738–743, 1989.
208. Garcia-Elias, M., Cooney, W.P., An, K.N., Linscheid, R.L., and Chao, E.Y.S.: Wrist Kinematics After Limited Intercarpal Arthrodesis. J. Hand Surg., 14A:791–799, 1989.
209. Garcia-Elias, M., Dobyns, J.H., Cooney, W.P., and Linscheid, R.L.: Traumatic Axial Dislocations of the Carpus. J. Hand Surg., 14A :446–457, 1989.
210. Garcia-Elias, M., Vall, A., Salo, J.M., and Lluch, A.L.: Carpal Alignment After Different Surgical Approaches to the Scaphoid: A Comparative Study. J. Hand Surg., 13A:604–612, 1988.
211. Gartland, J.J. Jr., and Werley, C.W.: Evaluation of Healed Colles' Fractures. J. Bone Joint Surg., 33A:895–907, 1951.
212. Gasser, H.: Delayed Union and Pseudarthrosis of the Carpal Navicular: Treatment by Compression-Screw Osteosynthesis: A Preliminary Report of Twenty Fractures. J. Bone Joint Surg., 47A:249–266, 1965.
213. Gelberman, R.H., Bauman, T.D., Menon, J., and Akeson, W.H.: The Vascularity of the Lunate Bone and Kienbock's Disease. J. Hand Surg., 5:272–278, 1980.
214. Gelberman, R.H., and Menon, J.: The Vascularity of the Scaphoid Bone. J. Hand Surg., 5:508–513, 1980.
215. Gelberman, R.H., Salamon, P.B., Jurist, J.M., and Posch, J.L.: Ulnar Variance in Kienböck's Disease. J. Bone Joint Surg., 57A:674–676, 1975.
216. Gelberman, R.H., Taleisnik, J., Panagis, J.S., and Baumgaertner, M.: The Arterial Anatomy of the Human Carpus: I. The Extraosseous Vascularity: II. The Intra-osseous. J. Hand Surg., 8:367–375, 1983.
217. Gellman, H., Caputo, R.J., Carter, V., Aboulafia, A., and McKay, M.: Comparison of Short and Long Thumb-Spica Casts for Non-Displaced Fractures of the Carpal Scaphoid. J. Bone Joint Surg., 71A:354–357, 1989.
218. Gellman, H., Schwartz, S.D., Botte, M.J., and Feiwell, L.: Late Treatment of a Dorsal Transscaphoid, Transtriquetral Perilunate Wrist Dislocation With Avascular Changes of the Lunate. Clin. Orthop., 237:196–203, 1988.
219. Fernandez, D.L., and Geissler, W.B.: Treatment of Displaced Articular Fractures of the Radius. J. Hand Surg. 16A(3):375–384, 1991.
220. Gibson, P.H.: Scaphoid-Trapezium-Trapezoid Dislocation. Hand, 15:267–269, 1983.
221. Gilford, W.W., Bolton, R.H., and Lambrinudi, C.: The Mechanism of the Wrist Joint: With Special Reference to Fractures of the Scaphoid. Guy's Hosp. Rep., 92:52–59, 1943.
222. Gilula, L.A.: Carpal Injuries: Analytic Approach and Case Exercises. A.J.R., 133:503–517, 1979.
223. Gilula, L.A., Destoutet, J.M., Weeks, P.M., Young, L.V., and Wray, R.C.: Roentgenographic Diagnosis of the Painful Wrist. Clin. Orthop., 187:52–64, 1984.
224. Gilula, L.A., Totty, W.G., and Weeks, P.M.: Wrist Arthrography: The Value of Fluoroscopic Spot Viewing. Radiology, 146:555–556, 1983.
225. Glickel, S.Z., and Millender, L.H.: Ligamentous Reconstruction for Chronic Intercarpal Instability. J. Hand Surg., 9A:514–527, 1984.
226. Goldman, S., Lipscomb, P.R., and Taylor, W.F.: Immobilization for Acute Carpal Scaphoid Fractures. Surg. Gynecol. Obstet., 129:281–284, 1969.
227. Goldner, J.L.: Treatment of Carpal Instability Without Joint Fusion—Current Assessment. J. Hand Surg., 7:325–326, 1982.
228. Gomez, W., and Grantham, S.A.: Radial Carpal-Volar Lunate Dislocation: A Case Report. Orthopedics, 11:937–940, 1988.
229. Green, D.P.: Dislocations and Ligamentous Injuries of the Wrist. *In* Surgery of the Musculoskeletal System, 2nd ed., vol. I, pp. 449–515. New York, Churchill Livingstone, 1990.
230. Green, D.P.: Pins and Plaster Treatment of Comminuted Fractures of the Distal End of the Radius. J. Bone Joint Surg., 57A:304, 1975.
231. Green, D.P.: The Effect of Avascular Necrosis on Rüsse Bone Grafting for Scaphoid Nonunion. J. Hand Surg., 10A:597–605, 1985.
232. Green, D.P., and O'Brien, E.T.: Classification and Management of Carpal Dislocations. Clin. Orthop., 149:55–72, 1980.
233. Green, D.P., and O'Brien, E.T.: Open Reduction of Carpal Dislocations: Indications and Operative Techniques. J. Hand Surg., 3:250–265, 1978.
234. Green, J.T., and Gay, F.H.: Colles' Fracture—Residual Disability. Am. J. Surg., 91:636–642, 1956.

235. Greene, M.H., Hadied, A.M., and LaMont, R.L.: Scaphoid Fractures in Children. J. Hand Surg., 9A:536–541, 1984.
236. Guimberteau, J.C., and Panconi, B.: Recalcitrant Non-Union of the Scaphoid Treated With a Vascularized Bone Graft Based on the Ulnar Artery. J. Bone Joint Surg., 72A:88–97, 1990.
237. Gunn, R.S.: Dislocation of the Hamate Bone. J. Hand Surg., 10B:107–108, 1985.
238. Gunther, S.F.: Dorsal Wrist Pain and the Occult Scapholunate Ganglion. J. Hand Surg., 10A:697–703, 1985.
239. Gunther, S.F., and Bruno, P.D.: Divergent Dislocation of the Carpometacarpal Joints: A Case Report. J. Hand Surg., 10A:197–201, 1985.
240. Haddad, R.J., and Riordan, D.C.: Arthrodesis of the Wrist: A Surgical Technique. J. Bone Joint Surg., 49A:950–954, 1967.
241. Hamlin, C.: Traumatic Disruption of the Distal Radioulnar Joint. Am. J. Sports Med., 5:93–96, 1977.
242. Hanel, D.P., and Scheid, D.K.: Irreducible Fracture–Dislocation of the Distal Radioulnar Joint Secondary to Entrapment of the Extensor Carpi Ulnaris Tendon. Clin. Orthop., 234:56–60, 1988.
243. Hankin, F.M., Amadio, P.C., Wojtys, E.M., and Braunstein, E.M.: Carpal Instability With Volar Flexion of the Proximal Row Associated With Injury to the Scaphotrapezial Ligament: Report of Two Cases. J. Hand Surg., 13B:298–302, 1988.
244. Hankin, F.M., White, S.J., Braunstein, E.M., and Louis, D.S.: Dynamic Radiographic Evaluation of Obscure Wrist Pain in the Teenage Patient. J. Hand Surg., 11A:805–811, 1986.
245. Hanks, G.A., Kalenak, A., Bowman, L.S., and Sebastianelli, W.J.: Stress Fractures of the Carpal Scaphoid. J. Bone Joint Surg., 71A:938–941, 1989.
246. Harper, W.M., and Jones, J.M.: Non-Union of Colles' Fracture: Report of Two Cases. Br. J. Hand Surg., 15B:121–123, 1990.
247. Hartz, C.R., and Beckenbaugh, R.D.: Long-Term Results of Resection of the Distal Ulna for Post-Traumatic Conditions. J. Trauma, 19:219–226, 1979.
248. Hastings, D.E., and Silver, R.L.: Intercarpal Arthrodesis in the Management of Chronic Carpal Instability After Trauma. J. Hand Surg., 9A:834–840, 1984.
249. Heim, U., Pfeiffer, K.M., and Meuli, H.C.: Small Fragment Set Manual: Technique Recommended by the ASIF Group (Swiss Association for Study of Internal Fixation). New York, Springer-Verlag, 1974.
250. Heiple, K.G., Freehafer, A.A., and Van't Hof, A.: Isolate Traumatic Dislocation of the Distal End of the Ulnar or Distal Radioulnar Joint. J. Bone Joint Surg., 44A:1287–1394, 1962.
251. Herbert, T.J.: Internal Fixation of the Carpus With the Herbert Bone Screw System. J. Hand Surg., 14A:397–400, 1989.
252. Herbert, T.J.: Scaphoid Fractures and Carpal Instability. Proc. R. Soc. Med., 67:1080, 1974.
253. Herbert, T.J., and Fisher, W.E.: Management of the Fractured Scaphoid Using a New Bone Screw. J. Bone Joint Surg., 66B:114–123, 1984.
253a. Herbert, T.J., Fisher, W.E., and Leicester, A.N.: The Herbert Bone Screw: A Ten Year Perspective Study. J. Hand Surg., 17B:409–419, 1992.
253b. Hertzberg, G., Comtet, J.T., Linscheid, R.L., Amadio, P.C., and Cooney, W.P.: Perilunate Dislocations and Fracture Dislocations: A Multicenter Study. J. Hand Surg., 18A:768–779, 1993.
254. Holdsworth, B.J., and Shackleford, I.: Fracture Dislocation of the Trapezio-Scaphoid Joint—The Missing Link? J. Hand Surg., 12B:40–42, 1987.
255. Hori, Y., Tamai, S., Okuda, H., Sakamoto, H., Takita, T., and Masuhara, K.: Blood Vessel Transplantation to Bone. J. Hand Surg., 4:23–33, 1979.
256. Horii, E., Garcia-Elias, M., An, K.N., et al.: Effect on Force Transmission Across the Carpus in Procedures Used to Treat Kienböck's Disease. J. Hand Surg., 15A:393–400, 1990.
256a. Horii, E., Nakamura, R., Watanabe, K., and Tsunoda, K.: Scaphoid Fracture as an "Puncher's Fracture." J. Orthop. Trauma, 8:107–110, 1994.
256b. Hove, L.M.: Simultaneous Scaphoid and Distal Radius Fractures. J. Hand Surg., 19B:384–388, 1994.
257. Howard, F.M.: Ulnar-Nerve Palsy in Wrist Fractures: Fracture of the Hamate Bone. J. Bone Joint Surg., 43A:1197–1201, 1961.
258. Howard, F.M., Fahey, T., and Wojcik, E.: Rotatory Subluxation of the Navicular. Clin. Orthop., 104:134–139, 1974.
258a. Huene, D.R., and Huene, D.S.: Treatment of Nonunions of the Scaphoid With the Enders Compression Blade Plate System. J. Hand Surg., 16A:913–922, 1991.
259. Hui, F.C., and Linscheid, R.L.: Ulnotriquetral Augmentation Tenodesis: A Reconstructive Procedure for Dorsal Subluxation of the Distal Radioulnar Joint. J. Hand Surg., 7:230–236, 1982.
260. Hultén, O.: Uber Anatomische Variationen der Handgelenkknochen: Ein Beitrag zur Kenntnis der Genese zwei verschiedener Mondbeinveranderungen. Acta Radiol., 9:155–168, 1928.
261. Hyman, G., and Martin, F.R.R.: Dislocation of the Inferior Radio-Ulnar Joint as a Complication of Fracture of the Radius. Br. J. Surg., 27:481–491, 1940.
261a. Imaeda, T., Nakamura, R., Miura, T., and Makino, N.: Magnetic Resonance Imaging in Scaphoid Fracture. J. Hand Surg., 17B:20–27, 1992.
262. Imbriglia, J.E., Broudy, A.S., Hagberg, W.C., and McKernan, D.: Proximal Row Carpectomy: Clinical Evaluation. J. Hand Surg., 15A:426–430, 1990.
262a. Inoue, G., Tanaka, T., and Nakamura, R.: Treatment of Transscaphoid Perilunate Dislocations by Internal Fixation With the Herbert Screw. J. Hand Surg., 15B:449–454, 1990.
263. Iwegbu, C.G., and Helal, B.: An Unusual Combination of Fractures at the Wrist. Hand, 12:173–175, 1980.
264. Jackson, W.T., and Protas, J.M.: Snapping Scapholunate Subluxation. J. Hand Surg., 6:590–594, 1981.
265. Jakob, R.P., and Fernandez, D.L.: The Treatment of Wrist Fractures With the Small AO External Fixation Device. *In* Uhthoff, H.K. (ed.): Current Concepts of External Fixation of Fractures, pp. 307–314. Berlin, Springer-Verlag, 1982.
266. James, E.T.R., and Burke, F.D.: Vibration Disease of the Capitate. J. Hand Surg., 9B:169–170, 1984.
267. Jasmine, M.S., Packer, J.W., and Edwards, G.S.: Irreducible Transscaphoid Perilunate Dislocation. J. Hand Surg., 13A:212–215, 1988.
268. Jeanne, L.A., and Mouchet, A.: Les Lesions Traumatiques Fermées du Poignet, pp. 149–165. 28th Congrès Français de Chirurgie, 1919.
269. Jenkins, N.H., Jones, D.G., Johnson, S.R., and Mintowt-Czyz, W.J.: External Fixation of Colles' Fractures: An Anatomical Study. J. Bone Joint Surg., 69B:207–211, 1987.
270. Jenkins, N.H., and Mintowt-Czyz, W.J.: Mal-Union and Dysfunction in Colles' Fracture. J. Hand Surg., 13B:291–293, 1988.
271. Jensen, B.V., and Christensen, C.: An Unusual Combination of Simultaneous Fracture of the Tuberosity of the Trapezium and the Hook of the Hamate. J. Hand Surg., 15A:285–287, 1990.
272. Johnson, R.P.: The Acutely Injured Wrist and Its Residuals. Clin. Orthop., 149:33, 1980.
273. Johnson, R.P., and Carrera, G.F.: Chronic Capitolunate Instability. J. Bone Joint Surg., 68A:1164–1176, 1986.
273a. Jones, R.S., and Kutty, S.: Intra-Articular Fractures of the Hamate. Injury, 24:272–273, 1993.
274. Jones, W.A.: Beware of the Sprained Wrist: The Incidence and Diagnosis of Scapholunate Instability. J. Bone Joint Surg., 70B:293–297, 1988.
275. Jones, W.A., and Ghorbal, M.S.: Fractures of the Trapezium: A Report on Three Cases. J. Hand Surg., 10B:227–230, 1985.
276. Jonsson, G.: Aseptic Bone Necrosis of the Os Capitatum. Acta Radiol., 23:562, 1942.
276a. Jonsson, K., Jonsson, A., Sloth, M., Kopglov, P., and Wingstrand, H.: Computed Tomography of the Wrist in Suspected Scaphoid Fracture. Acta Radiol., 33:500–501, 1992.
277. Jorgensen, E.C.: Proximal-row Carpectomy: An End-Result Study of Twenty-two Cases. J. Bone Joint Surg., 51:1104–1111, 1969.
278. Joseph, R.B., Linscheid, R.L., Dobyns, J.H., and Bryan, R.S.:

Chronic Sprains of the Carpometacarpal Joints. J. Hand Surg., 6:172–180, 1981.

278a. Jupiter, J., Rudor, J., and Roth, D.A.: Computer Generated Bone Models in the Planning of Osteotomy of Multidirectional Distal Radius Malunion. J. Hand Surg., 17A:406–415, 1992.

279. Kapandji, A.: Intra-Focal Pinning of Fractures of the Lower Extremity of the Radius: Ten Years After (in French). Ann. Chir. Main Memb. Super., 6:57–63, 1987.

280. Kapandji, I.A.: The Inferior Radioulnar Joint and Pronosupination. *In* Tubiana, R. (ed.): The Hand, pp. 121–129. Philadelphia, W.B. Saunders, 1981.

281. Kapandji, I.A.: Biomécanique du Carpe et du Poignet. Ann. Chir. Main Memb. Super., 6:147–169, 1987.

281a. Kaulesar-Sukal, D.M.K.S., and Johannes, E.J.: Transscaphotranscapitate Fracture Dislocations of the Carpus. J. Hand Surg., 17A:348–353, 1992.

282. Kauer, J.M.G.: Functional Anatomy of the Wrist. Clin. Orthop., 149:9–20, 1980.

283. Kauer, J.M.G.: The Articular Disc of the Hand. Acta Anat. 93:590–605, 1975.

284. Kauer, J.M.G.: The Mechanism of the Carpal Joint. Clin. Orthop., 202:16–26, 1986.

285. Kawai, H., Yamamoto, K., Yamamoto, T., Tadi, K., and Kaga, K.: Excision of the Lunate in Kienböck's Disease: Results After Long-Term Follow-Up. J. Bone Joint Surg., 70B:287–292, 1988.

286. Kessler, I., and Silberman, Z.: An Experimental Study of the Radiocarpal Joint by Arthrography. Surg. Gynecol. Obstet., 112:33–40, 1961.

287. Kienböck, R.: Uber Tramatische Malazie des Mondbeins und ihre Folgezustände: Entartungsformen und Kompressionsfrakturen. Fortschr. Geb. Roentgenstr. Nuklearmed. Erganzungsband, 16:78–103, 1910–1911.

288. Kimmel, R.B., and O'Brien, E.T.: Surgical Treatment of Avascular Necrosis of the Proximal Pole of the Capitate: Case Report. J. Hand Surg., 7:284, 1982.

289. King, G.J., McMurtry, R.Y., Rubenstein, J.D., and Ogston, N.G.: Computerized Tomography of the Distal Radioulnar Joint: Correlation With Ligamentous Pathology in a Cadaveric Model. J. Hand Surg., 11A:711–717, 1986.

290. King, G.J., McMurtry, R.Y., Rubenstein, J.D., and Gertzbein, S.D.: Kinematics of the Distal Radioulnar Joint. J. Hand Surg., 11A:798–804, 1986.

291. Kinnard, P., Tricoire, J.L., and Basora, J.: Radial Shortening for Kienböck's Disease. Can. J. Surg., 3:261–262, 1983.

292. Kleinert, H.E.: Post-traumatic Sympathetic Dystrophy. Orthop. Clin. North Am., 4:917, 1973.

293. Kleinert, J.M., Stern, P.J., Lister, G.D., and Kleinhans, R.J.: Complications of Scaphoid Silicone Arthroplasty. J. Bone Joint Surg., 67A:422–427, 1985.

294. Kleinman, W.B.: Long-Term Study of Chronic Scapho-Lunate Instability Treated by Scapho-Trapezio-Trapezoid Arthrodesis. J. Hand Surg., 14A:429–445, 1989.

295. Kleinman, W.B.: Management of Chronic Rotary Subluxation of the Scaphoid by Scapho-Trapezio-Trapezoid Arthrodesis: Rationale for the Technique, Postoperative Changes in Biomechanics, and Results. Hand Clin., 3:113–133, 1987.

296. Kleinman, W.B., Steichen, J.B., and Strickland, J.W.: Management of Chronic Rotary Subluxation of the Scaphoid by Scapho-Trapezio-Trapezoid Arthrodesis. J. Hand Surg., 7:125–136, 1982.

297. Knapp, M.E.: Treatment of Some Complications of Colles' Fracture. J.A.M.A., 148:825–827, 1952.

297a. Kline, S.C., and Holder, L.E.: Segmental Reflex Sympathetic Dystrophy: Clinical and Scintigraphic Criteria. J. Hand Surg., 18A:853–859, 1993.

298. Knirk, J.L., and Jupiter, J.B.: Intra-Articular Fractures of the Distal End of the Radius in Young Adults. J. Bone Joint Surg., 68A:647–659, 1986.

299. Köhler, A., and Zimmer, E.A.: Borderlands of the Normal and Early Pathologic in Skeletal Rotengenology (3rd. American ed., based on 11th German ed.). New York, Grune & Stratton, 1968.

300. Kongsholm, J., and Olerud, C.: Plaster Cast Versus External Fixation for Unstable Intraarticular Colles' Fractures. Clin. Orthop., 241:57–65, 1989.

301. Korkala, O.L., and Antti-Poika, I.U.: Late Treatment of Scaphoid Fractures by Bone Grafting and Compression Staple Osteosynthesis. J. Hand Surg., 14A:491–495, 1989.

301a. Korkala, O.L., Kuokkanen, H.O., Eerola, M.S.: Compression-Staple Fixation for Fractures, Non-unions, and Delayed Unions of the Carpal Scaphoid. J. Bone Joint Surg., 74A:423–426, 1992.

302. Kristensen, S.S., Thomassen, E., and Christensen, F.: Ulnar Variance in Kienböck's Disease. J. Hand Surg., 11B:258–260, 1986.

303. Kristiansen, A., and Gjersoe, E.: Colles' Fracture: Operative Treatment, Indications and Results. Acta Orthop. Scand., 39:33–46, 1968.

304. Kuenz, C.L.: Les Geodes du Semi-Lunaire (Thesis). Lyon, 1923.

305. Kuhlmann, J.N., Fournol, S., Mimoun, M., and Baux, S.: Fracture of the Lesser Multangular (Trapezoid) Bone. Ann. Chir. Main Memb. Super., 5:133–134, 1986.

306. Kuhlmann, J.N., Mimoun, M., Boabighi, A., and Baux, S.: Vascularized Bone Graft Pedicled on the Volar Carpal Artery for Non-Union of the Scaphoid. J. Hand Surg., 12B:203–210, 1987.

307. Kuhlmann, N., Gallaire, M., and Pineau, H.: Déplacements du Scaphoide et du Semi-lunaire au Cours des Mouvements du Poignet. Ann. Chir., 32:543–553, 1978.

308. Lambrinudi, C.: Injuries to the Wrist. Guy's Hosp. Gazette, 52:107, 1938.

309. Landsmeer, J.M.F.: Studies in the Anatomy of Articulation: I. The Equilibrium of the "Intercalated" Bone. Acta Morphol. Neerl. Scand., 3:287–303, 1961.

309a. Lane, L.: The Scaphoid Shift Test. J. Hand Surg., 18A:366–368, 1993.

310. Lange, R.H., Engber, W.D., and Clancy, W.G.: Expanding Applications for the Herbert Scaphoid Screw. Orthopedics, 9:1393–1397, 1986.

311. Larson, B., Light, T.R., and Ogden, J.A.: Fracture and Ischemic Necrosis of the Immature Scaphoid. J. Hand Surg., 12:122–127, 1987.

311b. Larsen, C.F., Mathiesen, F.K., and Lindequist, S.: Measurement of Carpal Bone Angles on Lateral Wrist Radiographs. J. Hand Surg., 16A:888–893, 1991.

311c. Lavernea, C.J., Cohen, M.S., and Taleisnik, J.: Treatment of Scapholunate Dissociation by Ligamentous Repair and Capsulodesis. J. Hand Surg., 17A:354–539, 1992.

312. Lee, M.L.H.: The Intraosseous Arterial Pattern of the Carpal Lunate Bone and Its Relation to Avascular Necrosis. Acta Orthop. Scand., 33:43–55, 1963.

313. Lentino, W., Lubetsky, H.W., Jacobson, H.G., and Poppel, M.H.: The Carpal Bridge View: A Position for the Roentgenographic Diagnosis of Abnormalities in the Dorsum of the Wrist. J. Bone Joint Surg., 39A:88–90, 1957.

314. Leung, K.S., Shen, W.Y., Tsang, K.H., Chiu, K.H., Leung, P.C., and Hung, L.K.: An Effective Treatment of Comminuted Fractures of the Distal Radius. J. Hand Surg., 15A:11–17, 1990.

315. Levinsohn, E.M., and Palmer, A.K.: Arthrography of the Traumatized Wrist. Radiology, 146:647–651, 1983.

316. Levy, M., Fischel, R.E., Stern, G.M., and Goldberg, I.: Chip Fractures of the Os Triquetrum: The Mechanism of Injury. J. Bone Joint Surg., 61B:355–357, 1979.

317. Lewis, O.J.: The Hominoid Wrist Joint. Am. J. Phys. Anthropol., 30:251–267, 1969.

318. Lewis, O.J., Hamshere, R.J., and Bucknill, T.M.: The Anatomy of the Wrist Joint. J. Anat., 106:539–552, 1970.

319. Lichtman, D.M., Alexander, A.H., Mack, G.R., and Gunther, S.F.: Kienböck's Disease—Update on Silicone Replacement Arthroplasty. J. Hand Surg., 7:343–347, 1982.

320. Lichtman, D.M., Noble, W.H., and Alexander, C.E.: Dynamic Triquetrolunate Instability: Case Report. J. Hand Surg., 9A:185–188, 1984.

321. Lidstrom, A.: Fractures of the Distal End of the Radius: A

Clinical and Statistical Study of End Results. Acta Orthop. Scand., 41(Suppl.):1–118, 1959.
322. Lindström, G., and Nyström, A.: Incidence of Post-traumatic Arthrosis After Primary Healing of Scaphoid Fractures: A Clinical and Radiological Study. J. Hand Surg., 15B:11–13, 1990.
323. Linscheid, R.L.: Kinematic Considerations of the Wrist. Clin. Orthop., 202:27–39, 1986.
324. Linscheid, R.L., and Dobyns, J.H.: Les Types d'Instabilité Anterieure du Carpe. *In* Razemon, J.-P., and Fisk, G.-R. (eds.): Le Poignet; Monographies du Groupe d'Etude de la Main, pp. 142–146. Paris, Expansion Scientifique Française, 1983.
325. Linscheid, R.L., and Dobyns, J.H.: Physical Examination of the Wrist. *In* Post, M. (ed.): Physical Examination of the Musculoskeletal System, pp. 80–94. Chicago, Year Book Medical Publishers, 1987.
326. Linscheid, R.L., and Dobyns, J.H.: Radiolunate Arthrodesis. J. Hand Surg., 10A:821–829, 1985.
327. Linscheid, R.L., and Dobyns, J.H.: The Unified Concept of Carpal Injuries. Ann. Chir. Main Memb. Super., 3:35–42, 1984.
328. Linscheid, R.L., and Dobyns, J.H.: Wrist Sprains. *In* Tubiana, R. (ed.): The Hand, vol. 2, pp. 970–985. Philadelphia, W.B. Saunders, 1985.
329. Linscheid, R.L., Dobyns, J.H., Beabout, J.W., and Bryan, R.S.: Traumatic Instability of the Wrist: Diagnosis, Classification and Pathomechanics. J. Bone Joint Surg., 54A:1612–1632, 1972.
330. Linscheid, R.L., Dobyns, J.H., Beckenbaugh, R.D., Cooney, W.P., and Wood, M.B.: Instability Patterns of the Wrist. J. Hand Surg., 8:682–686, 1983.
331. Linscheid, R.L., Dobyns, J.H., and Cooney, W.P.: Volar Wedge Grafting of the Carpal Scaphoid: Non-Union Associated With Dorsal Instability Patterns. Orthop. Trans., 6:464, 1982.
332. Linscheid, R.L., Dobyns, J.H., and Younge, D.K.: Trispiral Tomography in the Evaluation of Wrist Injury. Bull. Hosp. Jt. Dis. Orthop. Inst., 44:297–308, 1984.
332a. Linscheid, R.L., and Dobyns, J.H.: Treatment of Scapholunate Dissociation: Rotatory Subluxation of the Scaphoid. Hand Clin., 8:645–652, 1992.
333. Logan, S.E., Nowak, M.D., Gould, P.L., and Weeks, P.M.: Biomechanical Behavior of the Scapholunate Ligament. Biomed. Sci. Instrum., 22:81–85, 1986.
334. Loth, T.S., and McMillan, M.D.: Coronal Dorsal Hamate Fractures. J. Hand Surg., 13A:616–18, 1988.
335. Louis, D.S., Hankin, F.M., Greene, T.L., Braunstein, E.M., and White, S.J.: Central Carpal Instability: Capitate Lunate Instability Pattern: Diagnosis by Dynamic Displacement. Orthopedics, 7:1693–1696, 1984.
336. Louis, D.S.: Barton's and Smith's Fractures. Hand Clin., 4:399–402, 1988.
337. Lowrey, D.G., Moss, S.H., and Wolff, T.W.: Volar Dislocation of the Capitate: Report of a Case. J. Bone Joint Surg., 66:611–613, 1984.
338. Lowry, W.E., and Cord, S.A.: Traumatic Avascular Necrosis of the Capitate Bone: Case Report. J. Hand Surg., 6:254, 1981.
339. Lugnegard, H.: Resection of the Head of the Ulna in Posttraumatic Dysfunction of the Distal Radio-Ulnar Joint. Scand. J. Plast. Reconstr. Surg., 3:65–69, 1969.
340. Lynch, A.C., and Lipscomb, P.R.: The Carpal Tunnel Syndrome and Colles' Fractures. J.A.M.A., 185:363, 1963.
341. MacConaill, M.A.: The Mechanical Anatomy of the Carpus and Its Bearings on Some Surgical Problems. J. Anat., 75:166–175, 1941.
342. Mack, G.R., Bosse, M.J., Gelberman, R.H., and Yu, E.: The Natural History of Scaphoid Non-Union. J. Bone Joint Surg., 66A:504–509, 1984.
343. Macksoud, W.S., Dobyns, J.H., and Linscheid, R.L.: Nondissociative Collapse of the Proximal Carpal Row. Presented at 98th Annual Meeting of the American Orthopaedic Association, Coronado, CA, June 10–13, 1985.
344. Malgaigne, J.F.: A Treatise on Fractures (Packard, J.H. [trans.]). Philadelphia, J.B. Lippincott, 1859.
345. Manaster, B.J., Mann, R.J., and Rubenstein, S.: Wrist Pain: Correlation of Clinical and Plain Film Findings With Arthrographic Results. J. Hand Surg., 14A:466–473, 1989.
346. Manske, P.R., McCarthy, J.A., and Strecker, W.B.: Use of the Herbert Bone Screw for Scaphoid Nonunions. Orthopedics, 11:1653–1661, 1988.
347. Marck, K.W., and Klasen, H.J.: Fracture–Dislocation of the Hamatometacarpal Joint: A Case Report. J. Hand Surg., 11A:128–130, 1986.
348. Marsh, A.P., and Lampros, P.J.: The Naviculocapitate Fracture Syndrome. A.J.R., 82:255–256, 1959.
349. Masquelet, A.C.: Clinical Examination of the Wrist. Ann. Chir. Main Memb. Super., 8:159–175, 1989.
350. Mathoulin, C., Saffar, P., and Roukoz, S.: Luno-Triquetral Instabilities. Ann. Chir. Main Memb. Super., 9:22–28, 1990.
351. Matti, H.: Uber die Behandlung der Navicularefrakture und der Refractura Patellae durch Plombierung mit Spongiosa. Zentrabl. Chir., 64:2353–2359, 1937.
352. Matthews, L.S.: Acute Volar Compartment Syndrome, Secondary to Distal Radius Fracture in Athlete. Am. J. Sports Med., 11:6–7, 1983.
353. Maudsley, R.H., and Chen, S.C.: Screw Fixation in the Management of the Fractured Carpal Scaphoid. J. Bone Joint Surg., 54B:432–441, 1972.
354. Mayfield, J.K.: Mechanism of Carpal Injuries. Clin. Orthop., 149:45–54, 1980.
355. Mayfield, J.K., Johnson, R.P., and Kilcoyne, R.K.: Carpal Dislocations: Pathomechanics and Progressive Perilunar Instability. J. Hand Surg., 5:226–241, 1980.
356. Mayfield, J.K., Johnson, R.P., and Kilcoyne, R.K.: Carpal Injuries: An Experimental Approach: Anatomy, Kinematics and Perilunate Injuries. J. Bone Joint Surg., 57A:725, 1975.
357. Mayfield, J.K., Johnson, R.P., and Kilcoyne, R.F.: The Ligaments of the Human Wrist and Their Functional Significance. Anat. Rec., 186:417–428, 1976.
358. Mazet, R. Jr., and Hohl, M.: Fractures of the Carpal Navicular: Analysis of Ninety-One Cases and Review of the Literature. J. Bone Joint Surg., 45A:82–112, 1963.
359. McClain, E.J., and Boyes, J.H.: Missed Fractures of the Greater Multangular. J. Bone Joint Surg., 48A:1525–1528, 1966.
360. McMurtry, R.Y., Axelrod, T., and Paley, D.: Distal Radial Osteotomy. Orthopedics, 12:149–155, 1989.
361. McMurtry, R.Y., Youm, Y., Flatt, A.E., and Gillespie, T.E.: Kinematics of the Wrist: II. Clinical Applications. J. Bone Joint Surg., 60A:955–961, 1978.
362. Melone, C.P. Jr.: Open Treatment for Displaced Articular Fractures of the Distal Radius. Clin. Orthop., 202:103–111, 1986.
363. Menon, J., Wood, V.E., Schoene, H.R., Frykman, G.K., Hohl, J.C., and Bestard, E.A.: Isolated Tears of the Triangular Fibrocartilage of the Wrist: Results of Partial Excision. J. Hand Surg., 9A:527–530, 1984.
364. Mestdagh, H.: The Blood Supply of the Lunate. Ann. Chir. Main Memb. Super., 1:246–248, 1982.
365. Meyn, M.A. Jr., and Roth, A.M.: Isolated Dislocation of the Trapezoid Bone. J. Hand Surg., 5:602–604, 1980.
366. Meyerdierks, E.M., Mosher, J.F., and Werner, F.W.: Limited Wrist Arthrodesis: A Laboratory Study. J. Hand Surg., 12A:526–529, 1987.
367. Meyrueis, J.P., Schernberg, F., and Gerard, Y.: Radiological Investigation of Instability of the Wrist. *In* Tubiana, R. (ed.): The Hand, vol. 2, pp. 621–634. Philadelphia, W.B. Saunders, 1985.
368. Michon, J.: Kienböck's Disease and Complications of Injuries to the Lunate Bone. *In* Tubiana, R. (ed.): The Hand, vol. 2, pp. 1106–1116. Philadelphia, W.B. Saunders, 1985.
368a. Missakian, M., Cooney, W.P, Amadio, P.C., and Glidewell, H.: Open Reduction and Internal Fixation for Distal Radius Fractures. J. Hand Surg., 17A:745–755, 1992.
369. Mikic, Z.D.: Age Changes in the Triangular Fibrocartilage of the Wrist Joint. J. Anat., 126:367–384, 1978.
370. Mikic, Z.D.: Detailed Anatomy of the Articular Disc of the Distal Radioulnar Joint. Clin. Orthop., 245:123–132, 1989.

371. Mikic, Z.D.: Galeazzi Fracture–Dislocations. J. Bone Joint Surg., 57A:1071, 1975.
372. Milch, H.: Cuff Resection of the Ulna for Malunited Colles' Fracture. J. Bone Joint Surg., 23:311–313, 1941.
373. Milch, H.: Fracture of the Hamate Bone. J. Bone Joint Surg., 16:459–462, 1934.
373a. Milankov, M., Somer, T., Jovanovic, A., and Brankov, M.: Isolated Dislocation of Carpal Scaphoid. J. Trauma, 36:752–754, 1994.
374. Minami, A., Ogino, T., Ohshio, I., and Minami, M.: Correlation Between Clinical Results and Carpal Instabilities in Patients After Reduction of Lunate and Perilunar Dislocations. J. Hand Surg., 11B:213–220, 1986.
375. Minami, M., Yamazaki, J., Chisaka, N., Kato, S., Ogino, T., and Minami, A.: Nonunion of the Capitate. J. Hand Surg., 12A:1089–1091, 1987.
376. Minami, M., Yamazaki, J., and Ishii, S.: Isolated Dislocation of the Pisiform: A Case Report and Review of the Literature. J. Hand Surg., 9A:125–127, 1984.
377. Mino, D.E., Palmer, A.K., and Levinsohn, E.M.: The Role of Radiography and Computerized Tomography in the Diagnosis of Subluxation and Dislocation of the Distal Radioulnar Joint. J. Hand Surg., 8:23–31, 1983.
377a. Mintzer, C., and Waters, P.M.: Acute Open Reduction of a Displaced Scaphoid Fracture in a Child. J. Hand Surg. 19A:760–761, 1994.
378. Mirabello, S.C., Rosenthal, D.I., and Smith, R.J.: Correlation of Clinical and Radiographic Findings in Kienböck's Disease. J. Hand Surg., 12A:1049–1054, 1987.
379. Mitchell, S.W.: Injuries of Nerves and Their Consequences. Philadelphia, J.B. Lippincott, 1872.
380. Miyaji, N.: Treatment of Lunatomalacia With Vascular Bundle Transplantation (in Japanese). Seikei Geka (Orthopedic Surgery) 31:1591–1594, 1980.
381. Mizuseki, T., Ikuta, Y., Murakami, T., and Watari, S.: Lateral Approach to the Hook of Hamate for Its Fracture. J. Hand Surg., 11B:109–111, 1986.
382. Moberg, E.: Shoulder-Hand-Finger Syndrome, Reflex Dystrophy, Causalgia. Acta Chir. Scand., 125:523–524, 1963.
383. Moberg, E.: Treatment of Kienböck's Disease by Surgical Correction of the Length of the Radius or Ulna. *In* Tubiana, R. (ed.): The Hand, vol. 2, pp. 117–1120. Philadelphia, W.B. Saunders, 1985.
384. Mogan, J.V., Newberg, A.H., and David, P.H.: Intraosseous Ganglion of the Lunate. J. Hand Surg., 6:61–63, 1981.
384a. Mody, B.S., Belliappa, P.P., Dias, J.J., and Barton, N.J.: Nonunion of Fractures of the Scaphoid Tuberosity. J. Bone Joint Surg. 75B:423–425, 1993.
385. Monahan, P.R.W., and Galasko, C.S.B.: The Scapho-Capitate Fracture Syndrome: A Mechanism of Injury. J. Bone Joint Surg., 54B:122–124, 1972.
386. Moneim, M.S.: The Tangential Posteroanterior Radiograph to Demonstrate Scapholunate Dissociation. J. Bone Joint Surg., 63A:1324–1326, 1981.
387. Moneim, M.S., Hofammann, K.E., and Omer, C.E.: Transscaphoid Perilunate Fracture–Dislocation: Result of Open Reduction and Pin Fixation. Clin. Orthop., 190:227, 1984.
388. Monsivais, J.J., Nitz, P.A., and Scully, T.J.: The Role of Carpal Instability in Scaphoid Nonunion: Casual or Causal? J. Hand Surg., 11B:201–206, 1986.
389. Moran, R., and Curtin, J.: Scaphoid Fractures Treated by Herbert Screw Fixation. J. Hand Surg., 13B:453–455, 1988.
390. Mori, T., et al: Revitalization of the Osteonecrotic Lunate Bone by Vascular Bundle Transplantation (in Japanese). Seikei Geka (Orthopedic Surgery), 28:1556–1560, 1977.
391. Morrissy, R.T., and Nalebuff, E.A.: Dislocation of the Distal Radioulnar Joint: Anatomy and Clues to Prompt Diagnosis. Clin. Orthop., 144:154–158, 1979.
392. Mortier, J.P., Baux, S., Uhl, J.F., Mimoun, M., and Mole, B.: The Importance of the Posteromedial Fragment and Its Specific Pinning in Fractures of the Distal Radius. Ann. Chir. Main Memb. Super., 2:219–229, 1983.
393. Mouchet, A.: Fractures Isolées du Scaphoide Carpien. Presse Med., 6:122, 1934.
394. Moutet, F., Chapel, A., Cinquin, P., Rose-Pitet, L.: Three-Dimensional Imaging of the Carpus. Ann. Chir. Main Memb. Super., 9:32–37, 1990.
395. Mulder, J.D.: The Results of 100 Cases of Pseudarthrosis in the Scaphoid Bone Treated by the Matti–Rüsse Operation. J. Bone Joint Surg., 50B:110–115, 1968.
396. Mullan, G.B., and Lloyd, G.J.: Complete Carpal Disruption of the Hand. Hand, 12:39–43, 1980.
397. Müller, M.E., Algöwer, M., Schneider, R., and Willengger, H.: Manual of Internal Fixation, 2nd ed. Berlin, Springer-Verlag, 1979.
398. Murakami, Y.: Dislocation of the Carpal Scaphoid. Hand, 9:79–81, 1977.
399. Murakami, Y., and Todani, K.: Traumatic Entrapment of the Extensor Pollicis Longus Tendon in Smith's Fracture of the Radius: Case Report. J. Hand Surg., 6:238–240, 1981.
400. Murray, G.: End Results of Bone-Grafting for Non-Union of the Carpal Navicular. J. Bone Joint Surg., 28:749–755, 1946.
401. Nakamura, R., Hori, M., Horii, E., and Miura, T.: Reduction of the Scaphoid Fracture With DISI Alignment. J. Hand Surg., 12A:1000–1005, 1987.
402. Nakamura, R., Hori, M., Imamura, T., Horii, E., and Miura, T.: Method for Measurement and Evaluation of Carpal Bone Angles. J. Hand Surg., 14A:412–416, 1989.
403. Nakamura, R., Horii, E., Tanaka, Y., Imaeda, T., and Hayakawa, N.: Three Dimensional CT Imaging for Wrist Disorders. J. Hand Surg., 14B:53–58, 1989.
404. Nakamura, R., Imaeda, T., and Miura, T.: Radial Shortening for Kienböck's Disease: Factors Affecting the Operative Result. J. Hand Surg., 15B:40–45, 1990.
405. Nakata, R.Y., Chand, Y., Matiko, J.D., Frykman, G.K., and Wood, V.E.: External Fixators for Wrist Fractures: A Biomechanical and Clinical Study. J. Hand Surg., 10A:845–851, 1985.
405a. Nakamura, R., Horri, E., Watanabe, K., Tsunoda, K., Miura, T.: Scaphoid Nonunion: Factors Affecting the Functional Outcome of Open Reduction and Wedge Grafting With Herbert Screw Fixation. J. Hand Surg., 18B:219–224, 1993.
405b. Nakamura, R., Imaeda, T., Horii, E., Miura, T., and Hayakawan, N.: Analyses of Scaphoid Fracture Displacement by 3-D Computed Tomography. J. Hand Surg., 16A:485–492, 1991.
405c. Nakamura, R., Tsuge, S., and Watanabe, K.: Radial Wedge Osteotomy for Kienböck's Disease. J. Bone Joint Surg., 73A:1391–1396, 1991.
406. Nathan, P.A., and Meadows, K.D.: Ulna-Minus Variance and Kienböck's Disease. J. Hand Surg., 12A:777–778, 1987.
407. Navarro, A.: *In* Scaramuzza, R.F. (ed.): El Movimiento de Rotacion en el Carpo y sie Relacion con la Fisio Pathologica de sus Lesiones Traumaticas. Bull. Trabojos Soc. Argentina Orthop. Traumatol., 34:337–386, 1969.
408. Neviaser, R.J.: Proximal Row Carpectomy for Posttraumatic Disorders of the Carpus. J. Hand Surg., 8:301–305, 1983.
409. Neviaser, R.J., and Palmer, A.K.: Traumatic Perforation of the Articular Disc of the Triangular Fibrocartilage Complex of the Wrist. Bull. Hosp. Jt. Dis. Orthop. Inst., 44:376–380, 1984.
410. Newman, J.H., and Watt, I.: Avascular Necrosis of the Capitate and Dorsal Dorsi-Flexion Instability. Hand, 12:176–178, 1980.
411. Nielsen, P.T., Hedeboe, J., and Thommesen, P.: Bone Scintigraphy in the Evaluation of Fracture of the Carpal Scaphoid Bone. Acta Orthop. Scand., 54:303–306, 1983.
412. Nigst, H., and Buck-Gramcko, D.: Luxationen und Subluxationen des Kahnbeines. Handchir. Mikrochir. Plast. Chir., 7:81–90, 1975.
413. Norbeck, D.E., Larson, B., Blair, S.J., and Demos, T.C.: Traumatic Longitudinal Disruption of the Carpus. J. Hand Surg., 12A:509–514, 1987.
414. O'Brien, E.T.: Acute Fractures and Dislocations of the Carpus. *In* Lichtman, D.M. (ed.): The Wrist and its Disorders, pp. 129–159. Philadelphia, W.B. Saunders, 1988.
415. Ogunro, O.: Fracture of the Body of the Hamate Bone. J. Hand Surg., 8:353–355, 1983.
416. Ohshio, I., Ogino, T., and Miyake, A.: Dislocation of the Ha-

mate Associated With Fracture of the Trapezial Ridge. J. Hand Surg., 11A:658–660, 1986.
417. Olsen, N., Schousen, P., Dirksen, H., and Christoffersen, J.K.: Regional Scintimetry in Scaphoid Fractures. Acta Orthop. Scand., 54:380–382, 1983.
418. Omer, G.E., Jr., and Thomas, S.R.: The Management of Chronic Pain Syndromes in the Upper Extremity. Clin. Orthop., 104:37, 1974.
419. Ovesen, J.: Shortening of the Radius in the Treatment of Lunatomalacia. J. Bone Joint Surg., 63B:231–232, 1981.
420. Paley, D., McMurtry, R.Y., and Murray, J.F.: Dorsal Dislocation of the Ulnar Styloid and Extensor Carpi Ulnaris Tendon into the Distal Radioulnar Joint: The Empty Sulcus Sign. J. Hand Surg., 12A:1029–1032, 1987.
421. Palmer, A.K.: Trapezial Ridge Fractures. J. Hand Surg., 6:561–564, 1981.
422. Palmer, A.K.: Triangular Fibrocartilage Complex Lesions: A Classification. J. Hand Surg., 14A:594–606, 1989.
423. Palmer, A.K., Dobyns, J.H., and Linscheid, R.L.: Management of Post-Traumatic Instability of the Wrist Secondary to Ligament Rupture. J. Hand Surg., 3:507–532, 1978.
424. Palmer, A.K., Glisson, R.R., and Werner, F.W.: Relationship Between Ulnar Variance and Triangular Fibrocartilage Complex Thickness. J. Hand Surg., 9A:681–683, 1984.
425. Palmer, A.K., Glisson, R.R., and Werner, F.W.: Ulnar Variance Determination. J. Hand Surg., 7:376–379, 1982.
426. Palmer, A.K., Werner, F.W., Glisson, R.R., and Murphy, D.J.: Partial Excision of the Triangular Fibrocartilage Complex. J. Hand Surg., 13A:391–394, 1988.
427. Palmer, A.K., and Werner, F.W.: Biomechanics of the Distal Radioulnar Joint. Clin. Orthop., 187:26–35, 1984.
428. Palmer, A.K., and Werner, F.W.: The Triangular Fibrocartilage Complex of the Wrist—Anatomy and Function. J. Hand Surg., 6:153–162, 1981.
429. Panagis, J.S., Gelberman, R.H., Taleisnik, J., and Baumgaertner, M.: The Arterial Anatomy of the Human Carpus: II. The Intraosseous Vascularity. J. Hand Surg., 8:375–382, 1983.
430. Papilion, J.D., DePuy, T.E., Aulicino, P.L., Bergfield, T.G., and Gwathmey, F.W.: Radiographic Evaluation of the Hook of the Hamate: A New Technique. J. Hand Surg., 13A:437–439, 1988.
431. Parisien, S.: Settling in Colles' Fracture: A Review of the Literature. Bull. Hosp. Jt. Dis. Inst., 34:117–125, 1973.
432. Pattee, G.A., and Thompson, G.H.: Anterior and Posterior Marginal Fracture Dislocations of the Distal Radius: An Analysis of the Results of Treatment. Clin. Orthop., 231:183–195, 1988.
433. Peimer, C.A., Medige, J., Eckert, B.S., Wright, J.R., and Howard, C.S.: Reactive Synovitis After Silicone Arthroplasty. J. Hand Surg., 11A:624–638, 1986.
433a. Perlik, P.C., and Guildford, W.B.: MRI to Assess Vascularity of Scaphoid. J. Hand Surg., 16A:479–484, 1991.
434. Persson, M.: Causal Treatment of Lunatomalacia: Further Experiences of Operative Ulna Lengthening. Acta Chir. Scand., 100:531–544, 1950.
435. Peyroux, L.M., Dunaud, J.L., Caron, M., Ben Slamia, I., and Kharrat, M.: The Kapandji Technique and Its Evolution in the Treatment of Fractures of the Distal End of the Radius: Report on a Series of 159 Cases. Ann. Chir. Main Memb. Super., 6:109–122, 1987.
436. Pilcher, L.S.: Fractures of the Lower Extremity or Base of the Radius. Ann. Surg., 65:1, 1917.
437. Poirier, P., and Charpy, A.: Traite d'Anatomie Humaine (Arthrologie). Paris, Masson et Cie, 1897.
438. Posner, M.A., and Greenspan, A.: Trispiral Tomography for the Evaluation of Wrist Problems. J. Hand Surg., 13A:175–181, 1988.
439. Pouteau, C.: Oeuvres Posthumes de M. Pouteau, vol. 2, p. 251. Paris, P.D. Pierres, 1783.
440. Preiser, G.: Zur Frage der Typischen Traumatischen Ernahrungsstorungen der Kurzen Hand- und Fusswurzelknochen. Fortschr. Geb. Roentgenstrahlen. Nuklearmed. Erganzungsband., 17:360–362, 1911.
441. Primiano, G.A., and Reef, T.C.: Disruption of the Proximal Carpal Arch of the Hand. J. Bone Joint Surg., 56A:328–332, 1974.
442. Pring, D.J., Hartley, E.B., and Williams, D.J.: Scaphoid Osteosynthesis: Early Experience With the Herbert Bone Screw. J. Hand Surg., 12B:46–49, 1987.
442a. Proctor, M.T.: Nonunion of the Scaphoid: Early and Late Management. Injury, 25:15–20, 1994.
443. Prosser, A.J., Brenkel, I.J., and Irvine, G.B.: Articular Fractures of the Distal Scaphoid. J. Hand Surg., 13B:87–91, 1988.
443a. Pruitt, D.L., Gilula, L.A., Manske, P.R., and Vannier, M.W.: Computed Tomography Scanning With Image Reconstruction in Evaluation of Distal Radius Fractures. J. Hand Surg., 19A:720–727, 1994.
443b. Radford, P.J., Matthewson, M.H., and Meggitt, B.F.: The Herbert Screw for Delayed and Nonunion of Scaphoid Fractures. J. Hand Surg., 15B:455–459, 1990.
444. Rahme, H.: Idiopathic Avascular Necrosis of the Capitate Bone—Case Report. Hand, 15:274–275, 1983.
444a. Rafert, J.A., and Long, B.W.: Technique for Diagnosis of Scaphoid Fracture. Radiol. Technol., 63:16–20, 1991.
445. Ralston, E.L.: Handbook of Fractures. St. Louis, C.V. Mosby, 1967.
446. Rand, J.A., Linscheid, R.L., and Dobyns, J.H.: Capitate Fractures: A Long-Term Follow-Up. Clin. Orthop., 165:209–216, 1982.
446a. Rankin, G., Kuschner, S.H., Orlando, C., McKellop, H., and Brien, W.N.: A Biomechanical Evaluation of a Cannulated Compressive Screw for use in Fractures of the Scaphoid. J. Hand Surg., 16:1002-1010, 1991.
447. Rayhack, J.M., Linscheid, R.L., Dobyns, J.H., and Smith, J.H.: Posttraumatic Ulnar Translation of the Carpus. J. Hand Surg., 12A:180–189, 1987.
448. Razemon, J.P.: Pathogenic Study of Kienböck's Disease. Ann. Chir. Main Memb. Super., 1:240–242, 1982.
449. Reagan, D.S., Linscheid, R.L., and Dobyns, J.H.: Lunotriquetral Sprains. J. Hand Surg., 9A:502–514, 1984.
450. Reider, J.J.: Fractures of the Capitate Bone. U.S. Armed Forces J., 9:1513–1516, 1958.
451. Reinus, W.R., Hardy, D.C., Totty, W.G., and Gilula, L.A.: Arthrographic Evaluation of the Carpal Triangular Fibrocartilage Complex. J. Hand Surg., 12A:495–503, 1987.
452. Rhoades, C.E., and Reckling, F.W.: Palmar Dislocation of the Trapezoid: Case Report. J. Hand Surg., 8:85–88, 1983.
452a. Richards, R.R., Patrick, C.B., and Bell, R.S.: Internal Fixation of a Capitate Fracture With Herbert Screws. J. Hand Surg., 15A:885–887, 1990.
452b. Richards, R.R., and Regan, W.D.: Treatment of Scaphoid Nonunion by Radical Curettage, Trapezoidal Iliac Crest Graft, and Internal Fixation With a Herbert Screw. Clin. Orthop. Rel. Res. 262:148–158, 1991.
453. Riggs, S.A. Jr., and Cooney, W.P.: External Fixation of Complex Hand and Wrist Fractures. J. Trauma, 23:332–336, 1983.
454. Riis, J., and Fruensgaard, S.: Treatment of Unstable Colles' Fractures by External Fixation. J. Hand Surg., 14B:145–148, 1989.
455. Rogers, W.D., and Watson, H.K.: Radiol Styloid Impingement After Triscaphe Arthrodesis. J. Hand Surg., 14A:297–301, 1989.
456. Rongieres, M., Mansat, M., Devallet, P., Bonnevialle, P., and Railhac, J.J.: An Experimental Study of Partial Intercarpal Arthrodesis. Ann. Chir. Main Memb. Super., 6:269–275, 1987.
457. Rose-Innes, A.P.: Anterior Dislocation of the Ulna in the Inferior Radio-Ulnar Joint: Case Reports, With a Discussion of the Anatomy of Rotation of the Forearm. J. Bone Joint Surg., 42B:515–521, 1960.
458. Roth, J., and Haddad, R.G.: Radiocarpal Arthroscopy and Arthrography in the Diagnosis of Ulnar Wrist Pain. J. Arthroscopy, 2:234–243, 1986.
459. Roullet, J., and Walch, G.: Technique of the Elongation of Ulna in the Kienböck's Disease: Results After Ten Years. Ann. Chir. Main Memb. Super., 1:268–272, 1982.
460. Ruby, L.K., An, K.N., Linscheid, R.L., Cooney, W.P., and

Chao, E.Y.S.: The Effect of Scapholunate Ligament Section on Scapholunate Motion. J. Hand Surg., 12A:767–771, 1987.

461. Ruby, L.K., Cooney, W.P., An, K.N., Linscheid, R.L., and Chao, E.Y.S.: Relative Motion of Selected Carpal Bones: A Kinematic Analysis of the Normal Wrist. J. Hand Surg., 13A:1–10, 1988.
462. Ruby, L.K., Stinson, J., and Belsky, M.R.: The Natural History of Scaphoid Non-Union. J. Bone Joint Surg., 67:428–432, 1985.
463. Rüsse, O.: Fracture of the Carpal Navicular: Diagnosis, Non-Operative Treatment and Operative Treatment. J. Bone Joint Surg., 42A:759–768, 1960.
464. Russell, T.B.: Inter-Carpal Dislocations and Fracture–Dislocations: A Review of Fifty-Nine Cases. J. Bone Joint Surg., 31B:524–531, 1949.
465. Saffar, P.: Carpal Dislocations and Sequelar Instability. Ann. Chir. Main Memb. Super., 3:349–352, 1984.
466. Saffar, P.: Replacement of the Lunate by the Pisiform Bone. Ann. Chir. Main Memb. Super., 1:276–279, 1982.
467. Saffar, P., and Gentaz, R.: Comparison Between Surgical and Medical Management of Kienböck's Disease. Ann. Chir. Main Memb. Super., 1:250–252, 1982.
468. Sanders, W.E.: Evaluation of the Humpback Scaphoid by Computed Tomography in the Longitudinal Axial Plane of the Scaphoid. J. Hand Surg., 13A:182–187, 1988.
469. Sarmiento, A., Pratt, G.W., Berry, N.C., and Sinclair, W.F.: Colles' Fractures: Functional Bracing in Supination. J. Bone Joint Surg., 57A:311–317, 1975.
470. Sarrafian, S.K., and Breihan, J.H.: Palmar Dislocation of Scaphoid and Lunate as a Unit. J. Hand Surg., 15A:134–139, 1990.
471. Sarrafian, S.K., Melamed, J.L., and Goshgarian, G.M.: Study of Wrist Motion in Flexion and Extension. Clin. Orthop., 126:153–159, 1977.
472. Saunier, J., and Chamay, A.: Volar Perilunar Dislocation of the Wrist. Clin. Orthop., 157:139–142, 1981.
473. Schernberg, F.: Midcarpal Instability. Ann. Chir. Main Memb. Super., 3:344–348, 1984.
474. Schernberg, F.: Static and Dynamic Radioanatomy of the Wrist. Ann. Chir. Main Memb. Super., 3:301–312, 1984.
475. Schoenecker, P.L., Gilula, L.A., Shively, R.A., and Manske, P.R.: Radiocarpal Fracture–Dislocation. Clin. Orthop., 197:237–244, 1985.
476. Schuhl, J.F., Leroy, B., and Comtet, J.J.: Biodynamics of the Wrist: Radiologic Approach to Scapholunate Instability. J. Hand Surg., 10A:1006–1008, 1985.
477. Schuind, F., Donkerwolcke, M., Rasquin, C., and Burny, F.: External Fixation of Fractures of the Distal Radius: A Study of 225 Cases. J. Hand Surg., 14A:404–407, 1989.
478. Sebald, J.R., Dobyns, J.H., and Linscheid, R.L.: The Natural History of Collapse Deformities of the Wrist. Clin. Orthop., 104:140–148, 1974.
479. Seimon, L.P.: Compound Dislocation of the Trapezium: A Case Report. J. Bone Joint Surg., 54A:1297–1300, 1972.
480. Seitz, W.H. Jr., Putnam, M.D., and Dick, H.M.: Limited Open Surgical Approach for External Fixation of Distal Radius Fractures. J. Hand Surg., 15A:288–293, 1990.
481. Sennwald, G.: The Wrist, Anatomical and Pathophysiological Approach in Diagnosis and Treatment. Berlin, Springer-Verlag, 1987.
482. Sennwald, G., and Segmüller, G.: Arthrodèse de la Colonne Centrale du Carpe. Int. Orthop., 13:147–152, 1989.
483. Sennwald, G., and Segmüller, G.: Base Anatomique d'un Noveau Concept de Stabilité du Carpe. Int. Orthop., 10:25–30, 1986.
484. Seradge, H., Sterbank, P.T., Seradge, E., and Owens, W.: Segmental Motion of the Proximal Carpal Row: Their Global Effect on the Wrist Motion. J. Hand Surg., 15A:236–239, 1990.
485. Seitz, W.H., Froimson, A.I., Brooks, D.B., Postak, P.D., Parker, R.D., LaPorte, J.M., and Greenwald, A.S.: Biomechanical Analysis of Pin Placement and Pin Size for External Fixation of Distal Radius Fractures. Clin. Orthop., 251:207–212, 1990.
486. Sherlock, D.A.: Traumatic Dorsoradial Dislocation of the Trapezium. J. Hand Surg., 12A:262–265, 1987.
487. Short, W.H., Palmer, A.K., Werner, F.W., and Murphy, D.J.: A Biomechanical Study of Distal Radial Fractures. J. Hand Surg., 12A:529–534, 1987.
488. Siegel, M.W., and Hertzberg, H.: Complete Dislocation of the Greater Multangular (Trapezium): A Case Report. J. Bone Joint Surg., 51A:769–772, 1969.
489. Siegert, J.J., Frassica, F.J., and Amadio, P.C.: Treatment of Chronic Perilunate Dislocations. J. Hand Surg., 13A:206–212, 1988.
490. Smith, D.K., An, K.N., Cooney, W.P., Linscheid, R.L., and Chao, E.Y.S.: Effects of a Scaphoid Waist Osteotomy on Carpal Kinematics. J. Orthop. Res., 7:590–598, 1989.
491. Smith, D.K., Cooney, W.P., An, K.N., Linscheid, R.L., and Chao, E.Y.S.: The Effects of Simulated Unstable Scaphoid Fractures on Carpal Motion. J. Hand Surg., 14A:283–291, 1989.
491a. Smith, D.K., Gilula, L.A., and Amadio, P.C.: Dorsal Lunate Tilt (DISI Configuration): Sign of Scaphoid Fracture Displacement. Radiology, 176:497-499, 1990.
492. Smith, F.M.: Late Rupture of Extensor Pollicis Longus Tendon Following Colles' Fracture. J. Bone Joint Surg., 28:49–59, 1946.
492a. Smith, K., Helm, R., and Tonkin, M.A.: The Herbert Screw for Treatment of Scaphoid Fracture. Ann. Chir. Main Memb. Super., 10:556–563, 1991.
493. Smith, P., Wright, T.W., Wallace, P.F., and Dell, P.C.: Excision of the Hook of the Hamate: A Retrospective Survey and Review of the Literature. J. Hand Surg., 13A:612–615, 1988.
494. Smith, R.W.: A Treatise on Fractures in the Vicinity of Joints, and on Certain Forms of Accidental and Congenital Dislocations. Dublin, Hodges & Smith, 1854.
495. Snook, G.A., Chrisman, O.D., Wilson, T.C., and Wietsma, R.D.: Subluxation of the Distal Radio-Ulnar Joint by Hyperpronation. J. Bone Joint Surg., 51A:1315–1323, 1969.
496. Sowa, D.T., Holder, L.E., Patt, P.G., and Weiland, A.J.: Application of Magnetic Resonance Imaging to Ischemic Necrosis of the Lunate. J. Hand Surg., 14A:1008–1116, 1989.
497. Speed, J.S., and Knight, R.A.: Treatment of Malunited Colles's Fractures. J. Bone Joint Surg., 27:361–367, 1945.
498. Spinner, M., and Kaplan, E.B.: Extensor Carpi Ulnaris: Its Relationship to the Stability on the Distal Radio-ulnar Joint. Clin. Orthop., 68:124–129, 1970.
499. Stahl, F.: On Lunatomalacia (Kienböck's Disease): A Clinical and Roentgenological Study, Especially on Its Pathogenesis and the Late Results of Immobilization Treatment. Acta Chir. Scand., 45(Suppl. 126):1–133, 1947.
500. Stamm, T.T.: Excision of the Proximal Row of the Carpus. Proc. R. Soc. Med., 38:74–75, 1944.
500a. Stanciu, C., and Dumont, A.: Changing Patterns of Scaphoid Fractures in Adolescents. Can. J. Surg., 37:214–216, 1994.
501. Stark, A., Brostrom, L., and Svartengren, G.: Scaphoid Nonunion Treated With the Matti-Rüsse Technique: Long-Term Results. Clin. Orthop., 214:175–180, 1987.
502. Stark, H.H., Chao, E.K., Zemel, N.P., Rickard, T.A., and Ashworth, C.R.: Fracture of the Hook of the Hamate. J. Bone Joint Surg., 71A:1202–1207, 1989.
503. Stein, F., and Siegel, M.W.: Naviculocapitate Fracture Syndrome: A Case Report, New Thoughts on the Mechanism of Injury. J. Bone Joint Surg., 51A:391–393, 1969.
504. Stern, P.J.: Multiple Flexor Tendon Ruptures Following an Old Anterior Dislocation of the Lunate: A Case Report. J. Bone Joint Surg., 63A:489–490, 1981.
505. Stevanovic, M.V., Stark, H.H., and Filler, B.C.: Scaphotrapezial Dislocation. J. Bone Joint Surg., 72A:449–452, 1990.
506. Stewart, M.J.: Fractures of the Carpal Navicular (Scaphoid): A Report of 436 Cases. J. Bone Joint Surg., 36A:998–1006, 1954.
507. Sudeck, P.: Uber die Akute (Reflektorische) Knochenatrophie nach Entzündungen und Verletzungen an den Extremitäten und ihre Klinischen Erscheinungen. Fortschr. Geb. Roentgenstrahlen. Nuklearmed. Erganzungsband., 5:277–297, 1901–1902.

508. Sundberg, S.B., and Linscheid, R.L.: Kienböck's Disease: Results of Treatment With Ulnar Lengthening. Clin. Orthop., 187:43–51, 1984.
509. Sutro, C.J.: Bilateral Recurrent Intercarpal Subluxation. Am. J. Surg., 72:110–113, 1946.
510. Sutro, C.J.: Hypermobility of Bones Due to "Over-Lengthened" Capsular and Ligamentous Tissues. Surgery, 21:67, 1947.
511. Swanson, A.B.: Flexible Implant Resection Arthroplasty in the Hand and Extremities. St. Louis, C.V. Mosby, 1973.
512. Tachakra, T.: A Case of Trapezio-scaphoid Subluxation. Br. J. Clin. Pract., 31:162–165, 1977.
513. Tajima, T.: An Investigation of the Treatment of Kienböck's Disease. J. Bone Joint Surg., 48A:1649–1655, 1966.
514. Taleisnik, J.: Carpal Instability: Current Concepts Review. J. Bone Joint Surg., 70A:1262–1268, 1988.
515. Taleisnik, J.: Clinical and Technologic Evaluation of Ulnar Wrist Pain. J. Hand Surg., 13A:801–802, 1988.
516. Taleisnik, J.: The Ligaments of the Wrist. J. Hand Surg., 1:110–118, 1976.
517. Taleisnik, J.: Triquetrohamate and Triquetrolunate Instabilities (Medial Carpal Instability). Ann. Chir. Main Memb. Super., 3:331–343, 1984.
518. Taleisnik, J., Gelberman, R.H., Miller, B.W., and Szabo, R.M.: Extensor Retinaculum of the Wrist. J. Hand Surg., 9A:459–501, 1984.
519. Taleisnik, J., and Kelly, P.J.: Extraosseous and Intraosseous Blood Supply of the Scaphoid Bone. J. Bone Joint Surg., 48A:1125–1137, 1966.
520. Taleisnik, J., Malerich, M., and Prietto, M.: Palmar Carpal Instability Secondary to Dislocation of Scaphoid and Lunate: Report of a Case and Review of the Literature. J. Hand Surg., 7:606–612, 1982.
521. Taleisnik, J., Watson, H.K.: Midcarpal Instability Caused by Malunited Fractures of the Distal Radius. J. Hand Surg., 9A:350–357, 1984.
522. Teisen, H., and Hjarbaek, J.: Classification of Fresh Fractures of the Lunate. J. Hand Surg., 13B:458–462, 1988.
523. Testut, L., and Latarget, A.: Traite d'Anatomie Humaine. Paris, Doin, 1949.
524. Thomas, F.B.: Reduction of Smith's Fracture. J. Bone Joint Surg., 39B:463–470, 1957.
525. Thompson, T.C., Campbell, R.D. Jr., and Arnold, W.D.: Primary and Secondary Dislocation of the Scaphoid Bone. J. Bone Joint Surg., 46B:73–82, 1964.
525a. Tiel-Von Buol, M.M., Van Beek, E.J., Gubler, F.M., Braekhuizen, A.H., and Von Rayen, E.A.: The Value of Radiographs and Bone Scintigraphy in Suspected Scaphoid Fracture. J. Hand Surg., 18B:403–406, 1993.
525b. Tiel-Von Buol, M.M., Van Beek, E.J., Dijkstra, P.F., and Bakker, A.J.: Significance of a Hot Spot on the Bone Scan After Carpal Injury: Evaluation by CT. Eur. J. Nucl. Med., 20:159–164, 1993.
526. Tillberg, B.: Kienböck's Disease Treated With Osteotomy to Lengthen Ulna. Acta Orthop. Scand., 39:359–368, 1968.
527. Trevor, D.: Rupture of the Extensor Pollicis Longus Tendon After Colles' Fracture. J. Bone Joint Surg., 32B:370, 1950.
528. Trumble, T., Bour, C.J., Smith, R.J., and Edwards, G.S.: Intercarpal Arthrodesis for Static and Dynamic Volar Intercalated Segment Instability. J. Hand Surg., 13A:384–390, 1988.
529. Trumble, T., Glisson, R.R., Seaber, A.V., and Urbaniak, J.R.: A Biomechanical Comparison of the Methods for Treating Kienböck's Disease. J. Hand Surg., 11A:88–93, 1986.
530. Trumble, T.E., Bour, C.J., Smith, R.J., and Glisson, R.R.: Kinematics of the Ulnar Carpus Related to the Volar Intercalated Segment Instability Pattern. J. Hand Surg., 15A:384–392, 1990.
530a. Trumble, T.E., Benerschke, S.K., and Vedder, N.B.: Ipsilateral Fractures of the Scaphoid and Radius. J. Hand Surg., 18A:8–13, 1993.
530b. Trumble, T.E., Schmitt, S.R., and Vedder, N.B.: Factors Affecting Functional Outcome of Displaced Intra-Articular Distal Radius Fractures. J. Hand Surg., 19A:325–340, 1994.
531. Vahvanen, V., and Westerlund, M.: Fracture of the Carpal Scaphoid in Children: A Clinical and Roentgenological Study of 108 Cases. Acta Orthop. Scand., 51:909–913, 1980.
532. Vance, R.M., and Gelberman, R.H.: Acute Ulnar Neuropathy With Fractures at the Wrist. J. Bone Joint Surg., 60A:962, 1978.
533. Vance, R.M., Gelberman, R.H., and Evans, E.F.: Scaphocapitate Fractures: Patterns of Dislocation, Mechanism of Injury, and Preliminary Results of Treatment. J. Bone Joint Surg., 62A:271–276, 1980.
534. Varodompun, N., Limpivest, P., and Prinyaroj, P.: Isolated Dorsal Radiocarpal Dislocation: Case Report and Literature Review. J. Hand Surg., 10A:708–710, 1985.
535. Vasilas, A., Grieco, R.V., and Bartone, N.F.: Roentgen Aspects of Injuries to the Pisiform Bone and Pisotriquetral Joint. J. Bone Joint Surg., 42A:1317–1328, 1960.
536. Vender, M.I., and Watson, H.K.: Acquired Madelung-like Deformity in a Gymnast. J. Hand Surg., 13A:19–21, 1988.
537. Verdan, C.: Fractures of the Scaphoid. Surg. Clin. North Am., 40:461–464, 1960.
537a. Vidal, M.A., Linscheid, R.L., Amadio, P.C., and Dobyns, J.H.: Preiser's Disease. Ann. Chir. Main Memb. Super., 10:227–235, 1991.
538. Viegas, S.F., Patterson, R.M., Peterson, P.D., et al.: Ulnar-Sided Perilunate Instability: An Anatomic and Biomechanic Study. J. Hand Surg., 15A:268–278, 1990.
539. Viegas, S.F., Tencer, A.F., Cantrell, J., et al.: Load Transfer Characteristics of the Wrist: I. The Normal Joint. J. Hand Surg., 12A:971–978, 1987.
540. Viegas, S.F., Tencer, A.F., Cantrell, J., et al.: Load Transfer Characteristics of the Wrist: II. Perilunate Instability. J. Hand Surg., 12A:978–985, 1987.
540a. Viegas, S.F., Patterson, R.M., Holkanson, J.A., and Davis, J.: Wrist Anatomy: Incidence Distribution and Correlation of Anatomy Variations, Tears and Arthrosis. J. Hand Surg., 18A:463–475, 1993.
541. Volkmann, R.: Die Ischaemischen Muskellähmungen und Kontrakturen. Zentralbl. Chir., 8:801–805, 1881.
542. Volz, R.G., Lieb, M., and Benjamin, J.: Biomechanics of the Wrist. Clin. Orthop., 149:112–117, 1980.
543. Von Lanz, T., and Wachsmuth, W.: Praktische Anatomi: Ein Lehrund Hilfsbuch der anatomischen Grundlagen ärztlichen Handelns, 2nd ed., vol. 1. Berlin, Springer-Verlag, 1938.
544. Voorhees, D.R., Daffner, R.H., Nunley, J.A., and Gilula, L.A.: Carpal Ligamentous Disruptions and Negative Ulnar Variance. Skeletal Radiol., 13:257–262, 1985.
545. Wahlstrom, O.: Treatment of Colles' Fracture: A Prospective Comparison of Three Different Positions of Immobilization. Acta Orthop. Scand., 53:225, 1982.
546. Watson, H.K.: Limited Wrist Arthrodesis. Clin. Orthop., 149:126–136, 1980.
546a. Watson, H.K., Pitts, E.C., Ashmead, D., Marklouf, M.V., and Kauer, J.: Dorsal Approach to Scaphoid Nonunions. J. Hand Surg. 18A:359–365, 1993.
546b. Watson, H.K., Ottani, L., Pitts, E.C., and Handal, A.G.: Rotatory Subluxation of the Scaphoid: A Spectrum of Instability. J. Hand Surg. 18B:62-64, 1993.
547. Watson, H.K., and Ballet, F.L.: The SLAC Wrist: Scapholunate Advanced Collapse Pattern of Degenerative Arthritis. J. Hand Surg., 9A:358–365, 1984.
547a. Watson, H.K., and Hempton, R.F.: Limited Wrist Arthrodeses: I. The Triscaphoid Joint. J. Hand Surg., 5:320–327, 1980.
548. Watson, H.K., Goodman, M.L., and Johnson, T.R.: Limited Wrist Arthrodesis: II. Intercarpal and Radiocarpal Combinations. J. Hand Surg., 6:223–233, 1981.
549. Watson, H.K., and Rogers, W.D.: Nonunion of the Hook of the Hamate: An Argument for Bonegrafting the Nonunion. J. Hand Surg., 14A:486–490, 1989.
550. Watson, H.K., Ryu, J., and Akelman, E.: Limited Triscaphoid Intercarpal Arthrodesis for Rotatory Subluxation of the Scaphoid. J. Bone Joint Surg., 68A:345–349, 1986.
551. Watson, H.K., Ryu, J., and DiBella, A.: An Approach to Kienböck's Disease: Triscaphe Arthrodesis. J. Hand Surg., 10A:179–187, 1985.
552. Weber, E.R.: Concepts Governing the Rotational Shift of the

Intercalated Segment of the Carpus. Orthop. Clin. North Am., 15:193–207, 1984.

553. Weber, E.R., and Chao, E.Y.: An Experimental Approach to the Mechanism of Scaphoid Waist Fractures. J. Hand Surg., 3:142–148, 1978.

554. Weber, S.C., and Szabo, R.M.: Severely Comminuted Distal Radial Fracture as an Unsolved Problem: Complications Associated With External Fixation and Pins and Plaster Techniques. J. Hand Surg., 11A:157–165, 1986.

555. Weeks, P.M., Vannier, M.W., Stevens, W.G., Gayou, D., and Gilula, L.A.: Three-Dimensional Imaging of the Wrist. J. Hand Surg., 10A:32–39, 1985.

556. Weiss, C., Laskin, R.S., and Spinner, M.: Irreducible Radiocarpal Dislocation: A Case Report. J. Bone Joint Surg., 52A:562–564, 1970.

557. Werner, F.W., Palmer, A.K., and Glisson, R.R.: Forearm Load Transmission: The Effect of Ulnar Lengthening and Shortening. J. Hand Surg., 17A:423–428, 1992.

557a. Whalen, J.L., Bishop, A.T., and Linscheid, R.L.: Nonoperative Treatment of Acute Hamate Hook Fractures. J. Hand Surg., 17A:507–511, 1992.

558. White, S.J., Louis, D.S., Braunstein, E.M., Hankin, F.M., and Green, T.L.: Capitate-Lunate Instability: Recognition by Manipulation under Fluoroscopy. A.J.R., 143:361–364, 1984.

559. Wilson, J.N.: Profiles of the Carpal Canal. J. Bone Joint Surg., 36A:127–132, 1954.

559a. Wozasek, G.E., and Maser, K.D.: Percutaneous Screw Fixation for Fractures of the Scaphoid. J. Bone Joint Surg., 73B:138–142, 1991.

559b. Yanne, D., and Lieppins, L.M.: Fractures of the Carpal Scaphoid: A Critical Study of Standard Splint. J. Bone Joint Surg., 73B:600–602, 1991.

560. Youm, Y., and Flatt, A.E.: Kinematics of the Wrist. Clin. Orthop., 149:21–32, 1980.

561. Youm, Y., McMurtry, R.Y., Flatt, A.E., and Gillespie, T.E.: Kinematics of the Wrist: I. An Experimental Study of Radial-Ulnar Deviation and Flexion-Extension. J. Bone Joint Surg., 60A:423–431, 1978.

562. Zaidenberg, C., Siebert, J.W., and Angiogiane, C.: A New Vascularized Bone Graft for Scaphoid Nonunion. J. Hand Surg., 16A:474–478, 1991.

Rockwood and Green's Fractures in Adults, Fourth Edition,
edited by Charles A. Rockwood, David P. Green, Robert W. Bucholz and James D. Heckman.
Lippincott-Raven Publishers, Philadelphia © 1996.

CHAPTER 13

Fractures of the Shafts of the Radius and Ulna

Robin R. Richards and Fred G. Corley, Jr.

Fractures of Both Bones of the Forearm

Robin R. Richards

The forearm serves an important role in upper extremity function, facilitating positioning the hand in space and thus helping to provide the upper extremity with its unique mobility. In particular, the forearm, in combination with the proximal and distal radioulnar joints, allows pronation and supination, movements that are important to all of us in the usual activities of daily living. Exacting and aggressive management is required after fractures of the shafts of the radius and ulna if function is to be restored.

Chapter 12 includes a discussion of fractures of the distal radius and ulna, and Chapter 14 deals with fractures of the olecranon and radial head. This chapter, therefore, is limited to a discussion of fractures of the shaft of both bones of the forearm, single bone fractures of the radius, and single bone fractures of the ulna in adults. Also included is a discussion of fracture-dislocations involving fractures of the radius associated with distal radioulnar joint injury (Galeazzi fracture) and fractures of the ulna associated with proximal radioulnar joint injury (Monteggia fracture).

SURGICAL ANATOMY

As has been well described in the literature on the treatment of forearm fractures,[72,78,106] the surgical anatomy of the forearm creates problems in fracture treatment not found in the treatment of diaphyseal fractures of other long bones. The radius and ulna function as a unit but come into contact with each other only at the ends. They are bound proximally by the capsule of the elbow joint and the annular ligament and distally by the capsule of the wrist joint, the dorsal and volar radioulnar ligaments, and the fibrocartilaginous articular disc. As Palmer and Werner[68] have shown, the principal stabilizer of the distal radioulnar joint is the triangular fibrocartilage complex. The proximal and distal joints are very complex in both function and structure and relate closely to the ulnohumeral, radiocapitellar, and radiocarpal joints.

The ulna is a relatively straight bone, but the radius is much more complex. One frequently hears reference to the ulna moving about the radius. In fact, the ulna is a relatively fixed strut around which the radius rotates in pronation and supination.[60] In a study of 100 radii from cadavers, Sage[79] pointed out the complexity of the angles and curves in this bone (Fig. 13-1) and the importance of maintaining them, especially the lateral bow of the radius. A study by Schemitsch and Richards has confirmed the importance of restoration of the radial bow to forearm function after fracture.[86] If this is not done, the patient may not be able to achieve full pronation and supination after fracture (Fig. 13-2).

Between the shafts of the ulna and radius is the interosseous space. The fibers of the interosseous membrane run obliquely across the interosseous space from their distal insertion on the ulna to their proximal origin on the radius. The central portion of the interosseous membrane is thickened and measures about 3.5 cm in width (Fig. 13-3). Experimental studies by Hotchkiss and associates[43] showed that incision of the triangular fibrocartilage complex alone decreased relative stability by 8%. Incision of the triangular fibrocartilage complex and interosseous membrane proximal to the central band decreased stability by only 11%. Incision of the central band, however, reduced stability by 71%. The thickened central band of the interosse-

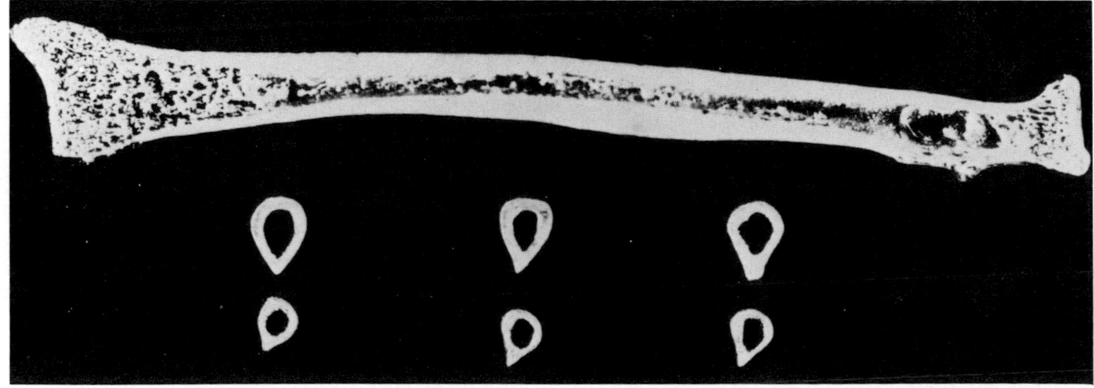

FIGURE 13-1. Cross-section configuration of the medullary canal of two radii at three points along the diaphysis. (*Sage, F.P.: Medullary Fixation of Fractures of the Forearm: A Study of the Medullary Canal of the Radius and a Report of Fifty Fractures of the Radius Treated with a Prebent Triangular Nail. J. Bone Joint Surg., 41A:1489–1516, 1959.*)

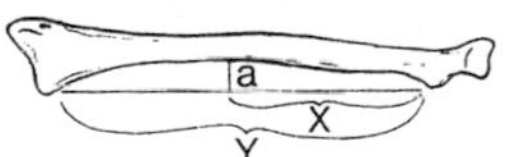

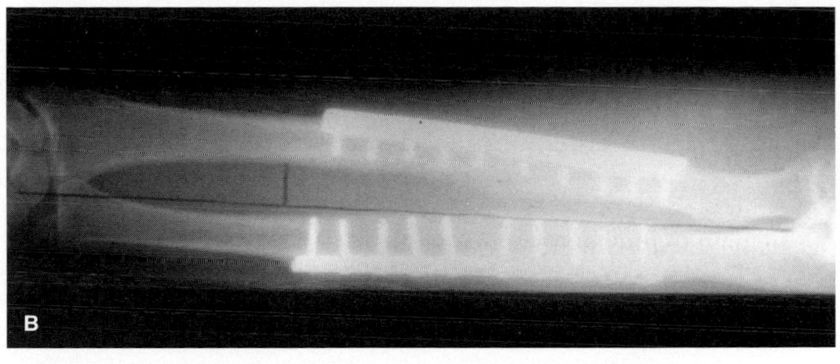

FIGURE 13-2. (**A**) Technique for measuring the amount and location of the maximum radial bow. The maximum radial bow is determined by drawing a line from the bicipital tuberosity to the most ulnar aspect of the radius at the wrist. A perpendicular line is drawn from this line to the radius at the point of maximum radial bow, and the distance is measured in millimeters. The location of maximum radial bow is determined by dividing the distance from the bicipital tuberosity to the point of maximum bow by the length of the entire bow. The value is expressed as a percentage. This measurement correlates with outcome following treatment of fractures of both bones of the forearm. (**B**) An anteroposterior radiograph of the radius and ulna with the forearm in neutral rotation. A line has been drawn from the bicipital tuberosity to the most ulnar aspect of the distal radius to measure the location and amount of maximum radial bow. The forearm fracture has healed after fixation with two 3.5-mm dynamic compression plates. (*Schemitsch, E.H., and Richards, R.R.: The Effect of Malunion on Functional Outcome After Plate Fixation of Fractures of Both Bones of the Forearm in Adults. J. Bone Joint Surg. 74A:1068–1078, 1992.*)

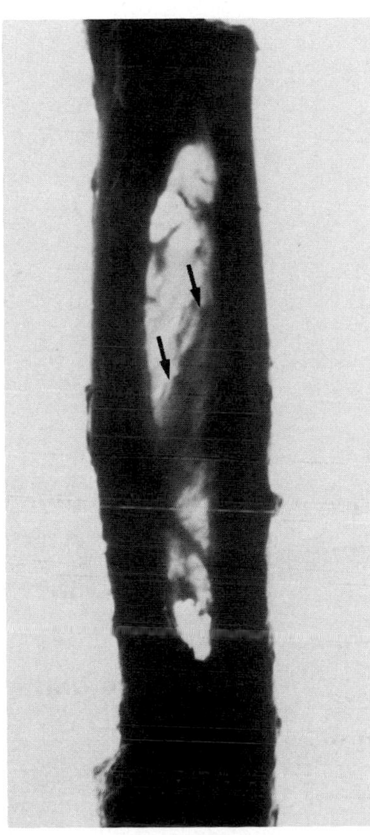

FIGURE 13-3. Backlighted photograph of a forearm specimen. The central band of the interosseous membrane is indicated by arrows. (*Hotchkiss, R.N., An, K., Sowa, D.T., Basta, S., and Weiland, A.J.: An Anatomic and Mechanical Study of the Interosseous Membrane of the Forearm: Pathomechanics of Proximal Migration of the Radius. J. Hand Surg., 14A:256–261, 1989.*)

ous membrane is a constant structure and accounts for most of the longitudinal support of the radius if the radial head is injured and requires resection. Proximal migration of the radius may occur, following radial head resection, resulting in painful ulnocarpal impingement. This phenomenon is more fully discussed in Chapter 14.

Not only are the forearm bones themselves and their associated joints complex, but the muscle groups acting across the forearm cause complex deforming forces when fractures are present. The radius and ulna are joined by three muscles—the supinator, pronator teres, and pronator quadratus—which take origin on one bone and insert on the other. In addition to their named functions, when there is a fracture, these muscles tend to approximate the radius and ulna and decrease the interosseous space. As Sage[78] has pointed out, the forearm muscles that take origin on the ulnar aspect of the forearm and insert on the radial side of the wrist or hand, such as the flexor carpi radialis, tend to exert a pronating force. In a similar manner, muscles such as the abductor pollicis longus and brevis and the extensor pollicis longus, which have their origins on the ulna and interosseous membrane on the dorsal side and are inserted on the radial side of the dorsum of the wrist, tend to exert a supinating force.

In addition to the supinator muscle itself, the biceps brachii is a powerful supinator of the radius. In fractures of the upper radius below the insertion of the supinator and above the insertion of the pronator teres, two strong muscles (the biceps and the supinator) exert an unopposed force that supinates the proximal radial fragment (Fig. 13-4). In fractures of the radius located distal to the pronator teres, the combined force of the biceps and supinator is somewhat neutralized. In these fractures the proximal fragment of the radius is usually in a slightly supinated or neutral position (Fig. 13-5). In closed treatment of forearm fractures, therefore, the location of the fracture of the radius helps to determine the degree of supination of the distal fragment needed to correct rotational alignment.

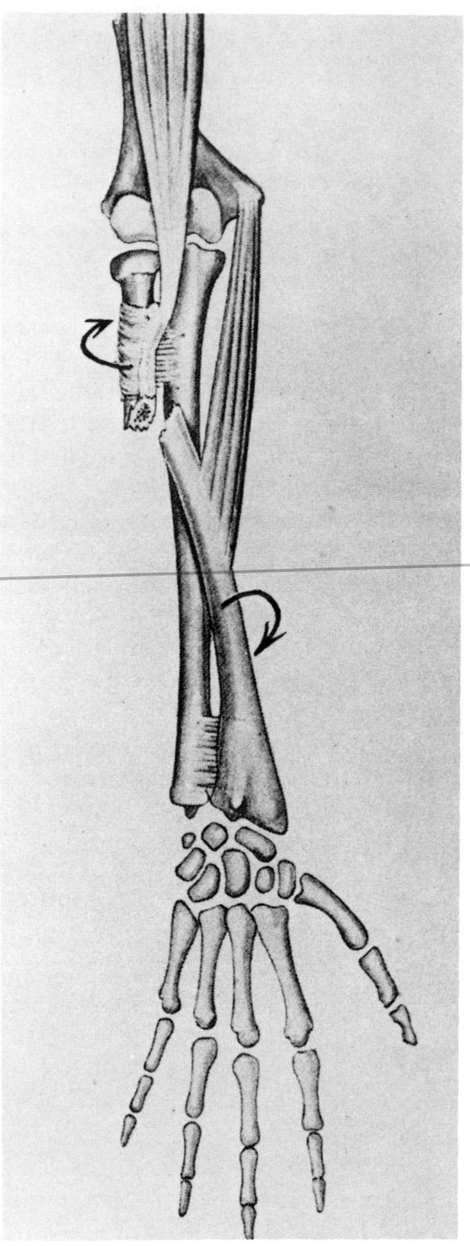

FIGURE 13-4. In a fracture of the upper shaft of the radius between the insertion of the supinator and pronator teres, the proximal fragment is supinated and the lower fragment is pronated. (*Watson-Jones, R.: Fractures and Joint Injuries, 4th ed., vol. 2. Edinburgh, E & S Livingstone, 1955.*)

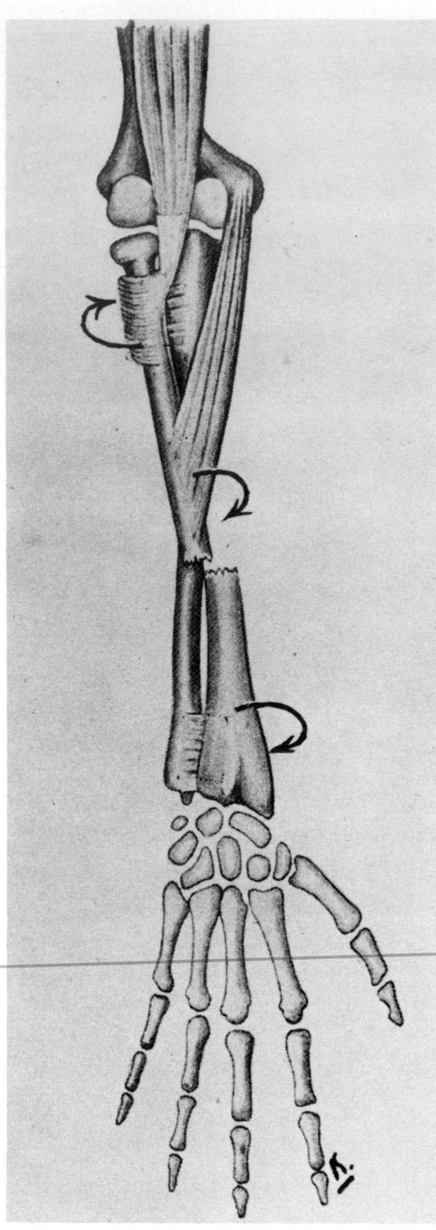

FIGURE 13-5. In a fracture of the middle or lower shaft of the radius between the insertions of the pronator teres and the pronator quadratus, the proximal fragment is in midposition (neutral rotation). (*Watson-Jones, R.: Fractures and Joint Injuries, 4th ed., vol. 2. Edinburgh, E & S Livingstone, 1955.*)

If satisfactory functional results are to be achieved in the treatment of fractures of the forearm, it is not sufficient merely to maintain the length of each bone. Axial and rotational alignment must be achieved as well, and the radial bow must be maintained.[81,86] With the complexity of the bones and joints involved, and the many and varied deforming muscle forces, it is extremely difficult to obtain union with sufficient restoration of the anatomy to ensure good functional results by closed treatment (Fig. 13-6). For these reasons some form of open reduction and internal fixation is

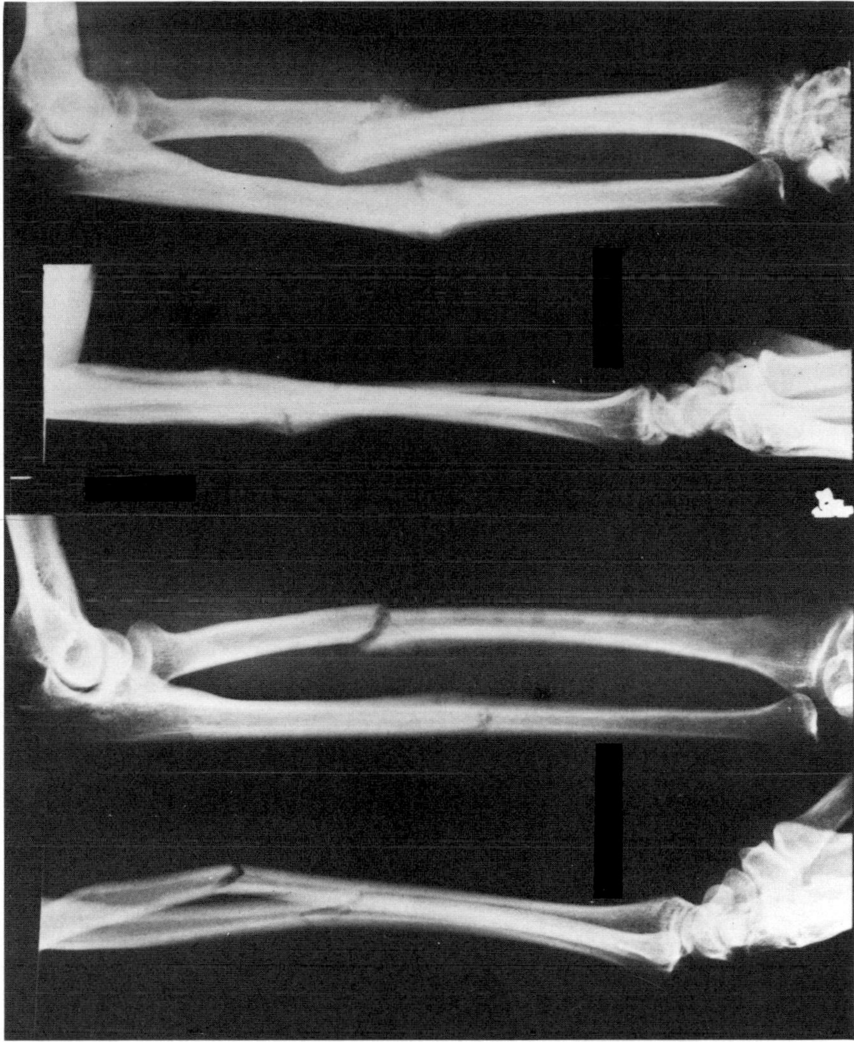

FIGURE 13-6. A fracture of the proximal shaft of the radius and midshaft of the ulna treated by closed reduction and cast immobilization. Three months later, the fracture healed with loss of the radial bow and ulnar angulation. Pronation and supination were severely limited.

recommended for most displaced diaphyseal fractures of the forearm in adults.

FRACTURES OF BOTH THE RADIUS AND ULNA

MECHANISM OF INJURY

The mechanisms of injury that cause fractures of the radius and ulna are myriad. By far the most common is some form of vehicular accident (Fig. 13-7), especially automobile and motorcycle accidents. Frequently the patient is unable to recount the exact mechanism of injury owing to the sudden nature of the accident. Probably most of these vehicular accidents result in some type of direct blow to the forearm. Other causes of direct blow injuries include fights in which one of the adversaries is struck on the forearm with a stick. Monteggia and nightstick fractures frequently result from this kind of blow, but fractures of both bones are often caused by this mechanism as well. The person throws the forearm up to protect his or her head, and the forearm is the recipient of the violence.

Gunshot wounds can cause fracture of both bones of the forearm. Such injuries are commonly associated with nerve or soft-tissue deficits and frequently have significant bone loss. Pathologic fractures of the forearm bones are not common. If they are excluded, most of the remainder of these fractures result from some type of fall. The force generated is usually much greater than that required to cause Colles' fracture. Most forearm shaft fractures resulting from falls occur in athletics or in falls from heights.

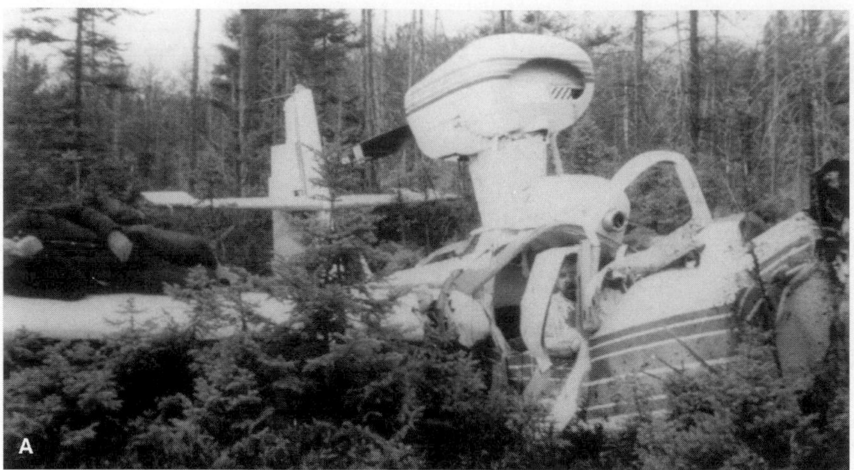

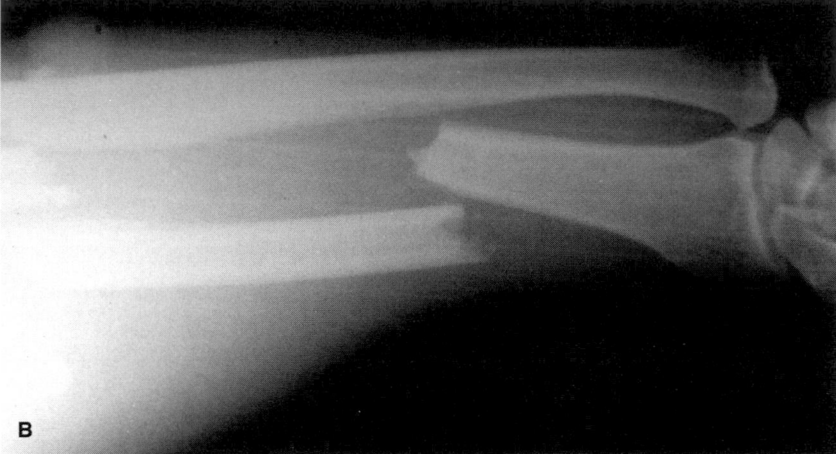

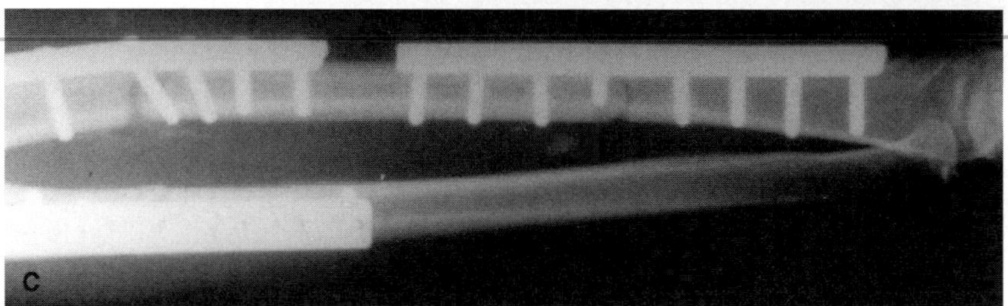

FIGURE 13-7. (**A**) The pilot of this aircraft sustained bilateral forearm fractures as he braced his arms against the dashboard during the crash. He had complex bipolar fracture dislocations with proximal and distal radioulnar joint injuries in association with fractures of both bones of the forearm. (**B**) Anteroposterior radiograph showing a displaced fracture of the distal radial diaphysis. There were proximal fractures of the radius and ulna as well. (**C**) Early (within 24 hours of injury) fixation of all fractures with 3.5-mm dynamic compression plates. Fixation was sufficiently rigid that early motion could be initiated while fracture union occurred. The patient returned to work as a dentist several months after the accident.

CLASSIFICATION

Fractures of both bones of the forearm are usually classified according to the level of fracture, the pattern of the fracture, the degree of displacement, the presence or absence of comminution or segment bone loss, and whether they are open or closed. Each of these factors may have some bearing on the type of treatment to be selected and the ultimate prognosis. For descriptive purposes it is useful to divide the forearm into thirds, based on the linear dimensions of the radius and ulna. Disruption of the proximal or distal radioulnar joints is of great significance to treatment and prognosis. It is imperative to determine whether the fracture is associated with joint injury because effective treatment demands that both the fracture and the joint injury be treated in an integrated fashion.

SIGNS AND SYMPTOMS

In adults, nondisplaced diaphyseal fractures of the shafts of both bones of the forearm are rare. An injury of sufficient force to break both the radius and the ulna is almost always sufficient to cause displacement. Because shaft fractures of both the radius and ulna are usually displaced, the signs and symptoms frequently make the diagnosis obvious. They include pain, deformity, and loss of function of the forearm and hand. Palpation along the subcutaneous border of the ulna usually elicits tenderness at the level of the fracture. Some degree of swelling is almost always present and is usually related to both the force causing the injury and the time since the injury. The examiner should not attempt to elicit crepitus, because this is painful and may cause additional soft-tissue damage. However, it may be noted when the forearm is aligned for splinting.

The physical examination should include a careful neurologic evaluation of the motor and sensory functions of the radial, median, and ulnar nerves. Neurologic deficits are not common in closed fractures of the shafts of the radius and ulna, but they do occur. One should also check the vascular status of the forearm as well as the amount of swelling. If the forearm is swollen and tense, a compartment syndrome may be present or may be developing. The extremity must be carefully examined for the presence or absence of this potentially devastating condition. The most valuable clinical test to diagnose a compartment syndrome is passive stretch of the fingers. If pain in the forearm is present when the fingers are passively extended, a compartment syndrome is probably present. If the patient is obtunded or otherwise noncooperative, compartment pressures should be measured to rule out the possibility of compartment syndrome. Immediate treatment by fasciotomy is required when a compartment syndrome is diagnosed (see Chapter 8).

Open fractures, especially those caused by gunshot wounds, frequently have associated nerve and major blood vessel involvement. This involvement must be carefully evaluated. Urgent treatment is required for open fractures (see Chapter 6). A sterile dressing should be placed over the wound. In open fractures it is a mistake to probe the wound while the patient is in the emergency department. This may carry contamination deeper into the wound and increase the risk of infection. The soft-tissue damage can be evaluated more objectively and more safely at the time of formal debridement in the operating room.

RADIOGRAPHIC FINDINGS

Just as the clinical signs and symptoms are usually obvious in shaft fractures of both bones of the forearm, so are the radiologic signs. The configuration of midshaft fractures of the radius and ulna varies depending on the mechanism of injury and the degree of violence involved. Low-energy fractures tend to be transverse or short oblique, whereas high energy injuries are frequently extensively comminuted or segmented, often with extensive soft-tissue injuries.[60]

A minimum of two views (anteroposterior and lateral) are mandatory in all suspected forearm fractures, and additional oblique views may be required. It is important to note the degree of offset and angulation as well as the amount of shortening and comminution. It is absolutely imperative to include the elbow and wrist joints in x-rays of the forearm to ascertain if there is an associated dislocation or articular fracture. Adequate visualization may require multiple (anteroposterior, lateral, and oblique) views of either the proximal or the distal radioulnar joints to determine the presence or absence of joint subluxation or dislocation. A line drawn through the radial shaft, neck, and head should pass through the center of the capitellum on any projection.[63] Associated injury to these joints is important to diagnose because it impacts heavily on prognosis and treatment.

The rotational alignment of the forearm is difficult to determine in ordinary anteroposterior and lateral x-rays. The bicipital tuberosity view recommended by Evans[32] is often helpful (Fig. 13-8). Because the surgeon has no control over the proximal radial fragment with closed methods, the distal radial fragment must be brought into correct relationship with the proximal

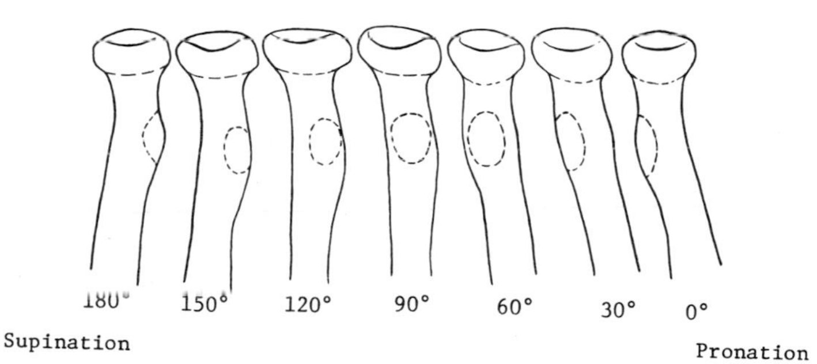

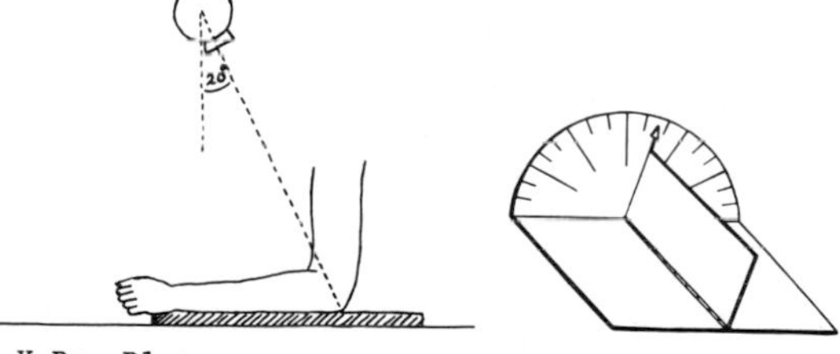

FIGURE 13-8. The tuberosity view. The position of the humeral condyles should be at equal distance from the x-ray film. The appearance of the bicipital tuberosity of the radius is shown at the top in different degrees of pronation and supination. The protractor for measuring rotation is shown at the bottom right. The hand is laid against the vertical plate, and the degree of rotation is read from the calibrated scale. (*Evans, E.M.: Rotational Deformity in the Treatment of Fractures of Both Bones of the Forearm. J. Bone Joint Surg., 27:373–379, 1945.*)

fragment. Ascertaining the rotation of the proximal fragment from the tuberosity view before reduction gives some idea of how much pronation or supination of the distal fragment is needed. The tuberosity view is made with the x-ray tube tilted 20° toward the olecranon, with the subcutaneous border of the ulna flat on the cassette. The x-ray can then be compared with a diagram showing the prominence of the tubercle in various degrees of pronation or supination. As an alternative, a film of the opposite elbow can be made in a given degree of rotation for comparison.

FRACTURE EPONYMS

There is no eponym associated with fractures of both bones of the forearm. The fracture of the shaft of the ulna with associated dislocation of the radial head was first described by Monteggia[73] in 1814 and has been known as the Monteggia fracture since then (see the discussion later in this chapter). The single-bone fracture of the ulna without dislocation of the radial head is often called a nightstick fracture, an obvious reference to one of the mechanisms of injury. The single-bone fracture of the radius in the distal third associated with dislocation of the radioulnar joint has several eponyms. Galeazzi,[73,116] of Italy, called attention to this treacherous injury in 1934, and since then it has been referred to as Galeazzi's fracture (see the discussion later in this chapter).

TREATMENT

The clinician has a variety of options for treating the patient with a fracture of both bones of the forearm. Cast immobilization, plate fixation, intramedullary nail fixation, and external fixation all have appropriate indications. However, it is fair to say that the vast majority of fractures of both bones of the forearm can be most effectively treated by accurate anatomical reduction, rigid plate fixation, and early mobilization of the soft tissues. Few other fractures are as amenable to treatment by this means as fractures of the shafts of the radius and ulna. The education of trainees and the emphasis by surgeons who only occasionally deal with this fracture should be directed toward perfecting this method of treatment.

Operative Versus Nonoperative Treatment

The treatment of displaced fractures of the shafts of the radius and ulna is primarily operative. Closed treatment of displaced fractures of the radius and ulna should not be considered "conservative," but should only be undertaken if there is a specific contraindication to operative treatment. The authors' indications for open reduction are summarized in Table 13-1. Nondisplaced fractures of the shafts of *both* the radius and the ulna are rare in adults.

Methods of Treatment

Cast Immobilization

The rare nondisplaced fracture of both bones of the forearm in adults can usually be treated by immobilization in a well-molded, long-arm cast in neutral pronation-supination with the elbow flexed to 90°. The completed cast should extend from the axilla to the midpalm, trimming the cast sufficiently to allow full motion of the fingers. Angulation of the fracture can occur in the cast. As Patrick[69] has pointed out, angulation may occur because much of the weight of the cast is taken by the collar-and-cuff sling. If the sling is attached to the cast distal to the level of the fractures, the cast may sag in this area as atrophy of the proximal forearm muscles occurs. Distally there is less soft tissue, so the forearm bones are still held firmly by the cast. As a result, angulation can occur (Fig. 13-9).

Angulation can be prevented by incorporating a wire or plaster loop on the radial side of the cast proximal to the level of the fractures. Suspending the cast from the patient's neck with a sling through this loop helps prevent angulation of the fractures by keeping the cast firmly against the ulna (Fig. 13-10). The loop should never be placed distal to the fracture, because this increases the chance of angulation. Despite good technique, an initially nondisplaced fracture can become displaced while immobilized in plaster. For this reason, x-rays should be made in both anteroposterior and lateral planes at weekly intervals for the first 4 weeks. If the fracture does displace, it should be treated as though it were displaced initially.

Plastic Deformation

In 1982, Greene[35] reported a case of a 24-year-old woman with plastic deformation of both bones of the forearm after a conveyor belt injury. Because little or no remodeling occurs in diaphyseal fractures in adults,

TABLE 13-1
Authors' Indications for Open Reduction of Fractures of the Shafts of the Radius and Ulna

All displaced fractures of radius and ulna in adults
All isolated displaced fractures of the radius
Isolated fractures of the ulna with angulation greater than 10°
All Monteggia fractures
All Galeazzi fractures
Open fractures
Fractures associated with a compartment syndrome, regardless of the degree of displacement.

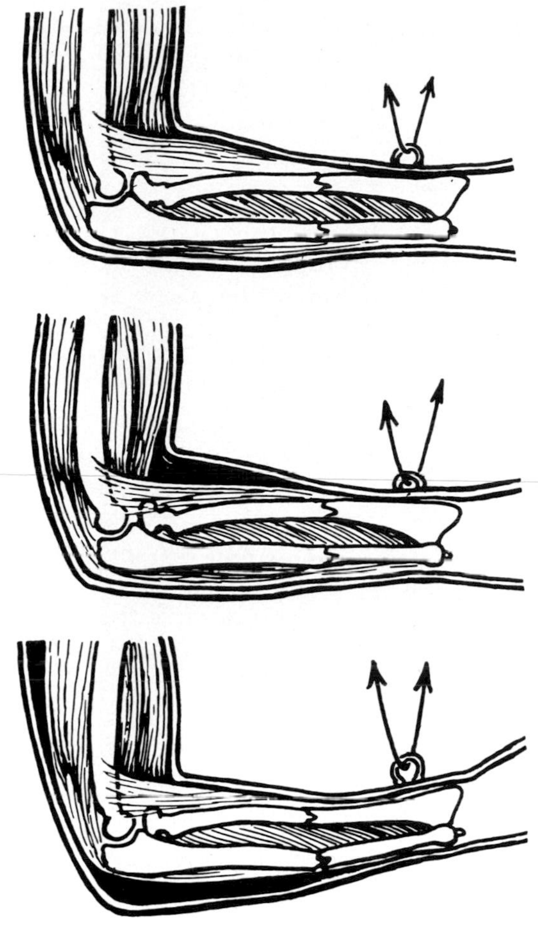

FIGURE 13-9. Angulation of the radius and ulna during the period of cast immobilization. (*Top*) Immediately after reduction the cast fits snugly. (*Center*) Swelling has subsided with consequent loosening of the cast in the upper half of the forearm. (*Bottom*) The cast has sagged while still holding the distal fragment firmly, thus causing angulation of the radius and ulna. (*Knight, R.A., and Purvis, G.D.: Fractures of Both Bones of the Forearm in Adults. J. Bone Joint Surg., 31A:755–764, 1949.*)

he recommended closed manipulation under anesthesia, noting that considerable force is required for correction. Scheuer and Pot[87] reported a similar case in 1986 in which the radius and ulna were forcibly fractured by closed manipulation. Their patient required a fasciotomy. They pointed out that the bowing of the bone due to plastic deformation is often subtle, and if this feature is suspected, a comparison view of the uninjured arm may be helpful. They concluded that incompletely reduced plastic deformities in older children and young adults resulted in significant loss of forearm rotation and, therefore, they recommended closed reduction under general anesthesia with stabilization by intramedullary nailing if necessary.

Closed Reduction and Cast Immobilization

For the reasons outlined in the discussion of surgical anatomy, it is difficult to reduce and maintain satisfactory position of the fragments by closed methods. Therefore, closed reduction and cast immobilization is *not* recommended for most displaced fractures of both bones of the forearm in adults. Knight and Purvis[49] analyzed 100 adults with shaft fractures of both bones of the forearm treated at the Campbell Clinic, of which approximately half had been treated by closed methods. Of those treated closed, 71% had unsatisfactory results, and the incidence of nonunion and malunion was high. Closed reduction is most successful for fractures of both the radius and ulna when the fractures are located in the distal third (Fig. 13-11). However, closed reduction should *not* be undertaken unless there is a contraindication to open treatment. If closed treatment is undertaken, the patient must be advised that he or she may require open reduction and internal fixation at any time to ensure solid union in an acceptable position.

Most series[44,49,69] report a high percentage of unsatisfactory results with closed treatment. However, the report of Sarmiento and associates[82] in 1975 and the excellent book by Sarmiento and Latta[83] on the use of early functional bracing for forearm fractures are significant exceptions. Sarmiento reported treatment of 44 fractures of both bones of the forearm. The fractures were initially reduced with the patient under

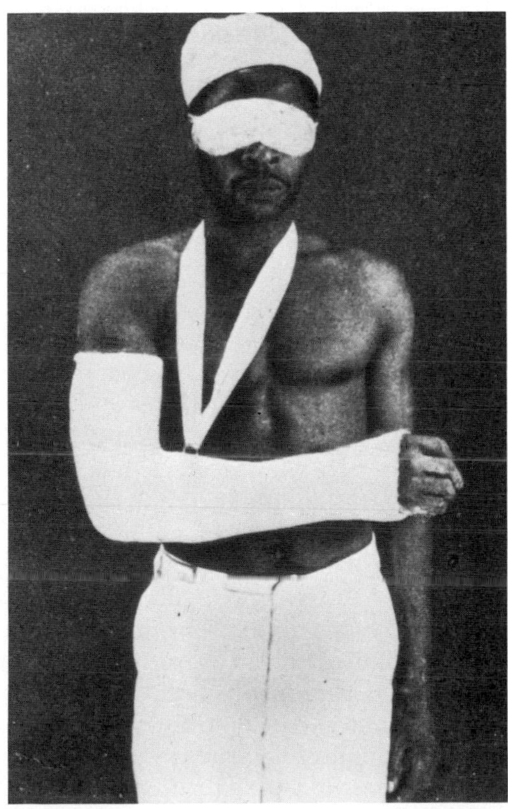

FIGURE 13-10. The proper method of suspending a cast by a sling so that the ulnar border of the cast is kept snugly against the forearm to prevent ulnar angulation. (*Knight, R.A., and Purvis, G.D.: Fractures of Both Bones of the Forearm in Adults. J. Bone Joint Surg., 31A:755–764, 1949.*)

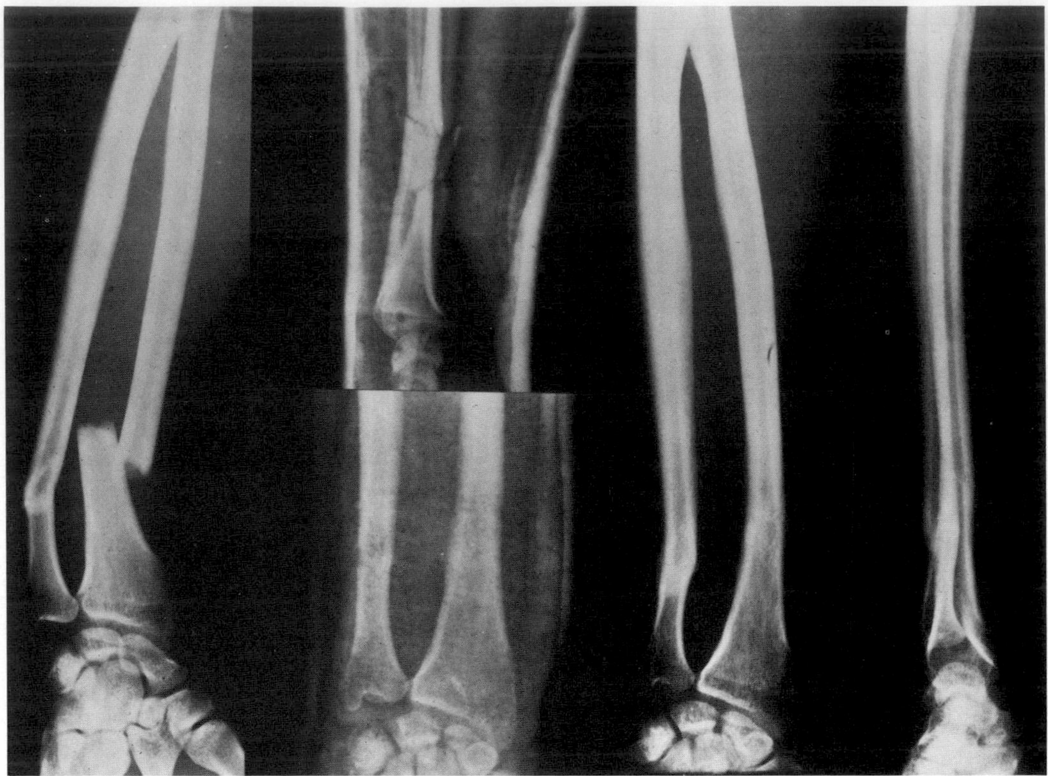

FIGURE 13-11. Satisfactory closed reduction and cast immobilization in fractures of the distal third of the radius and ulna. The fractures united with only mild narrowing of the interosseous space. (*Sage, F.P.: Fractures of the Shafts of the Radius and Ulna in the Adult. In Adams, J.P.* [*ed.*]*: Current Practice in Orthopaedic Surgery, vol. 1. St. Louis, C.V. Mosby, 1963.*)

anesthesia and the forearms placed in long-arm casts. Reduction was lost in four patients, and open reduction and internal fixation was carried out. The initial long-arm casts were replaced after an average of 18 days with a functional brace that limited pronation and supination but permitted flexion and extension of the elbow. Active exercise of the fingers was encouraged. The results were surprisingly good. In 39 patients the fractures united, and there was only one nonunion. Sarmiento found that 10° malalignment in any plane resulted in only a few degrees' loss of pronation and supination. This finding was supported by the laboratory work of Tarr, Garfinkel, and Sarmiento[96] and Matthews and coworkers.[62] They demonstrated on fresh cadaver specimens that angular and rotatory deformities of *10° or less* resulted in minimal limitation of pronation-supination and were readily acceptable to the patient in clinical practice. The healing time averaged 16 weeks for the entire series, including the one nonunion. Some of the patients had less than anatomical reductions, but despite this, good functional results were obtained. Over many years, Sarmiento and his associates have demonstrated considerable skill in the use of functional bracing. However, it must be emphasized that their results have not been duplicated by others, to the best of my knowledge. The reader is referred to the book by Sarmiento and Latta[83] for details of treatment by this method.

As a practical matter, I rarely attempt closed treatment for displaced fractures of both bones of the forearm in adults, unless some other condition of the patient precludes surgical treatment. The results are much too uncertain, and the period of immobilization is too long with this method of treatment.

Technique of Closed Reduction. Relaxation of the muscles is mandatory for closed reduction, and general anesthesia is usually the best choice. With the patient under anesthesia, the image intensifier is used to obtain a tuberosity view if that has not already been done. Finger traps or clove hitches of gauze are then placed on the thumb, index finger, and middle finger to suspend the extremity from an overhead frame or intravenous stand with the elbow flexed 90°. Countertraction is applied by means of a loop of muslin, stockinette, or other suitable material that is placed over the distal arm about 3 inches above the elbow. This is tied at a convenient height from the floor so that the surgeon's foot can be placed in it for countertraction. (An alternative method is to suspend 10 to 15 lb of weight from the loop.) The loop over the distal humerus is padded to prevent excessive pressure.

Traction and countertraction are applied, and an attempt is made to reduce the ulna under direct palpation. The radius usually cannot be palpated in the proximal half of the forearm because of swelling and overlying muscles. The forearm is placed in the appropriate amount of supination, as determined by the tuberosity view. When the fractures seem reduced and the alignment of the forearm appears satisfactory, a single layer of padding is applied from the midpalm to above the elbow with an extra layer over the bony prominences. A sugar-tong splint is then applied and molded well as it sets. Anteroposterior and lateral x-rays are taken to evaluate the reduction. Anything less than near anatomical reduction should not be accepted. If the reduction is not acceptable, the sugar tong is removed and the fractures are remanipulated.

If an acceptable reduction is achieved, the muslin loop is removed from the upper arm and the sugar tong is converted into a well-molded, long-arm cast while the extremity is still suspended. As the cast hardens, the posterior aspect of the cast plaster is flattened from the olecranon proximally to prevent the cast from slipping distally. Final x-rays are taken after the cast is completed. The cast should be suspended from the neck by a sling passed through a loop on the radial side of the cast. As mentioned in the discussion of nondisplaced fractures (see above), this loop should be at or proximal to the level of the fracture.

Aftercare

The circulation and function of the hand must be observed carefully until the swelling begins to decrease. During this period, the arm should be elevated by suspending it from an overhead frame with the fingers uppermost. The elbow should rest on the bed. Active flexion and extension of the fingers should be encouraged at frequent intervals to help reduce edema. If at any time the circulation appears in jeopardy, the cast should be split from the axilla to the hand on both sides, including the padding. Loss of reduction is not nearly as catastrophic as gangrene or Volkman's ischemic contracture.

Radiographs in two planes should be made at weekly intervals through the cast for the first month and every 2 weeks thereafter until union is solid. Each new set of films should be compared with the *original postreduction films that were accepted.* A common error is to compare the most recent films with the films from the previous visit. If this is done, a gradual loss of reduction goes undetected until it is too late. The cast should be changed at intervals of 4 to 6 weeks. Each new cast must be applied as carefully as the first one. The fractures can angulate even after some callus is present. There is no margin for error due to a sloppily applied cast.

Open Reduction and Internal Fixation

Over the years many methods of open reduction and internal fixation have been advocated. Open reduction without internal fixation has all the disadvantages of both open and closed treatment and has no place in the modern treatment of fractures of the shaft of the radius and ulna in adults.

Timing of Surgery

Displaced fractures of both bones of the adult should be fixed as soon as practicable, preferably within the first 24 to 48 hours of injury. The majority of patients in the series of Schemitsch and Richards[86] were operated on within 24 hours of injury. Mallin[60] believes that forearm fractures are best internally fixed as soon after injury as practical, preferably before the onset of swelling. In Hadden and colleagues AO series,[39] 44% of open and 23% of closed fractures were plated during the first 24 hours. Their reasons for delaying open treatment included patients with polytrauma in whom other injuries took priority, lack of availability of experienced personnel, and awaiting wound healing in open fractures (early in the series). Their current recommendation is primary fixation of open fractures. Chapman and colleagues[19] also recommend fixation of open fractures on the day of injury in most cases, unless other injuries preclude fixation.

We recommend open reduction and internal fixation on an emergent basis for open fractures of both bones of the forearm. Closed fractures of both bones of the forearm are best treated in the same manner on an urgent basis, if possible within 24 hours of injury.

Fixation with Plates and Screws

Historical Review. In the early 1900s, Lane,[8,54,55] in London, and Lambotte,[8,52,53] in Belgium, reported the use of plates for treating diaphyseal fractures. However, metal reaction led to frequent failures until modern metals for implantation were introduced in 1937 after the work of Venable and associates[103] on electrolysis. Campbell and Boyd[18] used autogenous tibial grafts fixed to the radius and ulna with bone pegs or screws for acute fractures as well as nonunions. Some of these attempts were successful, but unless external immobilization was prolonged, the grafts often developed fatigue fractures before they were revascularized.[49]

Even after better metals became available, many of the early plates used for fractures of the radius and ulna were poorly designed. Failures were common because adequate fixation was not achieved (Fig. 13-12). For a time, the use of plates and screws for the internal fixation of diaphyseal fractures fell into disfavor. Many surgeons treating fractures thought that fixation with a plate and screws held the fracture distracted and caused delayed union and nonunion. This belief was still common in the early 1960s.

Plate-and-screw fixation slowly began regaining favor after Eggers and associates[28–31] introduced the slotted plate or "contact splint," as he preferred to call it. The plate was designed with slots rather than round holes so that, theoretically, the longitudinal muscle

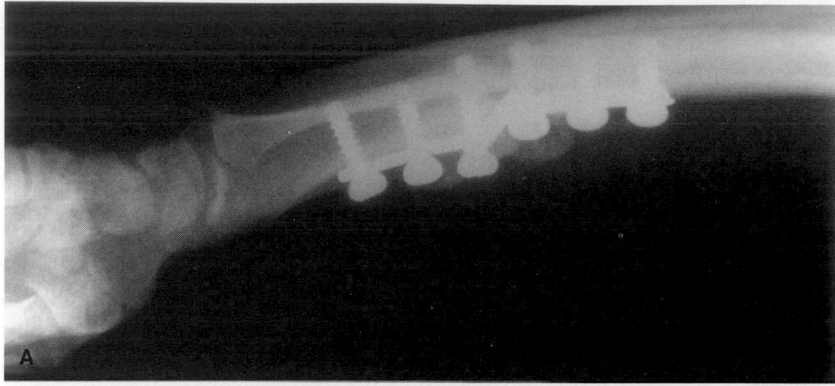

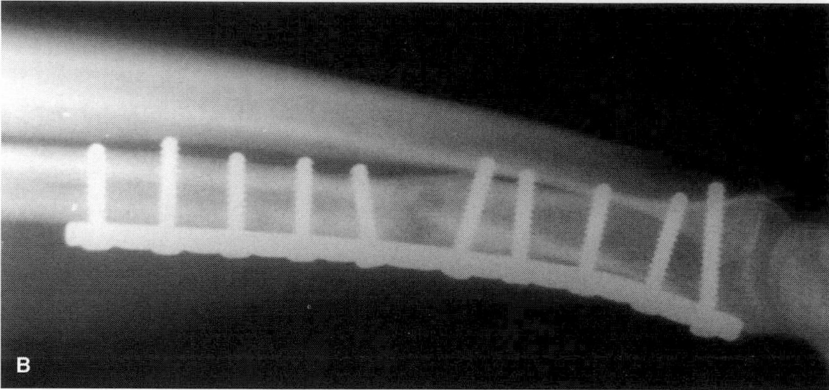

FIGURE 13-12. (**A**) Nonunion of a distal radius fracture due to inadequate fixation. The surgeon used a one-third tubular (small fragment) plate with large fragment screws. Predictably, a nonunion occurred, with breakage of the plate. (**B**) The nonunion was repaired with a contoured 10-hole 3.5-mm dynamic compression plate without bone grafting. The nonunion healed once adequate fixation was achieved without the need for supplementary external immobilization or bone grafting. The nonunion rate after plate fixation is very low if proper technique is used.

pull acting across the fracture would keep the bones in contact and promote union. Whether this actually happened was debatable. After the first few days, fibrous tissue and callus probably grew into the slots so that sliding was no longer possible. In any case, the Eggers plate was a much stronger plate than those used previously, and it provided better fixation. In 1960, Jinkins and coworkers[46] reported a series of 165 forearm fractures in which 145 slotted plates and 20 medullary nails had been used. The overall nonunion rate was only 4.2%. They concluded that the results were best when a slotted plate was used for the ulna and either a slotted plate or a Rush pin was used for the radius.

The idea of using plates through which active compression could be applied began with Danis[21] of Belgium. He published a book in 1949 in which the use of such plates was described. Danis revealed that diaphyseal fractures treated with these plates healed with very little peripheral callus, a phenomenon that he referred to as *primary fracture healing.* The plate used by Danis had a coapting screw at one end through which compression was applied.

Venable[102] described a similar plate in 1951. Boreau and Hermann[9] introduced a plate with two parts in which a cylindrical bolt forced the fragments together. Bagby and Janes[7] modified a Collison plate with oval holes, allowing compression to be achieved by eccentric placement of the screws. In 1958, Müller, Allgöwer, and Willenegger developed what is now known as the ASIF (AO*) compression plate (Fig. 13-13). The technique for using this plate and other techniques of the AO group were published in 1965.[66]

In 1975 Anderson and associates reported clinical experience from the Campbell Clinic with the AO compression plate for forearm fractures over the period from 1960 to 1970.[6] During this time, 258 adults with displaced fractures of the radius and ulna were treated with compression-plate fixation. Fourteen of these patients were lost to follow-up before the outcome was known. The remaining 244 were followed an average of 13.2 months: 112 had fractures of both bones of the forearm, 82 had single fractures of the radius, and 50 had single fractures of the ulna. All 132 patients with single-bone fractures of the radius or ulna were treated with compression plates. Of the 112 patients with both bones fractured, 86 had both fractures fixed with compression plates (Fig. 13-14). Of the remainder, 25 had the fracture of the radius fixed with a compression plate and the fracture of the ulna fixed with some other device (usually a Sage triangular nail). In 1 other patient, the ulna was fixed with a compression plate and the radius with a Sage nail. Thus, 137 fractures of the ulna and 193 fractures of the radius were treated by this method, a total of 330 forearm bones.

* ASIF (Association for the Study of Internal Fixation) is the English translation of AO (Arbeitgemeinschaft für Osteosynthesefragen).

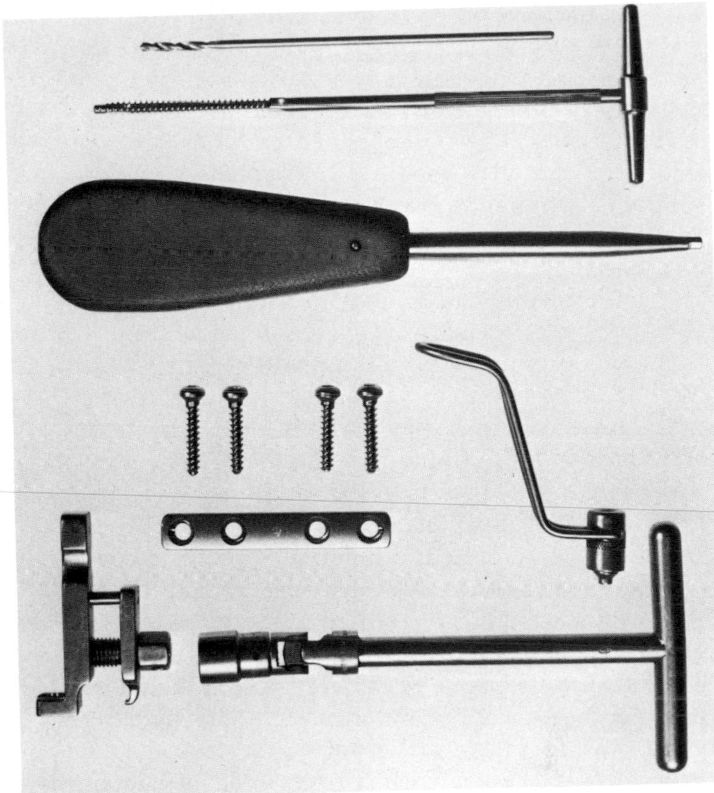

FIGURE 13-13. The original AO (ASIF) compression instruments. The 4.5-mm four-hole plate originally recommended for the human forearm was subsequently recognized as being too heavy and too short. The screws had small cores with large threads and were not self-tapping. The drill bit shown at the top had the same diameter as the core of the screws. The tap seen just below the drill bit was used to cut threads in the bone exactly matching those of the screws. The drill guide seen to the right of the screws was used to center the drill exactly so that the heads of the screws countersunk accurately into the plate. The compression device (shown at the bottom left with the wrench for tightening this device at the lower right) is rarely used now, having been supplanted by the dynamic compression plate. (*Anderson, L.D.: Compression Plate Fixation and the Effect of Different Types of Internal Fixation on Fracture Healing. J. Bone Joint Surg., 47A:191, 1965.*)

Twenty-eight patients (11.4%) had open fractures, and 216 patients (88.6%) had closed fractures. Campbell Clinic policy at that time was to delay internal fixation in most open fractures. The period of delay in these 28 patients ranged from 1 to 3 weeks. The average time of delay was 10.6 days. Autogenous iliac bone grafts were used if one third or more of the circumference of the bone was comminuted. Also, in two-bone fractures, if one bone was grafted because of comminution, the other bone was also grafted regardless of its comminution. In accordance with this policy, 63 of the 244 patients (25.9%) had bone grafts applied. The overall results of the Campbell Clinic Study are shown in Table 13-2 for fractures of the ulna and in Table

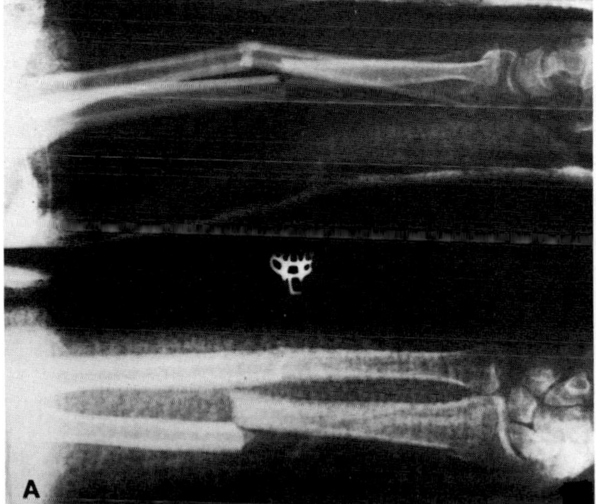

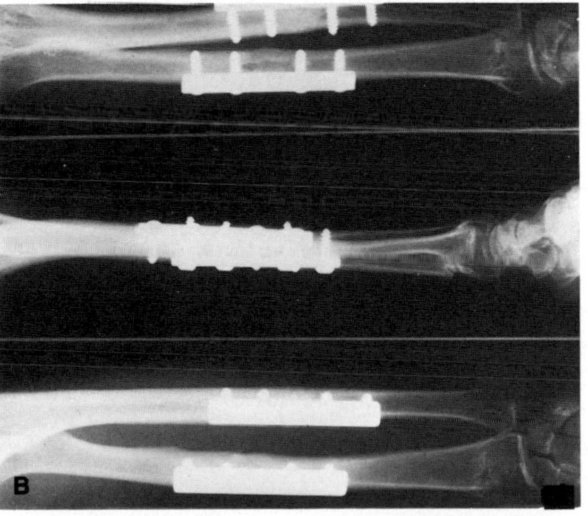

FIGURE 13-14. (**A**) Fractures of the radius and ulna in the middle third temporarily immobilized in a cast before surgery. Note that there is also a fracture of the distal radius. (**B**) Two years after open reduction and internal fixation with compression plates the radial bow is well maintained and the fractures show good union. The fracture of the distal radius was treated by cast immobilization for 6 weeks.

13-3 for fractures of the radius.[6] The nonunion rate was 3.7% for the ulna and 2.1% for the radius. The percentage of fractures that united compares favorably with that of other reports in the literature.

The functional results obtained by Anderson and associates were very good. Of 223 patients for whom sufficient information was available to determine the degree of function restored, the results were considered excellent in 131, satisfactory in 69, and fair in 16. The results in 7 patients who required additional operations for nonunion were considered failures.

The proportion in whom nonunion occurred when bone grafts were used was almost identical to that when grafts were not used (Table 13-4).[6] Schemitsch and Richards[86] also found that the use of bone grafts was not correlated with a higher influence of bone union after plate fixation of either forearm bone. These facts can be interpreted in different ways. One could conclude that bone grafting did not promote union. However, since grafts were used in the more comminuted fractures, a more reasonable conclusion seems to be that, when bone grafts are used, comminuted fractures heal as well as noncomminuted fractures. Obviously this is not a proven fact; to do so, one would have to prospectively treat a large series of patients with and without bone grafts and then determine whether the rate of nonunion could be correlated with the degree of comminution or the use of bone grafts.

Naiman and coworkers[67] and Dodge and Cody[25] reported a series of diaphyseal fractures of the radius and ulna treated by compression plates. In Naiman and coworkers' series, all 30 fractures united. Dodge and Cody also encountered no nonunions in their 78 patients in whom compression plates were used. However, ten infections occurred; the incidence was 3% in closed fractures and 36% in open fractures.

In 1980, Teipner and Mast[98] published a study comparing double plating with single compression plating for diaphyseal fractures of the forearm. Their double-plating technique was the one described by Jergensen in 1960.[45] The single compression (tension band) was carried out using the recommendations of the AO group.[66] Fifty-five patients with 84 fractures were treated using the double-plating technique. In this group there were 82 unions and 2 nonunions. They used a single compression plate in 48 patients with 70 fractures. All 70 of these fractures progressed to union. The authors concluded that both double plating and single compression plating are very effective methods of treating fractures of the diaphysis of the radius and ulna. However, they found that AO compression plating provided a shorter operative time and, at least theoretically, less stress protection of the bone and less devitalization of tissue from exposure. For these reasons, they reverted to the single compression-plate technique almost entirely.

In 1981, Rosacker and Kopta[77] reported 54 patients with two-bone fractures of the forearm treated with various fixation devices. Three major types of fixation were used: conventional plates, compression plates, and intramedullary rods. There were 108 fractures in the 54 patients. These workers found that their best results occurred when the fractures were reduced anatomically. The highest percentage of fractures that were anatomically reduced were those treated with compression plates. The authors suggested that it may be more difficult to apply a compression plate without reducing the fracture anatomically than it is to use a medullary rod or conventional plate with a suboptimal reduction. The authors used the criteria of Anderson and coworkers[6] to assess function. Excellent functional results were obtained in 56% of their patients and satisfactory results in 31%. This total of 87% acceptable results is very comparable to the results achieved by the Campbell Clinic group. The single factor most often associated with an excellent result was the adequacy of the reduction.

Rosacker and Kopta found delayed surgery to be a favorable factor in obtaining primary union. This phenomenon has been observed by others.[50,51,93] In Rosacker and Kopta's series, 19 patients with 38 fractures had their surgery delayed from 1 to 3 weeks

TABLE 13-2
Results of Compression Plate Fixation for Fractures of the Ulna

	Fractures	Union	Nonunion	Rate of Union
Ulna only	50	48	2	96
Ulna and radius	87	84	3	96.5
Total	137	132	5	96.3

Anderson, L.D., Sisk, T.D., Tooms, R.E., and Park, W.I., III: Compression-plate Fixation in Acute Diaphyseal Fractures of the Radius and Ulna. J. Bone Joint Surg., 57A:287–297, 1975.

TABLE 13-3
Results of Compression Plate Fixation for Fractures of the Radius

	Fractures	Union	Nonunion	Rate of Union
Radius only	82	80	2	97.5
Radius and ulna	111	109	2	98.2
Total	193	189	4	97.9

Anderson, L.D., Sisk, T.D., Tooms, R.E., and Park, W.I., III: Compression-plate Fixation in Acute Diaphyseal Fractures of the Radius and Ulna. J. Bone Joint Surg., 57A:287–297, 1975.

TABLE 13-4
Results of Compression Plate Fixation With and Without Bone Grafting

	Fractures	Union	Nonunion	Rate of Union
Radius without graft	149	146	3	97.3
Radius with graft	44	43	1	97.8
Ulna without graft	91	87	4	95.6
Ulna with graft	46	45	1	97.8
Total	330	321	9	97.3

Anderson, L.D., Sisk, T.D., Tooms, R.E., and Park, W.I., III: Compression-plate Fixation in Acute Diaphyseal Fractures of the Radius and Ulna. J. Bone Joint Surg., 57A:287–297, 1975.

for a variety of reasons. All of these fractures healed primarily. However, the authors pointed out that the economic factors associated with prolonged hospitalization and delayed surgery probably offset the healing benefit of postponing surgery, factors that are even more true today. In addition, early motion is beneficial to the soft tissues and tends to facilitate and maximize the range of motion that patients recover after fractures of both bones of the forearm.

In contrast to Anderson and associates,[5] Rosacker and Kopta[77] did not advocate primary bone grafting for comminution involving more than one third the circumference of the bone. However, 11 of their 54 patients required subsequent bone grafting for delayed union of their forearm fractures. This is 19%, compared with 2.7% in Anderson's series. Whether to use bone grafting primarily for comminuted fractures is a matter of judgment and opinion. The individual surgeon must decide whether it is better to primarily use bone grafting for all fractures that are significantly comminuted while the patient is under an anesthetic and the forearm bones are exposed or to defer bone grafting until a second operation only if nonunion or delayed union occurs.

Schemitsch and Richards[86] observed 55 adult patients with fractures of both bones of the forearm treated by plating for a mean of 6 years (range, 1–16 years). A complete functional and radiographic assessment was performed at follow-up. Malunion was quantified by measuring the amount and location of the maximum radial bow in relation to the opposite, normal forearm. Fifty-four of the radial and 54 of the ulnar fractures united. Eighty-four percent of the patients achieved an excellent, good, or acceptable functional result. Seven patients had bone grafts taken from the iliac crest. The indications of bone graft were major bone loss or comminution or both. However, not all the fractures with these features were bone grafted. Bone grafting did not affect the rate of union according to a chi-square test. Restoration of the normal radial bow was related to functional outcome. A good functional result (greater than 80% of normal forearm rotation) was associated with restoration of the normal amount and location of the radial bow ($p < .05$ and $p < .005$, respectively) (Figs. 13-15 and 13-16). Similarly, the recovery of grip strength was associated with the restoration of the location of the radial bow toward normalcy ($p < .005$).

Compression-plate fixation of forearm fractures is the preferred technique of most authors.[2,19,39,40,56,60,90] Sisk[90] pointed out that plates and screws are especially useful for fractures of the distal third or proximal fourth of the radial shaft and of the proximal third of the ulnar shaft. Fractures at these levels are poorly fixed with any other device. Chapman and associates[19] suggested that compression plates are indicated in all closed forearm fractures in adults in whom the radius or ulna is angulated greater than 10°. All authors now use the dynamic compression plate rather than the original AO plate with an outrigger (Fig. 13-17). This has the advantage of requiring less surgical exposure and has been shown by Anderson and Bacastow[2] to produce results comparable to those with the older-style plate.

Authors' Preferred Method of Treatment

Technique of Compression Plating. The technique of compression plating of forearm fractures has been described in detail in other texts.[4,65,66,90] Also, the principles of the AO (ASIF) techniques are presented in Chapter 3. However, some important points deserve emphasis here. Most failures in reported series of fractures of the forearm treated with compression plates have been due to errors in technique or to infection. Before compression plating is undertaken, the surgeon must be thoroughly familiar with the technique and, ideally, should have practiced it in a bioskills laboratory. A complete set of equipment must be available, and rigid aseptic technique must be enforced in the operating room.

Surgical Approach. Patients are positioned supine on the operating table with the extremity extended out on a hand table. A tourniquet is used unless

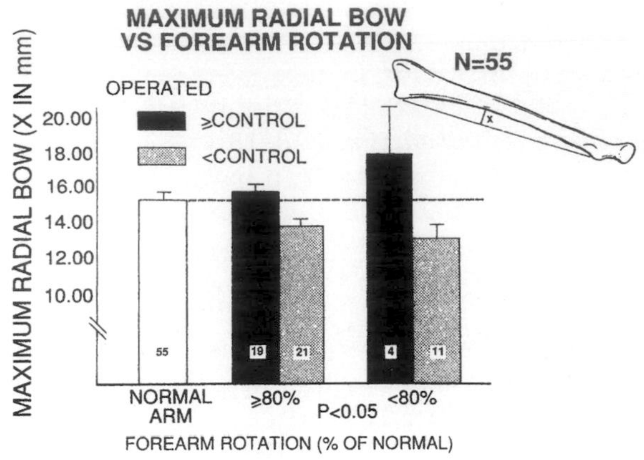

FIGURE 13-15. A histogram demonstrating the correlation between the amount of radial bow and forearm rotation after fixation of fractures of both bones of the forearm with plates. Both increased and decreased amounts of radial bow were associated with a significant reduction in the amount of forearm rotation. (*Schemitsch, E.H., and Richards, R.R.: The Effect of Malunion on Functional Outcome After Plate Fixation of Fractures of Both Bones of the Forearm in Adults. J. Bone Joint Surg., 74A:1068–1078, 1992.*)

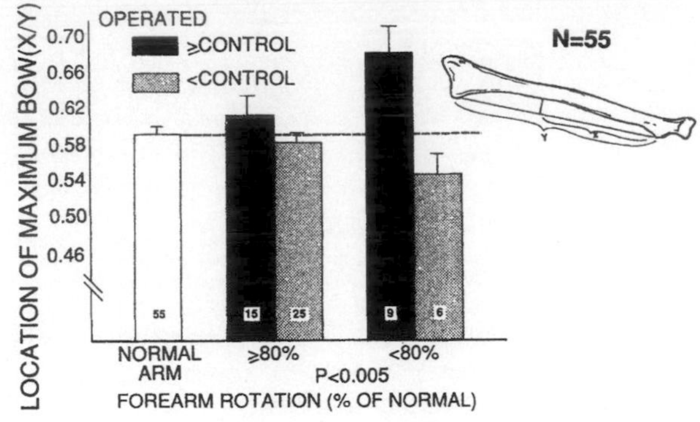

FIGURE 13-16. A histogram showing a similar correlation between the location of maximum radial bow and forearm rotation. (*Schemitsch, E.H., and Richards, R.R.: The Effect of Malunion on Functional Outcome After Plate Fixation of Fractures of Both Bones of the Forearm in Adults. J. Bone Joint Surg., 74A:1068–1078, 1992.*)

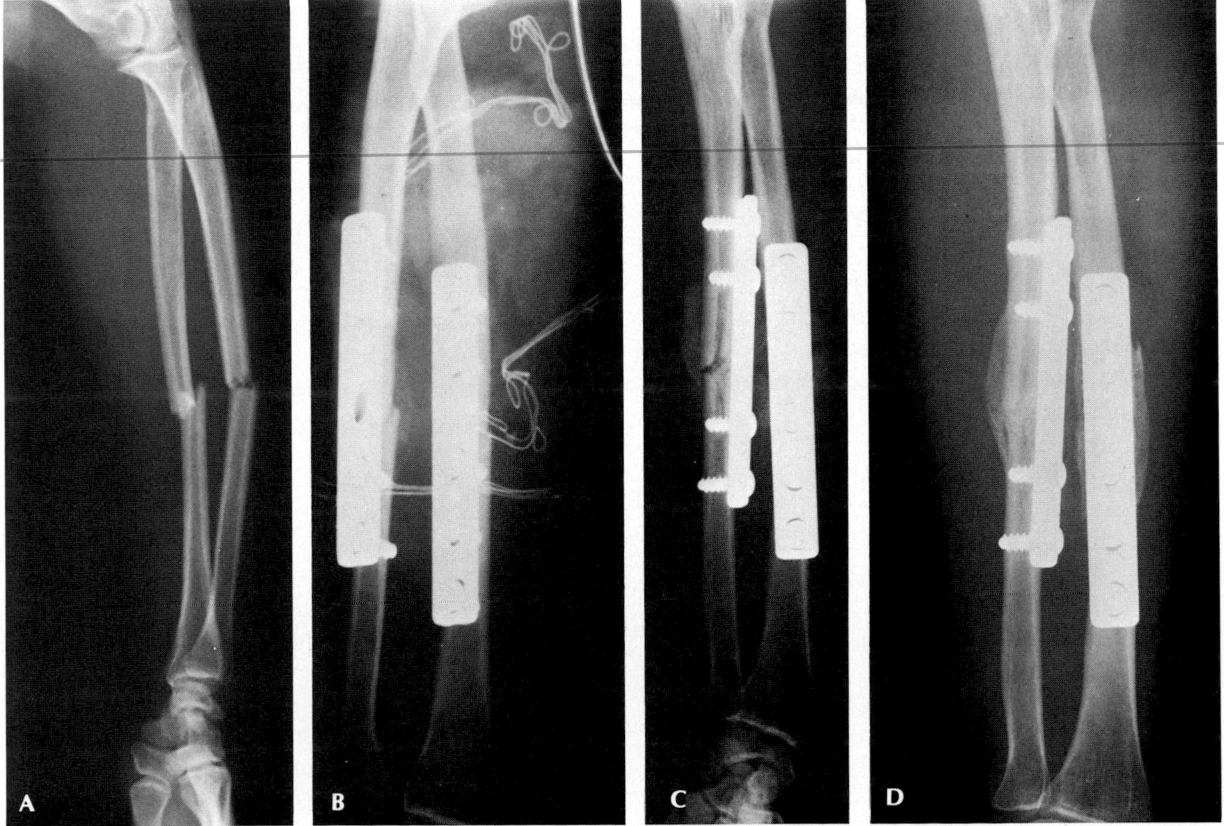

FIGURE 13-17. (**A**) Fractures of both bones of the forearm in the middle third. (**B**) Radiographs at the time of surgery. Fixation was achieved with two five-hole dynamic compression plates. Because of comminution, one hole in the ulnar plate was left empty and both fractures were bone-grafted. (**C**) At 6 weeks the comminution of the ulna and the iliac bone grafts are easily seen. (**D**) At 1 year the fractures are well united and the bone grafts have been incorporated. The patient had full range of motion in all planes.

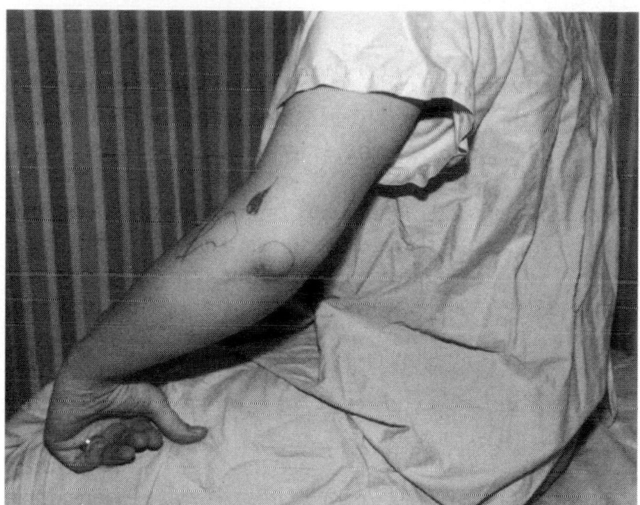

FIGURE 13-18. The posterior interosseous nerve crosses over the radial neck in the proximal forearm, where it is at risk of injury in posterior approaches to the radius in the proximal forearm. The authors recommend the volar approach to the radius to reduce the risk of injury to this nerve when plating fractures of the radius.

there has been a vascular injury. Two separate incisions are made. When the fracture of the radius is located in the distal half of the bone, most authors approach the radius through a volar Henry incision.[6,13,19,20,42] Anderson and associates[6] emphasized that although this is contrary to the principle of placing the plate on the tension side (dorsal radius), the soft-tissue coverage on the volar surface is better and the bone contour is flat, making it easier to apply the plate there. Also, there is less soft-tissue irritation and, thus, presumably, less likelihood of the need for subsequent plate removal. For fractures of the proximal half of the radius the dorsal Thompson approach has been recommended in the past,[6,13,20,99] positioning the plate on the dorsal surface. I recommend using the anterior (Henry) approach for *all* fractures of the radius, including very proximal fractures, so that the risk of posterior interosseous nerve injury is minimized (Figs. 13-18 and 13-19).[86] On occasion, a single incision can be used to approach fractures of the proximal ulna associated with dislocation of the radial head (see the section on Monteggia fractures).[14] If a posterior approach is used for very proximal fractures, the posterior interosseous nerve should be exposed and retracted. There is a great hazard of injuring the posterior interosseous nerve with a posterior approach, at the time of plate insertion and even more so during plate removal.[111] For this reason the posterior approach is not recommended.

For fractures of the ulna, the plate may be placed on either the volar or dorsal surface. The surface to be used is determined by which surface the plate fits better and the location of the comminuted fragments. If there is a butterfly fragment, it is reduced as accurately as possible and the plate is placed over the fragment to hold it in place.

Exposure of the Fracture Site. It was thought previously that exposure of the bone should be extraperiosteal. However, the work of Whiteside and Lesker,[109,110] demonstrated decreased blood flow to damaged muscle and impaired healing of osteotomies after extraperiosteal dissection. Therefore, most authors[19] now prefer subperiosteal exposure of the fracture minimizing of the amount of periosteal stripping. Only the fracture site and the surface on which the plate is to be applied should be stripped. Anderson preferred to place the plate on top of the periosteum because this was the technique used in his large series of forearm fractures in which the success rate was 97%.[6] However, this technique can compromise the accuracy of the reduction and I do not recommend it.

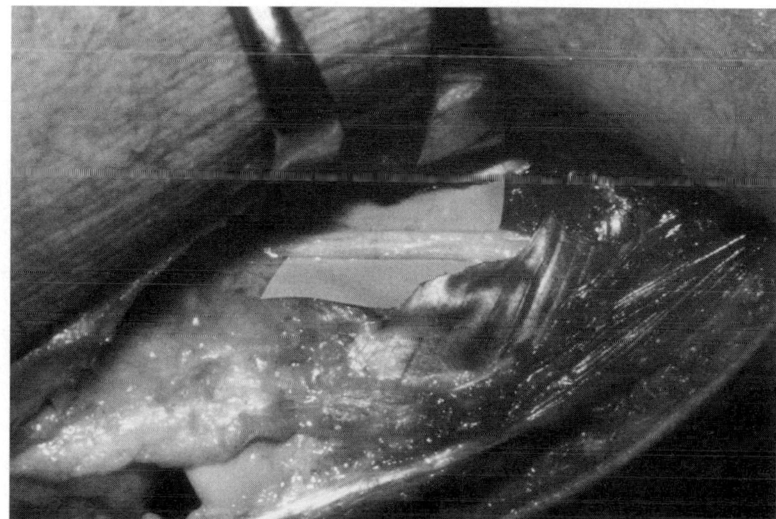

FIGURE 13-19. If a posterior approach to the radius is used, the posterior interosseous nerve should be identified. The nerve is small and difficult to safely dissect, particularly in the presence of a fracture, with the hemorrhage and edema that accompany fractures. The risk of injury to the nerve is minimized by the use of a volar (Henry) approach. The volar approach can be used to expose the entire radius.

Choice of Plate and Screws. The ideal length for the plate varies with the size of the plate, the amount of comminution, and the configuration of the fracture. An increasing number of authors[19,39,40] have advocated the use of 3.5-mm dynamic compression plates. In general, semitubular plates are not recommended for use in the forearm. However, in a patient with a very small ulna, Green (Green, D.P., personal communication, 1995) has used two semitubular plates stacked one on top of the other to provide improved strength. Chapman has shown no statistically significant difference in the rates of fracture union between the 4.5- and 3.5-mm dynamic compression plates. However, even in a transverse fracture, when 3.5-mm dynamic compression plates are used, it is usually necessary to use an eight-hole plate. Stern and Drury[94] reported a higher incidence of nonunion when four-hole plates were used. A longer plate must be used in very unstable or comminuted fractures. If the 3.5-mm dynamic compression plate is used, use of 3.5-mm cortical screws with 1.25-pitch threads allows the screw to grip the cortex of the bone with additional threads, which improves the pull-out strength. It is important to center the plate over the fracture so that no screw will be closer than 1 cm to the fracture line. If screws are placed closer than this, a crack may develop between the screw hole and the fracture as compression is applied and fixation will be compromised. It is therefore better to select a longer plate and leave one or two holes empty than to have screws too close to the fracture. In oblique fractures, either an additional lag screw is inserted in a different plane or an interfragmentary lag screw is used through the plate itself. Lag screw fixation across the fracture and any associated fragments increases the strength of the construct up to 40%. Most often, these screws are applied before axial compression of the fracture by the plate (Figs. 13-20 and 13-21).

Reduction of the Fracture. Whenever possible, comminuted fragments should be secured to the main fragments with lag screws to produce interfragmentary compression. When both the radius and ulna are fractured, both fractures should be exposed and reduced temporarily before a plate is applied to either; otherwise, fixation and reduction of one may be lost while an attempt is being made to reduce the other.

After the fracture is reduced and any comminuted fragments are fitted into place, a radial reduction clamp or bone-holding (eg, Lane) forceps is placed at each end of the plate to secure it temporarily to the bone. The third Lane forceps is placed directly over the fracture at right angles to the other two. Its purpose is to lock the comminuted fragments into place and to prevent shortening of oblique fractures as compression is applied. In unstable fractures, it is technically much easier to fix the plate to one fragment with a single screw before reduction. The fracture is then reduced to the plate-bone combination. This technique necessitates less soft-tissue dissection and makes it relatively easy to handle intercalary comminuted bone fragments as well. I frequently use this technique since it is often awkward to hold the fracture reduced and the plate applied with clamps.

Contouring the radial plate may prevent iatrogenic

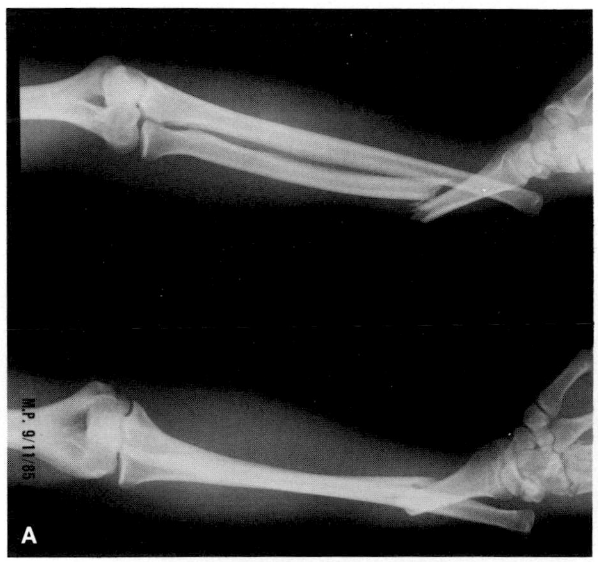

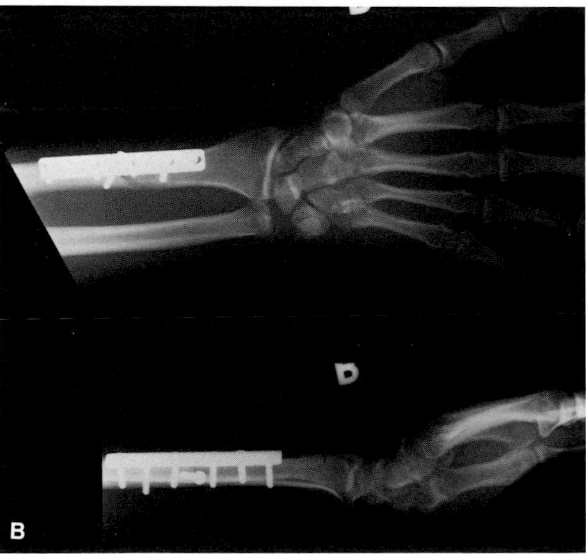

FIGURE 13-20. (**A**) Preoperative anteroposterior and lateral radiographs of a 25-year-old man with a closed Galeazzi fracture. (**B**) Postoperative radiographs showing primary fixation with a six-hole, 3.5-mm dynamic compression plate. Note the bicortical screws in the end holes and the separate interfragmentary screw. (*Chapman, M.W., Gordon, E.J., and Zissimos, A.G.: Compression-Plate Fixation of Acute Fractures of the Diaphyses of the Radius and Ulna. J. Bone Joint Surg., 71A:159–169, 1989.*)

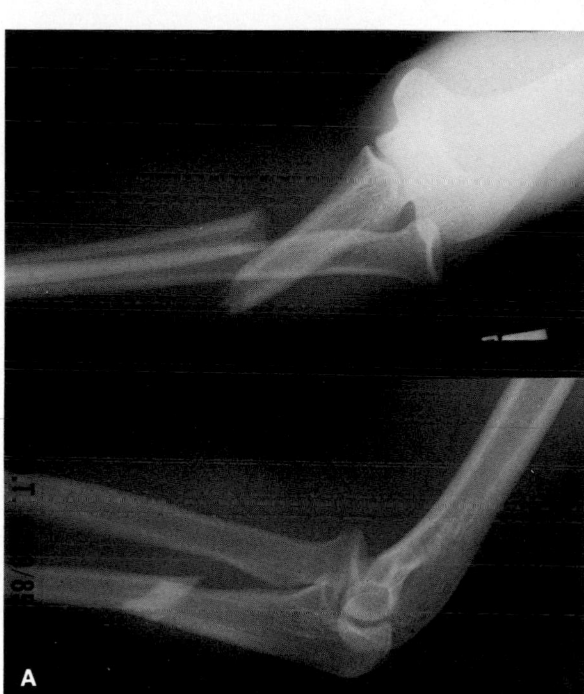

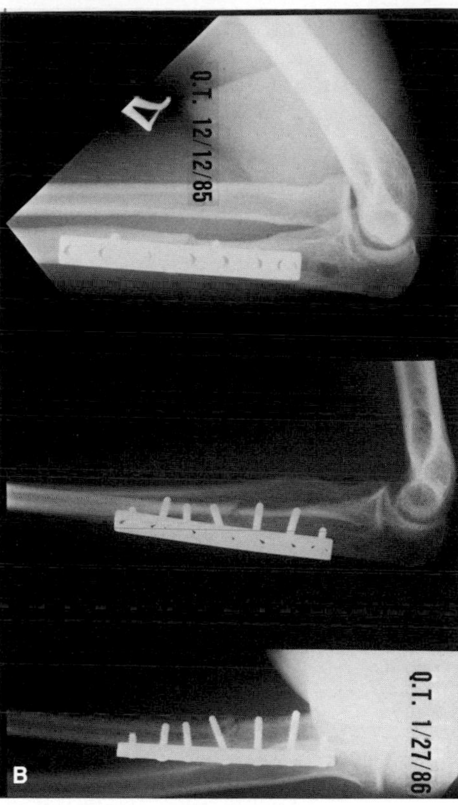

FIGURE 13-21. (**A**) Preoperative radiographs of an 18-year-old man with a closed Monteggia fracture. (**B**) Postoperative radiographs showing primary fixation with a seven-hole, 3.5-mm dynamic compression plate augmented by an olecranon bone graft. Note the unicortical screws on each end of the plate and the use of the center hole as the site for an interfragmentary screw. (*Chapman, M.W., Gordon, E.J., and Zissimos, A.G.: Compression-Plate Fixation of Acute Fractures of the Diaphyses of the Radius and Ulna. J. Bone Joint Surg., 71A:159–169, 1989.*)

loss of the radial bow (Fig. 13-22). The amount and exact location of plate contour required to produce an anatomical reduction of a radial fracture varies according to the location of the fracture, the magnitude of normal radial bow in the individual patient, and the surface of the radius to which the plate is being applied.[86] Less contour is required for volar, as opposed to radial or dorsoradial, plate placement. However, even when a plate is applied to the volar surface of the radius, care must be taken to be certain that the radius is not iatrogenically straightened by bone-holding clamps before screw placement. Since the amount of contouring required is variable, the surgeon must be exacting in critically assessing the quality of the radial reduction during plate application. Slight obliquity of the plate in relation to the bone can be acceptable if it is required to maintain the normal radial bow. Plate configuration must also be altered if interfragmentary screws have been used outside the plate to maintain the reduction of large cortical fragments.

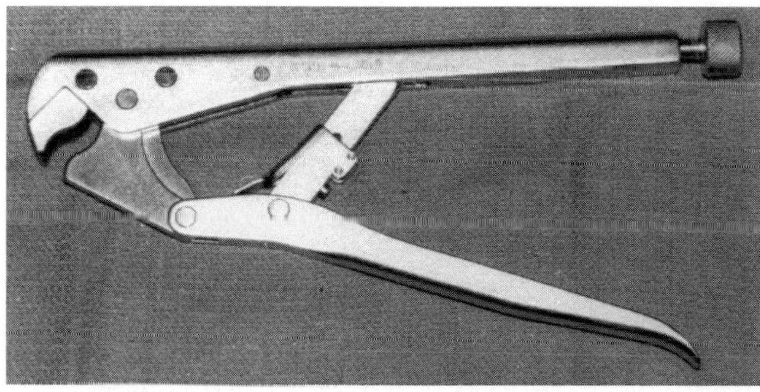

FIGURE 13-22. AO hand-held plate bending forceps. This instrument is very useful in contouring the radial plate at the time of surgery to maintain the radial bow. Application of either a straight plate or an overcontoured plate to the radius may not restore the radial bow anatomically. In most radial fractures at least a portion of the plate must be contoured to maintain the radial bow. Occasionally, a straight plate can be applied to the radius if the plate traverses the radius obliquely.

The external AO tension device (Fig. 13-23A) is no longer used routinely in treating forearm fractures, and the reader is referred to the AO *Manual of Internal Fixation*[65,66] for more information about this technique. This device may be useful as an adjunct in difficult reductions, especially for shortened and overlapped fragments. In such cases, the plate is applied to one of the major fragments; the articulated tension device is then used to distract the fragments by placing the hook so that it *pushes* against the opposite end of the plate.

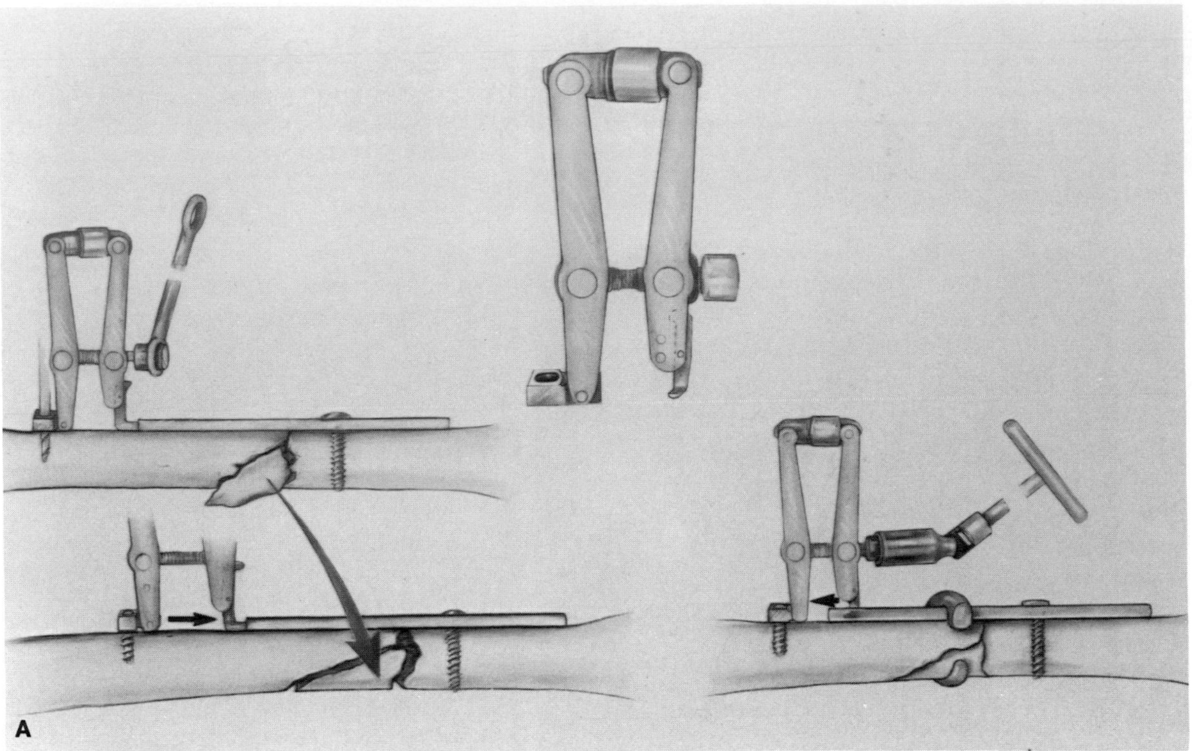

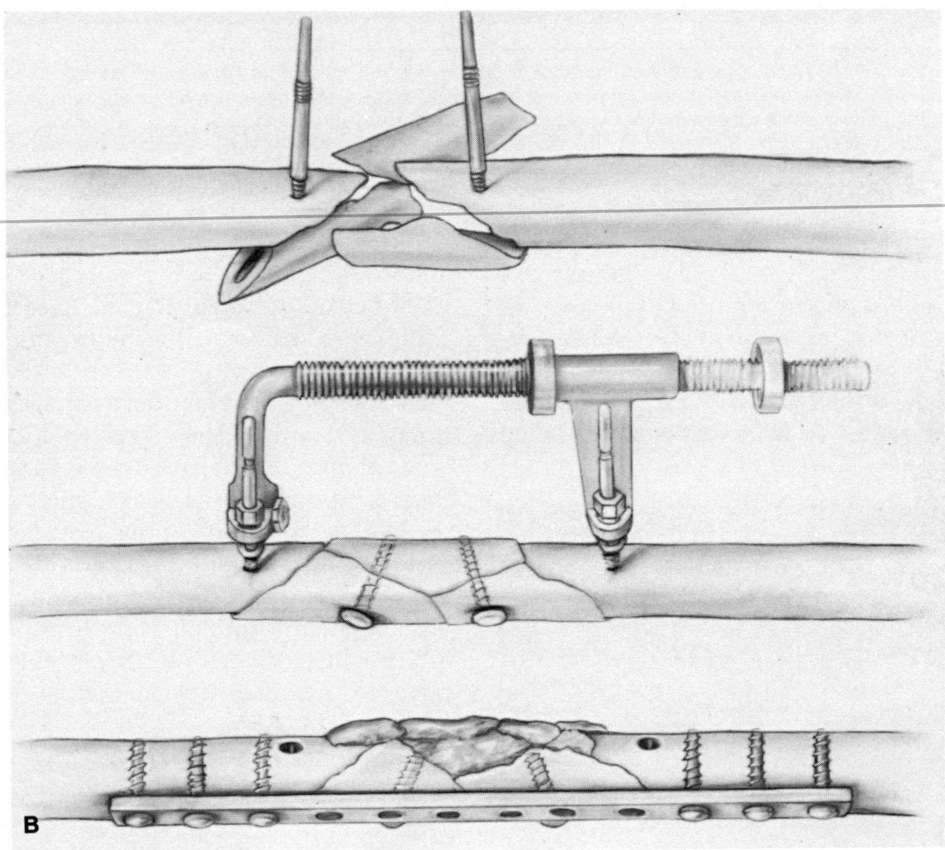

FIGURE 13-23. (**A**) Use of the AO articulated tension device to assist in initial reduction. See text for description of this device, which can be used as a distractor to faciltate reduction of difficult comminuted fractures, especially those with shortening or overlapping. (**B**) Use of the AO distracter to assist with reduction and preliminary stabilization of comminuted fractures. (*After Müller, M.E., Algöwer, M., Schneider, P., and Willenegger, H.: Manual of Internal Fixation, 2nd ed., pp. 121 and 123. New York, Springer-Verlag, 1979.; Mallin, B.A.: Principles of Management of Forearm Fractures. In Chapman, M.W.* [*ed.*]*: Operative Orthopaedics, vol. 1, pp. 263–271. Philadelphia, J.B. Lippincott, 1988.*)

This facilitates reduction. The hook is then reversed to apply tension to the plate (and to compress the fracture).[60]

Another situation in which distraction is helpful is when comminution may make it impossible to achieve perfect alignment and good screw fixation in the comminuted area. The "no touch" technique is used for reduction of the comminuted fragments as follows. The AO distractor (see Fig. 13-23*B*) is applied to 4.5-mm pins inserted at sites remote from the comminuted or segmental portion. The fragments are distracted sufficiently to obtain good alignment. The comminuted or defect areas are bridged by attaching a well-contoured plate over the intact extreme ends of the fracture. The plate acts as a strut over the comminuted area, to which bone graft is added. I usually use autogenous iliac bone graft if a significant degree of comminution is present. Significant comminution is arbitrarily defined as comminution that involves one third or more of the circumference of the bone.

Closure. It is of utmost importance to close only the subcutaneous tissue and skin. The deep fascia of the forearm is very dense. If it is sutured tightly, edema and hemorrhage may cause increased pressure in the forearm compartments, which can lead to ischemic contracture. Obviously, leaving the deep fascia unsutured is important not only with compression plating but also with other forms of internal fixation. I recommend that a closed drainage system be used to decrease the hematoma and resultant swelling. It is removed after 24 hours.

Aftercare. Care after compression-plate fixation is tailored to each patient. If the patient is reliable, if the fracture is not significantly comminuted, and if stable fixation has been achieved, no external immobilization is necessary (Fig. 13-24). A pressure dressing is applied, and the forearm is elevated until the swelling begins to subside. As soon as the patient has recovered from the anesthetic, gentle active exercises are begun for the elbow, wrist, and hand. By the end of 10 days, such patients have usually regained nearly normal ranges of motion.

Different aftercare is required if the fracture is not comminuted and stable fixation has been obtained but the patient's reliability is questionable, or if the fracture is comminuted and stable fixation has not been obtained. In such situations, I prefer to use a compression dressing with a sugar-tong splint for 10 to 12 days, at which time the sutures are removed and a long-arm splint is fabricated. The splint is removed for supervised sessions of physiotherapy but is otherwise worn full time until the fracture is radiographically united, usually after about 6 weeks.

Fixation With Intramedullary Nails

Historical Review. After intramedullary nailing became popular for fractures of the femur in the late 1940s, various devices for medullary fixation of the

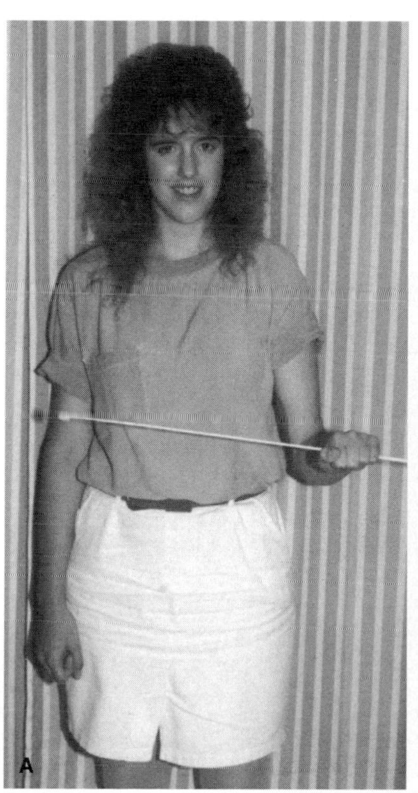

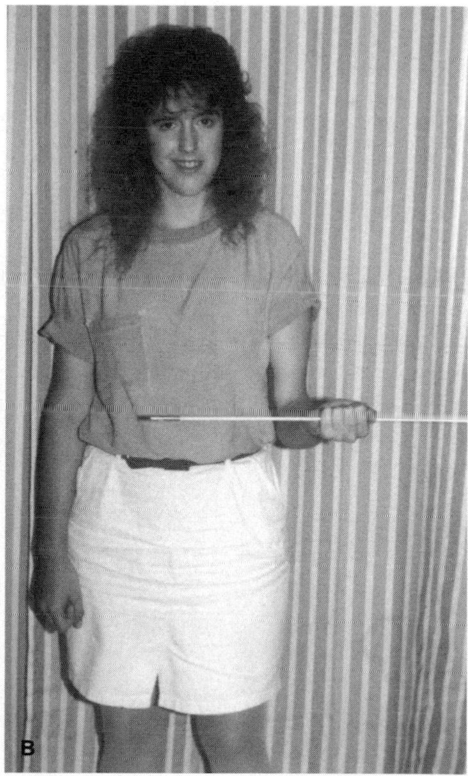

FIGURE 13-24. An 18-year-old patient after fixation of fractures of both bones of the forearm, repaired with 3.5-mm dynamic compression plates. One year after injury both fractures have healed and there is a full range of pronation (**A**) and supination (**B**). The patient started range of motion exercises within a few days of the injury.

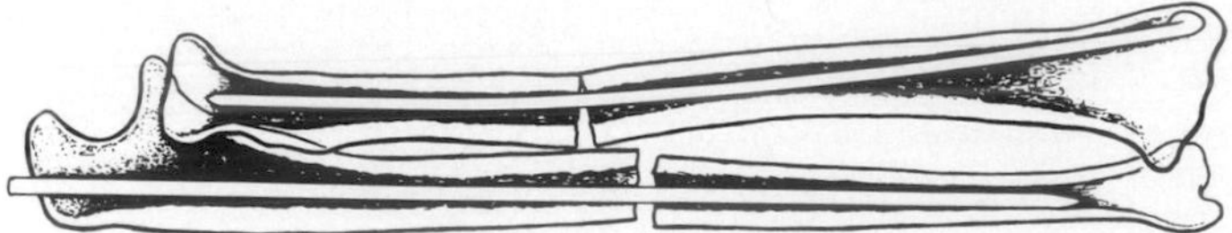

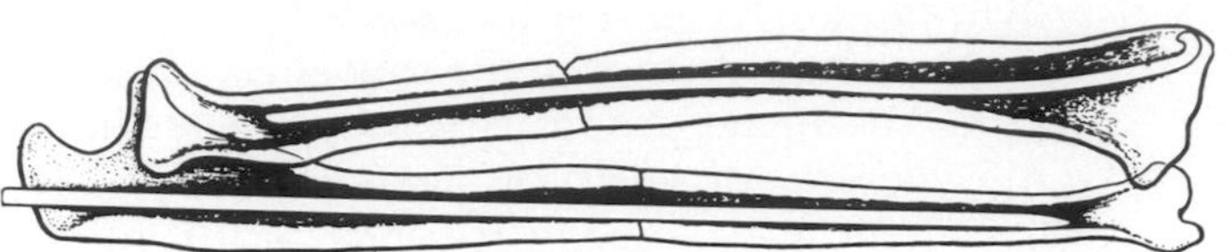

FIGURE 13-25. When intramedullary pins are used in both bones, fixation of the radius must be sufficiently stable to prevent collapse of the radial arch; otherwise, there will be a relative elongation of the radius with distraction of the ulnar fracture, and nonunion may result in one or both bones. (*Smith, H., and Sage, F.P.: Medullary Fixation of Forearm Fractures. J. Bone Joint Surg., 39A:91–98, 1957.*)

radius and ulna were used. In 1957, Smith and Sage[92] reported a series of 555 fractures collected from all over the country in which some form of intramedullary fixation had been used. The devices included Rush pins, Kirschner wires, Steinmann pins, Lottes nails, and Küntscher V-nails. The results were discouraging. Nonunion resulted in over 20% of the fractures, and malunion and poor function were common in those that did unite. The radial bow was not maintained, and the use of a round pin in a round medullary canal could not control rotation of the fragments (Fig. 13-25). Caden[17] reported a nonunion rate of 16.6% in forearm fractures treated with Rush pins.

In 1959, Sage[79] published his study of the anatomy of the radius and introduced Sage triangular forearm medullary nails. The nail for the ulna was straight and was inserted in a retrograde manner. The nail for the radius was bent to aid in maintaining the radial bow (Fig. 13-26). It was introduced from the radial styloid and driven proximally (Fig. 13-27). The ulnar nail was relatively easy to insert, but the technique for inserting the radial nail was more difficult and exacting. Sage reported good results with his nails. Nonunion occurred in only 6.2% of fractures and delayed union in 4.9%. Other triangular or diamond-shaped nails for the forearm bones were introduced by Ritchey and colleagues[76] and by Street.[95] These also gripped the cortex well and controlled rotation but did not preserve the radial bow as well as the Sage nail. Sage nails were not recommended for fractures of the distal third of the radius beyond the area where the medullary canal has begun to enlarge. Also their use was not advised if the medullary canal was less than 3 mm in diameter. When his nails were used, Sage[78] recommended the routine use of autogenous iliac bone grafting. Schemitsch and associates[85] demonstrated that in-

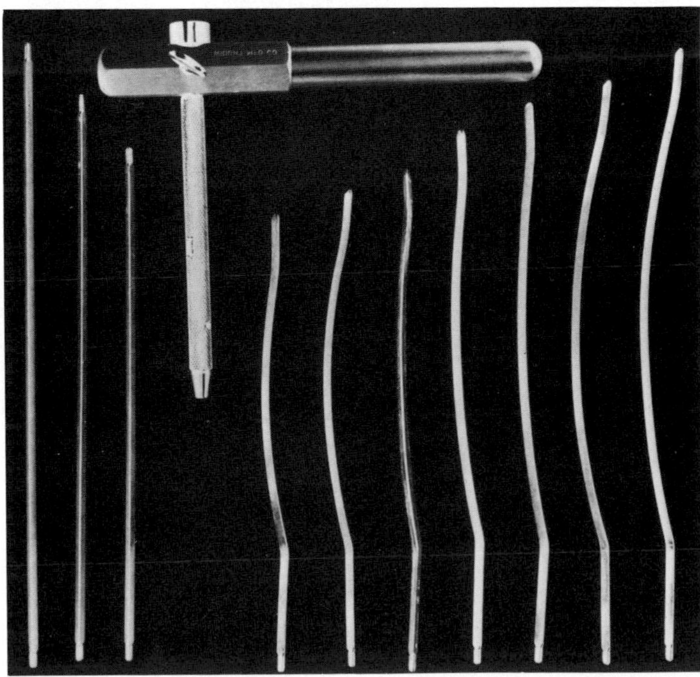

FIGURE 13-26. The Sage driver-extractor and full complement of Sage nails for the radius and ulna. (*Sage, F.P.: Medullary Fixation of Fractures of the Forearm: A Study of the Medullary Canal of the Radius and a Report of Fifty Fractures of the Radius Treated with a Prebent Triangular Nail. J. Bone Joint Surg., 41A:1489–1516, 1959.*)

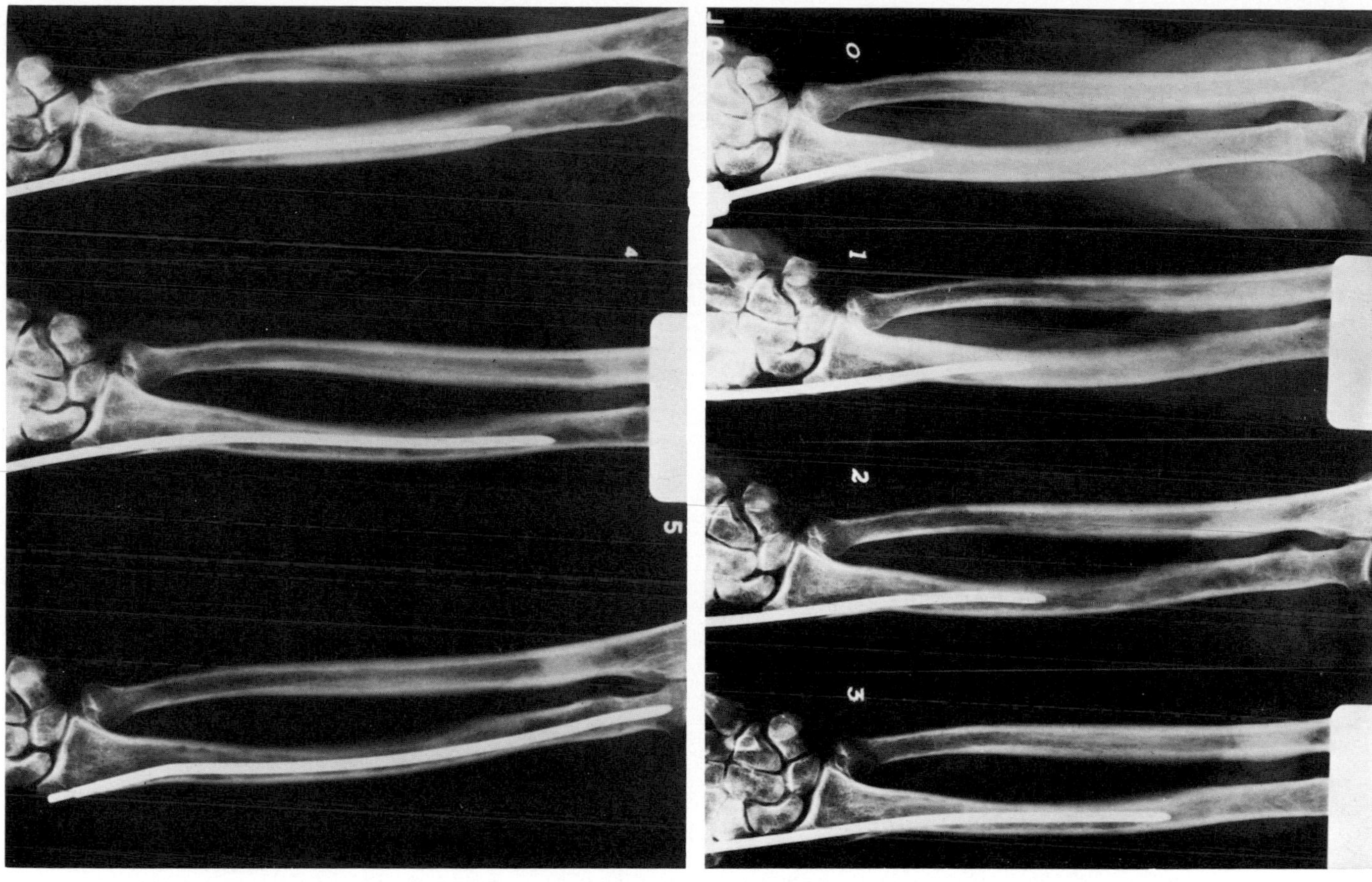

FIGURE 13-27. Serial radiographs to show a Sage radial nail being driven up the radius of an amputated specimen. The nail must bend as it traverses the canal and then finally spring back to its original shape. (*Sage, F.P.: Medullary Fixation of Fractures of the Forearm: A Study of the Medullary Canal of the Radius and a Report of Fifty Fractures of the Radius Treated with a Prebent Triangular Nail. J. Bone Joint Surg., 41A:1489–1516, 1959.*)

tramedullary nails can maintain a forearm reduction, although not as well as accurate plating.

In 1986, Street[95] published a report on a series of 137 forearm fractures treated with a square, reamed, intramedullary nail. Nailings were done by either closed or open technique, with the radial nail being introduced distally and the ulnar nail being introduced proximally. Postoperatively, the fractures were immobilized in a long-arm cast for 4 weeks, after which the patient was encouraged to use the arm normally regardless of the radiographic appearance of the fracture. Street reported a nonunion rate of only 7%. In addition, there were two delayed unions. Street believed that the most likely cause for these failures was either the selection of a nail that was too small or the presence of a butterfly fragment that was devascularized during open reduction. He believed that the technique could be used safely in open fractures but noted that the results were also good for primary debridement and delayed nailing after about 2 weeks. The advantages of this method, especially when done by closed technique, included early union, low incidence of refracture, low infection rate, relatively short operating time, minimal surgical trauma, and less scar than with other methods such as plate fixation.

Considerations in the Choice of Forearm Nails. According to Sisk,[90] when medullary fixation is used for any forearm fracture, errors in selection of the proper length and diameter of the nail, in operative technique, and in aftertreatment contribute to poor results. Disproportion between the size of the nail and the medullary canal is a common problem. If the nail is too small in diameter, side-to-side and rotatory movements occur. If the diameter is too large, it may explode the shaft of the radius or ulna. Triangular or diamond-shaped nails are preferred for control of rotation.

Technique for Sage Forearm Nails.[78] The straight Sage ulnar nail may be used for almost any diaphyseal fracture of the ulna, although it may be necessary to ream the medullary canal. The pre-bent Sage radial nail may be used for diaphyseal fractures of the radius unless the fracture is in the proximal one fourth or distal one third of the shaft. The radial nail should not be used when the medullary canal is less than 3 mm in diameter at its narrowest point. The nail must engage the cortex firmly; and if the cortex is too thin from reaming, the nail may split the shaft.

Before beginning the operation, it is imperative that a complete set of Sage nails and insertion equipment be available. This includes a full set of radial and ulnar nails, a combination driver and extractor, a 3-mm drill, and two reamers. When the ulna alone is to be nailed, the arm is positioned across the chest. When the radius or both bones are to be nailed, the arm is placed on a side table or arm board.

Usually, the ulna should be nailed first. The fracture is exposed through a short longitudinal incision over the subcutaneous border. Little or no periosteal stripping is required. The fracture is reduced with bone clamps and traction. Special care is taken to obtain exact rotatory reduction. The proximal fragment is delivered into the wound, and an ulnar nail is inserted into the medullary canal to test for fit. If the canal is too small, it is first enlarged with a 3.2-mm drill and then with a reamer. When the reamer passes the smallest diameter of the canal, resistance suddenly ceases. The proximal fragment is reamed until the tip of the reamer is felt beneath the skin at the tip of the olecranon.

After reaming both fragments, the surgeon selects an ulnar nail of correct length by placing it along the ulnar side of the forearm. With the driver threaded on the nail and the elbow flexed to 90°, the nail is driven retrograde up the proximal fragment of the ulna. A small incision is made in the skin over the end of the nail, and the nail is driven farther proximally until its distal end is at the fracture. The driver is then reversed, reducing the fracture, and the nail is driven down the distal fragment until the driver is within 1.3 cm of the olecranon. Final seating of the nail is delayed until the radius is fixed and radiographs are made confirming the adequacy of reduction.

The radius is then exposed through an appropriate incision. The volar Henry approach is preferred. Once exposed, the fracture is reduced with care to correct any deformity of rotation. The size of the medullary canal is checked with a radial nail, and the proximal and distal segments are reamed if necessary. The fracture is reduced, and the nail is placed along the radial border of the forearm to determine length. The nail should extend from the tip of the radial styloid to within 1.3 cm of the radial head or 3.8 cm of the lateral epicondyle of the humerus.

The wrist is flexed over a folded towel and deviated ulnarward so that the radial styloid is accessible. A longitudinal incision 2.5 cm long is made over the radial styloid and carried down to bone at its proximal end but only through the skin distally. Care must be taken to avoid the superficial branch of the radial nerve. The periosteum is reflected, and a hole is drilled with a 3.2- or 4.8-mm drill through the exposed cortex of the radial styloid. The hole is begun with the drill perpendicular to the cortex, and gradually the handle of the drill is angled distally until the drill is directed toward the lateral epicondyle of the humerus. The drill is advanced 5 or 6 cm, thus producing an oval hole at the point of insertion and a channel that nearly parallels the medullary canal.

The point of the nail is inserted with the nail rotated so that its dorsal or long bow parallels the long arc of the radius. With the wrist in flexion and ulnar deviation, the nail is inserted by hand in a proximal direction as far as possible. If the nail cannot be pushed in for 6 cm, the angle of insertion is too acute. The nail is withdrawn and the channel of insertion drilled more obliquely. The driver is threaded on the nail, and while the left hand exerts pressure to depress the nail toward the ulna, the nail is driven in with the right hand. If marked resistance is met, the nail is angled back and forth a few degrees and then driven with moderate blows until it reaches the fracture. When there is a nondisplaced butterfly fragment, it is held with a clamp, the fracture is reduced, and the nail is driven into the proximal fragment leaving 1.3 cm exposed at the radial styloid.

The position of the fracture and the position and length of the nail are checked with anteroposterior and lateral x-rays. If the nails are the correct length, they are then fully seated. The fractures are observed under direct vision to be sure that no distraction occurs. A wire loop is used around a butterfly fragment when it is large and loose. As recommended by Sage, autogenous iliac bone grafts are placed about all fractures of the radius and ulna fixed with medullary nails.

Aftercare. A long-arm cast is applied with the elbow at 90° flexion and neutral rotation. The cast is worn for 8 to 12 weeks until enough bridging callus is noted on the x-ray. The nails should be removed once union is present but not before 1 year.

Technique for Street Forearm Nails.[95] Whenever possible, the proper nail size should be determined before surgery. The required length may be determined either by measuring the involved limb or by measuring the bone on x-rays. To avoid the risk of driving the nail through the end of the bone, 1 cm should be subtracted from the measurement. The nail diameter is determined during surgery. As with the Sage nail, a full range of sizes should be available.

When performing open nailing techniques, separate subcutaneous approaches are important to avoid continuity of the hematoma of the two fracture sites, which can possibly contribute to the formation of radioulnar synostosis. After the fracture sites are exposed, the fragments are mobilized to displace the bone ends sufficiently to ream the canals. It is advisable to expose and ream both bones before nailing either one. The radius is nailed from the distal end. A 1- to 1.5-cm incision is made, extending distally from the dorsal margin of the joint surface at a precise point just lateral to Lister's tubercle; here there is a low ridge on the radius between the extensor carpi radialis longus and brevis tendons.

After the skin is incised, the deeper layers are spread gently to avoid damaging terminal divisions of the superficial branch of radial nerve and the dorsal branch of radial artery. The entry portal is directly in line with the medullary canal. At the dorsal margin of the joint, a drill and reamer are introduced at a 45° angle to the joint surface. After the bone is entered 1 to 1.5 cm, with care not to go through the palmar cortex, the angle of the drill is dropped to the axis of the bone and continued another 2 to 4 cm. Before the nail is inserted, it must usually be slightly bent to approximate the bow of the radius, which is mainly lateral but also slightly dorsal. It will be easier to drive the nail if the fracture has been reduced and held with bone-holding forceps. With proper reaming, the nail should meet some resistance but not require considerable force. When the insertion is almost complete, the driver is removed and reapplied to engage only four turns of the thread. The nail is then driven until the driver abuts the bone.

The nail for the ulna is inserted into the olecranon. A 1-cm longitudinal incision is made over the end of the olecranon, and the insertion of the triceps tendon is split. The reamer is introduced at a point 5 to 8 mm from the dorsal cortex to avoid entering the trochlear notch and 5 mm from the lateral cortex to compensate for the lateral bow. The reamer is then aimed at the fracture site and observed to appear in the canal. The ulna should be reamed all the way to its distal end, because although the canal is wide in this region, the resistance of the cancellous bone may cause distraction of the fracture as the nail is driven home. It may be necessary to withdraw and advance the nail several times while the wrist is held in ulnar deviation to close the gap.

An image intensifier is required in the technique of closed nailing. It is best to position the arm on an arm board, which allows good visualization with the C-arm. Nail selection and insertion are the same as for open nailing. The nail is inserted into the distal radial and proximal ulnar fragments before reduction. Once this has been done, reduction is obtained as described in the discussion of closed reduction. The nail is then driven home. It is important that the nail fit snugly because this proper fit enhances fracture healing and prevents overriding of oblique and comminuted fractures. Since the actual reduction can take considerable time, the surgeon must be aware of the amount of radiation exposure he or she is receiving. Comminuted and segmental fractures are more difficult to treat by closed techniques, but with perseverance, reduction and fixation can be achieved.

Aftercare. X-rays confirming the adequacy of reduction and nail placement are taken before the wounds are closed in the operating room. A long-arm cast is worn for 4 weeks. The position of the forearm in the cast depends on the level of the fracture. Fractures in the proximal third of the forearm are immobilized in supination, fractures in the middle third in neutral, and fractures in the distal third in pronation. Regardless of the radiographic appearance, the cast is removed after 4 weeks, and the patient is encouraged to resume normal activities

Complications of Intramedullary Nails

Most complications result from improper selection of nail size. A nail that is too long may be driven through the bone end. One that is too short may not adequately stabilize the fracture. A nail with too great a diameter may split the cortex, and one with a smaller diameter may not adequately control rotation, resulting in delayed union or nonunion of the fracture.

OPEN FRACTURES OF THE RADIUS AND ULNA

INCIDENCE

The ratio of open (compound) fractures to closed fractures is higher for the forearm bones than for any other bone except the tibia.[12] The high incidence of open fractures in the forearm attests to the degree of trauma required to break both bones of the forearm, the frequency of high energy trauma as the mechanism of injury when these fractures occur, and the relatively superficial location of the radius and ulna beneath the skin.[57]

CLASSIFICATION

In assessing open fractures of both bones of the forearm, I use the classification originally described by Smith[91] and modified by Gustilo and Anderson.[36] Open fractures are classified into three types.

Type I is an open fracture with a clean wound less than 1 cm long. Type II is an open fracture with a laceration more than 1 cm long without extensive soft-tissue damage, flaps, or avulsions. Type III is either an open segmental fracture, an open fracture with extensive soft-tissue damage, or a traumatic amputation. In 1984, Gustilo and colleagues[37,38] further divided type III injuries into A, B, and C. Type III-A injuries are gunshot injuries with adequate coverage of the fractured bone despite extensive soft-tissue lacerations, flaps, or high-energy trauma regardless of the size of the wound. Type III-B injuries are farm injuries with extensive soft-tissue injury with periosteal stripping and bony exposure, usually associated with massive contamination. Type III-C injuries are open fractures with associated vascular damage requiring repair. Fortunately, type I and type II wounds are more common in the forearm than are type III injuries. The usual cause is a sharp spike of bone compounding from within to without.

TREATMENT

Meticulous and extensive debridement under general anesthesia followed by primary open reduction and internal or external fixation for open injuries is recommended.[19,27,39,48,60,64,86] If this is to be done, meticulous technique is necessary. After wound cultures have been obtained, cefazolin is administered intravenously in the emergency department. The patient is then taken to the operating room, where the open fracture wound and limb are prepared with povidone-iodine solution (Betadine). The wound is copiously irrigated with sterile saline solution (bacitracin added) using pulsatile lavage. The ends of the bone are exposed using either extensile incisions from the open wound or separate incisions. The traumatic wounds should be incorporated into the surgical incision *only* if they lie in the line of a standard operative approach. Otherwise, entirely separate incisions should be made, ignoring the traumatic wounds. Soft-tissue dissection and periosteal stripping are kept to the minimum necessary for adequate exposure. A methodical debridement beginning with the skin and working layer by layer down to the bone is performed. All necrotic tissue is excised. Bone fragments with no soft-tissue attachments are usually discarded. The wound is again irrigated with pulsatile saline lavage until up to a total of 6 to 10 L of saline solution has been used. Final cultures are taken.

Internal fixation is performed as previously described. Traumatic wounds are not closed primarily but left open for 5 to 10 days and then covered with split-thickness skin grafts. If the open wound is small and minimal swelling occurs, skin grafting is not required. Surgical incisions can be closed primarily.

Antibiotics are given for 2 days postoperatively if there is no evidence of infection. On an empirical basis, I often prescribe oral therapy with a cephalosporin for another 5 to 7 days, especially if split-thickness skin grafts have been required.

If the wound is clean without signs of infection,

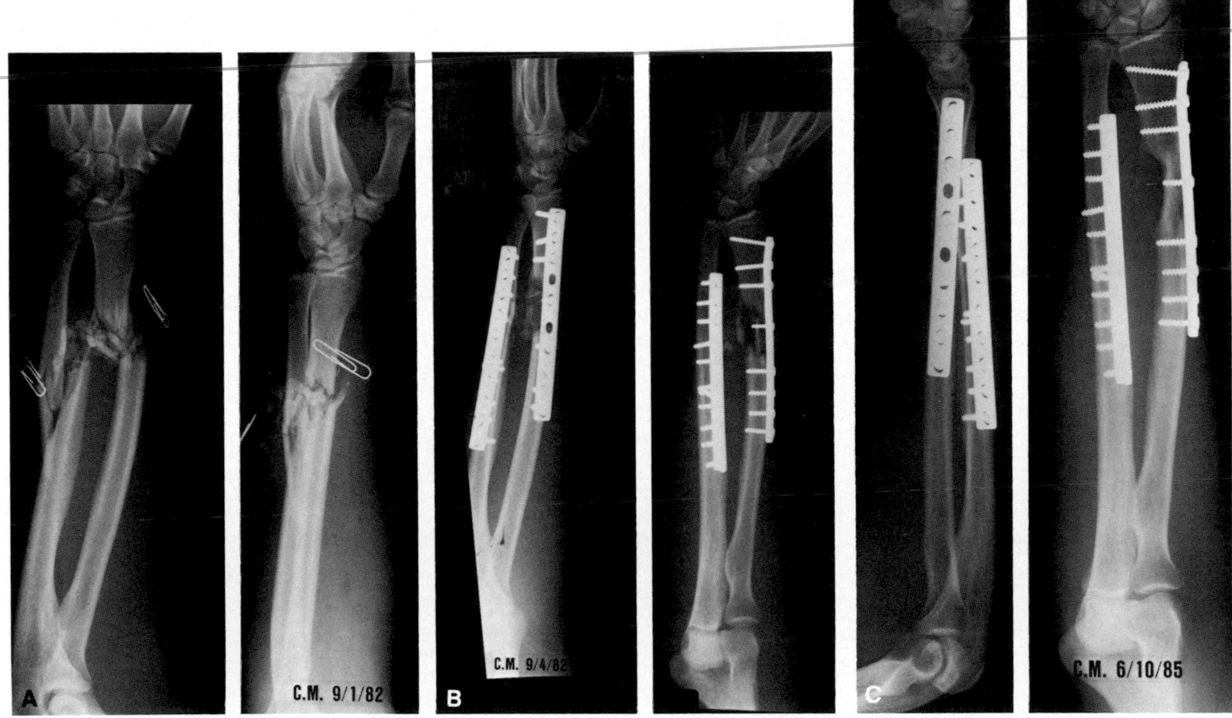

FIGURE 13-28. (**A**) Preoperative radiographs in a 32-year-old man with a type III-A open fracture of the radius and ulna secondary to a high-velocity gunshot wound. (**B**) Postoperative radiographs showing primary fixation with 10-hole, 3.5-mm dynamic compression plates on the radius and ulna. These were augmented by an iliac-crest bone graft at the time of delayed primary closure, 3 days after injury. (**C**) Radiographs showing union at 33 months. A normal range of motion was achieved. (*Chapman, M.W., Gordon, E.J., and Zissimos, A.G.: Compression-Plate Fixation of Acute Fractures of the Diaphyses of the Radius and Ulna. J. Bone Joint Surg., 71A:159–169, 1989.*)

bone grafting can be performed at the time of closure or coverage (Fig. 13-28). In the past, Anderson recommended delayed fixation for open fractures. He followed 28 patients with 38 open fractures in whom internal fixation was delayed. None developed infection. Currently, most authors believe that primary fixation can be safely undertaken provided that a vigorous debridement is performed.[47,86]

Concomitant Soft-Tissue Injury

With type III-B and type III-C injuries, management of soft-tissue injury is extremely difficult without the use of some form of internal fixation or external fixator. I have found that an external fixator provides good stable fixation of fractures while soft-tissue reconstruction is carried out (Fig. 13-29). Godina,[34] of the former Yugoslavia, advocated early soft-tissue reconstruction. He reviewed the results of 532 patients who had undergone microsurgical reconstruction after extremity trauma. Patients were divided into three groups based on the time from injury to the time of microsurgical reconstruction. Free flap transfer was used in group 1 within 72 hours of injury, in group 2 between 72 hours and 3 months after injury, and in group 3 between 3 months and 12.6 years after injury. In group 1, the flap failure rate was 0.75% and the infection rate was 1.5%. The average time to fracture healing was 6.8 months with an average hospital stay of 27 days. This was a significant improvement in all categories over patients who had undergone later reconstruction. (See Chapter 7 for a more thorough discussion of soft-tissue management of open fractures.)

External Fixators

The use of external fixation devices has grown in popularity as a method of initial management of severe open fractures of the radius and ulna with soft-tissue loss, bone

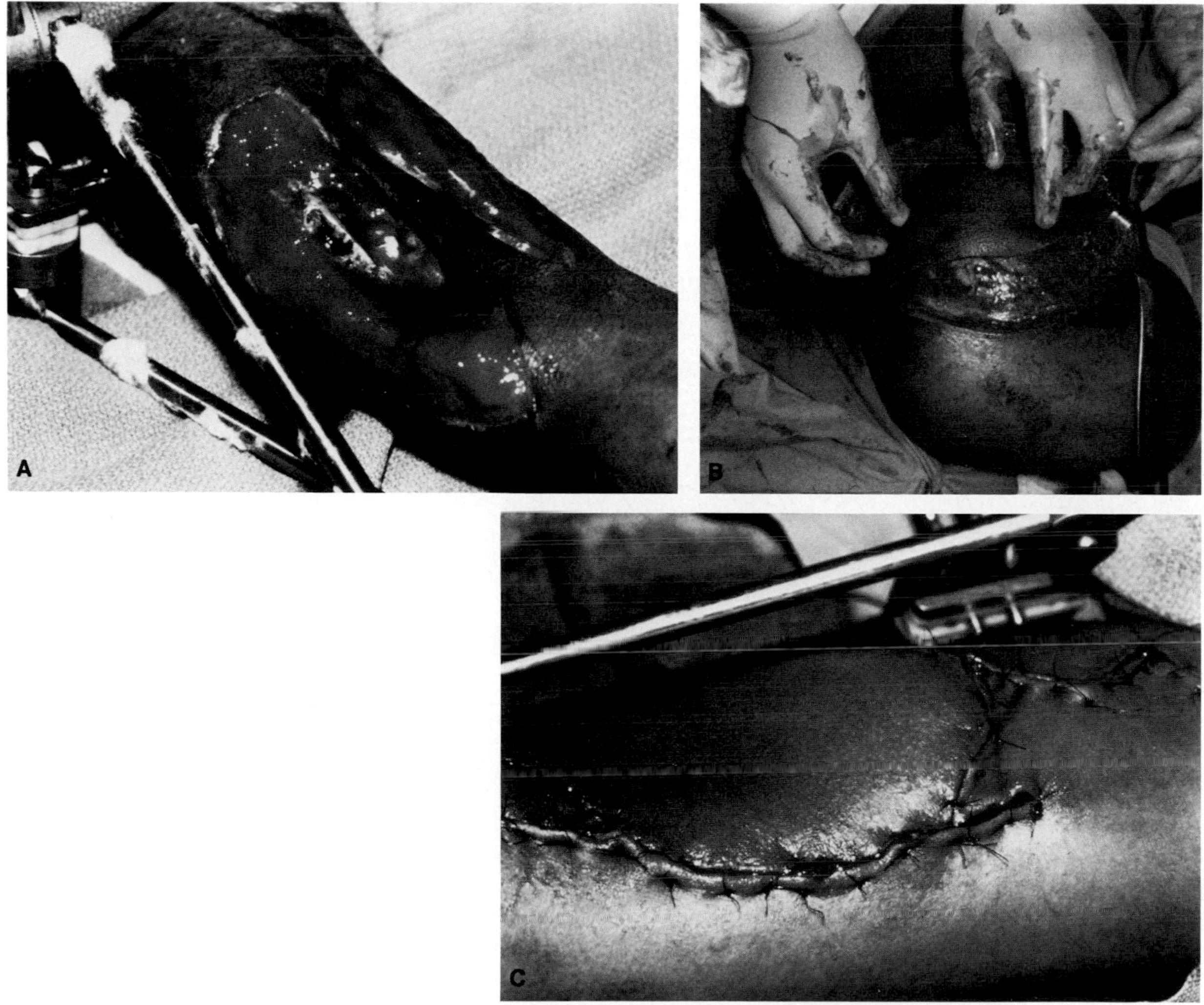

FIGURE 13-29. (**A**) A 16-year-old boy with extensive bone and soft-tissue loss secondary to a gunshot wound of the forearm. (**B** and **C**) After initial stabilization of the forearm with an external fixator, a free scapular flap was used to provide coverage.

loss, or severe comminution. Their use has been reported by Weiland and associates,[108] DeLee,[22] Heiser and Jacobs,[41] and Schuind and associates (Fig. 13-30).[88] DeLee noted that there are basically three types of external fixation devices for the forearm bones: the single Hoffmann half-pin frame (Fig. 13-31); the double Hoffmann half-pin frame; and the Hoffmann-Vidal frame with completely transfixing pins. It was DeLee's opinion that the indications for the use of *complete* transfixing pins in the forearm are very limited because of the risk of the pins damaging adjacent neurovascular tissue. Therefore, although the Hoffmann-Vidal frame is the most stable, either the single or the double Hoffmann frame is most often used with half-pins. DeLee suggested the following indications for the use of external fixation in the upper extremity: (1) the presence of severe open wounds with skin and soft-tissue loss and a fracture of the radius or ulna; (2) the need to maintain length in cases with bone loss or comminution; (3) open elbow fracture-dislocations with soft-tissue loss, in which internal fixation is not advisable; (4) certain unstable distal intra-articular radius fractures; and (5) infected nonunions (Fig. 13-32).

External Versus Internal Fixation in Open Fractures

Whether one chooses internal fixation or some form of external fixation, the device must be individualized. In some cases internal fixation of one bone, combined with external fixation of the same or the other bone may be in the best interest of the patient. This is particularly true of proximal and distal fractures. When internal fixation is chosen, an adequate amount of metal must always be used to stabilize the forearm for wound care. When treating open fractures both bones should be fixed by one method or the other. As in all open fractures, copious irrigation and meticulous debridement of the wound is of the utmost importance. Antibiotic therapy should be started intravenously in the emergency department after the wound has been cultured and should be continued during and after surgery. Tetanus prophylaxis should be provided.

Authors' Preferred Method of Treatment

For most displaced fractures of the radius and ulna in adults I prefer open reduction and internal fixation using AO dynamic compression plates. Closed treatment of these fractures generally yields a high incidence of poor results. On the other hand, the overall results of compression-plate fixation in my experience have been good or excellent. The incidence of nonunion has been low, and the functional results have been excellent in most cases. A longitudinal incision is made directly over the ulna, and a volar Henry ap-

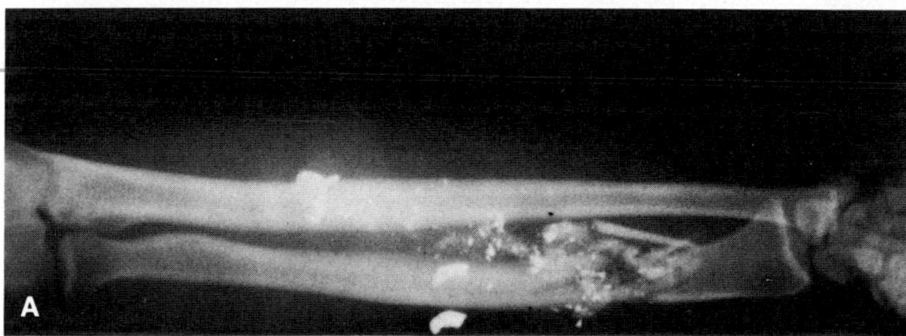

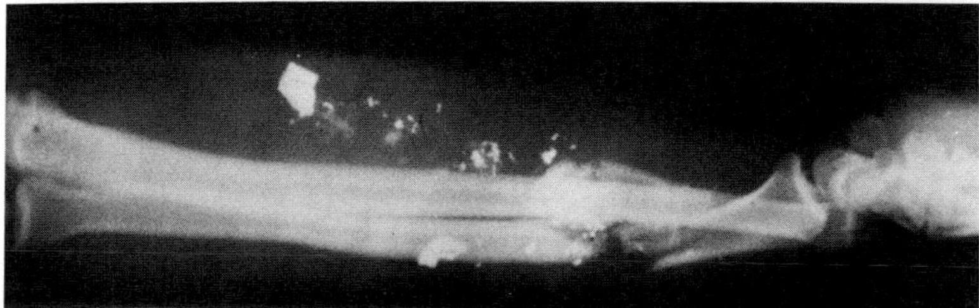

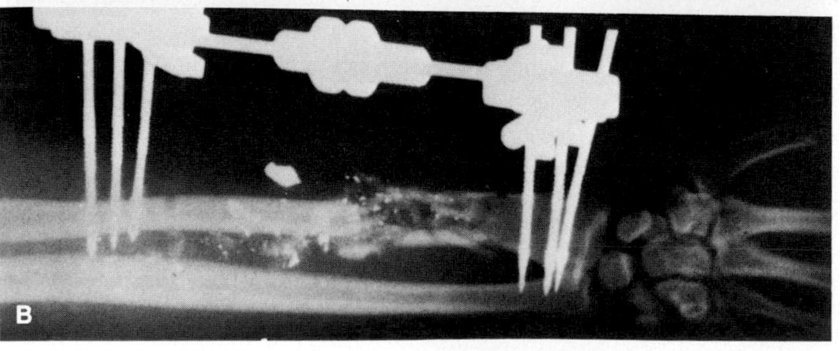

FIGURE 13-30. (**A**) A gunshot wound of the distal radius with shortening and disruption of the distal radioulnar joint. (**B**) A single Hoffmann half-pin frame has restored length to the radius and reduced the distal radioulnar joint. (*DeLee, J.C.: External Fixation of the Forearm and Wrist. Orthop. Rev., 6:43–48, 1981.*)

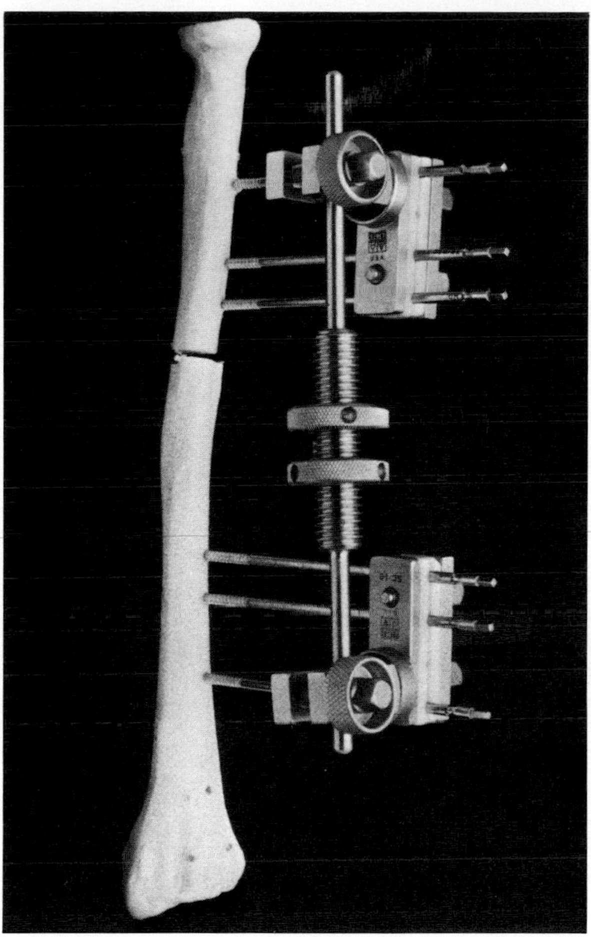

FIGURE 13-31. Single Hoffmann half-pin frame. Three pins above and three pins below the fracture site are connected by a single compression-distraction rod. (*DeLee, J.C.: External Fixation of the Forearm and Wrist. Orthop. Rev., 6:43–48, 1981.*)

proach is used for the radius. The preferred plate is the eight hole dynamic compression plate with 3.5-mm cortical screws. For segmental fractures of the radius I use two separate plates applied, if possible, in different planes. Moderate degrees of comminution can generally be handled with interfragmentary compression screws followed by plate application. Autogenous iliac crest bone grafts are not routinely used unless there is an intercalary (segmental) bone defect. Small (less than 6 cm) segmental defects are treated by application of a plate that is long enough to obtain six cortices of fixation on either side of the fracture, supplemented with autogenous iliac bone graft. I prefer to delay bone grafting in open fractures until definitive wound coverage is obtained (see below).

I cannot overemphasize the importance of meticulous attention to the details of operative technique. The need for strict asepsis in the operating room is absolute. Infection and errors in technique are the principal causes of failure. The time required for external immobilization after use of this method is usually less than that with other forms of internal fixation, and in appropriate cases I frequently use no cast at all.

Primary internal fixation is used for most open fractures of the shafts of the radius and ulna except in patients with major soft-tissue loss. In most instances, when the wound is relatively small and not too contaminated, the traumatic wound is irrigated, debrided, and left open. The operative wound is closed primarily. If a compartment syndrome has been diagnosed, or if the operative wound cannot be closed without tension, portions of the wound proximally and distally are closed to cover the desiccation-sensitive structures (vessels, nerves, and tendons), particularly when not covered by paratenon. The remainder of the wound is left open and covered with antibiotic ointment impregnated gauze. The wound is closed secondarily with split-thickness skin grafts 3 to 5 days after the primary surgery. Parenteral antibiotics are used liberally before, during, and after surgery. External fixation is used when there is extensive bone loss or when severe soft-tissue loss and contamination would make it difficult to cover a plate. Free tissue transfer may be required in these cases if there is segmental bone loss greater than 6 cm.

PROGNOSIS

The prognosis for adults with fractures of the radius and ulna depends on many factors. Was the fracture open, and if so, how extensive was the damage and how great was the contamination? Was the fracture displaced or nondisplaced, and what was the degree of comminution? The surgeon has no control over these and many other factors; they are decided at the time of injury. To be sure, the prognosis related to these factors may be affected by the surgeon's actions and decisions, including early and appropriate treatment. There are other factors over which the surgeon has more direct control. These include the choice of treatment method (open vs closed reduction), the timing of internal fixation in open fractures, and attention to the details of technique, including gentle soft-tissue handling, the prevention of infection, and restoration of the fracture fragments to their anatomical position.

The prognosis for displaced fractures of the radius and ulna in adults treated with closed reduction is generally considered poor in an unacceptably high percentage of patients. For fractures treated with open reduction and rigid internal fixation, the prognosis for achieving union is about 95%. In his series, Sage[79] reported union of 93.8% of the fractures treated with triangular medullary nails; and in Anderson's series[4] of forearm fractures treated with compression plates, 97.3% of the fractures united. Approximately 90% had satisfactory or excellent function, with only 10% having unsatisfactory or poor function after the first operation. Other articles concerning forearm fractures

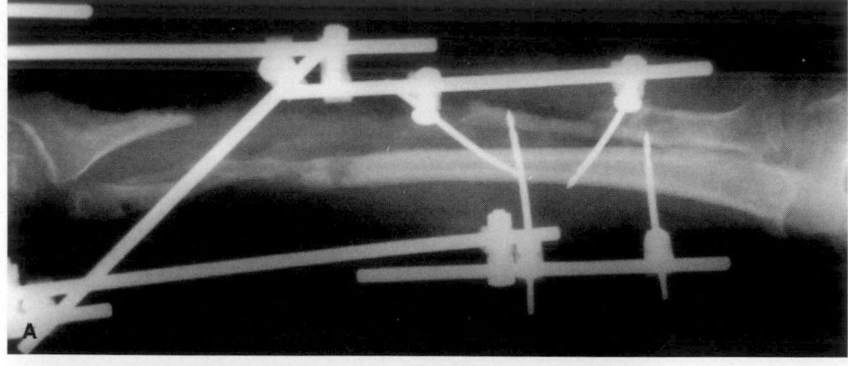

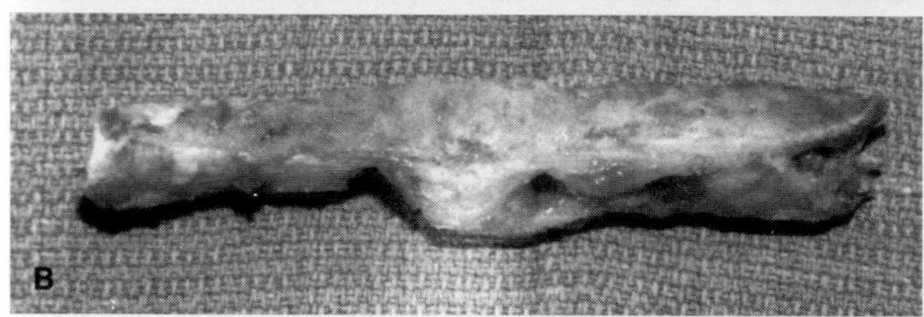

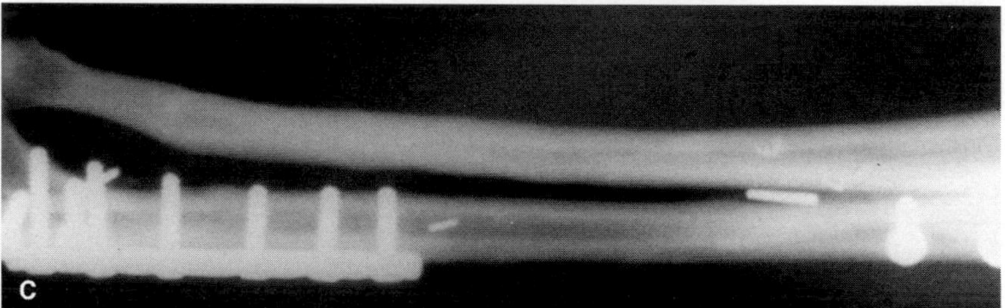

FIGURE 13-32. (**A**) Infected nonunion of both the radius and ulna after plate fixation of open fractures of both the radius and the ulna in a third world country. If plate fixation is used to treat open fractures of the forearm, debridement must be meticulous and thorough and rigid aseptic technique must be used. If these conditions do not exist, consideration should be given to the use of external fixation, a technique used to salvage the forearm in this case. (**B**) A nonviable, devascularized segment of the radius spontaneously extruded during debridement of the infected nonunion. The radial diaphysis had become sequestered. (**C**) A vascularized fibular bone graft was used to reconstitute the radius. Although union was achieved there was very little forearm rotation. The infection was eradicated.

treated with compression plates report similar results.[2–6,19,25,39,40,67,80,89,97,98]

In a group of forearm shaft fractures treated primarily with slotted plates by Jinkins and coworkers,[46] 95.8% united. Caden[17] reported a union rate of 92.5% with slotted plates. Other surgeons have reported similar good results with rigid fixation both with plates and with medullary nails.[16,76] The important feature common to all these reports in which over 90% of the fractures united was the rigidity of fixation. If intramedullary nails are used, they must control rotation of the fragments and be sturdy enough to resist angulatory forces. If plates and screws are used, they must be long enough and strong enough to resist loosening and breakage of the fixation.

The prognosis for union and good function is much poorer if round medullary nails or inadequate plates are used. Semitubular plates are not recommended. Neither are round medullary nails, which have been reported to lead to nonunion in 14% to 16% of cases.[17,92] Kirschner wire fixation was reported by Smith and Sage[92] to produce nonunion in 38% of forearm fractures.

Schemitsch and Richards[86] performed a multivariate analysis to evaluate the prognostic influence of such variables as patient age, the mechanism of injury, an ipsilateral upper extremity injury, an open injury, the time to treatment, and the presence of a complication. Although forearm rotation was reduced by the occurrence of a complication, rotation was not adversely affected by ipsilateral upper extremity injury or grade II and III open fractures. Similarly, reduced grip strength resulted from an industrial injury or by grade II and III open fractures, as well as from loss of radial bow. These findings demonstrate the importance of the accuracy of the reduction at the time of fixation in determining prognosis.

For open fractures of the shaft of the radius and ulna with major skin and soft-tissue loss, the prognosis must be more guarded.[24] In these cases, several operative procedures may be necessary, including the initial debridement and stabilization, skin grafting or pedicle or free flap applications, late reconstruction of the bones, and, frequently, the transfer of tendons. Occasionally, skeletal reconstruction requires creating a one-bone forearm, which provides the patient with a stable link between elbow and wrist but without forearm rotation. The position I prefer is 30° pronation. It is usually necessary to use a combination of bone grafting and internal fixation to achieve a one-bone forearm. If infection develops, excision of all nonviable bone and institution of irrigation-suction may be necessary. Usually, enough function can be preserved to make all this worthwhile, but the result is generally far from normal. Rarely, infection, fibrosis of the soft tissues, or loss of neurovascular function may necessitate amputation.

COMPLICATIONS

Nonunion and Malunion

Anderson's series of forearm fractures treated with compression plates included nine cases of nonunion (2.7%) and four delayed unions (1.2%) in 330 fractures. Seven of the 244 patients developed significant infection (2.9%) (Fig. 13-33). In 4 of these patients the infections cleared with antibiotic therapy and caused no further difficulty. In the other 3 patients the fractures failed to unite and subsequent operations were required. Almost all of the nonunions and delayed unions appeared to have been caused by infection or errors in technique.

Nonunion of fractures of the shafts of the radius and ulna is relatively uncommon (9.3% in Stern and Drury's series,[94] 2.7% in Anderson and associates' series[6]). It is most often seen when infection is present, when fixation after open reduction is inadequate, and when adequate reduction was not achieved and maintained after closed treatment (Fig. 13-34). Accurate open reduction and rigid internal fixation will prevent most of these complications (Fig. 13-35). The various methods of treating nonunion are discussed in Chapter 8.

Infection

Despite all attempts to prevent infection, some open fractures and closed fractures treated by open reduction inevitably become infected. The incidence is higher in patients with extensive soft-tissue injury. Stern and Drury[94] reported only a 3.1% incidence (2/87) of osteomyelitis; both occurred in patients with massive crush injuries. With good technique and operating facilities, this percentage should be small. If infection develops, the wound should be surgically drained, debrided, and copiously irrigated. Cultures of the wound are taken and sensitivity of the organism determined. Appropriate antibiotic therapy must be

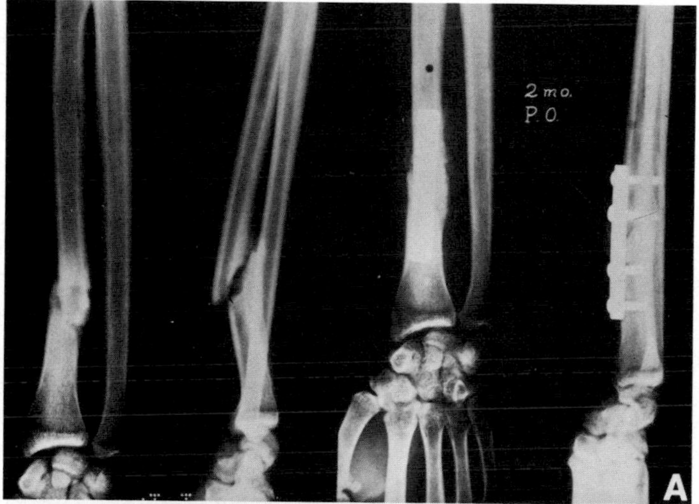

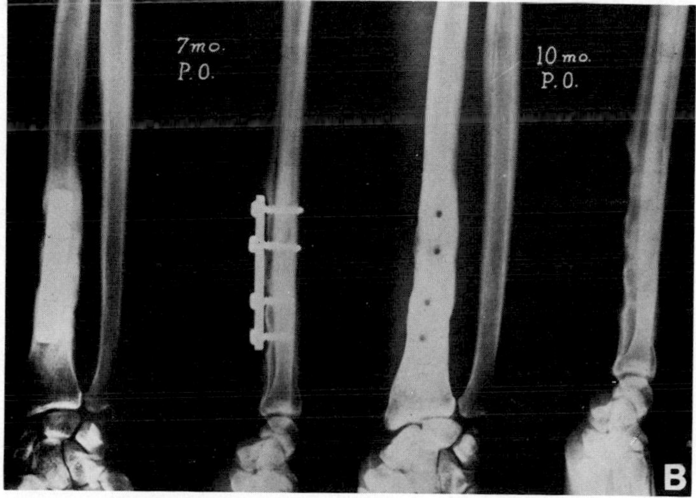

FIGURE 13-33. (**A**) A 20-year-old man with an untreated fracture at the junction of the middle and distal thirds of the radius incurred 6 weeks earlier. He was treated with a compression plate applied to the palmar surface of the radius. (**B**) The patient was lost to follow-up but returned at 7 months, at which time he had developed drainage secondary to a *Staphylococcus aureus* infection. Note the periosteal reaction present at the proximal end of the plate and the resorption about the screws in the distal end. The infection resolved when the plate was removed and irrigation-suction treatment was carried out.

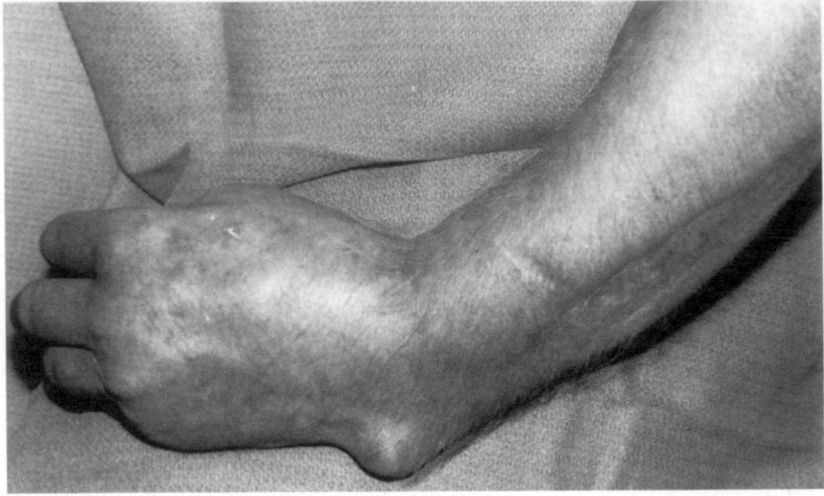

FIGURE 13-34. Malunion of the forearm. The patient developed an infected nonunion of the radius after fractures of both bones of the forearm. Due to the severe shortening of the radius it was necessary to create a single-bone forearm by centralizing the ulna and performing a wrist arthrodesis with a 12-hole 3.5-mm dynamic compression plate.

initiated. Superficial infections frequently respond to this treatment alone. If the infection appears to be deep, the wound should be opened to provide drainage; and if the arm is not already immobilized in a cast, a cast or thermoplastic splint should be applied. If internal fixation is in place and the fixation device has not loosened, it should not be removed. A fairly high percentage of fractures that have been fixed internally unite in spite of infection with antibiotic treatment and drainage. After the fracture has healed, the metal can be removed.

Aggressive treatment is required for late infections, when fixation has been lost and nonunion has developed. The metal should be removed along with any nonviable bone. The wound can be left open for dressing changes, or an irrigation-suction system can be instituted. The principle of treatment is that union of the fracture must be obtained even in the presence of infection. A radical debridement may be required, including removal of necrotic and infected diaphyseal bone. If an intercalary defect results, it can be spanned with a long plate and bone grafted when the wound is healthy after a period of dressing changes. Serial examinations of the wound are required to determine when bone grafting can be performed safely. The surgeon must be certain that all necrotic bone has been removed from the wound. Only after this has been accomplished and the wound has a healthy appearance should bone grafting be done. Alternatively, an external fixator can be used. If the intercalary defect is greater than 6 cm, a vascularized fibular bone graft may be required to bridge the defect. Appropriate antibiotics should be given before, during, and after the reconstructive surgery, although the most important element in the treatment of an infected nonunion is surgical.

Nerve Injury

Nerve injuries associated with fractures of both bones of the forearm are uncommon in closed fractures or those with only minor compounding wounds. Prosser

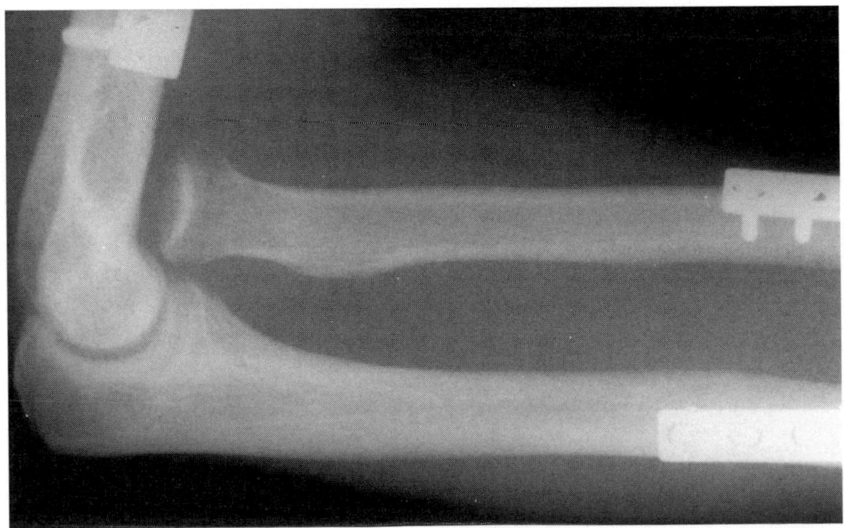

FIGURE 13-35. Anterior dislocation of the radial head after fixation of multiple upper extremity fractures. The radius was fixed with a straight plate and the dislocation of the radial head was missed initially. Patients with forearm fractures must have radiographs of both the proximal and distal radioulnar joints.

and Hooper[70] reported a case in which the ulnar nerve was trapped between the bone ends of a greenstick fracture of the ulna. Return of function was complete after removal of the nerve from the bone. Nerve injuries are more common in the major compound wounds with extensive soft-tissue loss, such as shotgun injuries. In such an injury, if one of the major nerves is found not to be functioning, it should be explored at the time of debridement to determine whether it is intact or divided. If it is divided, the ends should be tagged together with sutures to prevent retraction and facilitate later repair. If the wound is clean, the nerve cleanly transected, and the soft-tissue bed adequate, primary nerve repair at the time of wound closure is probably the appropriate treatment.

If the nerve injury occurs as the result of treatment, my recommendations for management are as follows. Incomplete iatrogenic nerve injuries can be observed for several weeks or months to determine if recovery will occur. If there is no evidence of recovery by 3 months, exploration is probably indicated. Complete iatrogenic nerve injuries should be explored early (within a few hours or days) if the nerve was not observed at the time of the primary operation. Early exploration is desirable in such cases to be certain that the nerve was not damaged by plating or suture placement. If the nerve had in fact been exposed and visualized throughout the operation (including just before closure) and the surgeon is confident that the nerve was not damaged, then observation with expectation of recovery is the appropriate management.

Vascular Injury

If the collateral circulation of the forearm is good, and if either the radial or the ulnar artery is functioning, viability of the hand and forearm is usually not in jeopardy. When either vessel is patent, the other can simply be ligated. Animal experiments by Gelberman and coworkers[33] and by Trumble and coworkers[100] showed low patency rates if one artery in the forearm is repaired when the other is intact. These researchers thought that this phenomenon was due to backpressure from the intact vessel and dilation of collateral vessels. It is rare to have both vessels lacerated except in open fractures in which a traumatic near-amputation has occurred. Here the damage to nerves, tendons, and bone is sometimes so severe that amputation may be necessary, although replantation or revascularization using microsurgical techniques is a reasonable alternative in selected cases.[75]

Compartment Syndrome

Compartment syndrome in the forearm is associated with supracondylar fractures, knife wounds of the forearm, soft-tissue crush injuries, and osteotomy of the radius and ulna in addition to fractures of both bones of the forearm. Compartment syndromes can occur in the forearm either after trauma or after surgery. In 1975, Eaton and Green[26] reported 19 patients with Volkmann's ischemia, which they considered to be a volar compartment syndrome of the forearm. They found the most important diagnostic physical finding to be palpable induration of the flexor compartment. Another important early sign is pain on passive extension of the fingers. Presence of the radial pulse is *not* a reliable diagnostic indicator; the radial pulse was absent in only 5 of their 19 patients. All clinicians should be aware that the presence of a palpable radial pulse does *not* rule out the presence of a volar compartment syndrome. Eaton and Green emphasized early decompression not only of the compartment but also of each muscle that shows vascular impairment.

Throughout the course of a compartment syndrome it is possible to have a palpable forearm pulse despite increased pressure in the forearm compartments sufficient to obliterate the capillary circulation to the muscles and nerves. This may confuse the picture and delay diagnosis and treatment. In such cases there may be decreased sensation in the fingers, little or no function in the forearm muscles, and deep, boring pain in the forearm disproportionate to what one would expect. Pain on passive extension of the fingers is also a very important sign of ischemia in the forearm muscles. One should not hesitate to make the diagnosis of a compartment syndrome in this clinical situation.

Compartment pressures can be measured to confirm the diagnosis of compartment syndrome, provided treatment is not delayed. It is only necessary to measure compartment pressures in unconscious or obtunded patients to make the diagnosis of a compartment syndrome. In a conscious patient the diagnosis of a compartment syndrome can be made on clinical grounds alone. The treatment is early and wide fasciotomy from the elbow to the wrist, including division of the lacertus fibrosis and transverse carpal ligament. At the time of operation, the muscles bulge into the wound. The incision should be allowed to separate, and delayed closure can be done later and usually requires split-thickness skin grafts.

Closed compartment syndromes that follow operations in the forearm are usually due to faulty hemostasis or closure of the deep fascia. They can usually be avoided by releasing the tourniquet before wound closure to make sure hemostasis is adequate and by closing only the subcutaneous tissue and skin. I know of three patients in whom compartment syndromes developed after open reduction and internal fixation of forearm fractures. In all three, the deep fascia had been closed. This complication is usually avoidable. In 1980, Matsen[61] published a comprehensive (and highly recommended) book providing a summation of knowledge of this subject, including etiology, measurement of compartmental pressures, and treatment. (Compartment syndromes are discussed in more detail in Chapter 8.)

Post-Traumatic Radioulnar Synostosis

Synostosis of the radius and ulna following fracture is relatively uncommon. In Anderson's series of forearm fractures treated with compression plates, only 3 of 112 patients with fractures of both the radius and the ulna developed this complication.[5] All 3 had badly displaced and comminuted fractures of both bones at the same level. Stern and Drury[94] reported a 9.4% incidence (6/87) of synostosis in their series. Patients in whom a synostosis develops frequently have a history of either a crushing injury of the forearm or a head injury.[94] If a synostosis develops and the position of the forearm is relatively functional, it is usually best to do nothing. If the rotational alignment of the forearm is poor, an osteotomy to position the hand in a more functional position can be considered. Alternatively, an attempt can be made to resect the synostosis.

A few cases of successful resection of synostoses have been reported. In 1983, Breit[15] reported good results in a 28-year-old woman who underwent resection of a post-traumatic synostosis, obliteration of the dead space with muscle, prevention of hematoma formation, and early mobilization. Maempel[59] reported two cases of successful excision of a traumatic radioulnar synostosis in which he had used a Silastic sheet interposed between the forearm bones after resection.

Vince and Miller[105] reported their results in the treatment of 28 adults with a post-traumatic radioulnar synostosis. They developed a classification system based on the anatomical location of the synostosis (Fig. 13-36). Type 1 involves the distal intra-articular part of the radius and ulna; this was the least common type in their series. Type 2 involves the nonarticular portion of the distal third and the middle third of the shafts of the radius and ulna; this was their most common type. Type 3 involved the proximal third (Fig. 13-37). Seventeen of 28 synostoses were excised. Three of 4 type 1, none of 10 type 2, and 2 of 3 type 3 cross-unions recurred after surgical treatment. Their results suggest that resection of a nonarticular post-traumatic synostosis in the distal or the middle third of the forearm has a good chance of success, but this is not the case if the synostosis is in the proximal third. Abrams and associates[1] report on the successful use of surgery combined with low-dose radiation therapy to prevent recurrent heterotopic ossification.

Refracture

Two other complications that have been seen with compression plates are refracture (if the plate is removed too early) and fracture at the end of the plate

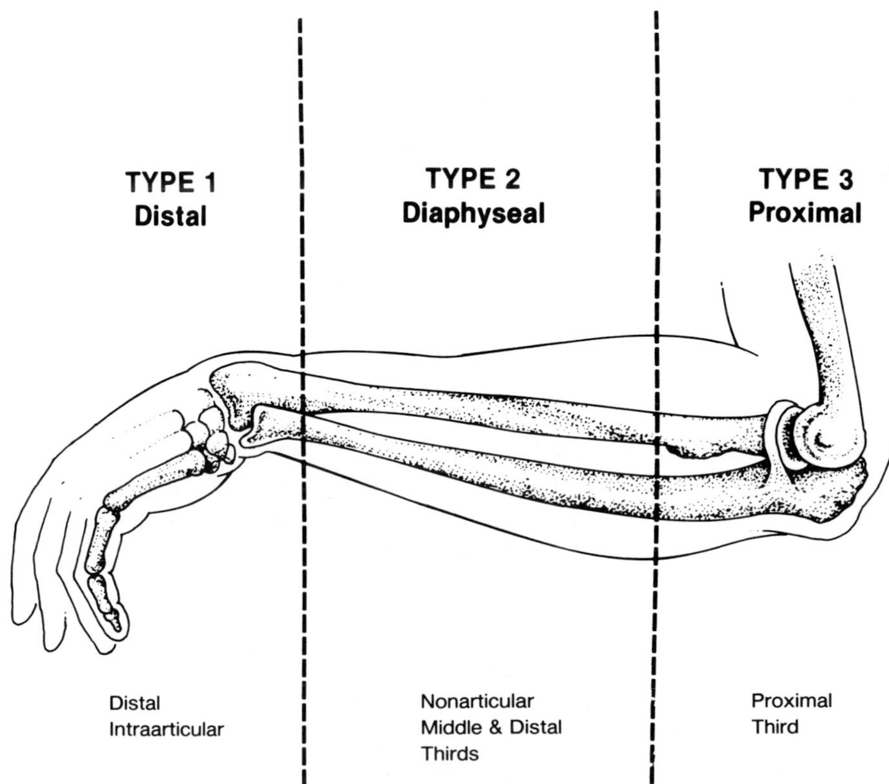

FIGURE 13-36. Classification system for cross-unions complicating fractures of the forearm. Type 1 (distal) is located in the distal intra-articular part of the forearm. Type 2 (diaphyseal) occurs in the middle and nonarticular distal thirds of the forearm and type 3 (proximal) in the proximal third, as determined by the length of the ulna. (*Vince, K.G., and Miller, J.E.: Cross-union Complicating Fracture of the Forearm: I. Adults. J. Bone Joint Surg., 69A:641, 1987.*)

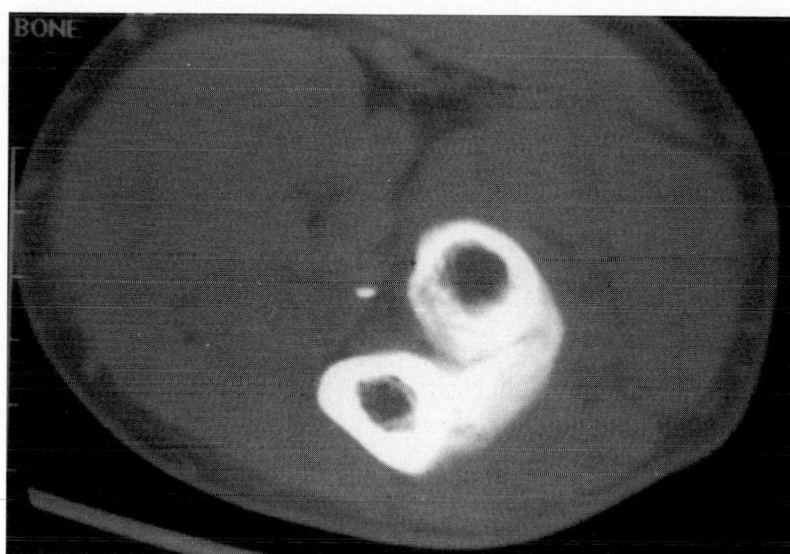

FIGURE 13-37. Cross-sectional CT scan of the proximal forearm demonstrating a post-traumatic synostosis. The patient was treated by resection of the synostosis supplemented with indomethacin and early motion. Approximately one half of the normal range of forearm rotation was regained.

from additional trauma. Anderson noted that these plates provide very rigid fixation, and the normal stresses acting over the bone beneath the plate are reduced. If the plate is removed early, minor trauma can cause a refracture at or near the site of the original fracture. Anderson did not advocate routine removal of plates; his specific indications for removal were (1) a prominent plate lying subcutaneously that causes the patient discomfort and (2) the intention of the patient to return to contact sports.

Anderson recommended that plates be left in for at least 18 months. After plate removal the extremity should be protected from impact-type activity for at least 8 weeks. I agree with these indications for plate removal.

In 1988, Deluca and coworkers[23] reported refractures in 7 of 67 patients. Refracture occurred between 42 and 121 days after plate removal. In their series, fracture always occurred through the original fracture site. The average time from original injury to plate removal in refractures was 16 months. No refractures were seen in patients if the plates were removed after 24 months. Of seven refractures, only one had adequate compression. Refracture should be included among the risks of removal.[104] Patients should be informed that refracture can occur for several months after plate removal and that they should avoid impact-type activities during this period, especially if they have any of the risk factors discussed below.

To help identify patients who are at risk, the physician should consider several factors: (1) the nature of the original injury (a disproportionate number of refractures occurred in patients in whom the initial fracture was due to high-energy trauma or a crush injury or was open or associated with other fractures in the extremity); (2) failure to achieve adequate initial compression or reduction in a comminuted fracture; or (3) radiographic determination that the site of the original fracture has remained radiolucent (in other words, the fracture never healed completely).

Chapman and associates[19] believe that the incidence of refracture can be reduced by the use of 3.5-mm dynamic compression plates. They reported only two refractures in their series and pointed out that both had occurred in fractures in which 4.5-mm plates had been used. In two cases, however, there was early failure of fixation. In one patient a 3.5-mm dynamic compression plate was used, and in the other a semitubular plate was used.

Radin and Rose[71] reported a fracture of a semitubular plate within a long-arm cast. The fracture was thought to be due to fatigue caused by the forces generated by the finger flexors. Semitubular plates are not recommended for treatment of forearm fractures except very rarely on the proximal radius or distal ulna. Schemitsch and Richards had a refracture rate of 17% (4/24) after plate removal. Refracture was not observed in their patients who did *not* undergo plate removal. The mean interval between fracture and plate removal in the patients who sustained a refracture was 10 months (range, 8–12 months). The mean interval between fracture and plate removal in the patients who did not sustain a refracture was 16 months (range, 8–26 months). I remove hardware only if there is significant irritation of the overlying soft tissues. Ideally, plates should be left in place *at least* 18 months because refracture is more common if removal is performed sooner than this. Bostman[10] reported on the use of absorbable material to avoid the need for implant removal.

Muscle and Tendon Entrapment and Adherence

Rayan and Hayes[74] reported a case in which the flexor digitorum profundus of the ring finger was trapped between the ends of the ulna in a two-bone forearm fracture. This was not recognized until 2 years later, after the fracture had healed. Release of the entrapped muscle belly resulted in return of full active extension of the ring finger. Littlefield and associates[58] reported on five patients with digital flexion contractures after healed forearm fractures that were initially diagnosed as mild Volkmann ischemic contractures. Lysis of adhesions and lengthening of the contracted muscles corrected the deformities.

FRACTURES OF THE RADIUS ALONE

Fractures of the shaft of the radius alone can be divided into two groups: (1) fractures in the proximal two thirds of the bone not associated with injury to the distal radioulnar joint and (2) those at the junction of the middle and distal thirds that are, to a greater or lesser extent, associated with injury to the distal radioulnar joint.

FRACTURES OF THE PROXIMAL RADIUS ALONE

Fractures of the upper two thirds of the radial shaft alone are not common in adults. The radial shaft in the proximal two thirds is relatively well padded by the forearm muscles. Most injuries severe enough to fracture the radius at this level will also fracture the ulna. Also, the anatomical position of the radius in most positions of function makes it less likely than the ulna to receive a direct blow.

The rare *nondisplaced* fracture of the shaft of the radius in the proximal two thirds should be immobilized in a long-arm cast with the forearm in mild or full supination, depending on whether the fracture is located above or below the insertion of the pronator teres. The reasons for placing the forearm in supination are outlined in the sections of this chapter dealing with surgical anatomy and fractures of both the radius and ulna. Nondisplaced fractures can become displaced, and frequent x-rays must be made during the first few weeks. Cast immobilization must be maintained until healing has occurred.

Displaced fractures of the proximal one fifth of the radius are probably best treated by open reduction and internal fixation. Internal fixation with a plate is challenging, owing to the small size of the proximal fragment. It is usually possible to obtain two or three screws in the proximal fragment, which is less than the ideal number. An anterior Henry approach is recommended. In the proximal forearm the incision must be extended proximal to the elbow to adequately visualize neurovascular structures. The radial recurrent vessels must be identified and divided. The radial nerve and its superficial and deep (posterior interosseous) branches should also be identified and protected. The supinator should be reflected from its ulnar border to reduce the risk of injury to the posterior interosseous nerve. If the annular ligament has to be divided to obtain exposure it should be repaired before closure of the wound (Fig. 13-38). The aftertreatment is the same as for fractures of both bones of the forearm treated with open reduction and internal fixation.

FRACTURES OF THE DISTAL RADIAL SHAFT (GALEAZZI'S FRACTURE)

The solitary fracture of the radius at the junction of the middle and distal thirds has several eponyms. The French, at least as early as 1929, referred to this lesion as a reverse Monteggia fracture.[101] Galeazzi[73] described the fracture in 1934 and called attention to the associated dislocation or subluxation of the distal radioulnar joint. He pointed out that subluxation of this joint may be present initially or may occur gradually during treatment. Galeazzi advocated treating the fracture with strong traction through the thumb. Campbell is said to have called this lesion "the fracture of necessity," by which he meant that open reduction and internal fixation was necessary if a good result were to be obtained (Anderson, L., personal communication, 1975).

An excellent description of the fracture of the distal shaft of the radius associated with dislocation of the distal radioulnar joint is that published by Hughston[44] in 1957. He collected 41 cases from members of the Piedmont Orthopaedic Society and reported a very high incidence of poor results, although his criteria for a satisfactory result were very strict. These included union with perfect alignment, no loss of length, no subluxation of the distal radioulnar joint, and full pronation and supination. Of the 38 fractures treated initially by closed reduction and immobilization, Hughston reported that poor results occurred in 35 (92%). Only three patients had a satisfactory result.

As pointed out by Hughston, four major deforming factors can contribute to loss of reduction:

1. Gravity acting through the weight of the hand, even in a cast, tends to cause subluxation of the distal radioulnar joint and dorsal angulation of the fractured radius.
2. The insertion of the pronator quadratus on the palmar surface of the distal fragment rotates it

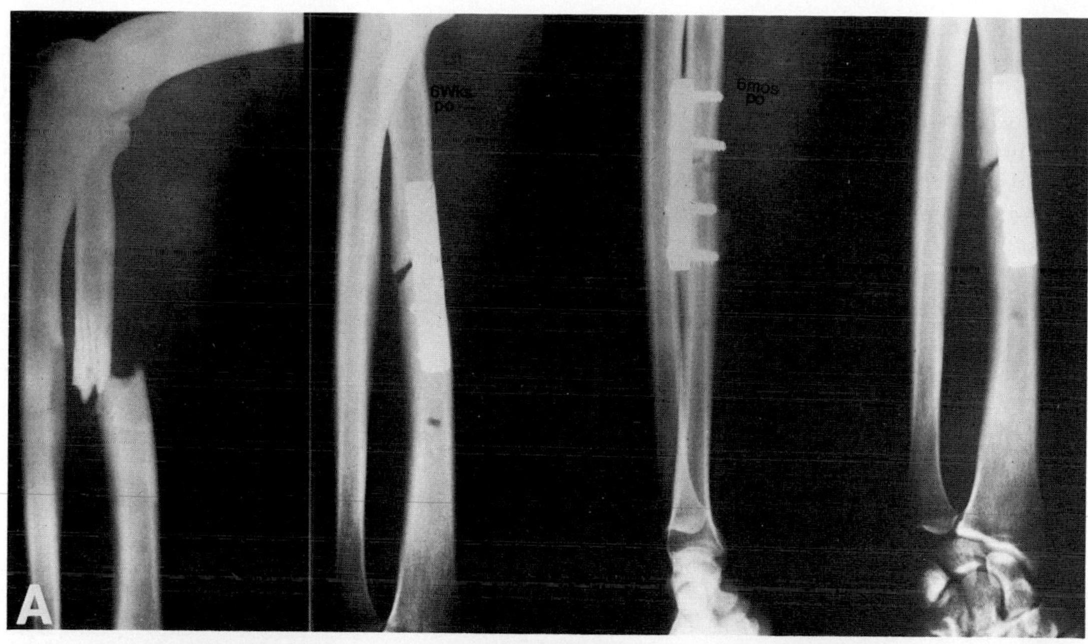

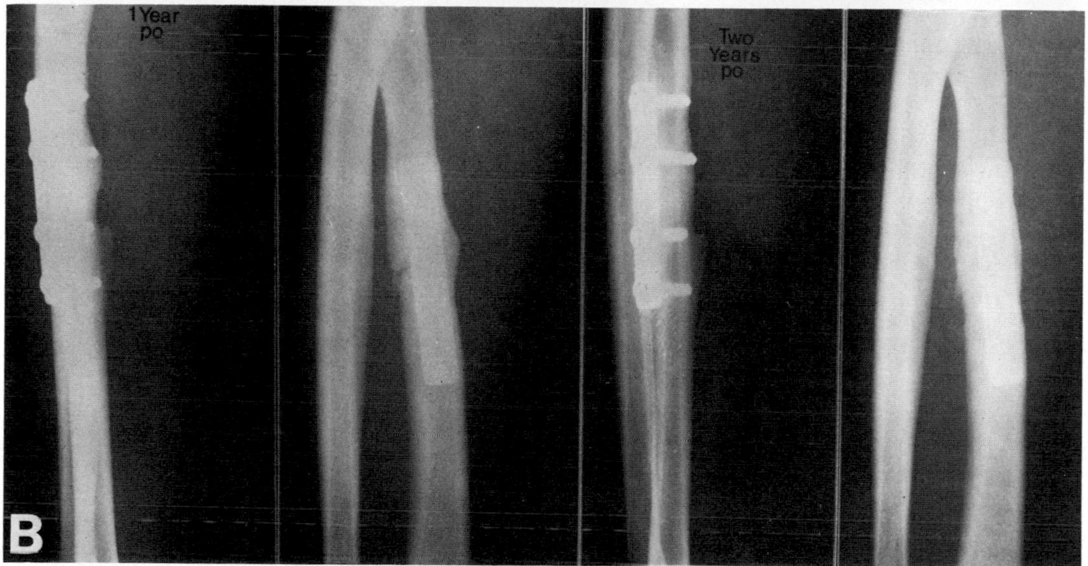

FIGURE 13-38. (**A**) A fracture of the shaft of the radius at the junction of the proximal and middle thirds with an intact ulna. Open reduction and internal fixation with a four-hole compression plate were performed. Note that the plate was placed on the dorsal aspect of the radius. At 6 months, a portion of the fracture line is still visible. A five-hole plate would have been better, and bone grafts probably should have been applied. (**B**) Radiographs at 1 year and 2 years show union. The patient regained full range of motion.

toward the ulna and pulls it in a proximal and palmar direction.

3. The brachioradialis tends to use the distal radioulnar joint as a pivot point on which to rotate the distal fragment of the radius and at the same time causes shortening.
4. The abductors and extensors of the thumb cause shortening and relaxation of the radial collateral ligament so that one is not able to keep the soft-tissue bridge on stretch, even though the wrist is placed in ulnar deviation.

MECHANISM OF INJURY

The two principal causes of Galeazzi's fracture are direct blows on the dorsolateral side of the wrist, and falls. Mikic[120] thought that the most probable mechanism of injury in Galeazzi's fracture is a fall on the outstretched hand combined with marked pronation of the forearm. According to Galeazzi,[116] this lesion is approximately three times as common as the Monteggia fracture.

SIGNS AND SYMPTOMS

The signs and symptoms vary with the severity of injury and the degree of displacement. In nondisplaced or relatively nondisplaced fractures, the only deformity may be swelling and tenderness about the fracture. If the displacement is greater, there will be shortening of the radius and posterolateral angulation. Subluxation or dislocation will be evident in the distal radioulnar joint with prominence of the head of the ulna and tenderness over the joint.[112] Rarely, a dislocation of the radial head can occur in association with a radial shaft fracture.[126] Most of these are closed fractures. In open fractures, the wound is usually a small puncture wound from within where the distal end of the proximal fragment has protruded through the skin. Nerve and vascular damage are rare.

RADIOGRAPHIC FINDINGS

The fracture at the junction of the middle and distal thirds of the radius usually has a transverse or short oblique configuration (Fig. 13-39). Most do not have significant comminution. If there is much displacement of the fractured radius, the distal radioulnar joint will be dislocated or subluxated. On the anteroposterior film the radius appears relatively shortened, with an increase in the space between the distal radius and ulna where they articulate. In the lateral view, the fractured radius is usually angulated dorsally and the head of the ulna is prominent dorsally. The injury to the radioulnar joint may be purely ligamentous, or the ligaments may remain intact and the ulnar styloid may be avulsed.

TREATMENT

From the above introductory discussion, it should be apparent that the results of closed treatment are poor. The deforming forces are so great that even if the fracture is nondisplaced initially or if good position is obtained by closed reduction, displacement in the cast is the rule (Fig. 13-40). To obtain functional pronation and supination and to avoid derangement and arthritic changes in the distal radioulnar joint, the fracture must unite in an anatomical position. For these reasons, open reduction and internal fixation is almost always the preferred form of treatment.

In their book, Sarmiento and Latta[83] stated that not all isolated fractures of the distal third of the radius have associated distal radioulnar joint pathology or damage to the interosseous membrane. Moore, Lester, and Sarmiento[122] created Galeazzi fractures in cadavers. They found that up to 5 mm of radial shortening

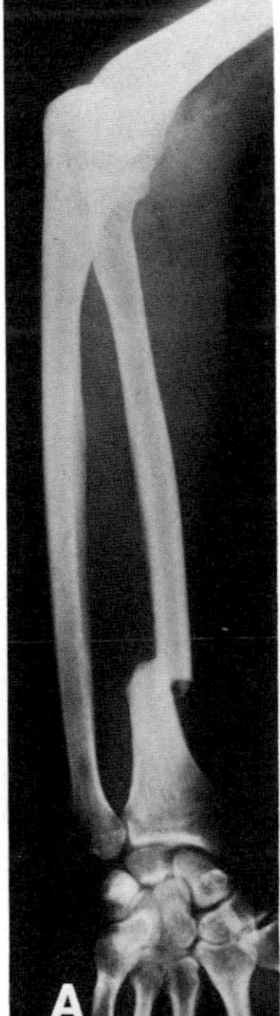

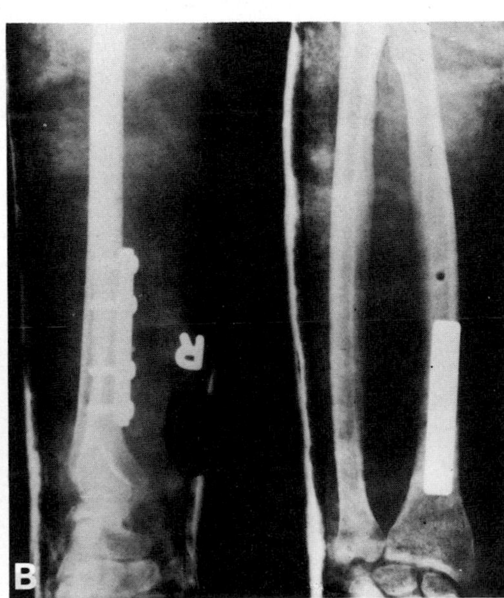

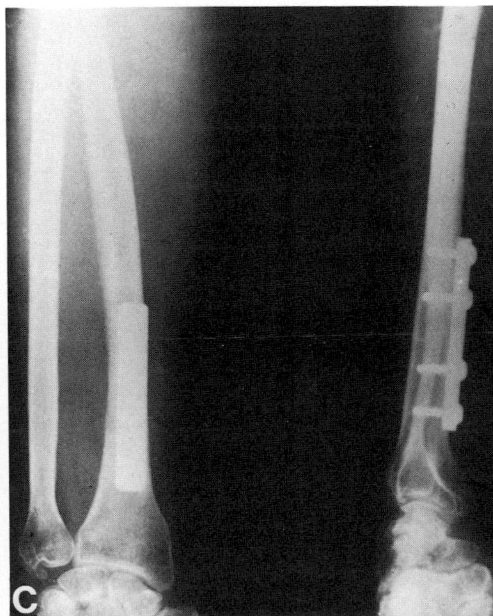

FIGURE 13-39. (**A**) A Galeazzi fracture of the distal radial shaft with dislocation of the distal radioulnar joint. (**B**) Successful internal fixation using a four-hole compression plate. Note that the plate was applied on the palmar surface of the radius where the bone is flatter. Compression was applied proximally. (**C**) One year later, union is complete and function is normal. A six or eight hole plate is now preferred (see text).

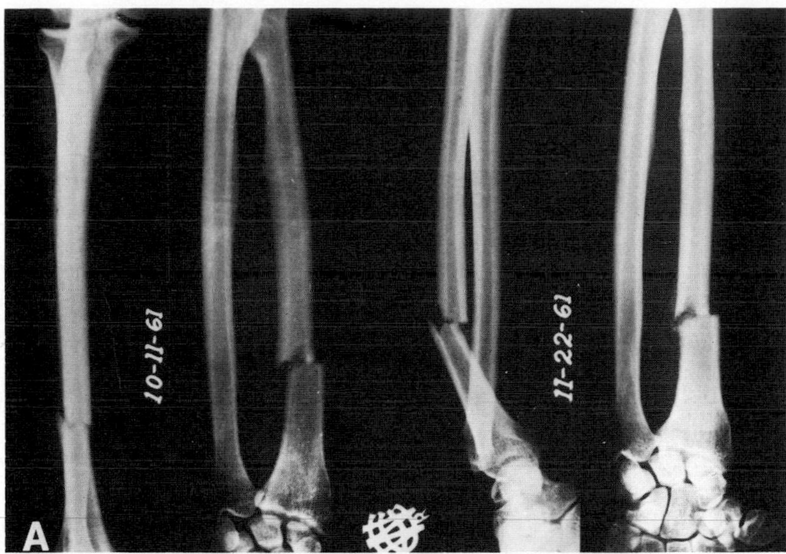

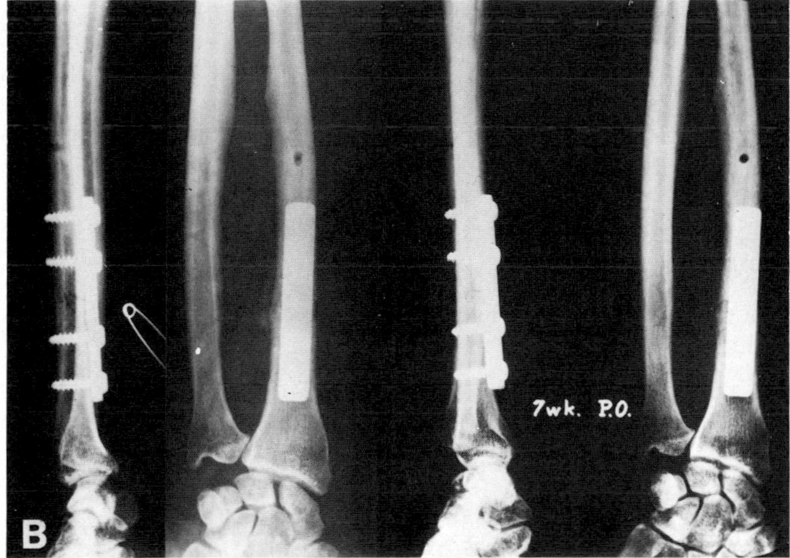

FIGURE 13-40. (**A**) Solitary fracture of the distal third of the radial shaft with minimal displacement (*first and second frames*). After 6 weeks' immobilization (by the family physician) in a long-arm cast, the fracture has angulated dorsally and the distal radioulnar joint is seen to be dislocated (*third and fourth frames*). (**B**) Immediate postoperative radiographs showing the fracture fixed with a four-hole compression plate applied to the palmar surface of the radius (*first and second frames*). Seven weeks later, the fracture has united (*third and fourth frames*). (*Anderson, L.D.: Fractures. In Crenshaw, A.H.* [*ed.*]*: Campbell's Operative Orthopaedics, 5th ed., vol. 1. St. Louis, C.V. Mosby, 1971.*)

occurred after osteotomy alone. Shortening of over 10 mm did not occur unless both the interosseous ligament and the triangular ligament were sectioned. They believe that isolated fractures of the distal third of the radius resulting from axial loading are more likely to be associated with distal radioulnar pathology and injury to the interosseous membrane. Sarmiento recommended that this type of injury be treated with open reduction and internal fixation. On the other hand, he believed that a similar fracture of the distal third of the radius resulting from a direct blow perpendicular to the bone, that displaces the radial fragment ulnarward does not necessarily have associated distal radioulnar joint pathology or injury to the interosseous membrane. He suggested that if this latter fracture were transverse and well reduced, it might not require internal fixation and was amenable to his functional bracing method.

Intramedullary nails do not provide satisfactory fixation for these fractures. The medullary canal at the level of the fracture is large and continues to enlarge distally. The nail does not prevent medial offset of the distal fragment and shortening of the radius. Also, the medullary canal of the distal fragment is too large for the nail to control rotation. Plate-and-screw fixation is by far the best method, but if good results are to be expected, the plate must be long enough and the screws must obtain good purchase in both cortices.

In 1975, Mikic[120] reported a large series of 125 patients with Galeazzi type fracture-dislocations of the forearm. Many of his patients in whom the radius alone was internally fixed had a poor result because of failure to maintain reduction of the distal radioulnar joint. For this reason he advocated pinning the ulna to the radius with one or two percutaneously placed Kirschner wires. The Kirschner wires are removed after a few weeks. Liang and coworkers[119] also advocated temporary, percutaneous, transradioulnar

Kirschner wire fixation for 4 weeks. However, Mikic advocated the Rush pin as his method of treatment for fracture of the radius, which as outlined previously, has been ineffective because it does not control rotation and allows shortening of the radius. Thus, redislocation of the distal radioulnar joint is almost inevitable with this type of fixation.

Once the radius has been anatomically reduced and rigidly fixed, the position and stability of the distal radioulnar joint must be critically assessed. Although much has been written advocating internal fixation of the radius in Galeazzi fractures, little has been said about the assessment and treatment of the distal radioulnar joint injury associated with the fracture.[114,118,121,123,124] My approach to this component of the injury complex is described below.

Authors' Preferred Method of Treatment

I prefer to treat fractures of the junction of the middle and distal thirds of the radius with compression-plate fixation, and I have had excellent results with this method. The details of the technique are reported elsewhere,[4,66,127] but a few points about using this technique to treat this particular fracture should be emphasized.

Surgical Approach

The anterior approach of Henry[13,20,42] is preferred. With the use of a hand table and tourniquet control, a 5- or 6-inch longitudinal incision is made, centered over the fracture in the plane between the flexor carpi radialis and the brachioradialis muscles. The radial artery and its venae comitantes are identified and retracted to the ulnar side. The brachioradialis and superficial radial nerve are retracted radially. All other structures are retracted ulnarly. The fracture is almost always located just above the proximal border of the pronator quadratus. The insertion of the pronator quadratus is detached from the radius and reflected ulnarward. The palmar surface of the proximal fragment is then exposed for a distance long enough to allow placement of the plate.

Fracture Reduction

With the use of self-retaining bone-holding forceps or a radial reduction clamp the fracture is reduced anatomically. Usually, there is little or no comminution; but if there is, the surgeon should try to fit each fragment anatomically into place. Butterfly fragments should be fixed to the major fragments with interfragmentary compression screws. A plate of appropriate length is selected, depending on the obliquity of the fracture and the degree of comminution. Reduction should only be attempted when the comminuted fragments have been lagged to the major fracture fragments, when the drill and screws are ready, and when the appropriate plate has been selected.

Plate Application

The volar cortex of the radius is flat and provides a good surface for the plate. In pure transverse fractures a six-hole 3.5-mm plate is adequate, but an eight-hole plate is preferred, particularly if there is any comminution or obliquity. The plate is centered accurately so that *at least* three 3.5-mm screws can be placed in both the proximal and distal fragments with no screw closer than 1 cm to the fracture, even if this means leaving a hole in the plate empty. The plate is clamped to the proximal and distal fragments with two bone-holding forceps or radial clamps. A third clamp is placed at right angles to the first two and secured to prevent angulation and shortening when compression is applied. If the fracture is oblique, compression can be obtained with an interfragmentary compression screw. The screws are inserted into the distal fragment first. Cancellous screws with large threads are used if the standard cortical screws do not gain adequate purchase, especially in the distal fragment. It may be necessary to contour the plate distally to accommodate the concavity of the distal radius. Inaccurate contouring of the radius can cause subluxation or dislocation of the distal radioulnar joint (Fig. 3-41).[117]

If open reduction and internal fixation are done properly, strong compression can usually be applied to the fracture without disturbing the distal relationship of the radius to the ulna. Occasionally, however, the fracture may be so comminuted or oblique that the radius shortens when compression is applied, and the distal relationship is disturbed. In this situation compression cannot be used and the plate is applied with neutralization technique. If there is significant comminution (there usually is if compression cannot be applied without causing the radius to shorten), autogenous iliac bone graft is added.

Assessment of Reduction and Distal Radioulnar Joint Stability

At this point, x-rays are taken in anteroposterior and lateral planes to be certain that the relationship at the distal radioulnar joint is anatomical. Distal radioulnar joint stability is assessed by ballottement of the distal ulna relative to the distal radius. Several possible scenarios exist at this point in the procedure, each of which demands a different course of action.

Distal Radioulnar Joint Reduced and Stable

This is the most common situation. In this situation the wound is closed and a padded plaster splint applied for 48 hours. At that point in time the forearm, wrist,

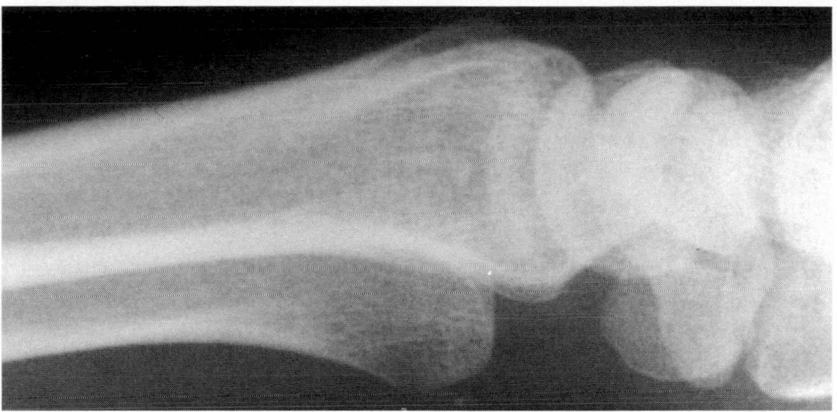

FIGURE 13-41. Lateral radiograph of the wrist demonstrating volar dislocation of the distal radioulnar joint. In this radiograph the scaphoid, lunate, and triquetrum are collinear. Accordingly the radiograph represents a "true" lateral of the wrist. The distal ulna is clearly dislocated in a volar direction. The proximal and distal radioulnar joints must be critically assessed clinically and radiographically when treating patients with fractures of both bones of the forearm.

and hand can be mobilized with no specific limitation. X-rays are taken on a regular basis until fracture union occurs, and distal radioulnar joint stability is reassessed at each clinic visit.

Distal Radioulnar Joint Reducible But Unstable

In this situation it is usually possible to find a point of forearm rotation where the distal radioulnar joint is stable. Usually this position is full supination.[113] If this is the case, the forearm is splinted in full supination and splintage is continued with a thermoplastic splint after the postoperative dressing is removed. Supination splinting is maintained for 4 weeks after the injury when mobilization of the forearm to neutral rotation is allowed. Six weeks after injury full rotation is allowed, although supination splinting at night is continued until 3 months after injury.

If no stable position can be found, the distal radioulnar joint is stabilized with a radioulnar pin. The radioulnar pin is passed just *proximal* to the radioulnar joint and left in place for 3 weeks. I use a 2-mm K-wire that is left long so that it can easily be removed in the clinic. Alternatively a "diastasis" screw can be used, using neutralization technique, by a method similar to that used in the ankle (Roth, J., personal communication, 1993). The advantage of the "diastasis" screw is that it provides more stable fixation than a smooth pin. The disadvantage is that it is more difficult to remove a screw a few weeks later.

Distal Radioulnar Joint Not Reducible

This is an uncommon scenario. The usual cause of an irreducible distal radioulnar joint is either malreduction of the radius or soft-tissue interposition within the joint. Assuming that the reduction of the radius is acceptable, open reduction of the distal radioulnar joint is required.

Exposure of the Distal Radioulnar Joint[125]

A separate, dorsal incision is made beginning 3 cm distal to the ulnar styloid. The incision is carried proximally at 45° to the long axis of the forearm in a radial direction until it reaches the dorsal aspect of the distal radius at the sigmoid notch. At this point the incision is angled sharply (90°) toward the ulna, and as it reaches the ulnar border of the forearm it is angled (45°) in a proximal direction.

The subcutaneous tissues are spread, taking care to preserve the dorsal sensory branch of the ulnar nerve. The dorsal sensory branch of the ulnar nerve passes onto the dorsum of the hand about 1 to 2 cm distal to the ulnar styloid, where it divides into multiple smaller branches. Care must be taken when dissecting the subcutaneous tissues to avoid injury to this sensory nerve, which will leave the patient with a painful neuroma. After the skin flaps have been raised the subcutaneous tissues are elevated from the extensor retinaculum. The key to identifying the important soft-tissue structures is the extensor digiti minimi tendon.

The supratendinous extensor retinaculum is elevated from the dorsum of the distal radioulnar joint. The retinaculum is elevated by first creating a transverse incision at the junction of the retinaculum proximally with the fascia over the extensor aspect of the forearm. This transverse incision is made at the proximal border of the distal radioulnar joint over the fourth extensor compartment. The transverse incision extends to the supratendinous portion of the extensor carpi ulnaris. The incision then runs longitudinally to a point just short of the distal extent of the retinaculum. It is best to preserve a small portion of the distal retinaculum to prevent bowstringing of the extensor tendons. The distal transverse limb lies just proximal to the distal border of the extensor retinaculum. As the extensor retinaculum is elevated the tendon of the extensor digiti minimi is visualized. An umbilical tape is placed around the extensor digiti minimi tendon, retracting it in a radial direction.

Exposure of the distal radioulnar joint is completed by making a dorsal capsulotomy. The limbs of the dorsal capsulotomy are similar to those created in the extensor retinaculum. The base of the dorsal capsulotomy lies along the extensor carpi ulnaris tendon. The transverse limbs of the capsular flap lie along the proximal margin of the distal radioulnar joint and the dorsal surface of the triangular fibrocartilage (TFC), respectively. The vertical incision used to create the capsular flaps lies over the dorsum of the sigmoid notch, leaving a small cuff of dorsal distal radioulnar joint capsule to repair at the conclusion of the procedure.

The most common form of distal radioulnar joint instability is dorsal instability. This disorder is associated with attenuation or complete rupture of the dorsal soft-tissue structures. Stabilization of the distal radioulnar joint can be accomplished by direct repair of the soft tissue or a dorsal capsulorrhaphy. The joint is inspected for loose bodies, traumatic chondromalacia, and any other pathologic conditions. Similarly, TFC should be inspected and probed for deficiencies. Peripheral tear of TFC can be repaired. Intra-articular abnormalities may require debridement. The dorsal capsule is imbricated with interrupted horizontal mattress sutures of 3-0 braided polyester suture on a tapered needle. It is usually possible to place three or four sutures. It is important to supinate the forearm when tying these sutures and to maintain the forearm in supination as closure proceeds. Supination approximates the dorsal soft-tissue structures and allows them to be repaired in a shortened position. Forceful pronation of the forearm before healing of the soft tissues can disrupt their repair.

Closure

The pronator quadratus is allowed to fall back into position over the plate but not reattached to the radius. The fascia should not be closed, for the reasons discussed previously. The subcutaneous tissue and skin are closed, and a well-molded sugar-tong splint is applied. Final films are made after the cast is in place to confirm that the distal radioulnar joint is reduced anatomically.

Aftercare

The length of postoperative immobilization is dependent on distal radioulnar joint stability (see the discussion on page 908 for assessment of stability).

Supination splinting is the mainstay of postoperative management if there is demonstrable instability of the distal radioulnar joint after fixation of the radial fracture. If the distal radioulnar joint is stable after fixation of the radial fracture, splinting is not required and early motion is encouraged. The vast majority of patients with distal radioulnar joint instability have dorsal instability that is evident on provocative testing. In the operating room the wrist and forearm are placed in a padded dressing with the forearm in full supination and the elbow at 90°. This position is maintained over the first 10 to 14 days until the patient returns for suture removal and x-rays. After removal of the sutures a thermoplastic splint is constructed. The splint holds the elbow at 90° and the forearm in full supination. Velcro straps are used to maintain the position of the forearm. The forearm is kept in full supination for 4 weeks. During this time the splint can be removed for bathing.

After 4 weeks the splint is removed for short periods of time. Night splinting is maintained and the patient wears the splint when outside the home. At 4 weeks a program of active forearm rotation is begun. Passive assisted motion is begun 6 weeks after surgery. Night splinting is maintained for 3 months. The object of the rehabilitation program is to progressively recover the range of forearm rotation while maintaining the reduction of the distal radioulnar joint (see p. 909). During the splinting program active finger and thumb motion is encouraged. Resistive exercises are avoided until a near-normal range of active motion is recovered. The program of rehabilitation is discontinued when the patient's progress plateaus.

Because the plate is well covered with soft tissue, it is seldom necessary to remove it, except in young athletes. If it is removed, the precautions noted to prevent refracture should be followed.

PROGNOSIS

Some of the older articles emphasized the poor prognosis for regaining good function after Galeazzi's fracture.[44,107] However, these articles were published before rigid fixation with compression plates was available. The points made by Campbell and Hughston were totally appropriate. Closed treatment gives poor results, as does inadequate internal fixation. The reduction of both the radial fracture and the distal radioulnar joint must be anatomical and stable. Since the advent of compression-plate fixation for this fracture, the results have been excellent.

COMPLICATIONS

The complications of Galeazzi's fracture are those incident to all forearm fractures: nonunion, malunion, and infection. In addition, subluxation and dislocation of the distal radioulnar joint can occur. In patients with acute fractures, these complications are largely avoidable with skillful surgical technique and rigid fixation. Much of the discussion in the section on complications after fracture of both bones of the forearm is applicable to complications occurring after isolated fractures of the radius.

In 1977, Cetti[115] described an unusual case of blocked reduction of Galeazzi's lesion. He reported two cases in which the extensor carpi ulnaris tendon was caught in the distal radioulnar joint, preventing reduction. In the first case, the fracture of the distal radius was internally fixed with a plate. Two months later, the fracture was healed, but there was marked restriction of pronation and supination. Additional radiographic examination suggested that the inferior radioulnar dislocation was still present or had recurred. At a second operation done 5 months after the first, the distal radioulnar joint was explored. The extensor carpi ulnaris tendon was found to be trapped between the radius and the ulna. The tendon was extracted, and the distal end of the ulna was excised with a good result.

In his second case, attempted closed reduction with the patient under general anesthesia was unsuccessful. The lower end of the ulna was then exposed through a dorsal vertical incision, revealing that the distal ulna had erupted dorsally through the capsule of the joint. There was complete separation of the ulnar styloid process, which, with the triangular fibrocartilage, remained in its normal relationship to the distal radius. The tendon of the extensor carpi ulnaris was found trapped between the ulna and the capsule. To reduce the dislocation, the capsule of the distal radioulnar joint had to be incised distally. The tendon could then be displaced and the dislocation of the distal radioulnar joint reduced.

In patients with nonunion and malposition presenting for treatment late (after 6 weeks), it is usually best to realign the radius and apply a bone graft.[128] If there has been much resorption of bone at the fracture, a full-thickness iliac graft from the crest may be used to regain radial length, restore the distal radioulnar relationship, and obtain reasonably good function.

In patients with mild to moderate degrees of malunion of the radius, pronation and supination will be limited and painful. In these, distal ulnar reconstruction can be considered after the radius is solidly united. Even if the distal ulna must be resected, I believe that it is better to allow the radial fracture to heal before doing so. Ulnar shortening can be considered if the radius unites in a shortened position and symptomatic ulnocarpal impaction occurs. More complex intra-articular deformities can be treated by hemiresection interposition arthroplasty as described by Bowers.[11] I prefer to avoid simple resection of the distal ulna if possible. If the distal ulna is resected, it should be done subperiosteally, and care should be taken to preserve the ulnar collateral ligament complex. (For more details about resection of the distal ulna, see Chapter 12.) Another alternative to resecting the distal ulna is the Sauve-Kapandji procedure,[84] an operation in which the distal radioulnar joint is fused and combined with the creation of a pseudarthrosis proximal to the fusion (Fig. 13-42). The technique for this procedure is well described elsewhere.[11]

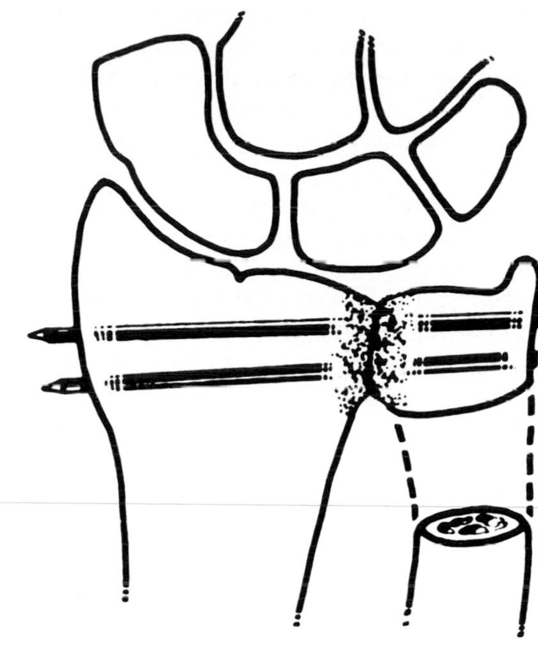

FIGURE 13-42. The Sauve-Kapandji procedure as described by Taleisnik. (*Bowers, W.H.: The Distal Radioulnar Joint. In Green, D.P. [ed.]: Operative Hand Surgery, 2nd ed., pp. 939–989. New York, Churchill Livingstone, 1988.*)

Isolated Fractures of the Ulnar Shaft and Monteggia Fractures

Fred G. Corley

ISOLATED FRACTURES OF THE ULNAR SHAFT

Isolated fractures of the ulnar shaft that are not associated with a dislocation of the radial head are common injuries. They are usually the result of a direct blow to the forearm and are frequently nondisplaced or only minimally displaced. The eponym "nightstick fracture" has been applied to those fractures caused by direct blows. Stress fractures in athletes have been reported by Bell[134] and by Patel,[161] unrelated to acute trauma.

NONDISPLACED FRACTURES

The effectiveness of "casual" treatment of isolated ulnar shaft fractures has been evaluated by Pollock[164] and by Hoffer.[149] Pollock[164] treated two comparable groups of patients with isolated ulnar fractures. One group was treated with a long-arm cast and the other with either a short-arm splint or no immobilization. No nonunions were reported in either group, and the average healing time was 6.7 weeks. Hoffer[149] noted three failures using "casual" treatment of ulnar shaft fractures, and he therefore recommended plaster immobilization or a functional brace as described by Sarmiento.[167,168]

A number of series have been reported in which nondisplaced or minimally displaced fractures of the ulna have been treated initially with a plaster cast followed by a functional brace (see Fig. 13-43). Sarmiento and associates[167,168] reported over 200 cases of minimally displaced isolated fractures of the ulna that were treated with an initial long-arm cast followed by a functional brace. The original plaster is removed when the acute swelling and symptoms resolve, and all subsequent treatment is with an orthoplast splint similar to the one shown in Figure 13-44. The functional brace allows elbow and wrist motion. The forearm is protected for at least 8 weeks or until the tenderness at the fracture site resolves clinically and callus is present radiographically.

Zych[181] pointed out that those fractures treated by Sarmiento's method must be limited to fractures that are angulated less than 10°. The patient should be reliable, and any fracture with a vascular or neurologic deficit should be considered for open reduction.

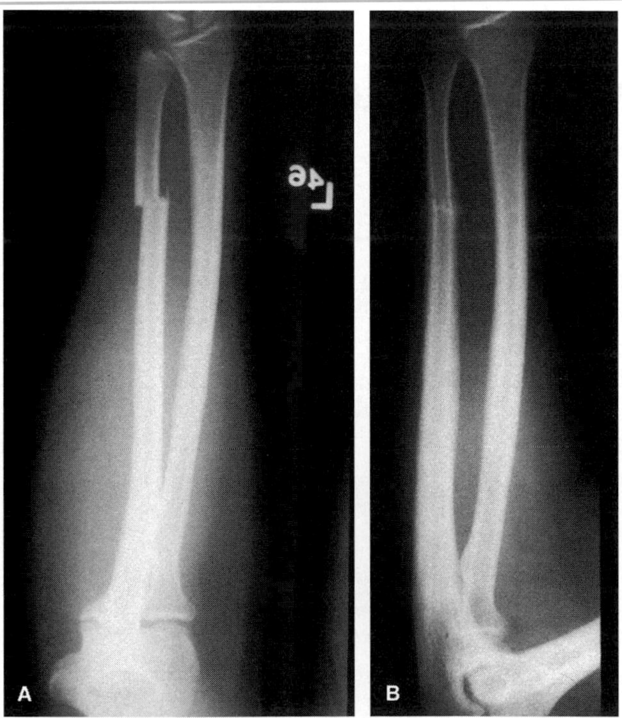

FIGURE 13-43. (**A**) Minimally displaced ulnar shaft fracture in a 26-year-old man. (**B**) This "nightstick" fracture was treated with a long-arm cast followed by a functional brace and was solidly healed at 8 weeks.

DISPLACED FRACTURES

Fractures of the ulnar diaphysis that are angulated more than 10° in any plane or displaced more than 50% of the diameter of the diaphysis were classified as displaced fractures by Dymond.[142] These displaced fractures are more unpredictable than nondisplaced fractures and should be approached with more caution for the following reasons:

1. Displaced ulnar fractures are often associated with radial head instability.
2. Displaced fractures of the ulnar diaphysis are prone to angulate, probably because of the loss of the supporting stability of the interosseous membrane.
3. Diaphyseal fractures of the distal ulna can shorten and cause symptoms in the distal radioulnar joint (Fig. 13-45).

AUTHORS' PREFERRED METHOD OF TREATMENT

In nondisplaced ulnar shaft fractures as classified by Dymond,[142] it has been my practice to treat the initial injury with a sugar-tong splint for 7 to 10 days or until swelling and pain subsides. After the swelling has resolved, a functional brace is worn by the patient until the fracture is clinically healed, usually 4 to 6 weeks. Close radiographic follow-up is necessary for the first 3 weeks to detect any displacement that might alter the treatment plan.

Technique for fabrication of the functional brace is outlined in Table 13-5. In isolated diaphyseal fractures with displacement more than 50% of the diameter (which are not associated with a dislocation of the radial head), I prefer to do an open reduction and internal fixation with a 3.5-mm dynamic compression plate. An attempt is made to obtain at least eight cortices on either side of the fracture site, if possible.

In displaced fractures of the distal ulna, it may be possible to secure only four cortices in the distal fragment. I advise bone grafting if comminution involving more than 50% of the shaft diameter is present.

Segmental fractures are plated with a single long plate or two overlapping 3.5-mm dynamic compression plates on the ipsilateral surface of the ulna. I prefer to treat all open, displaced ulna shaft fractures with primary plate fixation if the wound permits. If there is significant contamination in an open fracture, secondary plating is done after the wound is judged acceptable.

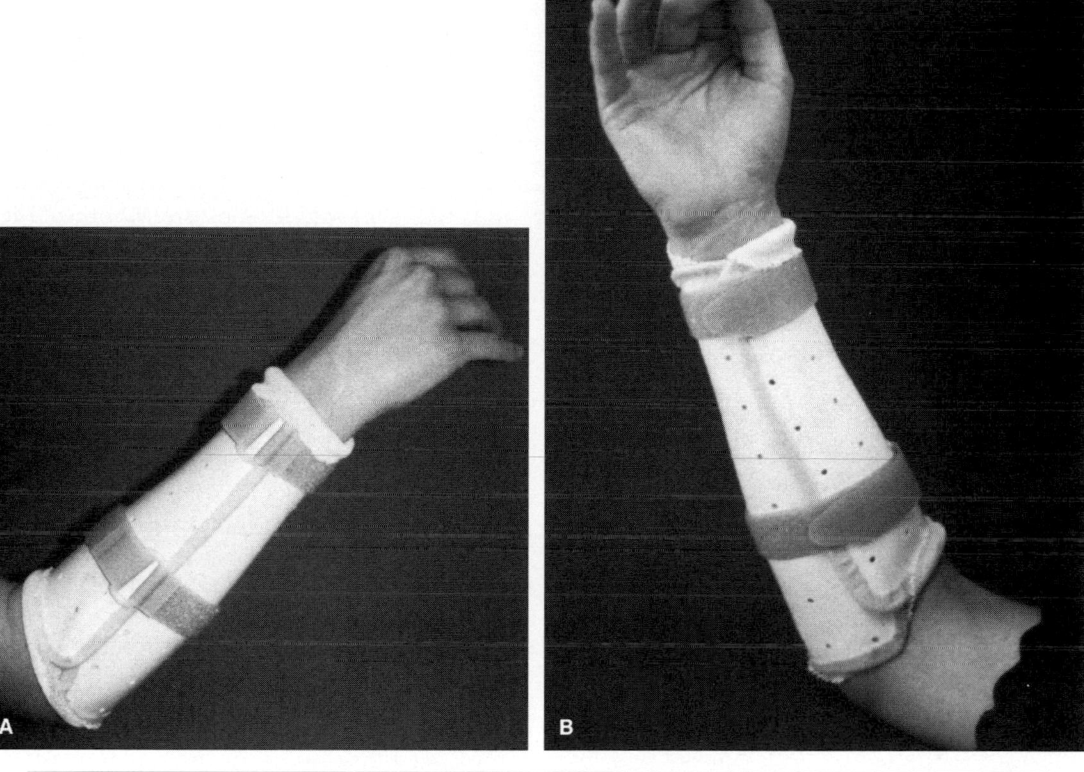

FIGURE 13-44. (**A** and **B**) A functional brace fabricated for a nondisplaced ulnar shaft fracture. This allows motion at the wrist and elbow while stabilizing the fracture site.

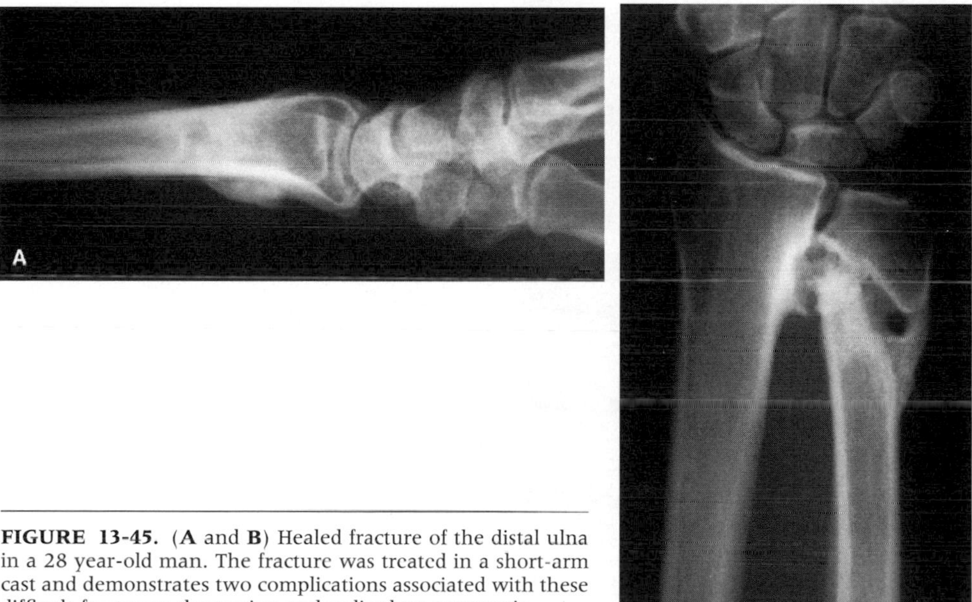

FIGURE 13-45. (**A** and **B**) Healed fracture of the distal ulna in a 28 year-old man. The fracture was treated in a short-arm cast and demonstrates two complications associated with these difficult fractures: shortening and radioulnar synostosis.

MONTEGGIA FRACTURES

CLASSIFICATION

Fractures of the ulna with associated dislocation of the radial head are rare injuries that compromise less than 5% of all forearm fractures.[153,163,166,169]

TABLE 13-5
Forearm Clamshell Fracture Brace/Splint for Ulnar Fractures

Skilled hand therapists are able to fabricate fracture braces/splints with thermoplastic materials for treatment of minimally nondisplaced ulnar fractures as well as healing fractures of the radius and ulna.

ADVANTAGES

Thermoplastic orthoses allow a well-contoured fit of the brace/splint to maintain fracture reduction and limit forearm rotation. They are lightweight and are easily removable for skin care. The thermoplastic fracture brace/splint also has the benefit of being more adjustable than plaster or fiberglass casts and thus may be more cost effective for the patient.

SPECIAL CONSIDERATIONS

1. Identify the fracture site. If the fracture is in the proximal third of the ulna, the brace should be formed over the humeral condyles, leaving the elbow joint as free as possible. It may be necessary to sacrifice the final range of elbow flexion to obtain adequate fracture support. If the fracture is in the distal third of the ulna, it may be necessary to mold the plastic as well as possible over the radial and ulnar styloids.
2. Obtain x-rays with the splint on. X-rays with the splint in place are important to ensure satisfactory reduction.

POTENTIAL PROBLEMS

1. The presence of severe edema or obesity may compromise a well contoured fit. Also, edema may develop distal to the fracture brace, necessitating edema control measures.
2. Pinching of the skin in the seam of the brace. Stockinette worn under the brace can prevent or minimize this problem.

FABRICATION

The splint consists of radial and ulnar based components. It can be made with thermoplastic materials such as Orthoplast, Orfit, Ezeform, etc. The ulnar-based gutter component is measured, cut out from the plastic, and molded to be well conformed to the ulnar aspect of the forearm from just proximal to the ulnar styloid to the tip of the olecranon. The ulnar gutter should cover approximately 3/4 the forearm circumference. (See Fig. 13-44*A*).

The radial-based gutter component is then measured, cut out from the plastic, and molded over the ulnar gutter so that it overlaps by approximately 3/4 inch (see Fig. 13-44*B*). Stockinette should be applied over the ulnar gutter component prior to application and molding of the radial gutter component to prevent them from bonding to each other.

Moleskin is then applied to the edges of the splint. The two components are held together with D-string straps, which may be riveted to the edge of the radial gutter. The D-ring straps allow the patient to adjust the compression of the splint to accommodate for changes in edema and to provide firm, but non-restrictive, compression of the forearm and fracture site.

In 1814, Monteggia described the injury as a fracture of the proximal third of the ulna and a concomitant anterior dislocation of the radial epiphysis.[132,133,156,158] In 1967, Bado[132] suggested the term *Monteggia lesion*, noting that Monteggia's original description was a fracture between the proximal third of the ulna and the base of the olecranon associated with an anterior dislocation of the radial head. In his series, Bado described four distinct variations of the Monteggia lesion:

Type I: Fracture of the ulnar diaphysis at any level with anterior angulation at the fracture site and an associated anterior dislocation of the radial head

Type II: Fracture of the ulnar diaphysis with posterior angulation at the fracture site and a posterolateral dislocation of the radial head

Type III: Fracture of the ulnar metaphysis with a lateral or anterolateral dislocation of the radial head

Type IV: Fracture of the proximal third of the radius and ulna at the same level with an anterior dislocation of the radial head (Fig. 13-46).

Bado[132,133] thereby extended Monteggia's original description to include any fracture of the ulna with an associated dislocation of the radial head. In his series, the type I lesion was the most common, type III and type II lesions were next in frequency, and type IV lesions were the rarest.

Jupiter and Kellam[153] noted that most large series of Monteggia fractures have included both adults and children, making it difficult to assess the relative incidence of each type in adults from those series previously reported in the literature. Speed and Boyd,[173] in 1940, and Bruce and Harvey,[139] in 1974, both reported the type I injury as being the most common, but, again, these studies included both pediatric and adult injuries.

Reports by Pavel,[162] Penrose,[163] and Jupiter[152] have emphasized that the posterior lesion is more common than originally thought, and it can present problems with treatment if the mechanism of injury and potential complications of treatment are not fully appreciated.

Jupiter and colleagues[152] found four different subgroups of the posterior Monteggia lesion, based on the location of the ulnar fracture:

Type IIA: The ulnar fracture involves the distal olecranon and coronoid process.

Type IIB: The ulnar fracture is at the metaphyseal and diaphyseal juncture, distal to the coronoid.

Type IIC: The ulnar fracture is diaphyseal.

Type IID: The ulnar fracture extends along the proximal third to half of the ulna (Fig. 13-47).

According to Jupiter and colleagues,[152] these subgroups of the Bado type II lesions with a comminuted

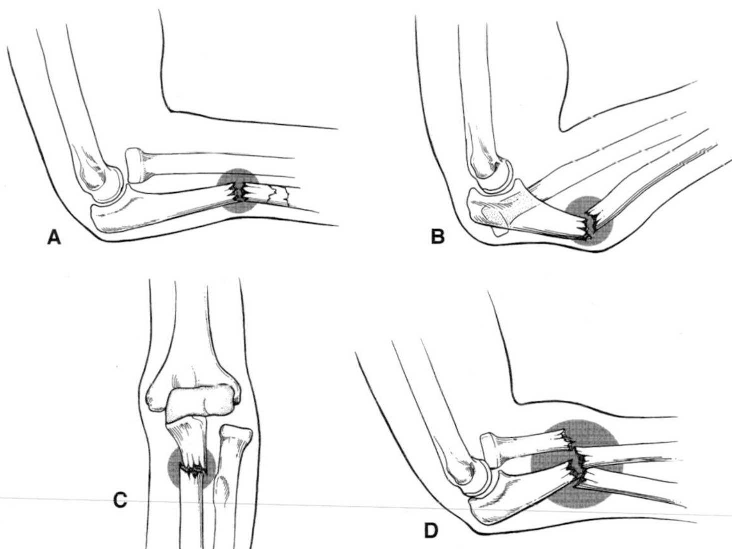

FIGURE 13-46. Bado's classification of Monteggia fractures. (**A**) Type I. An anterior dislocation of the radial head with associated anteriorly angulated fracture of the ulna shaft. (**B**) Type II. Posterior dislocation of the radial head with a posteriorly angulated fracture of the ulna. (**C**) Type III. A lateral or anterolateral dislocation of the radial head with a fracture of the ulnar metaphysis. (**D**) Type IV. Anterior dislocation of the radial head with a fracture of the radius and ulna. (Bado, J.L.: The Monteggia Lesion. Clin. Orthop. 50:70–86, 1967.)

anterior surface of the ulna are unstable injuries. Stable reconstruction and fixation of the ulna are necessary to prevent subsequent anterior angulation at the fracture site.

MECHANISM OF INJURY

Evans[144,145] postulated that in type I injuries the mechanism of injury is forced pronation of the forearm. He postulated this mechanism because in his series the type I injuries showed neither the bruising over the subcutaneous border of the ulna nor comminution of the fracture that one would expect to see in a direct blow injury.

Evans[144] further supported his theory with experimental studies. He produced fractures of the ulna with anterior dislocations of the radial head by stabilizing a cadaver humerus in a visc and slowly pronating the forearm. The ulna fractured, and as the pronation continued, the radial head was forced anteriorly out of the stabilizing capsular structures of the elbow.

Type II lesions were described by Penrose in 1951.[163] After observing this variation of fracture, he stabilized a cadaver humerus with the elbow flexed, and applied a force to the distal radius, causing a posterior dislocation of the elbow. He then weakened the proximal ulna by drilling the bone and again directed a force on the distal radius, causing what was later called a Bado type II lesion. This produced a posterior angulated fracture of the ulna with comminution anteriorly and a posterior dislocation of the radial head with a marginal fracture of the articular surface of the proximal radius. Penrose[163] concluded from these findings that the type II lesion is a variation of an elbow dislocation in which the ulnar shaft fails before the medial ligament of the elbow ruptures.

Type III lesions were studied by Mullick[160] in 1977, who postulated that the primary force on the elbow was an abduction force. If the forearm were supinated, the radial head dislocated posterolaterally. If the forearm were pronated, the radial head dislocated anterolaterally.

Type IV lesions were thought by Bado[132,133] to be type I lesions with an associated radial shaft fracture.

SIGNS AND SYMPTOMS

Swelling about the elbow, deformity, and bony crepitus and pain with movement at the site of the fracture are all signs of the Monteggia lesion. Often one can palpate the dislocated radial head. A careful neurologic examination is critical, because nerve injuries, especially of the radial nerve, are not uncommonly associated with Monteggia fractures. Boyd and Boals,[135] Bruce,[139] Mestdagh,[156] and Jessing[151] all reported acute injuries of the radial nerve or its terminal branch, the posterior interosseous nerve. Most of the nerve injuries have been associated with Bado type II lesions. Spar[172] reported *entrapment* of the posterior interosseous nerve, preventing closed reduction of the radial head. This occurred in a Bado type III lesion with an anterolateral dislocation of the radial head. The anterior interosseous nerve was reported by Engber[143] to be injured following a Bado type I lesion. Ulnar nerve lesions have been reported but are much less common than those involving the radial nerve. I have seen a patient with a malunion of a Monteggia fracture who presented with a tardy radial nerve palsy similar to

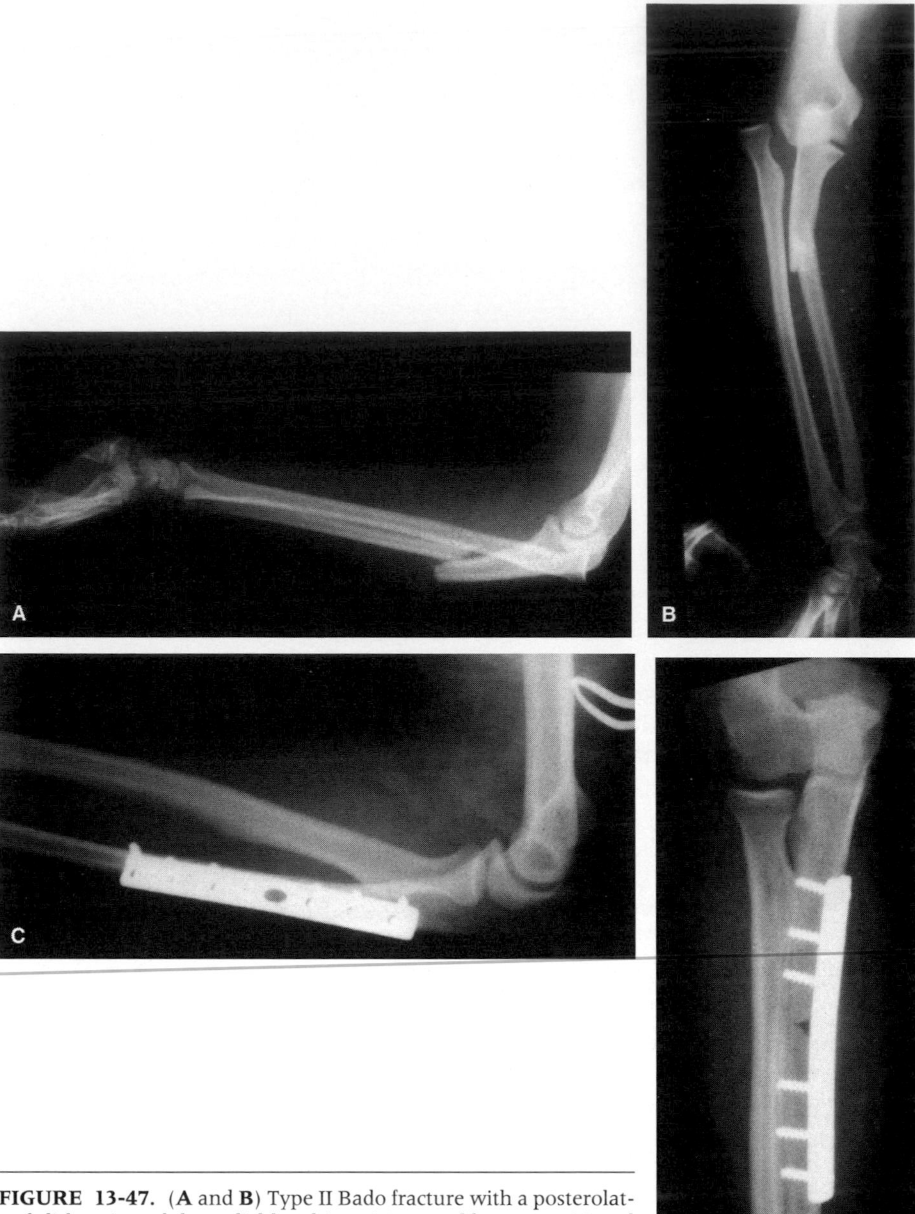

FIGURE 13-47. (**A** and **B**) Type II Bado fracture with a posterolateral dislocation of the radial head in a 26-year-old woman. (**C** and **D**) The ulna was fixed with a seven-hole dynamic compression plate, and the radial head was closed reduced with satisfactory stability to permit early motion at 7 days.

previous cases reported by Austin,[131] Holst-Nielsen,[150] and Lichter[154] (Fig. 13-48).

The clinical appearance of the patient and the physical examination should provide clues to the diagnosis. It is important, with any injury to the forearm, to examine the joints above and below the fracture. Any tenderness in either the wrist or elbow should arouse suspicion of associated joint injuries.

RADIOGRAPHIC FINDINGS

True anteroposterior and lateral x-rays of the elbow must be included in any upper extremity injury that involves a displaced fracture of the ulna. A true lateral view of the elbow can only be obtained if both the humerus and the forearm lie flat on the x-ray cassette. With both the humerus and forearm lying flat on the cassette in near 90° of flexion, a true lateral film of the elbow can be obtained regardless of whether the forearm is pronated, supinated, or neutral.

McLaughlin[155] recognized that to ensure proper alignment of the radiocapitellar joint, a line drawn down the shaft of the radius through the radial head should bisect the capitellum regardless of the position of the forearm.

Timely diagnosis of the Monteggia lesion depends on the experience and suspicions of the examiner and insistence on proper x-rays views of the elbow.

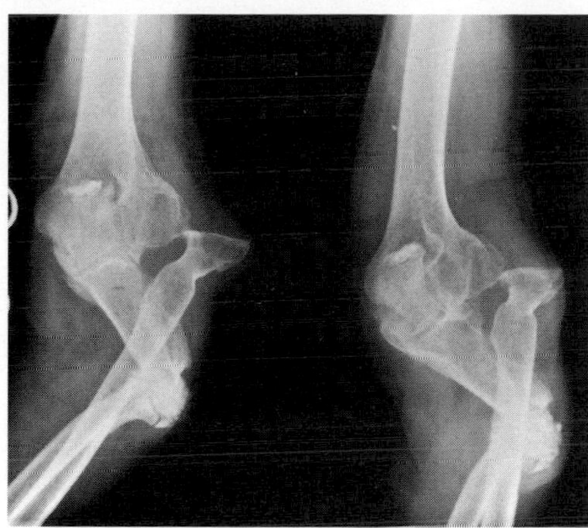

FIGURE 13-48. A 10-year-old malunion of a Monteggia fracture in a 60-year-old man. The patient was quite functional with this malunion until he developed a slowly progressive posterior interosseous nerve palsy that required surgical decompression.

TREATMENT

Although historically Monteggia injuries have been treated by closed manipulations and casting, closed methods are now considered to be satisfactory only in pediatric patients. Watson-Jones,[179] Bado,[132,133] Smith,[171] and Evans[144,145] all used closed reduction and casting, but Speed and Boyd[173] found that this method did not produce optimal results in adults. Most recent authors, including Anderson,[129] Boyd,[135,136] Reckling,[165,166] and Bruce[139] recommend open reduction and compression-plate fixation of the fracture of the ulna and closed reduction of the radial head dislocation. Smith and Sage[170] had good results after medullary fixation of forearm fractures, but most authors today believe that compression-plate fixation provides more rigid support than intramedullary fixation of the ulna.

 Authors' Preferred Method of Treatment

As noted by Anderson[130] in previous editions of this text, good results in Monteggia fractures depend on the following:

1. Early accurate diagnosis
2. Rigid fixation of the ulna
3. Accurate reduction of the radial head
4. Postoperative immobilization to allow ligamentous healing about the dislocated radial head.

In my experience with 40 Monteggia fractures, I have found that a 3.5-mm dynamic compression plate and a 3.5-mm pelvic reconstruction plate are equally suitable implants for stabilization of the fractured ulna.

Timing

Monteggia fractures should be treated as an urgent problem. If possible, closed reduction of the dislocation is accomplished in the emergency department and early operative intervention is advocated. Open fractures should be addressed as an emergency.

Operating Room Environment

It is important, in arranging the surgical suite, that free access for radiographic equipment be maintained. Although the image intensifier is suitable for preliminary x-rays and testing for radial head stability, I prefer permanent x-rays of the elbow, which are usually more reliable and subject to better interpretation than those taken with an image intensifier.

Positioning

These fractures can be approached with the patient supine and the arm extended over a hand table, but I prefer to position the patient in a lateral decubitus position, supported by a bean bag with the affected extremity draped free from the shoulder. This arrangement allows access to the entire upper extremity with full motion of, and access, to both the shoulder and elbow. If the radius is fractured, it can be approached by merely pronating or supinating the forearm. True anteroposterior and lateral x-rays of the elbow can be taken quite easily from this position.

Use of the Tourniquet

I prefer to use a sterile tourniquet so that the shoulder can be draped free, allowing full mobility of the upper extremity. Sustained tourniquet time should be no longer than 1 hour and 30 minutes. Any evidence of forearm ischemia before the surgery or questionable tissue viability may contraindicate prolonged tourniquet use.

Approach and Reduction

After adequate sterile prepping and draping, a closed reduction of the radial head is performed using distal traction and direct pressure over the radial head. I believe that this maneuver may lessen the likelihood of damage to the posterior interosseous nerve during the subsequent open reduction of the ulna.

After the reduction of the radial head, the forearm is draped over a roll of sheets. The skin incision is made as shown in Figure 13-49*A*, and a straight surgical approach is made to the ulna. The fracture site is exposed by subperiosteally dissecting around the fracture lines so that key fragments can be used in reducing the ulna to its appropriate length. Care must be taken to avoid any injury to the dorsal sensory branch of the ulnar nerve if the incision extends distally over the ulnar shaft (see Fig. 13-49).

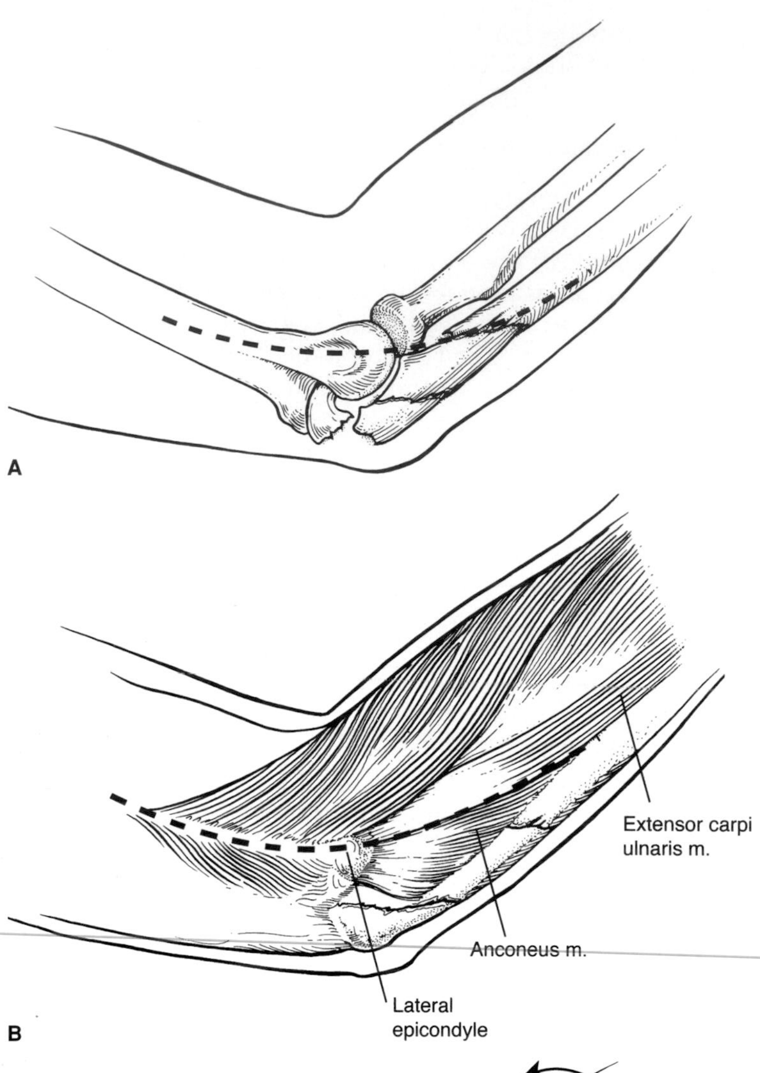

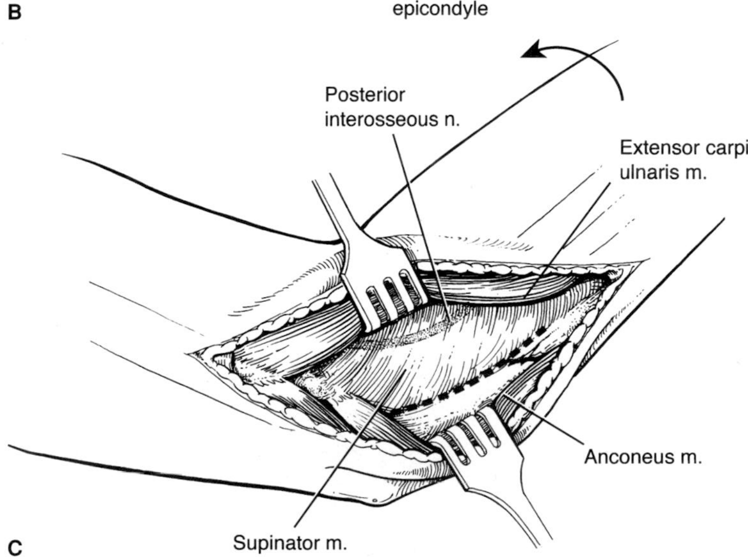

FIGURE 13-49. (**A** through **F**) Technique for open reduction of Monteggia fracture-dislocations. An incision is planned using the lateral epicondyle, radial head, and ulnar shaft as landmarks. The incision is centered over the lateral border of the humerus proximally, over the lateral epicondyle, and bisecting the interval between the radial head and the ulnar shaft distally. The interval proximally is between the extensors of the wrist superiorly and the triceps inferiorly and distally between the extensor carpi ulnaris and the anconeus. In this interval the anconeus and the extensor carpi ulnaris can be quite distorted with significant swelling. Often it is easier to find the interval distally where the anconeus inserts on the ulna rather than trying to find it proximally from its origin on the lateral epicondyle. (**C**) Deep to the anconeus, the fibers of the supinator are exposed. The supinator can be dissected off the ulna with minimal likelihood of harming the posterior interosseous nerve. Pronating the forearm displaces the posterior interosseous nerve farther from the plane of dissection, adding additional protection.

continues

Only the area where the plate is to be placed should be stripped of periosteum to ensure adequate blood supply to the ulnar shaft. I prefer to place the plate on the bare subcutaneous surface of the ulna for two reasons:

1. In proximal fractures, mobilization of the ulnar nerve is avoided when the plate is placed on the extensor surface.
2. If the radial head needs to be exposed, it is easy to continue the incision along the extensor surface,

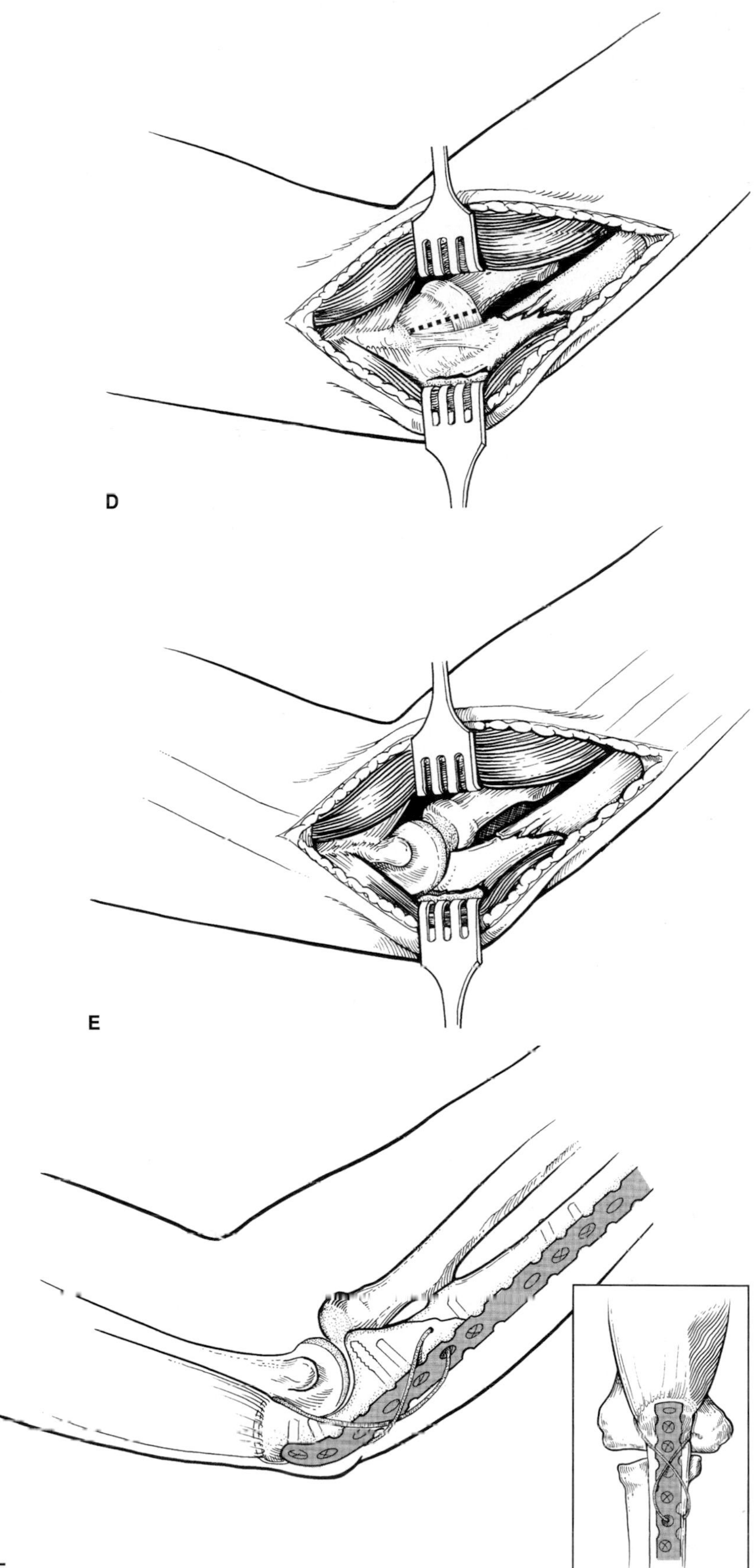

FIGURE 13-49. (continued) (**D**) The capsule is exposed, planning the capsular incision so as to spare the lateral collateral ligament arising from the ulna. (**E**) The fracture site and radial head are exposed. (**F**) The fracture here has been fixed with a pelvic reconstruction plate. With comminution proximally and inadequate screw fixation, a tension band can be used as a supplement to secure the proximal fragments displaced by the insertion of the triceps. (*Boyd, H.B.: Surgical Exposure of the Ulna and Proximal Third of the Radius Through One Incision. Surg. Gynecol. Obstet. 71:87–88, 1940.*)

proximally over the elbow joint, and expose the radial head by reflecting the supinator (see Fig. 13-49*B* and *C*).

After the ulna has been reduced, a 3.5-mm dynamic compression plate (or, alternatively, a 3.5-mm pelvic reconstruction plate; see Fig. 13-49*F*) is placed on the ulna and held with bone clamps, stabilizing the reduction.

X-rays are taken at this time to ensure that the radial head is reduced and the ulna is out to length. If the x-rays show accurate reduction, the plate is applied with the appropriate 3.5-mm screws.

After stabilization of the ulna, the elbow is passively ranged to assess the stability of the radial head. Often, the C-arm is used to assess radial head stability at this time. Permanent x-rays are taken to document the reduction and fixation.

The fascia is not closed. The skin and subcutaneous tissues are closed, and a drain is left deep in the wound. A long-arm posterior splint is applied to the forearm in neutral rotation.

POSTOPERATIVE CARE

The original dressing and splint are removed at 5 to 7 days and replaced with a long-arm cast or brace, depending on the assessment of stability at the time of surgery. If the patient is reliable and the fracture was stable through a full range of motion at the time of surgery, after 7 to 10 days the patient is allowed to remove the posterior splint and do active flexion/extension, pronation/supination exercises of the elbow, supervised initially by a therapist.

If at the time of surgery there is some question about fracture site stability or stability of the radial head, a long-arm cast is recommended for 6 weeks before motion is allowed.

X-rays are taken at 2 weeks, 4 weeks, and 6 weeks. After 6 weeks, if fixation is adequate and there is evidence of early healing at the fracture site, all external support and protection (except possibly a sling) is discontinued.

TECHNICAL TIPS

Preoperative Radial Nerve Deficit. If the radial or posterior interosseous nerve is absent at the time of injury and the radial head easily reduces, I do not recommend exploration of the radial or posterior interosseous nerve at the time of surgery. This is usually a neurapraxia, and function will return within 6 to 12 weeks after injury in the majority of cases. If the nerve is not functioning at 3 months, diagnostic studies are indicated, and, depending on the results, exploration of the nerve may be considered.

Open Fractures. Open fractures should be treated as emergencies, and I advocate early open reduction and plating if the wound permits. I do not close the skin primarily but recommend multiple debridements until a tidy wound is obtained. External fixation is used only in severely contaminated wounds that would prohibit plating the fracture. In less severely contaminated wounds, I have used a metacarpal pin with side-arm traction to allow wound care and maintain reduction. This allows adequate wound care so that one can do a delayed plating of the forearm when wound conditions are suitable.

Comminution. Extensive comminution of the ulnar shaft extending proximally into the olecranon can present problems with regaining anatomical length of the ulna. If the radial head is reduced and is stable, this often facilitates reconstruction of the length of ulna so that it can be plated to its normal anatomical length. If the radial head is unstable, it is important to open the elbow joint, ensure the reduction of the radial head under direct vision, and then restore the length to the ulna.

One or two 3.5-mm pelvic reconstruction plates can be used in comminuted proximal ulna fractures to match the contour of the olecranon (Fig. 13-50). If necessary, a tension band wire through the tip of the olecranon can be incorporated through a drill hole in the pelvic reconstruction plate to further aid in stability (see Fig. 13-49*F*).

Fractures of Both Radius and Ulna. With a type IV Bado lesion (fractures of both the radius and the ulna), it is much easier to plate the ulna first, which usually reduces the radial head before open reduction of the radial shaft fracture. Again, if reduction of the radial head is in question, the elbow joint can be opened through either the approach of the radius or the approach of the ulna. I do not recommend approaching both bones through one surgical incision.

The Radial Head Does Not Reduce Closed. If closed reduction is not successful in reducing the radial head, open reduction is indicated. This can be done through a separate approach to the radial head or by extending the approach to the ulna proximally so that the elbow joint can be visualized. The usual impediments to reduction are the anterior capsule and, at times, the annular ligament. With an arthrotomy of the elbow joint, the radial head can be easily reduced and the capsular structures can be repaired if this aids in the stability of the radial head. If there is sufficient annular ligament tissue present, the ligament is repaired, but I do not advocate reconstructing the annular ligament as described by Boyd and Boals.[135]

Radial Head Fracture. If x-rays show that there is a significant fracture of the radial head, I recommend open reduction and internal fixation of the radial head

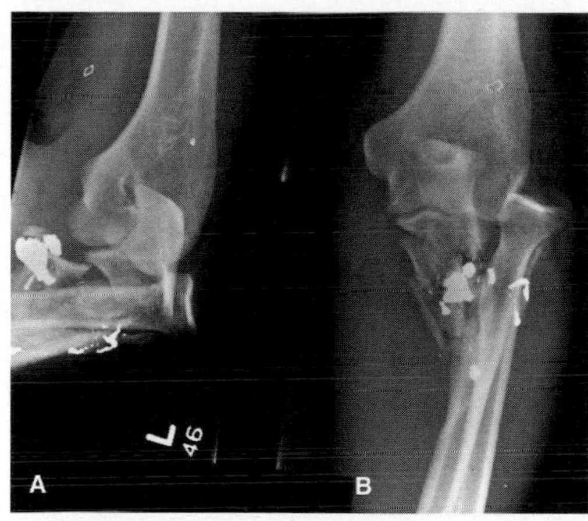

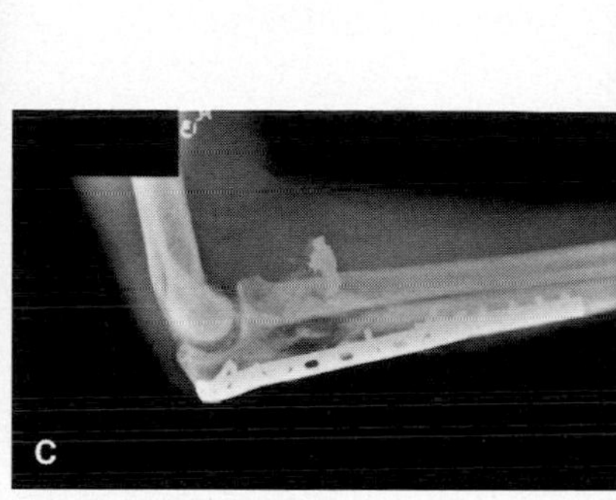

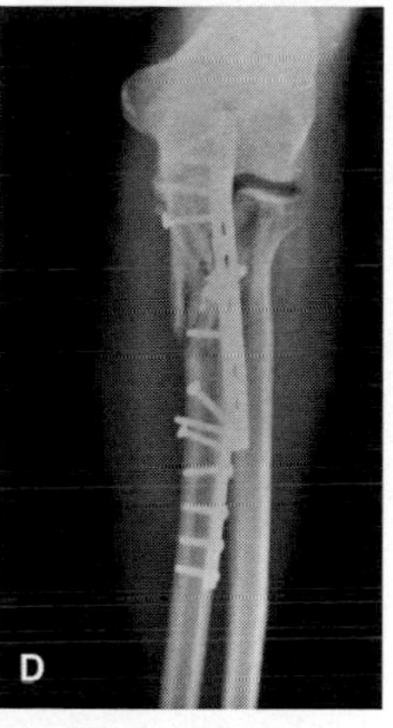

FIGURE 13-50. (**A** and **B**) Bado type II Monteggia fracture secondary to a gunshot wound in a 35-year-old man. (**C** and **D**) Adequate fixation required use of overlapping plates because of extensive comminution.

if possible (Fig. 13-51) or excision of the radial head if the fracture cannot be reconstructed (Fig. 13-52). If elbow stability is jeopardized by excision of the radial head, one can consider placement of a radial head prosthesis or repair of the medial collateral ligament of the elbow. The radial head prosthesis improves varus–valgus stability, but does not enhance anterior or posterior stability.

Bone Grafting. In fractures of the ulnar shaft that involve more than 50% comminution that cannot be anatomically restored or in those ulnar shaft fractures that are open with some compromise of the blood supply, I recommend cancellous bone grafting. It is important, in lesions of the proximal forearm, that the bone grafting not be placed so that it forms a continuous bridge between the radius and ulna. I prefer to place the graft if both radius and ulna need bone grafts on opposite sides of the interosseous membrane if possible.

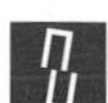 COMPLICATIONS

Monteggia fractures can develop complications that are the same as those seen with other fractures, including infection, implant failure, nonunion, and malunion.[129,130,136,140,141,147,148,153,157,165,166,171,176] Most of these complications can be attributed to severity of the injury, tissue viability, adequacy of fixation, and errors in technique.

Monteggia fractures also have a variety of complications that are peculiar to this unique lesion, including errors in diagnosis, nerve injuries, redislocation of the radial head, and radioulnar synostosis.

Errors in Diagnosis. Experience and an understanding of the relationship of the elbow–forearm unit can reduce the number of errors in diagnosis. Giustra and associates[146] emphasized that it is essential to obtain proper x-rays of the elbow in any displaced ulnar fracture or any forearm fracture with elbow tenderness.

Nerve Injuries. Acute nerve injuries must be documented at the time of injury by a thorough physical examination, paying particular attention to the terminal branches of the radial and median nerves (ie, the posterior interosseous and the anterior interosseous nerves).[143,151,159,172,174,175]

Nerve deficits occurring after surgical procedures that were not present preoperatively nearly always involve either the radial or median nerve. These injuries are usually due to pressure over the radial head during reduction or overzealous retraction. Rarely are these injuries due to laceration or direct injury.

The incidence of postoperative nerve injury can be decreased by gentle reduction of the radial head and an awareness of the proximity of the posterior interosseous nerve and the anterior interosseous nerve during open reduction.

Postoperative nerve palsies should be observed for at least 12 weeks before any surgical exploration is undertaken. Most will recover spontaneously without surgical intervention.

Radial Head Instability. Dislocation of the radial head after surgical repair in Monteggia fractures is uncommon if the fracture is reduced anatomically. If the radial head does dislocate after surgical repair, one must assess the quality of the reduction of the ulna. If the ulna is anatomically reduced, the radial head can be manipulated under anesthesia and held in a long arm cast. This maneuver can be successful up to 4 weeks after the initial surgery. If the ulna is not anatomically reduced and the radial head dislocates, one must consider removing the fixation

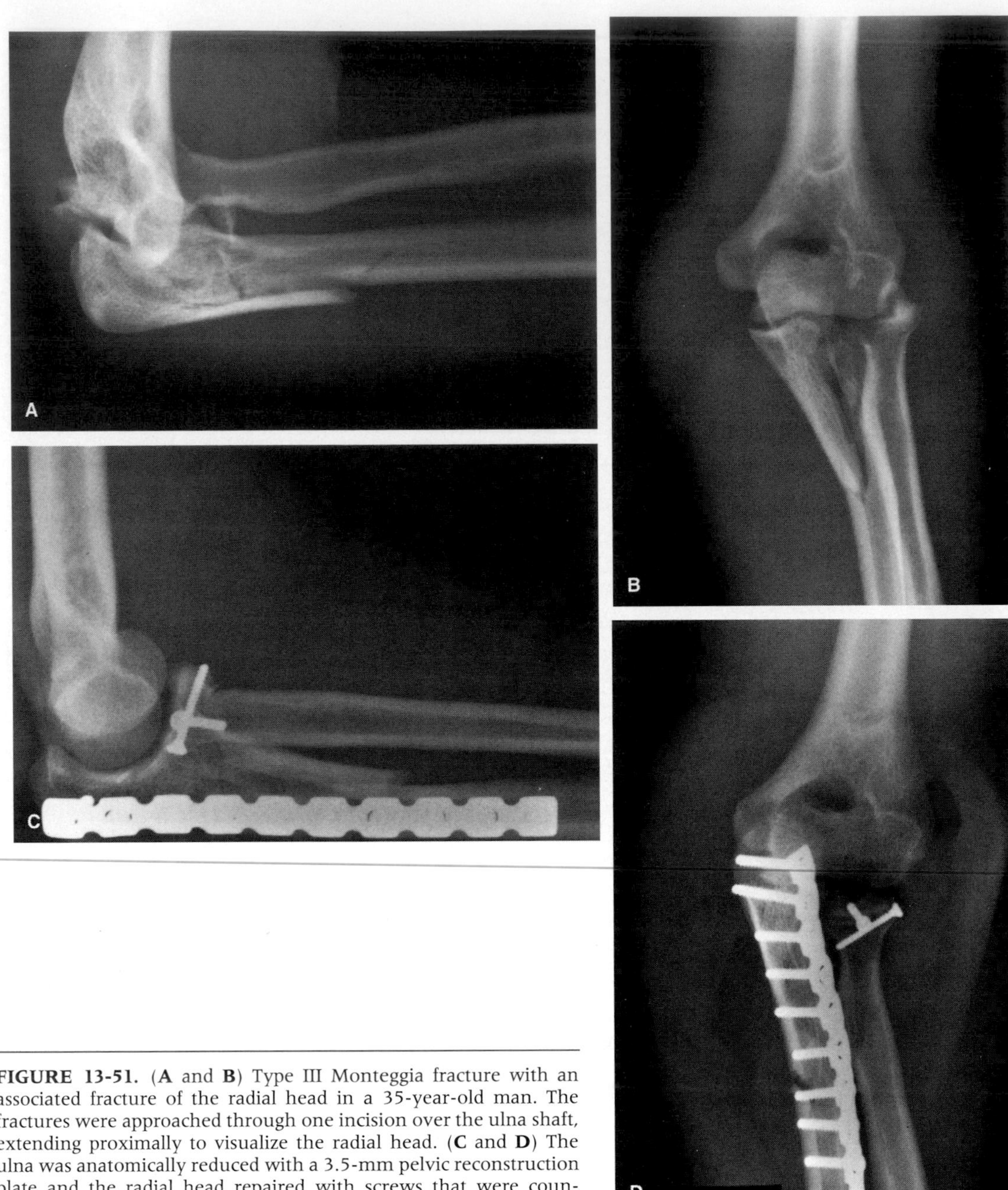

FIGURE 13-51. (**A** and **B**) Type III Monteggia fracture with an associated fracture of the radial head in a 35-year-old man. The fractures were approached through one incision over the ulna shaft, extending proximally to visualize the radial head. (**C** and **D**) The ulna was anatomically reduced with a 3.5-mm pelvic reconstruction plate and the radial head repaired with screws that were countersunk below the articular surface.

and anatomically reducing the ulna with an open reduction of the radial head. Dislocation of the radial head recognized more than 6 weeks after surgery is best treated by radial head excision (Fig. 13-53).

Radioulnar Synostosis. In my series of 40 patients, I have seen two post-traumatic synostoses of the proximal forearm. These were open injuries with significant soft-tissue damage that required bone grafting. The nature of these injuries and the pattern of synostosis were similar to those reported by Breit,[138] Vince and Miller,[177] and Watson and Eaton.[178]

In an attempt to avoid synostosis, I prefer to place the bone grafts along the border of the ulnar shaft opposite the interosseous membrane. Indomethacin (Indocin), given postoperatively, has also been used, but neither of these methods have been proven to be effective in all instances. Resection of the synostosis in the proximal forearm is beset with problems (see p. 902). I have resected two proximal forearm synostoses with placement of a Silastic sheet as a spacer, with moderate success (improved but still limited forearm rotation without re-formation of the synostosis). Yong-Hing and Tchang[180] recommended resection of the synostosis and an interposition of a

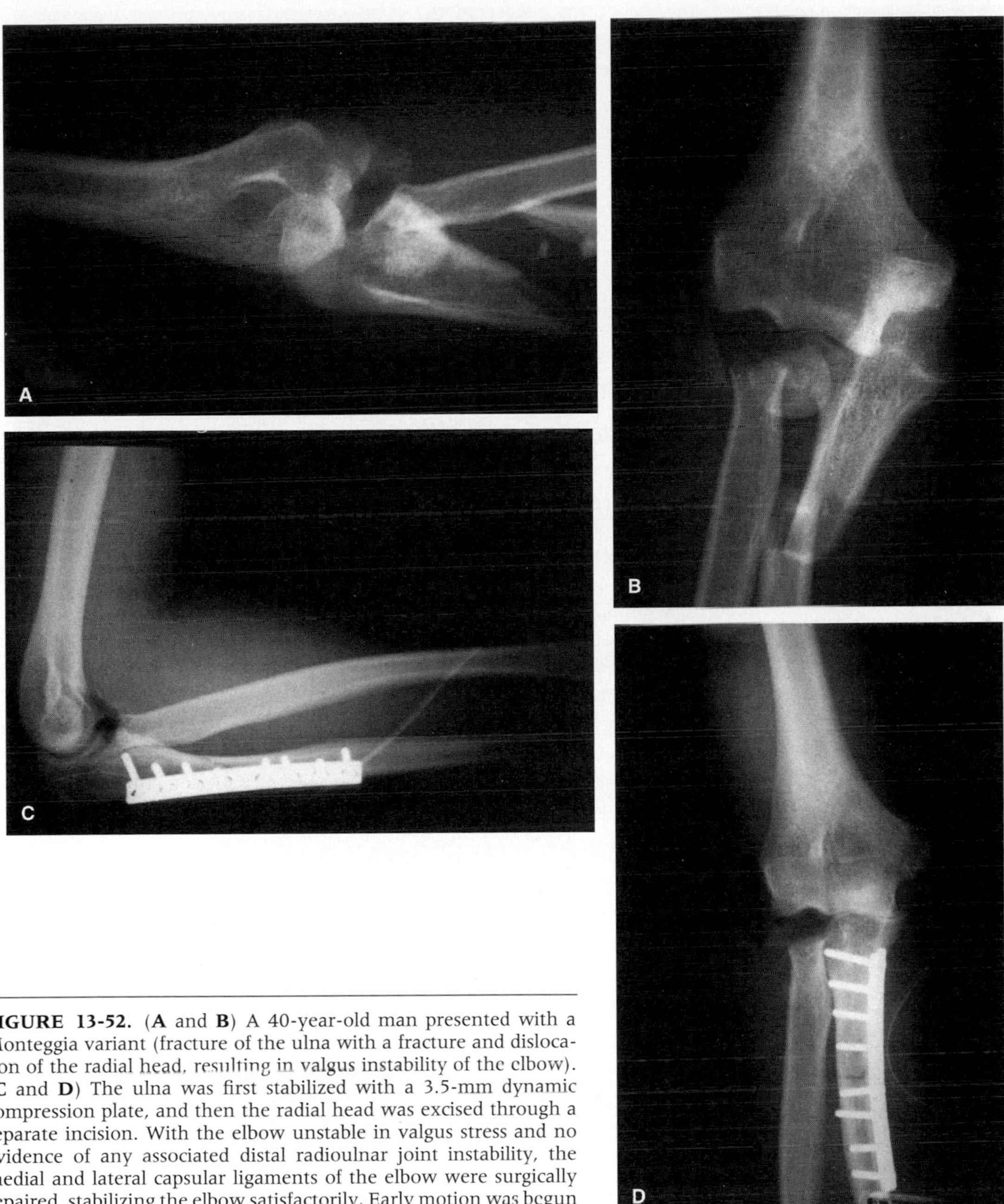

FIGURE 13-52. (**A** and **B**) A 40-year-old man presented with a Monteggia variant (fracture of the ulna with a fracture and dislocation of the radial head, resulting in valgus instability of the elbow). (**C** and **D**) The ulna was first stabilized with a 3.5-mm dynamic compression plate, and then the radial head was excised through a separate incision. With the elbow unstable in valgus stress and no evidence of any associated distal radioulnar joint instability, the medial and lateral capsular ligaments of the elbow were surgically repaired, stabilizing the elbow satisfactorily. Early motion was begun in a hinged brace at 10 days.

free fat graft with good results, but only a small series of patients were followed.

PROGNOSIS

Anderson's[129] criteria for evaluation of forearm fractures are shown in the following list:

Excellent: Union with less than 10° loss of elbow and wrist flexion/extension
Satisfactory: Union with less than 20° loss of elbow or wrist flexion/extension; less than 50% loss of forearm rotation
Unsatisfactory: Union with greater than 30° loss of elbow or wrist flexion/extension and with greater than 50% loss of forearm rotation
Failure: Malunion, nonunion, or unresolved chronic osteomyelitis

Although these criteria, when used to evaluate large series of fractures by Anderson[129] and by Chapman,[140] involved diaphyseal fractures as well as Monteggia lesions, satisfactory results were obtained in more than 90% of the cases surveyed.

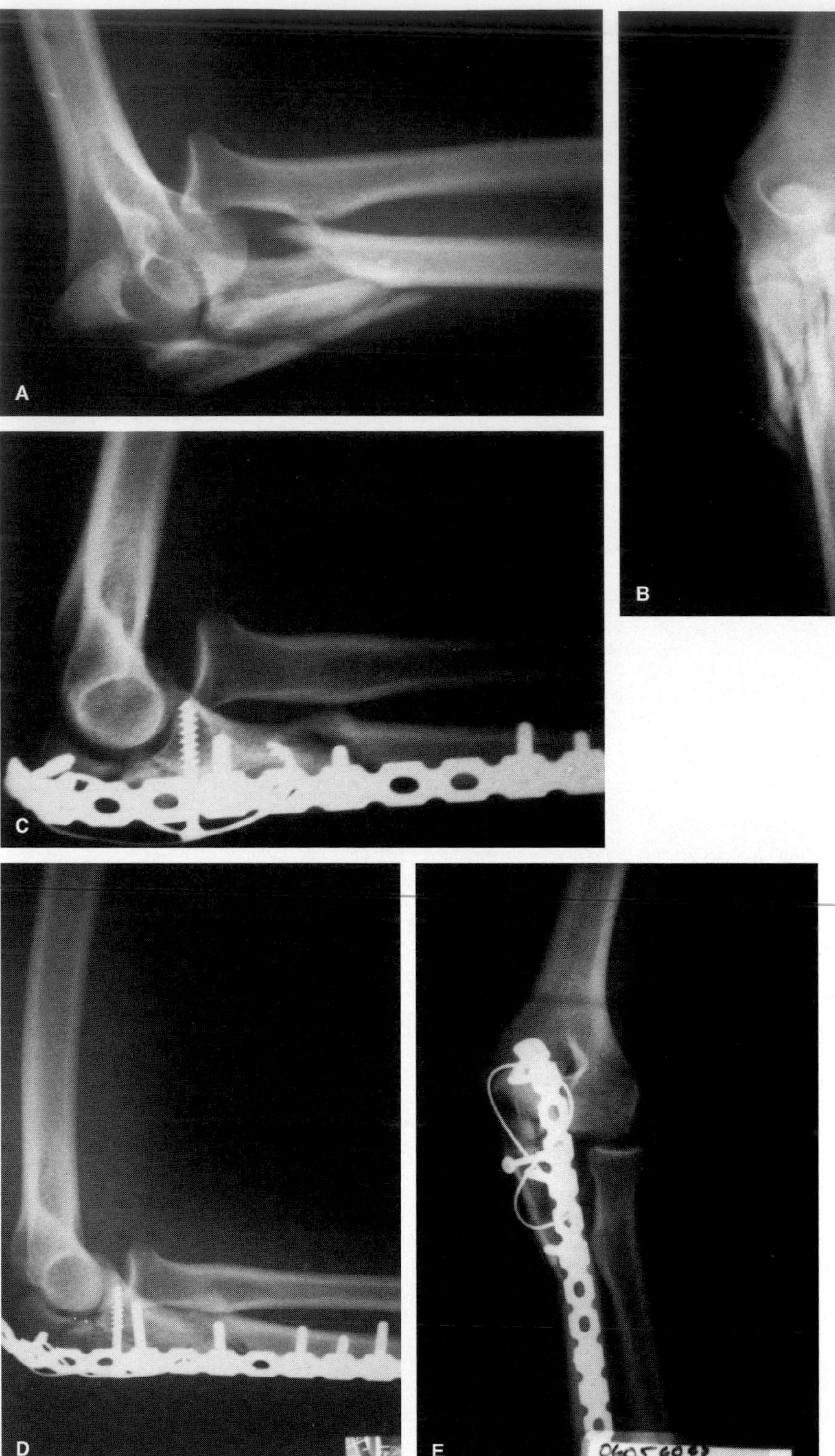

FIGURE 13-53. (**A** and **B**) A 24-year-old woman presented with a comminuted type I Monteggia fracture. (**C**) Open reduction was done with a pelvic reconstruction plate. Two weeks after surgery the radial head was noted to be anteriorly dislocated. (**D** and **E**) The radial head could not be reduced closed and required a repeat osteosynthesis of the ulna with adequate reduction and stability of the radial head.

In my series of 40 adult patients with Monteggia fractures, including 20 with at least a 2-year follow-up, satisfactory results were obtained according to the Anderson[129] criteria in 82% of the cases. Unsatisfactory results included two synostoses and one ulnar nonunion that was subsequently bone grafted.

Treatment of this rare injury can be expected to give reasonable results in 80% of adult fractures if attention is paid to accurate diagnosis, adequate reduction, and stable fixation at surgery. Attention to detail is of primary importance in successful outcomes.

REFERENCES

FRACTURES OF BOTH BONES OF THE FOREARM

1. Abrams, R.A., Simmons, B.P., Brown, R.A., Botte, M.J.: Treatment of Posttraumatic Radioulnar Synostosis With Excision and Low-dose Radiation. J. Hand Surg., 18A:703–707, 1993.
2. Anderson, L.D., and Bacastow, D.W.: Treatment of Forearm Shaft Fractures With Compression Plates. Contemp. Orthop., 8(6):17, 1984.
3. Anderson, L.D.: Compression Plate Fixation and the Effect of Different Types of Internal Fixation on Fracture Healing. J. Bone Joint Surg., 47A:191–208, 1965.
4. Anderson, L.D.: Fractures. *In* Crenshaw, A.H. (ed): Campbell's Operative Orthopaedics, 5th ed, vol. 1, pp. 477–691. St. Louis, C.V. Mosby, 1971.
5. Anderson, L.D., Sisk, T.D., Park, W.I., III, and Tooms, R.E.: Compression Plate Fixation in Acute Diaphyseal Fractures of the Radius and Ulna (Proceedings). J. Bone Joint Surg., 54A:1332–1333, 1972.
6. Anderson, L.D., Sisk, T.D., Tooms, R.E., and Park, W.I., III.: Compression-Plate Fixation in Acute Diaphyseal Fractures of the Radius and Ulna. J. Bone Joint Surg., 57A:287–297, 1975.
7. Bagby, G.W., and Janes, J.M.: The Effect of Compression on the Rate of Healing Using a Special Plate. Am. J. Surg., 95:761–771, 1958.
8. Bick, E.M.: Source Book of Orthopaedics, 2nd ed. Baltimore, Wilkins & Wilkins, 1948.
9. Boreau, J., and Hermann, P.: Plague d'Osteosynthèse Permettant I'Impaction des Fragments. Presse Med., 60:356, 1952.
10. Böstman, O.: Economic Considerations on Avoiding Implant Removals After Fracture Fixation by Using Absorbable Devices. Scand. J. Soc. Med., 22(1):41–45, 1994.
11. Bowers, W.H.: The Distal Radioulnar Joint. *In* Green, D.P. (ed.): Operative Hand Surgery, 2nd ed., pp. 939–989. New York, Churchill Livingstone, 1988.
12. Boyd, H.B., Lipinski, S.W., and Wiley, J.H.: Observations on Non-unions of the Shafts of the Long Bones, With a Statistical Analysis of 842 Patients. J. Bone Joint Surg., 43A:159–168, 1961.
13. Boyd, H.B.: Surgical Approaches. *In* Crenshaw, A.H. (ed.): Campbell's Operative Orthopaedics, 5th ed., vol. 1, pp. 58–137. St Louis, C.V. Mosby, 1971.
14. Boyd, H.B.: Surgical Exposure of the Ulna and Proximal Third of the Radius Through One Incision. Surg. Gynecol. Obstet., 71:86–88, 1940.
15. Breit, R.: Post-traumatic Radioulnar Synostosis. Clin. Orthop., 174:149–152, 1983.
16. Burwell, H.N., and Charnley, A.D.: Treatment of Forearm Fractures in Adults With Particular Reference to Plate Fixation. J. Bone Joint Surg., 46B:404–425, 1964.
17. Caden, J.G.: Internal Fixation of Fractures of the Forearm. J. Bone Joint Surg., 43A:1115–1121, 1961.
18. Campbell, W.C., and Boyd, H.B.: Fixation of Onlay Bone Grafts by Means of Vitallium Screws in the Treatment of Ununited Fractures. Am. J. Surg., 51:748–756, 1941.
19. Chapman, M.W., Gordon, J.E., and Zissimos, A.G.: Compression-Plate Fixation of Acute Fractures of the Diaphyses of the Radius and Ulna. J. Bone Joint Surg., 71A:159–169, 1989.
20. Crenshaw, A.H.: Surgical Approaches. *In* Crenshaw, A.H., (ed.): Campbell's Operative Orthopaedics, 7th ed., vol. 3, pp. 23–107. St. Louis, C.V. Mosby, 1987.
21. Danis, R.: Uncles Theorie et Practique de l'Osteosynthèse. Paris, Masson & Cie, 1949.
22. DeLee, J.C.: External Fixation of the Forearm and Wrist. Orthop. Rev., 6:43–48, 1981.
23. Deluca, P.A., Newington, R.W.L., and Ruwe, P.A.: Refracture of Bones of the Forearm After the Removal of Compression Plates. J. Bone Joint Surg., 70A:1372–1376, 1988.
24. Duncan, R., Geissler, W., Freeland, A.E., and Savoie, F.H.: Immediate Internal Fixation of Open Fractures of the Diaphysis of the Forearm. J. Orthop. Trauma, 6:25–31, 1992.
25. Dodge, H.S., and Cady, G.W.: Treatment of Fractures of the Radius and Ulna With Compression Plates: A Retrospective Study of 119 Fractures in 78 Patients. J. Bone Joint Surg., 54A(6):1167–1176, 1972.
26. Eaton, R.G., and Green, W.T.: Volkmann's Ischemia: A Volar Compartment Syndrome of the Forearm. Clin. Orthop., 113:58–64, 1975.
27. Edwards, C.C.: Management of Open Fractures in the Multiply Injured Patient. Instr. Course Lect., 37:257–273, 1988.
28. Eggers, G.W.N., Shindler, T.O., and Pomerat, C.M.: The Influence of the Contact-Compression Factor on Osteogenesis in Surgical Fractures. J. Bone Joint Surg., 31A:693–716, 1949.
29. Eggers, G.W.N., Ainsworth, W.H., Shindler, T.O., and Pomerat, C.M.: Clinical Significance of the Contact-Compression Factor in Bone Surgery. Arch. Surg., 62:467–474, 1951.
30. Eggers, G.W.N.: Internal Contact Splint. J. Bone Joint Surg., 30A(1):40–52, 1948.
31. Eggers, G.W.N.: The Internal Fixation of Fractures of the Shafts of Long Bones. *In* Carter, B.N. (ed.): Monographs on Surgery. Baltimore: Williams & Wilkins, 1952.
32. Evans, E.M.: Rotational Deformity in the Treatment of Fractures of Both Bones of the Forearm. J. Bone Joint Surg., 27:373–379, 1945.
33. Gelberman, R.H., Gould, R.N., Hargens, A.R., and Vande Berg, J.S.: Lacerations of the Ulnar Artery: Hemodynamic, Ultrastructural, and Compliance Changes in the Dog. J. Hand Surg., 8:306–309, 1983.
34. Godina, M.: Early Microsurgical Reconstruction of Complex Trauma of the Extremities. Plast. Reconstr. Surg., 78:285–292, 1986.
35. Greene, W.B.: Traumatic Bowing of the Forearm in an Adult. Clin. Orthop., 168:31–34, 1982.
36. Gustilo, R.B., and Anderson, J.T.: Prevention of Infection in the Treatment of One Thousand and Twenty-five Open Fractures of Long Bones: Retrospective and Prospective Analyses. J. Bone Joint Surg., 58A:453–458, 1976.
37. Gustilo, R.B.: Current Concepts in the Management of Open Fractures. Instr. Course Lect., 36:359–366, 1987.
38. Gustilo, R.B., Mendoza, R.M., and Williams, D.M.: Problems in Management of Type III Open Fractures: A New Classification of Type III Open Fractures. J. Trauma, 24:742, 1984.
39. Hadden, W.A., Reschauer, R., and Seggl, W.: Results of AO Plate Fixation of Forearm Shaft Fractures in Adults. Injury, 15:44–52, 1984.
40. Heim, U., and Pfeiffer, K.M.: Small Fragment Set Manual, 2nd ed., p. 119. New York, Springer-Verlag, 1982.
41. Heiser, T.M., and Jacobs, R.R.: Complicated Extremity Fractures: The Relation Between External Fixation and Nonunion. Clin. Orthop., 178:89–95, 1983.
42. Henry, A.K.: Extensile Exposure, 2nd ed. Baltimore, Williams & Wilkins, 1957.
43. Hotchkiss, R.N., An, K., Sowa, D.T., Basta, S., and Weiland, A.J.: An Anatomic and Mechanical Study of the Interosseous Membrane of the Forearm: Pathomechanics of Proximal Migration of the Radius. J. Hand Surg., 14A:256–261, 1989.
44. Hughston, J.C.: Fracture of the Distal Radial Shaft: Mistakes in Management. J. Bone Joint Surg., 39A:249–264, 402, 1957.
45. Jergensen, F.: Diaphyseal Fractures of the Major Long Bones (Proceedings). J. Bone Joint Surg., 42A:1446–1447, 1960.
46. Jinkins, W.J., Jr., Lockhart, L.D., and Eggers, G.W.N.: Fractures of the Forearm in Adults. South. Med. J., 53:669–679, 1960.
47. Jones, J.A.: Immediate Internal Fixation of High-Energy Open Forearm Fractures. J. Orthop. Trauma, 5:272–279, 1991.

48. Jupiter, J.B., Kour, A.K., Richards, R.R., Nathan, J., and Meinhard, B.: The Floating Radius in Bipolar Fracture-Dislocation of the Forearm. J. Orthop. Trauma, 8:99–106, 1994.
49. Knight, R.A., and Purvis, G.D.: Fractures of Both Bones of the Forearm in Adults. J. Bone Joint Surg., 31A:755–764, 1949.
50. Lam, S.J.S.: The Place of Delayed Internal Fixation in the Treatment of Fractures of the Long Bones. J. Bone Joint Surg., 46B:393–397, 1964.
51. Lam, S.J.S.: Delayed Internal Fixation for Fractures of the Radial Shaft. Guy's Hosp. Rep., 114:391–400, 1965.
52. Lambotte, A.: Chirurgie Operatorie Dans les Fractures. Paris, Masson & Cie, 1913.
53. Lambotte, A.: L'Intervention Operatorie Dans les Fracture de Vue de l'Osteosynthes Avec la Description des Plusieurs Techniques Nouvelles. Paris, A. Maloine, 1907.
54. Lane, W.A.: A Lecture on the Operative Treatment of Simple Fractures. Lancet, 1:1489–1493, 1900.
55. Lane, W.A.: The Operative Treatment of Fractures. London, Medical Publishing Co., 1905.
56. Langkamer, V.G., and Ackroyd, C.E.: Internal Fixation of Forearm Fractures in the 1980s: Lessons to be Learnt. Injury, 22:97–102, 1991.
57. Lenihan, M.R., Brien, W.W., Gellman, H., Itamura, J., and Kuschner, S.H.: Fractures of the Forearm Resulting From Low-Velocity Gunshot Wounds. J. Orthop. Trauma, 6:32–35, 1992.
58. Littlefield, W.G., Hasting, H., II, and Strickland, J.W.: Adhesions Between Muscle and Bone after Forearm Fracture Mimicking Mild Volkmann's Ischemic Contracture. J. Hand Surg., 17A:691–693, 1992.
59. Maempel, F.Z.: Post-traumatic Radioulnar Synostosis: A Report of Two Cases. Clin. Orthop., 186:182–185, 1984.
60. Mallin, B.A.: Principles of Management of Forearm Fractures. *In* Chapman, M.W., and Madison, M. (eds.): Operative Orthopaedics, vol. 1, pp. 263–271. Philadelphia, J.B. Lippincott, 1988.
61. Matsen, F.A.: Compartmental Syndromes. New York, Grune & Stratton, 1980.
62. Matthews, L.S., Kaufer, H., Graver, D.F., and Sonstegard, D.A.: The Effect on Supination-Pronation of Angular Malaignment of Fractures of Both Bones of the Forearm: An Experimental Study. J. Bone Joint Surg., 64A:14–17, 1982.
63. McLaughlin, H.L.: Trauma. Philadelphia, W.B. Saunders, 1959.
64. Moed, B.R., Kellam, J.F., Foster, R.J., Tile, M., and Hansen, S.T., Jr.: Immediate Internal Fixation of Open Fractures of the Diaphysis of the Forearm. J. Bone Joint Surg., 68A:1008–1017, 1986.
65. Müller, M.E., Allgöwer, M., Schneider, R., and Willenegger, H.: Manual of Internal Fixation, 2nd ed. Berlin, Springer-Verlag, 1979.
66. Müller, M.E., Allgöwer, M., and Willenegger, H.: Technique of Internal Fixation of Fractures. New York, Springer-Verlag, 1965.
67. Naiman, P.T., Schein, A.J., and Siffert, R.S.: Use of ASIF Compression Plates in Selected Shaft Fractures of the Upper Extremity. Clin. Orthop., 71:208–216, 1970.
68. Palmer, A.K., and Werner, F.W.: The Triangular Fibrocartilage Complex of the Wrist–Anatomy and Function. J. Hand Surg., 6:153–162, 1981.
69. Patrick, J.: A Study of Supination and Pronation, With Especial Reference to the Treatment of Forearm Fractures. J. Bone Joint Surg., 28B:737–748, 1946.
70. Prosser, A.J., and Hooper, G.: Entrapment of the Ulnar Nerve in a Greenstick Fracture of the Ulna. J. Hand Surg., 11B:211–212, 1986.
71. Radin, E.L., and Rose, R.R.: Fatigue Fracture of a Forearm Plate Within a Long-arm Cast. Clin. Orthop., 207:142–145, 1986.
72. Ralston, E.L.: Handbook of Fractures. St. Louis, C.V. Mosby, 1967.
73. Rang, M.: Anthology of Orthopaedics. Edinburgh, E & S Livingstone, 1968.
74. Rayan, G.M., and Hayes, M.: Entrapment of the Flexor Digitorum Profundus in the Ulna With Fracture of Both Bones of the Forearm: Report of a Case. J. Bone Joint Surg., 68A:1102–1103, 1986.
75. Richards, R.R.: Principles of Limb Salvage. *In* McMurtry R.Y., McLellan B.A. (eds.): Management of Blunt Trauma. Baltimore, Williams and Wilkins, 1990.
76. Ritchey, S.J., Richardson, J.P., and Thompson, M.S.: Rigid Medullary Fixation of Forearm Fractures. South. Med. J., 51:852–856, 1958.
77. Rosacker, J.A., and Kopta, J.A.: Both Bone Fractures of the Forearm: A Review of Surgical Variables Associated With Union. Orthopaedics, 4:1353–1356, 1981.
78. Sage, F.P.: Fractures of the Shaft of the Radius and Ulna in the Adult. *In* Adams, J.P. (ed.): Current Practice in Orthopaedic Surgery, vol. 1, pp. 152–173. St. Louis, C.V. Mosby, 1963.
79. Sage, F.P.: Medullary Fixation of Fractures of the Forearm: A Study of the Medullary Canal of the Radius and a Report of Fifty Fractures of the Radius Treated With a Prebent Triangular Nail. J. Bone Joint Surg., 41A:1489–1516, 1525, 1959.
80. Sargent, J.P., and Teipner, W.A.: Treatment of Forearm Shaft Fractures by Double Plating: A Preliminary Report. J. Bone Joint Surg., 47A:1475–1490, 1965.
81. Sarmiento, A., Ebramzadeh, E., Brys, D., and Tarr, R.: Angular Deformities and Forearm Function. J. Orthop. Res., 10:121–133, 1992.
82. Sarmiento, A., Cooper, J.S., and Sinclair, W.F.: Forearm Fractures: Early Functional Bracing—A Preliminary Report. J. Bone Joint Surg., 57A:297–304, 1975.
83. Sarmiento, A., and Latta, L.: Closed Functional Treatment of Fractures. Berlin, Springer-Verlag, 1981.
84. Sauve, L., and Kapandji, M.: Nouvelle Technique Traitement Chirurical des Luxations Récidivantes Isolées de l'extrémité Inférieure du Cubitus. J. Chir. (Paris), 47:589–594, 1936.
85. Schemitsch, E.H., Jones, D., Henley, M.B., and Tencer, A.F.: A Comparison of Malreduction After Plate and Intramedullary Nail Fixation of Forearm Fractures. J. Orthop. Trauma, 9:8–16, 1995.
86. Schemitsch, E.H., and Richards, R.R.: The Effect of Malunion on Functional Outcome After Plate Fixation of Fractures of Both Bones of the Forearm in Adults. J. Bone Joint Surg., 74A:1068–1078, 1992.
87. Scheuer, M., and Pot, J.H.: Acute Traumatic Bowing Fracture of the Forearm. Neth. J. Surg., 38:158–159, 1986.
88. Schuind, F., Andrianne, Y., and Burny, F.: Treatment of Forearm Fractures by Hoffman External Fixation: A Study of 93 Patients. Clin. Orthop., 266:197–204, 1991.
89. Sisk, D.T.: Fractures of Upper Extremity and Shoulder Girdle. *In* Crenshaw, A.H. (ed.): Campbell's Operative Orthopaedics. 7th ed., vol. 3, pp. 1557–2118. St. Louis, C.V. Mosby, 1987.
90. Sisk, D.T.: Internal Fixation of Forearm Fractures. *In* Chapman, M.W., and Madison, M. (eds.): Operative Orthopaedics, vol. 1, pp. 273–285. Philadelphia, J.B. Lippincott, 1988.
91. Smith, H.: Fractures. *In* Speed, J.S., and Smith, H. (eds.): Campbell's Operative Orthopedics, 2nd ed., p. 375. St. Louis, C.V. Mosby, 1949.
92. Smith, H., and Sage, F.P.: Medullary Fixation of Forearm Fractures. J. Bone Joint Surg., 39A:91–98, 188, 1957.
93. Smith, J.E.M.: Internal Fixation in the Treatment of Fractures of the Shafts of the Radius and Ulna in Adults. J. Bone Joint Surg., 41B:122–131, 1959.
94. Stern, P.J., and Drury, W.J.: Complications of Plate Fixation of Forearm Fractures. Clin. Orthop., 175:25–29, 1983.
95. Street, D.M.: Intramedullary Forearm Nailing. Clin. Orthop., 212:219–230, 1986.
96. Tarr, R.R., Garfinkel, A.I., and Sarmiento, A.: The Effects of Angular and Rotational Deformities of Both Bones of the Forearm. J. Bone Joint Surg., 66A:65–70, 1984.
97. Teasdall, R., Savoie, F.H., Hughes, J.L.: Comminuted Fractures of the Proximal Radius and Ulna. Clin. Orthop. 292:37–47, 1993.
98. Teipner, W.A., and Mast, J.W.: Internal Fixation of Forearm Fractures: Double Plating Versus Single Compression (Tension Band) Plating—A Comparative Study. Orthop. Clin. North Am., 11:381–391, 1980.
99. Thompson, J.E.: Anatomical Methods of Approach in Operations on the Long Bones of the Extremities. Ann. Surg., 68:309–329, 1918.
100. Trumble, T., Seaber, A.V., and Urbaniak, J.R.: Patency After

Repair of Forearm Arterial Injuries in Animal Models. J. Hand Surg., 12A:47–53, 1987.
101. Valande, M.: Luxation en Arrière de Cubitus Avec Fracture de la Diaphse Radiale. Bull. Mem. Soc. Nat. Chir., 55:435–437, 1929.
102. Venable, C.S.: An Impacting Bone Plate to Attain Closed Coaptation. Ann. Surg., 133:808–813, 1951.
103. Venable, C.S., Stuck, W.G., and Beach, A.: The Effects on Bone of the Presence of Metals, Based Upon Electrolysis: An Experimental Study. Ann. Surg., 105:917–938, 1937.
104. Victor, J., Mulier, T., Fabry, G.: Refracture of Radius and Ulna in a Female Gymnast: A Case Report. Am J. Sports Med., 21:753–754, 1993.
105. Vince, K.G., and Miller, J.E.: Cross-Union Complicating Fracture of the Forearm: I. Adults. J. Bone Joint Surg., 69A:640–653, 1987.
106. Watson-Jones, R.: Fractures and Joint Injuries, 4th ed., vol. 1. Edinburgh, E & S Livingstone, 1956.
107. Watson-Jones, R.: Fractures and Joint Injuries, 4th ed., vol. 2. Edinburgh: E & S Livingstone, 1956.
108. Weiland, A., Robinson, H., and Futrell, J.W.: External Stabilization of a Replanted Upper Extremity: A Case Report. J. Trauma, 16:239, 1976.
109. Whiteside, L.A., and Lesker, P.A.: The Effects of Extraperiosteal and Subperiosteal Dissection: I. On Blood Flow in Muscle. J. Bone Joint Surg., 60A:23–26, 1978.
110. Whiteside, L.A., and Lesker, P.A.: The Effects of Extraperiosteal and Subperiosteal Dissection: II. On Fracture Healing. J. Bone Joint Surg., 60A:26–30, 1987.
111. Young C, Hudson A, Richards R: Operative Treatment of Palsy of the Posterior Interosseous Nerve of the Forearm. J. Bone Joint Surg., 72A:1215–1219, 1990.

ISOLATED FRACTURES OF THE RADIUS AND GALEAZZI INJURIES

112. Adams, B.D.: Effects of Radial Deformity on Distal Radioulnar Joint Mechanics. J. Hand Surg., 18A:492–498, 1993.
113. Beneyto, M.F., Arandes Renu, J.M., Ferreres Claramunt, A., and Ramon Soler, R.: Treatment of Galeazzi Fracture-Dislocations. J. Trauma, 36:352–355, 1994.
114. Bruckner, J.D., Lichtman, D.M., and Alexander, A.H.: Complex Dislocations of the Distal Radioulnar Joint: Recognition and Management. Clin. Orthop., 275:90–103, 1992.
115. Cetti, N.E.: An Unusual Cause of Blocked Reduction of the Galeazzi Injury. Injury, 9:59–61, 1977.
116. Galeazzi, R.: Uber ein Besonderes Syndrom bei Verltzunger im Bereich der Unterarmknochen. Arch. Orthop. Unfallchir., 35:557–562, 1934.
117. Gosselin, R.A., Contreras, D.M., Delgado, E., and Paiement, G.D.: Anterior Dislocation of the Distal End of the Ulna After Use of a Compression Plate for the Treatment of a Galeazzi Fracture: A Case Report. J. Bone Joint Surg, 75:593–596, 1993.
118. Kraus, B., and Horne, G.: Galeazzi Fractures. J. Trauma, 25:1093–1095, 1985.
119. Liang, S.C., Liang, C.L., and Liang, C.S.: Galeazzi's Fracture: Report of 22 Cases. Taiwan, Hsueh Hui Tsa Chih, 79:421–426, 1980.
120. Mikic, Z.D.: Galeazzi Fracture-Dislocations. J. Bone Joint Surg., 57A:1071–1080, 1975.
121. Mohan, K., Gupta, A.K., Sharma, J., Singh, A.K., and Jain, A.K.: Internal Fixation in 50 Cases of Galeazzi Fracture. Acta Orthop. Scand., 59:318–320, 1988.
122. Moore, T.M., Lester, D.K., and Sarmiento, A.: The Stabilizing Effect of Soft-tissue Constraints in Artificial Galeazzi Fractures. Clin. Orthop., 194:189–194, 1985.
123. Moore, T.M., Klein, J.P., Patzakis, M.J., and Harvey, J.P., Jr.: Results of Compression Plating of Closed Galeazzi Fractures. J. Bone Joint Surg., 67A:1015–1021, 1985.
124. Reckling, F.W.: Unstable Fracture-Dislocations of the Forearm (Monteggia and Galeazzi Lesions). J. Bone Joint Surg., 64A:857–863, 1982.
125. Richards R.R.: Disorders of the Distal Radioulnar joint. *In* Richards, R.R.: Soft Tissue Reconstruction on the Upper Extremity. New York, Churchill Livingstone, 1995.
126. Simpson, J.M., Andreshak, T.G., Patel, A., and Jackson, W.T.: Ipsilateral Radial Head Dislocation and Radial Shaft Fracture: A Case Report. Clin. Orthop., 266:205–208, 1991.
127. Strehle, J., and Gerber, C.: Distal Radioulnar Joint Function After Galeazzi Fracture-Dislocations Treated by Open Reduction and Internal Plate Fixation. Clin. Orthop., 293:240–245, 1993.
128. Tillman, R.M., and Smith, R.B.: Successful Bone Grafting of Fracture Nonunion at the Forearm Radial Flap Donor Site. Plast. Reconstr. Surg., 90:684–686, 1992.

ISOLATED FRACTURES OF THE ULNAR SHAFT AND MONTEGGIA FRACTURES

129. Anderson, L.D., Sisk, T.D., Tooms, R.E., and Park, W.I., III.: Compression-Plate Fixation in Acute Diaphyseal Fractures of the Radius and Ulna. J Bone Joint Surg 57A:287–297, 1975.
130. Anderson, L.E., and Meyer, F.N. Fractures of the Shafts of the Radius and Ulna. *In* Rockwood, C.A., Green, D.P., and Bucholz, R. (eds): Fractures in Adults, 3rd ed., vol. 1, pp. 719–728. Philadelphia, J.B. Lippincott, 1991.
131. Austin, R: Tardy Palsy of Radial Nerve From a Monteggia Fracture. Injury, 7:202–204, 1976.
132. Bado, J.L.: The Monteggia Lesion. Clin. Orthop., 50:71–86, 1967.
133. Bado, J.L.: The Monteggia Lesion. Springfield, IL, Charles C Thomas, 1962.
134. Bell, R.H., and Hawkins, R.J.: Stress Fracture of the Distal Ulna: A Case Report. Clin. Orthop., 209:169–171, 1986.
135. Boyd, H.B., and Boals, J.C.: The Monteggia Lesion: A Review of 159 Cases. Clin. Orthop., 66:94–100, 1969.
136. Boyd, H.B., Lipinski, S.W., and Wiley, J.H.: Observations on Nonunion of the Shafts of the Long Bones, With a Statistical Analysis of 842 Patients. J Bone Joint Surg 43A:159–168, 1961.
137. Boyd, H.B.: Surgical Exposure of the Ulna and Proximal Third of the Radius Through One Incision. Surg. Gynecol. Obstet., 71:87–88, 1940.
138. Breit, R.: Post-Traumatic Radioulnar Synostosis. Clin. Orthop., 174:149–152, 1983.
139. Bruce, H.E., Harvey, J.P., and Wilson, J.C.: Monteggia Fractures. J. Bone Joint Surg., 56A:1563–1576, 1974.
140. Chapman, M.W., Gordon, J.E., and Zissimos, A.G.: Compression-Plate Fixation of Acute Fractures of the Diaphysis of the Radius and Ulna. J. Bone Joint Surg., 71A:159–169, 1989.
141. Dodge, H.S., and Cady, G.W.: Treatment of Fractures of the Radius and Ulna With Compression Plates: A Retrospective Study of One Hundred and Nineteen Fractures in Seventy-eight Patients. J. Bone Joint Surg., 54A:1167–1176, 1972.
142. Dymond, I.W.D.: The Treatment of Isolated Fractures of the Distal Ulna. J. Bone Joint Surg., 66B:408–410, 1984.
143. Engber, W.D., and Keene, J.S.: Anterior Interosseous Nerve Palsy Associated With a Monteggia Fracture. Clin. Orthop., 174:133–137, 1983.
144. Evans, E.M.: Pronation Injuries of the Forearm With Special Reference to Anterior Monteggia Fractures. J. Bone Joint Surg., 31B:578–588, 1949.
145. Evans, E.M.: Rotational Deformities in the Treatment of Fractures of Both Bones of the Forearm. J. Bone Joint Surg., 27:373–379, 1945.
146. Giustra, P.E., Killoran, P.J., Furman, R.S., and Root, J.A.: The Missed Monteggia Fracture. Radiology, 110:45–47, 1974.
147. Grace, T.G., and Eversmann, W.W. Jr.: Forearm Fractures: Treatment by Rigid Fixation With Early Motion. J. Bone Joint Surg., 62A:433–438, 1980.
148. Hadden, W.A., Reschauer, R., and Seggl, W.: Results of AO Plate Fixation of Forearm Shaft Fractures in Adults. Injury, 15:44–52, 1983.
149. Hotter, M.M., and Schobert, W.: The Failure of Casual Treatment for Nondisplaced Ulna Shaft Fractures. J. Trauma, 24:771–773, 1984.
150. Holst-Nielsen, F., and Jensen, V.: Tardy Posterior Interosseous Nerve Palsy as a Result of an Unreduced Radial Head Dislocation in Monteggia Fractures: A Report of Two Cases. J. Hand Surg., 9A:572–575, 1984.
151. Jessing, P.: Monteggia Lesions and Their Complicating Nerve Damage. Acta Orthop. Scand., 46:601–609, 1975.
152. Jupiter, J.B., Leibovic, S.J., Ribbans, W., and Wilk, R.M.: The

Posterior Monteggia Lesion. J. Orthop. Trauma, 5:395–402, 1991.

153. Kellam, J.F., and Jupiter, J.B.: Diaphyseal Fractures of the Forearm. *In* Browner, B.D. (ed.): Skeletal Trauma, vol. 1, pp. 1075–1125. Philadelphia, W. B. Saunders, 1992.
154. Lichter, R.L., and Jacobsen, T. Tardy Palsy of the Posterior Interosseous Nerve With a Monteggia Fracture. J. Bone Joint Surg., 57A:124–125, 1975.
155. McLaughlin, H.L.: Trauma. Philadelphia, W. B. Saunders, 1959.
156. Mestdagh, H., Vigier, J.E., and Mairesse, J.L. La Fracture de Monteggia Chez l'Adult. Ann. Chir., 33:417–423, 1979.
157. Moed, B.R., Kellam, J.F., Foster, R.J., Tile, M., and Hansen, S.T. Jr.: Immediate Internal Fixation of Open Fractures of the Diaphysis of the Forearm. J. Bone Joint Surg., 68A:1008–1017, 1986.
158. Monteggia, G.B.: Instituzioni Chirrugiche, vol. 5. Milan, Maspero, 1814.
159. Morris, A.H.: Irreducible Monteggia Lesion With Radial-Nerve Entrapment: A Case Report. J. Bone Joint Surg., 56A:1744–1746, 1974.
160. Mullick, S.: The Lateral Monteggia Fracture. J. Bone Joint Surg., 59A:543–545, 1977.
161. Patel, M.R., Irizarry, J., and Stricevic, M.: Stress Fracture of the Ulnar Diaphysis: A Review of the Literature and Report of a Case. J. Hand Surg., IIA:443–445, 1986.
162. Pavel, A., Pitman, J.M., Lance, E.M., and Wade, P.A.: The Posterior Monteggia Fracture: A Clinical Study. J. Trauma, 5:185–199, 1965.
163. Penrose, J.H.: The Monteggia Fracture With Posterior Dislocation of the Radial Head. J. Bone Joint Surg., 33B:65–73, 1951.
164. Pollock, F.H., Pankovich, A.M., Prieto, J.J., and Lorenz, M.: The Isolated Fracture of the Ulnar Shaft. J. Bone Joint Surg., 65A:339–342, 1983.
165. Reckling, F.W., and Cordell, L.D.: Unstable Fracture-Dislocations of the Forearm: The Monteggia and Galeazzi Lesions. Arch. Surg., 96:999–1007, 1968.
166. Reckling, F.W.: Unstable Fracture-Dislocation of the Forearm (Monteggia and Galeazzi Lesions). J. Bone Joint Surg., 64A:857–863, 1982.
167. Samiento, A., Cooper, J.S., and Sinclair, W.F. Forearm Fractures: Early Functional Bracing—A Preliminary Report. J. Bone Joint Surg., 51A:297–304, 1975.
168. Sarmiento, A., and Latta, L.L.: Closed Functional Treatment of Fractures. New York, Springer-Verlag, 1981.
169. Schatzker, J., and Tile, M. The Rationale of Operative Fracture Care. Berlin, Springer-Verlag, 1987.
170. Smith, H., and Sage, F.P. Medullary fixation of forearm fractures. J. Bone Joint Surg., 39A:91–98, 1957.
171. Smith, F.M.: Monteggia Fractures: An Analysis of Twenty-five Consecutive Fresh Injuries. Surg. Gynecol. Obstet., 85:630–640, 1947.
172. Spar, I.: A Neurologic Complication Following Monteggia Fracture. Clin. Orthop., 122:207–209, 1977.
173. Speed, J.S., and Boyd, H.B.: Treatment of Fracture of the Ulna With Dislocation of the Head of the Radius (Monteggia Fracture). J.A.M.A., 115:1699–1705, 1940.
174. Spinner, M., Freundlich, B.D., and Teicher, J.: Posterior Interosseous Nerve Palsy as a Complication of Monteggia Fractures in Children. Clin. Orthop., 58:141–145, 1968.
175. Stein, F., Grabias, S.L., and Deffer, P.A.: Nerve Injuries Complicating Monteggia Lesions. J. Bone Joint Surg., 53A:1432–1436, 1971.
176. Stern, P.J., and Drury, W.J.: Complications of Plate Fixation of Forearm Fractures. Clin. Orthop., 175:25–29, 1983.
177. Vince, K.G., and Miller, J.E.: Cross-Union Complicating Fractures of the Forearm: I. Adults. J. Bone Joint Surg., 69A:640–653, 1987.
178. Watson, F.M. Jr., and Eaton, R.G.: Post-traumatic Radio-ulnar Synostosis. J. Trauma, 18:467–468, 1978.
179. Watson-Jones, R.: Fractures and Joint Injuries, 4th ed., vol. 1. Edinburgh: E & S Livingstone, 1956.
180. Yong-Hing, K., and Tchang, S.P.K.: Traumatic Radio-ulnar Synostosis Treated by Excision and a Free Fat Transplant: A Report of Two Cases. J. Bone Joint Surg., 65B:433–435, 1983.
181. Zych, G.A., Latta, L.L., and Zagorski, J.B.: Treatment of Isolated Ulnar Shaft Fractures With Prefabricated Functional Fracture Braces. Clin. Orthop., 219:194–200, 1987.

Rockwood and Green's Fractures in Adults, Fourth Edition,
edited by Charles A. Rockwood, David P. Green, Robert W. Bucholz and James D. Heckman.
Lippincott-Raven Publishers, Philadelphia © 1996.

CHAPTER 14

Fractures and Dislocations of the Elbow

Robert N. Hotchkiss

Injuries of the elbow that lead to chronic pain and permanent restriction of motion limit use of the hand in most activities. Positioning of the hand for grip and prehension is dominated by freedom of motion at the elbow. Basic daily activities, from eating to perineal hygiene, require a wide range of positions and movement at the elbow in both flexion and extension and forearm rotation. Any restricted motion of the neck, shoulder, or wrist magnifies impairment of the elbow. More complex tasks, at the workplace or in recreation, require even greater functional demands.

Traditional salvage procedures after trauma, such as arthrodesis and arthroplasty, are poor alternatives for the post-traumatic elbow at this time. Except for rare occupational circumstances, there is no ideal position for fusion, and replacement arthroplasty has not yet stood the test of time or durability in the young, active patient. For these reasons, diligent and thoughtful management of the injured elbow, to maximize painless, effective motion, is compelling.

Operative procedures for repair and reconstruction of the injured elbow are technically demanding and require careful planning. Because of the proximity of crucial neurovascular structures, a thorough knowledge of the anatomy and extensile exposures is essential. Accurate reduction and stable fixation of bony injuries can often optimize ultimate function and limit long-term disability.

In the literature, the most notable evolution in the management of elbow injuries has been an increasing emphasis on early motion. Irrespective of the specifics of the injury, the importance of early active motion for restoration of effective function cannot be overstated. With this principle in mind, the optimal management of specific fractures and dislocations provides protection, stabilizing those structures damaged, while permitting as much active motion as pain and swelling allow.

ANATOMY AND BIOMECHANICS

Topographic Anatomy

Several bony landmarks of the elbow can be palpated readily. With the elbow in full extension, both epicondyles and the olecranon process lie in the same horizontal plane on the posterior aspect of the elbow. When the elbow is flexed 90°, these points form a nearly equilateral triangle in a plane parallel to the posterior surface of the humerus. In flexion, a fourth bony prominence, the outer border of the capitellum, becomes more evident on the lateral aspect of the humerus. It lies distal and anterior to the lateral epicondyle and should not be confused with it. Just distal to the capitellum the radial head can be palpated; it is most easily found by passively rotating the forearm. A familiarity with the bony prominences of the elbow and their relationships to one another greatly assists the surgeon in perceiving subtle abnormalities during examination of the injured elbow.

When the elbow is flexed, the anconeus muscle lies just distal and posterior to the radiohumeral joint in a triangular area outlined by the radial head, the lateral epicondyle, and the tip of the olecranon. The main portion of the radial collateral ligament extends anteriorly and distally, leaving only the fibrous capsule of the elbow joint underlying this rather small, thin muscle. Any distention of the joint with fluid can best be detected here, and this is the preferred site for aspiration of the joint.

Bones

Lower End of the Humerus

The distal aspect of the humerus divides into medial and lateral columns (Fig. 14-1). Each of these columns is roughly triangular and is bound on its outer border

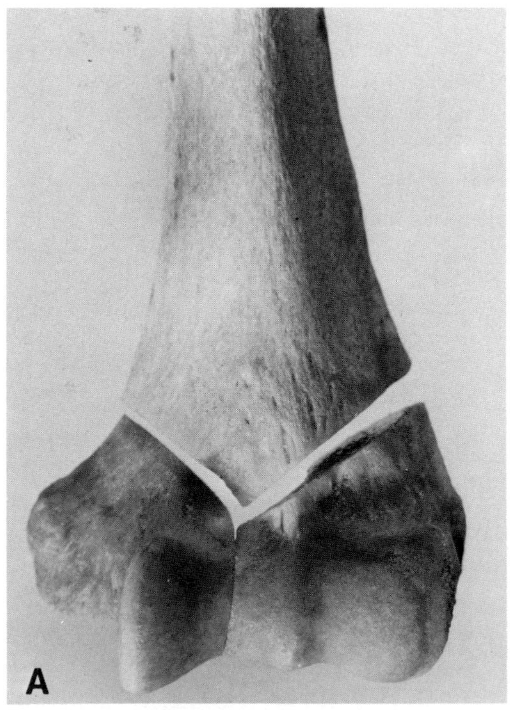

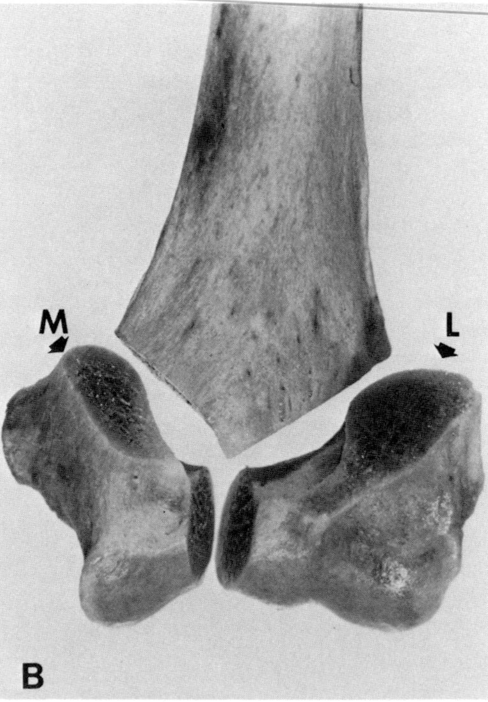

FIGURE 14-1. Internal structure of the distal humerus. (**A**) The anterior surface of a normal distal humerus with cuts through the medial and lateral supracondylar columns. (**B**) Rotation of the medial (*M*) and lateral (*L*) supracondylar columns demonstrates their internal structure. The diameter of the medial column (*M*) is smaller than that of the lateral column (*L*).

by a supracondylar ridge. The divergence of these two columns increases the diameter of the distal humerus in the mediolateral plane. From structural and functional standpoints, the distal humerus is divided into separate medial and lateral components, called condyles, each containing an articulating portion and a nonarticulating portion. Included in the nonarticulating portions are the epicondyles, which are the terminal points of the supracondylar ridges. The lateral epicondyle contains a roughened anterolateral surface from which the superficial forearm extensor muscles arise. The medial epicondyle is larger than its lateral counterpart and serves as the origin of the forearm flexor muscles. The posterior distal portion of the medial epicondyle is smooth and in contact with the ulnar nerve as it crosses the elbow joint. When a condyle loses continuity from its supporting column, as in a fracture, displacement can occur, because no muscles are attached to the condyles to oppose those attached to the epicondyles.

The articulating surface of the lateral condyle is hemispherical and projects anteriorly; it is called the capitellum (capitulum), or "little head." The capitellum is much smaller than the trochlea, and its convex surface articulates with the reciprocally concave head of the radius. These surfaces are in contact throughout only a small portion of the full range of elbow motion.

The articular surface of the medial condyle, the trochlea, is more cylindrical or spool-like (Fig. 14-2). It has very prominent medial and lateral ridges, which Milch believed are important in maintaining medial and lateral stability of the elbow. Between these ridges is a central groove that articulates with the greater sigmoid (semilunar) notch of the proximal ulna. The diameter of the trochlea at this groove is approximately half that of the medial ridge, and the groove occupies nearly the entire circumference of the trochlea. It originates anteriorly in the coronoid fossa and terminates posteriorly in the olecranon fossa. On the posterior surface of the trochlea the groove is directed slightly laterally. This obliquity of the trochlear groove produces the valgus carrying angle of the forearm when the elbow is extended. Between the lateral ridge of the trochlea and the hemispheric surface of the capitellum, a sulcus separates the medial and lateral condyles. This capitulotrochlear sulcus articulates with the peripheral ridge of the radial head.

Proximal to the condyles on the anterior surface of the humerus lie the coronoid and radial fossae. They receive the coronoid process and radial head, respectively, when the elbow is flexed. Posteriorly, the olecranon fossa is a deep hollow for the reception of the olecranon, making it possible for the elbow to go into full extension. The bone that separates these anterior and posterior fossae is extremely thin, usually translucent, and occasionally even absent. The presence of extraneous material in the olecranon fossa, such as fracture fragments or an internal fixation device, necessarily impedes full extension of the elbow.

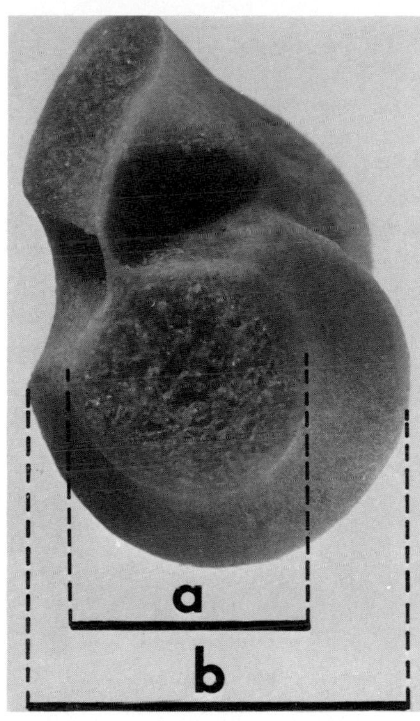

FIGURE 14-2. Cross section of the medial condyle through the trochlear groove. The diameter of the bony portion of the center of the groove (*a*) is slightly more than one half that of the medial trochlear ridge (*b*).

The articular cartilage surface of the capitellum and trochlea projects downward and forward from the end of the humerus at an angle of approximately 30°.[3] The centers of the arcs of rotation of the articular surfaces of each condyle lie on the same horizontal line through the distal humerus. Thus, malalignment of the relationship of one condyle to the other changes their arcs of rotation, limiting flexion and extension (Fig. 14-3).[9]

A bony spine, called the supracondylar process (Fig. 14-4), occasionally projects downward from the anteromedial surface of the humerus. It arises approximately 5 cm superior to the medial epicondyle and is attached to the medial epicondyle by a fibrous band. The process, the shaft of the humerus, and the fibrous band form a foramen through which the median nerve and the brachial artery pass. The spur gives origin to a part of the pronator teres muscle and may receive a lower portion of the insertion of the coracobrachialis muscle.

Upper End of the Radius

The proximal end of the radius consists of the disk-shaped head, the neck, and the radial tuberosity; the head and part of the neck lie within the joint. The

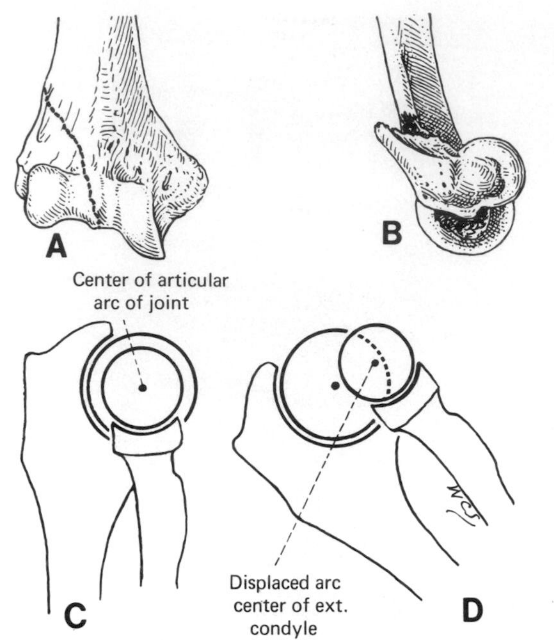

FIGURE 14-3. Effects of condylar malalignment. The centers of the articular arc of the separate condyles are located on the same horizontal line through the distal humerus (**A, C**). When there is malalignment of one condyle with another (**B, D**), flexion and extension of the elbow are blocked. *(Magnuson, P.B., and Stack, J.K.: Fractures, 5th ed. Philadelphia, J.B. Lippincott, 1949.)*

radial head is not perfectly round; rather, one diameter is consistently 1.5 to 3 cm larger than the other.[22] The shallow concavity of the head articulates with the convex surface of the capitellum, and the border of the head articulates with the lateral side of the coronoid process in the lesser sigmoid (radial) notch. The tuberosity, which is extra-articular, has a rough posterior portion for the insertion of the tendon of the biceps and a smooth anterior surface over which lies a bursa that separates the tuberosity from the tendon.

Upper End of the Ulna

The proximal end of the ulna consists of the olecranon and coronoid processes, which together form the greater sigmoid (semilunar) notch, although their articular surfaces may not always be continuous.[23] The articulation of this notch with the trochlea of the humerus provides inherent bony stability to the hinge joint of the elbow. Both the medial and lateral collateral ligaments attach to the proximal portion of the ulna.

The triceps inserts by a broad tendinous expansion into the olecranon posteriorly. On the anterior surface, the brachialis muscle inserts distal to the coronoid process. This insertion is broad and more distal on the ulna than is often thought (Fig. 14-5). Fractures of the coronoid are not usually avulsion fractures, but rather impact fractures.

The head of the radius rests within the lesser sigmoid (radial) notch on the lateral side of the coronoid process. The orbicular (annular) ligament consists of bands of strong fibers, which are intimately and inseparably connected with, but somewhat thicker than, the capsule of the elbow joint. The ligament encircles the head of the radius, retaining it within the radial notch but allowing it enough freedom to rotate easily.

Collateral Ligaments

The collateral ligaments of the elbow supplement the natural stability of the elbow joint.[1,7,14,18–20] The fan-shaped radial (lateral) collateral ligament originates from the lateral epicondyle and inserts into the orbicular (annular) ligament of the radius. Some posterior fibers go to the ulna just proximal to the posterior origin of the orbicular ligament. The thicker and stronger ulnar (medial) collateral ligament consists of two portions, both arising from the medial epicondyle. The anterior portion attaches to a tubercle (sublime tubercle) on the medial surface of the coronoid. The posterior portion attaches to the medial surface of the olecranon process.

Biomechanics

Unique in the body's collection of diarthrodial joints, the elbow contains two functionally independent articulations that share a synovial compartment but determine motion in two independent axes. The ulnotrochlear articulation directs flexion and extension, and the radiocapitellar joint governs forearm rotation. The ulnohumeral articulation is highly constrained and approximates a hinge with little deviation out of the frontal plane. The instant centers of rotation have been studied and demonstrate little deviation from a true hinge with a single axis.[8,10,17,25]

Forearm rotation is centered at the radiocapitellar joint. In forearm rotation, the radius rotates about the ulna, as the ulna is fixed by its articulation at the trochlea. By using these independent axes of motion, the hand can be positioned over a large area in a variety of attitudes. Morrey and colleagues[16] have shown that most activities of daily living require a relatively large range of motion: for flexion and extension, 30° to 130°, and for pronation and supination, 50° each. If a patient loses motion for any reason, he or she must adapt by using the uninjured extremity or changing shoulder, neck, or body position.

The anteroposterior stability of the elbow results from the static hemicircumferential articulation at the ulnohumeral joint and the dynamic tension provided by the biceps and brachialis anteriorly and the triceps

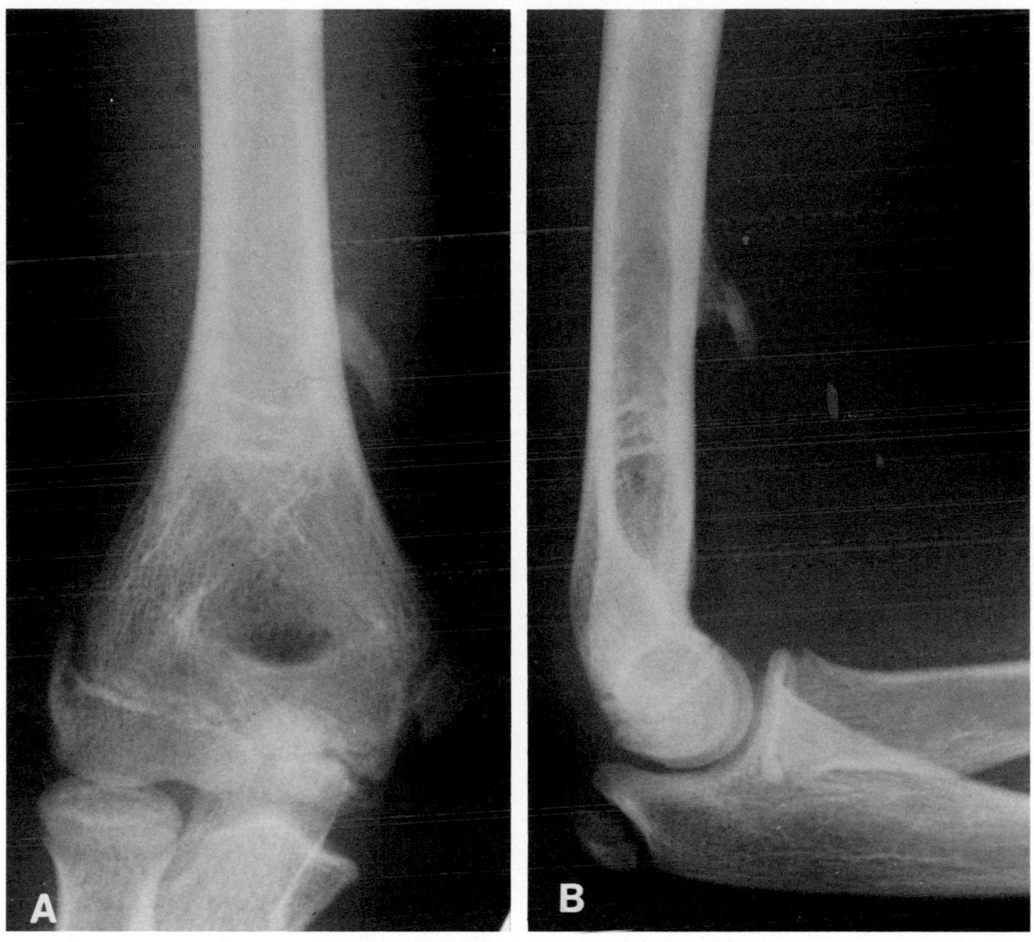

FIGURE 14-4. Anteroposterior (**A**) and lateral (**B**) views of a distal humerus that has a supracondylar process.

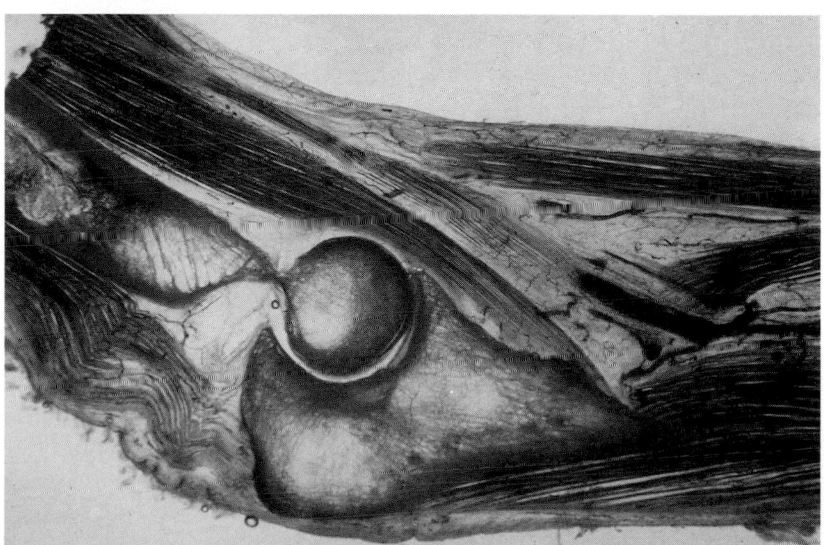

FIGURE 14-5. This sagittal anatomical section of the elbow demonstrates the insertion of the brachialis distal to the coronoid process. Also note the thin bone at the level of the olecranon fossa.

posteriorly. The dynamic stability provided by the flexors and extensors should not be underestimated. The anteromedial ligament and the lateral collateral ligament both provide anteroposterior support in combination with the articular surfaces. A clinical study[404] has shown that up to 50% of the proximal olecranon can be removed without creating instability. In a related biomechanical study,[1] there was a linear decline in stability with each section of the olecranon removed; however, there was no tension in the flexors or triceps. Both authors emphasized the importance of conserving the insertion of the anteromedial collateral ligament.

Most stressful activities such as lifting or throwing exert valgus stress at the elbow. Valgus forces are resisted primarily by a combination of ligaments and joint surfaces and minimally by muscle forces. The anterior portion of the medial collateral ligament is the primary stabilizer to valgus stress in most positions of flexion.[7,13,14,18–20,24] The radial head assists valgus stability by providing a broader base of support and increasing the mechanical advantage of the medial ligament (Fig. 14-6). In full extension, the anterior capsule becomes taut and resists valgus stress. The posterior portion of the medial collateral ligament is thin and contributes little to stability.[7]

Varus stress about the elbow is less problematic. The lateral collateral ligaments and the anconeus muscle confer a combination of static and dynamic stability.[4] The clinical relevance of the lateral ligaments has been studied by O'Driscoll and colleagues.[336,337] Osborne and Cotterill[338] believed that in cases of recurrent posterior dislocation, the lateral ligaments were paramount and required reconstruction. O'Driscoll and associates[336,337] have identified a group of patients with posterolateral instability who have demonstrated injury to the lateral ulnohumeral collateral ligament. Experimental sectioning of this structure has led to instability in the laboratory as well.

Joint reaction forces of the elbow have been calculated to reach two to three times body weight during strenuous lifting.[2,11,21] Lifting over the large lever of the forearm magnifies small weight in the hand. Position of the elbow also influences the joint reaction force. As the elbow moves into flexion, the joint reaction force decreases.

When the forearm or hand is loaded in grip or lifting, presumably some load sharing occurs between the ulnohumeral joint and the radiocapitellar joint, but the exact ratio and position dependence are not known. Morrey and coworkers[15] have shown in the cadaver that as the forearm rotates there is a measurable change in the contact at the radiocapitellar joint. The central portion of the interosseous ligament may also play a role in load distribution, because stiffness to longitudinal compression increases from pronation to supination, but the specific relationship in vivo is not known (see Surgical Anatomy section in Chapter 13).[6]

Radiographic Anatomy

Routine X-rays

Proper x-rays are vital when evaluating the elbow after trauma. True lateral projections are important when imaging the distal humerus and radiocapitellar joint. Anteroposterior views are also important, but often the elbow is held in the flexed position, causing over-

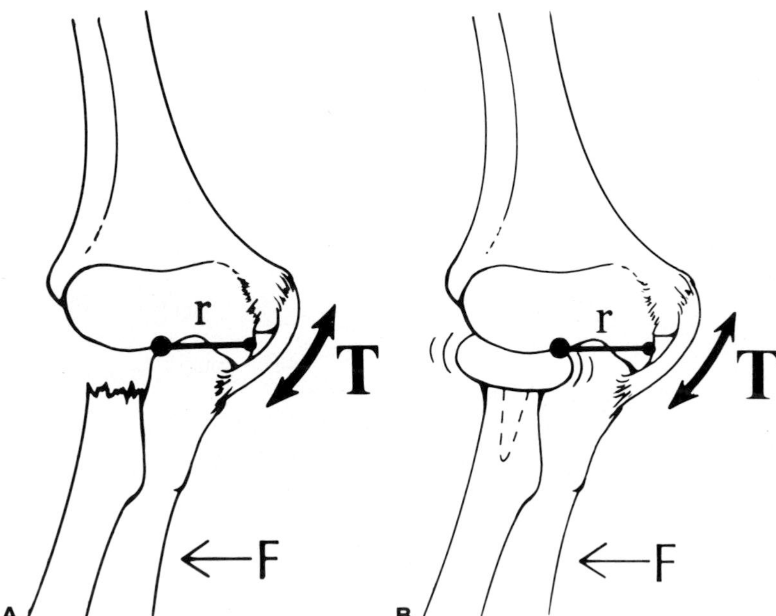

FIGURE 14-6. When the radial head is excised, the base of support to valgus stress (*F*) decreases and greater tension (*T*) is experienced by the medial ligaments (**A**). Silicone radial head replacement has not been shown in the laboratory to measurably increase valgus stability (**B**). *(Hotchkiss, R.N., and Weiland, A.J.: Valgus Stability of the Elbow. J. Orthop. Res., 5:372–377, 1987.)*

lap of the bones. The radial head should be aligned with the capitellum in all views, irrespective of position.

The presence of a so called fat pad sign can be indicative of trauma (Fig. 14-7).[28–30] The radiographic lucency posterior to the distal humerus is the displaced posterior fat from the olecranon fossa, not visible in the normal elbow. If the elbow is extended, the fat pad may be visible simply because of laxity of the triceps. Distention from a hemarthrosis can also displace the anterior fat pad but this may not be apparent.

Special Studies

Computed tomography (CT scanning) and magnetic resonance imaging have improved significantly and are now useful tools in the evaluation of the injured elbow. As these techniques evolve, the specific indications will become more refined. I use CT scans of the elbow to evaluate fractures of the radial head or capitellum when I am planning an open reduction and am concerned about the degree of fragmentation. Magnetic resonance imaging is becoming more useful in the assessment of the ligamentous structures, including the interosseous ligament of the forearm (Fig. 14-8). The use of improved surface coils and acquisition sequences has improved resolution and tissue identification.[26,27] With these methods and the advent of arthroscopy, the role of arthrography has become very limited.

FRACTURES OF THE DISTAL HUMERUS

Supracondylar Fractures

Supracondylar fractures are, by definition, extra-articular. If the joint is involved, they should be classified as intercondylar or transcondylar with proximal extension. Most often the point of fracture is the thin bone between the medial and lateral columns of the distal humerus.[60]

If the distal fragment is displaced posteriorly, it is usually the result of an extension force.[36,41] Anterior displacement reflects a flexion-type injury.[40] Roberts and Kelly[56] credited Kocher with describing four types of fractures, adding adduction and abduction to the flexion and extension types. However, pure displace-

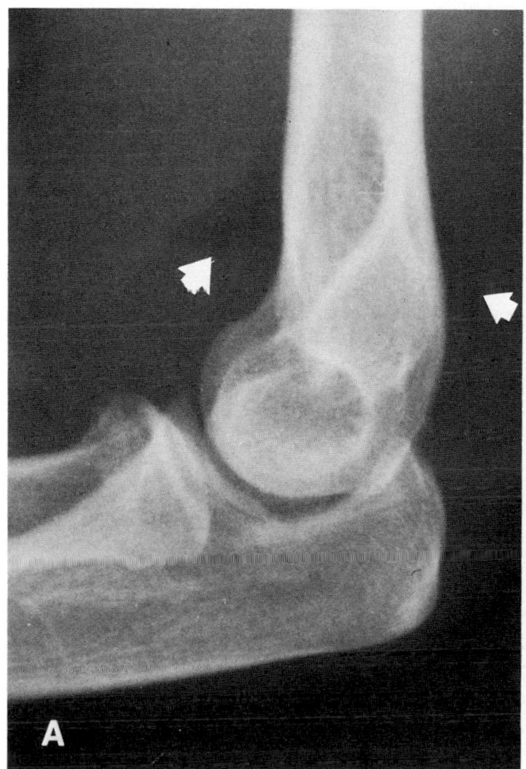

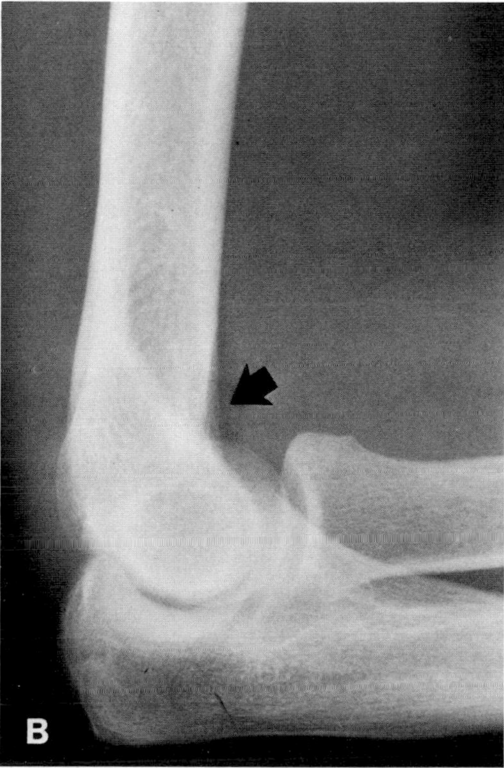

FIGURE 14-7. Fat pad sign. (**A**) A lateral view of the elbow joint shows a joint effusion secondary to a minimally displaced fracture of the radial head. There is anterior and superior displacement of the anterior fat pad in the presence of an effusion (*anterior arrow*), and the posterior fat pad is very prominent as well (*posterior arrow*). (**B**) Lateral x-ray of a normal elbow for comparison. The anterior fat pad is barely visualized (*arrow*); the posterior fat pad is not seen.

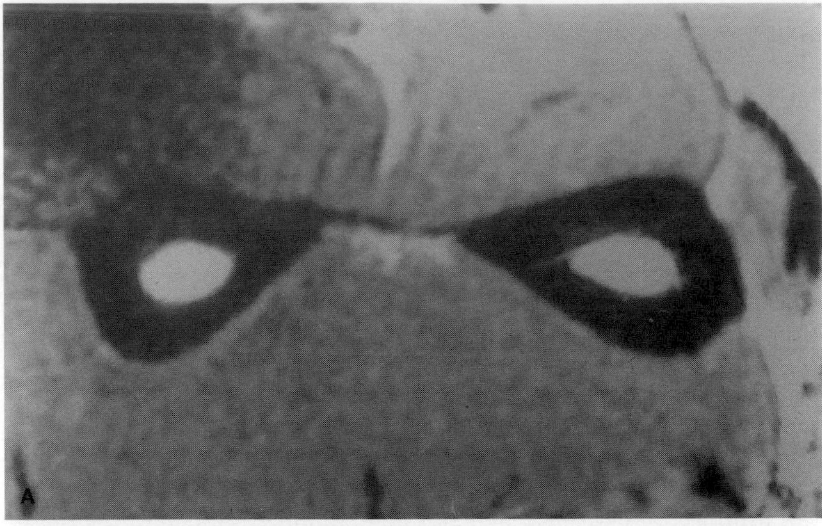

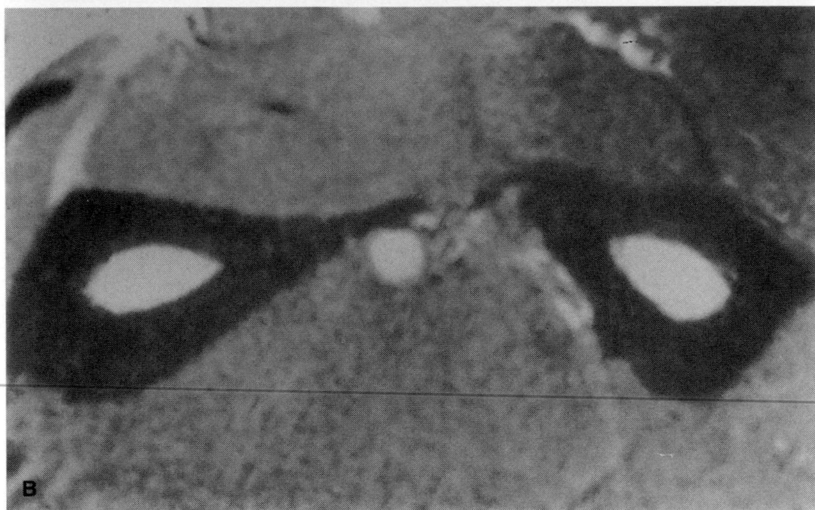

FIGURE 14-8. (**A**) MRI of the central portion of the interosseous ligament of the forearm. (**B**) The same view in a patient with a tear of this ligament after fracture of the radial head (Essex-Lopresti fracture).

ment in the lateral plane is not seen. I have included these with extension-type fractures.

Extension-Type Supracondylar Fractures

Mechanism of Injury

In Kocher's original classification of supracondylar fractures, the abduction and adduction fractures were thought to be due to pure abduction and adduction forces while the elbow was in extension.[31] Hyperextension (secondary to a fall on the outstretched hand) is often the mechanism.[31] However, the authors[56,64] cite direct violence to the elbow as a common cause. Most patients, in spite of careful questioning, cannot recall how they fell and the position of the arm at the time of injury. In addition, many attempts have been made to mimic fractures of the distal humerus in the laboratory by direct blows. None of the fracture patterns seen, using these methods, resemble those seen clinically. The active muscle forces probably play a crucial role at the time of injury.

In the lateral view, the fracture usually extends obliquely upward from the anterior distal aspect to posterior proximal aspect. In the extension type, the distal fragment is displaced posteriorly and proximally by the force of the initial injury and by the triceps acting on the proximal ulna. The distal fragment is also usually flexed at the elbow because of the pull of the origins of the forearm muscles on the epicondyles. The sharp, fractured end of the proximal fragment projects forward into the antecubital fossa, where it may contuse or even impale the brachial artery or median nerve.[40] Even if the artery escapes direct injury, vascular impairment may result from massive swelling of the elbow secondary to the frequently severe associated soft-tissue injury.[59] Neurovascular complications are an ever-present threat to the management of these difficult injuries.

Signs and Symptoms

The findings in an extension-type supracondylar fracture vary with both the degree of swelling and the displacement of the fracture. Open fractures, although rare, do occur and are usually secondary to direct trauma.[59]

When the patient is seen immediately after the injury, there is little swelling about the elbow, which makes it possible to palpate the bony landmarks.[32] More commonly, however, the patient is seen only after considerable swelling has developed, when the landmarks are not palpable.[59] With posterior displacement of the distal fragment, this fracture may be easily confused with a posterior elbow dislocation. Malgaigne's early emphasis on differentiating it from a dislocation[42] led to the association of the fracture with his name (the Malgaigne fracture).[44] In a supracondylar fracture the three bony landmarks, the medial and lateral epicondyles and the olecranon, maintain their normal spatial relationships.[32] The plane of the equidistant triangle that these points form now lies farther back and not necessarily parallel to the long axis of the humerus.[61] In a posterior dislocation of the elbow the relationship of these three points is disrupted. The tip of the olecranon is posterior to the two epicondyles.

Although Dupuytren[42] pointed out that another pathognomonic sign of this fracture was crepitus, no attempt should be made to elicit it. Uncontrolled manipulation can cause neurovascular damage and unnecessary pain. The extension-type supracondylar fracture is usually grossly unstable.

Careful initial neurovascular evaluation of the injured arm is essential.[59] Acute injury of the brachial artery and later development of a volar compartment syndrome must be suspected both initially and during the postreduction period.[33–40] Associated injury of all three major nerves has been reported with supracondylar fractures, although apparently the radial nerve is most frequently involved.[35]

Radiographic Findings

The radiographic findings depend on the degree of displacement. In the anteroposterior view, the fracture line is usually transverse in the minimally or displaced or nondisplaced fracture, lying just proximal to the articular capsule. In moderately displaced fractures, the distal fragment can lie either medially or laterally in relation to the humeral shaft. In cases of marked displacement there may be either axial rotation of the fragment or angulation in the mediolateral plane as well. In the lateral view, if the fracture is nondisplaced, there may be only a positive fat sign. In minimally displaced fractures, there may be only a decrease in the angulation of the articular surface with the long axis of the humerus. With marked displacement, the distal fragment is displaced posteriorly and proximally.

Methods of Treatment

The course of treatment of extension-type supracondylar fractures is influenced greatly by the presence of associated bone and soft-tissue injuries (especially neurovascular) in the same limb. In all cases, prompt reduction of the fracture is desirable, but impairment of circulation constitutes a surgical emergency.

Nonoperative Treatment. In nondisplaced or minimally displaced fractures, treatment consists of posterior plaster splint immobilization for 1 to 2 weeks, after which gentle motion exercise is started. The splint can be discontinued when the fracture is healed at 6 weeks.[36,51]

Closed Reduction. Closed reduction of displaced fractures is usually reserved for the pediatric patient. In the rare situation in adults in which reduction is attempted, this is usually done under anesthesia.

Muscle relaxation relieves tension on the vital neurovascular structures anterior to the elbow joint. First, however, the surgeon must thoroughly examine the x-rays and plan the manipulative maneuvers carefully. The degree of displacement of the distal fragment must be determined, especially the extent of abduction, adduction, medial or lateral displacement, and rotation. Reduction of markedly displaced fractures requires an anesthetic that can give both adequate relaxation and pain relief. This requires, at the minimum, a proximal regional block of the entire extremity or, preferably, if the condition of the patient permits, a general anesthetic. An assistant applies countertraction by grasping the upper arm and holds the proximal fragment steady while the surgeon manipulates the distal portion. This is usually best performed by applying traction at the wrist with one hand and guiding the distal fragment during manipulation with the other hand. The proximal pull of the triceps and biceps must first be overcome by longitudinal traction with the elbow extended.[32,49] Smith[62] cautioned against flexion before reduction is obtained, because this may impale the anteriorly placed neurovascular structures between the sharp ends of the fracture fragments. Once length has been restored by traction—a finding confirmed by a lateral x-ray, the elbow may be hyperextended slightly if extreme care is taken not to overstretch the anterior structures. This tends to unlock the fracture fragments. Once the fragments are free, forward pressure is applied to the distal fragment and backward pressure is applied to the proximal one. At the same time medial or lateral angulation can be corrected.[32,49]

With the fracture fragments now in their proper relationship, the elbow can be flexed gradually.[32] This usually locks the fracture fragment securely in place. The degree of flexion obtainable is usually limited by the amount of swelling about the elbow. The arm must be immobilized in sufficient flexion to maintain fracture reduction. Too much flexion prevents adequate venous return and may even cause occlusion of the brachial artery.[32] The elbow may be flexed just to the point where the radial pulse disappears, and then it should be extended 5° to 10° to accommodate additional swelling. The arm is immobilized in this position with a posterior splint. Patients who have displaced fractures or considerable swelling must be hospitalized after reduction. This allows close observation for the development of any delayed vascular complications.

The decision whether to immobilize the forearm in supination or in pronation is somewhat controversial.[5] Smith[61] pointed out that during reduction the hand must be supinated and directed toward the anterior portion of the shoulder. This helps to obtain adequate rotational alignment. In the past, various authors[56,61] had maintained this position of supination with flexion (the so-called natural splint technique) after reduction had been obtained. Others placed no special emphasis on the position of the forearm.[37,49,58,61,66] DePalma recommended that the forearm be in neutral position.[40] More recent thinking is that the position of the forearm does influence the position of the distal fragment. This is important because the angulation of the distal fragment is responsible for the cubitus valgus or varus deformities more frequently seen in children.[50,52,62] Böhler[32] recommended that the forearm be in pronation to prevent the more common varus angulation. On the basis of his cadaver and clinical studies, he believed that the varus angulation of the distant fragment resulted from the unopposed pull on the fragment by the pronators of the forearm. Placing the forearm in pronation relaxes these muscles. In full pronation, the rotation of the radius has been exhausted; thus all the forces directed to the forearm are transmitted through the ulna to the humerus. Full pronation tenses the medial collateral ligament, correcting the varus angulation of the distal fragment. Salter,[57] in treating this fracture in children, determined the intact periosteum by the location of the distal fragment in the mediolateral plane. He then used this intact periosteum as a hinge to secure the fragments. If there is medial displacement (intact medial periosteum), he recommends that the forearm be pronated. For lateral displacement (intact lateral periosteum), the forearm is supinated. Although the periosteum of adults is not as strong as that of children, these general principles can be useful. D'Ambrosia[38] also confirmed with cadaver studies (on the basis of ligament tension) that these fractures were more stable in pronation.

In extension-type fractures with minimal or moderate displacement the principles are essentially the same as for the severely displaced fractures. In many of these there is only loss of the normal condylar angulation.[47] If less than 20° of the condyle shaft angulation is lost, the position can be accepted.[61] This may result in some decrease of total flexion, but the patient should be able to reach his or her hand to the mouth. In fractures in which the angulation loss is greater than 20°, manipulation with open reduction and internal fixation should be considered.

In cases involving considerable swelling and difficult reduction, the extremity can be placed in Dunlop's[41] side-arm traction or overhead olecranon pin traction[61,62] until the swelling subsides and a reduction can be attempted with greater ease.

Care After Reduction. X-rays must be taken immediately after reduction. They should then be repeated on about the third and seventh days because occasionally loss of reduction occurs. Special attention must be given to the recognition of varus or valgus angulation of the distal fragments. Varus or valgus angulation can be visualized on a tangential view of the distal humerus through the flexed elbow. The alignment of the distal articular surface with the long axis of the humerus is then measured and compared with that on a similar x-ray of the opposite elbow.

Postoperative immobilization is accomplished by the use of a posterior plaster slab in the proper amount of flexion. This slab can be suspended by a collar-and-cuff arrangement or a sling. A posterior slab probably should be used even in nondisplaced fractures, instead of a collar and cuff alone. This provides protection for the tender injured elbow. Circular casts should never be used as the initial method of immobilization. The period of immobilization after reduction lasts from 4 to 6 weeks.[36] Periodic active motion out of the protective splint can be initiated as soon as the fracture is clinically stable. Active motion is facilitated by the application of heat. Passive stretching exercises should never be attempted.

Olecranon Traction. In some fractures, skeletal pin traction through the olecranon may be the treatment of choice (Fig. 14-9).[36] Smith[61] listed four types of severe supracondylar fractures for which Kirschner-wire traction is indicated: (1) when it is impossible to reduce the fracture by other closed methods; (2) when it is possible to reduce the fracture but impossible to maintain the reduction by flexion without compromising the circulation; (3) when swelling is excessive, circulatory impairment is present, or Volkmann's ischemia already threatens; and (4) when associated lesions such as gross contamination are present and external fixation is not available.

The main advantage of this method is that skeletal traction is easier to apply and adjust than skin traction (Fig. 14-10). Either side-arm or overhead skeletal traction can be used. Overhead skeletal traction facilitates edema control, and motion of the elbow can be started early with gravity assisting in flexion. Dressing changes are easily accomplished. Smith[61] suggested that angulation of the distal fragment could be better controlled as well. D'Ambrosia[38] reported no cubitus varus deformities after closed reduction and overhead olecranon pin traction in children. He believed this was be-

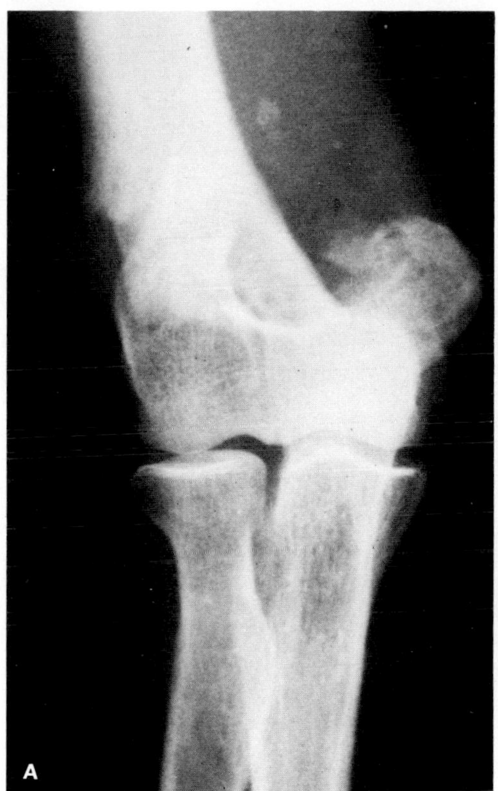

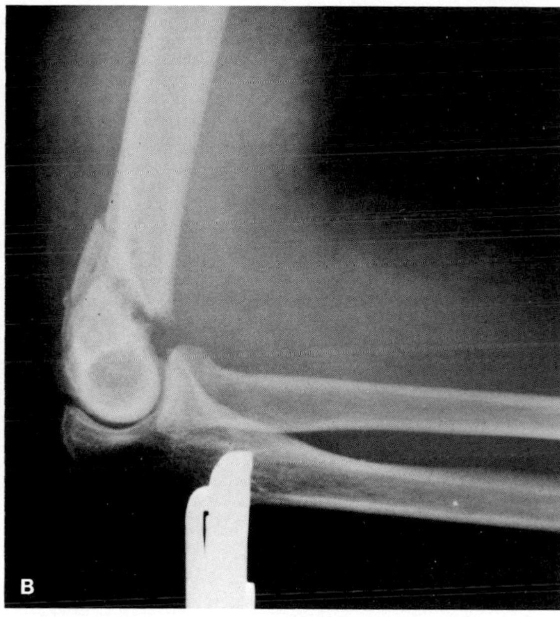

FIGURE 14-9. (**A**) Extension-type supracondylar fracture. (**B**) Lateral x-ray view demonstrating the fracture line running from posterior-proximal to anterior-distal. Olecranon pin traction resulted in satisfactory alignment of the fracture.

cause overhead skeletal traction keeps the forearm in pronation, whereas side-arm traction holds the forearm in the neutral or supinated position, which predisposes to varus deformity.[38] Conn and Wade[36] warned against some of the problems encountered with skeletal pin traction.

Too-early discontinuance of traction can result in a loss of reduction with poor results.[36] Problems with pin-tract infections have been reported.[36,39,53] Although the infection can be easily cleared, marked restriction of motion may result. A major disadvantage of this method is that it necessitates a lengthy hospitalization.

Operative Methods. Two operative techniques are available to the surgeon in the treatment of extension-type fractures. One is fixation of the distal fragment with percutaneously placed Kirschner wires after reduction has been obtained by closed methods. The second is primary open reduction and internal fixation. In adults, the latter is usually preferable.

Percutaneous Pin Fixation. Miller[54] first described percutaneous pinning of intercondylar fractures of the distal humerus in 1939. By directing the wires in a different direction, Swenson[65] adapted its use for supracondylar fractures in children. Although this technique has been used mainly for supracondylar fractures in children and adolescents, Jones reported its use in adults.[48] He modified the technique by allowing the pins to protrude through the skin to facilitate removal. He recommended leaving the pins in 4 to 5 weeks in the adult, followed by 1 to 2 weeks of plaster immobilization. This technique finds application in those fractures that are unstable except in extreme flexion. Stabilization of the fracture by this technique allows the arm to be immobilized in much less flexion.

In the adult, Kirschner wires are too small[48] and do not provide enough strength for mechanical rigidity, even with cast immobilization. Some authors have recommended small Steinman pins instead, hoping that the larger diameter provides greater stability. Percutaneous pin fixation should only be used when open reduction with rigid internal fixation is precluded. The danger of pin-related infection is significant. If local pin-tract infection occurs, the joint may also become infected. Pin fixation must not be done, of course, unless an adequate reduction can be accomplished. The technique relies heavily on the surgeon's ability to palpate the bony landmarks. Because both reduction and palpation may be difficult or even impossible

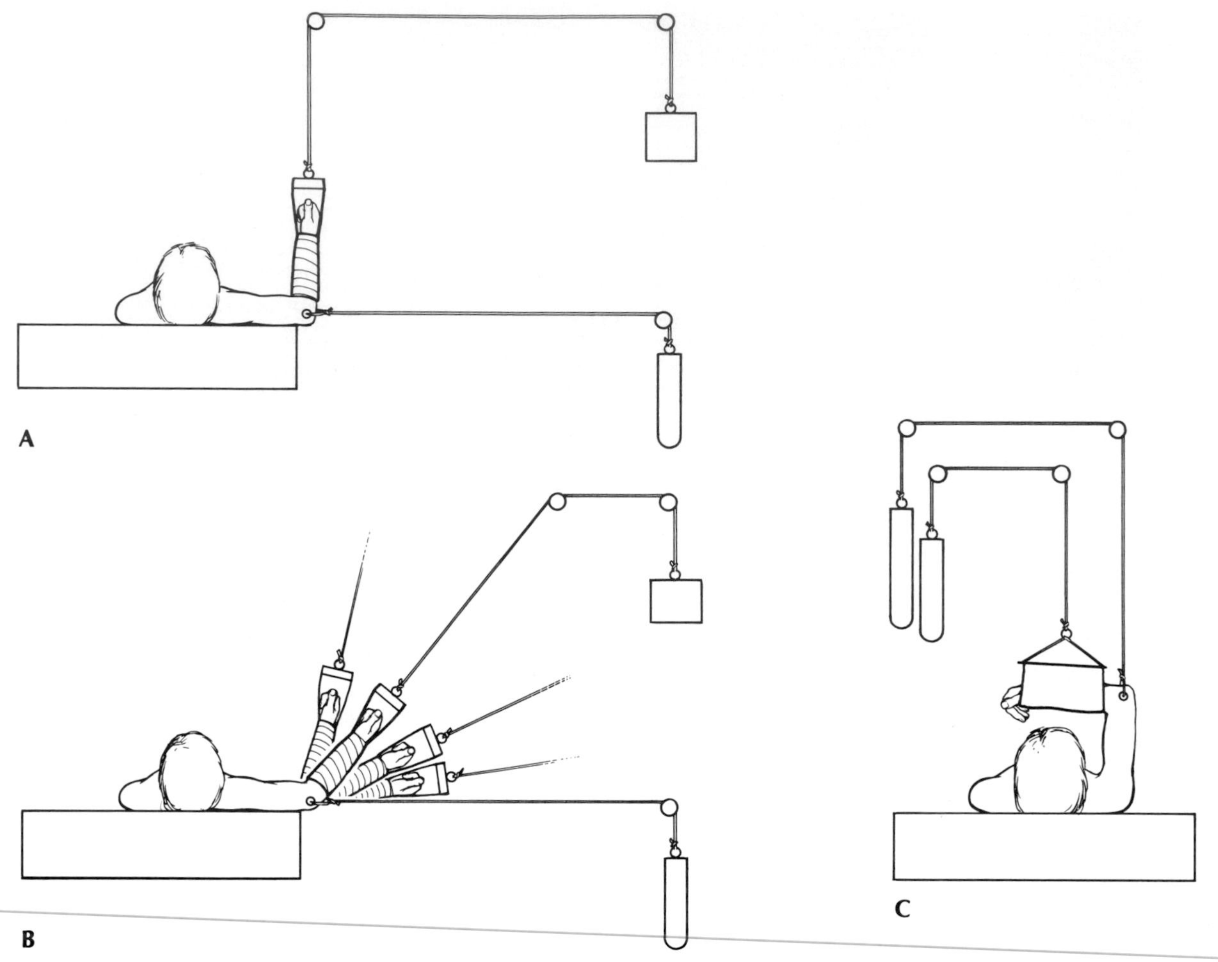

FIGURE 14-10. (**A**) Lateral skeletal olecranon pin traction. (**B**) Changing the position of the overhead pulley supporting the forearm (in skin traction) allows early institution of elbow motion. (**C**) Modification of skeletal olecranon pin traction in which the forearm is supported overhead is useful in the early postinjury phase to help decrease swelling.

in the severely swollen elbow, a preliminary period of traction may be necessary if this method of fixation is used. Power equipment for insertion of the pins greatly facilitates the procedure.

In the original descriptions,[48,65] the wires were passed medially and laterally through the epicondyles and continued proximally up the respective supracondylar columns. This technique entails some risk to the ulnar nerve during placement of the medial pin. In an effort to avoid this risk, Fowles and colleagues[43] used two pins laterally in children. One is passed laterally through the lateral epicondyle in the usual manner. A second pin traverses the joint just lateral to the olecranon in the region of the capitulotrochlear sulcus.

Some authors have recommended securing these fractures by pinning across the joint.[35] This should be avoided if at all possible. The stress across the joint can be great, even with a posterior splint in place. The large lever arm of the forearm leads to bending of the pin, or worse, cutting out at the fragile distal humerus or proximal ulna. In addition, the transarticular pin obviously prevents any flexion or extension motion until the pin is removed, leading to joint stiffness.

Open Reduction and Internal Fixation. The indications for primary open reduction are (1) those fractures in which there is inability to obtain a satisfactory closed reduction; (2) vascular injury; or (3) an associated fracture of the humerus or forearm in the same limb. In addition, Conn and Wade[36] believed that internal fixation may be the treatment of choice in selected elderly patients to hasten ambulation and joint mobilization.

In those cases in which reduction cannot be obtained, muscle, especially the brachialis, may be interposed between the fracture fragments. In rare instances the proximal humeral fragment may be buttonholed through the brachialis. Attempts at longitudinal traction only tighten the muscle around the protruding fragment. In those patients with vascular injury in whom arterial repair is necessary, the fracture must be stabilized as well. Access to both the antecubital fossa and the distal humerus can be accomplished by the surgical approach of Fiolle and Delmas as described by Henry.[45] In cases without associated vascular injury, the fracture can be approached through combined medial and lateral incisions[34] or through a posterior approach.[31,54]

In my experience the posterior approach provides better exposure and better access for internal fixation. After the underlying pathology is corrected, a reduction is obtained by direct visualization. Fracture stabilization has been reported using percutaneous pinning[35,43,48,65] or by direct internal fixation.[54] Bryan[33] recommended the use of a special Y-plate for internal fixation of these fractures. Müller and colleagues[55] recommend an AO semitubular or dynamic compression plate on the medial or lateral humeral column with as many screws as possible inserted as lag screws for internal fixation of supracondylar fractures. Helfet and Hotchkiss[104] demonstrated that the fatigue performance of two plates fixed at right angles was superior to a single posterior Y-plate or bicondylar screws.

Horne[46] noted that nonoperative treatment produced better results than operative treatment when stable fixation was not achieved, owing to comminution. However, this finding should not be used to justify nonoperative treatment for all displaced, comminuted fractures. More careful attention to the use of bone grafting and plate placement have improved results with internal fixation. The surgeon must remember, however, that although simple supracondylar fractures are suitable for internal fixation, conservative treatment has produced better results in patients in whom comminution at the fracture site prevents *stable* fixation.[46] Unstable internal fixation that necessitates prolonged cast immobilization to maintain the reduction combines the disadvantages of both closed and open treatment and produces the worst clinical results.[51] Early range of motion of the elbow is a major goal of treatment if open reduction is selected.

 **Author's Preferred Method of Treatment.** The initial evaluation of any serious elbow injury should include a careful assessment for signs of neurovascular injury. Most fractures in the adult distal humerus are intercondylar (not supracondylar), and one should suspect this when first seeing an adult patient with a "supracondylar" fracture.

Nondisplaced fractures are immobilized with a long-arm posterior splint for 1 to 2 weeks, and then active motion is begun. It is important to monitor the fracture radiographically for any sign of displacement during the first 2 weeks.

Fractures with displacement are usually unstable, and I seldom use closed manipulation and casting or olecranon pin traction in adults because of the difficulty in maintaining the reduction and prolonged immobilization required. If swelling is considerable, immobilization with external splinting is less reliable because adequate flexion is precluded. In certain patients, however, open reduction may be ill advised because of soft-tissue injury or other medical problems. In this situation, overhead olecranon pin traction may be a good alternative (see Fig. 14-9).

In most displaced fractures, I prefer open reduction with rigid internal fixation that allows motion in the first few days after injury. Several implants have been designed for use in the distal humerus; however, I believe that double plating offers the most stable configuration.[104] If there is significant comminution or bone loss, then iliac bone graft is added at the time of operation to reduce the likelihood of nonunion. Open reduction and internal fixation of a comminuted fracture of the distal humerus can be an exceedingly difficult procedure, and the surgeon should be experienced in the use of AO techniques before attempting to fix such a fracture. Poor technique, leading to nonunion, creates an even greater challenge, especially if plates and screws are already in place.

Open supracondylar fractures should be treated by debridement with the wounds left open and delayed wound closure, if grossly contaminated.[59] These open fractures are usually very unstable because of associated soft-tissue stripping at the fracture site. Therefore, primary reduction of the fracture and fixation with either rigid internal fixation or external fixation should be considered. Internal fixation should be used if an adequate debridement and cleansing of the tissue is performed.

Flexion-Type Supracondylar Fractures

This type of injury is quite rare.[37] In Smith's[61] series it occurred in less than 2% and in Siris'[59] series in only 4% of supracondylar fractures. The cause of this fracture is generally believed to be a force directed against the posterior aspect of the flexed elbow.[32,56,61,64] This results in anterior displacement of the distal fragments with the elbow joint. The posterior periosteum is torn, but the anterior periosteum may remain attached, having separated only from the anterior surface of the proximal fragment.[63] Because direct violence is usual in this injury, the fracture is often open, with the sharp proximal fragment piercing the triceps tendon and skin.[33,63] Vascular injuries are rare.

Signs and Symptoms

As in the extension-type fracture, the relationship between the epicondyles and the ulna remains the same, but the plane of their triangle is shifted anterior to the shaft of the humerus. The elbow is flexed, with resistance encountered on attempts at extension. The normal prominence of the posterior aspect of the elbow is absent.

Radiographic Findings

The obliquity of the fracture through the supracondylar region on the lateral view is from proximal anterior to distal posterior (opposite that seen in the extension type). The distal fragment lies anterior to the humerus and is flexed at the elbow. The fracture line, as a rule, is transverse on the anteroposterior projection.

Methods of Treatment

Nonoperative Treatment. Flexion-type supracondylar fractures are often difficult to manage.[39,53,63] Closed reduction can be obtained by first applying traction with the forearm flexed.[63] Applying traction with the forearm in extension before reduction is obtained increases the pull of the forearm muscles on the condyles, increasing the flexion of this fragment at the elbow joint. This inhibits reduction and can injure the anterior structures. As the traction is maintained, the distal humeral fragment is pushed posteriorly into position by pressure on its anterior aspect and counterpressure posteriorly on the proximal fragment. Once the fracture is reduced, the fracture fragments can be locked into place by extension of the elbow.

Opinions vary on the best method of immobilization after reduction.[37,40,66] If the anterior periosteum is intact, it can be used as a hinge to hold the distal fragment in place while pressure is applied to the anterior portion of the distal fragment in a posterior direction. This can be achieved by extension of the elbow with the posterior force being applied to the distal fragment through the anterior capsule and collateral ligaments. The usual obliquity of the fracture line also helps to buttress the posteriorly applied force on the distal fragment.

In children with an intact, strong, anterior periosteum, this fracture may be stable in extension. However, the thin periosteum present in adults (especially the elderly) offers little resistance and may allow gross displacement of the fracture.[63] In addition, I am opposed to immobilizing the elbow in the extended position for fear of not being able to regain flexion of the elbow after fracture union.[63]

A second method of reducing and holding the distal fragment, based on the fact that the humeral condyles behave as part of the forearm after a supracondylar fracture, was introduced by Soltanpur.[63] The surgeon grasps the humeral condyles in one hand and, with the other hand, maintains the elbow flexed with the forearm in supination. Traction is applied to the condyles to correct overriding and angulation. An assistant wraps the arm and hand in cast padding, and a circular cast is applied about the upper arm only. When the circular cast dries, the surgeon places one hand under the cast and with the other hand pushes posteriorly to reduce the fracture. The long-arm plaster cast is completed with the arm in this position. The cast is removed in 6 weeks, and elbow motion is instituted. Despite 6 weeks of immobilization, Soltanpur reported restoration of nearly complete elbow motion.

Operative Treatment. For those fractures that cannot be held by closed methods except by extremes of extension, open reduction with internal fixation using two plates is preferable. As mentioned earlier, attaining rigid fixation that permits motion in the first few weeks is highly desirable if open treatment is attempted.

Transcondylar (Dicondylar) Fractures

There is some controversy whether the transcondylar fracture should be classified as a separate entity. Although most of the earlier fracture texts distinguished it as a separate fracture, others did not.[76] Smith[76] classified transcondylar and supracondylar fractures as a single entity. He believed that for practical purposes the treatment, prognosis, and complications are essentially identical to those of a supracondylar fracture.

Bryan[68] emphasized that transcondylar fractures are particularly difficult to manage and should therefore be considered separately. He recognized several unique characteristics of these fractures. First, the distal fragment is small with only minimal extra-articular bony area to help control rotation. Second, this small distal fragment, being mainly intra-articular, may allow dislocation of the radiohumeral and ulnohumeral joints during attempted reduction. Third, the amount of bone contact available for union is small even when a perfect reduction is obtained.

Those fractures that pass through both condyles and are within the joint capsule should be classified as transcondylar fractures.[73] Kocher, Ashhurst, and Chutro are credited with distinguishing this fracture from supracondylar fractures.[67,69,74] There appear to be two types, extension and flexion, based on the position of the elbow when fractured.[77] The fracture line is characteristically crescent shaped or transverse, passing just proximal to the articular surface of the condyles.[74] It also enters the coronoid and olecranon fossae.[67,79] This fracture occurs just proximal to the old epiphyseal line. These fractures may be nondisplaced, or the lower fragment may be displaced posteriorly.[67,79] Anterior displacement is distinctly unusual.[67]

The mechanisms of injury and principles of treatment that apply to supracondylar fractures are basically the same in this fracture.[79] There are some differences that merit discussion, however. First, this type of injury is more common in elderly persons with fragile osteoporotic bone. Second, because this fracture lies within the joint cavity, excessive callus production can result in residual loss of motion.[71,73,79] This is especially true if callus develops in the olecranon or coronoid fossa.[68,70,78,79]

Bryan[68] recommended closed reduction (especially of minimally displaced fractures) followed by cast immobilization. If the fracture is not reducible, or if the reduction is unstable, he recommended percutaneous Kirschner-wire fixation. He emphasized the need to restore the normal forward tilt of the distal humerus to preserve a functional arc of elbow motion.

An unusual variation of the transcondylar fracture, recognized by Posadas in Buenos Aires in 1901, is the so-called Posadas fracture.[67,74,75,77] This injury was described in a monograph on elbow fractures by Chutro in 1904 in which he credited Posadas with the original description.[69] Chutro carefully distinguished between the transcondylar fracture of Kocher and Posadas' fracture. The latter consists of a transcondylar fracture, caused by trauma to the elbow in flexion, in which the distal (dicondylar) fragment is carried anteriorly and there is an associated dislocation of the radius and ulna from the dicondylar fragment. Clinically, the forearm presents in complete extension (and supination), lying along the longitudinal axis of the humerus.[69] The clinical appearance suggests a simple dislocation. The coronoid process appears to become wedged between the anteriorly displaced dicondylar fragment and the proximal supracondylar portion of the humeral diaphysis. Ashhurst[67] emphasized the need to recognize the associated dislocation of the radius and ulna to prevent ankylosis of the elbow. Scudder[75] described how, with improper treatment, the ulna can subsequently develop a pseudarthrosis with the distal portion of the humerus (ie, a type of traumatic arthroplasty). There is no consensus on the preferred method of treating this fracture. Although Chutro[69] reported the closed treatment of five such injuries, ankylosis in near-complete extension was the result. Ashhurst[67] presented a successful result after closed treatment. However, closed reduction is known to be difficult to obtain and maintain.[68,72] Grantham and Tietjen[72] recommended open reduction and internal fixation for this difficult fracture–dislocation.

Intercondylar T- or Y-Fractures

Intercondylar fractures represent one of the most complicated and challenging fractures in the upper extremity. Watson-Jones[138] wrote "Few fractures are more difficult to treat." The medial and lateral condyles are usually separate fragments, displaced in a T or Y configuration, and both are unconnected from the humeral shaft and rotated in the axial plane. The goal of treatment is to reestablish the articular congruity, obtain acceptable alignment, and provide rigid fixation to begin active motion as soon as possible. In most cases, open reduction with rigid internal fixation is preferred.

Mechanism of Injury

This particular fracture is probably caused by the impact of the ulna in the trochlear groove, forcing the condyles of the distal humerus apart.[82,87] The injury may occur in either flexion or extension.[95,110,143] In the flexion-type injury, Palmer[126] has speculated that the blow against the posterior elbow (olecranon), coupled with contraction of the forearm muscles, produces the fracture with less force than expected. In many instances, however, the forces applied to the posterior flexed elbow are violent, as in motor vehicle injuries. In the flexion-type fracture, the condyles are usually found anterior to the humeral shaft. In the extension-type injury, the ulna is directed anteriorly against the posterior aspect of the trochlea, separating the condyles at the same time as the supracondylar portion is fractured. Another mechanism is that proposed by Wilson and Cochrane,[143] who suggested that the separation of the condyles in this type of fracture may be created by the splitting effect of the humeral shaft as it is forced distally. In the extension-type injury, the condyles are usually found to lie behind the humeral shaft. Whatever the mechanism, there is usually considerable associated soft-tissue injury.[82] Some may have open lacerations extending into the fracture site.[82,131] Comminution of the bony fragments is not unusual.[126,131,139] Because of loss of bony continuity, the fracture fragments are displaced by unopposed muscle action.[131] In those with severe displacement, the origins of the forearm muscles pull the epicondyles distally, rotating the condyles so that their articular surfaces face a more proximal direction.[86,126] This converts the trochlear sulcus into a narrow inverted V, making it no longer congruous with the articular surface of the ulna. These actions of the biceps anteriorly and the triceps posteriorly pull the articular surface of the ulna proximally. In an opposing fashion the humeral shaft is forced distally between the rotated condyles.

Signs and Symptoms

Little can be added to points in diagnosis as outlined by Desault[96] in his original description of this injury:

> If the fingers, placed before or behind, press on the limb in the direction of the longitudinal fracture, the two condyles will be separated from each other, the one yielding in an outward, and the other in an inward direction, leaving a fissure or opening between them. The part at the same time expands in breadth. The forearm is almost constantly in a state of pronation. When we take hold of one of the condyles in each hand, and endeavor to make them move in opposite directions, they can be brought alternately forward or backward, and if their surfaces touch, a manifest crepitation is heard.

The key to distinguishing an intercondylar T- or Y-fracture from others is determining the presence of separation of the condyles from each other and from the humeral shaft. With proximal migration of the ulna the arm appears shortened. It is also widened by concomitant condylar separation. The independent mobility of the condyles can be determined by pressing the condyles between the index finger and the thumb. There is crepitus when the condyles are pressed together. Because they are still under the influence of the forearm muscles, the condyles tend to spring back into displacement when the pressure is released. Both the pressure and its release are a source of pain to the patient. The relationship of the epicondyles with the tip of the olecranon process has been disrupted. In those fractures with an extensive degree of displacement there is usually gross instability in all directions.

Radiographic Findings

Good-quality anteroposterior and lateral x-rays are essential in the evaluation of fracture displacement and comminution. One can usually assume that reality is worse than the x-ray appearance, that is, that comminution is worse than it appears on plain x-rays. Polytomography or CT scanning can also be helpful if the degree of comminution is in doubt. These films are particularly useful in preoperative planning.

In those fractures with considerable displacement of the fragments, the diagnosis is easy. Because of considerable comminution of the fracture fragments, it may be difficult to determine the origin of many small fragments. In those that are nondisplaced or minimally displaced, the surgeon must look carefully for the presence of a vertical intercondylar fracture to distinguish this from a simple supracondylar fracture.

Classification

Riseborough and Radin[129] devised a very useful classification of this type of fracture, based on its radiographic appearance (Fig. 14-11). This classification provides some guide to management and prognosis. They defined four types:

Type I. Nondisplaced fracture between the capitellum and trochlea

Type II. Separation of the capitellum and trochlea without appreciable rotation of the fragments in the frontal plane

Type III. Separation of the fragments with rotational deformity

Type IV. Severe comminution of the articular surface with wide separation of the humeral condyles

Müller and colleagues[125] have used a somewhat different classification, separating the fractures by the presence of a supracondylar extension or comminution.

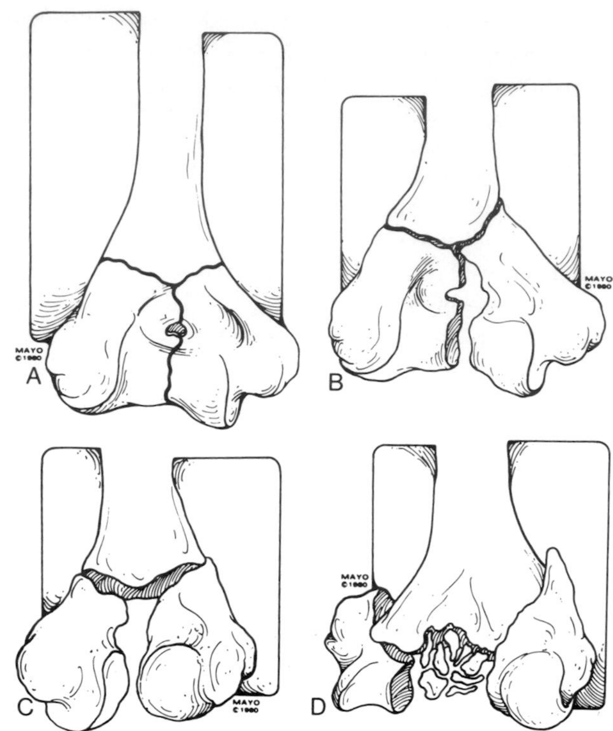

FIGURE 14-11. (**A**) Type I undisplaced condylar fracture of the elbow. (**B**) Type II displaced but not rotated T-condylar fracture. (**C**) Type III displaced and rotated T-condylar fracture. (**D**) Type IV displaced, rotated, and comminuted condylar fracture. *(Bryan, R.S.: Fractures About the Elbow in Adults. A.A.O.S. Inst. Course Lect. 30:200–223, 1981.)*

I believe that the classification of Riseborough and Radin is helpful for directing treatment and comparison of results. As with all current radiologically based classification systems, reliability and accuracy have not been tested. Nonetheless, if the surgeon carefully examines the x-rays of these fractures, looking for displacement, comminution, and bone loss (the primary focus of this classification), it is more likely that decisions and planning will be appropriate. Most authors[86,99,105,111,112,114,124,126,142] believe that the most important factor in determining outcome is the degree of displacement in the intra-articular component. In most instances, if there is either intra-articular malunion or nonunion, the functional results will be severely compromised. The supracondylar component may also be problematic, but some degree of displacement and angulation is acceptable as long as healing occurs.

Methods of Treatment

Closed Techniques

Because of the complexity and technical difficulty of operative treatment, some authors before the 1960s recommended closed treatment for all intercondylar fractures. More recently, closed treatment has been recommended for the elderly, for those whose fractures are deemed unsuitable for internal fixation, or for patients whose medical condition prohibits surgery.

Closed methods of treatment can be divided into three categories: (1) cast immobilization; (2) traction (skin, gravity, or skeletal); and (3) early motion without treatment, the "bag of bones" technique.

Cast Immobilization. It is difficult to find many advocates of closed manipulation and casting, because this technique usually represents the worst of both worlds: inadequate reduction and prolonged immobilization. Trynin[136] did report a case of closed manipulation and condylar compression in which a carpenter's clamp was used to hold the fracture for 4 weeks, although he emphasized the necessity of accurate reduction of the articular surface.

Riseborough and Radin[129] reported five patients treated with manipulation and casting; three had what they called a good outcome and two had a fair result. The degree of displacement in these fractures was minimal (type II), a rare fracture. If casting is used, most recommend starting motion at 3 weeks after injury, using a splint to protect the elbow between exercise sessions. Since their report in 1969, credible reports of cast immobilization for this fracture cannot be found in the literature.

Traction. The most popular method of closed treatment is some form of traction[94,95,108,113,116–118,129,130,134] used either to obtain reduction or to maintain position after manipulation. As late as the 1960s, many authors thought that traction should be used for *all* intercondylar fractures, but as surgical techniques improved, more authors began recommending its use only for complex type IV injuries or in cases in which open reduction was not feasible.[1134] In 1936, Reich[128] discussed the theoretical advantage of open reduction with anatomical restoration but recounted the failures of fixation. He believed that traction was a safer alternative. He applied an ice-tong device to the distal humerus and then used traction for 3 weeks or until callus formation was noted.

Olecranon Pin Traction. Reported by many authors, this method seems to provide the best line of pull to optimize the longitudinal position of the fracture fragments. In the overhead position, swelling rapidly subsides and the arm and hand are accessible during treatment. In addition, motion of the elbow can begin while in traction as the patient becomes more comfortable. Longitudinal traction alone, however, will not derotate the intercondylar fragments in the axial plane. Skin traction has been reported,[143] but it cannot be applied with more than 5 to 7 pounds because of potential skin slough. Other authors adapted olecranon pin traction to casts or frames that allowed the patient to leave the hospital. Unfortunately, these were often cumbersome or were incorporated into a long-arm cast, which precluded early motion.[127,128,135]

The outcome of displaced fractures treated with traction is difficult to glean from the literature. Riseborough and Radin[129] reported that 8 of their 12 patients with type III injuries had a good result when treated with traction, compared with 4 of 12 with a fair or poor result. Other advocates of traction treatment have reported somewhat similar results, but the numbers are smaller and reported methods inconsistent.

In most intra-articular fractures, accurate reduction of the joint surface is usually thought to be one of the most influential factors with respect to outcome. However, with this fracture, some authors have argued otherwise.[84,97,108] In 1932, Hitzrot[108] stated that "anatomic replacement is of secondary importance." Most other authors have disagreed with this position, especially in younger patients.[82,86,90,91,93,99,100,105,109,110,113–115,117,119,125,130,133,137,140,142,144]

Because of the relative rarity of this fracture, a reliable study comparing traction treatment with open reduction and rigid internal fixation has not been possible. The pressure to reduce the time of hospitalization, combined with improvement in fixation techniques and surgical approaches, has led to infrequent use of traction except in extraordinary circumstances. Series reporting a comparison of the methods contain patient selection bias or insufficient numbers to allow valid conclusions on a statistical basis.[84,86,129,144] In addition, many of the early series that employed open reduction with internal fixation used a myriad of implants ranging from multiple Kirschner wires to multiple plates and screws, preventing valid comparison with rigid fixation and early motion.[107,114] Techniques of exposure have also improved, with more attention given to preservation of the triceps mechanism.[86]

"Bag of Bones" Technique. Eastwood,[97] who popularized this method in England during the 1930s, credited Hugh Owen Thomas as being its originator. It involves simply placing the arm in a collar and cuff, initially in as much flexion as possible. The initial position of flexion is chosen because extension will improve over several months with exercise whereas flexion usually will not.[84,97] The elbow is left hanging free, which is an important point. The effect of gravity on the dependent elbow is thought to enable the fracture fragments to settle into a more natural alignment. Some attempt at initial reduction is made, but the permanent success of this maneuver is questionable.[84] Hand and finger motion are started immediately. Pendulum shoulder motion begins at 7 to 10 days. As the swelling and pain subside, the patient is allowed to actively extend the elbow gradually. The fracture is usually united in 6 weeks, at which time the sling is discarded. However, with intensive exercises, the range of motion will improve for 3 to 4 months. In a series reported by Brown and Morgan,[84] the patients achieved an average of 70° of elbow motion. It is significant that in the x-rays presented by both Eastwood[97] and Brown and Morgan,[84] adequate reductions of the fractures were noted. However, the relationship of fracture reduction to results is not mentioned by either author. One author[136] modified this method by the application of a large padded wooden carpenter's clamp to the condyles, suspending it from the neck. The clamp was tightened as the swelling subsided. In addition to the inherent dangers implied with such treatment, patients might not accept this modification.

Watson-Jones[138] noted that many of the patients treated with this method had residual loss of extension from excessive anterior tilting of the condyles. Evans[98] believed that although many of his patients treated in this manner had a satisfactory range of motion, a significant number complained of weakness and instability in the elbow. Bickel and Perry[82] also believed that this method does not produce the strong, stable elbow required by a young patient. Therefore, the "bag of bones" technique appears to be suitable perhaps for the elderly patient in whom early ambulation is desired.[95,117] It does require a good deal of patient motivation and cooperation to achieve a satisfactory result.

Operative Methods

The operative methods are (1) pins in plaster, (2) open reduction and internal fixation, (3) distal humeral replacement (prosthetic or allograft), and (4) arthroplasty.

Pins in Plaster. Pins in plaster was originally called blind nailing by Miller.[123] He initially placed the upper extremity in traction with a Kirschner wire in the olecranon. The condyles were then manually reduced and transfixed percutaneously with a second Kirschner wire. A third wire was likewise passed percutaneously through the proximal fragment. While the fracture was maintained in traction, a long-arm cast was applied, incorporating all three wires. Böhler[83] appears to be one of the few other surgeons to have used this technique. Although this method may facilitate maintaining alignment, it contains no provision for elbow motion. The presence of at least two pins penetrating the fracture site greatly enhances the chances of infection and its resultant disability.

Limited Open Reduction and Internal Fixation. In the performance of limited open reduction and internal fixation, two distinct methods have been reported. Both employ limited surgery to reestablish articular congruity between the humeral condyles. In one method, this is followed by postoperative traction[82,86,98,117] or closed manipulation and casting of the remaining supracondylar component of the fracture.[82,89,98,115,117] In 1953, Evans[98] reported this method in five cases, emphasizing the importance of articular congruity. Once the joint was reconstructed using open reduction and internal fixation between the condyles, the supracondylar portion was managed with splint or cast immobilization. Motion was started after 4 weeks.

Knight[118] reported using olecranon traction once the intercondylar portion was stabilized. Outcome from this technique is difficult to judge. In Evans'[98] series, four of the five patients had flexion contractures of 60° or more.

Open Reduction and Internal Fixation. Open reduction with internal fixation has evolved as the preferred method of treatment for most type II and III fractures.[86–88,91,99,103,105–107,109–115,118,119,125,129,130,133,140,141] Several authors in the 1930s were attracted to the idea of anatomical restoration with early motion, but they were discouraged by the disruptive surgical exposures and the lack of adequate implants.[123,128,142] Since then, improvements in both areas have engendered more confidence in this technique.

Surgical Exposure. To address the problem of exposure, Van Gorder[137] (who credited Campbell with the idea) described a posterior approach to the distal humerus by incising the triceps as a tongue of fascia and folding this distally to the level of the olecranon. Although helpful, this approach still does not permit good exposure of the anterior and distal portions of the joint. In addition, the incision in the triceps mechanism deterred early active motion for fear of rupture.

In 1969, Kelly and Griffin[115] advocated an anterior approach for open reduction. The biceps was retracted medially and the brachialis tendon transected at the level of the coronoid process. No attempt was made to secure the condylar fragments to the shaft of the humerus. There have been no other reports of this approach.

Olecranon osteotomy for exposure of the distal humerus was described for treatment of the ankylosed elbow by MacAusland[120] in 1915. Cassebaum[90,91] subsequently adopted this osteotomy for distal humeral fracture exposure. Müller[125] later modified the olecranon osteotomy by directing the bone cut so that the joint was not entered. The most recent recommendation of the AO group is a chevron or V-shaped osteotomy (Fig. 14-12), which enters the joint directly opposite the trochlea. Advocates of olecranon osteotomy suggest that better distal exposure is achieved and that there is no requirement for tendon-to-tendon healing. Rigid fixation of the osteotomy allows immediate active motion. Disadvantages, however, are that another "fracture" is created, bearing the risks of technical complication, implant failure, or nonunion.

In 1982, Bryan and Morrey[86] described a triceps-sparing posterior approach to the elbow (Fig. 14-13),

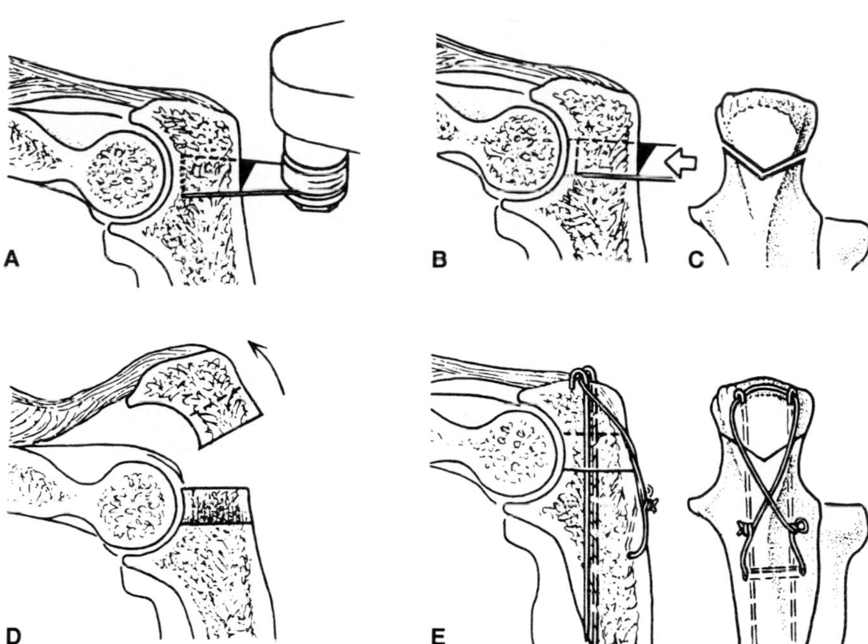

FIGURE 14-12. A chevron-shaped olecranon osteotomy can be used for exposure of the distal humerus. *(Heim, U., and Pfeiffer, K.M.: Internal Fixation of Small Fractures, 3rd ed. Berlin, Springer-Verlag, 1988.)*

initially used for total elbow replacement. The medial border of the triceps and the medial fascia of the forearm are elevated subperiosteally as a single unit in continuity. The ulnar nerve must be identified and protected. Excellent access to the joint is gained without osteotomy or transverse disruption of the triceps mechanism. No studies have compared this approach to olecranon osteotomy or have reported its use in trauma, but it has been successfully used in fractures of the distal humerus (see Author's Preferred Method of Treatment).

Methods of Fixation. There are two components of the T-type intercondylar fracture that must be secured, the intercondylar and the supracondylar. Because of the interest in articular congruity, more attention initially was given to the intercondylar portion of the fracture.[82,89,98,115,118] As techniques of exposure improved, emphasis on supracondylar fixation increased because of stiffness resulting from the prolonged immobilization required because of inadequate stability of this portion of the fracture.

The intercondylar portion of the fracture has been usually secured with screws, appropriate to the size of the fragments and their alignment. Multiple Kirschner wires have been reported for fixation,[82,98] but the use of smooth wires should be reserved for temporary (provisional) fixation, during assembly of the fragments. Without threaded compression, fatigue failure and loss of position is likely.[103,110,114] Regardless of the implant used, it is important to avoid any impingement in the olecranon fossa or trochlea (Fig. 14-14). If bone is missing, Heim and Pfeiffer[103] and others[99,105,111,113,119] have emphasized the importance of bone grafting any defects within the trochlea to maintain normal width.

Because the distal condylar portion of the humerus sits like a barrel on the end of a forked stick, rigid fixation of the supracondylar component without interference with elbow motion has been difficult to achieve. Screws directed from each condyle into the humeral shaft have been used, but the stiffness and fatigue properties of this construct can be low,[104] leading to supracondylar displacement or nonunion.[80,113] A posterior Y-shaped plate has also been used for fixation with good results,[85] but it has the disadvantage of single-plane fixation.[104]

Dual-plate fixation has been used by several authors and seems to provide the most secure fixation. As Gabel and colleagues[99] emphasized in their study of ten patients, no nonunions occurred and active motion was started on the second postoperative day. The recommendations of the AO group[103] are for placement of a semitubular plate medially and a 3.5-mm reconstruction plate posterolaterally (Fig. 14-15). Helfet and Hotchkiss[104] studied the rigidity and fatigue performance of several methods of fixation in the laboratory, including dual-plate fixation. They concluded that the dual-plate technique, with the plates oriented in two planes at 90° angles to each other, offered the most rigid and fatigue-resistant construct, especially in cases of comminution in which interfragmentary compression was precluded. There was no meaningful difference between the use of semitubular plates, reconstruction plates, or a combination of the two as recommended by the AO group.

Most recent reports have documented the suc-

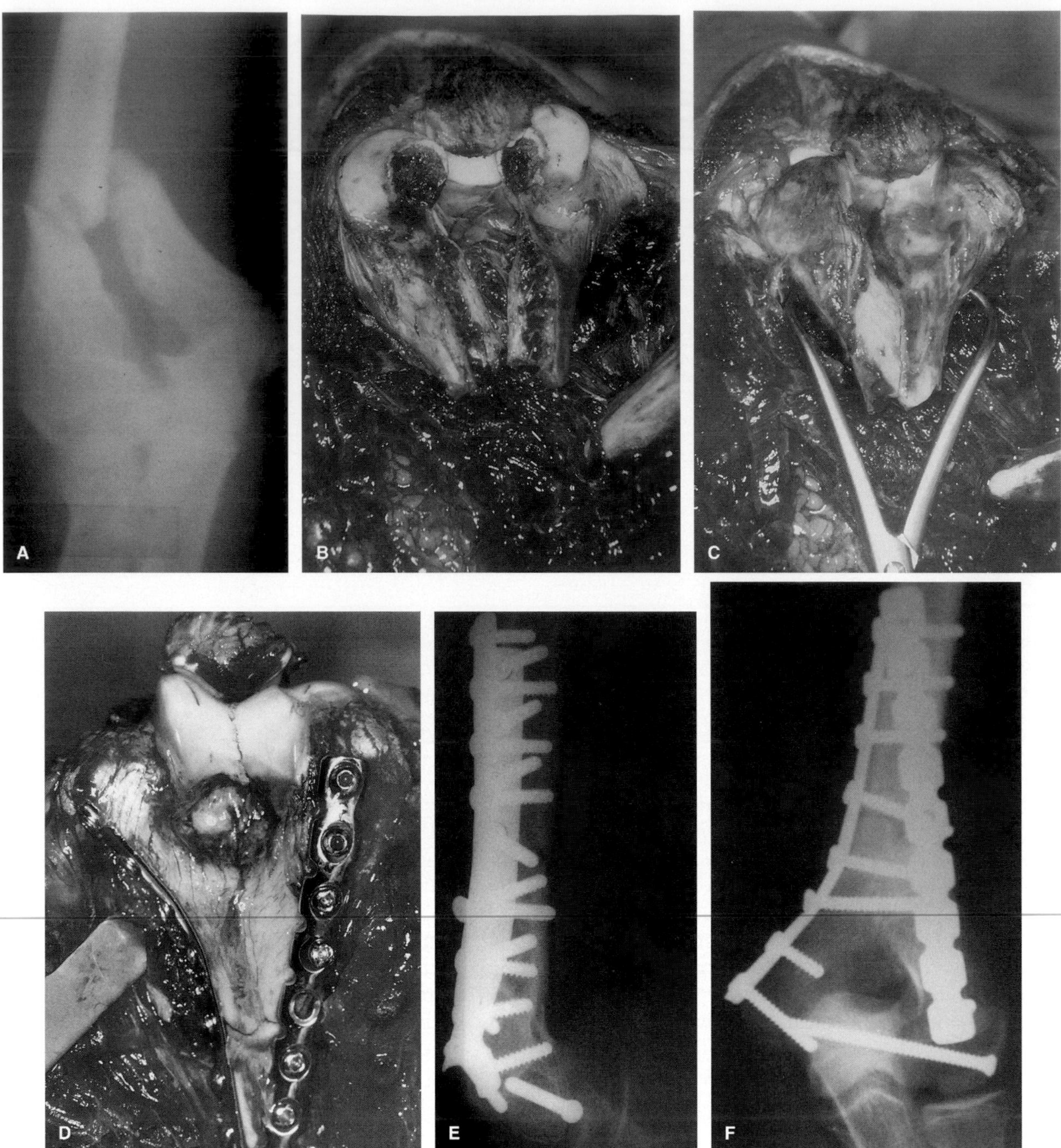

FIGURE 14-13. (**A**) A type II intercondylar fracture with displacement of the supracondylar portion. (**B**) Exposure achieved using the Bryan-Morrey approach. Sequence of assembly of the intercondylar (**C**), followed by supracondylar (**D**), dual plate fixation. (**E** and **F**) X-rays showing the two plates in different planes, plus the single screw holding the two articular fragments together.

cess of rigid fixation with early mobilization.[107,109,132,156,374,477,535] Sodergard and coauthors[370] have emphasized, as others, that the mechanical failure with nonunion is usually due to poor technique (Fig. 14-16). Jupiter[113] has also emphasized the importance of using plates and screws as dictated by the fracture configuration and bone stock available.

Alternatives to Fracture Repair: Distal Humeral Replacement and Total Elbow Replacement

In 1947, Mellen and Phalen[121] replaced the distal humerus in three patients with a customized acrylic prosthesis. Each patient had a nonunited, painful fracture of the distal humerus. They reported follow-up of several months with improved function. In 1954, Mac-

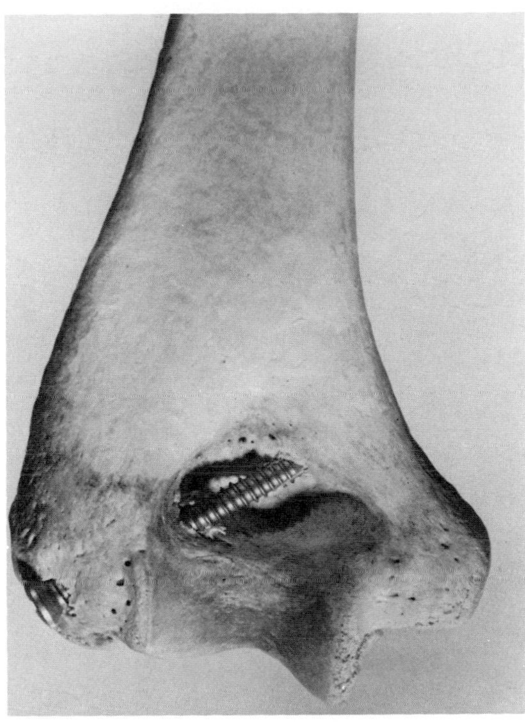

FIGURE 14-14. Improper placement of a screw into the lateral supracondylar column can result in its entering the olecranon fossa, which blocks extension of the elbow.

Ausland[120] reported good results in four patients with a nylon prosthesis. Venable[154] and others[145,148,152] have used Vitallium with some short-term success. Unfortunately, none of these materials or designs has demonstrated longevity or durability.

Breen and coworkers[146] reported using allograft replacement of the distal humerus in four patients. One allograft became infected and one developed a nonunion; both required removal.

Total elbow replacement for severely comminuted fractures in the elderly should be strongly considered. Although success has been reported with the "bag-of-bones" technique, I have seen many elderly patients with painful and disabling nonunions of the distal humerus. If the fragments are quite small and the patient has low demand, total elbow replacement is an excellent solution. The surgeon should be familiar with prosthetic designs that are "linked" but not fully constrained (sloppy hinge). The axle that links the ulnar and humeral components is usually vital in these cases because of the amount of avascular or missing bone (Fig. 14-17). Morrey and colleagues[151] and Figgie and associates[149] have documented both the functional improvement and longevity of total elbow replacement using their respective designs.

Distraction Arthroplasty. Arthroplasty of the elbow using distraction interpositional materials or simple resection is a highly specialized technique that requires special instrumentation and expertise.[147,150,153,155] The primary indication, irrespective of technique, is disabling pain in a young patient. There is seldom a reason to consider these procedures in the treatment of an acute fracture.

Author's Preferred Method of Treatment

Selection of the proper treatment for intercondylar fractures requires careful consideration. Each case must be individualized. In the young adult it is important to obtain as near an anatomical reduction of the articular surface as possible. In the older patient with an excessively comminuted fracture in osteoporotic bone, fixation is often poor or even impossible to achieve. In these patients early restoration of joint motion by total elbow replacement should be strongly considered. It must be emphasized that any method of treatment that requires prolonged immobilization is likely to result in fibrosis or ankylosis of the joint. The final radiographic appearance does not always coincide with the functional result, especially in the elderly.[116]

Type I. This fracture pattern is very rare in adults. For nondisplaced fractures of the distal humerus, I splint the elbow at 90° until swelling subsides. A long-arm cast can be applied, but because active motion is started between the second and third weeks after injury, a bivalved splint or clamshell Orthoplast splint can be used. It is helpful to warn the patient that occasionally displacement can occur. Extension, as with most other injuries of the elbow, is the slowest to return.

Types II and III. For displaced, unstable fractures, open reduction with rigid internal fixation is the optimal treatment for maximizing function. Adequate exposure is essential for accurate reduction and implant placement. Although the transolecranon approach is recommended by the AO group, I prefer the Bryan approach (see Fig. 14-13) for exposure. As Bryan and Morrey[86] have pointed out, it is usually necessary to remove the proximal tip (1 cm) of the olecranon to improve access.

Isolation and protection of the ulnar nerve are also important. If the fracture extends more proximally, it may be necessary to expose the radial nerve as well. It is helpful to warn the patient and the family preoperatively that retraction alone can cause temporary palsy of these nerves.

Operative Technique of Fixation of Distal Humerus Fractures. Careful planning of the operative reconstruction decreases operative time and improves the chances of achieving anatomical reduction with rigid fixation. Below is listed the equipment often used in operative reconstruction of complex fractures of the distal humerus:

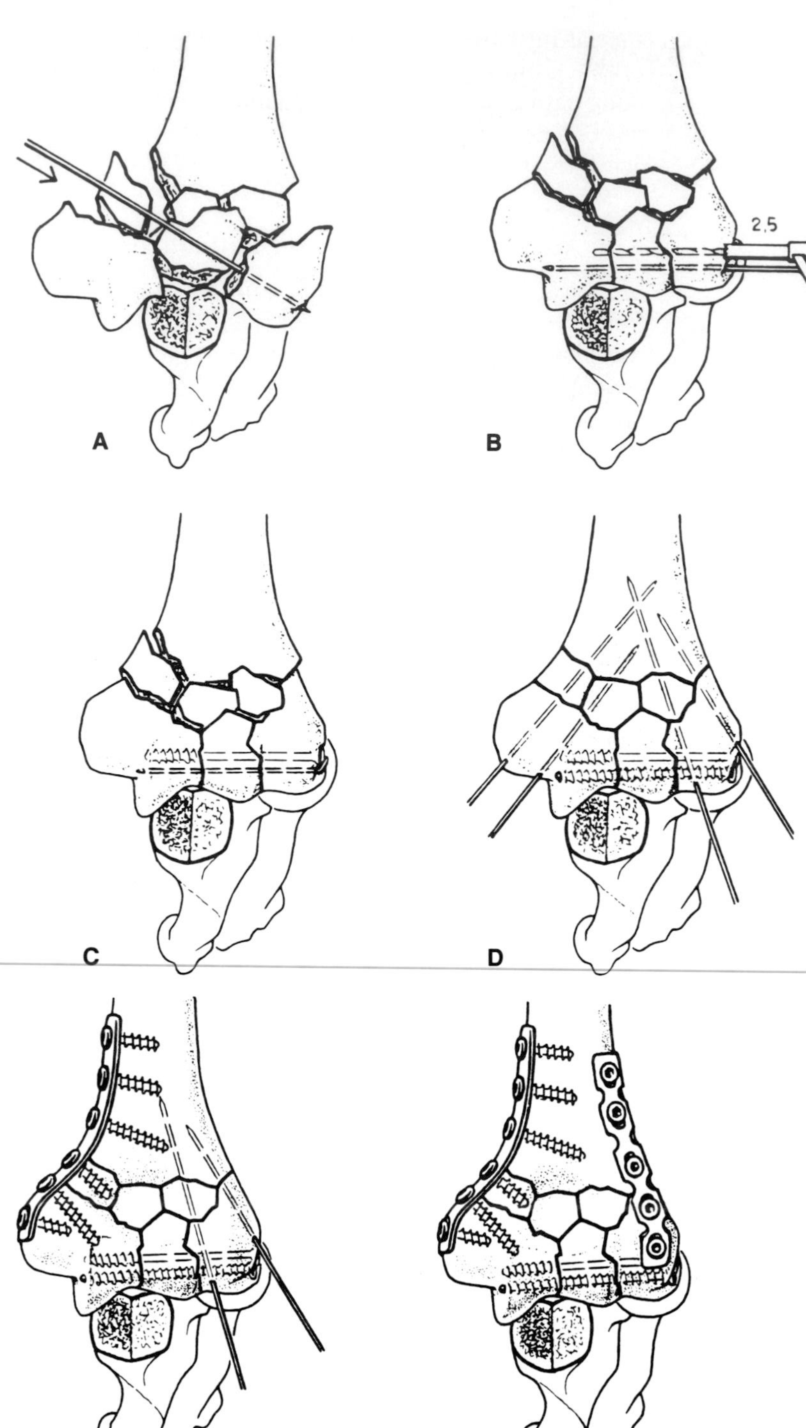

FIGURE 14-15. A useful sequence of reconstruction of the distal humerus. (**A** to **C**) First, the articular portions are reassembled with provisional K-wire fixation followed by screw fixation. (**D**) K-wires can then also be used to provide temporary fixation of the distal humerus. (**E**) A one-third tubular plate is attached to the medial side (**F**) followed by a 3.5 pelvic reconstruction plate on the posterolateral border. *(Heim, U., and Pfeiffer, K.M.: Internal Fixation of Small Fractures, 3rd ed. Berlin, Springer-Verlag, 1988.)*

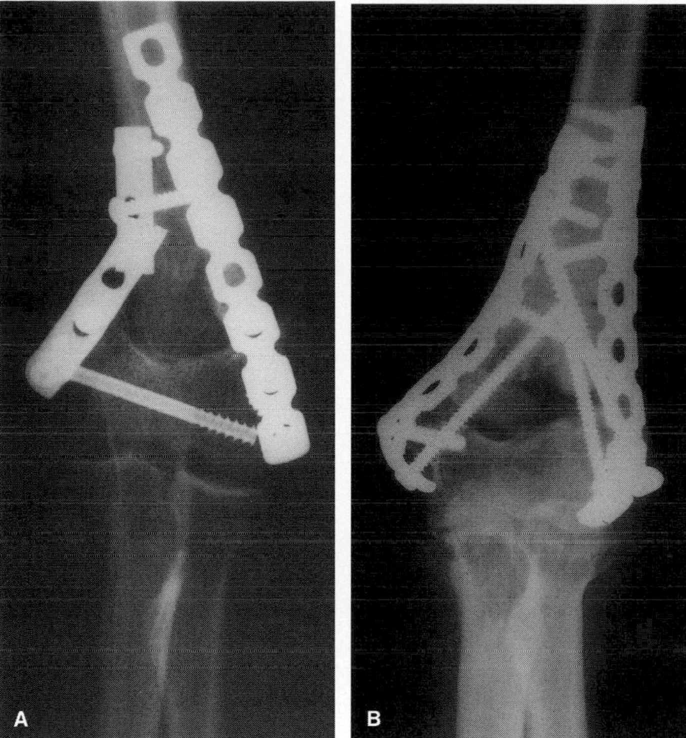

FIGURE 14-16. (**A**) Despite use of two plates, the medial plate (one-third tubular) along the posterior surface failed in fatigue. (**B**) The fracture was replated and bone grafted. Note the plates wrapping the distal condyles with long pelvic lag screws into the shaft.

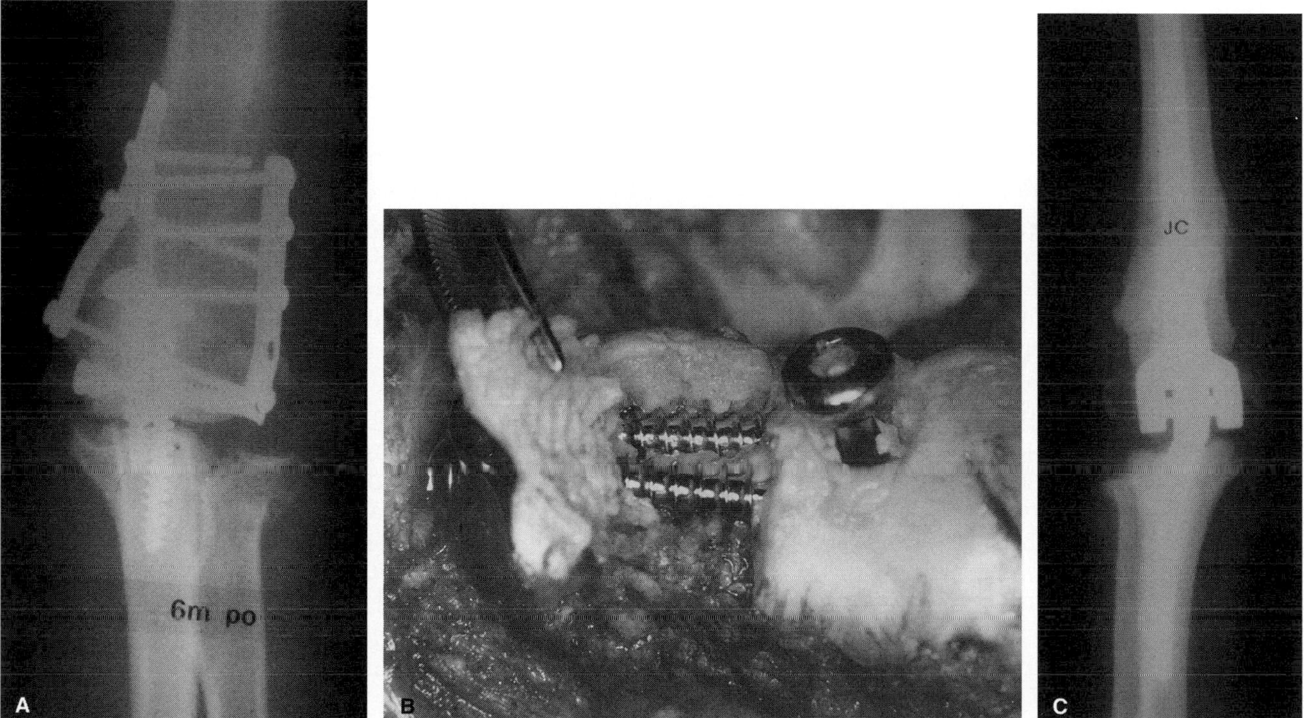

FIGURE 14-17. (**A**) An attempt was made to repair a severely displaced fracture. (**B**) Avascular necrosis and fragmentation resulted. (**C**) A total elbow replacement was done 2 years later with excellent function.

Sterile tourniquet (18 inch)
Internal fixation equipment (usually required)
Small fragment set
Reconstruction plates (3.5 mm)
Long screw set (pelvic) (3.5 mm)
Bone holding clamps
Oscillating saw
Stainless steel wire (olecranon osteotomy repair)
(Optional equipment)
Cannulated screw set
Herbert screw set (for small articular fragments)
Mini—fragment set (for small articular fragments)
Iliac bone graft preparation

In the operating room, the patient is placed in a semilateral position. A posterior (midline) skin incision is made to expose and release the ulnar nerve. The distal humerus is exposed by either of two methods: (1) a medial triceps sparing approach (see Fig. 14-13)[86] or a chevron—shaped olecranon osteotomy (see Fig. 14-12).[406] Fracture assembly is done as follows (1) distal reconstruction (articular surface restoration) with interfragmentary lag screws and (2) reassembly of the joint to the distal humerus with plates. Either repair of olecranon osteotomy or reattachment of triceps is done (depending on exposure used).

Before surgical reconstruction is done, it is helpful to remember some anatomical points regarding the distal humerus. When transcondylar fixation is obtained, the diameter of the trochlear sulcus is much smaller (approximately one half) than that of the medial trochlear ridge and the lateral condyle (see Fig. 14-2). The transfixation device must be centered exactly, or it may enter the articular surface.

The order of reassembly of the distal humerus is dictated by the individual fracture pattern. The intra-articular portion is usually assembled first (see Fig. 14-15), followed by reduction and fixation of the distal humeral component. However, there are times when one of the columns is minimally comminuted and it is simpler to secure this column first to the distal humerus, then reassemble the joint. Loss of articular cartilage can be accepted, but incongruity cannot. As the AO group[103] has taught, lag screws across the condyles can be used only if there is no bone missing and no comminution between them (Fig. 14-18). When reassembling the fragments, it is helpful to use K-wires for provisional fixation before applying the plates or screws. This portion of the operation requires the greatest patience and attention to detail. Each screw must be carefully directed to avoid the joint, secure solid purchase and not collide with another of its mates.

Although a single screw across the condyles has potential to allow the fragments to rotate, once the con-

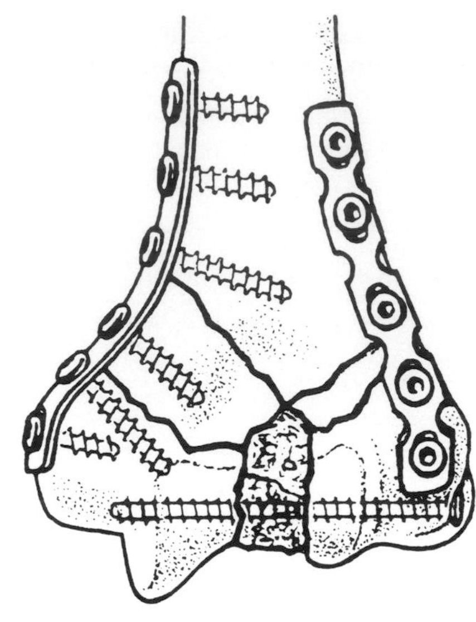

FIGURE 14-18. If bone is missing in the intercondylar portion, a corticocancellous bone graft is interposed to reestablish the anatomical proportions. *(Heim, U., and Pfeiffer, K.M.: Internal Fixation of Small Fractures, 3rd ed. Berlin, Springer-Verlag, 1988.)*

dylar portions are securely fixed to the shaft with neutralization plates, this will not happen. The AO cannulated screw system can be especially useful in assembling the distal humerus. Fractures judged by x-ray to be type III without comminution may turn out to be type IV fractures requiring bone graft. I therefore prepare the patient for iliac bone grafting in most cases.

Once the intercondylar portion of the fracture is fixed, the supracondylar component is addressed. If there is adequate bone stock that allows interfragmentary compression of the condylar portion of the fracture to the humeral shaft, multiple lag screws can occasionally be used. The placement of these screws is crucial and must be within the centers of the supracondylar columns, engaging the opposite cortex as a lag screw. Inaccurate placement of these screws will result in impingement within the olecranon fossa, and the olecranon will not fit into the fossa, limiting elbow extension (see Fig. 14-14).

In most cases I prefer dual-plate fixation oriented at right angles to one another (see Fig. 14-15). A 3.5-mm reconstruction plate (five or six holes, depending on fracture configuration) is fixed to the medial column. The posterolateral column is fixed with a 3.5-mm reconstruction plate (five or six holes). If there is any bone gap at the supracondylar junction from comminution, liberal amounts of cancellous bone graft should be added. For fractures with more proximal extension, longer plates can be used.

The fixation of the supracondylar portion can be improved if the most distal portion of the medial plate is bent around the medial epicondyle (see Fig. 14-16).

Not all fractures require this, but for comminution of the medial column, the foot of the plate serves to increase the surface of compression. In addition, a long screw can be directed up the shaft of the humerus to preload the plate. After this screw is placed, the more proximal screws can be placed, providing a very rigid construct. Jupiter[111,113] has recommended a third plate, if needed, to provide more plate contact and secure fixation. The use of this third plate is to increase the surface contact of the plate construct when comminution precludes interfragmentary lag.

The outcome from this injury greatly depends on postoperative rehabilitation. The elbow is splinted, and active motion is started during the first week after operation. If the gains in extension begin to plateau in the first 6 weeks, it is sometimes useful to add dynamic splinting in the form of a turnbuckle splint, especially if extension is regained slowly.

Type IV. Fractures with excessive comminution precluding reconstruction require individualized treatment. In younger patients, every effort should be made to restore as much of the articular surface of the distal humerus as possible. Unlike the weight-bearing joint of the lower extremity, surprisingly good function can sometimes be achieved with less than optimally appearing surfaces. Revascularization of the detached fragments can, and often does, occur. The surgeon should be prepared to place bone grafts wherever defects exist and to use internal fixation as dictated by the fracture pattern. Implants of a wide variety of sizes and types should be available (see previous list).

In the elderly patient, I sometimes prepare to perform a total elbow replacement acutely, if stable restoration of the articular surface is not possible. Total elbow replacement in the elderly should not be viewed with the same degree of nonchalance as endoprosthetic replacement of the femoral head fracture. Each patient must be carefully assessed preoperatively. Total elbow replacement should only be considered after discussion with the patient and finding a fracture that is not reconstructable. If total elbow replacement is a possibility, the medial triceps–sparing approach should be used for exposure, rather than olecranon osteotomy. The results of this total elbow replacement for complex fractures of the distal humerus can be gratifying (see Fig. 14-17).[149,151] Eastwood's[97] technique of early motion without surgery should be strongly considered for many elderly patients. However, my experience with the use of this technique has not been as predictable as originally presented.

Fractures of the Humeral Condyles

Anatomy and Classification

There appears to be some confusion about the nomenclature of the various anatomical structures of the distal humerus. Some standard anatomy texts[81,101,102] do not differentiate between medial and lateral condyles as separate entities. In *Gray's Anatomy*[102] the distal end of the humerus is described as being basically a condyle with articular and nonarticular surfaces. The articular portion is divided into two areas, the capitulum and the trochlea (Fig. 14-19). I will use the term *capitellum* instead of *capitulum* because it is more common in the orthopaedic literature. In this discussion the lateral condyle and the capitellum are not synonymous. The same is true for the terms *trochlea* and *medial condyle.*

In the discussion of fractures, separation of the distal humerus into medial and lateral condyles is widely accepted.[122,169] The capitulotrochlear sulcus is the terminal dividing point for these condyles.[122] Each condyle contains an articular and a nonarticular portion. The epicondyle is considered part of the nonarticular portion. The articulating portion of the lateral condyle is called the capitellum (capitulu rotuli humeri, eminentia capitata). The articular surface of the medial condyle is called the trochlea. It must be appreciated at this point that fractures of the condyles do not always follow these anatomical boundaries. For example, in a fracture of the lateral condyle or capitellum, a portion of the trochlea is often involved.[169]

During growth there are four separate ossification centers in the distal humerus.[101] The ossification center in the lateral condyle appears during the first year. It forms the bulk of the lateral condyle and a portion of the bone underlying the lateral aspect of the trochlea. The ossification of the medial condyle does not appear until the ninth or tenth year. The epicondyles also have separate ossification centers. The lateral epicondyle center appears at about age 12 years and fuses 1 or 2 years later with the main lateral condylar center. The center for the medial epicondyle appears at about age 4 to 6 years. Fusion with the main condylar segment does not occur until about the 20th year. In rare instances, fusion never occurs.[163] These separate ossification centers have considerable significance in the discussion of fractures of the distal humerus in children. In adults, however, there does not appear to be any residuum in the trabecular pattern within the distal humerus from these separate ossification centers. Thus, it would appear that in adults fractures of the distal humerus depend on the external contour of the bone and the forces applied rather than on intrinsic weakness due to physeal lines.

Distinction between the condyles and their various portions is important in the diagnosis and treatment of these fractures. Fractures of the condyle include separation of both the articular and nonarticular portions, including the epicondyle. There can be isolated fractures of either the articular portion or the epicondylar portion of the condyle. In this instance the remainder of the condyle is still attached to the shaft and to the opposite condyle.

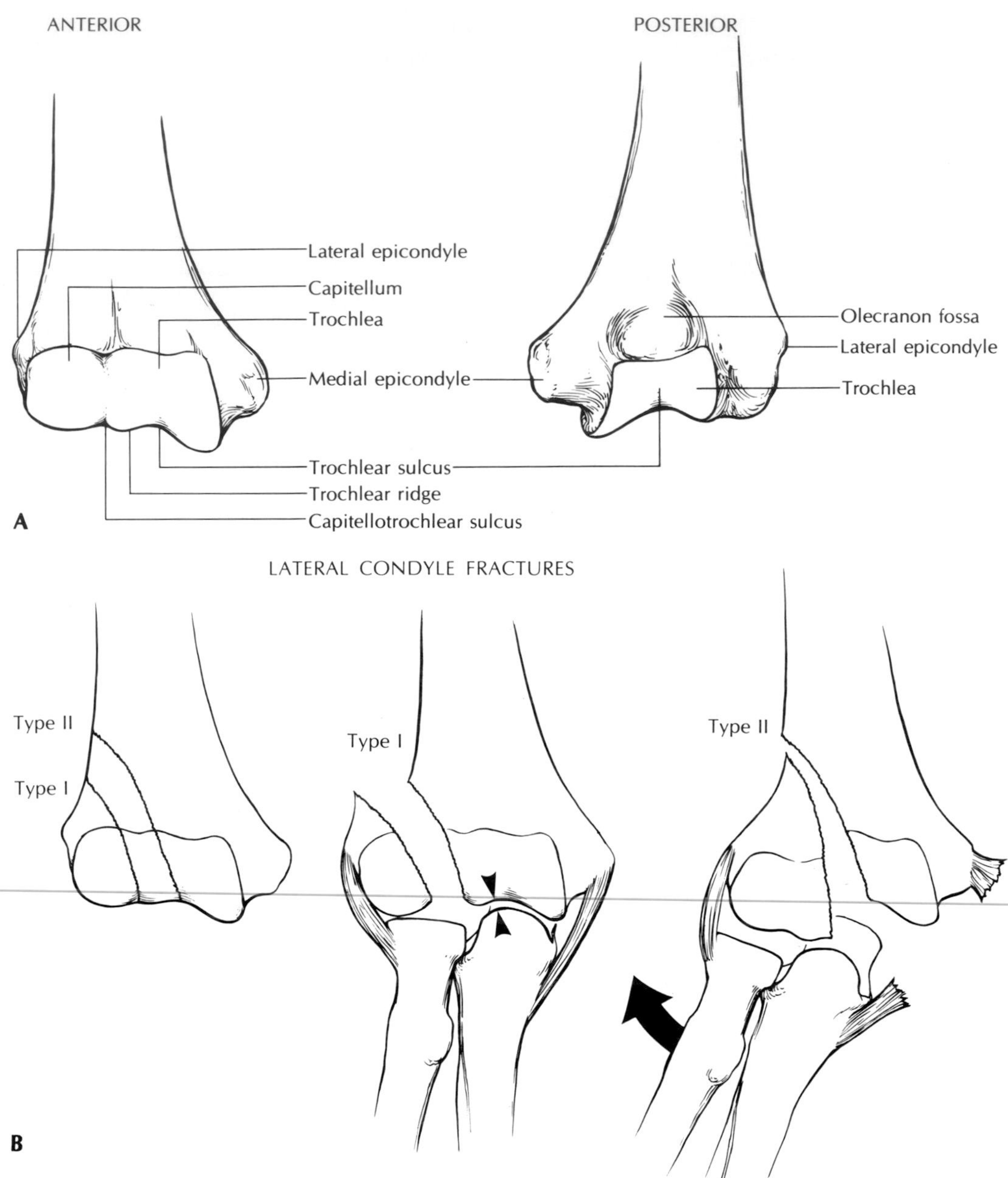

FIGURE 14-19. Classification of condylar fractures according to Milch[12] and the location of the common fracture lines seen in type I and II fractures of the lateral (**B**) and medial (**C**) condyles. (**A**) Anterior view of the anatomy of the distal articular surface of the humerus. The capitellotrochlear sulcus divides the capitellar and trochlear articular surfaces. The lateral trochlear ridge is the key to analyzing humeral condyle fractures. In type I fractures, the lateral trochlear ridge remains with the intact condyle, providing medial to lateral elbow stability. In type II fractures, the lateral trochlear ridge is a part of the fractured condyle, which may allow the radius and ulna to translocate in a medial to lateral direction with respect to the long axis of the humerus. (**B**) Fractures of the lateral condyle. In type I fractures, the lateral trochlear ridge remains intact, therefore preventing dislocation of the radius and ulna. In type II fractures, the lateral trochlear ridge is a part of the fractured lateral condyle. With capsuloligamentous disruption *medially,* the radius and ulna may dislocate. (**C**) Fractures of the medial condyle. In type I fractures, the lateral trochlear ridge remains intact to provide medial to lateral stability of the radius and ulna. In type II fractures, the lateral trochlear ridge is a part of the fractured medial condyle. With *lateral* capsuloligamentous disruption, the radius and ulna may dislocate medially on the humerus.

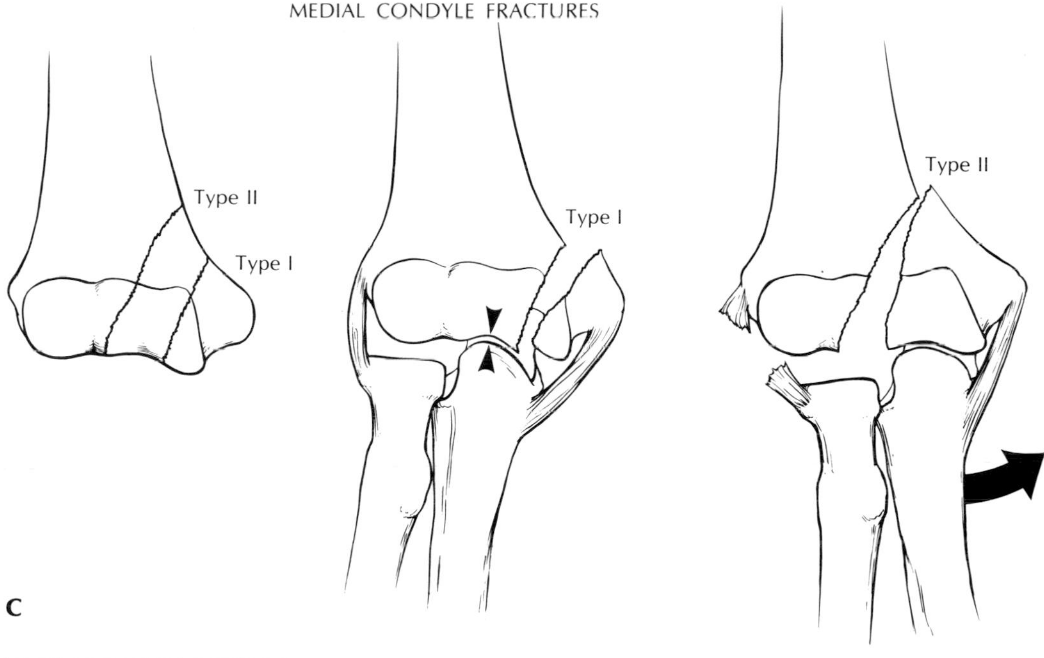

FIGURE 14-19. (continued)

This distinction has practical significance for both treatment and prognosis.[161,163] Fractures that extend beyond the capsule and joint line have attached muscle, capsule, and ligament and are therefore influenced by these attachments. Purely intra-articular fractures (see p. 958) by definition have no muscular attachments and can only be positioned by direct pressure of the opposing articular surface or by direct open reduction. Fractures of the entire condyle usually result in both restriction of motion and instability and require secure fixation to restore stability.[166]

Mechanism of Injury

Several external forces act on the distal humerus.[166] Avulsion forces are usually applied through tension on the collateral ligaments. The tension forces on these collateral ligaments can be increased by leverage through the forearm with the elbow in extension. Abduction or adduction of the extended forearm concentrates these forces to one side of the distal humerus. In addition, compressive forces can be applied to the articular surface. These forces may be indirect, being transmitted axially through the radius or ulna from forces applied to the distal portion of the extremity. There are specific areas of the articular surface where greater concentration of force can occur (eg, by the wedge-shaped articular portion of the ulna against the groove of the trochlea or by the rim of the radial head in the capitulotrochlear sulcus). Abduction or adduction of the forearm in extension can further concentrate the force in a given area. Direct forces can be applied to the elbow as well. This usually occurs on the posterior aspect of the flexed elbow. In this position the lateral condyle is more exposed on the lateral side, while medially the epicondyle is more vulnerable to injury from a direct force. Forces applied directly to the posterior border of the proximal ulna are concentrated in the trochlear groove. If force is applied centrally, both condyles may be wedged apart, producing an intercondylar fracture. If the force is applied eccentrically, fracture of an isolated condyle is produced.[92] Rarely are the forces applied during an injury pure. They are often mixed, resulting in a variety of fracture patterns.

Milch[122] emphasized the importance of differentiating isolated fractures of the humeral condyles from condylar fractures associated with dislocation of the elbow. He pointed out the importance of the lateral trochlear ridge in providing stability of the elbow after fracture of a single condyle. He divided fractures of either condyle into two classes, based on the preservation or loss of the integrity of this ridge. Type I fractures are simple fractures. In this type of fracture the lateral trochlear ridge remains with the intact condyle. Thus, mediolateral stability refers to the mediolateral translocation of the ulna with respect to the distal humerus. Varus or valgus instability secondary to associated contralateral ligament and joint capsule disruption can be present in a type I fracture.[161] Displacement of the fractured condyle can be proximal or distal, depending on the type of injury involved. In the type II fracture the lateral trochlear ridge is a part of the fractured condyle. This allows the radius and ulna to translocate in a mediolateral direction with respect to the long axis of the humerus if the contralateral collateral ligament and joint capsule are torn.[116,161,169] Therefore, the type II fracture is called a fracture–dislocation. This classification has therapeutic application. Some type I fractures can be treated by closed methods. All type II fractures require open reduction and internal fixation.[122]

Incidence

Fractures of the humeral condyles or their components are uncommon in adults.[130,158,160,163,168] In Knight's series,[167] fractures of a single condyle accounted for only about 5% of fractures of the distal humerus in adults. Fracture of the lateral condyle is more common than fracture of the medial condyle.[160,169] Bryan[158] emphasized the frequent association of humeral condyle fractures with other injuries, such as fractures of both bones of the forearm, which must be considered in planning treatment.

Fractures of the Lateral Condyle

Signs and Symptoms

Fracture of the lateral condyle is recognized by the presence of independent motion of the lateral condyle from the medial condyle and humeral shaft. The condyle may be proximal or distal to the main portion of the humerus, depending on the type of force that created the fracture. As the arm hangs at the side, the carrying angle may be lost.[171] Crepitus is usually present. Radial rotation may accentuate the crepitus.[172] Although intercondylar distance may be widened, the arm does not appear shortened as in intercondylar fractures. Medial elbow swelling and tenderness are present in patients with associated medial collateral ligament injury.

Radiographic Findings

The fracture line extends obliquely from either the capitulotrochlear sulcus or the lateral border of the trochlear groove up to the supracondylar ridge. Depending on the type of fracture, there may be lateral translocation of the ulna with respect to the shaft of the humerus. Displacement of the fragment by the action of extensor muscle origin is often present.[158] Lateral condylar fractures must be differentiated from fractures of the capitellum. A fracture of the lateral condyle has both articular and nonarticular components (Fig. 14-20). A fracture of the capitellum involves only the articular surface and its supporting bone. Smith[170] emphasized, however, that in some patients fracture of the lateral condyle is associated with a fracture of the capitellum, the two being separate fragments.

More recent reports have emphasized the importance of anatomical reduction, rigid internal fixation, and the need for early motion.[156,164,165]

Methods of Treatment

Nonoperative Treatment. Lateral condyle fractures may be nondisplaced or only minimally displaced. These usually can be treated by simple immobilization until stable.[122] Occasionally, percutaneous pinning of such nondisplaced fractures allows earlier institution of elbow motion.[158] Although some authors[171] believe that closed reduction is seldom successful, Conwell and Reynolds[160] described a method of closed reduction for displaced fractures. With the elbow extended and the forearm supinated, manual pressure is applied directly over the fragment for reduction. Adduction of the forearm opens up the lateral aspect of the joint to facilitate the reduction.[157] Anatomical reduction of the condyle is essential, because any displacement interferes with elbow motion.[122] The supinated forearm is then gradually flexed at the elbow. A long-arm cast is applied with lateral molding. There is some question about which position provides maximum stability after reduction. On the basis of the precedents set by Jones, Smith, and Lund, Cotton[161] believed that the best stability was achieved by the splinting effect of the triceps tendon in acute flexion. Milch believed that these fractures are more stable in extension.[122] In extension the olecranon is locked into its opposing fossa of the humerus, which affords mediolateral stability.[163] Although this position may be tolerated for a brief period by a child, it can result in considerable disability in the adult.[161] I prefer to immobilize these fractures in flexion with the forearm supinated and the wrist dorsiflexed slightly to relieve extensor muscle forces on the fragment.

Operative Treatment. The goals of operative intervention appear to be twofold. First, condylar alignment must be reestablished so that the axes of rotation of the condyles are the same.[167] Second, in the type II fracture the integrity of the lateral trochlear wall must be reestablished. Surgery is best performed as soon after the injury as possible.[168] Either the posterior or the lateral approach may be used.[157,168] Fixation is usually achieved with screws.[122,159] Care must be taken to preserve the soft-tissue attachments to the condylar fragment to protect its vascularity. Smith[169] recommended repairing the medial collateral ligament, if it is torn, through a separate medial approach. I reserve medial collateral ligament repair for the younger patient engaged in heavy labor when joint stability is not restored by reduction and internal fixation of the lateral condyle.

Complications and Prognosis

The result depends on the degree of comminution of the condyle, accuracy of reduction, and stability of internal fixation. Stable anatomical reduction and early motion help prevent traumatic arthritis and limitation of joint motion. Improper reduction or loss of fixation in a type

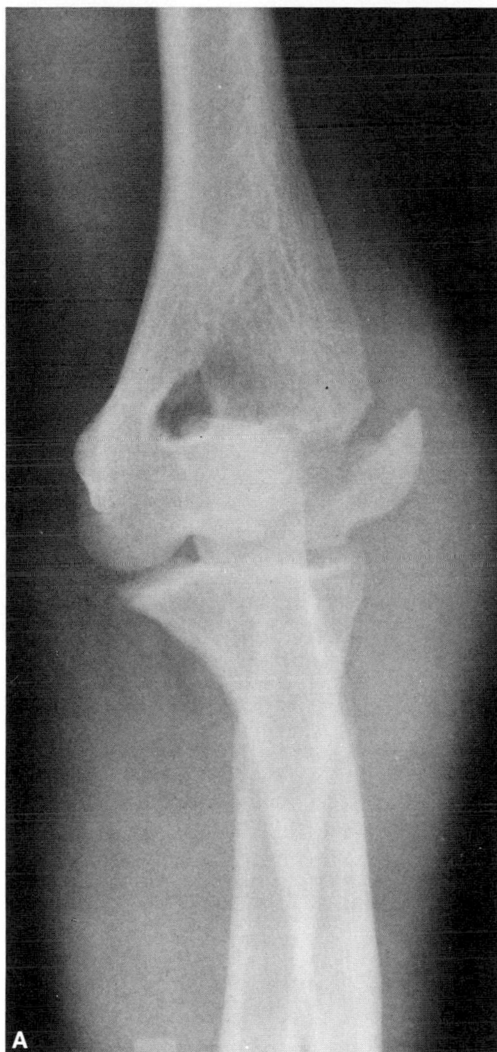

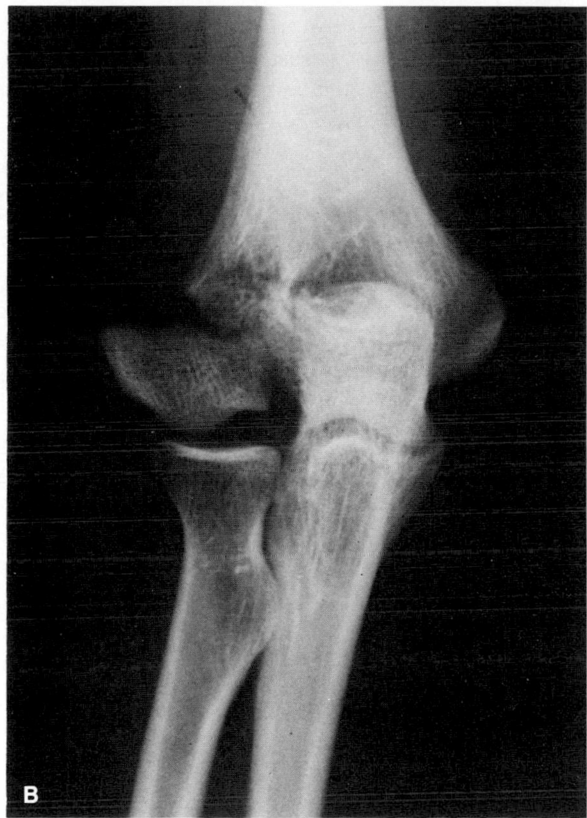

FIGURE 14-20. (**A**) This type I fracture of the lateral condyle involves both the articular surface of the capitellum and the nonarticular surface, including the lateral epicondyle. The distal portion of the fracture line emerges just lateral to the capitulotrochlear sulcus. (**B**) Anteroposterior x-ray of a type II fracture of the lateral condyle that involves both the articular surface of the capitellum and the nonarticular surface of the lateral condyle. The distal portion of the fracture line emerges medial to the capitellotrochlear sulcus.

I fracture can lead to cubitus valgus. In a type II fracture, cubitus valgus and lateral subluxation of the ulna may occur. This risk is increased if an associated fracture of the capitellum was removed.[169] This results in a greater deformity because the prominence of the medial condyle is accentuated. No matter what the cause, cubitus valgus may lead to ulnar nerve symptoms, which may require nerve transposition later.[169]

Fractures of the Medial Condyle

Isolated fracture of the medial condyle is a rare injury in the adult. It is noted much less frequently than the lateral condyle fracture, probably because direct blows to the medial side of the elbow more often fracture the prominent medial epicondyle than the deeper medial condyle.[157,161–163,169,171]

The mechanism of injury is thought to be either a fall on the outstretched arm with the elbow forced into varus[162] or a fall on the apex of the flexed elbow. The action of the flexor muscles of the forearm tends to displace the fracture distally. Generally, the fracture originates at the depth of the trochlear groove and ascends obliquely to end at the supracondylar ridge. If the primary wedging force on the articular surface is applied by the rim of the head of the radius, then the fracture may originate in the capitulotrochlear sulcus, producing a type II injury. Because it usually involves the trochlear groove, fracture of this condyle may have more disability associated with it.

Signs and Symptoms

Motion of the entire condyle occurs when the medial epicondyle is manipulated. If the radial head is displaced medially with the ulnar and medial condyle fragment, there may be an apparent increased prominence of the lateral condyle and capitellum. Extension of the elbow tends to produce motion of the fragment owing to increased tension on the origin of the forearm flexor muscles.

Signs of ulnar nerve injury or irritation may be present.[122] Lateral joint tenderness and swelling are present in patients with associated injury to the lateral collateral ligament.

Methods of Treatment

Nonoperative Treatment. In nondisplaced fractures, satisfactory treatment can be achieved with a posterior splint. Aspiration of the joint to relieve the hemarthrosis will improve patient comfort.[169] The elbow is flexed and the forearm is pronated with some wrist flexion to relax the muscles that originate on the medial epicondyle. Closed reduction of displaced fractures is difficult to achieve and maintain.[169] X-rays must be taken at frequent intervals to ensure that late displacement of the fragment does not occur.

Operative Treatment. Although some displaced fractures can be reduced closed, it is virtually impossible to maintain a reduction that will prevent a step-off in the articular surface. The joint surface should be restored by open reduction and internal fixation (Fig. 14-21). Our goal is to restore joint congruity with stable internal fixation that allows early institution of joint motion.[169] When the fragment is approached, the ulnar nerve must be carefully exposed and protected. Conwell and Reynolds[160] recommended anterior transposition of the nerve if the ulnar groove is involved in the fracture or if the nerve is injured. Firm fixation may be difficult to obtain.[164] The medial supracondylar column is long and narrow. Placement of screws up this column or through the narrow central portion of the trochlear groove may be difficult. Also, it is more difficult to obtain initial purchase of the screws on the pointed medial epicondyle than on the flattened surface of the lateral condyle.

Repair of the lateral collateral ligament is considered only if joint stability is not restored by reduction and fixation of the displaced condyle. Even in this situation, consideration of the patient's age and occupation is critical because repair of the collateral ligament may result in loss of joint motion secondary to scarring. If the fixation is not solid after operation, the extremity should be immobilized as with closed reduction (ie, with the elbow and wrist flexed and the forearm pronated).

Complications and Prognosis

Because of involvement of the trochlear groove, there is more chance for residual incongruity of critical articular surfaces. This increases the risk of posttraumatic arthritis. In addition, residual displacement of the medial condyle can restrict joint motion.[169] Malunion with the condyle displaced proximally results in cubitus varus. Tardy ulnar nerve symptoms may arise secondary to malunion or excess callus formation.[167]

Fractures of the Articular Surface of the Distal Humerus

Fractures of the distal humeral articular surface include fractures of the capitellum or trochlea, or both. These fracture lines occur in the coronal plane, parallel to the anterior surface of the humerus.[190–192] The fracture fragments therefore consist of the articular surfaces of the capitellum and trochlea with little or no soft-tissue attachment.[209] Mehne and Jupiter[112] have proposed another anatomical classification scheme that attempts to account for fracture patterns of the distal humerus that include coronal and sagittal splits in the articular surface of the distal humerus. The utility of these classification lies in recognition of differing fracture patterns and the varying spatial relationships. The requirements of joint restoration and secure fixation are still paramount.

Compressive wedging or shearing forces are usually involved in producing these fractures. Because of the lack of soft-tissue attachment, avulsion forces do not play a role in the production of these fractures.[169] The initial displacement is produced by the causative force. However, further displacement can occur because the fragment has no soft-tissue attachments and lies free within the joint cavity.[183,184,209,220,223]

The fracture fragments consist primarily of articular cartilage with varying amounts of associated subchondral bone.[213,220] Although I consider fractures of the capitellum and trochlea as separate entities for the purpose of discussion, often both articular surfaces are actually involved.

Fractures of the Capitellum

Although the first case was described by Hahn[194] in 1853, Kocher[202] is credited with calling attention to this fracture in his classic monograph *Fractura Rotuli Humeri.*[182,204,209] Thus, fractures of the capitellum are often called Kocher fractures.[218] Fractures of the capitellum are rare. The incidence of this fracture in the numerous series reported in the literature[178,181,188,212,217,223] varies from 05% to 1% of all elbow injuries seen.

Both Kocher and Lorenz recognized two types of fractures of the capitellum (Fig. 14-22).[202,206] The type I, or Hahn-Steinthal,[194,221] type involves a large part of the osseous portion of the capitellum and may contain part of the adjacent lip of the trochlea.[173,175,192,200,203,205,209] The type II, or Kocher-Lorenz,[202,206] type involves articular cartilage with very little bone attached.[193] Mouchet has described type II fractures as an "uncapping of the condyle.[193,211,213] Type II frac-

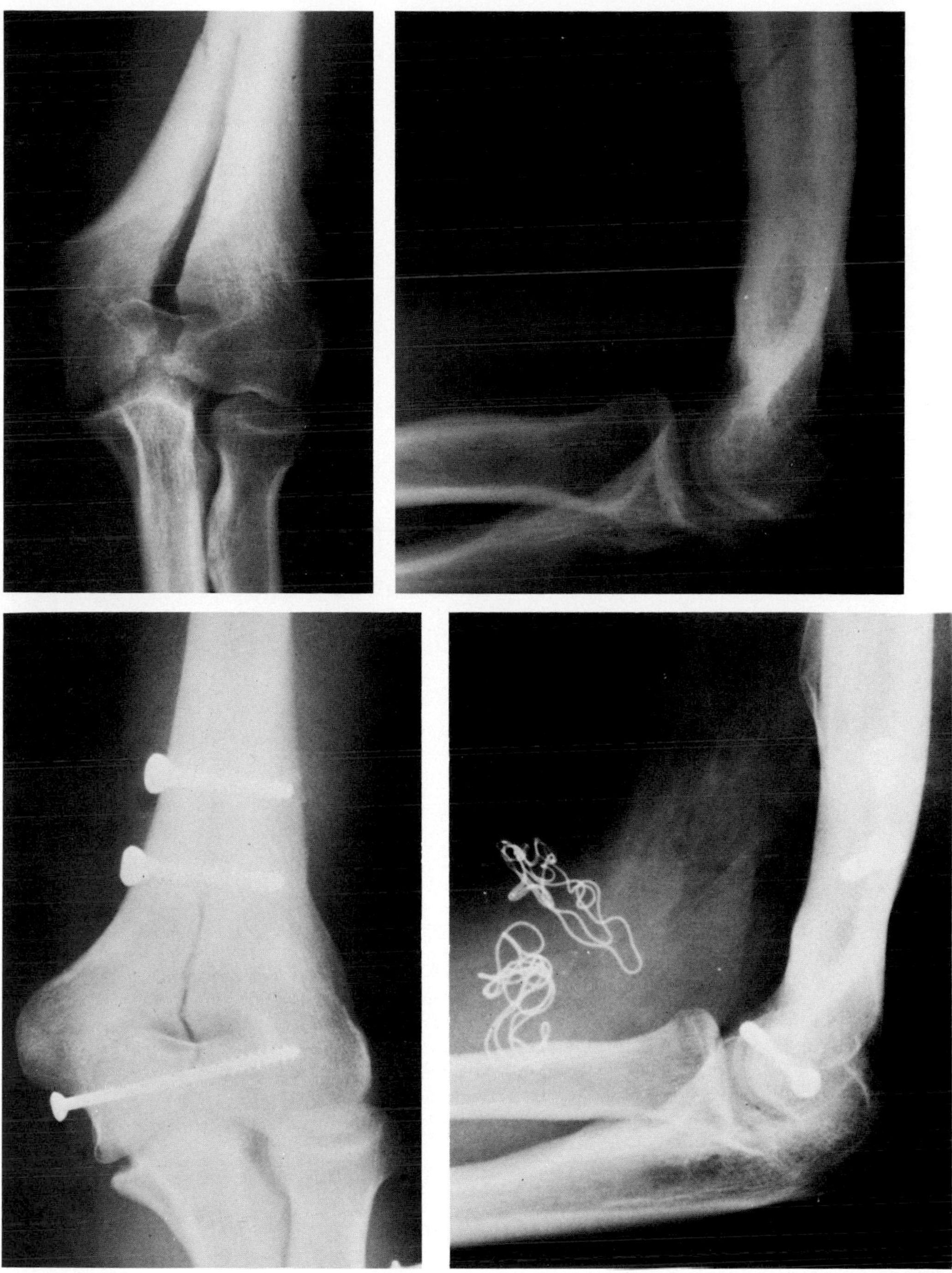

FIGURE 14-21. Anteroposterior and lateral x-rays of a fracture of the medial condyle. Open reduction and stable internal fixation of the type I medial condyle fracture allows early range of motion. Lag screw fixation was sturdy enough to permit motion. Use of a plate should be considered if secure lag fixation is not achieved with each screw.

tures are reported much less frequently than type I fractures.[191,192,199] Wilson[223] described a third type in which the articular surface is driven proximally and impacted into the osseous portion.

Johansson[198] reported rupture of the ulnar collateral ligament in 8 of 13 cases of capitellar fracture. Collert[180] suggested that restricted mobility after capitellar fracture partly depends on such associated capsular and ligamentous injury.

Emphasis must again be placed on the differentiation between fractures of the capitellum and lateral condyle.[191] A fracture of the capitellum involves only the intra-articular portion of the lateral condyle and does not include the epicondyle or metaphysis. A frac-

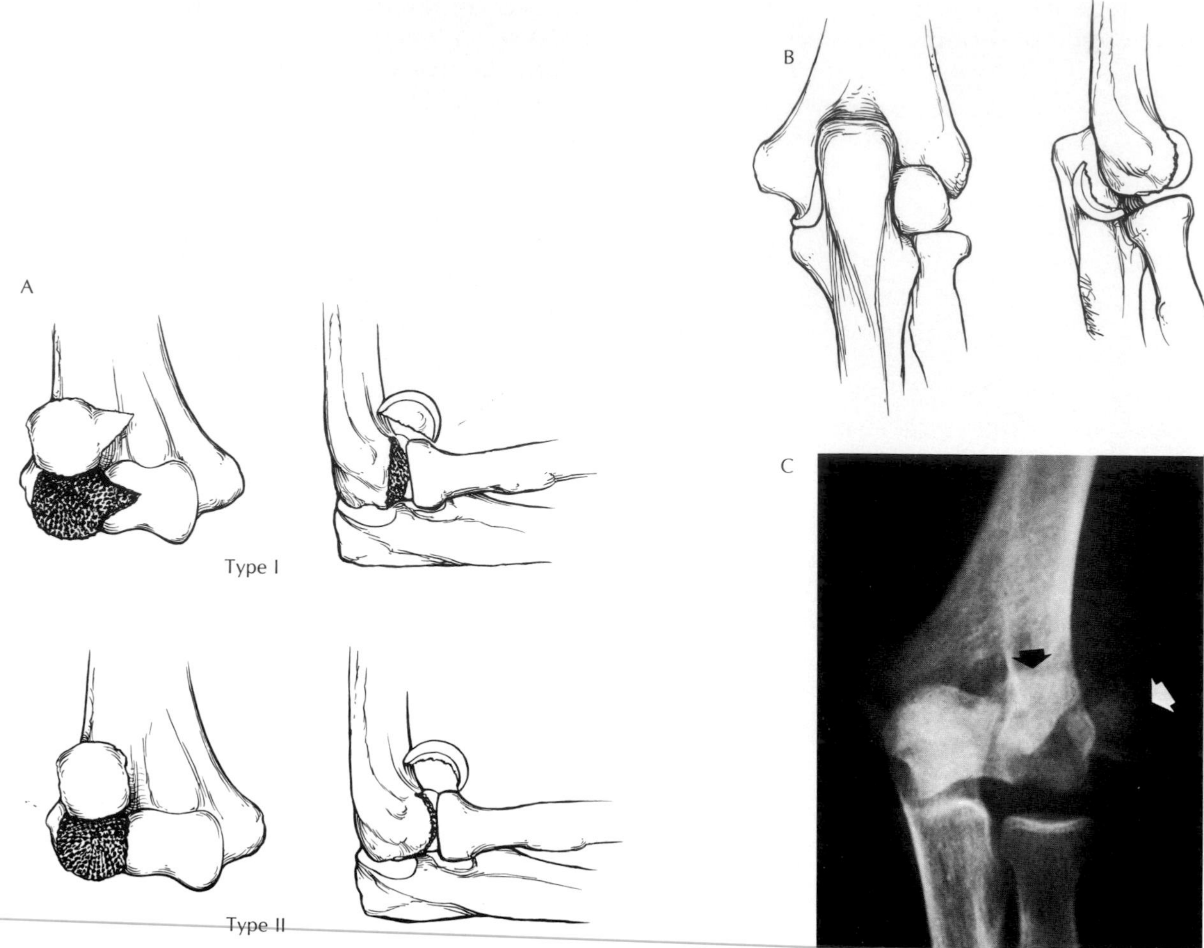

FIGURE 14-22. (**A**) The type I (Hahn-Steinthal) capitellar fracture. A portion of the trochlea may be involved in this fracture. The type II (Kocher-Lorenz) capitellar fracture. Very little subchondral bone is attached to the capitellar fragment. There is no fracture through the lateral condyle in the *sagittal* plane in either the type I or II capitellar fracture. (**B**) Although most often the capitellar fragment is displaced anteriorly, occasionally the fracture fragment may be displaced posteriorly. In this instance, an obstruction to extension is noted on physical examination. (**C**) The anteroposterior x-ray is often useful in demonstrating the degree of trochlear involvement. The *arrows* point to two fragments off the capitellotrochlear surface. This may be difficult to recognize on a lateral view.

ture of the lateral condyle involves the capitellum plus the nonarticular portion, which often includes the epicondyle.[191]

Anatomical Considerations

The capitellum presents an anterior and inferior articular surface but does not extend posteriorly.[173] The radial head articulates with the anterior surface when the elbow is flexed and with the inferior surface in extension. The radial fossa, a depression on the anterior humerus just above the capitellum, accommodates the margin of the radial head when the elbow is acutely flexed. The radial fossa must be cleared of all fracture fragments for the elbow to regain a full range of flexion.

Mechanism of Injury

This fracture is usually produced by the transmission of forces through the radial head, which acts like a piston to shear off the capitellum.[173,200,223] Thus, some authors use the term *anterior shear fracture of the capitellum.*[171,174,192,202,204] This mechanism also helps to explain the occasional association of radial head fractures.[178,189,201,204,210,215,223]

The mechanism most commonly results when one tries to break a fall and lands on the hand with the elbow in some degree of flexion or falls directly on the elbow in a position of full flexion.[180,193,222]

Bryan[176] suggested that type I fractures result from a force passing from the radius to the humerus in extension, thereby shearing off the capitellum anteriorly, or from a direct lateral blow in flexion. Type II fractures are the result of shearing forces across the joint in varying degrees of flexion.[176]

Milch[210] believed that the location of the fragment gives a clue to the position of the elbow when injured. If the elbow is in extension, the anterior surface of the capitellum is sheared off and the fragment is displaced anteriorly. Injury with the elbow flexed results in the fragment lying in the posterior aspect of the joint. Kocher originally suggested that in the type I fracture the anterior capsule avulsed the fragment when the elbow was forced into hyperextension.[190,204] There are no recent supporters of this mechanism. Because the lateral surface of the capitellum is exposed when the elbow is in a position of semiflexion and semipronation, some authors believe that type I injuries can result from a direct blow to this area.[190,204]

In some instances, especially in the type I fracture, a portion of the lateral trochlear ride may be included. Robertson and Bogart reported a fracture "en masse" of both articular surfaces.[217] This type of fracture may be confused with the Posadas type of transcondylar fracture, which extends through both condyles to their posterior borders. The fracture en masse, however, involves only articular surfaces (Fig. 14-23).

The preponderance of women in most series of capitellar fractures led Grantham and colleagues[193] to suggest a biomechanical-anatomical vulnerability based on the valgus conformation of the female elbow or a metabolic susceptibility because of osteoporosis.

There is a fair amount of consistency in the reported clinical findings. Because most of the acute symptoms are due to the distention of the joint with blood, there may be a silent interval between the time of injury and the development of symptoms.[213] Anterior displacement of the fragment results in its impingement on the radial or coronoid fossa, producing a bone block.[183] With posteriorly placed fragments there is no bone block, only pain with flexion as the fragment is forced against the capsule.[182,204]

Range of motion of the elbow is usually limited.[202,210] Alvarez and colleagues[173] found that type I fractures result in a mechanical block to flexion, whereas type II fractures usually demonstrate a block to extension. Pronation and supination are characteristically not limited by this injury.[190,192,199,202,210,222]

Crepitus may be present. Often, the fragments can be palpated anterior to the radial head when the elbow is extended. Because the external bony landmarks maintain their normal relationship, the clinical findings often do not correlate with the acute disability displayed with fracture of the capitellum.[209] Even though concomitant fractures of both the radial head and capitellum are rare, they do occur (Fig. 14-24). Milch[210] emphasized that dual tenderness on the lateral side of the elbow may be an important sign of fractures in both areas.

Tenderness and swelling medially, with or without valgus instability, indicate associated ulnar collateral ligament injury.[180,198,201]

Radiographic Findings

Because the fracture fragments consist largely of cartilage, x-rays do not reveal their true size.[174] The anteroposterior view is often misleading because the outline of the distal humerus is unaffected, and the fracture fragment may not be recognized against the background of the distal humerus.[173] Gejrot[192] and Jopson[199] emphasized, however, that the anteroposterior view is useful in demonstrating the degree of associated trochlear involvement.

Lindem[205] pointed out that the radiographic signs are best appreciated on the lateral x-ray. However, if the lateral x-ray is even slightly oblique, the fragment will be hidden by the humerus and the diagnosis may be missed.[191] The fragment most commonly lies anterior and proximal to the main portion of the capitellum.[209] The articular surface usually faces anteriorly. There may be a lack of the normal cortical margin in the area of the defect on the surface of the capitellum. If the defect is seen later, there may be union of the fragment with the humerus in the area of the radial fossa. It must be remembered that occasionally the fragment may be displaced posteriorly, as reported by Kocher and Lorenz.[202,206,209] The rare instances of dorsal fractures of both the radial head and the capitellum must always be kept in mind.[178,189,201,204,210,215,223] In all fractures of the capitellum the radial head must be carefully evaluated, clinically and radiographically. This is especially important when closed reduction is to be used, with pressure from the radial head to secure the fragment. The opposite is also true; that is, in evaluation of an isolated radial head fracture, the capitellum should be checked carefully for the presence of a fracture as well.[215] In Milch's[210] experience, fracture fragments from a comminuted radial head are rarely displaced in a proximal direction. Thus, if a large fragment is seen in the joint anterior and proximal to the radial head, it should be suspected to have originated from the capitellum rather than from the comminuted radial head.

Accurate diagnosis of the size, origin, and displacement of a fracture of the capitellum (or trochlea) may be difficult or even impossible by plain x-rays alone. If such a fracture is suspected, a CT scan may provide considerably more precise information.

Methods of Treatment

There is considerable controversy regarding the appropriate treatment of capitellar fracture. Methods available include nonoperative treatment (with and without closed reduction),[179,192,200,201,209,210] open reduction (with[171,180,183,185,187,190,191,193,196,203,214,219,224] and with-

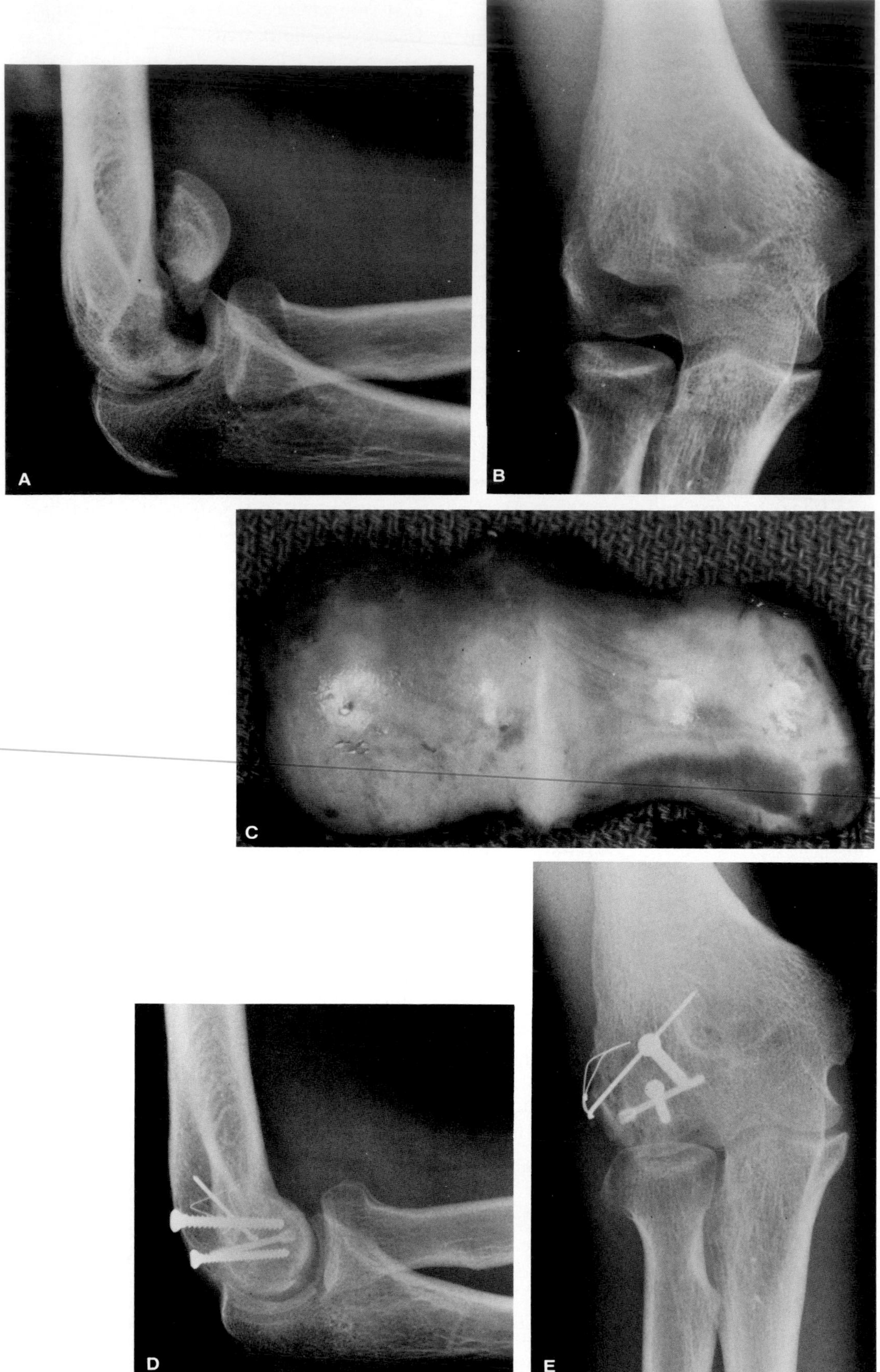

FIGURE 14-23. (**A** to **C**) A completely displaced and detached intra-articular fracture of the distal humerus of both the capitellum and trochlea. (**D**, **E**) One year after open reduction and internal fixation, there is no sign of ischemic necrosis or collapse.

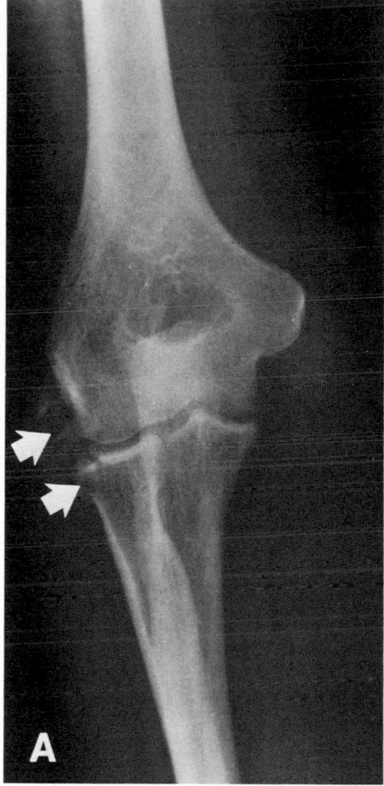

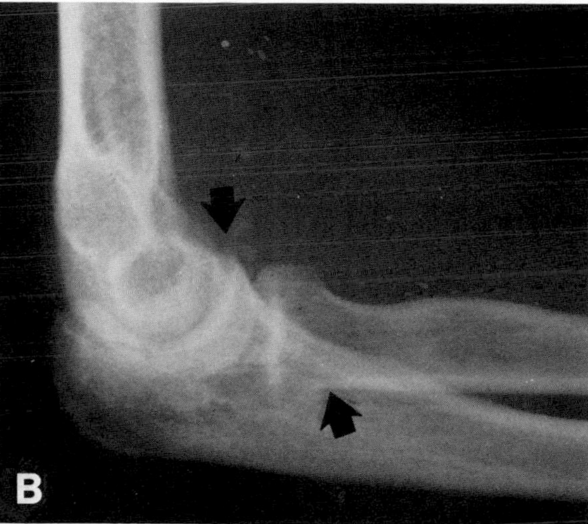

FIGURE 14-24. Concomitant fractures of the capitellum and radial head. This injury, sustained by a direct blow, shows fractures of both the capitellum and radial head (*arrows*): (**A**) anteroposterior and (**B**) lateral x-rays. The fragments from the capitellum (*upper arrow*) characteristically lie in the anterior aspect of the joint proximal to the radial head.

out[192,200] internal fixation), excision,[191,192,199,204,212] and prosthetic arthroplasty.[197] Union of capitellar fractures has been reported after both closed and open reduction even though the capitellar fragment has little soft-tissue attachment and vascularity.[208] If reduction (by either closed or open means) is selected, it must be anatomical, because even the slightest displacement is believed to interfere with joint motion.[176,220] Additionally, irrespective of the type of treatment used, supervision of the aftercare is essential if a good result is to be expected.

Nonoperative Treatment. Smith[220] recommended nonoperative treatment in a posterior splint for 3 weeks for nondisplaced fractures only. He did not recommend closed reduction of displaced fractures in adults but suggested that such treatment in children and young adults might be efficacious because of more rapid and complete bone healing in these patients.[220] Several authors have emphasized that the lack of soft-tissue attachment to the displaced fragment makes closed reduction difficult to achieve and maintain.[169,173,191,192] Because even the slightest residual displacement will limit the elbow function,[175,191,192] Bryan[176] also believe that the usefulness of closed reduction is limited. Other authors, however, strongly endorsed closed reduction.[201] Kleiger and Joseph[201] and Rhodin[213] emphasized that if closed reduction is achieved, excellent results can be anticipated. These authors reserved open reduction for those patients in whom closed reduction fails. The type I injury is the most amenable to closed reduction, if at all possible. Reduction must be very accurate, because the smallest amount of displacement can restrict motion of the radiohumeral joint. Most surgeons prefer to manipulate the fracture with the elbow extended.[175,179,182,201] Traction is applied to the forearm with the elbow extended.[179] Pressure is then placed directly over the fracture fragment to effect reduction.[179] Placing a varus stress on the forearm opens the lateral side of the elbow and facilitates replacement of the fracture fragment. Once reduction is accomplished, it is maintained by holding the elbow flexed. The fragment is held in place by the head of the radius. Although Kleiger and Joseph[201] emphasized the need for immobilization in maximum elbow flexion to maintain reduction, Rhodin[213] warned that flexion must be decreased in patients with severe associated swelling to avoid ischemic contracture. Pronation of the forearm seems to secure the radial fixation of the fragment. The ability of the radius to hold the fragment in place has been confirmed at the time of open reduction by Rhodin and Darrach.[185,213] The elbow should be immobilized for 4 to 6 weeks after the reduction.[175,179,201,220]

Operative Treatment. Open reduction and internal fixation can be very difficult, and unless stable fixation is achieved,[192] excision should be considered. Even with early postoperative motion, partial or complete joint ankylosis may occur despite an anatomical reduction.[177] The posterolateral approach has been described for the treatment of this fracture,[177,199,207,213] though I prefer to enter the joint anterior to the anconeous. A thorough understanding of the location of the posterior interosseous nerve is needed before using this approach. The principle advantage to staying anterior is that the posterior ulnohumeral ligament can be preserved, decreasing the chance of posterolateral rotatory instability after surgery.

Keon-Cohen[200] found that once an open reduction is obtained, the fragment may be stable and can thus be held in place with the opposing radial head, similar to a closed reduction. Most other authors fix the fragment with a screw.[171,180,183,185,187,190,191,193,196,203,214,219,224] The screw is usually inserted from the posterior aspect of the condyle. The tip engages the bony portion of the fragment, securing it to the condyle. The articular cartilage is therefore not penetrated. Bryan[176] and MacAusland and Wyman[207] suggested fixation with Kirschner wires buried beneath the articular surface. These can be removed later from the posterior aspect of the arm without the joint being reentered. These authors emphasized that early motion (2 to 3 weeks after fracture) is needed and that the radial fossa must be free of all fracture debris to ensure a good result. Collert[180] reported excellent results in 7 of 20 patients treated with internal fixation and open reduction. In the remaining patients, he excised the fragment or simply performed the open reduction without internal fixation. Even when the fracture fragment was devoid of all soft-tissue attachment, no avascular necrosis was evident by x-ray.

Simpson and Richards[219] used two Herbert screws in one patient, with a good result. Richards and associates[214] also reported good results using this device in four patients. The advantage of this implant is that the proximal screw head can be countersunk beneath the articular surface.

If the capitellar fragment is comminuted or has little subchondral bone for fixation, excision may be a better alternative.[191,192,199,204,212] Smith noted that functional recovery after excision and early motion is superior to that after either closed or open reduction of displaced fractures.[220] He recommended excision early rather than 4 to 5 days after injury when hemorrhage and exudate have begun to organize. Splinting is for only 2 to 3 days postoperatively, after which exercise and range of motion are instituted. Smith specifically noted that proximal migration of the radius with distal radioulnar disconformity is unusual.[220]

Alvarez and colleagues[173] advocated primary excision based on experience with 14 patients. However, only one patient in their series was treated with internal fixation (using Kirschner wires), and only two patients were followed for more than 2 years.

Wilson[223] and MacAusland and Wyman[207] mentioned the association of capitellar fractures with other fractures of the elbow and with dislocation of the joint. In these instances, care should be taken to avoid excision lest the stability of the entire elbow joint be compromised.[207]

Additionally, associated fractures of the true lateral condyle may be present.[217,223] Smith[220] believed that the articular fragments (capitellum) should be removed and the associated condylar fractures fixed internally. In his opinion, the lateral instability that is present has not led to ulnar nerve problems or disability. Attempting to replace such multiple fragments necessitates extensive dissection and prolonged postoperative immobilization that may combine to result in stiffness and ankylosis.[174] On the other hand, simple excision allows early motion and less morbidity.[197,203] Anderson[174] used the epicondyles as the point for deciding on retention or excision of the fragments.

Jakobsson[197] reconstructed the humeral articular surface with an alloy prosthesis in an effort to avoid avascular necrosis of the capitellar fragment and to maintain elbow stability. This approach required two surgical procedures and has not gained popularity.

A difficult problem in management arises when there are multiple fragments involving both articular surfaces. When both the radial head and capitellum are fractured, MacAusland and Wyman[207] recommended reduction and fixation of the capitellum and excision of the radial head. They warned against fixation of the radial head with excision of the capitellum. They also emphasized that in no instance should both fractures be excised. Despite this warning, there are instances where both sides of the joint are comminuted and require excision of loose fragments. Instability is usually the result of the violence of the injury and the associated ligamentous injury. Excision of either the radial head or capitellum will eliminate articular contact and stabilizing joint reaction force.[7,13] If the capitellum is excised, care must be taken to not disturb the posterolateral ligament complex.[336] In addition, the lateral capsule should be repaired and suture anchors used, if needed, to secure the capsule to bone.

In the late diagnosed and unreduced capitellar fracture, the displaced fragment may block flexion. In these cases, excision is the treatment of choice[174,175,186,200,220] with improvement in flexion and extension, even when excision is delayed for up to 6 months.[204,205,221]

Avascular Necrosis. Unlike the femoral head, complete separation of the capitellum from its blood supply does not usually lead to collapse and arthrosis. Several series have documented healing of the capitellar fragment without collapse, despite its being completely separated from soft tissue at the time of surgery.[180,187,193,201,203,214,219] Even when avascular necrosis is suggested on x-ray, the function of the elbow may not be impaired.[201,203]

Presumably, revascularization of the subchondral bone occurs with creeping substitution, but load across the radiocapitellar joint is insufficient during this period to cause collapse and disconformity, as commonly seen in the hip. Therefore, the frightful appearance of the capitellar fragment, completely devoid of soft-tissue attachment, should not discourage the surgeon from open reduction with internal fixation.

Author's Preferred Method of Treatment

Fractures of the capitellum usually occur in the same manner as fractures of the radial head. Therefore, it is important to look for associated injuries of the radial head, wrist, and ligaments of the elbow. The lateral condyle of the distal humerus may also be fractured.

Nondisplaced fractures of the capitellum are best treated with a posterior splint in approximately 90° of elbow flexion and neutral rotation. Gentle active-motion exercises, avoiding extremes of motion, can be started in as few as 10 days. I concentrate first on forearm rotation but avoid full extension and full pronation, because Morrey and colleagues[15] have demonstrated that radiocapitellar force transmission is greatest in this position.

If there is any initial displacement of the fracture, then operative intervention will probably be necessary. In my experience, closed reduction is usually impossible and the reduction, if achieved, is difficult to maintain. In addition, the prolonged immobilization necessary to maintain the reduction may lead to disabling contracture.

For displaced fractures, the goal of operation is anatomical restoration of the articular surface with rigid fixation that permits elbow motion in the immediate postoperative period (see Fig. 14-23). If this cannot be achieved because of comminution or fragment size, then the fragment or fragments should be excised. Before operation, the patient is informed of both possibilities.

Adequate exposure of the fracture is necessary for reduction, because the fragment is often embedded in joint capsule and rotated 90°. As mentioned earlier, the surgical exposure should not damage or compromise the posterolateral ligament complex. If this structure is compromised at surgery or because of the injury, primary repair with suture anchors to bone should be performed. In addition, the forearm should be splinted in pronation in the immediate postoperative period to protect this repair.

Once reduction is achieved, temporary fixation with Kirschner wires is used. Sometimes, the fragment carries a small but sufficient piece of lateral periarticular bone that permits fixation with standard AO (ASIF) screws from the mini-fragment set or the newer cannulated system. The Herbert screw can also be used, with insertion directly into the articular surface. Although insertion using the jig has been described, using the device "freehand" may be simpler. Even with careful technique, fragmentation can occur, necessitating excision.

Whether primary excision or open reduction is performed, active motion is begun within the first week. Even with an appropriately vigorous rehabilitation program, extension often returns slowly. After bony union is achieved, a turnbuckle orthosis or dynamic splinting may improve extension.

Fractures of the Trochlea

Isolated fractures of the trochlea are extremely rare.[85,111,188,220,222] Stimson[222] credited the original description to Laugier in 1853, hence the term *Laugier's fracture*. Very few authors report having seen it as an isolated fracture.[111,188,195,216,220]

The very structure of the trochlea probably contributes to its rarity as an isolated injury. The capitellum is subject to shear and compressive forces from the head of the radius. It can also be fractured by a direct blow. The trochlea, on the other hand, is deep within the elbow joint and thus protected from direct injury.[176] The transmitted force of the ulna against the trochlea tends to produce more of a wedging action than a tangential shearing force.[176,220] Bryan[176] noted that the shearing forces that may produce a trochlear fracture can be generated in an elbow dislocation, hence, he warned of the association between these two entities.

When the surgeon makes the clinical diagnosis, the signs of effusion, pain, restriction of motion, and crepitus indicate that an intra-articular fracture is probably present. The one finding that should lead the surgeon to suspect a fracture of the trochlea is a fragment lying on the medial side of the joint just distal to the medial epicondyle.[225]

The fracture may extend from the trochlea into the distal portion of the epicondyle.[225] If the fragment is nondisplaced, Smith recommended a posterior splint for 3 weeks followed by exercises and soaks.[225] If the fracture is displaced, the joint should be opened. Large fragments should be replaced and fixed with either a screw or Kirschner wires.[188,225] If internal fixation is used the elbow should be immobilized only 10 to 11 days before range of motion is begun. If the fragments are too small for fixation, excision and early motion is the treatment of choice.[188,225]

Fractures of the Epicondyles

Each epicondyle has its own ossification center.[231] This has special significance in children, because with tension on the collateral ligaments the point of weakness is at the epiphyseal growth plate rather than the ligaments. Thus, fractures of the epicondyles in children are usually epiphyseal separations most often caused by avulsion.[231,232,239] As primary isolated fractures in adults, they are uncommon.[176,232,239]

Fractures of the Lateral Epicondyle

Fracture of the lateral epicondyle is extremely rare. In fact, many authors have doubted that it even exists as an isolated fracture in adults.[239–241] The ossification center of the lateral epicondyle is small and appears in about the 12th year. After it fuses with the main portion of the lateral condyle at puberty, avulsion fractures are even more rare.[231] The lateral epicondyle is almost level with the flattened outer surface of the lateral condyle. Thus, it has only minimal exposure to a direct blow. Treatment involves simple immobilization until the pain subsides, then early motion, similar to the treatment for a nondisplaced lateral condyle (Fig. 14-25).

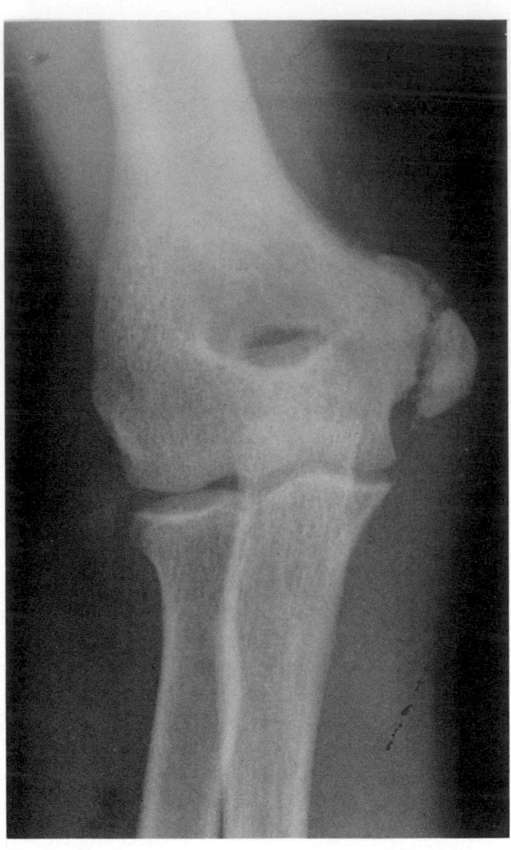

FIGURE 14-26. This fracture of the medial epicondyle is relatively undisplaced. There is evidence of periosteal new bone formation proximally along the supracondylar ridge.

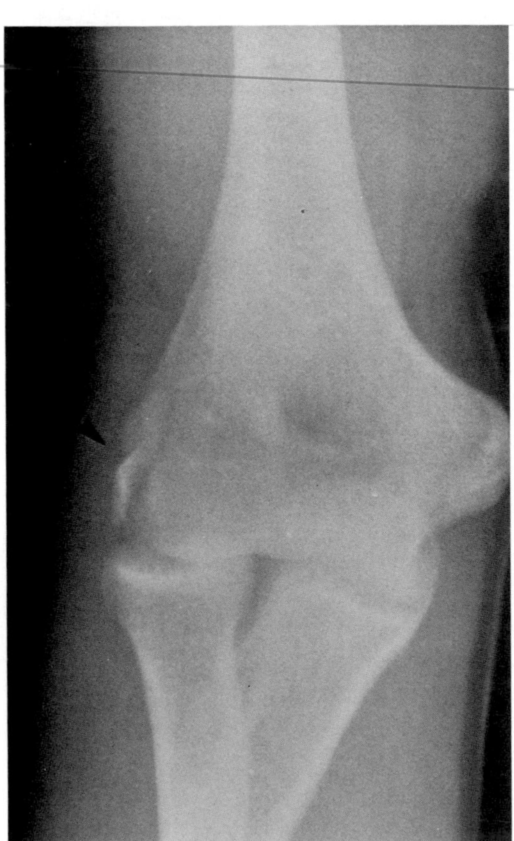

FIGURE 14-25. Fracture of the lateral epicondyle (*arrow*) with a small portion of the capitellum as well.

Fractures of the Medial Epicondyle

Fracture of the medial epicondyle or epitrochlea (Fig. 14-26) is more common than fracture of the lateral epicondyle.[231,239] Granger first reported fractures of the medial epicondyle in 1818.[226,231,239] In a series of ten cases, he outlined the pertinent anatomy, recognized the difficulty in regaining motion, and noted the favorable results after nonoperative treatment.[226]

Fusion of the ossification center of the medial epicondyle with the distal humerus does not occur until about the 20th year.[230] However, in some adults fusion may never occur, perhaps setting the stage for avulsion fractures of the medial epicondyle.[231]

Mechanism of Injury

In the child and adolescent this fragment is commonly avulsed from the humerus during a posterior dislocation of the elbow (Fig. 14-27).[231,239] The epicondylar fragment may be carried into the joint and remain lodged there when the elbow is reduced (Fig. 14-28).[232,234–236] The ulnar nerve can also become trapped with this fragment. After the age of 20 it

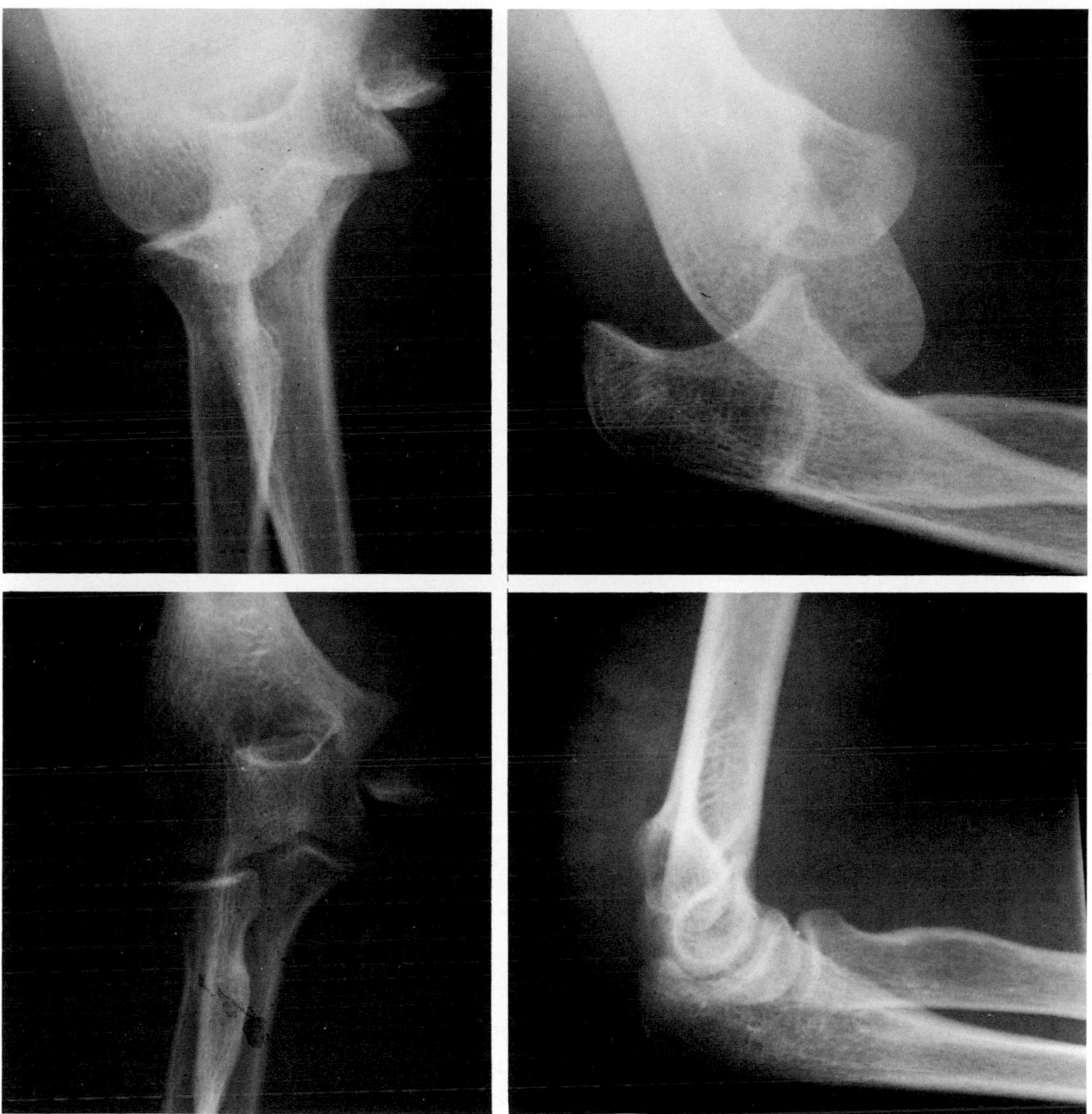

FIGURE 14-27. (**Top**) A posterolateral dislocation of the elbow with avulsion of the medial epicondyle. (**Bottom**) Closed reduction of the elbow dislocation was successful, but the position of the medial epicondyle remained unchanged. The patient was managed with simple immobilization for ten days, followed by early range of motion. The patient currently has a full range of motion in the elbow, no ulnar nerve symptoms, no elbow instability, and no complaints of deformity about the joint.

rarely occurs as a single fracture or associated with a dislocation.[232]

In a series of 143 patients with medial epicondyle fractures, Smith[239] found only two adults in whom the fracture was not associated with other fractures or dislocations of the elbow.

Because there is no residua of the old epiphyseal plate if fusion with the distal humerus occurs, avulsion forces are unlikely to cause this fracture in the adult. Fractures in the adult are not necessarily limited to the area originating from the medial epicondylar ossification center. They can extend into part of the main medial condylar mass as well.[231] These isolated fractures in the adult are most commonly caused by a direct blow to the epicondyle.[231,232,239] Its prominence on the medial aspect of the elbow makes it especially vulnerable to this type of force.

Signs and Symptoms

In displaced fractures the fragment is usually pulled anterior and distal by the forearm flexor muscles.[226,231] Local tenderness and crepitus over the medial epicon-

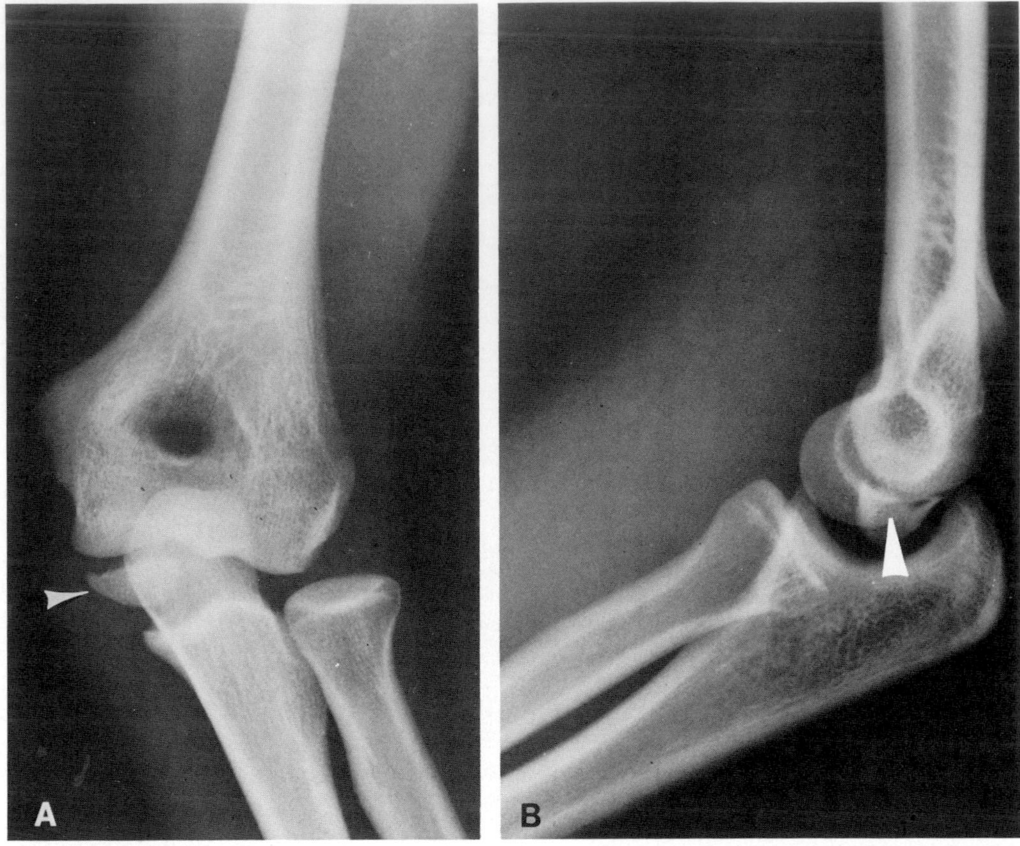

FIGURE 14-28. Avulsion of the medial epicondyle with displacement into the joint. (**A**) The epicondyle (*arrow*) is lodged between the medial articular surface of the trochlea and ulna, inhibiting reduction. (**B**) Lateral view of the same patient demonstrating intra-articular location of the medial epicondyle (*arrow*). If the fragment is seen this far distally, it must be assumed to be within the joint.

dyle are characteristic. Active flexion of the elbow and wrist along with pronation of the forearm will accentuate the pain.[225] Because of the proximity of the ulnar nerve to the epicondyle, ulnar nerve evaluation is critical in the physical examination.

Radiographic Findings

There may be a tendency to confuse the normal radiolucent epiphyseal growth plate with an acute fracture of the epicondyle in the adolescent patient. Comparison x-rays of the opposite elbow may be helpful.[226] In those cases in which the epicondylar fragment has been avulsed during a posterolateral dislocation, its presence within the joint must be ruled out.[238] Patrick[234] demonstrated a radiographic clue to its lodgment within the joint. With simple avulsion of the epicondyle, the fragment never migrates distally as far as the joint level. Thus, if the fragment is seen lying *at* the level of the joint, its intra-articular entrapment must be ruled out (see Fig. 14-28).

Methods of Treatment

General agreement exists on the proper method of treatment of either the minimally displaced fractures or those lodged within the joint.[228,229,232,238] In the minimally displaced fracture, the generally accepted method of treatment is short-term immobilization (7 to 10 days) with the elbow and wrist flexed and the forearm pronated.[227] Likewise, those fragments lying within the joint that cannot be extracted by the closed methods advocated by Patrick[234] must be removed operatively.

There is a difference of opinion on the subject of moderately to severely displaced fragments. Three methods of treatment are available to the surgeon: (1) manipulation and short-term immobilization, (2) open reduction with internal fixation, and (3) excision of the fragment.

Smith[239,240] advocated nonoperative treatment with early motion in nearly all cases. In his extensive review of patients with this injury, he was unable to confirm the presence of any previously described disabilities resulting from persistent displacement of the fragment.[239] None of those with fibrous union had pain or disability. Distal displacement of the epicondyle did not result in loss of elbow function or weakness of the flexor-pronator muscles. Only 1 in the 116 patients in his series treated by nonoperative means had any delayed ulnar nerve problems. It was his conclusion that the results with either bony or fibrous union were the same.

Proponents of operative treatment cite the possibility of ulnar nerve symptoms,[227,232,233,239] instability of the elbow with valgus stress testing,[236] wrist flexor weakness, and nonunion of the displaced epicondyle as reason for primary reattachment or excision of the fragment. Sisk's[238] indication for open reduction and internal fixation was displacement of greater than 1 cm. However, Bernstein and colleagues[226] and Wilson[223] found no patients with ulnar nerve symptoms or wrist flexor weakness when displaced fractures were treated nonoperatively.

In my experience, elbow instability has not been a problem in patients with medial epicondyle fractures associated with elbow dislocation when these injuries are managed nonoperatively. On the contrary, unless early motion is instituted, significant stiffness, not instability, will result.

Additionally, an interesting complication was reported by Roaf,[237] who described a case in which the median nerve had become trapped between the fracture fragments. With healing, two foramina were created through which the median nerve passed. With time and continued motion of the elbow the nerve became frayed at the distal foramen. Total disruption of the nerve resulted.

Author's Preferred Method of Treatment

As in other elbow injuries, early resumption of motion is essential to recovery of elbow function. Thus, these fractures are treated by manipulation and immobilization with the forearm pronated and the elbow and wrist flexed in a posterior splint for 10 to 14 days. Active motion is then allowed.

The surgeon must remember that patients with medial epicondyle fractures, especially those associated with an elbow dislocation, may require up to 1 year to regain elbow motion. Should the displaced fragment be unsightly or painful, or if ulnar nerve problems develop, the fragment can be excised later with minimal operative morbidity. Treatment of the entrapped fragment is discussed later in the section on dislocation of the elbow.

Fractures of the Supracondylar Process

The supracondylar (supracondyloid) process, a congenital variation of the distal end of the humerus, is a bony (or cartilaginous) projection that arises from the anteromedial surface of the humerus approximately 5 cm above the medial epicondyle (Fig. 14-29).[243–247] This process varies greatly in size from a small projection in the middle of a prominent ridge to an actual bony hook.[247] After arising from the anteromedial surface of the humerus, the process is directed downward, forward, and inward toward the medial epicondyle.[243,247] From the tip of the supracondylar process may extend a fibrous arch (which in rare cases may be ossified), the ligament of Struthers, which connects the supracondylar process with the medial epicondyle.[242,245,247] The upper fibers of the pronator teres and some of the lower fibers of the coracobrachialis may arise from the supracondylar process or the ligament of Struthers. Through this small arch formed by the supracondylar process, the ligament of Struthers, and the medial epicondyle passes the median nerve and frequently the brachial artery.[242–246]

Fracture of this uncommon process is of clinical significance and bears discussion. The incidence of this process is very low, ranging from 0.6% to 2.7%.[242–246] Because of its long, thin structure and muscle attachments, it is easily fractured.[243] The fracture itself may be quite painful, and the close proximity of the median nerve and brachial artery may result in symptoms of compression of these two structures.[243] One should always suspect its presence in the patient with high median nerve dysfunction.

The mechanism of injury is suspected to be direct trauma to the area, resulting in a fracture through the supracondylar process.[246] The palpation of a painful bony projection on the anteromedial aspect of the distal humerus approximately 5 cm above the elbow should suggest the presence of a fractured supracondylar process.[242] Active extension of the elbow with pronation or supination of the forearm may accentuate the pain of the fracture site, median nerve paresthesias, and brachial artery compression.

Although the diagnosis is often made by palpation, radiographic confirmation is essential. Routine anteroposterior and lateral x-rays may fail to demonstrate the bony process because of its origin on the anteromedial humerus. An oblique x-ray may be required to place the process in sharp profile.[242,243]

Treatment of fractures of the supracondylar process varies.[242–247] Most heal spontaneously and become asymptomatic with simple immobilization until pain free; then early elbow motion and muscle-strengthening exercises are instituted. In those that remain painful or produce median nerve dysfunction, surgical excision is indicated. Kolb and Moore[246] were more cautious in recommending surgical resection. They reported one case of myositis ossificans after removal of the fractured process. Barnard and McCoy[242] emphasized that when surgical excision is performed, removal of the periosteum of the process and the fibers

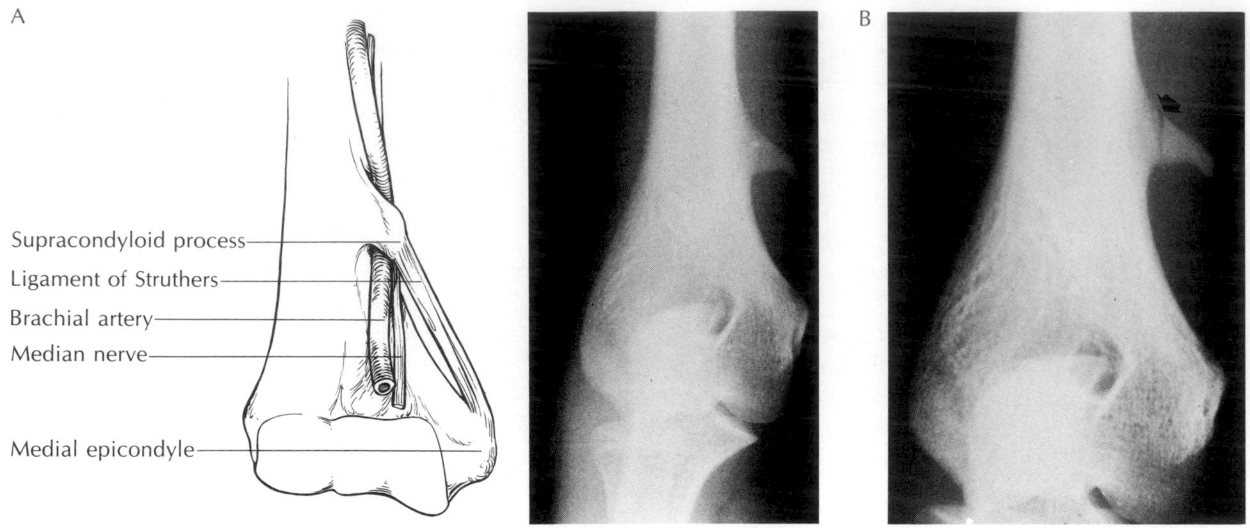

FIGURE 14-29. (**A**) The supracondylar process arises from the anteromedial aspect of the distal humerus. It is connected to the medial epicondyle by the ligament of Struthers, which forms a fibro-osseous arch through which pass the median nerve and usually the brachial artery. (**B**) A nondisplaced fracture of a supracondylar process.

of the pronator teres origin is essential to prevent reformation of the spur.

DISLOCATIONS

The elbow is one of the more highly constrained and stable joints in the body; yet dislocation is not uncommon. Because of this intrinsic stability, redislocation is rare in the elbow in contrast to the shoulder. The opposing tension of the triceps and flexors, coupled with the hinge-like articulation, confers stability that permits capsular healing even during active motion. The important medial and lateral stabilizing ligaments also seem capable of healing with enough mechanical integrity that repair for acute instability is seldom necessary.

Elbow dislocation has the highest incidence among the 10- to 20-year-old population and is often associated with sports injuries.[263] The injury can also occur in the elderly after a fall.

For dislocation to occur without fracture, a combination of levering forces and loading must be applied in a manner that first "unlocks" the olecranon from the trochlea and then translates the articular surfaces out of position. Once dislocation is recognized, prompt reduction with careful attention to the neurovascular status of the arm and hand should be carried out.

Classification

Because most acute elbow dislocations in adults occur at the ulnohumeral joint, most classifications refer to the position of the ulna relative to the humerus after injury. Desault, in 1811, described four types of ulnohumeral elbow dislocations.[254] Stimson's classification,[281] which included nearly every possible anatomical position, was adopted by most subsequent authors.[251,280] Unreduced (old) and recurrent dislocations require entirely different treatment and are classified and discussed separately in this section.

Most acute elbow dislocations are posterior (Fig. 14-30) and involve both the radius and ulna.[264,285] The distinction between posterior, posterolateral, and posteromedial is sometimes difficult to determine and seldom influences treatment. The other positions of dislocation—anterior, medial, lateral, and divergent—are rare and require alternative treatment. Pure lateral and medial dislocations are distinct and may require open reduction because of entrapped muscle or nerve. Isolated dislocations of the proximal radius are uncommon in adults, unlike in the pediatric population.

Mechanism of Injury

Posterior dislocations of the elbow are commonly caused by a fall on the hand or wrist. The precise mechanism of dislocation is not known because many patterns of injury share this frequent antecedent. Several authors have speculated that the position of greatest vulnerability is slight hyperextension or at least full extension. As force is transmitted from the fall to the extended elbow, a resultant anterior force is generated that levers the ulna out of the trochlea. As the joint continues to hyperextend, the anterior capsule and collateral ligaments are placed under increasing tension and eventually fail. In addition to hyperextension,

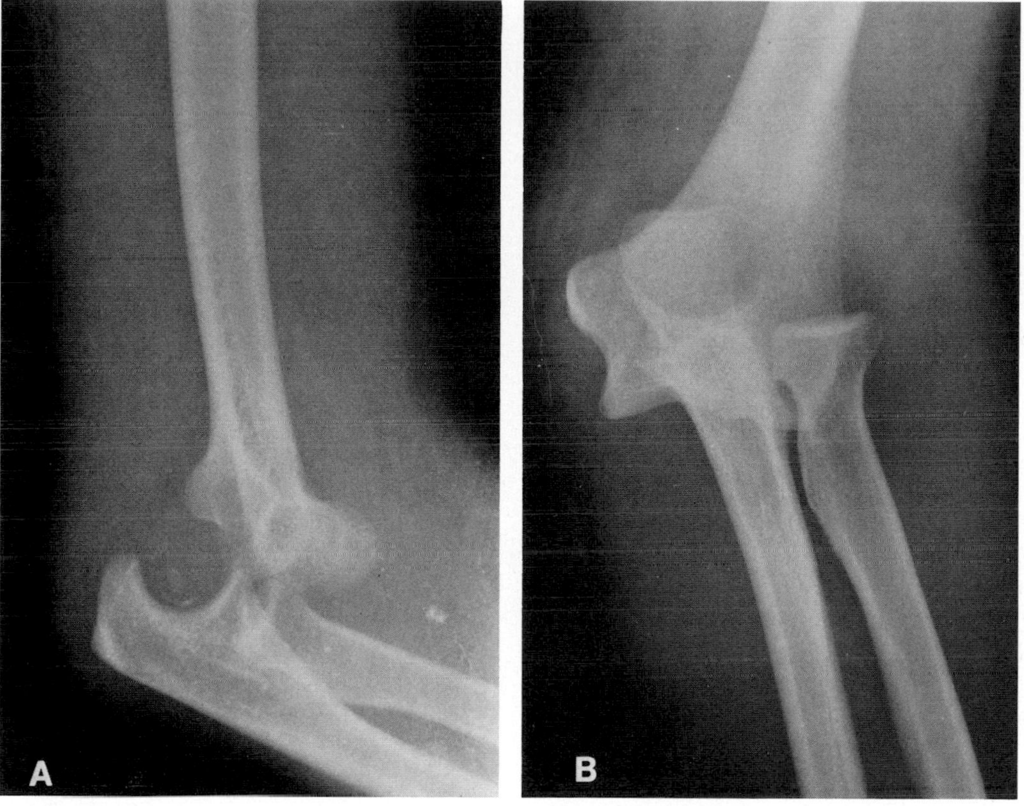

FIGURE 14-30. (**A**) A posterior dislocation of the elbow. Note that the coronoid process is adjacent to the olecranon fossa. (**B**) In the anteroposterior view, note the slight lateral displacement of the radius and ulna.

a valgus stress usually occurs. In patients who have undergone exploratory surgery immediately after posterior dislocation, nearly all have ruptured the medial collateral ligaments and some have even ruptured the origin of the flexor mass at the medial epicondyle.[259,260,262,282] This valgus stress is not unexpected, given the usual position of the arm away from the body at the time of the fall. In the child, this sudden valgus load can instead cause a fracture of the medial epicondyle through the growth plate.

Anterior dislocations are uncommon and are thought to be caused by impact on the posterior forearm in a slightly flexed position.

Initial Assessment

The first priority of care is to assess the neurovascular status of the hand and forearm *before* manipulation. The physician must attempt to document the status of the brachial artery and median and ulnar nerves because these are most vulnerable and can be entrapped during manipulation. Often, the patient is in great pain and is uncooperative, but nevertheless an attempt should be made. The x-rays must also be scrutinized for associated fractures at the distal humerus, radial head, and coronoid process. One should not hesitate to admit the patient for 24 hours of observation if there is any concern about excessive swelling, vascular injury, or the risk of compartment syndrome.

Vascular Injury

Many authors have reported injuries of the brachial artery associated with elbow dislocation.[280,287,288,294,299–303,306,307,311,313–315,318,319] In 1913, Sherill[314] repaired the brachial artery "(by) the method described by Carrel and employed by Crile" with good result. In 1937, Eliason and Brown[294] reported ligating the radial and ulnar arteries without repair and reported good results. Spear and Janes[315] also treated four patients with ligation, but their results were not as satisfying, because one patient demonstrated persistent ischemia in the hand. These authors thought that collateral circulation was adequate in the upper extremity in most cases.

Disputing this, many others have stated strongly that arterial repair with or without reversed saphenous vein grafting should be the standard of care.[284,286–289,295,296,303,304,311,318] Louis and colleagues[303] noted no cold intolerance or claudication in the patients with open and functioning arterial repairs but did find ischemic symptoms in the hand of the patient whose graft clotted. In addition, anatomical studies demonstrated that in dislocation much of the collateral circulation can be disrupted at the time of injury. DeBakey and Simeone's[293] analysis of World War II vascular injuries in the upper extremity also challenged the safety of ligation.

Early recognition of vascular injury is imperative. Loss of pulse does not preclude attempted closed reduction. If, however, arterial flow is not reestablished after reduction and the hand is poorly perfused, the patient should be prepared for immediate arterial reconstruction with saphenous vein grafting. Angiography, if used, should be performed in the operating room, especially if use of the angiography suite delays prompt treatment. If perfusion of the forearm and hand has been poor because of delayed treatment, volar forearm fasciotomy should be performed to reduce the chance of Volkmann's contracture.

A spectrum of arterial injury exists, and vigilance for loss of circulation after reduction due to intimal injury is important. The presence of pulses alone does not ensure adequate circulation to the hand or perfusion of the forearm musculature. It is necessary to examine for signs of increased compartment pressure in the forearm and hand. Pain with gentle passive extension of the digits is the most important early indicator of ischemia. The other clinical features and treatment of compartment syndromes are discussed in Chapter 8 and should be reviewed.

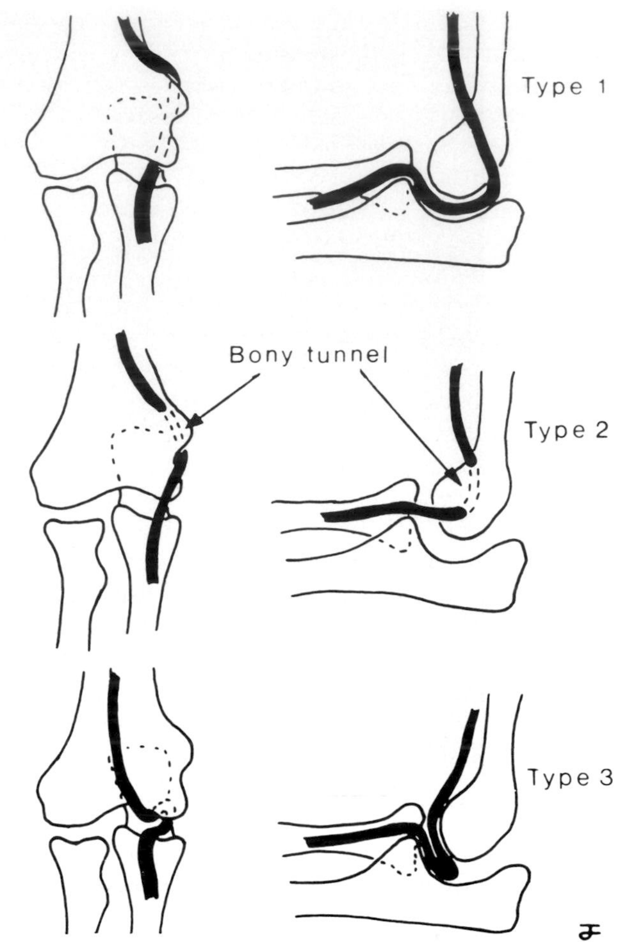

FIGURE 14-31. Hallet described three ways in which the median nerve can become entrapped in the elbow. *(Hallet, J.: Entrapment of the Median Nerve After Dislocation of the Elbow. A Case Report. J. Bone Joint Surg., 63B:408–412, 1981.)*

Nerve Injury

The median, ulnar, radial, and anterior interosseous nerves can be injured at the time of elbow dislocation. The relative incidence cannot be derived from the mere volume of case reports, but the radial nerve seems to be the least vulnerable and injury to it the most rarely reported.[320] Injury to the ulnar nerve with entrapment anterior to the joint has also been reported. The valgus displacement that occurs during dislocation can also put the ulnar nerve under stretch.

The median nerve can be injured both at the time of dislocation,[270,297,320] being stretched and attenuated, or during reduction, becoming entrapped in the joint[270,289–292,297,298,305,308–310,312,316,317,320] (Fig. 14-31).

It is therefore important to examine the patient *before* and *after* manipulation for the independent function of each nerve. The most difficult diagnosis is probably the isolated anterior interosseous nerve palsy, because no sensory loss is noted.[290] In cases in which the deficit was present both before and after reduction, it is best for the surgeon to wait and watch for signs of resolving palsy, counseling the patient that exploration may still be necessary. If there is a decline in function or severe pain in the distribution of the nerve, exploration and decompression are indicated.

After the initial phase of treatment, electromyographic studies demonstrate signs of denervation, but recovery may not be evident. Careful serial clinical examinations are the most helpful. Spontaneous recovery usually occurs, but if none is noted after 3 months, operation should be considered.

Posterior Dislocation of the Elbow

Methods of Treatment

Closed Reduction

After the initial examination of the neurovascular function of the hand and forearm is complete, manipulation and reduction are performed. Many techniques of manipulation have been described[258,264,266,267,269,272] for closed reduction of the posterior dislocation. All the methods employ some form of distraction followed by anterior translation. The principal controversy surrounds the use of hyperextension to "unlock" the olecranon from the distal humerus (Fig. 14-32). Some have advocated this as useful and necessary[267] in certain cases to achieve reduction. There is some danger, however, when full extension or hyperextension is used. Matev[308] and Hallett[298] suggested that hyperextension was responsible for entrapment of the median nerve after elbow dislocation in the cases they reported. Loomis[266] condemned extension and especially hyperextension because of the increased trauma to the brachialis muscle. He recommended reduction in flexion with distal traction on the forearm.

Starkloff positioned the patient prone with the arm hanging over the side of the stretcher, then applied traction with weights hung from the wrist. After 15 to 20 minutes, forward pressure on the olecranon was applied, gently effecting reduction. Parvin[272] also used the prone position (Fig. 14-33), but he used traction applied by the surgeon rather than with weights. Again, after several minutes of traction, the olecranon slipped into reduction with gentle flexion. Meyn and Quigley[269] used a similar technique, except that only the forearm dangles from the edge of the stretcher rather than the whole arm (Fig. 14-34). Lavine[264] used a similar method over the back of a chair. Hankin[258] has described a method of reduction that gently levers the olecranon over the distal humerus in the flexed position while applying traction. The advantage of these methods is that they require no assistant.

Open Reduction

The need for open reduction after acute dislocation is rare. Pawlowski and coworkers[274] and Greiss and Messias and colleagues[257] described patients who had irreducible dislocations because soft tissue was entrapped, blocking reduction. Durig[255] recommended that loose intra-articular fragments be removed, but the results of treatment were comparable to those of closed management. Occasionally in the adult (and more often in children), the medial epicondyle can be entrapped, preventing reduction. Purser[276] and Linscheid and Wheeler[265,284] reported adult patients who required open reduction with extraction of the entrapped medial epicondyle from the joint.

Repair of Ligaments

Some authors have advocated surgical repair of the associated ligamentous injuries.[255,282] However, Josefsson[260] studied 30 patients in a randomized, prospective study designed to compare the outcome of surgical

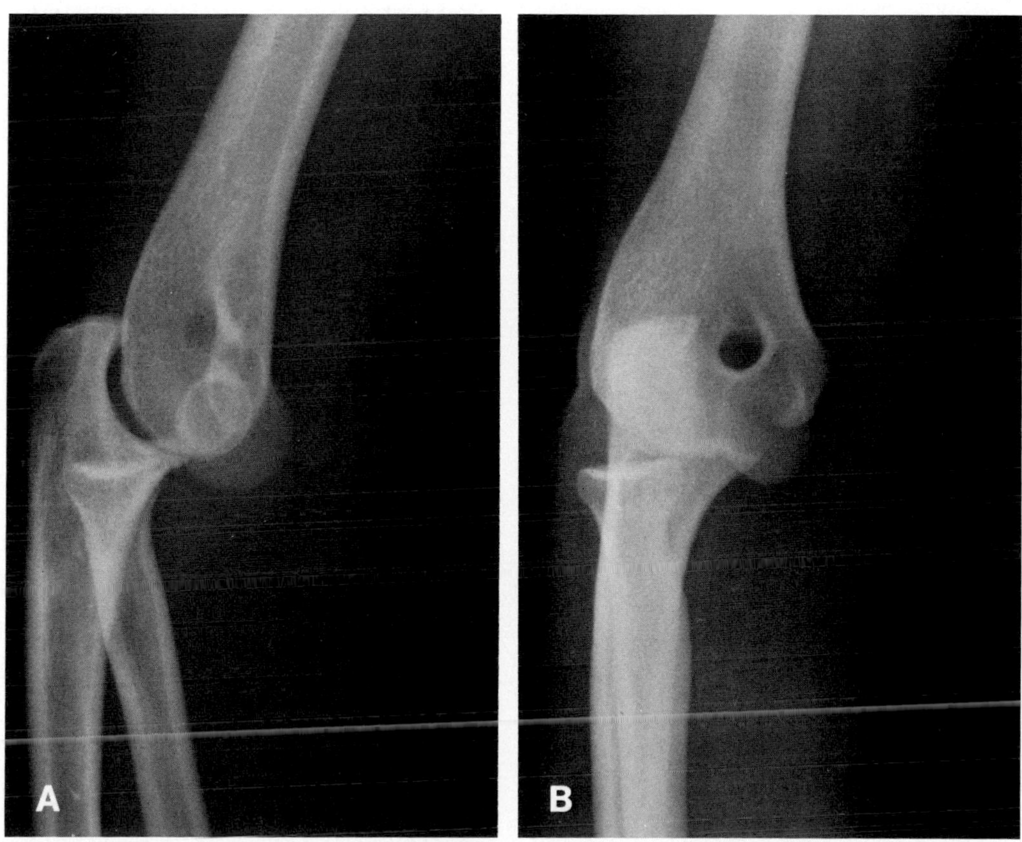

FIGURE 14-32. Lateral (**A**) and anterior (**B**) views of a posterior dislocation of the elbow in which the coronoid is impaled into the trochlea. In this injury, the coronoid could fracture from the impact.

versus nonsurgical treatment. They concluded that irrespective of the degree of acute instability when the patients were examined under anesthesia, no benefit was derived from open treatment and repair of the medial ligaments in simple posterior elbow dislocation.

Care After Reduction

There is disagreement in the literature concerning the duration of immobilization after reduction. Loomis and Wadsworth thought that 3 to 4 weeks of immobilization in a cast was mandatory to reduce ectopic calcification and allow healing.[266,283] Protzman and later Mehloff and colleagues associated greater contractures and dysfunction with immobilization and recommended motion within the first week after injury.[268,275] O'Driscoll and Linscheid also recommended gentle active motion in the first week.[271]

Author's Preferred Method of Treatment

As emphasized, the first step in treatment is a careful assessment of any associated neurovascular injuries and concomitant fractures. The vascular status of the hand is paramount. I assess both the radial and ulnar pulses and evaluate the perfusion of the hand. It is important to evaluate capillary refill in the volar fingertips rather than in the nail beds and compare it with that in the uninjured extremity.

The median, radial, and ulnar nerves can usually be tested in the hand independently without excessive discomfort to the patient. Both the sensory and motor components of each nerve should be checked.

If the dislocation occurred less than 2 hours before treatment, closed manipulation with sedation is usually successful. If the dislocation occurred more than 4 hours before treatment, the task becomes more difficult but still is usually possible without general or axillary block anesthesia. Forceful attempts should be avoided, and if spasm and pain preclude adequate relaxation, general anesthesia can be used. The disadvantage of axillary block is the inability to immediately assess the neurologic function after manipulation and reduction.

The simplest reduction maneuver requires gentle countertraction on the humerus by an assistant while the surgeon applies distal traction on the wrist and proximal forearm. Medial or lateral displacement is corrected first, and then distal traction is continued as the elbow is flexed. Downward pressure by the surgeon on the proximal forearm to disengage the coronoid from the olecranon fossa may be helpful. Hyperextension should be avoided.

When an assistant is unavailable or muscle spasm is more pronounced, Parvin's gravity method[272] (see Fig. 14-33), or that of Meyn and Quigley[269] (see Fig. 14-34), can be used to gradually overcome the

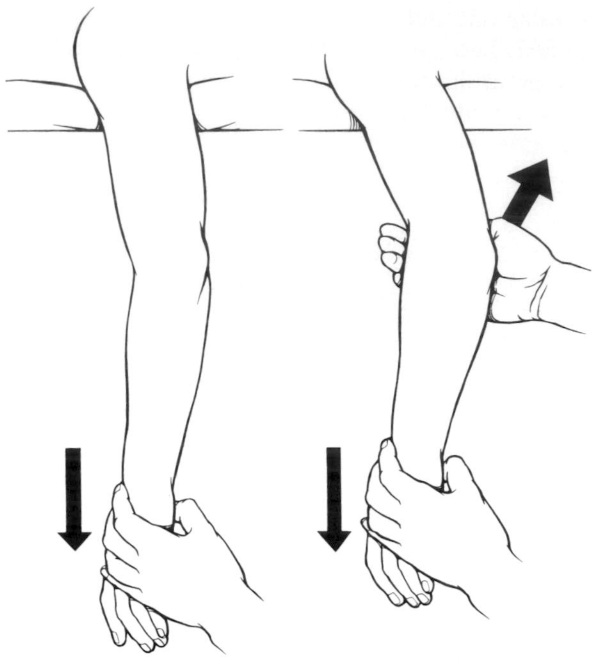

FIGURE 14-33. Parvin's method of closed reduction of an elbow dislocation. The patient lies prone on a stretcher, and the physician applies gentle downward traction on the wrist for a few minutes. As the olecranon begins to slip distally, the physician lifts up gently on the arm. No assistant is required, and if the maneuver is done gently, no anesthesia is required. *(Redrawn from Parvin, R.W.: Closed Reduction of Common Shoulder and Elbow Dislocations Without Anesthesia. Arch. Surg., 75:972–975, 1957.)*

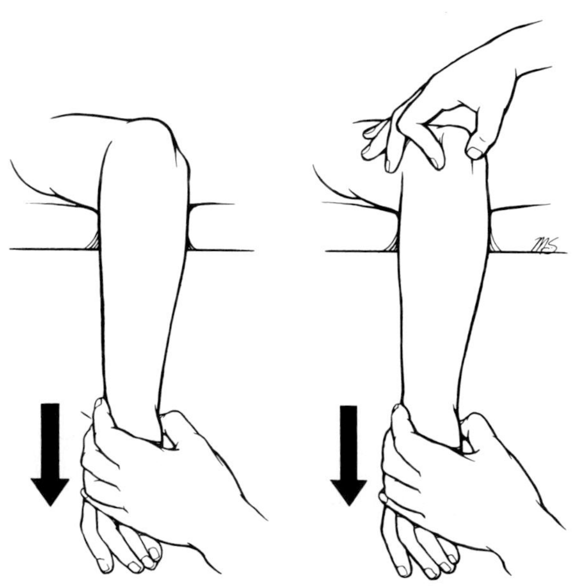

FIGURE 14-34. In Meyn and Quigley's method of reduction, only the forearm hangs from the side of the stretcher. As gentle downward traction is applied on the wrist, the physician guides reduction of the olecranon with the opposite hand. *(Redrawn from Meyn, M.A., and Quigley, T.B.: Reduction of Posterior Dislocation of the Elbow by Traction on the Dangling Arm. Clin. Orthop., 103:106–108, 1974.)*

spasm.[269,272] I have no personal experience with Hankin's method,[258] but he reported excellent results with no complications.

After manipulation and reduction, the elbow should be gently ranged passively to test the stability of reduction. Most elbows are stable and do not redislocate at 30° short of full extension. Pronation and supination should also be stable. If passive range of motion is not complete or smooth, postmanipulation x-rays should be carefully scrutinized for an associated fracture or entrapment of the medial epicondyle. The presence of valgus laxity is common immediately after reduction, especially if the patient is anesthetized. However, the medial ligaments are extracapsular and probably heal satisfactorily if protected from valgus stress during the healing process.

I usually apply a posterior splint with the elbow in 90° flexion, with loose circumferential wraps. The hand should be accessible for repeated examination for neurovascular dysfunction or compartment syndrome. Most elbows are stable enough after dislocation to permit gentle active motion exercises in both flexion and extension and forearm rotation during the first week after injury.

If the elbow has no tendency to dislocate at a position of 30° of flexion, I usually place the patient's arm in a sling rather than a posterior splint. Active motion in the sling can be started without delay, and the sling prevents extension without adding unneeded weight to the arm. A light splint can be used in conjunction with a sling for comfort, but it should be removed in the first week to reduce the amount of impending stiffness.

A complete dislocation probably disrupts both the medial and lateral collateral ligaments.[260] The medial side is protected adequately by restricting activities that create valgus stress. The posterolateral ligaments can be protected by avoiding full supination in extension with axial load. Injury to the posterolateral ligament complex can result in posterolateral rotatory instability. If this form of instability is possible or suspected, I recommend a careful rehabilitation program. As the patient begins supination of the forearm in rehabilitation, recurrent dislocation can be prevented by having the patient lie in the supine position with the arm overhead during treatment. This position uses the weight of the arm to maintain reduction of the joint.

If the unanesthetized patient exhibits instability immediately after reduction or redislocates the elbow in the splint, I carefully reexamine the patient in the operating room under fluoroscopy to determine the point of instability. If there are no associated fractures of the coronoid process or radial head, the patient can be fitted with a hinged brace with extension stops set to limit extension before the angle of instability is reached. Active motion can then be begun. At 3 weeks, the amount of extension allowed in the splint can be increased gradually. Forced passive motion should be avoided, because this can lead to pathologic heterotopic ossification.

The use of formal physical therapy should be determined on an individual basis. Some patients progress with little supervision, whereas others require more comprehensive instruction and surveillance. The shoulder, especially in the elderly, can become stiff and painful if not included in the exercise program.

The presence of some heterotopic calcification is not unusual and is seldom of clinical significance.[355,356] Ectopic bone formation is usually seen in the distal brachialis and the medial or lateral ligaments. Widespread heterotopic ossification can occur in more severe trauma and is discussed in more detail later.

Outcome

The outcome after simple posterior elbow dislocation has been reported in several series.[248,249,259–261,268,270,280] Josefsson[260] and coworkers studied 52 patients and found little long-term disability. Most had a slight flexion contracture (10° to 15°) and occasional pain. Recurrent dislocation did not occur; valgus instability was present in a few patients but was usually not symptomatic. Full recovery of motion and strength takes 3 to 6 months in most patients. Some patients do not do well, however, especially those with associated fractures or high-velocity trauma.

Recurrent dislocation without associated fracture, congenital deformity, or systemic ligamentous laxity is rare.

Unreduced Posterior Dislocation of the Elbow

Unreduced posterior dislocations are seen primarily in less developed regions of the world. The precise temporal definition of "old" or (in the more pejorative) *neglected* posterior dislocation is unclear.[321–329]

Treatment is complicated by the presence of an incipient or established contracture of the joint. According to Allende and Freytes,[321] if the joint is unreduced for more than 7 days, the chance for closed reduction, even after preliminary traction, is low. Both open reduction of the joint and release of the incipient contracture is required to restore function.

The operative treatment of this condition creates a therapeutic paradox. To reduce the joint, all soft tissue encapsulating the joint must be released. This includes stripping the capsule and ligaments both anteriorly and posteriorly. However, once this expansive release is completed, the joint becomes grossly unstable, easily dislocating back to the posterior position. The temptation is to pin the joint reduced 3 to 4 weeks and then begin active motion.

In addition, the triceps tendon becomes functionally shortened the longer the joint remains dislocated. This shortening creates increased resting tension in the triceps, making reduction and flexion after reduction difficult. Although the risk of heterotopic bone formation is theoretically significant, these joints must be operatively reduced, regardless of the time of discovery.

For these late-treated dislocations, I have used hinged external fixation to maintain joint reduction, permit motion, and enhance muscle-tendon stretching (Fig. 14-35). The hinge is applied after a complete open release and reduction is performed, including ulnar nerve transposition. It is not possible to reduce these joints, especially those longer than 3 to 4 weeks, without arthrotomy. The joint surfaces are covered with a well-organized hematoma that requires careful stripping. Once the cartilaginous surfaces are exposed and the capsule released both anteriorly and posteriorly, the joint can be gently reduced without undue force. The radiocapitellar joint also requires thorough debridement. I usually do not perform ligament repair or reconstructions at the time of open reduction. The hinge is left in place for 8 weeks, during which time active and passive motion is carried out. No cases of late instability or significant heterotopic bone have yet been encountered, but this is a rare condition.

Anterior Dislocation of the Elbow

Anterior dislocation usually occurs after a fall, with a force striking the posterior forearm in the flexed position.[342,343] In 1922, Cohn[342] credited Everts with the original description in 1787. Since then, about 30 cases have been reported in the literature.[341–347] Because of the blow posteriorly, a fracture of the olecranon can also occur.[342]

Signs and Symptoms

Because brachial artery injury can occur, the same careful assessment for neurovascular injury is recommended. Before reduction, the arm appears shortened, with the forearm held in supination. The distal humerus is prominent posteriorly. The biceps tendon tents the skin anteriorly.

Methods of Treatment

The reduction maneuver is essentially the reverse of the posterior dislocation. Gentle traction is first applied to the forearm to relax the contracted muscles. Posterior and downward pressure is then applied to the forearm with gentle anterior pressure on the distal humerus. Again, after the reduction, a careful examination for neurocirculatory deficit must be done.

The triceps insertion may be stripped and detached in this type of dislocation, and the examiner should test active extension of the elbow.

The elbow is splinted in slightly less than 90° of flexion, depending on the amount of swelling and the status of the triceps. If there is an associated olecranon fracture, open reduction with rigid fixation is probably necessary for stability.

Medial and Lateral Dislocations of the Elbow

Medial and lateral dislocations present with a widened appearance of the elbow and normal relative lengths of the arm and forearm. In the anteroposterior x-ray, a pure medial or lateral dislocation shows the greater sigmoid notch of the ulna in the plane of the distal humerus (Fig. 14-36).

In a pure lateral dislocation the greater sigmoid notch may articulate in the capitulotrochlear sulcus (Fig. 14-37), allowing some degree of flexion and extension. This motion may lead the unsuspecting surgeon astray in recognizing the dislocation, especially if there is considerable swelling.

Medial and lateral dislocations are reduced by countertraction on the arm, distal traction on the forearm in mild extension, and then straight medial or lateral pressure. Care should be taken to avoid converting this type into a posterior dislocation, causing further soft-tissue damage. The medial dislocation is usually a subluxation rather than a complete dislocation, and soft-tissue damage is not as extensive as in the more severe lateral dislocation. Exarchou[256] reported a lateral dislocation that required operative treatment because the anconeus muscle was interposed in the joint, blocking closed reduction.

Divergent Dislocation of the Elbow

In divergent dislocation of the elbow, a rare type of dislocation, the radius and ulna dislocate in diverging directions. Two types are seen: anteroposterior and mediolateral (transverse).

The more common anteroposterior type (Fig. 14-38) was first described by Bulley in 1841.[281] It involves a posterior dislocation of the ulna with the coronoid process lodged in the olecranon fossa. The radial head is dislocated anteriorly into the coronoid fossa. Cadaver studies demonstrated that this dislocation could be produced by forced pronation of the forearm after the medial collateral ligament had been cut. Thus, with the forearm in forced pronation and extension, the humerus is forced distally, separating the radius and ulna.[281] It can be appreciated that, in addition to rupture of the orbicular and collateral ligaments, the interosseous membrane is torn. Clinically, this type of dislocation resembles a posterior dislocation, except that the radial head is palpable in the antecubital fossa. Reduction is accomplished first by reduction of the ulna in a manner similar to reduction of a posterior dislocation. As the ulnar dislocation is being reduced, simulta-

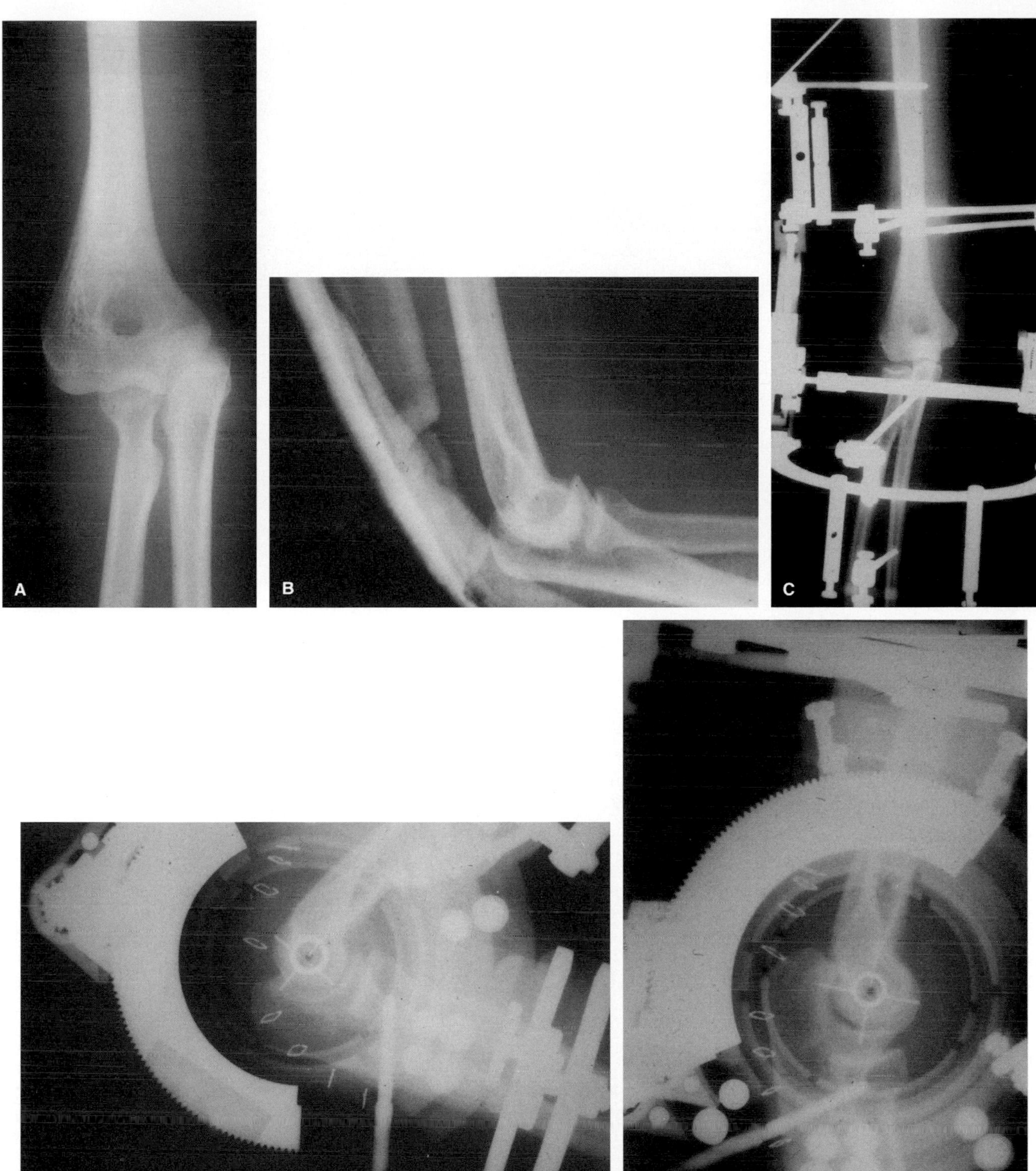

FIGURE 14-35. (**A** and **B**) A late-discovered (6 weeks) medial elbow dislocation. (**C** and **D**) After open reduction with complete exposure of joint from the medial side, a hinged external fixation was applied without ligament repair or reconstruction. (**E**) The device is well-centered on the axis of the elbow. (**F** and **G**) Motion after 18 months without instability.

continues

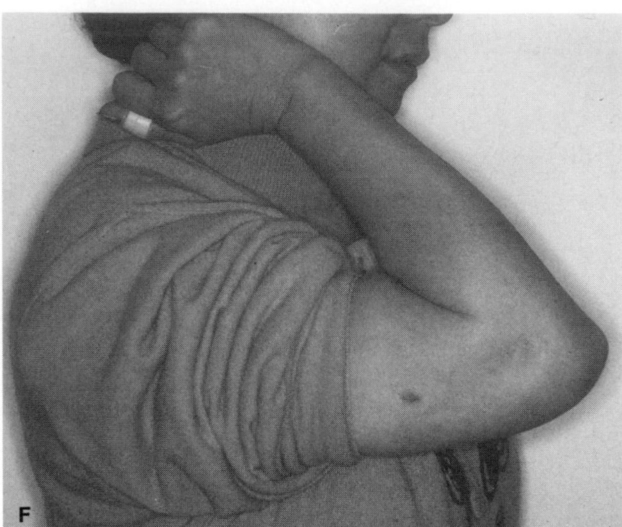

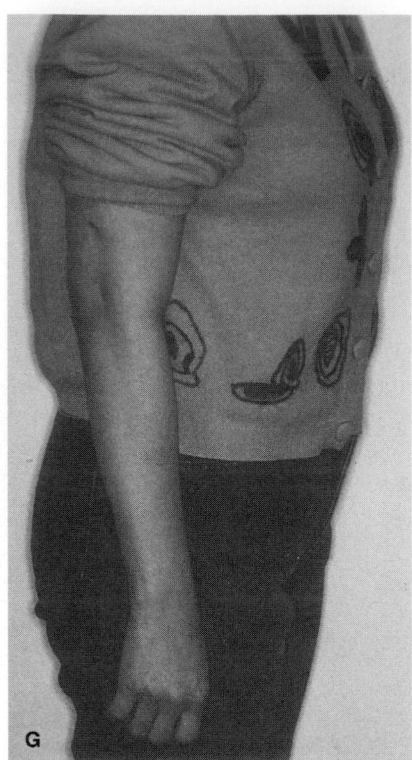

FIGURE 14-35. (continued)

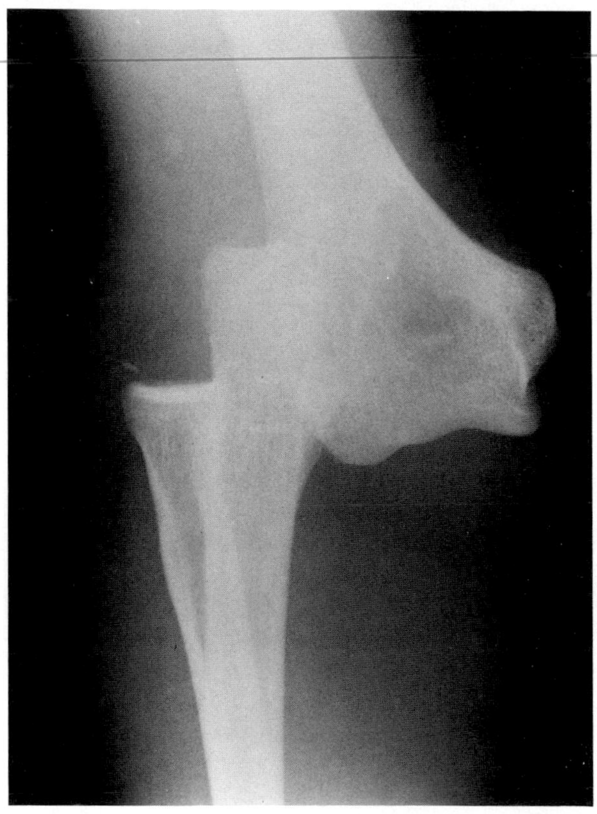

FIGURE 14-36. Anteroposterior view of a lateral dislocation in which the olecranon is completely displaced from the trochlea (This is less common than subluxation, which is shown in Fig. 14-37).

neous pressure is applied directly over the radial head to reduce it as well. Smith[279] warned that maintenance of reduction of the radial head may be difficult and may require operative intervention. Most authors recommend that after this injury the elbow should be immobilized in flexion with the forearm supinated.[250–252]

The mediolateral (transverse) type is considered by many to be so rare as to be listed as a surgical curiosity.[251,252,279] In Warmont's description of Guersant's original case in 1854, the distal humerus was found to be wedged between the radius laterally and the ulna medially.[346] This lesion should be easily recognized clinically. The elbow appears markedly widened. The articular surface of the trochlea can be palpated readily on the posterior surface of the elbow. Conwell and Reynolds[250] recommended reducing the transverse type by applying traction with the elbow in extension while pressing the proximal radius and ulna together.

Dislocation of the Ulna Alone

Isolated dislocation of the ulna can occur in either an anterior or a posterior direction. Stimson[281] described how the ulna can dislocate while the radius remains in position. The radial head serves as the pivot. The medial collateral ligament is torn, whereas the lateral collateral and orbicular ligaments remain intact. The mechanism requires a

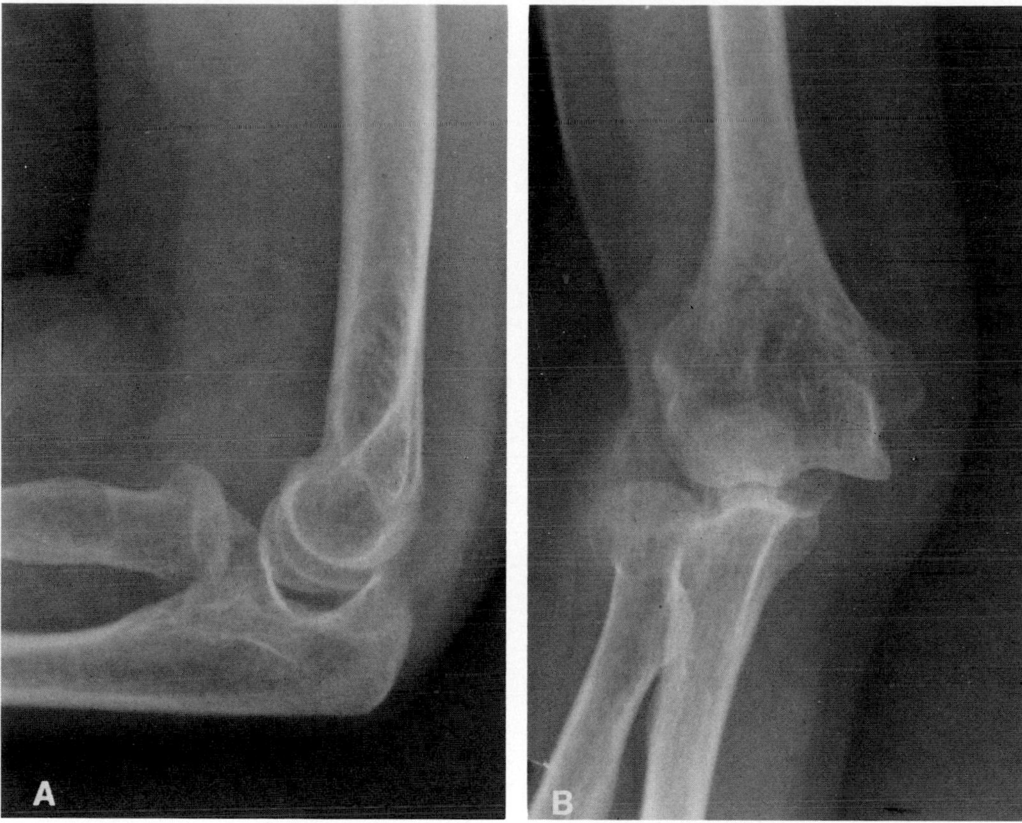

FIGURE 14-37. (**A**) Lateral view of a lateral subluxation of the elbow. The semilunar notch appears to be articulating with the distal humerus. There is no anterior or posterior displacement of the proximal ulna. (**B**) The anteroposterior view shows that the proximal radius and ulna have shifted laterally as a unit. The semilunar notch of the ulna is articulating in the capitulotrochlear sulcus. This may allow some limited flexion and extension.

combination of both angular and axial divergence of the forearm with the humerus. In normal supination with the proximal ulna secure, only the distal forearm can rotate with the radius. In this injury, proximal fixation of the ulna is lost, allowing the whole forearm, including the proximal ulna, to rotate with the radius. With adduction and posterior rotation of the forearm, the coronoid process becomes displaced posterior to the trochlea. Patients with this injury hold their elbows extended. The forearm loses its normal carrying angle and appears to be in varus. Reduction is achieved by applying traction in extension to the supinated forearm. The addition of a valgus force to the forearm facilitates the reduction.[279]

The anterior dislocation is much more rare. In this type, the ulna rotates anteriorly and the forearm is abducted. Again, the radius remains as a fixed pivot. The olecranon is carried forward and becomes locked in the coronoid fossa. Patients with this injury are said to keep the elbow flexed.[281] There is also an increase in the carrying angle. Reduction is achieved by direct pressure applied in a posterior direction over the proximal ulna while the forearm is adducted and pronated.

Dislocation of the Radial Head Alone

Isolated dislocations of the radial head are very rare. If the radial head appears to be dislocated anteriorly, a Monteggia fracture should be suspected. If the dislocation appears to be posterior, posterolateral rotatory instability (see p. 981) is a more likely prospect.[336,337]

In 1974, Wiley and coworkers[352] described two cases but provided no details other than that the direction of the dislocation was lateral. In 1982, Heidt and Stern[349] reported a posterior dislocation, discovered late, treated with radial head excision. In 1984, Burgess and Sprague[348] reported two cases of posterior subluxation after posterior radial head dislocation. In 1984, Ryu and colleagues[350] described closed reduction of an acute posterior dislocation. On the basis of these three reports, it is difficult to ascertain any single mechanism of injury or consistent method of treatment. In two of the reports,[348,349] the radius was reduced and stable in pronation, but in the other, supination was preferred.[350]

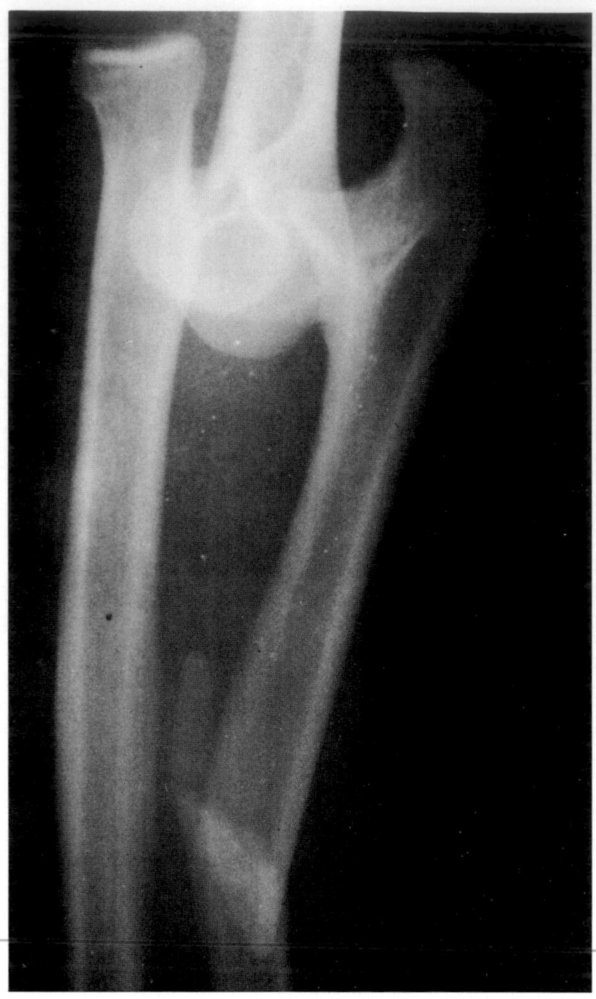

FIGURE 14-38. Anteroposterior divergent dislocation of the elbow. The ulna is dislocated posteriorly and the radius anteriorly. This patient also had a fracture of the ulna that required open reduction and internal fixation with an AO (ASIF) plate. The divergent dislocation was reduced closed, and the patient regained nearly full range of painless motion in the elbow.

Salama[351] reported anterior dislocation after a patient experienced a violent contracture after an electric shock. The dislocation was discovered late, and radial head excision was required.

The diagnosis of radial head dislocation should be made only after excluding a Monteggia fracture or congenital dislocation of the radial head. Forced pronation with impact may be the most likely mechanism of injury in isolated posterior radial head dislocation. If the injury occurs, the patient loses some pronation and supination. Dislocation of the radial head is present if a line drawn along the axis of the radial head does not pass through the center of the capitellum in any view (Fig. 14-39). It is important to distinguish isolated traumatic radial head dislocation, which is rare, from congenital dislocation of the radial head, which is more common. The adult with congenital radial head dislocation can feel pain after a fall and be reluctant to rotate the forearm as before. In addition, because of growth retardation of the radius, x-rays of the wrist will often demonstrate radioulnar inequality, mimicking acute radioulnar dissociation. However, in congenital radial head dislocation, the radial head is dome shaped and the capitellum flattened. There is no instability of the wrist and no pain or swelling of the forearm.

Recurrent Dislocation of the Elbow

Acute Recurrent Dislocation—The Grossly Unstable Elbow

Recurrent dislocation of the elbow in the acute setting usually occurs in the face of severe trauma where the radial head and coronoid process are fractured, and a widely displaced dislocation has occurred—*the terrible triad* of the elbow. The resting muscle tension, necessary for maintenance of joint coaptation, is minimal. Atonia or hypotonia of the musculature surrounding an injured joint has also been noted at the knee and shoulder. In most circumstances, the acute recurrent dislocation can be protected by increasing the position of flexion for several days as the patient regains muscle tone. Extension can be increased slowly and incrementally by using a hinged locking brace. During the first few days, redislocation can easily occur and must be suspected. X-rays should be taken at frequent intervals to ensure that the joint remains reduced during motion, especially as extension is increased.

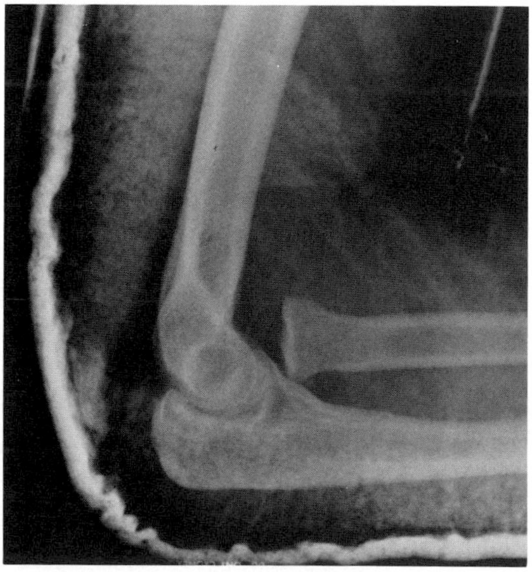

FIGURE 14-39. Anterior dislocation of the radial head. The axis of the radial head passes superior to the capitellum. In all dislocations of the radial head, a concomitant fracture of the ulna must be sought.

If these simpler measures are insufficient to maintain the reduction other measures should be considered, such as (1) internal fixation of the radial head or coronoid, (2) hinged external fixation of the elbow, and (3) prosthetic replacement of the radial head.

It is difficult to prioritize the measures listed previously in this complex injury. There are no large series of patients reported with this condition. Whatever method used, the elbow must be made stable enough to permit early motion. Pinning across the joint, even on a temporary (3 to 5 weeks) basis will usually result in stiffness and heterotopic bone formation. The minimal requirements for stability in the acute setting is sufficient muscle tendon tension and a competent ulnohumeral articulation. It may also be helpful to repair or reconstruct the medial and lateral ligaments.

Hinged external fixation may be the most important element in treatment, allowing motion without loss of a congruent reduction (see Fig. 14-35).[427] I have used this method in high-energy trauma, where all soft tissue was stripped from the joint. The hinged fixation was left in place for 8 weeks. If possible, the lateral capsule should be repaired at the time of open reduction using suture anchors into the lateral epicondyle.

The sequence of repair is also important. The joint should first be reduced and the hinged fixator applied. The sutures are placed in the lateral capsule and through the suture anchors but are not tied until after the hinge is in place. Care should also be taken to repair the lateral capsule as isometrically as possible. The medial side repair is more difficult and, in my opinion, is not always needed. Although Steinmann pins can be used to pin the joint in a reduced position, the risk of hertertopic bone and stiffness is considerable.

Chronic Recurrent Dislocation

Chronic instability of the elbow leading to recurrent dislocation is very rare after simple posterior elbow dislocation. Milch, in 1936, and Wainwright, in 1947, reported cases with recurrent instability caused by bony insufficiency of the proximal ulna, both of which were treated with an anterior bone block procedure.[335,340] Gosman reported a 15-year old with recurrent instability with hyperextensible joints, and many of the other reported cases were in children.[332,338,339] Others reported cases were in the mentally retarded or institutionalized patients.[331,334] No cases of recurrent dislocation have been reported in more recent series after simple posterior dislocation in adults.[261]

The principal pathology that leads to chronic instability and recurrent dislocation is not known. Although anatomical and biomechanical studies have recognized the importance of the anterior portion of the medial ligament, Osborne and Cotterill[338] and O'Driscoll[337] have suggested that laxity on the lateral side was the principal deficit (analogous to a Bankart lesion in anterior recurrent dislocation of the shoulder). Hassmann and colleagues[333] reported four patients, two of whom were treated with lateral advancement alone and two with both lateral and medial reconstructions. Dryer and associates[330] thought that avulsion of the brachialis and anterior capsule was contributory. Fractures of the coronoid process with displacement may also contribute to instability.

O'Driscoll and coworkers[336,337] have made the most significant contribution to elucidating the mechanism of recurrent instability and subluxation. As Osbourne and Cotterill[338] noted the importance of the lateral side clinically, O'Driscoll and colleagues[336,337] have identified the structure and pathoanatomy of the lateral ligaments. With the reconstruction of the posterolateral ligament complex using tendon graft, most patients do not experience redislocation or subluxation. It is important to rehabilitate these patients slowly as directed,[336,337] limiting supination in the early stages of therapy.

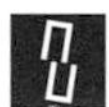

Complications and Associated Conditions of Elbow Dislocations

Associated Fractures

In the adult elbow, the coronoid process, radial head, or medial epicondyle may be fractured at the time of dislocation. In the case of radial head fractures and coronoid process fractures, the designation of one component of the injury as *primary* and the other as an *associated condition* is arbitrary. The relative incidence of associated fractures in previously reported series of elbow dislocations has ranged from 12% to 62%.[265,268,270,277,285] The most commonly recognized fracture has been that of the medial epicondyle, but this does not necessarily reflect the incidence of osteochondral fractures, which may not be recognized unless the joint is explored.[255,339]

Radial Head Fractures

Marginal radial head fractures occur frequently with posterior elbow dislocation. Often these fragments are small and are of no mechanical significance. There are other settings in which the radial head fracture requires operative attention, either excision or internal fixation. The acute stability of the elbow may depend on sufficient radial head–capitellar contact. This is especially true in cases of the *terrible triad,* in which the dislocation is accompanied by a radial head and coronoid process fracture. The subsequent section on radial head fractures provides more detail on this specific entity.

Olecranon Fractures

Fracture–dislocation of the elbow (fracture of the olecranon and anterior dislocation of the radial head) is distinctly different from a pure dislocation, and it is discussed in the section on fractures of the olecranon.

Medial Epicondyle Fracture (Entrapped)

A common pitfall of the unwary in the management of posterior dislocation of the elbow is failure to recognize an associated fracture of the medial epicondyle that becomes trapped within the joint after reduction.[273,276,278] Immediately after a closed reduction, the elbow should be taken through a full range of motion. If smooth, unrestricted motion is not possible or if there appears to be any type of mechanical block to motion, entrapment of the medial epicondyle should be suspected as the culprit. If lateral x-rays reveal the avulsed fragment to lie *at* the level of the joint, it should be assumed that the fragment lies *within* the joint.[272]

Although the entrapped medial epicondyle is more common in children, the possibility should be considered with each posterior dislocation. Failure to recognize this complication and to remove the fragment rapidly leads to severe destruction of the articular cartilage.[278]

The entrapped epicondyle can occasionally be extricated by manipulation, either by valgus stress of the forearm accompanied by supination and extension of the wrist and fingers to pull on the flexor muscles or by adduction of the elbow associated with flexion and extension movements of the elbow to express the epicondyle from the joint.[273]

Patrick[273] described a method of attempting to extricate the entrapped epicondyle by simultaneous valgus stress on the elbow and faradic stimulation of the flexor-pronator group of muscles. Usually, however, arthrotomy is necessary to remove the bone, which may then be secured to its normal location with Kirschner wires or screws. Alternatively, the bone can be excised and the common flexor origin reattached directly to bone.

Fractures of the Coronoid

Fractures of the coronoid process usually reflect severe trauma to the elbow. Although these fractures were thought to be avulsive in the past, they most likely occur due to *impact* against the trochlea of the distal humerus. The brachialis inserts much more distally than the tip of the coronoid, making avulsion less likely as a mechanism (see Fig. 14-5). Nonetheless, for larger fragments distal to the coronoid process, a significant portion of the brachialis may be attached (Fig. 14-40). Displacement of a large fragment of the coronoid has been associated with recurrent dislocation, and some authors recommend that these dislocations be immobilized in as much flexion as possible.[253,279,285]

Regan and Morrey[427] have classified, retrospectively, fractures of the coronoid into three types. Their retrospective study of patients was helpful in identifying the complexity of these fractures and the associated injuries. It is not, however, clear that the size of the fragment was the cause of instability. The fractures that sheared off the larger pieces were also associated with greater force and concomitant dislocations and fractures. Nonetheless, the presence of a significant coronoid fracture should evoke concern for acute instability requiring measures beyond simple closed treatment. (See sections on acute recurrent dislocation and radial head fractures.)

The period of immobilization should be 3 to 4 weeks, which is longer than for routine dislocations. Operative intervention appears to be limited to those fractures that interfere with joint motion. This can occur if the fragment is intra-articular or if it unites proximally and forms a significant bone block to flexion.

Ectopic Calcification and Heterotopic Bone Formation

The formation of bone around the elbow is common after trauma and surgery.[353,355,356,359–361,363,366–368] As Coventry[356] pointed out, it is important to distinguish between ectopic calcification, heterotopic bone formation (or ossification), and myositis ossificans. Unfortunately, these terms are often interchanged to describe any extra bone formed about the elbow after trauma.

Ectopic calcification is mineralization of soft-tissue structures, where calcification should not occur or is "out of place." For example, calcification of the collateral ligaments is very common after elbow dislocation[355] and presents no functional limitation and requires no treatment.

Heterotopic bone or ossification refers to the formation of trabecular bone at a location other than where it belongs.[353,356] Unlike ectopic calcification, this bone forms not necessarily by mineralizing a definable structure but by forming new bone in areas of previous hematoma and fibroblast activity. The capsule of the joint may be quite thick and lie adjacent to the heterotopic bone, but the capsule itself is not calcified. In its primitive and early state, the material is woven bone without discernable borders on x-ray. I use the term *heterotopic ossification* to refer to bone formed around the joint that is blocking motion and is, therefore, pathologic. *Myositis ossificans* is a subset of heterotopic bone formation. Myositis ossificans is a specific histopathologic condition that occurs in striated muscle, not simply around the capsule or around the joint.

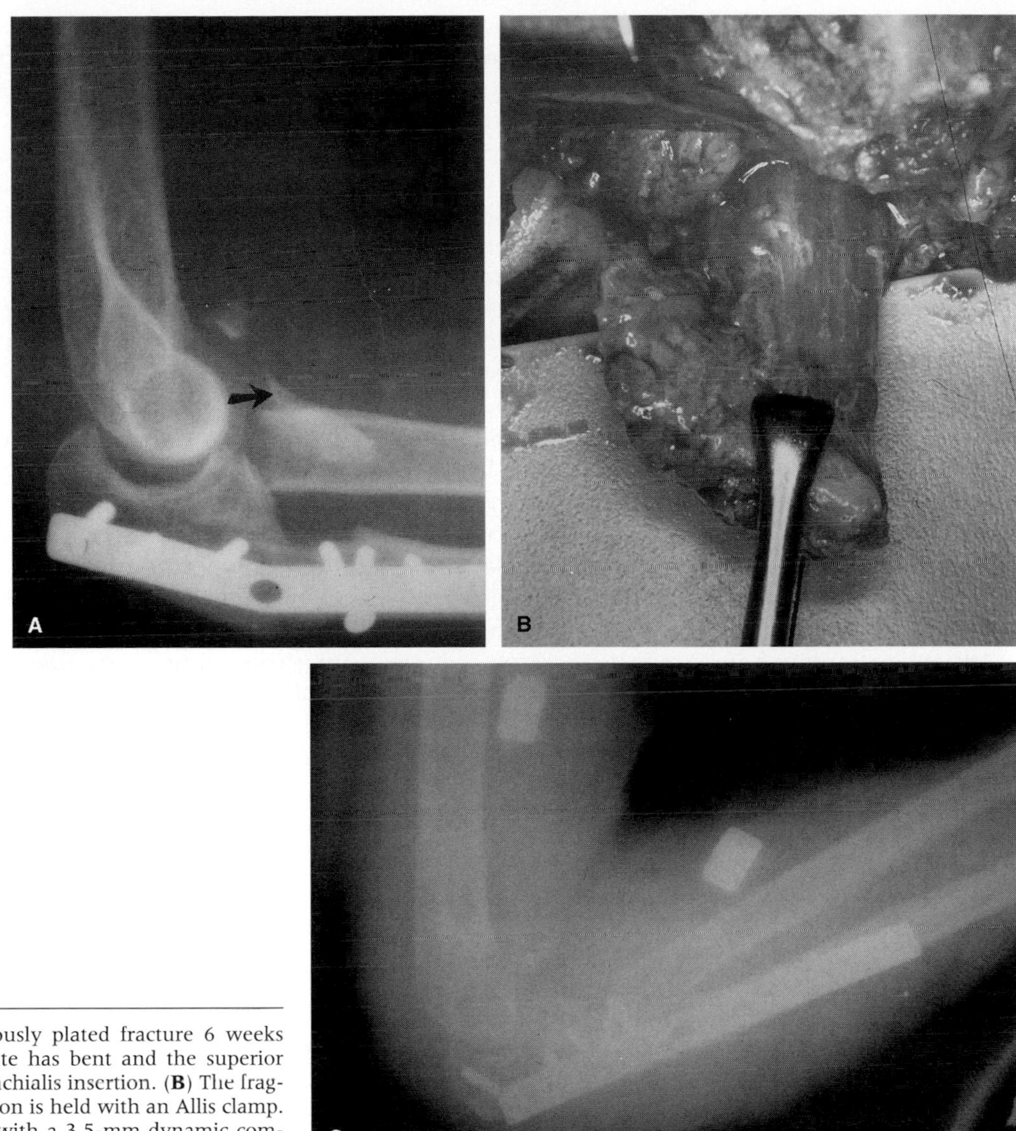

FIGURE 14-40. (**A**) A previously plated fracture 6 weeks after initial operation. The plate has bent and the superior fragment (*arrow*) carries the brachialis insertion. (**B**) The fragment with the brachialis insertion is held with an Allis clamp. (**C**) The fracture was replated with a 3.5-mm dynamic compression plate and a lag screw through the brachialis insertion

Several factors have been associated with the formation of pathologic heterotopic ossification:

Head trauma[359,360]
Burns[367]
Massive trauma
Immobilization
Ill-timed surgery?[503]
Passive mobilization?

The most important of these are head trauma and burns. Neither of these two factors is under the control of the orthopaedic surgeon. Often, the global injuries to the patients are so overwhelming that initiating motion or using indomethacin prophylaxis is out of the question. Massive trauma often leads to prolonged immobilization of the elbow (Fig. 14-41). Even attempts to move these patients early is difficult, leading to the opportunity for metaplastic differentiation of the fibroblast to an osteoblast.

Two of the factors that have been erroneously associated with heterotopic bone formation are ill-timed surgery and passive motion. Based on observations by Gaston and colleagues[475] and promulgated by McLaughlin[503] in his important book on trauma, a misconception has arisen about the role of the ill-timed surgical intervention. I have now performed over 30 operations in the past 5 years from 2 weeks to 3 months after injury and have not seen significant heterotopic bone formation (see Figs. 14-35 and 14-40). All of these patients began immediate active and gentle passive range of motion. Many were also treated with indomethacin, though compliance with taking the drug was not monitored. Undoubtedly, motion-limiting heterotopic ossification will occur frequently in patients who undergo extensive surgery after trauma and are immobilized for a sustained period of 2 or more weeks. However, there is no striking evidence that the surgery performed later than 3 days condemns a patient to heterotopic ossification. I believe it is the combination of extensive surgery and *immobilization* that leads to heterotopic ossification.

Passive mobilization does not necessarily contribute to the formation of heterotopic ossification. Several authors[370,374–376,378,380] have used passive motion after the treatment of the contracted elbow and have not noted any significant incidence. *Forceful passive manipulation,* followed by a period of immobilization would probably lead to heterotopic ossification and should be avoided. No *forceful* attempt should be made to improve motion in the weeks after injury or surgery.

For late excision of heterotopic ossification, the role of technetium bone scanning has been overemphasized. In the traumatized elbow, the bone scan will remain active in the delayed phase for many months. The maturity of the heterotopic ossification can be effectively assessed by plain x-ray or, in a few cases, by CT scans. As originally suggested by O'Brien,[364] if the bone demonstrates trabeculation and a mature rim, the heterotopic ossification can be effectively excised without undue fear of recurrence (Fig. 14-41), usually at 6 to 8 months. However, I believe motion in the postoperative period is crucial to limiting the recurrence.

Prophylaxis and Treatment. The most important factors to prevent formation of heterotopic ossification are early active motion, gentle passive mobilization, and use of indomethacin. Other treatments have been mentioned in the past, including the use of diphosphonates[354,358] and radiation.[357] I have not used either of these. Diphosphonates have not demonstrated efficacy once the medication was discontinued. Radiation, useful about the hip,[356,357] may also be useful at the elbow. Many of these patients are young, and the use of radiation, despite extremely low doses, is met with fear. Because the incidence of occurrence or recurrence has been so low using early motion and indomethacin, I have not seen fit to recommend radiation for use in injuries about the elbow.

The role of indomethacin treatment for the elbow is unknown.[356,359,360,362,365] The efficacy of postoperative administration of indomethacin has been documented in surgery about the hip.[362] Although there have been no studies with appropriate controls for injury to the elbow, I use indomethacin in all cases of late fracture reconstruction or contracture release. The dosage is 25 mg, three times a day or, for the slow-release form, 75 mg/once a day.

The duration of therapy is usually 4 to 6 weeks after operation. Several patients have been unable to tolerate the medication due to headache or gastrointestinal disturbance. Despite this, they have not demonstrated any significant formation of heterotopic ossification.

FRACTURES OF THE OLECRANON

Anatomy

The olecranon process is a large curved eminence comprising the proximal and posterior portions of the ulna. It lies in a subcutaneous position, which makes it espe-

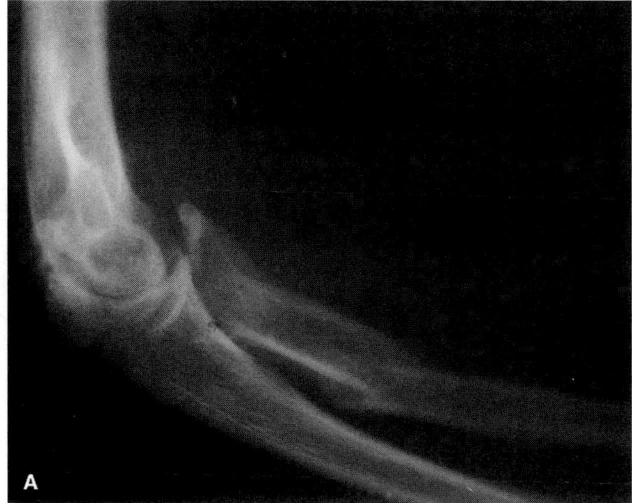

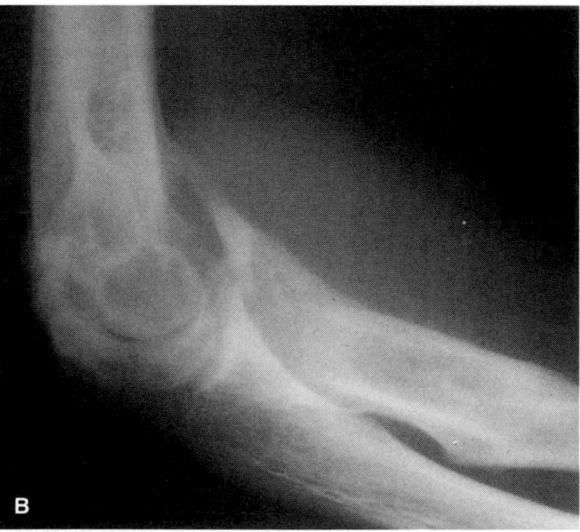

FIGURE 14-41. (**A**) Early heterotopic bone formation. (**B**) Mature heterotopic bone formation demonstrating a trabecular bone and a well-defined margin 5 months later.

cially vulnerable to direct trauma. Together with the proximal portion of the coronoid process, the olecranon forms the greater sigmoid (semilunar) notch of the ulna, a deep depression that serves as the articulation with the trochlea, which allows motion only in the anteroposterior plane and provides stability to the elbow joint. The articular cartilage surface is interrupted by a transverse line of bone, "a bare area," located midway between the tip of the olecranon and the coronoid process. If this is not recognized during reconstruction of the fractured olecranon, there is a temptation to eliminate any area uncovered by cartilage.

The ossification center for the olecranon appears at 10 years of age and is generally fused to the proximal ulna by the age of 16. There are reports of persistent physes in adults; these are usually bilateral and tend to occur in families.

This is not to be confused with patella cubiti, which is a true accessory ossicle located in the triceps tendon at its insertion into the olecranon.[415] Both of these entities may be confused with a fracture, especially if there has been local trauma. A comparison film may be helpful and prevent unneeded treatment.

Posteriorly, the triceps tendon covers the joint capsule before it inserts into the olecranon. The fascia overlying the triceps muscle spreads out medially and laterally like the retinaculum of the quadriceps in the knee. These expansions and the triceps aponeurosis insert into the deep fascia of the forearm and into the periosteum of the olecranon and proximal ulna. When using the Bryan-Morrey approach, this relationship need to be understood.[86]

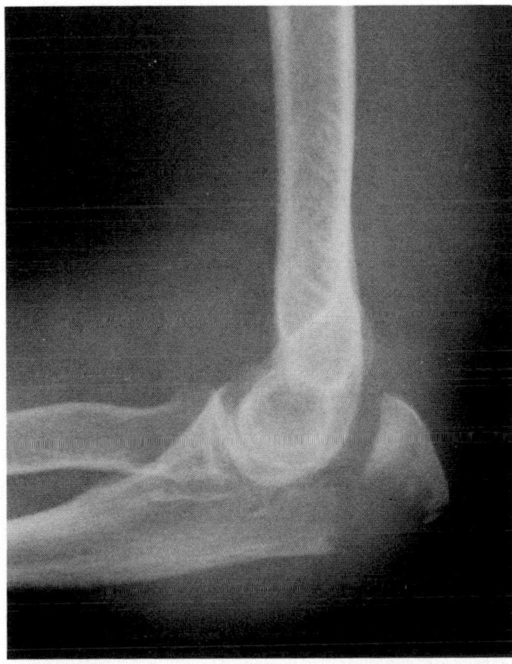

FIGURE 14-42. Fracture of the olecranon. Note the comminution and disruption of the articular surface; a true lateral view is necessary to visualize this adequately. The pull of triceps tendon is the displacing force on the proximal fragment.

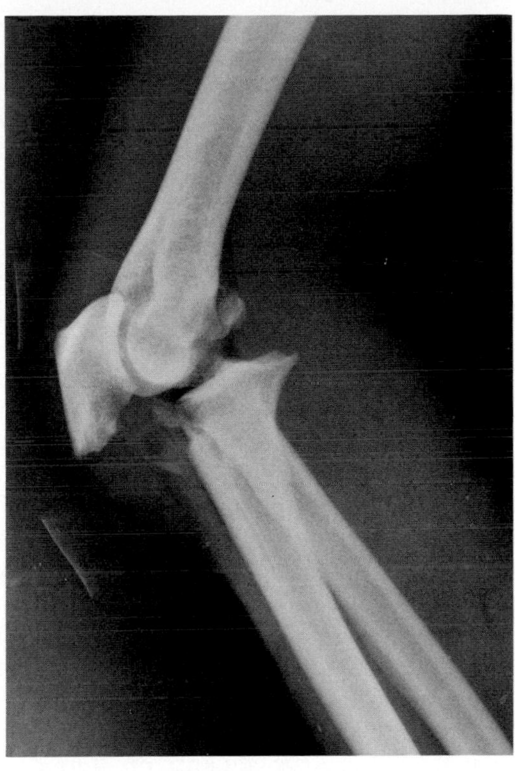

FIGURE 14-43. Fracture–dislocation of the elbow (fracture of the olecranon and anterior dislocation of the radius and ulna).

Mechanism of Injury

Fractures of the olecranon probably occur in response to direct impact at the posterior surface of the elbow and to falls on the upper limb that indirectly load the joint.[386,395,426,428,439,441] Undoubtedly, muscle–tendon tension, both resting and active, creates forces that determine the fracture pattern and displacement (Fig. 14-42).

In cases of extreme violence to the elbow, the proximal olecranon fragment often displaces posteriorly, whereas the distal ulnar fragment, together with the head of the radius, may displace anterior to the humerus, resulting in the so-called fracture–dislocation (Fig. 14-43). A fracture–dislocation is far more serious than the isolated olecranon fracture, and persistent or recurrent deformity is likely to occur if the olecranon is not stabilized adequately.

Signs and Symptoms

Because all fractures of the olecranon process have some intra-articular component, there is generally a hemorrhagic effusion of the elbow joint. This results in swelling and pain over the olecranon.[386] There may also be a palpable sulcus at the fracture site, accompanied by a painful and limited range of motion.

Inability to extend the elbow actively against gravity is the most important sign to be elicited; it indicates discontinuity of the triceps mechanism. The presence or absence of this sign often determines the plan of treatment of these fractures. A careful neurologic evaluation should be done, because ulnar nerve injuries may accompany fractures of the olecranon, especially in the extensively comminuted fracture that results from direct trauma.[433]

Radiographic Findings

Probably the most common pitfall in the initial evaluation of a fracture of the olecranon is failure to insist on a true lateral x-ray of the elbow. The slightly oblique view, which is frequently obtained in the emergency department, is inadequate to identify precisely the extent of the fracture, the degree of comminution, the amount of disruption of the articular surface in the semilunar notch, and any displacement of the radial head, if present. An anteroposterior x-ray is also important to delineate a fracture line in the sagittal plane. If the radial head is also fractured, significant shortening along this fracture line can occur without angular displacement in the lateral view.

Classification

The classification of fractures of the olecranon has been attempted by several groups.[390,391,406,409] Each of these schemes has merit, but none of these necessarily guide treatment and the proper selection of internal fixation.

Colton's classification[391] can be simplified to reflect displacement and the shape of the fracture:

I. Nondisplaced and stable
II. Displaced
    A. Avulsion fractures
    B. Transverse fractures
    C. Comminuted fractures
    D. Fracture/dislocations

To be considered nondisplaced and stable, the fractures must be displaced less than 2 mm, exhibit no change in position with gentle flexion to 90° with extension against gravity. Displaced fractures must be treated operatively.

Avulsion Fractures

A transverse fracture line separates a small proximal fragment of the olecranon process from the rest of the ulna. This fracture is most common in elderly patients.[426,430,434,444]

Oblique and Transverse Fractures

The fracture line runs obliquely, starting near the deepest part of the semilunar notch and running dorsally and distally to emerge on the subcutaneous crest of the proximal part of the ulna. This fracture may be a single oblique line, or it may have an element of comminution caused by a fracture in the sagittal plane or a central area of depression in the articular surface.

Comminuted Fractures

This group includes all the severely comminuted fractures of the olecranon, which usually result from direct trauma to the posterior aspect of the elbow. There are multiple fracture planes, often with severe crushing of many fragments. There may be associated fractures of the distal end of the humerus, the shafts of the forearm bones, or the head of the radius.

Fracture–Dislocations

The olecranon fracture is at or near the level of the tip of the coronoid process, so that a plane of instability is located through the fracture site and the radiohumeral joint as well, resulting in an anterior dislocation of the ulna and radius.[426,430,434,444] This fracture is usually secondary to a severe injury, such as a blow to the posterior aspect of the elbow. Most often, the configuration of this particular fracture requires plate fixation rather than tension-band wire methods.

Methods of Treatment

The historical treatment of fractures of the olecranon has run the gamut from early range of motion of the elbow without regard for the fracture[399,426] to precise and open anatomical reduction of the fracture site.[385,386,389–391,397,398,405,406,408,409,412,414,417,420]

Olecranon fractures were mentioned only occasionally in the very early treatises on fracture treatment. Before the era of aseptic surgery, these fractures were splinted in full extension for 4 to 6 weeks.[410] This usually resulted in a stiff elbow with loss of flexion and was the prime reason that early practitioners slowly began to use the position of mid-flexion.[396] This frequently led to nonunion of the olecranon because of separation of fracture fragments, resulting in decreased power of the triceps mechanism.[426]

In 1894, Sachs[399] reported excellent results with rapid restoration of function by dispensing with any form of splinting, allowing the arm to hang in extension, and instituting early massage. After 2 weeks, active movements were started; Sachs reported that full function returned in 6 weeks. This article was written before the discovery of roentgenography, and most of these cases probably represented fibrous union with resultant decreased strength of the olecranon. However, Eliot[399] reported rapid return to relatively normal flexion and extension of the elbow after this treatment regimen, regardless of whether fibrous or bony union resulted. In 1933, Daland[395] presented the first substantial series of olecranon fractures, in which he delineated the signs and symptoms and first recognized the need for accurate reduction of any displaced fracture.

Watson-Jones[439] believed that reduction by closed manipulation could often be achieved with the elbow in full extension with firm pressure over the fragment. He believed that conservative treatment was justified only if the position was accurate. Immobilization was continued for 5 weeks. He noted also that full flexion would be delayed for a year and that the elbow frequently required gentle manipulation at intervals for maximum return.

Nondisplaced Fractures

Most authors believe that nondisplaced fractures as defined previously are best treated by immobilization in a long-arm cast with the elbow in 45° to 90° of flexion for a short time.[383,386] The elbow should not be placed in full extension for immobilization because stiffness is likely and because, in general, if a fracture is not stable in partial flexion, it will not be stable in full extension.[396]

A follow-up x-ray should be obtained within 5 to 7 days after cast application to make certain that displacement has not occurred. Union of bone is usually not complete for 6 to 8 weeks, but generally there is adequate stability at 3 weeks to remove the cast and allow protected range-of-motion exercises, avoiding flexion past 90° until bone healing is complete radiographically. In elderly patients, the period of immobilization should be even less than 3 weeks. A sling can be used for a few days until the patient is comfortable enough to begin active range of motion of the elbow.[425]

Displaced Fractures

Open reduction and internal fixation or primary excision has generally become accepted as the treatment of choice for displaced fractures of the olecranon.[385,386,389–391,397,398,405,406,408,409,412,414,417,420] There are several disadvantages of nonoperative treatment:

1. Failure to reduce the fracture may allow it to heal in an elongated position by means of a fibrous union; this shortens the distance between the origin and insertion of the triceps muscle, which effectively decreases its power of extension.[426]
2. Articular incongruity secondary to inadequate reduction can lead to post-traumatic arthritis.[400,443]
3. A displaced olecranon fragment can block full extension of the elbow joint.[344,426]
4. Immobilization in full extension for a period sufficient to allow bone healing frequently results in failure to regain flexion of the elbow.

Despite these factors, Perkins[426] and Rowe[430] both suggested conservative treatment of displaced olecranon fractures in elderly patients because the loss of full extension and the decreased triceps power are not important in this age group. Rowe[430] stated that simple sling immobilization is all that is needed in these patients.

In an active patient, the aims of treatment of displaced fractures of the olecranon are (1) to maintain power of extension of the elbow, (2) to avoid incongruity of the articular surface, (3) to restore stability of the elbow, and (4) to prevent stiffness of the joint. To achieve this final, and perhaps most important, goal, any mode of internal fixation selected should, ideally, allow the patient to resume protected range of motion reasonably soon after open reduction.

Internal Fixation

The dilemma of nonunion versus stiffness led Lister in 1884 to choose the fracture of the olecranon to be the first fracture treated by open reduction and internal fixation using his method of antisepsis.[410] Lister provided fixation of the fragment with a wire loop (Fig. 14-44). This method of treatment was modified somewhat as the wire was placed in the form of a ring by Berger in 1902[387] and was later adopted by Böhler in 1929.[388] Modifications of this technique, which was the forerunner of the tension-band wiring technique advocated by the AO group, are now in use.[396,422]

Multiple methods of internal fixation have been proposed for olecranon fractures. The mechanical advantage that exists in favor of the triceps pull on the small proximal fragment dictates the need for strong internal fixation to prevent displacement of the fracture postoperatively[428] The surgical principles used in the internal fixation of olecranon futures include the following:[443]

1. Realignment of the longitudinal axis of the olecranon as accurately as possible and with sufficient stability to allow early controlled motion
2. Preservation of an adequately large coronoid process to form the distal limit of the articular surface
3. Anatomical restoration of the articular surface of the olecranon with the use of cancellous bone grafts to fill in defects in the articular surface

After internal fixation of the fracture, exact surgical repair of the medial and lateral triceps expansion is essential for a good result.

Biomechanics. Two studies[403,424] have attempted to compare the mechanical stability of methods of internal fixation for olecranon fractures. Fyfe and colleagues[403] tested stiffness of the configuration. Based on that criterion, the two-knot tension-band technique, as described in the AO technique manual,[422] was optimal. The one-third tubular plate was also quite

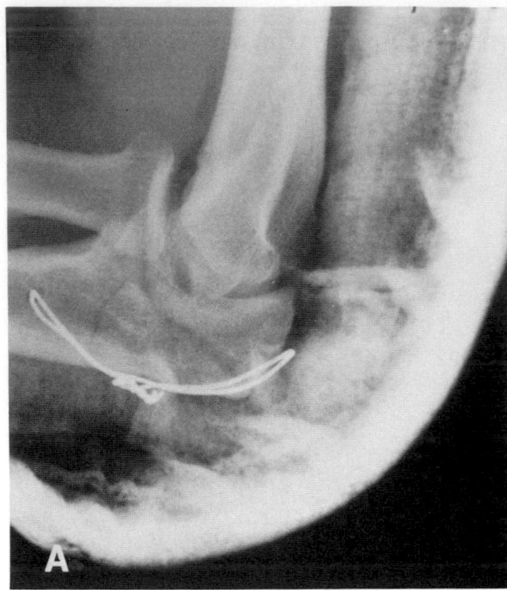

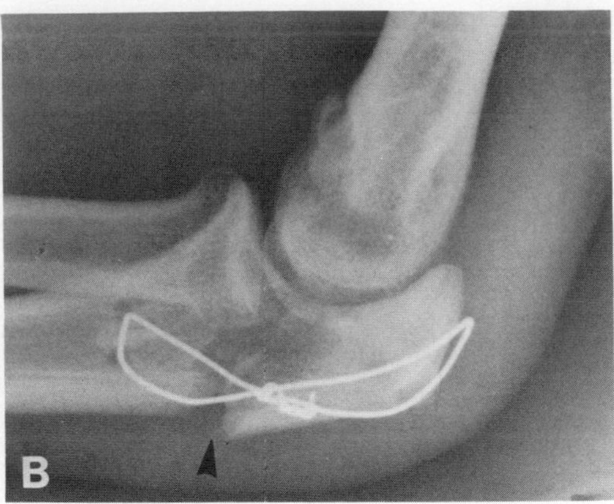

FIGURE 14-44. (**A**) Good approximation of a large olecranon fragment by means of a figure-of-eight wire. (**B**) Two months later there is considerable displacement at the fracture site (*arrow*), indicating inadequate fixation by the wire.

rigid and optimal in fractures with simulated comminution. Clinically, however, this plate may lack enough rigidity to sustain the reduction during motion (see Fig. 14-40). Murphy and colleagues[424] used a rapid tension method of testing, measuring energy-to-failure, and concluded that the tension-band wiring according to the AO technique[422] and the combination of a 6.5-mm cancellous screw with tension-band wire were essentially equal and optimal. They did not test one-third tubular plate fixation. The method of testing in both of these studies did not include *fatigue analysis,* which is probably the most common mode of failure of any fixation device.

Internal Suture. Rombold[429] was the first to publish a description of the use of the fascial strip suture to repair displaced olecranon fractures. In 1969, Bennett[386] also recommended the use of a fascial strip for internal fixation to avoid the use of metallic internal fixation and its inherent problems. Approximation of the fragments has been attempted with a variety of materials, including fascia, wire, catgut, and nonabsorbable suture.[386,394,410,413,429,440] In general, these do not provide true internal fixation that is rigid enough to allow early motion, and their use is not recommended.

Intramedullary Fixation. Fixation of displaced olecranon fractures by the use of an intramedullary screw was introduced by MacAusland in 1942.[417] Many types of intramedullary devices have also been used, including Rush rods,[432] cancellous (wood) screws,[417,428] large threaded Steinmann pins,[405] and several types of screws designed especially for olecranon fractures (Fig. 14-45).[393,405] The Leinbach screw, which is long enough to gain adequate purchase in the distal fragment, has been known to break at the shank-screw junction. Indeed, Rettig and colleagues[428] reported that 50% of patients in whom a malleable screw was used had significant complications. Therefore, if an intramedullary screw is used, these authors recommended that it be long enough to obtain purchase in the medullary canal of the distal ulna and strong enough to resist breakage. They suggested a rigid cancellous compression screw for this purpose.[428] McAtee[393] designed a special compression screw that provides stable internal fixation and permits early range of motion. Johnson and coworkers[412] treated 16 patients with an intramedullary 6.5-mm cancellous AO (ASIF) screw with good results. They also emphasized the importance of a screw of sufficient length to engage the distal intramedullary canal for adequate fixation.

Bicortical Screw Fixation. In 1969, Taylor and Scham[435] described a modified method of screw fixation for fractures of the olecranon. They advocated its use particularly in transverse and oblique fractures, which occur most frequently at or near the junction of the olecranon and the coronoid processes. Their method uses a posteromedial surgical approach, which allows direct visualization not only of the fracture site but also of the coronoid process. A cortical bone screw is passed from the posterior tip of the olecranon obliquely to engage the anterior cortex of the coronoid process near the sublime tubercle (near the insertion of the medial collateral ligament) (Fig. 14-46). Wadsworth[437] designed a special screw to obtain this type of bicortical fixation of olecranon fractures. The strong internal fixation achieved with this method allows active range of motion by the patient within 10 to 14 days after operation.

Tension-Band Wiring. Tension-band wiring, a method of internal fixation developed by the AO group,[406,414,422] differs significantly in technique and principle from con-

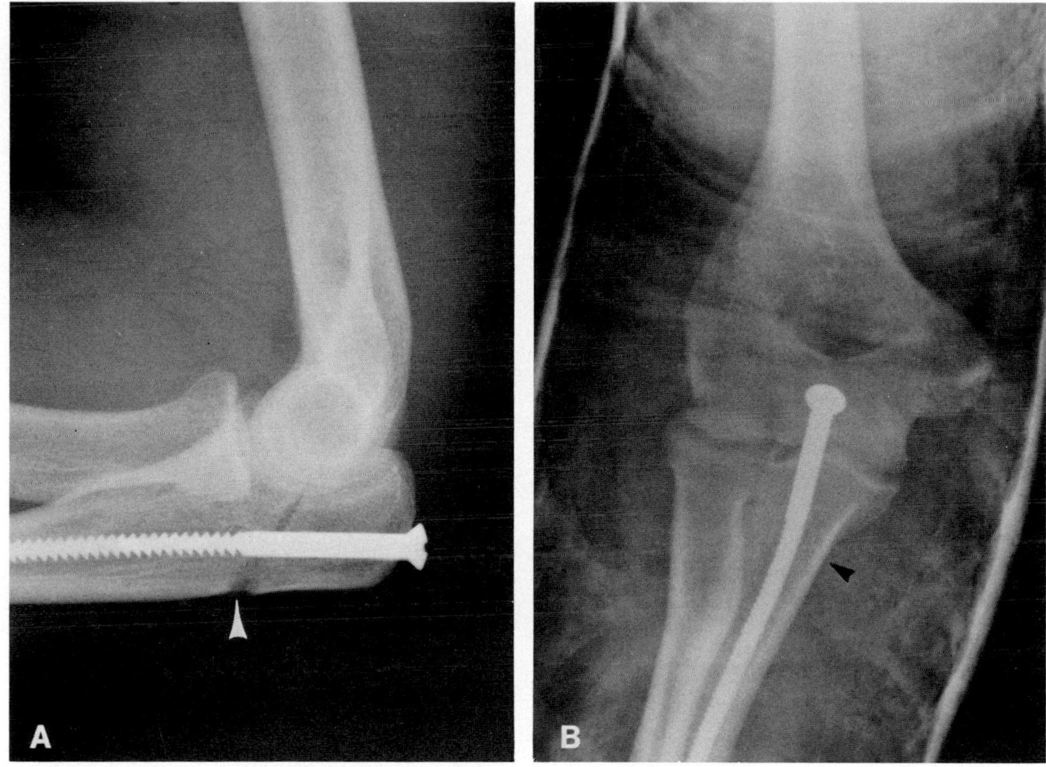

FIGURE 14-45. (**A**) An olecranon fracture transfixed with a Leinbach screw. Note the proximity of the fracture site and the junction of the thread and shank of the screw (*arrow*). (**B**) The anteroposterior view shows angulation of the threaded portion of the screw in the medullary canal (*arrow*). Breakage of the screw at the point of angulation and loss of fixation are likely.

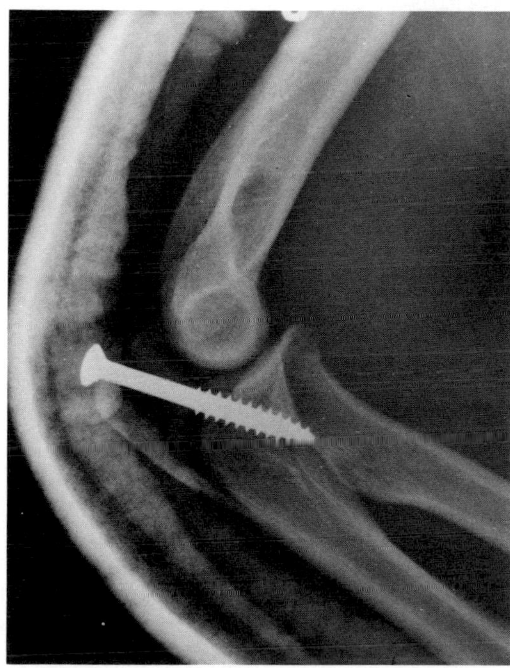

FIGURE 14-46. Bicortical fixation of an olecranon fracture. In this case, the threads of the screw cross the fracture site, which is undesirable unless the proximal fragment is overdrilled to give a lag effect.

ventional cerclage wiring. It is particularly useful in treatment of avulsion fractures. The basic principle is to counteract the tensile forces that act across the fracture site and convert them into compressive forces. To accomplish this, the wire is passed in figure-of-eight fashion around the insertion of the triceps tendon and then distally beyond the fracture site into a transverse drill hole on the posterior (subcutaneous) border of the olecranon (Fig. 14-47). Improved alignment and greater stability can be provided by introducing two parallel Kirschner wires across the fracture site before applying the tension band.[389,390,396,406,420,422] It might seem that this posterior position of the wire would cause the fracture site to gape at the articular surface in the semilunar notch. At the time of operation this may occur, but the counterpressure of the trochlea under tension by the triceps muscle causes a compression force across the fracture site sufficiently strong to allow immediate active range of motion.[406] As an alternative, Rowland[431] has suggested placing the tension-band wire volar to the long axis and longitudinal pins. A modification of this technique in which both limbs of the figure-of-eight are twisted has been introduced to allow the wire to be tightened from both sides of the fracture and thereby achieve equal compression.[390,396,406,414]

Several authors have reported problems associated with wire protrusion and pain after tension-band wir-

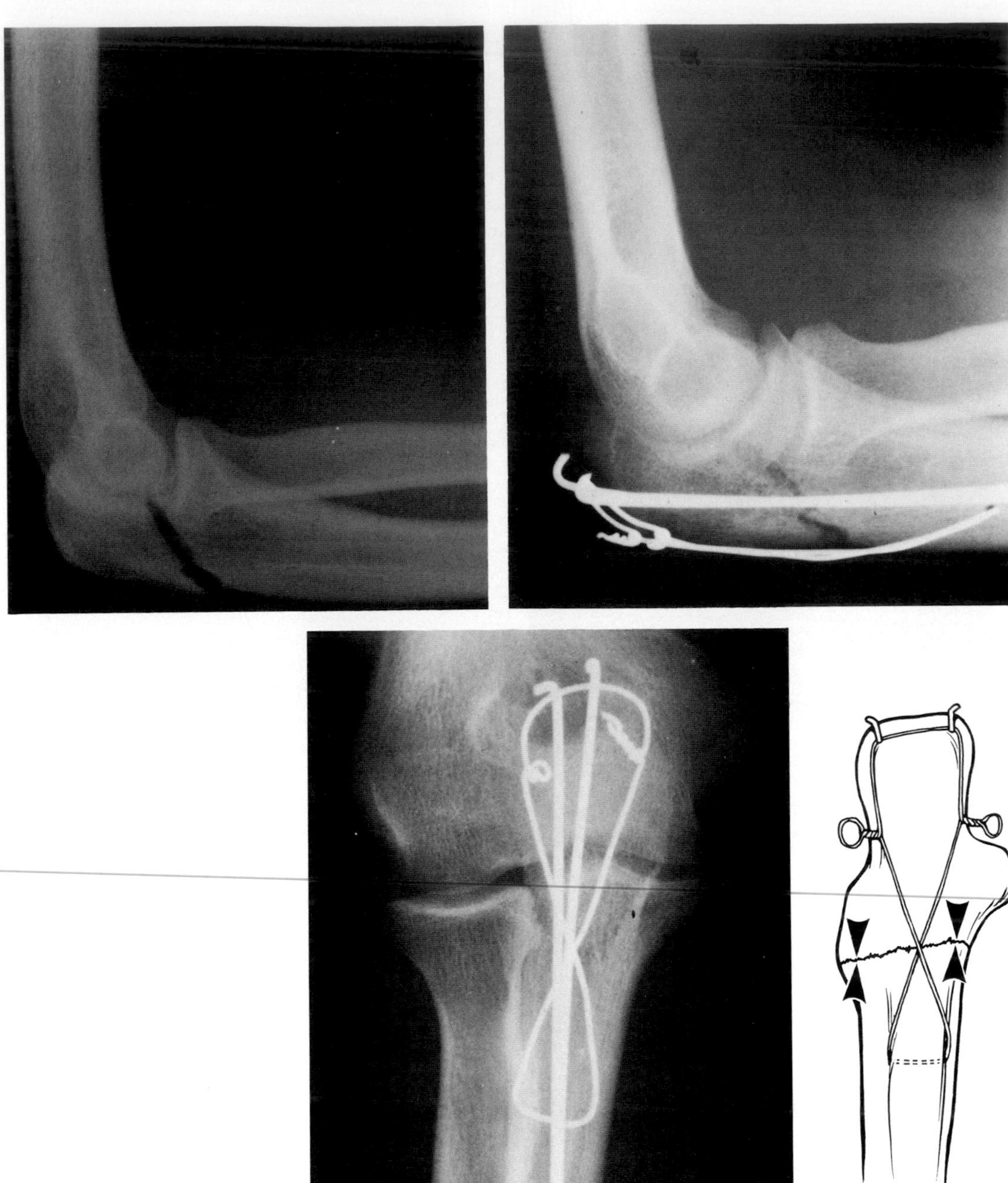

FIGURE 14-47. (**Top left**) Oblique fracture of the olecranon. (**Top right**) Open reduction and internal fixation using the AO tension band wiring method of fixation. (**Bottom**) Anteroposterior view demonstrating a modification of the tension band wiring technique in which both limbs of the figure-of-eight wire are twisted. This permits the wire to be tightened on both sides of the fracture to achieve equal compression (note the *arrows*).

ing.[401,411,419,445] Macko and Szabo[419] noted that patients had pain even without proximal migration of the pins. Most authors have emphasized the importance of placing the tension wire deep to the triceps and curling the longitudinal pins so that they are embedded in bone. Even with these measures, many patients require hardware removal.

Murphy and associates[423] reported the use of a 6.5-mm cancellous screw with tension-band wiring in ten patients. In this series, there were fewer complications with prominent hardware as compared with the use of Kirschner wires at the same institution, although removal was still necessary in some.

Zuelzer Plate. In 1951, Zuelzer first reported the use of a hook plate for fixation of fractures in which one small fragment was separated from the principal part of the bone.[446] This device has since been recommended for fixation of olecranon fractures.[396,442] Wesley and colleagues[442] reported uniformly good results regardless of the degree of comminution, obliquity of the fracture, or age of the patient. They believed that the advantage of the Zuelzer plate over the tension-band wiring technique was that it did not require supplemental fixation, which is often needed when tension-band wiring is applied to comminuted olecranon fractures.

AO Plate. A one-third tubular plate can be a very useful implant in cases of comminution or oblique longitudinal fractures.[403,406] Where there is comminution with bone loss, the tension-band technique tends to compress and shorten the olecranon. With the use of the plate posteriorly (Fig. 14-48) or on the posterolateral border, adequate rigidity can usually be achieved with restoration of the anatomy. Bone grafting to compensate for bone loss can also be incorporated with the construct.

Since the introduction of the 3.5-mm reconstruction plate, some have found this implant to be a more reliable and more versatile than the one-third tubular plate. The 3.5-mm plate can be placed directly posteriorly or along the lateral face of the ulna, depending on the specific needs of the fracture configuration.

Excision. Excision of the proximal fragment and repair of the triceps tendon for a fractured olecranon (Fig. 14-49) was first suggested by Fiolle[402] in 1918. Dunn,[398] in 1939, and Wainwright,[438] in 1942, each described several cases using this technique; excellent results were reported. Excision of the proximal fragment and triceps repair were popularized in the United States by McKeever and Buck[421] in a classic article in 1947. Their indications for this method of treatment

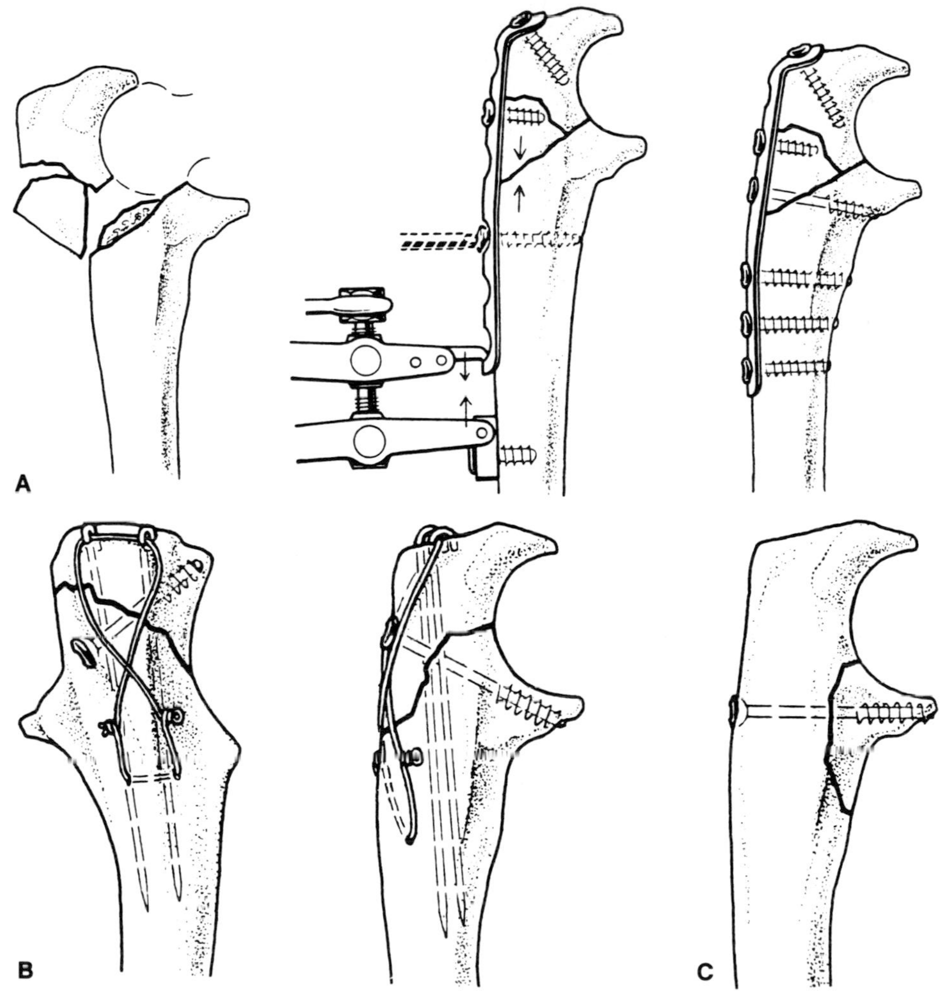

FIGURE 14-48. (**A**) Plate fixation can be used to stabilize comminuted fractures of the proximal ulna. (**B**) A combination of screws and wires can also be used. (**C**) Lag screw fixation of the coronoid may be crucial to stability if the fracture is associated with elbow dislocation. *(Heim, U., and Pfeiffer, K.M.: Internal Fixation of Small Fractures, 3rd ed. Berlin, Springer-Verlag, 1988.)*

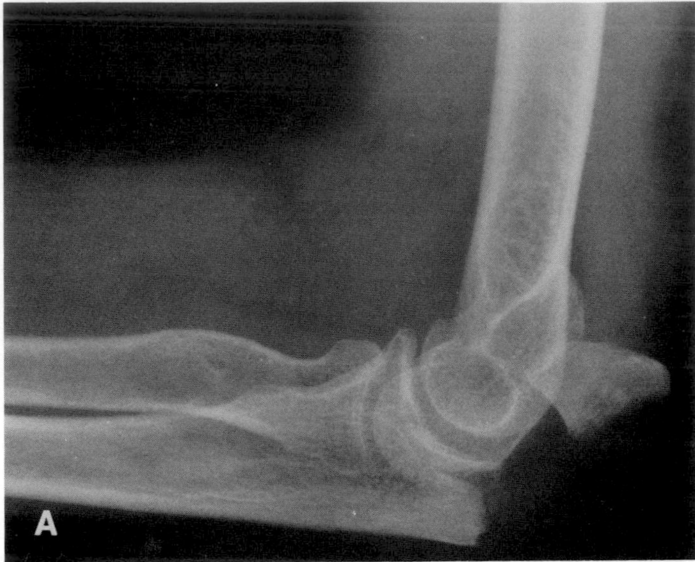

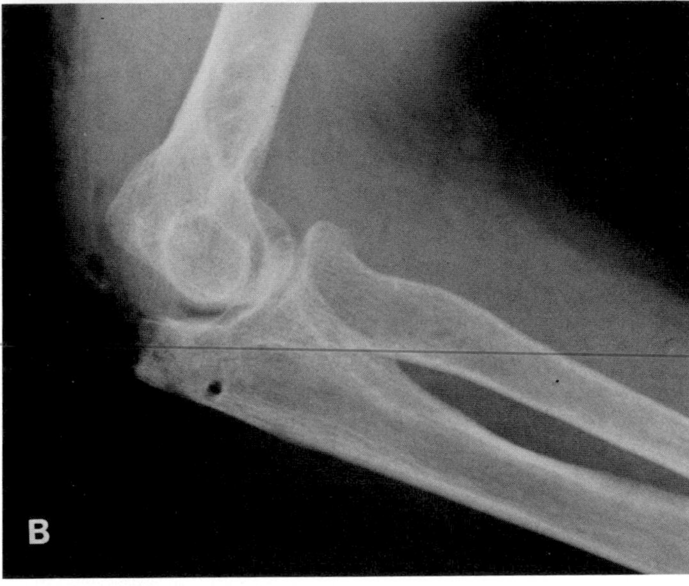

FIGURE 14-49. Fracture of the olecranon with rotation of the proximal fragment. (**A**) Lateral view shows wide retraction of the proximal fragment with the elbow in flexion. (**B**) This patient was treated by primary resection of the olecranon fragment and reattachment of the triceps tendon.

in olecranon fractures were (1) old nonunited fractures, (2) extensively comminuted fractures, (3) fractures in elderly persons, and (4) any fracture that did not involve the trochlear notch. They were the first to investigate and substantiate the idea that instability of the elbow joint does not result as long as the coronoid process and distal surface of the semilunar notch of the ulna remain intact. They stated that as much as 80% of the olecranon can be removed without danger of producing instability of the elbow joint.[392,421] Lou[416] later reported good results with this technique if the excised fragment was small.

MacAusland and Wyman[418] studied fractures of the olecranon extensively, with particular attention to excising the proximal fragments.[383,384] On the basis of these studies, they made several useful points, as follows, regarding excision of the olecranon:

1. Much of the olecranon process can be excised as long as the coronoid and anterior soft tissues are intact.
2. The triceps tendon should be securely reattached to the distal fragment with nonabsorbable sutures; wire is not recommended, because motion of the elbow will cause it to break.[385]
3. Excision is indicated only for isolated fractures of the olecranon. If there is evidence of damage to the anterior structures of the elbow (ie, if there is anterior dislocation of the radial head and shaft of the ulna—a fracture–dislocation of the elbow), primary excision should be considered as contraindicated. If the fragment, with the attachment of the triceps, is excised, stability of the entire joint would be much harder to maintain.

MacAusland further pointed out that occasionally during attempted internal fixation, comminution of the olecranon proves more extensive than was initially anticipated, and the surgeon's inability to achieve rigid internal fixation becomes apparent. In such cases, he believes it is better to admit defeat, as it were, and primarily excise the olecranon rather than persist, achieving poor fixation and an unstable repair.[384,418]

The advantages of excision are that it is an easy and rapid procedure and it eliminates the possibility of delayed or nonunion and post-traumatic arthritis.[383,384,386,409,421,436] The disadvantages of excision are said to be triceps weakness, elbow instability, and loss of elbow motion.[386,407,409,417] However, Rettig and colleagues[428] found elbow motion to be equal after internal fixation or excision. In addition, Gartsman and associates[404] found range of motion, elbow stability, and strength to be equal in patients who underwent open reduction compared with those who underwent excision. However, patients who underwent internal fixation had a much higher incidence of postoperative complications.

During excision, it is important to retain the insertion of the collateral ligaments for stability. The triceps tendon should also be sutured to the remaining bone flush with the articular surface and not to its original insertion point.[390]

 Author's Preferred Method of Treatment

Nondisplaced and Stable Fractures. For nondisplaced and stable fractures, a somewhat rare combination, the elbow can be splinted at 90° for approximately a week, to allow pain and swelling to diminish. At that point, gentle active flexion and extension exercises can be begun in a supervised environment. All of these fractures should be carefully followed for any sign of displacement during the early weeks of treatment. X-rays at 1 week, 2 weeks, and 4 weeks are mandatory.

Avulsion Fractures. These fractures are usually amenable to tension-band wiring. Because the fracture was caused by an avulsive force, no comminution should be present. The fracture fragment may be too small to accept a long screw as part of the tension band construct. In these cases, Kirschner wires should be used. For larger fragments, the combination of the screw and wire work well.[424]

Excision of the fragment with reattachment of the triceps tendon can also be used. Usually there is still some attachment of the triceps, overlying the displaced fracture fragment. The triceps can be sutured to the remaining tendon as well as into the distal tip with suture anchors as needed.

Transverse Fractures Without Comminution. Pure transverse fractures without comminution are ideally suited to tension-band wiring. The patient is positioned in the operating room with the affected side up in an semi-lateral position. This permits a posterior exposure of the elbow, over the patient's chest. In these cases it is usually helpful to incise the superficial aponeurotic expansion of the overlying fascia, taking care to maintain the triceps insertion in the proximal segment.

The fracture can generally be reduced by extending the elbow and holding the fracture together temporarily by reduction clamps. Longitudinal incisions in the triceps are needed to attain the needed exposure for the Kirschner wires. Where the fragment is large enough, a single 6.5-mm cancellous screw with washer may be used to secure the longitudinal component of the fracture reduction. If the fragment is too small, the screw can further fragment the proximal piece. If in doubt, two Kirschner wires work well, as detailed in Figure 14-48.

Transverse Fractures with Comminution. Transverse fractures with comminution may require plate fixation, depending on the configuration. With comminution, the tension-band technique will by its very nature collapse the fragments together. Some collapse (or shortening) is tolerable. However, if the width of the olecranon articulation narrows significantly, the joint will not track properly, leading to impingement or loss of motion. A combination of techniques may also be helpful, using longitudinal wires and a supplementary plate (Fig. 14-50). Iliac bone grafting should also be considered to fill in any gaps. I will also use a bicortical segment to fill the gap created by the comminution. The cortical bone of the iliac graft resists collapse.

Oblique Fractures With and Without Comminution. Although the use of tension-band techniques can occasionally be used with these fractures, it is important to recognize that a plate with lag screw fixation is preferable. If the two fracture fragments have no interdigitating spikes (see Fig. 14-47), compression along the tension band may displace the fracture, shortening along the inclined plane of the obliquity. In this circumstance, a reconstruction plate (3.5 mm) with lag screws across the fracture will provide better stability. As shown by the AO group (see Fig. 14-48), a one-third tubular plate can be used if soft-tissue coverage is a problem. The problem with this plate is fatigue failure (see Fig. 14-40). The increased thickness of the pelvic reconstruction plate may make the wound closure more difficult, especially if the plate is placed in a purely dorsal position. If the plate is placed along the lateral face of the ulna, wound closure is less of a challenge.

Any comminution present makes tension-band techniques even more undesirable. In this setting, bone graft and plating provide a more stable con-

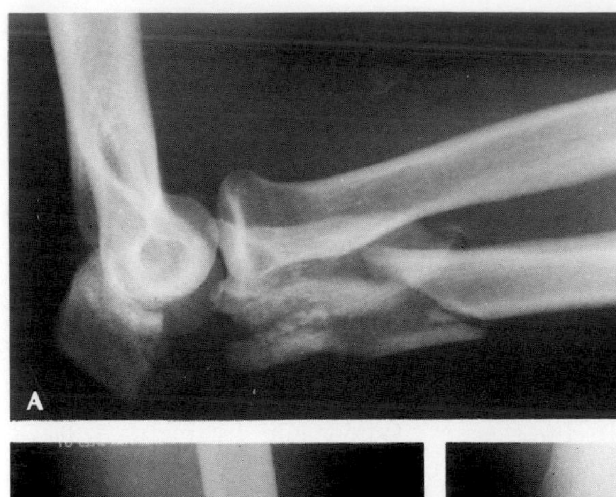

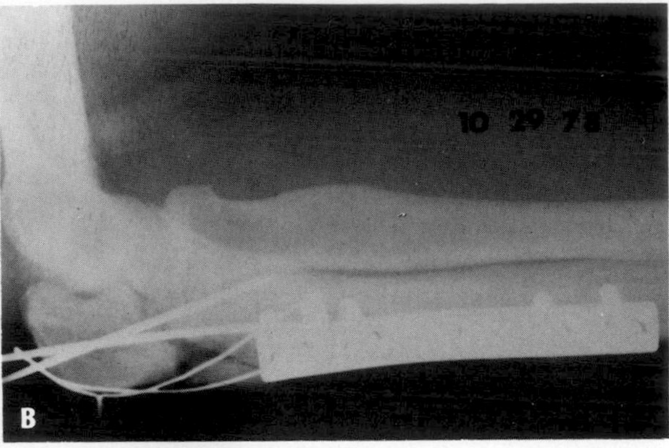

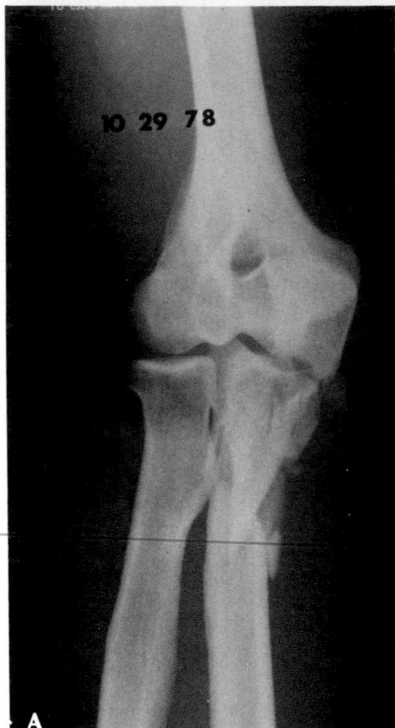

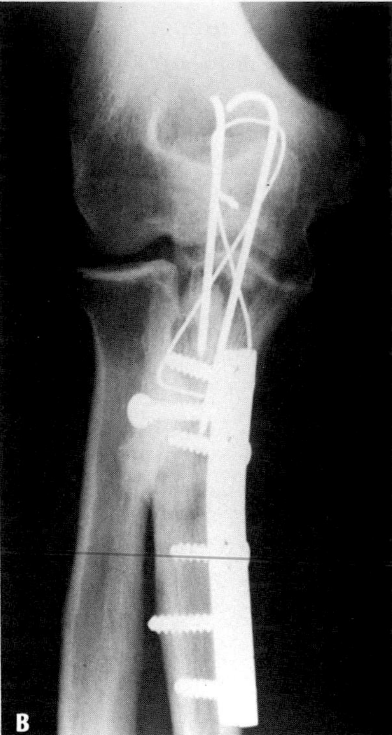

FIGURE 14-50. (**A**) Severely comminuted fracture of the olecranon. (**B**) The distal fracture has been stabilized using an AO plate. This essentially converts the comminuted fracture to an oblique fracture of the olecranon, which is then stabilized using the tension-band wiring technique. (**C**) A follow-up anteroposterior view demonstrates good maintenance of joint congruity.

continues

struct, permitting early motion. The placement of the pelvic reconstruction plate may be along the medial face, lateral face, or directly posterior. I use the position that provides the best control of the fracture and permits compression. All plate positions resist bending adequately. The 3.5-mm pelvic reconstruction plate provides greater strength than the one-third tubular plate and less bulk than the dynamic compression plate. Proximal fixation of the plate is the greatest challenge. The bone of the proximal ulna may be quite thin. For the most proximal fixation I will use cancellous screws rather than cortical screws. The screws must not protrude into the joint (Fig. 14-51).

Oblique Fractures. Oblique fractures lend themselves particularly well to lag screw fixation.[435] In most cases, I will use a plate as a neutralization implant or will place a lag screw through the plate. Carefully applied compression techniques can be used, using eccentric drilling and screw placement, but this method should be applied with a clear understanding of the pitfalls and limitations.

Isolated Comminuted Fractures (Proximal). Those fractures without dislocation of the ulna and radial head and without disruption of the anterior soft tissues are best treated by excision of the olecranon and secure reattachment of the triceps tendon with nonabsorbable suture to allow early active motion. It is important to retain the collateral ligaments, especially the anteromedial portion, for stability.

If the fracture includes part of the ulnar shaft and excision of the olecranon is not possible, AO plate stabilization of the distal fragment combined with tension-band wiring has proved very useful (see Fig. 14-50).[414] This technique is also applicable to fracture–dislocations. When comminution or instability precludes a standard

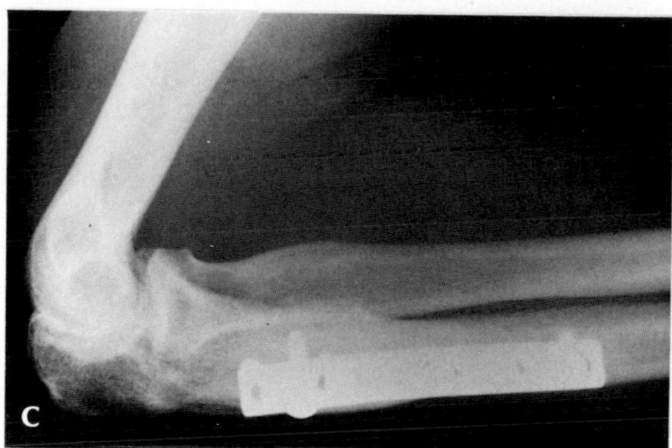

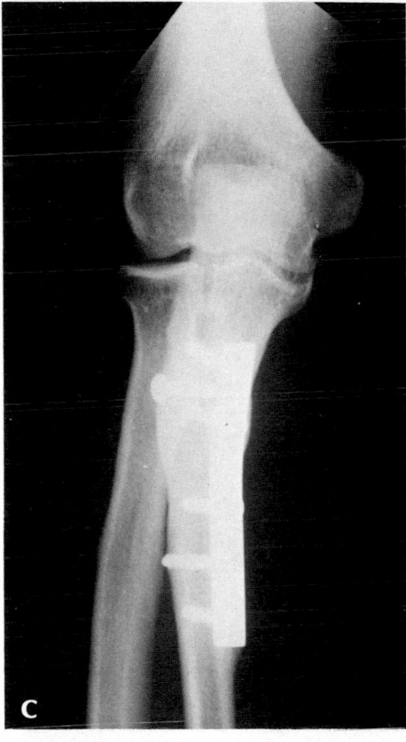

FIGURE 14-50. (continued)

approach, a creative combination of lag screws, wires, and plates should be considered. With comminution or bone loss, it is also helpful to have the patient prepared for iliac crest bone grafting if necessary.

Fracture–Dislocations. Fracture–dislocations present a challenging therapeutic problem because of the severe combination of bone and soft-tissue damage. Open reduction and internal fixation with restoration of alignment and stability of the ulna is the goal.[432,444] This can be achieved by using intramedullary wires or a long screw anchored in the distal medullary canal of the ulna.[444] Primary excision of the olecranon fracture must be carefully considered. As stated earlier, excision of the bone fragment that contains the triceps insertion makes the stabilization of the joint more difficult.

Open Fractures. Many fractures of the olecranon that require open reduction are open because of direct trauma. Internal fixation of these fractures is not contraindicated if there is no gross contamination and a thorough debridement is possible. However, if there is any question about the viability of soft-tissue coverage over the olecranon, local flaps or free tissue transfer should be considered (see Chapter 7). Antibiotic coverage should be started preoperatively and continued for 48 to 72 hours postoperatively. If there is concern about both contamination or skin viability, skeletal traction can be used for a few days, allowing a "second look," and time for the soft tissue to declare itself. Even 72 hours of elevation and wound care can make a helpful difference.

Complications

Complications of olecranon fractures are mainly decreased range of motion, post-traumatic arthritis, and nonunion.[392,400] It is hoped that loss of motion can be minimized by firm internal fixation and early range of motion of the joint.[414] Eriksson and colleagues[400] reported that up to 50% of patients have limited range of motion of the elbow after olecranon fractures, generally with loss of extension. However, in their series, the limitations were not great, and only 3% of the patients were aware of it.

Development of post-traumatic arthritis in the elbow is not as common (or perhaps not as noticeable) as in a weight-bearing joint. If reduction to less than 2-mm offset cannot be obtained, the possibility of arthritis developing later is significant. In the event of articular cartilage and bone loss, cancellous grafting in the defect may provide a fibrocartilaginous surface after graft revascularization.[443]

Nonunion of the olecranon has been reported to occur in 5% of olecranon fractures.[400] The treatment of a nonunion should be suited to the patient. In a young, active patient the pseudarthrosis may be taken down and the fracture site reapproximated and held with a tension-band wire or a suitable intramedullary device. Bone graft should be used to fill any defects in the fracture construct. Plate fixation may be needed, depending on the configuration of the fracture (see Fig. 14-51)

Excision of the proximal portion of the pseudarthrosis and repair of the triceps tendon is also an acceptable method of management, especially in older patients.

Ulnar nerve symptoms, generally in the form of numbness or paresthesias, have been reported in 10% of patients.[400] These symptoms usually clear spontaneously and require no definitive treatment.

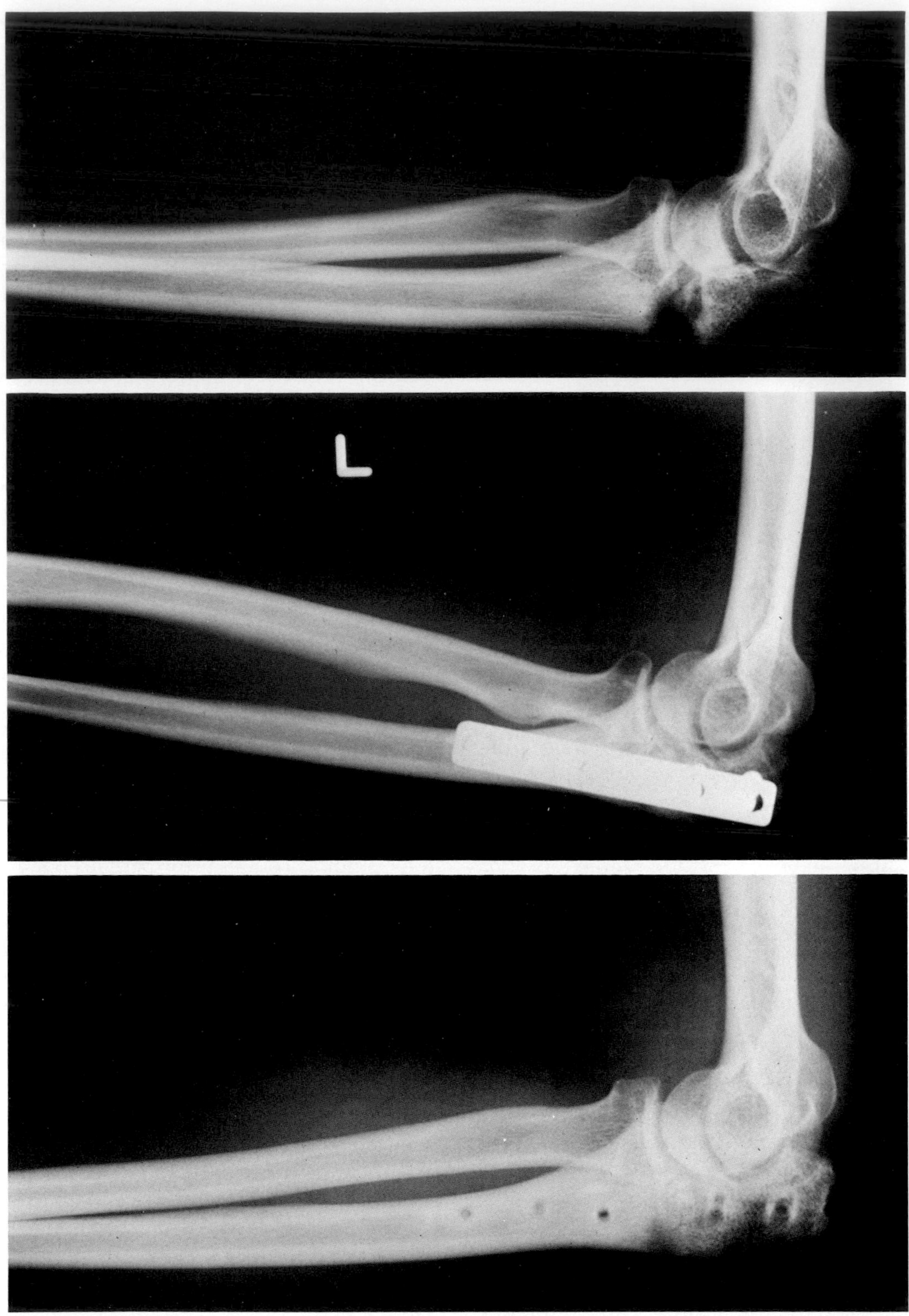

FIGURE 14-51. (**Top**) Established nonunion of the olecranon with a large proximal fragment. (**Center**) Articular congruity was reestablished and solid bony union achieved with an AO (ASIF) dynamic compression plate. (**Bottom**) Follow-up 1 year after plate removal.

RADIAL HEAD FRACTURES

The proper management of fractures of the radial head is difficult and controversial. The radial head is intra-articular and moves in both flexion and extension as well as with forearm rotation. With most other displaced intra-articular fractures, open reduction with internal fixation would be the rule. However, the radial head presents both a special technical challenge to fix securely and an incompletely understood mechanical role in the forearm. Given this, it is not surprising that the management of this injury is frequently controversial and uncertain.

The commonly asked questions are

1. Which fractures should be excised?
2. When should internal fixation be attempted?
3. Should a prosthetic replacement be used?

Because of increased recognition of the problems after radial head excision, there is more emphasis on preservation of the radial head after fracture, if technically possible. Ligamentous injury in the elbow and forearm may also be associated with radial head fracture. The decision to excise or internally fix is influenced by the presence of concomitant injury and its degree of severity. With the advent of more suitable implants for internal fixation of the radial head and neck, excision no longer needs to be the only operative alternative to closed treatment. However, the technical imperative of secure fixation using implants that do not interfere with motion may be difficult to achieve. A simple fracture can be made worse with poorly executed surgery. The indications for internal fixation must be considered carefully.

Anatomy and Biomechanics

The radial head is seated in the lesser sigmoid notch and maintains contact with the ulna throughout forearm pronation and supination. It was formerly believed that radiocapitellar contact was present only at extremes of flexion, but Morrey and colleagues,[15] using a more dynamic testing model, demonstrated force transmission at all angles, the greatest in full extension. In that same study, pronation also seemed to increase contact and force transmission.

Longitudinal force in grip or lifting activities is transmitted from the wrist to the elbow with load shared by both the radius and ulna. The specific load sharing between the ulna and radius is probably influenced by the position of the forearm in flexion and extension and pronation and supination. Unequal tension between the biceps and brachialis may also alter the load sharing proximally.

After radial head excision, the central bands of the interosseous ligament of the forearm help stabilize the radius resisting proximal translation of the radius relative to the ulna.[487,516]

Mechanical testing of prosthetic implants has questioned the efficacy of silicone prostheses. Valgus stability was not enhanced in vitro by silicone radial head implants in two independent studies.[488,514] Use of the silicone prosthesis to prevent proximal translation of the radius has also been challenged in the laboratory.[456,487]

The radial head also contributes to valgus stability when tested in the laboratory,[12,13,488] but the relative contribution in vivo is not known (see Fig. 14-6).

Mechanism of Injury

Fractures of the radial head are most frequently caused by direct longitudinal loading—a fall on the outstretched hand (Fig. 14-52). In addition, any injury that causes dislocation of the elbow can also result in fracture of the radial head.

Classification

In 1924, Speed[525] proposed a classification based on two factors—the amount of head involvement, marginal or complete, and the degree of displacement. In 1954, Mason[499] further subdivided the classification into three groups: type I—small or marginal fractures

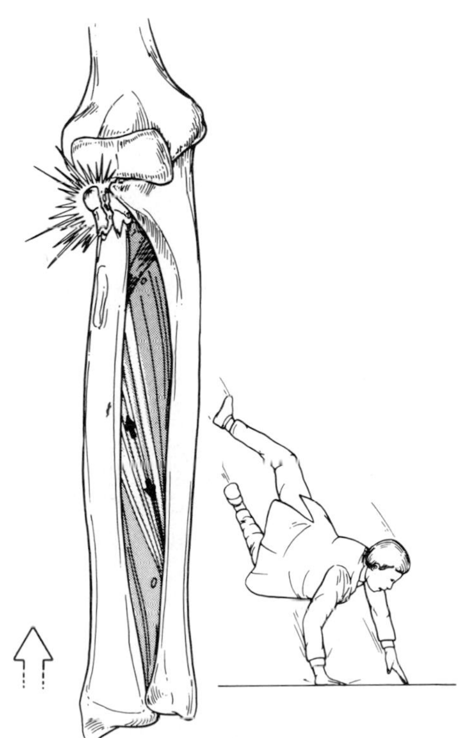

FIGURE 14-52. A fall that produces a ligament of the forearm also can strain or rupture the interosseous membrane (*black arrows*).

with minimal displacement; type II—marginal fractures with displacement; and type III—comminuted fractures of the head. This study was based on a retrospective examination of records and x-rays from 100 patients. Mason advocated closed treatment of type I fractures and radial head excision for type III fractures. The classification was less helpful in directing care for the type II fracture.

Is the Mason classification useful? As Thompson[531] had noted as early as 1905, fractures that were not displaced (type I) would do well without surgical intervention. Those fractures that were comminuted and displaced (described as Mason type III) required excision because of mechanical block to forearm rotation. Mason[499] himself stated that the presence of a mechanical block was an important factor in determining whether excision was indicated, irrespective of the x-ray appearance, but he did not include this feature in his classification system. Other important features of the injury (concomitant elbow dislocation and tear of the interosseous ligament of the forearm [so-called Essex-Lopresti]) were not included in the classification until Johnston's study in 1962.[490]

For fractures of the radial head, the presence of an acute mechanical block to rotation may be more important than the estimated amount of displacement on a plain x-ray. Associated injuries that include elbow dislocation or acute tears of the interosseous ligament of the forearm may also influence treatment beyond the simple radiographic appearance. For these reasons, the Mason classification alone, a purely radiologically based nominal classification, is insufficient to guide treatment. The idea of classifying or subdividing injuries has merit. However, the plain x-ray may be insufficient to reliably determine the amount of fragmentation, the degree of displacement, and the associated injuries.

For these reasons, I do not use the Mason classification as originally proposed but instead a modification based on the patient's radiologic fracture pattern, physical signs, and associated injuries.

Type I—Nondisplaced or minimally displaced fracture of head or neck
- Forearm rotation (pronation/supination) is limited only by acute pain and swelling
- Intra-articular displacement of the fracture is less than 2 mm

Type II—Displaced (greater than 2 mm) fracture of the head or neck
- Motion may be mechanically limited or incongruous
- Without severe comminution (may be repaired by open reduction with internal fixation)
- Fracture involves more than a marginal lip of the radial head

Type III—severely comminuted fracture of the radial head and neck
- Not reconstructable
- Requires excision for movement

Each of these radiologic patterns may be associated with posterior elbow dislocation, acute tear of the interosseous ligament of the forearm (Essex-Lopresti), fracture of the proximal ulna (Monteggia), and fracture of the coronoid. More than one of these conditions may also be present in combination.

In this system, type I fractures seldom require surgical treatment. Type II require careful consideration (see Author's Preferred Method of Treatment), and type III fractures should be strongly considered for excision. As in all clinical situations, rules and protocols provide a general framework that requires individualization, in this instance, for both the needs of the patient and the skills and experience of the surgeon.

Signs and Symptoms

Isolated fractures of the radial head usually cause pain on the lateral side of the elbow aggravated by forearm rotation. The examiner must be suspicious and palpate the radial head while passively rotating the forearm. Occasionally, motion elicits painful crepitus. When the fracture is associated with more massive trauma such as elbow dislocations, swelling and pain can be substantial, precluding adequate palpation or forearm rotation. The forearm and wrist should also be examined for pain and swelling. If wrist pain is present, acute radioulnar dissociation with injury to the interosseous ligament of the forearm and triangular fibrocartilage complex may have occurred.

Radiographic Examination

Plain Films

X-rays in the anteroposterior and lateral planes of the elbow are usually sufficient to diagnose the fracture. However, if a fat pad sign is present without a noticeable fracture, radiocapitellar views may be helpful. As described by Greenspan and Norman,[480] the radiocapitellar view is taken with the forearm in neutral rotation and the x-ray tube angled 45° cephalad. Posterior elbow dislocation or fracture of the capitellum should also arouse suspicion.[203,518,538] If wrist or forearm pain is present, x-rays of the wrist in the neutral-rotation view should also be taken.

Trispiral polytomography with 2-mm sections in the anteroposterior and lateral planes can be quite helpful, to assess comminution and displacement. However, the availability of this equipment is rapidly diminishing across the country. Improved CT scan techniques may eventually supplant traditional tomography.

Computed Tomography

CT scans of the radial head in axial, sagittal, and coronal cuts can be quite helpful in estimating the size, degree of fragmentation, and displacement. For fractures under consideration for open reduction and internal fixation, I usually request a CT scan to better visualize the fracture. The use of the CT scan has also dissuaded me from operating because the displacement was less than expected from the plain x-rays. Reconstructed images may also be helpful, but reorienting the elbow to obtain nonreformatted images in the sagittal and coronal planes is preferable (Fig. 14-56).

Historical Review—Methods of Treatment and Results

Type I—Nondisplaced Fractures

Retrospective studies of radial head fractures since that of Thomas in 1905 have concluded that nonoperative treatment of type I fractures (Fig. 14-53) is best.[447,448,450,455,460,465,468,471,474,475,478,481,483,489–491,493,498,499,503,507,508,515,517,521,525,531,534,537,539]

Some favored immobilization for 2 to 4 weeks in a cast.[491,521] In 1939, Eliason and North[471] advocated early motion, but it was Mason and Shutkin's[498] 1943 series with sling immobilization and active motion as early as tolerated that established this as the preferred method of treatment. Since then, few have questioned this practice. Most authors believe that early motion helps to shape and mold slight incongruities without substantial risk of greater displacement.

In addition to early active motion, Postlethwait[513] and others[447,475,484,492,503,512,515] advocated acute aspiration of the hemarthrosis and instillation of local anesthetic to reduce pain and assist early active motion. In a prospective study of 80 patients, Holdsworth and colleagues[484] demonstrated that aspiration and injection of local anesthetic increased comfort and improved the initial range of motion, but that this practice did not enhance the final outcome.

Most patients with type I fractures can expect good to excellent function after 2 to 3 months of active-motion exercises. Minimal loss of extension is not uncommon and some have occasional pain, aggravated by cold or stress. However, some patients with type I fractures do poorly. Contracture, pain, and inflammation can occur, despite what appears to be a well-aligned, minimally displaced fracture. Radin and Riseborough[517] attributed this to displacement of the fracture, which can occur but is rare.[528] Currey and colleagues[467] reported a patient with an inflammatory condition that histopathologically resembled rheumatoid-like arthritis after an isolated radial head fracture with minimal displacement.

In operating on radial head fractures, I have found a high incidence of concomitant osteochondral fractures of the capitellum that were not visible radiographically. This osteocartilaginous impact injury may contribute to a poor result in what otherwise appears to be a simple nondisplaced fracture.

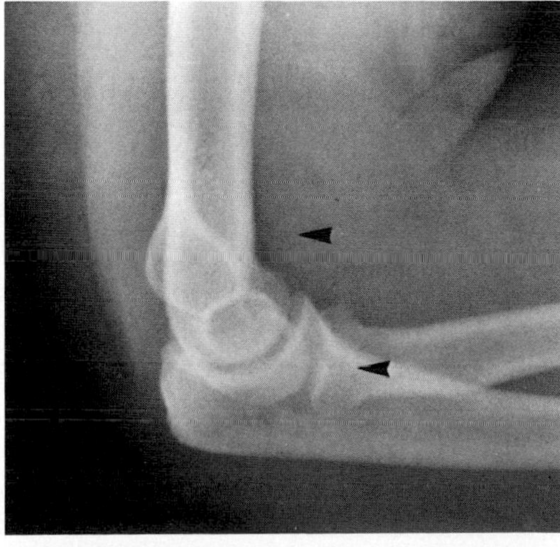

FIGURE 14-53. Type I (undisplaced) chisel fracture of the radial head (*lower arrow*). Note the elevation of the anterior fat pad (*upper arrow*), indicating hemarthrosis. The posterior fat pad is small but present.

Type II—Marginal Fractures With Displacement

The fracture with partial radial head involvement and displacement (Figs. 14-54 to 14-56) requires careful consideration. The decision to treat with early motion alone or operatively is difficult, and the literature is ambiguous. The principal limitation of the Mason classification is that it provides little guidance for patients with type II fractures. For these fractures, one can find advocates for total excision, partial excision, open reduction with internal fixation, and nonoperative care, each claiming good results. Unfortunately, these series are all retrospective, most affected by dropout bias, poor specificity of selection criteria, and inadequate measures of results.

When Mason[499] examined the results of treatment retrospectively, he concluded that if any tilt or displacement was present in fractures involving more than one fourth of the radial head, excision should be performed. If there was mechanical interference acutely, he recommended immediate excision but did not include this feature in his classification.

Adler and Shaftan and others advocated early motion without excision, even in cases of displacement and comminution.[447,498,537] Then suggested that if pain or a mechanical block were noted later, delayed excision could then be performed.

The timing of excision has been as controversial as

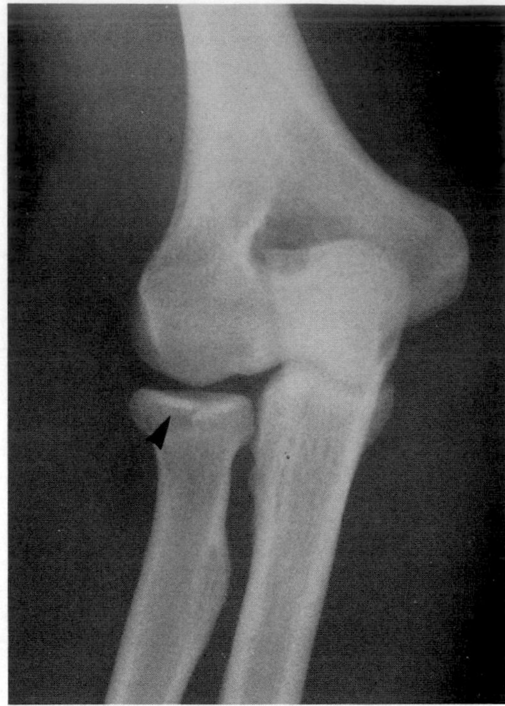

FIGURE 14-54. Minimally displaced central depression fracture of the radial head (*arrow*).

the practice itself. No prospective studies have adequately addressed the question on a comparative basis. Many authors[475,483,517,539] have argued that excision in the first 48 hours was obligatory and that delay would lead to contracture and ectopic calcification. Opposed to this position, Charnley[461] wrote that immediate excision was contraindicated, believing that the physician cannot properly assess the need for excision until 2 weeks after the injury. He recommended that if motion were restricted after 2 weeks, excision should be done at that time. He reported no incidence of ectopic calcification with delayed excision. Adler and Shaftan[447] could find no influence of the timing of excision on outcome. Broberg and Morrey[452] retrospectively evaluated four patients with type II fractures and documented pain relief and some improvement of motion with delayed excision.

Open reduction with internal fixation has become increasingly popular since reported in 1979.[454,469,473,476,477,501,509,511,520,522] Implants for internal fixation are now more varied in size and permit rigid fixation of head and neck fractures. Despite these improvements, great care must be taken to achieve rigid fixation without creating impingement in the proximal radioulnar joint. In the series published most recently,[469,473,476,477,520] larger implants have been used, including small plates as well as headed screws. The use of the Herbert screw for head fractures has also reported for head fractures alone.

Type III—Comminuted Fractures of the Whole Head

Unlike the controversy surrounding the treatment of the displaced but reparable type II fracture, the comminuted fracture involving the whole head usually requires excision and often does well (Fig. 14-57).[459,464,493,506,517,527,531,499] Excision and the immediate initiation of active and passive motion usually results in an optimal result. A delayed excision can be performed,[447,452] but this alternative is usually reserved for patients who exhibit no mechanical block to rotation or have other conditions that preclude immediate excision. As discussed later, excision of the radial head may lead to symptomatic proximal migration of the radius or instability of the elbow, and each patient should be carefully assessed and warned concerning this possibility.

Proximal Translation of the Radius: Acute and Chronic Longitudinal Radioulnar Dissociation

Proximal displacement of the radius after radial head fracture or radial head resection has been described by many investigators over the past 50 years.[449,452,464,466,470,472,495,502,506,517,524,525,527,529,530,533,532] Because of the variable nature of these reports, it is difficult to gauge the incidence of asymptomatic and symptomatic migration, but estimates range from 20% to 90% of patients after radial head resection. Ascertaining the natural history and timing of the proximal translation has not been possible because most reports addressing "proximal migration" did not specify the status of the wrist and forearm ligaments at the time of injury. In addition, it is unclear whether the proximal translation of the radius occurred over the first few weeks, months, or years.[486] Whatever the timing, the critical injury is the loss of mechanical support from radiocapitellar contact and the *interosseous ligament* of the fore-

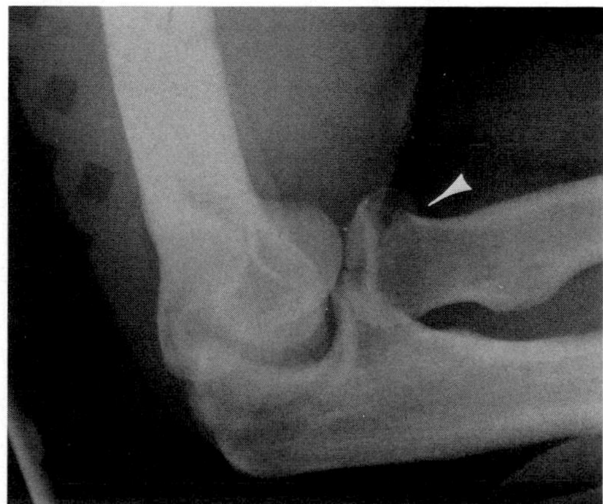

FIGURE 14-55. An isolated fracture of the radial head can involve more than 50% of the articular surface (type II) and not require excision if there is no mechanical block.

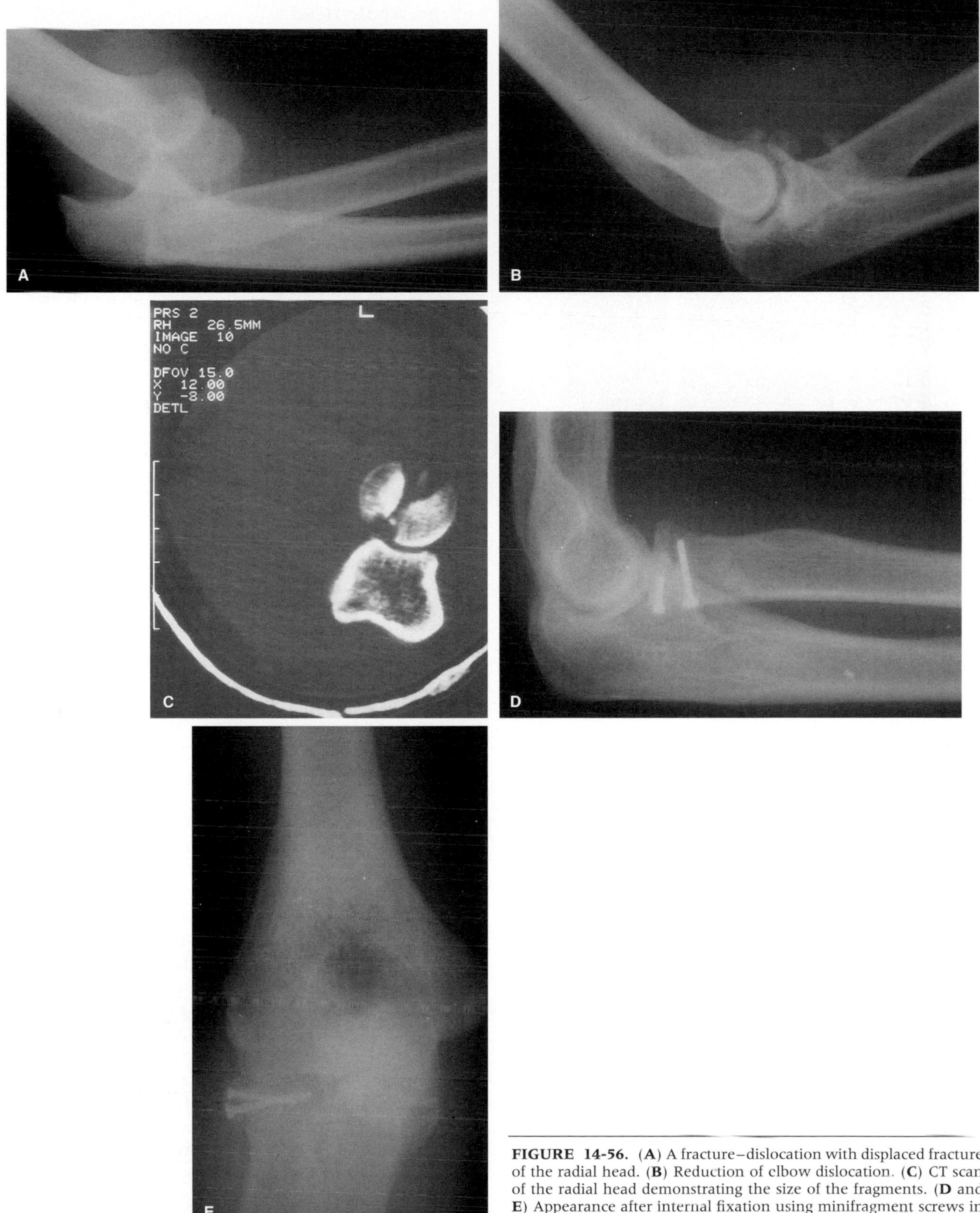

FIGURE 14-56. (**A**) A fracture–dislocation with displaced fracture of the radial head. (**B**) Reduction of elbow dislocation. (**C**) CT scan of the radial head demonstrating the size of the fragments. (**D** and **E**) Appearance after internal fixation using minifragment screws in the safe zone.

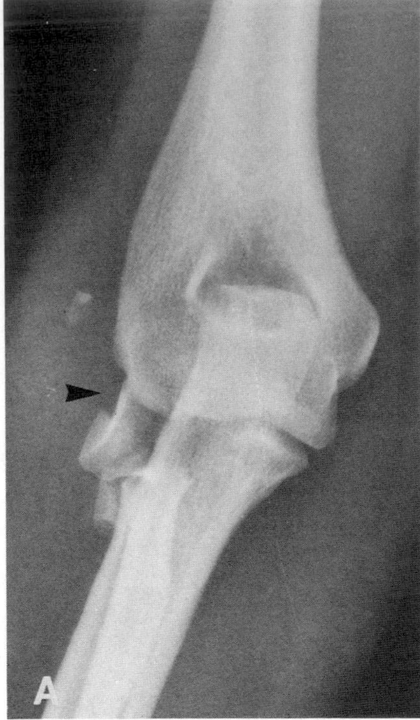

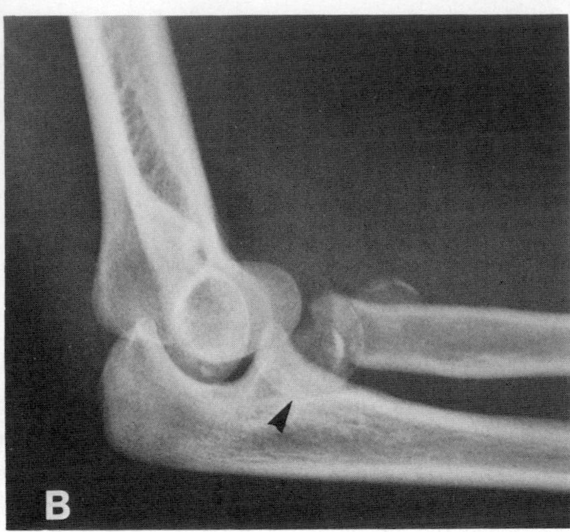

FIGURE 14-57. (**A**) A markedly comminuted and displaced fracture of the radial head (*arrow*) and neck. (**B**) The lateral view shows the fracture of the radial neck and rotation of the radial head (*arrow*).

arm (Figs. 14-58 and 14-59). In the past, the term *interosseous membrane* has been used, when, in fact, the central portion has the structure and function of a ligament.[487,516]

In 1930, Brockman[453] first reported two cases of radioulnar dissociation, the first noted 3 months after injury. Lewis and Thibodeau[495] reported eight patients with proximal translation, but seven of the eight were not skeletally mature at the time of radial head resection and growth retardation may have played a role. In 1941, Speed[526] suggested that radiocapitellar contact was important and attempted to employ the use of a ferrule cap to provide support. Since then, many investigators have attempted to quantify and gauge the clinical significance of the proximal translation. There are patients who, despite the radiologic confirmation of proximal translation 5 mm or greater, have minimal symptoms and acceptable function.[464] Other patients with similar findings on x-ray fare less well.[453,470,472,486,524,532]

In 1946, Curr and Coe[466] described a patient with *acute* proximal translation of the radius with disruption of the distal radioulnar joint combined with a radial head fracture. They described the clinical and surgical findings of complete dissociation between the radius and ulna and the difficulty in effectively treating the gross instability. In 1951, Essex-Lopresti[472] reported two cases with similar findings. For some reason, despite the earlier report by Curr and Coe, his name has been given eponymic prominence. He suggested that optimal treatment would include preservation of the radial head, if possible, or the use of a rigid prosthesis to maintain a proper longitudinal relationship. In 1988, Khurana and colleagues[492] reported a patient with acute radioulnar dissociation in which the interosseous ligament, visualized in the operating room, was noted to be completely disrupted. I have since shown the interosseous ligament of the forearm using magnetic resonance imaging, demonstrating the loss of continuity associated with this injury (see Fig. 14-8).[486]

The relationship between acute radioulnar dissociation as described by Curr and Coe[466] and more gradual proximal migration of the radius after radial head resection is not known. Most studies of proximal translation of the radius after radial head resection were done after trauma, making it difficult to separate the possible injury itself from the gradual attenuation of the interosseous ligament with longitudinal loading. Rymaszewski[519] did not note proximal translation in a series of 52 patients with rheumatoid arthritis who had undergone radial head resection for radiocapitellar arthrosis. Perhaps lower demand was a factor, though valgus instability of the elbow did develop in many of those patients. However, in a somewhat related study, this same group studied the efficacy of a metallic prosthesis for radial head replacement.[494] One patient required removal of the metallic replacement months after implantation, because of loosening. Within a short time, the radius translated a full centimeter, suggesting that the interosseous ligament does not heal with mechanical integrity, despite protection for months.

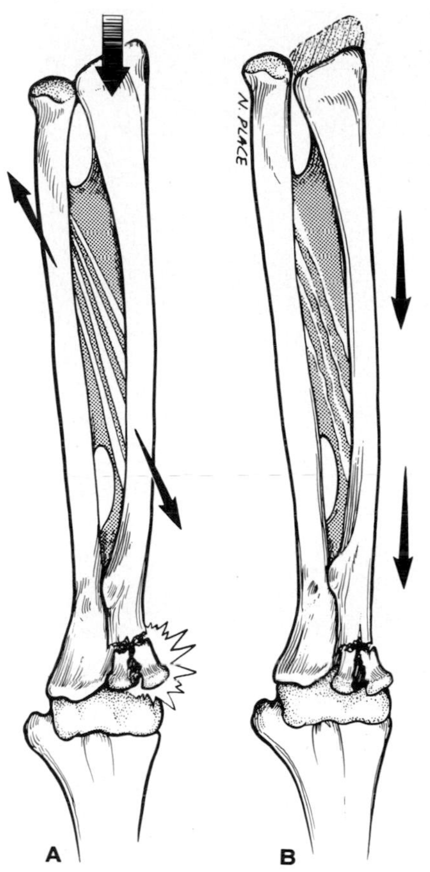

FIGURE 14-58. In acute longitudinal radioulnar dissociation (ALRUD), the ligamentous linkage between the radius and ulna may be injured to varying degrees. (**A**) There may be only a sprain without complete disruption. (**B**) Complete dissociation with longitudinal translation and distal radioulnar joint dislocation.

There is probably a continuum of injury, depending on the initial energy and force applied, that causes a partial or complete tear of the interosseous ligament and distal wrist ligaments.[516] If these structures are torn completely, then acute displacement can occur at the time of injury. If the ligaments are partially torn, no displacement may be initially present, but with use in grip and lifting activity, the radius can gradually displace.

There is no consistently effective treatment of established symptomatic proximal migration of the radius after radial head resection. If the radial head can be preserved by internal fixation and stabilization, proximal migration cannot occur. However, once the radiocapitellar contact is lost, relative radial shortening can occur (see Fig. 14-59).

Some authors have advocated the use of the silicone radial head prosthesis to provide support with radiocapitellar contact.[485,529,536] This concept was attractive as first suggested by Speed in 1941.[526] Others, however, have documented prosthetic failure and the inability of the silicone prosthesis to provide adequate mechanical support (Figs. 14-60 and 14-61).[470,524,536] Knight[494] reported the use of a vitallium prosthesis in 21 patients with favorable results at a mean follow-up of 4.5 years. It is unclear from the study if any of the patients had acute injury to the interosseous ligament of the forearm.

Shortening of the ulna has not been consistently helpful (Figs. 14-62 and 14-63). Temporary equality of length at the wrist is usually achieved, followed by continued proximal translation.[524] In many cases, as Brockman[453] first suggested in 1930, the creation of a radioulnar synostosis may be the only solution.

Despite continued controversy and intense study, most authors would support the following statement:

> Proximal translation after radial head fracture and resection occurs in many patients and is not always symptomatic, despite nonconformity at the distal radioulnar joint. When symptomatic, reliable treatment with restoration and maintenance of mobility and strength remains elusive.

Radial Head Excision and Prosthetic Replacement

Prosthetic replacement of the radial head was proposed by Speed[526] in 1941 in an attempt to restore radiocapitellar contact and prevent proximal translation of the radius. He implanted ferrule caps over the neck of the radius but found that they displaced and caused inflammation. Others authors have since reported the use of acrylic, metallic, and silicone radial head prostheses.[451,456–458,462,463,467,479,482,494,496,500,504,505,526,529,536,540]

The use of the silicone prosthesis began in the 1970s, and several reports of favorable results were published in a few patients.[496,497,536] Interestingly, Mackay and associates[496] noted that despite use of the prosthesis, 4 of the 16 patients demonstrated more than 4 mm of proximal translation of the radius. Sowa and associates[524] also reported several patients with continued proximal translation of the radius, despite use of the silicone prosthesis.

As experience grew with the prosthesis, more reports of material failure and dislocation were published.[451,496,500,505] In addition, particulate synovitis, which had been reported with carpal implants, was also seen in the radial head replacement.[479,540]

The theoretic value of the prosthesis was to improve valgus stability and prevent proximal translation of the radius. However, several independent biomechanical studies demonstrate the lack of mechanical efficacy of the silicone replacement in resisting valgus stress and proximal translation of the radius (see Fig. 14-61).[456,487,488,514,540]

A return to metallic prosthesis, in an attempt to improve load bearing, has also been attempted. There is not enough evidence at this time to recom-

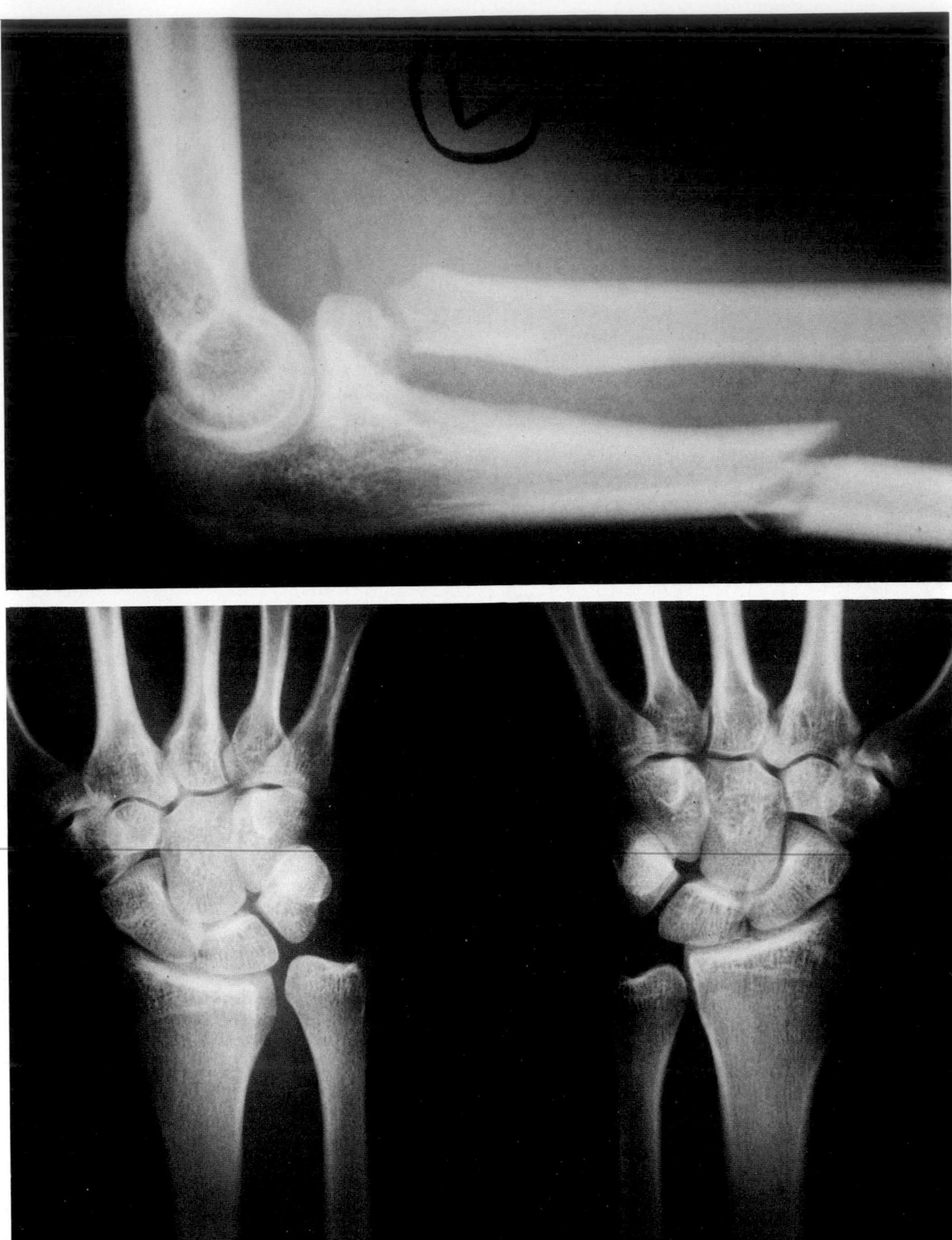

FIGURE 14-59. (**Top**) Essex-Lopresti fracture of the radial head (associated with a Monteggia fracture–dislocation in this patient). (**Bottom**) Comparison views of the wrist taken on the day of injury clearly demonstrate proximal migration of the radius and resulting length discrepancy in the radioulnar joint.

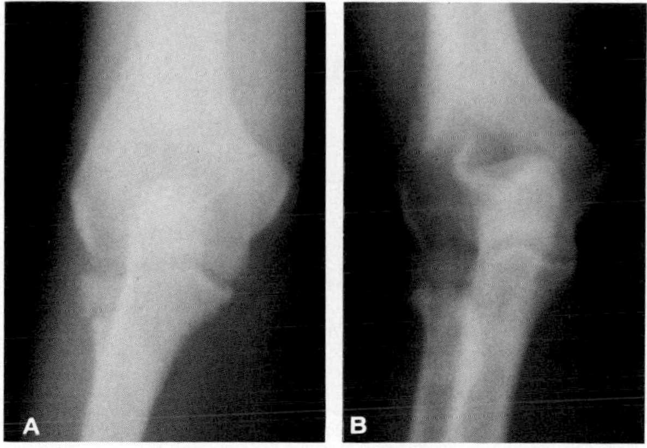

FIGURE 14-60. (**A**) A silicone radial head prosthesis was inserted at the time of injury to prevent proximal translation. (**B**) Two years later, symptomatic proximal translation was noted with compression of the prosthesis.

mend the routine use of the metallic radial head implant. Knight[494] and associates reported the use of a Vitallium prosthesis with encouraging results in 21 patients.

Factors Influencing Choice of Treatment

High or Low Demand Elbow. I first try to classify the patients into those with high-demand or low-demand elbows—the 26-year-old athlete versus the 72-year-old retired banker. There are obviously patients who do not easily fit into one of these two categories, but if you are considering preservation of the radial head with the use of internal fixation, the patient should fit into the high-demand group. Likewise, a low-demand patient is less likely to suffer the effects of proximal migration of the radius, after radial head resection; and excision, if needed, is usually well tolerated.

Associated Injuries. When first examining the patient with a reported radial head fracture, it is important to look for associated injuries of the elbow and forearm. Combination injuries are more common in high-energy trauma but can occur after a simple fall. The wrist, distal radioulnar joint, and interosseous ligament of the forearm should be examined for tenderness or swelling. If either is present, one should suspect acute radioulnar dissociation.

Acute Longitudinal Radioulnar Dissociation (ALRUD). The forearm should be inspected for signs of acute longitudinal radioulnar dissociation. The wrist must be palpated for tenderness over the distal radioulnar joint and the forearm examined for excessive swelling. If there is evidence of injury to the interosseous ligament and distal radioulnar ligaments, radial head preservation becomes more important.

Elbow Dislocation (Medial Ligament Disruption) and/or Fracture of the Coronoid. After examination of the forearm, the medial ligaments of the elbow should be gently palpated for swelling or tenderness. If these findings are present, the injury may have been a severe valgus stress causing both a medial ligament tear and radial head fracture. In such patients, there may be greater potential for instability, suggesting greater consideration for radial head preservation.

If there is an associated posterior dislocation (see Fig. 14-56), this is usually quite obvious. These injuries can be both deceptive and difficult to treat, once recognized. If there is an associated fracture of the coronoid, gross instability may be present. This combination injury—*the terrible triad* of the elbow—is discussed on p. 980.

Presence or Absence of Mechanical Block. A more complete examination with less discomfort to the patient can usually be achieved after anesthetizing the elbow joint with aspiration of the hemarthrosis and intra-articular injection of 0.5% bupivacaine (Marcaine) (Fig. 14-64). After intra-articular anesthesia is established using lidocaine (Xylocaine) or bupivacaine, the patient can be examined for the presence of crepitation or a mechanical block to forearm rotation. With the examiner's thumb or fingers over the radial head, gentle passive rotation of the forearm is attempted in several positions of elbow flexion. If there is a definite mechanical block, or

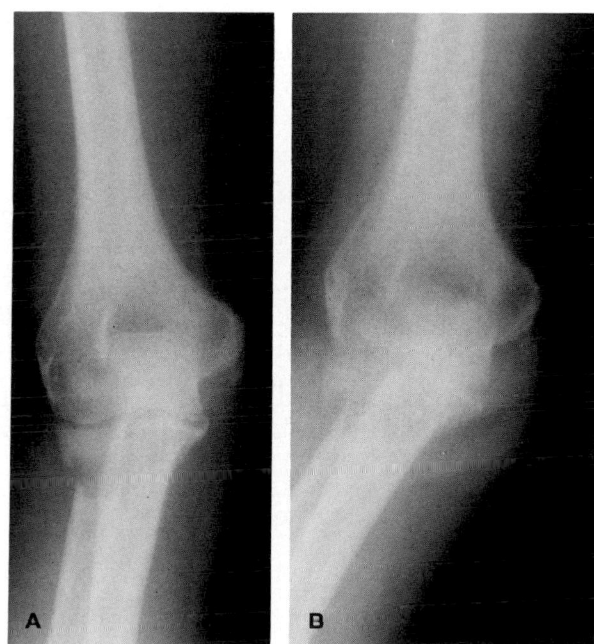

FIGURE 14-61. (**A**) A silicone radial head implant was used in this patient in an attempt to prevent valgus instability. (**B**) Six months after injury, stress films showed telescoping and compression of the implant, precluding effective capitellar contact. If the prosthesis is used, it is important to excise as little proximal radius as necessary and to use an implant that effectively fills the space.

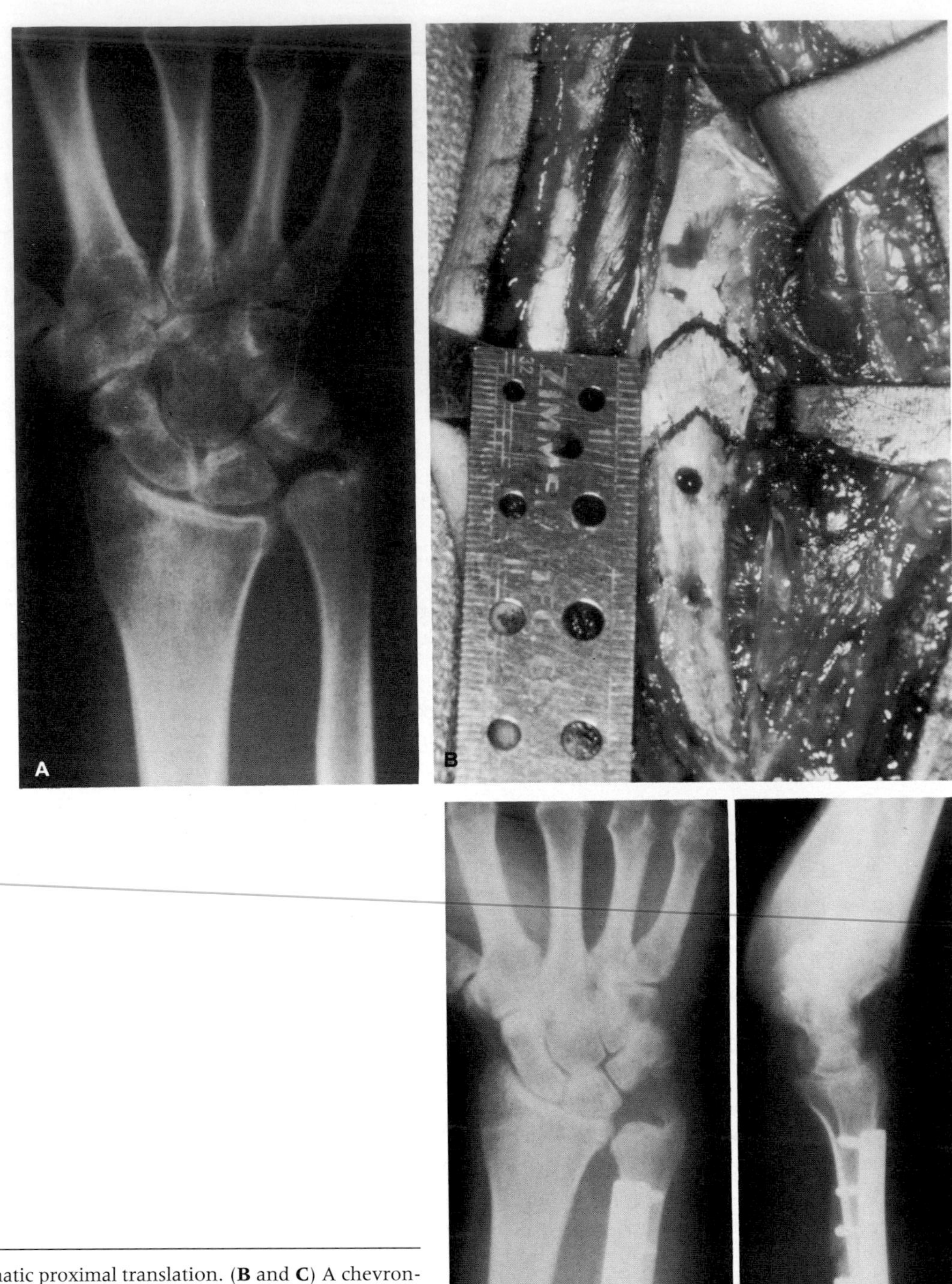

FIGURE 14-62. (**A**) Symptomatic proximal translation. (**B** and **C**) A chevron-type shortening osteotomy was performed with equalization of the radius and ulna at the wrist. (**D**) Several months later, further translation had occurred.

severe crepitus, this should be noted. For minimally displaced fractures, this portion of the examination is usually unnecessary.

Radiographic Findings X-ray interpretation of radial head fractures is difficult because of overlapping structures. Positioning of the patient is sometimes difficult because of pain, but a true lateral view is essential. Associated fractures of the capitellum can occur, and the lateral view should be examined for this. It is difficult to judge the degree of comminution and the position of the fragments in many fractures. X-rays of the wrist in the neutral posteroanterior view can also be helpful. Radiographic comparison with the uninjured side may be necessary (see Fig. 14-59).

CT scans of the radial head in axial, sagittal, and coronal cuts can be quite helpful in estimating the size, degree of fragmentation, and displacement (see Fig. 14-56). For fractures under consideration for open re-

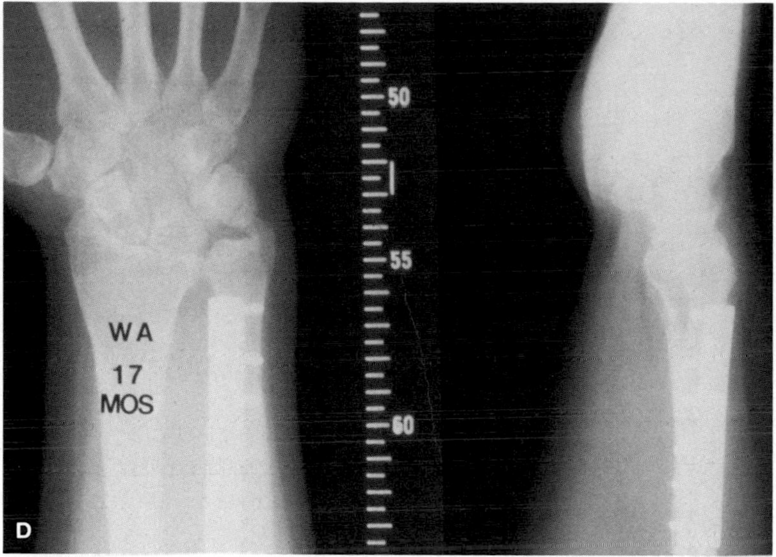

FIGURE 14-62. (continued)

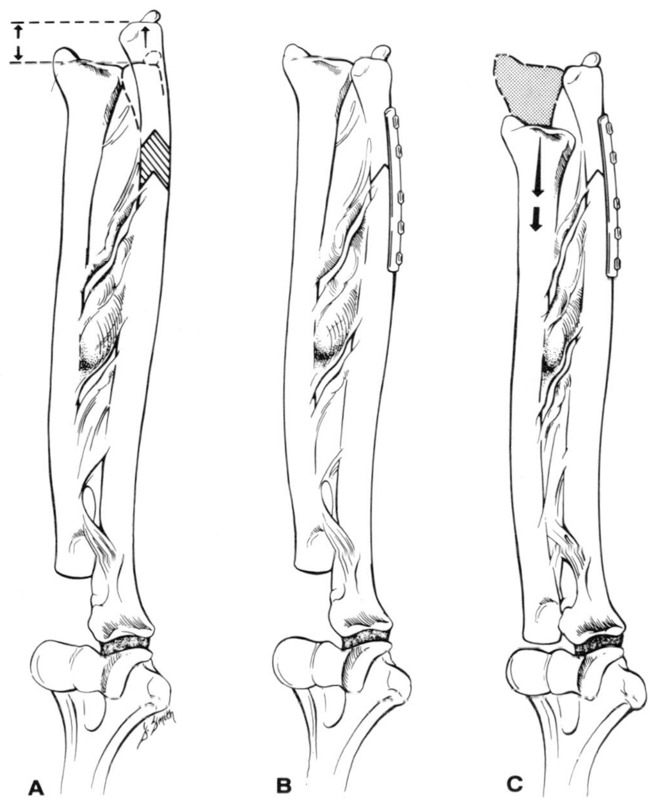

FIGURE 14-63. (**A** to **C**) Ulnar shortening usually fails to provide permanent equalization because the ligamentous linkage between the radius and ulna is completely disrupted.

duction and internal fixation, I usually request a CT scan to better visualize the fracture. The use of the CT scan has also dissuaded me from operating because the displacement was less than expected from the plain x-rays. Reconstructed images may also be helpful, but reorienting the elbow to obtain nonreformatted images in the coronal, sagittal, and axial planes is preferable.

AUTHOR'S PREFERRED METHOD OF TREATMENT

As stated earlier, before treating these fractures, a full and complete assessment of the patient's demands, other conditions, and associated injuries must be made. If internal fixation of the radial head is contemplated, CT scanning may be needed to fully assess the degree of comminution and displacement.

Type I

In nondisplaced or minimally displaced fracture of head or neck, forearm rotation (pronation/supination) is limited only by acute pain and swelling; there is no mechanical block. Intra-articular displacement of the fracture is less than 2 mm.

By definition, type I fractures are not displaced, require no reduction, and should not exhibit any mechanical block to passive forearm rotation. Substantial immediate relief of pain can be provided by aspirating the hematoma and injecting local anesthetic into the joint. The patient is given a sling, or the arm can be splinted but for no longer than 3 to 4 days. Active

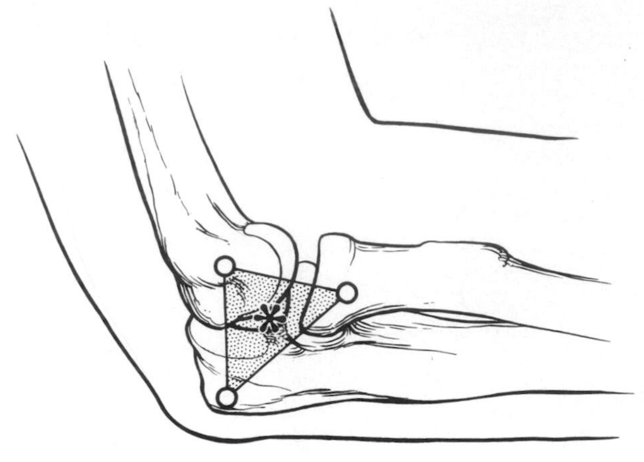

FIGURE 14-64. The landmarks for aspiration of the elbow joint are the radial head, lateral epicondyle, and tip of the olecranon. A needle inserted into the center of the triangle (*asterisk*) penetrates only the anconeus muscle and capsule before entering the joint.

forearm rotation is started as soon as tolerated. It is helpful to warn the patient that pain and stiffness can persist for some time and that occasionally the fracture can displace. If weekly gains in range of motion are not occurring, it may be helpful to recommend supervised physical therapy. Most patients should be encouraged to take responsibility for their own rehabilitation.

Most patients with type I fractures can expect good to excellent function after 2 to 3 months of active motion exercises. Some (10°–15°) loss of extension is not uncommon, and some patients have occasional pain, aggravated by cold or stress. There are a few patients with type I fractures who do poorly. Contracture, pain, and inflammation can occur, despite what appears to be a well-aligned, minimally displaced fracture.[467]

With Associated Injury (Elbow Dislocation)

If there was a concomitant posterior elbow dislocation, early motion is still recommended. The surgeon should determine, if possible, the safe limit of extension. This limitation of extension is usually only required during the first few weeks after injury. If there is any question about reduction, follow-up x-rays should be taken. The healing and rehabilitation process is usually protracted because of the additional trauma. This injury should be viewed as a posterior elbow dislocation with a radial head fracture, emphasizing care of the dislocation, because the fracture requires no specific intervention, except attention to forearm rotation. A hinged brace with mechanical stops may also be helpful, giving the patient reassurance without a strict limitation of motion.

Type II

In displaced (greater than 2 mm) fracture of the head or neck, motion *may* be mechanically blocked or incongruous. This type of fracture without severe comminution may be repaired by open reduction with internal fixation. Type II fracture involves more than a marginal lip of the radial head, and it may have associated injuries, such as interosseous ligament injury and posterior elbow dislocation.

Without Mechanical Block

Type II fractures without mechanical block or crepitus (and associated injury) should be treated similarly to type I fractures, especially in the low-demand patient. The patient should be warned that displacement can occur, though this is uncommon. The outcome of fractures of this type is similar to that of the type I fracture, although occasionally the incongruity can result in radiocapitellar arthrosis and pain. It is advisable to discuss with the patient the possibility of delayed radial head excision.

With Mechanical Block

For the high-demand patient, strong consideration should be given to open reduction with internal fixation. A careful discussion with the patient is needed. This procedure requires an understanding of the limits of hardware placement and the technical expertise to use a variety of implants that achieve rigid fixation and permit active motion (see later section on internal fixation of the radial head and neck.)

For the low-demand patient, complete excision should be performed. Although the idea of partial excision has been discussed, there are no studies that have long-enough follow-up to document the efficacy of this method. I have tried partial excision in an effort to retain some radial head contact but found that the remaining incongruity continued to cause crepitus and pain and required total excision. As Broberg and Morrey[452] have pointed out, if there is uncertainty about the amount of incongruity and mechanical block, a delayed excision is a viable option.

With Associated Injury

Interosseous Ligament Tear (Essex-Lopresti)
Preservation of radial head function may be of great value in this setting.[469,472] In fractures that do not demonstrate gross displacement of the radius relative to the ulna, there still may be injury to the interosseous ligament that would lead to symptomatic proximal translation if the radial head were excised. In this setting, open reduction with internal fixation of the radial head may be advantageous.

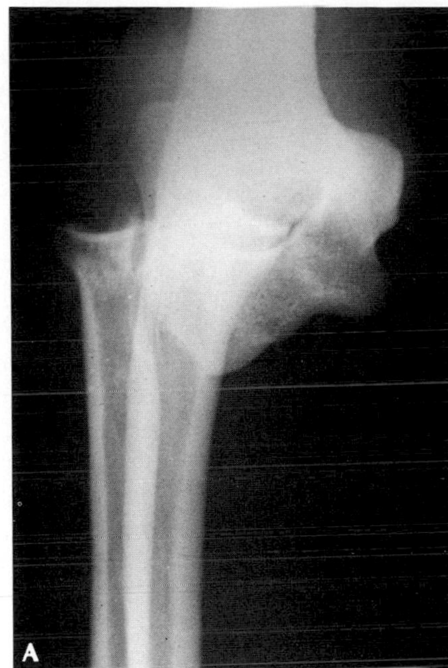

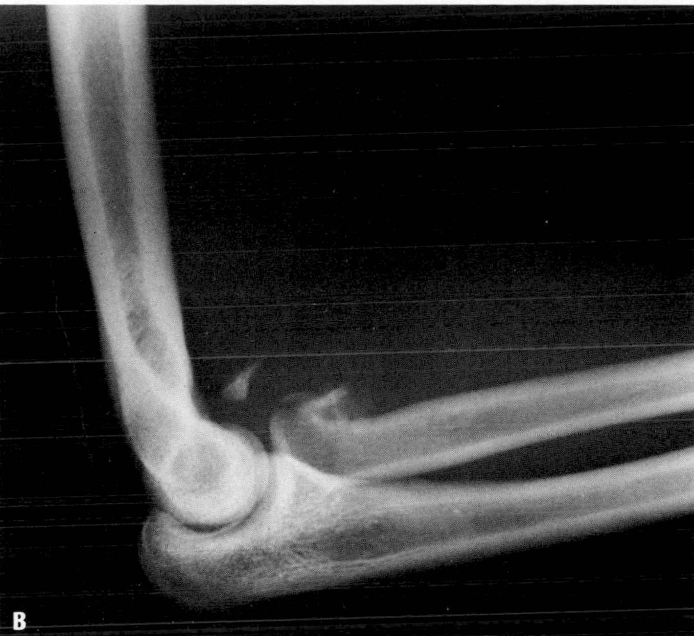

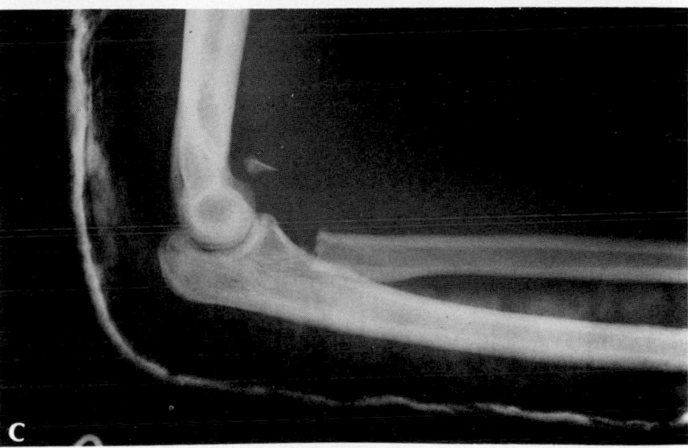

FIGURE 14-65. These x-rays illustrate the danger of excising the radial head when there is a concomitant fracture of the coronoid process, even if the coronoid is not removed. (**A**) The initial dislocation film showing a displaced, segmental fracture of the radial head. (**B**) Closed reduction of the elbow. The coronoid process is still markedly displaced. (**C**) The radial head was excised primarily, and the reduced elbow was immobilized in a long-arm splint. (**D**) Four days later the elbow resubluxated in the splint. (**E**) On the fifth day the elbow was reduced and held in more flexion.

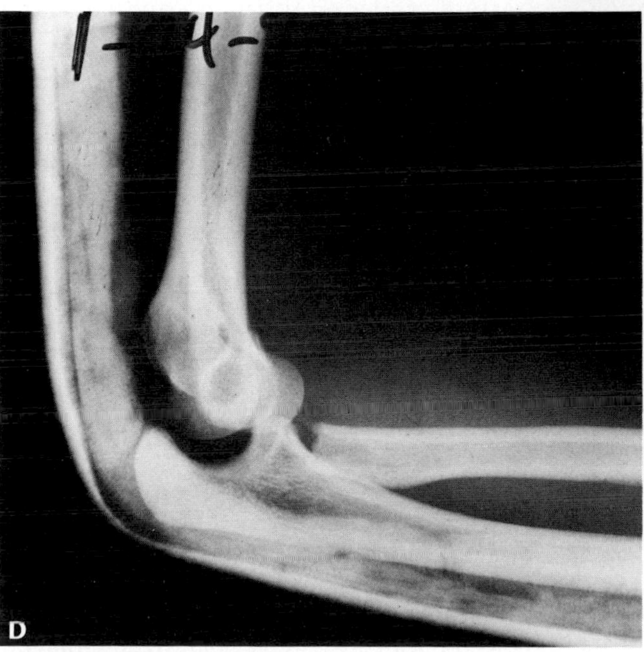

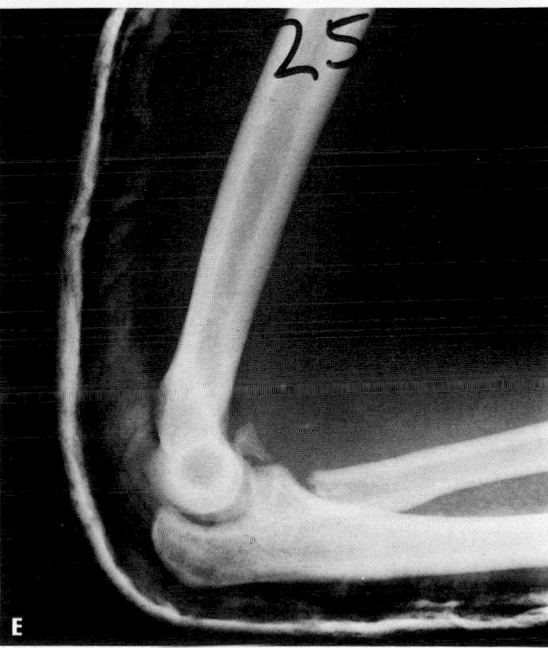

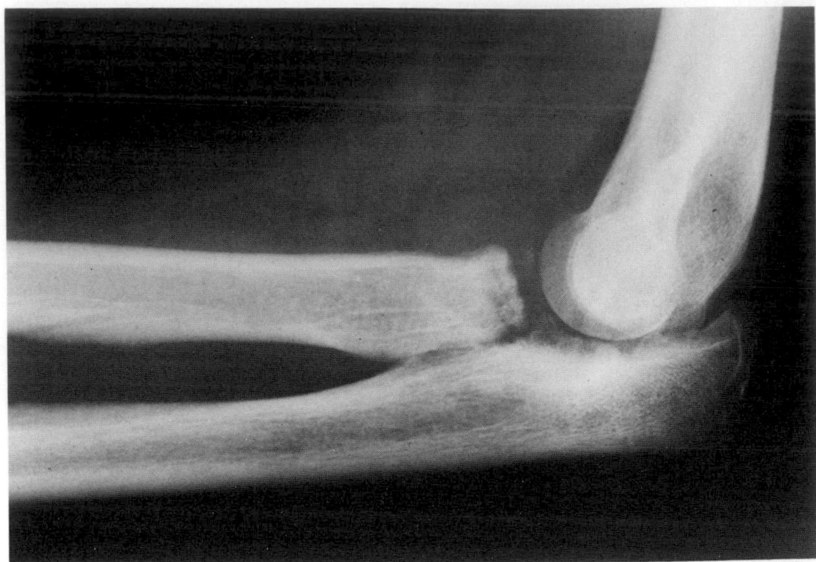

FIGURE 14-66. Concomitant excision of the radial head and coronoid process should rarely be done, because it may result in severe instability of the elbow joint, as in this patient.

Elbow Dislocation (With or Without Coronoid Fracture)

As noted earlier, preserving radiocapitellar contact in this setting may be helpful in stabilizing the joint in the acute setting. However, in most instances the combination of radial head fracture and dislocation does not result in gross instability or recurrent dislocation. If radial head fracture displacement requires open treatment, I prefer to preserve the radial head (see Fig. 14-56) if technically possible. In this situation, preservation and repair of the posterolateral ligament complex is paramount to maintain stability.[336,337] If the radial head requires excision, repair of the lateral ligament complex is also required. The forearm should be pronated during the repair. During rehabilitation, supination may need to be limited, gradually increasing the range of supination as healing permits.

A small fleck of the coronoid process may be fractured. In this setting, increasing flexion of the elbow may provide enough temporary stability. If the radial head cannot be saved and requires excision, the patient must be carefully observed for potential redislocation (Fig. 14-65). If a significant part of the coronoid is fractured (Regan-Morrey type III),[427] internal fixation of this fragment or the radial head or both could be helpful to stabilize the elbow acutely. These injuries may also be so unstable that external hinged fixation may be required (see Fig. 14-35). If the coronoid is excised and the radial head is absent, chronic and painful instability may result (Fig. 14-66).

Type III

Severely comminuted fracture of the radial head and neck is judged not reconstructable by x-ray and usually requires excision for movement. For fractures with extensive comminution and displacement without concomitant dislocation or longitudinal dissociation, early excision remains the treatment of choice. Prosthetic replacement should not be performed for this injury. After excision, the patient should begin early active motion with a passive assist as tolerated.

With Associated Injury

Interosseous Ligament Tear (Essex-Lopresti)

There is no ideal solution for this combination of injuries.[486] In a type III fracture, the degree of comminution usually requires excision with the subsequent loss of bony support. In rare instances, a two- or three-part fracture can be reconstructed and held with internal fixation. If excision is necessary and performed, continued proximal translation over weeks or months can occur, even with the use of a silicone radial head replacement.[451,496,500,505] The interosseous ligament has usually been torn and will not likely heal, despite immobilization. It is helpful to warn the patient that the injury is grave and that creation of a radioulnar synostosis with complete loss of forearm rotation may be the only ultimate solution in the months or years ahead. Cross-pinning the radius to the ulna for 6 to 8 weeks has not prevented proximal translation from occurring later.[524] However, without other alternatives, this measure is reasonable even though it is not likely to be beneficial.

The decision to excise the radial head in these patients is problematic and should be influenced by the amount of displacement. The radial head, once healed, could provide stability and potentially could prevent symptomatic proximal translation of the radius. Broberg and Morrey[452] have documented that delayed excision of the radial head can provide relief if pain develops, perhaps obviating immediate excision and near-certain chronic instability. However, with most type III fractures, the displacement of the fracture precludes any effective radiocapitellar contact for mechanical stability and the degree of displacement prevents early motion. In addition, if the initial proximal displacement is significant, the radius must be held out to length with cross-pinning of the radius to the ulna, preventing any motion and helpful remodeling of the radial head.

The use of the silicone radial head prosthesis is theoretically attractive but is not predictable in preventing proximal translation (see Fig. 14-60). With no acceptable alternative currently available, I recommend insertion of the silicone prosthesis with adequate size and firm seating on the proximal radius to act as effectively as possible. The development of a more effective metallic prosthesis remains elusive, though the latest incarnations of metallic prosthesis show some promise.[494] If the silicone prosthesis is used, the patient should be warned about material failure and continued proximal translation that may ultimately require radioulnar synostosis.

Operative Technique of Radial Head Excision

Excision of the radial head is more safely carried out through a lateral incision. As Strachan and Ellis[528] noted, the most vulnerable structure to inadvertent damage is the posterior interosseous nerve. They advised that the incision not extend more than 5 cm distal from the epicondyle and that the forearm be in full pronation during excision of the radial head. It is important, if possible, to preserve the posterolateral ligament complex in approaching the radial head. This can be achieved by entering the joint at the anterior edge of the anconeus border. In this exposure, the posterior interosseous nerve is more vulnerable, because it is closer to the area of the incision. A thorough understanding of the location of the nerve is needed.

The point of entry can also be more posterior, along the posterior border of the anconeus. Here the nerve is much less vulnerable to inadvertent injury. However, the posterior collateral ligament is usually incised through this approach. If the more posterior incision is used, a careful repair of the collateral complex is needed. If not repaired, posterolateral instability may occur.[336,337]

Open Reduction and Internal Fixation of the Radial Head—Operative Technique

Open reduction with internal fixation has become increasingly popular since reported in 1979.[454,469,473,476,477,501,509,511,520,522] Implants for internal fixation are now more varied in size and permit rigid fixation of head and neck fractures. Despite these improvements, great care must be taken to achieve rigid fixation without creating impingement in the proximal radioulnar joint. In the series published more recently,[469,473,476,477,520] larger implants have been used, including small plates as well as headed screws. The use of the Herbert screw for head fractures has also reported for head fractures alone. Before attempting operative repair of the fracture, the surgeon should be fully prepared to excise the radial head at the time of surgery if adequate restoration proves to be impossible, and the patient should be forewarned.

Insecure fixation, or implants that protrude into the proximal radioulnar joint, will generally do more harm than good.

Equipment and Technique

A complete supply of implants for internal fixation should be assembled preoperatively. It is helpful to have available an AO (ASIF) mini-fragment internal fixation set with reconstruction plates (including the mini-condylar) and a Herbert mini-screw set.

The surgical approach should be similar to that used for radial head excision, laterally, just anterior to the anconeus. As stated earlier, a thorough understanding of the location of the radial nerve and its posterior interosseous division is needed before attempting this operation.

The three major technical challenges are:

1. Reassembling the fractured radial head
2. Securing the fractured radial head to the radial neck
3. Ensuring that the implants do not interfere with pronation and supination

Once the fracture is thoroughly exposed, the pieces should be repositioned to reconstruct the radial head (Fig. 14-67). Although small Kirschner wires can be used to temporarily hold the fracture, I have sometimes found these to be more of an obstacle. There is so little room to place the implants that the wires are often in the way. Based on anatomical dissections, there is a safe zone of hardware placement comprising approximately 90°, centered about the equator in the neutral position (Fig. 14-68).[523] If this zone is used, both normally headed screws and plates can be placed without fear of impinging in the proximal radioulnar joint. If the fracture is limited to the radial head, without extension to the radial neck, the Herbert screw can be used and placed below the chondral surface. Absorbable pins have also been reported for this purpose.[510]

The radial head often requires plate fixation to the rest of the radial neck. In this instance the incision

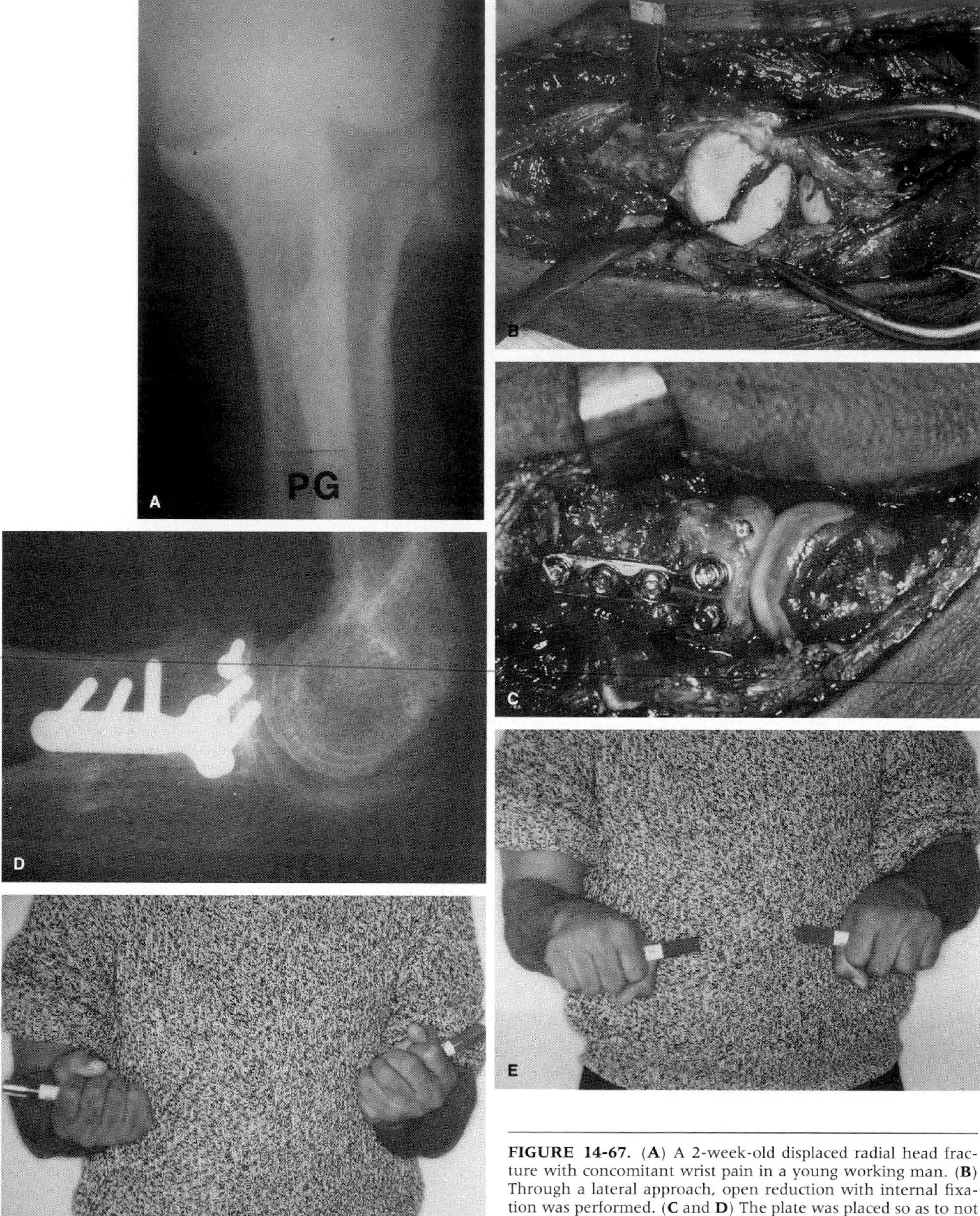

FIGURE 14-67. (**A**) A 2-week-old displaced radial head fracture with concomitant wrist pain in a young working man. (**B**) Through a lateral approach, open reduction with internal fixation was performed. (**C** and **D**) The plate was placed so as to not interfere with forearm rotation. (**E** and **F**) Eighteen months after injury, the patient retained excellent motion and function.

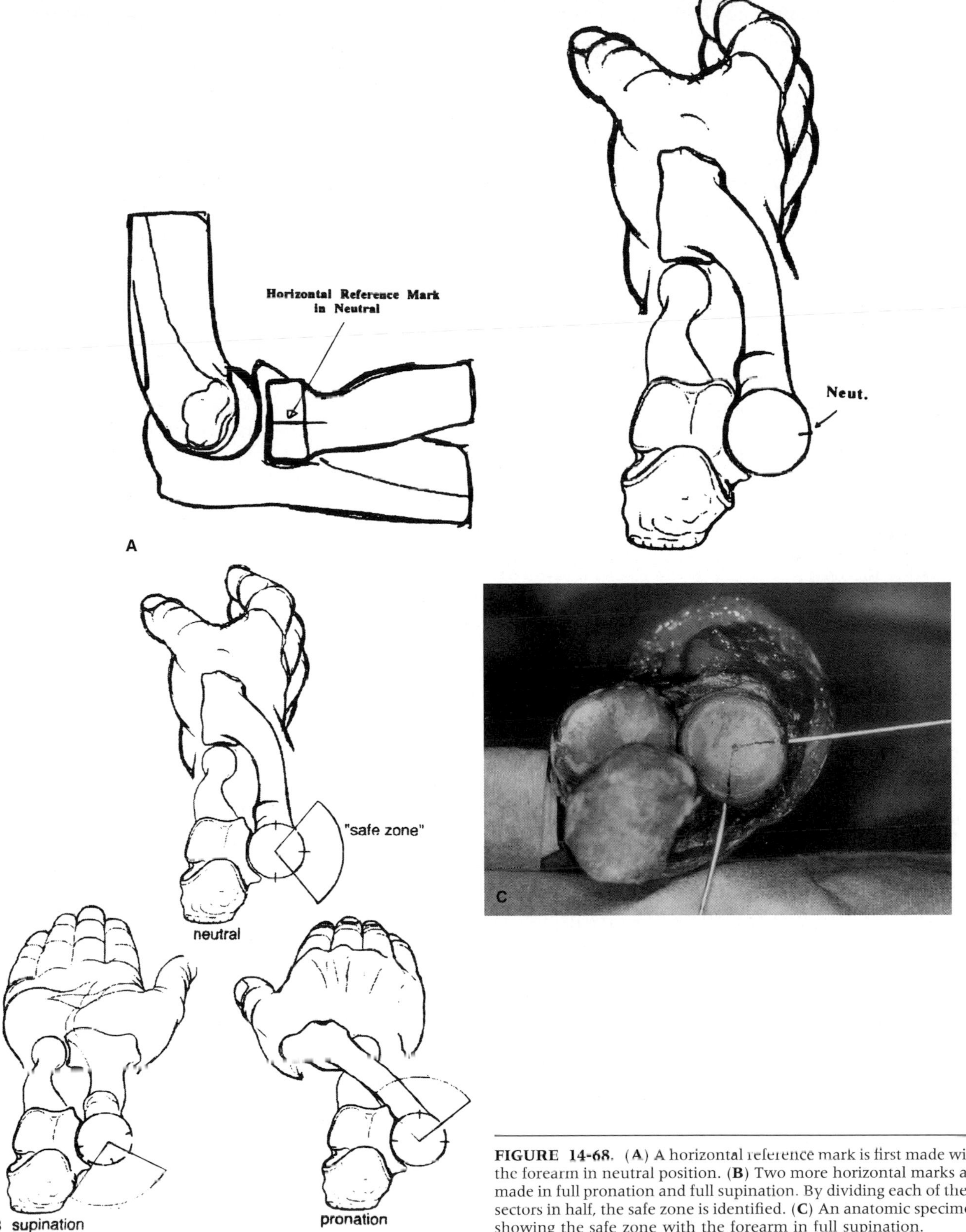

FIGURE 14-68. (**A**) A horizontal reference mark is first made with the forearm in neutral position. (**B**) Two more horizontal marks are made in full pronation and full supination. By dividing each of these sectors in half, the safe zone is identified. (**C**) An anatomic specimen showing the safe zone with the forearm in full supination.

must be extended distally. Again, the posterior interosseous nerve is vulnerable and should be identified if there is any question as to its location or safety. The 2.0- or 2.7-mm L-shaped plates can be carefully contoured to fit over the neck, providing excellent fixation. I have occasionally used a small amount of bone graft to fill any defects, especially in the area of the neck. The reduction should be checked by pronation and supination in several positions of flexion and extension. Despite detachment of all soft tissue from the head fragments, these fractures seem to heal without collapse from avascular necrosis.

The lateral capsular complex should be carefully repaired. Occasionally, suture anchors, fixed at the lateral epicondyle, are helpful to attain a sound repair of the posterolateral ligament complex. The annular ligament, a component of this structure, is usually secured into position by this repair. I do not try to repair the annular ligament as a separate structure. Active motion is initiated as soon as the patient is comfortable, usually within the first few days.

OPEN ELBOW INJURIES (SIDESWIPE INJURIES)

Sideswipe injuries[541–547] and massive open trauma to the elbow require a comprehensive team approach. Neurovascular injuries must be addressed, along with bone and soft-tissue injury. If the hand is not viable and nerve injury is extensive, primary amputation should be considered. An asensate, stiff hand is less useful than a prosthesis. Specific options for coverage of wounds about the elbow are discussed in Chapter 7. Skeletal stability and soft-tissue coverage are the primary goals of reconstruction. Although rigid internal fixation of all fractures is desirable, external fixation for wound care and soft-tissue management is often mandatory. As soon as feasible, the external fixator should be removed to initiate motion.

REHABILITATION

Proper and timely rehabilitation in the treatment of elbow injuries can reduce disabling contracture and pain. Although the inflammatory response to trauma in the elbow differs little in the initial phases from that in other major joints, one is often struck by the severity of swelling and stiffness from what seemed to be a minor blow or minimal fracture. More severe injuries, such as posterior dislocations or distal humeral fractures, commonly require formal supervised therapy to maximize outcome. The program of mobilization must be individualized to protect injured structures but permit maximal painless motion.

In the acute phase (1 to 6 weeks), the patient with a stable injury should be expected to begin active-motion exercise, both in flexion and extension and pronation and supination. During treatment and exercise, the maximal positions of flexion and extension should be sought and sustained, not rapid repetitions.

In operative cases, it is helpful to test range of motion of the elbow in the operating room to determine if there are any limits imposed by the particular fracture or ligamentous repair that would be jeopardized in any one position. One can then rationally design a program of rehabilitation with these constraints in mind. For example, in posterior dislocations, there is usually a safe zone in flexion and extension in which redislocation will not occur. One can then instruct the therapist to remain within that range of motion until healing occurs.

Active-motion exercises with attention to extension are emphasized in the first weeks after injury. If the patient is not showing progress, one can add a dynamic splinting program. Under no circumstances do I use passive manipulation to increase motion. This practice carries a very high risk for heterotopic bone formation and subsequent ankylosis.

The use of splints should be coordinated with the therapist and monitored closely. Turnbuckle orthoses, described by Green and McCoy,[372] can be effective at reducing flexion contractures. Although these were originally described using leather cuffs, Orthoplast can also be used. Commercially available dynamic splints are available,[372,373,377] but I have found that the patients tolerate this form of splinting less well than the turnbuckle orthosis.

Continuous passive motion is attractive and has been recommended by some,[369,370,376,378] but there is no evidence that the ultimate outcome is influenced by the use of these devices. Extremes of motion are difficult to achieve, and the continuous passive motion devices rarely allow the elbow to reach full extension or flexion.

If fixed contractures do occur, a number of studies have documented the improvement in motion after contracture release with the appropriate postoperative care.[369–371,374–376,379–382]

REFERENCES

ANATOMY AND BIOMECHANICS

1. An, K.N., Morrey, B.F., and Chao, E.Y.S.: The Effect of Partial Removal of the Proximal Ulna on Elow Constraint. Clin. Orthop., 209:270–279, 1986.
2. Askew, L.J., An, K.N., Morrey, B.F., and Chao, E.Y.: Isometric Elbow Strength in Normal Individuals. Clin. Orthop., 222:261–266, 1987.
3. Conwell, H.E. and Reynolds, F.C.: Key and Conwell's Management of Fractures, Dislocations and Sprains, 7th ed. St. Louis, C.V. Mosby, 1961.
4. Funk, D.A., An, K.N., Morrey, B.F., and Daube, J.R.: Electro-

myographic Analysis of Muscles Across the Elbow Joint. J. Orthop. Res., 5:529–538, 1987.
5. Goss, C.M.: Gray's Anatomy of the Human Body, 36th ed. Philadelphia, Lea & Febiger, 1954.
6. Hotchkiss, R.N., An, K.N., Sowa, D.T., Basta, S., and Weiland, A.J.: An Anatomic and Mechanical Study of the Interosseous Membrane of the Forearm: Pathomechanics of Proximal Migration of the Radius. J. Hand Surg., 14A:256–261, 1989.
7. Hotchkiss, R.N., and Weiland, A.J.: Valgus Stability of the Elbow. J. Orthop. Res., 5:372–377, 1987.
8. London, J.T.: Kinematics of the Elbow. J. Bone Joint Surg., 63A:529, 1981.
9. MacAusland, W.R.: Arthroplasty of the Elbow. N. Engl. J. Med., 236:97–99, 1947.
10. Milch, H.: Fractures of the External Humeral Condyle. J.A.M.A., 160:529–539, 1956.
11. Morrey, B.F.: Biomechanics of the Elbow. *In* Morrey, B.F. (ed.): The Elbow and Its Disorders, vol. 1, pp. 43–61. Philadelphia, W.B. Saunders, 1985.
12. Morrey, B.F.: Applied Anatomy and Biomechanics of the Elbow Joint. Instr. Course Lect., 35:59–68, 1986.
13. Morrey, B.F., and An, K.N.: Articular and Ligamentous Contributions to the Stability of the Elbow Joint. Am. J. Sports Med., 11:315–319, 1983.
14. Morrey, B.F., and An, K.N.: Functional Anatomy of the Ligaments of the Elbow. Clin. Orthop., 201:84–90, 1985.
15. Morrey, B.F., An, K.N., and Stormont, T.J.: Force Transmission Through the Radial Head. J. Bone Joint Surg., 70A:250–256, 1988.
16. Morrey, B.F., Askew, L.J., An, K.N., and Chao, E.Y.A.: Biomechanical Study of the Normal Elbow Motion. J. Bone Joint Surg., 63A:872–877, 1981.
17. Morrey, B.F., and Chao, E.Y.: Passive Motion of the Elbow Joint: A Biomechanical Analysis. J. Bone Joint Surg., 58A:501–508, 1976.
18. Olsen, B.S., Morten, G., Henriksen, G., Soibjerg, J.O., Helmig, P., and Sneppen, O.: Elbow Joint Instability: A Kinematic Model. J Shoulder Elbow Surg., 3:143–150, 1994.
19. Schwab, G.H., Bennett, J.B., Woods, G.W., and Tullos, H.S.: Biomechanics of Elbow Instability: The Role of the Medial Collateral Ligament. Clin. Orthop., 146:42–52, 1980.
20. Sojbjerg, J.O., Oversen, J., and Nielsen, S.: Experimental Elbow Instability After Transection of the Medial Collateral Ligament. Clin. Orthop., 218:186–190, 1987.
21. Solomonow, M., Guzzi, A., Baratta, R., Shoji, H., and D'Ambrosia, R.X.: EMG-force Model of the Elbows Antagonistic Muscle Pair: The Effect of Joint Position, Gravity, and Recruitment. Am. J. Phys. Med., 65:223–244, 1986.
22. Stone, C.A.: Subluxation of the Head of the Radius: Report of a Case and Anatomic Experiments. J.A.M.A., 67:28–29, 1916.
23. Taylor, T.K.F., and Scham, S.M.A.: Posteromedial Approach to the Proximal End of the Ulna for the Internal Fixation of Olecranon Fractures. J. Trauma, 9:594–602, 1969.
24. Tullos, H.S., Schwab, G., Bennett, J.B., and Woods, G.W.: Factors Influencing Elbow Instability. A.A.O.S. Instr. Course Lect., 8:185–199, 1982.
25. Volz, R.B.: Biomechanics Update #2. Basic Biomechanics: Lever Arm, Instant Center of Motion, Moment Force, Joint Reactive Force. Orthop. Rev., 15:677–684, 1986.

IMAGING

26. Franklin, P.D., Dunlop, R.W., Whitelaw, G., Jaquest, E., Jr., Blickman, J.G., and Shapiro, J.H.: Computed Tomography of the Normal and Traumatized Elbow. J. Comput. Assist. Tomogr., 12:817–823, 1988.
27. Herzog, R.J.: Magnetic Resonance Imaging of the Elbow. Magn Reson Q, 9(3):188–210, 1993.
28. Murphy, W.A., and Siegel, M.J.: Elbow Fat Pads With New Signs and Extended Differential Diagnosis. Radiology, 124: 659–665, 1977.
29. Norell, H.G.: Roentgenologic Visualization of Extracapsular Fat: Its Importance in the Diagnosis of Traumatic Injuries to the Elbow. Acta Radiol., 42.205–210, 1954.
30. Smith, D.N., and Lee, J.R.: The Radiological Diagnosis of Post-traumatic Effusion of the Elbow Joint and Its Clinical Significance: The "Displaced Fat Pad" Sign. Injury, 10:115–119, 1978.

SUPRACONDYLAR FRACTURES

31. Anderson, L.: Fractures. Campbell's Operative Orthopaedics, 5th ed. St. Louis, C.V. Mosby, 1971.
32. Bohler, L.: The Treatment of Fractures, vol. 5. Philadelphia, Grune & Stratton, 1956.
33. Bryan, R.S.: Fractures About the Elbow in Adults. A.A.O.S. Instr. Course Lect., 30:200–223, 1981.
34. Campbell, W.C.: Operative Orthopaedics. St. Louis, C.V. Mosby, 1939.
35. Childress, H.M.: Transarticular Pin Fixation in Supracondylar Fractures of the Elbow in Children. J. Bone Joint Surg., 54A:1548–1552, 1972.
36. Conn, J., and Wade, P.A.: Injuries of the Elbow (A Ten-Year Review). J. Trauma, 1:248–268, 1961.
37. Conwell, H.E., and Reynolds, F.C.: Key and Conwell's Management of Fractures, Dislocations, and Sprains, 7th ed. St. Louis, C.V. Mosby, 1961.
38. D'Ambrosia, R.D.: Supracondylar Fractures of the Humerus—Prevention of Cubitus Varus Deformity. J. Bone Joint Surg., 54A:60–72, 1972.
39. Decoulx, P., Decoulx, M., Hespeel, J., and Coulx, J.: Les Fractures de l'Extremité Inferieure de l'Humerus Chez l'Adulte. Rev. Chir. Orthop., 50:263–273, 1964.
40. DePalma, A.F.: The Management of Fractures and Dislocations. Philadelphia, W.B. Saunders, 1959.
41. Dunlop, J.: Transcondylar Fractures of the Humerus in Childhood. J. Bone Joint Surg., 21:59–73, 1939.
42. Dupuytren, B.G.: On the Injuries and Diseases of Bones. London, Syndeham Society, 1847.
43. Fowles, J.V., Kassab, M.T., and Said, K.: Supracondylar Fractures in Children, Stabilization by Two Lateral Percutaneous Pins. Presented at Canadian Orthopaedic Association Annual Meeting, Winnipeg, Manitoba, 1973.
44. Hamilton, F.H.: A Practical Treatise on Fractures and Dislocations, 8th ed. Philadelphia, Lea Brothers & Co, 1891.
45. Henry, A.K.: Extensile Exposure. Baltimore, Williams & Wilkins, 1945.
46. Horne, G.: Supracondylar Fractures of the Humerus in Adults. J. Trauma, 20:71, 1980.
47. Hoyer, A.: Treatment of Supracondylar Fractures of the Humerus by Skeletal Traction in an Abduction Splint. J. Bone Joint Surg., 34A:623–637, 1952.
48. Jones, K.G.: Percutaneous Pin Fixation of Fractures of the Lower End of the Humerus. Clin. Orthop., 50:53–69, 1967.
49. Keon-Cohen, B.T.: Fractures of the Elbow. J. Bone Joint Surg., 48A:1623–1639, 1966.
50. King, D., and Secor, C.: Bow Elbow (Cubitus Varus). J. Bone Joint Surg., 33A:572–576, 1951.
51. MacAusland, W.R., and Wyman, E.T.: Fractures of the Adult Elbow. A.A.O.S. Instr. Course Lect., 24:169–181, 1975.
52. Mann, T.S. Prognosis in Supracondylar Fractures. J. Bone Joint Surg., 45B:516–522, 1963.
53. Merle d'Aubigne, R., Meary, R., and Carlioz, J.: Fractures Sus et Intercondyliennes Recentes de l'Adulte. Rev. Chir. Orthop., 50:279–288, 1964.
54. Miller, O.L.: Blind Nailing of the T-Fracture of the Lower End of the Humerus Which Involves the Joint. J. Bone Joint Surg., 21:933–938, 1939.
55. Muller, M.E., Allgower, M., Schneider, R., and Willenggeı, H.: Manual of Internal Fixation. New York, Springer-Verlag, 1979.
56. Roberts, J.B., and Kelly, J.A.: Treatise on Fractures. Philadelphia, J.B. Lippincott, 1921.
57. Salter, R.B.: Problem Fractures in Children. A.A.O.S. Instr. Course Lect. Annual Meeting, Dallas, Texas, 1974.
58. Scudder, C.L.: Treatment of Fractures, 9th ed. Philadelphia, W.B. Saunders, 1923.
59. Siris, I.E.: Supracondylar Fractures of the Humerus. Gynecol. Obstet., 68:201–222, 1939.
60. Sisk, T.D.: Fractures of the Distal End of Humerus. In Crenshaw, A.H. (ed.): Campbell's Operative Orthopaedics, 6th ed., pp. 674–683, St. Louis, C.V. Mosby, 1980.

61. Smith, F.M.: Surgery of the Elbow, 2nd ed. Philadelphia, W.B. Saunders, 1972.
62. Smith, L.: Deformity Following Supracondylar Fracture of the Humerus. J. Bone Joint Surg., 42A:235–252, 1960.
63. Soltanpur, A.: Anterior Supracondylar Fracture of the Humerus (Flexion Type). J. Bone Joint Surg., 60B:383–386, 1978.
64. Speed, K.A.: Textbook of Fractures and Dislocation. Philadelphia, Lea & Febiger, 1935.
65. Swenson, A.L.: Treatment of Supracondylar Fractures of the Humerus by Kirschner-Wire Transfixation. J. Bone Joint Surg., 30A:993–997, 1948.
66. Watson-Jones, R.: Fractures and Joint Injuries, 3rd ed. Baltimore, Williams & Wilkins, 1946.

TRANSCONDYLAR FRACTURES

67. Ashurst, A.P.C.: An Anatomical and Surgical Study of Fractures of the Lower End of the Humerus. The Samuel D. Gross Prize Essay of the Philadelphia Academy. Philadelphia, Lea & Febiger, 1910.
68. Bryan, R.S.: Fractures About the Elbow in Adults. A.A.O.S. Instr. Course Lect., 30:200–223, 1981.
69. Chutro, P. Fracturas De La Extremidad Inferior Del Humero En Los Ninos. Theses J. Peuser, Buenos Aires, 1904.
70. Conwell, H.E., and Reynolds, F.C.: Key and Conwell's Management of Fractures, Dislocations, and Sprains, 7th ed. St. Louis, C.V. Mosby, 1961.
71. DePalma, A.F.: The Management of Fractures and Dislocations. Philadelphia, W.B. Saunders, 1959.
72. Grantham, S.A., and Tietjen, R.: Transcondylar Fracture–Dislocation of the Elbow. J. Bone Joint Surg., 58A:1030–1031, 1976.
73. Hamilton, F.H.: A Practical Treatise on Fractures and Dislocations, 8th ed. Philadelphia, Lea Brothers & Co., 1891.
74. Roberts, J.B., and Kelly, J.A.: Treatise on Fractures, 2nd ed. Philadelphia, J.B. Lippincott, 1921.
75. Scudder, C.L.: Treatment of Fractures, 9th ed. Philadelphia, W.B. Saunders, 1923.
76. Smith, F.M.: Surgery of the Elbow. Springfield, Ill., Charles C Thomas, 1954.
77. Speed, K.A.: Textbook of Fractures and Dislocations, 3rd ed. Philadelphia, Lea & Febiger, 1935.
78. Watson-Jones, R.: Fractures and Joint Injuries. Philadelphia, J.B. Lippincott, 1925.
79. Wilson, P.D., and Cochrane, W.A.: Fractures and Dislocations. Philadelphia, J.B. Lippincott, 1925.

INTERCONDYLAR FRACTURES

80. Ackerman, G., and Jupiter, J.B.: Non-union of Fractures and the Distal End of the Humerus. J. Bone Joint Surg., 70A:75–83, 1988.
81. Anson, B.J., and Maddock, W.B.: Callander's Surgical Anatomy. Philadelphia, W.B. Saunders, 1958.
82. Bickel, W.E., and Perry, R.E.: Comminuted Fractures of the Distal Humerus. J.A.M.A., 184:553–557, 1963.
83. Bohler, L.: The Treatment of Fractures. Vienna, Wilhelm Maudrich, 1929.
84. Brown, R.F., and Morgan, R.G.: Intercondylar T-shaped Fractures of the Humerus. J. Bone Joint Surg., 53B:425–428, 1971.
85. Bryan, R.S., and Bickel, W.H.: "T" Condylar Fractures of the Distal Humerus. J. Trauma, 11:830–835, 1971.
86. Bryan, R.S., and Morrey, B.F.: Extensive Posterior Exposure of the Elbow. Clin. Orthop., 166:188–192, 1982.
87. Burri, C., Henkemyer, H., and Spier, W.: Results of Operative Treatment of Intra-articular Fractures of the Distal Humerus. Acta Orthop. Belg., 41:227–234, 1975.
88. Bush, L.F., and McClain, E.J.: Operative Treatment of Fractures of the Elbow in Adults. Instr. Course Lect., 16:265–277, 1959.
89. Campbell, W.C.: Operative Orthopaedics. St. Louis, C.V. Mosby, 1939.
90. Cassebaum, W.H.: Operative Treatment of T- and Y-Fractures of the Lower End of the Humerus. Am. J. Surg., 83:265–270, 1952.
91. Cassebaum, W.H.: Open Reduction of T- and Y-Fractures of the Lower End of the Humerus. J. Trauma, 9:915–925, 1969.
92. Chacha, P.B.: Fracture of the Medial Condyle of the Humerus With Rotational Displacement: Report of Two Cases. J. Bone Joint Surg., 52A:1453–1458, 1970.
93. Conn, J., and Wade, P.A.: Injuries of the Elbow: A Ten-Year Review. J. Trauma, 1:248–268, 1961.
94. Conwell, H.E., and Reynolds, F.C.: Key and Conwell's Management of Fractures, Dislocations, and Sprains, 7th ed. St. Louis, C.V. Mosby, 1961.
95. DePalma, A.F.: The Management of Fractures and Dislocations. Philadelphia, W.B. Saunders, 1959.
96. Desault, P.J.: A Treatise on Fractures, Luxations and Other Affections of the Bones, 2nd ed. Philadelphia, Kimber & Conrad, 1811.
97. Eastwood, W.J.: The T-Shaped Fractures of the Lower End of the Humerus. J. Bone Joint Surg., 19:364–369, 1937.
98. Evans, E.M.: Supracondylar Y-Fractures of the Humerus. J. Bone Joint Surg., 35B:381–385, 1953.
99. Gabel, G.T., Hanson, G., Bennett, J.B., Noble, P.C., and Tullos, H.S.: Intraarticular Fractures of the Distal Humerus in the Adult. Clin. Orthop., 216:99–108, 1987.
100. Godette, G.A., and Gruel, C.R.: Percutaneous screw fixation of intercondylar fracture of the distal humerus. Orthop. Rev., 22:466–468, 1993.
101. Goss, C.M.: Gray's Anatomy of the Human Body, 26th ed. Philadelphia, Lea & Febiger, 1954.
102. Grant, J.C.B.: A Method of Anatomy, 5th ed. Baltimore, Williams & Wilkins, 1952.
103. Heim, U., and Pfeiffer, K.M.: Elbow. In: Internal Fixation of Small Fractures, vol. 3, pp. 107—109. Berlin, Springer-Verlag, 1976.
104. Helfet, D.L., and Hotchkiss, R.N.: Internal Fixation of the Humerus: A Biomechanical Comparison of Methods. J. Orthop. Trauma, 4:260–264, 1990.
105. Helfet, D.L., and Schmeling, G.J.: Bicondylar Intraarticular Fractures of the Distal Humerus in Adults. Clin. Orthop., 292:26–36, 1993.
106. Henley, M.B.: Intra-articular Distal Humeral Fractures in Adults. Orthop. Clin. North. Am., 18:11–23, 1987.
107. Henley, M.B., Bone, L.B., and Parker, B.: Operative Management of Intra-articular Fractures of the Distal Humerus. J. Orthop. Trauma, 1:24–35, 1987.
108. Hitzrot, J.M.: Fractures at the Lowest End of the Humerus in Adults. Surg. Clin. North Am., 12:291–304, 1932.
109. Holdsworth, B.J., and Mossad, M.M.: Fractures of the Adult Distal Humerus: Elbow Function After Internal Fixation. J. Bone Joint Surg., 72B:362–365, 1990.
110. Johansson, H., and Olerud, S.: Operative Treatment of Intercondylar Fractures of the Humerus. J. Trauma, 11:836–843, 1971.
111. Jupiter, J.B., Barnes, K.A., Goodman, L.J., and Saldana, A.E.: Multiplane Fracture of the Distal Humerus. J. Orthop. Trauma, 7:216–220, 1993.
112. Jupiter, J.B., and Mehne, D.K.: Fractures of the Distal Humerus. Orthopedics, 15:825–833, 1992.
113. Jupiter, J.B. and Morrey, B.F.: Fractures of the Distal Humerus. *In* Morrey, B.F. (ed.): The Elbow and Its Disorders, Philadelphia, W.B. Saunders, 1993.
114. Jupiter, J.B., Neff, U., Holzach, P., and Allgöwer, M.: Intercondylar Fractures of the Humerus. J. Bone Joint Surg., 67A:226–239, 1985.
115. Kelly, R.P., and Griffin, T.W.: Open Reduction of T-Condylar Fractures of the Humerus Through an Anterior Approach. J. Trauma, 9:901–914, 1969.
116. Keon-Cohen, B.T.: Fractures at the Elbow. J. Bone Joint Surg., 48A:1623–1639, 1966.
117. Knight, R.A.: Fractures of the Humeral Condyles in Adults. South. Med. J., 48:1165–1173, 1955.
118. Knight, R.A.: Management of Fractures About the Elbow in Adults. A.A.O.S. Instr. Course Lect., 26:123–141, 1957.
119. Letsch, R., Schmit-Neuerburg, K.P., Sturmer, K.M., and Walz, M.: Intraarticular Fractures of the Distal Humerus: Surgical Treatment and Results. Clin. Orthop., 241:238–244, 1989.

120. MacAusland, W.R.: Ankylosis of the Elbow: With Report of Four Cases Treated by Arthroplasty. J.A.M.A., 64:312–318, 1915.
121. Mellen, R.H., and Phalen, G.S.: Arthroplasty of the Elbow by Replacement of the Distal Portion of the Humerus With an Acrylic Prosthesis. J. Bone Joint Surg., 23:348–353, 1947.
122. Milch, H.: Fractures and Fracture–Dislocations of the Humeral Condyles. J. Trauma, 4:592–607, 1964.
123. Miller, O.L.: Blind Nailing of the T Fracture of the Lower End of the Humerus Which Involves the Joint. J. Bone Joint Surg., 21:933–938, 1939.
124. Miller, W.E.: Comminuted Fractures of the Distal End of the Humerus in the Adult. J. Bone Joint Surg., 46A:1644–657, 1964.
125. Muller, M.E., Allgöwer, M., Schneider, R., and Willenegger, H.: Manual of Internal Fixation, 2nd ed. New York, Springer-Verlag, 1979.
126. Palmer, I.: Open Treatment of Transcondylar T-Fractures of the Humerus. Acta Chir. Scand., 121:486–490, 1961.
127. Patterson, R.F.: A Method of Applying Traction in T and Y Fractures of the Distal Humerus. J. Bone Joint Surg., 17:476–477, 1935.
128. Reich, R.S.: Treatment of Intercondylar Fractures of the Elbow by Means of Traction. J. Bone Joint Surg., 18:997–1004, 1936.
129. Riseborough, E.J., and Radin, E.L.: Intercondylar T Fractures of the Humerus in the Adult: A Comparison of Operative and Non-Operative Treatment in Twenty-nine Cases. J. Bone Joint Surg., 51A:130–141, 1969.
130. Scharplatz, D., and Allgöwer, M.: Fracture–Dislocations of the Elbow. Injury, 7:143–159, 1975.
131. Smith, F.M.: Surgery of the Elbow. Philadelphia, W.B. Saunders, 1972.
132. Sodergard, J., Sandelin, J., and Bostman, O.: Mechanical Failures of Internal Fixation in T and Y Fractures of the Distal Humerus. J. Trauma, 33:687–690, 1992.
133. Talha, A., Toulemonde, J.L., Cronier, P., Lorimier, G., Ghestem, P., and Guntz, M.: Supra and Intercondylar Fractures: Late Results Following Stable Osteosynthesis. J. Chir. (Paris), 126:217–224, 1989.
134. Thomas, T.T.: A Contribution to the Mechanism of Fractures and Dislocations in the Elbow Region. Ann. Surg., 89:108–121, 1929.
135. Thorton, L.: Fractures of the Humerus Treated by Means of the Hoke Plaster Traction Apparatus. J. Bone Joint Surg., 12:911–924, 1930.
136. Trynin, A.H.: Intercondylar T Fracture of Elbow. J. Bone Joint Surg., 23:709–711, 1941.
137. Van Gorder, G.W.: Surgical Approach in Supracondylar "T" Fractures of the Humerus Requiring Open Reduction. J. Bone Joint Surg., 22:278–292, 1940.
138. Watson-Jones, R.: Fractures and Joint Injuries. Baltimore, Williams & Wilkins, 1946.
139. Wickstrom, J., and Meyer, P.R.: Fractures of the Distal Humerus in Adults. Clin. Orthop., 50:43–51, 1967.
140. Willenegger, H.: Problems and Results in the Treatment of Comminuted Fractures of the Elbow. Reconstr. Surg. Traumatol, 11:118–127, 1969.
141. Wilson, P.D.: Fractures and Dislocations in the Region of the Elbow. Surg. Gynecol. Obstet., 56:335–359, 1933.
142. Wilson, P.D.: Experience in the Management of Fractures and Dislocations. Philadelphia, J.B. Lippincott, 1938.
143. Wilson, P.D., and Cochrane, W.A.: Fractures and Dislocations. Philadelphia, J.B. Lippincott, 1925.
144. Zagorski, J.B., Jennings, J.J., Burkhalter, W.E., and Uribe, J.W.: Comminuted Intraarticular Fractures of the Distal Humeral Condyles: Surgical vs. Nonsurgical Treatment. Clin. Orthop., 202:197–204, 1986.

DISTAL HUMERAL FRACTURES—RECONSTRUCTION

145. Barr, J.S., and Eaton, R.G.: Elbow Reconstruction With a New Prosthesis to Replace the Distal End of the Humerus. J. Bone Joint Surg., 47A:1408–1413, 1965.
146. Breen, T., Gelberman, R.H., Leffert, R., and Botte, M.: Massive Allograft Replacement of Hemiarticular Traumatic Defects of the Elbow. J. Hand Surg., 13A:900–907, 1988.
147. Deland, J.T., Walker, P.S., Sledge, C.B., and Faberov, A.A.: Treatment of Posttraumatic Elbows with a New Hinge Distractor. Orthopedics, 732–737, 1983.
148. Dunn, A.W.: A Distal Humeral Prosthesis. Clin. Orthop., 215:199–202, 1987.
149. Figgie, H.E., Inglis, A.E., Ranawat, C.S., and Rosenberg, G.M.: Results of Total Elbow Arthroplasty as a Salvage Procedure for Failed Elbow Reconstructive Operations. Clin. Orthop., 219: 185–193, 1987.
150. Morrey, B.F.: Post-Traumatic Contracture of the Elbow: Operative Treatment, Including Distraction Arthroplasty. J. Bone Joint Surg., 72A:601–618, 1990.
151. Morrey, B.F., Bryan, R.S., Dobyns, J.H., and Linscheid, R.L.: Total Elbow Arthorplasty: A Five Year Experience at the Mayo Clinic. J. Bone Joint Surg., 63A:1050–1063, 1981.
152. Ross, A.C., Sneath, R.S., and Scales, J.T.: Endoprosthetic Replacement of the Humerus and Elbow Joint. J. Bone Joint Surg., 69B:652–655, 1987.
153. Shahriaree, H., Sajadi, K., Silver, C., and Sheikholeslamzadeh, S.: Excisional Arthoplasty of the Elbow. J. Bone Joint Surg., 61A:922–927, 1979.
154. Venable, C.S.: An Elbow and an Elbow Prosthesis. Am. J. Surg., 83:271–275, 1952.
155. Volkov, M.V., and Oganesian, O.V.: Restoration of Function in the Knee and Elbow With a Hinge Distractor Apparatus. J. Bone Joint Surg., 57A:591–607, 1975.

CONDYLAR FRACTURES

156. Bodoky, A., Neff, U., and Regazzoni, P.: Intra-articular Unicondylar Humerus Fractures: Late Results Following Stable Osteosynthesis. Orthopade, 17:257–261, 1988.
157. Bohler, L.: The Treatment of Fractures, 5th ed. New York, Grune & Stratton, 1956.
158. Bryan, R.S.: Fractures About the Elbow in Adults. Instr. Course Lect., 30:200–223, 1981.
159. Conn, J., and Wade, P.A.: Injuries of the Elbow (A Ten-Year Review). J. Trauma, 1:248–268, 1961.
160. Conwell, H.E., and Reynolds, F.C.: Key and Conwell's Management of Fractures, Dislocations, and Sprains, 7th ed. St. Louis, C.V. Mosby, 1961.
161. Cotton, F.J.: Dislocations and Joint Fractures, 2nd ed. Philadelphia, W.B. Saunders, 1924.
162. Ghawabi, M.H.: Fracture of the Medial Condyle of the Humerus. J. Bone Joint Surg., 57A:677–680, 1975.
163. Hamilton, F.H.: A Practical Treatise on Fractures and Dislocations, 8th ed. Philadelphia, Lea Brothers & Co., 1891.
164. Jupiter, J.B., Neff, U., Regazzoni, P., and Allogöwer, M.: Unicondylar Fractures of the Distal Humerus: An Operative Approach. J. Orthop. Trauma, 2:102–109, 1988.
165. Kalenak, A.: Ununited Fractures of the Lateral Condyle of the Humerus: A 50 Year Follow-up. Clin. Orthop., 124:181–183, 1977.
166. Keon-Cohen, B.T.: Fractures of the Elbow. J. Bone Joint Surg., 46A:1623–1639, 1966.
167. Knight, R.A.: Fractures of the Humeral Condyles in Adults. South. Med. J., 48:1165–1173, 1955.
168. Niemann, K.M.W.: Condylar Fractures of the Distal Humerus in Adults. South. Med. J., 70:915–918, 1977.
169. Smith, F.M.: Surgery of the Elbow, 2nd ed. Phildelphia, W.B. Saunders, 1972.
170. Smith, F.M.: An Eighty-Four Year Follow-up on a Patient With Ununited Fracture of the Lateral Condyle of the Humerus. J. Bone Joint Surg., 55A:378–380, 1973.
171. Speed, J.S.: Surgical Treatment of Condylar Fractures of the Humerus. Instr. Course Lect., 7:187–194, 1950.
172. Wilson, P.D., and Cochrane, W.A.: Fractures and Dislocations, pp. 175–179. Philadelphia, J.B. Lippincott, 1925.

CAPITELLAR FRACTURES

173. Alvarez, E., Patel, M., Wimburg, G., and Pearlman, H.S.: Fracture of the Capitellum Humeri. J. Bone Joint Surg., 57A:1093–1096, 1975.
174. Anderson, L.: Fractures. *In* Crenshaw, A.H. (ed.): Campbell's Operative Orthopaedics, 5th ed. St. Louis, C.V. Mosby, 1971.

175. Bohler, L.: The Treatment of Fractures, 5th ed. New York, Grune & Stratton, 1956.
176. Bryan, R.S.: Fractures About the Elbow in Adults. Instr. Course Lect., 30:200–223, 1981.
177. Bush, L.F., and McClain, E.J.: Operative Treatment of Fractures of the Elbow in Adults. Instr. Course Lect., 16:265–277, 1959.
178. Buxton, S.J.D.: Fractures of the Head of the Radius and Capitellum Including External Condylar Fractures of Childhood. Br. Med. J., 2:665–666, 1936.
179. Christopher, F., and Bushnell, L.F.: Conservative Treatment of Fracture of the Capitellum. J. Bone Joint Surg., 17:489–492, 1935.
180. Collert, S.: Surgical Management of Fracture of the Capitellum Humeri. Acta Orthop. Scand., 48:603–606, 1977.
181. Conn, J., and Wade, P.A.: Injuries of the Elbow (A Ten-Year Review). J. Trauma, 1:248–268, 1961.
182. Conwell, H.E., and Reynolds, F.C.: Key and Conwell's Management of Fractures, Dislocations, and Sprains, 7th ed. St. Louis, C.V. Mosby, 1961.
183. Cotton, F.J.: Two Unusual Forms of Fracture: Fracture of the Capitellum; Fracture of the Fifth Metatarsal by Inversion. Boston Med. Surg. J., 149:734–736, 1903.
184. Cotton, F.J.: Dislocations and Joint Fractures. Philadelphia, W.B. Saunders, 1924.
185. Darrach, W.: Open Reduction of Fractures of the Capitellum. Ann. Surg., 63:487, 1916.
186. DePalma, A.F.: The Management of Fractures and Dislocations. Philadelphia, W.B. Saunders, 1959.
187. Dushuttle, R.P., Coyle, M.P., Zawadsky, J.P., and Bloom, H.: Fractures of the Capitellum. J. Trauma, 25:317–321, 1985.
188. Eliason, E.L., and North, J.P.: Fractures About the Elbow. Am. J. Surg., 44:88–99, 1939.
189. Flemming, C.W.: Fractures of the Head of the Radius. Proc. R. Soc. Med., 25:1011–1015, 1932.
190. Flint, C.P.: Fractures of the Eminentia Capitata. Surg. Gynecol. Obstet., 7:343–356, 1908.
191. Fowles, J.V., and Kassab, M.T.: Fracture of the Capitellum Humeri. J. Bone Joint Surg., 56A:794–798, 1974.
192. Gejrot, W.: On Intra-Articular Fractures of the Capitellum and Trochlea of the Humerus With Special Reference to the Treatment. Acta Chir. Scand., 71:253–270, 1932.
193. Grantham, S.A., Norris, T.R., and Bush, D.C.: Isolated Fractures of the Humeral Capitellum. Clin. Orthop., 161:262–269, 1981.
194. Hahn, N.F.: Fall von Cine Besonderes Varietat der Frakturen des Ellenbogens. Z. Wundarzte Geburtshilfe, 6:185–189, 1853.
195. Hamilton, F.H.: A Practical Treatise on Fractures and Dislocations, 8th ed. Philadelphia, Lea Brothers & Co., 1891.
196. Hendel, D., Aghasi, M., and Halperin, N.: Unusual Fracture–Dislocation of the Elbow Joint. Arch. Orthop. Trauma Surg., 104:187–188, 1985.
197. Jakobsson, A.: Fracture of the Capitellum of the Humerus in Adults: Treatment With Intra-Articular Chrome-Cobalt-Molybdenum Prosthesis. Acta Orthop. Scand., 26:184–190, 1957.
198. Johansson, O.: Capsular and Ligament Injuries of the Elbow Joint. Acta Chir. Scand. (Suppl.), 287:50–65, 1962.
199. Jopson, J.H.: Fracture of the Capitellum. Int. Clin. Series, 4:232–242, 1913.
200. Keon-Cohen, B.T.: Fractures at the Elbow. J. Bone Joint Surg., 48A:1623–1639, 1966.
201. Kleiger, B., and Joseph, H.: Fracture of the Capitellum Humeri. Bull. Hosp. Joint Dis., 25:64–70, 1964.
202. Kocher, T.: Beitrage zur Kenntniss Einiger Tisch Wichtiger Frakturformen, pp. 585–591. Basel, Sallman, 1896.
203. Lansinger, O., and Mare, K.: Fracture of the Capitellum Humeri. Acta Orthop. Scand., 52:39–44, 1981.
204. Lee, W.E., and Summey, T.J.: Fracture of the Capitellum of the Humerus. Ann. Surg., 99:497–509, 1934.
205. Lindem, M.C.: Fractures of the Capitellum and Trochlea. Ann. Surg., 76:78–82, 1922.
206. Lorenz, H.: Zur Kenntniss der Fractura humeri (eminentiae capitatae). Dtsch. Z. Chir., 78:531–545, 1905.
207. MacAusland, W.R., and Wyman, E.T.: Fractures of the Adult Elbow. Instr. Course Lect., 24:169–181, 1975.
208. MacDonald, J.A., and McGoey, P.F.: Fractures of the Articular Portion of the Capitellum of the Humerus in Adults. Can. Med. Assoc. J., 81:634–636, 1959.
209. Mazel, M.S.: Fracture of the Capitellum. J. Bone Joint Surg., 17:483–488, 1935.
210. Milch, H.: Unusual Fractures of the Capitellum Humeri and the Capitellum Radii. J. Bone Joint Surg., 13:882–886, 1931.
211. Mouchet, M.A.: Fractures de l'Extremité Inferieure de l'Humerus, p. 282. Paris, G. Steinheil, 1898.
212. Patterson, R.F.: Fracture of the Capitellum. J. Tenn. Med. Assoc., 22:277–282, 1929.
213. Rhodin, R.: On the Treatment of Fracture of the Capitellum. Acta Chir. Scand., 86:475–486, 1942.
214. Richards, R.R., Khoury, G.W., Burke, F.D., and Waddell, J.P.: Internal Fixation of Capitellar Fractures Using Herbert Screws: A Report of Four Cases. Can. J. Surg., 30:188–191, 1987.
215. Rieth, P.L.: Fractures of the Radial Head Associated With Chip Fracture of the Capitellum in Adults: Surgical Considerations. South. Surg., 14:154–159, 1948.
216. Roberts, J.B., and Kelly, J.A.: Treatise on Fractures, 2nd ed. Philadelphia, J.B. Lippincott, 1921.
217. Robertson, R.C., and Bogart, F.B.: Fracture of the Capitellum and Trochlea, Combined with Fracture of the External Humeral Condyle. J. Bone Joint Surg., 15:206–213, 1933.
218. Schultz, R.J.: The Language of Fractures. Baltimore, Williams & Wilkins, 1972.
219. Simpson, L.A., and Richards, R.R.: Internal Fixation of a Capitellar Fracture Using Herbert Screws. Clin. Orthop., 209:166–168, 1986.
220. Smith, F.M.: Surgery of the Elbow, 2nd ed. Philadlephia, W.B. Saunders, 1972.
221. Steinthal, D.: Die isolierte Fraktur der Eminentia capitata in Ellenbogengelenk. Zentralbl. Chir., 15:17–20, 1898.
222. Stimson, L.A.: A Treatise on Fractures. Philadelphia, Henry C. Lea's Son & Co., 1890.
223. Wilson, P.D.: Fractures and Dislocations in the Region of the Elbow. Gynecol. Obstet., 56:335–359, 1933.

TROCHLEAR FRACTURES

224. Noue, G., and Horli, E.: Combined Shear Fractures of the Trochlea and Capitellum Associated With Anterior Fracture–Dislocation of the Elbow. J. Orthop. Trauma, 6:373–375, 1992.
225. Smith, F.M.: Surgery of the Elbow, 2nd ed. Philadelphia, W.B. Saunders, 1972.

EPICONDYLAR FRACTURES

226. Bernstein, S.M., King, J.D., and Sanderson, R.A.: Fractures of the Medial Epicondyles of the Humerus. Contemp. Orthop., 3:637–642, 1981.
227. Conn, J., and Wade, P.A.: Injuries of the Elbow: A Ten-Year Review. J. Trauma, 1:248–268, 1961.
228. Conwell, H.E., and Reynolds, F.C.: Key and Conwell's Management of Fractures, Dislocations, and Sprains. St. Louis, C.V. Mosby, 7th ed. 1961.
229. DePalma, A.F.: The Management of Fractures and Dislocations. Philadelphia, W.B. Saunders, 1959.
230. Goss, C.M.: Gray's Anatomy of the Human Body, 26th ed. Philadelphia, Lea & Febiger, 1954.
231. Hamilton, F.H.: A Practical Treatise on Fractures and Dislocations, 9th ed. Philadelphia, Lea Brothers & Co., 1891.
232. Keon-Cohen, B.T.: Fractures at the Elbow. J. Bone Joint Surg., 48A:1623–1639, 1966.
233. Knight, R.A.: Fractures of the Humeral Condyles in Adults. South. Med. J., 48:1165–1173, 1955.
234. Patrick, J.: Fracture of the Medial Epicondyle With Displacement Into the Elbow Joint. J. Bone Joint Surg., 28:143–147, 1946.
235. Purser, D.W.: Dislocation of the Elbow and Inclusion of the Medial Epicondyle in the Adult. J. Bone Joint Surg., 36B:247–249, 1954.
236. Rang, M.: Children's Fractures. Philadelphia, J.B. Lippincott, 1974.

237. Roaf, R.: Foramen in the Humerus Caused by the Median Nerve. J. Bone Joint Surg., 39B:748–749, 1957.
238. Sisk, F.D.: Fractures. *In* Crenshaw, A.H. (ed.): Campbell's Operative Orthopaedics. St. Louis, C.V. Mosby, 1980.
239. Smith, F.M.: Medial Epicondyle Injuries. J.A.M.A., 142:396–402, 1950.
240. Stimson, L.A.: A Treatise on Fractures. Philadelphia, Henry C. Lea's Son & Co., 1890.
241. Watson-Jones, R.: Fractures and Joint Injuries, 3rd ed., vol. 2. Baltimore, Williams & Wilkins, 1946.

SUPRACONDYLAR PROCESS FRACTURES

242. Barnard, L.B., and McCoy, S.M.: The Supracondylar Process of the Humerus. J. Bone Joint Surg., 23:845–850, 1946.
243. Doane, C.P.: Fractures of the Supracondylar Process of the Humerus. J. Bone Joint Surg., 18:757–759, 1936.
244. Genner, B.A.: Fractures of the Supracondyloid Process. J. Bone Joint Surg., 41A:1333–1335, 1959.
245. Hollinshead, W.H.: Anatomy for Surgeons: The Back and Limbs, 2nd ed. New York, Harper & Row, 1969.
246. Kolb, L.W., and Moore, R.D.: Fractures of the Supracondylar Process of the Humerus: Report of Two Cases. J. Bone Joint Surg., 49A:532–534, 1967.
247. Lund, H.J.: Fracture of the Supracondyloid Process of the Humerus. J. Bone Joint Surg., 12:925–928, 1930.

DISLOCATIONS

248. Borris, L.C., Lassen, M.R., and Christensen, C.S.: Elbow Dislocation in Children and Adults: A Long-Term Follow-up of Conservatively Treated Patients. Acta Orthop. Scand., 58:649–651, 1987.
249. Broberg, M.A., and Morrey, B.F.: Results of Treatment of Fracture–Dislocations of the Elbow. Clin. Orthop., 216:109–119, 1987.
250. Conwell, H.E., and Reynolds, F.C.: Management of Fractures, Dislocations, and Sprains, 7th ed. St. Louis, C.V. Mosby, 1961.
251. Cotton, F.J.: Dislocations and Joint Fractures, 2nd ed. Philadelphia, W.B. Saunders, 1924.
252. DeLee, J.C.: Transverse Divergent Dislocation of the Elbow in a Child. J. Bone Joint Surg., 63A:322–323, 1981.
253. DePalma, A.F.: The Management of Fractures and Dislocations. Philadelphia, W.B. Saunders, 1959.
254. DeSault, P.J.: A Treatise on Fractures, Luxations and Other Affections of the Bones. Philadelphia, Kimber & Conrad, 1811.
255. Durig, M., Mueller, W., Ruedi, T.P., and Gauer, E.F.: The Operative Treatment of Elbow Dislocation in the Adult. J. Bone Joint Surg., 61A:239–240, 1979.
256. Exarchou, E.J.: Lateral Dislocation of the Elbow. Acta Orthop. Scand., 48:161–163, 1977.
257. Greiss, M., and Messias, R.: Irreducible Posterolateral Elbow Dislocation: A Case Report. Acta Orthop. Scand., 58:421–422, 1987.
258. Hankin, F.M.: Posterior Dislocation of the Elbow: A Simplified Method of Closed Reduction. Clin. Orthop., 190:254–256, 1984.
259. Josefsson, P.O., Gentz, C.F., Johnell, O., and Wendeberg, B.: Surgical Versus Nonsurgical Treatment of Ligamentous Injuries Following Dislocations of the Elbow Joint. Clin. Orthop., 214:165–169, 1987.
260. Josefsson, P.O., Gentz, C.F., Johnell, O., and Wendeberg, B.: Surgical Versus Non-Surgical Treatment of Ligamentous Injuries Following Dislocation of the Elbow Joint. J. Bone Joint Surg., 69A:605–608, 1987.
261. Josefsson, P.O., Johnell, O., and Gentz, C.F.: Long-Term Sequelae of Simple Dislocation of the Elbow. J. Bone Joint Surg., 66A:927–930, 1984.
262. Josefsson, P.O., Johnell, O., and Wendeberg, B.: Ligamentous Injuries in Dislocations of the Elbow Joint. Clin. Orthop., 214:221–225, 1987.
263. Josefsson, P.O., and Nilsson, B.E.: Incidence of Elbow Dislocation. Acta Orthop. Scand., 57:537–538, 1986.
264. Lavine, L.S.: A Simple Method of Reducing Dislocations of the Elbow Joint. J. Bone Joint Surg., 35A:785–786, 1953.
265. Linscheid, R.L., and Wheeler, D.K.: Elbow Dislocations. J.A.M.A., 194:1171–1176, 1965.
266. Loomis, L.K.: Reduction and After-Treatment of Posterior Dislocation of the Elbow. Am. J. Surg., 63:56–60, 1944.
267. McLaughlin, H.L.: Trauma, p. 225. Philadelphia, W.B. Saunders, 1959.
268. Mehlhoff, T.L., Noble, P.C., Bennett, J.B., and Tullos, H.S.: Simple Dislocation of the Elbow in the Adult. J. Bone Joint Surg., 70A:244–249, 1988.
269. Meyn, M.A., and Quigley, T.B.: Reduction of Posterior Dislocation of the Elbow by Traction on the Dangling Arm. Clin. Orthop., 103:106–108, 1974.
270. Neviaser, J.S., and Wickstrom, J.K. Dislocation of the Elbow: A Retrospective Study of 115 Patients. South. Med. J., 70:172–173, 1977.
271. O'Driscoll, S.W., and Linscheid, R.L.: Elbow Dislocations. *In* Morrey, B.F. (ed.): The Elbow and its Disorders. Philadelphia, W.B. Saunders, 1993.
272. Parvin, R.W.: Closed Reduction of Common Shoulder and Elbow Dislocations Without Anesthesia. Arch. Surg., 75:972–975, 1957.
273. Patrick, J.: Fracture of the Medial Epicondyle With Displacement Into the Elbow Joint. J. Bone Joint Surg., 28:143–147, 1946.
274. Pawlowski, R.F., Palumbo, F.C., and Callahan, J.J.: Irreducible Posterolateral Elbow Dislocation: Report of a Rare Case. J. Trauma, 10:260–266, 1970.
275. Protzman, R.R. Dislocation of the Elbow Joint. J. Bone Joint Surg., 60A:539–541, 1978.
276. Purser, D.W.: Dislocation of the Elbow and Inclusion of the Medial Epicondyle in the Adult. J. Bone Joint Surg., 36B:247–249, 1954.
277. Roberts, P.H.: Dislocation of the Elbow. Br. J. Surg., 56:806–815, 1969.
278. Smith, F.M.: Displacement of the Medial Epicondyle of the Humerus Into the Elbow Joint. Ann. Surg., 124:410–425, 1946.
279. Smith, F.M.: Surgery of the Elbow. Springfield, Ill., Charles C Thomas, 1954.
280. Speed, K.: Fractures and Dislocations. Philadelphia, Lea & Febiger, 1935.
281. Stimson, L.A.: A Treatise on Fractures. Philadelphia, Henry C. Lea's Son & Co. 1890.
282. Tullos, H.S., Bennett, J., Shepard, D., Noble, P.C., and Gabel, G.: Dislocations: Mechanism of Instability. Instr. Course Lect., 35:69–82, 1986.
283. Wadsworth, T.G.: The Elbow, pp. 216–222. New York, Churchill Livingstone, 1982.
284. Wheeler, D.K., and Linscheid, R.L.: Fracture–Dislocations of the Elbow. Clin. Orthop., 50:95–106, 1967.
285. Wilson, P.D.: Fractures and Dislocations in the Region of the Elbow. Surg. Gynecol. Obstet., 56:335–359, 1933.

NEUROVASCULAR INJURY

286. Amsallem, J.L., Blankstein, A., Bass, A., and Horoszowski, H.: Brachial Artery Injury: A Complication of Posterior Elbow Dislocation. Orthop. Rev., 15:379–382, 1986.
287. Ashbell, T.S., Kleinert, H.E., and Kutz, J.E.: Vascular Injuries About the Elbow. Clin. Orthop., 50:107–127, 1967.
288. Aufranc, O.E., Jones, W.N., and Turner, R.H.: Dislocation of the Elbow With Brachial Artery Injury. J.A.M.A., 197:719–721, 1966.
289. Ayala, H., Depablos, J., Gonzales, J., and Martinez, A.: Entrapment of the Median Nerve After Posterior Dislocation of the Elbow. Microsurgery, 4:215–220, 1983.
290. Beverly, M.C., and Fearn, C.B.: Anterior Interosseous Nerve Palsy and Dislocation of the Elbow. Injury, 6:126–128, 1984.
291. Boe, S., and Holst-Nielsen, F.: Intra-articular Entrapment of the Median Nerve After Dislocation of the Elbow. J. Hand Surg., 12B:356–358, 1987.
292. Danielsson, L.G.: Median Nerve Entrapment in Elbow Dislocation: A Case Report. Acta Orthop. Scand., 57:450–452, 1986.
293. DeBakey, M.E., and Simeone, F.A.: Battle Injuries of the Arteries in World War II: An Analysis of 2471 Cases. Ann. Surg., 123:534–579, 1946.
294. Eliason, E.L., and Brown, R.B.: Posterior Dislocation at the

Elbow With Rupture of the Radial and Ulnar Arteries. Ann. Surg., 106:1111–1115, 1937.
295. Friedmann, E.: Simple Rupture of the Brachial Artery Sustained in Elbow Dislocations. J.A.M.A., 177:208–209, 1961.
296. Grimer, R.J., and Brooks, S.: Brachial Artery Damage Accompanying Closed Posterior Dislocation of the Elbow. J. Bone Joint Surg., 67B:378–381, 1985.
297. Gurdjian, E.S., and Smathers, H.M.: Peripheral Nerve Injury in Fractures and Dislocations of Long Bones. J. Neurosurg., 2:202–219, 1945.
298. Hallett, J.: Entrapment of the Median Nerve After Dislocation of the Elbow. J. Bone Joint Surg., 63B:408–412, 1981.
299. Hennig, K., and Franke, D.: Posterior Displacement of Brachial Artery Following Closed Elbow Dislocation. J. Trauma, 20:96–98, 1980.
300. Jackson, J.A.: Simple Anterior Dislocation of the Elbow Joint With Rupture of the Brachial Artery. Am. J. Surg., 47:479–486, 1940.
301. Kerin, R.: Elbow Dislocations and Its Association With Vascular Disruption. J. Bone Joint Surg., 51A:756–758, 1969.
302. Kilburn, P., Sweeney, J.G., and Silk, F.F.: Three Cases of Compound Posterior Dislocation of the Elbow With Rupture of the Brachial Artery. J. Bone Joint Surg., 44B:119–121, 1962.
303. Louis, D.S., Ricciardi, J.E., and Spengler, D.M.: Arterial Injury: A Complication of Posterior Elbow Dislocation. J. Bone Joint Surg., 56A:1631–1636, 1974.
304. Mains, D.B., and Freeark, R.J.: Report on Compound Dislocation of the Elbow With Entrapment of the Brachial Artery. Clin. Orthop., 106:180–185, 1975.
305. Mannerfelt, L.: Median Nerve Entrapment After Dislocation of Elbow (Report of a Case). J. Bone Joint Surg., 50B:152–155, 1968.
306. Manouel, M., Minkowitz, B., Shimotsu, G., Haq, I., and Feliccia, J.: Brachial Artery Laceration With Closed Posterior Elbow Dislocation in an Eight Year Old. Clin. Orthop., 296:109–112, 1993.
307. Marnham, R.: Dislocation of the Elbow With Rupture of the Brachial Artery. Br. J. Surg., 22:181, 1934.
308. Matev, I.: Radiological Sign of Entrapment of the Median Nerve in the Elbow Joint after Posterior Dislocation: A Report of Two Cases. J. Bone Joint Surg., 58B:353–355, 1976.
309. Pritchard, D.J., Linscheid, R.L., and Svien, H.J.: Intraarticular Median Nerve Entrapment With Dislocation of the Elbow. Clin. Orthop., 90:100–103, 1973.
310. Rana, N.A., Kenwright, J., Taylor, R.G., and Rushworth, G.: Complete Lesion of the Median Nerve Associated with Dislocation of the Elbow Joint. Acta Orthop. Scand., 45:365–369, 1974.
311. Rubens, M.K., and Aulicino, P.L.: Open Elbow Dislocation With Brachial Artery Disruption. Orthopedics, 9:539–542, 1986.
312. Seddon, H.J.: Surgical Disorders of the Peripheral Nerves, 2nd ed. New York, Churchill Livingstone, 1975.
313. Sharma, R.K., and Covell, N.A.G.: An Unusual Ulnar Nerve Injury Associated With Dislocation of the Elbow. Injury, 8:145–147, 1976.
314. Sherrill, J.G.: Direct Suture of Brachial Artery Following Rupture: Result of Traumatism. Ann. Surg., 58:534–536, 1913.
315. Spear, H.C., and Janes, J.M.: Rupture of the Brachial Artery Accompanying Dislocation of the Elbow or Supracondylar Fracture. J. Bone Joint Surg., 33A:889–894, 1951.
316. Steiger, R.N., Larrick, R.B., and Meyer, T.L.: Median-Nerve Entrapment Following Elbow Dislocation in Children (A Report of Two Cases). J. Bone Joint Surg., 51A:381–385, 1969.
317. Strange, F.G.: Entrapment of the Median Nerve After Dislocation of the Elbow. J. Bone Joint Surg., 64B:224–225, 1982.
318. Strum, J.T., Rothenberger, D.A., and Strate, R.G.: Brachial Artery Disruption Following Closed Elbow Dislocation. J. Trauma, 18:364–366, 1978.
319. Sullivan, M.F.: Rupture of the Brachial Artery From Posterior Dislocation of the Elbow Treated by Veingraft (A Case Report). Br. J. Surg., 58:470–471, 1971.
320. Watson-Jones, R.: Primary Nerve Lesions in Injuries of the Elbow and Wrist. J. Bone Joint Surg., 12:121–171, 1930.

DISLOCATIONS—DELAYED

321. Allende, G., and Freytes, M.: Old Dislocation of the Elbow. J. Bone Joint Surg., 24:691–706, 1944.
322. Arafiles, R.P.: Neglected Posterior Dislocation of the Elbow. J. Bone Joint Surg., 69B:199–202, 1987.
323. Billett, D.M.: Unreduced Posterior Dislocation of the Elbow. J. Trauma, 19:186–189, 1979.
324. Bruce, C., Laing, P., Dorgan, J., and Klenerman, L.: Unreduced Dislocation of the Elbow: Case Report and Review of the Literature. J. Trauma, 35:962–965, 1993.
325. Kini, M.G.: Dislocations of the Elbow and Its Complications. J. Bone Joint Surg., 22:107–117, 1940.
326. Krishnamoorthy, S., Bose, K., and Wong, K.P.: Treatment of Old Unreduced Dislocation of the Elbow. Injury, 8:39–42, 1976.
327. Silva, J.F.: Old Dislocations of the Elbow. Ann. R. Coll. Surg. Engl., 22:363–381, 1953.
328. Speed, J.S.: An Operation for Unreduced Posterior Dislocation of the Elbow. South Med. J., 18:193–198, 1925.
329. Vangorder, G.W.: Surgical Approach in Old Posterior Dislocation of the Elbow. J. Bone Joint Surg., 14:127–143, 1932.

DISLOCATIONS—RECURRENT

330. Dryer, R.F., Buckwaltere, J.A., and Sprague, B.L.: Treatment of Chronic Elbow Instability. Clin. Orthop., 148:254–255, 1980.
331. Ejested, R., Christensen, F.A., and Nielsen, W.B.: Habitual Dislocation of the Elbow. Arch. Orthop. Trauma Surg., 105:187–190, 1986.
332. Gosman, J.A.: Recurrent Dislocation of the Ulna at the Elbow. J. Bone Joint Surg., 25:448–449, 1943.
333. Hassmann, G.C., Brunn, F., and Neer, C.S., II: Recurrent Dislocation of the Elbow. J. Bone Joint Surg., 57A:1080–1084, 1975.
334. Jacobs, R.L.: Recurrent Dislocation of the Elbow Joint. Clin. Orthop., 74:151–154, 1971.
335. Milch, H.: Bilateral Recurrent Dislocation of the Ulna at the Elbow. J. Bone Joint Surg., 18:777–780, 1936.
336. Nestor, B.J., O'Driscoll, S.W., and Morrey, B.F.: Ligamentous Reconstruction for Posterolateral Rotary Instability of the Elbow. J. Bone Joint Surg., 74A:1235–1241, 1992.
337. O'Driscoll, S.W., Bell, D.F., and Morrey, B.F.: Posterolateral Rotatory Instability of the Elbow. J. Bone Joint Surg., 73A:440–446, 1991.
338. Osborne, G., and Cotterill, P.: Recurrent Dislocation of the Elbow. J. Bone Joint Surg., 48B:340–346, 1966.
339. Spring, W.E.: Report of a Case of Recurrent Dislocation of the Elbow. J. Bone Joint Surg., 35B:55, 1953.
340. Wainwright, D.: Recurrent Dislocation of the Elbow Joint. Proc. Rev. Soc. Med. (Biol.), 40:33–34, 1947.

DISLOCATIONS—ANTERIOR

341. Caravias, D.E.: Forward Dislocation of the Elbow Without Fracture of the Olecranon. J. Bone Joint Surg., 39B:334, 1957.
342. Cohn, I.: Forward Dislocation of Both Bones of the Forearm at the Elbow. Surg. Gynecol. Obstet., 35:776–788, 1922.
343. Oury, J.H., Roe, R.D., and Laning, R.C.: A Case of Bilateral Anterior Dislocations of the Elbow. J. Trauma, 12:170–173, 1972.
344. Simon, M.M.: Complete Anterior Dislocation of Both Bones of the Forearm at the Elbow (Review of Recorded Cases and Literature With Report of a Case). Med. J. Rec., 133:333–336, 1931.
345. Staunton, F.W.: Dislocation Forwards of the Forearm Without Fracture of the Olecranon. Br. Med. J., 2:1520, 1905.
346. Tees, F.J., and McKim, L.H.: Case Reports: Anterior Dislocation of the Elbow. Can. Med. Assoc. J., 20:36–38, 1929.
347. Winslow, R.A.: Case of Complete Anterior Dislocation of Both Bones of the Forearm at the Elbow. Surg. Gynecol. Obstet., 16:570–571, 1913.

DISLOCATIONS—RADIAL HEAD

348. Burgess, R.C., and Sprague, H.H.: Post-traumatic Posterior Radial Head Subluxation—Two Case Reports. Clin. Orthop., 186:192–194, 1984.

349. Heidt, R.S., and Stern, P.J.: Isolated Posterior Dislocation of the Radial Head. Clin. Orthop., 168:136–138, 1982.
350. Ryu, J., Pascal, P.E., and Levine, J.: Posterior Dislocation of the Radial Head Without Fracture of the Ulna. Clin. Orthop., 183:169–172, 1984.
351. Salama, R.: Recurrent Dislocation of the Head of the Radius. Clin. Orthop., 125:156–158, 1977.
352. Wiley, J.J., Pegington, J., and Horwich, J.P.: Traumatic Dislocation of the Radius at the Elbow. J. Bone Joint Surg., 56B:501–507, 1974.

HETEROTOPIC OSSIFICATION

353. Ackerman, L.V.: Extra-Osseous Localized Non-Neoplastic Bone and Cartilage Formation (So-Called Myositis Ossificans). J. Bone Joint Surg., 40A:279–298, 1958.
354. Bijvoet, O.L.M., Nollen, A.J.G., Slooff, T.J.J.H., and Feith, R.: Effect of a Diphosphonate on Para-articular Ossification After Total Hip Replacement. Acta Orthop. Scand., 45:926–934, 1974.
355. Buxton, S.J.D.: Ossification in the Ligaments of the Elbow Joint. J. Bone Joint Surg., **20**:709–714, 1938.
356. Coventry, M.B.: Ectopic Ossification About the Elbow. *In* Morrey, B. F. (ed.): The Elbow and Its Disorders, pp. 464–471. Philadelphia, W.B. Saunders, 1985.
357. Coventry, M.B., and Scanlon, P.W.: The Use of Radiation to Discourage Ectopic Bone: A Nine Year Study in Surgery About the Hip. J. Bone Joint Surg., 63A:201–208, 1981.
358. Finerman, G.A.M., Krengel, W.F., Lowell, J.D., Murray, W.R., and Volz, R.: Role of Diphosphonate (EHDP) in the Prevention of Heterotopic Ossification After Total Hip Arthroplasty: A Preliminary Report. Proceedings of the Fifth Open Scientific Meeting Hip Society, pp. 222–234. St. Louis, C.V. Mosby, 1977.
359. Garland, D.E., Hanscom, D.A., Keenan, M.A., Smith, C., and Moore, T.: Resection of Heterotopic Ossification in the Adult With Head Trauma. J. Bone Joint Surg., 67A:1261–1269, 1985.
360. Garland, D.E., and O'Hollaren, R.M.: Fractures and Dislocations About the Elbow in the Head Injured Adult. Clin. Orthop., 168:38–41, 1982.
361. MacAusland, W.R.: Ankylosis of the Elbow: With Report of Four Cases Treated by Arthroplasty. J.A.M.A., 64:312–318, 1915.
362. McLaren, A.C.: Prophylaxis With Indomethacin for Heterotopic Bone After Open Reduction of Fracture of the Acetabulum. J. Bone Joint Surg., 72A:245–247, 1990.
363. Mohan, K.: Myositis Ossifications Traumatica of the Elbow. Int. Surg., 57:475–478, 1972.
364. O'Brien, E.T.: Personal communication, 1989.
365. Ritter, M.A., and Gio, J.J.: The Effect of Indomethacin or Para-Articular Ectopic Ossification Following Total Hip Arthroplasty. Clin. Orthop., 167:113–117, 1982.
366. Roberts, J.B., and Pankratz, D.G.: The Surgical Treatment of Heterotopic Ossification at the Elbow Following Long-Term Coma. J. Bone Joint Surg., 61A:760–763, 1979.
367. Seth, M.K.: Bony Ankylosis of the Elbow after Burns. J. Bone Joint Surg., 66B:747–749, 1985.
368. Thompson, H.C., III, and Garcia, A.: Myositis Ossificans: Aftermath of Elbow Injuries. Clin. Orthop., 50:129–134, 1967.

CONTRACTURE

369. Breen, T.F., Gelberman, R.H., and Ackerman, G.N.: Elbow Flexion Contractures: Treatment by Anterior Release and Continuous Passive Motion. J. Hand Surg., 13B:286–287, 1988.
370. Gates, H.S., Sullivan, F.L., and Urbaniak, J.R.: Anterior Capsulectomy and Continuous Passive Motion in the Treatment of Post-Traumatic Flexion Contracture of the Elbow. J. Bone Joint Surg., 74A:1229–1234, 1992.
371. Glynn, J.J., and Niebauer, J.: Flexion and Extension Contractures of the Elbow: Surgical Management. Clin. Orthop., 117:289–291, 1976.
372. Green, D.P., and McCoy, H.: Turnbuckle Orthotic Correction of Elbow-Flexion Contractures After Acute Injuries. J. Bone Joint Surg., 61A:1092–1095, 1979.
373. Hepburn, G.R., and Crivelli, K.: Use of Elbow Dynasplint for Reduction of Elbow Flexion Contracture: A Case Study. J. Orthop. Phys. Ther., 5:269–274, 1984.
374. Hotchkiss, R.N., An, K.N., Weiland, A.J., and O'Brien, E.T.: Treatment of the Severe Elbow Contracture Using the Concepts of Ilizarov (Abstract). Presented before the American Association of Orthopaedic Surgeons, New Orleans, 1994.
375. Husband, J.B., and Hastings, H.: The Lateral Approach for the Operative Release of Post-Traumatic Contracture of the Elbow. J. Bone Joint Surg., 72A:1353–1358, 1990.
376. Kaps, H.P., and Schmidt, E.: Arthrolysis and Arthroplasty of the Elbow Joint: A Comparison of Surgical Results Between Children and Adults. Z. Orthop. Ihre Grenzgeb, 131:335–339, 1993. In German.
377. Richard, R.L.: Use of the Dynasplint to Correct Elbow Flexion Burn Contracture: A Case Report. J. Burn Care Rehabil., 7:151–152, 1986.
378. Soffer, S.R., and Yahiro, M.A.: Continuous Passive Motion After Internal Fixation of Distal Humerus Fractures. Orthop. Rev., 19:88–93, 1990.
379. Stern, P.J., Law, E.J., Benedict, F.E., and Macmillan, B.G.: Surgical Treatment of Elbow Contractures in Postburn Children. Plast. Reconstr. Surg., 76:441–446, 1985.
380. Urbaniak, J.R., Hansen, P.E., Beissinger, S.F., and Aitken, M.S.: Correction of Post-traumatic Flexion Contracture of the Elbow by Anterior Capsulotomy. J. Bone Joint Surg., 67A:1160–1164, 1985.
381. Willner, P.: Anterior Capsulectomy for Contractures of the Elbow. 1948.
382. Wilson, P.D.: Capsulectomy for the Relief of Flexion Contractures of the Elbow Following Fractures. J. Bone Joint Surg., 26:71–86, 1944.

OLECRANON AND PROXIMAL ULNA (CORONOID) FRACTURES

383. Adler, S., Fay, G.F., and MacAusland, W.R.: Olecranon Fractures. J. Bone Joint Surg., 41A:1540, 1959.
384. Adler, S., Fay, G.F., and MacAusland, W.R., Jr.: Treatment of Olecranon Fractures: Indications for Excision of the Olecranon Fragment and Repair of the Triceps Tendon. J. Trauma, 2:597–602, 1962.
385. AuFranc, O.E., and Jones, W.N.: Open Fracture of the Olecranon. J.A.M.A., 202:427–429, 1967.
386. Bennett, G.S.: Fractures of the Olecranon and Its Repair. Am. J. Orthop. Surg., 11:121–123, 1969.
387. Berger, P.: Le Traitement de Fractures de l'Olecrane et Particulierment la Sutur de l'Olecrane par un Procede (Cedarg de l'Olecranon). Ga. Hebd. Med., 2:193–199, 1902.
388. Bohler, L.: The Treatment of Fractures. Vienna, Wilhelm Maudrich, 1929.
389. Bryan, R.S.: Fractures About the Elbow in Adults. Instr. Course Lect., 30:200–203, 1981.
390. Cabanela, M.E., and Morrey, B.F.: Fractures of the Proximal Ulna and Olecranon. *In* Morrey, B. F. (ed.): The Elbow and its Disorders, pp. 405–428. Philadelphia, W.B. Saunders, 1993.
391. Colton, C.L.: Fractures of the Olecranon in Adults: Classification and Management. Injury, 5:121–129, 1973.
392. Conn, J., and Wade, P.A.: Injuries of the Elbow (A Ten-Year Review). J. Trauma, 1:248–268, 1961.
393. Coughlin, M.J., Slabaugh, P.B., and Smith, T.K.: Experience With the McAtee Olecranon Device in Olecranon Fractures. J. Bone Joint Surg., 61A:385–388, 1979.
394. Crenshaw, A.H.: Campbell's Operative Orthopaedics, 5th ed. St. Louis, C.V. Mosby, 1971.
395. Daland, E.M.: Fractures of the Olecranon. J. Bone Joint Surg., 15:601–607, 1933.
396. Deane, M.: Comminuted Fractures of the Olecranon. An Appliance for Internal Fixation. Injury, 2:103–106, 1970.
397. Deliyannis, S.N.: Comminuted Fractures of the Olecranon Treated by Weber-Vasey Technique. Injury, 5:19–24, 1973.
398. Dunn, N.: Operation for Fracture of the Olecranon. Br. Med. J., 1:214–215, 1939.
399. Eliot, E., Jr.: Fracture of the Olecranon. Surg. Clin. North Am., 14:487–492, 1934.
400. Eriksson, E., Sahlen, O., and Sandahl, U.: Late Results of Conservative and Surgical Treatment of Fracture of the Olecranon. Acta Chir. Scand., 113:153–166, 1957.

401. Finlayson, D.: Complications of Tension-Band Wiring of Olecranon Fractures (Letter). J. Bone Joint Surg., 68A:951–952, 1986.
402. Fiolle, D.J.: Note sur les Fractures de Folecrane par Projectiles de Guerre. Marseille Med., 55:241–245, 1918.
403. Fyfe, I.S., Mossad, M.M., and Holdsworth, B.J.: Methods of Fixation of Olecranon Fractures: An Experimental Mechanical Study. J. Bone Joint Surg., 67B:367–372, 1985.
404. Gartsman, G.M., Sculco, T.P., and Otis, J.C.: Operative Treatment of Olecranon Fractures Excision or Open Reduction With Internal Fixation. J. Bone Joint Surg., 63A:718–721, 1981.
405. Harmon, P.H.: Treatment of Fractures of the Olecranon by Fixation With Stainless-Steel Screw. J. Bone Joint Surg., 27:328–329, 1945.
406. Heim, U., and Pfeiffer, K.M.: Elbow. *In* Heim, U., and Pfeiffer, K. M. (eds): Internal Fixation of Small Fractures, 3rd ed., pp. 107–109. Berlin, Springer-Verlag, 1988.
407. Hey-Groves, E.W.: Fracture of the Olecranon. Br. Med. J., 1:296, 1939.
408. Holdsworth, B.J., and Mossad, M.M.: Elbow Function Following Tension Band Fixation of Displaced Fractures of the Olecranon. Injury, 16:182–187, 1984.
409. Horne, J.G., and Tanzer, T.L.: Olecranon Fractures: A Review of 100 Cases. J. Trauma, 21:469–472, 1981.
410. Howard, J.L., and Urist, M.R.: Fracture-Dislocation of the Radius and the Ulna at the Elbow Joint. Clin. Orthop., 12:276–284, 1958.
411. Jensen, C.M., and Olsen, B.B.: Drawbacks of Traction-Absorbing Wiring (TAW) in Displaced Fracture of the Olecranon. Injury, 17:174–175, 1986.
412. Johnson, R.P., Roetker, A., and Schwab, J.P.: Olecranon Fractures Treated With AO Screw and Tension Bands. Orthopedics, 9:66–68, 1986.
413. Keon-Cohen, B.T.: Fractures at the Elbow. J. Bone Joint Surg., 48A:1623–1639, 1966.
414. Kiviluoto, O., and Santavirta, S.: Fractures of the Olecranon. Acta Orthop. Scand., 49:28–31, 1978.
415. Kohler, A., and Zimmer, E.A.: Borderlands of the Normal and Early Pathologic in Skeletal Roentgenology, 3rd ed. New York, Grune & Stratton, 1968.
416. Lou, I.: Olecranon Fractures Treated in the Orthopaedic Hospital, Copenhagen 1936–1947: A Follow-up Examination. Acta Orthop., 19:166–179, 1949.
417. MacAusland, W.R.: The Treatment of Fractures of the Olecranon by Longitudinal Screw or Nail Fixation. Ann. Surg. 116:293–296, 1942.
418. MacAusland, W.R., and Wyman, E.T.: Fractures of the Adult Elbow. Instr. Course Lect., 24:169–181, 1975.
419. Macko, D., and Szabo, R.M.: Complications of Tension-Band Wiring of Olecranon Fractures. J. Bone Joint Surg., 57B:399, 1975.
420. Mathewson, M.H., and McCreath, S.W.: Tension Band Wiring in the Treatment of Olecranon Fractures. J. Bone Joint Surg., 57B:399, 1975.
421. McKeever, F.M., and Buck, R.M.: Fracture of the Olecranon Process of the Ulna. J.A.M.A., 135:1–5, 1947.
422. Muller, M.E., Allgöwer, M., Schneider, R., and Willenegger, H.: Manual of Internal Fixation, 2nd ed. New York, Springer-Verlag, 1970.
423. Murphy, D.F., Greene, W.B., and Dameron, T.B., Jr.: Displaced Olecranon Fractures in Adults: Clinical Evaluation. Clin. Orthop., 224:215–223, 1987.
424. Murphy, D.F., Greene, W.B., Gilbert, J.A., and Dameron, T.: B., Jr.: Displaced Olecranon Fractures in Adults: Biomechanical Analysis of Fixation Methods. Clin. Orthop., 224:210–214, 1987.
425. Netz, P. and Stromberg, L.: Non-Sliding Pins in Traction Absorbing Wire of Fractures: A Modified Technique. Acta Orthop. Scand., 53:355–360, 1982.
426. Perkins, G.: Fractures of the Olecranon. Br. Med. J. (Clin. Res.), 2:668–669, 1936.
427. Regan, W., and Morrey, B.F.: Fractures of Coronoid Process of the Ulna. J. Bone Joint Surg., 71A:1348–1354, 1989.
428. Rettig, A.C., Waugh, T.R., and Evanski, P.M.: Fracture of the Olecranon: A Problem of Management. J. Trauma, 19:23–28, 1979.
429. Rombold, C.: A New Operative Treatment for Fractures of the Olecranon. J. Bone Joint Surg., 16:947–949, 1934.
430. Rowe, C.: The Management of Fractures in Elderly Patients is Different. J. Bone Joint Surg., 47A:1043–1959, 1965.
431. Rowland, S.A., and Burkhalter, S.S.: Tension Band Wiring of Olecranon Fractures—A Modification of the AO Technique. Clin. Orthop., 277:238–242, 1992.
432. Rush, L.V., and Rush, H.L.: A Reconstruction Operation for Comminuted Fractures of the Upper Third of the Ulna. Am. J. Surg., 38:332–333, 1937.
433. Scharplatz, D., and Allgöwer, M.: Fracture–Dislocation of the Elbow. Injury, 7:143–159, 1975.
434. Stug, L.H.: Anterior Dislocation of the Elbow with Fracture of the Olecranon. Am. J. Surg., 85:700–703, 1948.
435. Taylor, T.K.F., and Scham, S.M.: A Posteromedial Approach to the Proximal End of the Ulna for the Internal Fixation of Olecranon Fractures. J. Trauma, 9:594–602, 1969.
436. Van Derkloot, J.F.V.R.: Results of Treatment of Fractures of the Olecranon. Arch. Chir. Neerld., 16:237–249, 1964.
437. Wadsworth, T.G.: Screw Fixation of the Olecranon After Fracture or Osteotomy. Clin. Orthop., 119:197–201, 1976.
438. Wainwright, D.: Fractures of the Olecranon Process. Br. J. Surg., 29:403–406, 1942.
439. Watson-Jones, R.: Fractures and Joint Injuries, 3rd ed. Baltimore, Williams & Wilkins, 1946.
440. Watson-Jones, R.: Fractures and Joint Injuries, 4th ed. Edinburgh, E.S. Livingstone, 1952.
441. Waxman, A., and Geshelin, H.: Fracture of the Olecranon Process Due to Muscle Pull With the Forearm in Hyperextension. Calif. Med., 66:358–359, 1947.
442. Weseley, M.S., Barnefeld, P.A., and Eisenstein, A.L.: The Use of Zuelzer Hook Plate in Fixation of Olecranon Fractures. J. Bone Joint Surg., 58A:859–863, 1976.
443. Willenegger, H.: Problems and Results in the Treatment of Comminuted Fractures of the Elbow. Surg. Traumatol., 11:118–127, 1969.
444. Wilppula, E., and Bakalim, G.: Fractures of the Olecranon: III. Fractures Complicated by Forward Dislocation of the Forearm. Ann. Chir. Gynacol. Fenn., 60:105–108, 1971.
445. Wolfgang, G., Burke, F., Bush, D., Parenti, J., Perry, J., and LaFollette, B.: Surgical Treatment of Displaced Olecranon Fractures by Tension Band Wiring Technique. Clin. Orthop., 224:192–204, 1987.
446. Zuelzer, W.A.: Fixation of Small but Important Bone Fragaments With a Hook Plate. J. Bone Joint Surg., 33A:430–436, 1951.

RADIAL HEAD FRACTURES

447. Adler, J.B., and Shaftan, G.W.: Radial Head Fractures, Is Excision Necessary? J. Trauma, 4:115–136, 1964.
448. Arner, O., Ekengren, K., and Von Schreeb, T.: Fractures of the Head and Neck of the Radius: A Clinical and Roentgenographic Study of 310 Cases. Acta Chir. Scand., 112:115–134, 1957.
449. Aufranc, O.E., Jones, W.N., Turner, R.H., and Thomas, W.H.: Dislocation of the Elbow With Fracture of the Radial Head and Distal Radius. J.A.M.A., 202:131–134, 1967.
450. Bakalim, G.: Fractures of Radial Head and Their Treatment. Acta Orthop. Scand., 41:320–331, 1970.
451. Bohl, W.R., and Brightman, E.: Fracture of a Silastic Radial-Head Prosthesis: Diagnosis and Localization of Fragments by Xerography. J. Bone Joint Surg., 63A:1482–1483, 1981.
452. Broberg, M.A., and Morrey, B.F.: Results of Delayed Excision of the Radial Head After Fracture. J. Bone Joint Surg., 68A:669–674, 1986.
453. Brockman, E.P.: Two Cases of Disability at the Wrist Joint Following Excision of the Head of the Radius. Proc. R. Soc. Med., 24:904–905, 1930.
454. Bunker, T.D., and Newman, J.H.: The Herbert Differential Pitch Bone Screw in Displaced Radial Head Fractures. Injury, 16:621–624, 1985.
455. Burton, A.E.: Fractures of the Head of the Radius. Proc. R. Soc. Med., 35:764–765, 1942.

456. Carn, R.M., Medige, J., Curtain, D., and Koneig, A.: Silicone Rubber Replacement of the Severely Fractured Radial Head. Clin. Orthop., 209:259–269, 1986.
457. Carr, C.R.: Metallic Cap Replacement of the Radial Head (Abstract). J. Bone Joint Surg., 53A:1661, 1971.
458. Carr, C.R., and Howard, J.W.: Metallic Cap Replacement of Radial Head Following Fracture. West. J. Surg., 59:539–546, 1951.
459. Carstam, N.N.: Operative Treatment of Fracture of the Head and Neck of the Radius. Acta Chir. Scand., 19:502–526, 1951.
460. Castberg, T., and Thing, E.: Treatment of Fractures of the Upper End of the Radius. Acta Chir. Scand., 105:62–69, 1953.
461. Charnley, J.: The Closed Treatment of Common Fractures. Edinburgh, E & S Livingstone, 1950.
462. Cherry, J.C.: Use of Acrylic Prosthesis in the Treatment of Fracture of the Head of the Radius. J. Bone Joint Surg., 35B:70–71, 1953.
463. Cherry, J.C.: Fracture of the Head of the Radius Treated by Excision and Substitution of an Acrylic Head. J. Bone Joint Surg., 35B:486, 1953.
464. Coleman, D.A., Blaire, W.F., and Shurr, D.: Resection of the Radial Head for Fracture of the Radial Head. J. Bone Joint Surg. 69A:385–392, 1987.
465. Crawford, G.P.: Late Radial Tunnel Syndrome After Excision of the Radial Head. J. Bone Joint Surg., 70A:1416–1418, 1988.
466. Curr, J.F., and Coe, W.A.: Dislocation of the Inferior Radio-ulnar Joint. Br. J. Surg., 34:74–77, 1946.
467. Currey, J., Therkildsen, L.H., and Bywaters, E.G.: Monarticular Rheumatoid-like Arthritis of Seven Years' Duration Following Fracture of the Radial Head. Ann Rheum. Dis., 45:783–785, 1986.
468. Cutler, C.W.: Fractures of the Head and Neck of the Radius. Ann. Surg., 83:267–278, 1926.
469. Ebraheim, N.A., Skie, M.C., Zeiss, J., Saddemi, S.R., and Jackson, W.T.: Internal Fixation of Radial Neck Fracture in a Fracture–Dislocation of the Elbow: A Case Report. Clin. Orthop., 276:187–191, 1992.
470. Edward, G.S., and Jupiter, J.B.: Radial Head Fracture With Acute Distal Radioulnar Dislocation: Essex-Lopresti Revisited. Clin. Orthop., 234:61–69, 1988.
471. Eliason, E.L., and North, J.P.: Fractures About the Elbow. Am. J. Surg., 44:88–99, 1939.
472. Essex-Lopresti, P.: Fractures of the Radial Head With Distal Radial-Ulnar Dislocations. J. Bone Joint Surg., 33B:244–247, 1951.
473. Evans, C.D., and Kellam, J.F.: Open Reduction and Internal Fixation of Radial Head Frctures. J. Orthop. Trauma, 5:21–28, 1991.
474. Fleming, C.W.: Fractures of the Head of the Radius. Proc. R. Soc. Med., 25:1011–1015, 1932.
475. Gaston, S.R., Smith, F.M., and Baab, O.D.: Adult Injuries of the Radial Head and Neck. Am J. Surg., 78:631–635, 1949.
476. Geel, C.W., and Palmer, A.K.: Radial Head Fractures and Their Effect on the Distal Radioulnar Joint: A Rationale for Treatment. Clin. Orthop., 275:79–84, 1992.
477. Geel, C.W., Palmer, A.K., Ruedi, T., and Leutenegger, A.F.: Internal Fixation of Proximal Radial Head Fractures. J. Orthop. Trauma, 4:270–274, 1990.
478. Gerard, Y., Schernberg, F., and Nerot, C.: Anatomical, Pathological, and Therapeutic Investigation of Fractures of the Radial Head in Adults. J. Bone Joint Surg., 66B:141, 1984.
479. Gordon, M., and Bullough, P.G.: Synovial and Osseous Inflammation in Failed Silicone-Rubber Prosthesis. J. Bone Joint Surg., 64A:574–580, 1982.
480. Greenspan, A., and Norman, A.: Radial Head—Capitellum View: An Expanded Imaging Approach to Elbow Injury. Radiology, 164:272–274, 1987.
481. Grossman, J.: Fracture of the Head and Neck of the Radius. N.Y. Med. J., 117:472–475, 1923.
482. Harrington, I.J., and Tountas, A.A.: Replacement of the Radial Head in the Treatment of Unstable Elbow Fractures. Injury, 12:405–412, 1981.
483. Hein, B.J.: Fractures of the Head of the Radius. Indust. Med., 6:529–532, 1937.
484. Holdsworth, B.J., Clement, D.A., and Rothwell, P.N.: Fractures of the Radial Head: The Benefit of Aspiration: A Prospective Controlled Trial. Injury, 18:44–47, 1987.
485. Horne, G., and Sim, P.: Nonunion of the Radial Head. J. Trauma, 25:452–453, 1985.
486. Hotchkiss, R.N.: Injuries to the Interosseous Ligament of the Forearm. Hand Clin., 10:391–398, 1994.
487. Hotchkiss, R.N., An, K.N., Sowa, D.T., Basta, S., and Weiland, A.J.: Pathomechanics of Proximal Migration of the Radius: An Anatomic and Mechanical Study of the Interosseous Membrane of the Forearm. J. Hand Surg., 14A:256–261, 1989.
488. Hotchkiss, R.N., and Weiland, A.J.: Valgus Stability of the Elbow. J. Orthop. Res., 5:372–377, 1987.
489. Jacobs, J.E., and Kernodle, H.B.: Fractures of the Head of the Radius. J. Bone Joint Surg., 28:616–622, 1946.
490. Johnston, G.W.: A Follow-up of One Hundred Cases of Fractures of the Head of the Radius With a Review of the Literature. Ulster Med. J., 31:51–56, 1962.
491. Key, J.A.: Treatment of Fractures of the Head and Neck of the Radius. J.A.M.A., 96:101–104, 1931.
492. Khurana, J.S., Kattapuram, S.V., Becker, S., and Mayo-Smith, W.: Galeazzi Injury With an Associated Fracture of the Radial Head. Clin. Orthop., 234:70–71, 1988.
493. King, B.B.: Resection of the Radial Head and Neck. J. Bone Joint Surg., 21:839–857, 1939.
494. Knight, D.J., Rymaszewski, L.A., Amis, A.A., and Miller, J.H.: Primary Replacement of the Fractured Radial Head With a Metal Prosthesis. J. Bone Joint Surg., 75B::572–576, 1993.
495. Lewis, R.W., and Thibodeau, A.A.: Deformity of the Wrist Following Resection of the Radial Head. Surg. Gynecol. Obstet., 64:1079–1085, 1937.
496. Mackay, I., Fitzgerald, B., and Miller, J.H.: Silastic Replacement of the Head of the Radius in Trauma. J. Bone Joint Surg., 61B:494–497, 1979.
497. Martinelli, B.: Fractures of the Radial Head Treated by Substitution With the Silastic Prosthesis. Bull. Hosp. Joint Dis., 36:61–65, 1975.
498. Mason, J.A., and Shutkin, N.M.: Immediate Active Motion Treatment of Fractures of the Head and Neck of the Radius. Surg. Gynecol. Obstet., 76:731–737, 1943.
499. Mason, M.L.: Some Observations on Fractures of the Head of the Radius With a Review of One Hundred Cases. Br. J. Surg., 42:123–132, 1954.
500. Mayhall, W.S.T., Tiley, F.W., and Paluska, D.J.: Fractures of Silastic Radial-Head Prosthesis. J. Bone Joint Surg., 63A:459–460, 1981.
501. McArthur, R.A.: Herbert Screw Fixation of Fracture of the Head of the Radius. Clin. Orthop., 224:79–87, 1987.
502. McDougall, A., and White, J.: Subluxation of the Inferior Radio-Ulnar Joint Complicating Fracture of the Radial Head. J. Bone Joint Surg., 39B:278–286, 1957.
503. McLaughlin, H.L.: Fracture of the Head of the Radius in Trauma. *In* Trauma, pp. 221–225. Philadelphia, W.B. Saunders, 1959.
504. Mikic, Z.D., and Vukadinovic, S.M.: Late Results in Fractures of the Radial Head Treated by Excision. Clin. Orthop., 181:712–717, 1983.
505. Morrey, B.F., Askew, L., and Chao, E.Y.: Silastic Prosthetic Replacement for the Radial Head. J. Bone Joint Surg., 63A:454–458, 1981.
506. Morrey, B.F., Chao, E.Y., and Hui, F.C.: Biomechanical Study of the Elbow Following Excision of the Radial Head. J. Bone Joint Surg., 61A:63–68, 1979.
507. Murray, R.C.: Fractures of the Head and Neck of the Radius. Br. J. Surg., 28:106–118, 1940.
508. O'Connor, B.T., and Taylor, T.K.F.: The Conservative Approach to Radial Head Fractures (Abstract). J. Bone Joint Surg., 44B:743, 1962.
509. Odenheimer, K., and Harvey, J.P.: Internal Fixation of Fracture of the Head of the Radius. J. Bone Joint Surg., 61A:785–787, 1979.
510. Pelto, K., Hirvensalo, E., Bostman, O., and Rokkanen, P.: Treatment of Radial Head Fractures with Absorbable Polygly-

colide Pins: A Study on the Security of the Fixation in 38 Cases. J. Orthop. Trauma, 8:94–98, 1994.
511. Perry, C.R., and Tessier, J.E.: Open Reduction and Internal Fixation of Radial Head Fractures Associated With Olecranon Fracture or Dislocation. J. Orthop. Trauma, 1:36–42, 1987.
512. Pinder, J.M.: Fracture of the Head of the Radius in Adults (Abstract). J. Bone Joint Surg., 51B:386, 1969.
513. Postlethwait, R.W.: Modified Treatment for Fracture of the Head of the Radius. Am. J. Surg., 67:77–80, 1945.
514. Pribyl, C.R., Kester, M.A., Cook, S.D., Edmunds, J.O., and Brunet, M.E.: The Effect of the Radial Head and Prosthetic Radial Head Replacement on Resisting Valgus Stress at the Elbow. Orthopedics, 9:723–726, 1986.
515. Quigley, T.B.: Aspiration of the Elbow Joint in the Treatment of Fractures of the Head of the Radius. N. Engl. J. Med., 240:915–916, 1949.
516. Rabinowitz, R.S., Light, T.R., Havey, R.M., Gourineni, P., Patwardhan, A.G., Sartori, M.J., and Vrbos, L.: The Role of the Interosseous Membrane and Triangular Fibrocartilage Complex in Forearm Stability. J. Hand Surg., 19A:385–393, 1994.
517. Radin, E.L., and Riseborough, E.J.: Fractures of the Radial Head. J. Bone Joint Surg., 48A:1055–1064, 1966.
518. Rieth, P.L.: Fractures of the Radial Head Associated With Chip Fracture of the Capitellum in Adults: Surgical Considerations. South. Surg., 14:154–159, 1948.
519. Rymaszewski, L.A., MacKay, I., Amis, A.A., and Miller, J.H.: Long-term Effects of Excision of the Radial Head in Rheumatoid Arthritis. J. Bone Joint Surg., 66B:109–113, 1984.
520. Sanders, R.A., and French, H.G.: Open Reduction and Internal Fixation of Comminuted Radial Head Fractures. Am. J. Sports Med., 14:130–135, 1986.
521. Sever, J.W.: Fractures of the Head and Neck of the Radius: A Study of End Results. J.A.M.A., 84:1551–1555, 1925.
522. Shumeli, G., and Herold, H.Z.: Compression Screwing of Displaced Fractures of the Head of the Radius. J. Bone Joint Surg., 63B:535–538, 1981.
523. Smith, G.B., and Hotchkiss, R.N.: Radial Head and Neck Fractures: Anatomic Guidelines for Proper Placement of Internal Fixation. J. Shoulder Elbow, 1995. (In Press)
524. Sowa, D.T., Hotchkiss, R.N., and Weiland, A.J.: Symptomatic Proximal Translation of the Radius Following Radial Head Resection. Clin. Orthop., 317:106–113, 1995.
525. Speed, K.: Fracture of the Head of the Radius. Am. J. Surg., 38:845–850, 1924.
526. Speed, K.: Ferrule Caps for the Head of the Radius. Surg. Gynecol. Obstet., 73:845–850, 1941.
527. Stephen, I.B.M.: Excision of the Radial Head for Closed Fracture. Acta Orthop. Scand., 52:409–412, 1981.
528. Strachan, J.C.H., and Ellis, B.W.: Vulnerability of the Posterior Interosseous Nerve During Radial Head Resection. J. Bone Joint Surg., 53B:320–323, 1971.
529. Swanson, A.B., Jaeger, S.H., and Larochelle, D.: Comminuted Fractures of the Radial Head. J. Bone Joint Surg., 63A:1039–1049, 1981.
530. Taylor, T.K.F., and O'Connor, B.T.: The Effect Upon the Inferior Radio-ulnar Joint of Excision of the Head of the Radius in Adults. J. Bone Joint Surg., 46B:83–88, 1964.
531. Thomas, T.T.: Fractures of the Head of the Radius: An Experimental Study and Report of Cases. Univ. Penn. Med. Bull., 18:184–197, 1905.
532. Trousdale, R.T., Amadio, P.C., Cooney, W.P., and Morrey, B.F.: Radio-ulnar Dissociation: A Review of Twenty Cases. J. Bone Joint Surg., 74A:1486–1497, 1992.
533. Vichard, P., Tropet, Y., Dreyfus-Schmidt, G., Besancenot, J., and Menez, D.: Treatment of Isolated Fractures of the Proximal End of the Radius in Adults: Remarks Concerning 168 Cases. Ann Chir. Main., 6:189–194, 1987.
534. Wagner, C.J.: Fractures of the Head of the Radius. Am. J. Surg., 89:911–913, 1955.
535. Ward, W.G., and Nunley, J.A.: Concomitant Fractures of the Capitellum and Radial Head. J. Orthop. Trauma, 2:110–116, 1988.
536. Weingarden, T.L.: Prosthetic Replacement in the Treatment of Fractures of the Radial Head. J. Am. Osteopath. Assoc., 77:804–807, 1978.
537. Weseley, M.S., Barenfeld, P.A., and Eisenstein, A.L.: Closed Treatment of Isolated Radial Head Fractures. J. Trauma, 23:36–39, 1983.
538. Wheeler, D.K., and Linscheid, R.L.: Fracture-Dislocations of the Elbow. Clin. Orthop., 50:95–106, 1967.
539. Wilson, P.D.: Fractures and Dislocations in the Region of the Elbow. Surg. Gynecol. Obstet., 56:335–359, 1933.
540. Worsing, R.A., Engber, W.D., and Lange, T.A. Reactive Synovitis From Particulate Silastic. J. Bone Joint Surg., 64A:581–584, 1982.

OPEN ELBOW INJURIES (SIDESWIPE INJURIES)

541. Kuur, E., and Kjaersgaad-Anderson: Side-Swipe Injury to the Elbow. J. Trauma, 28:1397–1399, 1988.
542. Meals, R.A.: The Use of a Flexor Carpi Ulnaris Muscle Flap in the Treatment of an Infected Nonunion of the Proximal Ulna: A Case Report. Clin. Orthop., 240:168–172, 1989.
543. Nicholson, J.T.: Compound Comminuted Fractures Involving the Elbow Joint. J. Bone Joint Surg., 28:565–575, 1946.
544. Shitany, U., and Wray, R.C., Jr.: Use of the Rectas Abdominis Muscle Flap to Reconstruct an Elbow Defect. Plast. Reconstr. Surg., 77:988–989, 1986.
545. Shorbe, H.B.: Car Window Elbows. South. Med. J., 34:372–376, 1941.
546. Stern, P.J., and Carey, J.P.: The Latissimus Dorsi Flap for Reconstruction of the Brachium and Shoulder. J. Bone Joint Surg., 70A:525–535, 1988.
547. Wood, C.F.: Traffic Elbow. Kentucky Med. J., 39:78–81, 1941.

Rockwood and Green's Fractures in Adults, Fourth Edition,
edited by Charles A. Rockwood, David P. Green, Robert W. Bucholz and James D. Heckman.
Lippincott-Raven Publishers, Philadelphia © 1996.

CHAPTER 15

Fractures of the Shaft of the Humerus

Joseph D. Zuckerman and Kenneth J. Koval

Fractures of the humeral shaft are commonly encountered by orthopaedic surgeons, accounting for approximately 3% of all fractures.[25] Treatment of these injuries continues to evolve as advances are made in both nonoperative and operative management. Most humeral shaft fractures can be managed nonoperatively with anticipated good to excellent results. Appropriate nonoperative and operative treatment of patients with humeral shaft fractures, however, requires an understanding of humeral anatomy, the fracture pattern, and the patient's activity level and expectations.

ANATOMY

The shaft of the humerus extends proximally from the upper border of the pectoralis major insertion to the supracondylar ridge distally.[103] The proximal aspect of the humeral shaft is cylindrical on cross section; distally its anteroposterior diameter narrows.[49] The anterior border of the humerus extends from the anterior aspect of the greater tuberosity to the coronoid fossa. Its medial border extends from the lesser tuberosity to the medial supracondylar ridge. Its lateral border extends from the posterior aspect of the greater tuberosity to the lateral supracondylar ridge. The deltoid muscle inserts onto the deltoid tuberosity, located on the anterolateral surface of the proximal humeral shaft. The radial sulcus contains the radial nerve and the profunda artery. The posterior surface is the origin for the triceps and contains the spiral groove.

The medial and lateral intermuscular septa divide the arm into anterior and posterior compartments. The biceps brachii, coracobrachialis, and brachialis muscles are contained in the anterior compartment. The brachial artery and vein and the median, musculocutaneous, and ulnar nerves course along the medial border of the biceps. The posterior compartment contains the triceps brachii muscle and radial nerve.[49]

The blood supply to the humeral diaphysis arises from branches of the brachial artery.[66] The nutrient artery enters the medial humerus distal to its midshaft region. In some patients there is a second nutrient canal at the origin of the radial sulcus. The lateral intermuscular septum is perforated by the radial nerve and the deep branch of the brachial artery. The medial intermuscular septum is perforated by the ulnar nerve, the superior ulnar collateral artery, and a posterior branch of the inferior ulnar collateral artery.

The muscle forces that act on the humeral shaft produce characteristic fracture deformities (Fig. 15-1). A fracture proximal to the pectoralis major insertion results in abduction and internal rotation of the proximal fragment secondary to the pull of the rotator cuff, while the distal fragment is displaced medially by the pectoralis major. If the fracture is distal to the pectoralis major insertion and proximal to the deltoid insertion, the distal fragment is laterally displaced by the deltoid, while the pectoralis major, latissimus dorsi, and teres major displace the proximal fragment medially. When the fracture is distal to the deltoid insertion, the proximal fragment is abducted and flexed while the distal fragment is proximally displaced.

MECHANISM OF INJURY

Humeral shaft fractures result from direct and indirect trauma. Common mechanisms for humeral shaft fractures include falls on the outstretched hand, motor vehicle accidents, and direct loads to the arm.[33] Extreme muscle contraction may cause fracture of the humeral shaft;[3,5,40] there are reports of fracture of the humeral shaft occurring after throwing a ball or javelin.[40] Elderly patients who suffer a humeral shaft fracture as a result of a fall often have less comminuted fracture patterns. Greater amounts of comminution and soft tissue injury result from higher energy injuries. Experimental fractures of the humeral shaft have been produced by Klenerman.[61] Pure compressive forces result in proximal or distal humerus fractures; bending forces, however, typically result in transverse fractures of the humeral shaft. Torsional forces result in spiral fracture patterns. The combination of bending and torsion usually results in an oblique fracture, often with an associated butterfly fragment.

CLASSIFICATION

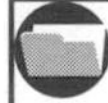

Classification of Humeral Shaft Fractures

- Fracture Location
  - Proximal
  - Middle
  - Distal
- Direction and Character
  - Transverse
  - Oblique
  - Spiral
  - Segmental
  - Comminuted
- Associated Soft Tissue Injury
- Associated Periarticular Injury
- Associated Nerve Injury
- Associated Vascular Injury
- Intrinsic Condition of Bone

There is no universally accepted classification system for humeral shaft fractures. Classically, humeral shaft fractures have been classified on the basis of various factors that influence treatment, such as (1) fracture location (proximal, middle, or distal third of the humeral shaft) and, additionally, whether the fracture is proximal to the pectoralis major insertion, distal to the

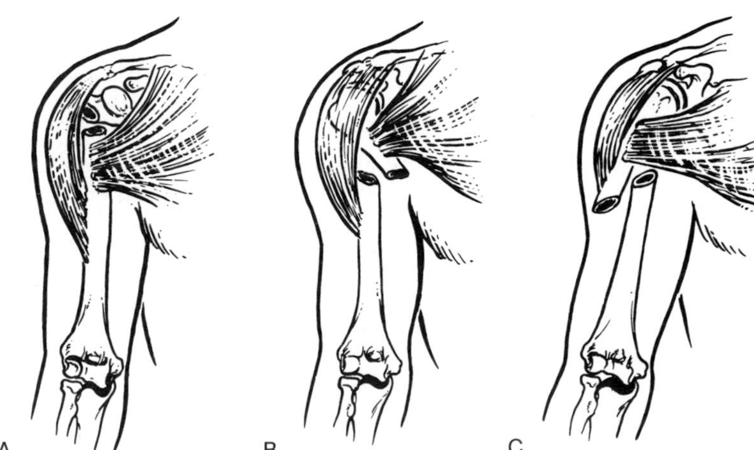

FIGURE 15-1. (**A**) A fracture proximal to the pectoralis major insertion results in abduction and internal rotation of the proximal fragment secondary to the pull of the rotator cuff, while the distal fragment is displaced medially by the pectoralis major. (**B**) If the fracture is distal to the pectoralis major insertion and proximal to the deltoid insertion, the distal fragment is laterally displaced by the deltoid while the pectoralis major, latissimus dorsi, and teres major displace the proximal fragment medially. (**C**) When the fracture is distal to the deltoid insertion, the proximal fragment is abducted and flexed while the distal fragment is proximally displaced.

pectoralis major insertion but proximal to the deltoid insertion, or distal to the deltoid insertion; (2) direction and character of fracture line (transverse, oblique, spiral, segmental, or comminuted); (3) associated soft-tissue injury (open or closed fracture); (4) associated periarticular injury involving the glenohumeral or elbow joints; (5) associated nerve injury involving either the radial, median, or ulnar nerves; (6) associated vascular injury involving either the brachial artery or vein; and (7) intrinsic condition of the bone (normal or pathologic).[32]

The AO/ASIF classification of humeral shaft fractures is based on fracture comminution: type A are simple (noncomminuted), type B have a butterfly fragment, and type C are comminuted (Fig. 15-2).[73] These fracture types are further divided according to fracture pattern.

SIGNS AND SYMPTOMS

Patients with humeral shaft fractures typically complain of arm pain, swelling, and deformity. The arm is shortened with gross motion and crepitus on gentle manipulation. The clinical signs may be more subtle with nondisplaced fractures. Because humeral shaft fractures may result from high-energy trauma, the physician should have a high index of suspicion for other associated injuries. The immediate objective of the clinical examination is to identify and treat life-threatening injuries. Secondary assessment should include a systematic inspection of the entire extremity. Soft-tissue abrasions must be differentiated from open fractures. Intra-articular extensions of puncture wounds around the shoulder and elbow can be determined by injection of saline into the joint away from the area of the puncture and noting extravasation of fluid. The neurovascular status of the extremity must be assessed. Doppler pulses and compartment pressure measurements should be made if indicated. Particular attention should be directed to areas of swelling or soft-tissue injury, since associated injuries are not uncommon. This is particularly important in the patient with polytrauma or in the obtunded patient.

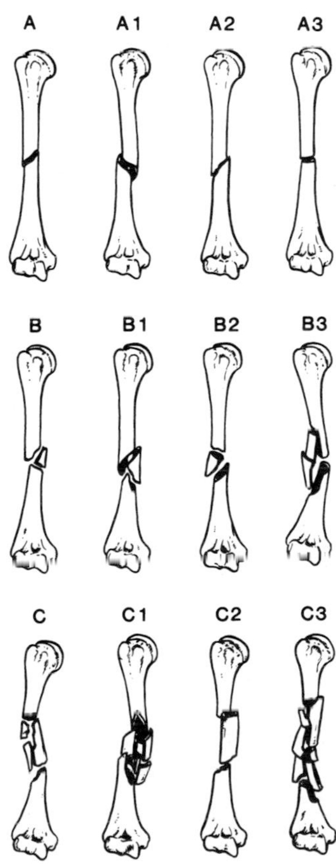

FIGURE 15-2. The AO/ASIF classification of humeral shaft fractures.

RADIOGRAPHIC FINDINGS

The standard radiographic views of the humerus include anteroposterior and lateral radiographs, taken at 90° to one another. The shoulder and elbow joint should be included on each view. This will identify associated dislocations or intra-articular fracture extension, which may interfere with intramedullary nailing. The radiographs are obtained by moving the patient rather than simply rotating the injured extremity. In highly comminuted or displaced fractures, traction radiographs may allow better fracture definition. Comparison radiographs of the contralateral humerus are helpful for preoperative planning. Tomograms and computed tomography are rarely indicated. In pathologic fractures, additional studies (technetium bone scan, computed tomography, and magnetic resonance imaging) may be necessary to delineate the extent of disease before fracture treatment.

METHODS OF TREATMENT

The goals of humeral shaft fracture management are to establish union with an acceptable humeral alignment and restore the patients to their prior level of function. Many methods have been described for the treatment of humeral shaft fractures.[11,32,101] Good to excellent results have been reported in most series of humeral shaft fractures treated closed or with open reduction and internal fixation. Both patient and fracture characteristics (patient age, presence of associated injuries, soft-tissue status, and fracture pattern) need to be considered to select the appropriate treatment option.

Nonoperative Treatment

Closed Treatment Methods

Most humeral shaft fractures can be managed nonoperatively with greater than a 90% expected union rate. The closed treatment methods available include (1) hanging arm cast; (2) coaptation or U-shaped brachial splint; (3) Velpeau dressing; (4) abduction humeral splint/shoulder spica cast; (5) skeletal traction; and (6) functional brace. Although good to excellent results have been reported using each of these different treatment modalities, functional fracture bracing has become the most common treatment for closed humeral shaft fractures.

The Hanging Arm Cast. The hanging arm cast, described by Caldwell in 1933, uses dependency traction provided by the weight of the cast to effect fracture reduction.[17,18] Therefore, for this technique to be effective, the patient must remain upright or semi-erect at all times. The hanging arm cast may be the definitive fracture treatment or can be exchanged for a functional fracture brace. A concern with use of the hanging arm cast is fracture distraction resulting in delayed union. The indications for use of the hanging arm cast include displaced midshaft humeral shaft fractures with shortening, particularly those fractures with an oblique or spiral pattern. Use of the hanging arm cast is not indicated for transverse fractures because of the potential for distraction and healing complications.

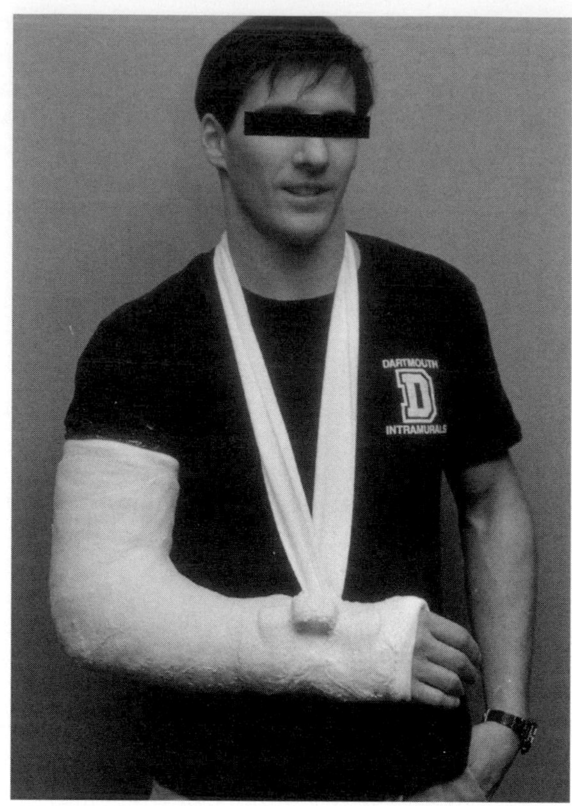

FIGURE 15-3. The hanging arm cast is applied with the elbow in 90° flexion and the forearm in neutral rotation. The supporting stockinette passes through one of three loops applied at the wrist.

Treatment with the hanging arm cast requires meticulous attention to detail.[97] The cast should be lightweight and applied with the elbow at 90° and the forearm in neutral rotation (Fig. 15-3). The cast should extend at least 2 cm proximal to the fracture. Three plaster or wire loops are applied at the distal forearm in dorsal, neutral, and volar positions; a stockinette is passed through one of these loops and around the patient's neck. Apex anterior angulation is corrected by shortening the sling; apex posterior angulation is corrected by lengthening the sling; apex medial angulation is corrected by using the volar loop; and apex lateral angulation is corrected by using the dorsal loop (Fig. 15-4).[41] The cast must hang free of the body with the arm in a dependent position to provide a traction force. The patient is instructed to sleep erect or semi-erect and to avoid supporting the elbow when seated. Initial radiographic evaluation of the fracture with the patient standing or sitting should be made at weekly intervals. Shoulder and hand range of motion exercises are instituted as pain permits; circumduction shoulder exercises are important to prevent a frozen shoulder. Isometric exercises are encouraged when discomfort subsides.

Careful patient and fracture selection and meticulous application of the hanging cast are necessary to maximize treatment success and minimize complications. Proper use of hanging arm cast has resulted in up to a 96% union rate.[95,98,104] It is probably best used as initial treatment for displaced spiral and oblique humeral shaft fractures with shortening followed by early functional brace application.

Coaptation Splint. The U-shaped coaptation splint with collar and cuff is indicated for the acute treatment of humeral shaft fractures with minimal shortening. A carefully molded plaster slab is placed around the medial and lateral aspects of the arm, extending around the elbow and over the deltoid and acromion (Fig. 15-5). Slippage of the cast can be prevented by contouring the slab over the shoulder or applying tincture of benzoin to the arm before the splint application. The forearm is suspended by a collar and cuff. The splint should hang free of the body. The patient is instructed in range of motion exercises of the shoulder, elbow, wrist, and hand. Disadvantages of the coaptation splint include loss of elbow extension, axillary irritation, patient discomfort, and the bulkiness of the device. It is not uncommon that the plaster slab will slip, requiring reapplication. Similar to the hanging arm cast, the coaptation splint is frequently exchanged

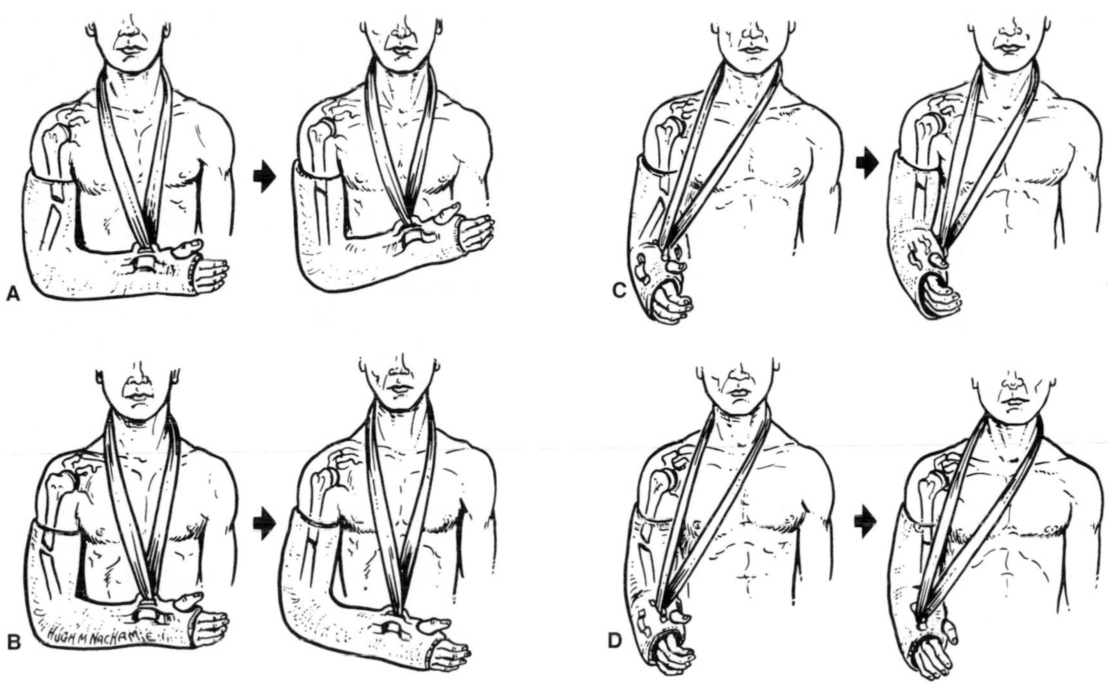

FIGURE 15-4. With use of the hanging cast, apex anterior angulation is corrected by shortening the sling (**A**), apex posterior angulation is corrected by lengthening the sling (**B**), apex medial angulation is corrected by using the volar loop (**C**), and apex lateral angulation is corrected by using the dorsal loop (**D**).

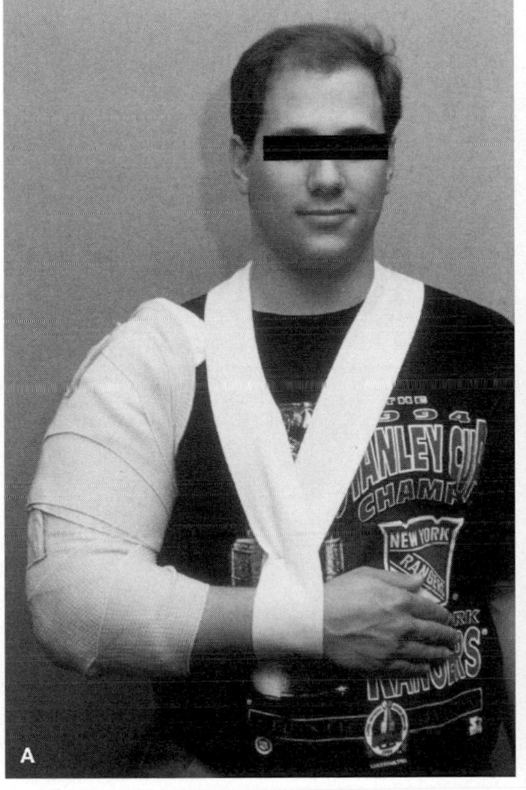

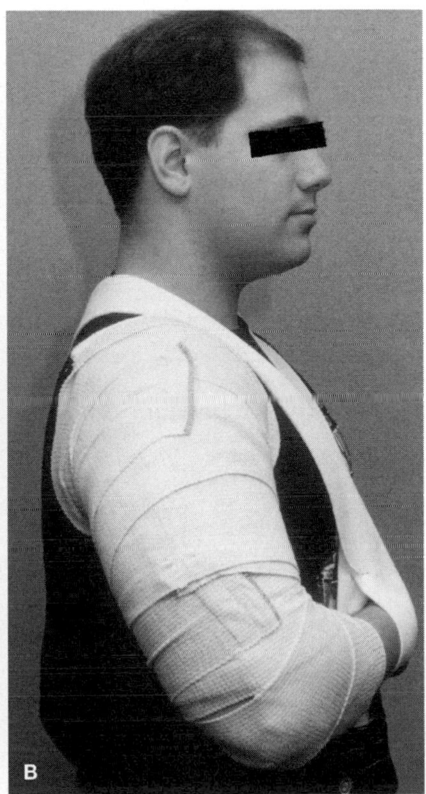

FIGURE 15-5. The U-shaped coaptation splint is placed around the medial and lateral aspects of the arm, extending around the elbow and over the deltoid.

for a functional cast brace 1 to 2 weeks after injury as the patient's pain permits.

Thoracobrachial Immobilization. A stockinette Velpeau shoulder dressing was described by Gilchrist for immobilization of the shoulder girdle.[38] This over-the-shoulder device is inexpensive, comfortable, and easily applied (Fig. 15-6). This device is most useful in nondisplaced or minimally displaced fractures in children or the elderly who are unable to tolerate other methods of management.[50] In these cases, patient comfort, not fracture reduction, is the critical consideration. An axillary pad may be used to abduct the distal fragment. The patient should be encouraged to perform shoulder pendulum exercises. Early humeral fracture brace application should be considered as well.

Shoulder Spica Cast. The indications for use of a shoulder spica cast are unclear. The primary indications may be when closed reduction of the fracture requires significant abduction and external rotation of the upper extremity. However, when this uncommon situation occurs, operative management is frequently performed. Disadvantages of the shoulder spica cast include difficulty in application, cast weight and bulkiness, skin irritation, and patient discomfort. It should be avoided in patients with significant pulmonary problems.

Skeletal Traction. Skeletal traction is rarely indicated for the treatment of closed or open humeral shaft fractures. The historical indications for use of skeletal traction (associated skeletal injuries requiring prolonged recumbency, open fractures) are now considered indications for operative intervention. When indicated, skeletal traction is applied through a transolecranon Kirschner wire or Steinmann pin. The pin should be inserted from medial to lateral to minimize the risk of ulnar nerve injury.

Functional Bracing. The humeral functional brace was first described by Sarmiento in 1977.[92] A functional brace is an orthosis that effects fracture reduction through soft-tissue compression.[108] Use of this device maximizes shoulder and elbow motion. This brace initially was custom made and designed as a wraparound sleeve. However, current braces are prefabricated and consist of an anterior shell (contoured for the biceps tendon distally) and a posterior shell (Fig. 15-7). These shells are circularized with Velcro straps, which can be tightened as swelling decreases. The proximal aspect of the brace approaches the acromion laterally and encircles the arm underneath the axilla medially. Distally, the sleeve is fashioned to avoid the medial and lateral epicondyles, permitting free elbow motion. Over-the-shoulder extensions are available but seldom necessary; they are most often used for comminuted fractures of the proximal humerus, but the associated restriction of shoulder motion is a significant disadvantage. Contraindications to use of the

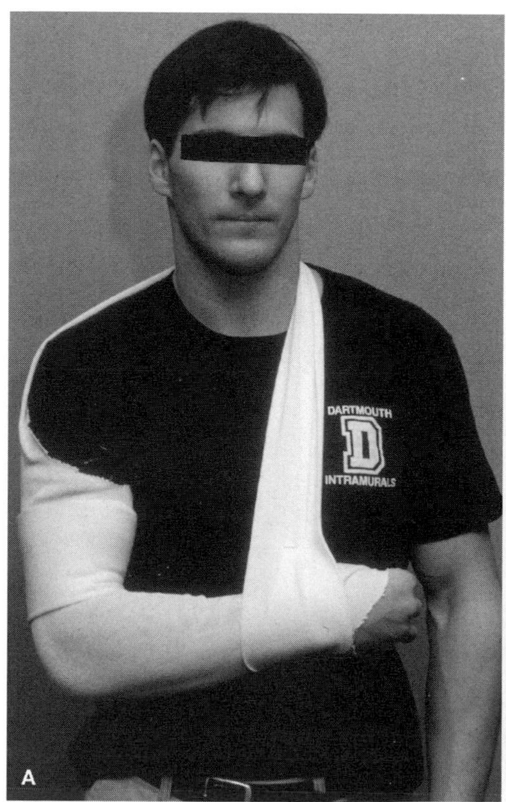

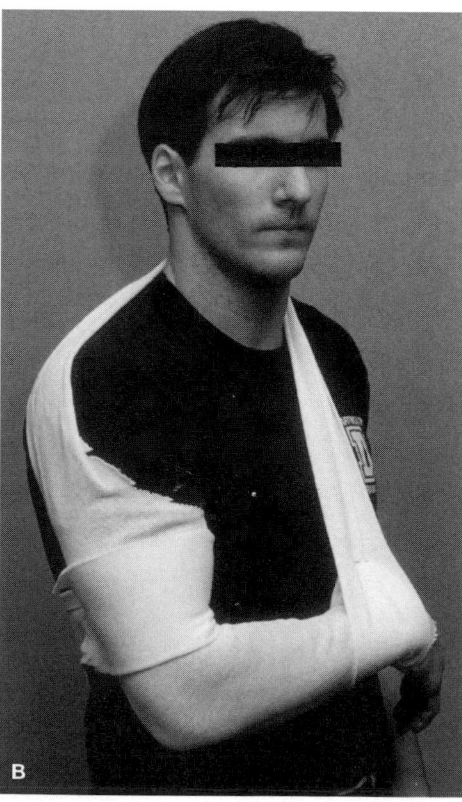

FIGURE 15-6. A Velpeau shoulder dressing can be made from a single piece of stockinette. It is inexpensive, comfortable, and easily applied.

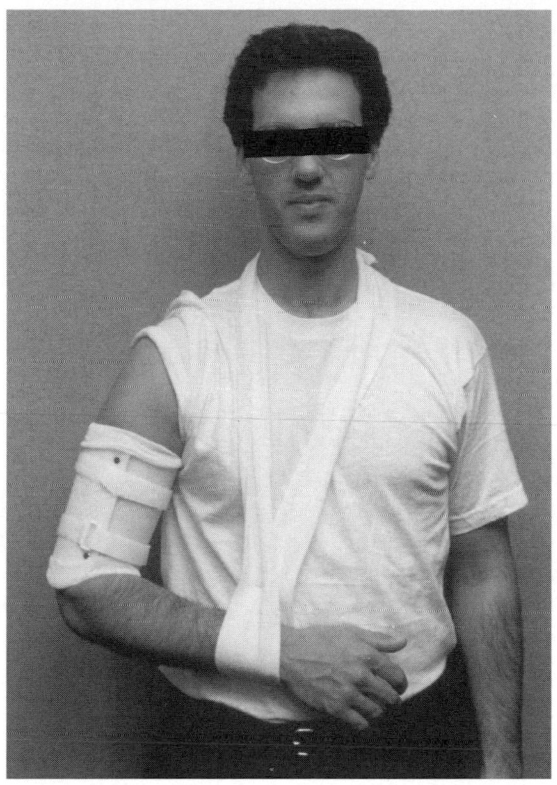

FIGURE 15-7. A functional brace consists of an anterior shell (contoured for the biceps tendon distally) and a posterior shell, held together with Velcro straps.

functional brace include (1) massive soft-tissue injury or bone loss; (2) an unreliable or uncooperative patient; and (3) an inability to obtain or maintain acceptable fracture alignment.[76]

The humeral fracture brace can be applied acutely or 1 to 2 weeks after application of a hanging arm cast or coaptation splint. If the fracture brace is applied acutely, the patient should be reevaluated the following day to assess the extremity's neurovascular status and amount of arm/forearm edema. The patient is instructed to keep the arm hanging free of the body; use of a sling may result in varus angulation. The patient is followed at weekly intervals for the first 3 to 4 weeks to assess fracture alignment and instructed in pendulum exercises and range of motion of the shoulder, elbow, wrist, and hand. The patient is encouraged to remain upright to allow gravity to assist fracture reduction. When patient comfort permits, the brace can be removed for hygiene. The brace is worn for a minimum of 8 weeks post fracture.

Operative Treatment

The indications for operative management of humeral shaft fractures are listed in Table 15-1. Open humerus fractures require emergent debridement. Fracture stabilization after soft-tissue and osseous debridement has been reported to reduce the incidence of infection.[23] The humeral shaft fracture with associated vascular injury is best managed with internal or external fixation, either before or after vascular repair depending on the viability of the limb. When vascular repair is needed, nonoperative management is contraindicated because fracture motion may jeopardize the repair. Nonoperative treatment of patients with a floating elbow (an ipsilateral fracture of the humerus and radius/ulna) has resulted in high rates of nonunion, malunion, and elbow stiffness.[67,86] Improved results have been reported after internal fixation of the humerus and radius/ulna fractures, followed by early range of elbow motion. Nonoperative treatment of a segmental humerus fracture is associated with increased risk of nonunion at one or both fracture sites.[35] Pathologic fractures should be internally stabilized to maximize patient comfort and to increase upper extremity function. Operative stabilization of bilateral humerus fractures significantly improves patient self-care.[60,93] The patient with polytrauma is often unable to remain in the semi-sitting position necessary to effect fracture reduction by nonoperative measures, and operative stabilization of the humerus is necessary to maximize the recovery and rehabilitation potential of this patient. Radial nerve dysfunction after fracture manipulation may be an indication for radial nerve exploration and fracture stabilization.[93] Neurologic loss after penetrating injury is an indication for nerve exploration. Fractures that cannot be maintained in acceptable alignment should be operatively stabilized. In the humeral shaft, one can accept up to 3 cm shortening, 20° of anterior or posterior angulation, and 30° of varus.[62] Significant varus can be cosmetically disfiguring in thin individuals, however, and in these patients fewer degrees of varus should be accepted. Humeral shaft fractures in obese patients and women

TABLE 15-1
Indications for Operative Management of Humeral Shaft Fractures

Open fracture
Associated vascular injury
Floating elbow
Segmental fracture
Pathologic fracture
Bilateral humerus fractures
Humerus fracture in polytrauma patient
Radial nerve dysfunction after fracture manipulation
Neurologic loss after penetrating injury
Fractures with unacceptable alignment
Intra-articular fracture extension

with large pendulous breasts are at increased risk of varus angulation. Malrotation is well tolerated secondary to compensatory shoulder motion. Finally, fractures of the humeral shaft associated with intra-articular fracture extension require operative treatment.[93]

Operative Approaches to the Humerus

Operative stabilization of humeral shaft fractures may be performed through an anterolateral, anterior, or posterior approach.[51]

Anterolateral Approach. The patient is positioned supine with the arm placed either on a hand table or arm board. An incision is made along the lateral border of the biceps, ending just proximal to the elbow flexion crease. The lateral border of the biceps is identified and the muscle retracted medially. The interval between the brachialis and brachioradialis is identified proximal to the elbow and the two muscles separated. The brachioradialis is retracted laterally and the brachialis and biceps muscles retracted medially. The radial nerve lies between the brachialis and brachioradialis and must be identified (Fig. 15-8). The radial nerve is traced proximally through the lateral intermuscular septum and protected throughout the remainder of the procedure. The periosteum is incised longitudinally at the lateral border of the brachialis muscle and the humerus subperiosteally dissected. The anterolateral approach can be extended proximally into an anterior approach to the shoulder and distally to an anterior approach to the elbow. This approach is preferred for proximal third humerus fractures.

Anterior Approach. The anterior approach to the humeral shaft is similar to the anterolateral approach. It cannot be extended distally, however, to the elbow. The patient is positioned supine with the arm on a hand table or arm board. A longitudinal incision is made from the coracoid process to the deltoid insertion and extended distally following the lateral border of the biceps. The distal limit of the incision is 5 cm proximal to the elbow flexion crease. The brachialis and biceps muscle interval is identified and the biceps retracted medially. The fibers of brachialis are separated longitudinally to expose the anterior surface of the humeral shaft. Proximally, the deltopectoral interval is entered, retracting the cephalic vein either medially or laterally. The periosteum lateral to the pectoralis major insertion is incised and the humerus subperiosteally dissected. The approach must remain subperiosteal to avoid radial nerve injury. The anterior approach can be extended into an anterior approach to the shoulder; since this approach cannot be extended distally, it is less useful than the anterolateral approach to the humerus.

Posterior Approach. The posterior approach provides excellent exposure to most of the humerus and is limited only in its most proximal extent. The patient is positioned either lateral or prone. A posterior longitudinal incision extends from 8 cm distal to the acromion to the olecranon. The interval between the lateral and long heads of the triceps is identified and these two muscles separated. The medial head of the triceps is identified; the radial nerve lies alongside its lateral border and is traced proximal and distal through the intermuscular septum (Fig. 15-9). The medial head of the triceps is incised longitudinally and the posterior aspect of the humerus subperiosteally dissected. Proximal dissection is limited by the axillary nerve and pos-

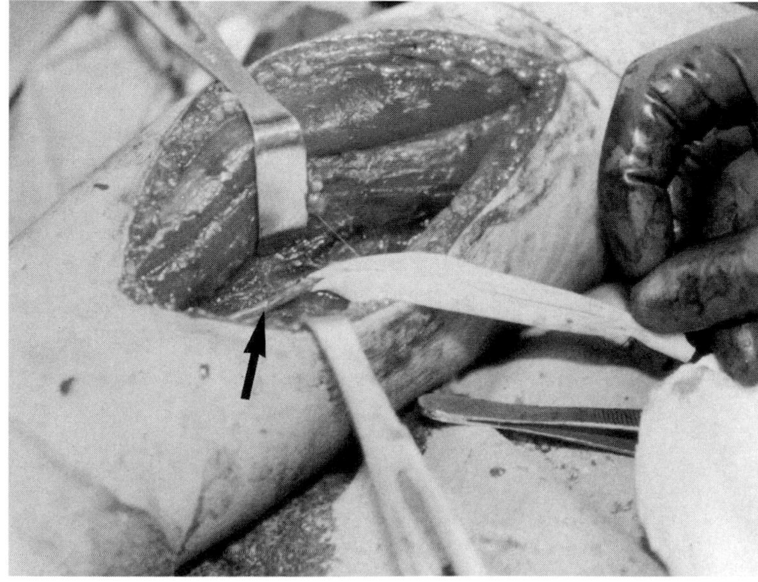

FIGURE 15-8. In the distal arm, the radial nerve (*arrow*) lies between the brachialis and brachioradialis muscles.

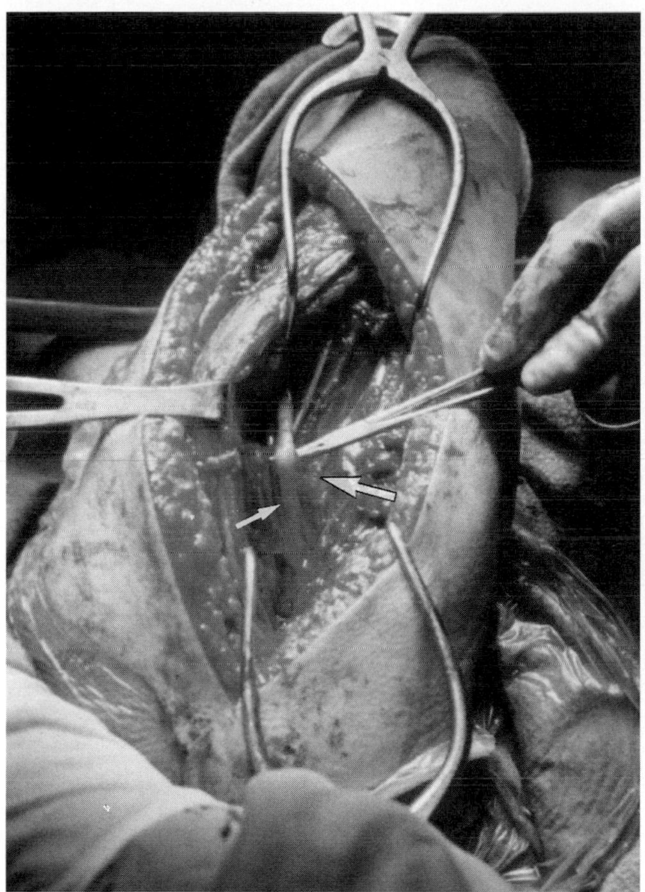

FIGURE 15-9. In the mid to upper arm the radial nerve (*small arrow*) lies along the lateral border of the medial head of the triceps (*large arrow*).

terior humeral circumflex vessels. The elbow can be exposed after performing an olecranon osteotomy.

Operative Fixation Using Plate and Screws

One can achieve anatomical fracture reduction and stable fixation of the humeral shaft without violation of the rotator cuff using plates and screws. The exact nature of the fracture, with identification of all major fracture fragments, should be determined before definitive surgical intervention is attempted.[70] Identification of the individual fragments is often facilitated with traction radiographs. Radiographs of the opposite, uninjured extremity serve as templates for preoperative planning; the individual fracture fragments, chosen implant, and surgical tactic are drawn on the intact humeral template (Fig. 15-10). This requires the surgeon to understand the "personality of the fracture" and to mentally prepare for the operative procedure.

At surgery, minimal stripping of soft tissue should be performed; butterfly fragments must not be devitalized. A 4.5-mm broad dynamic compression plate is usually selected for shaft fractures in average- to large-sized patients (Fig. 15-11).[89,93] In smaller patients, a 4.5-mm narrow dynamic compression plate may be used.[93] Proximal and distal humerus fractures require use of other types of implants (single or double reconstruction plates, T plates). Depending on the fracture level, one can use a precontoured plate as a reduction aid. If the fracture pattern permits, the plate should be applied in compression.[93] Lag screws should be inserted whenever possible. Fixation of eight to ten cortices proximal and distal to the fracture should be obtained. Fixation stability must be assessed before closure. The need for bone grafting is determined by the amount of comminution and stripping of soft tissue. In general, one should have a low threshold for cancellous bone grafting of these fractures when plates and screws are used.

External Fixation

The indications for external fixation of humeral shaft fractures include open fractures with extensive soft-tissue injury, fractures with overlying burns, and infected nonunions. Use of both unilateral frames with

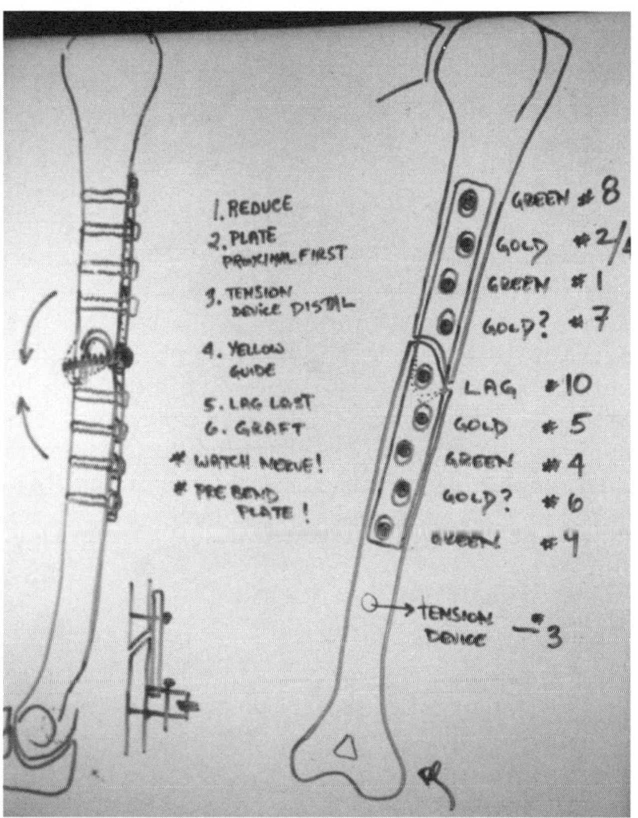

FIGURE 15-10. Preoperative plan of a midshaft humeral plating, including the order of screw placement. (*Courtesy of Roy Sanders, Florida Orthapaedic Institute, Tampa, FL.*)

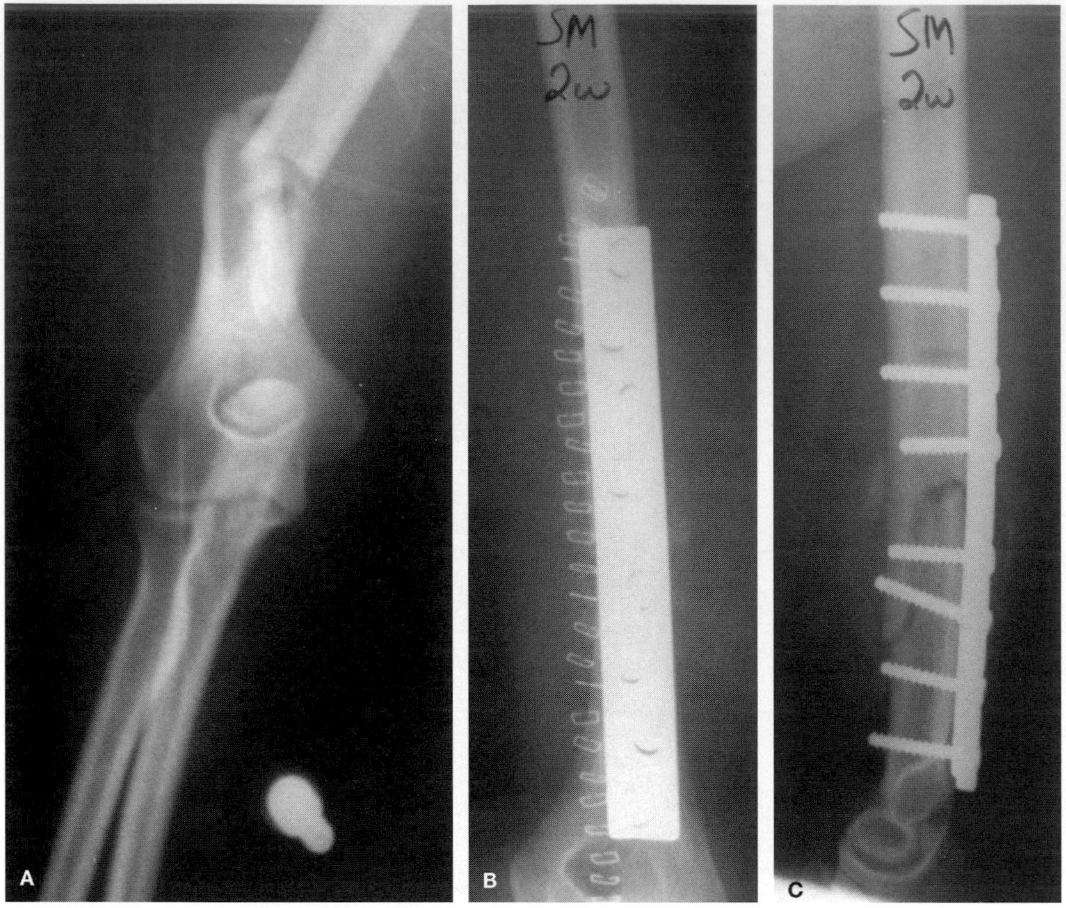

FIGURE 15-11. (**A** through **C**) Displaced distal humeral shaft fracture stabilized with a 4.5-mm broad dynamic compression plate and lag screws.

standard half pins (Fig. 15-12) and ring-type fixators with small-diameter tension wires (Fig. 15-13) have been described for humeral stabilization.[9,19,31] Complications of external fixators include pin tract infection; neurovascular, muscle, and tendon impalement; and nonunion.[39] Most of these complications can be avoided by meticulous attention to operative technique by the surgeon. Pin placement in the humeral shaft should be done under direct visualization to minimize the risk of neurovascular injury.[39]

Intramedullary Fixation

An intramedullary nail is satisfactory for most diaphyseal fractures of long bones.[16,21] Mechanically, intramedullary nails offer several advantages over plates and external fixators:

1. Because the intramedullary canal is closer to the mechanical axis than the usual plate position on the external surface of the bone, intramedullary nails are subjected to smaller bending loads than plates and are less likely to fail by fatigue.[2,16]
2. Intramedullary nails can act as load-sharing devices in fractures with cortical contact; if the nail is not locked at both proximal and distal ends, it will act as a gliding splint and allow fracture compression as the extremity is loaded.[2,16,21]
3. In midshaft fractures, nails that fill the medullary canal automatically reestablish osseous alignment.[16,21]
4. Stress shielding with resultant cortical osteopenia, commonly seen with plates and screws, is minimized with intramedullary nails.[16,65]
5. Refracture after implant removal is rare with the use of intramedullary nails, secondary to lack of cortical osteopenia, and the fewer stress risers created.[15,21]

Intramedullary nails also offer significant biological advantages over other fixation methods.[10,15,21,26,74,77,78,87,105] Although insertion can be technically demanding, intramedullary nails do not require the extensive exposure required for plate application. With the use of image intensification, these devices can be inserted in a closed manner, without exposing the fracture. These

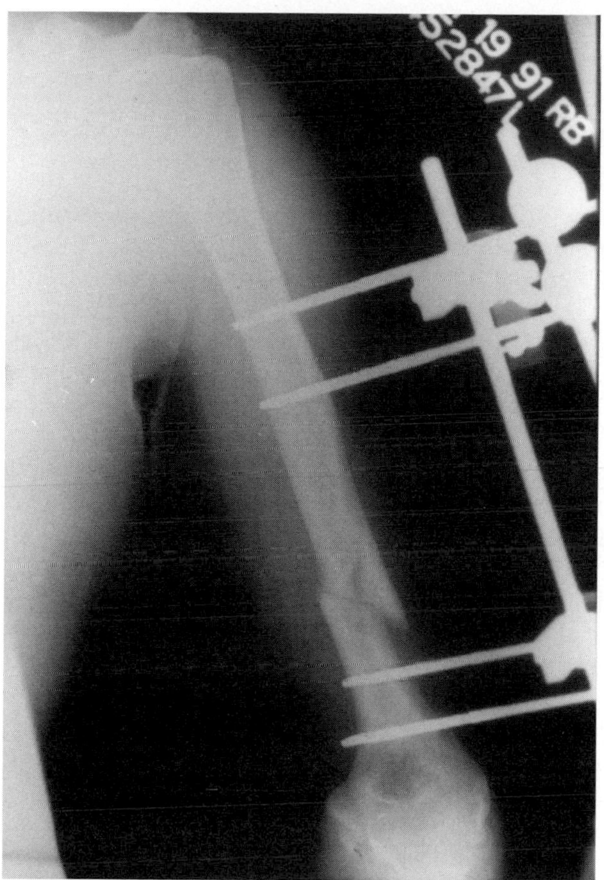

FIGURE 15-12. A unilateral half pin fixator used to stabilize an open humeral shaft fracture. (*Courtesy of Paul Tornetta, Downstate Medical Center, Brooklyn, NY.*)

closed techniques may result in a lower infection rate and higher union rate with minimal soft-tissue scarring.[10,15,16,26,74,77,78,87,105] Two types of intramedullary nails are available for use in humeral shaft fractures: flexible and interlocked nails.

Flexible Intramedullary Nails. Flexible intramedullary devices available for use in the management of humeral shaft fractures include Ender nails, Hackenthal nails, and Rush rods (Fig. 15-14). With these devices, multiple implants are required to achieve fracture stability. They can be inserted retrograde from the distal humerus or antegrade near the rotator cuff. Violation of the rotator cuff during insertion, however, especially if compounded by encroachment of the subacromial space, can result in loss of shoulder motion. In Hall and Pankovich's series of 89 humeral fractures stabilized with Ender nails, shoulder abduction at follow-up averaged only 91°.[45] In a series of 63 humeral shaft fractures stabilized with either Rush pins or Ender nails inserted antegrade or retrograde, Brumback and associates[14] reported the best results with retrograde insertion through an entry portal located proximal to the olecranon fossa. Flexible intramedullary nails do not provide rigid fixation; they do not prevent fracture shortening nor do they provide significant rotational control. Use of a functional fracture brace should be considered after flexible intramedullary nailing of the humerus if additional stability is needed.

Interlocked Nails. The success of interlocked nails for the treatment of unstable femur and tibia fractures has resulted in the design of several types of locked intramedullary humeral nails. These nails usually rely on proximal screw and distal screw or fin fixation to provide stability. Locked intramedullary nails are able to maintain alignment of unstable fracture patterns, preventing fracture shortening and rotation (Fig. 15-15). They can be used to stabilize fractures from 2 cm distal to the surgical neck to 3 cm proximal to the olecranon fossa. Interlocked humeral nails can be inserted antegrade through the rotator cuff/greater tuberosity or retrograde proximal to the olecranon fossa, with or without prior reaming. Reaming increases the length along which the nail contacts the endosteal surface of the intramedullary canal, thereby providing better fracture stability. Reaming also decreases the risk of nail incarceration and permits placement of a larger-diameter (and thus, stronger) nail. Finally,

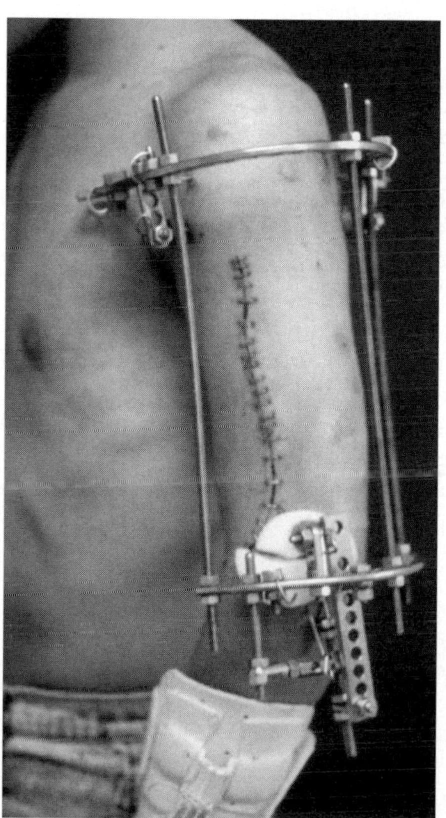

FIGURE 15-13. Ring fixator with small-diameter tensioned wires.

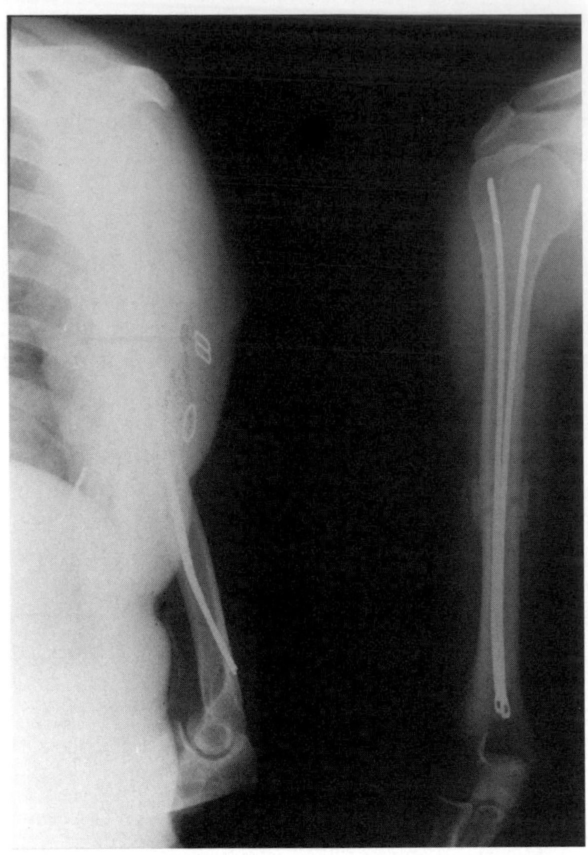

FIGURE 15-14. Midshaft humerus fracture stabilized with two retrograde-inserted Ender nails.

reaming results in the production of a large quantity of morselized bone chips that have osteoinductive effects.[20,24] The effect of reaming on the osseous blood supply, however, must be carefully considered. Intramedullary nailing, whether by reamed or nonreamed techniques, interferes with the endosteal blood supply.[1,22,30,82,84] Rhinelander[83] has shown that the endosteal blood supply rapidly reconstitutes itself after intramedullary nailing with nonreamed nails. Reaming obliterates the nutrient artery and endosteal blood supply, but this will reconstitute itself if the nail has channels along its length to permit revascularization.[22] Since the endosteal blood supply is inevitably damaged during intramedullary nailing, precautions must be taken to preserve the periosteal blood supply.[68]

With antegrade insertion, it is important to bury the humeral nail below the rotator cuff to prevent encroachment of the nail on the subacromial space. Oblique proximal locking screws inserted from superolateral to inferomedial may result in subacromial impingement if the screws are located proximal to the equator of the humeral head.[85] The axillary nerve is at risk during proximal locking screw insertion.[85] The distal locking screws can be inserted in either an anteroposterior or posteroanterior direction. However, dissection should be performed down to the cortex to minimize the possibility of soft-tissue injury.

 Authors' Preferred Method of Treatment

Most closed humeral shaft fractures can be managed nonoperatively with closed reduction and application of a coaptation splint with collar and cuff followed by a functional fracture brace 1 to 2 weeks after injury (if significant fracture shortening is present, a hanging arm cast can be used initially) (Fig. 15-16). The patient is instructed to sit in a semi-reclining position and not to lean on the elbow for support (Fig. 15-17). The patient is started on shoulder pendulum exercises as soon as discomfort allows as well as range of motion of the elbow, wrist, and hand (Fig. 15-18). Assisted shoulder range of motion is performed as tolerated. The functional brace is removed only for hygiene; it is tightened gradually as swelling subsides. Initially the patient is followed at weekly intervals for clinical and radiographic evaluation. The patient is slowly weaned from the brace as clinical and radiographic findings indicate progression of fracture union. This usually occurs 6 to 8 weeks after fracture.

When open reduction is indicated, an antegrade-inserted interlocked humeral nail is our implant of choice. The patient is positioned supine on a radiolucent operating room table (Fig. 15-19). A sandbag is placed between the patient's shoulder blades, and the patient's head is turned toward the contralateral side to maximize exposure of the proximal humerus. The patient is prepped from the base of the neck to the fingertips with the arm draped free. A 3- to 4-cm incision is made extending distally from the lateral acromion along the direction of the deltoid fibers. The deltoid muscle is incised in line with its fibers; the deltoid should not be incised farther than 4 to 5 cm distally to avoid injury to the axillary nerve. The rotator cuff is identified and an awl used to enter the intramedullary canal just medial to the greater tuberosity at the site of insertion of the rotator cuff. The direction of the awl should be in line with the anatomical axis of the humerus. A guide wire is inserted into the proximal humerus, the fracture reduced under fluoroscopic control, and the guide wire passed to the distal humeral metaphysis. If the fracture cannot be reduced by closed manipulation, a small incision can be made on the anterolateral aspect of the arm and a finger used to manipulate the fracture. Distal containment of the guide wire within the intramedullary canal is confirmed radiographically by rotation of the distal humerus. The selected humeral nail is usually 8 to 9 mm in diameter. Young patients often have a smaller-diameter intramedullary canal that requires reaming before nail placement; in older patients with a larger-

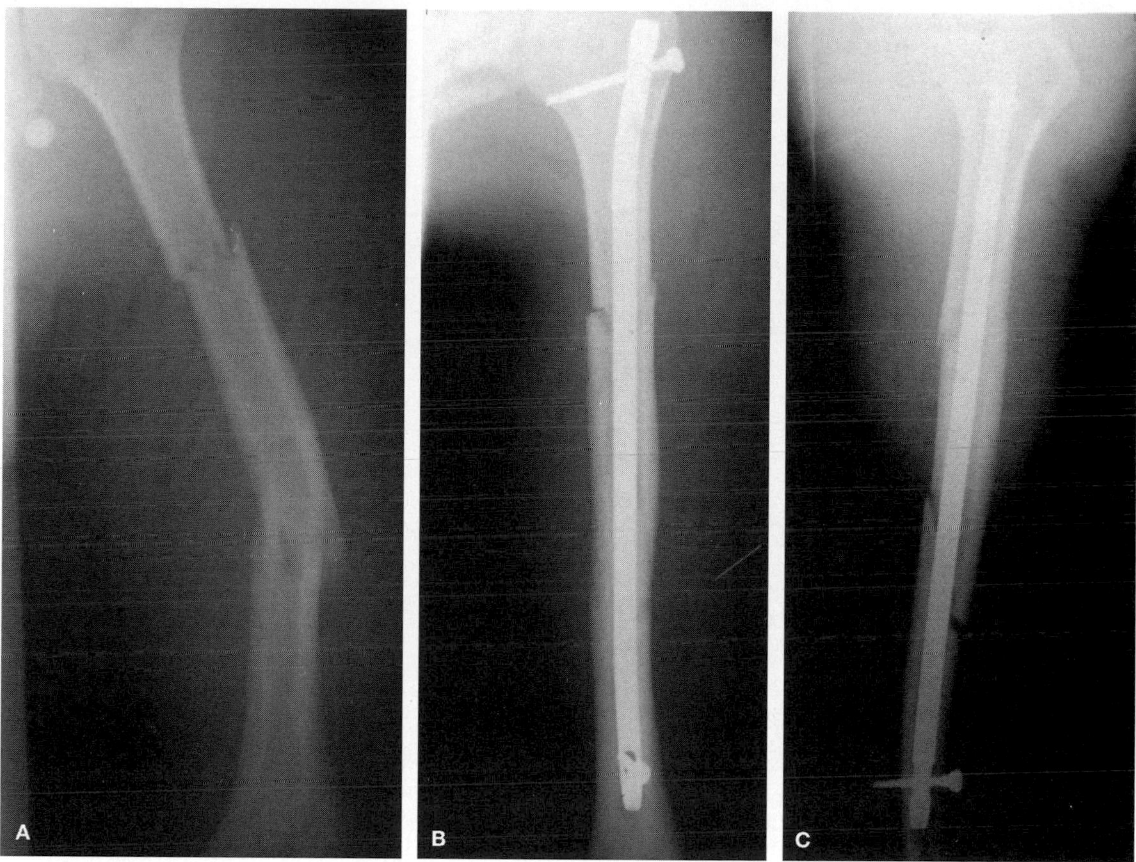

FIGURE 15-15. Segmental humerus fracture (**A**) stabilized with an antegrade-inserted locked intramedullary nail (**B** and **C**).

diameter intramedullary canal an unreamed 9-mm humeral nail can often be used. When reaming is performed, it is essential not to ream areas of comminution. This avoids increasing the amount of comminution and soft-tissue injury at the fracture site. Nail length is determined using a second guide wire of identical length; nail length can also be determined from the uninjured humerus. After guide wire exchange, the nail is hand inserted down the intramedullary canal and seated below the rotator cuff. Proximal locking is performed using a targeting device. The safest locking screw configuration is from superolateral to inferomedial.[85] One should use frequent radiographic imaging to avoid overpenetration of the medial humeral cortex.[85] Distal locking is performed using a free-hand technique. An incision is made over the distal locking hole and a hemostat used to spread the soft tissue down to the cortex. A trocar or drill bit can be used to penetrate the anterior and posterior humeral cortices and the locking screw inserted. One should assess fracture stability clinically and radiographically before wound closure. The upper extremity is then placed in a long-arm posterior splint. Active and active-assisted range of motion exercises for the elbow, wrist, and hand are initiated on the first postoperative day. Shoulder range of motion exercises should also be initiated on the first postoperative day. Resistive exercises are added when there is radiographic evidence of healing. We use a functional fracture brace in conjunction with intramedullary nailing if there are concerns about fracture stability.

REHABILITATION

Early institution of a closely monitored rehabilitation protocol is essential to maximize functional outcome after humeral shaft fracture. Range of motion exercises of the hand and wrist should be started immediately after injury. Range of motion exercises of the shoulder and elbow are instituted as discomfort subsides. Regardless of the method of treatment or immobilization, shoulder range of motion exercises should be emphasized to avoid postfracture stiffness.

The elbow requires special consideration. Elbow range of motion exercises should be limited to active exercises only. Passive exercises, particularly if forceful, can result in myositis ossificans. When fracture

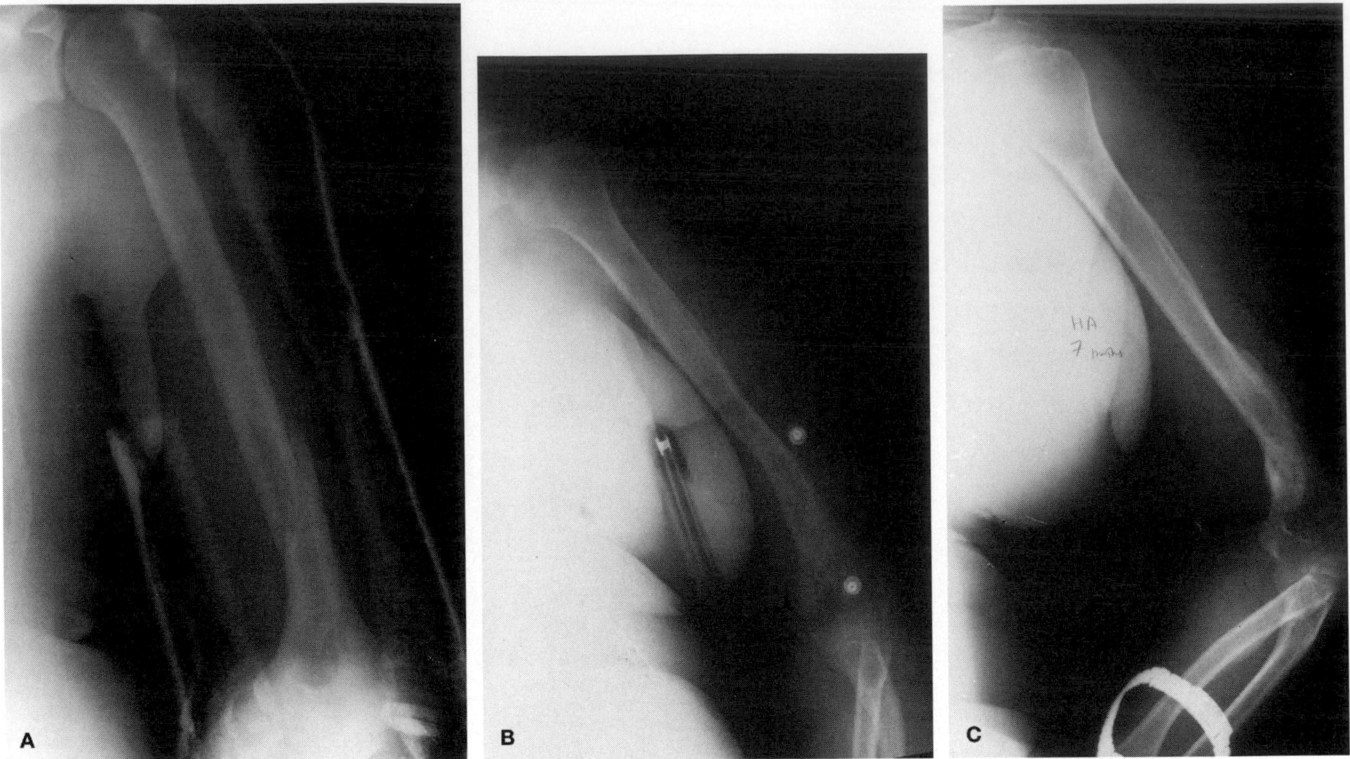

FIGURE 15-16. Humeral shaft fracture managed nonoperatively with a closed reduction and application of a coaptation splint (**A**) followed by a functional fracture brace at 1 to 2 weeks (**B**). (**C**) Radiograph of the healed fracture at 7-month follow-up.

healing is evident both clinically and radiographically, a shoulder and elbow strengthening program can be initiated, progressing from isometric to isotonic exercises.

PROGNOSIS

Nonoperative Treatment

Good to excellent results can be obtained with both nonoperative and operative treatment of patients with humeral shaft fractures. Winfield and coworkers[104] re-

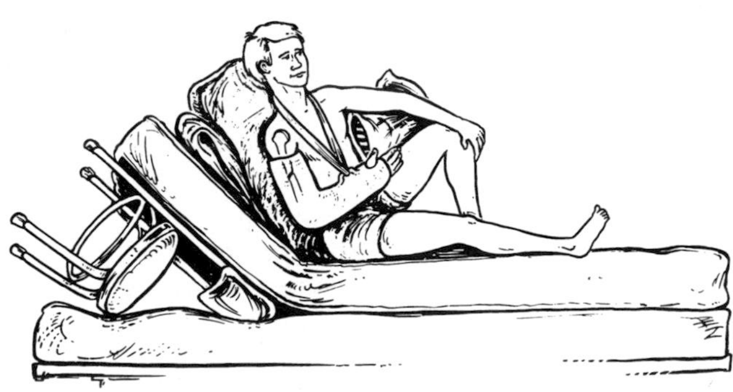

FIGURE 15-17. The patient is instructed to sleep in a semi-reclining position without the elbow supported.

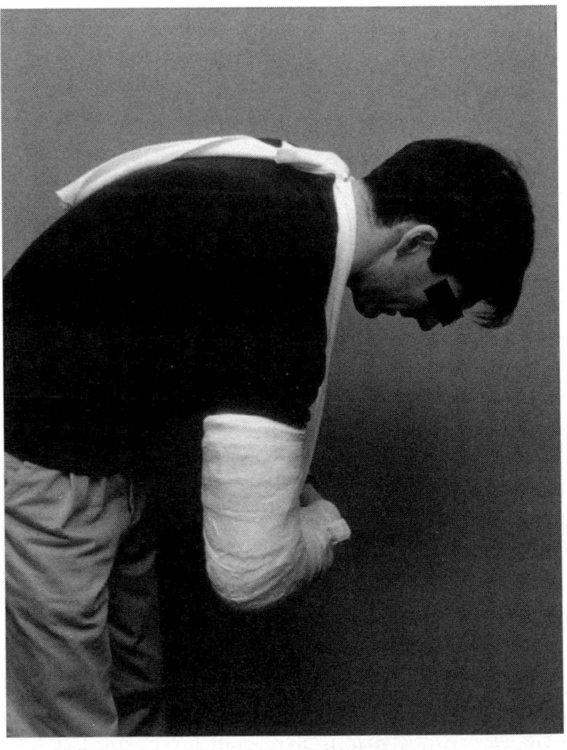

FIGURE 15-18. Circumduction shoulder exercises are important to prevent adhesive capsulitis.

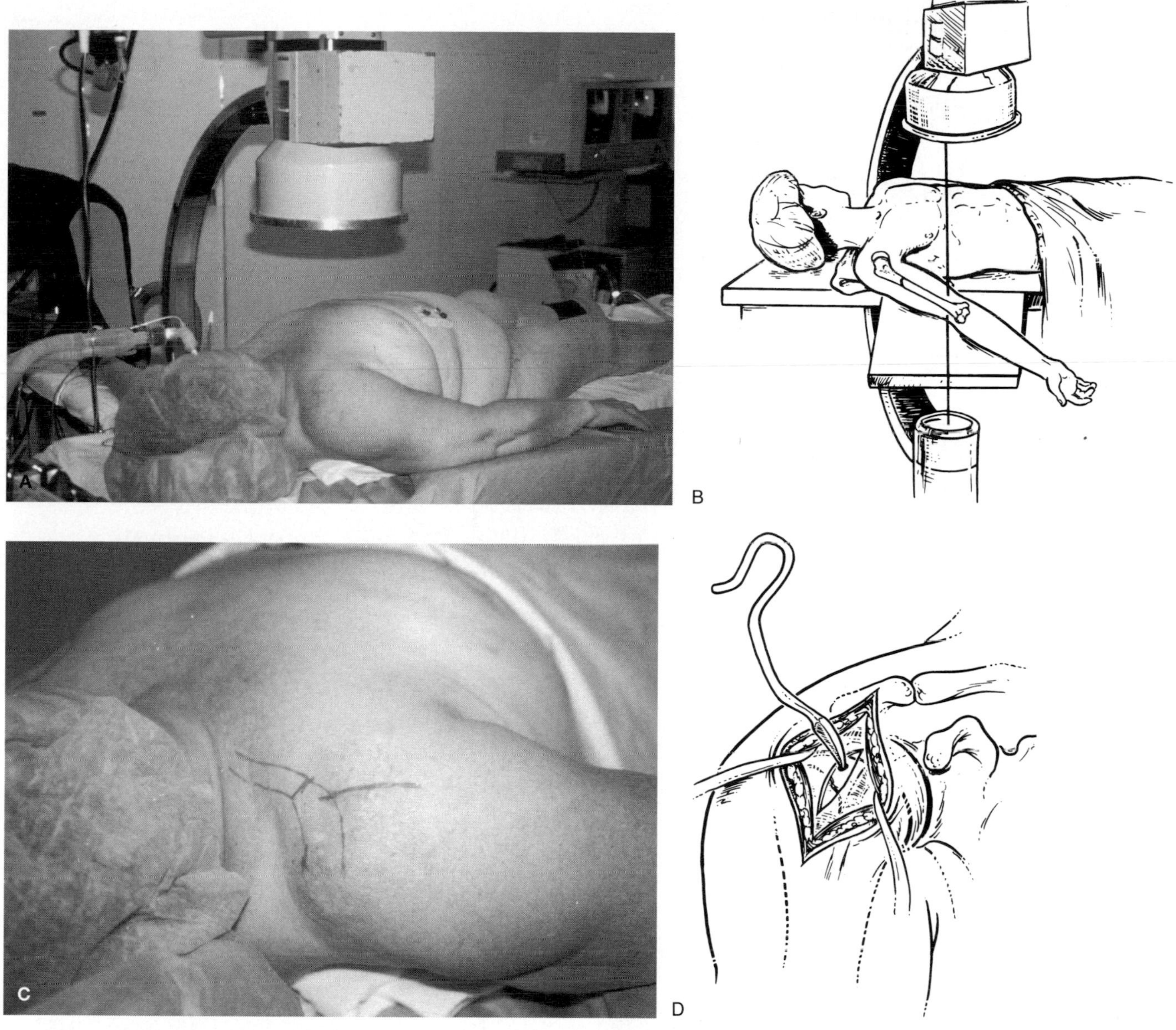

FIGURE 15-19. (**A** and **B**) For intramedullary nailing of the humerus, the patient is positioned supine on a radiolucent operating room table. A sandbag is placed between the shoulder blades, and the patient's head is turned toward the contralateral side to maximize exposure of the proximal humerus. (**C**) A 3- to 4-cm incision extends distally from the lateral acromium along the direction of the deltoid fibers. (**D**) The deltoid muscle is incised in line with its fibers; the deltoid should not be incised farther than 4 to 5 cm to avoid injuring the axillary nerve. The rotator cuff is identified, and an awl is used to enter the intramedullary canal medial to the tip of the greater tuberosity in line with the anatomical axis of the humerus.

continues

ported 136 humeral shaft fractures treated with a hanging arm cast; 103 were available for follow-up. There was one delayed union and one nonunion. Stewart and Hundley[98] reported 107 humeral shaft fractures also treated with a hanging cast: 93.5% of patients experienced an excellent or good result. The Pennsylvania Orthopaedic Society[95] reported a series of 159 fractures of the humeral shaft; 86 patients (54%) were treated with a hanging cast, and 96% of these patients achieved fracture union at an average of 10 weeks after injury.

Hunter[53] reported 60 humeral shaft fractures treated with a coaptation splint. The arm was suspended by a collar and cuff after application of the splint. Treatment success was based on fracture union, residual deformity, and limb function. Fifty-six fractures (93%) united; all had less than 30° angulation. The average time to union was 43 days for males and 45 days for

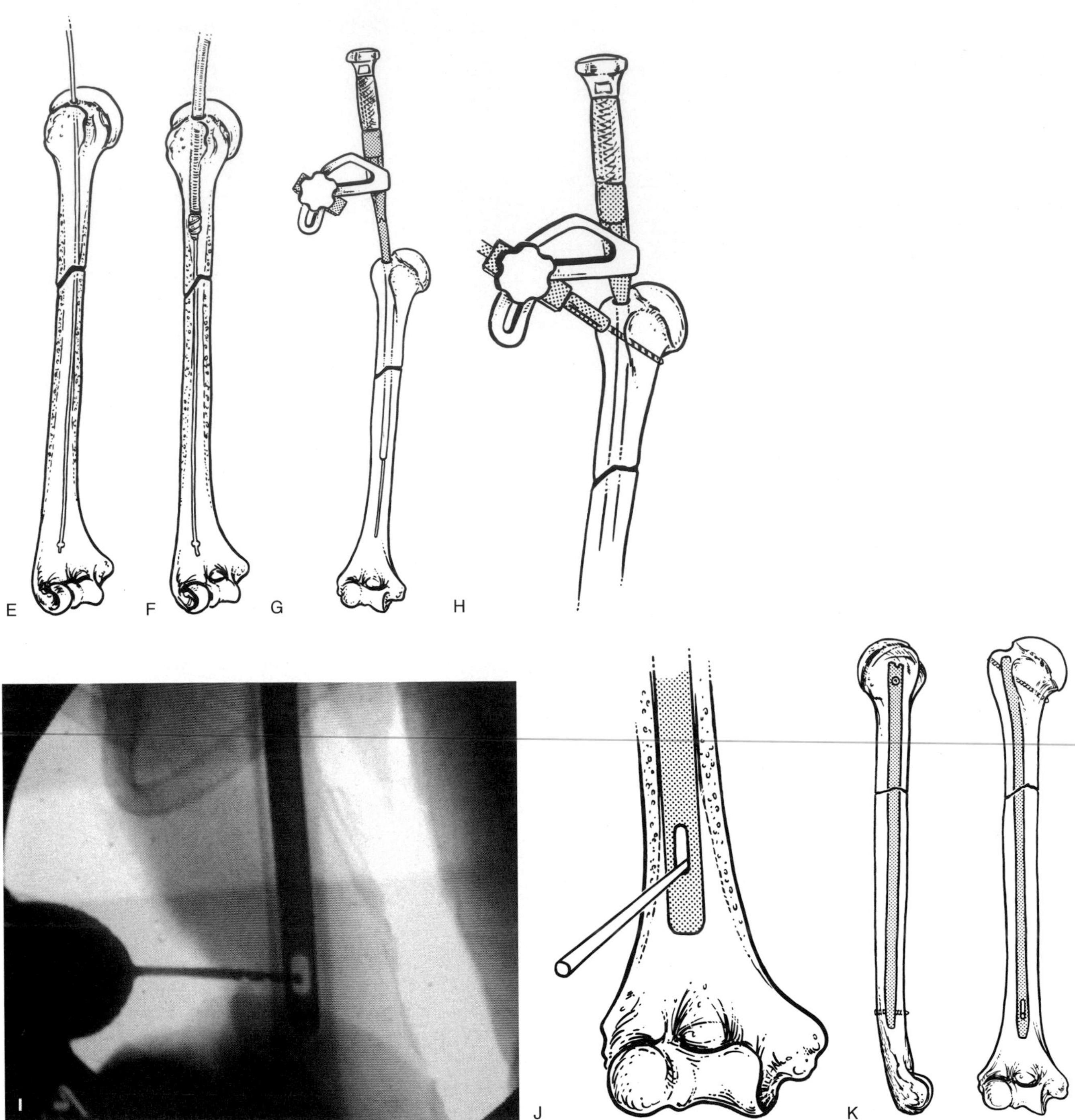

FIGURE 15-19. (*continued*) (**E**) A guide wire is inserted into the proximal humerus, the fracture reduced, and the guide wire passed to the distal humeral metaphysis. (**F**) Reaming of the medullary canal may be necessary before nail insertion. (**G**) Following guide wire exchange, the nail is hand inserted down the intramedullary canal and seated below the rotator cuff. (**H**) Proximal locking is performed using a targeting device. The safest locking screw configuration is from superolateral to inferomedial. (**I** and **J**) Distal locking is performed using a free-hand technique. (**K**) Anteroposterior and lateral diagrams of the humerus after nail insertion.

females. There was no correlation between healing and patient sex, fracture level, or need for fracture manipulation. With one exception, all patients younger than age 35 recovered full extremity function by 10 weeks. In older patients, functional return was slower and less complete. The authors concluded that a coaptation splint could be used effectively to treat patients with humeral shaft fractures.

Sarmiento[92] reported a series of 51 humeral shaft fractures treated with a plastic sleeve, either custom-molded or prefabricated. There were 9 proximal third, 26 middle third, and 16 distal third fractures of the humerus. Initial fracture stabilization involved use of either a hanging cast, sugar tong splint, Velpeau bandage, or skeletal traction. The functional brace was applied after acute pain and swelling had subsided. At first, the fracture sleeves were molded individually. However, as experience increased, a prefabricated polypropylene sleeve was used. Patients were encouraged to perform active and passive motion exercises of all joints of the fractured extremity. The brace was worn until there was clinical and radiographic evidence of fracture union; brace use averaged 8.5 weeks. One nonunion occurred in a patient with metastatic breast disease. Forty-two patients (82%) had full shoulder motion at brace removal. Eight patients (16%) had 10° to 20° angular deformity.

Zagorski and colleagues[107] reported a series of 233 patients who had a humeral shaft fracture treated with a prefabricated functional brace. There were 170 patients available for follow-up at an average of 28 weeks. Forty-three fractures were open, 35 of which were secondary to gunshot wounds. One hundred sixty-seven fractures (98%) united. The average time to union was 9.5 weeks for closed fractures and 13.6 weeks for open fractures. At follow-up, varus-valgus angulation averaged 5°, anteroposterior angulation averaged 3°, and shortening averaged 4 mm. One hundred fifty-eight patients (95%) had an excellent functional result with an essentially full range of motion of the shoulder and elbow.

Balfour and coworkers[6] reported 42 patients with a humeral shaft fracture treated with a functional brace. Forty-one fractures (97%) united. The time to union averaged 54 days. Varus deformity averaged 9°. Deformity in the anteroposterior plane averaged 6.2°. Thirty-eight patients (90%) had full motion of the shoulder and elbow 4 months after fracture. Sarmiento and associates[91] reported a series of 85 extra-articular comminuted distal third humeral shaft fractures in adults treated with a prefabricated fracture brace. Fifteen percent were open fractures; 18% had an associated radial nerve injury. The brace was applied an average of 12 days after injury and was worn for approximately 10 weeks. Seventy-two fractures were available for follow-up; 69 fractures (96%) united. There were no infections. All nerve injuries had resolved or were improving at latest examination. At union, 56 patients (81%) had varus deformity that averaged 9°; shortening averaged 5 mm. The most affected shoulder motion was external rotation; 26 patients (45%) lost 5° to 45°. The authors concluded that use of a functional brace gives satisfactory results for most comminuted, extra-articular distal-third fractures of the humerus.

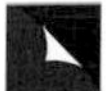

Operative Treatment

Plates and Screws

Bell and associates[8] reported 39 humeral shaft fractures in patients with multiple injuries stabilized using plates and screws. The average age was 31.5 years; 14 fractures were open fractures and 20 had significant comminution. Twenty-three fractures were stabilized within 24 hours of admission. Seven underwent primary bone grafting, and five had delayed bone grafting. Thirty-three of 34 fractures (97%) available for follow-up united; the time to union averaged 19 weeks. Thirty-three patients (97%) had a fully functional shoulder. No patient with an isolated humeral shaft fracture lost elbow motion. Complications included one nonunion, one fixation failure, and one infection. Dabezies and coworkers[29] reported 44 humeral shaft fractures stabilized using plates and screws. Patient age averaged 31 years. There were 11 open fractures and 15 with an associated radial nerve injury. Cancellous bone graft was used when significant comminution was present. Follow-up was available in all patients and averaged 50 months. Forty-three fractures (97%) united at an average of 12 weeks. One plate had loss of fixation and required revision with a longer plate and bone grafting, leading to subsequent union. At follow-up, range of motion of the shoulder and elbow was essentially normal. All 12 anatomically intact radial nerve palsies recovered in an average of 17 weeks after plate fixation. One lacerated radial nerve was repaired with full recovery. One nerve with segmental loss associated with an open fracture was not repaired, as was an avulsed radial nerve associated with a closed fracture. The authors concluded that plate fixation of humeral shaft fractures results in an excellent rate of osseous union. In addition, the dissection required for plate fixation provides information that may be used to determine appropriate treatment of an associated radial nerve injury and the prognosis for spontaneous recovery.

Heim and associates[47] reported 127 patients with humeral shaft fractures also stabilized using plates and screws. Patient age averaged 51 years. Nineteen patients had an associated radial nerve palsy; an additional four patients developed palsies after fracture manipulation. Nine fractures were open fractures; eighty-six were isolated injuries. Of the 127 patients, 102 were available for follow-up 1 year after fracture. Eighty-nine patients (87%) had full functional recovery of their upper extremity. Two patients had a transient postoperative radial nerve palsy, four developed a postoperative infection, five had early fixation failure, and two developed a nonunion.

Intramedullary Devices

Stern and colleagues[96] reported 70 humeral shaft fractures stabilized with several types of nonlocked intramedullary devices between 1970 and 1981. Complications developed in 47 (67%) of the fractures; 45 (64%) required at least one additional operative procedure. Of the 60 fractures that were surgically treated within 6 weeks of injury, nine (15%) developed a delayed union and five (8.3%) did not unite. Three of 10 fractures (10%) that had surgery more than 6 weeks after injury never united despite additional procedures. Delayed union and nonunion were more common in open fractures (33%) than in closed fractures (21%) and after an open nailing (39%) compared with closed or semi-open nailing (9%). Adhesive capsulitis of the shoulder developed in 56% of patients stabilized using an antegrade technique. However, elbow motion was not restricted in patients who were stabilized using a retrograde technique.

Hall and Pankovich[45] reported a prospective series of 89 humeral shaft fractures stabilized with Ender nails. Patient age averaged 36 years; 71 of the fractures were isolated. The operative time averaged 76 minutes. Fractures of the middle and proximal third of the humeral shaft had retrograde nail insertion from a distal portal. Fractures of the distal third had antegrade nail insertion from a proximal portal. Postoperative immobilization was not needed in any of the fractures. Eighty-six fractures were available for follow-up at an average of 21 months after injury. Eighty-five of 86 fractures (99%) united at an average of 7.2 weeks. There were no infections or malunions. Six of nine preoperative and both postoperative radial nerve palsies recovered spontaneously. All three preoperative radial nerves that did not recover had been disrupted by the original penetrating trauma and needed further attention. Nail back-out was reported in eight patients, five of whom required revision. Loss of elbow extension averaged 4°; elbow flexion averaged 132°. Average shoulder range of motion was 91° abduction, 54% external rotation, and 68° internal rotation. The authors concluded that closed intramedullary Ender nailing could be performed safely and effectively in selected fractures of the humeral shaft.

Brumback and colleagues[14] reported 63 humeral shaft fractures in patients with multiple trauma stabilized with either Rush rods or Ender nails. Both antegrade and retrograde entry portals were used as well as insertion through the distal humeral epicondyles. Most patients underwent closed intramedullary nailing within 24 hours of injury. Follow-up was available for 58 fractures and averaged 25 months. Fifty-five fractures (94%) united at an average of 10.5 weeks after surgery. Thirty-six patients (62%) had an excellent clinical result. Antegrade nailing gave excellent results if the entry portal did not violate the rotator cuff. Symptoms of subacromial impingement required early hardware removal in seven patients. All fractures that had retrograde nail insertion through the epicondyles had a poor result. However, retrograde insertion, with the portal of entry located proximal to the olecranon fossa, yielded excellent results.

Henley and associates[48] reported 48 consecutive humeral shaft fractures treated with stacked Hackethal intramedullary nails; patient age averaged 40 years. Four fractures were open; eight had an associated radial nerve injury. All fractures were reduced closed with the retrograde nail inserted through a posterior cortical window proximal to the olecranon fossa. Follow-up was available in 33 patients at an average of 4 years after surgery. Thirty-two fractures (97%) had united within 1 year; the average time to union was 7.5 weeks. No angular malunions greater than 10° in either the coronal or sagittal planes were identified. There were no iatrogenic nerve palsies. Loss of elbow extension averaged 5°; elbow flexion averaged 145°. There was one delayed union, one nonunion, one deep infection, and three occurrences of heterotopic ossification at the entry portal. One patient had proximal nail penetration through the humeral head, and two patients had distal nail migration that required removal.

Habernek and Orthner[44] reported 19 humeral shaft fractures stabilized with the Seidel interlocking nail. All nails were inserted using an antegrade technique after prior reaming. Eighteen of 19 nails were inserted in a static mode. The one fracture stabilized with a dynamically locked nail required secondary static locking a few days after surgery because of nail migration. There were no infections or iatrogenic radial nerve injuries. All 19 fractures united at an average of 2 months after surgery. Four fractures united with varus angulation up to 10° and three with recurvatum up to 5°. Eighteen of 19 patients regained full shoulder motion by 6 weeks. Return to work varied from 4 to 10 weeks. The authors recommended that proximal locking of the nail should always be performed to avoid proximal nail migration. They cautioned against use of the Seidel nail for distal humeral shaft fractures.

Jensen and associates[56] reported a series of 16 humeral shaft fractures also stabilized using the Seidel interlocking nail. The average patient age was 68 years.

All nail stabilizations were performed using an antegrade technique. Reaming was performed in 10 patients; the width of the medullary canal in six patients was considered sufficient to accommodate a 9-mm nail without reaming. Closed nailing could be performed in 12 patients. Thirteen of 14 patients (92%) available for follow-up had united fractures after an average of 6 weeks. Two patients with pathologic fractures died before radiologic union. One fracture in a patient with an atrophic pseudarthrosis did not unite. There were four patients with shoulder pain secondary to nail prominence.

Crolla and colleagues[28] reported a series of 46 Seidel interlocked humeral nailings in patients with an average age of 46 years. There were 30 acute fractures, seven pathologic fractures, and nine nonunions. All nails were inserted in an antegrade manner. All acute fractures united 6 to 12 weeks after surgery. Of the 27 patients with functional follow-up information, there were 18 excellent results, three satisfactory, two unsatisfactory, and four with a poor result based on the Neer rating scale. Six of nine nonunions united by 6 months. All seven patients with a pathologic fracture died within 8 months of surgery; however, all had been pain free before death. The authors concluded that the Seidel locked intramedullary humeral nail is an effective addition to the current methods available for the operative treatment of humeral shaft fractures.

Russell and associates[90] reported a prospective series of 51 consecutive interlocked humeral nailings performed with a closed section (Russell-Taylor) intramedullary nail. Forty-one patients with at least 6-month follow-up were available for evaluation. Union was achieved in all acute fractures and eight of ten nonunions; all pathologic fractures united or were asymptomatic. Complications included three transient brachial plexus neurapraxias, two infections, three cases of nail impingement, and two intraoperative fractures.

Ingman and Waters[55] reported 41 humeral shaft fractures stabilized using a modified 9-mm Grosse-Kempf reamed interlocking tibial nail. The average patient age was 53 years. There were 21 acute fractures, five nonunions, and 15 pathologic fractures. Four fractures were open, and six had an associated radial nerve injury. However, radial nerve exploration was not performed. Thirty-nine of 41 nails had static interlocking. The first 11 nails were inserted antegrade through the rotator cuff; the remainder were inserted retrograde through a portal proximal to the olecranon fossa. Twenty-nine nailings were performed using a closed technique. Twenty of 21 acute fractures (95%) united; 18 united within 3 months and two within 6 months. The remaining fracture united after bone grafting. Four of five nonunions (80%) united within 6 months of surgery. All seven pathologic fractures available for 3-month follow-up had united. The remaining eight patients with pathologic fractures died by 3-month follow-up. At 6-week follow-up, all patients who underwent antegrade insertion had significant restriction of active shoulder elevation. Twenty-nine of 30 patients (97%) who underwent retrograde insertion had less than 30° loss of elbow extension at 6 weeks. Seven of eight radial nerve palsies recovered; the remaining nerve deficit occurred in a patient with a pathologic fracture who died soon after surgery. The authors concluded that (1) closed, locked intramedullary humeral nailing can reliably provide secure fixation and acceptable clinical results; (2) locked intramedullary humeral nailing is the method of choice for internal fixation of osteoporotic and pathologic fractures; (3) the nail should be inserted retrograde from the olecranon fossa for middle and lower third humeral shaft fractures, and proximal fractures require antegrade insertion; and (4) a modified 9-mm tibial nail is suitable for fixation of virtually all humeral shaft fractures.

COMPLICATIONS

Radial Nerve Injury

Up to 18% of humeral shaft fractures have an associated radial nerve injury.[79,80] Although the Holstein-Lewis fracture (oblique, distal third) is best known for its association with neurologic injury (Fig. 15-20),[52] radial nerve palsy is most commonly associated with middle-third humeral shaft fractures.[59] Most nerve injuries represent a neurapraxia or axonotmesis; 90% will resolve in 3 to 4 months.[37,59] Electromyography and nerve conduction studies can aid in determining the degree of nerve injury and monitor the rate of nerve regeneration. Indications for early nerve exploration are radial nerve palsies associated with an open fracture or penetrating injury and possibly one that develops after fracture manipulation.

Management of radial nerve palsy associated with a humeral shaft fracture remains controversial. Postacchini and Morace[81] reported 42 cases treated with either observation or early or late surgical exploration. Of the 14 cases treated nonoperatively, 12 (86%) recovered fully. All 18 cases treated with early nerve exploration (within 30 days of injury) recovered; however, only six (33%) were found to have a lesion that clearly benefitted from surgical exploration (nerve trapped in fracture callus, nerve laceration). In comparison, all 10 late explorations (greater than 4 months after injury) had a lesion that required surgical intervention; however, functional recovery was noted in only 50%. The authors concluded that the decision whether to perform an early or late

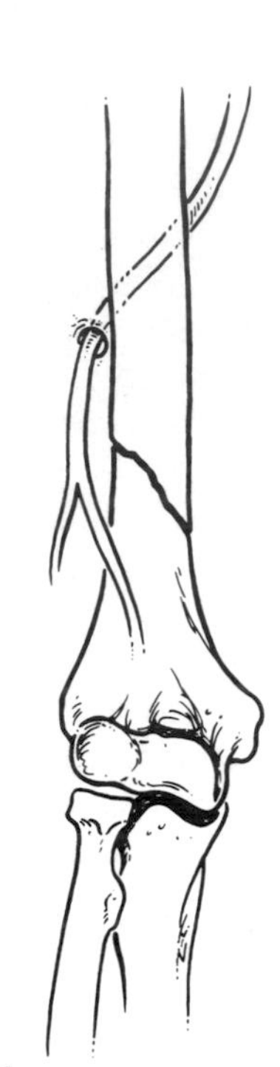

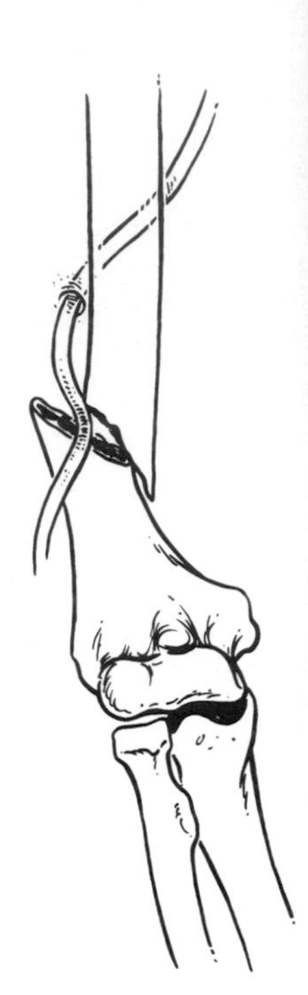

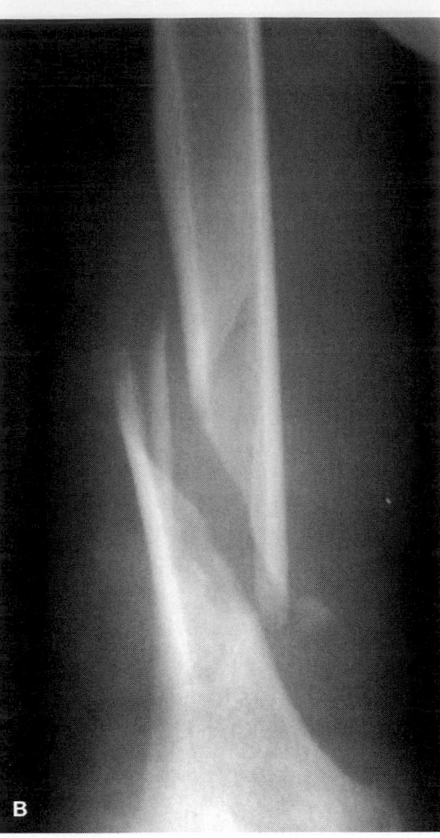

FIGURE 15-20. Diagram (**A**) and radiograph (**B**) of a typical Holstein-Lewis fracture.

nerve exploration should be based on four criteria: (1) the fracture level, (2) the degree of fracture displacement, (3) the nature of the soft-tissue injury (open fracture), and (4) the degree of neurologic deficit.

Other authors recommend surgical exploration 3 or 4 months after injury if there is no evidence of neurologic recovery. Advantages of late versus early nerve exploration include (1) enough time would have passed for recovery from neurapraxia or axonotmesis; (2) precise evaluation of the nerve lesion is possible; (3) the associated fracture will have united; and (4) the results of secondary repair are as good as primary repair. Pollock and coworkers[80] reported 24 humeral fractures associated with varying degrees of radial nerve deficit. Initial treatment was closed in all but one patient in whom debridement of an open fracture revealed a lacerated radial nerve. All 24 patients had complete return of radial nerve function. Only two patients required radial nerve exploration, one at 14 weeks for nerve entrapment in fracture callus and the other at 6 weeks for repair of the lacerated radial nerve. Pollack and coworkers suggested that lack of neurologic improvement at $3^1/_2$ to 4 months after injury was an indication for nerve exploration.

Amillo and associates[4] reported 12 patients who underwent surgical exploration of radial nerve injuries after humeral shaft fracture. Patient follow-up averaged 6 years; the mean time to full recovery was 19 months. The mean interval between the fracture and surgical exploration of the associated nerve injury was 6 months. Perineural fibrosis was observed in 4 patients, and three nerves were found to be trapped in callus. Partial lacerations were identified in two cases and complete lacerations in three cases. The techniques employed for nerve repair or reconstruction were microsurgical reconstruction with interfascicular grafting using sural nerve (six cases), neurolysis (five cases), and tendon transfers (one case). Good to excellent results were obtained in 11 patients (91%). The authors recommended nerve exploration if there are no clinical or electrophysiologic signs of nerve recovery after 3 months.

Foster and colleagues[36] reported 14 patients with an associated radial nerve palsy after open humeral shaft fracture. The average patient age was 29 years. In 9 of the patients (64%) the radial nerve was either lacerated or interposed between the fracture fragments. There was an equal incidence of radial nerve laceration versus entrapment regardless of the degree of soft-tissue injury (grade I, II, or III). Epineural radial nerve repair, performed primarily or secondarily, provided satisfactory return of radial nerve function at a minimum of 1-year follow-up. The authors concluded that radial nerve palsy in association with an open humerus fracture should have a nerve exploration at the time of initial fracture surgery.

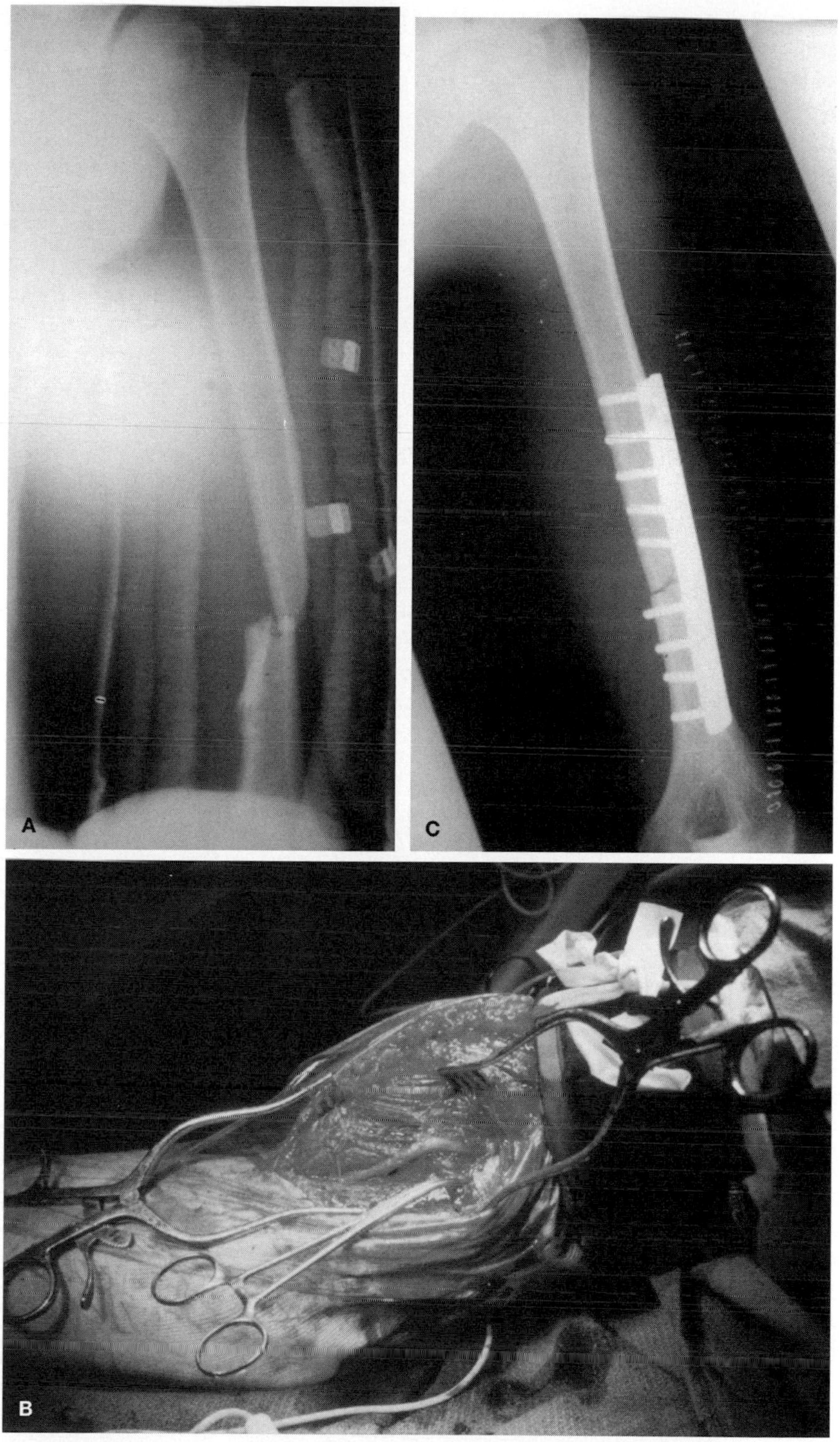

FIGURE 15-21. (**A**) Humeral shaft fracture that developed a radial nerve palsy after fracture manipulation. (**B**) An early radial nerve exploration was performed and the nerve found to be intact. (**C**) Postoperative radiograph after humeral plating.

Authors' Preferred Management With Radial Nerve Injury

We recommend early exploration for radial nerve palsies associated with an open fracture, penetrating injury, or one that develops after fracture manipulation (Fig. 15-21). Radial nerve palsies that occur at the time of closed humerus fracture should be observed; radial nerve exploration is performed at 3 $^1/_2$ to 4 months after injury if there is lack of neurologic improvement.

Vascular Injury

Although uncommon, injury or laceration of the brachial artery can be associated with fractures of the humeral shaft. Mechanisms of brachial artery injury include a gunshot wound, a stab wound, vessel entrapment between the fracture fragments, and occlusion secondary to hematoma or swelling in a tight fascial compartment. The brachial artery is at the greatest risk for injury in the proximal and distal thirds of the arm. The role of arteriography in evaluation of long-bone fractures with associated vascular compromise remains controversial. Some authors support use of the arteriogram as a diagnostic tool. However, the diagnosis of arterial injury can be clinically established in at least 50% of cases, particularly when associated with an open fracture. The major disadvantage in obtaining a formal preoperative arteriogram is the time delay before initiating definitive treatment. Unnecessary delays for studies of equivocal value are imprudent in the management of an ischemic limb. Arterial flow should be emergently reestablished in cases approaching an ischemic time of 6 hours.

Fractures complicated by vascular injury constitute an orthopaedic emergency. Primary control of the hemorrhage can usually be accomplished by direct pressure while the patient is prepared for surgery. At surgery, the vessel should be explored and repaired and the fracture stabilized. If limb viability is not in jeopardy, bony stabilization can be performed before vascular repair. If there is significant ischemic time without distal limb perfusion, the vascular surgeon should place a temporary intraluminal vascular shunt before the fracture is stabilized.[57] Stabilization of the fracture is mandatory to protect the vascular repair and minimize additional soft-tissue injury. The technique for definitive arterial repair is determined by the type and location of the vascular injury. Clean lacerations involving short segments of arterial wall can often be managed by direct repair. Jagged injuries and gunshot wounds may require excision of segments of artery followed by an end-to-end anastomosis or vein graft.[27,72]

Nonunion

The literature suggests that 4 months is a reasonable period of time for humeral shaft fractures to unite.[35,97,109] A nonunion is present when healing is no longer evident. The nonunion rate following

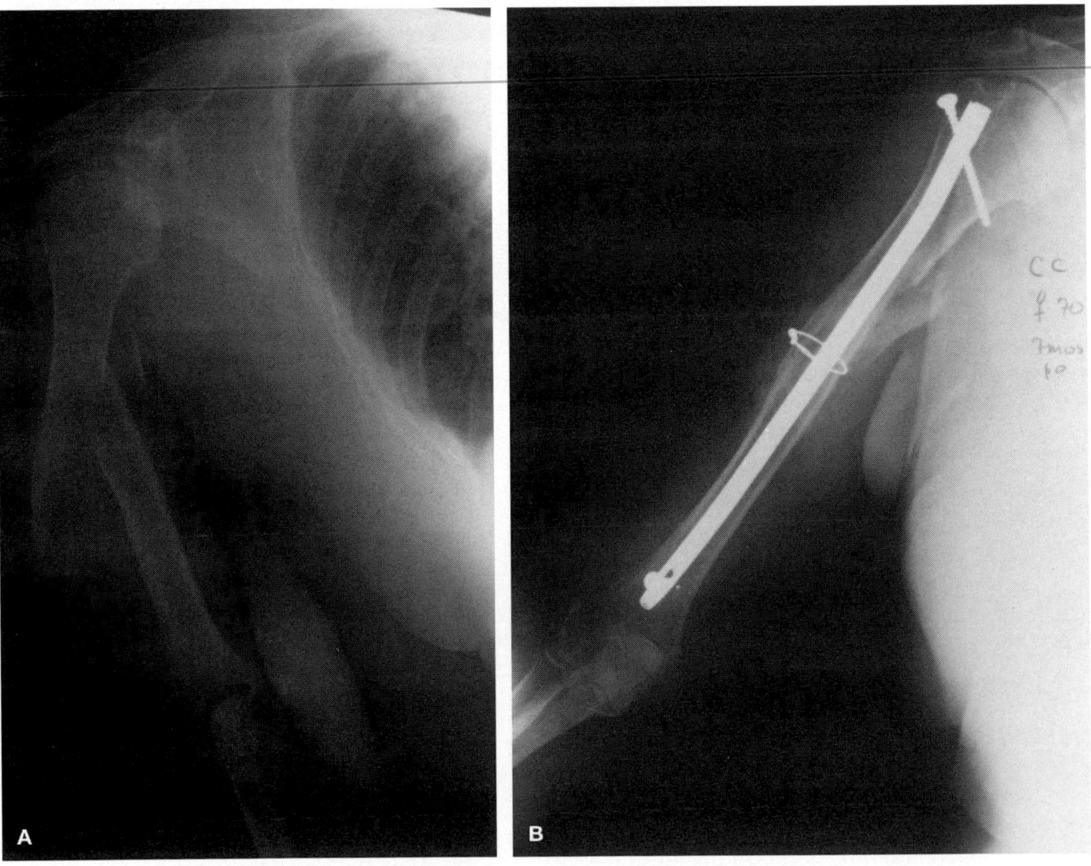

FIGURE 15-22. (**A**) Preoperative radiograph of a midshaft humeral nonunion with deformity. (**B**) Seven-month postoperative radiograph demonstrating union after placement of a reamed humeral interlocked nail and cerclage wire.

humeral shaft fracture ranges from 0 to 15%.[13] The proximal and distal thirds of the humerus are at increased risk of nonunion. Other factors associated with nonunion include a transverse fracture pattern, fracture distraction, soft-tissue interposition, and inadequate immobilization.[12,71,75,99] Limitation of shoulder motion also increases the risk of humeral nonunion. With loss of normal shoulder motion, increased stresses are transmitted to the fracture site. Medical factors that may predispose to nonunion include older age, poor nutritional status, obesity, diabetes mellitus, use of corticosteroids, anticoagulation, previous radiation, and fractures underlying a burn. Interestingly, higher rates of nonunion have been reported after operative treatment than nonoperative management.[46]

Evaluation of the patient with a humeral nonunion should include a thorough history and physical examination. Details of the initial injury and prior treatment are important. The physical examination should include the shoulder and elbow to identify significant restriction of motion. Flexion/extension lateral views of the humerus can be used to assess motion at the nonunion site. Nuclear medicine studies (bone, gallium, and indium scans) can be helpful in determining the biological capability of the nonunion, as well as evidence of infection.

Based on standard radiographs and bone scans, nonunions can be classified as either vascular or hypovascular.[102] Vascular nonunions are capable of biological reaction and have abundant callus, but have insufficient stability to unite. Hypovascular (avascular) nonunions are incapable of biological reaction and require, in addition to bony stability, some type of bone graft to stimulate a vascular response. When a pseudarthrosis is present, a false joint with synovial lining develops at the nonunion site. Each one of the nonunion types can be complicated by the presence of infection.

The treatment objectives for patients with a humeral shaft nonunion are to establish fracture union, limb alignment, and function and, when necessary, to eliminate infection. Treatment options include functional bracing, electrical stimulation, bone grafting, and internal or external fixation. Functional bracing may have a role in the treatment of delayed unions but will not be helpful in established nonunions. Electrical stimulation can be beneficial in combination with a functional brace. Contraindications to use of electrical stimulation are the presence of a gap greater than 1 cm, synovial pseudarthrosis, and infection. Compression plating with bone grafting and reamed intramedullary nailing are probably the most effective methods for the treatment of established nonunions (Fig. 15-22).[35] With use of either device, the basic principles of nonunion treatment must be followed: (1) obtain osseous stability, (2) eliminate nonunion gap, (3) maintain or restore osseous vascularity, and (4) eradicate infection.

Two series have reported effective treatment of humeral shaft nonunions using compression plating combined with cancellous bone grafting.[7,88] Barquet and coworkers[7] reported successful union in 24 of 25 (96%) aseptic humeral shaft nonunions. Rosen[88] reported a 97% healing rate after one surgical procedure in 32 humeral nonunions treated with plates and screws. Wu and Shih[106] reported 35 humeral shaft nonunions treated with either plates and screws (19 patients) or an antegrade-inserted interlocked nail (16 patients). Follow-up ranged from 12 to 52 months. Plate fixation resulted in a 89.5% union rate within 4.5 ± 1.7 months; antegrade nailing resulted in an 87.5% union rate within 4.4 ± 1.8 months. Patients who had plate fixation sustained more complications than those managed by interlocked nailing (21% vs 12%). The authors concluded that interlocked nailing is comparable to plating for the treatment of humeral shaft nonunions but may be associated with fewer complications.

Jupiter[58] reported four patients with complex nonunions of the humeral diaphysis treated with a medial approach, an anterior plate, and vascularized fibular graft. Patient age averaged 40 years and patient weight averaged 232 pounds. Each patient had one to five unsuccessful previous operations in an attempt to achieve union. At an average follow-up of 27 months, all four nonunions had united. Three patients regained full function of the shoulder and elbow. In one patient, a second plate was applied secondary to inadequate fixation of the original plate proximally.

Authors' Preferred Method of Treating Nonunion of Humeral Shaft

Our approach to humeral nonunions is based on the following principles: mobilization of the adjacent joint, realignment of the mechanical axis, debridement of infected tissue, pseudarthrosis stabilization, bone grafting of avascular fragments, and early range of motion (Fig. 15-23). Aseptic humeral nonunions that are in adequate alignment are stabilized with a reamed interlocked nail inserted without opening the nonunion site. Aseptic nonunions that require nonunion exposure to mobilize and reduce the proximal and distal fragments are stabilized with either a reamed interlocked nail or compression plate, depending on nonunion level, type of prior implant, and degree of osteopenia. Reamed interlocked nails are used for

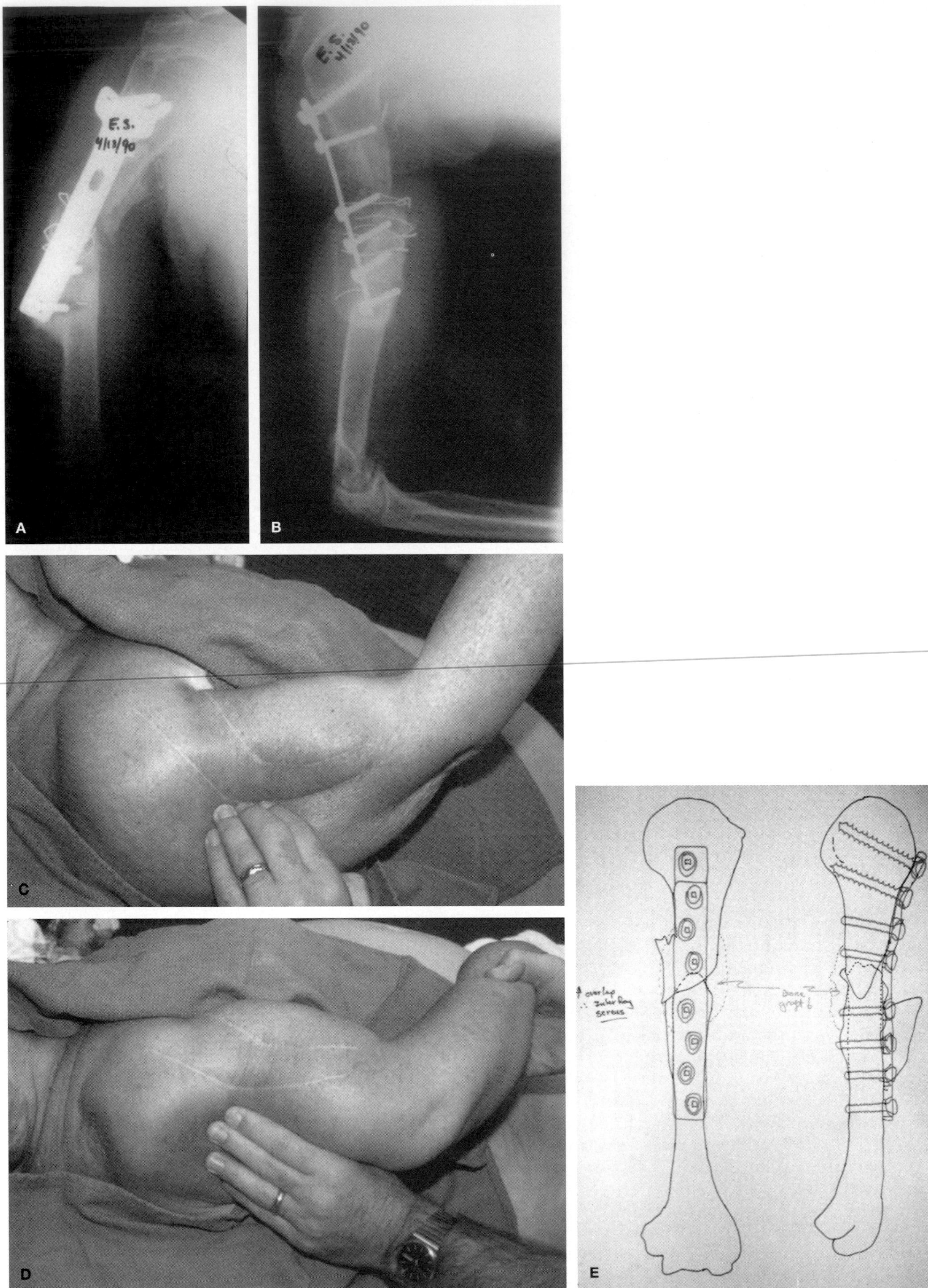

FIGURE 15-23.

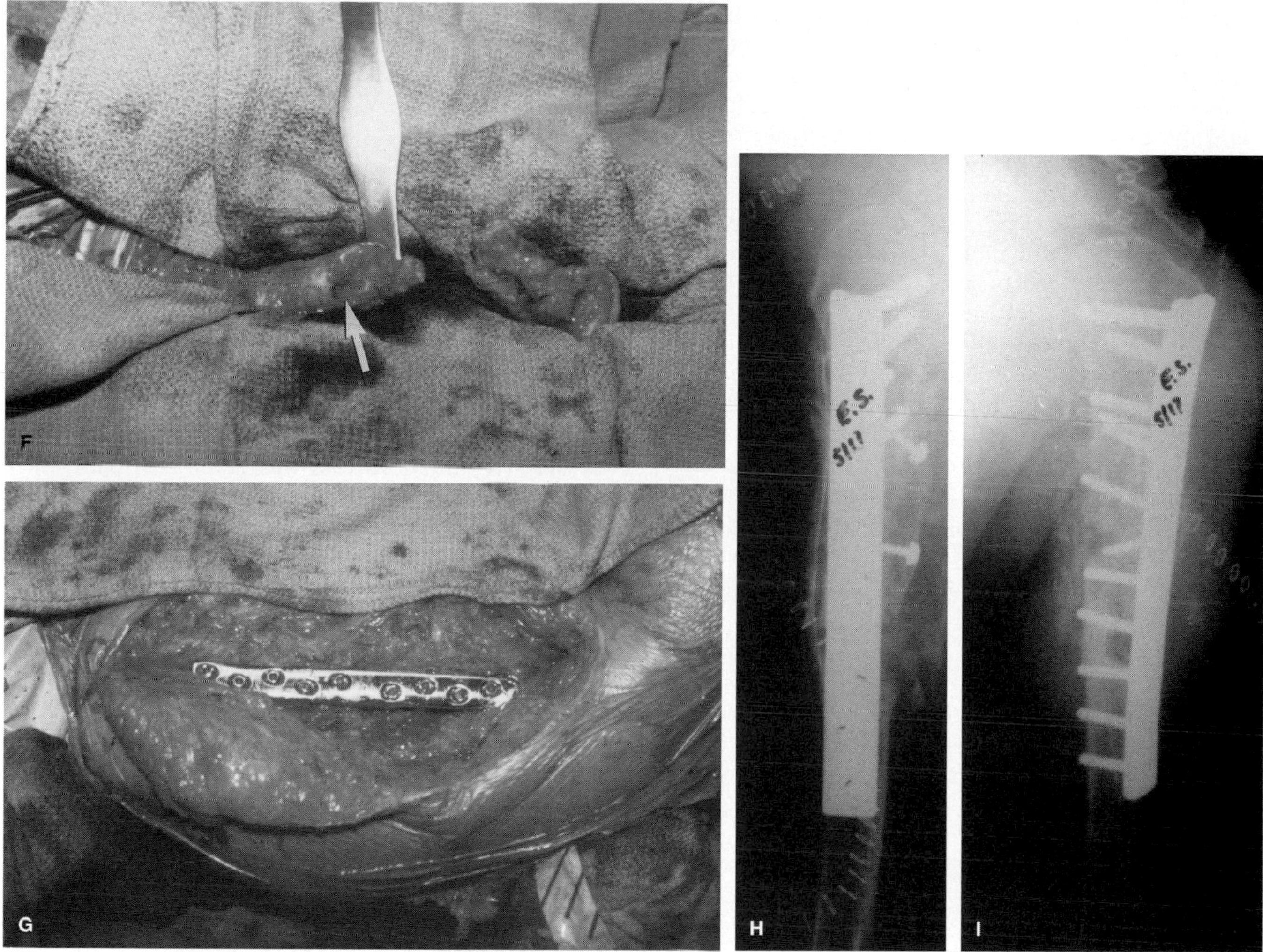

FIGURE 15-23. (**A** and **B**) Preoperative radiographs of a humeral shaft nonunion with failure of internal fixation. (**C** and **D**) Clinical photographs demonstrating gross motion at the nonunion. Note the multiple prior surgical incisions. (**E**) The preoperative plan. (**F**) Intraoperative photograph demonstrating exposure of the proximal and distal fragments and opening of the medullary canals (*arrow*). (**G**) Intraoperative photograph after placement of a 4.5-mm broad dynamic compression plate. (**H** and **I**) Postoperative radiographs after internal fixation and bone grafting. (*Courtesy of Roy Sanders, Florida Orthapaedic Institute, Tampa, FL.*)

nonunions located in the midshaft of the humerus while plates are chosen for those located in the proximal and distal regions. We also favor use of interlocked nails if the humerus is osteopenic or compromised from prior implants. Regardless of implant choice, one should open the medullary canal of both the proximal and distal fragments. The need for bone grafting is based on the vascularity of the nonunion; atrophic nonunions and those with bone loss require bone grafting. Infected nonunions without drainage for 3 months are debrided of all necrotic/infected tissue and then treated as atrophic nonunions with compression plating and bone graft. Infected nonunions with drainage are debrided and stabilized with an external fixator. Repeat debridements are performed until all necrotic/infected tissue has been excised. The patient may be treated to completion in the external fixator or later have exchange of the external fixator for plate and screws. Bone grafting is performed once there is no further evidence of infection.

MANAGEMENT OF SPECIAL PROBLEMS

Open Fracture

Open fractures of the humeral shaft should be managed using the same principles as for any open long-bone fracture.[42,43] A sterile dressing should be placed over the open wound, the arm splinted, and appropriate antibiotic coverage administered along with tetanus prophylaxis. The patient should be taken emergently to the operating room for a formal debridement with extension of the skin wound to completely expose the zone of injury. Debridement begins with the superficial tissue and extends to the deeper soft tissues and eventually to the fracture site. All necrotic and devascularized tissue must be excised and the wound irrigated using pulsatile lavage. Grade I open injuries can be treated as closed fractures after debridement, while fractures with more severe soft-tissue damage should be stabilized to allow better management of soft tissue. Both plates and screws and external fixators have been used successfully in the treatment of open humeral shaft fractures. More recently, there has been interest in the use of interlocked humeral nails; these nails should be inserted without prior reaming. Patients with higher energy soft-tissue and osseous injuries should return to the operating room within 48 hours for a "second-look" debridement. Early soft-tissue coverage is preferable; bone grafting can be performed, if necessary, once the wound is clean, closed, and dry.

Pathologic Fracture

The humeral shaft is a relatively common site for metastatic disease, and pathologic fracture may result. Although prophylactic internal fixation of impending humeral shaft fractures is not routinely recommended, operative stabilization of pathologic fractures is indicated for optimal pain relief, for ease of nursing care, and to maximize patient independence (Fig. 24).[34] Lewallen and associates[69] reported 55 cases of impending or established pathologic humeral shaft fracture; intramedullary Rush pin fixation provided significant pain relief and maintained patient function. Hyder and Wray[54] reported 16 pathologic humeral shaft fractures treated with multiple Ender nails inserted using a retrograde technique without exposing the fracture site. Follow-up in this group of patients was clinical rather than radiographic because a considerable number of patients entered hospice care within a few months and the majority were deceased within 1 year. Treatment success was defined as pain relief with return of upper extremity function. All patients were able to feed themselves after the operation, and all were able to dress themselves once the incision had healed. Although most patients lacked some elbow extension, overall elbow function was not compromised. In those cases in which radiographic follow-up was available, union occurred uneventfully. The authors concluded that closed retrograde Ender nailing is a satisfactory method of stabilizing pathologic fractures of the humerus. In the future, however, the inter-

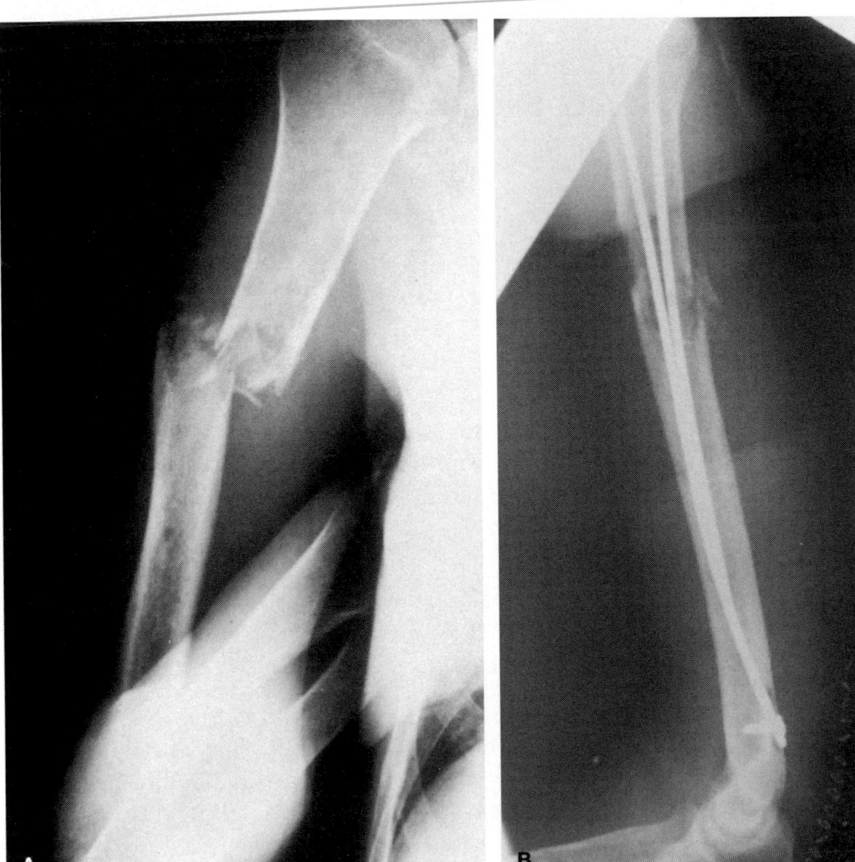

FIGURE 15-24. Pathologic humeral shaft fracture (**A**) stabilized with multiple Ender nails (**B**).

locked humeral nail may become the implant of choice for the treatment of these fractures.

Several authors have advocated the use of adjunctive polymethylmethacrylate in the treatment of pathologic fractures.[63,64] Local use of polymethylmethacrylate increases fixation in situations with a large bony defect from tumor. Schatzker and Ha'Eri[94] reported treatment success in a series of pathologic fractures stabilized with polymethylmethacrylate and compression plating. Vail and Harrelson[100] reported 22 pathologic humeral shaft fractures secondary to myeloma or metastatic disease. Nineteen of 22 fractures were treated with intramedullary stabilization and 12 of the 19 required adjunctive polymethylmethacrylate. Two patients underwent compression plating alone, and the remaining patients were treated nonoperatively. Postoperatively, 78% of the patients reported only mild to moderate pain. Both patients stabilized with plates and screws had failure of fixation. The authors concluded that intramedullary fixation of pathologic fractures with adjunctive polymethylmethacrylate is an excellent option for fixation and pain relief.

We recommend use of intramedullary fixation (either flexible or interlocked nails) for the treatment of pathologic humerus fractures. Interlocked nails should, however, be inserted without prior reaming. Plates are used for proximal and distal pathologic humerus fractures not amenable for intramedullary nailing. With plate and screws, one should be prepared to use adjunctive methylmethacrylate, if needed, for additional fixation.

REFERENCES

1. Aginsky, J., and Reis, N.D.: The Present State of Medullary Nailing of the Femur: Biomechanical Limitations and Problems of Blood Supply to the Fractures Due to Reaming. Injury, 11:109–197, 1980.
2. Allen, W.C., Piotrowski, G., Burstein, A.H., and Frankel, V.H.: Biomechanical Principles of Intramedullary Fixation. Clin. Orthop., 60:13–20, 1968.
3. American College of Surgeons Committee on Trauma: An Outline of the Treatment of Fracture, 8th ed. Philadelphia, W.B. Saunders, 1965.
4. Amillo, S., Barrios, R.H., Martinez-Peric, R., and Losada, J.I.: Surgical Treatment of the Radial Nerve Lesions Associated with Fractures of the Humerus. J. Orthop. Trauma, 7(3):211–215, 1993.
5. Baker, D.M.: Fractures of the Humeral Shaft Associated With Ipsilateral Fracture Dislocation of the Shoulder: Report of a Case. J. Trauma, 11:532–534, 1971.
6. Balfour, G.W., Mooney, V., and Ashby, M.E.: Diaphyseal Fractures of the Humerus Treated with a Ready-Made Fracture Brace. J. Bone Joint Surg., 64A:11–13, 1982.
7. Barquet, A., Fernandez, A., Luvizio, J., et al.: A Combined Therapeutic Protocol for Aseptic Nonunion of the Humeral Shaft: A Report of 25 Cases. J. Trauma, 29:95–98, 1989.
8. Bell, M.J., Beauchamp, C.G., Kellam, J.K., and McMurtry, R.Y.: The Results of Plating Humeral Shaft Fractures in Patients with Multiple Injuries: The Sunnybrook Experience. J. Bone Joint Surg., 67B:293–296, 1985.
9. Benedetti, G.B., and Argnani, F.: Fractures of the Humerus. *In* Maiocchi, A.B., and Aronson, J. (eds.): Operative Principles of Ilizarov, pp. 146-159. Baltimore, Williams & Wilkins, 1991.
10. Bohler, J.: Closed Intramedullary Nailing of the Femur. Clin. Orthop., 60:51–67, 1968.
11. Bone, L.B.: Fractures of the Shaft of the Humerus. *In* Chapman, M.W., and Madison, M. (eds.): Operative Orthopaedics, vol. 1, pp. 221–234. Philadelphia, J.B. Lippincott, 1988.
12. Boyd, H.B.: The Treatment of Difficult and Unusual Non-Unions. J. Bone Joint Surg., 25:535, 1943.
13. Boyd, H.B., Lipinski, S.W., and Wiley, J.H.: Observations on Non-union of the Shafts of the Long Bones, With a Statistical Analysis of 842 Patients. J. Bone Joint Surg., 43A:159, 1962.
14. Brumback, R.J., Bosse, M.J., Commander, Bosse, M.J., Poka, A., and Burgess, A.R.: Intramedullary Stabilization of Humeral Shaft Fractures in Patients with Multiple Trauma. J. Bone Joint Surg., 68A:960–969, 1986.
15. Bucholz, R.W.: Dilemmas and Controversies in Intramedullary Nailing. *In* Browner, B.D., and Edwards, C.C. (eds.): The Science and Practice of Intramedullary Nailing, pp. 85–89. Philadelphia, Lea & Febiger, 1987.
16. Bucholz, R.W., and Brumback, R.J.: Fractures of the Shaft of the Femur. *In* Rockwood, C.A., Jr., Green, D.P., and Bucholz, R.W. (eds.): Fractures in Adults, pp. 1653–1723. Philadelphia, J.B. Lippincott, 1991.
17. Caldwell, J.A.: Treatment of Fractures in the Cincinnati General Hospital. Ann. Surg., 97:161–176, 1933.
18. Caldwell, J.A.: Treatment of Fractures of the Shaft of the Humerus by Hanging Cast. Surg. Gynecol. Obstet., 70:421–425, 1940.
19. Catagni, M.A., Guerreschi, F., Probe, R.A.: Treatment of Humeral Nonunions with the Ilizarov Technique. Bull. Hosp. Joint Dis., 51(1):74–83, 1991.
20. Chapman, M.W.: Closed Intramedullary Bone Grafting and Nailing of Segmental Defects of the Femur. J. Bone Joint Surg., 62A:1004–1012, 1980.
21. Chapman, M.W.: Principles of Intramedullary Nailing. *In* Chapman, M.W. (ed.): Operative Orthopaedics, pp. 151–160. Philadelphia. J.B. Lippincott, 1988.
22. Chapman, M.W.: The Role of Intramedullary Nailing in Fracture Management. *In* Browner, B.D., and Edwards, C.D. (eds.): The Science and Practice of Intramedullary Nailing, pp. 17–23. Philadelphia, Lea & Febiger, 1987.
23. Chapman, N.W., and Mahoney, M.: The Role of Internal Fixation in the Management of Open Fractures. Clin. Orthop., 138:120–131, 1979.
24. Chester, S., Hallfeldt, K., Perren, S., and Schweiberer, L.: The Effects of Reaming and Intramedullary Nailing on Fracture Healing. Clin. Orthop., 212:18–25, 1986.
25. Christensen, S.: Humeral Shaft Fractures: Operative and Conservative Treatment. Acta Chir. Scand., 133:455, 1967.
26. Clawson, D.K., Smith, R.F., and Hansen, S.T.: Closed Intramedullary Nailing of the Femur. J. Bone Joint Surg., 53A:681–692, 1971.
27. Connolly, J.: Management of Fractures Associated with Arterial Injuries. Am. J. Surg., 120:331, 1970.
28. Crolla, M.P.H., de Veries, L.S., and Clevers, G.J.: Locked Intramedullary Nailing of Humeral Fractures. Injury 24:403–406, 1993.
29. Dabezies, E.J., Banta, C.J., II, Murphy, C.P., and d'Ambrosia, R.D.: Plate Fixation of the Humeral Shaft for Acute Fractures, With and Without Radial Nerve Injuries. J. Orthop Trauma, 6(1):10–13, 1992.
30. Danckwardt-Lilliestrom, G.: Reaming of the Medullary Cavity and its Effect on Diaphyseal Bone. Acta Orthop. Scand. (Suppl.), 128, 1969.
31. DeBastiani, G., Aldegheri, R., and Briviol, R: The Treatment of Fractures with a Dynamic Axial Fixator. J. Bone Joint Surg., 66B:53–545, 1984.
32. Epps, C.H., Jr., and Grant, R.E.: Fractures of the Shaft of the Humerus. *In* Rockwood, C.A., Green, D.P., and Bucholz, R.W. (eds.): Fractures in Adults, 3rd ed., pp. 843–869. Philadelphia, J.B. Lippincott, 1991.
33. Fenyo, G.: On Fractures of the Shaft of the Humerus. Acta Chir. Scand., 137:221–226, 1971.
34. Flemming, J.E., and Beals, R.K.: Pathologic Fracture of the Humerus. Clin. Orthop., 203:258–260, 1986.

35. Foster, R.J., Dixon, G.L., Bach, A.W., Appleyard, R.W., and Green, T.M.: Internal Fixation of Fractures and Non-Unions of the Humeral Shaft: Indications and Results in a Multi-Center Study. J. Bone Joint Surg., 67A:857–864, 1985.
36. Foster, R.J., Swiontkowski, M.F., Bach, A.W., and Sack, J.T.: Radial Nerve Palsy Caused by Open Humeral Shaft Fractures. J. Hand Surg. [Am.], 18:121–124, 1993.
37. Garcia, A., Jr., and Maeck, B.H.: Radial Nerve Injuries in Fractures of the Shaft of the Humerus. Am. J. Surg., 99:625-627, 1960.
38. Gilchrist, D.K.: A Stockinette-Velpeau for Immobilization of the Shoulder Girdle. J. Bone Joint Surg., 49A:750–751, 1967.
39. Green, S.A.: Complications of External Skeletal Fixation. *In* Uhthoft, H.K. (ed.): Current Concepts of External Fixation, pp. 43–52. Heidelberg, Springer-Verlag, 1982.
40. Gregersen, H.N.: Fractures of the Humerus From Muscular Violence. Acta Orthop. Scand., 42:506–512, 1971.
41. Griswold, R.A., Goldberg, H., Robertson, J.: Fractures of the Humerus. Arch Surg., 81:86, 1960.
42. Gustilo, R.B., and Anderson, J.T.: Prevention of Infection in the Treatment of 1025 Open Fractures of the Long Bones: Retrospective and Prospective Analysis. J. Bone Joint Surg., 58A:453–458, 1976.
43. Gustilo, R.B., Simpson, L., Nixon, R., and Ruiz, A.: Analysis of 511 Open Fractures. Clin. Orthop., 66:148–154, 1969.
44. Habernek, H., and Orthner, E.: A Locking Nail for Fractures of the Humerus. J. Bone Joint Surg., 73B:651–653, 1991.
45. Hall, R.F., Jr., and Pankovich, A.M.: Ender Nailing of Acute Fractures of the Humerus: A Study of Closed Fixation by Intramedullary Nails Without Reaming. J. Bone Joint Surg., 69A:558–567, 1987.
46. Healey, W., White, G., Mick, C., et al.: Nonunion of the Humeral Shaft. Clin. Orthop. 219:206–213, 1987.
47. Heim, D., Herkert, F., Hess, P., and Regazzoni, P.: Surgical Treatment of Humeral Shaft Fractures—The Basel Experience. J. Trauma, 35:226–232, 1993.
48. Henley, M.B., Chapman, J.R., and Claudi, B.F.: Closed Retrograde Hackethal Nail Stabilization of Humeral Shaft Fractures. J. Orthop. Trauma, 6:18–24, 1992.
49. Hollinshead, W.H.: Anatomy for Surgeons, vol. 3. New York, Hoeber-Harper, 1958.
50. Holm, C.L.: Management of Humeral Shaft Fractures: Fundamentals of Nonoperative Techniques. Clin. Orthop., 71:132–139, 1970.
51. Hoppenfeld, S., and deBoer, P.: The Humerus. *In* Hannon, B.C. (ed.): Surgical Exposures in Orthopaedics: The Anatomic Approach, 2nd ed., pp. 52–65. Philadelphia, J.B. Lippincott, 1984.
52. Holstein, A., and Lewis, G. B.: Fractures of the Humerus with Radial-Nerve Paralysis. J. Bone Joint Surg., 45A:1382–1388, 1963.
53. Hunter, S.G.: The Closed Treatment of Fractures of the Humeral Shaft. Clin. Orthop., 164:192–198, 1982.
54. Hyder, N., and Wray, C.C.: Treatment of Pathological Fractures of the Humerus with Ender Nails. J. R. Coll. Surg. Edinb., 38:370–372, 1993.
55. Ingman, A.M., and Waters, D.A.: Locked Intramedullary Nailing of Humeral Shaft Fractures: Implant Design, Surgical Technique, and Clinical Results. J. Bone Joint Surg., 76B:23–29, 1994.
56. Jensen, C.H., Hansen, D., and Jorgensen, U.: Humeral Shaft Fractures Treated by Interlocking Nailing: A Preliminary Report on 16 Patients. Injury, 23(4):234–236, 1992.
57. Johansen, K., Bandyk, D., Thiele, B., Hansen, S.T.: Temporary Intraluminal Shunts: Resolution of a Management Dilemma in Complex Vascular Injuries. J. Trauma, 22:395–402, 1982.
58. Jupiter, J.B.: Complex Non-Union of the Humeral Diaphysis: Treatment With Medial Approach, an Anterior Plate and a Vascularized Fibular Graft. J. Bone Joint Surg., 72A:701–707, 1990.
59. Kettlekamp, D.B., and Alexander, H.: Clinical Review of Radial Nerve Injury. J. Trauma, 7:424–432, 1967.
60. Kim, D.D., Sadr, B., and Grant, R.E.: Comminuted Bilateral Humeral Fractures Treated with Interlocking Humeral Nails: A Case Report. Contemp. Orthop. 23:607, 1991.
61. Klenerman, L.: Experimental Fractures of the Adult Humerus. Med. Biol. Eng., 7:357–364, 1969.
62. Klenerman, L.: Fractures of the Shaft of the Humerus. J. Bone Joint Surg., 48B:105–111, 1966.
63. Kunec, J.R., and Lewis, R.J.: Closed Intramedullary Rodding of Pathologic Fractures with Supplement Cement. Clin. Orthop., 188:183–186, 1984.
64. Kuntscher, G.: The Kuntscher Method of Intramedullary Fixation. J. Bone Joint Surg., 40A:17–26, 1958.
65. Kyle, R.F., Schaffhausen, J.M., and Bechtold, J.E.: Biomechanical Characteristics on Interlocking Femoral Nails in the Treatment of Complex Femoral Fractures. Clin. Orthop., 267:169–173, 1991.
66. Laing, P: The Arterial Supply of the Adult Humerus. J. Bone Joint Surg., 38A:1105, 1956.
67. Lange, R.H., and Foster, R.J.: Skeletal Management of Shaft Fractures Associated with Forearm Fractures. Clin. Orthop., 195:173–177, 1985.
68. Larson, R.L., Kelly, P.J., Jones, J.M., and Peterson, L.: Suppression of the Periosteal and Nutrient Blood Supply of the Femora of Dogs: A Histologic, Microangiographic and Roentgenologic Study. Clin. Orthop., 21:217, 1961.
69. Lewallen, R.P., Pritchard, D.J., and Sim, F.H.: Treatment of Pathologic Fractures or Impending Fractures of the Humerus with Rush Rods and Methylmethacrylate: Experience With 55 Cases in 54 Patients, 1968–1977. Clin. Orthop., 166:193, 1982.
70. Mast, J., Jakob, R., and Ganz, R.: Planning and Reduction Techniques in Fracture Surgery. New York, Springer-Verlag, 1989.
71. Mast, J.W., Spiegel, P.G., and Harvey, J.P.: Fractures of the Humeral Shaft: A Retrospective Study of 240 Adult Fractures. Clin. Orthop., 112:254–262, 1975.
72. McNamara, J.J., Brief, D.K., Stremple, J.F., and Wright, J.K.: Management of Fractures with Associated Arterial Injury in Combat Casualties. J. Trauma, 13:17–19, 1973.
73. Muller, M.E., Nazarian, S., Koch, P., and Schatzker, J.: The Comprehensive Classification of Fractures of Long Bones. Berlin, Springer-Verlag, 1990.
74. Murti, G.S., and Ring, P.A.: Closed Medullary Nailing of Fractures of the Femoral Shaft Using the AO Method. Injury, 14:318–323, 1983.
75. Naiman, P.T., Schein, A.J., and Siffert, R.S.: Use of ASIF Compression Plates in Selected Shaft Fractures of the Upper Extremity: A Preliminary Report. Clin. Orthop. 71:208, 1970.
76. Naver, L., and Aalberg, J.R.: Humeral Shaft Fractures Treated With a Ready-Made Fracture Brace. Arch. Orthop. Trauma Surg., 106:20–22, 1986.
77. Nichols, P.J.R.: Rehabilitation after Fractures of the Shaft of the Femur. J. Bone Joint Surg., 45B:96–102, 1963.
78. Ong, L.B., Satku, K., and Lim, P.H.C.: The Treatment of Femoral Shaft Fractures by Closed Kuntscher Nailing (Without Reaming). Injury, 12:466–470, 1981.
79. Parkes, A.R.: A Report on Traumatic Ischaemia of Peripheral Nerves with Some Observations on Volkmann's Ischaemic Contracture. Br. J. Surg., 32:403, 1945.
80. Pollock, F.H., Drake, D., Bovill, E.G., Day, L., and Trafton, P.G.: Treatment of Radial Neuropathy Associated with Fractures of the Humerus. J. Bone Joint Surg., 63A:239–243, 1981.
81. Postacchini, F., and Morace, G.: Fractures of the Humerus Associated with Paralysis of the Radial Nerve. Ital. J. Orthop. Traumatol., 14:455–464, 1988.
82. Rand, J.A., et. al.: A Comparison of the Effect of Open Intramedullary Nailing and Compression-Plate Fixation on Fracture-Site Blood Flow and Fracture Union. J. Bone Joint Surg., 63A:427–442, 1981.
83. Rhinelander, F.W.: Effects of Medullary Nailing on the Normal Blood Supply of Diaphyseal Cortex. A.A.O.S. Instructional Course Lectures. St. Louis, C.V. Mosby, 1973.
84. Rhinelander, F.W.: Tibial Blood Supply in Relation to Fracture Healing. Clin. Orthop., 105:34–81, 1975.
85. Riemer, B.L., and D'Ambrosia, R.: The Risk of Injury to the

Axillary Nerve, Artery, and Vein from Proximal Locking Screws of Humeral Intramedullary Nails. Orthopaedics, 15:697–699, 1992.

86. Rogers, J.F., Bennett, J.B., and Tullos, H.S.: Management of Concomitant Ipsilateral Fractures of the Humerus and Forearm. J. Bone Joint Surg., 64A:552–556, 1984.
87. Rokkanen, P., Slatis, P., and Vankka, E.: Closed or Open Intramedullary Nailing of Femoral Shaft Fractures: A Comparison with Conservatively Treated Cases. J. Bone Joint Surg., 51B:313–323, 1969.
88. Rosen, H.: The Treatment of Nonunions and Pseudarthrosis of the Humeral Shaft. Orthop. Clin. North Am., 21:725–742, 1990.
89. Ruedi, T., and Schweiberer, L.: Scapula, Clavicle and Humerus. *In* Muller, M.E., Allgower, M., Schneider, R., and Willenegger, H. (eds.): Manual of Internal Fixation: Techniques Recommended by the AO-ASIF Group, pp. 442–445. New York, Springer-Verlag, 1991.
90. Russell, T.A., LaVelle, D.G., Nichols, R.L., Simard, J., Taylor, J.C., and Walker, B.J.: Interlocking Intramedullary Nailing of Humeral Fractures. Presented before the annual meeting of the American Academy of Orthopaedic Surgeons, Washington, D.C., February 1992.
91. Sarmiento, A., Horowitch, A., Aboulafia, A., and Vangsness, C.T., Jr.: Functional Bracing for Comminuted Extra-articular Fractures of the Distal Third of the Humerus. J. Bone Joint Surg., 72B:283–287, 1990.
92. Sarmiento, A., Kinman, P.B., Galvin, E.G., Schmitt, R.H., and Phillips, J.G.: Functional Bracing of Fractures of the Shaft of the Humerus. J. Bone Joint Surg., 59A:596–601, 1977.
93. Schatzker, J.: Fractures of the Humerus. *In* Schatzker, J. and Tile, M.: The Rationale of Operative Fracture Care, pp. 61–70. New York, Springer-Verlag, 1987.
94. Schatzker, J., and Ha'Eri, E.B.: Methylmethacrylate as an Adjunct in the Internal Fixation of Pathologic Fractures. Can. J. Surg., 22:179, 1979.
95. Scientific Research Committee, Pennsylvania Orthopaedic Society: Fresh Midshaft Fractures of the Humerus in Adults. Penn. Med. J., 62:848–850, 1959.
96. Stern, P.J., Mattingly, D.A., Pomery, D.L., Zenni, E.J., Jr., and Kreig, J.K.: Intramedullary Fixation of Humeral Shaft Fractures. J. Bone Joint Surg., 66A:639–646, 1984.
97. Stewart, M.J.: Fractures of the Humeral Shaft. *In* Adams, J.P. (ed.): Current Practice in Orthopaedic Surgery. St. Louis, C.V. Mosby, 1964.
98. Stewart, M.J., and Hundley, J.M.: Fractures of the Humerus: A Comparative Study in Methods of Treatment. J. Bone Joint Surg., 37A:681–692, 1955.
99. Urist, M.R., Mazet, R., and McLean, F.C.: The Pathogenesis and Treatment of Delayed Union and Non-Union. J. Bone Joint Surg., 36A:931, 1954.
100. Vail, T.P., and Harrelson, J.M.: Treatment of Pathologic Fracture of the Humerus. Clin. Orthop., 268:197–202, 1991.
101. Ward, E.F., Savoie, F.H., and Hughes, J.L.: Fractures of the Diaphyseal Humerus. *In* Browner, B.D., Jupiter, J.B., Levine, A.M., and Trafton, P.G. (eds.): Skeletal Trauma, vol. 1, pp. 1177–1200. Philadelphia, W.B. Saunders, 1992.
102. Weber, B.G., and Cech, O. Pseudarthrosis: Pathophysiology, Biomechanics, Therapy and Results, pp. 29–44. New York, Grune & Stratton, 1976.
103. Williams, P.L., Warwick, R., Dyson, M., and Bannister, L.H. (eds.): Gray's Anatomy, 37th ed. New York, Churchill Livingstone, 1989.
104. Winfield, J.M., Miller, H., and LaFerte, A.D.: Evaluation of the "Hanging Cast" as a Method of Treating Fractures of Humerus. Am. J. Surg., 55:228–249, 1942.
105. Winquist, R.A., Hansen, S.T., Jr., and Clawson, D.K.: Closed Intramedullary Nailing of Femoral Fractures. J. Bone Joint Surg., 66A:529–539, 1984.
106. Wu, C.C., and Shih, C.H.: Treatment for Nonunion of the Shaft of the Humerus: Comparison of Plates and Seidel Interlocking Nails. Can. J. Surg., 35:661–665, 1992.
107. Zagorski, J.B., Latta, L.L., Zych, G.A., and Finnieston, A.R.: Diaphyseal Fractures of the Humerus: Treatment with Prefabricated Braces. J. Bone Joint Surg., 70A:607–610, 1988.
108. Zagorski, J.B., Zych, G.A., Latta, L.L., and McCollough, N.C.: Modern Concepts in Functional Fracture Bracing: The Upper Limb. *In* Instructional Course Lectures, vol. 36, pp. 377–401. Park Ridge, IL, American Academy of Orthopaedic Surgeons, 1987.
109. Zuckerman, J.D., Giordano, C., and Rosen, H.: Humeral Shaft Nonunions. *In* Bigliani, L.U. (ed.): Complications of Shoulder Surgery, pp. 173–189. Baltimore, Williams & Wilkins, 1993.

Rockwood and Green's Fractures in Adults, Fourth Edition,
edited by Charles A. Rockwood, David P. Green, Robert W. Bucholz and James D. Heckman.
Lippincott-Raven Publishers, Philadelphia © 1996.

CHAPTER 16

Fractures of the Proximal Humerus

Louis U. Bigliani, Evan L. Flatow, and Roger G. Pollock

HISTORICAL REVIEW

Fractures of the proximal humerus are challenging to diagnose and treat. Much information has been published in recent decades about these injuries, as new techniques of treatment have been developed and old ones rediscovered. Hippocrates[138] is credited with documenting the first fracture of the proximal humerus in 460 B.C. and describing a method of weight traction that aided in bone healing. However, little was written about this subject until the latter part of the 19th century.[26,42,59,123,189,192] These reports discussed treatment of most fractures by immobilization in a sling followed by range-of-motion exercises. This treatment was adequate for nondisplaced fractures; but the more complex fractures were not appreciated or understood, and the results of treatment were poor.

In 1896, Kocher[161] developed an anatomical classification in an attempt to improve diagnosis and treatment, but this simplified scheme was not thorough enough and lacked consistency. Other early attempts at overly simple classifications were confusing and incomplete.[39,42,68,105,108,142,150,153,155,177,

[198,209,252,268,279,285,307,315,326] Lack of consensus on fracture description and classification made it difficult to evaluate treatment adequately.

In 1934, Codman[52] made a significant contribution when he divided proximal humeral fractures into four basic parts. These parts were divided along the epiphyseal lines and consisted of the head, lesser tuberosity, greater tuberosity, and shaft. The subsequent four-part classification reported by Neer[228] in 1970 is based on this anatomical classification. Neer's classification is a comprehensive system that integrates fracture anatomy, biomechanics, and displacement, allowing for consistent diagnosis and treatment. It remains the most useful and common classification system for proximal humerus fractures.

In the early 20th century, methods of closed reduction,[4,285] traction,[58,108,153,307] casting,[97,114] and abduction splints[14,57,292,334] were developed to achieve and maintain accurate anatomical alignment of displaced fractures. Often, however, these closed techniques were not sufficient to allow an adequate anatomical reduction. In 1932, Roberts[268] reported that the use of an elaborate apparatus and prolonged immobilization was less satisfactory than treatment with simpler forms of fixation and early motion. Other authors also stressed the importance of early motion and avoidance of the abduction position.[35,97,142,152,158,336] Howard and Eloesser[142] developed a complex theoretic shoulder model simulating muscle forces and demonstrated that the abduction splint was not beneficial for reduction and control of muscle forces.

Open reduction of severely displaced fracture–dislocations gained popularity during the same period in an effort to provide better anatomical alignment.[19,47,50,68,252,262,279,285,300,314] Roberts[268] and Meyerding[211] suggested the use of open reduction early to improve alignment and avoid malunions that would limit motion. Also, in some instances, internal fixation was performed.[155,198] Suture material, wire, and screws were types of early fixation. In 1949, Widen[341] first reported on intramedullary nailing of a transcervical fracture, and he credited Palmer with the development of the technique. In 1955, Rush[281] described his method of intramedullary nailing for the treatment of displaced fractures, and it became quite popular. In the early 1970s, the ASIF group popularized the use of AO plates and screws for displaced fractures. However, more recent reports have stressed a high incidence of complications when this technique is used in more displaced fractures with osteoporotic bone.[169,248,310] Techniques of internal fixation, which emphasize less disruptive soft-tissue dissection and "minimal fixation" with wire and nonabsorbable sutures, have been successful with a low complication rate.[125,229,238]

In the early 1950s, interest grew in the use of a humeral head prosthesis for the treatment of severely displaced fracture–dislocations of the proximal humerus.[9,82,235,254,265] Closed reduction, open reduction and internal fixation, arthrodesis, and humeral head excision proved generally unsuccessful in the treatment of these injuries.[229] In 1955, Neer[226] reported good results with the use of a metal humeral head prosthesis in 27 patients with fracture–dislocations. In 1973, the prosthesis was redesigned to have a more anatomical head, and recent technical improvements have led to better results.[237] Several types of proximal humeral replacements are in use: some employ one-piece components and others employ two-piece or modular head components.

Complications of the treatment of proximal humeral fractures are not uncommon and are wide ranging, including avascular necrosis, malunion, nonunion, infection, and neurovascular injury. In this chapter a comprehensive approach to proximal humeral fractures that will aid in diagnosis and treatment is outlined.

ANATOMY

It is important to understand the complex anatomy of the shoulder, since optimum function of the glenohumeral joint is dependent on proper alignment and interaction of its anatomical structures. Malunion and nonunion of fractures disrupt the balance of forces across the shoulder, interfering with smooth scapulohumeral rhythm and causing impingement beneath the subacromial arch.

The shoulder has an almost global range of motion, more than any other major joint in the body. This degree of movement occurs because the glenoid cavity is a shallow socket approximately one third to one fourth the size of the humeral head.[282] The glenohumeral joint depends largely on capsule, ligaments, and muscle rather than on bone for stability. The capsule is quite loose and approximately double the size of the humeral head, allowing for a great deal of motion. The subdeltoid bursa lies on top of the rotator cuff and greatly facilitates movement of the cuff beneath the coracoacromial arch.

Proximal Humerus

The proximal humerus consists of the humeral head, lesser tuberosity, greater tuberosity, bicipital groove, and proximal humeral shaft (Fig. 16-1). It is important to differentiate between the anatomical neck, which is at the junction of the head and the tuberosities, and the surgical neck, which is below the greater and lesser tuberosities. The boundaries of the latter are somewhat variable without a distinct line. Anatomical neck fractures are rare and have a poor prognosis, since the

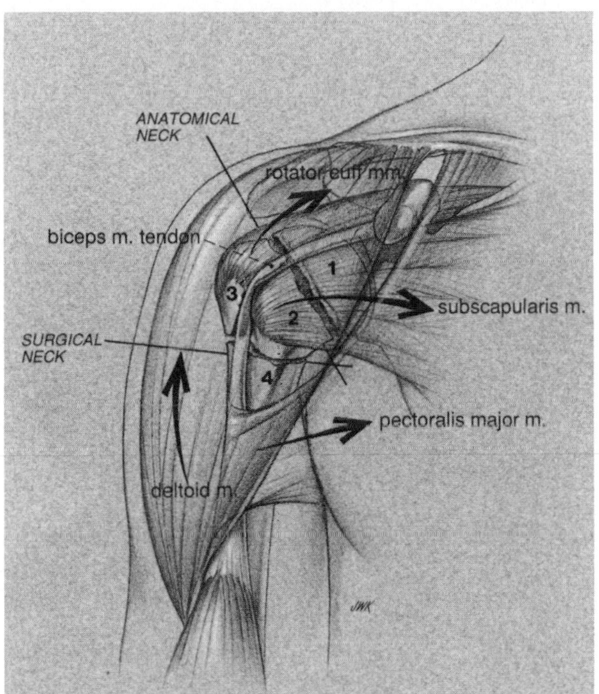

FIGURE 16-1. The anatomy of the shoulder is complex, and shoulder function depends on proper alignment and interaction of anatomical structures. Displacement of fracture fragments is due to the pull of muscles attaching to the various bony components. The four anatomical components of the proximal humerus are the head, lesser tuberosity, greater tuberosity, and shaft. The anatomical neck is at the junction of the head and tuberosities, and the surgical neck is below the greater and lesser tuberosities. The subscapularis inserts on the lesser tuberosity, causing medial displacement, whereas the supraspinatus and infraspinatus insert on the greater tuberosity, causing superior and posterior displacement. The pectoralis major inserts on the humeral shaft and displaces it medially.

blood supply to the head is completely disrupted (Fig. 16-2). On the other hand, surgical neck fractures are common and the blood supply to the head is preserved. The lesser tuberosity, the area of attachment for the subscapularis muscle, lies on the anterior aspect of the humerus and is smaller than the greater tuberosity. The bicipital groove lies between the greater and lesser tuberosities and is on the anterior aspect of the proximal humerus. There are considerable variations in both the height and depth of the groove.[70,139,140] The biceps tendon lies in the bicipital groove and is covered by the transverse humeral ligament. The greater tuberosity lies posteriorly and superiorly on the humeral shaft and provides an attachment site for the supraspinatus, infraspinatus, and teres minor muscles. The greater tuberosity does not protrude above the humeral head. The glenoid is a shallow, convex structure shaped like an inverted comma,[70] approximately one third to one fourth the surface area of the humeral head. It articulates with the humeral head and also provides attachment at its rim for the glenoid labrum and capsule.

Acromion

The acromion protects the superior aspect of the glenohumeral joint and provides origin and mechanical leverage for the deltoid muscle, which is a prime mover of the shoulder. It also forms the lateral component of the acromioclavicular joint. The acromion, together with the coracoacromial ligament and the coracoid process, forms the coracoacromial arch (see Fig. 16-2). This is a rather rigid structure, under which the proximal humerus, rotator cuff, and subacromial bursa must pass. Displaced fractures may disrupt the smooth flow of these structures below the coracoacromial arch, which may result in impingement and prevent normal glenohumeral motion. The subacromial (subdeltoid) bursa is a large synovial membrane. The roof is adherent to the undersurface of the coracoacromial ligament, acromion, and deltoid muscle laterally, and the floor is closely adherent to the rotator cuff and greater tuberosity.[140] It also extends anteriorly and posteriorly around the humerus, creating a gliding mechanism that facilitates the movement of the proximal humerus under the coracoacromial arch. This structure may be injured in even nondisplaced fractures, resulting in fibrotic thickening and loss of glenohumeral motion. Early institution of range-of-motion exercises after a fracture limits the formation of bursal adhesions.

Rotator Cuff and Muscles

The dynamic interplay of the rotator cuff and deltoid muscles is essential for glenohumeral function. The stability of the humeral head in the glenoid created by these muscles allows the deltoid muscle to function optimally. The rotator cuff consists of four muscles: the subscapularis, supraspinatus, infraspinatus, and teres minor. The long head of the biceps tendon is another important component of this complex (see Fig. 16-1). The subscapularis is a head depressor and in certain positions an internal rotator. The infraspinatus and teres minor are external rotators. These muscles work as a unit, rather than individually, to maintain dynamic glenohumeral stability.

Since the rotator cuff muscles are attached to the tuberosities, it is important to understand the direction of pull of their fibers, because this will facilitate an understanding of displacement of the tuberosity fragments. For example, in a fracture of the greater tuberosity, the fragment will be pulled superiorly and posteriorly because of the supraspinatus, infraspinatus, and teres minor muscles. On the other hand, in a fracture of the lesser tuberosity, the fragment will be pulled anteriorly and medially by the subscapularis muscle. The long head of the biceps attaches to the supraglenoid tubercle of the glenoid and has a stabilizing and

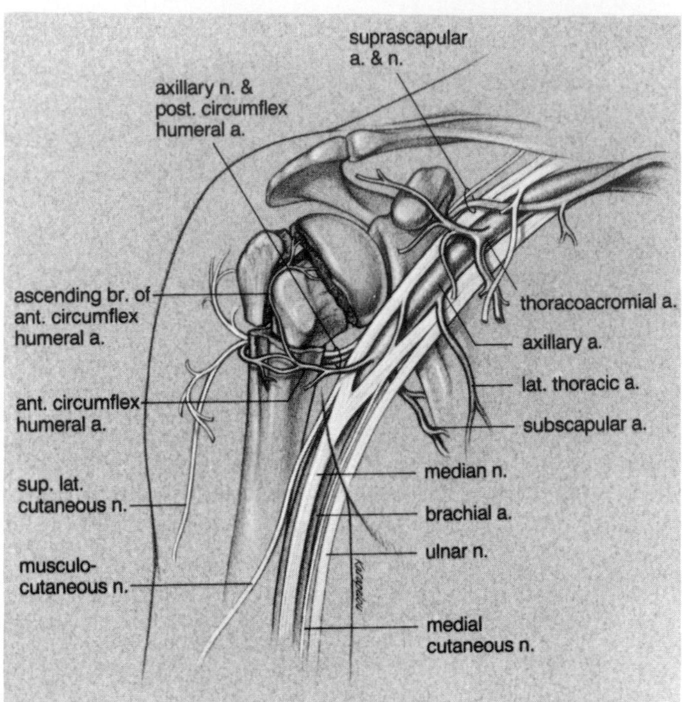

FIGURE 16-2. The brachial plexus and axillary artery lie adjacent to the coracoid process and can be injured with fractures of the proximal humerus. The major blood supply to the humeral head is through the ascending branch of the anterior humeral circumflex artery, which penetrates the head at the superior aspect of the bicipital groove and becomes the arcuate artery. There are three important nerves about the shoulder: the axillary, suprascapular, and musculocutaneous.

depressing action on the humeral head. It is a significant structure to consider in closed reductions, since it can act as a tether and block reduction. Also, during operative procedures, it is a useful landmark from which the rotator interval can be identified, so that bone fragments are properly identified and the rotator cuff muscles are preserved.

Two other important muscles must be considered in relation to the proximal humerus: the deltoid and pectoralis major. The deltoid is a prime mover in the shoulder and originates from the lateral one third of the clavicle, acromion, and spine of the scapula. It inserts at the deltoid tuberosity on the lateral shaft of the humerus and can cause displacement of fractures of the proximal humeral shaft. The pectoralis major is a large fan-shaped muscle that has a broad origin from the clavicle, upper ribs, and sternocostal area. It inserts on the lower portion of the lateral lip of the bicipital groove and can displace the proximal shaft of the humerus medially, as is usually seen in surgical neck fractures.

Blood Supply

It is important to consider the blood supply to the proximal humerus, because avascular necrosis is not uncommon after displaced fractures. The major blood supply to the humeral head is from the anterior humeral circumflex artery[165,170,178,224,262] (see Fig. 16-2). Laing[175] was the first to describe the arcuate artery, which is a continuation of the ascending branch of the anterior humeral circumflex as it penetrates the bone. This tortuous artery supplies blood to a large portion of the humeral head. It routinely enters the bone in the area of the intertubicular groove and gives branches to the lesser and greater tuberosities. Also, a small contribution to the humeral head blood supply comes from branches of the posterior circumflex artery and from the vascular rotator cuff through tendinous-osseous anastomoses.

Rothman and Parke[276] have outlined the blood supply to the rotator cuff as routinely derived from six arteries: the anterior humeral circumflex, posterior humeral circumflex, suprascapular, thoracoacromial, suprahumeral, and subscapular. The anterior humeral circumflex is the major supplier to the anterior cuff and the long head of the biceps, while the posterior humeral circumflex and suprascapular anastomosis supply the posterior cuff. The thoracoacromial artery supplies the supraspinatus, while the suprahumeral and subscapular arteries supply the anterior inferior aspect of the cuff. In one anatomical study, Gerber and associates[103] found that vascularization of the humeral head was possible only through the ascending branch of the anterior circumflex artery. When this artery is injured close to its entrance to the humeral head, it is likely that the blood supply to the humeral head will be compromised.

Nerve Supply

Injury to the nerves about the shoulder can occur with fractures. The brachial plexus and axillary arteries can be injured with anterior fracture–

dislocations and violent trauma to the proximal humerus (see Fig. 16-2). Isolated injuries to the major nerves innervating the muscles around the shoulder—the axillary, suprascapular, and musculocutaneous—can also occur.

The most commonly injured nerve is the axillary nerve. The axillary nerve is composed of fibers from the fifth and sixth cervical roots, in most cases, and takes its origin from the posterior cord at the level of the axilla. Then it crosses the anterior surface of the subscapularis muscle and dips back posteriorly under its inferior border. It passes along the inferior border of the capsule of the glenohumeral joint and then through the quadrangular space (see Fig. 16-2). After emerging from the quadrangular space, it gives off a branch to the teres minor and divides into anterior and posterior branches. The posterior branch supplies the posterior deltoid and gives off the superolateral brachial cutaneous nerve. The anterior branch supplies the middle and anterior deltoid muscles as it winds around the undersurface of this muscle. Owing to its relative fixation at the posterior cord and the deltoid, any abnormal downward motion of the proximal humerus can result in traction and injury to this nerve. Also, its close relationship to the inferior capsule makes it susceptible to injury with anterior dislocation and open repairs for anterior fracture–dislocations.

The suprascapular nerve can also be injured, but this is much less common. It is made up of fibers from the fifth and sixth cervical roots and originates from the upper trunk of the brachial plexus. It runs laterally deep to the omohyoid and trapezius, passing through the suprascapular notch (see Fig. 16-2). After giving off two branches to the supraspinatus, it passes around the lateral border of the scapular spine to the infraspinatus. The two points of fixation of the nerve are at its origin from the upper trunk and at the suprascapular notch, where it passes beneath the transverse scapular ligament, making it susceptible to traction injury.

Injury to the musculocutaneous nerve is rare. Composed of fibers from C5 to C6 with the occasional addition of C7 fibers, it originates from the lateral cord at the level of the pectoralis minor and passes obliquely distally through the coracobrachialis and between the biceps and brachialis (see Fig. 16-2). In the 93 cadaver shoulders we have dissected, the distance from the coracoid to the point of entrance into the coracobrachialis muscle has been between 3.1 and 8.2 cm, with a mean of 5.6 cm.[90] More importantly, 29% entered less than 5 cm from the coracoid, demonstrating that the frequently cited safe zone of 5 to 8 cm is inaccurate. The nerve terminates in the lateral antecubital brachial nerve, as it exits the deep fascia at the level of the elbow. Blunt trauma as well as traction injuries can result in injury to the musculocutaneous nerve.

MECHANISM OF INJURY

The most common mechanism of injury for proximal humeral fractures is a fall onto the outstretched hand from a standing height or less.[186] In most instances, severe trauma does not play a significant role. Rather, the trauma need only be minor to moderate in degree, because osteoporosis is usually present. In younger patients, high energy trauma is more frequently involved, and the resulting fracture is often more serious. These patients usually have fracture–dislocations with significant soft-tissue disruption and multiple trauma. When multiple trauma is treated, the proximal humeral fracture is commonly initially ignored, because attention is focused on more life-threatening problems. However, as the patient regains consciousness, complaints of pain in the shoulder may prove secondary to a fracture. Another mechanism of injury, first mentioned by Codman, is excessive rotation of the arm, especially in the abducted position. The humerus locks against the acromion in a pivotal position and a fracture can occur, especially in older patients with osteoporotic bone. Proximal humerus fractures may also result from a direct blow to the side of the shoulder. This usually occurs in the lateral position and may result in fracture of the greater tuberosity.

An often ignored cause of fracture–dislocations of the proximal humerus is electrical shock or a convulsive episode.[29,77,123,263,284,295,345] The fracture–dislocation may be anterior or posterior and is often overlooked. Metastatic disease may significantly weaken the bone, so that a pathologic fracture may occur with just trivial activity. Whenever a trivial event causes a fracture of the proximal humerus, a pathologic etiology should be considered.

CLASSIFICATION

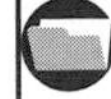

Classification of Fractures of the Proximal Humerus

- Nondisplaced
- Displaced
  - Neer four-part classification
  - AO classification

A workable classification system for fractures of the proximal humerus is necessary for proper manage-

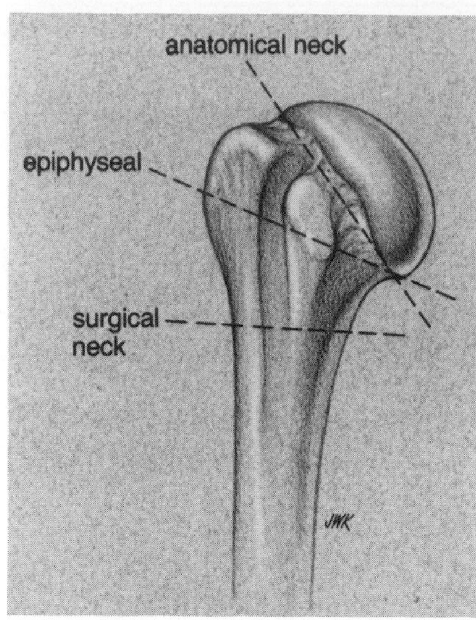

FIGURE 16-3. Kocher classification. This classification is based on three anatomical levels for fractures: anatomical neck, epiphyseal region, and surgical neck. This classification does not allow for differentiation of multiple fractures at two different sites, nor does it differentiate between displaced and undisplaced fractures. (*Adapted from Kocher, T.: Beitrage zur Kenntnis Einiger Praktisch Wichtiger Fracturenformen. Basel, Carl Sallman Verlag, 1896.*)

ment. A classification system must be comprehensive enough to encompass all factors, yet specific enough to allow accurate diagnosis and treatment. Also, it must be flexible enough to accommodate variations and allow logical deductions for treatment. Most proximal humeral fractures are nondisplaced or minimally displaced and must be differentiated from the more displaced fractures, since the treatment is significantly different. Inadequate diagnosis of complex fractures creates confusion and improper management.

The underpinnings of a fracture classification system are a thorough knowledge of the anatomy and accurate radiographic views to outline the anatomical structures. The most logical and commonly used classification is the four-part fracture classification developed by Neer[228] in 1970.

Neer Classification

Before the Neer classification, various other methods had been proposed, including anatomical level of the fracture,[35,52,149,153,161] mechanism of injury,[69,308,334] amount of contact by the fracture fragments,[80] degree of displacement,[159] and vascular status of the articular segment.[9,147] Furthermore, others have devised classifications using combinations of the preceding criteria that have resulted in confusion about the diagnosis and treatment of these complex fractures.[21,69,71,81,83,133,159,198,261,268]

In 1896, Kocher was the first to devise a classification of proximal humeral fractures.[161] His classification was based on different anatomical levels for fractures: anatomical neck, epiphyseal region, and surgical neck (Fig. 16-3). The problem with this type of classification is that it does not allow for multiple fractures at different sites, nor does it differentiate between displaced and nondisplaced fractures, which require different treatment. Classification according to the mechanism of injury can also be misleading, as in the Watson-Jones classification of an abduction or adduction type of fracture.[334] It has since been pointed out that the deformity in these fractures is anterior angulation; and depending on whether radiographs are obtained with the arm in internal or external rotation, the fracture can become either an abduction or an adduction fracture.[228,344]

In 1934, Codman[52] made a significant contribution to the understanding of proximal humeral fractures by proposing that fractures be separated into four distinct fragments, occurring roughly along the anatomical lines of epiphyseal union (Fig. 16-4). He was able to differentiate four major fragments: the anatomical head, the greater tuberosity, the lesser tuberosity, and the shaft. Codman's conclusion was that all fractures were some combination of these different fracture fragments. Furthermore, the musculotendinous cuff attaches to the more proximal fragments and can hold the fractured fragments together.

This was the cornerstone on which Neer,[228] in 1970, based his four-part classification (Fig. 16-5). This was

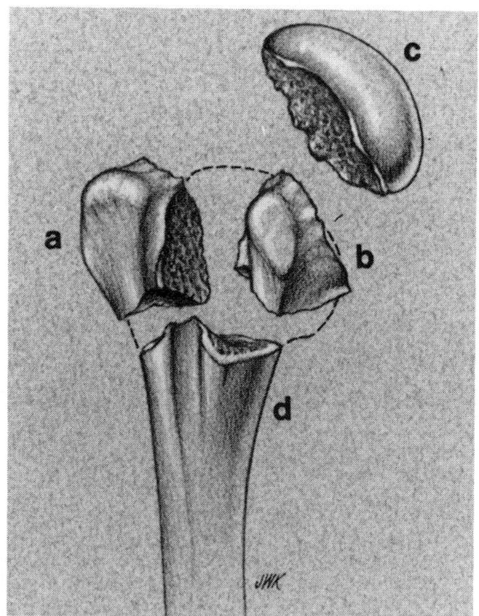

FIGURE 16-4. Codman divided the proximal humerus into four distinct fragments that occur roughly along anatomical lines of epiphyseal union. He differentiated the four major fragments as (**a**) greater tuberosity, (**b**) lesser tuberosity, (**c**) head, and (**d**) shaft. (*Adapted from Codman, E.A.: The Shoulder: Rupture of the Supraspinatus Tendon and Other Lesions in or About the Subacromial Bursa. Boston, Thomas Todd, 1934.*)

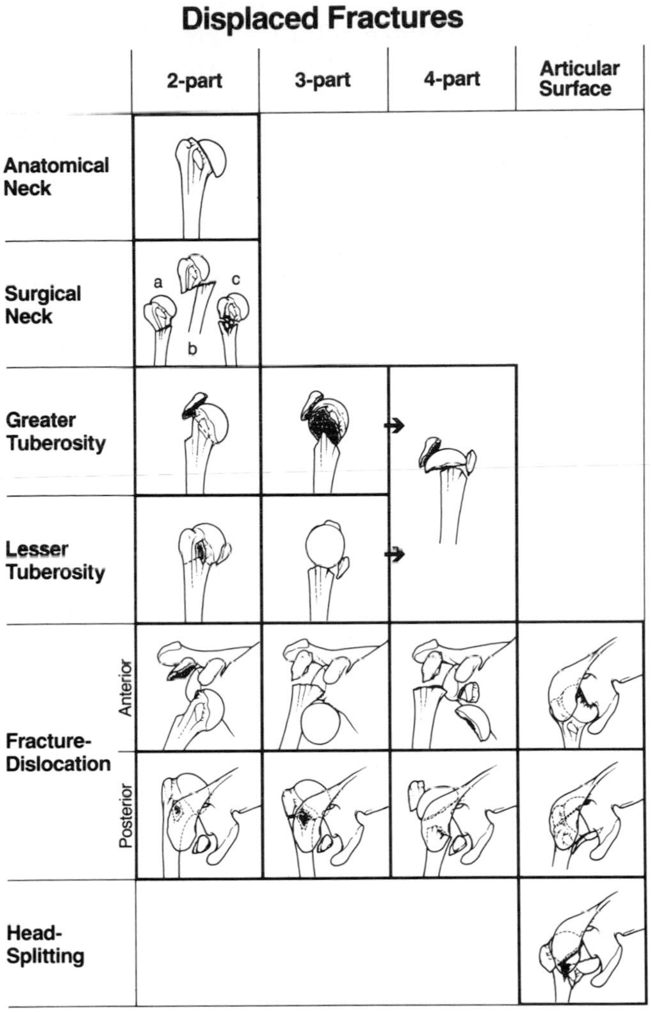

FIGURE 16-5. Neer classification. The most commonly used classification at present is the Neer four-part classification. It is a comprehensive system that encompasses anatomy and biomechanical forces that result in the displacement of fracture fragments. It is based on accurate identification of the four major fragments and their relationship to each other. A displaced fracture is either two-part, three-part, or four-part. In addition, there are fracture–dislocations that can be either two-part, three-part, or four-part. Fissure lines or hairline fractures are not to be considered displaced fragments. A fragment is considered displaced when there is more than 1 cm of separation or a fragment is angulated more than 45° from the other fragments. Impression fractures of the articular surface also occur and are usually associated with an anterior or posterior dislocation. Head-splitting fractures are usually associated with fractures of the tuberosities or surgical neck. (*After Neer, C.S.: Displaced Proximal Humeral Fractures: I. Classification and Evaluation. J. Bone Joint Surg., 52A:1077–1089, 1970.*)

the first truly comprehensive system that considered the anatomy and biomechanical forces resulting in the amount of displacement of fracture fragments and related these factors to diagnosis and treatment. It is the most commonly used classification for proximal humeral fractures and is used extensively in this chapter to identify fracture patterns.

The Neer classification of fractures of the proximal humerus is a system based on the accurate identification of the four major fragments and their relationship to each other. There is nothing to memorize, but an adequate knowledge of the anatomy and the insertions of the tendons of the rotator cuff is essential to its proper use (see Fig. 16-5). The identification of fragments can be accomplished only with proper radiographs, including the trauma series, which consists of anteroposterior and lateral views in the scapular plane, as well as an axillary view. This fracture system is a concept rather than a numerical classification and sets forth guidelines that are arbitrary and designed to be helpful in recognizing displaced fractures. Emphasis is placed on determining the vascular supply to the humeral head, since avascular necrosis is a common complication of displaced fractures.

Most fractures, over 80%,[238] are minimally displaced, although Rose and associates[272] in 1982 and Horak and Nilsson[141] in 1975 have reported lower incidences, 78% and 61%, respectively. (Minimally displaced fractures must be accurately identified so that they can be differentiated from the more serious displaced fractures.) In the Neer four-part classification, the four parts are the same as Codman has described: the articular segment or the head, the greater tuberosity, the lesser tuberosity, and the shaft (see Fig. 16-5). When any of the four major segments is displaced greater than 1 cm, or angulated more than 45°, the fracture is considered displaced. Fissure lines or hairline fractures are not considered displaced fragments. A fragment may have several undisplaced components: these should not be considered separate fragments since they are in continuity and are held together by soft tissue.

If the preceding criteria for displacement are not met, then the fracture should be considered minimally displaced, and there is only one part. In a two-part fracture, one fragment is displaced in reference to the other three fragments. In a three-part fracture, two fragments are displaced in relationship to each other and the other two undisplaced fragments, but the head remains in contact with the glenoid. In a four-part fracture, all four fracture fragments are displaced; the head is out of contact with the glenoid and angulated either laterally, anteriorly, posteriorly, inferiorly, or superiorly. Furthermore, it is detached from both tuberosities and is deprived of its blood supply. The central focus of this fracture classification is the status of the blood supply to the humeral head and the relationship of the humeral head to the displaced parts and the glenoid.

Neer[228] has also emphasized the term *fracture–dislocation* and the accurate diagnosis of this problem (see Fig. 16-5). A fracture–dislocation exists when the head is displaced outside the joint space, not merely rotated, and there is, in addition, a fracture. Fracture–

dislocations can be classified according to direction (anterior or posterior) as well as to the number of fracture fragments (two-part, three-part, or four-part). Head-splitting fractures and impression fractures of the articular surface are special fractures (see Fig. 16-5). Impression fractures of the articular surface are graded according to the percentage of the articular surface involved. The general guidelines that have been adopted for these are less than 20%, between 20% and 45%, and greater than 45% of the articular head. Fractures in which the articular surface is shattered into several fragments are termed *head-splitting fractures.* This term is not applicable to fractures in which a small portion of articular surface (<10% or 15%) is attached to a displaced greater tuberosity but rather is reserved for fractures with significant articular disruption. Head-splitting fractures are frequently involved with other fractures of the proximal humerus and are often the result of violent trauma.

Researchers have assessed interobserver reliability and intraobserver reproducibility for evaluating proximal humerus fractures using the Neer classification system.[43,168,298,299] Sidor and associates[298] found intraobserver reproducibility to be higher than interobserver reliability. The level of experience and expertise was a significant factor, with a shoulder specialist achieving the highest correlation coefficient. Observers in a second study pointed out that the main difficulties in fracture classification were assessment of the lesser tuberosity and determination of the exact amount of displacement of the fragments.[299] Because the Neer classification system is not a radiographic classification but a pathoanatomical classification of fracture displacements, accurate use of the system may require special radiographic studies, in addition to the routinely obtained views, or even operative assessment in difficult cases.[27,231,269]

AO Classification

On the basis of a review of 730 fractures, Jakob and colleagues[147] and the AO group have applied the AO system for classifying long-bone fractures to fractures of the proximal humerus and have emphasized the vascular supply to the articular segments. The vascular supply to the articular segment plays a pivotal role in the prognosis of a proximal humeral fracture, since avascular necrosis is such a common complication. The system is divided into three categories, according to the severity of injury. The least severe is the type A fracture, in which vascular isolation of the articular segment is not present and avascular necrosis is unlikely. It is extracapsular and involves two of the four primary segments. A type B fracture is more severe, and there is partial isolation of the articular segment with a low risk of avascular necrosis. It is partially intracapsular, and three of the four primary segments are involved. In a type C fracture, which is the most severe, total vascular isolation of the articular segment occurs with a high risk of avascular necrosis. It is intracapsular, and all four primary segments are involved. In addition, each alphabetical group is subgrouped numerically, with higher numbers generally reflecting greater severity. This more complicated system aims to create a framework for more detailed therapeutic and prognostic guidelines. However, the complex nature of this system has made it less attractive and less frequently used than the Neer system.

Rating System

A consistent method of evaluating results is important. Unless results from different series are reported in a uniform manner, it is difficult to draw valid comparisons. When Hagg and Lundberg[119] reported their series of fractures, they had 52% satisfactory results using Santee's criteria[285] and 35% satisfactory results using Neer's criteria.[229] Confusion persists because authors continue to use their own criteria for evaluation. The most commonly used rating system for fracture has been Neer's, based on 100 units. There are 35 units for pain, 30 units for function, 25 units for range of motion, and 10 units for anatomy. Pain is the most significant factor. An excellent result is greater than 89 units; satisfactory, greater than 80 units; unsatisfactory, greater than 70 units; and failure, less than 70 units.

In an effort to standardize results, the American Shoulder and Elbow Surgeons developed a form for assessment of the shoulder.[266] This assessment form has a patient self-evaluation section and a physician assessment section. In the patient self-evaluation section, there are subsections for pain, instability, and function. Pain and instability are graded using visual analogue scales. Ten activities of daily living are assessed on a four-point ordinal scale, from unable to do to not difficult to do. The physician assessment measures range of motion, strength, and stability and evaluates the presence or absence of various signs, such as impingement or localized tenderness. By using the patient evaluation form, a shoulder score can be derived from the visual analogue pain score (50%) and the cumulative activities of daily living score (50%). It is hoped that this method of evaluation will be used widely and will allow communication between investigators and provide meaningful comparison of treatment outcomes.

INCIDENCE

Fractures of the proximal humerus are not uncommon, especially in older age groups. They have previously been reported to account for 4% to 5% of all fractures, but this figure may be low.[186,228,309] An epidemiologic study reported by Bengner and colleagues[24] from Malmo, Sweden, of more than 2125 fractures has shown a steady and significant increase in the incidence of proximal humeral fractures. Lind and colleagues[186] noted a similar trend in Denmark and believed that the increased average lifespan was partially responsible. In two other comprehensive studies, one from Rochester, Minnesota,[272] and another also from Malmo, Sweden,[141] the age-adjusted incidence of proximal humeral fractures among adult residents was practically identical—105 and 104 per 100,000 person-years, respectively. Furthermore, it was correlated in the Minnesota study that proximal humeral fractures occur at nearly 70% of the reported rate of proximal femur fractures, all ages considered. A comparison with a previous study concerning proximal femur fractures in the same population was performed.[98] Based on the epidemiologic data available, it was concluded that most proximal humeral fractures are primarily related to osteoporosis and, like hip fractures, represent an important source of morbidity among the elderly population. Buhr and Cooke[38] also noted a strong similarity in the incidence and pattern of these two fractures.

Proximal humeral fractures were the most common humeral fractures (45%) in the study by Rose and colleagues, concerning the epidemiologic features of humeral fractures in Rochester, Minnesota.[272] In adults older than 40 years of age, the percentage of proximal humeral fractures increases to 76%. Osteoporosis was believed to be a major factor, and the amount of trauma responsible for the fracture was significantly less in the older age group. Shaft and distal humeral fractures are more common in the younger age groups in which more violent trauma is usually associated with the injury. Also, a higher incidence of proximal humeral fractures was noted in women than in men, by a rate of approximately 2 to 1. Horak and Nilsson[141] have also reported increased incidence with age and in females and the same frequency as fractures of the proximal end of the femur. The patients with proximal humeral fractures had an increased incidence of alcoholism and prior gastric resection. Furthermore, prevalence of other fractures was approximately doubled in patients who have had proximal humeral fractures. Rose and colleagues[272] and Horak and Nilsson[141] concluded that osteoporosis was a significant factor in these fractures.

SIGNS AND SYMPTOMS

Most fractures of the proximal humerus present acutely, and, therefore, the most common symptoms are pain, swelling, and tenderness about the shoulder, especially in the area of the greater tuberosity. Palpation of the bony contour of the shoulder may be difficult, since the soft-tissue covering of the shoulder is generous. Crepitus may be present with motion of the fracture fragments, if they are in contact. Ecchymosis generally becomes visible within 24 to 48 hours of the injury and may spread to the chest wall and flank and distally down the extremity. It is important to warn the patient that this development may occur, since it may cause alarm that further internal damage has occurred after the initial fracture. In most instances, patients find it difficult to initiate active motion and hold the arm closely against the chest wall. However, history and physical examination are only suggestive of a fracture; the definitive diagnosis is made with the proper radiographs.

A detailed neurovascular evaluation is essential in all fractures of the proximal humerus. The brachial plexus and axillary arteries are just medial to the coracoid process, and injury to these structures is not uncommon. It can occur even in undisplaced fractures.[128,302] It is important to test the peripheral pulses and question the patient about paresthesias and loss of sensation in the distal extremity. The easiest way to diagnose a neurovascular complication is to suspect the injury and test for it at the initial examination. The most common nerve that is injured with fractures about the shoulder is the axillary nerve. Sensation should be tested over the deltoid muscle, since testing for deltoid activity or weakness may be very difficult because of pain. Occasionally, in the immediate postfracture or postoperative period, there may be inferior subluxation of the humerus. In most instances, this is secondary to deltoid atony, rather than an injury to the axillary nerve.[63,69,87,317,333,343] The arm should be supported in the sling, and gentle isometric exercises will help recover deltoid tone. If this situation is severe and persists for more than 4 weeks, then it must be differentiated from a true axillary nerve palsy.

Examination of the chest should not be ignored, since complications involving the thoracic cavity have been reported after fractures of the proximal humerus. Although rare, they do occur, and several authors have reported intrathoracic penetration by the humeral head associated with fractures.[106,122,251,338] Also, a pneumothorax may occur, especially in patients who have multiple trauma.

Fracture–dislocations of the proximal humerus are difficult to diagnose and often are missed by the initial examiner (Fig. 16-6*A*).[125,126,137,205,327,328] This is especially true of posterior fracture–dislocations. It is estimated that more than 50% of these injuries are missed by the initial treating physician.[11,126,238] In a fracture–dislocation, there is loss of contour of the shoulder. With an anterior fracture–dislocation, there is an anterior bulge and the posterior aspect of the joint is flattened or hollow. The

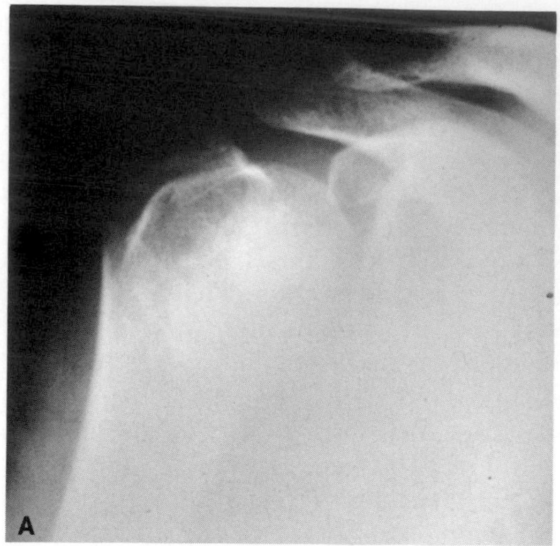

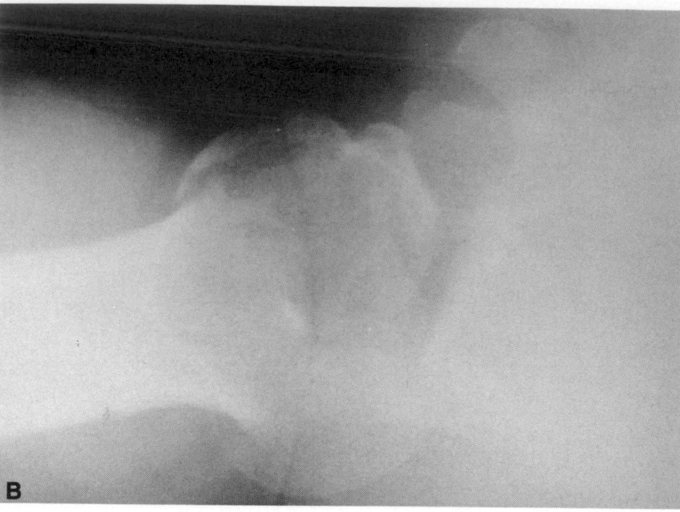

FIGURE 16-6. (**A**) An anteroposterior x-ray of an obese woman taken in the emergency department was initially read as a minimally displaced fracture. This poor-quality radiograph was the only view taken. The patient was started on early range-of-motion exercises but after 4 weeks had −30° of external rotation, forward elevation to 70°, and no abduction. (**B**) An axillary x-ray taken after 4 weeks reveals a missed posterior fracture–dislocation. An axillary x-ray is essential for diagnosis of posterior fracture–dislocations.

reverse is true with a posterior fracture–dislocation, in which the anterior aspect of the shoulder is flattened, the coracoid is more prominent, and there is a posterior bulge with the axis of the humerus pointing posteriorly. With a posterior dislocation, there will always be a loss of external rotation and abduction secondary to pain. However, if there is a surgical neck fracture component to the fracture, rotation and abduction through the fracture site can occur. This diagnosis must be confirmed by proper radiographs (ie, a lateral view in the scapular plane or an axillary view) (see Fig. 16-6*B*) or by computed tomography ([CT]).

When a patient has a convulsive episode or a history of an electrical shock accident and presents with pain and swelling about the shoulder, the patient must first be evaluated for a posterior dislocation or fracture–dislocation, as well as an anterior dislocation.[13,126,157,295] Although this seems obvious, there has been a case reported of bilateral posterior fracture–dislocations that were undiagnosed for 14 days after injury.[187] The patient had significant swelling and ecchymosis, as well as a fixed internal rotation contracture. The ecchymosis was attributed to a reaction to a drug prescribed by the initial physician. It cannot be overemphasized that a fixed posterior fracture–dislocation is commonly missed. To avoid this, the examining physician must have a high degree of suspicion, so that appropriate radiographs can be ordered.

RADIOGRAPHIC FINDINGS

Accurate radiographic evaluation of fractures of the proximal humerus is essential for diagnosis and treatment. Incorrectly positioned or oblique radiographs only misrepresent the fracture and create confusion.

Trauma Series

The trauma series remains the best initial method for diagnosing proximal humeral fractures.[228] This consists of anteroposterior and lateral radiographs in the scapular plane and an axillary view (Fig. 16-7). The lateral radiograph in the scapular plane is also called the tangential or Y-view of the scapula. This series allows evaluation of the fracture in three separate perpendicular planes, so that accurate assessment of fracture displacement can be achieved. The scapula sits obliquely on the chest wall, and the glenoid surface is tilted 35° to 40° anteriorly. Therefore, the glenohumeral joint does not lie in either the sagittal or the coronal plane. The anteroposterior and lateral radiographs in this scapular plane can be taken without removing the patient's arm from the sling. They can be done in either a sitting, standing, or prone position. For the anteroposterior radiograph in the scapular plane, the posterior aspect of the affected shoulder is placed against the x-ray plate and the opposite shoulder is rotated out approximately 40°. This gives a true anteroposterior view of the glenohumeral joint and avoids any superimposition of other tissues that will obscure bony detail. The lateral radiograph in the scapular plane is accomplished by placing the anterior aspect of the affected shoulder against the x-ray plate and rotating the other shoulder out approximately 40°. The x-ray tube is then placed posteriorly along the scapular spine, and this provides a true lateral view of the shoulder.

The axillary view allows for evaluation in the axial plane and is essential for evaluating the degree of tuberosity displacement, the glenoid articular surface,

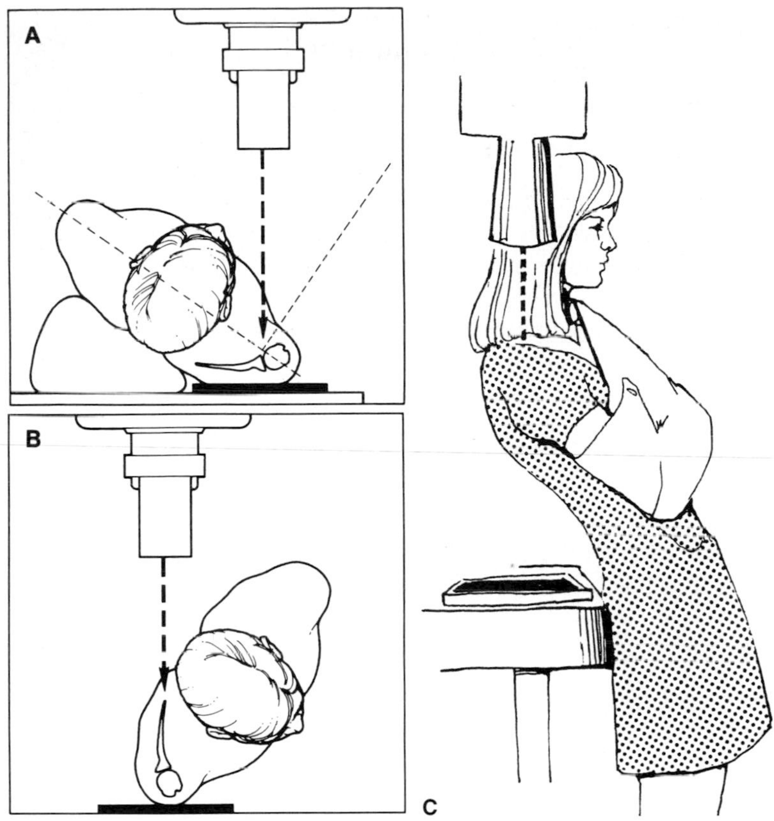

FIGURE 16-7. Trauma series. The trauma series consists of anteroposterior and lateral x-rays in the scapular plane as well as an axillary view. These views may be done sitting, standing, or prone. The lateral is called the tangential or Y-view of the scapula. This series allows evaluation of the fracture in three perpendicular planes so that the fracture displacement can be accurately assessed. The scapula sits obliquely on the chest wall, and the glenoid surface is tilted 35° to 40° anteriorly. Therefore, the glenohumeral joint is not in the sagittal or the coronal plane. (**A**) For the anteroposterior x-ray in the scapular plane, the posterior aspect of the affected shoulder is placed against the x-ray plate and the opposite shoulder is tilted forward approximately 40°. (**B**) For the lateral x-ray in the scapular plane, the anterior aspect of the affected shoulder is placed against the x-ray plate and the other shoulder is tilted forward approximately 40°. The x-ray tube is then placed posteriorly along the scapular spine. (**C**) The Velpeau axillary view is preferred after trauma when the patient can be positioned for this view, since it allows the shoulder to remain immobilized and avoids further displacement of the fracture fragments.

and the relationship of the humeral head to the glenoid (ie, whether or not a dislocation is present) (see Fig. 16-6*B*). Greater tuberosity fragments may be small and hard to see on poor radiographs, especially if they overlie the head. Many severely displaced greater tuberosity fractures have posterior rather than superior retraction, and this can only be appreciated on an axillary view or CT scan. This view is often not obtained, even though its importance has been stressed for years by several authors.[97,211,229,268,340] An axillary view may be obtained in either the standing, sitting, or prone position. If possible, the supine position is preferable. The arm can be held by a knowledgeable person in mild abduction, so that further displacement of the fracture does not occur. The x-ray plate is placed above the patient's shoulder, and the arm is gently abducted to 30°. The x-ray tube is placed slightly below the patient, and the beam goes from inferior to superior. It is helpful in these cases to rest the patient's shoulder on a soft cushion so that it is elevated off the table and bony pathology is not obscured. The Velpeau axillary view has also been described, in which the arm is not removed from the sling.[32] The patient is seated and tilted obliquely backward 45°. The plate is below and the x-ray tube above. This view is preferred in patients who can comply with the positioning required to obtain it, since the arm is left undisturbed in the sling.

In attempting to judge the amount of angular displacement at the surgical neck level, one must consider the neck shaft angle of the humerus in both the anteroposterior and lateral planes. On the anteroposterior projections, the neck shaft angle is the angle created at the intersection of lines that are perpendicular to the anatomical neck and parallel to the shaft of the humerus. On the lateral radiograph, the neck shaft angle is the angle formed at the intersection of the lines parallel to the anatomical neck and parallel to the shaft of the humerus. Keene and colleagues[156] have demonstrated that the neck shaft angle can vary with humeral rotation. Therefore, it is important to consider the position of the arm when evaluating radiographs and compare them to radiographs of the unaffected side, if necessary. In Keene and coworkers' studies of 25 control patients, the average neck shaft angle in the anteroposterior projection was 143°, with a range of 134° to 166°. This angle was less with external rotation and greater with internal rotation. Therefore, this angle can vary as much as 30° with rotation of the arm. The posterior angulation, which was measured on the lateral radiograph, averaged approximately 25° with a range from −9° to 59°. Supplemental radiographic views, such as transthoracic and various rotational views, can at times be useful to estimate the amount of displacement of specific segments. These can also be useful in malunions, especially of fractures of the greater tuberosity.

Other Techniques

Several other diagnostic tests are helpful, including tomograms and CT. Tomograms can be useful in evaluating a proximal humeral fracture for a nonunion or for assessing the amount of articular surface (glenoid and humeral head) involvement (Fig. 16-8). However, in most instances, CT has replaced tomography as the procedure of choice in these cases. Morris and associates have reported a series of patients in which CT was helpful in judging the amount of displacement of greater tuberosity fractures.[221] CT is also extremely helpful in evaluating the amount of articular involvement with head-splitting fractures, impression fractures, chronic fracture–dislocations (Fig. 16-9), and glenoid rim fractures. Magnetic resonance imaging can more easily image in multiple planes and show the relation of tuberosity fragments to the rotator cuff tendons, but it is less helpful for cortical bone and is usually not indicated.

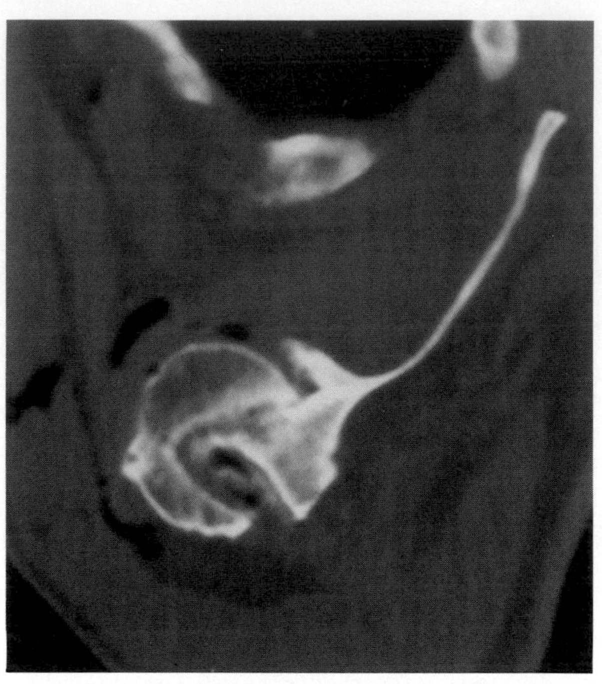

FIGURE 16-9. This 64-year-old man had a chronic anterior fracture–dislocation that was missed for approximately 1 year. This CT scan was helpful in evaluating the amount of head and glenoid involvement.

DIFFERENTIAL DIAGNOSIS

In most instances, the diagnosis of a fracture is readily made when proper and accurate radiographs of the shoulder are available. However, the patient may have acute pain, after a traumatic incident, with radiographs that rule out a fracture. The differential diagnosis of proximal humeral fractures includes any abnormality that causes acute pain, swelling, and loss of active motion. Acute hemorrhagic bursitis, a traumatic rotator cuff tear, a simple dislocation, an acromioclavicular separation, and calcific tendinitis may all present clinically with these symptoms. A fall on an outstretched hand may injure the soft tissues about the shoulder, causing hemorrhage into the subacromial space and leading to inflammation and scarring of the subacromial bursa. If this condition does not resolve several weeks after injury, then one must consider the possibility of a full-thickness rotator cuff tear, especially if the individual is older, if there was a previous anterior dislocation, or both. Greater tuberosity tenderness, weakness of forward elevation and external rotation, an arc of pain, and a positive impingement sign are usually present in these patients. If there is a high degree of suspicion, magnetic resonance imaging or an arthrogram is indicated. Calcific tendinitis may have been a preexisting problem that was activated by trauma. Patients with an acromioclavicular separation have direct tenderness over the acromioclavicular joint, and in more severe cases the distal clavicle is displaced superiorly. A careful history, in addition to radiographs, will help differentiate a spontaneously reduced dislocation.

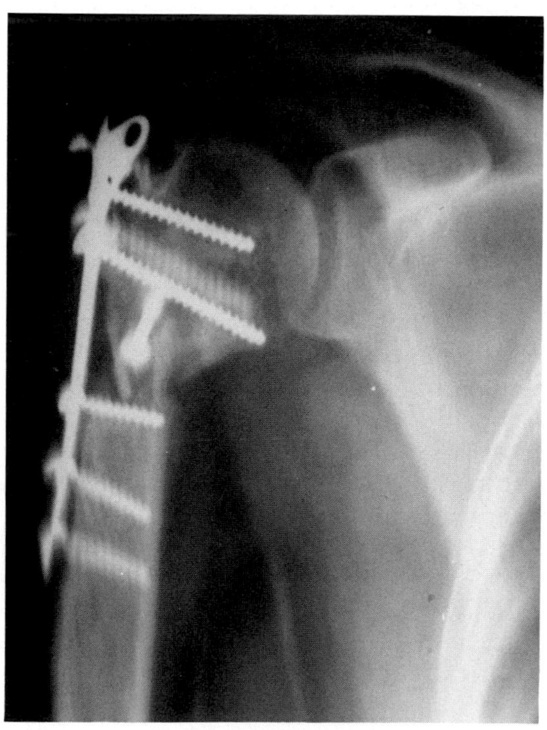

FIGURE 16-8. This patient had a nonunion of a comminuted proximal shaft fracture after buttress plate fixation. A tomogram was helpful in establishing a nonunion. Note that the plate is placed extremely high and impinging on the acromion. Also, the plate is distracting the fracture.

Another important factor to consider is the possibility of an underlying problem that may have contributed to the fracture. Treatment of a pathologic fracture is more complicated, and bone healing is usually compromised. One should suspect that a pathologic fracture may have occurred when a trivial incident is the cause. Metastatic carcinoma, metabolic bone disease, rheumatoid arthritis, osteonecrosis, and osteoporosis are some of the more common processes that may weaken bone and result in a pathologic fracture.

TREATMENT

Nonoperative Treatment

Many methods of treatment of proximal humeral fractures have been proposed through the years, creating a great deal of controversy and, at times, confusion. Fortunately, most proximal humeral fractures are minimally displaced and can be satisfactorily treated with a sling and early range-of-motion exercises. The controversy exists when the fractures are significantly displaced. Needless to say, it is imperative to make the appropriate diagnosis initially. Precise radiographs and a reproducible classification system are essential to achieve consistent treatment of displaced fractures. Through the years, various treatment methods have been proposed, including closed reduction, casts, splints, percutaneous pinning, open reduction and internal fixation, and the use of a humeral head prosthesis. However, one method does not fit all cases, and we must discriminate and use sound judgment to determine the appropriate treatment for each fracture.

Initial Immobilization and Early Motion

Initial immobilization and early motion has been described over the years as having a high degree of success, because most proximal humeral fractures are minimally displaced.[83,99,139,220,259,268,277,336] The shoulder has a large capsule, allowing a wide range of motion that can compensate for even moderate amounts of displacement. The arm is supported by a sling at the side or in the Velpeau position. A swathe may be needed in the immediate postfracture period to enhance immobilization and comfort. An axillary pad may also be useful. Gentle range-of-motion exercises can be started by 7 to 10 days after a fracture when the pain has diminished and the patient is less apprehensive. It is important to establish that the fracture is clinically stable and moves as a unit before exercises are started. Overly aggressive exercises may distract a minimally displaced fracture and result in a malunion or nonunion (Fig. 16-10). Intermittent radiographs in two perpendicular planes (anteroposterior and lateral in the scapular plane) are essential to determine if there have been any fractures. Bertoft and colleagues[25] have reported that the greatest amount of improvement in range of movement occurs between 3 and 8 weeks after injury. Therefore, it is very important to have an organized and supervised physiotherapy program in place during this period. The exercises can be performed by the patient at home, but supervision by a physical therapist is often beneficial. The exercises should be performed at least three to four times a day. The results of this treatment with complex displaced fractures are not as successful.

Closed Reduction

For years closed reduction has been a popular method of treatment for all types of displaced proximal humeral fractures.[101,114,153,213,268,334,350] However, it is important to differentiate between which fractures are suitable to closed reduction and which are not. Repeated and forcible attempts at closed reduction may complicate a fracture by causing further displacement, fragmentation, or neurovascular injury. Various other types of reduction maneuvers have been used with mixed results.[114,153,213,292,334]

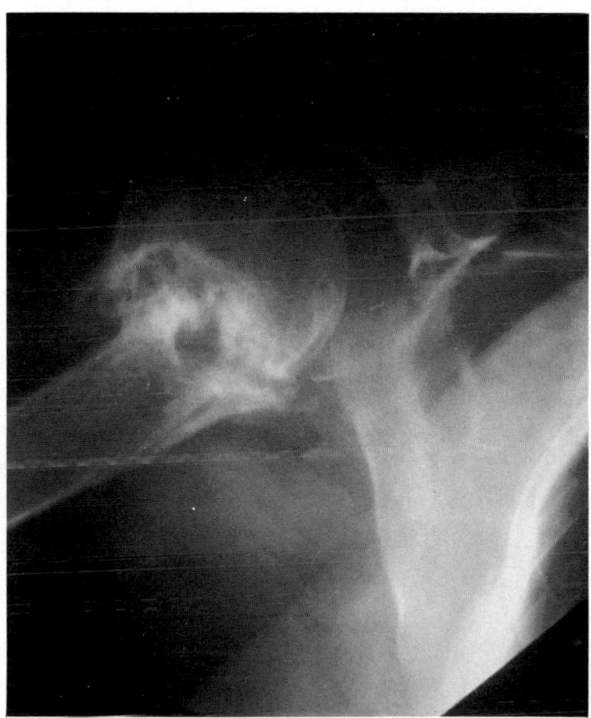

FIGURE 16-10. This minimally displaced surgical neck fracture progressed to a nonunion. Note the sclerotic margins of the fracture. This patient was started on overly aggressive physiotherapy and was not sufficiently supervised.

Before a closed reduction is performed, it is important to understand the type of deformity and the forces involved in the fracture. Watson-Jones[333] described a classic technique of hyperabduction and traction to achieve a closed reduction. This technique was thought necessary because in the surgical neck "abduction-type fracture" the proximal fragment was pulled into abduction. However, the deformity is anterior angulation and not hyperabduction; therefore, this type of reduction is not necessary. Also, in the displaced two-part surgical neck fracture, the deforming force is created by the pectoralis major muscle and other internal rotators pulling the shaft medially. This force must be neutralized by adducting the arm before an adequate reduction can be performed. Adequate relaxation is necessary for a closed reduction. The patient is usually more comfortable supine. An intravenous catheter should be in place in the contralateral arm; a muscle relaxant and narcotic should be given intravenously after a small test dose. Whenever possible, fluoroscopic C-arm visualization should be employed to enhance visualization of the reduction and precise location of the fracture fragments. Also, the stability of the fracture reduction can be tested in different positions. If a fracture after reduction is unstable, further operative stabilization may be necessary.

Two-Part Anatomical Neck Fracture

Displaced anatomical neck fractures are difficult to treat by closed reduction. The thickness of the head is quite small and the head may be rotated or angulated in the joint capsule, preventing adequate head and neck alignment. However, several other types of two-part fractures and fracture–dislocations are amenable to closed reduction.

Two-Part Surgical Neck Fracture

In the displaced two-part surgical neck fracture, both tuberosities are attached to the head, so that it remains in a neutral position. The shaft is usually displaced medially by the pull of the pectoralis major. The hyperabduction overhead technique is not required, nor is significant traction with weight needed. Gentle traction with flexion and some adduction is usually all that is required to reduce the shaft fragment, so that it can be impacted under the head. If reduction is not possible, there may be interposition of soft tissue, either muscle, capsule, or long head of the biceps tendon. Usually in these cases, the long head of the biceps is caught in the fracture site, creating a tether that will distract the fracture with repeated attempts at reduction (Fig. 16-11). This situation requires open reduction and internal fixation. An impacted but angulated two-part surgical neck fracture can also be improved with a closed reduction. If the anterior angulation is more than 45°, this will later limit forward elevation. The head should be disimpacted from the shaft; then the shaft is reduced and placed underneath the head with less anterior angulation. A comminuted fracture can be treated with a closed reduction if it is undisplaced and stable, but displaced and unstable fractures require open reduction and internal fixation to properly align the fragments.[51,53,61,216,229,280,291,305,311,350]

Two-Part Greater Tuberosity Fracture

Greater tuberosity fractures are usually retracted posteriorly and superiorly, and closed reduction is difficult. However, if this fracture is associated with an anterior

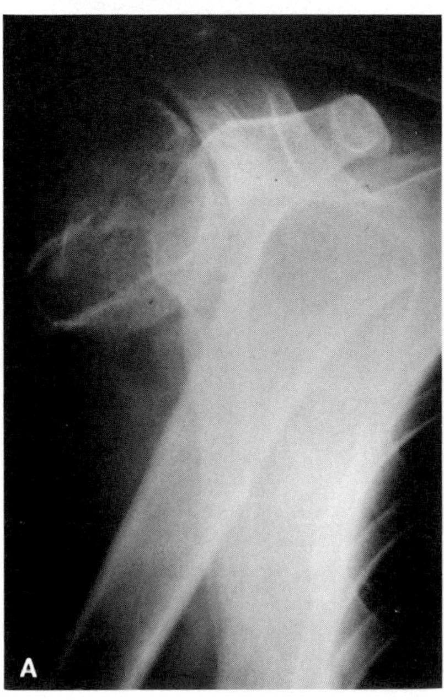

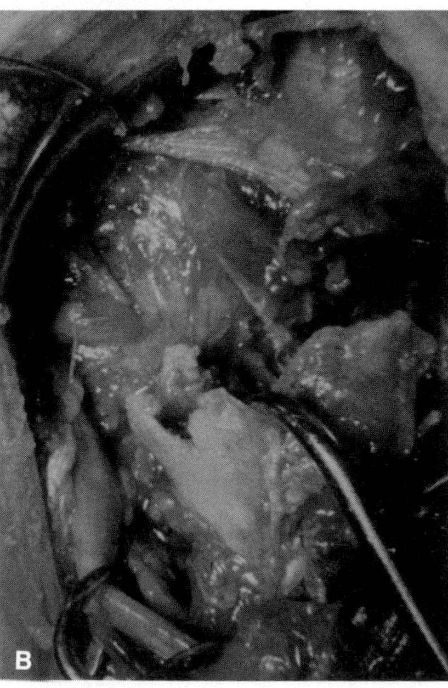

FIGURE 16-11. (**A**) An anteroposterior x-ray of a displaced two-part surgical neck fracture. The shaft is displaced medially by the pull of the pectoralis major muscle. Several attempts at closed reduction were performed both in the emergency department and in the operating room with the patient under general anesthesia and with the use of an image intensifier. However, the fracture could not be reduced. (**B**) Operative photograph at the time of surgery showing interposition of the biceps tendon between the proximal fragment and the shaft. The loop retractor is on the biceps tendon, which was tethering the head and wedged between the shaft and the head, preventing reduction.

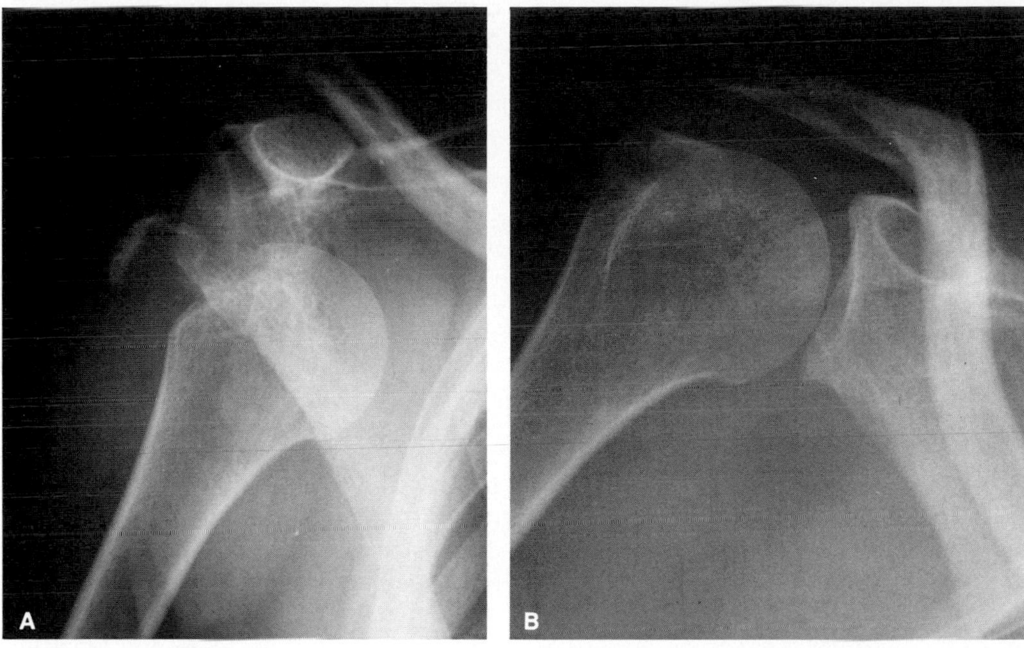

FIGURE 16-12. (**A**) An anteroposterior x-ray of a two-part anterior fracture–dislocation with a displaced greater tuberosity fracture. (**B**) After a closed reduction, the greater tuberosity fracture reduced and healed without further displacement. The patient achieved a normal range of motion without any further anterior dislocations.

dislocation, a closed reduction of the glenohumeral dislocation may successfully reduce the greater tuberosity fracture (Fig. 16-12). If the fracture heals in an adequate alignment, the chance of recurrent dislocation is low. However, there is a tendency for the greater tuberosity fragment to displace superiorly and posteriorly after a reduction (Fig. 16-13).[204] If this fragment is not properly reduced, a malunion can occur that will block glenohumeral motion (Fig. 16-14). One author[246] reported a case in which the fracture of the greater tuberosity blocked reduction of the anterior glenohumeral dislocation. Isolated greater tuberosity fractures are associated with an anterior dislocation in 5% to 8% of cases,[110,268,289] though higher rates (between 10% and 15%) have also been reported.[211,213,238,336]

Two-Part Lesser Tuberosity Fracture

If the fragment is small and does not block internal rotation, successful treatment by closed reduction of the rare two-part lesser tuberosity fracture has been reported.[147,238,274] Usually, this injury is associated with a posterior dislocation and may also be treated by closed reduction if the articular involvement is minimal and the injury occurred within 2 to 3 weeks (Fig. 16-15). The arm should be immobilized in neutral or slight external rotation.

Three-Part Fractures

Three-part fractures are quite unstable and difficult to treat by closed reduction. They have a tuberosity fragment as well as a surgical neck fragment. In three-

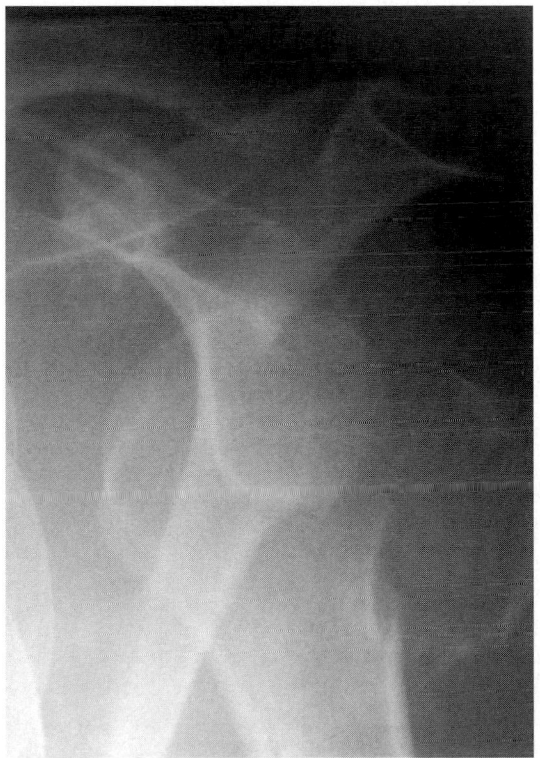

FIGURE 16-13. In this case, the greater tuberosity fragment remained displaced after closed reduction of the dislocation and required open reduction and internal fixation with nonabsorbable sutures.

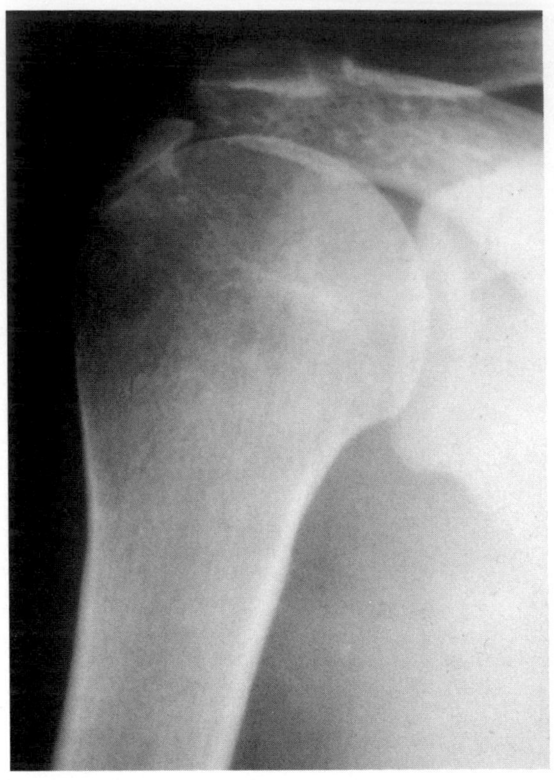

FIGURE 16-14. This greater tuberosity malunion resulted from the unopposed pull of the supraspinatus and infraspinatus muscles, which displaced the fragment superiorly and posteriorly. Several attempts at closed reduction were performed both in the emergency department and in the operating room with the patient under general anesthesia and with the use of an image intensifier. However, the fracture could not be reduced.

part lesser tuberosity fractures, the greater tuberosity is attached to the head, pulling it into external rotation (ie, the articular surface faces anteriorly). In a three-part fracture of the greater tuberosity, the lesser tuberosity remains attached to the head, pulling it into internal rotation (ie, the articular surface faces posteriorly). In addition, the shaft is pulled medially by the pectoralis major, adding another component to be considered during the closed reduction. These deforming forces would have to be considered if a closed reduction were to be attempted. The long head of the biceps tendon may also be caught between the fragments, obstructing the reduction. Repeated attempts at a closed reduction in these fractures should not be done, because most of them are in elderly persons with osteoporotic bone, and these reductions may result in further comminution of the fracture. However, several authors have reported good results with closed reduction of three-part fractures.[83,184,217,350] The better results were in older sedentary individuals with limited goals. The pain relief was adequate, but functional activity was limited. Dingley and Denham[78] have described a modified closed technique for fracture–dislocations. They use a percutaneous pin in the dislocated head to facilitate reduction and then remove the pin. Other literature has reported poor results with closed reduction, a high incidence of pain, malunion, and avascular necrosis.[51,101,119,159,235,311]

Four-Part Fractures

Closed reduction of four-part fractures of the proximal humerus generally produces poor results. In various series, there has been an extremely high incidence of avascular necrosis, between 13% and 34%.[101,119,159,229,253,288,305,311] Malunion and degenerative arthritis also occur. Lee and Hansen[180] have reported the only series of satisfactory results with closed reduction.

Impression Fractures

If a missed dislocation with an impression fracture is diagnosed within 2 to 3 weeks, and the impression fracture of the head is less than 20%, then an attempt at a closed reduction may be worthwhile. It is important to accurately assess the amount of the head impression fracture with a CT scan or axillary radiographic view to judge whether the reduction will be stable. An adequate result may be obtained with a closed reduction in some displaced fractures, because the shoulder has a great capacity to compensate within a restricted range of motion. Many functional activities involving the shoulder can be done with a restricted range of motion. However, an anatomical reduction should be the goal in the treatment of most displaced fractures of the proximal humerus. In older, sedentary individuals, who do not place great demands on the

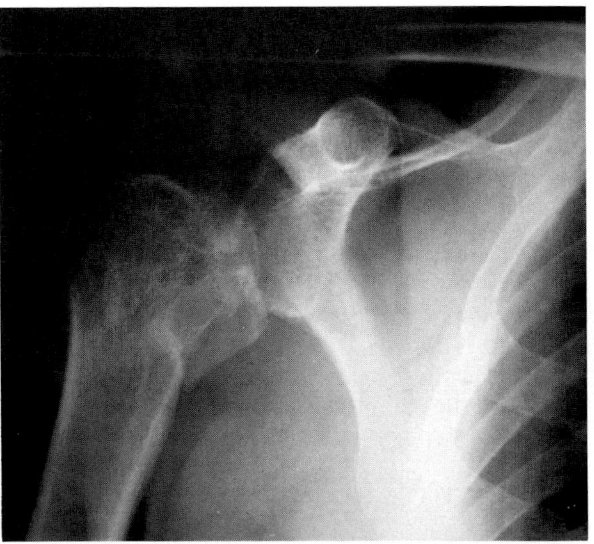

FIGURE 16-15. An anteroposterior x-ray of a two-part posterior fracture–dislocation after reduction. The lesser tuberosity fragment was minimally displaced and did not block medial rotation. This injury was treated closed with excellent return of function.

shoulder, one may accept a less than perfect reduction, especially in the nondominant extremity.

Percutaneous Pins and External Fixation

Percutaneous pinning may be used after a closed reduction if the reduction is unstable.[147,162,167,171,172] This technique is very useful in the treatment of unimpacted two-part surgical neck fractures. Jacob and coworkers[147] have outlined the technique and reported satisfactory results in 35 of 40 cases. In another more recent series of percutaneous stabilization of unstable fractures of the proximal humerus, Jaberg and associates[146] found good or excellent results in 34 of 48 patients (70%). This series included not only displaced surgical neck fractures but also fractures of a higher complexity (three and four parts). The authors suggested that this method of treatment is technically demanding but offers the advantage of less disruption of soft tissues and minimal fixation, thus reducing the prevalence of avascular necrosis.

In this technique, two 2.5-mm terminally threaded AO pins are placed into the proximal shaft near the deltoid insertion and are directed superiorly into the humeral head, using fluoroscopic guidance. A third pin is passed from the anterior cortex into the head fragment. In addition, if the greater tuberosity is displaced, two pins are inserted in a retrograde direction through the tuberosity to engage the medial cortex of the shaft. The pins are trimmed beneath the skin, and the arm is immobilized for 3 weeks in a Velpeau dressing.[146] The pins are removed when there is adequate stability of the fracture, and range of motion can progress without fear of displacement.

Kristiansen and Kofoed have reported satisfactory results with the use of transcutaneous pin reduction combined with external fixation for three- and four-part fractures.[171,172] In a series of 31 displaced proximal humeral fractures, this technique was compared with closed reduction and the results with percutaneous pinning were better. It is important to place the pins laterally to avoid injury to neurovascular structures, including the cephalic vein, and to avoid limitation of glenohumeral motion.[167]

Plaster Splints and Casts

Many types of splints and casts have been proposed through the years, with varying success, for the treatment of displaced proximal humerus fractures.[4,14,83,114,145,240,285,292,334,336,339,340,346] A sling and swathe or Velpeau sling are the most commonly used methods of immobilization for proximal humeral fractures, and more elaborate devices are generally not required. However, a plaster slab along the humeral shaft and superior aspect of the shoulder can be used for extra support and comfort.

Older literature suggested that reduction in an abducted and flexed position was essential for proper alignment. Milch[213,214] and others[292,334] thought that the abducted and overhead position better neutralized the muscle forces about the shoulder than the anatomical position of Kocher, with the arm at the side. The shoulder spica casts and braces needed to maintain this position were extremely cumbersome and uncomfortable for the patient. These devices began to lose popularity in the 1920s.[268] However, a shoulder spica cast with some degree of abduction (20° to 30°) may be needed to provide extra stability for a severely comminuted fracture of the proximal humerus. Jakob and coworkers[147] recommend the use of an abduction splint for the treatment of selected greater tuberosity fractures.

Good results have been reported with the hanging cast, especially with humeral shaft fractures.[44–46,113,143,145,174,258,340,346] However, a significant amount of patient cooperation is required, and frequent supervision is necessary to avoid angulation and distraction. The weight of a heavy cast may cause distraction of the fracture fragments. This is especially true of comminuted proximal shaft fractures in which there is inferior subluxation.[317] Stewart and Hundley[308] recommended supplementing a hanging cast with an abduction brace for extra support and comfort in the immediate postfracture period. In general, the use of hanging casts for fractures of the proximal humerus should be avoided, since there is a tendency for distraction of the fracture fragments, leading to nonunion or malunion. The hanging cast technique may be more applicable to the treatment of humeral shaft fractures.

Skeletal Traction

The use of traction is not commonly indicated but may be helpful in the management of a comminuted fracture.[158,230,238,240] Traction can be difficult to maintain and restricts patient mobility, especially if the patient has multiple injuries and requires other diagnostic and treatment procedures. However, it can provide temporary benefit until a more definitive procedure can be performed.

The arm should be held in a flexed position and in slight adduction to relax the pectoralis major, which is the most important deforming force. The abducted position should be avoided. The shoulder is flexed to 90°, and the elbow is also flexed to 90°. A threaded Kirschner wire, a Steinmann pin, or an AO screw should be placed in the ulna and the forearm and wrist suspended in a sling. This allows hand and elbow motion to avoid stiffness. The goal is to try to hold the shaft fragment in a neutral position, since in this fracture both tuberosities are attached to the head and the head is essentially in a neutral position. When there is sufficient callus formation, the traction can be discontinued and the patient's arm placed in a sling or spica cast.

Operative Treatment of Open Reduction and Internal Fixation

Open reduction of displaced fractures gained popularity in the early part of the 20th century.[19,47,52,110,155,252,268,279,285,314] In many instances, closed reduction and external fixation was unable to correct deformity and maintain reduction sufficiently. Various techniques and devices have been proposed to treat fractures of the proximal humerus. The choice of technique and device depends on several factors, including the type of fracture, quality of the bone and soft tissue, and age and reliability of the patient. The goal of internal fixation should be a stable reduction allowing for early motion of the shoulder. The current trend is toward limited dissection of the soft tissue about the fracture fragments and the use of a minimal amount of hardware required for stable fixation.[53]

Two-Part Anatomical Neck Fracture

Anatomical neck fractures are extremely rare, and very few cases are reported in the literature on which to base a discussion concerning treatment. The prognosis for survival of the humeral head is poor, since it has been completely separated from its blood supply. However, several authors recommend an attempt at open reduction and internal fixation, especially if the patient is young.[71,147,163,238] If the small humeral head cannot be secured to the proximal humerus, then excision of the humeral head and replacement with a prosthesis is indicated.

Two-Part Surgical Neck Fracture

Two-part displaced surgical neck fractures may require open reduction and internal fixation, either because interposition of soft tissue prevents a closed reduction or the reduction is not stable. Various devices have been proposed for fixation, including intramedullary nails or rods, plates and screws, staples, wire, nonabsorbable suture material, multiple pins, and combinations of these.

The Rush rod technique can be performed through a very limited incision and split in the deltoid and rotator cuff. The rod has been a very popular device, and several authors have reported good results.[183,281,317,337,344] However, the relative inability of this device to control rotation may be inadequate for some displaced surgical neck fractures. Furthermore, a second procedure may be required to remove the device, since it can impinge against the anterior or inferior acromion during forward elevation and rotation. This technique may be useful in older, debilitated patients in whom minimal surgery is indicated and the functional goals are limited. The use of an AO buttress plate and screws has been associated with good results, especially with two-part surgical neck fractures, but the soft-tissue dissection should be limited and the bone quality must be adequate for screw fixation. Yamano[348] has reported a high success rate with a hooked plate. The use of a figure-of-eight tension-band technique with wire or nonabsorbable sutures is also useful and usually provides adequate fixation (Fig. 16-16), although one series reported a loss of fixation with a modified tension band wiring technique in 27% (4 of 14 fractures).[164] If the quality of the bone is poor, then the sutures can be passed through the rotator cuff for proximal fixation, since it may be stronger than the bone. In cases involving comminution, intramedullary fixation with either a Rush rod or Enders nails will improve fixation and maintain length (Fig. 16-17). The Enders rod in Figure 16-18 has been adapted to have a more superior hole for the passage of sutures. This allows for deeper placement of the rod in the rotator cuff so that it is less prominent, avoiding impingement against the acromion.

Two-Part Greater Tuberosity Fracture

Greater tuberosity fractures that are displaced more than 1 cm may require open reduction and internal fixation because the posterior and superior displacement will cause impingement beneath the acromion (Fig. 16-19).[71,204,229] Screws, wire, and suture material have all been proposed as types of fixation of the greater tuberosity. The rent in the rotator cuff that occurs with displaced greater tuberosity fractures must also be repaired. Screws may not provide adequate fixation in osteoporotic bone (Fig. 16-20). Nonabsorbable sutures are probably a better choice of fixation.

Two-Part Lesser Tuberosity Fracture

Displaced isolated fractures of the lesser tuberosity are rare injuries and may require internal fixation with nonabsorbable sutures, especially if the fragment is quite large and blocks medial rotation.[8,116,147,173,203,238,274,296,344] Stangl[306] has described removal of the bone fragment and suture of the subscapularis tendon to the cortical edge of the fracture site. When the fragment is large, it may involve part of the articular surface.

Three-Part Fractures

Open reduction and internal fixation is the treatment of choice of displaced three-part fractures of the proximal humerus.[2,86,119,125,248,273,286] It is important to avoid extensive exposure and soft-tissue dissection of the fragments, which may compromise blood supply. Hagg and Lundberg[119] have reported a high rate of avascular

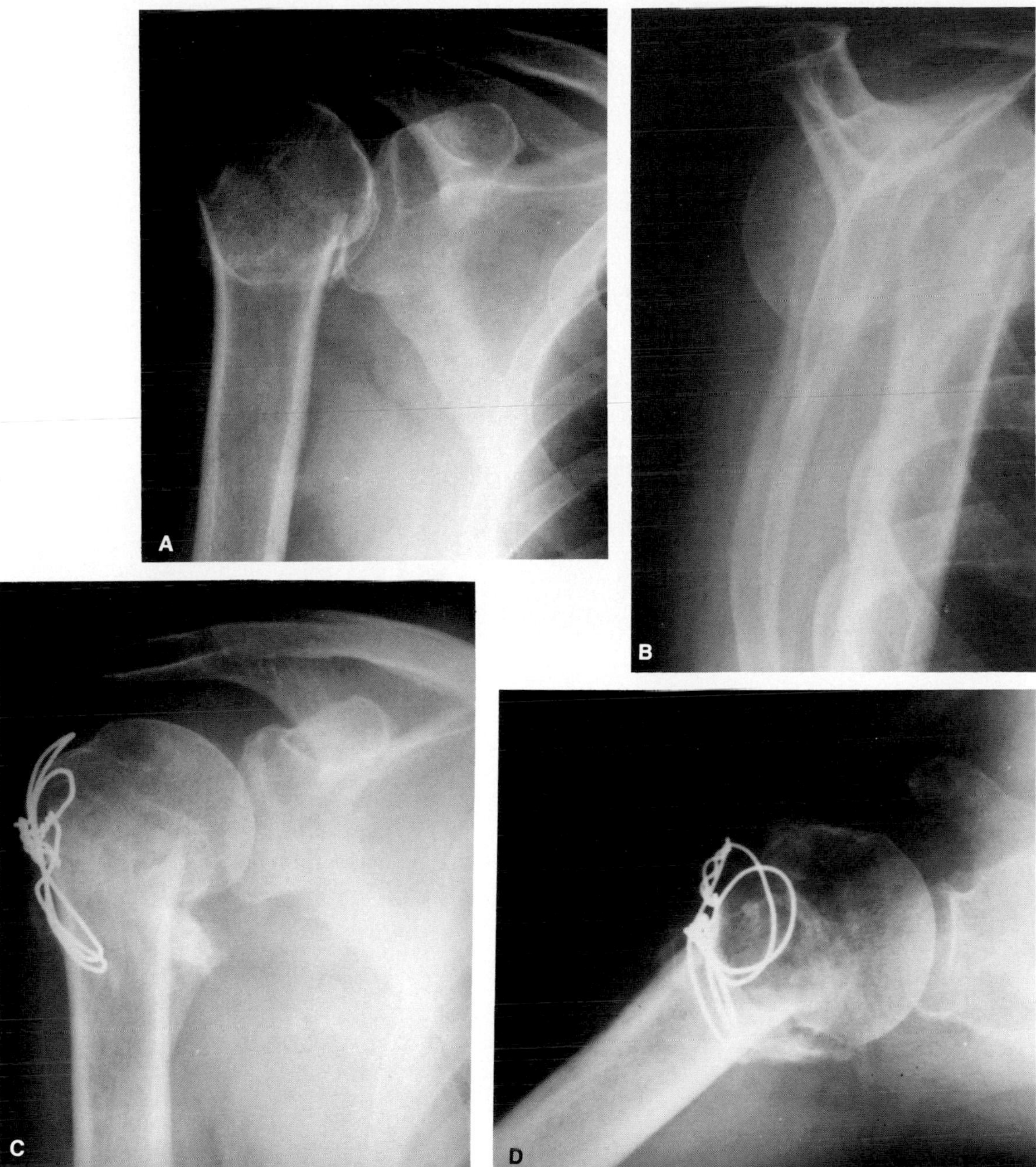

FIGURE 16-16. (**A**) Anteroposterior and lateral x-rays of a displaced surgical neck fracture. (**B**) This fracture was treated for 3 weeks as an undisplaced fracture on the basis of an anteroposterior x-ray only. The follow-up lateral x-ray in the scapular plane revealed a significant anterior shaft displacement. (**C** and **D**) Anteroposterior and lateral x-rays after open reduction and internal fixation with two figure-of-eight wires. The wires are placed through both the cuff and the tuberosities, as well as the proximal shaft. We now prefer the use of heavy nonabsorbable sutures over wire, when open reduction and internal fixation are chosen for displaced surgical neck fractures.

necrosis, between 12% and 25%, in a review of several series of open reduction and internal fixation of three-part fractures.

Regardless of the type of fixation used, it must secure the displaced tuberosity to both the humeral head and shaft. The use of intramedullary nails or rods is usually not adequate fixation to neutralize the deforming forces in this type of fracture and could result in a malunion (Fig. 16-21). Mouradian[223] developed an intramedullary nail with screw fixation for the head and tuberosities. However, the incidence of avascular necrosis was high and follow-up was short. The AO

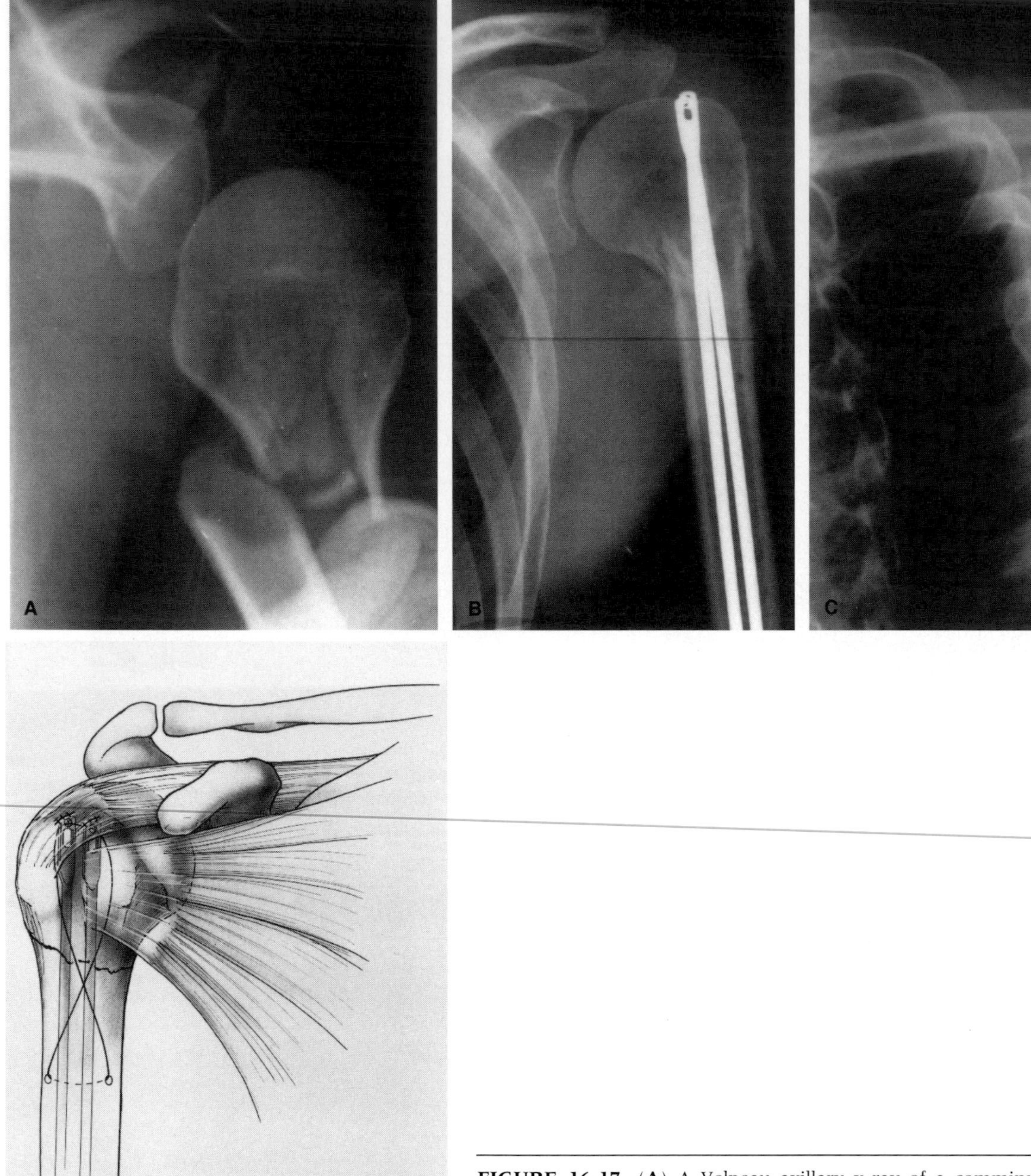

FIGURE 16-17. (**A**) A Velpeau axillary x-ray of a comminuted displaced surgical neck fracture. (**B** and **C**) Anteroposterior and lateral x-rays after open reduction and internal fixation with two Enders nails as well as heavy nonabsorbable sutures. (**D**) Schematic showing figure-of-eight suture configuration in combination with Enders rods.

buttress plate technique has been a popular procedure for this fracture, but reports from several authors have reflected poor results with the AO plate for both three- and four-part fractures.[169,170,248,310] The complications include avascular necrosis secondary to extensive soft-tissue dissection, superior placement of the plate leading to impingement, loss of plate fixation with screw loosening, malunion, and infection. Paavolainen and coworkers[248] reported that the most common technical error was placing the plate too high on the greater tuberosity, which restricted motion and reduced the fracture into a varus deformity (see Fig. 16-8). Kristiansen and Christensen[169] reported 55% unsatisfactory results in a series of 20 patients with two-, three-, and four-part fractures that were managed with plates and screws. Sturzenegger and colleagues[310] have reported a high incidence (34%) of avascular necrosis.

Neer[229] reported good results with internal fixation

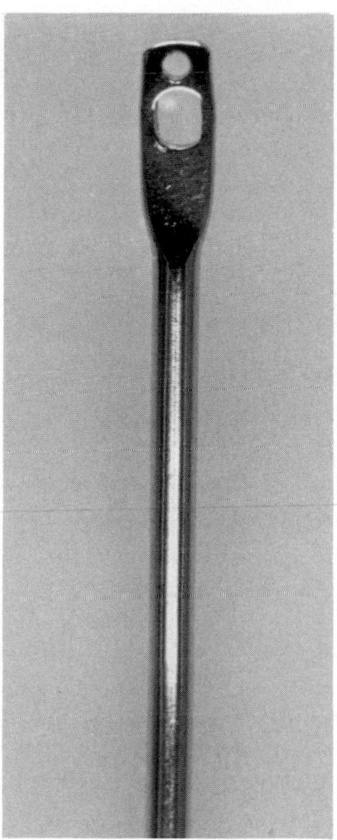

FIGURE 16-18. An Enders rod modified with a superior hole for passage of wire or suture. This allows for deeper seating of the rod into the rotator cuff.

of three-part fractures, if the displaced tuberosity is reattached to the shaft and head with either wire or, more recently, nonabsorbable suture. The poor results in his series were due to tuberosity displacement from failure of vertical fixation devices (Rush rods, Kirschner wires, splints) to hold the tuberosities in position. Hawkins and coworkers,[125] in 1986, reported in a series of 15 patients that good results were obtained in 14 patients with the use of a figure-of-eight wire for three-part fractures of the proximal humerus. The only early failure in their series occurred in a patient who had a T-plate and screws for fixation. In two patients, avascular necrosis developed, and one patient required a humeral head prosthesis. In osteoporotic bone, the soft tissues of the rotator cuff are stronger than the bone, and these can be incorporated into the fracture fixation to strengthen the construct. Wire or heavy nonabsorbable suture can be passed through the rotator cuff as well as the bone of the tuberosity and then attached to the shaft below. This method usually supplies sufficient stability to begin early motion.

Four-Part Fractures

Open reduction and internal fixation of four-part fractures generally yields unsatisfactory results, as confirmed by numerous reports.[119,155,169,216,229,248,305,310,312,313] The complications are essentially the same as with three-part fractures, just more severe and with a higher percentage of avascular necrosis and malunion.A significant number of four-part fractures occur in the elderly, in whom osteoporosis and poor bone quality are more common. This is not the ideal setting for internal fixation with pins, rods, or plate and screws. Jakob and associates[147,148] have reported that open reduction and internal fixation with multiple pins (minimal fixation techniques) of a subgroup of four-part fractures may be indicated (Fig. 16-22). In this group, which these authors have called "four-part valgus impacted fractures," the head is impacted on the shaft and the tuberosities are split but in close proximity to the head and shaft. The head is not dislocated or displaced laterally, and some contact with the glenoid is maintained. However, this type of fracture is not a true four-part displacement, according to the Neer classification. The humeral head is elevated, and the tuberosities are placed beneath it. Multiple pins are used to provide fixation and left under the skin subcutaneously. The pins are removed between the fourth and sixth weeks, when early healing and some stability occur. In a series of 19 "valgus impacted four-part fractures" treated by this method, Jakob and associates[147,148] reported 74% satisfactory results. The major reason for failure was avascular necrosis, which occurred in 5 cases (26%). As a rule, however, the results of internal fixation of four-part fractures are generally poor.

Replacement Prosthesis

The use of the humeral head prosthesis for fractures of the proximal humerus was first reported in the early 1950s. Several authors reported different designs that were being developed for use in displaced fracture–dislocations of the proximal humerus.[9,82,88,177,235,254,265,324,325] The design that has become the most commonly used was developed by Neer. In 1953, Neer[235] reported the first use of this prosthesis for complex fracture–dislocation of the proximal humerus.

At that time, treatment options for this fracture included closed reduction,[97] open reduction and internal fixation,[235,272,287] arthrodesis,[235] and humeral head excision.[150,151] The results were usually unsatisfactory for all these treatments. However, several authors earlier in this century reported satisfactory results with humeral head excision.[212,322] The use of this procedure yields a weakened, short, and painful extremity. In 1955 and 1970, Neer[229,232] reported on a series of patients successfully treated with the proximal humeral prosthesis. The original prosthesis (Fig. 16-23) was revised by Neer in 1973 to a more anatomical surface design (Fig. 16-24).

The prosthesis has two head sizes—15 and 22 mm in thickness. The larger gives better leverage and me-

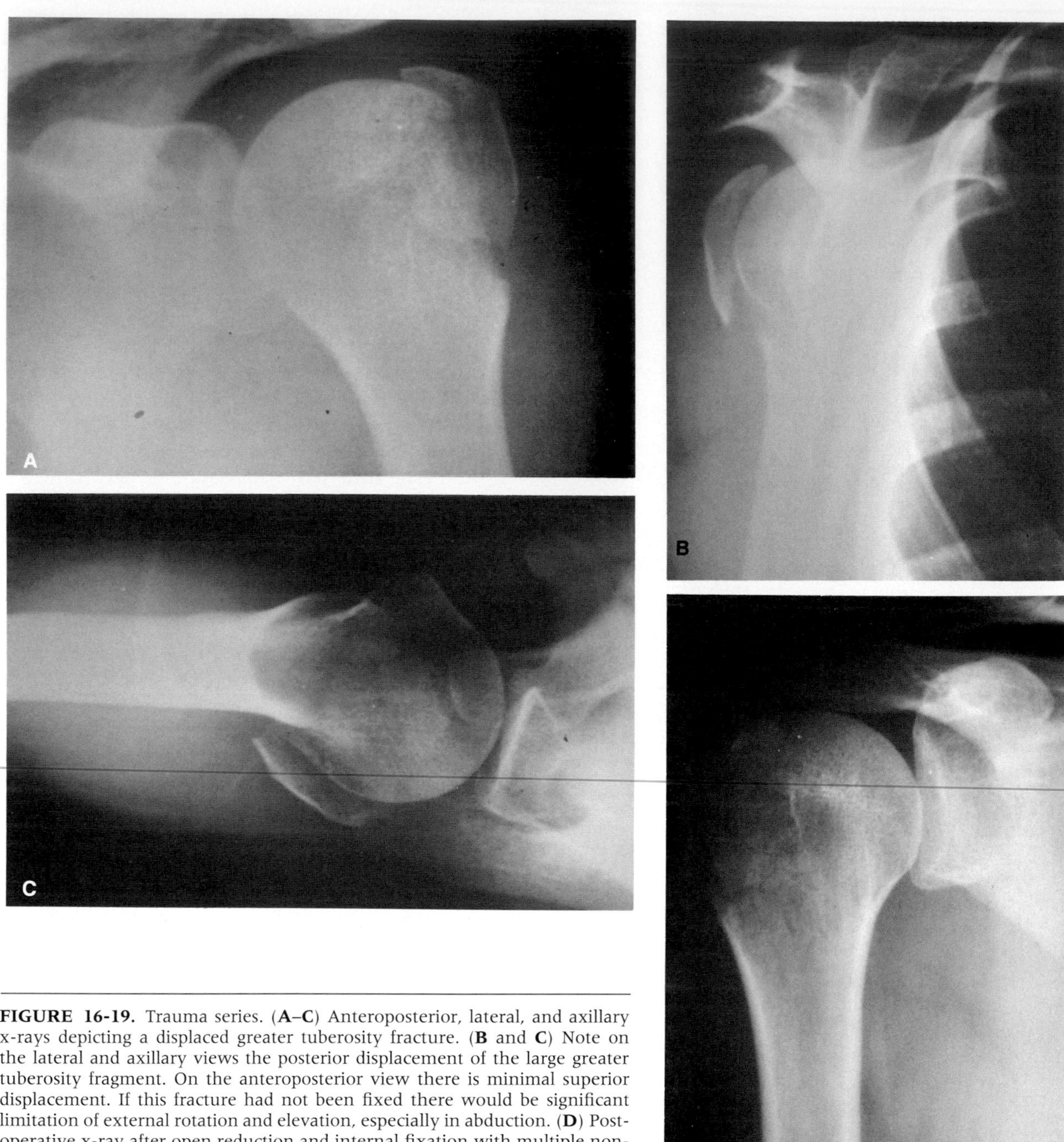

FIGURE 16-19. Trauma series. (**A–C**) Anteroposterior, lateral, and axillary x-rays depicting a displaced greater tuberosity fracture. (**B** and **C**) Note on the lateral and axillary views the posterior displacement of the large greater tuberosity fragment. On the anteroposterior view there is minimal superior displacement. If this fracture had not been fixed there would be significant limitation of external rotation and elevation, especially in abduction. (**D**) Postoperative x-ray after open reduction and internal fixation with multiple nonabsorbable sutures.

chanical advantage for forward elevation, but the smaller may be required for coverage by the rotator cuff. There are three stem sizes—7, 9.5, and 12 mm—and two stem lengths—125 and 150 mm (see Fig. 16-24). Longer stem lengths are available on special order if needed to bridge a shaft fracture.

The surgical technique has evolved over the past 30 years, and it is reliable for four-part fractures and fracture–dislocations of the proximal humerus. Most recently, Neer and McIlveen[237] have reported better results secondary to technical considerations concerning the anatomical approach, surgical technique, and rehabilitation. Results in 51 of the 61 patients in their series were rated excellent, nine satisfactory, and only one unsatisfactory. The technical considerations are outlined in the next section in the description of the technique. Several other series have reported good results using this prosthesis; pain relief and function were adequate.[72,73,96,127,313,321] Others have reported adequate pain relief but a higher incidence of unsatisfactory results secondary to postoperative stiffness and limitation of function.[81,166,197,217,342]

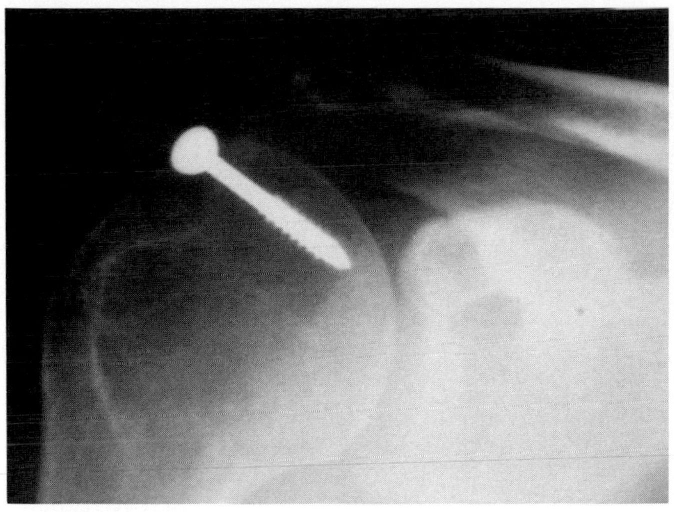

FIGURE 16-20. Anteroposterior x-ray of an AO screw that had migrated superiorly with the greater tuberosity fragment. This led to significant impingement and loss of motion. There was loss of fixation of the screw, since it was placed in the soft cancellous bone of the humeral head.

Modular hemiarthroplasty has been used in the treatment of complex fractures of the proximal humerus.[219] The modular humeral design offers greater flexibility in head sizes, perhaps allowing more precise tensioning of the soft tissue. Moreover, the ability to disassemble the component allows easier access to the glenoid if revision to a total shoulder replacement is later necessary. This eliminates the need to remove a well-fixed humeral component during revision surgery.[219,294] However, dissociation of modular components has also been reported.[30]

The surgical approach, care of the soft tissues, and postoperative rehabilitation are as important as the insertion of the prosthesis. A humeral head prosthesis may be required for an anatomical neck fracture if internal fixation is not feasible. Also, in certain comminuted osteoporotic three-part fractures in older individuals, a primary humeral head prosthesis may be a better choice than internal fixation, because the poor bone quality does not allow sufficient stability with internal fixation to allow early motion.[53,238,313] A humeral head prosthesis allows secure tuberosity fixation, so that rehabilitation can be started earlier and a more functional result can be achieved. A prosthesis is indicated in head-splitting fractures and also impression fractures in which more than 45% of the articular surface is involved. The results with prosthetic replacement in acute fractures are generally better than the results with humeral hemiarthroplasty in chronic fractures or from revisions of failed internal fixation. In the latter situations, tuberosity malunion, soft-tissue contracture and adhesions, and nerve injury make successful prosthetic reconstruction more difficult.

Fracture–Dislocation

Two- and three-part fracture–dislocations are readily treated by open reduction and internal fixation. In these fracture–dislocations, the vascular supply to the head is maintained by the soft-tissue attachments to the intact tuberosity, and, therefore, adequate fixation should be attained by the procedures that have been previously outlined. Redislocation is rare after adequate fracture healing. In two-part fracture–dislocations, a closed reduction may have adequately treated the glenohumeral dislocation; but if there is a persistent tuberosity displacement, this requires open reduction and internal fixation. The results from internal fixation of four-part fracture–dislocations have been poor, and a prosthesis is generally indicated in this type of lesion (Fig. 16-25).

Surgical Approaches

There are two basic surgical approaches for treatment of the proximal humeral fractures. The first is the superior deltoid approach (Fig. 16-26*A*).[238] The skin incision is made in Langer's lines just lateral to the anterolateral aspect of the acromion. Through this approach the deltoid can be split from the edge of the acromion distally for 4 to 5 cm (see Fig. 16-26*B*). The deltoid origin is not removed, allowing exposure of the supe-

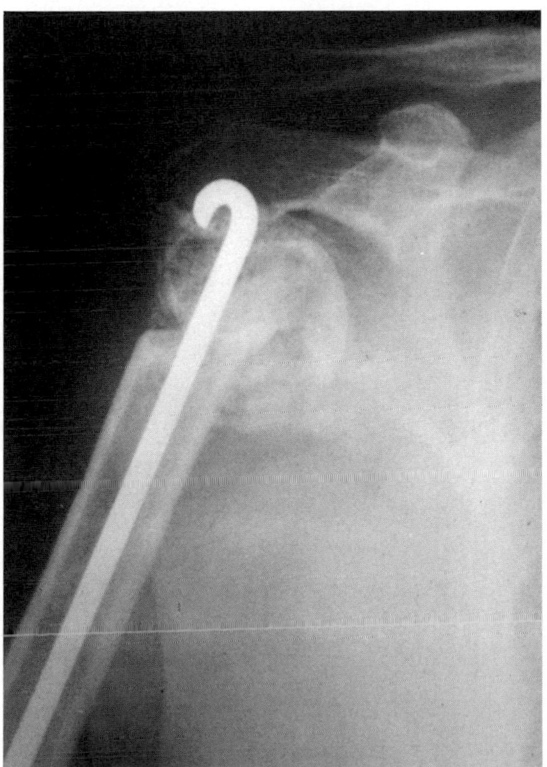

FIGURE 16-21. Anteroposterior x-ray of a malunion of a three-part fracture of the proximal humerus. The Rush rod alone was not sufficient to provide adequate fixation of the displaced fragments.

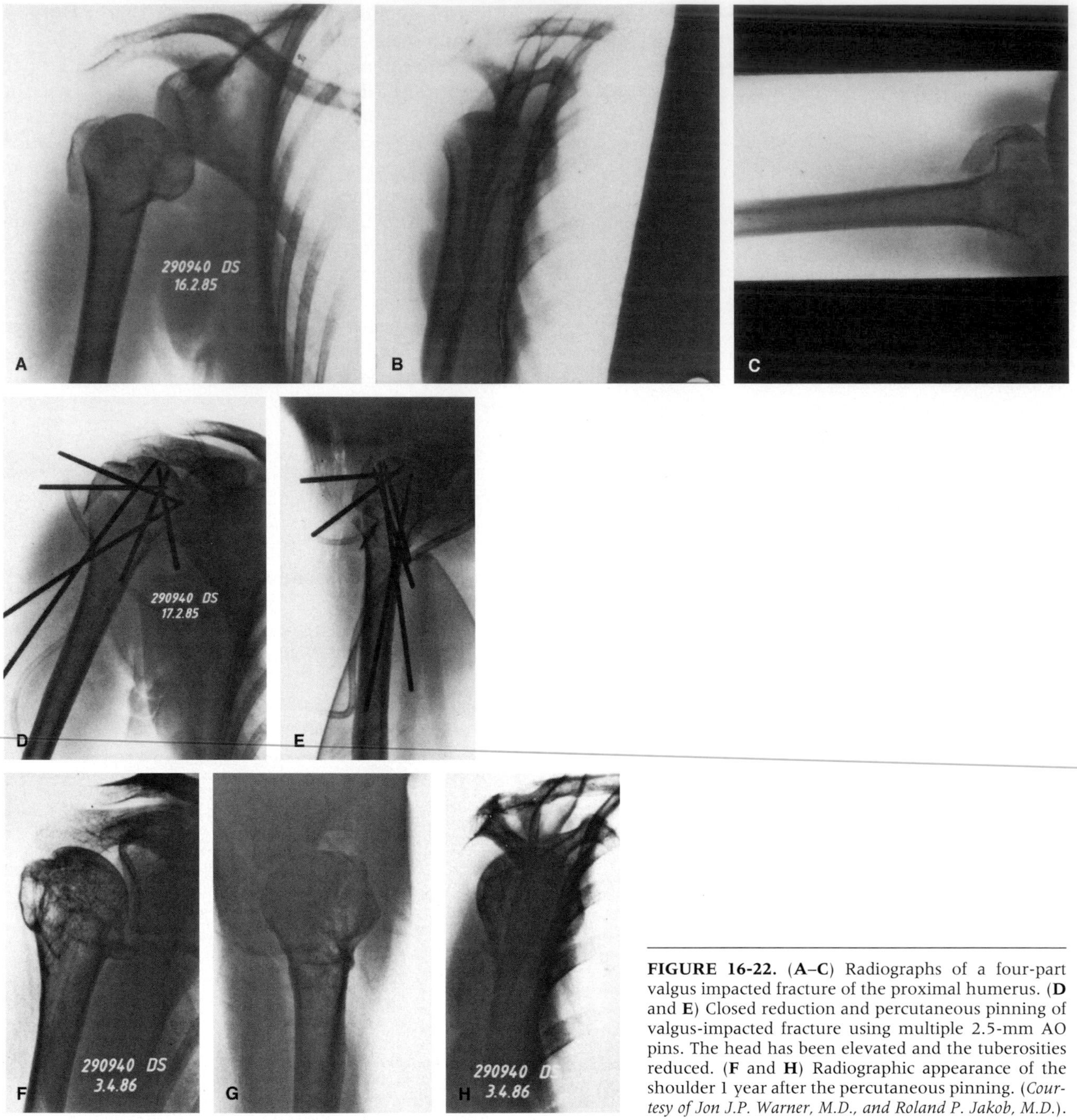

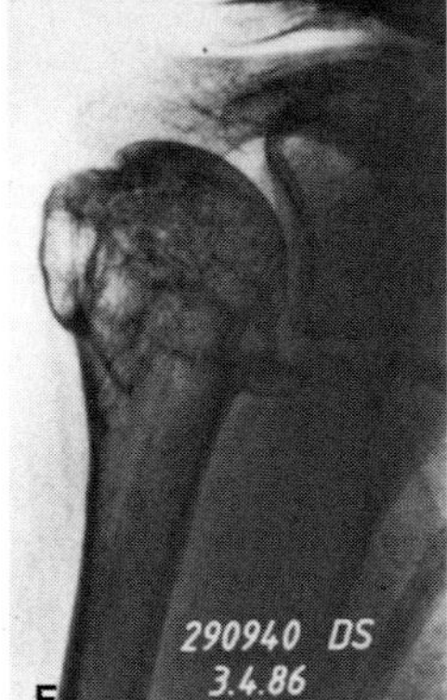

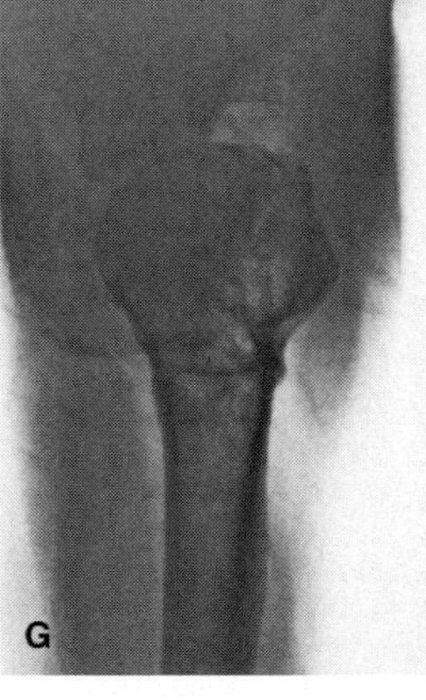

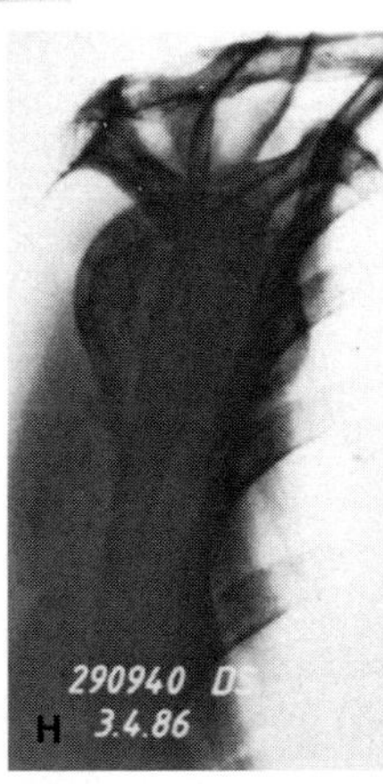

FIGURE 16-22. (**A–C**) Radiographs of a four-part valgus impacted fracture of the proximal humerus. (**D** and **E**) Closed reduction and percutaneous pinning of valgus-impacted fracture using multiple 2.5-mm AO pins. The head has been elevated and the tuberosities reduced. (**F** and **H**) Radiographic appearance of the shoulder 1 year after the percutaneous pinning. (*Courtesy of Jon J.P. Warner, M.D., and Roland P. Jakob, M.D.*).

rior aspect of the proximal humerus. This approach is useful for internal fixation of fractures of the greater tuberosity and is helpful for the insertion of a proximal intramedullary rod. Rotation, flexion, or extension of the humerus or all three greatly enhance exposure of the underlying structures.

The second approach is a long deltopectoral approach (Fig. 16-27*A*).[239] In this approach both the deltoid origin and insertion are preserved. The skin incision is started just inferior to the clavicle and extends across the coracoid process and down to the area of insertion of the deltoid. The cephalic vein should be preserved and retracted either laterally or medially, depending on which is the easiest direction. The deltopectoral interval is dissected proximally and distally (see Fig. 16-27*B*). If more exposure is needed, the superior part of the pectoralis major tendon insertion can be divided.

Procedures that split or remove the lateral part of the acromion are unnecessary and may lead to complications. Both of these approaches are extremely worthwhile because they preserve deltoid function,

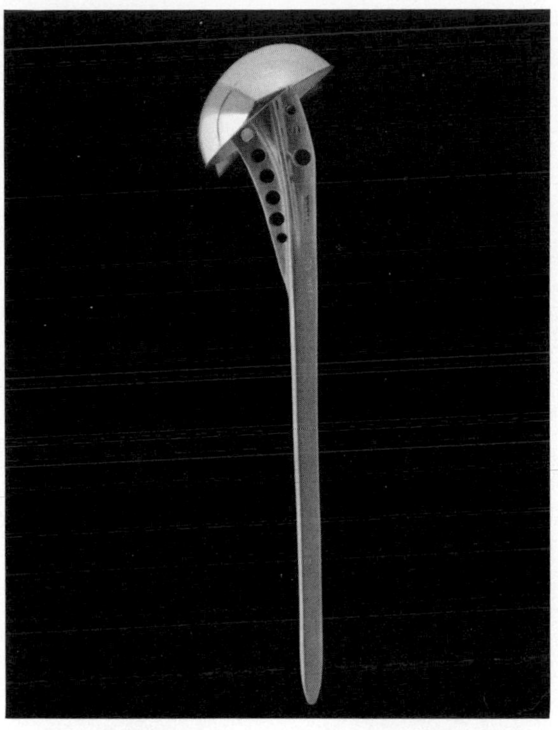

FIGURE 16-23. The original Neer I prosthesis, which was designed in 1951.

which allows a more rapid rehabilitation in the postoperative period. Removal of the deltoid origin is unnecessary because it seriously affects the function of this important muscle and slows the postoperative rehabilitation program. Splitting the middle deltoid beyond 5 cm from the edge of the acromion presents a high risk of injury to the axillary nerve.

 Authors' Preferred Method of Treatment

Minimally Displaced Fractures

Minimally displaced fractures are treated with a sling and swathe for comfort. The swathe can usually be removed after a few days. On rare occasions, if there is significant swelling and discomfort, we may use a plaster slab on the shaft of the humerus and the superior aspect of the shoulder. Elbow supination, pronation, and flexion can be started while the patient is in the sling.

If the fracture is stable, then range-of-motion exercises can be started early—within 10 days when the pain is tolerable. The physician must evaluate the fracture for clinical stability by standing on the side of the patient and supporting the elbow and forearm with

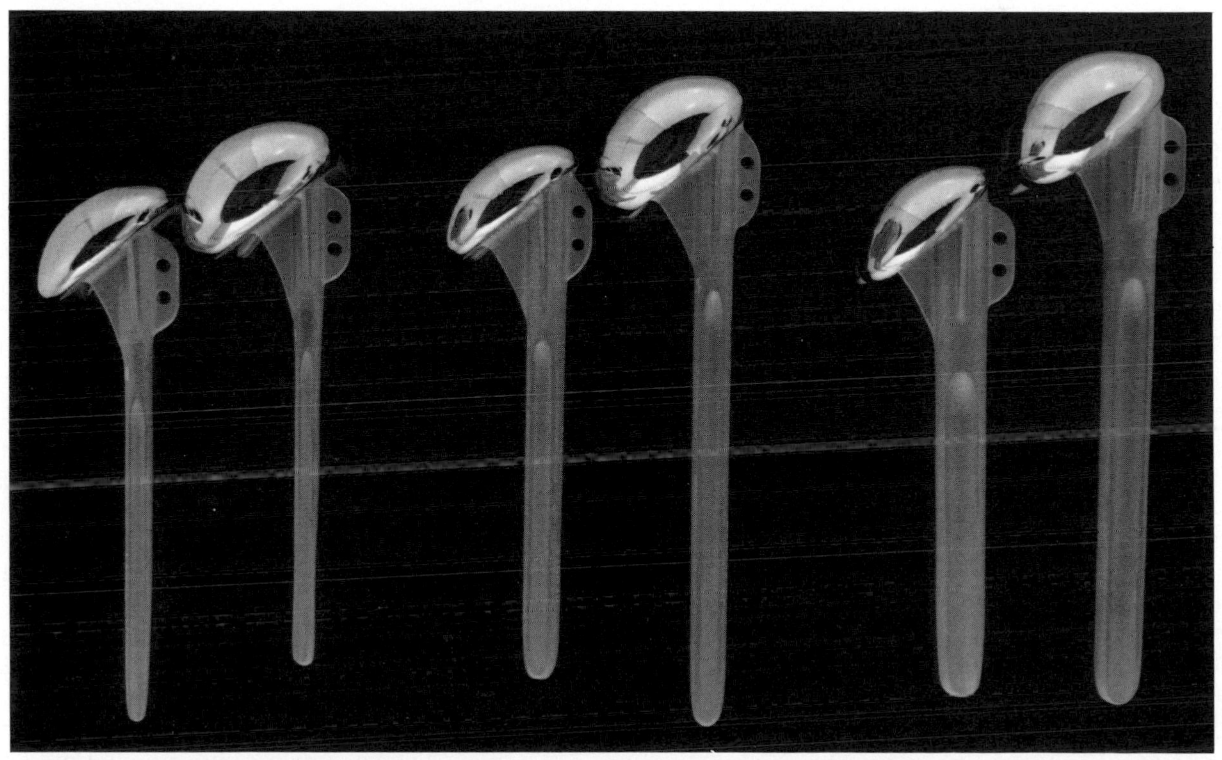

FIGURE 16-24. The Neer II prosthesis, which was redesigned in 1973. There are two head sizes (15 and 22 mm) as well as three stem sizes (7, 9.5, and 12 mm) and two stem lengths (125 and 150 mm).

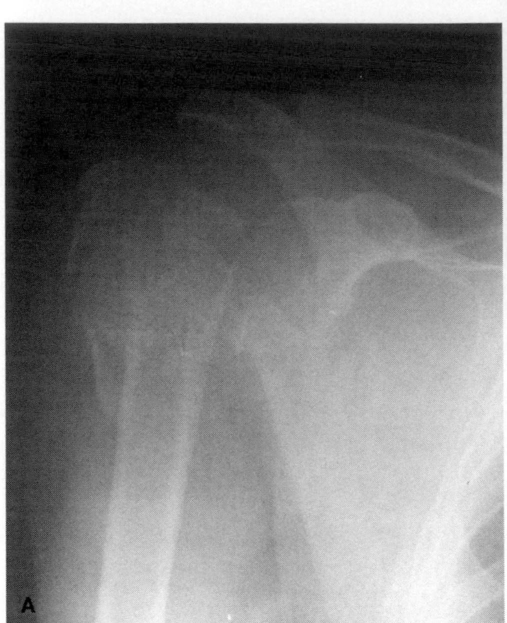

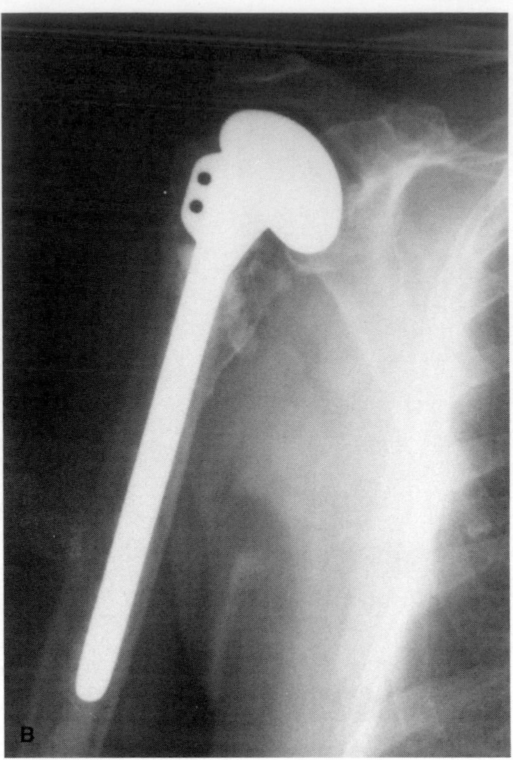

FIGURE 16-25. (**A**) Four-part fracture of the proximal humerus. (**B**) Humeral head replacement with fixation of the tuberosities using heavy nonabsorbable sutures as treatment for this four-part fracture. The tuberosities are carefully secured to the fin of the prosthesis and to the humeral shaft below the level of the articular surface. In general, the humeral prosthesis is cemented with fractures, to avoid spinning of the prosthesis in the medullary canal.

one hand and placing the other hand over the proximal humerus. Then the elbow and forearm are gently rotated. If the entire humerus appears to move as a unit, the fracture is stable and gentle and passive range-of-motion exercises can be started. The complete physical therapy regimen is outlined in the rehabilitation section. Frequent radiographic evaluation is needed to check for displacement of fracture fragments.

Two-Part Anatomical Neck Fracture

Anatomical neck fractures are extremely rare, and there are very few reports of treatment.[42,71,147,229] Certainly, no surgeon has treated large numbers of this type of fracture. In young patients, we recommend an attempt at open reduction and internal fixation. If there is some soft-tissue attachment to the head and if the quality of the bone is good, it may be possible to achieve fixation to the tuberosities and shaft. In older patients, a primary prosthesis is a better choice, allowing early motion and a more rapid recovery.

Two-Part Surgical Neck Fracture

Displaced two-part surgical neck fractures are divided into three distinct types: unimpacted, angulated impacted, and comminuted. Most of these fractures can be initially treated by closed reduction. The exception is the severely comminuted surgical neck fracture, in which there is little chance of improved alignment and stability is not possible.

In the displaced surgical neck fracture, the shaft is displaced medially by the pectoralis major and is in close proximity to the brachial plexus and axillary arteries. The head remains within the glenohumeral joint in a neutral position, since both tuberosities are attached. To achieve a closed reduction, gentle traction should be placed on the arm as it is brought out to the side and then gently flexed. Traction should be maintained, and flexion is increased as the arm is gradually adducted to gain reduction of the shaft beneath the head (Fig. 16-28). The adduction neutralizes the pull of the pectoralis major and other internal rotators, which are creating the deformity. Counterpressure by an assistant beneath the armpit or digital pressure on the proximal fragment may be needed to achieve stabilization. An attempt is made to hook the proximal

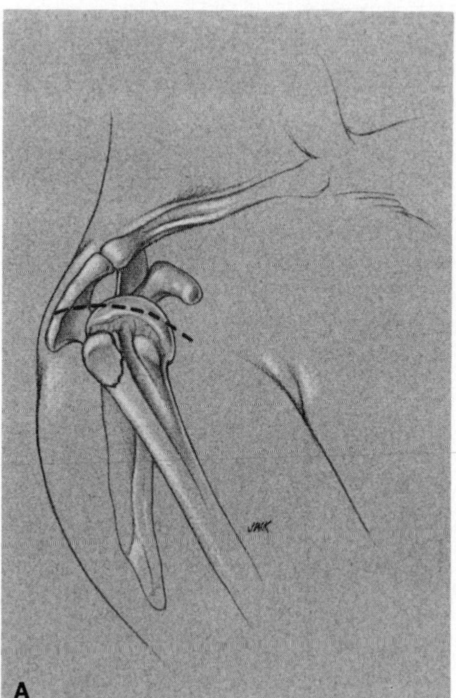

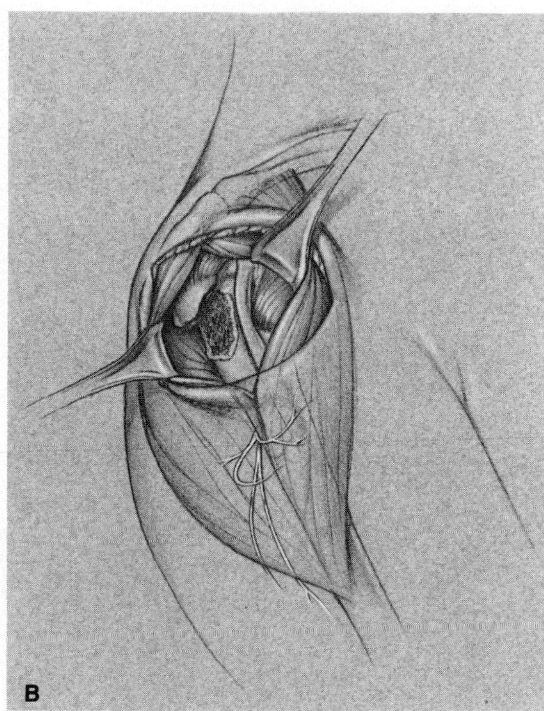

FIGURE 16-26. (**A**) Superior anterior approach to the shoulder. The skin incision for the superior anterior approach to the shoulder consists of an oblique incision in Langer's lines beginning on the anterolateral aspect of the acromion and extending down obliquely for 8 to 9 cm. (**B**) Two Richardson retractors are placed in the deltoid as it is split 4 to 5 cm from the tip of the acromion. This gives adequate exposure for greater tuberosity fractures. Great care is taken not to extend the split below 5 cm, since there may be injury to the axillary nerve. Rotation of the humerus allows for improved exposure of the different parts of the proximal humerus.

shaft beneath the humeral head, and then the arm is slightly abducted and the shaft is impacted beneath the head. To adequately perform this procedure, it is important to have good relaxation. This may not be possible in an emergency department situation with only intramuscular or intravenous analgesics and muscle relaxants. Multiple attempts at closed reduction in the emergency department without adequate relaxation are ill advised.

If the first attempt at closed reduction is unsuccessful, then we prefer to perform the next closed reduction in the operating room under adequate anesthesia and image intensifier control. This monitoring allows precise visualization of the fracture fragments. If a satisfactory reduction is achieved and it is stable, the arm is immobilized in a sling and swathe. However, if the reduction is unstable, then percutaneous pinning should be performed. The patient should be prepped and draped, and intravenous antibiotics should be given. The arm is then reduced and held in a stable position. Two pins are directed proximally, starting above the deltoid insertion through the shaft fragment and into the head and tuberosity fragment (Fig. 16-29). These pins should be 2.5-mm terminally threaded AO pins. The use of a power drill is important since it may be difficult to pierce the cortex of the proximal humerus. Each pin should be individually checked with the image intensifier in two perpendicular planes. A third pin is started proximally from above into the greater tuberosity and then proceeds distally into the shaft fragment. An additional fourth pin from distal to proximal through the anterior shaft into the head will achieve further stability, if required. Care must be taken not to enter the articular surface of the head. After this, the arm is rotated and stability is assessed. The pins are cut short beneath the skin and not removed until there is radiographic evidence of fracture stability, usually between 4 and 6 weeks.

If closed reduction is not possible, or if the reduction is unstable and percutaneous pinning is unsuccessful, then open reduction and internal fixation are required. There may be soft-tissue interposition. The long head of the biceps can act as a tether in between the fracture fragments and actually prevent reduction by causing distraction (see Fig. 16-11*B*).

The surgical exposure is a long deltopectoral approach in which the origin and insertion of the deltoid are preserved. It provides adequate exposure without injuring the deltoid muscle or axillary nerve. Care should be taken to avoid extensive dissection of the

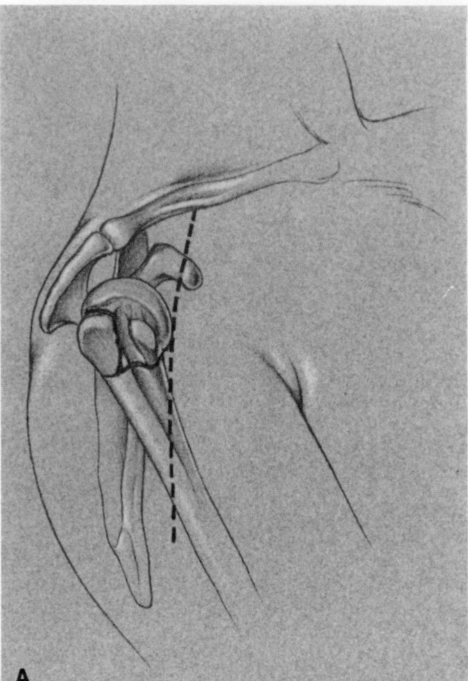

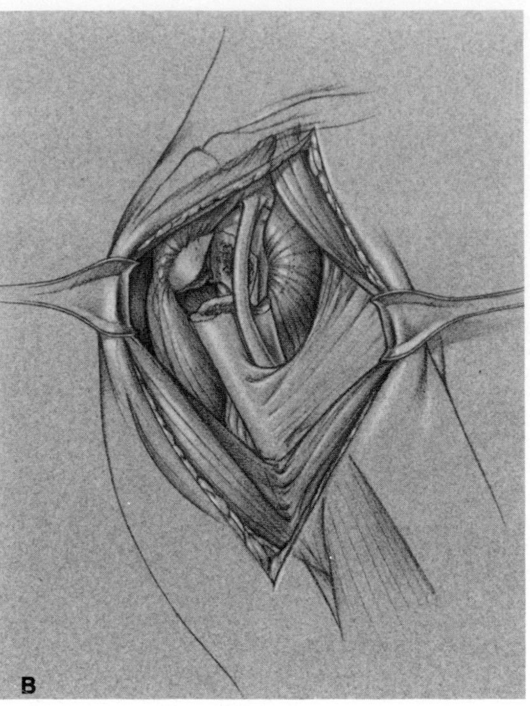

FIGURE 16-27. (**A**) A long deltopectoral approach is useful for two-, three-, and four-part fractures. The incision is made from the clavicle, passing over the coracoid and extending down to the shaft of the humerus near the deltoid insertion. (**B**) Exposure that can be achieved. The insertion of the pectoralis major can also be released to improve exposure. Care is taken never to remove the deltoid origin from the clavicle. If more exposure is needed, the deltoid insertion can be elevated, though this is rarely necessary.

soft tissue from the fracture fragments. We prefer to treat these fractures with a figure-of-eight wire (18-gauge) technique or No. 5 nonabsorbable braided suture. Wire provides greater stability but may be an irritant in the subacromial space and may also break or migrate. Therefore, we have tended to favor the heavy nonabsorbable sutures over wire for acute fracture fixation in most cases. The nonabsorbable sutures should be passed through and under the rotator cuff, as well as through the tuberosity. In many instances, the cuff may be better-quality tissue than the osteoporotic bone in the proximal humerus. A large 14- or 16-gauge spinal needle or plastic angiocath is helpful in passing suture through the cuff. A drill hole is made in the shaft of the humerus, approximately 1 inch below the fracture site, and the nonabsorbable sutures can be passed through the hole and then looped back in a figure-of-eight manner. Two separate sutures are used, one through the greater tuberosity and the other through the lesser tuberosity. Then, both sutures are placed through the same drill hole in the proximal humerus. Excellent stability can be achieved, allowing for early range-of-motion exercises. For surgical neck fractures that can be reduced and impacted, heavy sutures alone may be used for fixation. For comminuted surgical neck fractures, longitudinal fixation is supplemented with intramedullary rods placed in the nonarticular surface just inside the greater or lesser tuberosities. Small longitudinal incisions in the rotator cuff are used to place these nails. We prefer Enders nails, since they allow for three-point fixation and the eyelet of the nail allows passage of sutures to prevent proximal migration of the rod. We have modified the Enders nail by placing an additional hole above the eyelet for suture incorporation (see Fig. 16-18). This allows insertion of the nail deeper into the bone, so that its proximal tip is seated below the surface of the rotator cuff tendons. This has decreased the incidence of subacromial impingement due to the rod and thus the need for rod removal. Satisfactory results with these techniques has been reported in 18 of 22 patients (82%).[64]

Impacted surgical neck fractures angulated greater than 45° should be reduced. The deformity is usually in the anterior plane, and malunion will limit forward elevation. Multiple rotational radiographic views, as well as comparison radiographs of the normal shoulder, are important to judge the amount of angulation fully. The reduction maneuver includes abduction and flexion to the pivotal position. This usually distracts the fracture fragments and frees the shaft from under the head, allowing correction of the deformity. A hyperabduction maneuver is not indicated in this fracture because the proximal fragment is not abducted. The head may be reimpacted so that stability can be

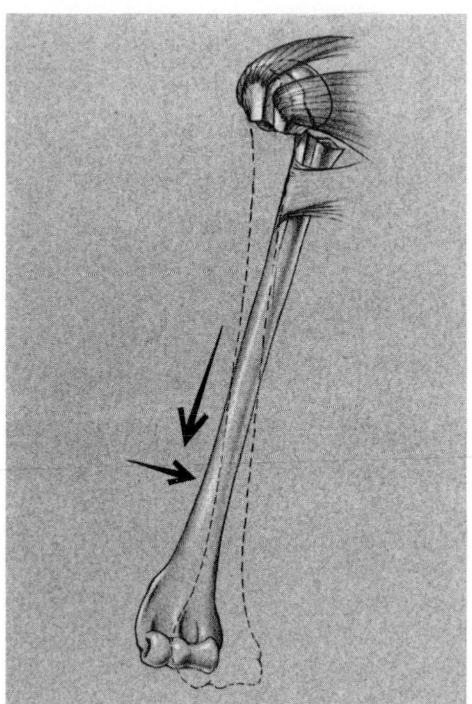

FIGURE 16-28. Closed reduction of a surgical neck fracture. To achieve a closed reduction, gentle traction should be placed on the arm as it is brought out to the side and gently flexed. Traction should be maintained and flexion is increased as the arm is gradually adducted to gain reduction of the shaft beneath the head. Adduction neutralizes the pull of the pectoralis major and other internal rotators that are creating the deformity. Counterpressure by the assistant may be needed beneath the armpit or digital pressure on the proximal fragment to achieve stabilization. The shaft should be beneath the head for a stable reduction.

achieved and early motion started. The arm is immobilized at the side in a sling and swathe.

Initially, comminuted proximal humeral fractures without significant displacement should be treated with a sling and swathe and a plaster splint applied along the shaft of the humerus and onto the top of the shoulder. Occasionally, a shoulder spica cast is helpful. Traction is difficult to maintain and tolerate and is a problem in patients with multiple injuries. If closed reduction is not successful, open reduction and internal fixation with Enders rods and multiple nonabsorbable sutures or wire is employed (see Fig. 16-17). Occasionally, in young patients, fixation can be achieved with a plate and screws (Fig. 16-30), although in older patients the osteoporotic proximal fragment will be less amenable to fixation with plates and screws. Fixation with a plate and screws and multiple sutures or wire, if necessary, is indicated (see Fig. 16-30). Although this fixation may not be rigid enough to allow early motion, it is adequate to maintain alignment until there is early healing and range of motion can be started. Addition of a shoulder spica cast can help to enhance fixation.

Two-Part Greater Tuberosity Fracture

Two-part greater tuberosity fractures displaced greater than 1 cm require open reduction and internal fixation. A closed reduction is difficult to achieve because there is a tear in the rotator cuff and the fragment is pulled posteriorly and superiorly. If left in this position, impingement will develop and the patient will lose motion (both elevation and external rotation) of the shoulder (see Fig. 16-14). The surgical approach for this type of fracture is a superior approach in Langer's lines (see Fig. 16-26). The deltoid is split a short distance from the acromion for 3 to 4 cm. We prefer to stabilize the bone fragment with multiple heavy nonabsorbable sutures (Fig. 16-31). The rotator cuff must also be repaired. Repairing the rent in the cuff offers stability and removes tension from the fracture repair. The greater tuberosity is anatomically replaced using several No. 5 nylon (Tevdek) sutures placed through drill holes in the tuberosity and shaft (Fig. 16-32). Bone fragments and hematomas may need to be removed from the fracture surface of the greater tuberosity to improve the reduction. Exercises are started early, on the first or second postoperative day. We have reported uniformly satisfactory results (six

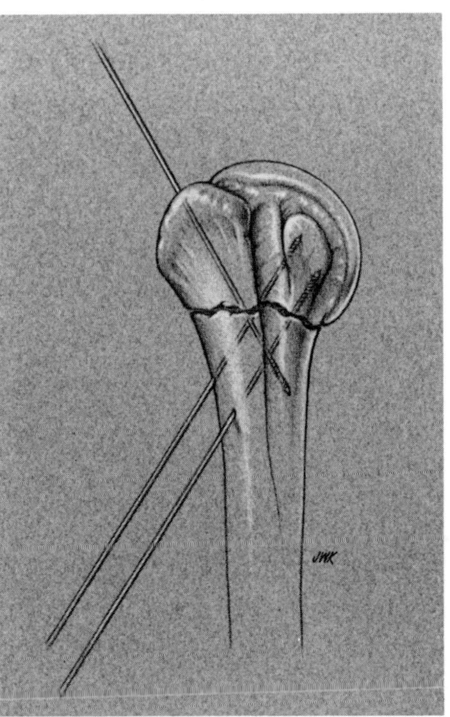

FIGURE 16-29. Technique of percutaneous pinning of surgical neck fractures. The fracture is reduced and held in a stable position. Two pins are then directed proximally, starting above the deltoid insertion through the proximal fragment and into the head and tuberosity fragment. These pins should be 2.5-mm terminally threaded AO pins. A power drill must be used because it may be difficult to pierce the cortex. The third pin is started proximally from above into the greater tuberosity and then into the shaft.

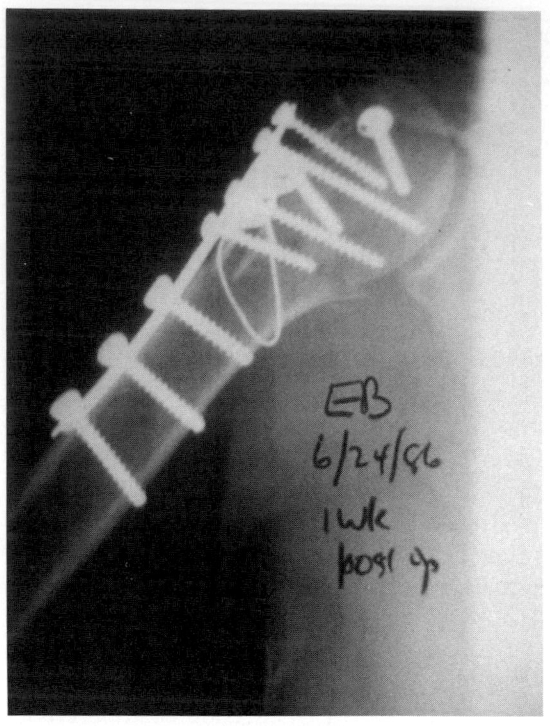

FIGURE 16-30. Anteroposterior x-ray of an open reduction and internal fixation with a plate and screws of a comminuted fracture of the proximal humerus. Excellent fixation was achieved, and the patient had excellent union and achieved a good functional result. (*Courtesy of Howard Rosen, M.D.*)

excellent and six good results) with this method of treatment in a series of 12 patients with displaced fractures of the greater tuberosity.[91]

Two-Part Lesser Tuberosity Fracture

Displaced isolated fractures of the lesser tuberosity are extremely rare. If the fragment is small and rotation is not affected, then the arm can be supported in a sling and the patient is instructed about range-of-motion exercises. If the fragment is large and blocks medial rotation, then open reduction and internal fixation with nonabsorbable sutures is needed. The fracture fragment may also be removed and the tendon of the subscapularis repaired back to the proximal humerus.

Three-Part Fractures

Most three-part fractures are quite unstable, and closed reduction is difficult. In general, open reduction and internal fixation is the treatment of choice in active patients, since a stable reduction can usually be achieved allowing early motion. Closed reduction is an option only in debilitated patients or patients in whom surgery is contraindicated. The surgical approach to this procedure is also deltopectoral.

Great care must be taken not to denude the fracture fragments of their blood supply, which may lead to avascular necrosis. In most cases, we prefer to use internal fixation of the fragments with No. 5 nonabsorbable sutures or 18-gauge figure-of-eight wires. The technique is similar to that previously described for two-part surgical neck fractures (Fig. 16-33). The displaced tuberosity should be attached to the humeral head and remaining tuberosity fragment as well as the shaft below (Fig. 16-34). Multiple sutures are necessary for stability. In selected cases, when there is significant osteoporosis and the quality of the bone is poor, not allowing internal fixation, a primary humeral head prosthesis is indicated. This allows earlier mobilization of the shoulder.

Four-Part Fractures

The treatment of choice for four-part fractures of the proximal humerus is a humeral head prosthesis, since other methods of treatment are associated with poor results. Occasionally, in patients younger than 40 years of age, without a dislocation, if the humeral head is still in continuity with the glenoid and there appears to be some soft-tissue attachment, open reduction may be attempted. Fixation of the head fragment is difficult and best achieved with multiple K-wires that are removed after adequate healing.[67] However, this type of fracture has a high incidence of avascular necrosis.

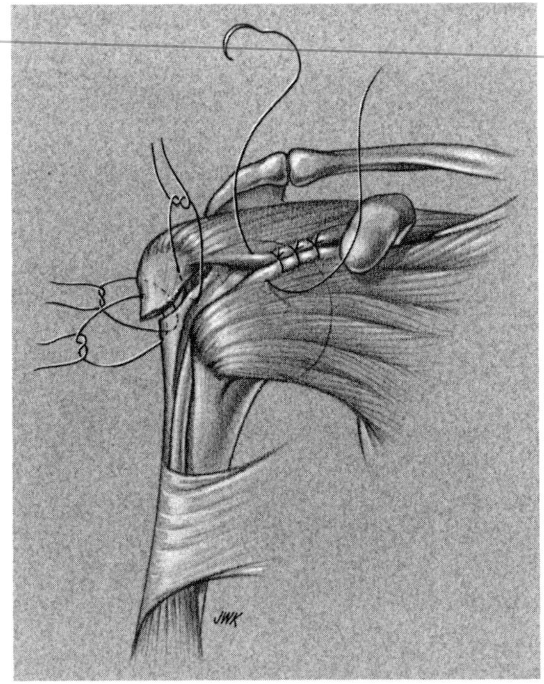

FIGURE 16-31. Technique of open reduction and internal fixation of the greater tuberosity fracture. Our preferred method of fixation for greater tuberosity fractures is multiple nonabsorbable nylon sutures. The cuff must also be repaired. It is advisable to repair the cuff first, since this reduces tension from the bony sutures and stabilizes the fracture fragment. Several drill holes are placed in the proximal shaft and through the greater tuberosity and the tuberosity fragment is secured with sutures.

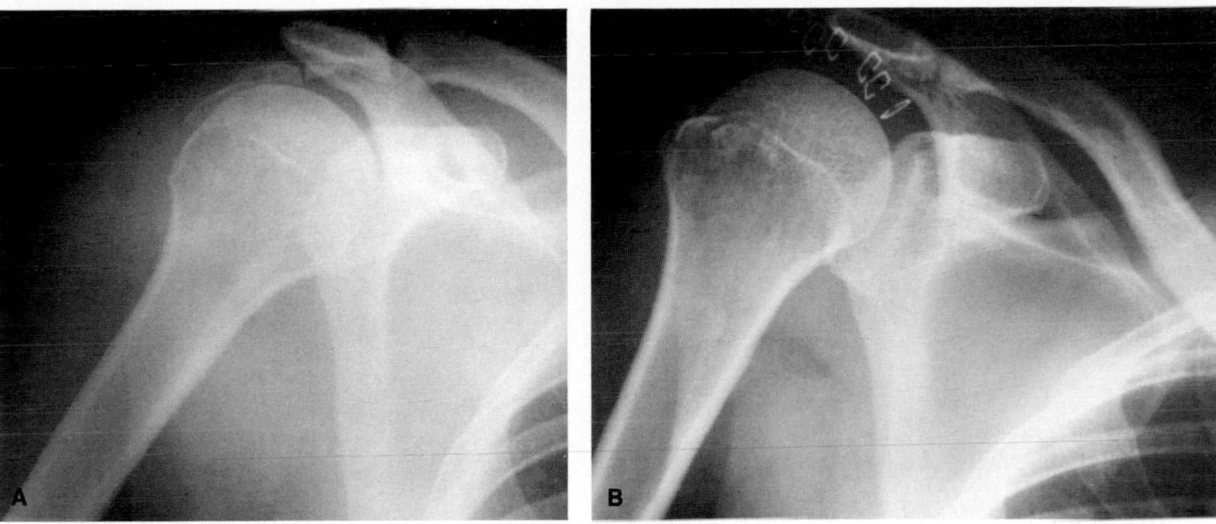

FIGURE 16-32. (**A**) Anteroposterior x-ray of the displaced greater tuberosity fracture, which is pulled posteriorly and superiorly by the supraspinatus and the infraspinatus. (**B**) Postoperative x-ray showing stabilization of the fracture with multiple nonabsorbable sutures.

Our preference is use of the Neer humeral head prosthesis.[89] It is available in various sizes. The surgical approach is important because the deltoid must be preserved to allow optimum postoperative shoulder function. The deltoid should not be detached from its origin because this will weaken it. A long deltopectoral approach avoids detachment of the deltoid origin but still allows adequate exposure (see Fig. 16-27). If more exposure is needed, the deltoid insertion may be slightly elevated, although this is rarely necessary. Another important technical aspect is to restore proper length to the humerus, with the prosthesis preserving proper tension in the myofascial sleeve. The tendency is to set the prosthesis against the remaining humeral shaft, which significantly shortens the humerus. This creates an unstable situation that leads to inferior subluxation of the prosthesis and inability to elevate the extremity. In this situation, the deltoid is shortened and its function is significantly compromised (Fig. 16-35). The addition of cement enhances stability, since there is usually inadequate bony support for the stem, and it allows for adjustment of the prosthesis to the proper length. Fixation with cement also prevents the prosthesis from spinning into malversion in the intramedullary canal. The prosthesis has to be set at the proper length and the proper degree of retroversion, which is generally between 30° and 40° (Fig. 16-36). The distal humeral condyles must be palpated to aid in estimating the amount of humeral head retroversion. This is performed with the elbow flexed and the prosthesis in position so that anterior and posterior stability can be assessed. A sponge can be placed into the medullary canal of the proximal humerus, which allows sufficient support of the prosthesis so that the chosen height and version can be maintained during the trial reduction. If part of the biceps groove is intact, then this can be a useful landmark. The lateral fin of the prosthesis, containing two holes through which

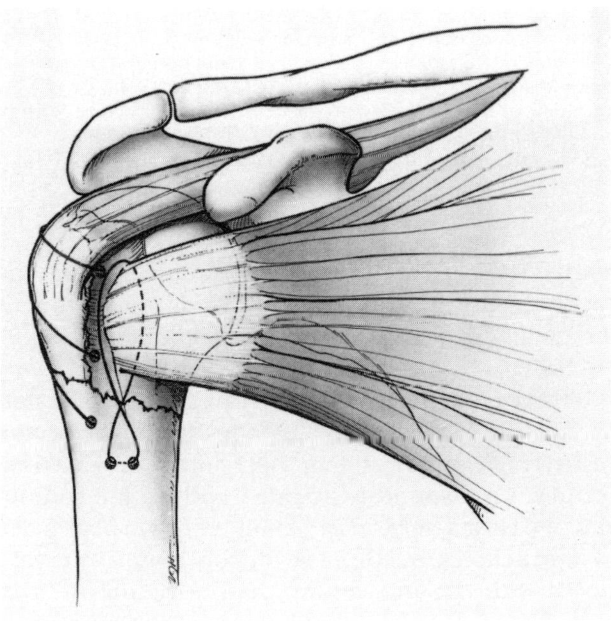

FIGURE 16-33. Schematic of technique for repair of three-part fractures using heavy nonabsorbable sutures. The suture fixation incorporates both bone and rotator cuff tendon into the repair. The displaced tuberosity is repaired to the proximal articular segment, as well as to the humeral shaft. Figure-of-eight suture fixation between the major proximal fragment and the humeral shaft is also employed.

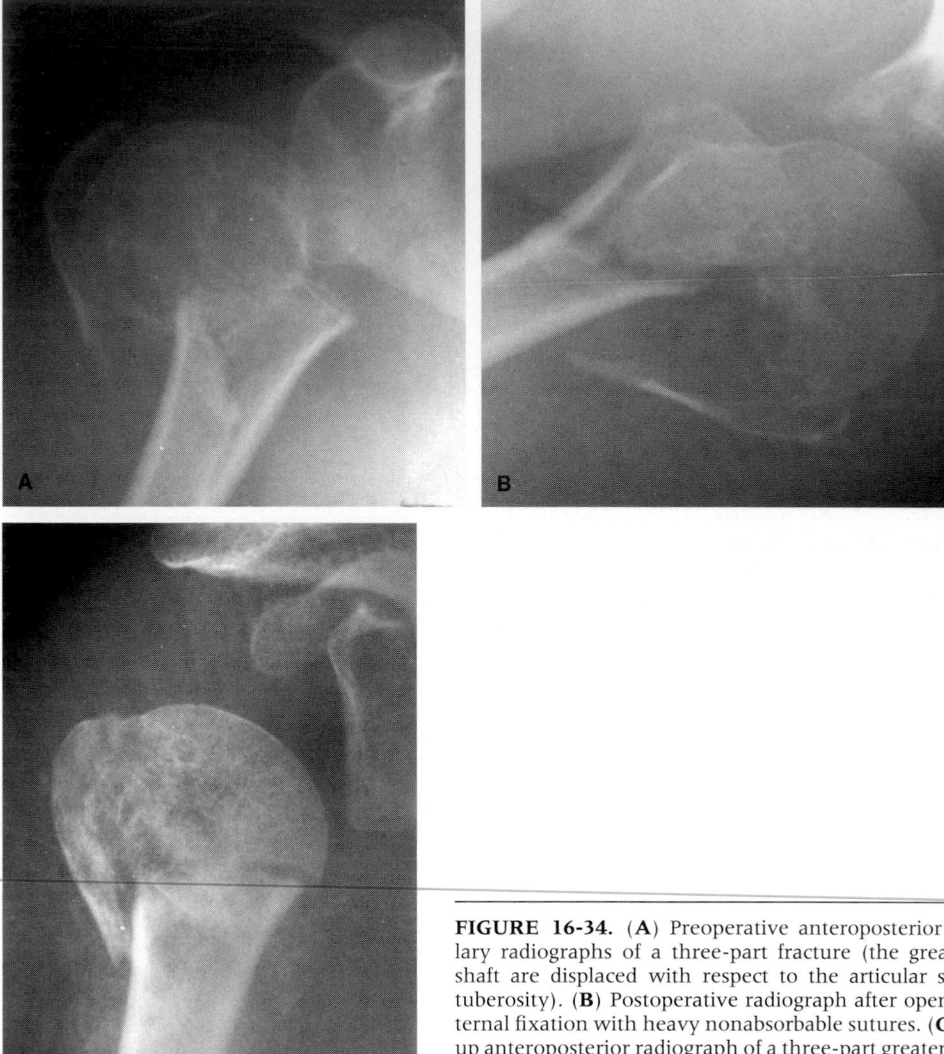

FIGURE 16-34. (**A**) Preoperative anteroposterior and Velpeau axillary radiographs of a three-part fracture (the greater tuberosity and shaft are displaced with respect to the articular segment and lesser tuberosity). (**B**) Postoperative radiograph after open reduction and internal fixation with heavy nonabsorbable sutures. (**C**) One-year follow-up anteroposterior radiograph of a three-part greater tuberosity fracture fixed with multiple nonabsorbable sutures. Healing was excellent, and the patient has a full range of motion with normal function.

sutures may be passed for tuberosity fixation, should sit just at the posterior aspect of the groove (Fig. 16-37).

Secure fixation of the tuberosities is essential to allow early postoperative motion of the shoulder. The tuberosities should be sutured with heavy nonabsorbable braided suture (eg, No. 2 or No. 5 Tevdek) to each other and to the shaft of the humerus through the fin of the prosthesis (Fig. 16-38). Two or three sutures should be placed from the greater tuberosity to the shaft, and two sutures should be placed from the greater tuberosity through the holes in the fin of the prosthesis to the lesser tuberosity. It is important to close the rent in the rotator cuff. One or two sutures are also passed from the lesser tuberosity to the shaft of the humerus. If possible, the long head of the biceps should be preserved by retracting it anteriorly or posteriorly and then replacing it into its groove in the humerus. The head of the prosthesis should be positioned above the greater tuberosity to avoid impingement of the greater tuberosity against the acromion (see Fig. 16-25*B*).

If there is a humeral shaft fracture, it should be stabilized before cementing the prosthesis. This can be done with a cerclage wire and multiple nonabsorbable nylon sutures. The wound is irrigated with saline solution, and two closed-suction irrigation tubes are placed deep to the deltoid muscle. The deltopectoral interval is closed with chromic sutures, and if the insertion has been elevated, this should be reattached. The skin is closed with a subcuticular Dexon or prolene suture. Prophylactic antibiotics are given preoperatively, intraoperatively, and postoperatively for 48 hours. Range-of-motion exercises are begun by the operating surgeon on the first postoperative day. To avoid the devastating complication of tuberosity pull-off, active

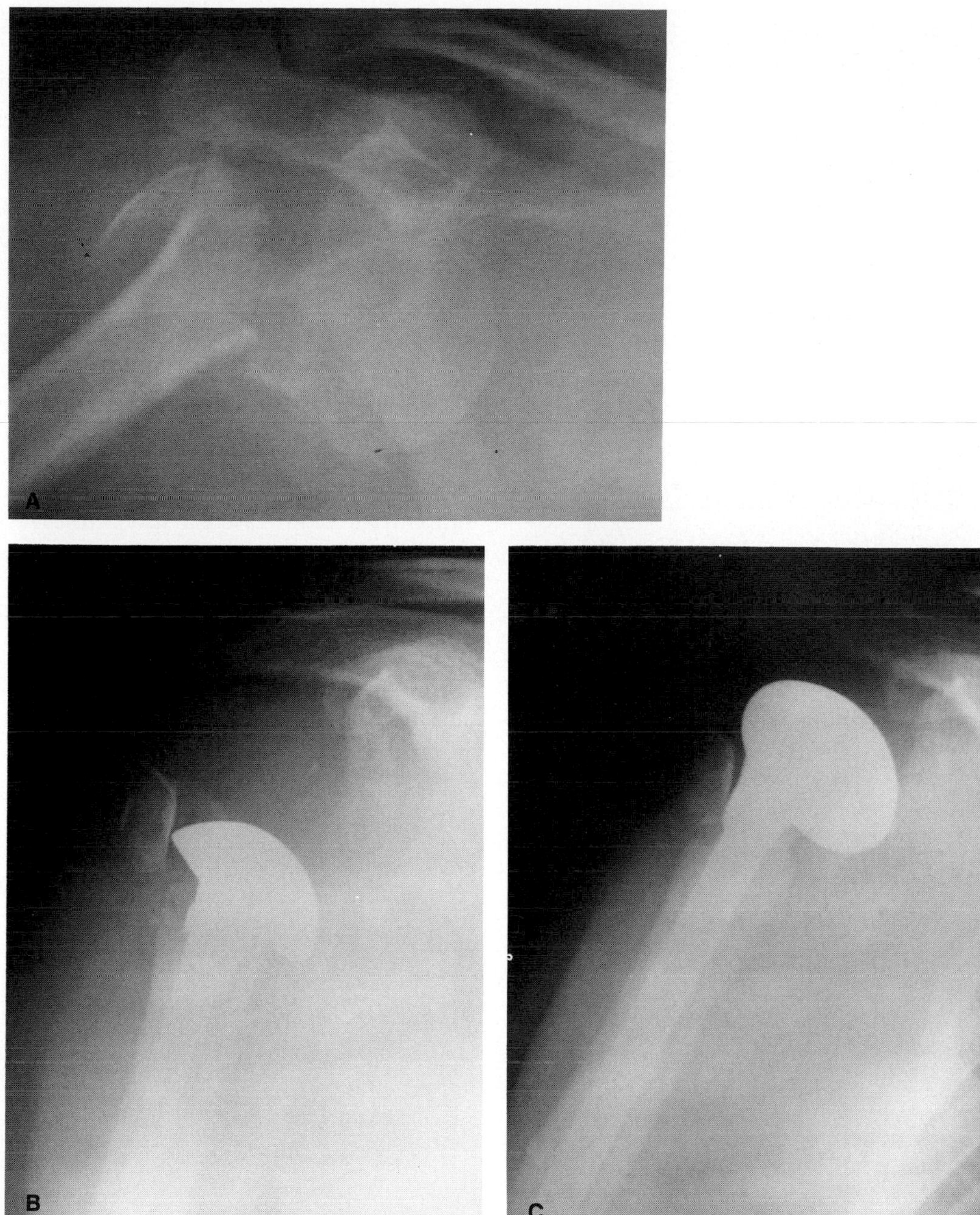

FIGURE 16-35. (**A**) Anterior four-part fracture–dislocation with head displaced beneath the coracoid. (**B**) Failed Neer I prosthesis in which the prosthesis was placed against the proximal shaft, creating an unstable situation leading to inferior subluxation. In addition, both tuberosities became detached as a result of inadequate fixation. (**C**) Revision of the prosthesis in which cement was used to elevate the prosthesis approximately 4 cm to achieve stability. Enough bone was left on the greater tuberosity to place it beneath the head. This patient, in addition, had a partial axillary nerve palsy. However, he did achieve a pain-free shoulder with approximately 80° of forward elevation and 30° of external rotation.

motion is deferred. Electromyographic studies of shoulder exercises have demonstrated that assistive exercises, such as pulley elevation, can involve significant active use of the rotator cuff and deltoid.[202] Several cases of early tuberosity pull-off in patients after humeral head replacement for acute fractures were thought to be related to pulley exercises. For this reason, we now limit early passive motion in these cases to pendulum and passive elevation by the surgeon, therapist, or a trained family member. The arm is raised in the plane of the scapula to a point determined at the time of surgery, depending on the security of tuberosity fixation (generally 130° to 140°). Active exercises are not performed until there is healing

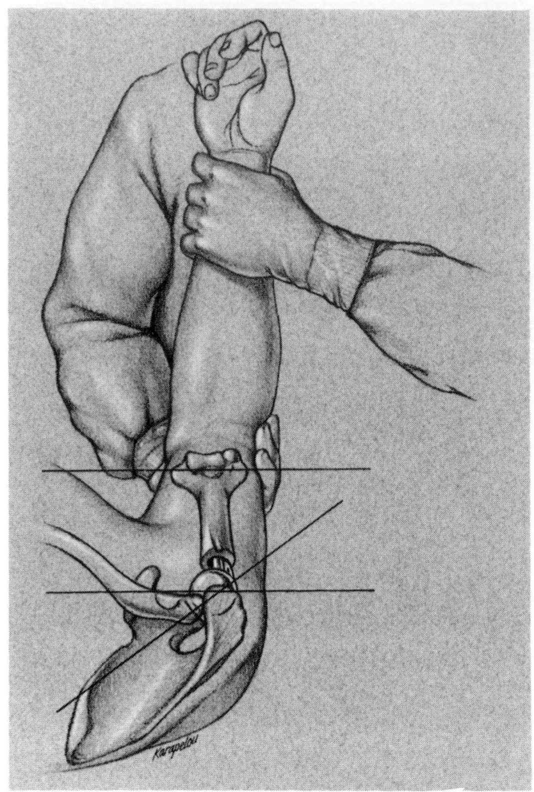

FIGURE 16-36. The humeral head prosthesis should be placed in 30° to 40° of retroversion. This can be accomplished by palpating the distal humeral condyles with the elbow flexed and estimating the amount of humeral head retroversion. Anterior and posterior stability should be assessed with the prosthesis in the shaft. A sponge can be stuffed into the medullary canal of the humerus with the trial prosthesis to allow sufficient support of the prosthesis. If part of the biceps groove is intact, then this can be used as a landmark. The fin of the prosthesis should sit at the posterior aspect of the groove.

of the tuberosities, generally by 6 weeks. After this, resistance is gradually added and terminal stretching exercises are emphasized.

Fracture–Dislocations

Two-Part Fracture–Dislocations. Two-part fracture–dislocations should initially be treated by a closed reduction. The head is attached to the shaft and, it is hoped, in most instances, that the displaced tuberosity fragment will be reduced to an acceptable position (see Fig. 16-12). Anterior two-part fracture–dislocations are immobilized at the side with a sling and swathe. Posterior fracture–dislocations are immobilized in neutral or slight external rotation with the arm in a cast or brace. There is a tendency for redisplacement of the tuberosity fragment, especially with greater tuberosity fractures. Therefore, frequent follow-up radiographs are essential in the postreduction period. If the tuberosities are displaced, these should be treated the same as two-part fractures.

Usually, with repair of the tuberosity, further glenohumeral dislocations do not occur. Two-part fracture–dislocations involving the anatomical or surgical neck are extremely rare. If an anatomical head fragment is outside the joint, we would use a humeral head prosthesis. With fracture–dislocation involving the surgical neck, we prefer open reduction and internal fixation.

Three-Part Fracture–Dislocations. We prefer open reduction and internal fixation of three-part fracture–dislocations. In anterior fracture–dislocation, it must remembered that the head is very close to the brachial plexus and axillary artery. Therefore, great care must be taken in an open reduction of an anterior three-part fracture–dislocation to gently reduce the head to avoid injury to the neurovascular structures. The glenoid surface should also be inspected for impression fractures. Open reduction and internal fixation using sutures is performed with the same technique as described for three-part fractures.

Four-Part Fracture–Dislocations. Four-part fracture–dislocations are treated with a humeral prosthesis.

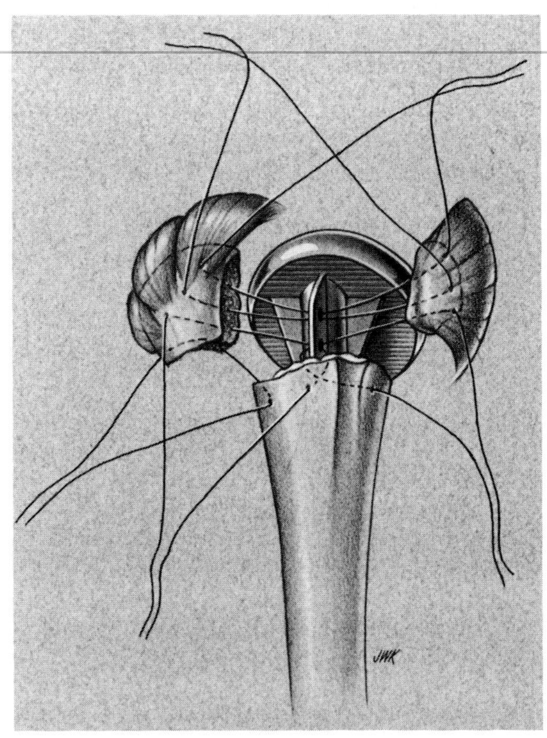

FIGURE 16-37. Prosthesis repair. The prosthesis has been cemented into place and is elevated off the shaft. Both tuberosities should be able to fit below the head. The tuberosities should be repaired superior to the head. Drill holes should be placed through both tuberosities and the shaft, and the tuberosities should be attached to each other through the fin of the prosthesis as well as to the shaft below.

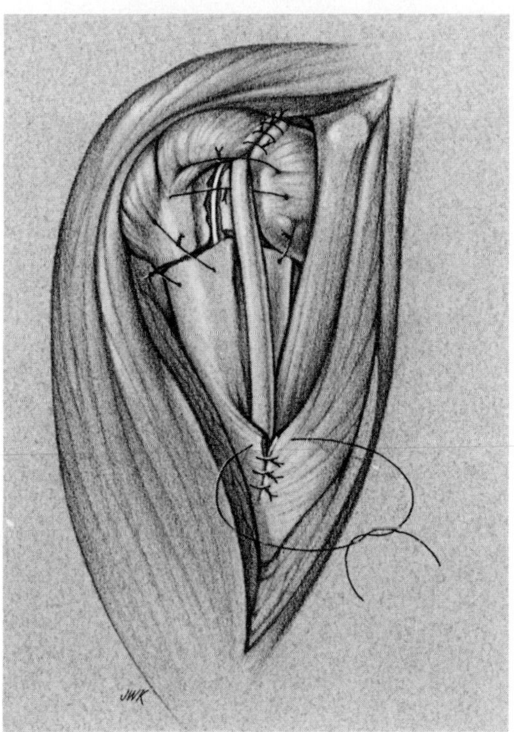

FIGURE 16-38. The completed repair of the tuberosities with the rotator cuff interval closed and the biceps preserved. In general, nonabsorbable sutures provide a firm repair, allowing for early motion.

The head is devoid of any soft-tissue attachment with fracture–dislocations and usually is a free-floating fragment. Once again, great caution should be used in trying to remove the humeral head in an anterior fracture–dislocation (Fig. 16-39), especially if surgery has been delayed for several weeks, because the dislocated head segment may be adherent to the axillary artery. With a posterior fracture-dislocation, there may be excessive posterior instability, and less retroversion may be required for the prosthesis. If the prosthesis is unstable posteriorly, then retroversion may be decreased by 10° to 15°, and this will usually create stability.

Impression and Head-Splitting Fractures.

Treatment of impression fractures of the articular surface varies according to the size of the defect and the time of the diagnosis. If head involvement is less than 20% of the articular surface and the treatment is within 2 to 3 weeks after injury, closed reduction may be adequate. The arm should be immobilized in external rotation after reduction, if the dislocation is posterior. For defects involving 20% to 45% of the anterior head that are associated with a posterior dislocation, we prefer to use a modification of the McLaughlin procedure as reported by Hawkins and associates.[126] The lesser tuberosity, with the attached tendon of the subscapularis, is transferred into the defect in the head and fixed with a screw through an anterior approach. For head defects greater than 45%, or when the dislocation is 6 months or more old and the head has softened or degenerated, we prefer to use a prosthesis.[126,331] If the glenoid is fractured, eroded, or worn, it may also require replacement. Generally, impression fractures occur with posterior fracture–dislocations.

Head-splitting fractures also require a prosthesis. These are usually associated with fractures of either tuberosities or the surgical neck (Fig. 16-40). In a young patient, if bone stock is adequate, open reduction and internal fixation may be attempted, but this is usually a very difficult procedure, associated with a high incidence of failure.

REHABILITATION

Rehabilitation of proximal humeral fractures is essential because adequate motion is needed for optimum function. If a fracture or fracture repair is stable, then

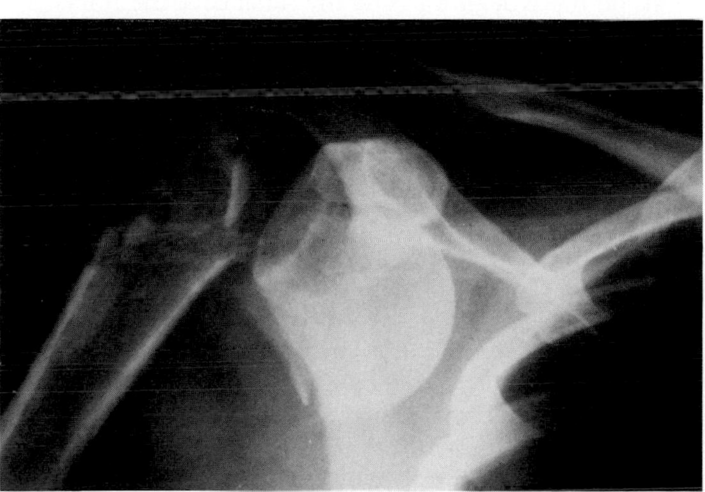

FIGURE 16-39. Anteroposterior x-ray of a four-part fracture–dislocation. The head is displaced below the coracoid and is adjacent to the neurovascular bundle.

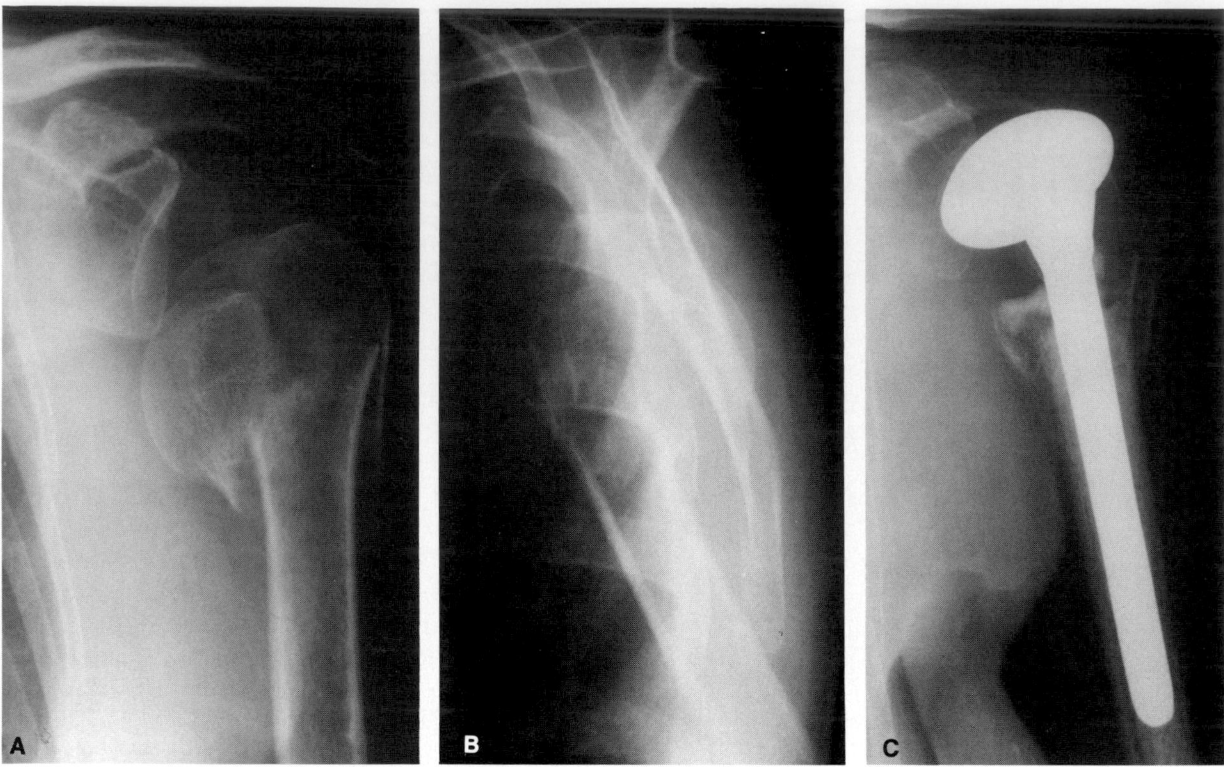

FIGURE 16-40. (**A**) Anteroposterior x-ray of a head-splitting fracture in which a significant portion of the articular surface is involved. The superior portion of the head is with the greater tuberosity fragment, and the inferior portion is with the lesser tuberosity fragment. There is also a surgical neck fracture. (**B**) Lateral x-ray in the scapular plane is a head-splitting fracture showing the superior fragment above. The inferior fragment below demonstrates the discontinuity of the articular surface. (**C**) Anteroposterior x-ray of a Neer prosthesis used to treat the head-splitting fracture.

therapy should be started early. The most useful rehabilitation protocol is the three-phase system that has been devised by Hughes and Neer[144] (Fig. 16-41). The first phase consists of passive-assistive exercises. In the second phase, active- and early-resistive exercises are started. The third phase is a maintenance program aimed at advanced stretching and strengthening exercises. Application of this system is variable and depends on the type of fracture, the stability of the fracture or fracture repair, and the ability of the patient to comprehend the exercise program. The exercises are performed three to four times per day for 20 to 30 minutes. A hot pack applied 20 minutes before the exercise session is beneficial. Early in the program an analgesic may be needed to control pain and thus allow sufficient stretching. Often it is advisable to involve a physical therapist for guidance and management of the exercise program.

Phase I exercises are started early in the postfracture or postoperative period. If a fracture is minimally displaced or has been treated by closed reduction and is stable, then exercises are generally started between days 7 and 10 after fracture. The first exercise is usually a pendulum exercise (Codman), in which the arm is rotated both outwardly and inwardly in small circles (see Fig. 16-41*A* and *B*). The second exercise is supine external rotation with a stick (see Fig. 16-41*C*). It is important to support the elbow and the distal humerus with either a folded towel or sheet because this will create a sense of security for the patient. A slight amount of abduction (15° to 20°) may also aid in performing this exercise.

Three weeks after fracture, assisted forward elevation (see Fig. 16-41*D*) as well as pulley exercises (see Fig. 16-41*E*) can be added. Extension can be added shortly later. Isometric exercises are generally started at 4 weeks (see Figs. 16-41*F* and *G*). After a secure surgical repair, passive exercises can be started by the physician within 24 to 48 hours. The physician should start elbow flexion and extension first and then gently assist the patient with pendulum exercises. Supine external rotation and assisted forward elevation, either supine or sitting, are also performed. These passive exercises may also be performed with the therapist shortly after surgery. As discussed earlier, we have avoided the use of assistive pulley exercises in the early postoperative period, to prevent the complication of tuberosity pull-off. These exercises can be added after there is radiographic evidence of tuberosity healing, usually after 6 weeks.

Phase II exercises involve early active, resistive, and stretching exercises. The first exercise is supine active forward elevation, since gravity is partially eliminated, making elevation easier (see Fig. 16-41*H–J*). The forward elevation exercise can then be performed in the erect position. The use of a stick in the unaffected arm assists the involved arm in forward elevation (see Fig. 16-41*K–M*). As the arm gains strength, active erect elevation can be performed unassisted. It is important initially to keep the elbow flexed and the arm close to the midline. Strips of rubber sheeting of various strengths (Therabands) are used to strengthen the internal rotators, the external rotators, and anterior, middle, and posterior deltoids (see Figs. 16-41*N* and *O*). Three sets of 10 to 15 repetitions are recommended at each exercise session. Stretching for forward elevation on the top of a door or wall is started, as well as stretching in the door jamb for external rotation (see Fig. 16-41*T*). Also, the arm is raised over the head with hands clasped, and then the hands are placed behind the head and the arms externally rotated and abducted (see Figs. 16-41*P–R*). This exercise is extremely important to achieve abduction and external rotation. "Wall climbing" is generally not performed because this does not promote stretching. Internal rotation is helped by using the normal arm to pull the involved arm into internal rotation (see Fig. 16-41*S*).

Phase III exercises are generally started at 3 months. Rubber tubing is substituted for the rubber strips to increase resistance. The arm is stretched higher on the wall by leaning the torso into the wall (see Fig. 16-41*T*). Also, stretching on the end of the door and prone stretching for forward elevation are extremely useful. A hot shower before stretching promotes relaxation. Light weights could be used after 3 months. These should be started at 1 pound and increased at 1-pound increments, with the limit being 5 pounds. If there is persistent pain after exercises with weights, then the weights should be decreased or eliminated. Strength can be achieved with functional activity. A well-supervised rehabilitation regimen is essential for successful fracture treatment. Even a perfect fracture reduction or surgical repair will not achieve a good result without proper rehabilitative efforts.

COMPLICATIONS

Displaced fractures of the proximal humerus are difficult to manage, and numerous complications have been reported after both closed and open treatment. Some of these include avascular necrosis, nonunion, malunion, hardware failure, frozen shoulder, infection, neurovascular injury, and pneumothorax or pneumohemothorax.

Vascular Injury

Vascular complications occurring after proximal humeral fractures are infrequent, but they do occur and can have profound consequences.[128,132,166,188,229,267,288,302,305,316] Injury to the axillary artery accounts for approximately 6% of all arterial trauma. It occurs secondary to fractures of the proximal humerus and is the most common vascular injury seen in these fractures. In a series of 81 fractures, Stableforth[305] reported a 4.9% incidence of arterial damage in displaced fractures. The injury is usually associated with penetrating or violent blunt trauma, resulting in a displaced fracture. However, it has also been reported with minimally displaced fractures. In addition, the risk is increased in older patients with arteriosclerosis, because the vessel walls have lost elasticity and cannot stretch in response to the trauma. Therefore, in the elderly, a trivial trauma can result in an arterial injury.

The most common site of injury to the axillary artery is proximal to the takeoff of the anterior circumflex artery. Reports have stressed the need to suspect vascular injury whenever there is a fracture near a major vessel because the key to successful treatment is early diagnosis and repair.[128,288,352] It is important to check the radial pulse in the injured extremity; however, the presence of peripheral pulses may be secondary to collateral circulation. Therefore, an intact radial pulse is not a guarantee that significant arterial injury has not occurred. Doppler ultrasonography can be helpful in detecting a pulse but can also be misleading because collateral circulation can create a pulse detectable by Doppler examination. Other signs include an expanding hematoma, pallor, and paresthesias. Paresthesias are probably the most reliable sign of inadequate distal circulation and should raise suspicion of a vascular injury.

If an arterial injury is not recognized, the results can be catastrophic, including gas gangrene, amputation, and compressive neuropathies of the brachial plexus, leading to permanent deficits unless there is early evacuation of the hematoma. Angiography should be performed to confirm the diagnosis and to establish the exact location and nature of the injury. Arterial repair should be performed without delay and, if necessary, coordinated with appropriate orthopaedic fracture repair.

Brachial Plexus Injury

Brachial plexus injuries also occur after fractures of the proximal humerus. Stableforth[305] reported an incidence of 6.1% after fractures of the proximal humerus. Any or all components of the brachial plexus may be involved. Isolated injury to the axillary nerve is not uncommon and has been reported.[34] This is especially true of anterior fracture–dislocations because the nerve courses on the inferior surface of the capsule and is susceptible to injury. Injury to the suprascapular and musculocutaneous

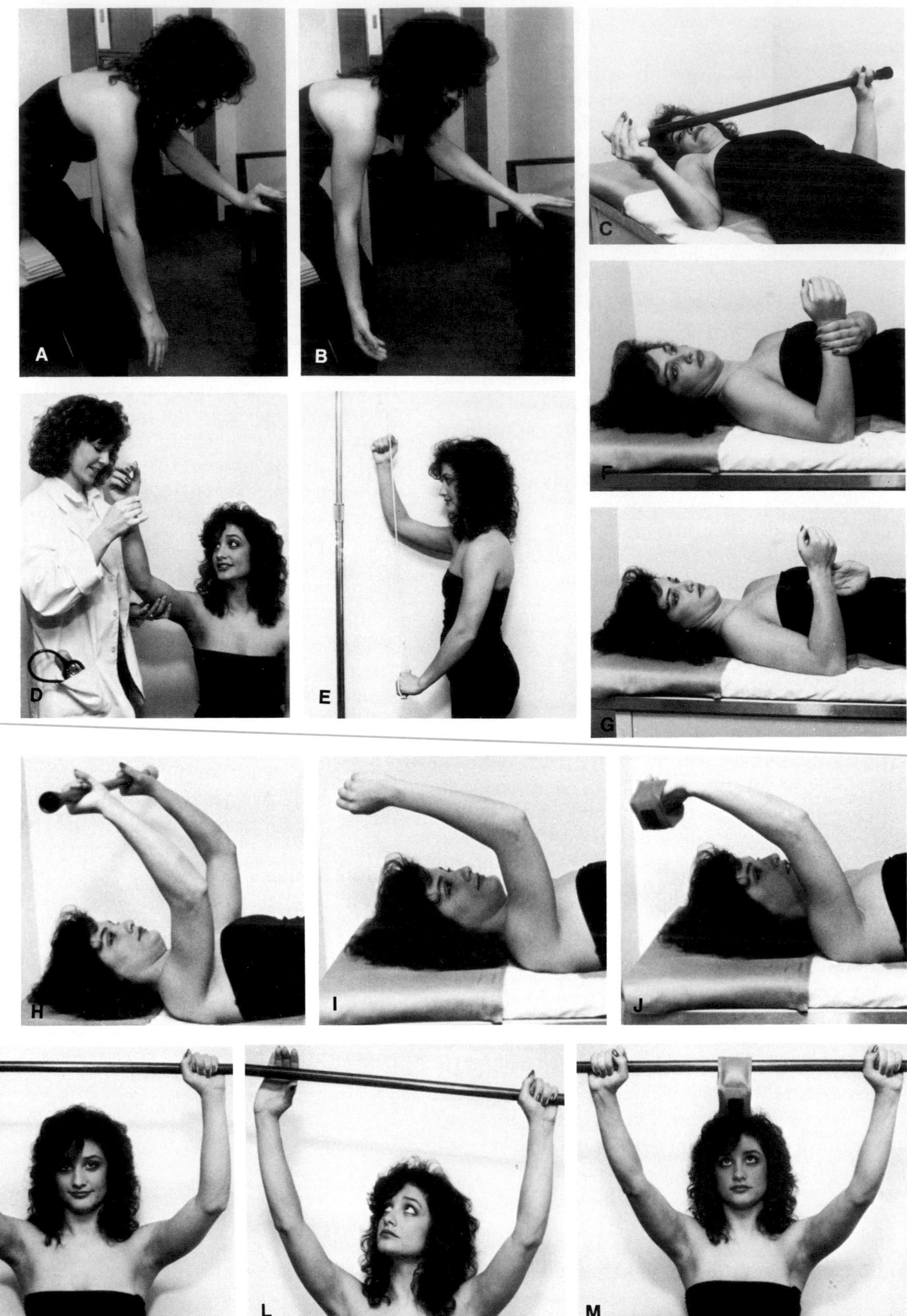

FIGURE 16-41.

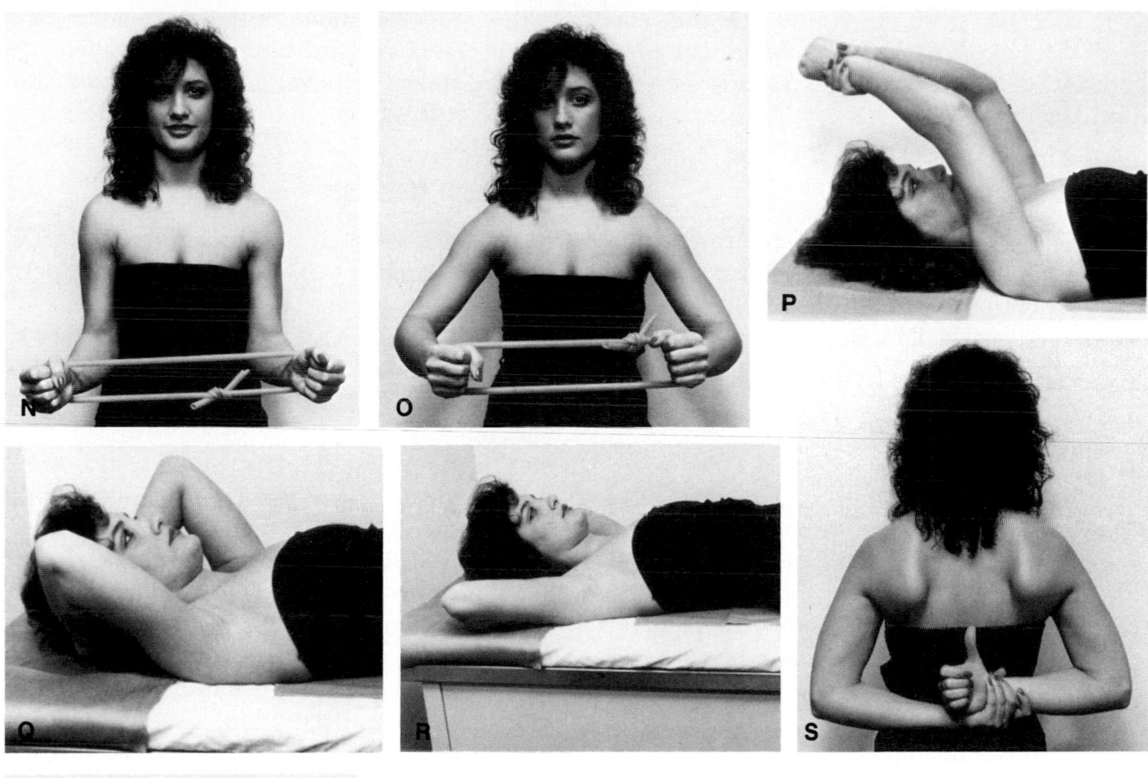

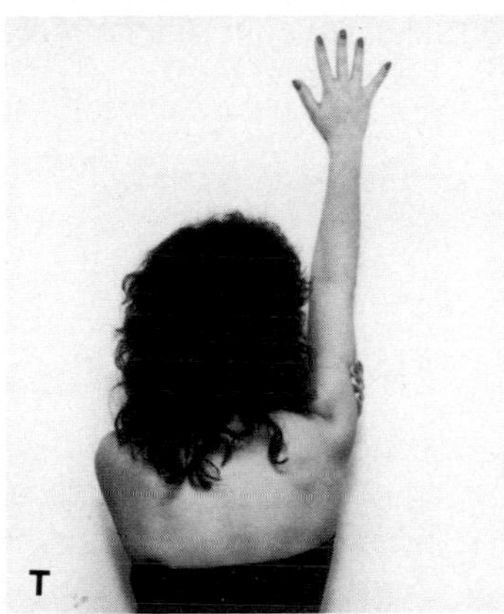

FIGURE 16-41. This exercise regimen should be done at least three to four times a day. It is best to warm up first with a hot shower, heating pad, or hot water bottle. The exercise regimen should take between 15 and 20 minutes. (**A** and **B**) Pendulum exercises are performed with the patient standing and bent over at the waist. Large circles are made with the entire arm with the palm forward and backward. (**C**) External rotation with a stick should be performed supine with the elbow abducted slightly from the side. The noninvolved arm pushes the involved arm out, supplying the power. (**D**) Assisted forward elevation is done by the therapist, with the patient either erect or supine. (**E**) Pulley exercises are performed with the uninvolved arm supplying the power for elevation of the involved arm. (**F** and **G**) Isometric exercises to strengthen both the external and internal rotators are started with the patient supine. (**H–J**) Active forward elevation with a stick is started supine with the elbow bent. As strength permits, this may be done with the arm unassisted. Later, a 1- or 2-pound weight can be added for strengthening. (**K–M**) Erect forward elevation can also be performed with a stick using the uninvolved arm to assist the involved arm.As the patient gets stronger, an attempt should be made to release the stick from the involved hand and to lower the arm on its own. Weights can be added for strengthening. (**N**) Strips of rubber sheeting of various strengths or rubber tubing can be used to strengthen the external rotators by placing the tubing around the wrist, keeping the elbows at the side, and externally rotating. (**O**) This can also be used to strengthen the deltoid by abducting the shoulders. In addition, if the rubber tubing is attached to a doorknob and used, the anterior and posterior deltoids can also be strengthened. (**P–R**) As healing permits, the arm is raised overhead with the help of the other arm and abduction can also be performed. (**S**) Internal rotation is done with the aid of the uninvolved arm or a towel over the shoulder. (**T**) Stretching for a forward elevation can be done against the wall or the end of a door. It is important to try to lean the weight of the body into the wall so as to stretch the shoulder in forward elevation.

nerves is less common. It is thus important to establish, at the time of initial evaluation, if there are any nerve injuries. This can be done clinically by testing skin sensation and motor power. If nerve injury is suspected, it should be explained to the patient and carefully followed. Electromyographic and nerve conduction studies should be used to follow the progress of the injury. In complete axillary nerve injuries that do not show any signs of improvement within 2 to 3 months of injury, early exploration may be indicated.

Chest Injury

Injury to the thorax can also occur after fractures of the proximal humerus.[228,305] There have been several reports of intrathoracic dislocation of the humeral head with surgical neck fractures of the humerus.[106,122,251] In addition, a pneumothorax or a hemopneumothorax can occur after fractures of the proximal humerus.

Myositis Ossificans

Myositis ossificans, especially after fracture–dislocations, has been reported by several authors.[71,229,255] It is unusual for this to occur with uncomplicated fractures but it is seen especially when there is a chronic unreduced fracture–dislocation.

Frozen Shoulder

A frozen shoulder may result if there is inadequate rehabilitation after a fracture or operative repair. It is essential to have a well-organized and monitored physiotherapy program. In general, the first step with a stiff shoulder is to start the patient on a progressive exercise program. However, in cases where the stiffness does not respond to a program of stretching exercises, we would consider performing an open release of adhesions. This is usually preferred to manipulation under anesthesia alone, because of the risk of refracture, particularly in patients with osteoporotic bone. If there is painful hardware or impingement of hardware and the patient does have fracture union, removal of hardware may also be performed at this time.

Avascular Necrosis

Avascular necrosis is not uncommon after three- and four-part fractures and has also been reported after some two-part fractures.[21,92,101,119,147,159,169,180,223,228,248,288,310,311] In reviewing several large series, Hagg and Lundberg[119] have reported an avascular necrosis rate of 3% to 14% after closed reduction of displaced three-part fractures and a rate of 13% to 34% after four-part fractures. The result is usually a stiff, painful joint. In addition to the avascular necrosis, malunion and glenohumeral arthritis may be present, resulting in significant pain and loss of glenohumeral motion. The example seen in Figure 16-42 is that of an active 72-year-old woman who had a painful stiff shoulder, secondary to avascular necrosis, and a malunion of a four-part fracture, which had been treated by closed reduction and early motion. Degenerative arthritis of the glenohumeral joint developed, and a total shoulder replacement was required for pain relief and improved

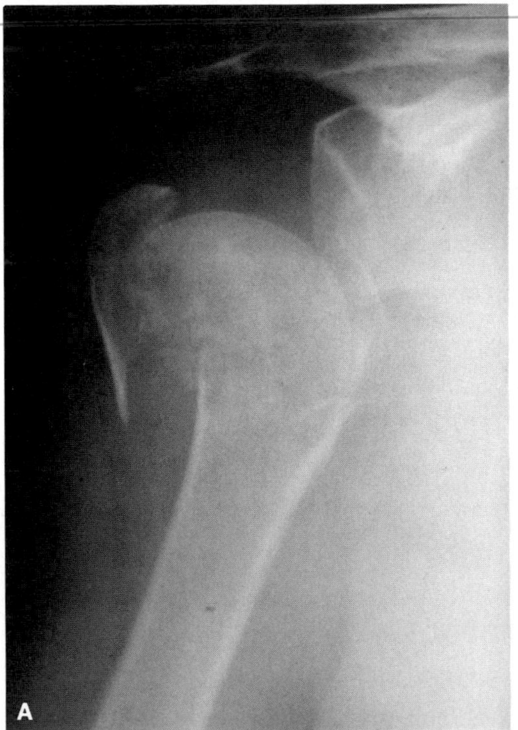

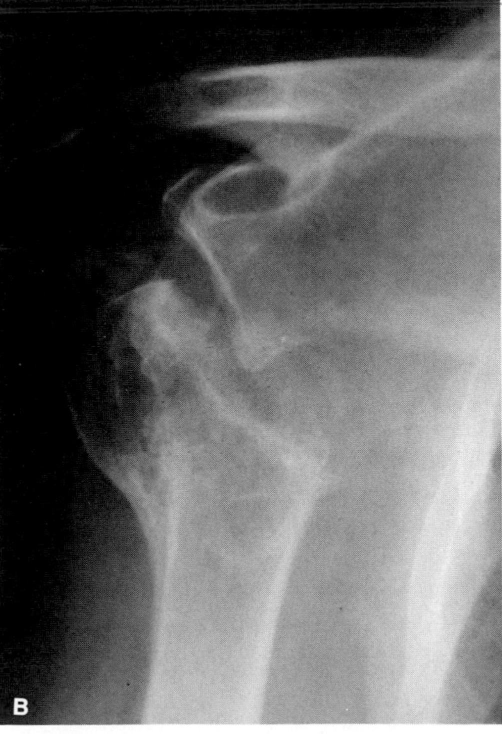

FIGURE 16-42. (**A**) An anteroposterior x-ray of a four-part fracture in an active 72-year-old woman. Her physician believed that there was sufficient congruity of the glenoid and head that early motion could be started and that the patient was too old for an operative procedure. (**B**) Ten months after the fracture, the patient has avascular necrosis and degenerative arthritis. She had significant pain and disability and could not use the upper extremity for even simple activities of daily living. The patient required a total shoulder replacement for pain relief and improved function.

function. This was an especially difficult procedure to perform, since there was joint incongruity and capsular, bursal, and tendon scarring with contracture and loss of bone. However, some reports have described adequate function if there is reasonable congruity of the glenohumeral joint, especially if the tuberosities were anatomically reduced at the initial operative repair.[104,222,223]

Besides the severity of the fracture, extensive dissection of soft tissue has been identified as a major contributing factor. Sturzenegger and associates[310] reported a 34% incidence of avascular necrosis in a series of 17 patients treated with a T-plate. The extensive soft-tissue exposure needed for plate fixation was thought to be a factor in this series (Fig. 16-43). The treatment of choice for avascular necrosis is a humeral head prosthesis or total shoulder replacement, if the glenoid is involved.

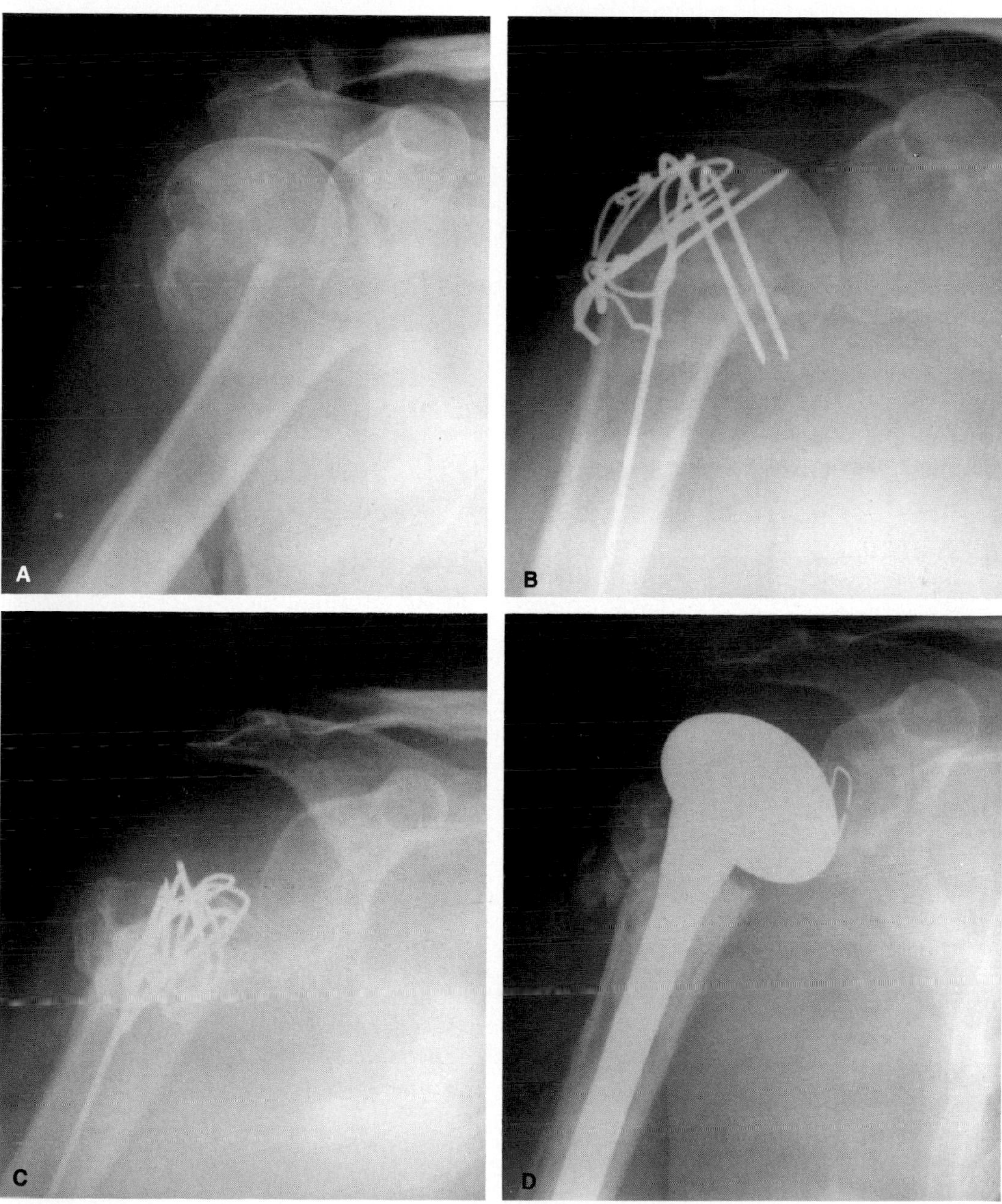

FIGURE 16-43. (**A**) Three-part fracture with avascular necrosis. Anteroposterior x-ray of a three-part greater tuberosity fracture. There is displacement of the shaft medially, and the greater tuberosity is rotated and separated from the head. (**B**) Open reduction and internal fixation achieved with numerous pins and wires. Extensive soft tissue dissection was needed for this repair. (**C**) Eight months postoperatively the head has disappeared due to avascular necrosis. (**D**) This failed fracture repair was salvaged with a total shoulder replacement, since the glenoid was also involved with degenerative disease.

Nonunion

Nonunions of the proximal humerus are not very common[65,80,178,199,229,271,287,304] and are usually associated with displaced fractures, but they can also occur after minimally displaced fractures (see Fig. 16-10). Unfortunately, treatment may be difficult because they often occur in older, debilitated patients with soft, osteoporotic bone. Also, loss of bone stock can occur. The literature on this subject is scarce. In 1964, Sorensen[304] reported on only seven cases, five found in the literature and two of his own. Neer[228,229] reported 16 cases of nonunions in his paper on displaced proximal humeral fractures in 1970 and later reported on an additional 50 cases of nonunion of the surgical neck of the humerus.[234] Some of the nonunions were secondary to a hanging cast or excessive overhead traction. Other causes after closed treatment include severe displacement; comminution; soft-tissue interposition such as capsule, deltoid muscle, or the long head of the biceps; systemic disease; a preexisting stiff glenohumeral joint; an uncooperative patient; and overly aggressive physiotherapy. Nonunion can also occur after open treatment secondary to poor bone quality, inadequate fixation, or infection (Fig. 16-44).

Neer has described a pathologic condition in nonunion of surgical neck fractures in which there is significant resorption of bone beneath the humeral head and a characteristic cavitation of the head fragment, which is produced by the upper end of the shaft. In this situation, there is constant motion because of the unopposed pull of the pectoralis major muscle. A pseudarthrosis with a synovial lining develops because of the communication with the joint and flow of joint fluid into this area. Internal fixation with heavy metal, such as screw and plate fixation, is impossible in this situation because of the poor quality of the remaining humeral head.

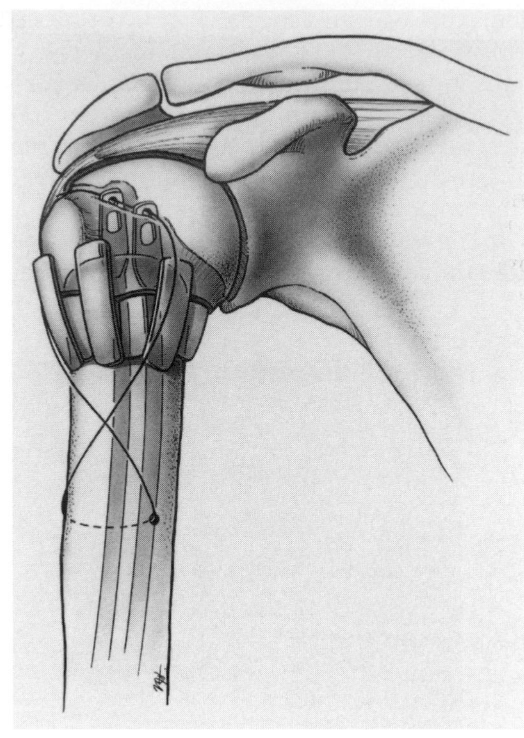

FIGURE 16-45. Schematic of repair of a nonunion of the surgical neck. Enders rods and figure-of-eight tension banding with wire or nonabsorbable sutures are used when the proximal bone can hold fixation and the glenohumeral articular surface is intact. Iliac bone grafting is routinely also performed.

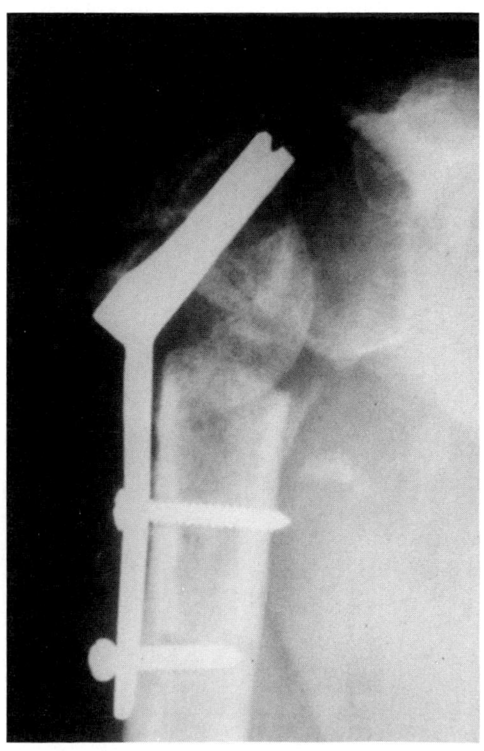

FIGURE 16-44. This patient had an open reduction and internal fixation of a four-part fracture with a baby Jewett nail. This hip device was not appropriate for the shoulder, and the patient went on to have a nonunion as well as an infection after this procedure.

The indications for surgical treatment are significant pain, loss of function, and deformity. Open reduction and internal fixation with the addition of autogenous iliac crest bone graft is the preferred treatment, if there is adequate remaining bone stock (especially of the proximal fragment) (Fig. 16-45). However, a humeral head prosthesis may be necessary if there is articular damage or inadequate bone in the humeral head to hold fixation (Fig. 16-46). Humeral head excision and arthrodesis should be avoided. The results of surgical reconstruction for nonunions of surgical neck fractures are mixed: pain relief is often satisfactory, but overall results are less satisfactory owing to persistent deficits in strength and function at or above shoulder level. Since this is a difficult reconstruction with a significant

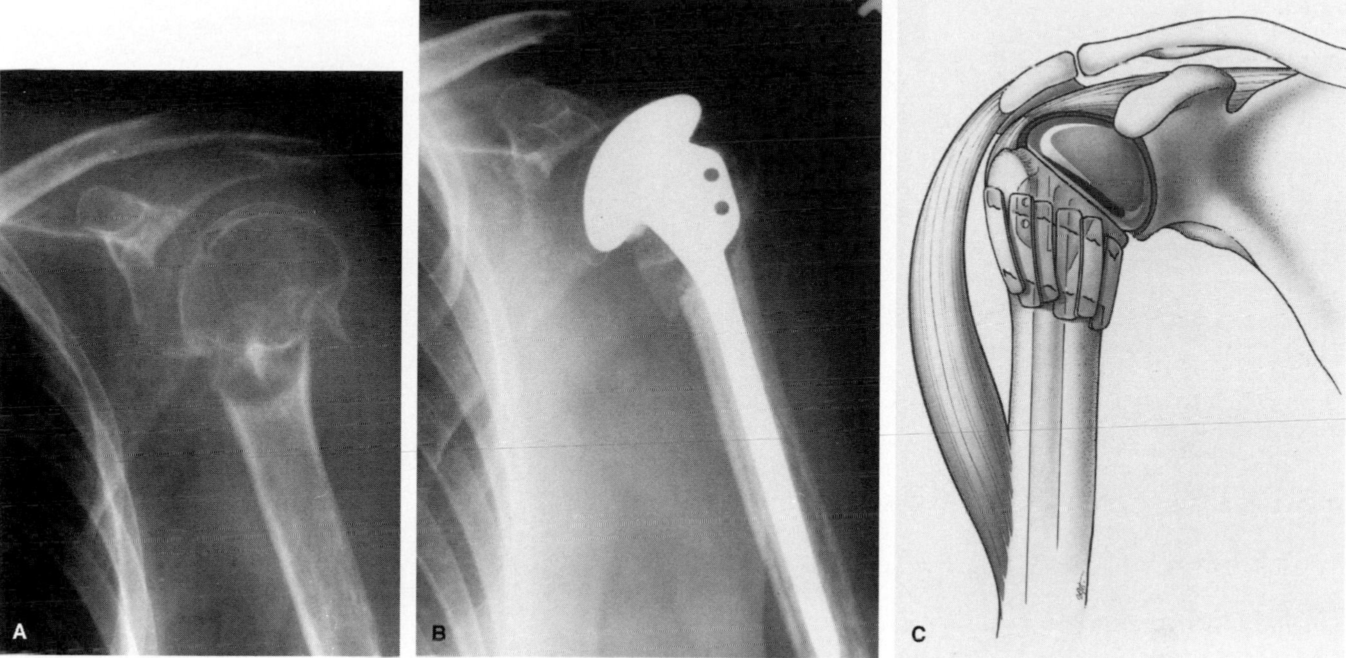

FIGURE 16-46. (**A**) Nonunions of a surgical neck fracture with considerable cavitation of the humeral head, making fixation problematic due to the proximal fragment. (**B**) Surgical reconstruction of the nonunions with humeral head replacement, bone grafting, and fixation of the tuberosities. (**C**) Schematic of reconstruction of a surgical neck nonunion with humeral head replacement and bone grafting. Such reconstructions are challenging with significant risks of complications and should be reserved for patients with disabling symptoms.

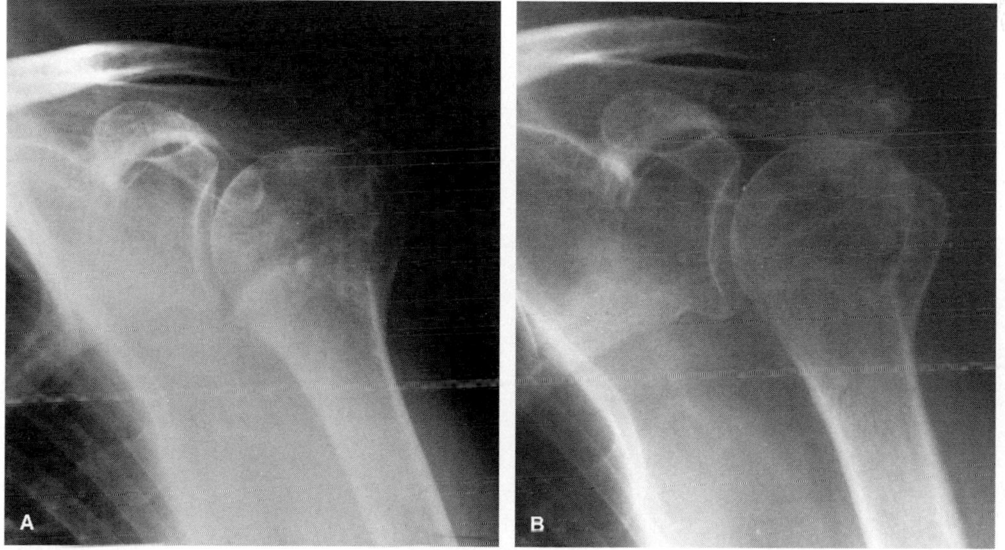

FIGURE 16-47. (**A**) Malunion of a greater tuberosity fracture with a lesser degree of tuberosity prominence superiorly. (**B**) Treatment consisted of an open release of adhesions, as well as an anterior acromioplasty and trimming of the prominent tuberosity fragment. A malunion with a greater degree of tuberosity displacement would require osteotomy, mobilization, and reduction of the tuberosity.

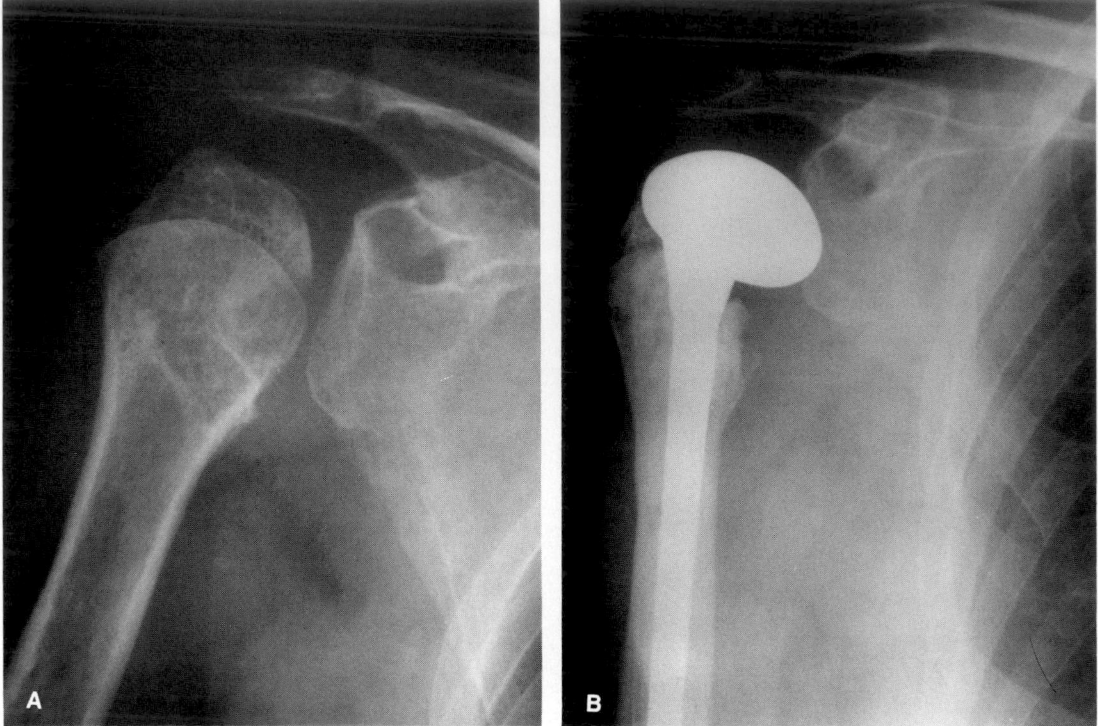

FIGURE 16-48. (**A**) Anteroposterior x-ray of a malunion of a four-part fracture in which the greater tuberosity has healed above the head. The patient's surgery was delayed for 8 months because of neurologic complications. (**B**) A prosthesis was eventually inserted, and the repair was quite difficult because of the malunion and scarring of the soft tissues. The patient eventually achieved 130° of forward elevation with 30° of external rotation. There is some discomfort and weather ache, but the patient does have a functional shoulder.

risk of postoperative complications and limited results, conservative treatment may be an option in older patients who are less symptomatic, especially those in whom the nondominant extremity is involved.[28]

When operative treatment is chosen and there is not a satisfactory quantity and quality of bone to allow open reduction and internal fixation, the choice of hardware should be either Enders rods and figure-of-eight wire or suture or a plate and screws. Rods and wire are preferred in surgical neck nonunions and when the bone is soft. A plate is more suited for proximal shaft nonunions with

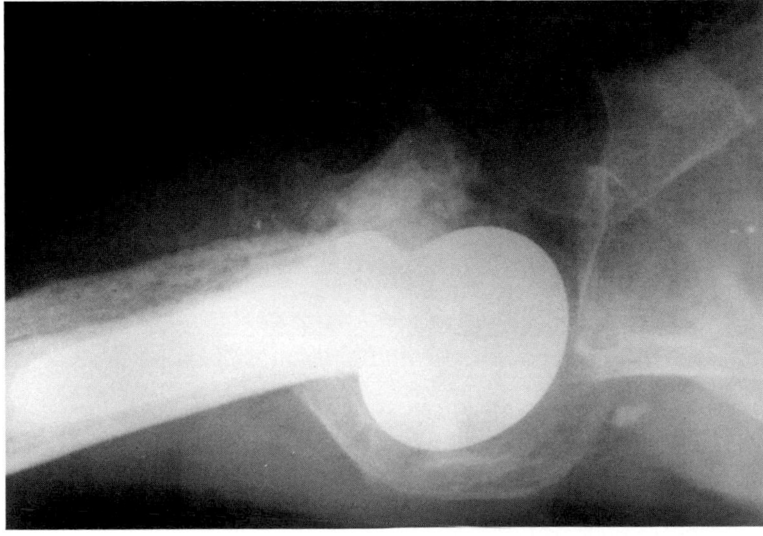

FIGURE 16-49. The patient had a posterior fracture–dislocation that was treated with a Neer prosthesis that also dislocated posteriorly. There was extensive myositis ossificans in the soft tissues.

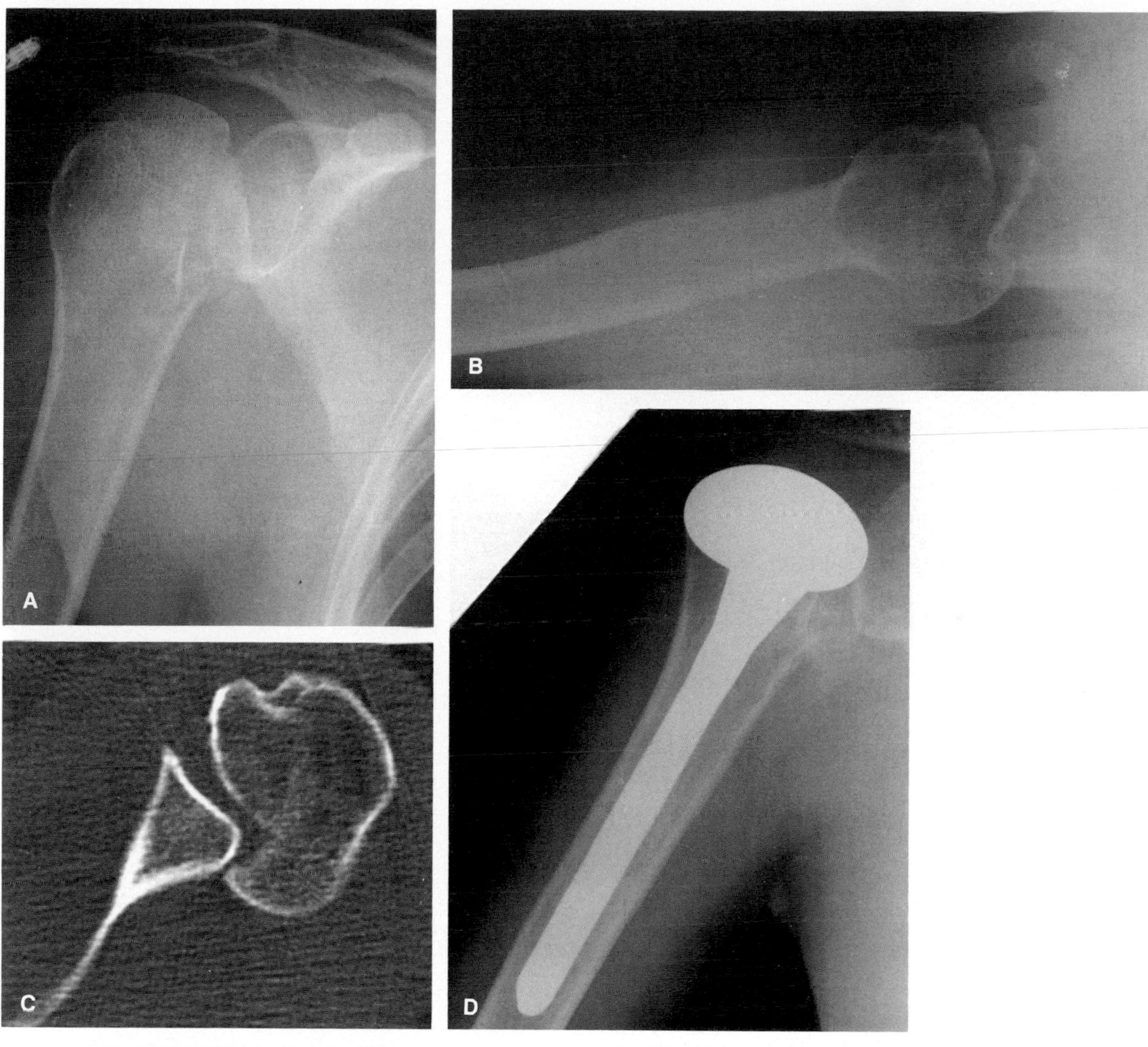

FIGURE 16-50. (**A**) Anteroposterior x-ray showing a posterior fracture–dislocation with involvement of the lesser tuberosity as well as a component of the articular surface. (**B**) Axillary radiograph shows significant involvement of the humeral head with a fracture of the lesser tuberosity. (**C**) CT scan of the head showing a greater than 50% involvement of the articular surface of the head. (**D**) A humeral head prosthesis was put in excessive retroversion and dislocated posteriorly. The patient had significant pain for approximately 8 months after surgery and had a fixed internal rotation contraction of approximately 30°. (**E**) Axillary x-ray shows the prosthesis dislocated posteriorly. (**F**) Anteroposterior x-ray shows a total shoulder replacement that was used to revise the failed humeral head prosthesis. The glenoid was also significantly degenerated. The humeral head was placed in less retroversion, approximately 20°, and this achieved satisfactory stability. In the postoperative period, the patient was held in a neutral position for approximately 2 weeks, and forward elevation was performed in the neutral position, with the patient sitting or standing.

good bone stock so that the screws can hold the cortex.[154] In most cases a spica cast is necessary for 6 to 8 weeks because of poor-quality bone. Electrical stimulation may be a helpful adjunct to promote healing. After the cast is removed, range-of-motion exercises are started and progressed if healing is sufficient. A second procedure may be needed to release adhesions and remove hardware, especially a prominent rod.

Malunion

Malunion occurs after an inadequate closed reduction or a failed open reduction and internal fixation. This problem is especially difficult to treat because there is excessive scar tissue with retraction of the tuberosities, displacement of the shaft, or both. In addition, neurologic and soft-tissue deficits may compromise surgical repair. Greater tuberosity malunions lead to impinge-

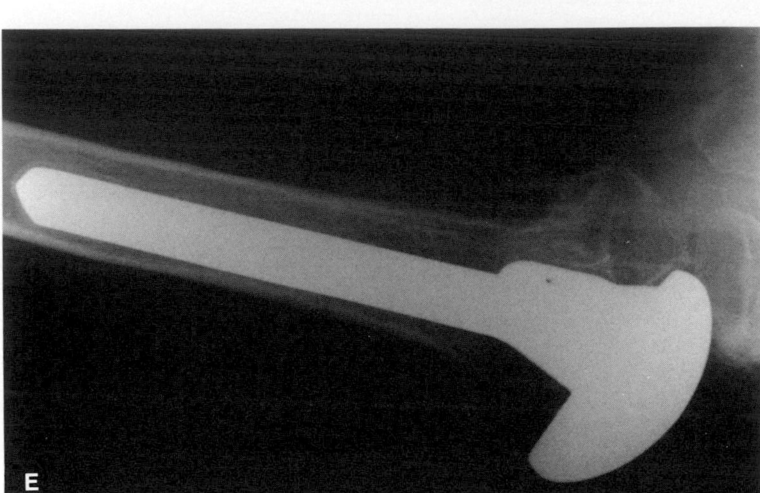

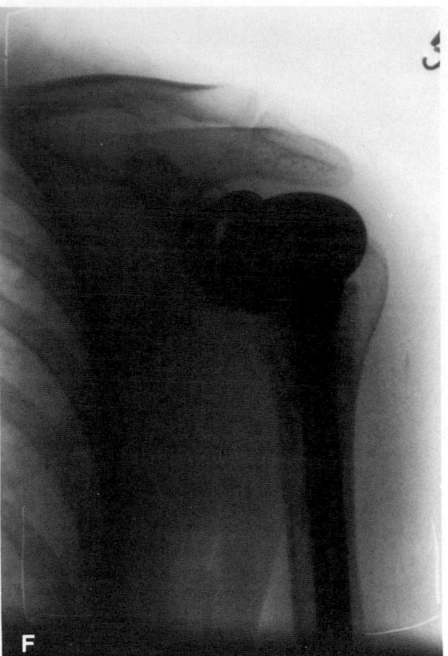

FIGURE 16-50.

ment against the acromion[317] (see Fig. 16-14), if the fragment is superiorly displaced, or abutment against the glenoid if there is posterior retraction. If the displacement of the malunited greater tuberosity is severe, then this problem is best managed through a superior approach in which the fragment is completely mobilized and replaced in its original position. It is important to also mobilize the rotator cuff and bring this tissue out to length. For greater tuberosity malunions that are symptomatic but have lesser amounts of displacement, then removal of the protuberance (exostectomy) along with anterior acromioplasty and a lysis of adhesions provides a satisfactory treatment alternative (Fig. 16-47).

Malunions of three-part fractures are more complex, and avascular necrosis or post-traumatic degenerative arthritis is generally also present. Thus, osteotomy of the displaced fracture components and internal fixation is usually not adequate, and prosthetic replacement is generally required. A glenoid component may be required if there is arthritis of the glenoid surface. Dissection is difficult, and it is important to always be aware of the position of the axillary, suprascapular, and musculocutaneous nerves. A malunion of a surgical neck fracture with increased anterior angulation can limit forward elevation, and osteotomy to correct the anterior angulation and the rotational deformities may be indicated.[117,303] However, seemingly dramatic degrees of surgical neck angulation can be compatible with good function if the joint is supple. Despite the dramatic appearance of radiographs in a surgical neck malunion, much of the functional loss is often due to soft-tissue scarring and adhesions. We have treated a series of patients with loss of motion and a surgical neck malunion with open release and trimming of any prominent spikes with good results.[270] We have reserved osteotomy and open reduction with internal fixation for severe angulation.

Malunion and avascular necrosis of a four-part fracture require a prosthesis. The humeral head is usually quite distorted, and often there is significant displacement of the tuberosities (Fig. 16-48). A tuberosity osteotomy must often be performed to allow adequate placement of the humeral head prosthesis. Unless the head is centered and the proper length of the humerus is maintained, function will be impaired. The results of these procedures are not as good as those of a primary prosthesis, since the scarring and retraction of the tuberosities and soft tissues often limit the range of motion and restrict overhead function. However, the pain relief is usually satisfactory.

Malunion of a fracture–dislocation is extremely difficult to treat because the head component may be totally out of the glenohumeral joint area and wedged against the anterior or posterior aspect of the glenoid. Mobilizing the head from the anterior subcoracoid area is especially dangerous because the neurovascular bundle may be attached to the scar tissue surrounding the head. A very careful dissection should be performed. Furthermore, there is an increased incidence of myositis ossificans after surgical reconstruction of fracture–dislocations (Fig. 16-49).

Revision of Failed Prosthesis

Revision of a failed prosthesis is especially difficult. There may be associated soft-tissue deficits and bone loss as well as nerve paralysis, which may complicate revision surgery. An electromyogram is helpful in the evaluation before any reconstruction. Revision of a prosthesis is indicated for pain relief, since it may be difficult to significantly improve function because of nerve and muscle damage (Fig. 16-50).

ACKNOWLEDGMENTS
Portions of the text and selected illustrations have been used with permission from *The Shoulder,* edited by Charles Rockwood and Frederick Matsen, published by W.B. Saunders Company, Philadelphia, 1990.

REFERENCES

1. Ahlgren, O., and Appel, H.: Proximal Humeral Fractures. Acta Orthop. Scand., 44:124–125, 1973.
2. Ahovuo, J., Paavolainen, P., and Bjorkenheim, J.: Fractures of the Proximal Humerus Involving the Intertubercular Groove. Acta Radiol., 30:373–375, 1989.
3. Aitken, A.P.: End Results of Fractures of the Proximal Humeral Epiphysis. J. Bone Joint Surg., 18:1036–1041, 1936.
4. Albee, F.H.: Juxta-epiphyseal Fracture of the Upper End of the Humerus. Med. Rec., 81:847–851, 1912.
5. Albee, F.H.: Restoration of Shoulder Function in Cases of Loss of Head and Upper Portion of the Humerus. Surgery, 32:11–19, 1921.
6. Alberts, K.A., and Engstrom, C.F.: Fractures of the Proximal Humerus. Opuscula Med., 24(4)121–123, 1979.
7. Aldredge, R.H., and Knight, M.P.: Fractures of the Upper End of the Humerus Treated by Early Relaxed Motion and Massage. New Orleans Med. Surg. J., 92:519–524, 1940.
8. Andreasen, A.T.: Avulsion Fracture of the Lesser Tuberosity of the Humerus. Lancet, 1:750, 1941.
9. De Anquin, C.L., and De Anquin, A.: Prosthetic Replacement in the Treatment of Serious Fractures of the Proximal Humerus. *In* Bayley, I., and Kessel, I. (eds.): Shoulder Surgery. New York, Springer-Verlag, 1965.
10. Ansorge, D.: Fracture Dislocation as a Result of a High Voltage Current Accident. Zentralbl. Chir., 105:465–467, 1980.
11. Arndt, J.H., and Sears, A.D.: Posterior Dislocation of the Shoulder. A.J.R., 94:639–645, 1965.
12. Aufranc, O.E.: Nonunion of Humerus. J.A.M.A., 175:1092–1095, 1961.
13. Aufranc, O.E., Jones, W. N., and Turner, R.H.: Bilateral Shoulder Fracture–Dislocations. J.A.M.A., 195:1140–1143, 1966.
14. Austin, M.D.: Fractures Hazards, Reporting 3 Uncommon Fracture Cases, With Use of Original Crucifixion Splint in Fracture of Surgical Neck of Humerus. Indiana Med., 16:129, 1923.
15. Autin, A.: Traitement des Fractures de l'ESH. Thèse Médicine no. 840 Paris, 1960.
16. Baker, D.M., and Leach, R.E.: Fracture–Dislocation of the Shoulder: Report of Three Unusual Cases With Rotator Cuff Avulsion. J. Trauma, 5:659–664, 1965.
17. Bandi, W.: Zur Operativen Therapie der Humeruskopf-undhalsfrakturen. Unfallheilkunde, 196:38–45, 1976.
18. Bandmann, F.: Beitrag fur Behandlung der Oberarmkopffrakturen. Zentralbl. Chir., 76:97–102, 1951.
19. Bardenheuer, F.H., cited by Hans Lorenz: Die Isolirte Fractur des Tuberculum Minus Humeri. Deut. Zeit. Chir., 58:593, 1900–1901, 1949.
20. Barrett, W.P., Franklin, H., Jackins, S.E., Wyss, C.R., and Matsen, F.A.: Total Shoulder Arthroplasty. J. Bone Joint Surg., 69A:865–872, 1987.
21. Baudin, P.: Intramedullary Nailing of Fractures of the Proximal Humerus. Thèse Médecine. Bordeaux, 1977.
22. Baxter, M.P., and Wiley, J.J.: Fractures of the Proximal Humeral Epiphysis: Their Influence on Humeral Growth. J. Bone Joint Surg., 68B:570–573, 1986.
23. Bell, H.M.: Posterior Fracture–Dislocation of the Shoulder: A Method of Closed Reduction: A Case Report. J. Bone Joint Surg., 47A:1521–1524, 1965.
24. Bengner, U., Johnell, O., and Redlund-Johnell, I.: Changes in the Incidence of Fracture of the Upper End of the Humerus During a 3-Year Period: A Study of 2125 Fractures. Clin. Orthop., 231:179–182, 1988.
25. Bertoft, E.S., Lundh, I., and Ringqvist, I.: Physiotherapy After Fracture of the Proximal End of the Humerus. Scand. J. Rehabil. Med., 16:11–16, 1984.
26. Bigelow, H.J.: A Memoir of Henry Jacob Bigelow. Boston, Little, Brown, 1900.
27. Bigliani, L.U., Flatow, E.L., and Pollock, R.G.: Fracture Classification Systems: Do They Work and Are They Useful? J. Bone Joint Surg., 76A:790–792, 1994.
28. Bigliani, L.U., Nicholson, G.P., Pollock, R.G., Duralde, X.A., Self, E.B., and Flatow, E.L.: Operative treatment of non-unions of the surgical neck of the humerus. Orthop. Trans. 18:937, 1994.
29. Blasier, R.B., and Burkus, J.K.: Management of Posterior Fracture Dislocations of the Shoulder. Clin. Orthop., 232:199–204, 1988.
30. Blevins, F.T., Warren, R.F., Deng, X., and Torzilli, P.A.: Dissociation of humeral shoulder arthroplasty components. J. Shoulder Elbow Surg., 3(Suppl.):S75, 1994.
31. Blom, S., and Dahlback, L.O.: Nerve Injuries in Dislocations of the Shoulder Joint and Fractures of the Neck of the Humerus: A Clinical and Electromyographical Study. Acta Chir. Scand., 136:461–466, 1970.
32. Bloom, M.H., and Obata, W.: Diagnosis of Posterior Dislocation of the Shoulder With Use of Velpeau Axillary and Angle-up Roentgenographic Views. J. Bone Joint Surg., 49A:943–949, 1967.
33. Boehler, J.: Les Fractures Recentes de l'Epaule. Acta Orthop. Belg., 30:235–242, 1964.
34. Bohler, L.: The Treatment of Fractures, 5th ed. New York, Grune & Stratton, 1956.
35. Bohler, L.: The Treatment of Fractures, 4th English ed. Baltimore: Williams Wood & Co., 1935.
36. Bohler, L.: Die Behandlung von Verrenkungsbruchen der Schulter. Dtsch. Z. Chir., 219:238–245, 1929.
37. Bosworth, D.M.: Blade Plate Fixation. J.A.M.A., 141:1111–1113, 1949.
38. Buhr, A.J., and Cooke, A.M.: Fracture Patterns. Lancet, 1:531–535, 1959.
39. Brickner, W.M.: Certain Afflictions of the Shoulder and Their Management. Int. Clin., 2:191–211, 1924.
40. Brighton, C.T., Friedenberg, Z.B., Zemsky, L.M., and Pollis, R.R.: Direct-Current Stimulation on Non-union and Congenital Pseudarthrosis. J. Bone Joint Surg., 57A:368–377, 1975.
41. Brostrom, F.: Early Mobilization of Fractures of the Upper End of the Humerus. Arch. Surg., 46:614–615, 1943.
42. Buchanan, J.J.: Fracture Through the Anatomical Neck of the Humerus With Dislocation of the Head. Ann. Surg., 47:659–671, 1908.
43. Burstein, A.H.: Fracture Classification Systems: Do They Work and Are They Useful? J. Bone Joint Surg., 75A:1743–1744, 1993.
44. Caldwell, G.A.: The Treatment of Fractures of the Upper End of the Humerus. Rocky Mountain Med. J., 40:33, 1943.
45. Caldwell, J.A.: Treatment of Fractures in the Cincinnati General Hospital. Ann. Surg., 97:174–177, 1933.
46. Caldwell, J.A., and Smith, J.: Treatment of Unimpacted Fractures of the Surgical Neck of the Humerus. Am. J. Surg., 31:141–144, 1936.
47. Callahan, D.J.: Anatomic Considerations. Closed Reduction of Proximal Humeral Fractures. Orthop. Rev., 13:79–85, 1984.
48. Carew-McColl, M.: Bilateral Shoulder Dislocations Caused by Electric Shock. Br. J. Clin. Pract., 34:251–254, 1980.
49. Cathcart, C.S.: Movements of the Shoulder Girdle Involved in

Those of the Arm on the Trunk. J. Anat. Physiol., 18:211–218, 1884.
50. Chalier, A.: Fracture de l'Epaule avec Luxation de la Tête Humerale et avec Section Tendineuse du long Biceps. Rep. Lyon Chir., 29:226, 1932.
51. Clifford, P.C.: Fractures of the Neck of the Humerus: A Review of the Late Results. Injury, 12:91–95, 1980.
52. Codman, E.A.: The Shoulder: Rupture of the Supraspinatus Tendon and Other Lesions in or About the Subacromial Bursa, pp. 262–293. Boston, Thomas Todd, 1934.
53. Cofield, R.H.: Comminuted Fractures of the Proximal Humerus. Clin. Orthop., 230:49–57, 1988.
54. Collin, I.: Brug og Misbrug af Massage hos Ulykkesforsikrede Patienter. *In* Kiaer, S. (ed.): Ulykkesforsikringsbogen. Copenhagen, Nordisk Forog, 1931.
55. Conforty, B.: The Results of the Boytchev Procedure for Treatment of Recurrent Dislocation of the Shoulder. Int. Orthop., 4:127–132, 1980.
56. Conforty, B.: Boytchev's Procedure for Recurrent Dislocation of the Shoulder (Proceedings). J. Bone Joint Surg., 56B:386, 1974.
57. Coonse, G.K.: An Improved Humerus Splint for Hospital Use. J. Bone Joint Surg., 13:374–375, 1931.
58. Coonse, G.K., and Moore, H.: Treatment of Fractures of the Humerus by Mobilization and Traction. N. Engl. J. Med., 203:829–832, 1930.
59. Cooper, A.: A Treatise in Dislocations and Fractures of the Joints. Philadelphia, H.C. Carey & I. Lea, 1825.
60. Cooper, A.: On the Dislocation of the Os Humeri Upon the Dorsum Scapulae and Upon Fractures Near the Shoulder Joint. Guy Hosp. Rep., 4:265–284, 1839.
61. Cornell, C.N., Levine, D., and Pagnani, M.J.: Internal fixation of proximal humerus fractures using the screw-tension band technique. J. Orthop. Trauma, 8:23–27, 1994.
62. Cotton, F.J.: Dislocations and Joint Fractures. Philadelphia, W.B. Saunders, 1910.
63. Cotton, F.J.: Subluxation of the Shoulder Downward. Boston Med. Surg. J., 185:405–407, 1921.
64. Cuomo, F., Flatow, E.L., Maday, M., Miller, S.R., McIlveen, S.J., and Bigliani, L.U.: Open Reduction and Internal Fixation of Two- and Three-Part Displaced Surgical Neck Fractures of the Proximal Humerus. J. Shoulder Elbow Surg., 1:287–295, 1992.
65. Coventry, M.B., and Laurnen, E.L.: Ununited Fractures of the Middle and Upper Humerus: Special Problems in Treatment. Clin. Orthop., 69:192–198, 1970.
66. Dameron, T.B.: Complications of Treatment of Injuries to the Shoulder. *In* Epps, C.H. (ed.): Complications in Orthopaedic Surgery, 2nd ed., pp. 247–275. Philadelphia, J.B. Lippincott, 1986.
67. Darder, A., Darder, A. Jr., Sanchis, V., Gastaldi, E., and Gomar, F.: Four-Part Displaced Proximal Humeral Fractures: Operative Treatment Using Kirschner Wires and a Tension Band. J. Orthop. Trauma, 7:497–505, 1993.
68. DeBernardi, L.: Sul Trattamento della Dussazione con Frattura dell'Estremita Superiore dell'Omero. Boll. Mem. Soc. Piemontese Chir., 11:193, 1932.
69. Dehne, E.: Fractures at the Upper End of the Humerus. Surg. Clin. North Am., 25:28–47, 1945.
70. DePalma, A.F.: Surgery of the Shoulder, 3rd ed., pp. 372–403. Philadelphia, J.B. Lippincott, 1983.
71. DePalma, A.F., and Cautilli, R.A.: Fractures of the Upper End of the Humerus. Clin. Orthop., 20:73–93, 1961.
72. Des Marchais, J.E., and Benazet, J.P.: Evaluation de l'Hemiarthroplastie de Neer dans le Traitement des Fractures de l'Humerus. Can. J. Surg., 26:469–471, 1983.
73. Des Marchais, J.E., and Morais, G.: Treatment of Complex Fractures of the Proximal Humerus by Neer Hemiarthroplasty. *In* Bateman, J.E., and Welsh, R.P. (eds.): Surgery of the Shoulder. Philadelphia, B.C. Decker, 1984.
74. Destree, C., and Safary, A.: Le Traitement des Fractures Humerales, Col et Diaphyse, par l'Enclouage Fascicule de Hackethal. Acta Orthop. Belg., 45:666–677, 1979.
75. Dewar, F.P., and Yabsley, R.H.: Fracture–Dislocation of the Shoulder: Report of a Case. J. Bone Joint Surg., 49B:540–543, 1967.
76. Dimon, J.H.: Posterior Dislocation and Posterior Fracture Dislocation of the Shoulder: A Report of 25 Cases. South. Med. J., 60:661–666, 1967.
77. Din, K.M., and Meggitt, B.F.: Bilateral Four-Part Fractures With Posterior Dislocation of the Shoulder: A Case Report. J. Bone Joint Surg., 65B:176–178, 1983.
78. Dingley, A., and Denham, R.: Fracture–Dislocation of the Humeral Head: A Method of Reduction. J. Bone Joint Surg., 55A:1299–1300, 1973.
79. Drapanas, T., Hewitt, R.L., Weichert, R.F., and Smith, A.D.: Civilian Vascular Injuries: A Critical Appraisal of Three Decades of Management. Ann. Surg., 172:351–360, 1970.
80. Drapanas, T., McDonald, J., and Hale, H.W.: A Rational Approach to Classification and Treatment of Fractures of the Surgical Neck of the Humerus. Am. J. Surg., 99:617–624, 1960.
81. Duparc, J., and Largier, A.: Les Luxations-Fractures de l'Extremitie Superieure de l'Humerus. Rev. Chir. Orthop., 62:91–110, 1976.
82. Edelman, G.: Immediate Therapy of Complex Fractures of the Upper End of the Humerus by Means of Acrylic Prosthesis. Presse Med., 59:1777–1778, 1951.
83. Einarsson, F.: Fracture of the Upper End of the Humerus. Acta Orthop. Scand. [Suppl.], 3:10–209, 1958.
84. Ekstrom, T., Lagergren, C., and von Schreeb, T.: Procaine Injections and Early Mobilization for Fractures of the Neck of the Humerus. Acta Chir. Scand., 130:18–24, 1965.
85. Elliot, J.A.: Acute Arterial Occlusion: An Unusual Cause. Surgery, 39:825–826, 1956.
86. Esser, R.D.: Treatment of Three- and Four-Part Fractures of the Proximal Humerus with a Modified Cloverleaf Plate. J. Orthop. Trauma. 8:15–22, 1994.
87. Fairbank, T.J.: Fracture–Subluxations of the Shoulder. J. Bone Joint Surg., 30B:454–460, 1948.
88. Fellander, M.: Fracture–Dislocations of the Shoulder Joint. Acta Chir. Scand., 107:138–145, 1954.
89. Fischer, R.A., Nicholson, G.P., McIlveen, S.J., McCann, P.D., Flatow, E.L., and Bigliani, L.U.: Primary Humeral Head Replacement for Severely Displaced Proximal Humeral Fractures. Orthop. Trans. 16:779, 1992.
90. Flatow, E.L., Bigliani, L.U., and April, E.W.: An Anatomic Study of the Musculocutaneous Nerve and Its Relationship to the Coracoid Process. Clin. Orthop., 244:166–171, 1989.
91. Flatow, E.L., Cuomo, F., Maday, M.G., Miller, S.R., McIlveen, S.J., and Bigliani, L.U.: Open Reduction and Internal Fixation of Two-Part Displaced Fractures of the Greater Tuberosity of the Proximal Part of the Humerus. J. Bone Joint Surg., 73A:1213-1218, 1991.
92. Fourrier, P., and Martini, M.: Post-traumatic Avascular Necrosis of the Humeral Head. Int. Orthop., 1:187–190, 1977.
93. Frankau, C.: A Manipulative Method for the Reduction of Fractures of the Surgical Neck of the Humerus. Lancet, 2:755, 1933.
94. Freg, E.K.: Zur Operation de Bruche am Oberen Ende des Oberarmes. Zentralbl. Chir., 61:851, 1934.
95. Frey, F.: Die Knocherne Heilung von Schienbeinschaftbruchen. Arch. Orthop. Unfallchir., 46:482–484, 1954.
96. Frich, L.H., Sojbjerg, J.O., and Sneppen, O.: Shoulder Arthroplasty in Complex Acute and Chronic Proximal Humeral Fractures. Orthopedics, 14:949–951, 1991.
97. Funsten, R.V., and Kinser, P.: Fractures and Dislocations About the Shoulder. J. Bone Joint Surg., 18:191–198, 1936.
98. Gallagher, J.C., Melton, L.J., Riggs, B.L., and Bergstrath, E.: Epidemiology of Fractures of the Proximal Femur in Rochester, Minnesota. Clin. Orthop., 150:163–171, 1980.
99. Garceau, G.J., and Cogland, S.: Early Physical Therapy in the Treatment of Fractures of the Surgical Neck of the Humerus. Indiana Med., 34:293–295, 1941.
100. Garraway, W.M., Stauffer, R.N., Kurland, L.T., and O'Fallon, W.M.: Limb Fractures in a Defined Population: I. Frequency and Distribution. Mayo Clin. Proc., 54:701–707, 1979.
101. Geneste, R., et al.: Closed Treatment of Fracture–Dislocations of the Shoulder Joint. Rev. Chir. Orthop., 66:383–386, 1980.

102. Gerard-Marchant, P.: Diagnostic et Traitement des Luxations de l'Epaule Compliques de Fracture de l'Humerus. J. Chir., 31:659–670, 1928.
103. Gerber, C., Schneeberger, A., and Vinh, J.S.: The arterial vascularization of the humeral head: An anatomic study. J. Bone Joint Surg., 72A:1486-1494, 1990.
104. Gerber, C., and Berberat, C.: The Clinical Relevance of Posttraumatic Avascular Necrosis of the Humeral Head. J. Shoulder Elbow Surg., 2:S30, 1993.
105. Gibbons, A.P.: Fracture of the Tuberculum Majus by Muscular Violence. Br. Med. J. [Clin. Res.], 2:1674, 1909.
106. Glessner, J.R.: Intrathoracic Dislocation of the Humeral Head. J. Bone Joint Surg., 43A:428–430, 1961.
107. Gold, A.M.: Fractured Neck of the Humerus With Separation and Dislocation of the Humeral Head. Bull. Hosp. Jt. Dis. Orthop. Inst., 32:87–99, 1971.
108. Gordon, D.: Fractures of the Upper End of the Humerus. J.A.M.A., 96:332–336, 1931.
109. Graham, J., and Wood, S.: Aseptic Necrosis of Bone Following Trauma. *In* Davidson, J.K. (ed.): Aseptic Necrosis of Bone, pp. 113–117, 136–137. Amsterdam, Excerpta Medica, 1976.
110. Greeley, P.W., and Magnuson, P.B.: Dislocation of the Shoulder Accompanied by Fracture of the Greater Tuberosity and Complicated by Spinatus Tendon Injury. J.A.M.A., 102:1835–1838, 1934.
111. Greenhill, B.J.: Persistent Posterior Shoulder Dislocation: Its Diagnosis and Its Treatment by Posterior Putti Platt Repair. J. Bone Joint Surg., 54B:763, 1972.
112. Grimes, D.W.: The Use of Rush Pin Fixation in Unstable Upper Humeral Fracture: A Method of Blind Insertion. Orthop. Rev., 9:75–79, 1980.
113. Griswold, R.A., Hucherson, D.C., and Strode, E.C.: Fractures of the Humerus Treated With Hanging Cast. South. Med. J., 34:777–778, 1941.
114. Gurd, F.B.: A Simple Effective Method for the Treatment of Fractures of the Upper Part of the Humerus. Am. J. Surg., 47:433–453, 1940.
115. Haas, K.: Displaced Proximal Humeral Fractures Operated by Rush Pin Technique. Opuscula Med., 23:100–102, 1978.
116. Haas, S.L.: Fracture of the Lesser Tuberosity of the Humerus. Am. J. Surg., 63:253–256, 1944.
117. Habermeyer, P., and Schweiberer, L.: Korrektureingriffe Infolge con Humeruskopffrakturen. Orthopade, 21(2):148-57, 1992.
118. Hackaethal, K.H.: Die Bundelnagelung. Berlin, Springer-Verlag, 1961.
119. Hagg, O., and Lundberg, B.: Aspects of Prognostic Factors in Comminuted and Dislocated Proximal Humeral Fractures. *In* Bateman, J.E., and Welsh, R.P. (eds.): Surgery of the Shoulder, pp. 51–59. Philadelphia, B.C. Decker, 1984.
120. Hall, M.C., and Rosser, M.: The Structure of the Upper End of the Humerus, With Reference to Osteoporotic Changes in Senescence Leading to Fractures. Can. Med. Assoc. J., 88:290–294, 1963.
121. Hall, R.H., Isaac, F., and Booth, C.R.: Dislocations of the Shoulder With Special Reference to Accompanying Small Fractures. J. Bone Joint Surg., 41A:489–494, 1959.
122. Hardcastle, P.H., and Fisher, T.R.: Intrathoracic Displacement of the Humeral Head With Fracture of the Surgical Neck. Injury, 12:313–315, 1981.
123. Hartigan, J.W.: Separation of the Lesser Tuberosity of the Head of the Humerus. N.Y. Med. J., 61:276, 1895.
124. Hawkins, R.J.: Unrecognized Dislocations of the Shoulder. A.A.O.S. Instr. Course Lect., 34:258–263, 1985.
125. Hawkins, R.J., Bell, R.H., and Gurr, K.: The Three-Part Fracture of the Proximal Part of the Humerus: Operative Treatment. J. Bone Joint Surg., 68A:1410–1414, 1986.
126. Hawkins, R.J., Neer, C.S., Pianta, R.M., and Mendoza, F.X.: Locked Posterior Dislocation of the Shoulder. J. Bone Joint Surg., 69A:9–18, 1987.
127. Hawkins, R.J., and Switlyk, P. Acute prosthetic replacement for severe fractures of the proximal humerus. Clin. Orthop. 289:156-60, 1993.
128. Hayes, M.J., and Van Winkle, N.: Axillary Artery Injury With Minimally Displaced Fracture of the Neck of the Humerus. J. Trauma, 23:431–433, 1983.
129. Hendenach, J.C.R.: Recurrent Posterior Dislocation of the Shoulder. J. Bone Joint Surg., 23:582–586, 1947.
130. Henderson, M.S.: The Massive Bone Graft in Ununited Fractures. J.A.M.A., 107:1104–1107, 1936.
131. Henderson, R.S.: Fracture–Dislocation of the Shoulder With Interposition of Long Head of the Biceps: Report of a Case. J. Bone Joint Surg., 34B:240–241, 1952.
132. Henson, G.F.: Vascular Complications of Shoulder Injuries: A Report of Two Cases. J. Bone Joint Surg., 38B:528–531, 1956.
133. Heppenstall, R.B.: Fractures of the Proximal Humerus. Orthop. Clin. North Am., 6:467–475, 1975.
134. Herbert, J.J., and Paillot, J.: Treatment of Complicated Fractures of the Upper End of the Humerus: Epiphysio-diaphysial Pegging. Rev. Chir. Orthop., 46:739–747, 1960.
135. Hermann, O.J.: Fractures of the Shoulder Joint With Special Reference to Correction of Defects. A.A.O.S. Instr. Course Lect., 2:359–370, 1944.
136. Heuget, L., LaLaude, J., and Vielpeau, C.: Bone Cement in the Treatment of Certain Fractures of the Proximal Humerus. Ann. Chir., 27:311–313, 1973.
137. Hill, N.A., and McLaughlin, H.L.: Locked Posterior Dislocation Simulating a 'Frozen Shoulder.' J. Trauma, 3:225–234, 1963.
138. Hippocrates: The Genuine Works of Hippocrates. Baltimore, Williams & Wilkins, 1939.
139. Hitchcock, H.H., and Bechtol, C.O.: Painful Shoulder: Observations on the Role of the Tendon of the Long Head of the Biceps Brachii in Its Causation. J. Bone Joint Surg., 30A:263–273, 1948.
140. Hollingshead, W.H.: Anatomy for Surgeons, Vol. 3. *In* The Back and Limbs, 3rd ed. Philadelphia, Harper & Row, 1982.
141. Horak, J., and Nilsson, B.: Epidemiology of Fractures of the Upper End of the Humerus. Clin. Orthop., 112:250–253, 1975.
142. Howard, N.J., and Eloesser, L.: Treatment of Fractures of the Upper End of the Humerus: An Experimental and Clinical Study. J. Bone Joint Surg., 16:1–29, 1934.
143. Hudson, R.T.: The Use of the Hanging Cast in Treatment of Fractures of the Humerus. South. Surgeon, 10:132–134, 1941.
144. Hughes, M., and Neer, C.S.: Glenohumeral Joint Replacement and Postoperative Rehabilitation. Phys. Ther., 55:850–858, 1975.
145. Hundley, J.M., and Stewart, M.J.: Fractures of the Humerus: A Comparative Study in Methods of Treatment. J. Bone Joint Surg., 37A:681–692, 1955.
146. Jaberg, H., Warner, J.J., and Jakob, R.P.: Percutaneous stabilization of unstable fractures of the humerus. J. Bone Joint Surg. 74A:508–515, 1992.
147. Jakob, R.P., Kristiansen, T., Mayo, K., Ganz, R., and Müller, M.E.: Classification and Aspects of Treatment of Fractures of the Proximal Humerus. *In* Batemen, J.E., and Welsh, R.P. (eds.): Surgery of the Shoulder. Philadelphia, B.C. Decker, 1984.
148. Jakob, R.P., Miniaci, A., Anson, P.S., Jaberg, H., Osterwalder, A., and Ganz, R.: Four-part valgus impacted fractures of the proximal humerus. J. Bone Joint Surg., 73B:295–298, 1991.
149. Johansson, O.: On Complications and Failures of Surgery in Various Fractures of the Humerus. Acta Chir. Scand., 120:469–478, 1961.
150. Jones, L.: Reconstructive Operation for Non-reducible Fractures of the Head of the Humerus. Ann. Surg., 97:217–225, 1933.
151. Jones, L.: The Shoulder Joint: Observations on the Anatomy and Physiology With Analysis of Reconstructive Operation Following Extensive Injury. Surg. Gynecol. Obstet., 75:433–444, 1942.
152. Jones, R.: On Certain Fractures About the Shoulder. Ir. J. Med. Sci., 78:282–291, 1932.
153. Jones, R.: Certain Injuries Commonly Associated With Displacement of the Head of the Humerus. B.M.J., 1:1385–1386, 1906.
154. Jupiter, J.B., and Mullaji, A.B.: Blade plate fixation of proximal humeral non-unions. Br. J. Accident Surg., 25:301–303, 1994.

155. Keen, W.W.: Fractures of the Tuberculum Majus. Ann. Surg., 45:938–949, 1907.
156. Keene, J.S., Huizenga, R.E., Engber, W.D., and Rogers, S.C.: Proximal Humeral Fractures: A Correction of Residual Deformity With Long-term Function. Orthopedics, 6:173–178, 1983.
157. Kelly, J.P.: Fractures Complicating Electroconvulsive Therapy and Chronic Epilepsy. J. Bone Joint Surg., 36B:70–79, 1954.
158. Key, J.A., and Conwell, H.E.: Fractures, Dislocations, and Sprains, 7th ed., pp. 348–431. St. Louis, C.V. Mosby, 1961.
159. Knight, R.A., and Mayne, J.A.: Comminuted Fractures and Fracture–Dislocations Involving the Articular Surface of the Humeral Head. J. Bone Joint Surg., 39A:1343–1355, 1957.
160. Knowleden, J., Buhr, A.J., and Dunbar, O.: Incidence of Fractures in Persons Over 35 Years of Age: A Report to the M.R.C. Working Party on Fractures in the Elderly. Br. J. Prev. Soc. Med., 18:130–141, 1964.
161. Kocher, T.: Beitrage zur Kenntnis Einiger Praktisch Wichtiger Fracturenformen. Basel, Carl Sallman Verlag, 1896.
162. Kocialkowski, A., and Wallace, W.A.: Closed Percutaneous K-Wire Stabilization for Displaced Fractures of the Surgical Neck of the Humerus. Br. J. Accident Surg., 21:209–212, 1990.
163. Kofoed, H.: Revascularization of the Humeral Head. Clin. Orthop., 179:175–178, 1983.
164. Koval, K.J., Sanders, R., Zuckerman, J.D., et al.: Modified-Tension Band Wiring of Displaced Surgical Neck Fractures of the Humerus. J. Shoulder Elbow Surg., 2:85–92, 1993.
165. Krakovic, M., et al.: Indications and Results of Operation in Proximal Humeral Fractures. Monatsschr. Unfallheilk., 78: 326–332, 1975.
166. Kraulis, J., and Hunter, G.: The Results of Prosthetic Replacement in Fracture–Dislocations of the Upper End of the Humerus. Injury, 8:129–131, 1976.
167. Kristiansen, B.: External Fixation of Proximal Humerus Fracture. Acta Orthop. Scand., 58:645–648, 1987.
168. Kristiansen, B., Andersen, U.L., Olsen, C.A., and Varmarken, J.E.: The Neer Classification of Fractures of the Proximal Humerus: An Assessment of Interobserver Variation. Skeletal Radiol. 17:420–422, 1988.
169. Kristiansen, B., and Christensen, S.W.: Plate Fixation of Proximal Humeral Fractures. Acta Orthop. Scand., 57:320–323, 1986.
170. Kristiansen, B., and Christensen, S.W.: Proximal Humeral Fractures. Acta Orthop. Scand., 58:124–127, 1987.
171. Kristiansen, B., and Kofoed, H.: External Fixation of Displaced Fractures of the Proximal Humerus. J. Bone Joint Surg., 69B:643–646, 1987.
172. Kristiansen, B., and Kofoed, H.: Transcutaneous Reduction and External Fixation of Displaced Fractures of the Proximal Humerus. J. Bone Joint Surg., 70B:821–824, 1988.
173. LaBriola, J.H., and Mohaghegh, H.A.: Isolated Avulsion Fracture of the Lesser Tuberosity of the Humerus: A Case Report and Review of the Literature. J. Bone Joint Surg., 57A:1011, 1975.
174. LaFerte, A.D., and Nutter, P.D.: The Treatment of Fractures of the Humerus by Means of Hanging Plaster Cast: "Hanging Cast." Ann. Surg., 114:919–930, 1955.
175. Laing, P.G.: The Arterial Supply of the Adult Humerus. J. Bone Joint Surg., 38A:1105–1116, 1956.
176. Lane, L.B., Villacin, A., and Bullough, P.G.: The Vascularity and Remodelling of Subchondral Bone and Calcified Cartilage in Adult Human Femoral and Humeral Heads: An Age- and Stress-Related Phenomenon. J. Bone Joint Surg., 59B:272–278, 1977.
177. Lasher, W.W.: Fracture–Dislocation of the Head of the Humerus. J.A.M.A., 84:356–358, 1925.
178. Leach, R.E., and Premer, R.F.: Nonunion of the Surgical Neck of the Humerus: Method of Internal Fixation. Minn. Med., 48:318–322, 1965.
179. LeBorgne, J., LeNeel, J.C., and Mitland, D.: Les Lesions de l'Artere Axillaire et ses Branches Consecutives a un Traumatisme Ferme de l'Epaule. Ann. Chir., 27:587–594, 1973.
180. Lee, C.K., and Hansen, H.R.: Post-traumatic Avascular Necrosis of the Humeral Head in Displaced Proximal Humeral Fractures. J. Trauma, 21:788–791, 1981.
181. Lee, C.K., Hansen, H.T., and Weiss, A.B.: Surgical Treatment of the Difficult Humeral Neck Fracture: Acromial Shortening Anterolateral Approach. J. Trauma, 20:67–70, 1980.
182. Leikkonen, O.: Osteosynthesis With Special Modified Plate in Fractures of the Proximal End of the Humerus. Ann. Clin. Gynaecol. Fenn., 49:309–314, 1960.
183. Lentz, W., and Meuser, P.: The Treatment of Fractures of the Proximal Humerus. Arch. Orthop. Trauma Surg., 96:283–285, 1980.
184. Leyshon, R.L.: Closed Treatment of Fractures of the Proximal Humerus. Acta Orthop. Scand. 55:48–51, 1984.
185. Lim, T.E., Ochsner, P.E., Marti, R.K., and Holscher, A.A.: The Results of Treatment of Comminuted Fractures and Fracture–Dislocations of the Proximal Humerus. Neth. J. Surg., 35:139–143, 1983.
186. Lind, T., Kroner, T.K., and Jensen, J.: The Epidemiology of Fractures of the Proximal Humerus. Arch. Orthop. Trauma Surg., 108:285–287, 1989.
187. Lindholm, T.S., and Elmstedt, E.: Bilateral Posterior Dislocation of the Shoulder Combined With Fracture of the Proximal Humerus: A Case Report. Acta Orthop. Scand., 51:485–488, 1980.
188. Linson, M.A.: Axillary Artery Thrombosis After Fracture of the Humerus: A Case Report. J. Bone Joint Surg., 62A:1214–1215, 1980.
189. Lorenz, H.: Die Isolirte Fractur des Tuberculum minus Humeri. Dtsch. Zeitschr. Chir., 58:593, 1900–1901.
190. Lorenzo, F.T.: Osteosynthesis With Blount Staples in Fracture of the Proximal End of the Humerus: A Preliminary Report. J. Bone Joint Surg., 37A:45–48, 1955.
191. Lovett, R.W.: The Diagnosis and Treatment of Some Common Injuries of the Shoulder Joint. Surg. Gynecol. Obstet., 34:437–444, 1922.
192. Lucas-Championniere, J.: Traitement des Fractures par le Massage et la Mobilisation. Paris, Rueff, 1895.
193. Lundberg, B.J., Svenungson-Hartwig, E., and Vikmark, R.: Independent Exercises Versus Physiotherapy in Non-displaced Proximal Humeral Fractures. Scand. J. Rehabil. Med., 11:133–136, 1979.
194. Luppino, D., Santangelo, G., Vicenzi, G., Innao, V., and Capelli, A.: Le Fratture dell'Estremita Prossimale dell'Omero de Interesse Chirurgico (Studio de 40 Casi). Chir. Organi Mov., 67:373–381, 1982.
195. MacDonald, F.R.: Intra-articular Fractures in Recurrent Dislocations of the Shoulder. Surg. Clin. North Am., 43:1635–1645, 1963.
196. Machmull, G., and Weeder, S.D.: Bilateral Fracture of the Anatomical and Surgical Necks of the Humeral Heads: Cases With Bilateral Fracture of the Anatomical and Surgical Necks of the Humeri Due to Convulsion. Radiology, 55:735–739, 1950.
197. Marotte, J.H., Lord, G., and Bancel, P.: L'Arthroplastie de Neer dans les Fractures et Fractures-Lexatons Complexes de l'Epaule: A Propos de 12 Cas. Chirurgie, 104:816–821, 1978.
198. Mason, J.M.: The Treatment of Dislocation of the Shoulder Joint Complicated by Fracture of the Upper Extremity of the Humerus. Ann. Surg., 47:672–705, 1908.
199. Mauclaire, M.: Bull. Mem. Soc. Chir. Paris, 46:572, 1920.
200. Mazet, R.: Intramedullary Fixation in the Arm and the Forearm. Clin. Orthop., 2:75–92, 1953.
201. McBurney, C., and Dowd, C.N.: Dislocation of the Humerus Complicated by Fracture at or Near the Surgical Neck With a New Method of Reduction. Ann. Surg., 19:399–415, 1894.
202. McCann PD, Wootten ME, Kadaba MP, Bigliani LU: A kinematic and electromyographic study of shoulder rehabilitation exercises. Clin. Orthop., 288:179-188, 1993.
203. McGuinness, J.P.: Isolated Avulsion Fracture of the Lesser Tuberosity of the Humerus. Lancet, 1:508, 1939.
204. McLaughlin, H.L.: Dislocation of the Shoulder With Tuberosity Fracture. Surg. Clin. North Am., 43:1615–1620, 1963.
205. McLaughlin, H.L.: Locked Posterior Subluxation of the Shoulder: Diagnosis and Treatment. Surg. Clin. North Am., 43:1621–1622, 1963.

206. McLaughlin, H.L.: Posterior Dislocation of the Shoulder. J. Bone Joint Surg., 34A:584–590, 1952.
207. McLaughlin, H.L.: Treatment of Shoulder Injuries. *In* American Academy of Orthopaedic Surgeons: Regional Orthopaedic Surgery and Fundamental Orthopaedic Problems. Ann Arbor, Mich., Edwards, 1947.
208. McQuillan, W.M., and Nolan, B.: Ischemia Complicating Injury: A Report of Thirty-seven Cases. J. Bone Joint Surg., 50B:482–492, 1968.
209. McWhorter, G.L.: Fractures of the Greater Tuberosity of the Humerus With Displacement. Surg. Clin. North Am., 5:1005–1017, 1925.
210. Mestdagh, H., Butruille, Y., Tillie, B., and Bocquet, F.: Resultats du Traitement des Fractures de l'Extremite Superieure de l'Humerus par Embrochage Percutané: A Propos de Cent Quarante-deux Cas. Ann. Chir., 38:5–13, 1984.
211. Meyerding, H.W.: Fracture–Dislocation of the Shoulder. Minn. Med., 20:717–726, 1937.
212. Michaelis, L.S.: Comminuted Fracture–Dislocation of the Shoulder. J. Bone Joint Surg., 26:363–365, 1944.
213. Milch, H.: The Treatment of Recent Dislocations and Fracture–Dislocations of the Shoulder. J. Bone Joint Surg., 31A:173–180, 1949.
214. Milch, H.: Treatment of Dislocation of the Shoulder. Surgery, 3:732–740, 1938.
215. Miller, S.R.: Practical Points in the Diagnosis and Treatment of Fractures of the Upper Fourth of the Humerus. Indust. Med., 9:458–460, 1940.
216. Mills, H.J., and Horne, G.: Fractures of the Proximal Humerus in Adults. J. Trauma, 25:801–805, 1985.
217. Mills, K.L.G.: Severe Injuries of the Upper End of the Humerus. Injury, 6:13–21, 1974.
218. Mills, K.L.G.: Simultaneous Bilateral Posterior Fracture–Dislocation of the Shoulder. Injury, 6:39–41, 1974.
219. Moeckel, B.H., Dines, D.M., Warren, R.F., and Altchek, D.W.: Modular Hemiarthroplasty for Fractures of the Proximal Part of the Humerus. J. Bone Joint Surg., 74A:884–889, 1992.
220. Moriber, L.A., and Patterson, R.L.: Fractures of the Proximal End of the Humerus. J. Bone Joint Surg., 49A:1018, 1967.
221. Morris, M.E., Kilcoyne, R.F., and Shuman, W.: Humeral Tuberosity Fractures: Evaluation by CT Scan and Management of Malunion. Orthop. Trans., 11:242, 1987.
222. Moseley, H.F.: The Arterial Pattern of the Rotator Cuff of the Shoulder. J. Bone Joint Surg., 45B:780–789, 1983.
223. Mouradian, W.H.: Displaced Proximal Humeral Fractures: Seven Years' Experience With a Modified Zickel Supracondylar Device. Clin. Orthop., 212:209–218, 1986.
224. de Mourgues, G., Razemon, J.-P., Leclair, H.P., Comtet, J.J., and Suares, H.: Fracture–Dislocations of the Shoulder Joint. Rev. Chir. Orthop., 51:151–156, 2185.
225. Murphy, J.B.: Nailing of Fracture of Surgical Neck of Humerus After an Unsuccessful Attempt to Secure Union by Bone Transplantation. Surg. Clin. Chicago, 3:531–536, 1914.
226. Neer, C.S.: Articular Replacement for the Humeral Head. J. Bone Joint Surg., 37A:215–228, 1955.
227. Neer, C.S.: Degenerative Lesions of the Proximal Humeral Articular Surface. Clin. Orthop., 20:116–125, 1981.
228. Neer, C.S.: Displaced Proximal Humeral Fractures: I. Classification and Evaluation. J. Bone Joint Surg., 52A:1077–1089, 1970.
229. Neer, C.S.: Displaced Proximal Humeral Fractures: II. Treatment of Three-Part and Four-Part Displacement. J. Bone Joint Surg., 52A:1090–1103, 1970.
230. Neer, C.S.: Four-Segment Classification of Displaced Proximal Humeral Fractures. A.A.O.S. Instr. Course Lect. 24:160–168, 1975.
231. Neer, C.S.: Fracture Classification Systems: Do They Work and Are They Useful? J. Bone Joint Surg., 76A:789–790, 1994.
232. Neer, C.S.: Indications for Replacement of the Proximal Humeral Articulation. Am. J. Surg., 89:901–907, 1955.
233. Neer, C.S.: Prosthetic Replacement of the Humeral Head: Indications and Operative Technique. Surg. Clin. North Am., 43:1581–1597, 1983.
234. Neer, C.S., II: Nonunion of the Surgical Neck of the Humerus. Orthop. Trans., 7:389, 1983.
235. Neer, C.S., Brown, T.H., and McLaughlin, H.L.: Fracture of the Neck of the Humerus With Dislocation of the Head Fragment. Am. J. Surg., 85:252–258, 1953.
236. Neer, C.S., McCann, P.D., Macfarlane, E.A., and Padilla, N.: Earlier Passive Motion Following Shoulder Arthroplasty and Rotator Cuff Repair: A Prospective Study. Orthop. Trans., 11:231, 1987.
237. Neer, C.S., and McIlveen, S.J.: Recent Results and Technique of Prosthetic Replacement for 4-part Proximal Humeral Fractures. Orthop. Trans., 10:475, 1986.
238. Neer, C.S., and Rockwood, C.A., Jr.: Fractures and Dislocations of the Shoulder. *In* Rockwood, C.A., and Green, D.P. (eds.): Fractures, 2nd ed., pp. 675–707, Philadelphia, J.B. Lippincott, 1984.
239. Neer, C.S., Watson, K.C., and Stanton, F.J.: Recent Experience in Total Shoulder Replacement. J. Bone Joint Surg., 64A:319–337, 1982.
240. Neviaser, J.S.: Complicated Fractures and Dislocations About the Shoulder Joint. J. Bone Joint Surg., 44A:984–998, 1982.
241. Newton-John, H.F., and Morgan, D.B.: The Loss of Bone With Age, Osteoporosis, and Fractures. Clin. Orthop., 71:229–252, 1970.
242. Nicola, F.G., Ellman, H., Eckardt, J., and Finerman, G.: Bilateral Posterior Fracture–Dislocation of the Shoulder Treated With a Modification of the McLaughlin Procedure. J. Bone Joint Surg., 63A:1175–1177, 1981.
243. Nissen-Lie, H.S.: Pseudarthroses of Humerus. Acta Orthop. Scand., 21:22–30, 1951.
244. North, J.P.: The Conservative Treatment of Fractures of the Humerus. Surg. Clin. North Am., 20:1633–1643, 1940.
245. O'Flanagan, P.H.: Fracture Due to Shock From Domestic Electricity Supply. Injury, 6:244–245, 1975.
246. Oni, O.O.A.: Irreducible Acute Anterior Dislocation of the Shoulder Due to a Loose Fragment From an Associated Fracture of the Greater Tuberosity. Injury, 15:138, 1983.
247. Ostapowicz, G., and Rahn-Myrach, A.: The Functional Treatment of Fractures of the Head of the Humerus. Bruns. Butr. Klin. Chir., 202:96–114, 1981.
248. Paavolainen, P., Bjorkenheim, J.-M., Slatis, P., and Paukku, P.: Operative Treatment of Severe Proximal Humeral Fractures. Acta Orthop. Scand., 54:374–379, 1983.
249. Palmer, I.A.: A Dualistic Method of Treatment Pseudoarthrosis. Acta Chir. Scand., 107:261–268, 1954.
250. Palmer, I.: On the Complications and Technical Problems of Medullary Nailing. Acta Chir. Scand., 101:491–492, 1951.
251. Patel, M.R., Pardee, M.L., and Singerman, R.C.: Intrathoracic Dislocation of the Head of the Humerus. J. Bone Joint Surg., 45A:1712–1714, 1983.
252. Phemister, D.B.: Fractures of the Greater Tuberosity of the Humerus. Ann. Surg., 37:440–449, 1912.
253. Pilgaard, S., and Och Oster, A.: Four-Segment Fractures of the Humeral Neck. Acta Orthop. Scand., 44:124, 1973.
254. Poilleux, F., and Courtois-Suffit, M.: Des Fractures du Col Chirurgical de l'Humerus. Rev. Chir., 133–158, 1954.
255. Post, M.: Fractures of the Upper Humerus. Orthop. Clin. North Am., 11:239–252, 1980.
256. Prillaman, H.A., and Thompson, R.C.: Bilateral Posterior Fracture–Dislocation of the Shoulder: A Case Report. J. Bone Joint Surg., 51A:1627–1630, 1989.
257. Proximal Humeral Fractures. What Price History? Editorial. Injury, 12:89–90, 1981.
258. Raney, R.B.: The Treatment of Fractures of the Humerus With the Hanging Cast. N. C. Med. J., 6:88–92, 1945.
259. Rasmussen, S., Hvass, I., Dalsgaard, J., Christensen, B.S., and Holstad, E.: Displaced Proximal Humerus Fractures: Results of Conservative Treatment. Br. J. Accident Surg., 23(1):1–3, 1992.
260. Rathbun, J.B., and Macnab, I.: The Microvascular Pattern of the Rotator Cuff. J. Bone Joint Surg., 52B:540–553, 1970.
261. Razemon, J.P., and Baux, S.: Fractures and Fracture–Dislocations of the Proximal Humerus. Rev. Chir. Orthop., 55:387–396, 1965.

262. Rechtman, A.M.: Open Reduction of Fracture–Dislocation of the Humerus. J.A.M.A., 94:1656–1657, 1930.
263. Reckling, F.W.: Posterior Fracture–Dislocation of the Shoulder Treated by a Neer Hemiarthroplasty With a Posterior Surgical Approach. Clin. Orthop., 207:133–137, 1986.
264. Rendlich, R.A., and Poppel, M.H.: Roentgen Diagnosis of Posterior Dislocation of the Shoulder. Radiology, 36:42–45, 1941.
265. Richard, A., Judet, R., and Rene, L.: Reconstruction Prothetique Acrylique de l'Extremite Superieure de l'Humerus Specialement au Cours des Fratures-Luxations. J. Chir., 68:537–547, 1952.
266. Richards, R.R., An, K-N., Bigliani, L.U., et al: A Standardized Method for the Assessment of Shoulder Function. J. Shoulder Elbow Surg., 3:347–352, 1994.
267. Rob, C.G., and Standeven, A.: Closed Traumatic Lesions of the Axillary and Brachial Arteries. Lancet, 1:597–599, 1956.
268. Roberts, S.M.: Fractures of the Upper End of the Humerus: An End-Result Study Which Shows the Advantage of Early Active Motion. J.A.M.A., 98:367–373, 1932.
269. Rockwood, C.A., Jr.: Fracture Classification Systems: Do They Work and Are They Useful? J. Bone Joint Surg., 76A:790, 1994.
270. Rodosky, M.W., Duralde, X.A., Pollock, R.G., Flatow, E.L., and Bigliani, L.U.: Operative Treatment of Malunions of Proximal Humerus Fractures. Presented at the American Shoulder and Elbow Surgeons Tenth Open Meeting, New Orleans, Louisiana, Feb. 27, 1994.
271. Rooney, P.J., and Cockshott, W.P.: Pseudarthrosis Following Proximal Humeral Fractures: A Possible Mechanism. Skeletal Radiol., 15:21–24, 1986.
272. Rose, S.H., Melton, L.J., Morrey, B.F., Ilstrup, D.M., and Riggs, L.B.: Epidemiologic Features of Humeral Fractures. Clin. Orthop., 168:24–30, 1982.
273. Rosen, H.: Tension Band Wiring for Fracture Dislocation of the Shoulder. *In* Proceedings of the 12th Congress of the International Society of Orthopaedic Surgery and Traumatolgie, pp. 939–941. Tel Aviv, October 9–12, 1972.
274. Ross, J., and Lov, J.B.: Isolated Evulsion Fracture of the Lesser Tuberosity of the Humerus: Report of Two Cases. Radiology, 172:833–834, 1989.
275. Rothman, R.H., Marvel, J.P., and Heppenstall, R.B.: Anatomic Considerations in the Glenohumeral Joint. Orthop. Clin. North Am., 6:341–352, 1975.
276. Rothman, R.H., and Parke, W.W.: The Vascular Anatomy of the Rotator Cuff. Clin. Orthop., 41:176–186, 1985.
277. Rowe, C.R., and Colville, M.: The Glenohumeral Joint. *In* Rowe, C.R. (ed.): The Shoulder, pp. 331–358. New York, Churchill Livingstone, 1988.
278. Rowe, C.R., and Marble, H.: Shoulder Girdle Injuries. *In* Cave, E.F. (ed.): Fractures and Other Injuries, pp. 250–289. Chicago: Year Book Medical Publishers, 1958.
279. Royster, H.A.: Management of Dislocations of the Humerus Complicated by Fracture of the Neck of the Humerus. J.A.M.A., 49:487–491, 1907.
280. Ruedi, T.: Treatment of Displaced Metaphyseal Fractures With Screw and Wiring Systems. Orthopaedics, 12:55–59, 1989.
281. Rush, L.V.: Atlas of Rush Pin Techniques. Meridian, Mich., Beviron Co., 1959.
282. Saha, A.K.: The Zero Position of the Glenohumeral Joint: Its Recognition and Clinical Importance. Ann. R. Coll. Surg. Engl., 22:223, 1958.
283. Sakai, K., Hattori, S., Kawai, S., Saiki, K., et al.: One Case of the Fracture at the Attachment of the Subscapularis Muscle. Shoulder Joint, 7:58, 1981.
284. Salem, M.I.: Bilateral Anterior Fracture–Dislocation of the Shoulder Joints Due to Severe Electric Shock. Injury, 14:361–363, 1983.
285. Santee, H.E.: Fractures About the Upper End of the Humerus. Ann. Surg., 80:103–114, 1924.
286. Savoie, F.H., Geissler, W.B., and Vander Griend, R.A.: Open Reduction and Internal Fixation of Three-Part Fractures of the Proximal Humerus. Orthopaedics, 12:65–70, 1989.
287. Scheck, M.: Surgical Treatment of Nonunions of the Surgical Neck of the Humerus. Clin. Orthop., 167:255–259, 1982.
288. Schubl, J.F.: Fracture–Dislocations of the Proximal Humerus. Thèse Médecine. Lyon, 1973.
289. Schweiger, G., and Ludolph, E.: Fractures of the Shoulder Joint. Unfallchir 6, 1980.
290. Scudder, C.L.: The Treatment of Fractures, 11th ed., pp. 564–603. Philadelphia, W.B. Saunders, 1939.
291. Sehr, J.R., and Sazabo, R.M.: Semitubular Blade Plate for Fixation of the Proximal Humerus. J. Orthop. Trauma, 2:327–332, 1989.
292. Sever, J.W.: Fracture of the Head of the Humerus: Treatment and Results. N. Engl. J. Med., 216:1100–1107, 1937.
293. Sever, J.W.: Nonunion in Fracture of the Shaft of the Humerus: Report of Five Cases. J.A.M.A., 104:382–386, 1935.
294. Shaffer, B.S., Giordano, C.P., andZuckerman, J.D.: Revision of a loose glenoid component facilitated by a modular humeral component: A technical note. J Arthroplasty 5(Suppl.):S579–S581, 1990.
295. Shaw, J.L.: Bilateral Posterior Fracture–Dislocation of the Shoulder and Other Trauma Caused by Convulsive Seizures. J. Bone Joint Surg., 53A:1437–1440, 1971.
296. Shibuya, S., and Ogawa, K.: Isolated Avulsion Fracture of the Lesser Tuberosity of the Humerus: A Case Report. Clin. Orthop., 211:215–218, 1986.
297. Shuck, J.M., Omer, G.E., and Lewis, C.E.: Arterial Obstruction Due to Intimal Disruption in Extremity Fractures. J. Trauma, 12:481–489, 1972.
298. Sidor, M.L., Zuckerman, J.D., Lyon, T., Koval, K., Cuomo, F., and Schoenberg, N.: The Neer Classification System for Proximal Humeral Fractures: An Assessment of Interobserver Reliability and Intraobserver Reproducibility. J. Bone Joint Surg. 75A:1745—1750, 1993.
299. Siebenrock, K.A., and Gerber, C.: The Reproducibility of Classification of Fractures of the Proximal End of the Humerus. J. Bone Joint Surg., 75A:1751—1755, 1993.
300. Silverskoild, N.: On the Treatment of Fracture–Dislocations of the Shoulder-Joint: With Special Reference to the Capability of the Head-Fragment, Disconnected From Capsule and Periosteum to Enter Into Bony Union. Acta Chir. Scand., 64:227–293, 1928.
301. Sjovall, H.: A Case of Spontaneous Backward Subluxation of the Shoulder Treated by the Clairmont-Ehrlich Operation. Nord. Med. (Hygeia), 21:474–476, 1944.
302. Smyth, E.H.J.: Major Arterial Injury in Closed Fracture of the Neck of the Humerus: Report of a Case. J. Bone Joint Surg., 51B:508–510, 1989.
303. Solonen, K.A., and Vastamaki, M.: Osteotomy of the Neck of the Humerus for Traumatic Varus Deformity. Acta Orthop. Scand., 56:79–80, 1985.
304. Sorensen, K.H.: Pseudarthrosis of the Surgical Neck of the Humerus: Two Cases, One Bilateral. Acta Orthop. Scand., 34:132–138, 1964.
305. Stableforth, P.G.: Four-Part Fractures of the Neck of the Humerus. J. Bone Joint Surg., 66B:104–108, 1984.
306. Stangl, F.H.: Isolated Fracture of the Lesser Tuberosity of the Humerus. Minn. Med., 16:435–437, 1933.
307. Stevens, J.H.: Fracture of the Upper End of the Humerus. Ann. Surg., 69:147–160, 1919.
308. Stewart, M.J., and Hundley, J.M.: Fractures of the Humerus: A Comparative Study in Methods of Treatment. J. Bone Joint Surg., 37A:681–692, 1955.
309. Stimson, B.B.: A Manual of Fractures and Dislocations, 2nd ed., pp. 241–260. Philadelphia, Lea & Febiger, 1947.
310. Sturzenegger, M., Fornaro, E., and Jakob, R.P.: Results of Surgical Treatment of Multifragmented Fractures of the Humeral Head. Arch. Orthop. Trauma Surg., 100:249–259, 1982.
311. Svend-Hansen, H.: Displaced Proximal Humeral Fractures: A Review of 49 Patients. Acta Orthop. Scand., 45:359–364, 1974.
312. Szyszkowitz, R., Seggl, W., Schleifer, P., and Cundy, P.J.: Proximal Humeral Fractures: Management Techniques and Expected Results. Clin. Orthop., 292:13–25, 1993.
313. Tanner, M.W., and Cofield, R.H.: Prosthetic Arthroplasty for Fractures and Fracture–Dislocation of the Proximal Humerus. Clin. Orthop., 179:116–128, 1983.

314. Tanton, J.: Fractures de l'Extremite Superiere de l'Humerus. *In* LeDentu, A., and Delbet, P. (eds.): Noveau Traite de Chirurgie, Fase 4. Paris, Bailliere et Fils, 1915.
315. Taylor, H.L.: Isolated Fracture of the Greater Tuberosity of the Humerus. Ann. Surg., 54:10–12, 1908.
316. Theodorides, T., and Dekeizer, G.: Injuries of the Axillary Artery Caused by Fractures of the Neck of the Humerus. Injury, 8:120–123, 1976.
317. Thompson, F.E., and Winant, E.M.: Comminuted Fracture of the Humeral Head With Subluxation. Clin. Orthop., 20:94–97, 1981.
318. Thompson, F.R., and Winant, E.M.: Unusual Fracture Subluxations of the Shoulder Joint. J. Bone Joint Surg., 32A:575–582, 1950.
319. Thompson, J.E.: Anatomical Methods of Approach in Operations on the Long Bones of the Extremities. Ann. Surg., 68:309–329, 1918.
320. Tondeur, G.: Les Fractures Recentes de l'Epaule. Acta Orthop. Belg., 30:1–144, 1984.
321. Tonino, A.J., and van de Werf, G.J.I.M.: Hemiarthroplasty of the Shoulder. Acta Orthop. Belg., 51:625–631, 1985.
322. Trotter, E.: A Propos d'un Cas de Resection de la Tête de l'Humerus. J. l'Hotel-dieu Montreal, 11:368, 1933.
323. Vainio, S.: Observation on Serious Fractures of the Proximal End of the Humerus. Ann. Clin. Gynaecol. Fenn., 49:302–308, 1980.
324. Valls, J.: Acrylic Prosthesis in a Case With Fracture of the Head of the Humerus. Bal. Soc. Orthop. Trauma, 17:61, 1952.
325. Vander-Ghirst, M., and Houssa, R.: Acrylic Prosthesis in Fractures of the Head of the Humerus. Acta Chir. Belg., 50:31–40, 1951.
326. Van Hook, W.: Fracture–Dislocations of the Humeral Head. Boston Med. Surg. J., 187:960–962, 1922.
327. Vastamaki, M., and Solonen, K.A.: Posterior Dislocation and Fracture–Dislocation of the Shoulder. Acta Orthop. Scand., 51:479–484, 1980.
328. Vastamaki, M., and Solonen, K.A.: Posterior Dislocation and Posterior Fracture–Dislocation of the Shoulder. Acta Orthop. Scand., 50:124, 1979.
329. Veseley, D.G.: Use of the Split Diamond Nail for Fractures of the Humerus, 1958–2181. Clin. Orthop., 41:145–156, 1985.
330. Vichard, P.H., and Bellanger, P.: Ascending Bipolar Nailing Using Elastic Nails in the Treatment of Fractures of the Upper End of the Humerus. Nouv. Presse Med., 7:4041–4043, 1978.
331. Walch, G., Boileau, P., Martin, B., and Dejour, H.: Luxations et Fractures-Luxations Posterieures Inveterées de l'Epaule: A Propos de 30 Cas. Rev. Chir. Orthop., 76:546–558, 1990.
332. Wallace, W.A.: The Dynamic Study of Shoulder Movement. *In* Bayley, I., and Kessel, L. (eds.): Shoulder Surgery, pp. 139–143. New York, Springer-Verlag, 1982.
333. Watson-Jones, R.: Fractures and Joint Injuries, 4th ed., pp. 473–476. Baltimore, Williams & Wilkins, 1955.
334. Watson-Jones, R.: Fractures and Joint Injuries, 3rd ed., pp. 460–461. Baltimore, Williams & Wilkins, 1943.
335. Weise, K., Meeder, P.J., and Wentzensen, A.: Indications and Operative Technique in Osteosynthesis of Fracture–Dislocations of the Shoulder Joint in Adults. Langenbecks Arch. Chir., 351:91–98, 1980.
336. Wentworth, E.T.: Fractures Involving the Shoulder Joint. N.Y. State J. Med., 40:1282–1288, 1940.
337. Weseley, M.S., Barenfeld, P.A., and Eisenstein, A.I.: Rush Pin Intramedullary Fixation for Fractures of the Proximal Humerus. J. Trauma, 17:29–37, 1977.
338. West, E.F.: Intrathoracic Dislocation of the Humerus. J. Bone Joint Surg., 31B:61–62, 1949.
339. Whitman, R.: A Treatment of Epiphyseal Displacements and Fractures of the Upper Extremity of the Humerus Designed to Assure Definite Adjustment and Fixation of Fragments. Ann. Surg., 47:706–708, 1908.
340. Whiston, T.B.: Fractures of the Surgical Neck of the Humerus: A Study in Reduction. J. Bone Joint Surg., 36B:423–427, 1954.
341. Widen, A.: Fractures of the Upper End of Humerus With Great Displacement Treated by Marrow Nailing. Acta Chir. Scand., 97:439–441, 1949.
342. Willems, W.J., and Lim, T.E.A.: Neer Arthroplasty for Humeral Fracture. Acta Orthop. Scand., 56:394–395, 1985.
343. Wilson, G.E.: Fractures and Their Complications. New York, Macmillan, 1931.
344. Wilson, J.N. (ed.): Watson-Jones Fractures and Joint Injuries, 6th ed., pp. 533–545. New York, Churchill Livingstone, 1982.
345. Wilson, J.C., and McKeever, F.M.: Traumatic Posterior (Retroglenoid) Dislocation of the Humerus. J. Bone Joint Surg., 31A:160–172, 180, 1949.
346. Winfield, J.M., Miller, H., and LaFerte, A.D.: Evaluation of the "Hanging Cast" as a Method of Treating Fractures of the Humerus. Am. J. Surg., 55:228–249, 1942.
347. Wood, J.P.: Posterior Dislocation of the Head of the Humerus and Diagnostic Value of Lateral and Vertical Views. U.S. Naval Med. Bull., 39:532–535, 1941.
348. Yamano, Y.: Comminuted Fractures of the Proximal Humerus Treated With Hook Plate. Arch. Orthop. Trauma Surg., 105:359–363, 1986.
349. Yano, S., Takamura, S., and Kobayshi, I.: Use of the Spiral Pin for Fractures of the Humeral Neck. J. Jpn. Orthop. Assoc., 55:1607, 1981.
350. Young, T.B., and Wallace, W.A.: Conservative Treatment of Fractures and Fracture–Dislocations of the Upper End of the Humerus. J. Bone Joint Surg., 67B:373–377, 1985.
351. Zadik, F.R.: Recurrent Posterior Dislocation of the Shoulder. J. Bone Joint Surg., 30B:531–532, 1948.
352. Zuckerman, J.D., Flugstad, D.L., Teitz, C.C., and King, H.A.: Axillary Artery Injury as a Complication of Proximal Humeral Fractures: Two Case Reports and a Review of the Literature. Clin. Orthop., 189:234–237, 1984.

Rockwood and Green's Fractures in Adults, Fourth Edition,
edited by Charles A. Rockwood, David P. Green, Robert W. Bucholz and James D. Heckman.
Lippincott-Raven Publishers, Philadelphia © 1996.

CHAPTER 17

Fractures of the Clavicle

Edward V. Craig

Although clavicular fractures usually are readily recognizable and unite uneventfully with treatment, they occur frequently and can be associated with difficult early and late complications. The fact that the clavicle is the most commonly fractured bone in childhood,[44,255] and that it has been estimated that 1 of every 20 fractures involves the clavicle,[175] underscores the clinical relevance of these injuries. In fact, fractures of the clavicle may account for up to 44% of all shoulder girdle injuries.[222]

HISTORICAL REVIEW

The clavicle is entirely subcutaneous and, thus, easily accessible to inspection and palpation. This may account for its inclusion in some of the earliest descriptions of injuries of the human skeleton and their treatment. As early as 400 B.C., Hippocrates recorded several observations about clavicular fractures:

1. With a fractured clavicle, the distal fragment and arm sag, whereas the proximal fragment—held securely by the sternoclavicular joint attachments—points upward.
2. It is difficult to reduce and maintain the reduction. Hippocrates noted, "They act imprudently who think to depress the projecting end of the bone. But it is clear that the underpart ought to be brought to the upper, for the former is the moveable part, and that which has been displaced from its natural position."

3. Union usually occurs rapidly and produces prominent callus; despite the deformity, healing generally proceeds uneventfully.

Hippocrates also noted:

> *A fractured clavicle like all other spongy bone, gets speedily united; for all such bone forms callus in a short time. When, then, a fracture has recently taken place, the patients attach much importance to it, as supposing the mischief greater than it really is . . . ; but, in a little time, the patients having no pain, nor finding any impediment to their walking or eating, become negligent, and the physicians, finding they cannot make the parts look well, take themselves off, and are not sorry at the neglect of the patients, and in the mean time the callus is quickly formed.*[2]

The Edwin Smith Papyrus provides what is probably the earliest description of the now-accepted method of fracture reduction, indicating that an unknown Egyptian surgeon in 3000 B.C. recommended treating fractures of the clavicle thus:

> *Thou shouldst place him prostrate on his back with something folded between his shoulder-blades, thou shouldst spread out with his two shoulders in order to stretch apart his collarbone until that break falls into place.*[44,77,175]

Paul of Aegina, a 17th-century Byzantine, reported that all that could ever be written about fractures of the clavicle had been written; he noted that treatment options included supine positioning as well as the application of potions of olive oil, pigeon dung, snake oil, and other essences.[158]

Some of the earliest documented cases resulted from reports of riding accidents. In 1702, William III died from a fracture of the clavicle 3 days after his horse shied at a mole hill. Sir Benjamin Brodi described a "diffuse false venous aneurysm" complicating a fracture of the clavicle in Sir Robert Peel, who fell from his horse in 1850 on the way to Parliament. As he lapsed into unconsciousness, a pulsatile swelling rapidly developed behind the fracture and his arm was paralyzed. The *Lancet* defended the physicians' handling of the case when many skeptics doubted that death could occur from a clavicular fracture.[51,135,283]

Dupuytren, a keen though controversial anatomist and observer, noted in 1839 that the cumbersome devices used to maintain reductions of the clavicle often were unnecessary, and he advocated simply placing the arm on a pillow until union occurred. He observed that some of the devices in use appeared to aggravate the fractures or create new problems. He described one case on which he consulted where bleeding could not be arrested: "When I was summoned I merely removed the apparatus (the pressure of which was the cause of the mischief) and placed the arm on a pillow. The bleeding immediately ceased."[54,283] He railed against cumbersome and painful treatment methods.

Malgaigne, in 1859, concluded that most treatment methods led to healing with residual clavicular deformity,

> *. . . but while for a century and a half we see the most celebrated surgeons striving to prefer, or perhaps more strictly to complicate, the contrivances for treating fractured clavicle we may follow parallel to them another series of no lest estimable surgeons, who disbelieving in these so-called improvements, return to the simplest means, as to Hippocrates before them. If now we seek to judge of all these contrivances by their results we see that most of them are extolled as producing cures without deformity; but we see also that subsequent experience has always falsified these promises. I therefore, regard the thing (absence of deformity) as not impossible, although for my own part I have never seen such an instance.*[151]

This well summarizes the results of most conservative therapies for fractured clavicles. That is, most of the fractures unite uneventfully with one of several treatment methods, many of the patients have residual deformity (ie, some shortening and a lump), yet interference with function, cosmesis, activity level, and satisfaction appears to be minimal. In the late 1860s, the present-day ambulatory treatment was described by Lucas-Championniere, who advocated the use of a figure of eight dressing and suggested that recumbency, popular in his day, be abandoned in favor of early mobilization of the patient.[84] In 1891, Sayer, recognizing the difficulty of maintaining the reduction, advocated an ambulatory treatment that involved a rigid dressing to maintain the reduction and support the extremity. This method was echoed and taught in the textbooks of his time, and still has many advocates today.[229]

Ambulatory treatment with support of the arm, while maintaining satisfactory and acceptable alignment of the fracture fragments, remains the mainstay of care for clavicular fractures.

ANATOMY

The embryology of the clavicle is unique in that it is the first bone in the body to ossify (fifth week of fetal life), and the only long bone to ossify by intramembranous ossification without going through a cartilaginous stage.[80,165,166] The ossification center begins in the central portion of the clavicle, and this area is responsible for growth of the clavicle up to about 5 years of age.[44,69] Although epiphyseal growth plates develop at both the medial and lateral ends of the clavicle, only the sternal ossification center is evident on radiography.[44,262] This medial growth plate is responsible for most of the longitudinal growth of the clavicle—contributing up to 80% of its length.[185] The appearance and fusion of the sternal ossification center occur relatively late, with ossification occurring between 12 and

19 years of age and fusion to the clavicle occurring between 22 and 25 years of age.[113,271] Thus, many so-called sternoclavicular dislocations in young adults actually are epiphyseal fractures; this is a potential source of confusion, unless the late sternoclavicular epiphyseal closure is remembered.

Because the clavicle is subcutaneous along its entire length, the only structures that cross it are the supraclavicular nerves.[12] In most people, it is possible to grasp the bone and manipulate it, which can be helpful in producing crepitus if an acute fracture is suspected or movement if a nonunion is suspected.

The clavicle is the sole bony strut connecting the trunk to the shoulder girdle and arm, and it is the only bone of the shoulder girdle that forms a synovial joint with the trunk.[143] Its name is derived from the Latin word for "key"—*clavis*—the diminutive of which is *clavicula,* referring to the musical symbol of similar shape.[165]

The shape and configuration of the clavicle are important to its function. They also help explain the pattern of fractures encountered in this bone.

In 1993, Harrington and colleagues described an image-processing system that was used to evaluate the histomorphometric properties of 15 adult male and female human clavicles.[99a] Variations in porosity, cross-sectional area, and anatomic and principal moments of inertia were assessed at 2.5% to 5% increments along the length of the bones. The clavicle's biomechanical behavior (axial, flexural, and torsional rigidity and the critical force for buckling) was modeled from these data using beam theory. More than three-fold variations in porosity and moments of inertia were found along the length of the S-shaped clavicle; the greatest porosity and moments of inertia were located in the variably shaped sternal and acromial thirds of the bone, in contrast to the denser, smaller, and more circular central third of the bone. Clavicle orientation, as indicated by the direction of greatest resistance to bending (maximum principal moment of inertia), was found to rotate from a primarily craniocaudal orientation at the sternum to a primarily anteroposterior orientation at the acromion. Based on cross-sectional geometry, section moduli, and estimates of flexural and torsional rigidity, the clavicle was found to be weakest in the central third of its length. These data concur with the fracture location most commonly reported clinically. Analysis by Euler predicted a minimum critical force for buckling during axial loading of about 2 to 3 body weights for an average adult. Thus, buckling, or a combination of axial loading and bending or torsional loading, must be considered as possible failure mechanisms for this commonly injured bone.

Although the clavicle appears nearly straight when viewed from the front, from above, it appears as an S-shaped double curve that is concave ventrally on its outer half and convex ventrally on its medial half (Fig. 17-1). Although some authors have noted differences in the shape and size of the clavicle between males and females and between dominant and nondominant arms, others have not found this to be so, or have discounted its clinical significance.[50,70,143,185] DePalma found that the outer third of the clavicle exhibited varying degrees of anterior torsion, and suggested that

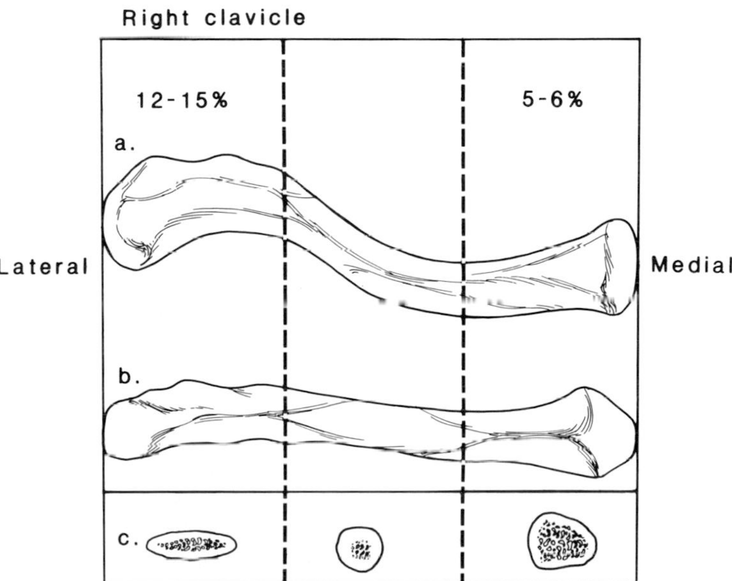

FIGURE 17-1. The clavicle appears nearly straight when viewed from the front (**b**), but as an S-shaped double curve when viewed from above (**a**). The lateral end of the clavicle is flat in cross section (**c**), whereas the medial aspect is more tubular.

changes in torsion might alter stresses and lead to primary degenerative disease in the acromioclavicular joint.[50] The cross section of the clavicle differs in shape along its length, varying from flat along the outer third to prismatic along the inner third. The exact curvature of the clavicle and, to a high degree, its thickness, vary according to the attachments of the muscles and ligaments.[143] The flat outer third is most compatible with pull from muscles and ligaments, whereas the tubular medial third is compatible with axial pressure or pull. The junction between the two cross sections varies in its precise location with the middle third of the clavicle. This junction is a weak spot, particularly to axial loading.[143] This may be one reason why fractures occur so commonly in the middle third. Another may be that the area is not reinforced by muscles and ligaments and is just distal to the subclavius insertion.[102,108,175] It is curious that nature has strengthened, through ligaments or muscular reinforcement, every part of the clavicle except the end of the outer part of the middle third—which is the thinnest part of the bone.[16]

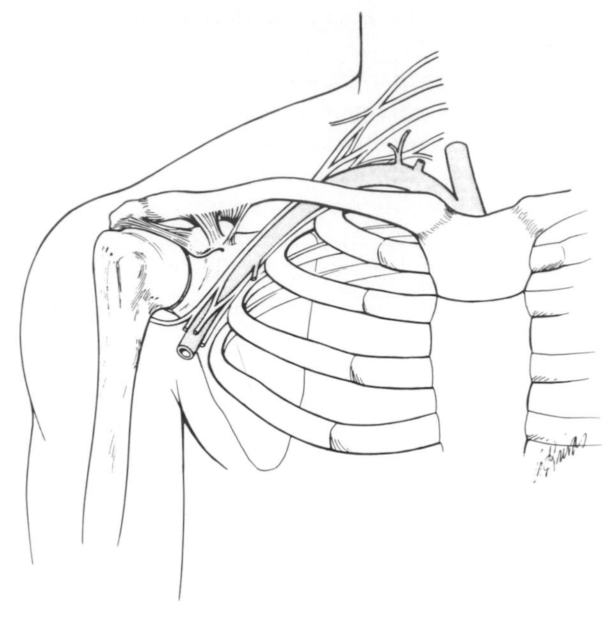

FIGURE 17-2. The clavicle is bound securely by ligaments at both the sternoclavicular and acromioclavicular joints. It is the only bony strut from the torso to the extremity. The brachial plexus and greater vessels are seen posterior to the medial third of the clavicle between the clavicle and the first rib.

The clavicle articulates with the sternum through the sternoclavicular joint; this joint has little actual articular contact, but surprisingly strong ligamentous attachments. The medial end of the clavicle is moored firmly against the first rib by the intra-articular sternoclavicular joint cartilage (which functions as a ligament), the oblique fibers of the costoclavicular ligaments, and, to a lesser degree, the subclavius muscle.[50] The scapula and clavicle are bound securely through both the acromioclavicular and coracoclavicular ligaments; the mechanism and function behind this have been reported extensively, and contribute significantly to the movement and stability of the entire upper extremity[78,268] (Fig. 17-2). The clavicle in the adult is dense, honeycombed, and lacks a well-defined medullary cavity. The bone of the clavicle has been described as "thick compacta,"[80] and its main nutrient vessel enters just medial to the attachment of the coracoclavicular ligaments.[185]

The tubular third of the clavicle, thicker in cross section, offers protection for the important neurovascular structures that pass beneath the medial third of the clavicle. The intimate relationship between these structures and the clavicle assumes great importance both in acute fractures, in which direct injury may occur, and in the unusual fracture sequelae of malunion, nonunion, or excessive callus, in which compression may lead to late symptoms. The brachial plexus, at the level where it crosses beneath the clavicle, comprises three main branches (see Fig. 17-2). Of these, two are anterior. The lateral anterior branch originates from the fifth, sixth, and seventh cervical roots and forms the musculocutaneous nerve and a branch of the median nerve; the medial anterior branch originates from the eighth cervical and first thoracic roots and forms another branch of the median nerve, the entire ulnar nerve, and the medial cutaneous nerve. The single posterior branch of the plexus forms the axillary and radial nerves. The cord of the brachial plexus, which contains the first components of the ulnar nerve, crosses the first rib directly under the medial third of the clavicle. The other two cords are situated farther to the lateral side and more posteriorly. Therefore, the ulnar nerve is involved more frequently in complications arising from fractures of the medial third of the clavicle.

The space between the clavicle and the first rib has been called the *costoclavicular space.* This space has been measured in gross anatomical studies, and often appears adequate. However, the costoclavicular space is not as large in living subjects as in cadavers, possibly because the vessels are distended in living subjects and the dimensions of the cords of the brachial plexus are larger than in cadavers. In addition, the space is diminished in living subjects as the first rib elevates owing to contraction of the scalenus anticus. Hence, when the inner end of the outer fragment of the fractured clavicle is depressed, there is much less space between the first rib and the clavicle, the result being that the vessels (especially the subclavian and axillary vessels) and the nerves (especially the ulnar nerve) may be subjected to injury, pressure, or irritation.[16] The internal jugular, adjacent to the sternoclavicular joint (see Fig. 17-2), usually is not injured with middle-third fractures, but has the potential for injury in more medial trauma involving the sternum and sternoclavicular joint.

Surgical Anatomy

The surgical anatomy relative to the fascial arrangements about the clavicle has been detailed extensively by Abbott and Lucas.[1] Knowledge of these structures decreases the risk of damage to the neurovascular structures during surgical dissection.[219] It is useful to divide the fascia into the areas above, below, and behind the clavicle.

Superior to the Clavicle

At the sternal notch, a layer of cervical fascia splits into two layers: a superficial layer attached to the front of the manubrium and a deep layer attached to the back. The space between these layers contains lymphatics and a communicating vessel between the two anterior jugular veins. The two layers of fascia proceed laterally to enclose the sternocleidomastoid before passing down to the clavicle. For an inch above the clavicle, they are separated by some loose fat. The superficial layer is ill defined and is continuous with the fascia covering the undersurface of the trapezius muscle. A prolongation from the deep layer forms an inverted sling for the posterior belly of the omohyoid muscle; this layer continues to blend with the fascia enclosing the subclavius muscle. Medially, the omohyoid fascia covers the sternohyoid muscle.

Inferior to the Clavicle

Two layers, consisting of muscle and fascia, form the anterior wall of the axilla. The pectoralis major and pectoral fascia form the superficial layer, whereas the pectoralis minor and clavipectoral fascia form the deep layer. The pectoral fascia closely envelops the pectoralis major. Above, it is attached to the clavicle, and laterally, it forms the roof of the superficial infraclavicular triangle (formed by the pectoralis major, a portion of the anterior deltoid, and the clavicle). The deep layer, the clavipectoral fascia, extends from the clavicle above to the axillary fascia below. At the point where it attaches to the clavicle, it consists of two layers, which enclose the subclavius muscle. The subclavius muscle arises from the manubrium and first rib and inserts at the inferior surface of the clavicle. At the lower border of the subclavius, the two fascial layers join to form the costocoracoid membrane. This membrane fills a space between the subclavius above and the pectoralis minor below. This membrane is attached medially to the first costal cartilage and laterally to the coracoid process. Below, it splits into two layers, which ensheathe the pectoralis minor. The costocoracoid membrane is pierced by the cephalic vein, the lateral pectoral nerve, and the thoracoacromial artery and vein.

Deep to the Clavicle

A continuous myofascial layer, which has not been commonly appreciated in surgical anatomy, lies in front of the large vessels and nerves as they pass from the root of the neck of the axilla. From above to below, this layer consists of the following: (1) the omohyoid fascia enclosing the omohyoid muscle, and (2) the clavipectoral fascia, which encloses the pectoralis minor and subclavius muscles.[1] Behind the medial clavicle and the sternoclavicular joint, the internal jugular and subclavian veins join to form the innominate vein. These veins are covered by the omohyoid fascia and by its extension medially over the sternohyoid and sternal thyroid muscle. Behind the clavicle, at the junction between the middle and medial thirds, the junction of the subclavian and axillary veins lies close to the clavicle and is protected by this myofascial layer.

Between the omohyoid fascia posteriorly and the investing layer of cervical fascia anteriorly is a space, described by Grant, in which the external jugular vein usually joins the subclavian vein at its confluence with the internal jugular vein.[90] Before this junction, the external jugular vein is joined on its lateral aspect by the transverse cervical and scapular veins, and on its medial aspect by the anterior jugular vein. This anastomosis usually lies just behind the fascial envelope and the angle formed by the posterior border of the sterno mastoid muscle and the clavicle.[1]

FUNCTION OF THE CLAVICLE

The function of the clavicle can be inferred, in part, by some study of comparative anatomy. Codman has stated, "We are proud that our brains are more developed than the animals: we might also boast of our clavicles. It seems to me that the clavicle is one of man's greatest skeletal inheritances, for he depends to a greater extent than most animals except the apes and monkeys on the use of his hands and arms."[30] Mammals that depend on swimming, running, or grazing have no clavicles, whereas those species that have clavicles appear to be predominantly flyers or climbers. Codman theorized that animals with strong clavicles need to use their arms more in adduction and abduction. The long clavicle may facilitate the placement of the shoulder in a more lateral position, so the hand can be more effectively positioned to deal with the three-dimensional environment.[191] The teleologic role of the clavicle has been disputed, however, because there have been reports of entirely normal function of the upper limb after complete excision of the clavicle.[36,97,106] These reports, combined with observations in patients with congenital absence of the clavicle (cleidocranial dysostosis) who appear not to show any impairment of limb function, probably are responsible for the often-stated belief that this bone is a surplus part that can be excised without disturbance of function. However, others have noted drooping of the shoulder, weakness, and loss of motion after clavicular excision and have used these observations to attribute to the clavicle its important role in normal extremity function[220,244] (Fig. 17-3).

The clavicle does have several important functions, each of which can be expected to be altered not only by excision of the bone, but also by fracture, nonunion, or malunion.

Power and Stability of the Arm

The clavicle, by serving as a bony link from the thorax to the shoulder girdle, provides a stable linkage in the arm–trunk mechanism, and contributes significantly to the power and stability of the arm and shoulder girdle, especially in movement above shoulder level.[166] Through the coracoclavicular ligaments, the clavicle transmits the support and force of the trapezius muscle to the scapula and arm.

Although patients with cleidocranial dysostosis and absence of the clavicle do not appear to have significantly decreased motion, and actually may have increased protraction and retraction of the scapula, they may exhibit some weakness in supporting a load overhead; this further suggests that the clavicle adds stability to the extremity under load in extreme ranges of motion.[106]

The clavicle is supported and stabilized predominantly by passive structures,[143] particularly the sternoclavicular ligaments.[13,14] Although it has been reported that there is electromyographic evidence of trapezius muscle activity at rest, suggesting a role for that muscle in support of the clavicle,[1] others have not been able to demonstrate that such activity plays any role in clavicular support.

Motion of the Shoulder Girdle

When the arm is elevated 180°, the clavicle angles upward 30° and backward 35° at the sternoclavicular joint. It also rotates upward on its longitudinal axis

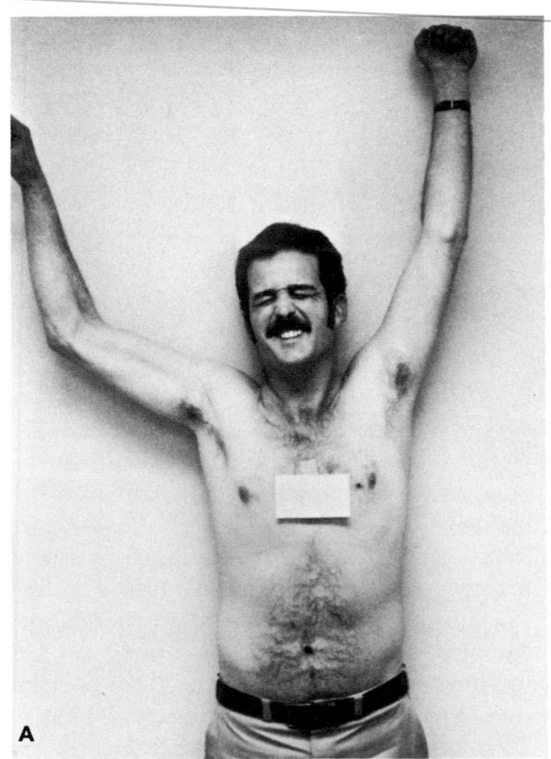

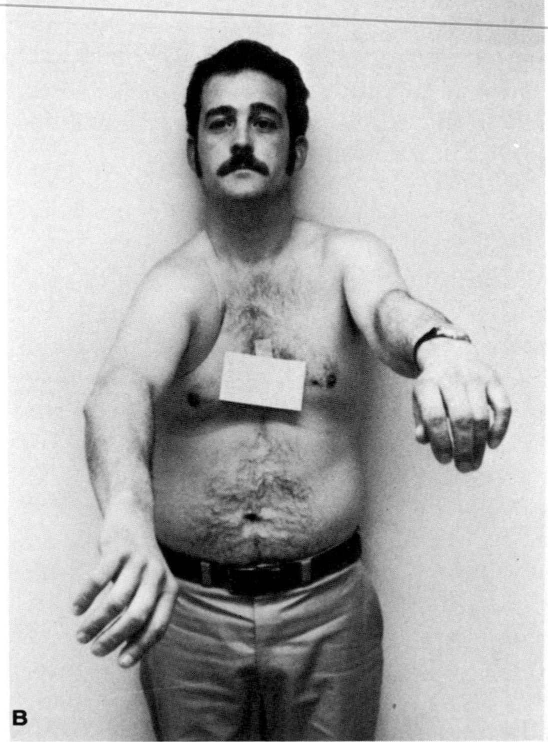

FIGURE 17-3. (**A**) A patient who had his right clavicle excised. Eight years after resection, the patient has a painful and limited range of shoulder motion. (**B**) During flexion, the shoulder collapses medially. The patient has no strength in abduction or flexion. He has significant drooping of the upper extremity, which has produced a traction brachial plexitis. (*Courtesy of C. Rockwood, M.D.*)

about 50°. During combined glenohumeral, acromioclavicular, and sternoclavicular movement, the humerus moves about 120° at the glenohumeral joint and the scapula moves along the chest wall about 60°. These complex and combined movements of the joints and their articulating bony structures (ie, scapula, humerus, clavicle) simultaneously, seem to imply an important role for the clavicle in range of motion of the arm. There is some debate about this, however. It has been observed by some that loss of the clavicle does not impair abduction of the arm and may allow full range of motion.[1,281] However, Rockwood observed loss of the clavicle to result in disabling loss of function, weakness, drooping of the arm, and pain secondary to brachial plexus irritation[220] (see Fig. 17-3).

It has been stated that contribution to motion may be the most important function of the clavicle, and that this is related to its curvature—especially the lateral curvature. The 50° rotation of the clavicle on its axis appears to be important for free elevation of the extremity. Direct relationships have been found among the line of attachment of the coracoclavicular ligaments, the amount of clavicular rotation, the extent and relative lengthening of the ligaments, and scapular rotation. Of the total 60° of scapular rotation, the first 30° are related to elevation of the clavicle as a whole by movement of the sternoclavicular joint, whereas the next 30° are permitted through the acromioclavicular joint by clavicular rotation and elongation of the coracoclavicular ligaments. Thus, the lateral curvature of the clavicle permits the clavicle to act as crank shaft, effectively allowing half of the scapular movement.[142]

The smooth, rhythmic movement of the shoulder girdle is a complex interaction of muscle groups acting on joints and both subacromial and scapulothoracic spaces. Although it is difficult to break down all the contributions of the clavicle to the total motion, it appears that its geometric and kinematic design, by permitting rotation, maximizes the stability of the upper limb against the trunk while permitting mobility, particularly of the scapula along the chest wall. The practical result of this is that the glenoid fossa moves continually, facing and contacting the humeral head as the arm is used overhead.[106]

Muscle Attachments

The clavicle also acts as a bony framework for muscle origins and insertions. The upper third of the trapezius inserts on the superior surface of the outer third of the clavicle, opposite the origin of the clavicular head of the deltoid along its anterior edge. The clavicular head of the sternocleidomastoid muscle arises from the posterior edge of the inner third of the clavicle. The clavicular head of the pectoralis major muscle arises from the anterior edge of the clavicle. During active elevation of the arm, these muscles contract simultaneously. It has been suggested, in theory, that the muscles above the clavicle may be attached directly to those below the clavicle as a continuous muscular layer without an interposed bony attachment,[1] but the stable bony framework clearly provides the advantage of a solid foundation for muscle attachment.

The subclavius muscle is the other muscle that inserts on the clavicle. After it arises from the first rib anteriorly at the costochondral junction, it proceeds obliquely and posteriorly into a groove on the undersurface of the clavicle. It appears to aid in depressing the middle third of the clavicle. Fractures of the clavicle often occur at the distal portion of its insertion. In midclavicular fractures, this muscle may offer some protection to the neurovascular structures beneath.

Protection of the Neurovascular Structures

The clavicle also acts as a skeletal protection for adjacent neurovascular structures and for the superior aspect of the lung. The subclavian and axillary vessels, the brachial plexus, and the lung are directly behind the medial third of the clavicle. As noted earlier, the tubular cross section of the medial third of the clavicle increases its strength and adds to its protective function at this level. The anterior curve of the medial two thirds of the clavicle provides a rigid arch beneath which the great vessels pass as they move from the mediastinum and thoracic outlet to the axilla. It has been shown that during elevation of the arm, the clavicle, as it rotates upward, also moves backward, the curvature providing increased clearance for the vessels.[259] Loss of the clavicle eliminates this bony protection from external trauma.[1]

Respiratory Function

Elevation of the lateral part of the clavicle results in increased pull on the costoclavicular ligament and subclavius muscle. Because of the connections between the clavicle and the first rib and between the first rib and the sternum, elevation of the shoulder girdle brings about a cephalad motion of the thorax, corresponding to an inspiration. This relationship is made use of in some breathing exercises and in some forms of artificial respiration.[1]

Cosmesis

By providing a graceful curve to the base of the neck, a cosmetic function is served by the smooth subcutaneous bony clavicle. In some patients, after surgical excision, the upper limb falls downward and forward, giving a foreshortened appearance to this area. In addition, the cosmetic function of the clavicle is noted by many concerned patients with excessive formation of callus after clavicular fracture or with deformity secondary to clavicular malunion.[1]

CLASSIFICATION

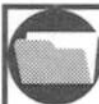

Authors' Classification

Group I—middle-third fractures
Group II—distal-third fractures
- Type I—minimal displacement (interligamentous)
- Type II—displacement secondary to fracture medial to the coracoclavicular ligaments
  - A. Conoid and trapezoid attached
  - B. Conoid torn, trapezoid attached
- Type III—articular surface fractures
- Type IV—ligaments intact to periosteum (children), with displacement of the proximal fragment
- Type V—comminuted, with ligaments not attached proximally nor distally, but to an inferior, comminuted fragment

Group III—proximal-third fractures
- Type I—minimal displacement
- Type II—significant displacement (ligaments ruptured)
- Type III—intra-articular
- Type IV—epiphyseal separation (children and young adults)
- Type V—comminuted[39]

Although clavicular fractures have been classified by fracture configuration (ie, greenstick, oblique, transverse, comminuted),[236] the usual classification is by fracture location. Allman classified the fractures into three groups:[5]

Group I—Fractures of the middle third
Group II—Fractures of the distal third
Group III—Fractures of the medial third

This appears to better compartmentalize our understanding of the fracture anatomy, mechanism of injury, clinical presentation, and alternative methods of treatment.[5,59,67,173,194] Neer,[170a,172,173] as well as Jäger and Breitner, have a specific classification for fractures of the distal third of the clavicle.[110a]

Fractures of the Middle Third of the Clavicle

Group I fractures (middle third) are the most common in both adults and children. The middle third of the clavicle is the point at which the bone changes from a prismatic cross section to a flattened cross section. The force of the traumatic impact follows the curve of the clavicle and disperses on reaching the lateral curve.[178–180,243] In addition, the proximal and distal segments of the clavicle are mechanically secured by ligamentous structures and muscular attachments, whereas the central segment is relatively free. Group I fractures account for 80% of all clavicular fractures[175,222] (Figs. 17-4 through 17-6).

Fractures of the Distal Third of the Clavicle

Group II fractures account for 12% to 15% of clavicular fractures and are subclassified according to the location of the coracoclavicular ligaments relative to the fracture fragments.[100] Neer first pointed out the importance of these fractures, and subdivided them into

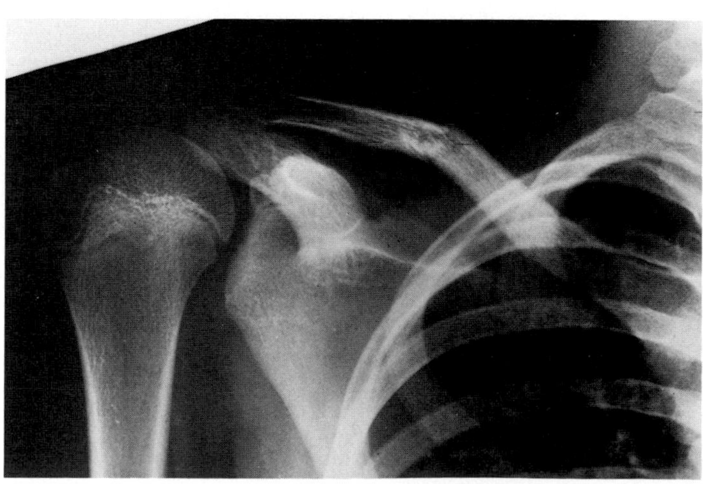

FIGURE 17-4. Typical location for a nondisplaced group I fracture of the clavicle.

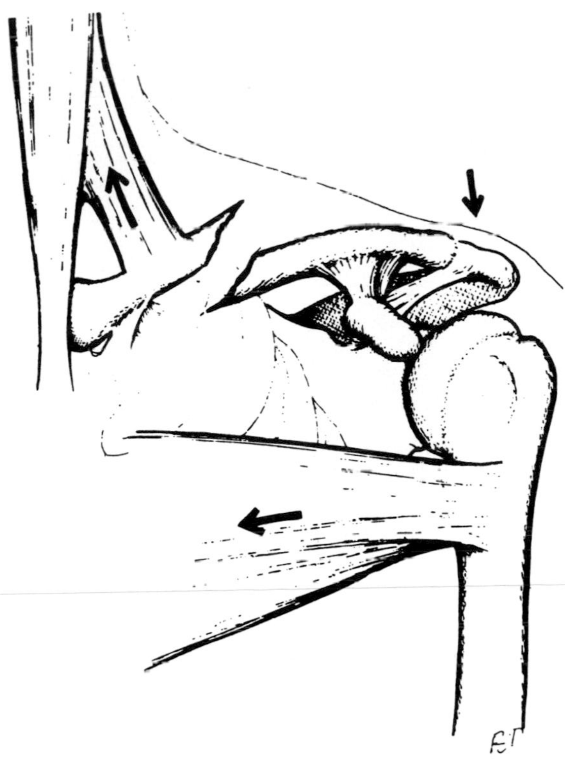

FIGURE 17-5. When displacement occurs, the proximal fragment is pulled superiorly and posteriorly by the pull of the sternocleidomastoid, whereas the distal segment droops forward as a result of gravity and the pull of the pectoralis.

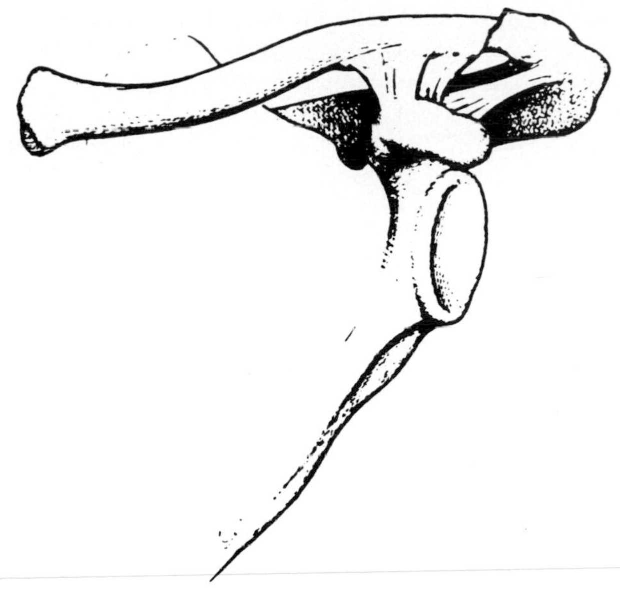

FIGURE 17-7. A type I fracture of the distal clavicle (group II). The intact ligaments hold the fragments in place.

three types. The type I fracture is the most common distal fracture, by a ratio of 4:1. In this fracture, the ligaments remain intact to hold the fragments together and prevent rotation, tilting, or significant displacement. This is an interligamentous fracture occurring between the conoid and trapezoid or the coracoclavicular and acromioclavicular ligaments[172] (Figs. 17-7 and 17-8).

In type II distal clavicular fractures, the coracoclavicular ligaments are detached from the medial segment. Both the conoid and the trapezoid may be on the distal fragment (type IIA; Fig. 17-9), or the conoid ligament may be ruptured while the trapezoid ligament remains attached to the distal segment[44] (type IIB; Fig. 17-10). Four forces act on this fracture; these may impair healing and may contribute to the high incidence of nonunion. These forces are as follows:

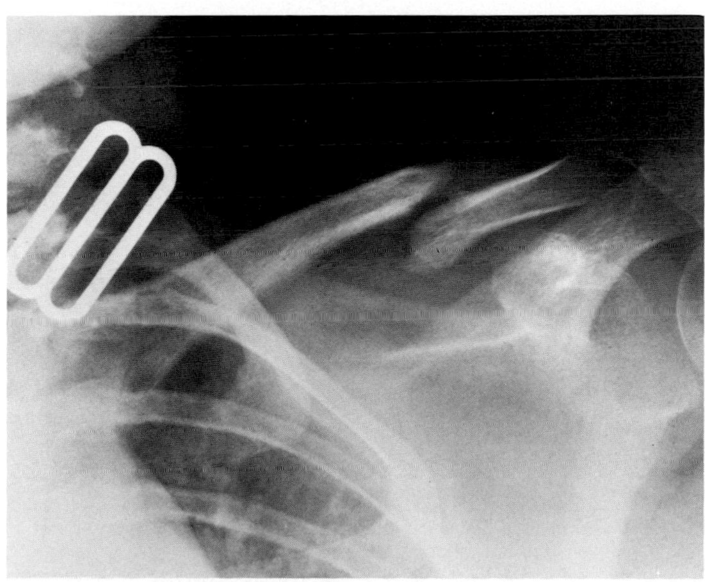

FIGURE 17-6. Radiographic appearance of the displacement in a typical group I fracture of the clavicle.

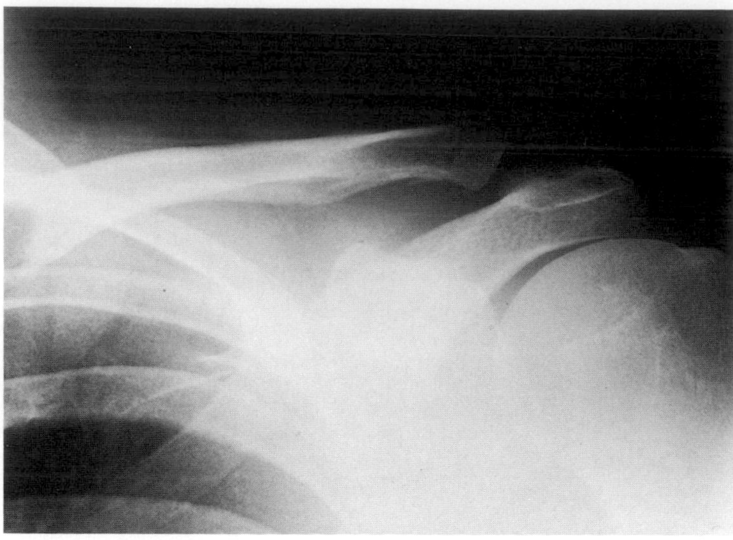

FIGURE 17-8. A type I fracture of the distal clavicle seen radiographically. The fragments are held in place securely by intact coraclavicular and acromioclavicular ligaments.

1. Weight of the arm—When the patient is erect, the outer fragment, retaining the attachment of the trapezoid ligament to the scapula through the intact acromioclavicular ligaments, is pulled downward and forward.
2. Pectoralis major, pectoralis minor, and latissimus dorsi—These structures draw the distal segment downward and medially, causing overriding.
3. Scapular rotation—The scapula may rotate the distal segment as the arm is moved.
4. Trapezius and sternocleidomastoid muscles—The trapezius muscle attaches on the entire outer two thirds of the clavicle, whereas the sternocleidomastoid attaches to the medial third. Thus, these muscles draw the clavicular segment superior and posterior, often into the substance of the trapezius muscle.[173]

Type III distal clavicular fractures involve the articular surface of the acromioclavicular joint alone (Fig. 17-11). Although type II fractures may have intra-articular extension (Fig. 17-12), in type III fractures, there is a break in the articular surface without a ligamentous injury. The type III injury may be subtle, may be confused with a first-degree acromioclavicular separation, and may require special views to visualize. It actually may present as late degenerative arthrosis of the acromioclavicular joint. In addition, it has been suggested that "weight-lifter's clavicle"—resorption of the distal end of the clavicle—may result from increased vascularity secondary to microtrauma or microfractures.[26,175,210]

It appears logical to add two more types of distal clavicular fractures, because in some cases, bone displacement occurs secondary to deforming muscle forces, yet the coracoclavicular ligaments remain attached to bone or periosteum. Type IV fractures oc-

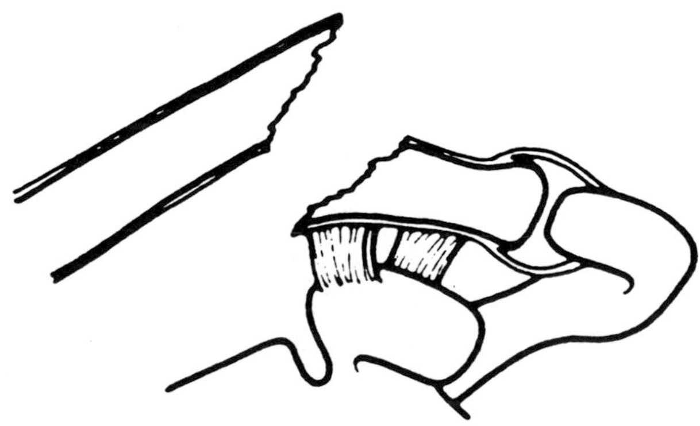

FIGURE 17-9. A type IIA distal clavicle fracture. In type IIA, both conoid and trapezoid ligaments are on the distal segment, whereas the proximal segment, without ligamentous attachments, is displaced. (*Courtesy of C. Rockwood, M.D.*)

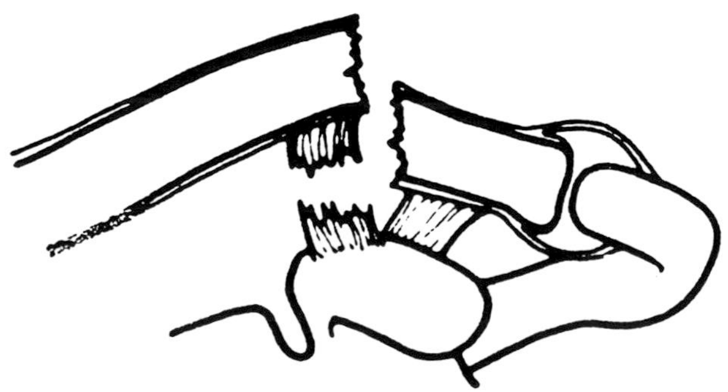

FIGURE 17-10. A type IIB fracture of the distal clavicle. The conoid ligament is ruptured, whereas the trapezoid ligament remains attached to the distal segment. The proximal fragment is displaced. (*Courtesy of C. Rockwood, M.D.*)

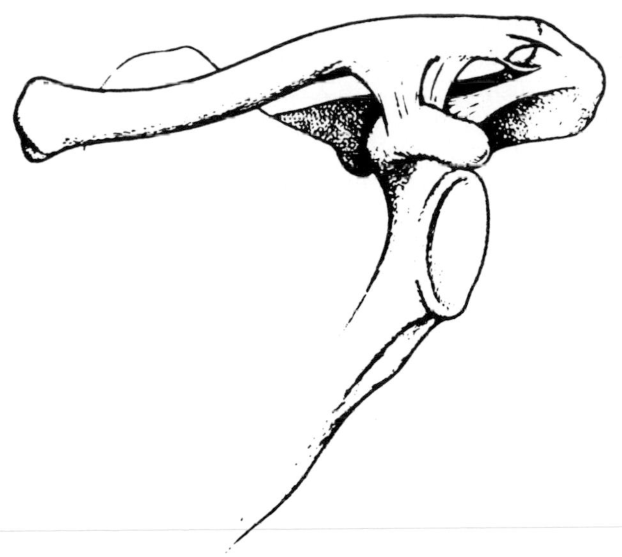

FIGURE 17-11. A type III distal clavicle fracture, involving only the articular surface of the acromioclavicular joint. There is no ligamentous disruption or displacement. These fractures present as late degenerative changes of the joint.

cur in children and may be confused with complete acromioclavicular separation. Called "pseudodislocation" of the acromioclavicular joint, these injuries typically occur in children younger than 16 years of age.[219] The distal clavicle fractures, but the acromioclavicular joint remains intact. In children and young adults, there is a relatively loose attachment between bone and periosteum. The proximal fragment ruptures through the thin periosteum, and may be displaced upward by muscular forces. The coracoclavicular ligaments remain attached to the periosteum or are avulsed with a small piece of bone.[59,67,219] Clinically and radiographically, it may be impossible to distinguish between a grade III acromioclavicular separation, a type II fracture of the distal clavicle, and the type IV fracture with rupture of the periosteum.[172,173,175]

In type V fractures, which occur in adults, neither of the main fracture fragments has functional coracoclavicular ligaments. These fragments are displaced by the deforming muscles, as in type I distal clavicular fractures, but the coracoclavicular ligaments are intact and remain attached to a small, third, comminuted intermediary segment.[194] This fracture is thought to be more unstable than the type II distal clavicular fracture (see Fig. 17-12).

Fractures of the Medial Third of the Clavicle

Group III fractures, or fractures of the inner third of the clavicle, comprise 5% to 6% of clavicular fractures. As with distal clavicular fractures, these can be subdivided according to the integrity of the ligamentous structures. If the costoclavicular ligaments remain intact and attached to the outer fragment, there is little or no displacement.[5,125,204] Satisfactory x-rays are crucial, because these fractures often are overlooked as a result of bony overlap. When these lesions occur in children, they usually are epiphyseal fractures[44] (Fig. 17-13). In adults, articular surface injuries also can lead to degenerative changes.[175,282]

One additional injury to consider is the panclavicular dislocation ("traumatic floating clavicle").[15,81,111,202,226a] This is not actually classified as a clavicular fracture, but neither is it an isolated sternoclavicular or acromioclavicular separation. In this injury, both sternoclavicular ligaments and coracoclavicular ligamentous structures are disrupted.

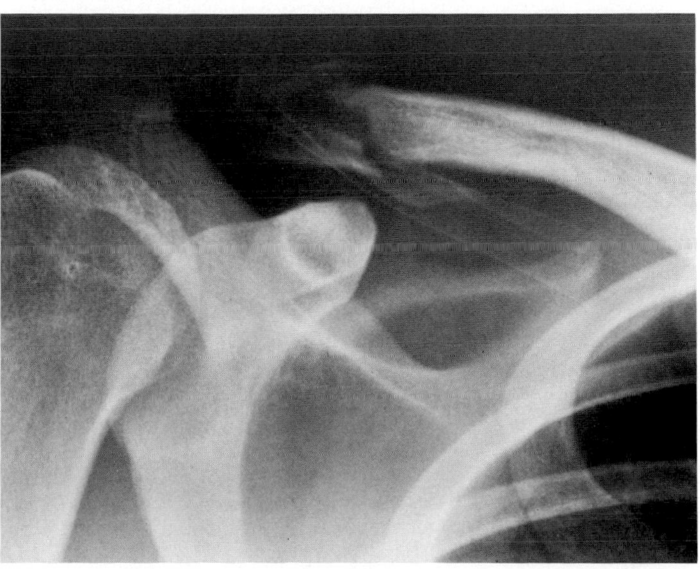

FIGURE 17-12. Although there is an intra-articular component to this fracture, it is not a type III fracture, but a type II fracture with intra-articular extension.

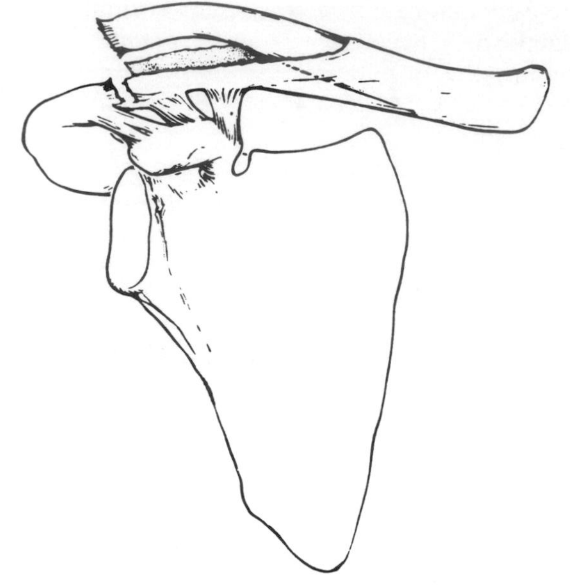

FIGURE 17-13. A type IV fracture, which occurs in children and has been called a "pseudodislocation" of the acromioclavicular joint. The coracoclavicular ligaments remain attached to the bone or the periosteum, whereas the proximal fragment ruptures through the thin superior periosteum and may be displaced upward by muscle forces. (*Dameron, T.B., Jr., and Rockwood, C.A., Jr.: Fractures and Dislocations of the Shoulder. In Rockwood C.A., Jr., Wilkins, K.E., King, R.E. (eds.): Fractures in Children, p. 635. Philadelphia, J.B. Lippincott, 1984.*)

MECHANISMS OF INJURY

Because the clavicle is the most frequently fractured bone, many mechanisms of injury—both traumatic and nontraumatic—have been reported.[60]

Traumatic Injuries

The mechanisms of injury of clavicular fractures in adults have been widely reported to consist of either direct or indirect forces. It has generally been assumed that the most common mechanism is a fall on an outstretched hand.[50] However, Allman, when dividing clavicular fractures into three groups, proposed different mechanisms of injury for each fracture group.[5] He believed that in group I (middle-third) fractures, the most common mechanism was a fall on an outstretched hand, with the force being transmitted up the arm and across the glenohumeral joint and dispersing along the clavicle. He found group II (distal) fractures most likely to result from a fall on the lateral shoulder, driving the shoulder and scapula downward. In group III (proximal) fractures, he cited indirect force applied from the lateral side as the most likely mechanism.[204]

Fowler[73] pointed out that almost all clavicular injuries follow a fall or a blow on the point of the shoulder, whereas a blow to the bone itself rarely is the cause (except in athletics, particularly stick sports such as lacrosse or hockey).[239] In a series of 342 patients with clavicular fractures studied by Sankarankuty and Turner, 91% had a fall or sustained a blow to the point of the shoulder, whereas only 1% had a fall on the outstretched hand.[228]

Stanley and associates studied 150 consecutive patients with clavicular fractures, 81% of whom provided detailed information regarding the mechanism of injury.[246] These investigators found that 94% of the patients had sustained a direct blow to the shoulder, whereas only 6% had fallen on an outstretched hand. Further biomechanical analysis revealed that a direct injury produces a critical buckling load, which is exceeded at a compression force equivalent to the body weight, resulting in fracture of the bone. When the force is applied along the axis of the arm, the buckling force rarely is reached in the clavicle. These investigators recorded fractures at every site along the clavicle with a direct injury to the point of the shoulder, and found that little support could be produced for Allman's concept that fractures at different anatomic sites had different mechanisms of injury. In addition, they theorized that a direct blow to the shoulder might even be the mechanism of injury in patients who described falling on an outstretched hand, for as the hand makes contact with the ground, the patient's body weight and falling velocity are such that movement does not stop, but the fall continues, with the shoulder becoming the upper limb's next contact point with the ground.

Another indirect mechanism of middle-third clavicular fractures occurs from a direct force on the top of the shoulder, which forces the clavicle against the first rib and often produces a spiral fracture of the middle third.[50]

Traumatic fractures of the clavicle also have been reported in association with seizures.[71]

Nontraumatic Fractures

It is well recognized that the clavicle can be the site of neoplastic or infectious destruction of bone. Fracture also can result from relatively minor trauma or from radiation to a neoplastic area (Fig. 17-14). Dambrain and colleagues have described the osteolytic osteolysis of bone that can occur after radiation therapy.[42a] Lack of a traumatic episode should cause the clinician to consider the possibility of a pathologic bone. In addition to both malignant and benign lesions,[17] pathologic fractures of the clavicle also have been described in association with arteriovenous malformation, an entity that may mimic neoplasm.[162]

Atraumatic stress fractures also have been reported in the clavicle.[124] In addition, spontaneous fractures

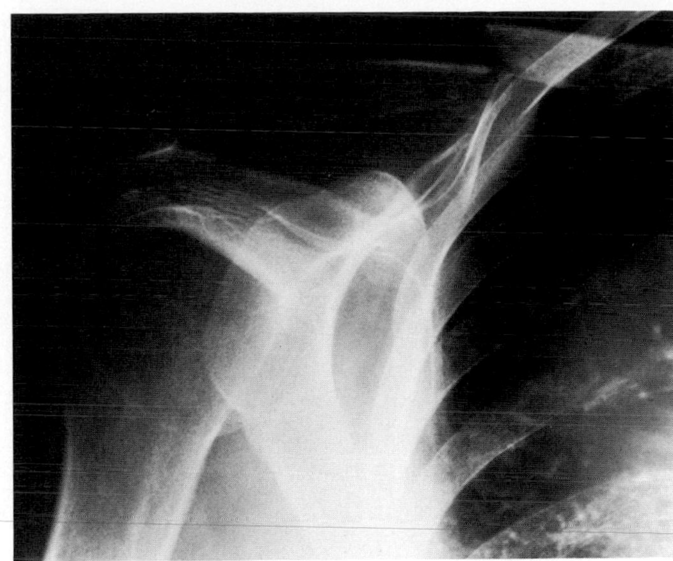

FIGURE 17-14. A pathologic fracture of the clavicle from metastatic thyroid carcinoma. The patient presented without a traumatic episode.

of the medial end of the clavicle have been reported as "pseudotumors" after radical neck dissection.[41,72,187,253]

Synthetic material used for coracoclavicular disruption also has been reported to produce stress fractures in the clavicle, with subsequent nonunion.[55] Martell described a nonunion of the clavicle after the use of Mersilene tape to repair a grade III dislocation of the acromioclavicular joint.[154a]

INCIDENCE OF INJURY

The incidence of clavicular injuries in adults appears to be increasing as a result of several factors, including the rise in high-velocity vehicular injuries and the increased popularity of contact sports for adults.[50,76,183a]

In 1994, Nordqvist and Petersson reviewed the incidence of fractures of the clavicle.[183a] They reviewed 2035 fractures that occurred between 1952 and 1987.

The fractures were classified in three groups according to the Allman system. Each group was divided further into undisplaced and displaced fracture subgroups, with an extra subgroup of comminuted midclavicular fractures in group I. Seventy-six percent of the fractures were classified as Allman group I. The median age of the patients in this group was 13 years. There were significant differences in age- and gender-specific incidence between the undisplaced, displaced, and comminuted fracture subgroups. Twenty-one percent of the fractures were classified as Allman group II. The median age of these patients was 47 years, and there was no difference in age between the undisplaced and displaced fracture subgroups. Three percent of the fractures were classified as Allman group III, and the median age of the patients in this group was 59 years. All three groups were characterized by a significant preponderance of men.

CLINICAL PRESENTATION

Because of their characteristic clinical presentation in adults, displaced fractures of the clavicle present little difficulty with diagnosis if the patient is seen soon after injury. There usually is a clear history of some form of either direct or indirect injury to the shoulder. Clinical deformity is obvious and may be out of proportion to the amount of discomfort the patient experiences.[12] The proximal fragment is displaced upward and backward, and may tent the skin. Although compounding of this fracture is unusual, it can occur[213] (Fig. 17-15). The patient usually exhibits splinting of the involved extremity at the side, because any movement elicits pain. The involved arm droops forward and downward (Fig. 17-16). Although the initial deformity may be obvious later, with acute swelling of soft tissue and hemorrhage, the deformity can be obscured. With a fracture near the ligamentous structures (ie, the acromioclavicular or sternoclavicular joints), the deformity may mimic a purely ligamentous injury.

Physical examination reveals tenderness directly over the fracture site and pain with any movement of the arm. There may be ecchymosis over the fracture site, especially if severe displacement of the bony fragments has produced associated tearing of soft tissue. The patient may angle the head toward the injury, attempting to relax the pull of the trapezius on the fragment. As in children, the patient may be more comfortable with the chin tilted to the opposite side.

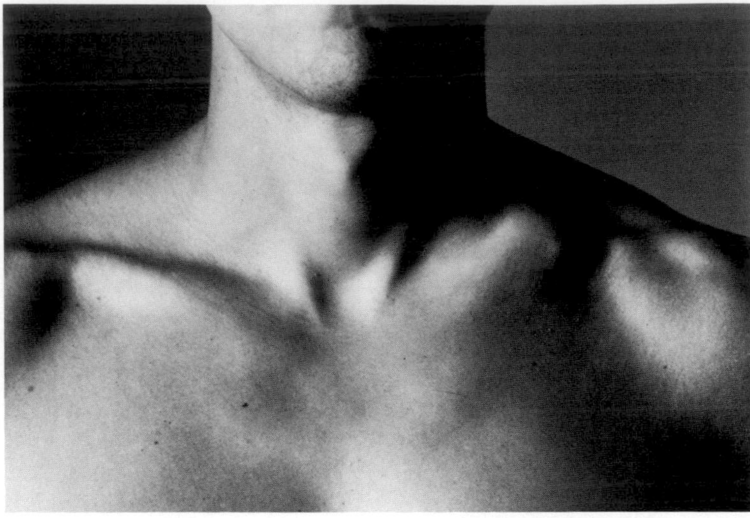

FIGURE 17-15. An adult clavicle fracture showing prominence of the proximal fragment, which is displaced upward and backward. This may tent the skin, although compounding is unusual.

Gentle palpation and manipulation usually produce crepitus and motion, and the site of the fracture is easily palpable because of the subcutaneous position of the bone. The skin over the clavicle, the scapula, or the chest wall may provide a clue to the mechanism of injury and may indicate other areas to be evaluated for associated injuries. The lungs must be examined for the presence of symmetric breath sounds, and the whole extremity should be examined carefully.

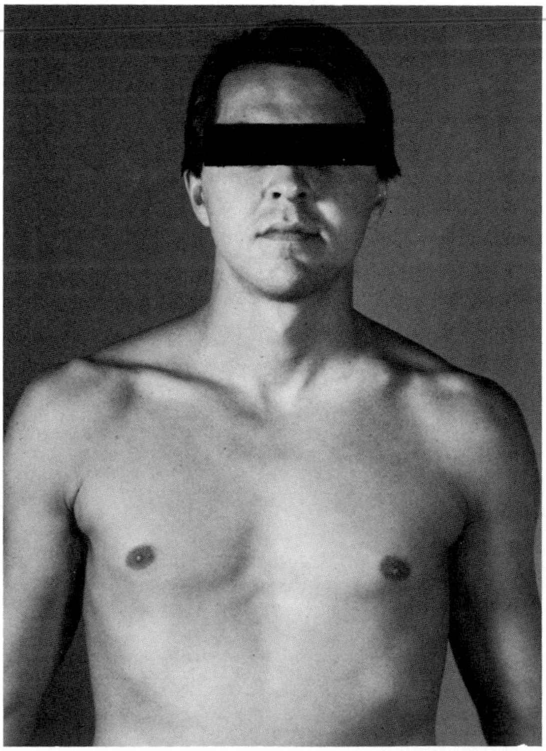

FIGURE 17-16. With an adult clavicle fracture, the arm may droop forward and downward to varying degrees.

Undisplaced fractures or isolated fractures of the articular surfaces may not cause deformity, and these can be overlooked unless they are sought specifically using radiography. If the diagnosis is in doubt, special x-ray views or a second x-ray film of the clavicle in 7 to 10 days may be indicated.

The panclavicular dislocation typically is produced by extreme and forceful protraction of the shoulder. This injury usually is the result of a major traumatic episode, such as a high-speed traffic accident, a fall from a height, or the impact of a heavy object on the shoulder,[81] although it has been reported after a minor fall at home.[111] Clinically, there usually is bruising over the spine of the scapula, and swelling and tenderness at both ends of the clavicle. This injury is associated with anterosuperior sternoclavicular dislocation and either posterosuperior or subjacent displacement of the clavicle. The whole clavicle may be freely mobile and may feel as if it is floating. X-rays usually confirm this injury.

ASSOCIATED INJURIES

Note: The reader also should review the section regarding complications that can occur with fractures of the clavicle.

In 1830, Gross reported that, "Fractures of the clavicle usually assume a mild aspect, being seldom accompanied by any serious accident."[92] Although, statistically, most clavicular fractures are relatively innocuous, serious associated injuries can occur. A delay in treating these injuries can be life-threatening.[53] Therefore, it is critical in a patient with a clavicular fracture that a careful examination of the entire upper extremity be performed, with particular emphasis on the neurovascular status and, as already mentioned, a careful examination of the lungs.[53] Herscoviei and coworkers recommended internal fixation of only the clavicle.[100b]

Associated injuries accompanying acute fractures of the clavicle can be divided into (1) associated skeletal injuries, (2) injuries to the lungs and pleura, (3) brachial plexus injuries, and (4) vascular injuries.

Associated Skeletal Injuries

Associated skeletal injuries include separations or fracture dislocations of the sternoclavicular or acromioclavicular joints[25,119,137,260,282a] (Fig. 17-17). As might be anticipated with ipsilateral sternoclavicular or acromioclavicular joint injuries, closed reduction of the ligamentous injury usually is impossible because of the accompanying clavicular fracture.[119] Baccarani and colleagues reported a fracture of the coracoid process associated with a fracture of the clavicle that they treated by open reduction and internal fixation of the coracoid.[7a]

Head and neck injuries may be present,[279] especially with displaced distal clavicular fractures; in one series, 10% of patients were comatose.[172]

Fractures of the first rib are common but easily overlooked.[3,277] These rib fractures may be directly responsible for accompanying lung, brachial plexus, or subclavian vein injuries. Underrecognition of rib fractures may be related to the fact that they are not easily seen on standard chest x-rays. Weiner and O'Dell recommended an anteroposterior view of either the cervical spine or the thoracic spine, plus a lateral view of the thoracic spine to detect rib fractures.[277] The location of a first rib fracture may be either the ipsilateral or contralateral rib to the clavicular fracture. Weiner outlined how several of these rib fractures occur. The scalenus anticus muscle attaches on a tubercle of the first rib. On each side of this tubercle lies a groove for the subclavian vein anteriorly and the subclavian artery posteriorly. Posterior to the groove for the subclavian artery lies a roughened area for the attachment of the scalenus medius muscle. These two muscles elevate the rib during inspiration. The serratus anterior muscle arises from the outer surfaces of the upper eight ribs and fixes the ribs posteriorly during inspiration. These structures may interact to contribute to fractures of the first rib as the clavicle is fractured. Three mechanisms have been theorized to be responsible for this combination of injuries: (1) indirect forces transmitted through the manubrium; (2) avulsion fracture at the weakest portion of the rib by the scalenus anticus; and (3) injury to the lateral clavicle, which causes an acromioclavicular separation that produces indirect force from the subclavius muscle on the costal cartilage and anterior aspect of the first rib.[203,277]

Fractures of the clavicle also may be associated with scapulothoracic dissociation—disruption of the scapulothoracic articulation presenting with swelling of the shoulder, lateral displacement of the clavicle, severe neurovascular injury, and fracture of the clavicle or the acromioclavicular or sternoclavicular joint.[56]

Fractures of the Clavicle and Scapula (The Floating Shoulder)

Some authors suggest that the "floating shoulder" be treated by open reduction and fixation of both fractures.[131a,139a]

Rockwood surveyed members of the American Shoulder and Elbow Surgeons and concluded that treatment should be directed primarily at stabilization of the clavicle. The primary indication for internal fixation of the scapula is to reduce and internally stabilize a grossly displaced intra-articular fracture of the glenoid fossae (Rockwood, C.A., personal communication, 1995).

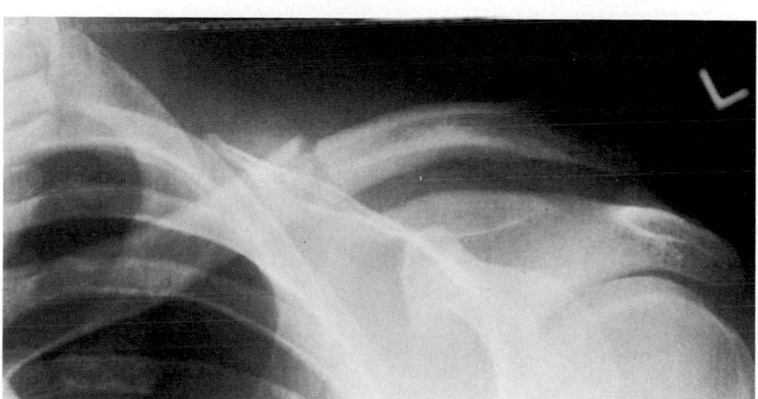

FIGURE 17-17. An unusual clavicular fracture associated with a complete acromioclavicular separation. The associated clavicular fracture makes treatment of the ligamentous injury very difficult.

Injuries to the Lungs and Pleura

Many authors have commented on the potentially serious complication of pneumothorax or hemothorax associated with fracture of the clavicle.[53,109,150,247,250,283] This is a concern because the apical pleura and upper lung lobes lie adjacent to the clavicle (Fig. 17-18). Rowe reported a 3% incidence of pneumothorax in a series of 690 clavicular fractures, although he did not comment on how many had associated rib or scapular fractures.[222] Although it is easy to see how a severely displaced fracture may puncture the pleura with a sharp shard of bone, the x-ray appearance can be misleadingly benign, with little evidence to suggest what might have been significant fragment displacement at the time of injury.[53] Careful physical examination of the lung at the time of the initial presentation is essential, searching for the presence and symmetry of breath sounds. In addition, an upright chest film appears to be important in the assessment of all patients with clavicular fractures who have decreased breath sounds or other physical findings suggestive of a pneumothorax; particular attention should be paid to the lung outline on the chest film.[150] This is especially true in multiply traumatized or unconscious patients who have neither obvious blunt chest trauma nor any external signs of trauma to the chest that might yield a clue to lung or pleural complications.

Tears of the trachea or main bronchi from blunt chest trauma also have been associated with fractures of the clavicle. These usually present either as abnormalities in the appearance of the endotracheal tube (cuff overdistention or extraluminal position of the tip) or as the radiographic appearance of lung collapse toward the lateral chest wall and away from the midline.[267]

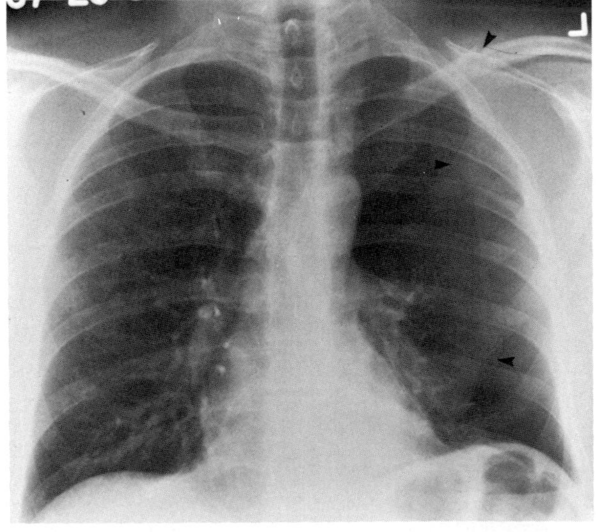

FIGURE 17-18. A fracture of the left clavicle associated with a left pneumothorax. The lung markings are absent on the left side. There also is a fracture of the second rib.

Brachial Plexus Injuries

Although nerve injuries with clavicular fractures are rare, acute injuries to the brachial plexus do occur. The neurovascular bundle emerges from the thoracic outlet under the clavicle on top of the first rib.[214,276] As it passes under the clavicle, the neurovascular bundle is protected to a certain extent by the thick, medial clavicular bone. Thus, considerable trauma usually is necessary to damage the brachial plexus and break the clavicle at the same time. When the force is severe enough to do this, a subclavian vascular injury often occurs concomitantly (Fig. 17-19). Forces resulting in nerve injury usually come from above downward or from the front downward. As the force is applied, the nerves may be stretched, with the fulcrum of maximum tension being the transverse process of the cervical vertebra.[156] The roots also can be torn above the clavicle or avulsed from their attachment to the spinal cord.[11] Although the posterior periosteum, subclavius muscles, and bone offer some protection to the underlying plexus, the plexus can be injured directly by bone fragments. This is especially important, because manipulation of clavicular fragments should not be done without adequate x-ray studies of the position of these fracture fragments.[270]

If the brachial plexus is injured directly, the ulnar nerve usually is involved, because this portion of the plexus lies adjacent to the middle third of the clavicle.

Vascular Injuries

Acute vascular injuries are unusual because of many of the same local anatomic factors that protect the nerves from direct injury. The subclavius muscle and thick deep cervical fascia also act as barriers to direct injury to the vessels. After initial displacement of the fracture fragment occurs, if the adjacent vessels are intact, they are unlikely to be injured further because the distal fragment is pulled downward and forward by the weight of the limb, whereas the proximal fragment is pulled upward and backward by the pull of the trapezius. Thus, as with acute nerve injury, a major trauma usually is required to produce an acute vascular insult.[196] Nevertheless, injuries have been reported, even with a greenstick fracture.[161] In addition, acute vascular compression resulting from fracture angulation has been described.[47]

Potential vascular injuries include laceration, occlusion, spasm, and acute compression. The vessels most commonly injured are the subclavian artery, subclavian vein, and internal jugular vein.[112,129,141,155] The subclavian vein is particularly vulnerable to tearing,

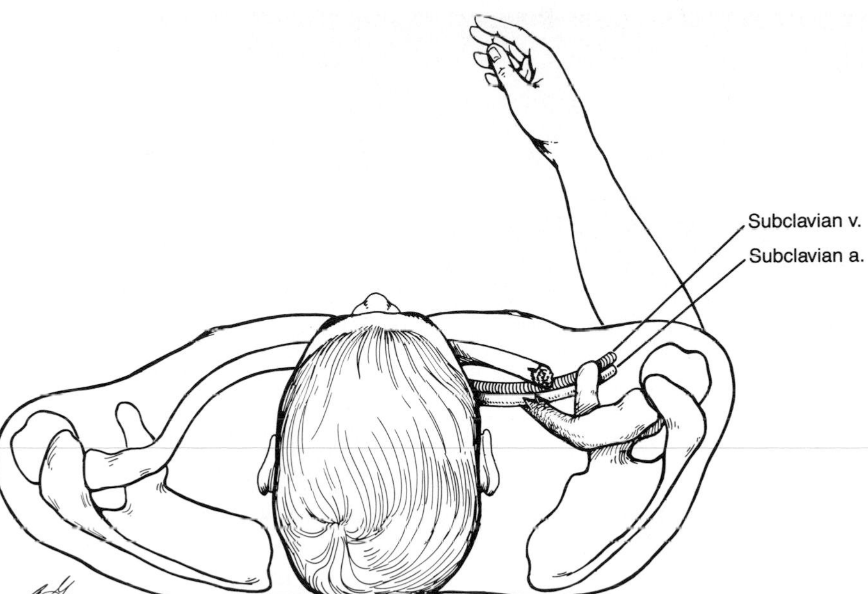

FIGURE 17-19. As the clavicle fractures and displaces, the subclavian vessels immediately posterior to the clavicle may be injured by sharp shards of bone.

because it is fixed to the clavicle by fascial aponeurosis.[93,249] Injuries to the suprascapular artery and axillary artery also have been reported.[107,265] Laceration can result in life-threatening hemorrhage, whereas arterial thrombus and occlusion can lead to distal ischemia. Damage to the arterial wall can lead to aneurysm formation and late embolic phenomena. Venous thrombosis also can present a problem; although its clinical presentation typically is not life- or limb-threatening, there is a potential for pulmonary embolism, which certainly can be.[230] Clinical recognition of an acute vascular injury can be difficult, particularly in a patient who is unconscious or in shock. Although a complete laceration may present with a life-threatening hemorrhage or an extremity that is cold, pulseless, and pale, a partial laceration is more likely to present with uncontrolled, life-threatening bleeding. The color and temperature of the extremity may be normal, but the absence of a pulse, the presence of a bruit, or the development of a pulsatile hematoma (as the hematoma is walled off or produces a false aneurysm) should raise strong suspicion of a major vascular injury.[265] If there is a significant obstruction to blood flow, the injured limb usually is colder than the uninjured limb, and the blood pressure also may be different in the two limbs.[283] Vascular contusion or spasm can result in thrombotic and later thromboembolic phenomena.[278] It sometimes is difficult to recognize the difference between arterial spasm and interruption or occlusion. It may be reasonable to consider a sympathetic block to help distinguish a spasm from more serious injury.

Although penetrating trauma often focuses attention on the clinical diagnosis of vascular injury, blunt trauma may produce as many as 9% of subclavian artery injuries. In one series, all 15 patients with distal subclavian artery involvement from blunt trauma had fractures of the clavicle and absent radial pulses. Eight of the patients had critical ischemia of the hand.[38]

If major injury to a vessel is suspected, an arteriogram should be performed.[283] In the rare event of a torn large vessel, surgical exploration is mandatory. To gain adequate exposure, as much of the clavicle should be excised as needed to isolate and repair the injured major vessel. Although the vessel can be ligated in some cases, ligation of a major vessel in an elderly patient can be dangerous because of inadequate remaining circulation to the extremity. In any event, a surgeon who is skilled in the choice and performance of vascular repair techniques is essential if a major injury has occurred.

RADIOGRAPHIC FINDINGS

Shaft Fractures

In most cases of clavicular shaft fracture, because of the clinical deformity, the diagnosis is not in doubt and x-rays are confirmatory. Nevertheless, to get an accurate evaluation of the fragment position, two projections of the clavicle typically are used—an anteroposterior and a 45° cephalic tilt view. In the anteroposterior view, the proximal fragment usually is displaced upward and the distal fragment downward (Fig. 17-20). In the 45° cephalic tilt view, the tube is directed from below upward and more accurately assesses the anteroposterior relationship of the two

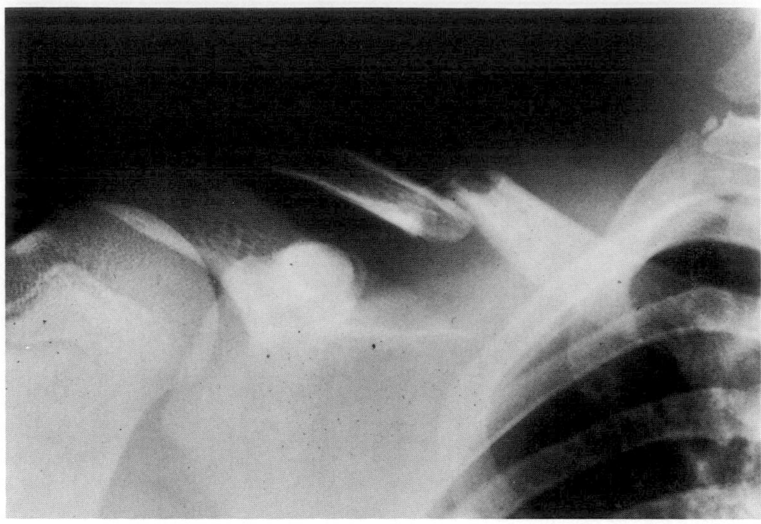

FIGURE 17-20. An anteroposterior view of a right clavicle fracture, showing the typical deformity with a proximal fragment displaced superiorly.

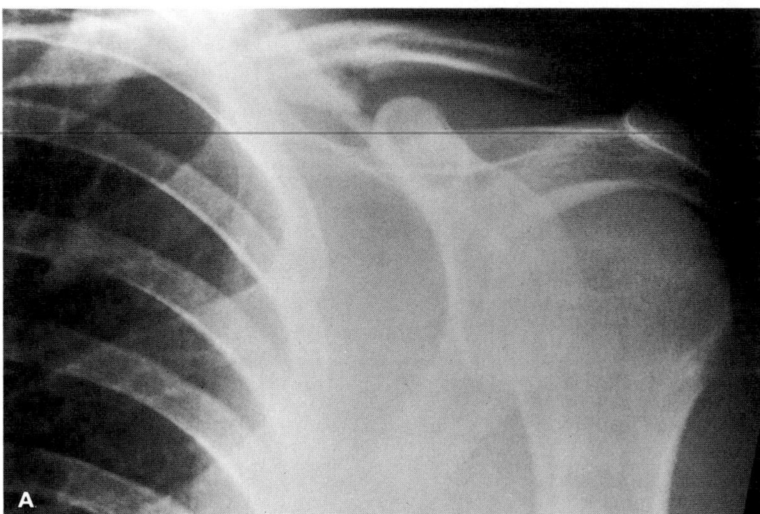

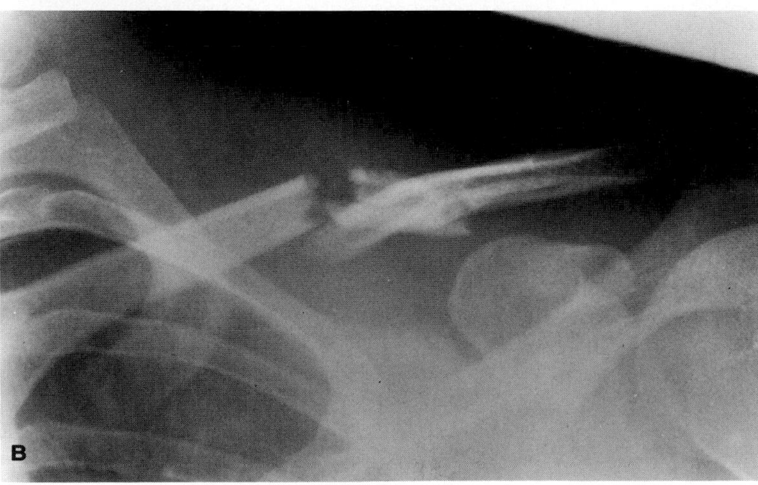

FIGURE 17-21. (**A**) An anteroposterior view of a left comminuted clavicular fracture poorly defines and identifies the fracture fragments because of overlying bone in the area of the fragments. (**B**) However, when a 20° to 45° cephalic tilt view is obtained, the fracture anatomy is more clearly delineated.

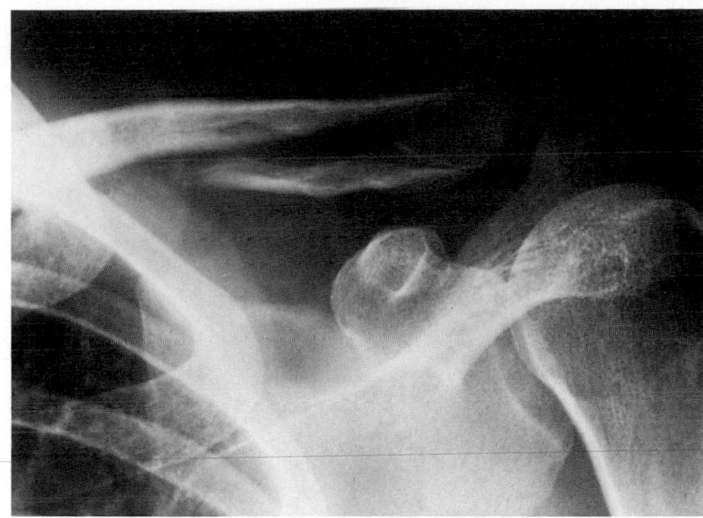

FIGURE 17-22. An anteroposterior view of a distal clavicle fracture. This cephalic tilt view (about 15°) brings the clavicle and acromioclavicular joint away from the overlying bony anatomy.

fragments[278] (Fig. 17-21). Quesana recommended two views at right angles to each other, a 45° angle superiorly and a 45° angle inferiorly, to assess the extent and displacement of clavicular fractures.[207]

Rowe suggested that when ordering an anteroposterior study, the film should include the upper third of the humerus, the shoulder girdle, and the upper lung fields, so that other shoulder girdle fractures and pneumothorax can be identified more quickly.[222] The configuration of the fracture also is important, because it may provide a clue to associated injuries. Although the usual clavicular shaft fracture in the adult is slightly oblique, if it is more comminuted, and especially if the middle spike is projecting from superior to inferior, it probably has resulted from a greater force and may alert the surgeon to the potential for associated neurovascular or pulmonary injuries.

Fractures of the Distal Third

In both children and adults, the usual radiographic views obtained for shaft fractures are inadequate to completely assess distal clavicular fractures. The standard exposure for evaluation of shoulder or shaft fractures overexposes the distal clavicle. The usual exposure for the distal clavicle should be about one third that used for the shoulder joint. This is especially true if it is important to determine articular surface involvement.

Type II distal clavicular fractures can be particularly difficult to diagnose, because the usual anteroposterior and 40° cephalic tilt views typically do not reveal the extent of injury.[172] If the exposure is appropriate, a distal clavicular fracture can be identified on the anteroposterior and lateral views of the trauma series (Figs. 17-22 and 17-23), but to accurately assess the extent of injury and the presence or absence of associated ligamentous damage, Neer[172,173,175] recommended three views. A posteroanterior view of *both* shoulders should be obtained on one plate, with the patient erect and with a 10-lb weight strapped to each wrist (Fig. 17-24). If the distance between the coracoid and the medial fragment is increased compared with the normal side, ligamentous detachment from the medial fragment can be assumed to be present. However, because much of the fracture displacement is in the anteroposterior plane, Neer suggested two additional views. An anterior 45° oblique view, with the patient erect and the injured shoulder against the plate, pro-

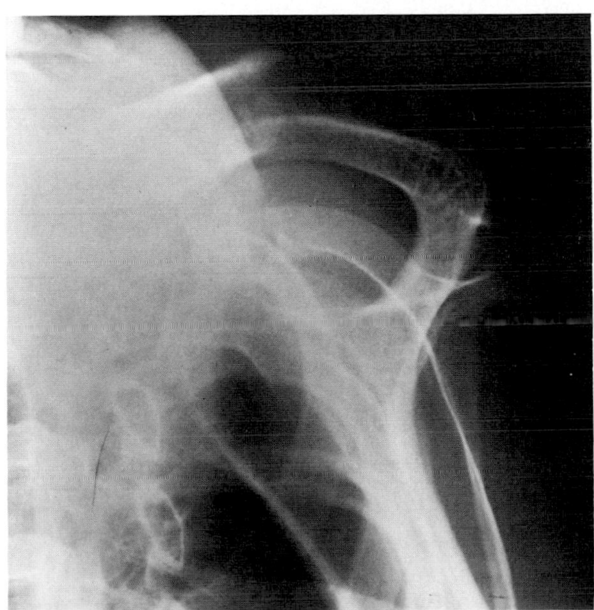

FIGURE 17-23. A lateral view of a distal clavicular fracture. The displacement of the proximal segment is identified, but the fracture detail may be obscured by bony and soft-tissue anatomy.

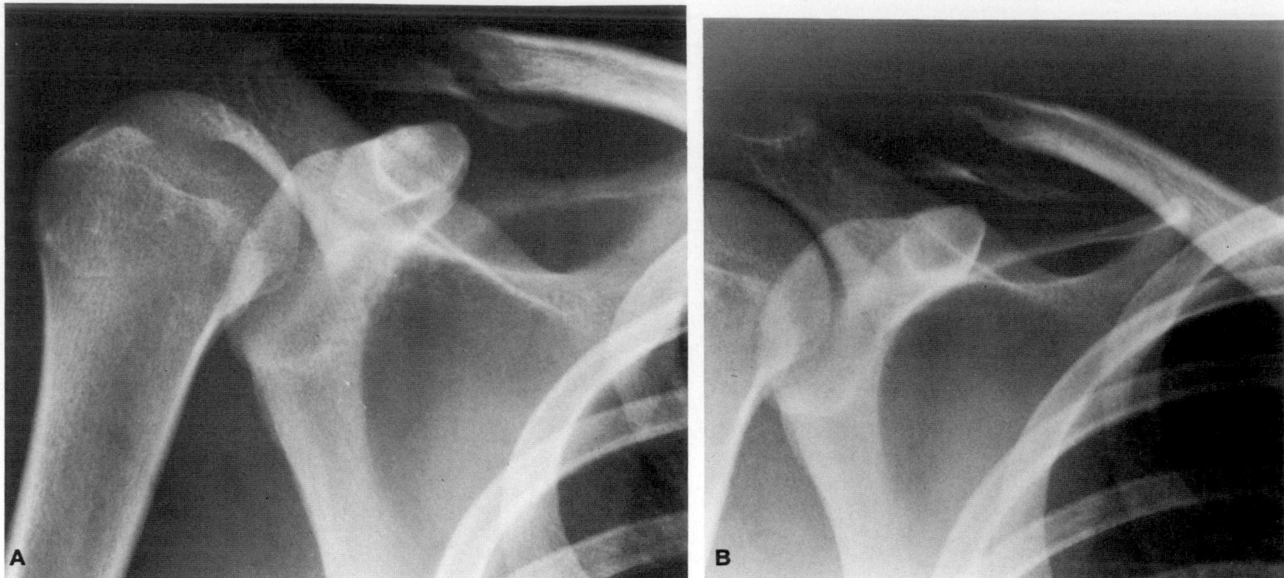

FIGURE 17-24. (**A**) A fracture of the right distal clavicle. In an anteroposterior view, the fracture location is suggestive of ligamentous involvement, with the ligaments attached to the distal fragment. (**B**) The extent of ligamentous involvement is confirmed on a weighted view, where there is a widening of the coracoclavicular distance. The coracoclavicular ligaments are attached to the distal clavicular segment.

vides a lateral view of the scapula and shows the medial fragment posteriorly with the outer fragment displaced anteriorly. A posterior 45° oblique view, with the patient erect and the injured shoulder against the plate, also demonstrates the extent of separation of the two fragments.

In a type II distal clavicular fracture, if x-ray views at right angles and with cephalic tilt show good bony overlap and proximity of the fragments, and if crepitation confirms contact between the fragments, stress radiographic views with weights probably are not necessary; in fact, the use of weights may further displace otherwise minimally displaced fracture fragments (Figs. 17-25 through 17-27).

Articular surface fractures of the distal clavicle are easily overlooked unless high-quality x-rays are obtained. If the fracture is not seen on a plain x-ray view and the clinical suspicion is strong, tomography or computed tomography may reveal the presence and extent of an articular surface injury (Fig. 17-28).

Fractures of the Medial Third

Fractures of the medial third can be particularly difficult to detect on routine x-rays because of the overlap of ribs, vertebrae, and mediastinal shadows. However, a cephalic tilt view of 40° to 45° often reveals the fracture in both children and adults. In children, particularly, fractures of the medial end of the clavicle often are misdiagnosed as sternoclavicular dislocations, when they actually are usually epiphyseal injuries. As with distal clavicular injuries, tomography or computed tomography may be useful to demonstrate the intra-articular or epiphyseal nature of injuries in this location.

DIFFERENTIAL DIAGNOSIS

In adults, fractures of the shaft of the clavicle usually are not confused with other diagnoses, although pathologic fractures occasionally are difficult to recog-

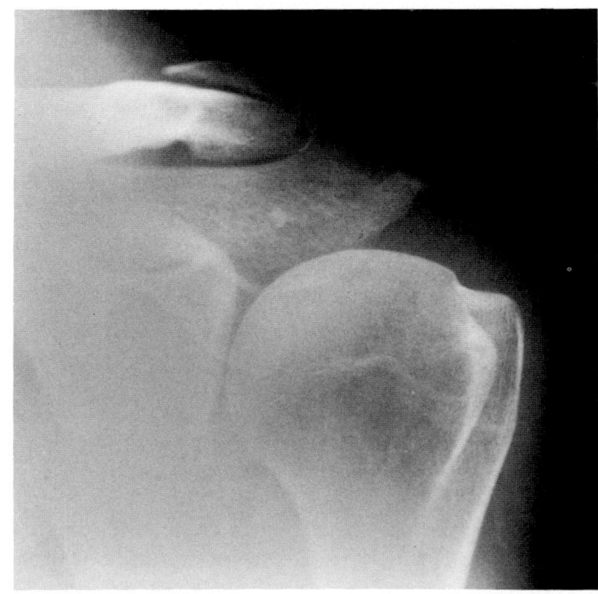

FIGURE 17-25. A distal clavicular fracture. The proximal fragment has all the coracoclavicular ligaments attached to it, but there is good bony contact between the two segments.

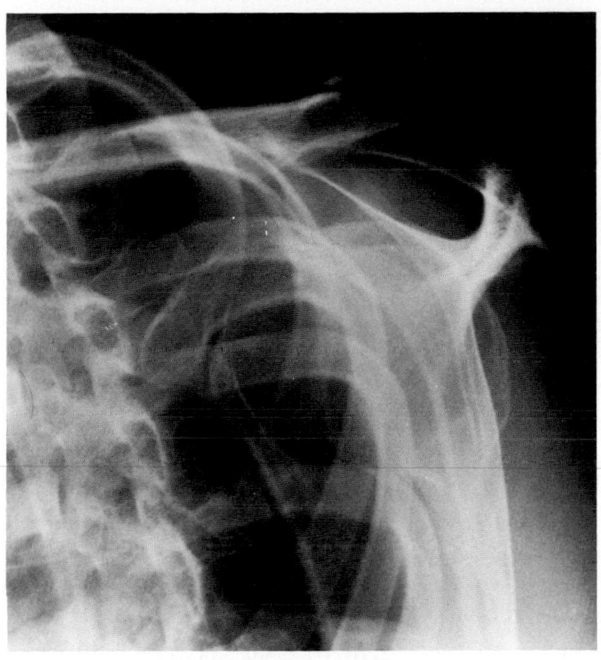

FIGURE 17-26. With good bony contact in perpendicular views, weighted views usually are not necessary, and may cause distraction of the fragments.

nize. However, fractures of the distal or medial end of the clavicle may appear clinically to be complete acromioclavicular or sternoclavicular separations, although these rarely present confusion once proper radiographic studies are performed.

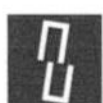

COMPLICATIONS

Nonunion

Despite the frequency of clavicular fractures, nonunion of unoperated shaft fractures is rare, with a reported incidence of 0.9% to 4%.*

* References 7, 62, 114, 130, 154, 231, 258, 271.

In a study of 235 consecutive patients, Neer reported nonunion rates of 0.1% after conservative treatment and 4.4% after operative treatment.[171] Rowe reported nonunion rates of 0.8% after conservative treatment and 3.7% after operative treatment.[222] Although there is some debate in the literature regarding the definition of clavicular nonunion, most authors consider it to be characterized by failure to show clinical or radiographic progression of healing at 4 to 6 months.[116,142,206,225,280] There are some temporal differences between atrophic and hypertrophic nonunion. Manske and Szabo reported that tapered, sclerotic, atrophic bone ends at 16 weeks were unlikely to unite and, thus, could be assumed to be a nonunion, but they classified other fractures as delayed unions after 16 weeks as long as there were some signs of healing.[152] Bilateral post-traumatic pseudarthrosis also has been reported in an adult.[99]

Although nonunion of the clavicle occurs predominantly in adults, it has been described in children.[183] However, when nonunion is seen in children, it is likely to be congenital pseudarthrosis.

Predisposing Factors

Several factors appear to predispose to nonunion of the clavicle:

1. Inadequate immobilization
2. Severity of trauma
3. Refracture
4. Distal-third fracture
5. Marked displacement
6. Primary open reduction.

Inadequate Immobilization

It long has been recognized that the clavicle is one of the most difficult bones to immobilize properly and completely after fracture while providing the patient with the simplicity and comfort that are ideal and prac-

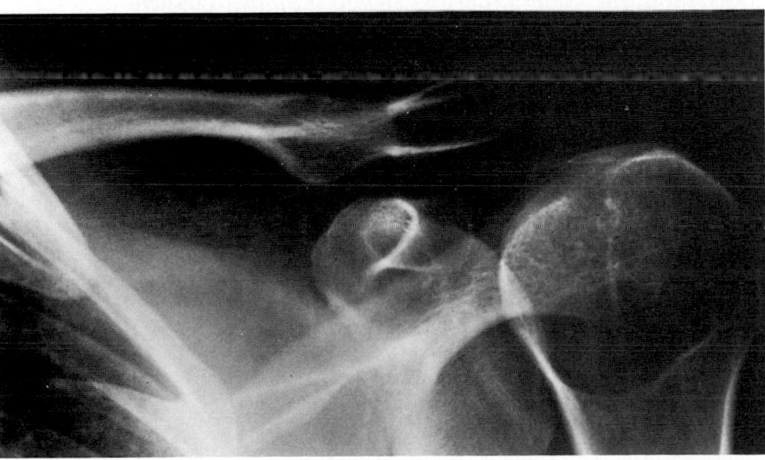

FIGURE 17-27. This distal clavicle fracture healed uneventfully with nonoperative treatment.

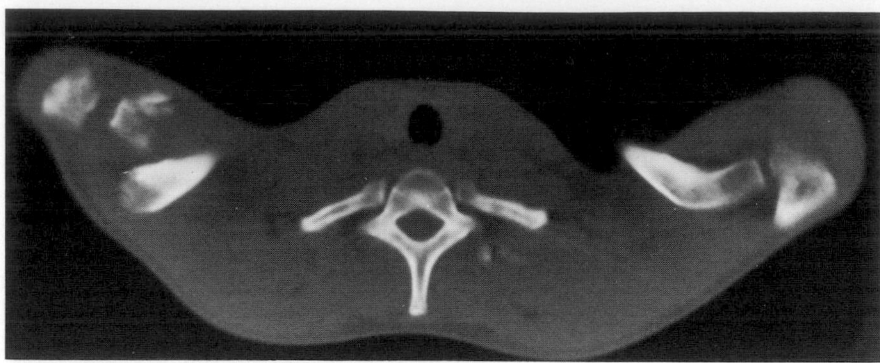

FIGURE 17-28. CT scan of a right clavicular fracture. Not only does this image confirm the site of the clavicular fracture as the distal clavicle, but it identifies a previously unsuspected intra-articular extension of the distal clavicle fracture.

tical in fracture treatment. Immobilization, by whatever means, should be continued until union is complete, although it may be difficult to determine this time with certainty. Rowe suggested that the usual healing periods for fractures of the middle third of the clavicle were 2 weeks for infants, 3 weeks for children, 4 to 6 weeks for young adults, and 6 weeks or more for older adults.[222] Moreover, it has been recognized that radiographic union may progress more slowly than clinical union, with x-ray evidence of union not appearing for 12 weeks or more.[222] When in doubt, immobilization probably should be continued. It has been suggested that once a fracture is clinically united, with no motion or tenderness at the fracture site, a gradual increase in activity can be permitted safely, even if radiographic union is incomplete.[222]

Severity of Trauma

Up to half of all clavicular fractures that result in nonunion follow severe trauma.[117] Wilkins and Johnston reviewed a series of 33 nonunited clavicle fractures.[280] Many of these patients had severe trauma, manifest by the degree of displacement of the fracture fragments, the amount of soft-tissue damage, and associated injuries (eg, multiple long-bone, spine, pelvic, and rib fractures). The authors pointed out the similarities between the clavicle and the tibia, another subcutaneous long bone that is prone to nonunion, and emphasized that the subcutaneous position of the clavicle predisposes it to more severe trauma, more severe soft-tissue damage, and, thus, nonunion.[280] As with other bones, open fractures have been implicated as a factor in nonunion of the clavicle.[142] Late perforation of the skin with a free compounding fragment also has been reported.[213]

It should be noted that many factors associated with clavicular nonunion, such as the degree of displacement, compounding, operative management, poor immobilization, and soft-tissue interposition, may simply reflect cases associated with more severe trauma to the clavicle. Thus, the independent statistical importance of some these associations with nonunion may be questioned.

Refracture

Some authors have identified refracture of previously healed clavicular fractures as contributing to nonunion.[117,154] In the series of Wilkins and Johnston, 7 of 31 nonunions occurred in such patients.[280] There appears to be no relationship between nonunion after refracture and the length of time between injuries, the age of the patient, the duration of immobilization of the original fracture, or the severity of the initial or subsequent traumatic injuries. It has been theorized that because the vascular anatomy of fractured bone remains altered for a long period, even after fracture union,[215] reinjury in some way might prevent this altered blood supply from reacting to the new fracture.[280]

Distal-Third Fracture

About 85% of nonunions of the clavicle occur in the middle third of the bone.[211] Despite this, it appears that distal-third clavicular fractures are much more prone to nonunion than are shaft fractures. In his series on clavicular nonunions, Neer noted that distal clavicular fractures accounted for more than half of nonunited clavicles after closed treatment.[171] He found several reasons for this. First, distal clavicular fractures are unstable, and the muscle forces and weight of the arm tend to displace the fracture fragments.[241] Second, because distal clavicular injuries often result from severe trauma, there is extensive local soft-tissue injury, and other associated injuries may affect generalized biologic and specific fracture healing.[172] Finally, distal fractures are difficult to secure adequately with external immobilization.

Even in fractures where union might occur with closed methods, the union time for distal clavicular fractures often is lengthy, and this long healing time, combined with soft-tissue trauma, may lead to stiffness and prolonged disability from disuse. For these reasons, Neer advocates early open reduction and internal fixation for this injury.[172,173]

Marked Displacement

In a large series reported by Jupiter and Leffert, the degree of displacement was the most significant factor in producing a nonunion.[117] However, in many clavicular fractures, marked displacement is associated with other factors that delay fracture healing, such as severe trauma, soft-tissue damage, open fractures, and soft-tissue interposition. Manske and Szabo believed that soft-tissue interposition alone was a major contributing factor in fractures that failed to heal, and at surgery, they frequently found a fracture fragment impaled in the trapezius muscle.[152] They particularly implicated soft-tissue interposition in the development of atrophic nonunions. However, others have reported that muscle interposition is uncommon.[117]

Primary Open Reduction

Some authors have associated primary open reduction of acute clavicular shaft fractures with an increased incidence of nonunion, whereas others have reported nonunion after osteotomy of the clavicle or radiation therapy.[131,214] Rowe reported a 0.8% incidence of nonunion in fractures treated without surgery and a 3.7% incidence in those treated with surgery.[222] Neer had a similar experience, with nonunion rates of 0.1% in fractures treated without surgery compared with 4.6% in those treated with surgery.[171] Schwartz and Leixnering reported a nonunion rate of 13% in patients with primary open reduction of clavicular fractures, although they suggested that inadequate internal fixation may have played a prominent role in this high incidence.[234] Poigenfürst and associates reported a complication rate of 10%, with four nonunions in 60 fresh clavicular fractures treated with internal plate fixation.[200b]

Poor internal fixation, rather than the surgery itself, may play the primary role in the increased incidence of nonunion in clavicular fractures treated with primary surgery (Fig. 17-29). Zenni and colleagues reported a series of 25 acute clavicular fractures treated with primary open reduction using an open intramedullary pin or cerclage suture and bone grafting; all of the fractures healed without complications.[286] In some reports citing an increased incidence of nonunion with open reduction, it is probable that the operative fractures included difficult cases (ie, those with severe trauma, soft-tissue damage, and associated injuries), thus contributing to the poor results. Nevertheless, the excellent results obtained with nonoperative treatment are undeniable, and primary open reduction of clavicular fractures rarely is indicated.

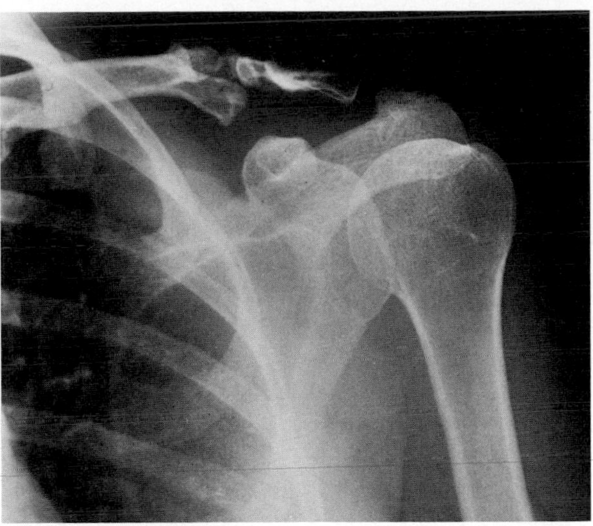

FIGURE 17-29. A radiographic view of a nonunited distal clavicular fracture after primary open reduction and internal fixation using an intramedullary pin. Inadequate internal fixation may be a contributing factor in nonunion of surgically treated acute fractures.

Radiographic Evaluation

Although nonunion often can be demonstrated clinically by motion at the fracture site, radiographic confirmation should be obtained on anteroposterior and 45° cephalic tilt views. The radiographic signs of nonunion are not always clear. If there is minimal displacement of the fracture fragments and no gross motion, tomography (or even a bone scan) may be useful to demonstrate the presence of a nonunion in a symptomatic patient (Figs. 17-30 and 17-31). As with other fractures, nonunion of the clavicle may present with hypertrophic or atrophic bone ends. There may be real or apparent bone loss, particularly if there has been comminution. It is particularly helpful in evaluating nonunion to obtain an anteroposterior film of both clavicles on a single large cassette. In this way, the distance from sternum to acromion can be measured on the normal side and compared with the symptomatic side. This may help in deciding whether primary osteosynthesis with bone grafting will be adequate, or whether an intercalary segment of bone will be needed to span the area of segmental bone loss.

Symptoms

About 75% of patients with nonunited clavicular fractures have symptoms, including moderate to severe pain.[117,152] However, there is some evidence that patients with atrophic nonunion, although symptomatic initially, become less so with time.[280] Nonunion pain can radiate to the neck, down into the forearm, or even into the hand, especially if there is nerve irritation.[225] Patients may complain of grating or crepitation, which often is palpable. The shoulder may appear to sag forward, inward, and medially, and the apex of the medial fragment may be observed angling upward underneath the trapezius. Twenty-five percent or more of patients are affected by neurologic symptoms, often as a result of compromise of the brachial plexus by overabundant callus.[117,225] Likewise, chronic vascu-

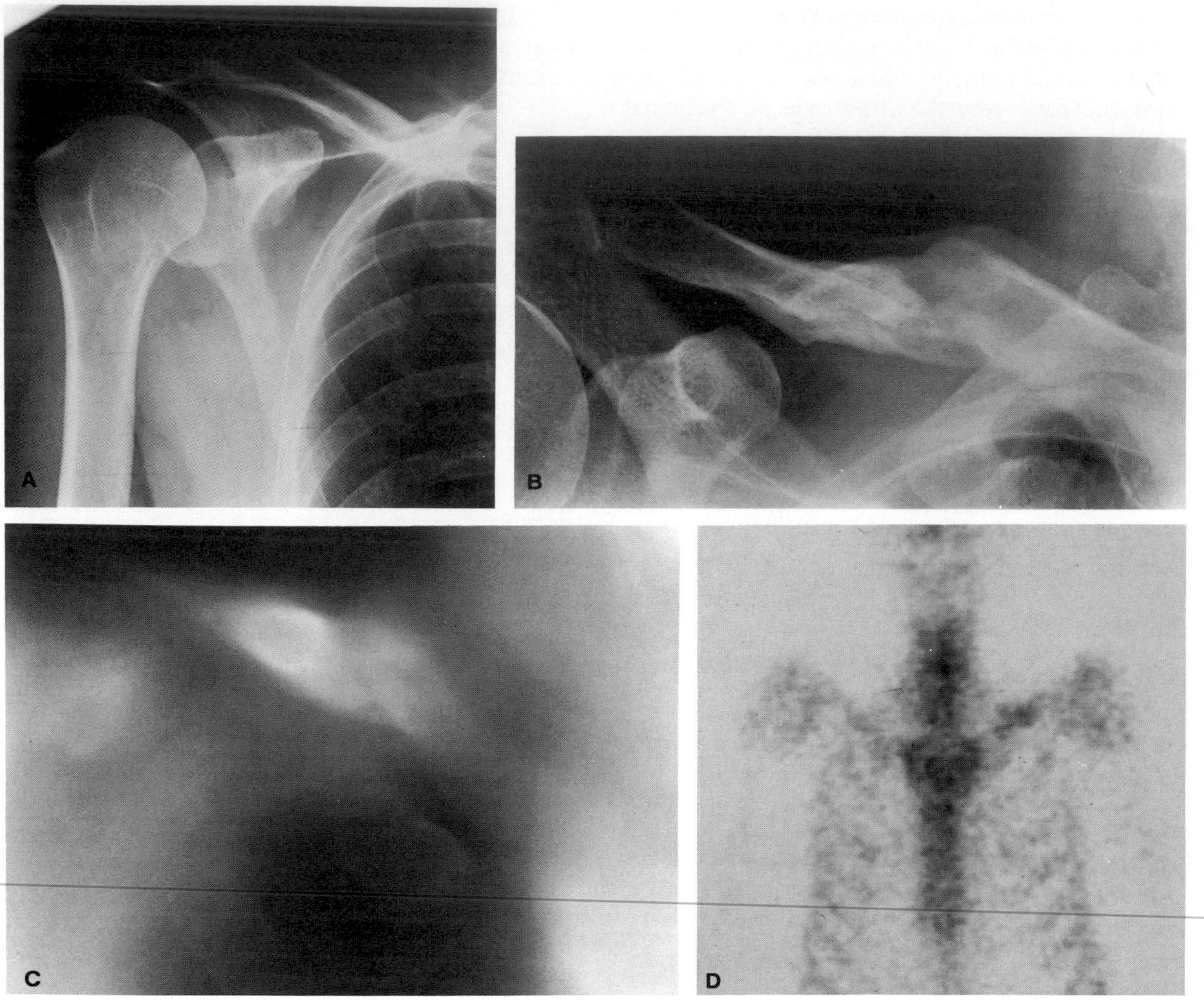

FIGURE 17-30. (**A**) An anteroposterior view of the right shoulder in a patient with pain after a clavicle fracture. The fracture area is poorly seen on this view. (**B**) A 45° cephalic tilt view shows the clavicle much more clearly, but it is still uncertain whether there is clear bridging of the fracture site. (**C**) Tomography suggests a lucent line in the area of the fracture that occurred 4 years earlier. (**D**) A bone scan shows increased activity in the right clavicle, which confirms the presence of a clavicular nonunion.

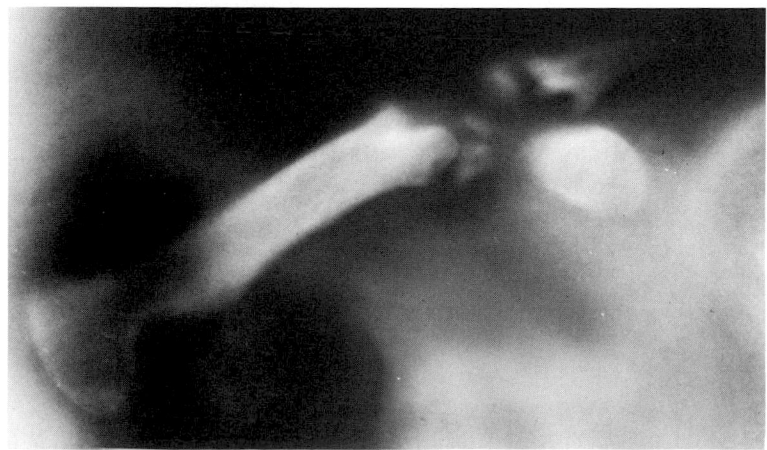

FIGURE 17-31. A tomogram showing bone fragmentation in a clear-cut nonunion of the clavicle.

lar symptoms can result from pressure on the subclavian vein, producing symptoms of thoracic outlet syndrome.[9,33,117,198]

It must be emphasized that when considering nonunion as the cause of a patient's painful symptoms, nonunion may be an incidental finding. A careful history and physical examination must be obtained, because many soft-tissue and bony abnormalities around the shoulder, including post-traumatic arthrosis of either the sternoclavicular or acromioclavicular joint, mimic the symptoms of a nonunion; these degenerative changes in the joint can appear several years after the injury.[280]

Physical Examination

Physical examination may reveal motion as the clavicle is manipulated, or pain on pressure at a nonunion site. Prominent bone of comminuted fragments may be palpable. Occasionally, there is limited range of motion at the shoulder joint, but this often is associated with soft-tissue, subacromial, or glenohumeral joint disease rather than resulting directly from the clavicular nonunion. If there are neurologic symptoms, these often are referred to the ulnar nerve distribution, and intrinsic weakness may occur.[83,225]

Malunion

In children with clavicular fractures, foreshortening is frequent but has not been reported to be a problem, and the angular deformity often remodels. However, in adults, there is no remodeling potential, and shortening or angulation may occur. This has been described by some as being purely a cosmetic deformity with little interference with function.[12] However, Eskola and associates reported that patients with shortening of the clavicular segments of more than 15 mm at follow-up examination had statistically significantly more pain than did those without these findings, and these authors recommended taking care to avoid the acceptance of a shortened clavicle.[63]

If the malunited fracture is a significant cosmetic or functional problem, simply shaving down the bone may be inadequate.[175] Several authors have recommended osteotomy, internal fixation, and bone grafting.[12] The patient must be made aware, however, that nonunion can be a sequela, and that the cosmetic appearance of the surgical scar may be more troublesome than the bump from the malunited bone.

Neurovascular Complications

The large amount of callus that follows healing of a clavicular fracture in a child rarely causes compression of the costoclavicular space, and the callus mass usually decreases with time.[44] In adults, however, late neurovascular sequelae can follow both united and nonunited fractures.[27,82,168,235,252,262]

Normally, the sternoclavicular angle and anterior bow of the clavicle provide abundant room for the brachial plexus and subclavian vessels in the costoclavicular space. Although there is some normal variability in the width and space between the clavicle and the first rib, this room usually is adequate.[104] Occasionally, a congenital anomaly such as a bifid clavicle or a straight clavicle with no medial or anterior angulation (Fig. 17-32) narrows the costoclavicular space and causes neurovascular compression.[221] Thus, it is not surprising that abundant callus or significant fracture deformity in some patients narrows this space enough to cause symptoms, which most frequently involve the subclavian vessels, the carotid artery, or the brachial plexus.[31,45,105,120] Although these compression phenomena are infrequent, they are important, because their clinical presentation can be confusing to the clinician and challenging for the patient until definitive treatment is instituted. Several vascular structures have been reported to be involved in compression syndromes.

Eilenberger and coworkers described a patient in whom cardiac arrest occurred after a fracture of the medial clavicle.[59a] They explained the complication as vagus nerve irritation secondary to hematoma of the fracture.

Carotid Artery

Obstruction of the carotid artery can lead to symptoms of syncope. This would be expected to be associated with fracture deformity or callus at the medial end of the clavicle.

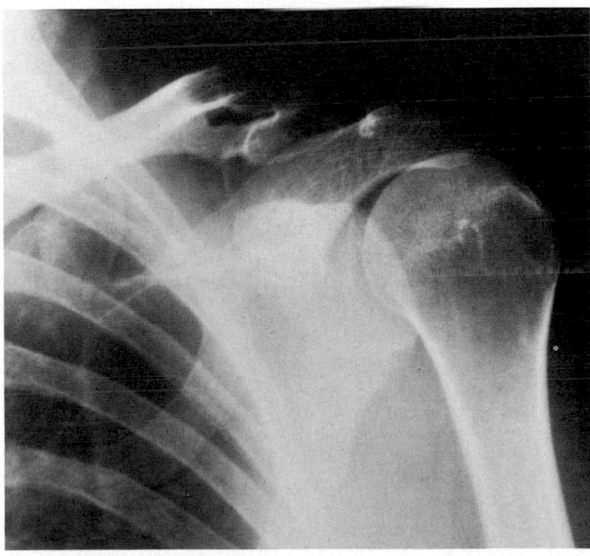

FIGURE 17-32. A partial or complete bifid clavicle may narrow the normal space between the clavicle and the first rib, leading to neurovascular compression syndromes.

Subclavian Vein

Compression of the subclavian vein between the clavicle and first rib, with subsequent obstruction, probably is the most common late vascular complication and can be accompanied by plexus and subclavian artery involvement.[132] The point of this obstruction has been shown by Lusskin and colleagues to be the site where the vein crosses the first rib and passes beneath the subclavius muscle and costoclavicular ligament.[148] Some authors have emphasized the role of the subclavius muscle and the condensation of the clavipectoral fascia known as the costocoracoid ligament in producing venous obstruction and subsequent thrombosis.[148] The syndrome is characterized by dilatation of the veins of the upper extremity and anterior chest on the affected side, produced by congestion of the collateral venous network. This compression is relieved by a downward thrust of the shoulder.[66,146,226,251] Lusskin and colleagues reported that this costoclavicular syndrome could be distinguished from the typical anterior scalene, cervical rib, and thoracic outlet compression syndromes, which also can produce arterial and neurologic symptoms but typically are reproduced by the Adson maneuver. The other syndromes generally are not accentuated by shoulder girdle extension.[47,95,104,238] The treatment depends on the offending structure. If it is overabundant callus, addressing the surgery to the clavicle may be necessary. However, if the clavicle is more normal, it might make more sense to resect the first rib.

Subclavian Artery

Subclavian artery compression was reported by Guilfoil and Christiansen, who described a case of thrombosis secondary to a clavicular nonunion.[95] Although injury to this artery is well recognized in acute clavicular injuries,[93,170] it is unusual as a late complication secondary to overabundant clavicular callus or nonunion. However, Yates and Guest recorded a case of death from embolus to the basilar artery, which originated from a thrombosis in the subclavian artery after a nonunited clavicular fracture.[284]

Aneurysm

Both traumatic aneurysms[28,49,176] and pseudoaneurysms[236] have been reported after clavicular fractures. These can present as pulsatile masses or soft-tissue densities in the area of the clavicular fracture or nonunion, and also can be the source of thrombi.

Hansky and associates reported a case of aneurysm of the subclavian artery that produced compression on the brachial plexus.[98a]

Brachial Plexus

Several neurologic symptoms have been described relating to late complications of clavicular fractures.† Symptoms can involve the entire brachial plexus or a single nerve. Suso and coworkers reported an injury to the anterior interosseous nerve secondary to a fracture of the distal clavicle.[253a] Bartosh and associates reported a case of an injury to the musculocutaneous nerve after a refracture of the midshaft of the clavicle that occurred 3 weeks after the original injury.[9a]

Because the onset of symptoms varies from the time of fracture to the establishment of nonunion, the late sequelae can be confused with nerve injuries occurring at the time of acute injury. Thus, it is particularly important to perform a careful neurologic examination of the patient with an acute fracture. Rumball and colleagues suggest that a patient with a displaced fracture of the medial clavicle be advised to report immediately the development of any new symptoms.[223a]

Although an early nerve injury usually is a traction neurapraxia, involves the lateral cord, and has a guarded prognosis, late compression neuropathies typically affect the medial cord, produce ulnar nerve symptoms, and have more benign prognoses. Typically associated with middle-third fractures, the proximal tip of the distal nonunited fragment is pulled downward and posteriorly, bringing it into contact with the neurovascular bundle, which is squeezed by the nonunited site above and the first and second ribs below. As would be expected, this problem is more common with hypertrophic than atrophic nonunions (Fig. 17-33). Ivey and associates reported a case of reflex sympathetic dystrophy of the anterior chest wall after an injury to the supraclavicular nerve that was associated with a midshaft clavicle fracture.[106a]

The diagnosis of late compression syndrome usually is made through a careful history, physical examination, and electrical studies such as electromyography and nerve conduction velocities.‡ Magnetic resonance imaging may be helpful to outline the relationship between the brachial plexus and hypertrophic callus or clavicular fragments (Fig. 17-34). Della Santa reported that in 16 cases of clavicular fracture, 2 patients had early neurovascular complications and 14 had late symptoms of the costoclavicular syndrome.[49a,49b]

Post-traumatic Arthritis

Post-traumatic arthritis may occur after intra-articular injuries of both the sternoclavicular and acromioclavicular joints, although degenerative disease of the dis-

† References 9a, 16, 31, 49A, 61, 94, 104, 106a, 123, 148, 160, 179, 223a, 225, 253a.

‡ References 16, 61, 104, 123, 148, 160, 179, 225.

tal clavicle is much more common. Often, this is the result of an unrecognized intra-articular (type III) fracture. The patient may have symptoms specifically related to pain at the acromioclavicular joint, or symptoms of impingement secondary to an inferior protruding osteophyte of the acromioclavicular joint causing extrinsic pressure on the subacromial bursa and rotator cuff.[174] On radiography, there may be cystic changes, spur formation, or narrowing of the acromioclavicular joint, or there may be resorption of the distal clavicle.[110] Further radiologic studies may be needed to define the lesion, especially in the area of the sternoclavicular joint, and additional tomograms or computed tomography may be indicated. The symptoms often decrease after a diagnostic injection of 1% lidocaine (Xylocaine) into the affected joint. If appropriate nonoperative treatment, including nonsteroidal medications or a steroid injection, does not provide lasting relief, surgical excision of the joint may be indicated. If the outer clavicle is to be resected, the distal 2 cm of bone is removed, lateral to the coracoclavicular ligaments, and the deltoid is repaired to the trapezius fascia. If resection of the sternoclavicular joint is indicated, the clavicular head of the sternocleidomastoid muscle can be used to fill in the area of resection.[175]

TREATMENT

As early as the late 1920s, more than 200 treatment methods already had been described for fractures of the clavicle[133,139] (Fig. 17-35). In general, excellent results have been reported with nonoperative treatment of these fractures.

The exact method of therapy used for a fractured clavicle depends on several factors, including the age and medical condition of the patient, the location of the fracture, and associated injuries.

Essentially all the authors who have written on the treatment of fractures of the clavicle have recommended a conservative approach. In adults with clavicular fractures, as with other fractures, the goal of treatment is to achieve bone healing with minimum morbidity, minimal loss of function, and minimal residual deformity. Keeping this in mind, some traditional, and cumbersome, methods of clavicular immobilization deserve reevaluation.

The main principles of nonoperative treatment historically have included several points: (1) to brace the shoulder girdle to raise the outer fragment upward, outward, and backward; (2) to depress the inner fragment; (3) to maintain reduction; and (4) to enable the

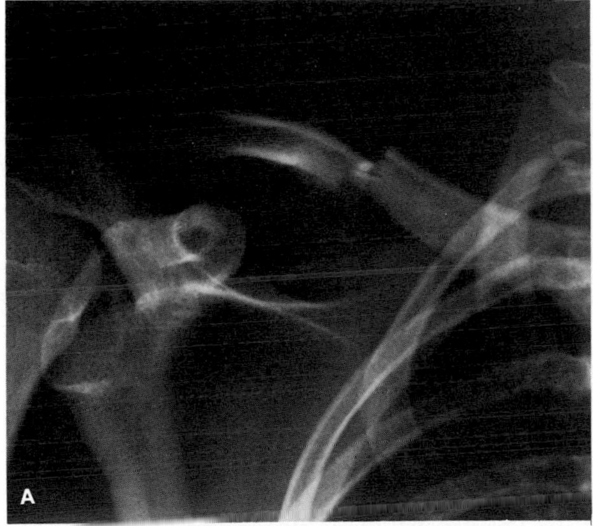

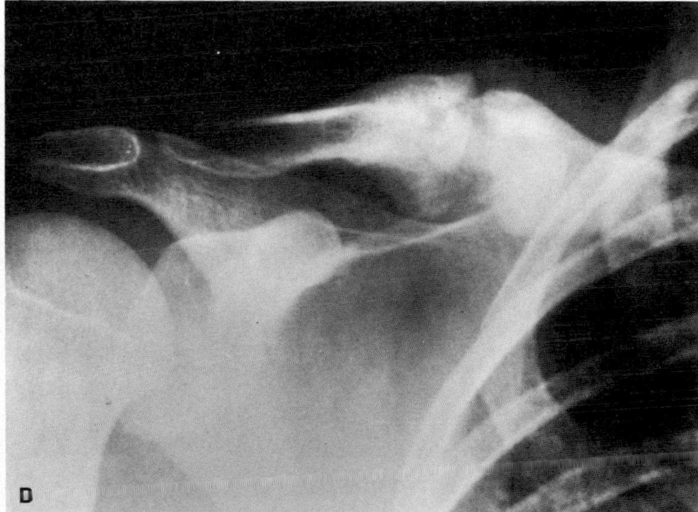

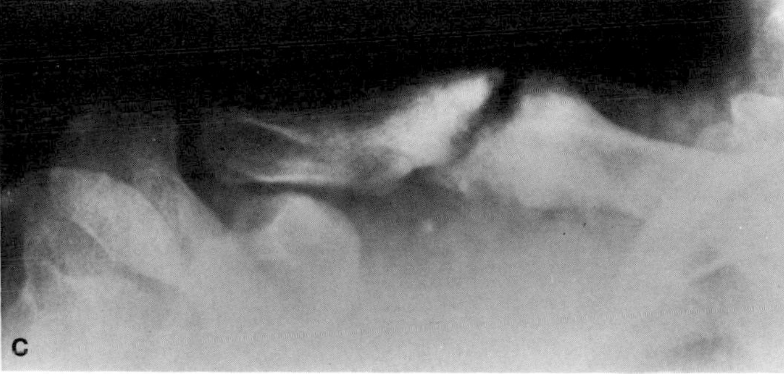

FIGURE 17-33. (**A**) A mid-clavicular fracture in an adult, with a mild degree of displacement. This was treated with a figure of eight splint, which was discontinued early so motion could be started. (**B**) An anteroposterior view showing abundant callus formation. It is unclear whether the fracture has united. (**C**) A cephalic tilt view confirms the presence of a nonunion with hypertrophic callus. The patient had symptomatic paresthesias, suggestive of irritation of the brachial plexus.

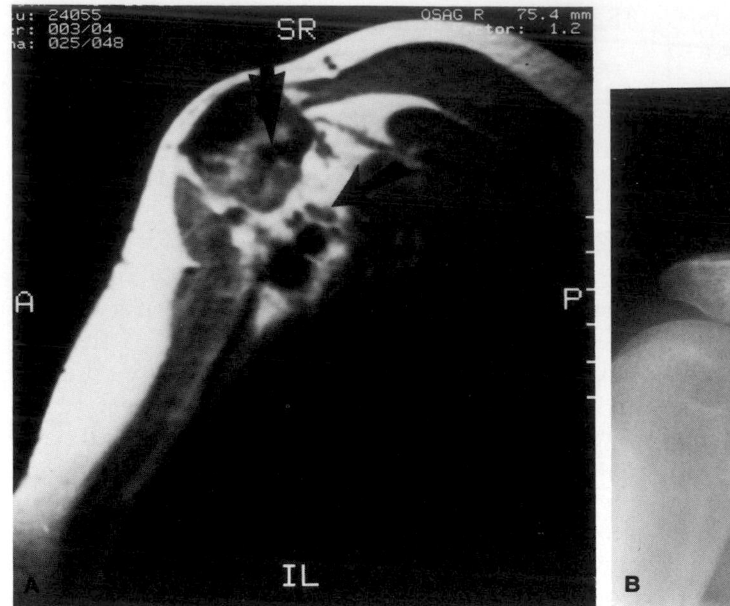

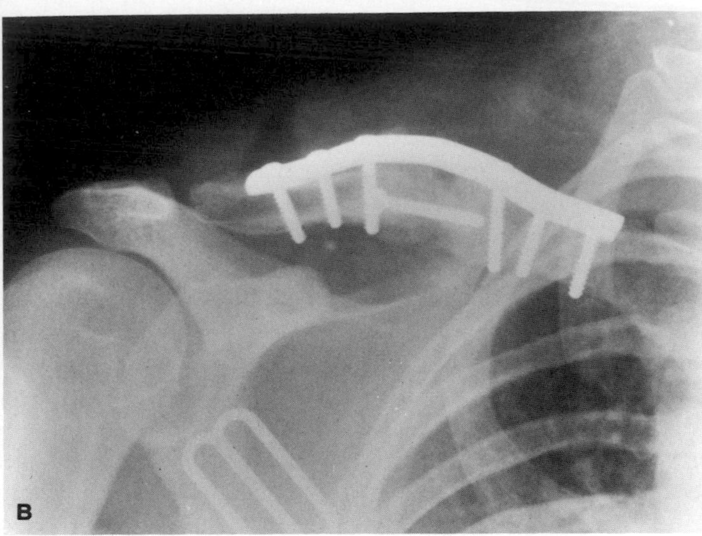

FIGURE 17-34. (**A**) An MRI scan showing the location of a hypertrophic callus (*large arrow*) and brachial plexus (*small arrow*). MRI can image actual encroachment on the brachial plexus, which was minimal in this case. (**B**) The patient was treated with a dynamic compression plate and bone grafting for this symptomatic, hypertrophic nonunion, with debulking of the callus.

ipsilateral elbow and hand to be used so that associated problems with immobilization can be prevented.

An extensive review of the literature would lead one to conclude that immobilization is nearly impossible to achieve, that deformity and shortening are usual, and that even if some shortening occurs, it generally does not interfere with function. The literature is replete with methods of various complexity to immobilize the clavicle, and treatment has been described ranging from long-term recumbency alone[12,208] to ambulatory treatment[34] to internal fixation methods.[§]

Treatment of Shaft Fractures

Simple Support

The simplest form of treatment is to provide support for the arm (Fig. 17-36). This might include a sling alone, a sling-and-swathe bandage, a Sayre bandage, or a Velpeau bandage.[139] No attempt is made to maintain a clavicular reduction, provided that satisfactory positioning of the bone appears to be present and union might be anticipated.[199] Although sling treatment is the simplest way to treat the fractured clavicular shaft, it often is unsettling to the orthopaedic surgeon who wishes to effect realignment of the fracture fragments. This probably explains the popularity of the many methods used to effect and maintain closed reduction.

Closed Reduction

A closed reduction is followed by an attempt to maintain reduction by bringing the distal fragment up and back. This may involve the use of a bandage alone (including the figure-of-eight bandage),[18,208] a bandage with plaster reinforcement,[35,285] or full immobilization of the shoulder in a spica cast[127,175,192,222,264] (Figs. 17-37 and 17-38). A variety of materials have been described to maintain the closed reduction, including metal, leather, plastic, plaster, and muslin.[175] The position required to reduce the fracture and maintain reduction (upward, lateral, and backward) is difficult to achieve, often is uncomfortable for the patient, and occasionally has been reported to cause symptoms of either neurovascular compression or even displacement of the fragment if careful attention is not paid to placing the external immobilization precisely.[222] Few studies have attempted, in a controlled fashion, to evaluate whether vigorous efforts to effect and maintain reduction provide a greater chance for a better outcome than does simple arm support. In two studies directly comparing figure-of-eight dressings to sling support, it was noted that figure-of-eight dressings were time-consuming, required frequent adjustments, might have contributed to other problems, and had

[§] References 21, 108, 122, 136, 138, 164, 169, 182, 193, 197, 224, 286.

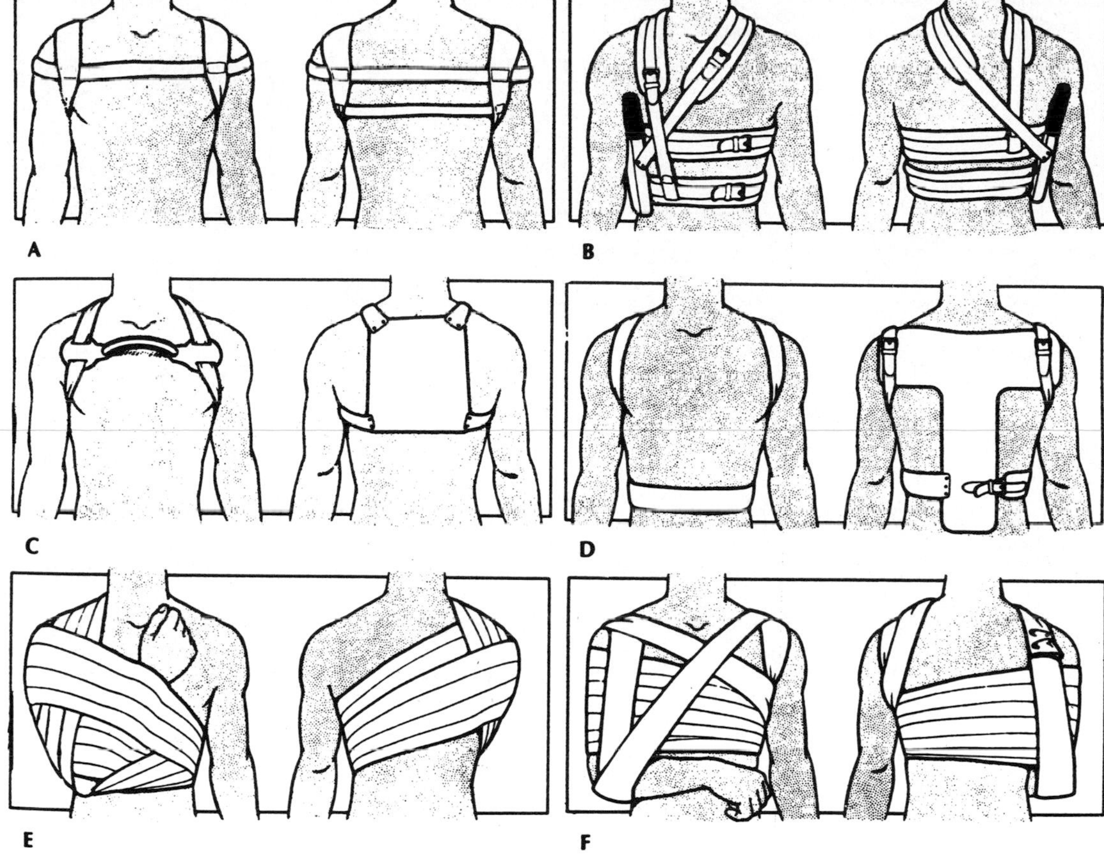

FIGURE 17-35. A variety of closed treatment methods have been used for fractures of the clavicle. Several of these are illustrated: (**A**) the Parham support; (**B**) the Böhler brace; (**C**) the Taylor clavicle support; (**D**) unidentified support; (**E**) a Velpeau wrap; and (**F**) a modified Velpeau wrap. (*Dameron, T.B., Jr., and Rockwood, C.A., Jr.: Fractures and Dislocations of the Shoulder. In Rockwood C.A., Jr., Wilkins, K.E., King, R. E. (eds.): Fractures in Children, p. 609. Philadelphia, J.B. Lippincott, 1984.*)

more complications than did simple sling treatment. The authors concluded that the functional and cosmetic sequelae of the two methods were identical, with alignment of the healed fracture unchanged from the initial displacement.[6,159] Another group studied the recovery time after conservative treatment of clavicular fractures in 140 patients. There was no difference in the speed of recovery between those treated with the sling and those treated with the figure-of-eight bandage, although patient age at the time of fracture

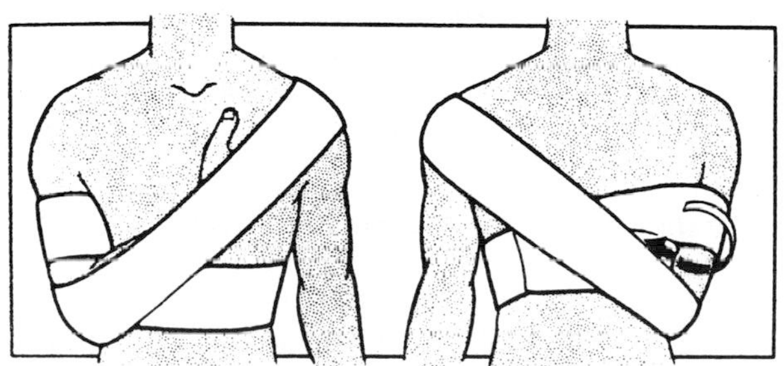

FIGURE 17-36. Modification of a Sayre bandage, which is intended not to reduce the fracture, but simply to support the arm. (*Dameron, T.B., Jr., and Rockwood, C.A., Jr.: Fractures and Dislocations of the Shoulder. In Rockwood C.A., Jr., Wilkins, K.E., King, R.E. (eds.): Fractures in Children, p. 617. Philadelphia, J.B. Lippincott, 1984.*)

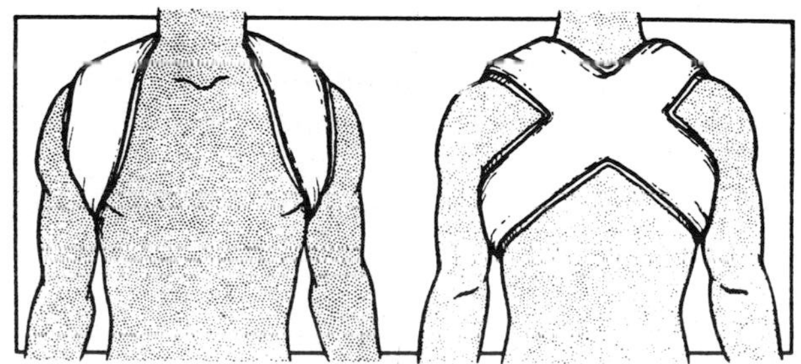

FIGURE 17-37. A Billington yoke, used to maintain a reduction, consists of a plaster figure-of-eight. (*Dameron, T.B., Jr., and Rockwood, C.A., Jr.: Fractures and Dislocations of the Shoulder. In Rockwood C.A., Jr., Wilkins, K.E., King, R.E. (eds.): Fractures in Children, p. 617. Philadelphia, J.B. Lippincott, 1984.*)

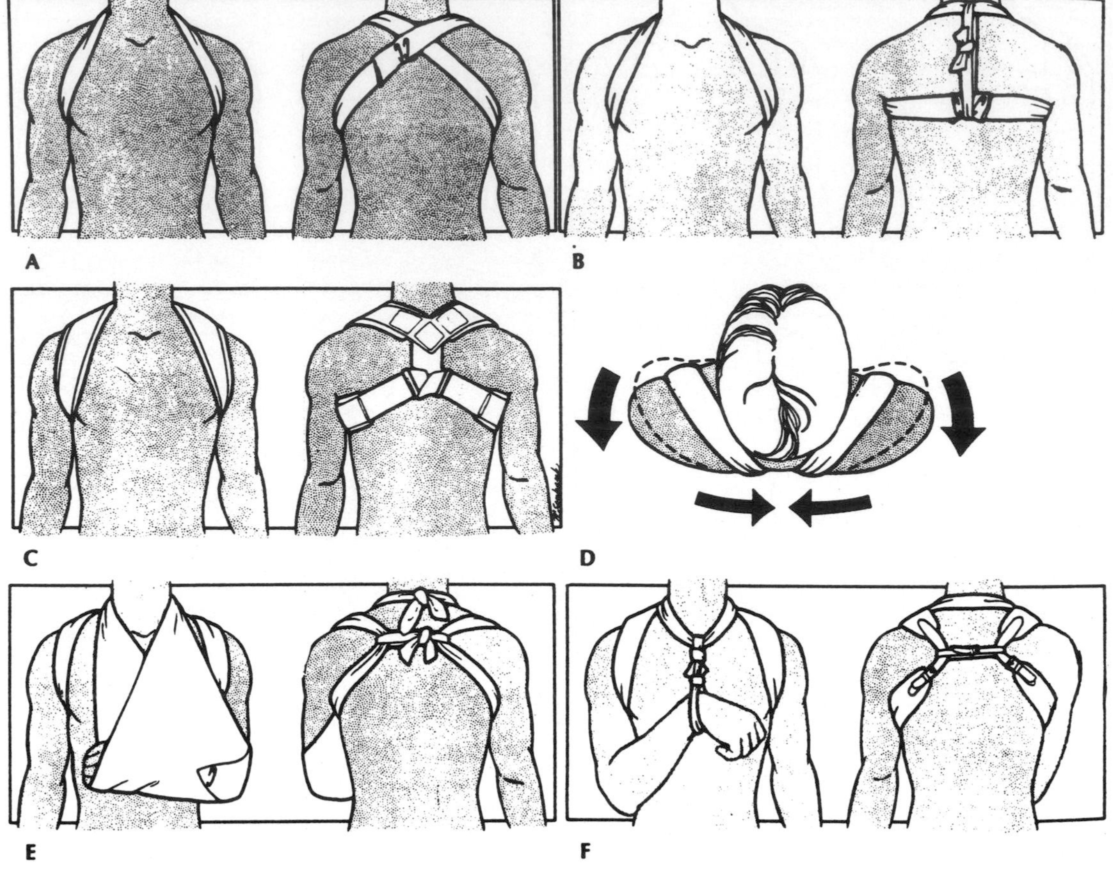

FIGURE 17-38. Other types of figure-of-eight bandages. These are intended to maintain reductions achieved by closed means. (**A**) Stockinette padded with three layers of sheet wadding and held in place with safety pins. (**B**) Padded stockinette with the upper and lower borders tied to one another; this knot is tightened daily, increasing tension to maintain the reduction. (**C**) A commercial figure-of-eight support. (**D**) Superior view of the patient, showing how the figure-of-eight support pulls the shoulder up and backward. (**E**) A modified figure-of-eight bandage with a sling. (**F**) A figure-of-eight support used with a collar and cuff. (*Dameron, T.B., Jr., and Rockwood, C.A., Jr.: Fractures and Dislocations of the Shoulder. In Rockwood C.A., Jr., Wilkins, K.E., King, R. E. (eds.): Fractures in Children, p. 618. Philadelphia, J.B. Lippincott, 1984.*)

did affect the recovery, with 33% of patients older than 20 years still having symptoms 3 months after injury.[245]

Open Reduction With Internal Fixation

Many devices have been described for the treatment of clavicular fractures through internal fixation.[98,188,240] These devices have included cerclage sutures[264]; intramedullary devices (eg, Steinmann pins, Hagie pins,[18a] Kirschner wires, Knowles pins, Rush rods)[||]; plate fixation[130,167]; and Küntscher nails.[182a]

Open or Closed Reduction With External Fixation

In some cases, such as open fractures or septic nonunions, external fixation can be considered. In one study using the Hoffmann device, the average time for the external fixator to be left on was 51 days; there were no pleural or vascular complications, and all fractures united.[233] However, this is not a technique with which there is extensive experience, and there is a potential for complications with this procedure.[43] Xiao reported on a new external fixation device that produced near-anatomical reduction in 87.4% of his patients.[282b]

Treatment of Fractures of the Distal Clavicle

Fractures of the distal third of the clavicle may heal with nonoperative immobilization.[183b,183c,218,219] However, the deforming forces and high incidence of nonunion have led many authors to recommend primary open reduction and internal fixation,[#] using either an

|| References 21, 24, 138, 164, 169, 182, 193, 197, 224, 237, 286.

References 8a, 24a, 64, 88a, 97a, 164a, 200.

intramedullary pin[172,173] or some method of dynamic fixation to bring the proximal clavicular segment to the distal segment[122] (Figs. 17-39 and 17-40). Others have used a coracoclavicular screw.[286]

Complications have been reported with each of these methods, including migration of intramedullary wires. Plate fixation often is impractical because of the small distal segment. Some type of intramedullary device that is not prone to migration might offer the safest method of therapy for distal clavicular fractures. Poigenfürst and associates reported on 25 fractures of the distal clavicle. Only two patients who were treated without surgery had a successful result.[200] These authors recommended the use of a coracoclavicular lag screw for simple fractures associated with rupture of the coracoclavicular ligament and plating for fragmented fractures. Brunner and coworkers reported 237 clavicular fractures, 75 of which (33%) involved the lateral third of the bone.[24a] At 5-year follow-up after exclusively conservative treatment, good results were found in Neer type I and III fractures and there was a 31% rate of pseudarthrosis in Neer type II (Jäger/Breitner type IIA) fractures. These authors described a new bandage to prevent posterior and upward displacement of the proximal fragment.[24a] However, they recommended open reduction and internal fixation for Neer type II fractures and Jäger/Breitner fractures, using extra-articular implants. Nordqvist and colleagues described 110 patients with fractures of the lateral end of the clavicle who were treated without surgery.[183b,183c] After an average follow-up period of 15 years, they reported on 73 undislocated Neer type I fractures, 23 dislocated type II fractures, and 14 intra-articular type III fractures. The average age of the patients at the time of injury was 36 years (range, 2 to 71 years). At follow-up, 95 shoulders were asymptomatic. Fifteen shoulders had moderate pain and dysfunction and were rated as fair. No patient had severe residual shoulder disability. There were 10 cases of nonunion, 8 of which were asymptomatic. These authors concluded that fracture of the lateral end of the clavicle does not require operation.

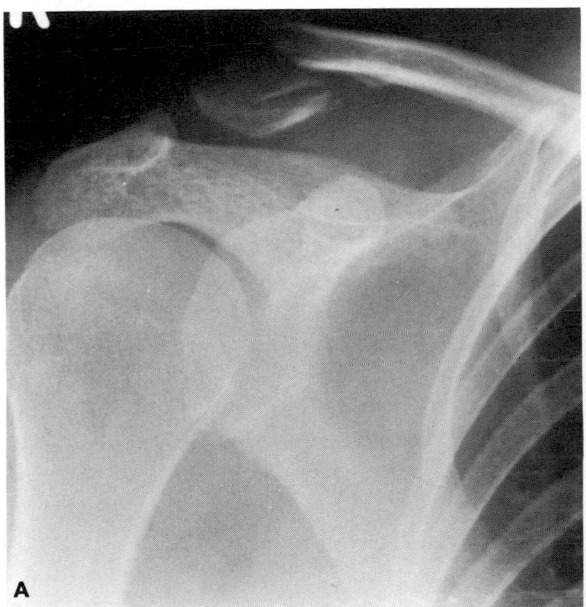

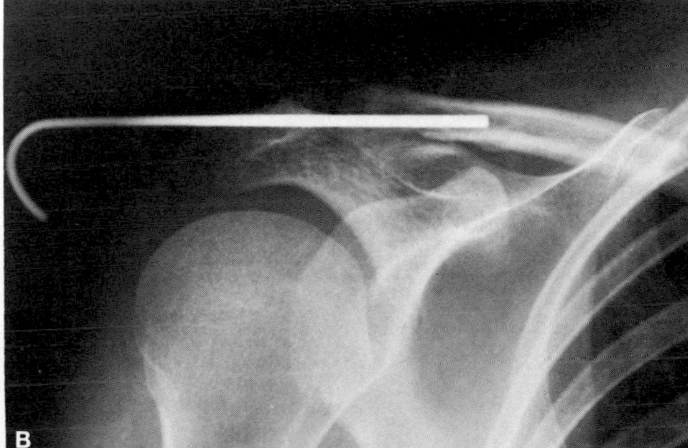

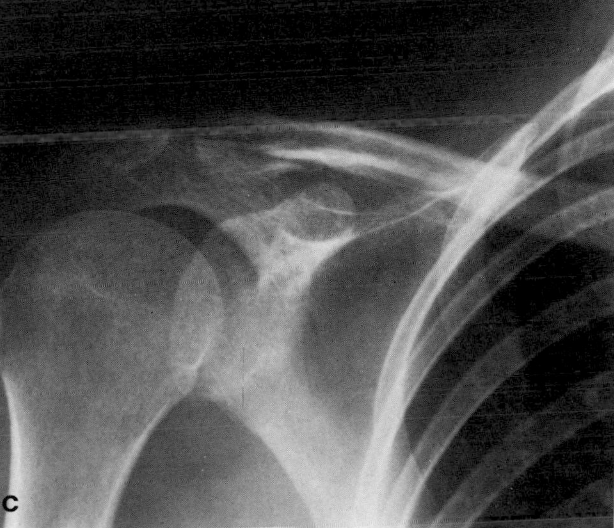

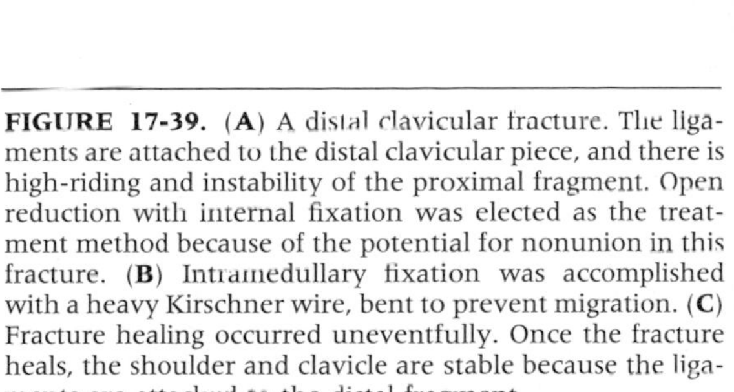

FIGURE 17-39. (**A**) A distal clavicular fracture. The ligaments are attached to the distal clavicular piece, and there is high-riding and instability of the proximal fragment. Open reduction with internal fixation was elected as the treatment method because of the potential for nonunion in this fracture. (**B**) Intramedullary fixation was accomplished with a heavy Kirschner wire, bent to prevent migration. (**C**) Fracture healing occurred uneventfully. Once the fracture heals, the shoulder and clavicle are stable because the ligaments are attached to the distal fragment.

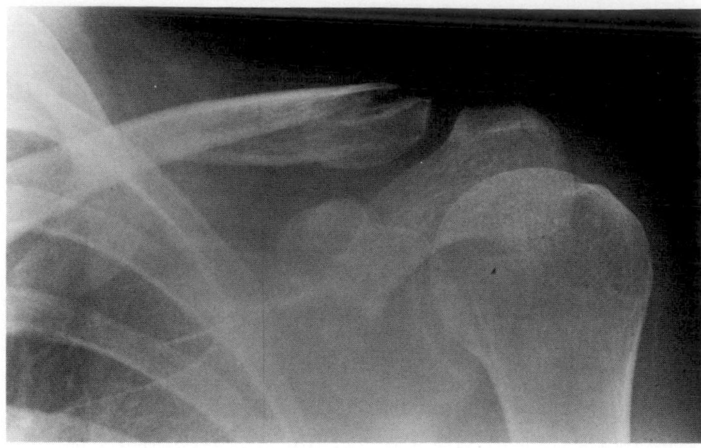

FIGURE 17-40. Distal clavicular fractures heal well without surgical treatment in some instances, as evidenced by this radiograph. The view is in an adult who had an oblique distal clavicular fracture treated without surgery. Clinical and radiographic union have occurred.

Treatment of Nonunion

Asymptomatic clavicular nonunion need not be treated. In addition, nonunion in the elderly probably should be considered for nonoperative treatment. Nonoperative methods to obtain union have been reported, particularly the use of electrical stimulation. However, there have been only a few documented cases of healing of clavicular nonunion by pulsed electromagnetic fields,[22,48] and most authors share the view that there is little role for electrical stimulation in the treatment of this complication. This is especially true because operative methods have shown such high degrees of success.[10,32]

Indications for surgical treatment are (1) pain or aching clearly attributable to the nonunion; (2) shoulder girdle dysfunction, weakness, or fatigue; and (3) neurovascular compromise.[193]

Although bone drilling has been suggested as a means of stimulating a delayed union to progress,[205] there is little role for this in established nonunion.

Partial claviculectomy, with excision of the nonunion site, has been reported as a means of treating nonunited clavicular fractures.[222a] In the short term, this may alleviate the crepitus and often eliminates the pain.[152] However, many patients treated in this manner remain mildly to moderately symptomatic;[117,280] the stabilizing function of the clavicle is lost, and neurogenic symptoms can be a problem.[142,280] In contrast, resection of the nonunion and filling of the defect with cancellous bone chips may stimulate regeneration of the clavicle as well as decompress the neurovascular structures if nonunion is accompanied by symptoms of thoracic outlet syndrome.[33] Surgical treatment most commonly consists of an attempt to gain union through some means of internal fixation with bone grafting. Techniques for the surgical treatment of nonunion have evolved, as have internal fixation techniques for other long-bone fractures and nonunions.

Several open treatment methods have been detailed. Some authors have used wire sutures through the ends of either clavicular fragment and through iliac crest graft.[12,83,171] Sutures of other materials, including catgut, braided suture, and even loops of kangaroo tendon, also have been used.[175] Simple intrafragmen-

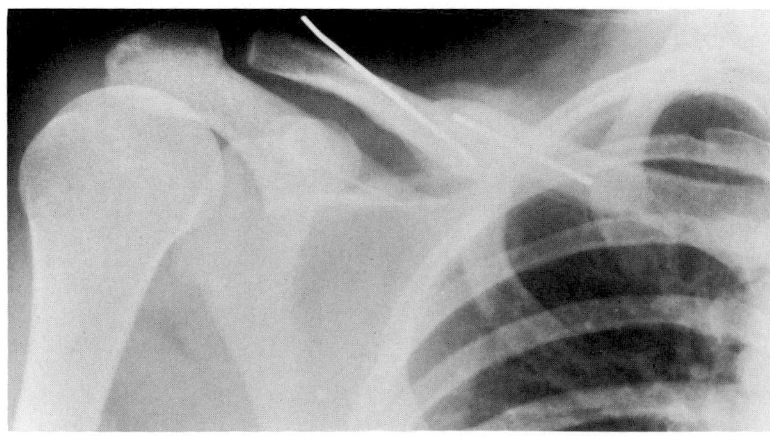

FIGURE 17-41. A complication of intramedullary fixation with a Kirschner wire or Steinmann pin. Insufficient bone purchase combined with motion can lead to hardware failure and migration of pins, with potentially catastrophic results.

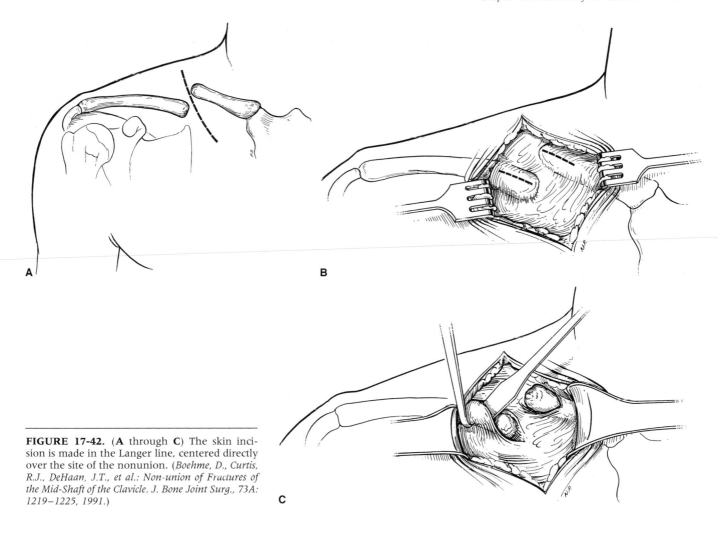

FIGURE 17-42. (**A** through **C**) The skin incision is made in the Langer line, centered directly over the site of the nonunion. (*Boehme, D., Curtis, R.J., DeHaan, J.T., et al.: Non-union of Fractures of the Mid-Shaft of the Clavicle. J. Bone Joint Surg., 73A: 1219–1225, 1991.*)

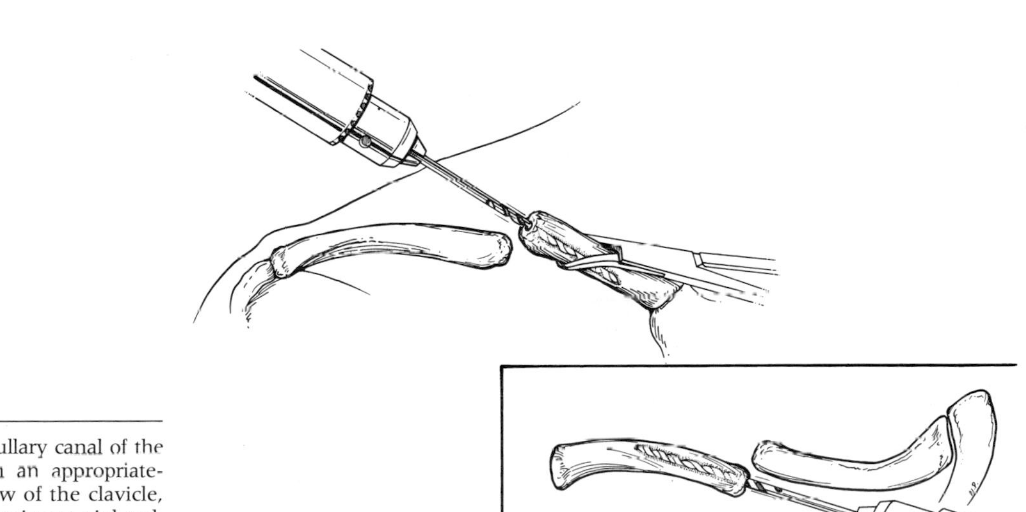

FIGURE 17-43. The intramedullary canal of the medial fragment is drilled with an appropriate-size drill bit. Inset: superior view of the clavicle, showing that the anterior cortex is not violated. (*Boehme, D., Curtis, R.J., DeHaan, J. T., et al.: Non-union of Fractures of the Mid-Shaft of the Clavicle. J. Bone Joint Surg., 73A: 1219–1225, 1991.*)

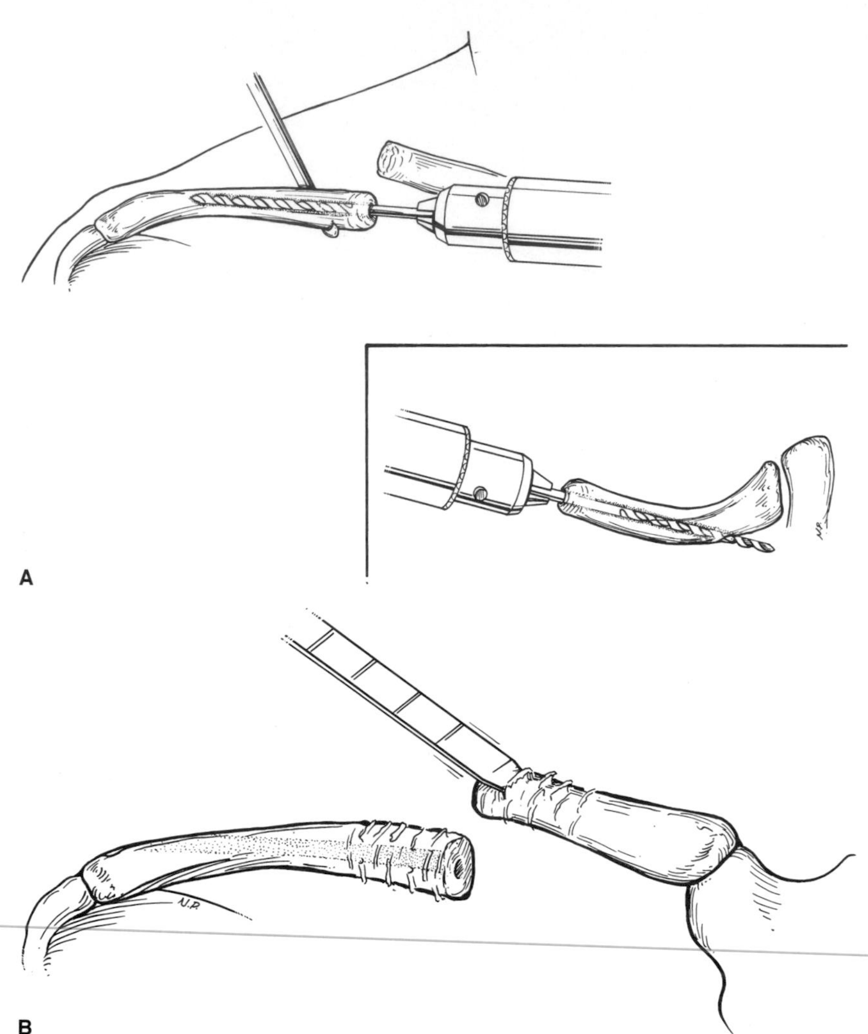

FIGURE 17-44. Frontal view. (**A**) The intramedullary canal of the lateral fragment is drilled with the same size drill bit used for the medial fragment. Inset: Superior view. The drill bit exits the lateral end of the clavicle medial and posterior to the acromioclavicular joint, secondary to the S-shaped configuration of the clavicle. (**B**) The drilling should continue until the bit is palpable beneath the skin on the posterolateral aspect of the shoulder. (*Boehme, D., Curtis, R.J., DeHaan, J.T., et al.: Non-union of Fractures of the Mid-Shaft of the Clavicle. J. Bone Joint Surg., 73A: 1219–1225, 1991.*)

tary screw fixation has been advocated, with fixation of the iliac bone as onlay graft and cancellous bone grafting at either junction.[157,225] However, because the clavicle exhibits so much movement in multiple planes, and because these methods control rotation poorly, neither suture nor screw fixation is secure enough to be reliable without additional protection. External cast or brace support is necessary to prevent screw or wire breakage and possible wire fragment migration, which can produce disastrous results.[134,148a,158,184]

Open reduction with intramedullary fixation is popular. Fixation is achieved with Kirschner wires** (with or without screws), screws,[49a] Steinmann pins,[27a,126,173,222] Knowles pins,[34,182,180] or modified Hagie pins.[18a,217] Although reports of these methods have been encouraging, rotation is poorly controlled under most circumstances, the intramedullary fixation can be difficult to insert if there are atrophic bone ends

** References 131a, 147, 154, 175, 181, 234, 258, 263, 273.

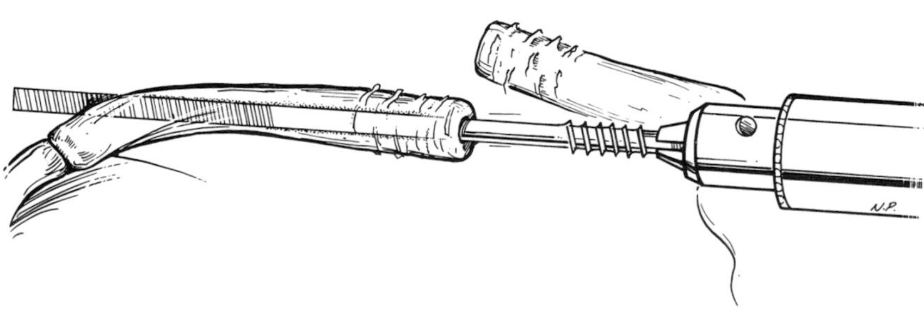

FIGURE 17-45. The fine-threaded end of the Hagie pin is drilled out through the lateral fragment. Petalling of the ends of the site of the nonunion was accomplished with an osteotome. (*Boehme, D., Curtis, R.J., DeHaan, J.T., et al.: Non-union of Fractures of the Mid-Shaft of the Clavicle. J. Bone Joint Surg., 73A: 1219–1225. 1991.*)

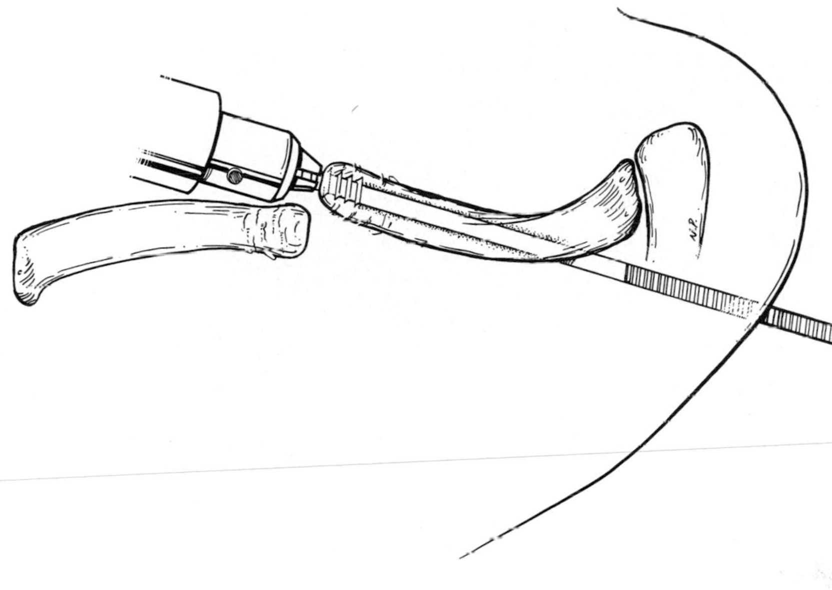

FIGURE 17-46. Superior view. The Hagie pin is drilled out through the skin on the posterolateral aspect of the shoulder. (*Boehme, D., Curtis, R.J., DeHaan, J.T., et al.: Non-union of Fractures of the Mid-Shaft of the Clavicle. J. Bone Joint Surg., 73A: 1219–1225. 1991.*)

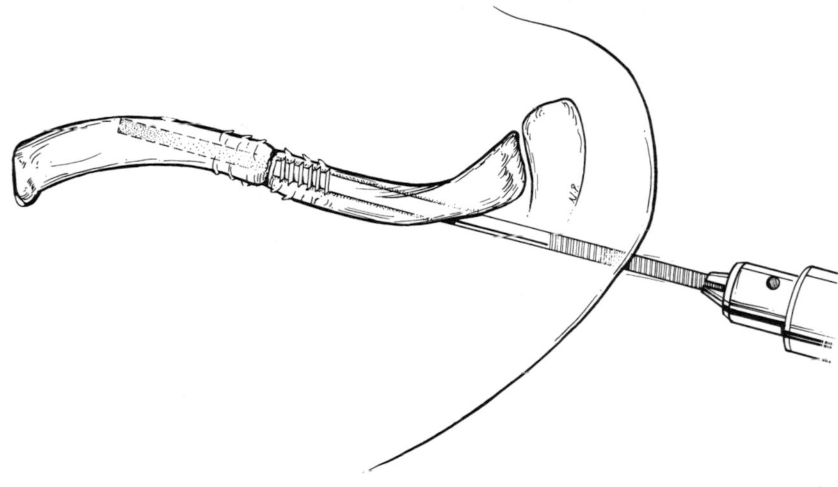

FIGURE 17-47. Superior view. With the sharp point of the trocar of the modified Hagie pin removed and with the fracture held reduced, the hand drill is placed on the distal end of the pin. The pin is extracted until the blunt end is at the level of the site of the nonunion. Bone-holding forceps are used to align the segments of the clavicle. The pin then is drilled down into the medial fragment of the clavicle. (*Boehme, D., Curtis, R.J., DeHaan, J.T., et al.: Non-union of Fractures of the Mid-Shaft of the Clavicle. J. Bone Joint Surg., 73A: 1219–1225, 1991.*)

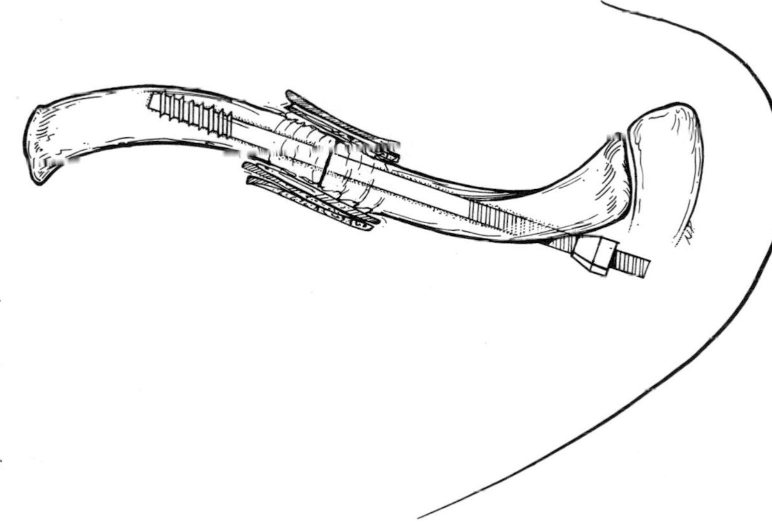

FIGURE 17-48. Superior view. If sufficient compression at the site of the nonunion is not obtained, the Hagie nut can be applied to the fine-threaded end of the pin and tightened, which will produce additional compression. The bone graft is applied superiorly, inferiorly, and posteriorly about the site of the fracture. (*Boehme, D., Curtis, R.J., DeHaan, J.T., et al.: Non-union of Fractures of the Mid-Shaft of the Clavicle. J. Bone Joint Surg., 73A: 1219–1225, 1991.*)

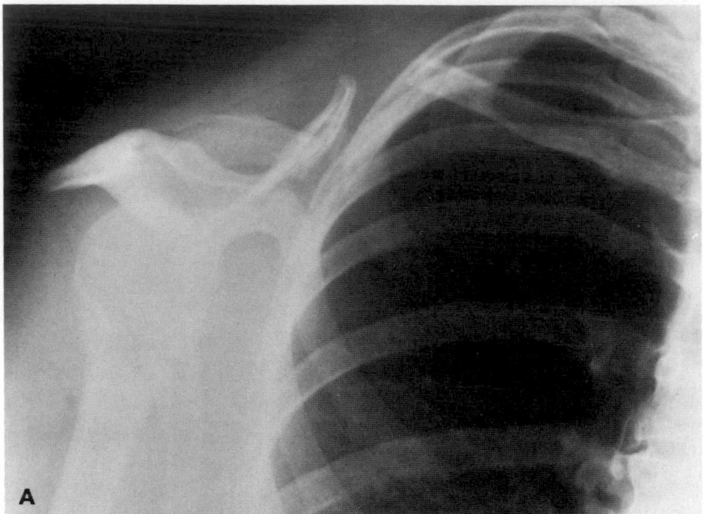

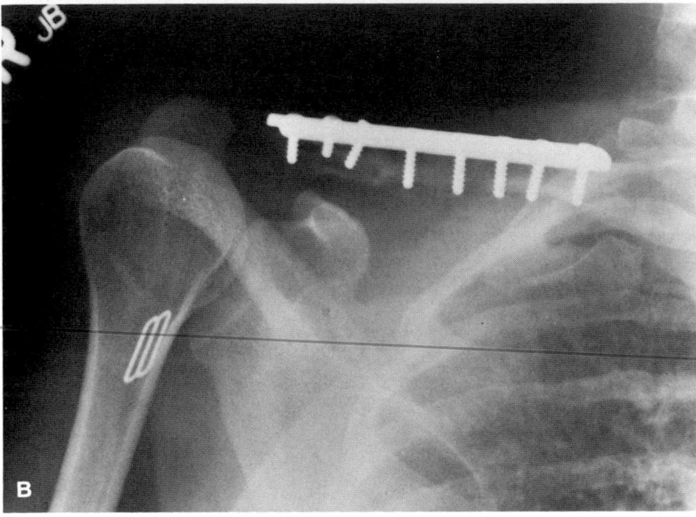

FIGURE 17-49. (**A**) Radiograph in a 26-year-old woman who fractured her clavicle 5 years previously. A painful nonunion was present, with an intermediate gap and atrophic ends. (**B**) Rigid internal fixation was accomplished using a dynamic compression plate with an intercalary bone graft. Clinical and radiographic union occurred.

(especially with the flat, curved clavicle), and external plaster support often is required. In addition, distraction of the fracture at the nonunion site can occur with threaded pins.[126] The intramedullary device can bend or break, and several complications have been reported with pin migration[134,158,184] (Fig. 17-41). Despite reports of success,[261] the complication rate can be high with intramedullary fixation—as high as 75% in one series.[280]

In 1991, Rockwood and associates described a series of 21 patients with nonunion of the clavicle who were treated successfully with an intramedullary pin. These patients underwent open reduction, internal fixation with a modified Hagie intramedullary pin, and autogenous bone grafting. The average duration of follow-up was 35 months (range, 5 months to 11 years). Healing occurred in 20 (95%) of the 21 patients. Compared with other treatments, such as fixation with a plate and screws, intramedullary fixation has several advantages. The intramedullary pin can be inserted through a cosmetically acceptable incision in a Langer line, it requires less dissection of the soft tissues, and, after healing, it can be removed through a small incision under local anesthesia (Figs. 17-42 through 17-48).[††]

The use of rigid internal fixation for acute fractures has facilitated the management of many traditionally difficult fractures, and the concept of rigidly immobilizing fragment ends has had natural applications in the treatment of nonunion as well. Although rigid internal fixation techniques using A-O plates without bone grafting have been reported to be successful in clavicular nonunion,[101,206,248] the addition of supplemental bone graft to rigid plating has been the most popular approach to this complication. With this

[††] A set of four different sizes of Hagie pins along with the proper size drill bits, self-retaining screwdriver, and depth gauge are available in a set of instruments from DePuy Orthopaedic Company.

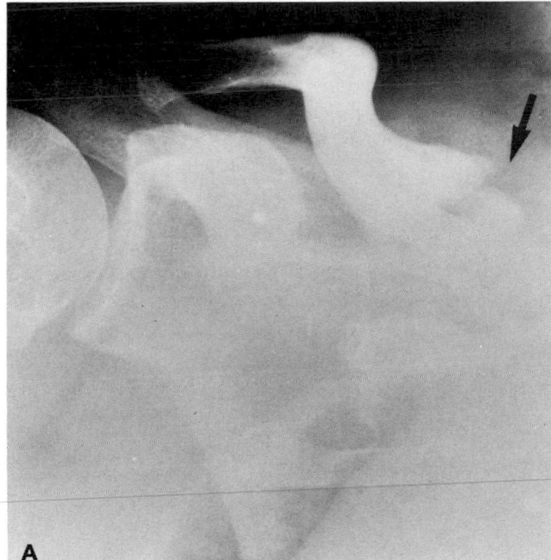

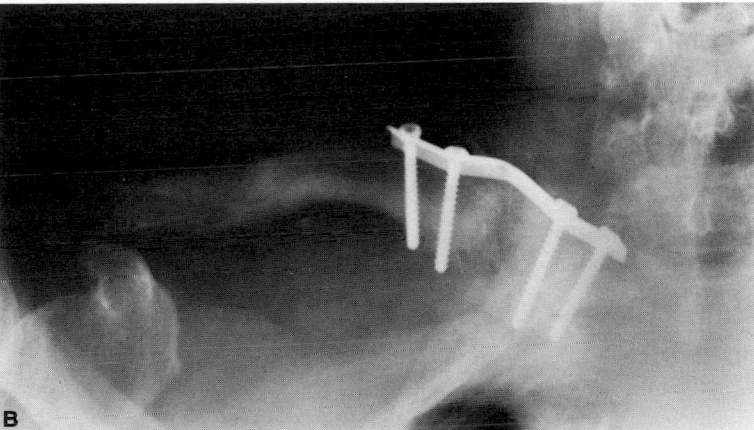

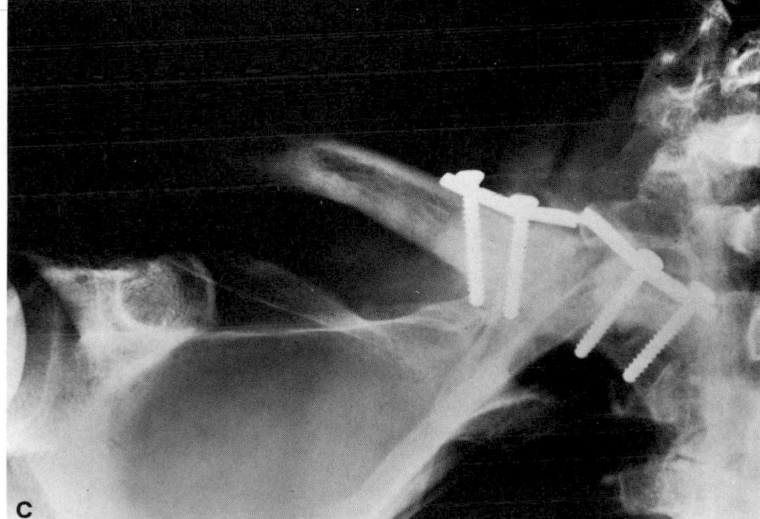

FIGURE 17-50. (**A**) A medial clavicular nonunion (*arrow*) may be difficult to treat with internal fixation. It is a dangerous area for intramedullary fixation, and it often is difficult to obtain six cortices with plate fixation. (**B**) This medial clavicular nonunion was treated with plate fixation. Only four cortices could be obtained for purchase on the medial fragment, so a semitubular plate was used. (**C**) A small plate with inadequate rigidity, when combined with poor postoperative protection, can lead to hardware failure in a medial clavicular fracture.

method of treatment, union rates of nearly 100% have been achieved.[‡‡] Using open reduction and internal fixation with compression plating and bone grafting, Manske and Szabo reported a 100% incidence of union by 10 weeks after surgery with no complications.[152] Jupiter and Leffert reported on 23 cases of clavicular nonunion, including 2 resulting from clavicular osteotomy for surgical access, with an overall success rate of 89% in achieving union.[117] However, 93.7% of those treated with grafting and dynamic compression plating achieved union. Eskola and associates reported healing in 20 of 22 clavicular nonunions treated with rigid plate fixation and bone grafting, but warned against shortening the clavicle to achieve union.[62] For this reason, if resection of the sclerotic edges of the atrophic margin to achieve primary osteosynthesis would result in significant clavicular shortening, many authors recommend intercalary bone grafting along with plate fixation[16,142,234a] (Fig. 17-49). Plate fixation with bone grafting is reliable, safe, and has few complications; in addition, the internal fixation usually is so secure that no postoperative external cast immobilization is needed and a sling alone is adequate. The plate does have the disadvantage of requiring a second operation to remove the hardware if it irritates the skin.[52] In addition, screw holes weaken the bone, and protection is needed after hardware removal. The advent of the low-contact dynamic compression plate enables further refinement of well-established principles of plating. Its structured undersurface allows the preservation of blood supply to plated bone segments, and avoidance of stress risers produced at implant removal reduces the possibility of refracture after plate removal. The excellent biocompatibility of titanium ensures superb tissue tolerance and increases the possibility of leaving plates in situ, thus obviating a second procedure.[168a]

There is one instance in which intramedullary fixation probably is the treatment of choice. In nonunion of the distal third of the clavicle, particularly type II distal clavicu-

‡‡ References 57, 58, 118, 168a, 206, 212, 261, 275.

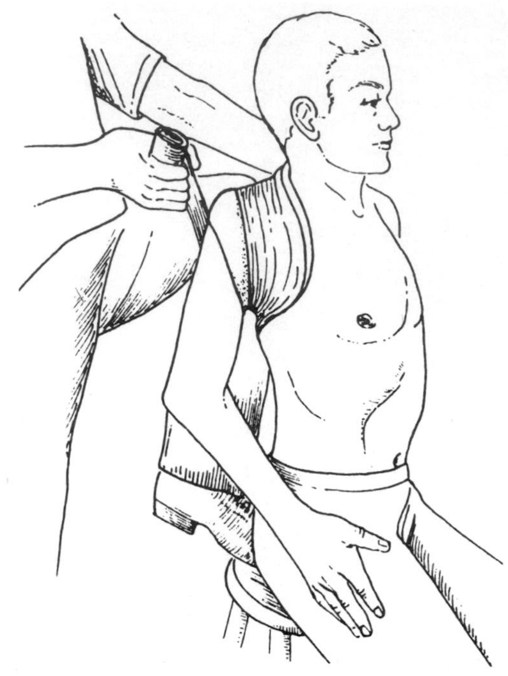

FIGURE 17-51. A method of reducing the clavicle and applying a figure-of-eight bandage. The physician's knee is placed between the scapulae, both outer edges of the shoulder are held securely, and the shoulders are pulled upward, outward, and backward.

lar fractures, the distal fragment usually is too small for adequate plate and screw fixation; excellent success has been achieved using intramedullary fixation with bone grafting for this specific nonunion.[172]

Medial clavicular nonunion, although rare, is particularly troublesome to treat (Fig. 17-50). The proximity to the sternoclavicular joint and vital structures makes intramedullary fixation worrisome, and there often is little proximal bone with which to secure a standard dynamic compression plate. Thinner plates frequently are prone to breakage. A postoperative spica cast may be required.

Treatment of Neurovascular Complications

The treatment of late neurovascular lesions depends on the cause of the compromised structures. After a fracture of the middle third of the clavicle, if there is neurovascular compromise secondary to massive callus formation and callus debulking is risky, if internal fixation with bone grafting of pseudarthrosis is impractical because of comminution, or if there is a malunion with a severe deformity and realignment osteotomy cannot be achieved, then resection of the middle third of the clavicle may be the best choice. Abbott and Lucas outlined the areas of the clavicle that can be resected without untoward sequelae, as well as the areas that do less well with resection.[1] Although some authors advocate total claviculectomy, it probably is wiser to perform careful subtotal resection when possible.

If there is excessive callus build-up or malunion of the clavicle, and the lesion is amenable to bone grafting and plate fixation, then removal of the hypertrophic callus and realignment osteotomy (with or without segmental interposition of bone graft and cancellous bone grafting) often relieves the neurovascular symptoms.

If the clavicle has a satisfactory appearance and is stable, enlargement of the costoclavicular space and, thus, neurovascular decompression can be accomplished by resecting the first rib and partially excising the scalene muscle or subclavius muscle.[47,235]

Author's Preferred Method of Treatment

Shaft Fractures

Despite the broad range of treatment methods available for clavicular shaft fractures, in adults, I prefer a commercially available figure-of-eight splint after closed reduction. To reduce the clavicle, the patient is seated on a stool with the surgeon standing behind. After meticulous preparation, the fracture area and

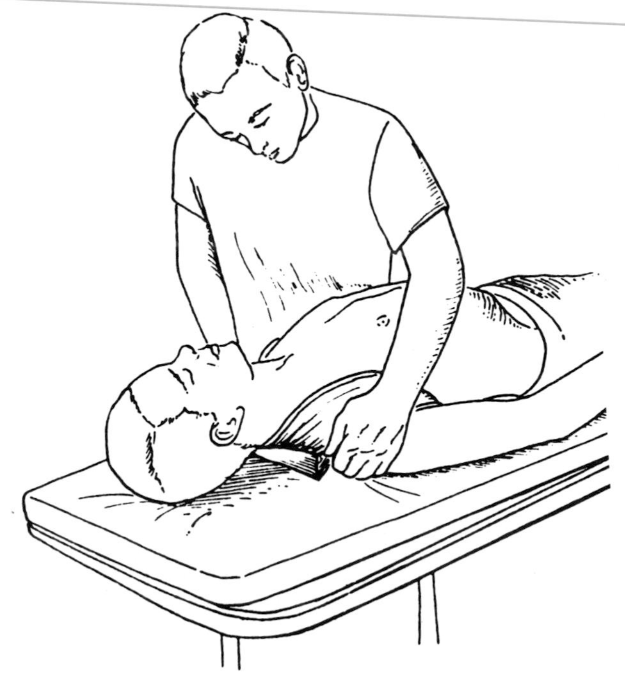

FIGURE 17-52. Recumbency has been described as one of the treatment methods for clavicular fractures, especially in patients with multiple injuries. A bump or pillow is placed between the scapulae, allowing the weight of the arm to reduce the fracture. A multiply traumatized patient may be managed by reduction and rigid internal fixation.

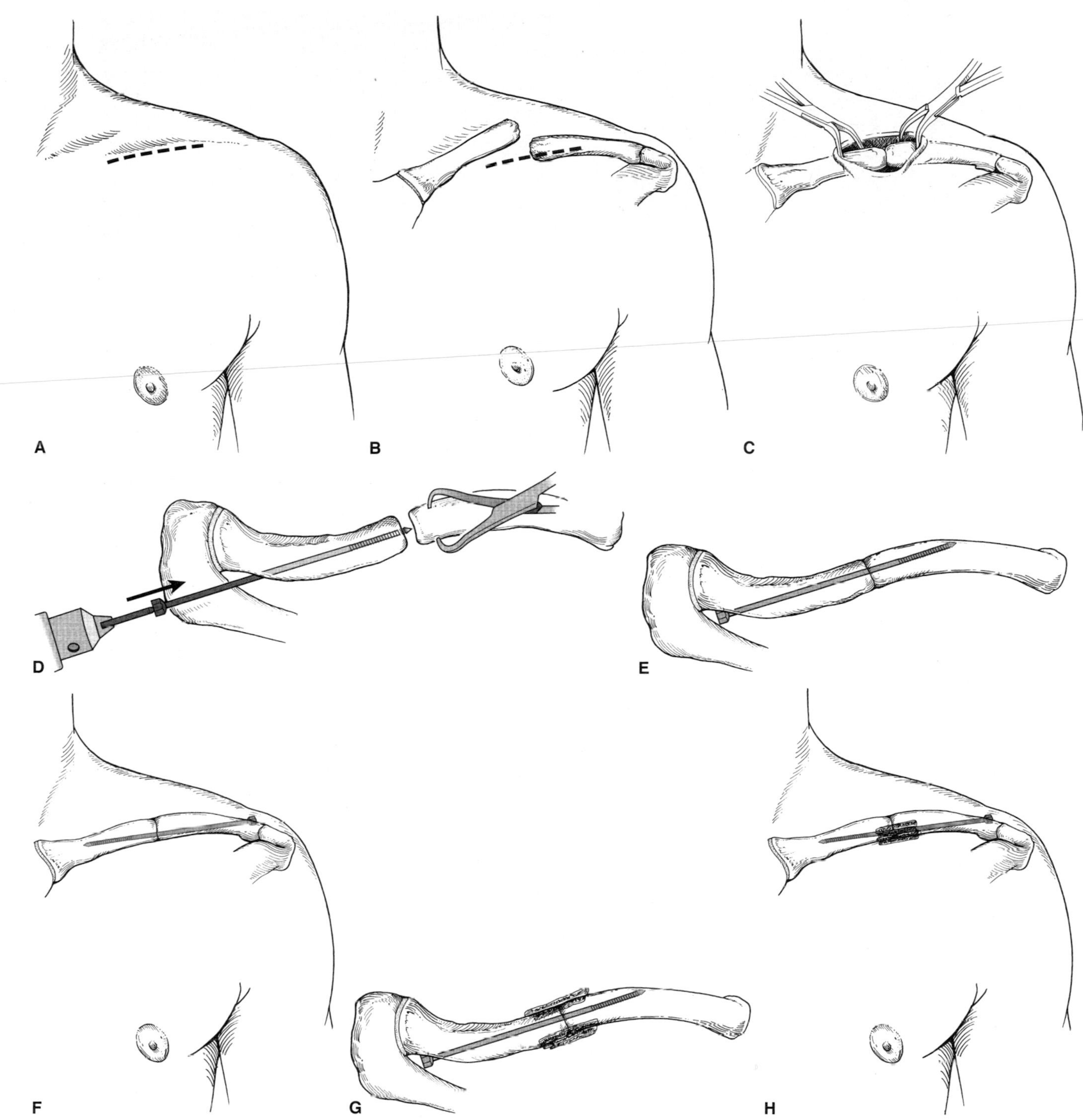

FIGURE 17-53. (**A** and **B**) The patient is positioned on the operating room table and a small horizontal incision is made at the level of the fracture. (**C**) The fracture is reduced and held with two towel clips. (**D** through **F**) A Knowles pin is drilled into the posterior fragment and down into the medullary canal of the medial clavicle. The pin should avoid the acromioclavicular joint. (**G** and **H**) Bone graft added to the site of nonunion.

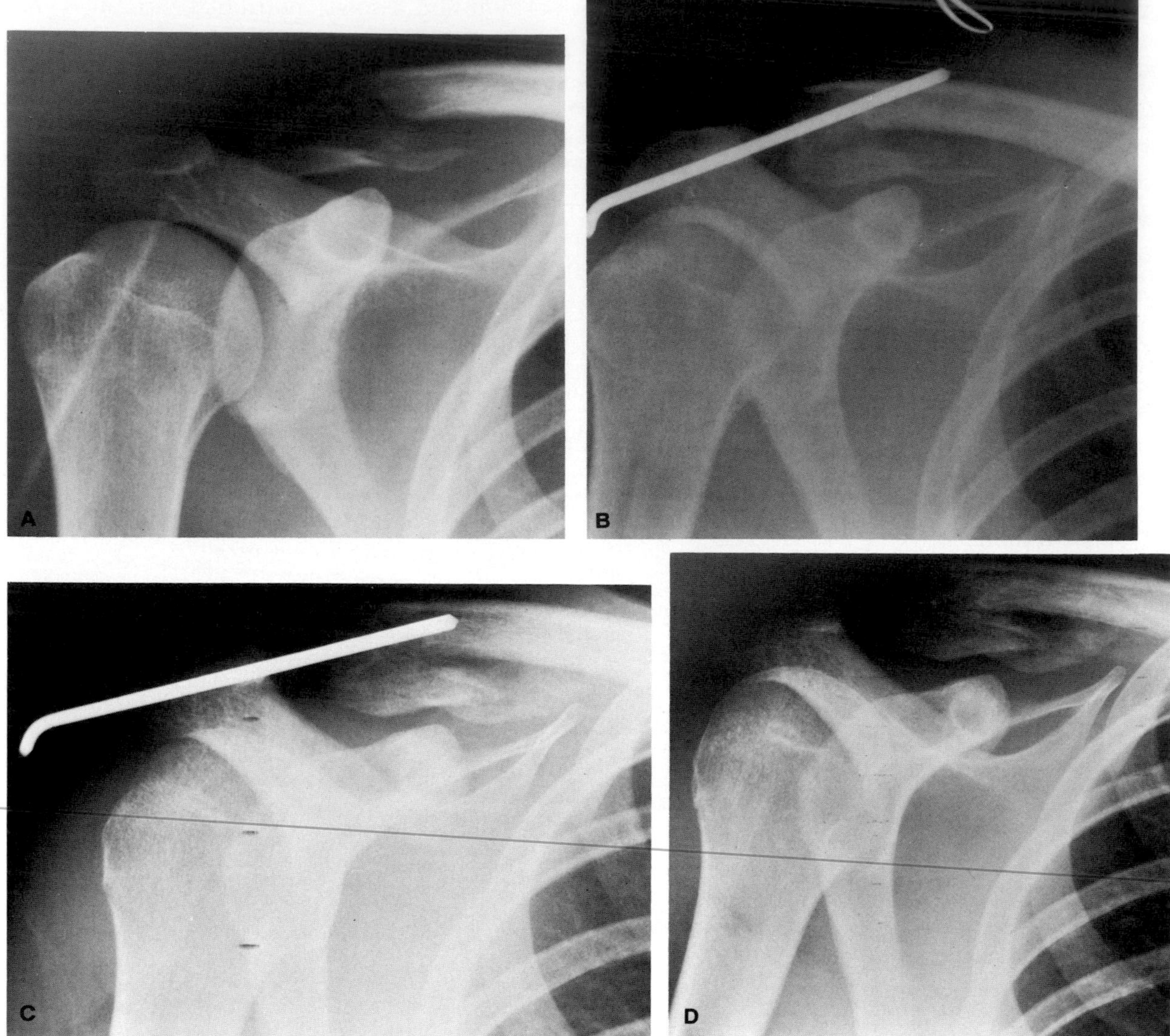

FIGURE 17-54. (**A**) A distal clavicular fracture—probably a type V, comminuted fracture. (**B**) Treatment consisted of intramedullary fixation using a heavy Steinmann pin. (**C**) Early healing. (**D**) Internal fixation is removed, and radiographic union has occurred.

fracture hematoma are infiltrated with 8 to 12 mL of 1% lidocaine (Xylocaine). The physician's knee is placed between the scapulae, both outer edges of the shoulder are held securely, and the shoulders are pulled upward, outward, and backward (Fig. 17-51). The fracture then can be manipulated into place. In a patient with multiple injuries, the fracture can be reduced in a supine position (Fig. 17-52).

The commercially available figure-of-eight bandage, usually with an ABD pad for the area of the axilla, is preferred because it is more comfortable, less cumbersome, and more cosmetic than options such as a plaster spica cast. In addition, with the figure-of-eight bandage, immobilization of the fracture is achieved as adequately as in more drastic and bulky forms of external fixation. The figure-of-eight bandage has the added advantage of keeping both hands and elbows free. If some patients feel more comfortable, a sling can be added to provide additional support for the arm; this also may make sleeping more comfortable. Because adults usually have more trouble with fracture healing than do children, immobilization must be maintained for 6 to 8 weeks. Although I permit rotation of the arm at the side in any direction and to any extent, I limit active use of the arm until clinical union takes place. If refracture occurs during treatment, continued immobilization is appropriate. Participation in athletic activities is not permitted for at least 6 weeks after clinical and radiographic union has been achieved. At 6 to 8 weeks, the patient is taken out of the figure-of-eight bandage and placed in a sling for an additional 3 to 4 weeks for added protection, while gentle isometric and mobilization exercises are begun.

Indications for Primary Open Fixation

My indications for operative treatment of acute clavicular fractures are as follows:

1. Neurovascular injury or compromise that is progressive or fails to reverse with closed reduction of the fracture
2. Severe displacement caused by comminution with resulting severe angulation and tenting of the skin (enough to threaten its integrity) that fails to respond to closed reduction
3. An open fracture that requires operative debridement
4. Multiple trauma, in which patient mobility is desirable and closed methods of immobilization are impractical or impossible
5. A "floating" shoulder, with a displaced clavicular fracture and an unstable scapular fracture
6. Many type II distal clavicular fractures (see later)
7. Inability of the patient to tolerate closed immobilization (eg, neurologic problems of parkinsonism, seizure disorders, or other neurovascular disorders)[257]
8. The rare patient in whom the cosmetic lump over the healed clavicle is intolerable, and the patient is willing to exchange this for a potentially equally noncosmetic surgical scar and the possibility of a nonunion.

Although there are many relative and absolute indications for surgery, few fractures of the shaft need to be treated with primary open reduction and internal fixation.[175,179]

If surgery for a fractured clavicle is to be undertaken, historically the choice has been between plate fixation (A-O) and intramedullary fixation.[158,168] I prefer intramedullary fixation for acute fractures for the following reasons: (1) less exposure of the fracture is required, so there is a smaller skin incision; (2) little periosteal stripping is needed, so there is less interference with the healing potential of the fracture; (3) removal of hardware is easier and usually can be done with a local anesthetic; and (4) no screw holes remain to act as potential areas of weakness of the bone.

Although the use of a threaded Steinmann pin, bent at the lateral end to prevent migration, has been well described, I prefer to use a Knowles pin in a method described by Neviaser. The Knowles pin has a hub that is large enough to prevent pin migration and is easily palpable beneath the skin for removal. The threaded distal end of the pin also helps prevent migration. To insert this pin, the patient is seated in a beach-chair position and a small, horizontal incision is made at the level of the fracture, which is then exposed. The fracture is reduced and held with towel clips. The Knowles pin is drilled from lateral to medial, entering the clavicle at the posterolateral aspect of the acromion (avoiding the acromioclavicular joint, if possible). It then is directed toward the medial fragment of the clavicle and down the intramedullary portion of the medial fragment (Fig. 17-53).

Alternatively, a 4-mm Steinmann pin can be drilled retrograde from medial to lateral after the fracture is exposed, entering the lateral fragment at the fracture site and emerging at the posterolateral aspect of the acromion. At the point of egress of the pin, a Knowles pin is drilled antegrade through the acromion, following the Steinmann pin as the pin is withdrawn. At the fracture site, the fracture is reduced and held with towel clips, and the Knowles pin is drilled into the medullary canal. If the Knowles pin penetrates the anterior cortex, and the tip of the pin is excessively prominent, it can be cut even with the anterior edge of the clavicle to prevent prominence under the skin. In addition, the subacromial space must be palpated to ensure that the intramedullary pin is not in the subacromial space, but actually passes through the acromion.

I also prefer to add bone graft acutely, along with internal fixation, when any acute shaft fracture is treated with open reduction and internal fixation.

Distal Clavicular Fractures

In type I distal clavicular fractures, the ligaments are intact, displacement is minimal, and the patient can be treated with a sling for comfort, early isometric

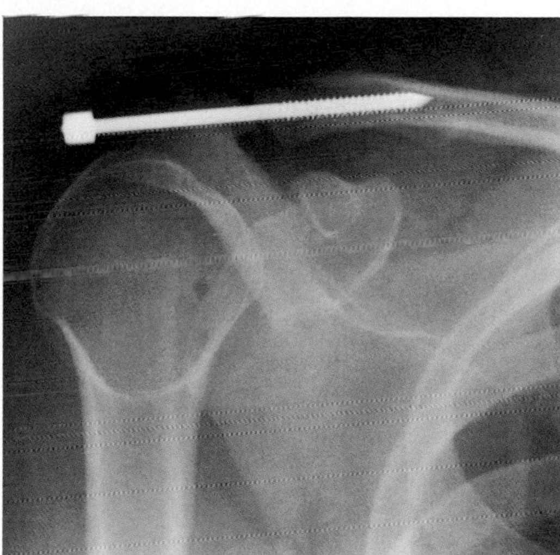

FIGURE 17-55. A Knowles pin often is a preferable method of internal fixation, because the hub prevents migration and is easily palpable for later removal. It can be buried underneath the skin.

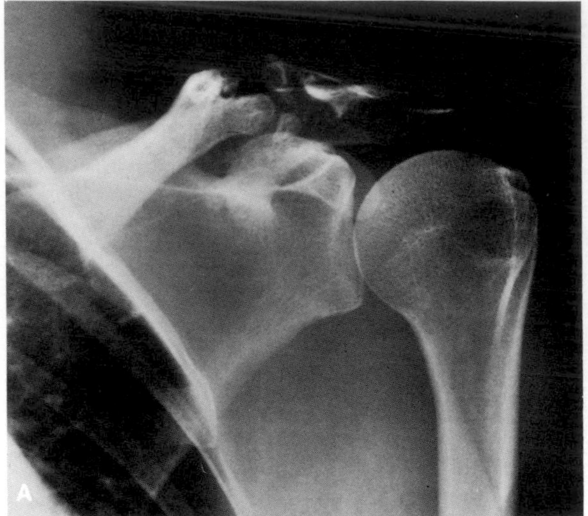

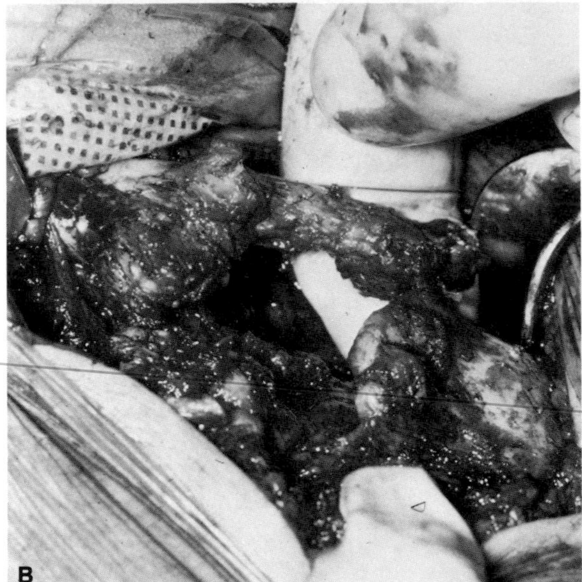

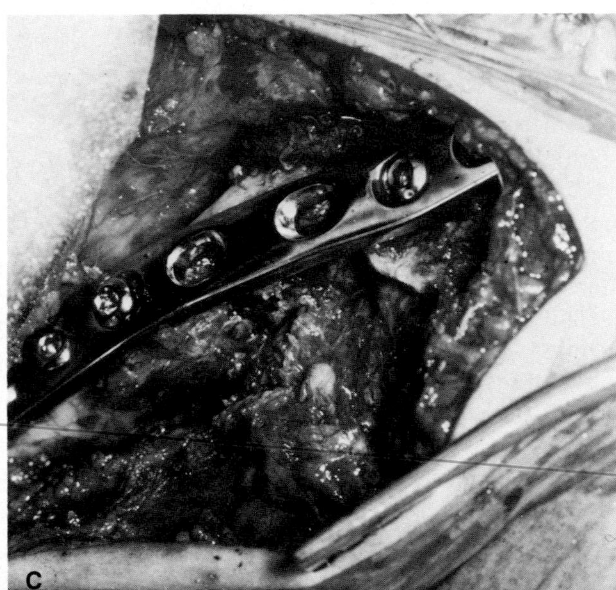

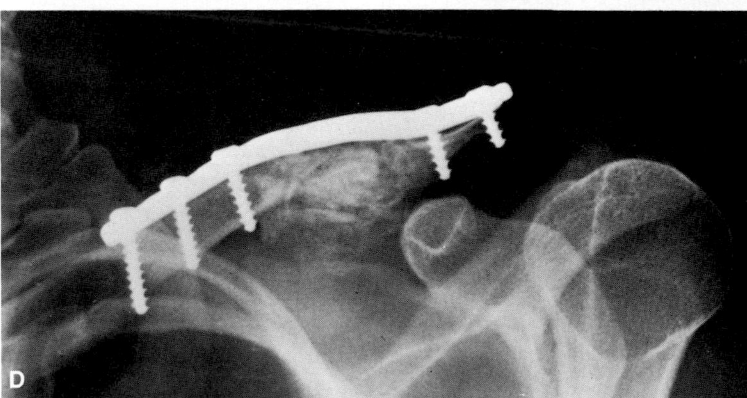

FIGURE 17-56. (**A**) Three years after a clavicle fracture, this patient has a symptomatic left clavicular nonunion. The ideal treatment is bone grafting and rigid internal fixation, preferably with a dynamic compression plate (DCP). (**B**) Intraoperative photograph showing small, thin, tapered sclerotic edges of the nonunion. (**C**) A seven-hole DCP was used with massive cortical cancellous grafting. Only two screws could be placed in the small lateral segment. (**D**) Healing has occurred. A disadvantage of plate fixation for nonunion is that the plate may need to be removed if it causes subcutaneous irritation.

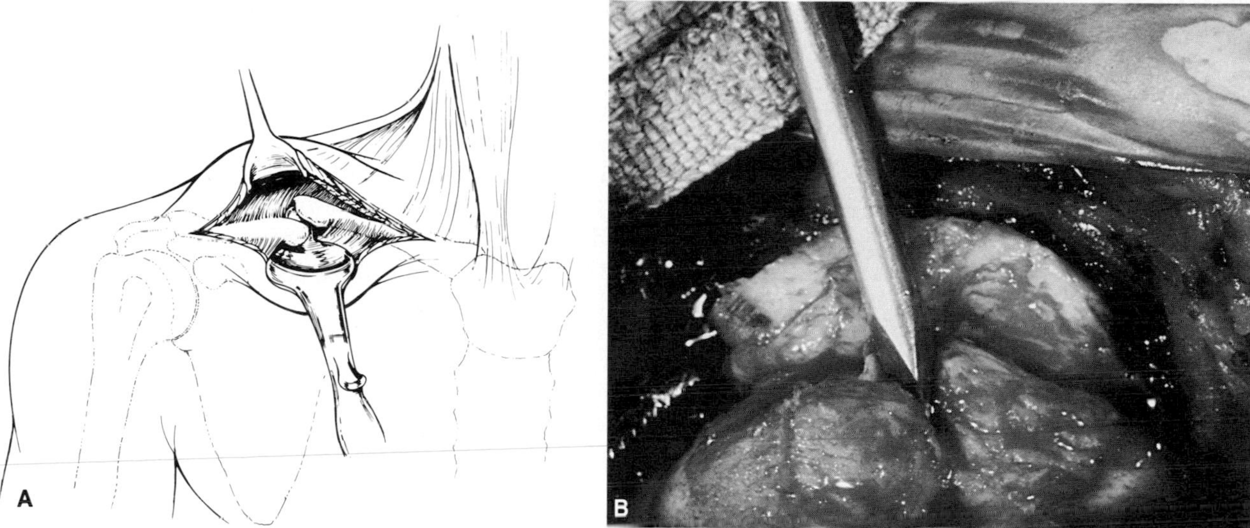

FIGURE 17-57. Surgical treatment of symptomatic nonunion. (**A**) Operative approach. A horizontal incision is made. The trapezius and deltoid are elevated off the clavicle and the nonunion is exposed. Blunt retractors protect the retroclavicular vital structures. (**B**) The nonunion is exposed. Sclerotic edges are trimmed and fibrous tissue is removed. Usually, the fragments are large enough to take six cortices on each side of the fracture.

exercises, and discontinuation of the immobilization as symptoms permit.

Type II distal clavicular fractures, as discussed previously, are difficult to treat without surgery. Immobilization is difficult to achieve, the fragments are distracted by muscle forces and the weight of the arm, the proximal fragment is unstable and has no ligamentous attachment, and nonunion occurs all too frequently. The usual sling does not reduce the deformity, and the use of a figure-of-eight bandage actually can increase the deformity by holding the proximal fragment posteriorly. Although closed treatment has been successful,[219] union often is delayed and shoulder stiffness may increase morbidity. However, if there is obvious bony contact, as manifested by crepitus and a radiographic bone wedge, nonoperative treatment should be considered. Patients with type II distal fractures probably are treated best with immediate open reduction and internal fixation if the fragments are displaced and the fracture is unstable. The operative treatment depends on the size of the lateral fragment and on the position and integrity of the coracoclavicular ligaments relative to the fragments.

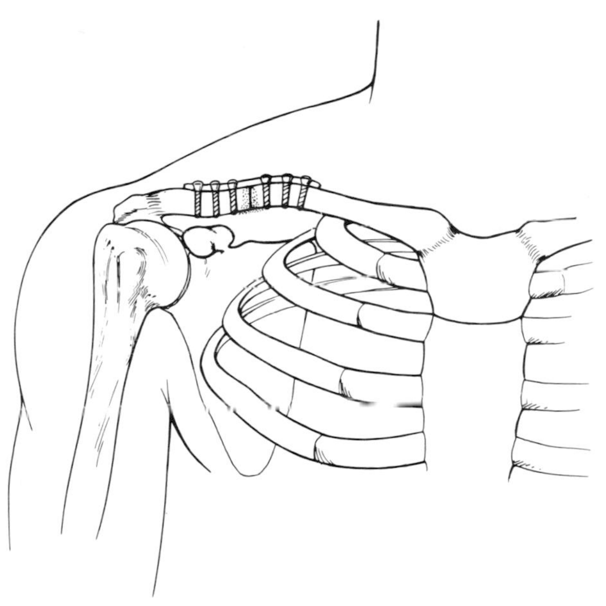

FIGURE 17-58. Illustration of internal fixation and bone grafting of a nonunited middle-third clavicular fracture. At least six cortices should be incorporated into the dynamic compression plate. Care must be taken so the screws do not project too far inferiorly. The bone graft should be packed in the nonunion site and inferiorly, but *not* in the retroclavicular space.

Although a variety of encircling wires,[179,180] pins (Fig. 17-54), and sutures[172] binding the proximal fragment to the coracoid process have been described, I prefer open intramedullary fixation with a Knowles pin (Fig. 17-55; see Fig. 17-53). It must be remembered that, because of the fracture anatomy, the coracoclavicular ligaments usually are attached to the distal fragment, with the proximal fragment pulled upward by contraction of the trapezius muscle. Therefore, if fracture union can be achieved, the acromioclavicular joint and clavicle are stable.

With the patient in the beach-chair position and the head turned away from the side of the fracture, a small vertical incision is made at the fracture site. The deltoid–trapezius interval is split horizontally, and the fracture site is exposed. I often place a very heavy nonabsorbable suture or tape around the coracoid process and proximal clavicular segment to secure the reduction. This is passed before reduction of the fracture. In addition, before reduction, a Knowles pin is drilled from the posterolateral aspect of the acromion to emerge from the medullary canal of the distal clavicular segment. Once the pin is seen and the subacromial space is palpated to make certain that the pin has not violated it, the fracture is reduced. Reduction can be maintained with towel clips, and the Knowles pin is advanced through the intramedullary canal of the proximal clavicular fragment. If the pin penetrates the anterior cortex, this usually is not a problem, and any excessive pin length can be cut flush with the anterior clavicle. The nonabsorbable suture or tape from the coracoid to the clavicle then is tied securely for added fixation. Although both the conoid and trapezoid ligaments can be attached to the distal clavicular segment, the conoid ligament frequently is torn, with the trapezoid alone attached to the distal segment. If this is the case, the conoid ligament can be sutured into the clavicular periosteum or into the clavicular insertion of the trapezoid ligament. With adequate internal fixation of an acute fracture of the lateral clavicle, I typically do not add bone graft because union usually ensues; however, bone graft can be added. The patient then is placed in a sling-and-swathe bandage, and isometric exercises are begun in the early postoperative period. The Knowles pin is removed after radiographic signs of early fracture healing are noted (6 weeks). Because the coracoclavicular sutures contribute to security, early healing generally has occurred by this time, and removal is especially helpful if the hub of the Knowles pin is irritating the skin.

Type III fractures of the distal clavicle often are not recognized acutely. When they are seen acutely, if they are unstable, or if they appear as an extension of a type II injury into the joint, they should be treated as type II injuries. If they lead to symptomatic late degeneration of the acromioclavicular joint, the distal 2 cm of the clavicle can be excised with little morbidity and excellent results. When a type III distal fracture is treated surgically in the acute stage, the distal fragment should be retained because of its attachment to the coracoclavicular ligaments, unless there is hopeless damage of the articular surface or severe comminution. In extremely rare instances, if it is necessary to excise the distal segment, the proximal clavicular segment must be stabilized, usually with an intramedullary pin, and the ligaments transferred from the distal fragment to the proximal fragment. Occasionally, the coracoacromial ligament can be secured to the proximal fragment acutely.[274]

Medial Clavicular Fractures

Fractures of the medial clavicle require symptomatic support only, unless there is severe neurovascular compromise or injury. If this occurs, and the fracture must be operated on, open reduction should be considered. However, even if this fracture is openly reduced, I prefer to avoid intramedullary fixation because of the difficulty of securing and positioning the fragment and the danger of pin migration, which has the potential for catastrophic results.

Nonunion

Fortunately, clavicular nonunions are rare. When they do occur, 75% are in the shaft (30% atrophic, 70% hypertrophic) and 25% are in the distal third.[117,152]

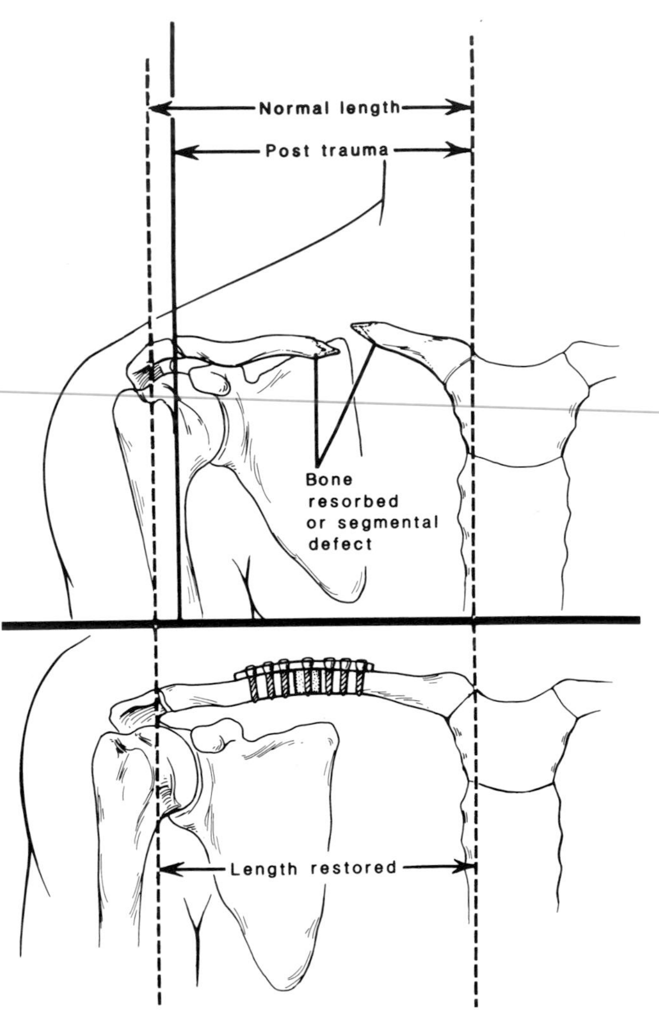

FIGURE 17-59. In an atrophic clavicular nonunion, there often are tapered sclerotic edges, and an intercalary bone graft may be needed between the two ends of the nonunion. The normal manubrial acromial length is demonstrated. The post-traumatic manubrial acromial length decreased because of bone resorption or a segmental defect. To restore the normal length of the clavicle, an intercalary bone graft can be placed between the two sides of the nonunion. It often is helpful to internally fix the intercalary segment (fibula or iliac crest) with a cortical screw.

Nonunion of Shaft Fractures

My preference for the treatment of a symptomatic clavicular shaft nonunion is to use a compression plate and bone graft; ideally, I use a six- or seven-hole dynamic compression plate (3.5 mm) with at least six cortices secured on each clavicular segment. I prefer a dynamic compression plate because it uses small fragment screws, as compared with the 4.5-mm screws used for the semitubular plate. In addition, compression appears to be less difficult to achieve (Fig. 17-56).

The surgical technique requires that the patient be in a semiseated or beach-chair position with the head turned toward the opposite shoulder. A horizontal incision is made parallel to the medial clavicular segment along its superior border. The interval between the deltoid and the trapezius is found, and a horizontal incision is made in this interval. The ends of the clavicle are exposed subperiosteally and any interposed soft tissue is removed (Figs. 17-57 and 17-58). In a hypertrophic nonunion, the extra callus build-up and excessively hypertrophic bone can be shaved down to a more normal clavicular size to facilitate fitting of the plate. In an atrophic nonunion, if the sclerotic ends need to be resected, an intercalary segment of iliac crest graft is fashioned to fit between the two clavicular segments. If it is anticipated that an intercalary bone graft will be needed, it is useful to be able to palpate the distance from the acromial tip to the midsternum on both the injured and uninjured sides (Figs. 17-59 and 17-60). In addition, before surgery, the distance between the acromion and the sternum on each side can be measured on an x-ray taken on a large cassette. This helps in judging how much clavicular length will need to be made up by intercalary graft.

Blunt retractors (ie, Darrach, Bennett) are used to protect the infraclavicular structures during drilling of the plate holes. I prefer to place the plate superiorly and have not found this to be a problem in terms of cosmesis or symptoms. I use a 3.5-mm, six- or seven-hole (depending on the fracture configuration) dynamic compression plate, and I attempt to place three screws in each clavicular segment as bicortical fixation. Occasionally, an interfragmentary screw can be used if the bony anatomy warrants it and the nonunion anatomy is oblique enough (see Fig. 17-34**B**). The plate is contoured to the clavicle and secured to the bone. If an intercalary iliac crest segment is to be used, the middle hole of a seven-hole plate can be used to place a screw from the plate directly into the intercalary segment. After secure plate fixation, iliac crest bone is placed at the fracture site along the superior and inferior clavicular borders. Excessive bone should not be placed posteriorly and inferiorly, to prevent late irritation or crowding of the neurovascular structures. The trapezius and deltoid fascia are repaired and the patient is placed in a sling-and-swathe bandange after surgery.

Nonunion of Lateral Fractures

For lateral clavicular nonunions, I prefer the same method of internal fixation as for acute fractures (ie, use of a Knowles pin). However, iliac crest graft is always added (Fig. 17-61). In addition, I usually place a piece of Mersilene tape or heavy nonabsorbable suture from the coracoid around the proximal fragment of the clavicle. In this type of procedure, the fracture site is exposed as with an acute fracture, the Knowles pin is passed from the posterolateral corner of the clavicle through the small distal segment, and, after the nonunited edges are trimmed to satisfactory bone, the Knowles pin is advanced across the nonunion site. Coracoclavicular fixation then is tightened and bone graft is added. As with an acute fracture, the Knowles pin is taken out after 6 to 8 weeks.

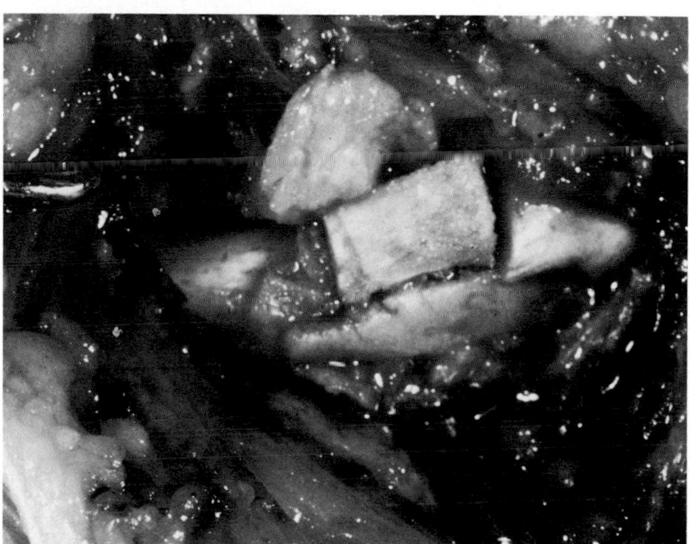

FIGURE 17-60. Operative photograph of an intercalary bone graft segment placed between the two sides of a nonunion.

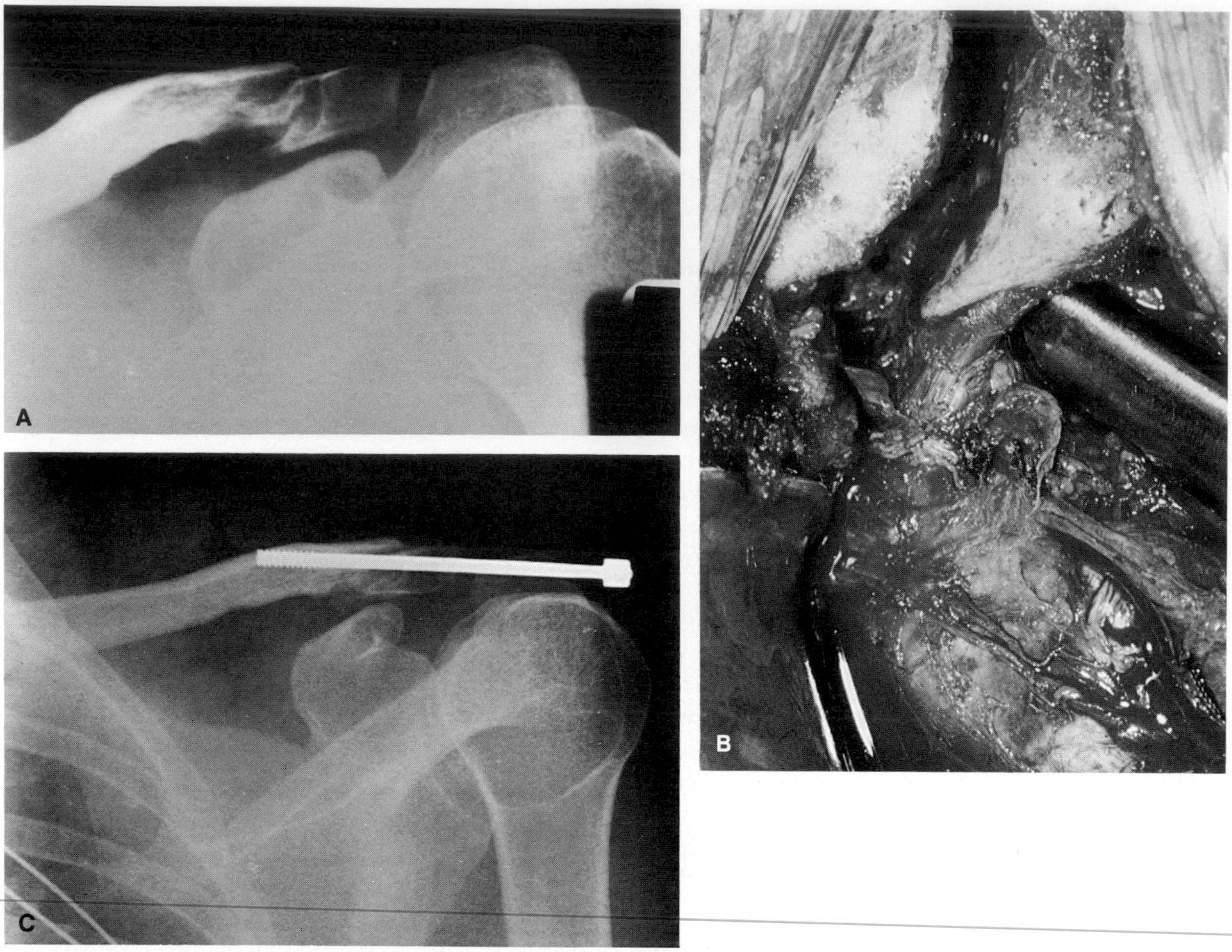

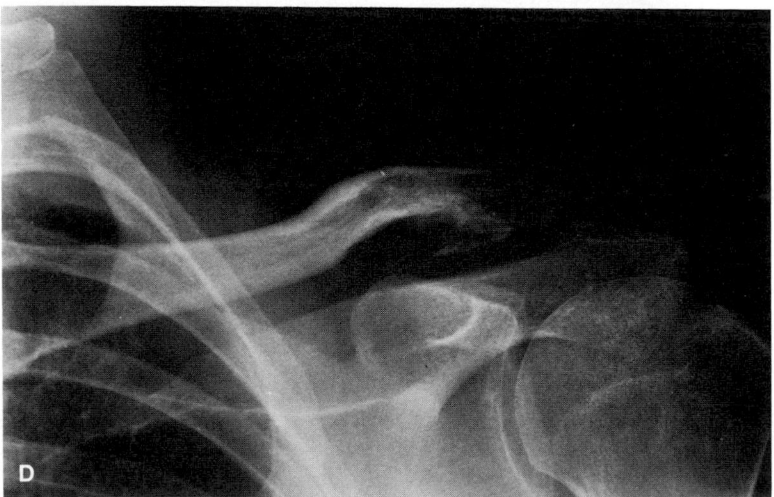

FIGURE 17-61. (**A**) Two years after a type II distal clavicle fracture, a painful nonunion has occurred. (**B**) Exposure of the nonunion reveals the ligaments on the small distal segment and fibrous tissue between the bone ends. (**C**) Internal fixation with a Knowles pin (which has been cut off where it protruded past the anterior cortex) and bone grafting of the nonunion site were performed. Ligament reconstruction is not ordinarily needed, because the ligaments remain attached to the distal fragment. (**D**) Clinical and radiographic union have occurred.

Nonunion of Medial Fractures

For medial clavicular nonunions, my preference is for plate fixation and grafting rather than intramedullary devices. However, obtaining purchase on the medial fragment can be difficult, compromising the thickness and size of the plate that can be used. If less than six-cortex purchase must be accepted, a supplementary spica cast is recommended.

It must be remembered that healing takes longer for a nonunion than for an acute fracture in an adult clavicle. It often requires a period of 3 to 6 months, and the patient should be protected until radiographic signs of union are present. A sling usually provides adequate immobilization for at least 6 to 8 weeks, and gentle range of motion can be instituted once immobilization is discontinued. Removal of the plate is optional after healing of the fracture, whereas the intramedullary Knowles pin is removed after about 6 weeks.

In the rare instance involving a previously excised lateral clavicular segment and an unstable proximal segment after a type II distal clavicle fracture, I use Mersilene tape around the proximal segment to secure the segment to the coracoid, then transfix the proximal segment with an intramedullary Knowles pin after reduction, and transfer the coracoacromial ligament into the end of the clavicle.[177,274]

POSTOPERATIVE CARE

After operative treatment of a nonunion or an acute fracture, the patient is placed in a sling-and-swathe bandage in the operating room. The postoperative x-ray should include not only the fracture site and internal fixation, to verify fracture alignment and hardware placement, but also enough of the lung to ensure that no injury has occurred during surgery. When comfortable, the patient is discharged from the hospital and wound care is the same as for any shoulder surgery.

If the glenohumeral joint and the subacromial bursa have not been violated surgically and are not otherwise diseased, there appears to be no need for early range-of-motion exercises, because shoulder range of motion, if normal before surgery, usually remains so. Thus, the patient can be kept safely supported in a sling or immobilizer until radiographic signs of union occur without fear of producing a frozen shoulder.

Early postoperative isometric exercises for the rotator cuff can be initiated, although isometric strengthening of the trapezius and deltoid muscles is delayed until their suture junction is healed securely (3 to 4 weeks). Range of motion after surgery is not permitted past 45° of flexion in the plane of the scapula until there are clinical signs of union, usually at 4 to 6 weeks.

When clinical or radiographic union is present, the patient can begin full range of motion, particularly forward elevation (using an overhead pulley) and external rotation (using a cane or stick); hyperextension–internal rotation also can be added. Resistive exercises of the deltoid, trapezius, cuff, and scapular muscles are added gradually to the rehabilitation program. When radiographic union is present, full active use of the arm is permitted.

The patient is not permitted to return to full, strenuous work or athletic activities until there is a nearly full range of shoulder motion, strength has returned to near normal, and bone healing is presumed to be solid. In adults, this usually is 4 to 6 months after surgery.

ACKNOWLEDGMENT

The author wishes to thank Dr. Cesar Restrepo for his contribution to the preparation of this manuscript.

REFERENCES

1. Abbott, L.C., and Lucas, D.B.: The Function of the Clavicle: Its Surgical Significance. Ann. Surg., 140:583–599, 1954.
2. Adams, C.F.: The Genuine Works of Hippocrates. Baltimore, Williams & Wilkins, 1939.
3. Aitken, A.D., and Lincoln, R.E.: Fractures of the First Rib Due to Muscle Pull: Report of Case. N. Engl. J. Med., 220:1063–1064, 1939.
4. Alldred, A.J.: Congenital Pseudoarthrosis of the Clavicle. J. Bone Joint Surg., 45B:312–319, 1963.
5. Allman, F.L.: Fractures and Ligamentous Injuries of the Clavicle and Its Articulation. J. Bone Joint Surg., 49A:774–784, 1967.
6. Anderson, K., Jensen, P.O., Lauritzen, J.: Treatment of Clavicular Fractures: Figure-of-Eight Bandage Vs. a Simple Sling. Acta Orthop. Scand., 57:71–74, 1987.

6a. Andrews, J.R., and Wilk, K.E. (eds.): The Athlete's Shoulder. New York, Churchill Livingstone, 1994.

7. Apeli, L., and Burch, H.B.: Study on the Pseudoarthrosis of the Clavicle. *In* Chapcal, G. (ed.): Pseudarthroses and Their Treatment. Eighth International Symposium on Topical Problems in Orthopaedic Surgery, pp. 188–189. Stuttgart, Thieme, 1979.

7a. Baccarani, G., Porcellini, G., Brunetti, E.: Fracture of the Coracoid Process Associated With Fracture of the Clavicle: A Description of a Rare Case. Chir. Organi. Mov., 78:49–51, 1993.

8. Balata, A., Olzai, M.G., Porcu, A., Spano, B., Ganau, R., Corchia, C.: Fractures of the Clavicle in the Newborn. Ital. Ped., 6:125–129, 1984.

8a. Ballmer, F.T., and Gerber, C.: Coracoclavicular Screw Fixation for Unstable Fractures of the Distal Clavicle. A Report of Five Cases. J. Bone Joint Surg., 73:291–294, 1991.

9. Bargar, W.L., Marcus, R.E., Ittleman, F.P.: Late Thoracic Outlet Syndrome Secondary to Pseudoarthrosis of the Clavicle. J. Trauma, 24:857–859, 1984.

9a. Bartosh, R.A., Dugdale, T.W., Nielsen, R.: Isolated Musculocutaneous Nerve Injury Complicating Closed Fracture of the Clavicle. A Case Report. Am. J. Sports Med., 20:356–359, 1992.

10. Basom, W.C., Breck, L.W., Herz, J.R.: Dual Grafts for Nonunion of the Clavicle. South Med. J., 40:898–899, 1987.
11. Bateman, J.E.: Nerve Injuries About the Shoulder in Sports. J. Bone Joint Surg., 49A:785–792, 1967.
12. Bateman, J.E.: The Shoulder and Neck. Philadelphia, W.B. Saunders, 1978.
13. Bearn, J.G.: An Electromyographic Study of the Trapezius, Deltoid, Pectoralis Major, Biceps, and Triceps Muscles During Static Loading of the Upper Limb. J. Anat., 140:103–108, 1961.
14. Bearn, J.G.: Direct Observation in the Function of the Capsule to the Sternoclavicular Joint in Clavicular Support. J. Anat., 10:159–170, 1967.
15. Beckman, T.: A Case of Simultaneous Luxation of Both Ends of the Clavicle. Acta Chir. Scand., 56:156–163, 1934.
16. Berkheiser, E.J.: Old Ununited Clavicular Fractures in the Adult. Surg. Gynecol. Obstet., 64:1064–1072, 1937.
17. Bernard, T.N., and Haddad, R.J.: Enchrondroma of the Proximal Clavicle: An Unusual Cause of Pathologic Fracture Dislocation of the Sternoclavicular Joint. Clin. Orthop., 167:239–241, 1982.
18. Billington, R.W.: A New (Plaster Yoke) Dressing for Fracture of the Clavicle. South. Med. J., 24:667, 1931.

18a. Boehme, D., Curtis, R.J., DeHaan, J.T., Kay, S.P., Young, D.C., Rockwood, C.A., Jr.: Non-union of Fractures of the Mid-Shaft of the Clavicle. Treatment With a Modified Hagie Intramedullary Pin and Autogenous Bone-Grafting. J. Bone Joint Surg., 73A:1219–1226, 1991.
19. Bonnett, J.: Fracture of the Clavicle. Arch. Chir. Neerlandicum, 27:143–151, 1975.
20. Bowen, A.D.: Plastic Bowing of the Clavicle in Children: A Report of Two Cases. J. Bone Joint Surg., 65A:403–405, 1983.
21. Breck, L.: Partially Threaded Round Pins With Oversized Threads for Intramedullary Fixation of the Clavicle and the Forearm Bones. Clin. Orthop., 11:227–229, 1958.
22. Brighton, C.T., and Pollick, S.R.: Treatment of Recalcitrant Nonunion With a Capacatively Coupled Electrical Field. A Preliminary Report. J. Bone Joint Surg., 67A:577–585, 1985.
23. Brooks, A.L., and Henning, G.D.: Injuries to the Proximal Clavicular Epiphysis. J. Bone Joint Surg., 54A:1347, 1972.
24. Bronz, G., Heim, D., Posterla, C.: Die stabile Clavicula Osteosynthese. Unfallheilkunde, 84:319–325, 1981.
24a. Brunner, U., Habermeyer, P., Schweiberer, L.: Die Sonderstellung der lateralen Klavikulafraktur. Orthopade, 21: 163–171, 1992.
25. Butterworth, R.D., and Kirk, A.A.: Fracture Dislocation Sternoclavicular Joint. Virgina M. Month. 79:98–100, 1952.
26. Cahill, B.R.: Osteolysis of the Distal Part of the Clavicle in Male Athletes. J. Bone Joint Surg., 64A:1053–1058, 1982.
27. Campbell, E., Howard, W.B., Breklund, C.W.: Delayed Brachial Plexus Palsy Due to Ununited Fracture of the Clavicle. J.A.M.A., 139:91–92, 1949.
27a. Capicotto, P.N., Heiple, K.G., Wilbur, J.H.: Midshaft Clavicle Nonunions Treated With Intramedullary Steinmann Pin Fixation and Onlay Bone Graft. J. Orthop. Trauma, 8:88–93, 1994.
28. Caspi, I., Ezra, E., Nerubay, J., Horoszovski, H.: Musculocutaneous Nerve Injury After Coracoid Process Transfer for Clavicle Instability. Acta Orthop. Scand., 58:294–295, 1987.
29. Cayford, E.H., and Tees, F.J.: Traumatic Aneurysm of the Subclavian Artery as a Late Complication of Fractured Clavicle. Can. Med. Assoc. J., 25:450–452, 1931.
30. Codman, E.A.: The Shoulder—Rupture of the Supraspinatus Tendon and Other Lesions in or About the Subacromial Bursa. Boston, T. Todd Co., 1934.
31. Coene, L.N.: Mechanisms of Brachial Plexus Lesions. Clin. Neurol. Neurosurg., 95(Suppl):S24–29, 1993.
31a. Cohen, A.W., and Otto, S.R.: Obstetric Clavicular Fractures. J. Reprod. Med., 25:119–122, 1980.
32. Connolly, J.F.: Electrical Treatment of Nonunion: Its Use and Abuse in 100 Consecutive Fractures. Orthop. Clin. North Am., 15:89–106, 1984.
32a. Connolly, J.F.: Fractures and Dislocations of the Clavicle. J. Musculoskel. Med., 9:135–148, 1992.
33. Connolly, J.F., and Dehne, R.: Delayed Thoracic Outlet Syndrome From Clavicular Non-Union: Management by Morseling. Nebr. Med. J., 71:303–306, 1986.
34. Connolly, J.F., and Dehne, R.: Nonunion of the Clavicle and Thoracic Outlet Syndrome. J. Trauma, 29:1127–1132, 1989.
35. Conwell, H.E.: Fractures of the Clavicle, J.A.M.A., 90:838–839, 1928.
36. Cook, T.: Reduction and External Fixation of Fractures of the Clavicle in Recumbency. J. Bone Joint Surg., 36A:878–880, 1954.
37. Copeland, S.M.: Total Resection of the Clavicle. Am. J. Surg., 72:280–281, 1946.
38. Costa, M.C., and Robbs, J.V.: Nonpenetrating Subclavian Artery Trauma. J. Vasc. Surg., 8:71–75, 1988.
39. Craig, E.V.: Fractures of the Clavicle. *In* Rockwood, C.A. Jr., and Matsen, F.A., III (eds.): The Shoulder, pp. 367–412. Philadelphia, W.B. Saunders, 1990.
40. Cumming, W.A.: Neonatal Skeletal Fractures: Birth Trauma, or Child Abuse? J. Canad. Assoc. Rad., 30:30–33, 1979.
41. Cummings, C.W., and First, R.: Stress Fracture of the Clavicle After a Radical Neck Dissection. Case Report. Plast. Reconstr. Surg., 55:366–367, 1975.
42. Curtis, R.J., Jr.: Operative Treatment of Children's Fractures of the Shoulder Region. Orthop. Clin. North Am., 21:315–324, 1990.
42a. Dambrain, R., Raphael, B., Dhem, A., Lebeau, J.: Radiation Osteitis of the Clavicle Following Radiotherapy and Radical Neck Dissection of Head and Neck Cancer. Bull. Group. Int. Rech. Sci. Stomatol. Odontol., 33:65–70, 1990.
43. Dameron, T.B., Jr.: External Fixation of the Clavicle for Fracture or Nonunion in Adults. (Letter) J. Bone Joint Surg., 71A:1272, 1989.
44. Dameron, T.B., Jr., and Rockwood, C.A., Jr.: Fractures of the Shaft of the Clavicle. *In* Rockwood, C.A., Jr., Wilkins, K.E., King, R.E. (eds.): Fractures in Children, pp. 608–624. Philadelphia, J.B. Lippincott, 1984.
45. Dannohl, C., Meeder, P.J., Weller, S.: Costoclavicular Syndrome: A Rare Complication of Clavicular Fracture. Aktuel. Taumatol., 18:149–151, 1988.
46. Das, N.K., and Deb, H.K.: Synovioma of the Clavicle. Report of a Case. J. Int. Coll. Surg., 35:776–780, 1961.
47. Dash, U.N., and Handler, D.: A Case of Compression of Subclavian Vessels by a Fractured Clavicle Treated by Excision of the First Rib. J. Bone Joint Surg., 42A:798–801, 1960.
48. Day, L.: Electrical Stimulation in the Treatment of Ununited Fractures. Clin. Orthop., 161:54–57, 1981.
49. De Bakey, E., Beall, C., Jr., Ukkasch, D.C.: Recent Developments in Vascular Surgery With Particular Reference to Orthopaedics. Am. J. Surg., 109:134–142, 1965.
49a. Della Santa, D.R., and Narakas, A.O.: [Fractures of the Clavicle and Secondary Lesions of the Brachial Plexus]. Z. Unfallchir. Versicherungsmed., 85:58–65, 1992.
49b. Della Santa, D., Narakas, A., Bonnard, C.: Late Lesions of the Brachial Plexus After Fracture of the Clavicle. Ann. Hand Surg., 10:531–540, 1991.
50. DePalma, A.: Surgery of the Shoulder, 3rd ed., pp. 348–362. Philadelphia, J.B. Lippincott, 1983.
51. Dickson, J.W.: Death Following Fractured Clavicle. B.M.J., 2:666, 1952.
52. Dolin, M.: The Operative Treatment of Midshaft Clavicular Nonunions. (Letter) J. Bone Joint Surg., 68A:634, 1986.
52a. Domingo-Pech, J.: El Enclavado a Compresión de las Fracturas de Clavícula, con Tornillo de Esponjosa. Barcelona Quirurgica, 15:500–520, 1971.
53. Dugdale, T.W., and Fulkerson, J.B.: Pneumothorax Complicating a Closed Fracture of the Clavicle: A Case Report. Clin. Orthop., 221:212–214, 1987.
54. Dupuytren, Le Baron: On the Injuries and Diseases of Bone (Clark, L., trans.). London, Sydenham Society, 1847.
55. Dust, W.N., and Lenczner, A.M.: Stress Fracture of the Clavicle Leading to Nonunion Secondary to Coracoclavicular Reconstruction With Dacron. Am. J. Sports Med., 17:128–129, 1989.
55a. Eberle, C., Fodor, P., Metzger, U.: [Hook Plate (So-Called Balser Plate) or Tension Banding With the Bosworth Screw in Complete Acromioclavicular Dislocation and Clavicular Fracture]. Z. Unfallchir. Versicherungsmed., 85:134–139, 1992.
56. Ebraheim, N.A., An, H.S., Jackson, W.T., et al.: Scapulothoracic Dissociation. J. Bone Joint Surg., 70:428–432, 1988.
57. Echtermeyer, V., Zwipp, H., Oestern, H.J.: Fehler und Gefahren in der Behandlung der Fracturen und Pseudarthrosen des Schlusselbeins. Langenbecks Arch. Chir., 364:351–354, 1984.
58. Edvardsen, P., and Odegard, O.: Treatment of Posttraumatic Clavicular Pseudoarthrosis. Acta Orthop. Scand. 48:456–457, 1977.
58a. Edwards, D.J., Kavanagh, T.G., Flannery, M.C.: Fractures of the Distal Clavicle: A Case for Fixation. Injury, 23:44–46, 1992.
59. Eidman, D.K., Siff, S.J., Tullos, H.S.: Acromioclavicular Lesions in Children. Am. J. Sports Med., 9:150–154, 1981.
59a. Eilenberger, K., Janousek, A., Poigenfurst, J.: [Heart Arrest as a Sequela of Clavicular Fracture]. Unfallchirurgie, 18:186–188, 1992.

60. Elliott, A.C.: Tripartite Injury of the Clavicle: A Case Report. S. Afr. Med. J., 70:115, 1986.
61. Enker, S.H., and Murthy, K.K.: Brachial Plexus Compression by Excessive Callus Formation Secondary to a Fractured Clavicle: A Case Report. Mt. Sinai J. Med., 37:678–682, 1970.
62. Eskola, A., Vainionpaa, S., Myllyen, P.: Surgery for Ununited Clavicular Fracture. Acta Orthop. Scand., 57:366–367, 1986.
63. Eskola, A., Vainionpaa, S., Myllynen, P., Patiala, H., Rokkanen, P.: Outcome of Clavicular Fracture in 89 Patients. Arch. Orthop. Trauma Surg., 105:337–338, 1986.
64. Eskola, A., Vainionpaa, S., Patiala, H., et al.: Outcome of Operative Treatment in Fresh Lateral Clavicle Fracture. Ann. Chir. Gynaecol., 76:167–168, 1987.
65. Fairbank, H.: Cranio-Cleido-Dysostosis. J. Bone Joint Surg., 31B:608, 1949.
66. Falconer, M.A., and Weddell, G.: Costoclavicular Compression of the Subclavian Artery and Vein. Lancet, 2:539, 1943.
67. Falstie-Jensen, S.: Pseudodislocation of the Acromioclavicular Joint. J. Bone Joint Surg., 64B:368–369, 1982.
68. Farkas, R., and Levine, S.: X-Ray Incidence of Fractured Clavicle in Vertex Presentation. Am. J. Obstet. Gynecol., 59:204–206, 1950.
69. Fawcett, J.: The Development and Ossification of the Human Clavicle. J. Anat., 47:225–234, 1913.
70. Fich, R.: Handbuch der Anatomie und Mechanic der Galanke. *In* Bvdeleben, V. (ed.): Handbuch der Anatomie des Menschen, Vol. 2, Section 1, pp. 163–187. Jema, Gustava Discher, 1910.
71. Finelli, P.F., and Cardi, J.K.: Seizure as a Cause of Fracture. Neurology, 39:858–860, 1989.
72. Fini-Storchi, O., LoRusso, D., Agostini, V.: "Pseudotumors" of the Clavicle Subsequent to Radical Neck Dissection. J. Laryngol. Otol., 99:73–83, 1985.
73. Fowler, A.W.: Fractures of the Clavicle. J. Bone Joint Surg., 44B:440, 1962.
74. Freedman, M., Gamble, J., Lewis, C.: Intrauterine Fracture Simulating a Unilateral Clavicular Pseudarthrosis. J. Assoc. Radiol., 33:37–38, 1982.
74a. Freeland, A.: Unstable Adult Midclavicular Fracture. Orthopedics, 13:1279–1281, 1990.
75. Friedman, R.J., and Gordon, L.: False Positive Indium-111 White Blood Cell Scan in Enclosed Clavicle Fracture. J. Orthop. Trauma, 2:151–153, 1988.
76. Frobenius, H., and Betzel, A.: Injuries and Their Causes in Bicycle Accidents. Unfallchirurgie, 13:135–141, 1987.
77. Fry, J.: Photo of the "Edwin Smith Surgical Papyrus." *In* Rockwood, C.A., Wilkins, K.E., King, R.E. (eds.): Fractures in Children, p. 679. Philadelphia, J.B. Lippincott, 1984.
78. Fukuda, K., Craig, E.V., An, K.N., Cofield, R.H., Chao, E.Y.: Biomechanical Study of the Ligamentous System of the Acromioclavicular Joint. J. Bone Joint Surg., 68A:434–440, 1986.
79. Gardner, E.: The Embryology of the Clavicle. Clin. Orthop., 58:9–16, 1968.
80. Gardner, E.D., Grey, D.J., Orahilly, R.: Anatomy, p. 108. Philadelphia, W.B. Saunders, 1960.
81. Gearen, P.F., and Petty, W.: Panclavicular Dislocation: Report of a Case. J. Bone Joint Surg., 64A:454–455, 1982.
82. Gebuhr, P.: Brachial Plexus Involvement After Fractures of the Clavicle. Ugeskr Laeger, 150:105–106, 1988.
83. Ghormley, R.K., Black, J.R., Cherry, J.H.: Ununited Fractures of the Clavicle. Am. J. Surg., 51:343–349, 1941.
84. Gibbon, J.H.: Lucas-Championnierer and Mobilization in the Treatment of Fractures. Surg. Gynecol. Obstet., 43:271–278, 1926.
85. Gibson, D.A., and Carroll, N.: Congenital Pseudoarthrosis of the Clavicle. J. Bone Joint Surg., 52B:629–643, 1970.
86. Gilbert, W.M., and Tchabo, J.G.: Fractured Clavicle in Newborns. Int. Surg., 73:123–125, 1988.
87. Gitsch, V.G., and Schatten, C.: Frequenz und potentielle Faktoren in der Genese der geburtstraumatisch bedingten Klavicula fraktur. Zentralbl. Gynakol., 109:909–912, 1987.
88. Goddard, N.J., Stabler, J., Albert, J.S.: Atlanto-Axial Rotatory Fixation in Fracture of the Clavicle: An Association and a Classification. J. Bone Joint Surg., 72B:72–75, 1990.
88a. Golser, K., Sperner, G., Thoni, H., Resch, H.: [Early and Intermediate Results of Conservatively and Surgically Treated Lateral Clavicular Fractures]. Aktuel. Traumatol., 21:148–152, 1991.
89. Gonik, B., Allen, R., Sorab, J.: Objective Evaluation of the Shoulder Dystocia Phenomenon: Effect of Maternal Pelvic Orientation on Bone Reduction. Obstet. Gynecol., 74:44–48, 1989.
90. Grant, J.C.B.: A Method of Anatomy, 5th ed. Baltimore, Williams & Wilkins, 1952.
91. Gresham, E.L.: Birth Trauma. Pediatr. Clin. North Am., 22:317, 1975.
92. Gross, S.D.: The Anatomy, Physiology, and Diseases of the Bones and Joints, p. 67. Philadelphia, John Grigg, 1830.
93. Gryska, P.F.: Major Vascular Injuries. N. Engl. J. Med., 266:381–385, 1982.
94. Guattieri, G., and Frassi, G.: Late Truncal Paralysis of the Brachial Plexus in Sequela of Fracture of the Clavicle. Arch Ortopedia., 74:840–848, 1961.
95. Guilfoil, P.H., and Christiansen, T.: An Unusual Vascular Complication of Fractured Clavicle. J.A.M.A., 200:72–73, 1967.
96. Guillemin, A.: Dechrune de la Vein Sous-Claviere par Fracture Fermie de la Clavicule. Bull. Mem. Soc. Nat. Chir., 56:302–304, 1930.
97. Gurd, F.B.: The Treatment of Complete Dislocation of the Outer End of Clavicle: A Hitherto Undescribed Operation. Ann. Surg., 113:1094–1097, 1941.
97a. Hackenbruch, W., Regazzoni, P., Schwyzer, K.: [Surgical Treatment of Lateral Clavicular Fracture With the "Clavicular Hooked Plate"]. Z. Unfallchir. Versicherungsmed., 87:145–152, 1994.
98. Hackstock, H., and Hackstock, H.: Surgical Treatment of Clavicular Fracture. Unfallchirurg, 91:64–69, 1988.
98a. Hansky, B., Murray, E., Minami, K., Korfer, R.: Delayed Brachial Plexus Paralysis Due to Subclavian Pseudoaneurysm After Clavicular Fracture. Eur. J. Cardiothorac. Surg., 7:497–498, 1993.
99. Hargan, B., and Macafee, A.L.: Bilateral Pseudoarthrosis of the Clavicles. Injury, 12:316–318, 1981.
99a. Harrington, M.A., Jr., Keller, T.S., Seiler, J.G., III, Weikert, D.R., Moeljanto, E., Schwartz, H.S.: Geometric Properties and the Predicted Mechanical Behavior of Adult Human Clavicles. J. Biomech., 26:417–426, 1993.
100. Heppenstall, R.B.: Fractures and Dislocations of the Distal Clavicle. Orthop. Clin. North Am., 6:447–486, 1975.
100a. Hersovici, D., Jr., Fiennes, A.G.T., Allgöwer, M., Ruëdi, T.P.: The Floating Shoulder: Ipsilateral Clavicle and Scapular Neck Fractures. J. Bone Joint Surg., 74B:362–364, 1992.
100b. Herscovici, D., Jr., Fiennes, A.G.T.W., Ruedi, T.P.: The Floating Shoulder: Ipsilateral Clavicle and Scapular Neck Fractures. (Abstract) J. Orthop. Trauma, 6:499, 1992.
101. Hicks, J.H.: Rigid Fixation as a Treatment for Hypertrophic Nonunion. Injury, 8:199–205, 1976.
102. Hoyer, H.E., Kindt, R., Lippert, H.: Zur Biomechanik der menschlichen Claveula. Z. Orthop. Ihre Grenzgeb., 118:915–922, 1980.
103. Houston, H.E.: An Unusual Complication of Clavicular Fracture. J. Ky. Med. Assoc., 75:170–171, 1977.
104. Howard, F.M., and Schafer, S.J.: Injuries to the Clavicle With Neurovascular Complications: A Study of Fourteen Cases. J. Bone Joint Surg., 47A:1335–1346, 1965.
105. Hughes, A.W., and Sherlock, D.A.: Bilateral Thoracic Outlet Syndrome Following Nonunion of Clavicles Associated With Radio-osteodystrophy Injury. J. Bone Joint Surg., 19:40–41, 1988.
106. Inman, V.T., and Saunders, J.B.: Observation on the Function of the Clavicle. Calif. Med., 65:158–165, 1946.
106a. Ivey, M., Britt, M., Johnston, R.V.: Reflex Sympathetic Dystrophy After Clavicle Fracture: Case Report. J. Trauma, 31:276–279, 1991.

107. Iqbal, O.: Axillary Artery Thrombosis Associated With Fracture of the Clavicle. Med. J. Malaysia, 26:68–70, 1971.
108. Jablon, M., Sutker, A., Post, M.: Irreducible Fractures of the Middle Third of the Clavicle. J. Bone Joint Surg., 61A:296–298, 1979.
108a. Jackson, D.W. (ed.): Shoulder Surgery in the Athlete. Rockville, Md, Aspen Publications, 1985.
109. Jackson, W.J.: Clavicle Fractures: Therapy Is Dictated by the Patient's Age. Consultant, 177, 1982.
110. Jacobs, P.: Post-traumatic Osteolysis of the Outer End of the Clavicle. J. Bone Joint Surg., 46B:705–707, 1964.
110a. Jäger, M., Breitner, S.: [Therapy Related Classification of Lateral Clavicular Fracture]. Unfallheilkunde, 87:467–473, 1984.
111. Jain, A.S.: Traumatic Floating Clavicle: A Case Report. J. Bone Joint Surg., 66B:560–561, 1984.
112. Javid, H.: Vascular Injuries of the Neck. Clin. Orthop., 28:70–78, 1963.
113. Jit, I., and Kulkrani, M.: Times of Appearance and Fusion of Epiphysis at the Medial End of the Clavicle. Indian J. Med. Res., 64:773–792, 1976.
114. Johnson, E.W., Jr., and Collins, H.R.: Nonunion of the Clavicle. Arch. Surg., 87:963–966, 1963.
115. Joseph, P.R., and Rosenfeld, W.: Clavicular Fractures in Neonates. Am. J. Dis. Child., 144:165–167, 1990.
116. Joukainen, J., and Karaharju, E.: Pseudoarthrosis of the Clavicle. Acta Orthop. Scand., 48:550, 1977.
117. Jupiter, J.B., and Leffert, R.D.: Nonunion of the Clavicle. J. Bone Joint Surg., 69A:753–760, 1987.
118. Kabaharjve, E., Joukainen, J., Peltonen, J.: Treatment of Pseudoarthrosis of the Clavicle. Injury, 13:400–403, 1982.
119. Kanoksikarin, S., and Wearne, W.N.: Fracture and Retrosternal Dislocation of the Clavicle. Aust. N. Z. J. Surg., 48:95–96, 1978.
120. Karwasz, R.R., Kutzner, M., Krammer, W.G.: Late Brachial Plexus Lesion Following Clavicular Fracture. Unfallchurg., 91:45–47, 1988.
121. Katz, R., Landman, J., Dulitzky, F., Bar-Ziv, J.: Fracture of the Clavicle in the Newborn: An Ultrasound Diagnosis. J. Ultrasound Med., 7:21–23, 1988.
122. Katznelson, A., Nerubay, J., Oliver, S.: Dynamic Fixation of the Avulsed Clavicle. J. Trauma, 16:841–844, 1976.
123. Kay, S.P., and Eckardt, J.J.: Brachial Plexus Palsy Secondary to Clavicular Nonunion: A Case Report and Literature Survey. Clin. Orthop., 206:219–222, 1986.
124. Kaye, J.J., Nance, E.P., Jr., Green, N.E.: Fatigue Fracture of the Medial Aspect of the Clavicle: An Academic Rather Than Athletic Injury. Radiology, 144:89–90, 1982.
125. Key, J.A., and Conwell, E.H.: The Management of Fractures, Dislocations, and Sprains, 2nd ed., p. 437. St. Louis, C.V. Mosby, 1937.
126. Khan, M.A.A., and Lucas, H.K.: Plating of Fractures of the Middle Third of the Clavicle. Injury, 9:263–267, 1978.
127. Kini, M.G.: A Simple Method of Ambulatory Treatment of Fractures of the Clavicle. J. Bone Joint Surg., 23:795–798, 1941.
128. Kite, J.H.: Congenital Pseudoarthrosis of the Clavicle. South. Med. J., 761:703–710, 1968.
129. Klier, I., and Mayor, P.B.: Laceration of the Innominate Internal Jugular Venous Junction: Rare Complication of Fracture of the Clavicle. Orthop. Rev., 10:81–82, 1981.
130. Koch, F., Papadimitriou, G., Groher, W.: Die Clavicula pseudoarthroseihse Entstehung und Behandlung. Unfallheilkunde, 74:330–337, 1971.
131. Koelliker, F., and Ganz, R.: Results of the Treatment of Clavicular Pseudarthrosis. Unfallchirurg, 92:164–168, 1989.
131a. Kohler, A., Kach, K., Platz, A., Friedl, H.P., Trentz, O.: [Extended Surgical Indications in Combined Shoulder Girdle Fracture.] Z. Unfallchir. Versicherungsmed., 85:140–144, 1992.
131b. Kona, J., Bosse, M.J., Staeheli, J.W., Rosseau, R.L.: Type II Distal Clavicle Fractures: A Retrospective Review of Surgical Treatment. J. Orthop. Trauma, 4:115–120, 1990.
132. Koss, S.D., Giotz, H.T., Redler, N.R., et al.: Nonunion of a Midshaft Clavicle Fracture Associated With Subclavian Vein Compression: A Case Report. Orthop. Rev., 18:431–434, 1989.
133. Kreisinger, V.: Sur le Traitement des Fractures de le Clavicule. Rev. Chir., 43:376, 1927.
134. Kremens, V., and Glauser, F.: Unusual Sequelae Following Pinning of Medial Clavicular Fracture. A.J.R. Am. J. Roentgenol., 74:1066–1069, 1956.
135. Lancet (editorial): Sir Robert Peel's Death. Lancet, 2:19, 1850.
136. Lee, H.G.: Treatment of Fracture of the Clavicle by Internal Nail Fixation. N. Engl. J. Med., 234:222–224, 1946.
137. Lemire, L., and Rosman, M.: Sternoclavicular Epiphyseal Separation With Adjacent Clavicular Fracture. J. Pediatr. Orthop., 4:118–120, 1984.
138. Lengua, F., Nuss, J., Lechner, R., Baruthio, J., Veillon, F.: The Treatment of Fracture of the Clavicle by Closed Medio-Lateral Pinning. Rev. Chir. Orthop. Reparatrice Appar. Mot., 73:377–380, 1987.
139. Lester, C.W.: The Treatment of Fractures of the Clavicle. Ann. Surg., 89:600–606, 1929.
139a. Leung, K.S., and Lam, T.P.: Open Reduction and Internal Fixation of Ipsilateral Fractures of the Scapular Neck and Clavicle. 75A:1015–1018, 1993.
140. Liechtl, R.: Fracture of the Clavicle and Scapula. *In* Weber, B.G., Brunner, C., Freuler, F. (eds.): Treatment of Fractures in Children and Adolescents, pp. 88–95. New York, Springer-Verlag, 1988.
141. Lim, E., and Day, L.J.: Subclavian Vein Thrombosis Following Fracture of the Clavicle: A Case Report. Orthopedics, 10:349–351, 1987.
142. Lipton, H.A., and Jupiter, J.B.: Nonunion of Clavicular Fractures: Characteristics and Surgical Management. Surg. Rounds Orthop., 1988.
143. Ljunggren, A.E.: Clavicular Function. Acta Orthop. Scand., 50:261–268, 1979.
144. Lloyd-Roberts, G.C., Apley, A.G., Owen, R.: Reflections Upon the Etiology of Congenital Pseudoarthrosis of the Clavicle. J. Bone Joint Surg., 57B:24–29, 1975.
145. Lombard, J.J.: Pseudoarthrosis of the Clavicle: A Case Report. S. Afr. Med. J., 66:151–153, 1984.
146. Lord, J.W., and Rosati, J.M.: Neurovascular Compression Syndromes of the Upper Extremity. CIBA Found. Symp., 10, 1958.
147. Lukin, A.V., and Grishken, V.A.: Two Cases of Successful Treatment of Fracture Dislocation of the Clavicle. Ortop. Travmatol. Protez., 11:35, 1987.
148. Lusskin, R., Weiss, C.A., Winer, J.: The Role of the Subclavius Muscle in the Subclavian Vein Syndrome (Costoclavicular Syndrome) Following Fracture of the Clavicle. Clin. Orthop., 54:75–84, 1967.
148a. Lyons, F.A., and Rockwood, C.A.: Migration of Pins Used in Operations on the Shoulder. J. Bone Joint Surg., 72A:1262–1267, 1990.
149. Madsen, E.T.: Fractures of the Extremities in the Newborn. Acta Obstet. Gynecol. Scand., 34:41–74, 1955.
150. Malcolm, B.W., Ameli, F.N., Simmons, E.H.: Pneumothorax Complicating a Fracture of the Clavicle. Can. J. Surg., 22:84, 1979.
151. Malgaigne, J.F.: A Treatise on Fractures, pp. 374–401. (Transl. by Packard, J.H.) Philadelphia, J.B. Lippincott, 1859.
152. Manske, D.J., and Szabo, R.M.: The Operative Treatment of Mid-Shaft Clavicular Non-Unions. J. Bone Joint. Surg., 67A:1367–1371, 1985.
153. Marie, P., and Sainton, P.: On Hereditary Cleidocranial Dysostosis. Clin. Orthop., 58:5–7, 1968.
154. Marsh, H.O., and Hazarian, E.: Pseudoarthrosis of the Clavicle. (Abstract) J. Bone Joint Surg., 52B:793, 1970.
154a. Martell, J.R.: Clavicular Nonunion—Complication With the Use of Mersilene Tape. Am. J. Sports Med., 20:360–362, 1992.
155. Matry, C.: Fracture de la Clavicule Gauche au Tiers Interne: Blessure de la Vein Sous-Claviere. Osteosynthese Bull. Mem. Soc. Nat. Chir., 58:75–78, 1932.
155a. Matsen, F.A., III, Fu, F., Hawkins, R.J. (eds.): The Shoulder:

A Balance of Mobility and Stability. Chicago, The American Academy of Orthopaedic Surgeons, 1993.
155b. Matsen, F.A., Lippitt, S.B., Sidles, J.A., Harryman, D.T., II (eds.): Practical Evaluation and Management of the Shoulder. Philadelphia, W.B. Saunders, 1994.
156. Matz, S.O., Welliver, P.S., Welliver, D.I.: Brachial Plexus Neuropraxia Complicating a Comminuted Clavicle Fracture in a College Football Player: Case Report and Review of the Literature. Am. J. Sports Med., 17:581–583, 1989.
157. Mayer, J.H.: Nonunion of Fractured Clavicle. Proc. Roy. Soc. Med., 58:182, 1965.
158. Mazet, R.: Migration of a Kirschner Wire From the Shoulder Region Into the Lung: Report of Two Cases. J. Bone Joint Surg., 25:477–483, 1943.
159. McCandless, D.N., and Mowbray, M.: Treatment of Displaced Fractures of the Clavicle. Sling Vs. Figure-of-Eight Bandage. Practitioner, 223:266–267, 1979.
159a. Meeks, R.J., and Riebel, G.D.: Isolated Clavicle Fracture With Associated Pneumothorax: A Case Report. Am. J. Emerg. Med., 9:555–556, 1991.
160. Miller, D.S., and Boswick, J.A.: Lesions of the Brachial Plexus Associated With Fractures of the Clavicle. Clin. Orthop., 64:144–149, 1969.
161. Mital, M.A., and Aufranc, O.E.: Venous Occlusion Following Greenstick Fracture Clavicle. J.A.M.A., 206:1301–1302, 1968.
162. Mnaymneh, W., Vargas, A., Kaplan, J.: Fractures of the Clavicle Caused by Arteriovenous Malformation. Clin. Orthop., 148:256–258, 1980.
163. Moir, J.C., and Myerscough, P.R.: Operative Obstetrics, 7th ed. Baltimore, Williams & Wilkins, 1964.
164. Moore, T.O.: Internal Pin Fixation for Fracture of the Clavicle. Am. Surg., 17:580–583, 1951.
164a. Moschiniski, D., Baumann, G., Linke, R.: Osteosynthesis of Distal Clavicular Fracture With Reabsorptive Implant. Aktuel. Chir., 27:33–35, 1992.
165. Moseley, H.F.: The Clavicle: Its Anatomy and Function. Clin. Orthop., 58:17–27, 1968.
166. Moseley, H.F.: Shoulder Lesions, pp. 207–235. New York, Churchill Livingstone, 1972.
167. Mueller, M.E., Allgower, N., Willenegger, H.: Manual of Internal Fixation. New York, Springer-Verlag, 1970.
168. Mulder, D.S., Greenwood, F.A., Brooks, C.E.: Post-Traumatic Thoracic Outlet Syndrome. J. Trauma, 13:706–713, 1973.
168a. Mullaji, A.B., and Jupiter, J.B.: Low Contact Dynamic Compression Plating of the Clavicle. Injury, 25:41–45, 1994.
169. Murray, G.: A Method of Fixation for Fracture of the Clavicle. J. Bone Joint Surg., 22:616–620, 1940.
170. Natali, J., Maraval, M., Kieffer, E., Petrovic, P.: Fractures of the Clavicle and Injuries of the Subclavian Artery: Report of 10 Cases. J. Cardiovasc. Surg. (Torino), 16:541–547, 1975.
170a. Neer, C.S. (ed): Shoulder Reconstruction. Philadelphia, W.B. Saunders, 1990.
171. Neer, C.S., II: Nonunion of the Clavicle, J.A.M.A., 172:1006–1011, 1960.
172. Neer, C.S., II: Fracture of the Distal Clavicle With Detachment of Coracoclavicular Ligaments in Adults. J. Trauma, 3:99–110, 1963.
173. Neer, C.S., II: Fractures of the Distal Third of the Clavicle. Clin. Orthop., 58:43–50, 1968.
174. Neer, C.S., II: Impingement Lesions. Clin. Orthop., 173:70–77, 1983.
175. Neer, C.S., II: Fractures of the Clavicle. *In* Rockwood, C.A., Jr., and Green, D.P. (eds.): Fractures in Adults, pp. 707–713. Philadelphia, J.B. Lippincott, 1984.
176. Nelson, H.P.: Subclavian Aneurysm Following Fracture of the Clavicle. St. Bartholomew (Hospital Report), 65:219–229, 1932.
177. Neviaser, J.S.: Acromioclavicular Dislocations Treated by Transference of the Coracoacromial Ligament. Bull. Hosp. Jt. Dis., 12:46–54, 1951.
178. Neviaser, J.S.: Injuries in and About the Shoulder Joint. Instr. Course Lect., 13:187–216, 1956.
179. Neviaser, J.S.: The Treatment of Fractures of the Clavicle. Surg. Clin. North Am., 43:1555–1563, 1963.
180. Neviaser, J.S.: Injuries of the Clavicle and Its Articulations. Orthop. Clin. North Am., 11:233–237, 1980.
181. Neviaser, R.J.: Injuries to the Clavicle and Acromioclavicular Joint. Orthop. Clin. North Am., 18:433–438, 1987.
182. Neviaser, R.J., Neviaser, J.S., Neviaser, T.J.: A Simple Technique for Internal Fixation of the Clavicle. Clin. Orthop., 109:103–107, 1975.
182a. Niemeier, U., and Zimmermenn, H.G.: Die offene Marknagelung der Clavicula nach Küntscher. Eine Alternative in der Behandlung alter Schlüsselbeinbrüche. Chirurg, 61:464–466, 1990.
183. Nogi, J., Heckman, J.D., Hakala, M., Sweet, D.E.: Nonunion of the Clavicle in the Child: A Case Report. Clin. Orthop., 110:19–21, 1975.
183a. Nordqvist, A., and Petersson, C.: The Incidence of Fractures of the Clavicle. Clin. Orthop., 300:127–132, 1994.
183b. Nordqvist, A., Petersson, C., Redlund-Johnell, I.: Fractures of the Lateral End of the Clavicle—A Long-Term Study. (Abstract) Acta Orthop. Scand., 62(Suppl.246):25–26, 1991.
183c. Nordqvist, A., Petersson, C., Redlund-Johnell, I.: The Natural Course of Lateral Clavicle Fracture. Acta Orthop. Scand., 64:87–91, 1993.
184. Noriel, H., and Llewelleyn, R.C.: Migration of a Threaded Steinmann Pin From an Acromioclavicular Joint Into the Spinal Canal: A Case Report. J. Bone Joint Surg., 47A:1024, 1965.
185. Ogden, J.A., Conologue, G.J., Bronson, N.L.: Radiology of Postnatal Skeletal Development: The Clavicle. Skeletal Radiol., 4:196–203, 1979.
186. Oppenheimer, W.L., David, A., Growdon, W.A., Dorey, F.J., Davlin, L.B.: Clavicle Fractures in the Newborn. Clin. Orthop., 250:176, 1990.
187. Ord, R.A., and Langon, J.D.: Stress Fracture of the Clavicle: A Rare Late Complication of Radical Neck Dissection. J. Maxillofac. Surg., 14:281–284, 1986.
188. O'Rourke, I.C., and Middleton, R.W.: The Place and Efficacy of Operative Management of Fractured Clavicle. Injury, 6:236–240, 1975.
189. Ostreich, A.E.: The Lateral Clavicle Hook—An Acquired as Well as a Congenital Anomaly. Pediatr. Radiol., 11:147, 1981.
190. Owen, R.: Congenital Pseudoarthrosis of the Clavicle. J. Bone Joint Surg., 52B:642–652, 1970.
191. Oxnard, C.E.: The Architecture of the Shoulder in Some Mammals. J. Morphol., 126:249–290, 1968.
192. Packer, B.D.: Conservative Treatment of Fracture of the Clavicle. J. Bone Joint Surg., 26:770–774, 1944.
193. Paffen, P.J., and Jansen, E.W.: Surgical Treatment of Clavicular Fractures With Kirschner Wires: A Comparative Study. Arch. Chir. Neerl., 30:43–53, 1978.
193a. Palarcik, J.: Clavicular Fractures (Group of Patients Treated in the Traumatological Research Institute in 1986–1989). Czech. Med., 14:184–190, 1991.
194. Parkes, J.C., and Deland, J.D.: A Three-Part Distal Clavicle Fracture. J. Trauma, 23:437–438, 1983.
195. Patel, C.V., and Audenwalla, H.S.: Treatment of Fractured Clavicle by Immediate Partial Subperiosteal Resection. J. Postgrad. Med., 18:32–34, 1972.
196. Penn, I.: The Vascular Complications of Fractures of the Clavicle. J. Trauma, 4:819–831, 1964.
197. Perry, B.: An Improved Clavicular Pin. Am. J. Surg., 112:142–144, 1966.
198. Pipkin, G.: Tardy Shoulder Hand Syndrome Following Ununited Fracture of Clavicle: A Case Report. J. Missouri Med. Assoc., 643–646, 1951.
199. Piterman, L.: "The Fractured Clavicle." Aust. Fam. Physician, 11:614, 1982.
200. Poigenfürst, J., Baumgarten-Hofmann, U., Hofmann, J.: Unstabile Bruchformen am äuBeren Schlüsselbeinende und Grundsätze der Behandlung. Unfallchirurgie, 17:131–139, 1991.
200a. Poigenfürst, J., Rappold, G., Fischer, W.: Plating of Fresh Cla-

vicular Fractures: Results of 122 Operations. Injury, 23:237–241, 1992.

200b. Poigenfürst, J., Reiler, T., Fischer, W.: Plating of Fresh Clavicular Fractures: Experience With 60 Operations. Unfallchirurgie, 14:26–37, 1988.

201. Pollen, A.G.: Fractures and Dislocations in Children. Baltimore, Williams & Wilkins, 1973.

202. Porral, A.: Observation d'une Double Luxation de la Clavicule Droite Juniva. Hibd. Med. Chir. Part., 2:78–82, 1831.

203. Post, M.: Injury to the Shoulder Girdle. *In* Post, M. (ed.): The Shoulder: Surgical and Non-surgical Management, pp. 432–447. Philadelphia, Lea & Febiger, 1988.

204. Post, M.: Current Concepts in the Treatment of Fractures of the Clavicle. Clin. Orthop., 245:89–101, 1989.

205. Pusitz, M.E., and Davis, E.V.: Bone-Drilling in Delayed Union of Fractures. J. Bone Joint Surg., 26A:560–565, 1944.

206. Pyper, J.B.: Nonunion of Fractures of the Clavicle. Injury, 9:268–270, 1978.

207. Quesana, F.: Technique for the Roentgen Diagnosis of Fractures of the Clavicle. Surg. Gynecol. Obstet., 42:4261–4281, 1926.

208. Quigley, T.B.: The Management of Simple Fracture of the Clavicle in Adults. N. Engl. J. Med., 243:286–290, 1950.

209. Quinlan, W.R., Brady, P.G., Regan, B.F.: Congenital Pseudoarthrosis of the Clavicle. Acta Orthop. Scand., 51:489–492, 1980.

210. Quinn, S.F., and Glass, T.A.: Post Traumatic Osteolysis of the Clavicle. South. Med. J., 76:307–308, 1983.

211. Rabenseifner, L.: Zur Atiologie und Therapie bei Schlusselbeinpsuedarthosen. Acta Traumatol., 11:130–132, 1981.

212. Raymakers, E., and Marti, R.: Nonunion of the Clavicle. *In* Pseudarthroses and Their Treatment. Eighth International Symposium on Topical Problems in Orthopaedic Surgery. Thieme, 1979.

213. Redmond, A.D.: A Complication of Fracture of the Clavicle. (Letter) Injury, 13:352, 1982.

214. Reid, J., and Kenned, J.: Direct Fracture of the Clavicle With Symptoms Simulating a Cervical Rib. B.M.J., 2:608–609, 1925.

215. Rhinelander, F.W.: Tibial Blood Supply in Relation to Fracture Healing. Clin. Orthop., 105:34–81, 1974.

216. Ring, M.: Clavicle. *In* Ring, M. (ed.): Children's Fractures, 2nd ed. Philadelphia, J.B. Lippincott, 1983.

217. Rockwood, C.A.: Fractures of the Outer Clavicle in Children and Adults. J. Bone Joint Surg., 64B:642, 1982.

218. Rockwood, C.A.: Management of Fracture of the Clavicle and Injuries of the SC Joints. Orthop. Trans., 6:422, 1982.

219. Rockwood, C.A.: Treatment of the Outer Clavicle in Children and Adults. Orthop. Trans., 6:472, 1982.

220. Rockwood, C.A.: "Don't throw away the clavicle". Orthop. Transactions, 16:763, 1992–1993.

220a. Rockwood, C.A., Jr., Matsen, F.A., III (eds.): The Shoulder. Philadelphia, W.B. Saunders, 1990.

221. Rosati, L.M., and Lord, J.W., Jr.: Neurovascular Compression Syndromes of the Shoulder Girdle. New York, Grune & Stratton, 1961.

222. Rowe, C.R.: An Atlas of Anatomy and Treatment of Mid-Clavicular Fractures. Clin. Orthop., 58:29–42, 1968.

222a. Rowe, C.R. (ed.): The Shoulder. New York, Churchill Livingstone, 1988.

223. Rubin, A.: Birth Injuries: Incidence, Mechanisms and End Result. Obstet. Gynecol., 23:218–221, 1964.

223a. Rumball, K.M., DaSilva, V.F., Preston, D.N., Carruthers, C.C.: Brachial-Plexus Injury After Clavicular Fracture: Case Report and Literature Review. Can. J. Surg. 34(3): 264–266, 1991.

224. Rush, L.V., and Rush, H.L.: Technique of Longitudinal Pin Fixation in Fractures of the Clavicle and Jaw. Miss. Doctor, 27:332, 1949.

225. Sakellarides, H.: Pseudoarthrosis of the Clavicle. J. Bone Joint Surg., 43A:130–138, 1961.

226. Sampson, J.J., Saunders, J.B., Capp, C.S.: Compression of the Subclavian Vein by the First Rib and Clavicle With Reference to Prominence of the Chest Veins as a Sign of Collaterals. Am. Heart J., 19:292–315, 1940.

226a. Sanders, A., and Rockwood, C.A., Jr.: Management of Dislocations of Both Ends of the Clavicle. J. Bone Joint Surg., 72A:399–402, 1990.

227. Sandford, H.N.: The Moro Reflex as a Diagnostic Aid in Fracture of the Clavicle and the Newborn Infant. Am. J. Dis. Child., 41:1304–1306, 1931.

228. Sankarankuty, M., and Turner, B.W.: Fractures of the Clavicle. Injury, 7:101–106, 1975.

229. Sayer, L.: A Simple Dressing for Fractures of the Clavicle. Am. Pract., 4:1, 1871.

230. Scarpa, F.J., and Levy, R.M.: Pulmonary Embolism Complicating Clavicle Fracture. Conn. Med., 43:771–773, 1979.

231. Schewior, T.: Die Durckpallenostesynthese bei Schlusselpein pseudarthrosen. Acta Traumatol., 4:113–125, 1974.

232. Schrocksnadel, H., Heim, K., Dapunt, O.: The Clavicular Fracture—A Questionable Achievement in Modern Obstetrics. Geburtshilfe Frauenheilkd., 49:481–484, 1989.

233. Schuind, F., Pay-Pay, E., Andrianne, Y., Donkerwolcke, M., Rasquin, C., Burny, F.: External Fixation of the Clavicle for Fracture or Nonunion in Adults. J. Bone Joint Surg., 70A:692–695, 1988.

233a. Schwarz, N., and Höcker, K.: Osteosynthesis of Irreducible Fractures of the Clavicle With 2.7 mm ASIF Plates. J. Trauma, 33:179–183, 1992.

234. Schwartz, V.N., and Leixnering, M.: Technik und Ergebienisse der Klavikula-markdrahtung. Zentralbl Chir., 111:640–647, 1986.

234a. Seiler, J.G., and Jupiter, J.B.: Intercalary Tri-cortical Iliac Crest Bone Grafts for the Treatment of Chronic Clavicular Nonunion With Bony Defect. J. Orthop. Tech., 1:19–22, 1993.

235. Shauffer, I.A., and Collins, W.V.: The Deep Clavicular Rhomboid Fossa. J.A.M.A., 195:778–779, 1966.

236. Shih, J., Chao, E., Chang, C.: Subclavian Pseudoaneurysm After Clavicle Fracture: A Case Report. J. Formos. Med. Assoc., 82:332–335, 1983.

237. Siebermann, R.P., Spieler, U., Arquint, A.: Rush Pin Osteosynthesis of the Clavicle as an Alternative to Conservative Treatment. Unfallchirurgie, 13:303–307, 1987.

238. Siffrey, and Aulong: Thrombose Post-Traumatique de l'Artere Sous-Claviere Gauche. Lyon Chir., 51:479–481, 1956.

239. Silloway, K.A., Mclaughlin, R.E., Edlich, R.C., Edlich, R.F.: Clavicular Fractures and Acromioclavicular Joint Injuries in Lacrosse: Preventable Injuries. J. Emerg. Med., 3:117–121, 1985.

240. Simpson, L.A., and Kellam, J.: Surgical Management of Fractures of the Clavicle, Scapula, and Proximal Humerus. Orthop. Update Series, 4:1–8, 1985.

241. Smith, R.W.: A Treatise on Fractures in the Vicinity of Joints, pp. 209–224. Dublin, Hodges & Smith, 1847.

242. Snyder, L.A.: Loss of the Accompanying Soft Tissue Shadow of Clavicle With Occult Fracture. South. Med. J., 72:243, 1979.

243. Sorrells, R.B.: Fracture of the Clavicle. J. Ark. Med. Soc., 71:253–256, 1975.

244. Spar, I.: Total Claviculectomy for Pathological Fractures. Clin. Orthop., 129:236–237, 1977.

245. Stanley, D., and Norris, S.H.: Recovery Following Fractures of the Clavicle Treated Conservatively. Injury, 19:162–164, 1988.

246. Stanley, D., Trowbridge, E.A., Norris, S.H.: The Mechanism of Clavicular Fracture. J. Bone Joint Surg., 70B:461–464, 1988.

247. Steenburg, R.W., and Ravitch, M.M.: Cervico-Thoracic Approach for Subclavian Vessel Injury From Compound Fracture of the Clavicle: Considerations of Subclavian Axillary Exposures. Ann. Surg., 1:839, 1963.

248. Steffelaar, H., and Heim, V.: Sekundare Plattenosteosynthesen an der Clavicula. Arth. Orthop. Unfallchir., 79:75, 1974.

249. Steinberg, I.: Subclavian-Vein Thrombosis Associated With Fractures of the Clavicle. Report of Two Cases. N. Engl. J. Med., 264:686–688, 1961.

250. Stimson, L.A.: A Treatise on Fractures, p. 332. Philadelphia, Henry A. Lea's Son, 1883.

251. Stone, P.W., and Lord, J.W.: The Clavicle and Its Relation to Trauma to the Subclavian Artery and Vein. Am. J. Surg., 98:834–839, 1955.
252. Storen, H.: Old Clavicular Pseudoarthrosis With Late Appearing Neuralgias and Vasomotor Disturbances Cured by Operation. Acta Chir. Scand., 94:187, 1946.
253. Strauss, M., Bushey, M.J., Chung, C., Baum, S.: Fractures of the Clavicle Following Radical Neck Dissection or Postoperative Radiotherapy: A Case Report and Review of the Literature. Laryngoscope, 92:1304–1307, 1982.
253a. Suso, S., Alemany, X., Combalia, A., Ramon, R.: Compression of the Anterior Interosseous Nerve After Use of a Robert-Jones Type Bandage for a Distal End Clavicle Fracture: Case Report. J. Trauma, 136(5):737–739, 1994.
254. Swischuk, L.E.: Radiology of Newborn and Young Infants, 2nd ed., p. 630. Baltimore, Williams & Wilkins, 1981.
255. Tachdjian, M.O.: Pediatric Orthopaedics. Philadelphia, W.B. Saunders, 1972.
256. Tanchev, S., Kolishev, K., Tanchev, P., Gramcheva, O., Asparukhov, A.: Etiology of a Clavicle Fracture Due to the Birth Process. Akush. Ginekol., 24:39–43, 1985.
257. Taylor, A.R.: Nonunion of Fractures of the Clavicle: A Review of 31 Cases. J. Bone Joint Surg., 51B:568–569, 1969.
258. Taylor, A.R.: Some Observations on Fractures of the Clavicle. Proc. Roy. Soc. Med., 62:1037–1038, 1969.
259. Telford, E.D., and Mottershead, S.: Pressure at the Cervicobrachial Junction: An Operative and an Anatomical Study. J. Bone Joint Surg., 30B:249, 1948.
260. Thomas, C.B., Jr., and Friedman, R.J.: Ipsilateral Sternoclavicular Dislocation and Clavicular Fracture. J. Orthop. Trauma, 3:355–357, 1989.
261. Thompson, A.G., and Batten, R.C.: The Application of Rigid Internal Fixation to the Treatment of Nonunion and Delayed Union Using AO Technique. Injury, 8:88, 1977.
262. Todd, T.W., and D'Errico, J., Jr.: The Clavicular Epiphysis. Am. J. Anat., 41:25–50, 1928.
263. Tregonning, G., and Macnab, I.: Post-Traumatic Pseudoarthrosis of the Clavicle. J. Bone Joint Surg., 58B:264, 1976.
264. Trynin, A.H.: The Bohler Clavicular Splint in the Treatment of Clavicular Injuries. J. Bone Joint Surg., 19:417–424, 1937.
265. Tse, D.H.W., Slabaugh, P.B., Carlson, P.A.: Injury to the Axillary Artery by a Closed Fracture of the Clavicle. J. Bone Joint Surg., 62A:1372–1373, 1980.
266. Tsou, P.N.: Percutaneous Cannulated Screw Coracoclavicular Fixation for Acute Acromioclavicular Dislocations. Clin. Orthop., 243:112–121, 1989.
267. Unger, J.M., Schuchmann, G.G., Grossman, J.E., Pellett, J.R.: Tears of the Trachea and Main Bronchi Caused by Blunt Trauma: Radiologic Findings. A.J.R. Am. J. Roentgenol., 153:1175–1180, 1989.
268. Urist, M.R.: Complete Dislocation of the Acromioclavicular Joint. J. Bone Joint Surg., 28A:813–837, 1946.
269. Valdes-Dopena, M.A., and Arey, J.B.: The Causes of Neonatal Mortality: An Analysis of 501 Autopsies on Newborn Infants. J. Pediatr., 77:366, 1970.
270. Van Vlack, H.G.: Comminuted Fracture of the Clavicle With Pressure on Brachial Plexus: Report of Case. J. Bone Joint Surg., 22A:446–447, 1940.
271. Wachsmudh, W.: Allgemiene und Specielle Operadion Slettie, pp. 375. Berlin, Springer-Verlag, 1956.
272. Wall, J.J.: Congenital Pseudoarthrosis of the Clavicle. J. Bone Joint Surg., 52A:1003–1009, 1970.
272a. Wang, S.J., Liang, P.L, Pai, W.M., Au, M.K., Lin, L.C.: Experience in Open Reduction and Internal Fixation of Mid-Shaft Fractures of the Clavicle. J. Surg. Assoc. ROC, 23:7–11, 1990.
273. Watson-Jones, R.: Fractures and Other Bone and Joint Injuries, pp. 90–91. Edinburgh, E. & S. Livingstone, 1940.
274. Weaver, J.K., and Dunn, H.K.: Treatment of Acromioclavicular Injuries, Especially Acromioclavicular Separation. J. Bone Joint Surg., 54A:1187–1198, 1972.
275. Weber, B.G.: Pseudoarthrosis of the Clavicle. *In* Pseudoarthrosis: Pathophysiology, Biomechanics, Therapy, Results, pp. 104–107. New York, Grune & Stratton, 1976.
276. Weh, L., and Torklus, D.Z.: Fracture of the Clavicle With Consecutive Costoclavicular Compression Syndrome. Z. Orthop. Ihre. Grenzgeb., 118:140–142, 1980.
277. Weiner, D.S., and O'Dell, H.W.: Fractures of the First Rib Associated With Injuries to the Clavicle. J. Trauma, 9:412–422, 1969.
278. Widner, L.A., and Riddewold, H.O.: The Value of the Lordotic View in Diagnosis of Fractured Clavicle. Rev. Int. Radiol., 5:69–70, 1980.
279. Wilkes, J.A., and Hoffer, M.: Clavicle Fractures in Head-Injured Children. J. Orthop. Trauma, 1:55–58, 1987.
280. Wilkins, R.M., and Johnston, R.M.: Ununited Fractures of the Clavicle. J. Bone Joint Surg., 65A:773–778, 1983.
281. Wood, V.E.: The Results of Total Claviculectomy. Clin. Orthop., 207:186–190, 1986.
282. Worcester, J.N., and Green, D.P.: Osteoarthritis of the Acromioclavicular Joint. Clin. Orthop., 58:69–73, 1968.
282a. Wurtz, L.D., Lyons, F.A., Rockwood, C.A., Jr.: Fracture of the Middle Third of the Clavicle and Dislocation of the Acromioclavicular Joint. J. Bone Joint Surg., 74:133–137, 1992.
282b. Xiao, X.Y.: [Treatment of Clavicular Fracture Patient With a Percutaneous Bone-Embracing External Clavicular Microfixer]. Chung Hua Wai Ko Tsa Chih, 31:657–659, 1993.
283. Yates, D.W.: Complications of Fractures of the Clavicle. Injury, 7:189–193, 1976.
284. Yates, A.G., and Guest, D.: Cerebral Embolus Due to Ununited Fracture of the Clavicle and Subclavian Thrombosis. Lancet, 2:225–226, 1928.
285. Young, C.S.: The Mechanics of Ambulatory Treatment of Fractures of the Clavicle. J. Bone Joint Surg., 13:299–310, 1931.
286. Zenni, E.J., Jr., Krieg, J.K., Rosen, M.J.: Open Reduction and Internal Fixation of Clavicular Fractures. J. Bone Joint Surg., 63A:147–151, 1981.

Rockwood and Green's Fractures in Adults, Fourth Edition,
edited by Charles A. Rockwood, David P. Green, Robert W. Bucholz and James D. Heckman.
Lippincott-Raven Publishers, Philadelphia © 1996.

CHAPTER 18

Fractures and Dislocations of the Scapula

Kenneth P. Butters

The scapula has an important role in arm function. It sits congruently against the ribs and stabilizes the upper extremity against the thorax. It also links the upper extremity and the axial skeleton through the glenoid, acromioclavicular, clavicle, and sternoclavicular joints. The scapula is subject to indirect injury through axial loading on the outstretched arm (scapular neck), through direct trauma—often high energy, from a blow or fall (body)—and through direct trauma to the point of the shoulder (acromion, coracoid). Shoulder dislocation may cause glenoid fracture. Traction by muscles or ligaments may cause avulsion fractures.

Fracture of the scapula occurs infrequently,[70] the incidence being 3% to 5% of shoulder girdle injuries[39,104] and 0.4% to 1% of all fractures.[86,122] This low incidence may be due to the scapula's thickened edges, its great mobility with recoil, and its position between layers of muscle. The mean age of patients with scapular fractures is 35 to 45.[3,69,119]

Associated injuries to other points in the shoulder girdle, the thoracic cage, and soft tissues are common and may lead to delayed diagnosis of the scapular fracture. Such problems as cervical spine fracture or vascular injury often require immediate attention. Operative surgical indications for scapular fracture are rare. Significant trauma is required to fracture the scapula, as evidenced by the cause of injury—motor vehicle accidents in about 50% of cases[49,69] and motorcycle accidents in 11% to 25%.

ANATOMY

The practice of orthopaedics is applied anatomy. Bony contour, muscle attachments, and the location of adjacent neurovascular structures should be understood in the evaluation of scapular fractures and certainly should be studied before surgery.

The anterior scapular surface is covered with the attachment of the subscapularis muscle, and the serratus anterior muscle attaches to the anterior medial border of the scapula (Figs. 18-1 and 18-2). The posterior scapula has on its surface the supraspinatus and infraspinatus muscles, and the trapezius muscle overlies the supraspinatus and attaches to the spine and clavicle (Fig. 18-3). The deltoid overlies a portion of the infraspinatus posteriorly and the lateral subscapularis anteriorly; its origin is from the scapular spine, acromion, and anterior clavicle. Many other muscles attach to the scapular margin—the levator scapulae and rhomboids to the medial border, the teres minor and teres major from the lateral border, and an inconsistent latissimus attachment to the inferior tip of the scapula. The pectoralis minor, the short head of the biceps, and the coracobrachialis attach to the coracoid; the long head of the biceps attaches to the superior glenoid; and the triceps attaches to the inferior glenoid (see Figs. 18-1 and 18-4).

The coracoid process projects upward, forward, and lateral from the superior border of the scapula. The brachial plexus and axillary artery run posterior to the pectoralis minor tendon, which inserts on the medial aspect of the base of the coracoid. Just medial to the coracoid base is the scapular notch, bridged by the transverse scapular ligament. The suprascapular nerve passes through the notch under the ligament, and the suprascapular artery passes over the ligament. The acromion continues laterally from the spine; a gap between it and the neck of the scapula constitutes the spinoglenoid notch, transmitting the suprascapular nerve and vessels to the infraspinatus. Figure 18-4*B* shows this relationship and the proximity of the axillary and suprascapular nerves and the brachial plexus to the scapula.

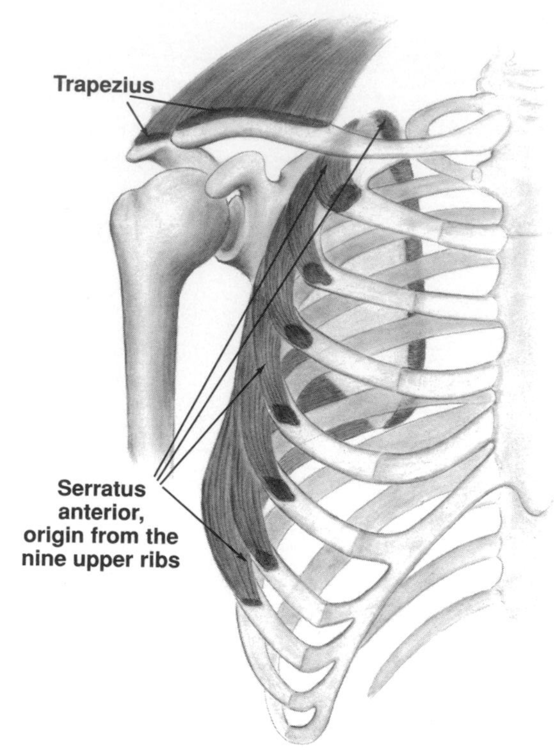

FIGURE 18-2. Schematic drawing showing the primary scapular stabilizing muscles. The serratus anterior passes deep to the scapula, attaching to the medial border holding the scapula against the chest wall.

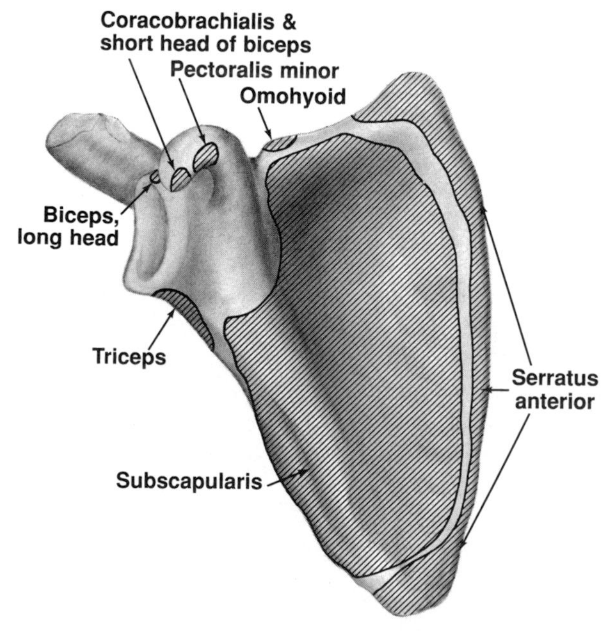

FIGURE 18-1. The muscle attachments to the anterior surface of the scapula.

The dorsal scapular and accessory nerves travel with the deep and superficial branches of the transverse cervical artery, respectively, parallel to and medial to the vertebral border of the scapula.

Most shoulder function involves simultaneous humeral and scapular movements with a definite rhythm. The scapula is a platform for the upper extremity. It rotates into abduction to assist the arm with forward elevation and undergoes abduction, elevation, or depression to help position the extremity. With all these movements, the scapula is in its bed against the chest wall. Scapular fracture malunion, soft-tissue scarring, and muscle and nerve injury can all affect rhythm and limit scapular excursion, decreasing shoulder motion.

CLASSIFICATION

Certain fracture patterns are seen in the scapula. They are described by anatomical area for ease of discussion (ie, body and spine, glenoid neck, intra-articular gle-

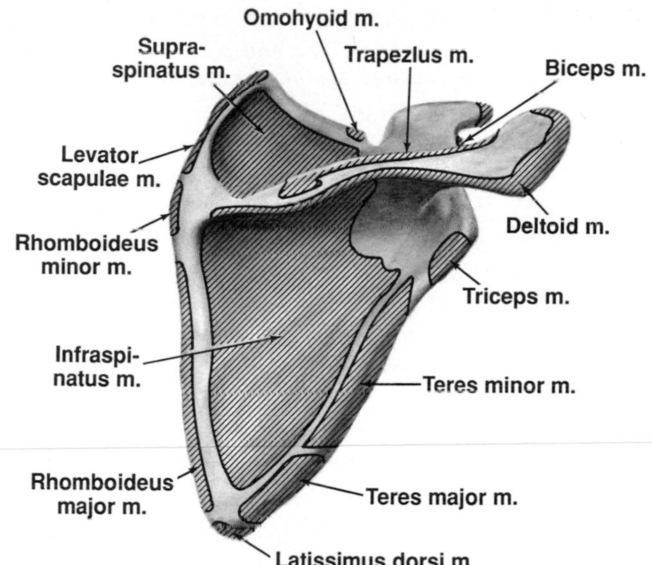

FIGURE 18-3. The muscle attachments to the posterior surface of the scapula.

noid, coracoid, and acromion). Several areas of the scapula are often involved, but the neck (10% to 60%) and body (49% to 89%) are most common.[3,49,69,121] Zdravkovic and Damholt[125] divided scapular fractures into three types: type I, fractures of the body; type II, fractures of the apophysis, including the coracoid and acromion; and type III, fractures of the superior lateral angle, including the neck and glenoid. This classification was devised to separate the type III fracture, which is generally considered the most difficult to treat. Displaced or comminuted type III (neck and glenoid) fractures constituted only 6% of this entire series of scapular fractures.

Thompson and colleagues,[119] in their trauma center series of wide-impact blunt trauma, classified scapular fractures into class I, the coracoid and acromion and small fractures of the body; class II, the glenoid and neck; and class III, major scapular body fractures. Class II and III fractures were much more likely to have associated injuries. Ideberg[48] has proposed a classification of six types of intra-articular glenoid fractures (described later in this chapter).

Goss[37c] described an alternative method of describing certain shoulder injuries, including some scapular fractures. He named the superior shoulder suspensory complex (SSSC) as a bony/soft-tissue ring composed

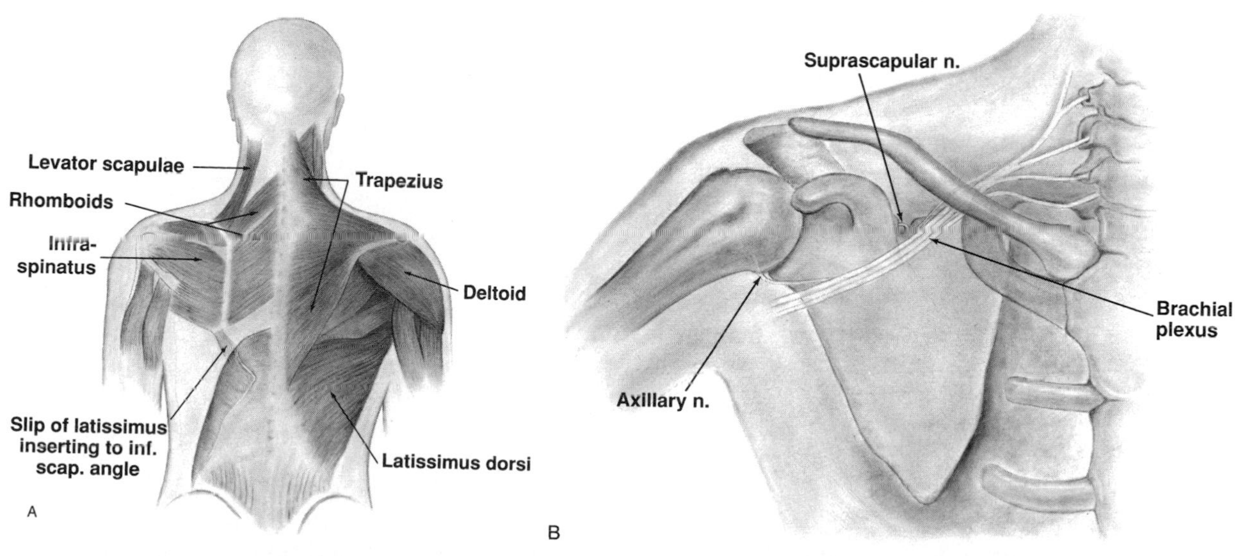

FIGURE 18-4. (A) The posterior torso musculature, superficial (*right*) and deep (*left*). (B) A schematic diagram showing the positions of the brachial plexus relative to the scapula.

of the glenoid, coracoid, acromion, distal clavicle, and the connecting ligaments. The complex maintains the stable relationship between the upper extremity and the axial skeleton. Single disruptions remain stable; double disruptions create a potentially unstable anatomical situation leading to later problems.

Displaced distal clavicle fractures and complete acromioclavicular separations would qualify as double disruptions but are usually treated nonoperatively unless there is "unacceptable displacement."

A glenoid neck fracture plus a disruption to the acromioclavicular joint or clavicle fracture would be an indication for surgery using this concept.

A glenoid fossa fracture type III (displaced intra-articular) through the upper glenoid plus a second disruption of the clavicle or acromion would be another good example. The treatment principles based on this anatomical description include indication for open reduction to be a double disruption plus displacement likely to lead to a delayed union or to adverse functional consequences for the shoulder girdle. Understanding the concept allows the surgeon to evaluate the scapular injury and recommend a treatment with which he or she is comfortable.

CLINICAL PRESENTATION

Throughout the literature, a classic clinical description of scapular fracture, that of the scapular glenoid neck, is noted. According to Hitzrot and Bolling,[45] Sir Astley Cooper described flattening of the shoulder and prominence of the acromion. When the deformity was reduced by supporting the elbow, the movement was associated with bony crepitus. Interestingly, two of his three cases proved to be humeral neck fractures. Some authors have tried to make a clinical diagnosis by measuring arm length or midline-to-coracoid distance[45] without finding that this offers consistent, accurate help in diagnosis.

The typical presentation is that the arm is held adducted and protected from all movements, with abduction especially painful. Local tenderness is present. The shoulder may appear flattened with a displaced neck or acromion fracture. Ecchymosis is less than expected from the degree of bony injury present, as opposed to fracture of the upper humerus. Pain with deep inspiration may be present with coracoid fracture (pectoralis minor) or body fracture (serratus anterior). One should always be aware of the possibility of associated pneumothorax, either immediate or delayed. With body fractures especially, deep swelling may be quite painful, producing "pseudorupture of the rotator cuff."[85] Neviaser[85] described the syndrome of weak cuff function and loss of active arm elevation, which is probably only inhibition of muscle contractions from intramuscular hemorrhage and which usually resolves within a few weeks. This syndrome can be differentiated from rotator cuff tear, since the fracture is seen on radiography and the swelling present with fracture and pseudorupture syndrome exceeds that normally seen with a cuff tear. As noted, a scapular fracture is often accompanied by associated injuries needing more urgent treatment.

ASSOCIATED INJURIES

Significant associated injuries occur in 35% to 98% of patients with scapular fractures. The higher incidence is attributed to admissions to trauma units for serious injuries.[3,30,49,69,119,121] This figure reflects the degree of trauma necessary to fracture the scapula.

Fischer and colleagues[30] and Thompson and associates[119] have stated that direct scapular trauma and resultant scapular body fracture from wide-impact trauma have a particularly high incidence of associated ipsilateral upper torso injuries, so these fractures should be regarded as warnings. Similarly, the diagnosis of scapular fracture is often delayed while more urgent care is provided.[3]

Pneumothorax was found in 16 of 30 patients in a prospective study of fractured scapulae.[71] Interestingly, 10 of the 16 pneumothoraces were delayed in onset from 1 to 3 days. A follow-up chest radiograph, physical examination, and blood gas determinations should therefore be considered in patients with scapular fractures. Other series have reported a lower overall incidence of pneumothorax (11% to 38%).[3,30,119]

Ipsilateral fractured ribs are present in 27% to 54% of cases.[119] Correlation with pneumothorax is probably strong enough to warrant a prophylactic chest tube before early surgery is done for other injuries.[30] Armstrong and Vanderspuy found a fracture of the scapula with an underlying first rib fracture a particularly severe injury.[3]

Pulmonary contusion, which can be a life-threatening associated injury, is present in 11% to 54% of scapular fractures.[30,119] This injury may result in marked oxygen desaturation requiring tracheal intubation and positive end-expiratory pressure ventilation. Figure 18-5 illustrates several common associated injuries. Fracture of the clavicle frequently (23% to 39%) is associated with a fracture of the glenoid or glenoid neck. This may represent a continuation of an impaction force. Brachial plexus injury (5% to 13%) is usually a supraclavicular type with a poor prognosis.[3,30,49,69,119] In their series, McGahan and colleagues noted the association of brachial plexus injury with injuries about the acromion. They postulated that this may be due to depression of the shoulder and contralateral neck flexion as a mechanism of injury.[67,82]

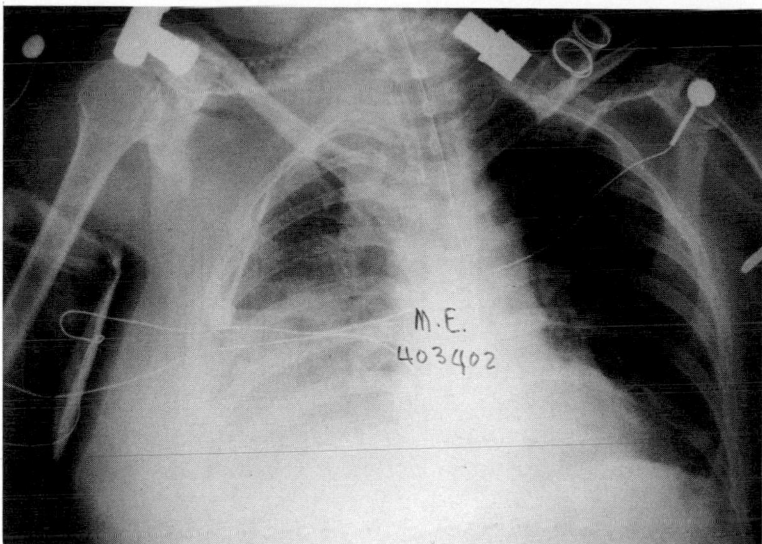

FIGURE 18-5. X-ray of a multiple trauma patient with a fractured neck of the scapula and associated upper extremity fractures and pulmonary contusion.

However, in Fischer and coworkers'[30] series of badly injured patients in the trauma unit, 70% of the brachial plexus injuries seen occurred with major body fracture caused by wide, blunt trauma. Also, 57% of those patients with scapular fracture and a brachial plexus injury also had arterial injury of the ipsilateral upper torso. A scapular fracture alone had an 11% incidence of arterial injury. Case reports in the literature of nerve and arterial injuries[69,89,114] with scapular fracture supplement the trauma studies and reinforce the importance of a complete neurovascular examination. Skull fractures, which occur in 24% of patients with scapular fractures, and closed head injuries, which occur in 20%, generate concern, especially with a history of loss of consciousness.[69] Folman and associates[31B] studied 25 cases of scapula fractures and traumatic paralysis. Seventy-six percent were in the thoracic spine, 20% in the lower cervical spine, and 4% in the lumbar spine.

Distal extremity and spinal injury, blunt abdominal trauma, and pelvic fracture are all reported to increase in occurrence with major scapular body fracture.

Associated injuries were responsible for the 15% mortality that occurred with scapular fracture in the patients reported by Fischer and colleagues[30] and in 10% of the patients reported by Armstrong and Vanderspuy.[3] Half of these deaths were from pulmonary contusion with sepsis. Landi and colleagues[58a] discussed compartment syndrome of the scapula and presented the Comolli sign, which is a triangular swelling on the posterior thorax overlying the scapula. They stated that the subscapularis can swell toward the thorax, but the fascia on the spinati is less yielding. One of their patients had a scapula fracture, presence of Comolli sign, and increased measured pressures in the spinati, improving with surgical decompression of the hematoma.

In summary, then, the presence of scapular fracture on initial anteroposterior chest radiograph is an indication for a good workup for additional torso and extremity trauma on the injured side. The converse is also true. The presence of fracture or soft-tissue injury about the thorax should lead one to search for a scapular fracture. In McGahan's and associates'[69] and Armstrong and Vanderspuy's[3] series, 50% of the fractures had grave associated injuries and no scapular surgery could even be carried out, indicating simple immobilization treatment followed by range-of-motion exercises. Harris and Harris[40a] published a study of chest radiographs from 100 patients with scapula fracture, and in only 57% was a fracture appreciated on the initial chest film. Also, in only 2 of 100 radiographs was a scapula fracture the only skeletal injury seen in the thorax.

RADIOGRAPHIC FINDINGS

Fracture of the scapula requires radiographic diagnosis, but visualization is not always easy. Superimposition of the thorax may cloud the structural details of the scapula; however, most scapular fractures can be adequately evaluated by multiple plane views. A single view cannot provide all the information. A true anteroposterior view of the shoulder and an axillary and true scapular lateral view (trauma series) show glenoid (Fig. 18-6), neck, body (Fig. 18-7), and acromion (Fig. 18-8) fractures. The axillary lateral view is helpful for acromial and glenoid rim fractures, and the cephalic tilt or Stryker notch view is useful for coracoid frac-

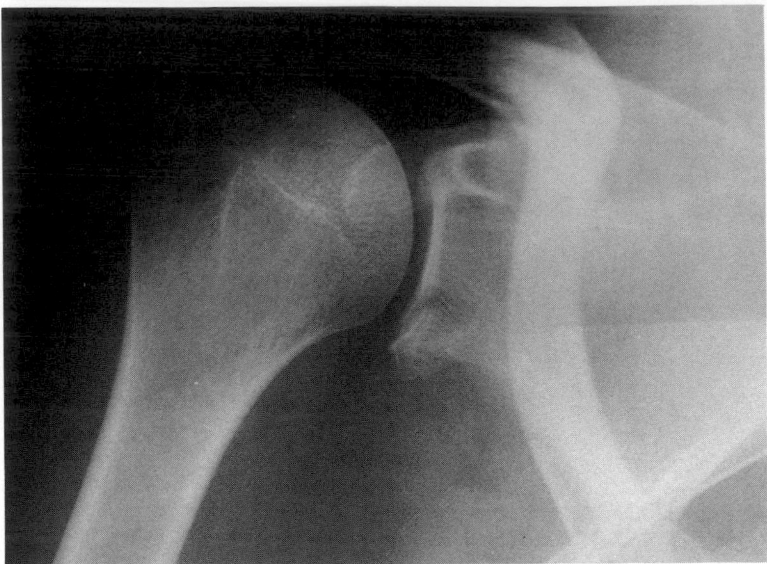

FIGURE 18-6. A true anteroposterior view of the glenoid showing an anteroinferior glenoid fracture.

tures (Fig. 18-9). Tomograms have not been very helpful in the overall evaluation of scapular fractures; they can be used in carefully chosen planes to evaluate union or displacement of the fracture; anteroposterior tomograms for intra-articular glenoid fracture are especially useful.

The oblique position of the scapula on the chest wall and its narrow width make tomographic evaluation difficult to interpret. Computed tomography (CT) in the standard transverse plane again may not allow a three-dimensional concept of the fracture. The CT scan can be used in evaluating a glenoid fracture to confirm

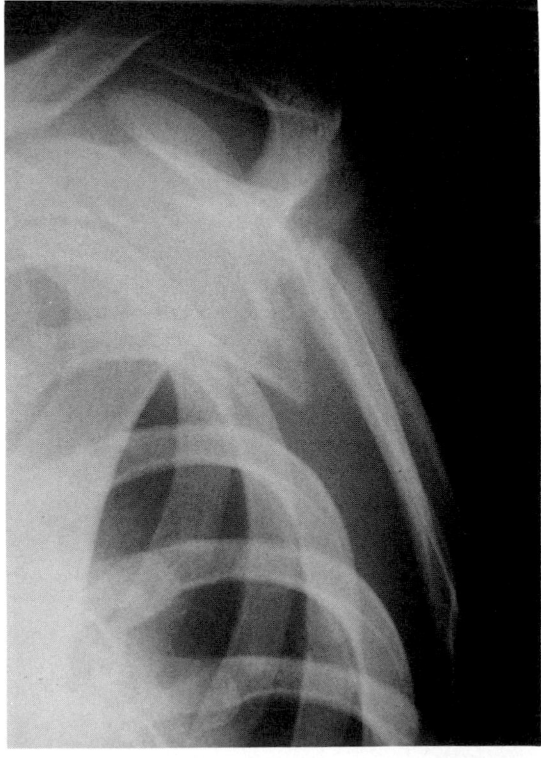

FIGURE 18-7. A true (tangential) scapular lateral view (trauma series lateral view) showing a displaced scapular body fracture with a bayonet position.

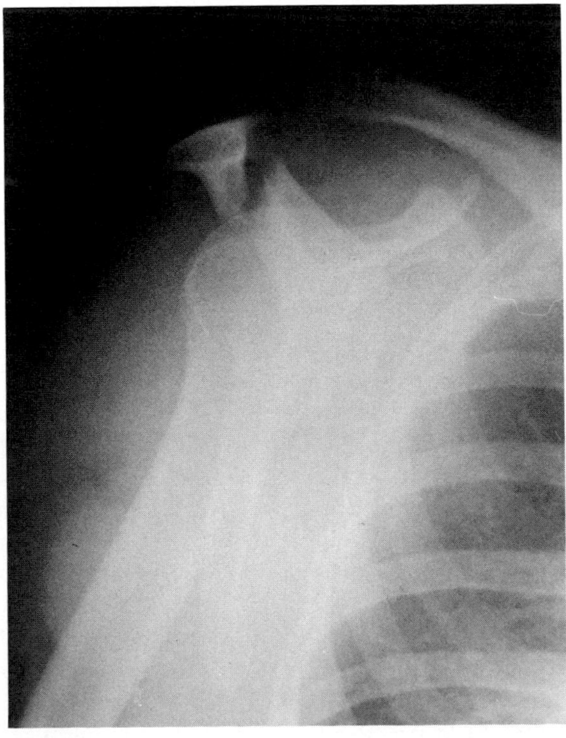

FIGURE 18-8. The fractured base of the acromion is well seen on a true (tangential) scapular lateral view.

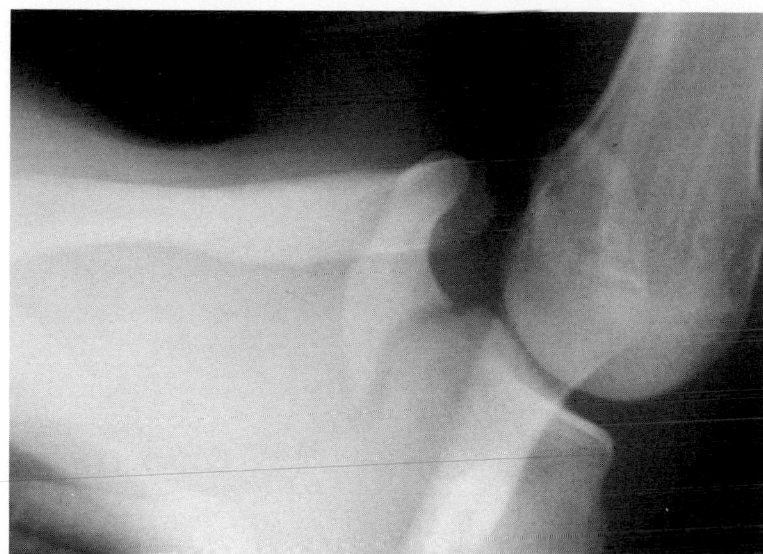

FIGURE 18-9. A fracture of the base of the coracoid is best seen on a Stryker notch view.

the reduced position of the humeral head. A three-dimensional reconstruction can be used to evaluate the shoulder girdle complex.[87]

DIFFERENTIAL DIAGNOSIS

Epiphyseal Lines

Most important in the discussion of differential diagnosis is understanding the development of the scapula and its ossification pattern.[67,90,117] At birth the body and spine form one ossified mass, and the coracoid, acromion, glenoid, and inferior angle are all cartilaginous. At 3 to 18 months of age, a center of ossification, which may be bipolar, appears at the midcoracoid. At 7 to 10 years of age, the coracoid base, including the upper third of the glenoid, appears. Sometimes called a subcoracoid bone, it joins the rest of the coracoid at 14 to 16 years of age (adolescence). An ossification center at the tip and a shell-like center at the medial apex of the coracoid may appear at the same time and go on to fusion at ages 18 to 25 (Figs. 18-10 and 18-11).

Two or three acromial centers form at ages 14 to 16, coalesce at age 19, and fuse to the spine at ages 20 to 25. Failure of this to occur, with persistence of one ossification center past age 25, is known as *os acromiale.*

The glenoid fossa ossifies from four sources: (1) the coracoid base (including the upper third of the glenoid); (2) the deep portion of the coracoid process; (3) the body; and (4) the lower pole (joining the body at ages 20 to 25 and deepening the glenoid cavity). At ages 8 to 13 the glenoid border may be dentate from irregular ossification.[54]

At the inferior angle of the scapula, an ossification center appears at age 15 and fuses at age 20; the vertebral border center appears at ages 16 to 18 and fuses by the 25th year. The ossification centers may be asymmetric, and comparison films may not be helpful.

Os Acromiale

Clinically, os acromiale is the best-known separate bone, resulting from failure of coalescence of the adjacent ossification centers. It simulates acromial fracture. The open epiphyseal line occurs at the level of the acromioclavicular joint (Fig. 18-12).[9] (Interestingly, Liberson's classic 1937 study was stimulated by a worker's compensation claim.[61]) The unfused apophysis is present in 2.7% of random patients and when present is bilateral in 60%.[61] Four ossification centers are present in the acromion, as seen in Figure 18-13. The most common site of nonunion is between the mesoacromion and the meta-acromion at the midacromioclavicular joint. An axillary lateral radiograph is essential for an accurate description. Factors favoring the diagnosis of os acromiale over fracture are bilateral occurrence, rounded borders with uniform space, and the position of the bony ossification center even with or above the posterior acromion on the anteroposterior view. Norris[88] has reported that the unfused physis has been mistaken for fracture and that there is an association between os acromiale and rotator cuff tear. Fracture separation, or at least some movement at this site, has been seen during acromioplasty, and bone graft plus surgical fixation with pins or screws at the time of cuff repair has been necessary.[82,83]

Glenoid Dysplasia

Scapular neck dysplasia (hypoplasia of the glenoid) resembling an impaction of the glenoid may have an associated acromial or humeral head abnormality. It

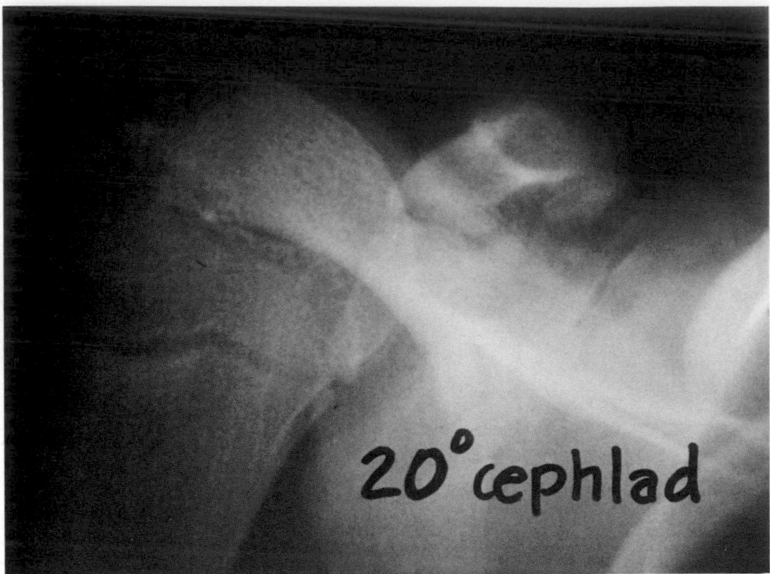

FIGURE 18-10. A normal ossification pattern at the base of the coracoid. A crescent-shaped center is seen at the apex of the coracoid.

usually has a benign course; many cases are found inadvertently, first being evaluated in the sixth or seventh decade of life.[95,99] Rockwood has seen glenoid dysplasia present in individuals of college age that become symptomatic with increased athletic use of the shoulder.[100] Wirth and associates[122b] reviewed the records of 16 patients, 15 to 62 years old, who had glenoid hypoplasia with or without an associated deformity of the humeral head. The patients were divided into three groups: (1) those who had bilateral glenoid hypoplasia without instability of the shoulder, (2) those who had bilateral glenoid hypoplasia with instability of the shoulder, and (3) those who had unilateral glenoid hypoplasia with deformity of the humeral head. When first seen, 13 of the 16 patients had pain in the shoulder, which they had noted after an increase in their previous level of activity. All were managed with a specific rehabilitation program for the shoulder. The patients were followed for an average of 5 years, and most were able to return to their previous level of activity with the resolution of the symptoms. One might suspect an increased incidence of impingement with medial head position and less rotator cuff lever arm. Figure 18-14 is a radiograph of a 60-year-old patient with mild shoulder pain and stiffness.

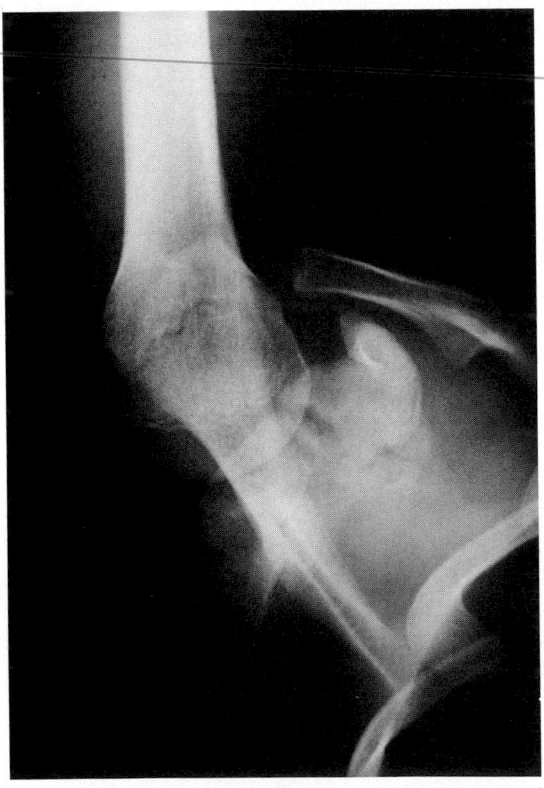

FIGURE 18-11. An epiphyseal line is seen across the upper third of the glenoid. It serves as a common growth plate for the upper portion of the glenoid and for the base of the coracoid process. This may be confused with a fracture and is the precise location of most type III glenoid fractures.

Normal Scapular Foramina

Scapular foramina[99] from disrupted ossification of the body and neck are common. They appear benign and are well circumscribed.

TREATMENT

Glenoid Neck (Extra-articular) Fracture

The literature of the early 20th century interestingly parallels that of today. A fractured scapula was thought to be produced by trauma, usually of great violence, with associated injuries. The treatment was usually

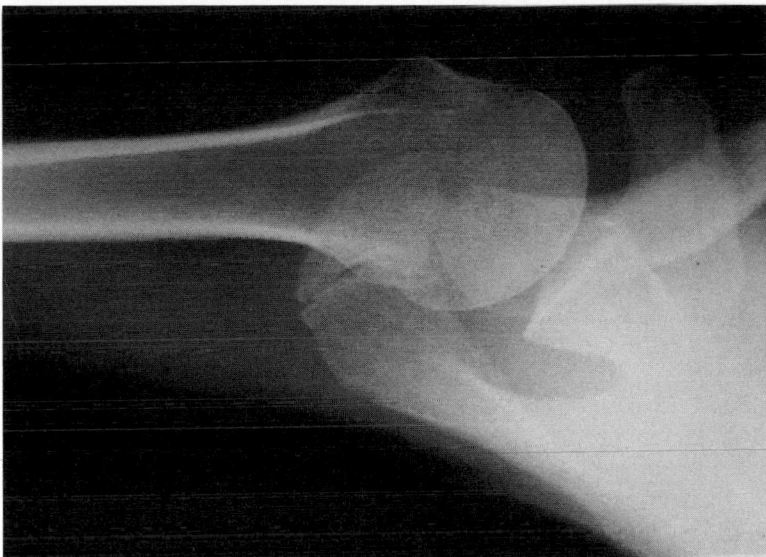

FIGURE 18-12. Os acromiale.

conservative. The published work focused on displaced scapular neck fractures. Scudder[112] believed that traction with abduction of the arm was helpful. In 1992, Van Wellen and coworkers[119A] published a case report using a traction suspension system for reduction of a displaced neck fracture. Cotton and Brickley[18] in 1921 described a closed reduction, using an axillary pad and 3 weeks of bed rest with "hypnotics" and a pillow placed between the scapulae. Hitzrot and Bolling,[45] in 1916, believed that manipulation and traction had no effect, and even with displaced fractures the results were satisfactory enough that reduction attempts were unnecessary. The posterior approach was used if surgery was done on intra-articular fractures. Findlay,[29] in 1931, kept his patients with scapular body fractures flat in bed for 10 days. Most authors agreed that "early motion" was important.

A fracture of the neck of the scapula is probably the second most common scapular fracture, occurring from direct trauma, a fall on the point of the shoulder, or a fall on the outstretched arm from impaction. True anteroposterior, tangential scapular lateral, and axillary lateral radiographs and often CT scans are necessary to confirm the extra-articular nature of the fracture and the reduced position of the humeral head.

With neck fracture, the glenoid articular surface is intact and the fracture pattern extends from the suprascapular notch area across the neck to the lateral border of the scapula. The glenoid and coracoid may be comminuted or remain as an intact unit. The glenoid neck fracture is often displaced, but an intact clavicle and acromioclavicular joint will limit this displacement and enhance stability as opposed to what occurs with the clavicle fracture seen in Figure 18-15.

Reduction of the scapular neck fracture and restoration of the glenoid to its anatomical position may not be necessary. Sling immobilization for comfort is probably enough. Further displacement is rare. In a study of neck and body fractures, Lindblom and Leven found

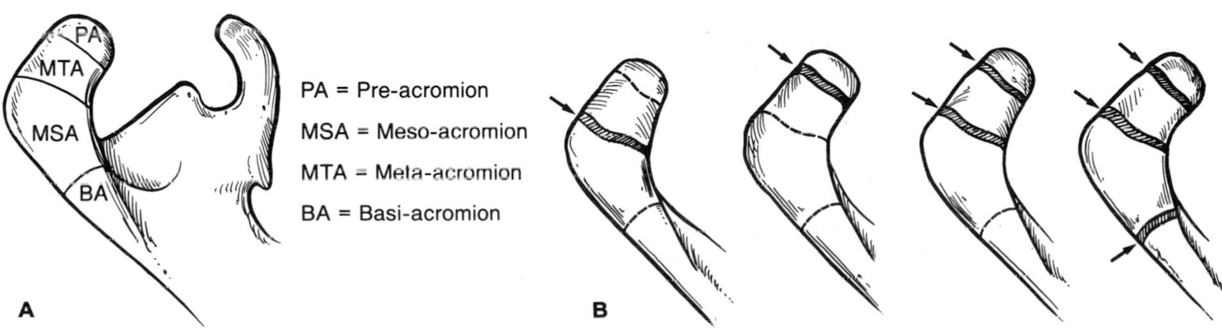

FIGURE 18-13. (A) The diagram represents the ossification centers of the acromion. (B) The most common site of failure of ossification is between the mesoacromion and the meta-acromion.

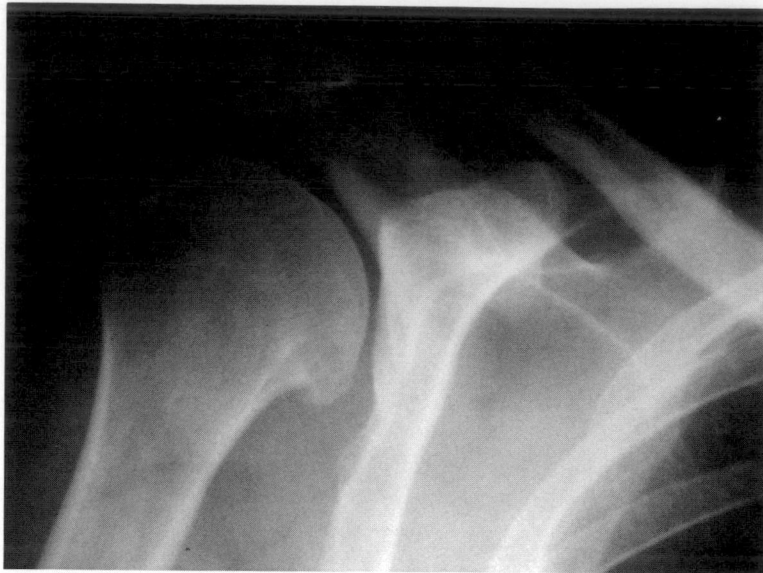

FIGURE 18-14. Scapular dysplasia.

that, if untreated, all healed in the position displayed at the time of the primary examination.[62]

For displaced fracture, DePalma[21] recommends closed reduction and olecranon pin traction for 3 weeks, followed by use of a sling. Bateman[6] favored closed reduction in a shoulder spica for 6 to 8 weeks in those cases in which "shortening of the neck is sufficient to favor subluxation or interfere with abduction." McLaughlin[70] believed that most neck fractures were impacted, making attempts at correction difficult. Neer[83a] believes that the functional result of glenoid neck fractures is not related to the radiographic appearance and open reduction is only necessary for the associated clavicle fracture.

Many series report good range of motion and function in follow-up of neck and body fractures (Fig. 18-16).[48,62,121] Armstrong and Vanderspuy[3] reported that some residual stiffness was present in six of seven neck fractures, but their patients had no functional disability. Zdravkovic and Damholt[125] came to the same conclusion in a study with an average follow-up of 9 years. Gagney and colleagues[34] found a good result in only 1 of 12 displaced fractures. They thought that the injury would "disorganize the coracoacromial arch" and recommended open reduction. A fractured surgical neck may be significantly displaced. Hardegger and coworkers[39] believed that the amount of displacement and stability depends on the presence of an associated fracture of the clavicle or a coracoclavicular ligament tear. The altered glenohumeral-acromial re-

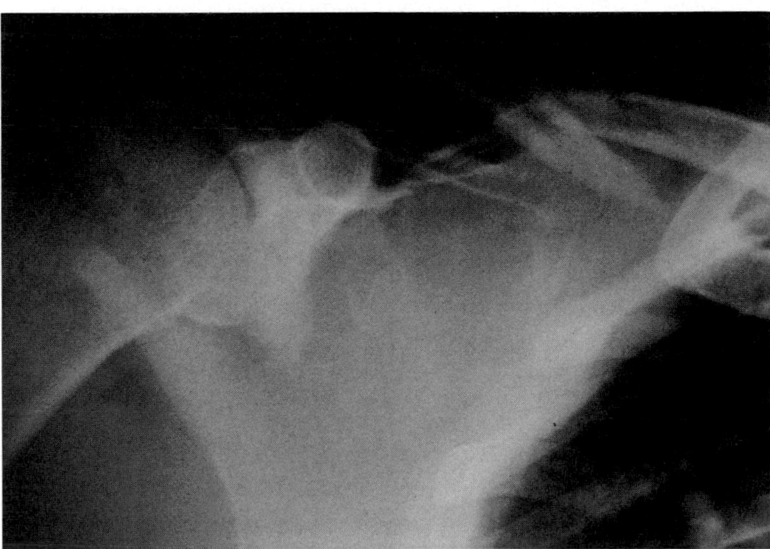

FIGURE 18-15. Scapular neck fracture with an associated body and clavicle fracture.

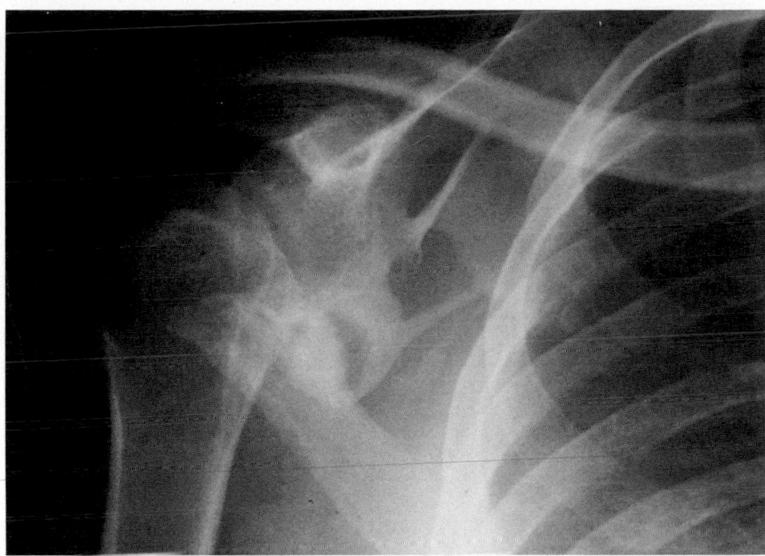

FIGURE 18-16. Healed glenoid neck fracture with marked medial displacement. The patient had a full range of shoulder motion.

lationship results in "functional imbalance." They recommended open reduction and scapular fixation of this fracture. Figure 18-17 is a radiograph of such a scapular neck fracture with an associated fractured clavicle, and Figure 18-18 shows the importance of an intact clavicle in glenoid fracture stability.

Ada and Miller[1] found, in 16 patients with displaced and glenoid neck fractures treated closed, 40% had weakness of abduction, 50% had subacromial and night pain, and 20% had decreased range of motion.

Eight patients treated surgically with open reduction through a posterior approach had no complications and no rest or night pain and what they described as greater than 85% of glenohumeral motion. They recommended open reduction of the fracture if the glenoid neck fracture is angulated at 40° or displaced greater than 1 cm.

Leung and Lam[60a] reported 15 cases of fractured clavicle and glenoid neck fractures, citing the indication "loss of the normal lever arm of the cuff." They recommended open reduction of both the clavicle and glenoid, stating this was better than fixation of the clavicle alone.

Wilkes and Halawa,[121a] in a case with limited abduction, reported on osteotomies to correct inferolateral angulation of the glenoid and clavicle malunion. Both osteotomies united and the range of motion improved.

Glenoid (Intra-articular) Fracture

Intra-articular glenoid fractures may lure the orthopaedist into choosing surgical treatment. In the past decade there was greater interest in open reduction of these glenoid fractures to lessen the possibility of

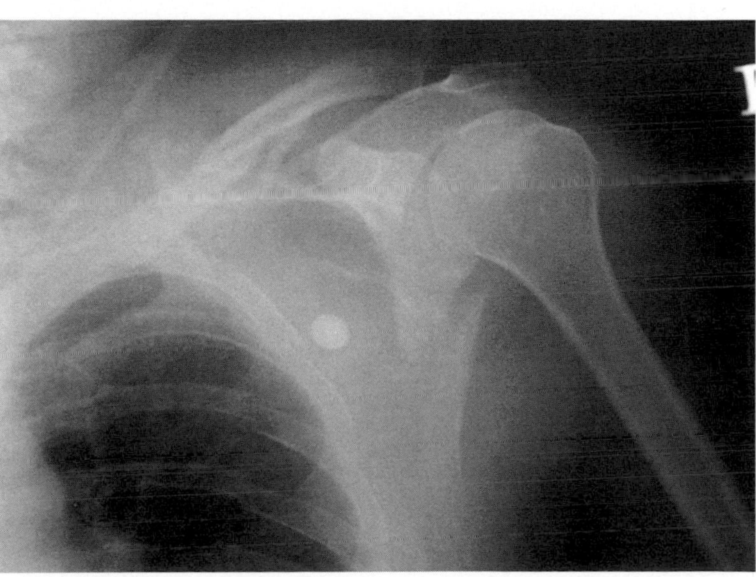

FIGURE 18-17. Surgical stabilization should be utilized for this unstable glenoid neck fracture associated with a fractured clavicle. The author has used clavicular plate fixation.

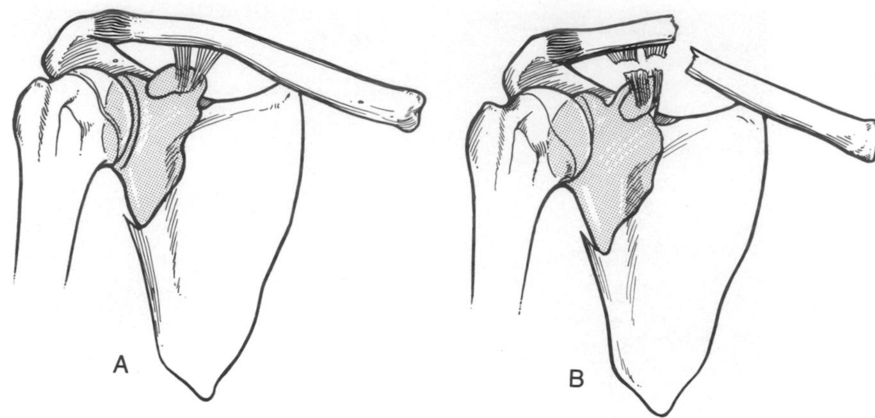

FIGURE 18-18. These diagrams show the distinction between stable (A) and unstable (B) scapular neck fractures. The association of a scapular neck fracture with either a fractured clavicle or disruption of the coracoclavicular ligament creates an unstable fracture.

traumatic arthritis.[37A,50a] True anteroposterior, axillary lateral, and West Point views, Stryker notch view, and often CT scans and anteroposterior tomograms are needed to assess these fractures. A direct force on the lateral shoulder or indirect axial compression of the extremity may cause a stellate glenoid fracture. Most of these require no reduction since the head remains centered (Figs. 18-19 and 18-20).

Ideberg[47,48] classified glenoid fractures into five types (Fig. 18-21), based on 300 cases: type I—fractures of the glenoid rim; type IA—anterior and type IB—posterior are distinct from the small avulsions occurring with traumatic instability; type II—transverse fracture through the glenoid fossa, with an inferior triangular fragment displaced with the humeral head; type III—oblique fracture through the glenoid exiting at the midsuperior border of the scapula, often associated with acromioclavicular fracture or acromioclavicular dislocation; type IV—horizontal, exiting through the medial border of the blade; and type V—which combines type IV with a fracture separating the inferior half of the glenoid. Goss[37e] included type VI, which is severe comminution of the glenoid surface.

Type I

A type I fracture is an anterior avulsion fracture occurring from traumatic instability or from direct injury. These fractures, if displaced, may predispose to instability. Usually, continuity is maintained between the capsule, labrum, and fracture fragment. Interestingly, however, a history of recurrent dislocation may precede the episode, causing a fracture of the anterior glenoid margin. Figure 18-22 shows such a fracture repaired with open reduction and AO screw fixation.

Ideberg believed that the size of the fragment is not prognostic for further instability. DePalma[21] thought that displacements greater than 10 mm, particularly if the size of the fragment is one fourth that of the glenoid, would indicate an open reduction. Late open reduction of the displaced fragment or reconstruction of the anterior gle-

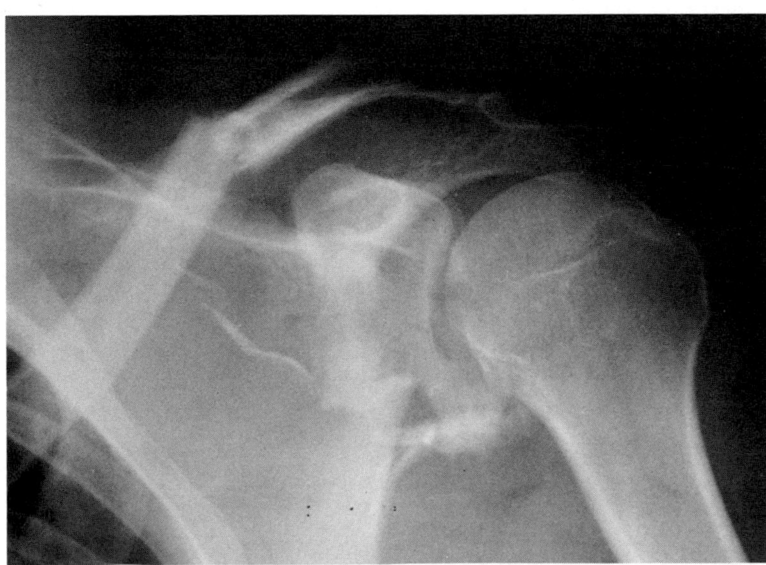

FIGURE 18-19. Comminuted glenoid articular surface fracture with satisfactory position.

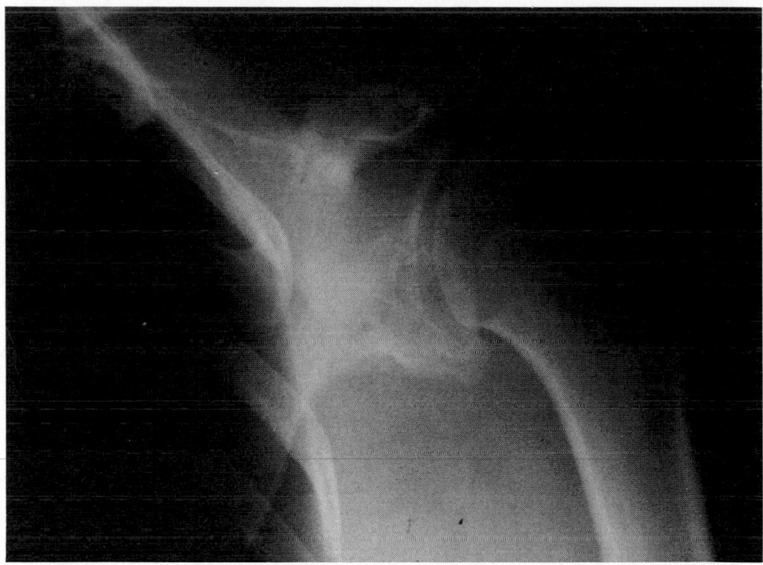

FIGURE 18-20. The fracture in Figure 18-19 healed well without problems and with good preservation of the joint surface.

noid is difficult, often requiring a bone graft or coracoid bone block. In their Bankart study, Rowe and colleagues[107] found that those fractures involving one fourth or even one third of the glenoid had equal success with repair compared with those in which one sixth or less of the glenoid was involved.

According to Rockwood,[100] a fracture involving one fourth of the glenoid fossa that is associated with shoulder instability is an indication for open reduction of the fragment with screw fixation. A CT scan is helpful in determining fragment size and humeral head position (Fig. 18-23). An anterior approach allows excellent exposure for type IA fractures and a posterior approach for type IB.

Ideberg's indication for operation is persisting subluxation or an unstable reduction (recurrent instability soon after reduction). No details were given, but 125 to 130 cases of glenoid avulsion in Ideberg's report had a satisfactory outcome. Of the 68 patients with associated dislocations, 11 had surgery, 5 with satisfactory results.

A distinction must be made between a glenoid type I fracture and a small glenoid rim or labrum avulsion fracture, which is commonly seen with traumatic anterior shoulder instability. These latter lesions are evidence of injury from traumatic anterior instability, not an indication for acute repair or reconstruction. Posterior rim fractures are much less common, and similar judgment is applied.

When the decision is made to treat a large anterior glenoid fracture nonsurgically, a follow-up radiograph must be taken and a physical examination done. A chronic dislocation may occur, especially in older patients, and postreduction resubluxation may go unnoticed.[57]

Type II

A type II fracture involves a transverse or oblique fracture through the glenoid with the inferior glenoid as a free fragment. The humeral head may subluxate inferiorly, with the fragment leading the surgeon to consider open reduction (Figs. 18-24 to 18-26).

Type III

A type III fracture involves the upper third of the glenoid and includes the coracoid; it may occur along the old epiphyseal line separating ossification centers. This fracture is often accompanied by a fractured acromion or clavicle or by acromioclavicular separation (Figs. 18-27 to 18-29). Goss[37e] recommends, as in all intra-articular fractures, open reduction for a step-off of 5 mm or greater.

Intact glenohumeral ligaments may keep the incongruity slight, and early motion may spontaneously improve fracture position. Open reduction is difficult, as it is in type II fractures. One technique uses an anterior arthrotomy (deltopectoral approach) as used for anterior reconstruction, plus superior exposure for a superior-to-inferior glenoid screw. Partial-thickness clavicle removal or even resection of the distal clavicle may need to be done to clear a path for the screw. These injuries may reduce nicely with open glenoid reduction and screw fixation, but additional stabilization of a superior suspensory complex disruption may be necessary. Such additional fixation may also be good treatment, improving the position of a comminuted glenoid fracture. Five of Ideberg's 17 cases of type III fractures had a poor result, usually with associated injuries. Only one of the 17 had open reduction.

Type IV

A type IV fracture is a horizontal glenoid fracture extending all the way through the body to the vertebral border. Four of Ideberg's 23 patients had poor results from an extra-articular origin, and 3 of the 23 had poor results from glenoid irregularity. Open reduction should be considered in the separated fracture or dis-

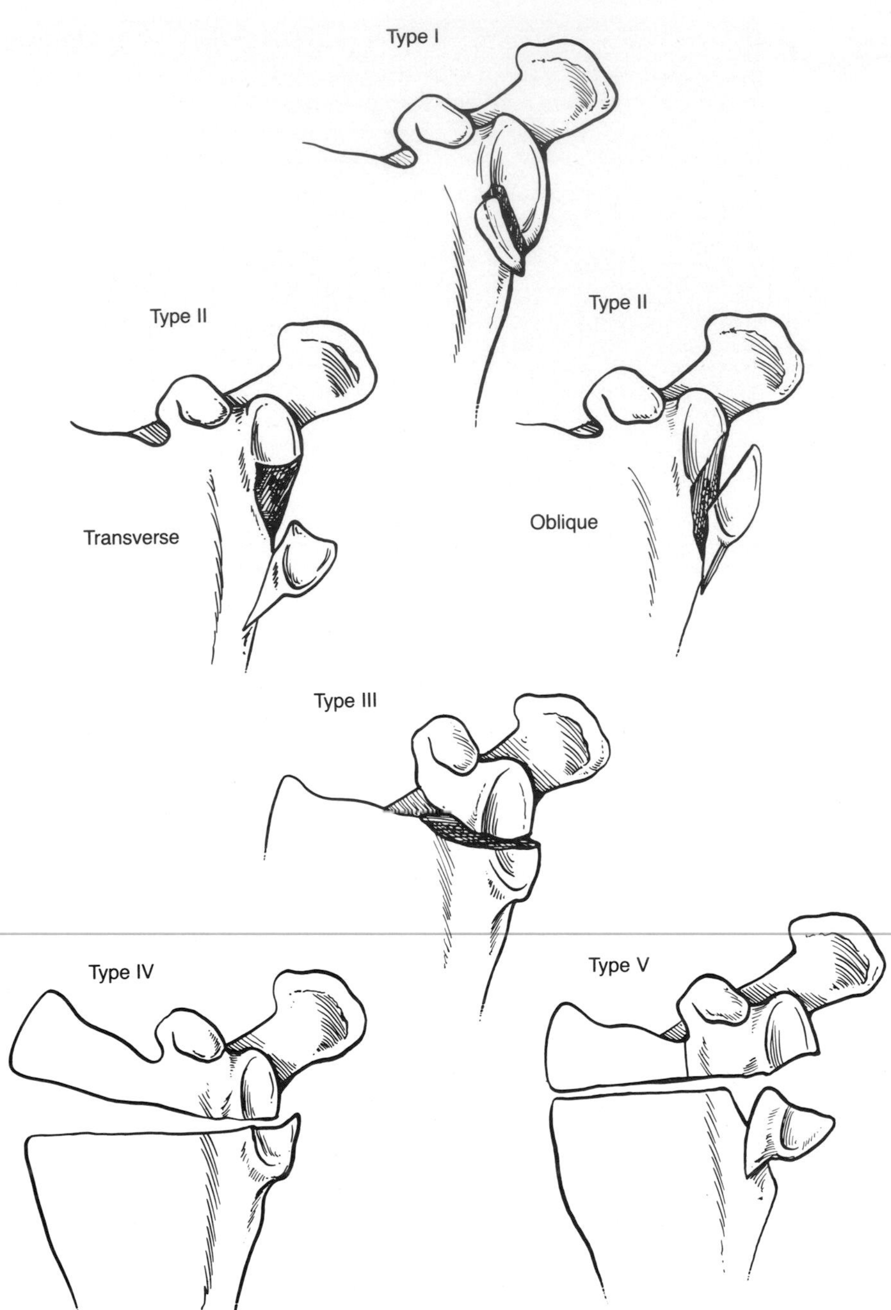

FIGURE 18-21. Ideberg's classification of intra-articular fracture of the glenoid into five types based on fracture patterns.

placed fracture, especially if the superior fragment of the glenoid is displaced laterally.

Type V

Type V fractures combine types II and IV. Direct violent trauma was the cause in most cases, often delaying scapular treatment and probably influencing the results. Interestingly, of the 7 patients of 20 who had poor results, all 7 had surgery, whereas only 1 of 13 with good results had open reduction (Figs. 18-30 and 18-31). The same judgment used for types II and III should be used in determining the need for open reduction, being more conservative if the humeral head is well centered. Type VI is a badly comminuted fracture best treated with early motion.

Ideberg's experiences with fractures of types II through V, which represent 40% of the total series, are summarized as follows. Closed reduction under anesthesia was always unsuccessful in improving fracture position at the time, but some late improvement in displacement was seen in most of the conservatively treated fractures. This improvement in fracture position may come from molding by muscle forces across the joint. A good result occurred in 75% of the cases

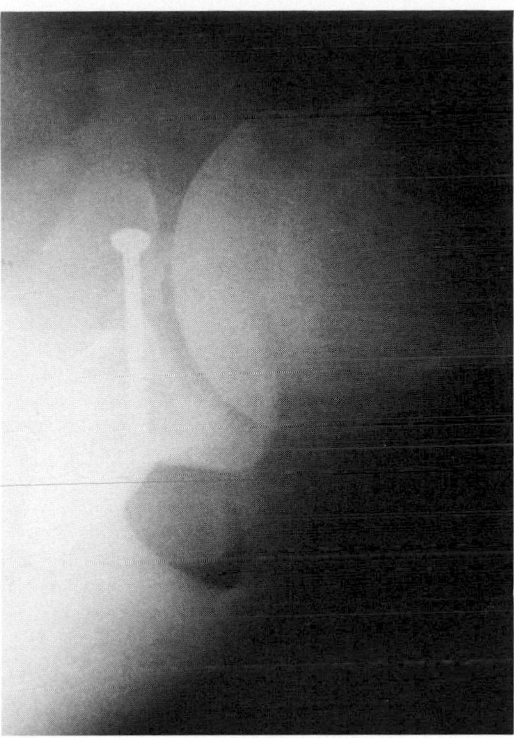

FIGURE 18-22. Anterior glenoid fracture seen on an axillary view after open reduction and internal fixation.

of types II to V and was obtained mainly by early mobilization. Open reduction, however, can also produce a good result. Associated problems, such as other fractures about the shoulder, nerve, or muscle lesions, may worsen the outcome.

Some European literature suggests a more aggressive surgical indication to treatment of scapular fractures. Basing their evaluation on true anteroposterior, tangential scapular lateral, and axillary lateral radiographs, Hardegger and coworkers[39] described eight varieties of fracture with some surgical indication: (1) fracture of the body with a lateral spike entering the joint; (2) fracture of the glenoid rim with instability after reduction of dislocation; (3) fracture of the glenoid fossa, displaced; (4) extra-articular fracture of the glenoid neck with lateral and distal displacement; (5) similar displaced neck fractures with a displaced clavicle fracture or coracoclavicular ligament rupture; (6) fracture of the acromion (if significant displacement is present, nonunion may develop or the deltoid may tilt the acromion fragment inferiorly, interfering with rotator cuff function); (7) fracture of the coracoid, displaced with neurovascular compression or with coracoclavicular ligament rupture; and (8) avulsion of the coracoid tip in an athlete.

The surgical approach is anterior for anterior glenoid rim and coracoid fractures. The posterior approach is employed for posterior glenoid rim, neck, and glenoid fossa fractures. The posterior approach is performed one of two ways: (1) a vertical incision with a deltoid split with minimal detachment, then entering the infraspinatus-teres minor interval and exposing the posterior glenoid neck and capsule with subsequent arthrotomy; and (2) reflecting the entire posterior deltoid off the spine, performing a vertical incision in the tendinous portion of the infraspinatus, and elevating the infraspinatus from its fossa and retracting it upward and retracting the teres minor downward. Fixation is with a cannulated screw or buttress plate. Kavanagh and colleagues[50A] reported good results with nine cases of intra-articular glenoid fracture, strongly recommending the posterior approach.

Scapular Body Fracture

Direct violence and sudden contraction of divergent muscles may cause fractures of the body of the scapula. Other reported causes include electrical shock treatments and accidental electrical shock causing seizures.[10,43,66,118] Of all scapular fractures, body fractures have the highest incidence of associated injury. Scapular fractures may be quite comminuted and displaced. True anteroposterior and trauma lateral (tangential scapular lateral) radiographs of the shoulder will show the scapular body fracture (Figs. 18-32 and 18-33). Axillary and cephalic tilt views may also be helpful in looking for other fractures, since injury often is not isolated to the body. CT is not usually helpful in treatment (Fig. 18-34). In the immediate treatment of these fractures, no reduction is attempted. The patient is

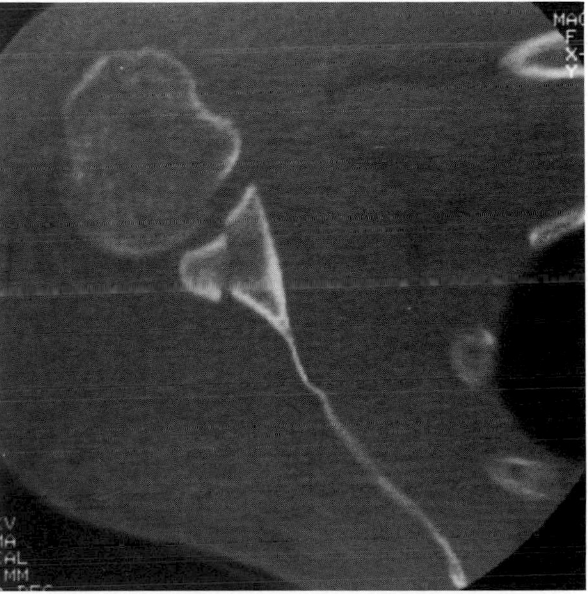

FIGURE 18-23. CT scan showing a large glenoid fracture with residual humeral head subluxation.

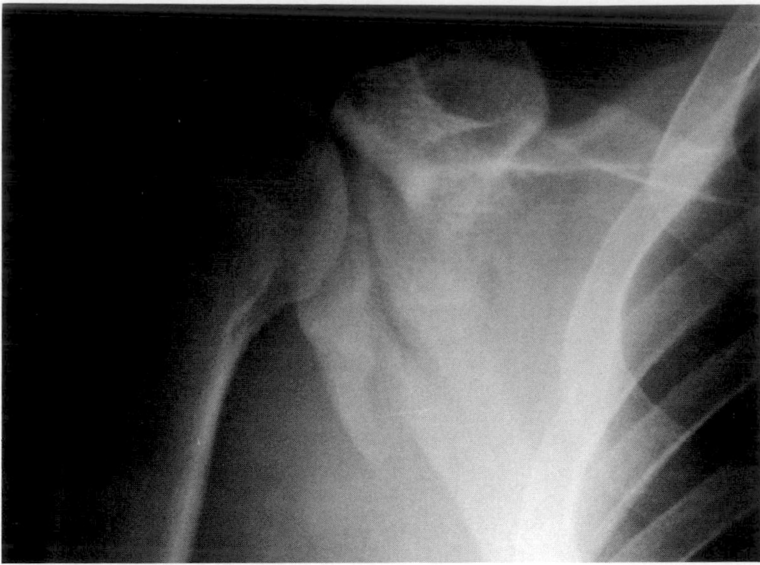

FIGURE 18-24. Type II (oblique) glenoid fracture treated with early rehabilitation.

given local ice and immobilization for comfort. Cross-strapping with adhesive moleskin to immobilize the scapula in a nonambulatory patient was described by Bateman and Neer.[6,83] Such immobilization may produce a stiff shoulder.[70] Pendulum exercises, use of overhead pulleys, and a further passive or active assisted range-of-motion program are begun within a week after injury. Multiple muscle attachments form an excellent environment for healing, and nonunion is rare. Pain may persist until the fracture is solid, but a full range of motion should be the goal in rehabilitation to mobilize the scapula, and progressive-resistance exercises to the rotator cuff and deltoid are essential.

Nordqvist and Petersson[88a] report that long-term results after scapular fracture are not uniformly favorable. They found only 3 of 7 good results in scapular body fractures with greater than 10 mm displacement and 29 of 34 good results in those with less than 10 mm displacement. Also significantly more symptoms were found in those shoulders with radiographic deformity.

Normal bony anatomy is not necessary for good function in a healed scapular body fracture. Perceived malunion with scapulothoracic irritation rarely restricts shoulder function; although when accompanied by associated scarring, it may impair scapular motion.

A stress fracture of the spine is reported by Ho and

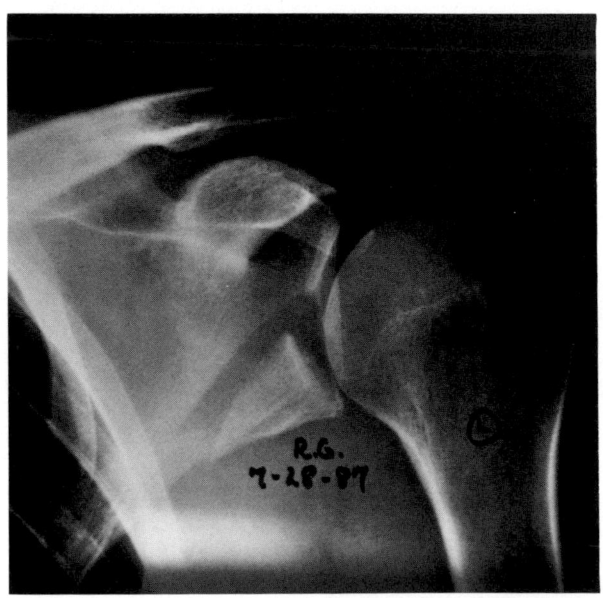

FIGURE 18-25. Type II glenoid fracture requiring fixation.

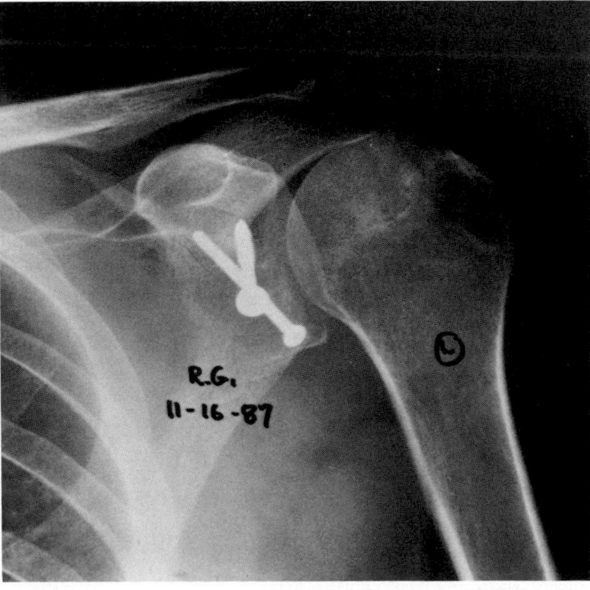

FIGURE 18-26. Anterior glenoid fracture fixed with open reduction and fixation with two screws.

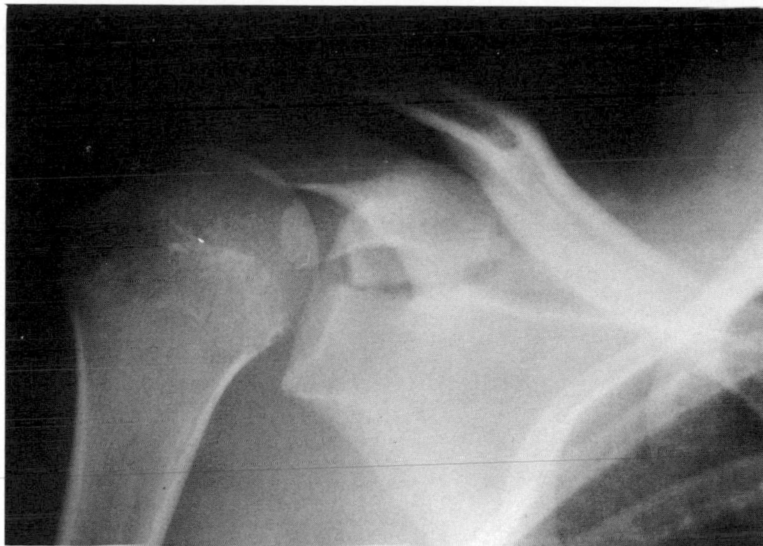

FIGURE 18-27. Type III glenoid fracture near the original epiphyseal line.

associates[45a] in a patient not undergoing radiation therapy. A nonunion of the scapular spine was reported by Robinson and Court-Brown,[99b] treated with AO plate and bone graft, and healed in 14 weeks.

The literature includes mention of operative treatments of body fractures. These include an acute excision of a displaced inferolateral fragment[40] and an open reduction for body fracture, which "interferes in unity of the scapula in performing function as adjunct to arm elevation."[31] Martin and Weiland[64b] published a case report of symptomatic scapular body malunion with removal of rib prominences and a portion of the scapula relieving symptoms and improving range of motion.

Acromion Fracture

The acromion commonly absorbs direct superior blows, and acromioclavicular separation is a much more common sequela than acromion fracture. Most acromial fractures have very little displacement. Commonly the fracture line is lateral to the acromioclavicular joint, causing confusion with os acromiale. In addition to the standard views, radiographic evaluation must include axillary and 30° caudal tilt views. A supraspinatus outlet view may be helpful, as well as radiographs of the contralateral shoulder to look for os acromiale (bilateral in 60% of patients) and to compare acromial configuration.

Another mechanism of acromial fracture is traumatic or superior displacement of the humeral head. This often causes an associated extensive rotator cuff tear. If the humeral head is displaced upward in the subacromial space (acromiohumeral distance is reduced), a rotator cuff tear should be suspected and an arthrogram obtained. A stress fracture can occur in association with the superior migration of the humeral head, as is seen with long-standing cuff disease (Fig.

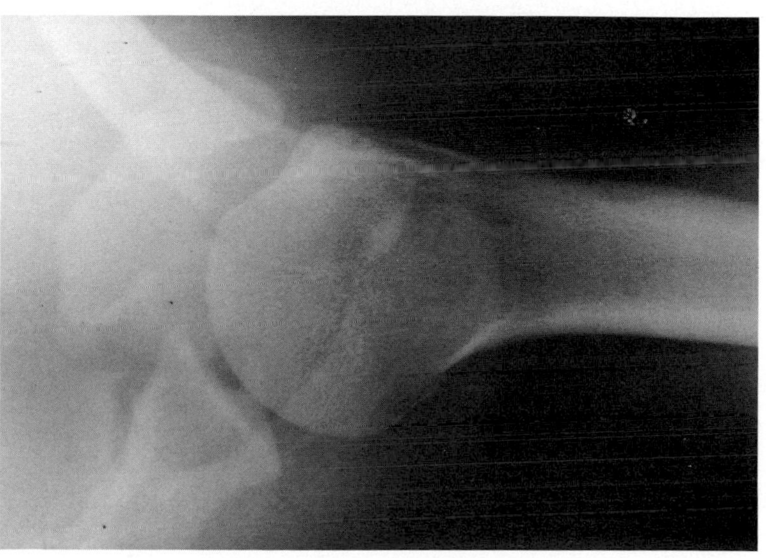

FIGURE 18-28. Type III glenoid fracture including the base of the coracoid and the upper third of the glenoid, seen on an axillary view.

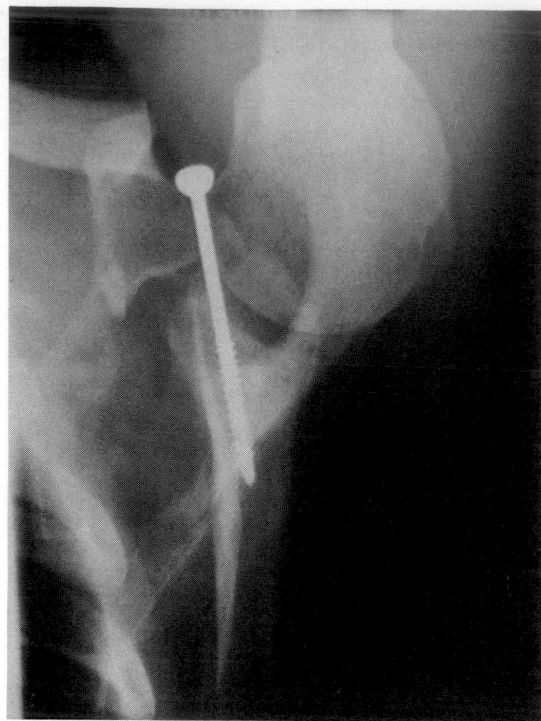

FIGURE 18-29. Type III nonunion, treated by open reduction through the anterior and superior approaches with resection of the distal clavicle.

18-35). Cuff repair and open reduction of the end of the acromion probably should be done. Acromionectomy should, as always, be avoided. An acromial avulsion by deltoid force has been reported.[58]

Kuhn and colleagues' proposed classification is helpful in determining treatment of acromion fractures.[56a] For type I minimally displaced and type II displaced (without decreasing subacromial space), Kuhn recommended nonsurgical treatment. Type II displaced (with reduction of the subacromial space), symptomatic stress fractures, and painful nonunions are all suggested as surgical problems. A tension band fixation or plating with screws is recommended.[18]

A nondisplaced fracture of the acromion should respond well to initial symptomatic treatment and the use of a sling for 3 weeks. Rehabilitation is begun immediately with range-of-motion exercises—passive initially—progressing to isometrics and an active program of rotator cuff and deltoid progressive-resistance exercises after fracture healing.

Results of simple acromial fracture treatment are generally good. Loss of motion, however, was noted by Wilbur and Evans,[121] who recommended cast immobilization in 60° of abduction, 25° of forward flexion, and 25° of external rotation for 6 weeks. Displaced fractures occasionally require elevation and Kirschner wire or screw fixation to eliminate impingement or to reduce the acromioclavicular joint (Fig. 18-36). Acromial nonunion is reported in isolated cases. I have experience with two cases of symptomatic nonunions of fracture of the acromion. One case became asymptomatic with prolonged protection, and the other healed after open reduction and fixation with Kirschner wire—tension band fixation and bone graft. Darrach[20] recommended open reduction, fixation, and immobilization. Ruther[110] used a bone graft and cast. Wong-Pack and associates used a plate across the clavicle to the acromion.[124] Mick and Weiland employed a lag screw and plate along the scapular spine.[75] Neer reminds us that no more than a small fragment of acromion should ever be excised.[83]

A fracture of the base of the acromion near the

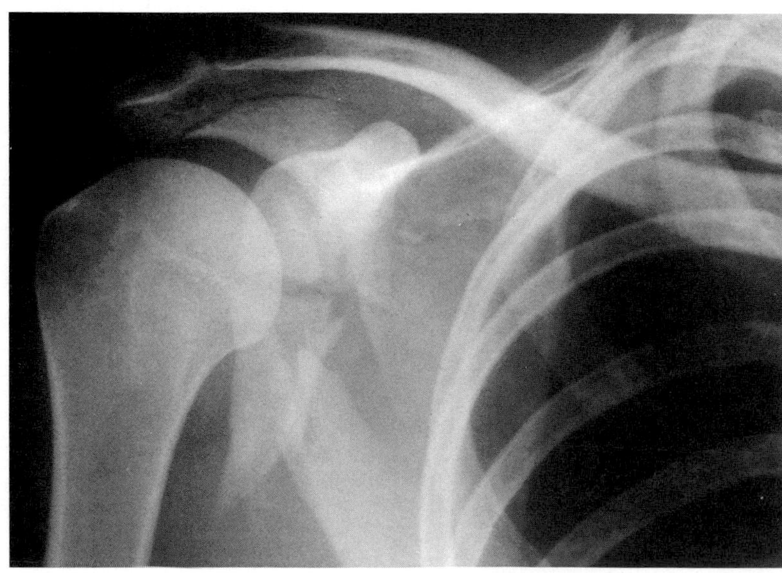

FIGURE 18-30. Type Va glenoid fracture.

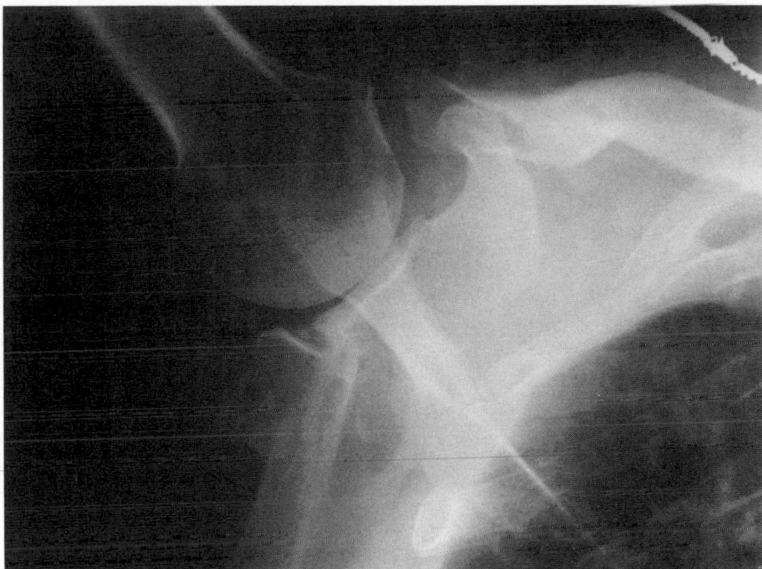

FIGURE 18-31. Type V glenoid fracture, well healed, with good functional motion without pain.

spine, if displaced, may progress to nonunion, and acute open reduction fixation is a good option (Figs. 18-37 to 18-39). As always, when early surgery for the scapular fracture is contemplated, the clinical picture, age, and occupation of the patient must be carefully considered. With the small cross section of contact area in acromion fractures, postoperative protection is necessary.

Stress fractures of the acromion have been described by Veluvolu and coworkers,[120a] Ward and associates,[120c] Warner and Port,[120d] and Marr and Misamore.[64a] These occur in athletes and after weakening of the acromion by arthroscopic subacromial decompression. Iatrogenic acromion fracture may also occur during arthroscopic acromioplasty and would benefit from fixation.

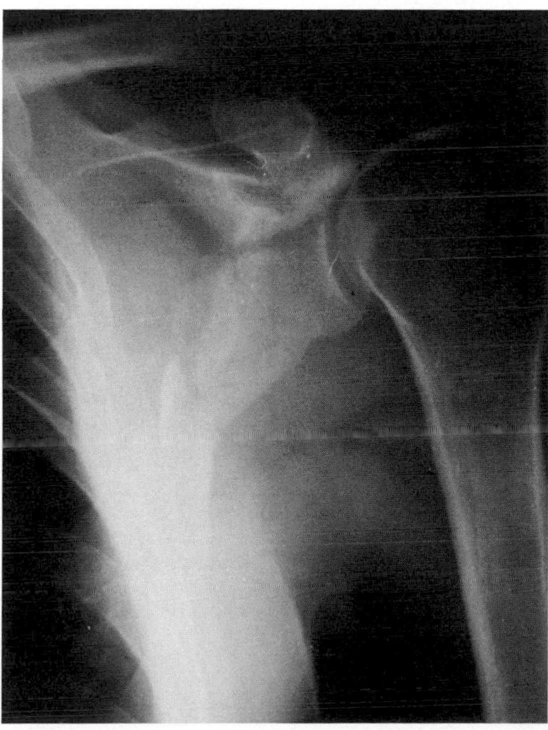

FIGURE 18-32. Comminuted fracture of the body of the scapula.

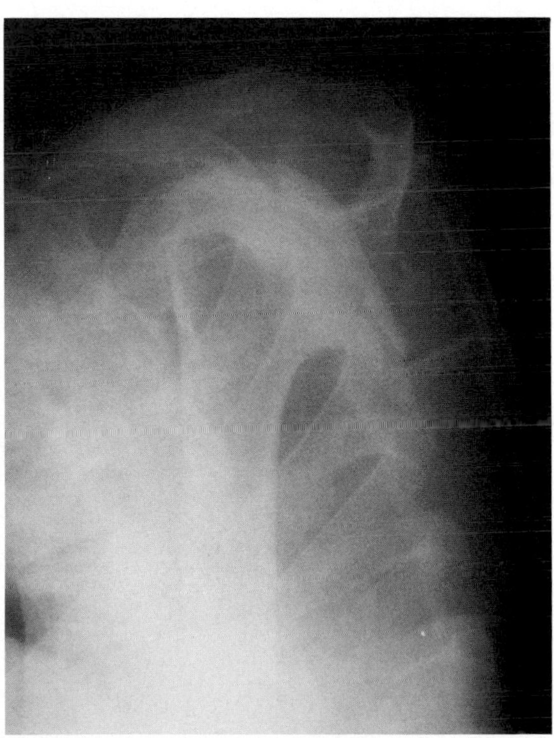

FIGURE 18-33. True (tangential) scapulolateral view showing a comminuted body fracture.

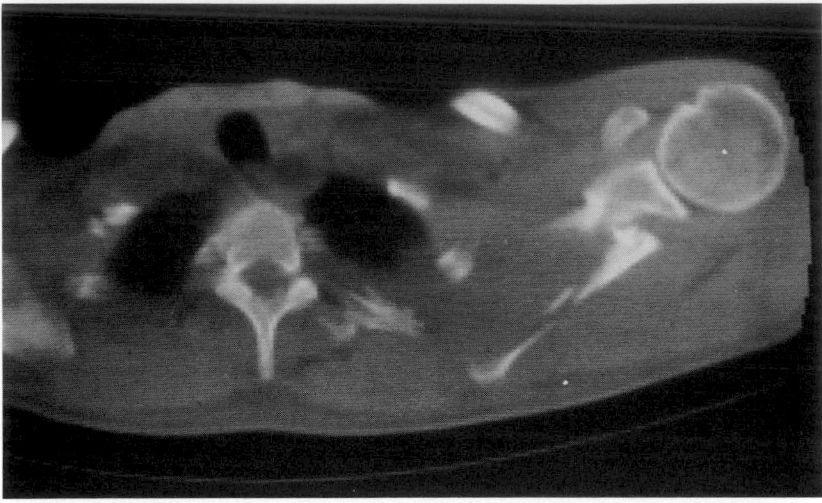

FIGURE 18-34. CT scan showing fracture of the body with an intact glenohumeral joint.

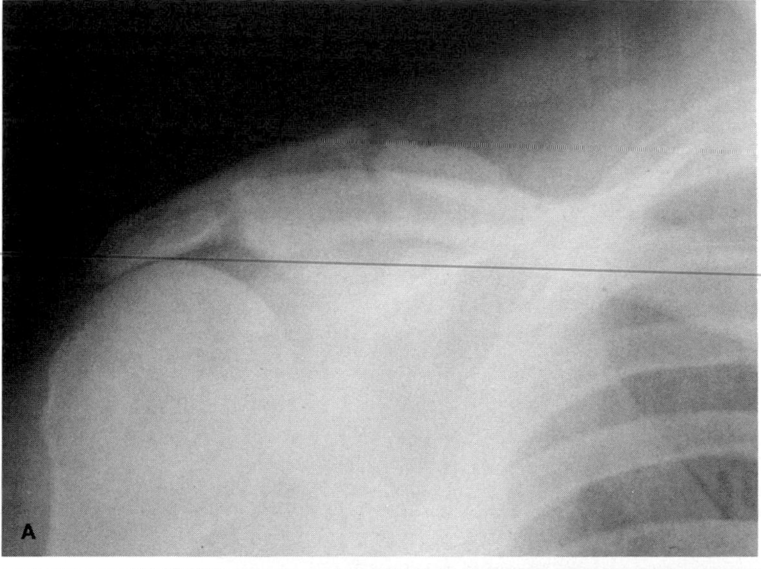

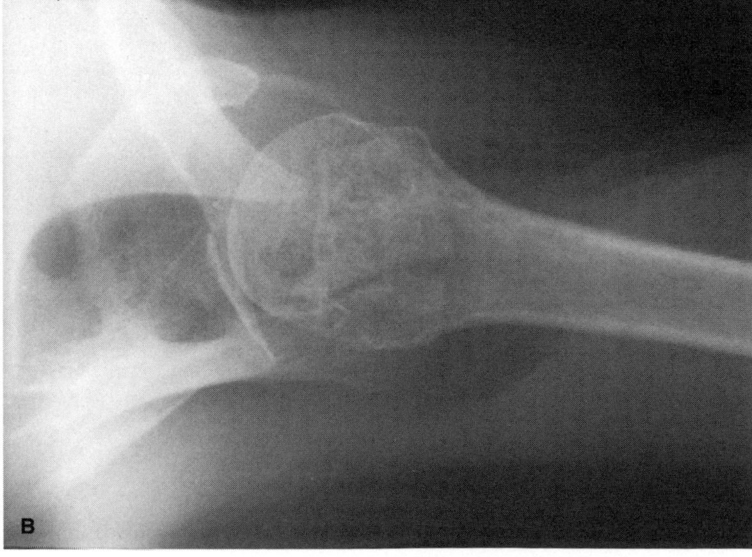

FIGURE 18-35. (**A** and **B**) Stress fractures of the acromion in two patients with cuff arthropathy.

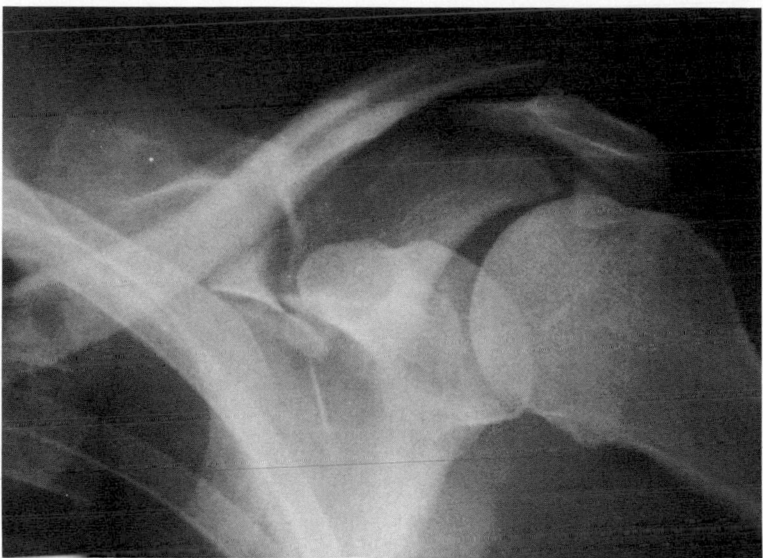

FIGURE 18-36. A patient with a displaced acromion fracture is a candidate for open reduction.

Coracoid Fracture

The coracoid is an important part of the attachment of the limb flexion muscles and ligaments, especially those stabilizing the clavicle. The coracoid is not readily visualized by an anteroposterior radiograph; an axillary view and an anteroposterior cephalic tilt view of 35° to 60° are needed (Fig. 18-40). A Stryker notch view[124] and Goldberg[37] posterior oblique 20° cephalic tilt views are also helpful. Weight-hanging films may also be helpful if an associated acromioclavicular separation is present. Fractures of the coracoid may be isolated, occurring from a direct blow to the coracoid or to the point of the shoulder. Coracoid fracture may also occur along with acromioclavicular dislocation, with the coracoclavicular ligaments remaining intact.[9,50,126] This occurs with traction exerted on the intact ligaments, avulsing the coracoid at its base or through an epiphyseal line. A radiographic clue to diagnosis is a normal and symmetric coracoclavicular distance on radiography and clinical evidence of third-degree acromioclavicular separation with a high-riding clavicle (Fig. 18-41). A cephalic tilt view, especially taken to evaluate the clavicle, may reveal the fracture. I believe the best view is the Stryker notch view. This coracoid fracture may be overlooked when attention is restricted to the obvious acromioclavicular separation. The coracoid tip may be avulsed by muscle pull of the biceps and coracobrachialis[103] or from direct contact from a dislocating humeral head.[35,70] Garcia-Elias and

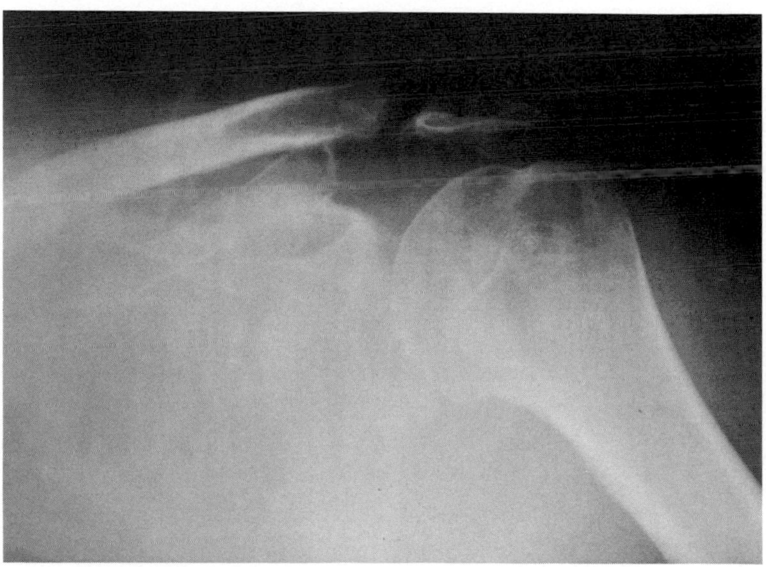

FIGURE 18-37. Nonunion of a fracture of the acromion.

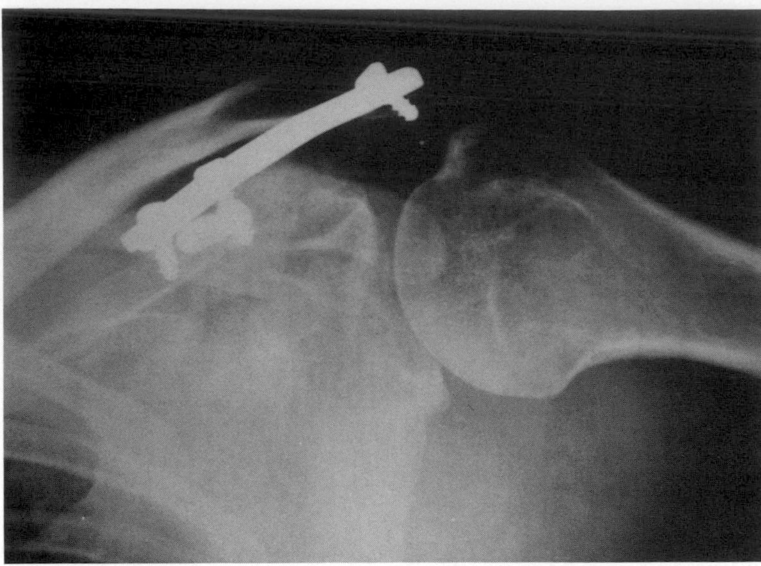

FIGURE 18-38. Nonunion of the acromion, fixed with an intercalary graft and AO plate anchored along the spine of the scapula.

Salo pointed out that this association is easily missed and that follow-up postreduction axillary lateral radiographic evaluation is necessary if pain continues in the shoulder (Fig. 18-42).[35] Fatigue fractures, such as trapshooter's shoulder,[11] have been reported. There are case reports of coracoid fractures with complications from surgical use of the coracoclavicular tape fixation[78] and from medial migration of the humeral head from cuff arthropathy (Fig. 18-43).

The fracture occurs most commonly through the base and is minimally displaced unless significant acromioclavicular separation occurs. A fracture line may extend across the suprascapular notch to the superior surface of the scapula or into the upper third of the glenoid. Confusion may exist concerning a normal accessory ossification center; such a center may be present at the ligament insertion at the site of an avulsion. (See the section on epiphyseal lines.)

Combined acromioclavicular separation with coracoclavicular ligament disruption and coracoid fracture is reported by Wilson and Colwill[121c] and Wang and colleagues.[120b] This probably occurs from two separate mechanisms—coracoclavicular ligament tear with acromioclavicular separation and coracoid muscle avulsion.

In the coracoid fracture with acromioclavicular separation, surgical and nonsurgical treatment appear to offer equally favorable results. The literature is unclear about the time required for union, but no nonunions are reported. Some authors believe that open reduction is indicated but only for treatment of the

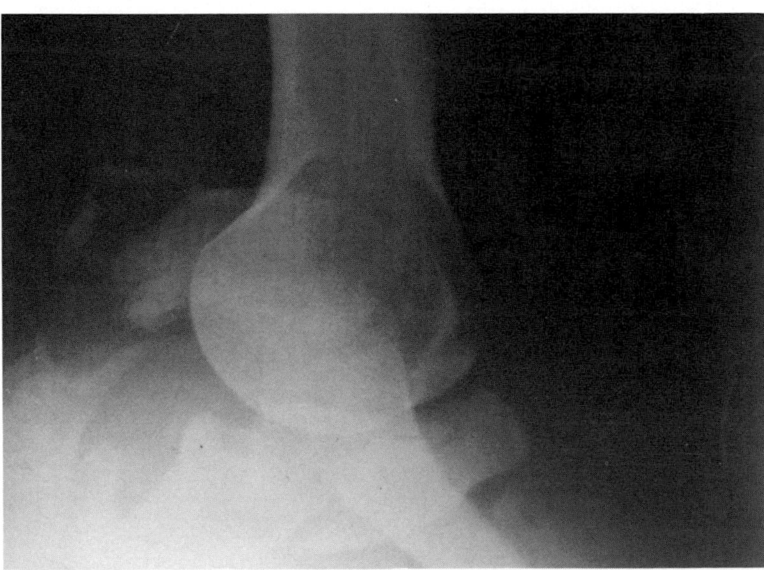

FIGURE 18-39. Nonunion of the acromion after a comminuted scapular fracture, well seen on an axillary view.

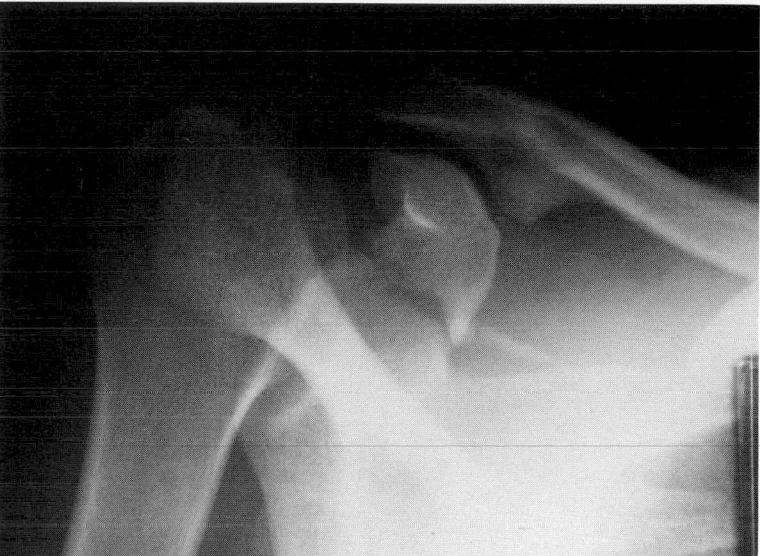

FIGURE 18-40. A 35° cephalic tilt view showing a fracture of the base of the coracoid.

acromioclavicular separation. Stability of the fractured coracoid is supplied by the coracoacromial and coracoclavicular ligaments superiorly and by the pectoralis minor and conjoined tendon inferiorly. For the isolated coracoid fracture, therefore, most authors believe that no specific treatment is needed since an anatomical alignment is not essential for adequate function or healing. For a displaced fracture, especially with associated acromioclavicular separation, Bateman[6] recommended shoulder spica or acromioclavicular fixation. Other authors' indications for surgery include "marked displacement,"[106] associated acromioclavicular separation,[59,64,83,113,121] and compression of the brachial plexus.[83] Neer also described suprascapular nerve paralysis with fracture in the area of the suprascapular notch. Electromyography is essential in the diagnosis, and early exploration is usually indicated.[83]

McLaughlin believed that fibrous union is not uncommon but is rarely symptomatic.[70] Garcia-Elias and Salo reported a painful coracoid nonunion, discovered late after shoulder dislocation, which did well after excision of the fragment.[35] Both Steindler[115] and Benton and Nelson[8] have reported that the tip of the coracoid can be excised and the conjoined tendons reattached to the remaining coracoid process.

Avulsion Fractures of the Scapula

Some of these injuries have been discussed within the anatomical groups, but they are mentioned here for completeness, owing to a common mechanism. Scapu-

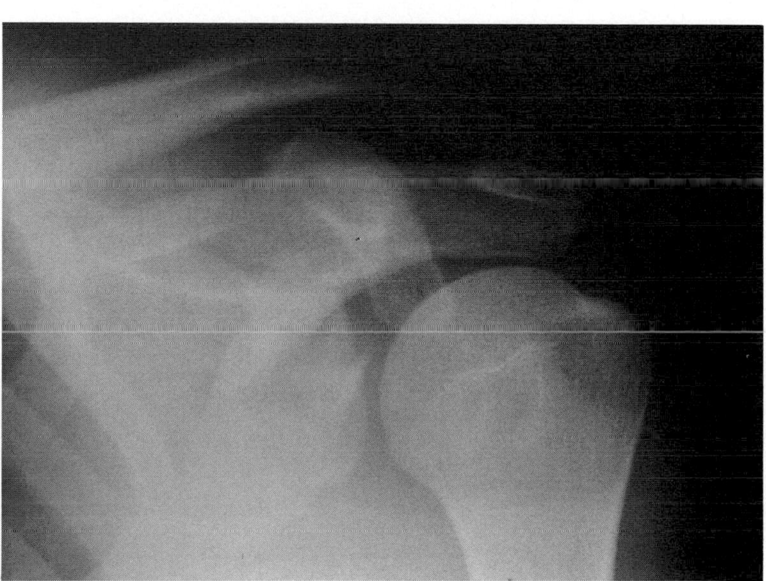

FIGURE 18-41. A third-degree acromioclavicular separation with fractured base of the coracoid and a comminuted glenoid fracture. Note the normal coracoclavicular distance, indicating intact ligaments.

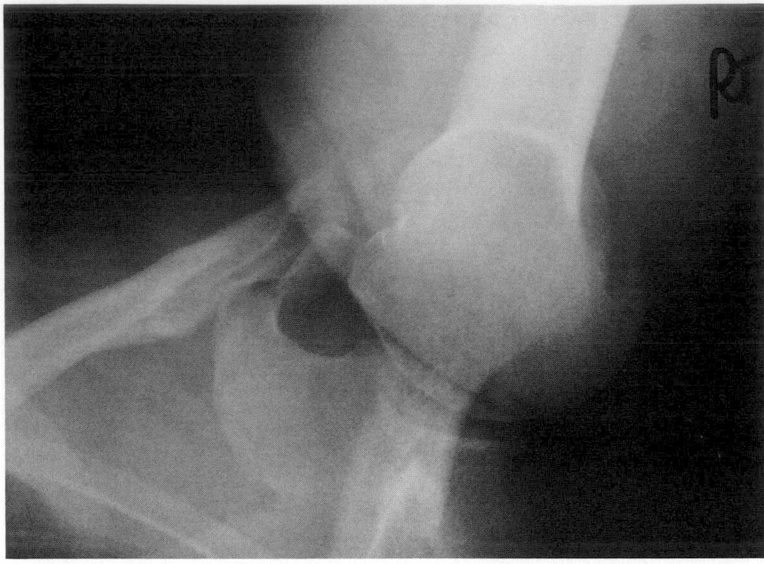

FIGURE 18-42. Fracture of the coracoid tip from a direct blow, seen on Stryker notch, cephalic tilt view.

lar fracture due to avulsion of its many muscular and ligament attachments is uncommon. Four mechanisms may be involved[44]: (1) uncoordinated muscle contraction due to electrical shock, electroconvulsive therapy, or seizures; (2) muscle pull as the result of trauma or unusual exertion; (3) ligamentous avulsion; and (4) stress fracture near a muscle attachment.

A coracoid fracture may occur by means of a coracoclavicular ligament avulsion associated with acromioclavicular separation,[50,83,113] resisted muscle force (coracobrachialis, short head of the biceps) with direct blow,[22,103] and stress fracture of the tip.[8,11] An electroshock treatment has caused an avulsion fracture.[52,97] A superior scapular border avulsion is seen as an extension of the fractured coracoid, created by the coracoclavicular ligament or possibly by avulsion of the omohyoid muscle and levator sequelae.[50] Deltoid avulsion of the acromion is seen in case reports[44,58,98] and can be confused with os acromiale.

Binazzi and associates[10a] reported eight cases of avulsion fracture, including lateral border of the scapula by teres major, infraglenoid tubercle by triceps, and medial spine by trapezius—all with good results with conservative management.

Nonoperative Treatment

Results of treatment of scapular fractures have been reported generally across the spectrum of injuries, and functional results have been satisfactory with conser-

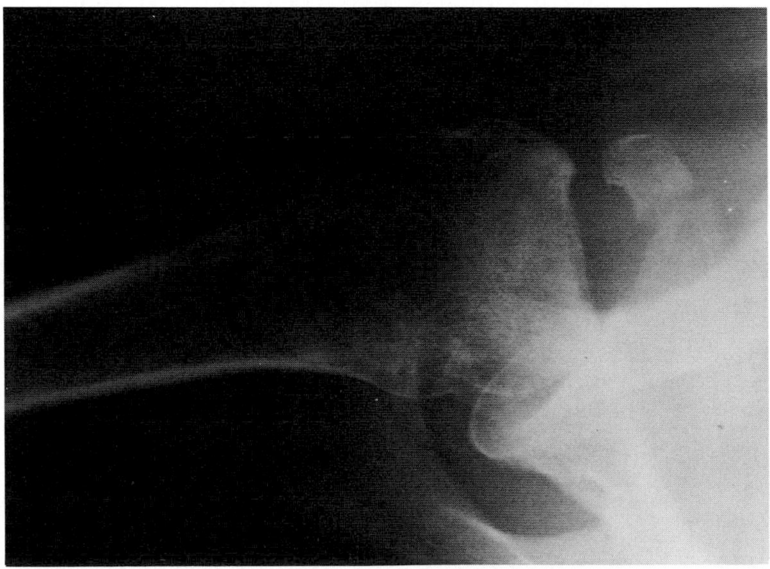

FIGURE 18-43. A stress fracture of the coracoid from medial humeral head migration in cuff arthropathy.

vative treatment. McGahan and coworkers,[69] Lindblom and Leven,[62] McLaughlin,[70] Zdravkovic and Damholt,[125] and Armstrong and Vanderspuy[3] all had series of patients with fractures of the scapula treated nonsurgically. Few patients had long-term disability of the shoulder. Steindler,[125] in 1946, reported insignificant disability associated with nonsurgical treatment and found occasional limitation of abduction in neck fractures with grating and limitation of motion due to surrounding scar in body fractures. He thought that intra-articular glenoid fracture, however, could lead to painful post-traumatic arthritis. Armstrong and Vanderspuy[3] found 6 of 11 extra-articular neck fractures to have residual stiffness but no functional disability. Three of their six patients with glenoid fractures, however, had restricted painful movement on follow-up. Wilbur and Evans[121] grouped acromion, glenoid, and coracoid fractures and found 10 of 11 to have a decreased range of motion, with poor results in only 2. Zdravkovic and Damholt[125] found 23 of 28 patients to have moderately severe deformity on radiography in follow-up, but only 2 had restricted elevation (both cases were intra-articular glenoid fractures). Only 2 patients changed occupation, and only 1 had severe osteoarthritis after 9 years. Nordqvist and Petersson[88a] studied long-term results in 68 cases, with those scapula fractures covered by muscle (body, neck, and spine) having 51 good, 15 fair, and 2 poor results. Scapular deformity was present in 20 patients, and 8 of these patients experienced pain.

McGinnis and Denton[69a] reviewed 39 patients with a variety of scapula fractures treated nonoperatively. In 33% results were fair to poor. His three poor results were related to multiple injuries or inadequate rehabilitation.

As stated earlier, Ada and Miller[1] found decreased range of motion in 20% to 45% and residual pain in 50% to 60% of neck and spine fractures.[1]

Again, older published results support conservative management of most scapular fractures, but newer literature presents a worse prognosis.

Author's Preferred Method of Treatment

Glenoid Neck Fracture

Reduction of displaced extra-articular scapular neck fractures is not necessary to obtain a good clinical result. Early experience with traction did not improve the position of the fracture and necessitated prolonged recumbency and hospital stay. Symptomatic local care, followed in a few days by passive exercises, allows satisfactory motion and does not interfere with fracture healing. When a displaced clavicle fracture accompanies a medially displaced glenoid neck fracture, an unstable segment that includes the glenoid, acromion, and lateral clavicle is created. Stabilization by plate fixation of the clavicle allows for much faster rehabilitation.

Body and Spine

Patients are examined for associated injuries, which are very common with body fractures. Symptomatic treatment is indicated. Application of ice and sling immobilization are followed by stretching exercises and later, after fracture healing, by scapular mobilization and shoulder girdle strengthening.

Glenoid, Intra-articular

Radiographic evaluation is important. Axillary and West Point views as well as CT and true anteroposterior tomograms are used to diagnose significant glenoid fractures involving 25% or more of the joint surface. One must separate these from a small avulsion fracture. If these larger fragments are displaced, open reduction with 3.5 mm cannulated AO screw fixation is indicated. If dislocation is the mechanism of injury, the chance for recurrent instability if these fractures are left untreated, especially in the younger age group, approaches 100%. The operative approach, although difficult, is easier than later reconstruction with fragment fixation, iliac bone graft, coracoid bone block, or Bankart repair. I start gentle motion at 7 days in these patients.

The other types of glenoid fractures (types II through VI) have less clear indications for operative treatment. If the humeral head is centered on the major portion of the glenoid and the shoulder joint is stable, then nonsurgical treatment is indicated as the head remains intracapsular. When the humeral head appears to be subluxated along with a major fragment, surgical treatment with capsular repair is indicated. Consideration should also be given to open reduction for a 5-mm intra-articular step-off, especially with the superior glenoid displaced laterally. Again, a workup with carefully positioned anteroposterior tomograms and CT gives the surgeon a three-dimensional view of the fracture. I usually prefer the anterior approach to reduce the type II fracture, combined with superior visualization to pass the screw. The path of the screw is cleared by partial-thickness clavicle removal or even by resection of the distal clavicle. It is critical to understand the obliquity of the fracture before surgery can be planned, and a posterior approach is better for many. This surgery is difficult, and the fixation often is not pleasing.

Acromion

As stated, most fractures of the acromion are without significant displacement. They should be protected in a supervised passive and active assisted exercise program with no resisted deltoid function until union occurs. If there has been upward movement of the humeral head, fracturing the acromion, then the rotator cuff must be investigated and repaired. The presence of os acromiale must be remembered as part of the differential diagnosis for fracture; its presence alone is associated with an increased incidence of cuff disease.[83] The use of a dorsal tension band wire is a good technique for fixation of acromial fractures.

I believe surgery is indicated for displaced fractures of the acromion that decrease the acromiohumeral space.

Coracoid

The Stryker notch or the 35° cephalic tilt view provides the information needed to assess the displacement of the coracoid fracture. Complete third-degree acromioclavicular separation combined with the significantly displaced coracoid fracture is an indication for open reduction of both injuries with transacromioclavicular Steinmann pin fixation (Fig. 18-44). I have experience with two late explorations of suprascapular nerve injury in association with coracoid and body fractures and agree with Neer, who favors early exploration of the nerve.

OTHER DISORDERS

Dislocation of the Scapula

Dislocation of the scapula between the ribs and into the thoracic cage is very rare. Ainscow describes one type with little violence and a preexisting factor such as generalized laxity or locking osteochondroma.[1A] The medial border is lodged between the third and fourth ribs or in the fourth to fifth intercostal space.[84] A second type is associated with more violent trauma involving chest injury. This is a rare variation of the injury and usually causes fracture of the scapula and ribs. The rhomboid muscles must be stretched or torn.[53] The diagnosis is suspected on examination of the upper extremity and inspection of the posterior chest wall but may be missed, owing to associated injuries, or may not be appreciated on anteroposterior views of the chest.

Nettrour and colleagues' series[84] had a case in which the displaced scapula was thought to be a chest wall hematoma on plain chest films. The Nettrour anterior oblique or tangential scapular lateral (trauma lateral) view or CT scan will confirm the diagnosis. Reduction under general anesthesia is accomplished by hyperabducting the arm and manually manipulating the axillary border, rotating the scapula forward and at the same time pushing it back, as described by DePalma.[21] Acute reduction is usually stable, but adhesive strapping plus collar and cuff is recommended by Key and Conwell.[53] Late discovery may require open reduction and soft-tissue reattachment to maintain reduction.[83]

Scapulothoracic Dissociation

Scapulothoracic dissociation is a violent, closed, lateral displacement of the scapula with associated clavicle fracture and severe soft-tissue injury. Usually included in the injury are brachial plexus and vascular disruption. It has been described by Ebraheim and coworkers[25] as "closed, traumatic forequarter amputation" and has been infrequently reported, since most patients have died. Soft-tissue injury includes complete

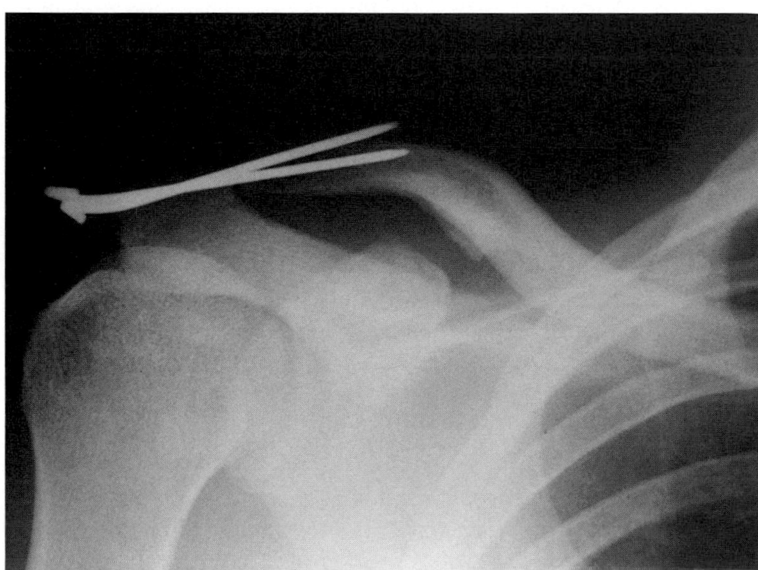

FIGURE 18-44. Open reduction of the acromioclavicular joint with transacromioclavicular joint pins.

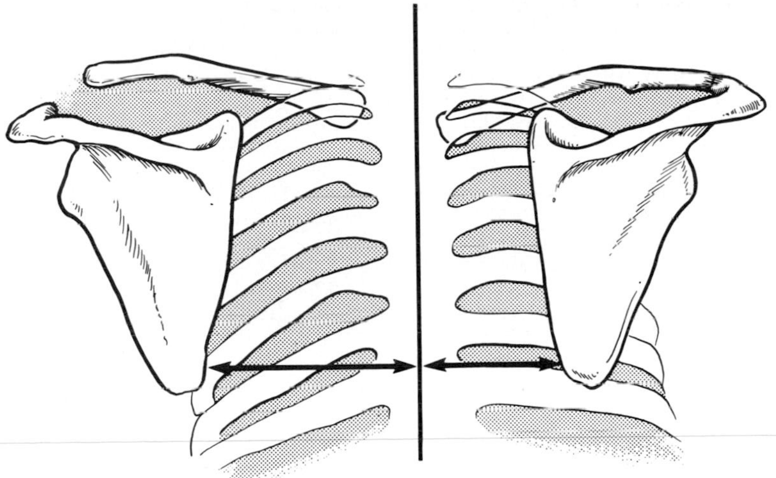

FIGURE 18-45. A diagram of scapulothoracic dissociation, demonstrating a lateral displacement of the scapula on the injured side (*left*) compared with the normal side (*right*) on a nonrotated chest x-ray.

or partial tears of the deltoid, pectoralis, and posterior scapular muscles. Vascular disruption occurs most frequently at the level of the subclavian artery. Most often there is complete avulsion of the brachial plexus, but incomplete neuropraxia is possible. Bony injury may appear as acromioclavicular or sternoclavicular separation or clavicle fracture. Ipsilateral upper extremity fractures are often also present. Associated injuries are usually discovered early, without full appreciation of the magnitude of the injury. The diagnosis is made when a nonrotated chest radiograph shows significant lateral displacement of the scapula as measured by the distance from the sternal notch to the coracoid, glenoid margin, or medial scapular border. Kelbel and associates[51] found the ratio of the medial border to spine distance to be 1.5 or greater. Figure 18-45 shows this measurement.

Leung and Lam[60a] believe there is a spectrum of neurovascular compromise ranging from normal to complete disruption. All of the factors satisfy the radiographic criteria for a scapulothoracic dissociation. They suggested a classification to reflect this variable clinical presentation. Oni and associates[90a,90b] suggest a classification based on the location of the associated clavicle injury.

The primary mode of injury is direct trauma occurring, for example, during a motorcycle, mill wheel, hay baler, or motor vehicle accident.[91] Extremities are flail and pulseless, but swelling from dissecting hematoma may be the only external signs. A more distal vascular injury may divert attention from the more severe proximal injury. After resuscitation of the patient, the chest radiograph should be carefully inspected and arteriography performed to delineate the vascular lesion. Exploration to restore vascular integrity and diagnose the level and severity of the brachial plexus injury is next. On the basis of this information and on assessment of scapular muscle damage, early above-elbow amputation and shoulder fusion are considered.[24,25] Rorabeck found no advantage to shoulder arthrodesis in this setting.[102] If parts of the brachial plexus remain intact, vascular and neurologic repair for limb salvage is indicated.

Sampson and coworkers[110a] presented a series of cases each with a diagnostic radiograph for scapulothoracic dissociation. They questioned the need for vascular repair in these patients, who had complete brachial plexus palsy, no radial pulse, and subclavian or axillary artery occlusion by arteriogram. In 11 cases, 6 were revascularized, 5 were not. All 11 remained viable, and none of the 11 patients have regained function.

REFERENCES

1. Ada, J.R., and Miller, M.E.: Scapular Fractures: Analysis of 113 Cases. Clin. Orthop., 269:174–180, June 1991.

1a. Ainscow, D.A.: Dislocation of the Scapula. J. Coll. Surg. Edinb., 27:56–57, 1982.

2. Anderson, L.D.: Fractures. *In* Crenshaw, A.H. (ed.): Campbell's Operative Orthopaedics, 6th ed., p. 662. St. Louis, C.V. Mosby, 1971.

3. Armstrong, C.P., and Vanderspuy, J.: The Fractured Scapula: Importance in Management Based on a Series of 62 Patients. Injury, 15:324–329, 1984.

4. Aston, J.W., and Gregory, C.F.: Dislocation of the Shoulder With Significant Fracture of the Glenoid. J. Bone Joint Surg., 55A:1531–1533, 1973.

4a. Baccarani, G., Porcellini, G., and Brunetti, E.: Fracture of the Coracoid Process Associated with Fracture of the Clavicle. Description of a Rare Case. Chir. Organi. Mov., 78:49–51, 1993.

5. Banerjee, A.K., and Field, S.: An Unusual Scapular Fracture Caused by a Water Skiing Accident. Br. J. Radiol., 58:65–467, 1985.

6. Bateman, J.E.: The Shoulder and Neck, 2nd ed. Philadelphia, W.B. Saunders, 1978.

7. Benchetrit, E., and Friedman, B.: Fracture of the Cricoid Process Associated With Subglenoid Dislocation of the Shoulder. J. Bone Joint Surg., 61A:295–296, 1979.

8. Benton, J., and Nelson, C.: Avulsion of the Coracoid Process in an Athlete. J. Bone Joint Surg., 53A:356–358, 1971.
9. Bernard, T.N., Brunet, M.E., and Haddad, R.J., Jr.: Fractured Coracoid Process in Acromioclavicular Dislocations. Clin. Orthop., 175:227–231, 1983.
10. Beswick, D.R., Morse, S.D., and Barnes, A.U.: Bilateral Scapular Fractures From Low Voltage Electrical Injury—A Case Report. Ann. Emerg. Med., 11:12–13, 1982.
10a. Binazzi, R., Assiso, J., Vaccari, V., and Felli, L.: Avulsion Fractures of the Scapula: Report of Eight Cases. J. Trauma, 33:785–789, 1992.
11. Boyer, D.W.: Trap Shooter's Shoulder: Stress Fracture of the Coracoid Process. J. Bone Joint Surg., 57A:862, 1975.
12. Caffey, J. (ed.): Pediatric X-ray Diagnosis, 7th ed., pp. 320–321. Chicago, Year Book Medical Publishers, 1978.
12a. Cain, T.E., and Hamilton, W.P.: Scapular Fractures in Professional Football Players. Am. J. Sports Med., 20:363–365, 1992.
13. Cameron, H.U.: Snapping Scapula: A Report of Three Cases. Eur. J. Rheumatol. Inflamm., 7:66–67, 1984.
13a. Carr, A.J., and Broughton, N.S.: Acromioclavicular Dislocation Associated with Fracture of the Coracoid Process. J. Trauma, 29:125–126, 1989.
14. Charlton, M.R.: Fracture, Neck of the Scapula. Northwest Medicine, 37:18–21, 1938.
15. Cigtay, O.S., and Mascatello, V.J.: Scapular Defects: A Normal Variation. A.J.R., 132:239–241, 1979.
16. Cockshott, W.P.: The Coracoclavicular Joint. Radiology, 132:313–316, 1979.
17. Cooley, L.H., and Torg, J.S.: "Pseudo-winging" of the Scapula Secondary to Subscapular Osteochondroma. Clin. Orthop., 162:119–124, 1982.
18. Cotton, F.J., and Brickley, W.J.: Treatment of Fracture of the Neck of the Scapula. Boston Med. Surg. J., 185:326–329, 1921.
19. Coues, W.P.: Fracture of the Coracoid Process of the Scapula. N. Engl. J. Med., 212:727–728, 1935.
20. Darrach, W.: Fractures of the Acromion Process of the Scapula. Ann. Surg., 59:455–456, 1914.
21. DePalma, A.F.: Surgery of the Shoulder, 3rd ed., pp. 366–367. Philadelphia, J.B. Lippincott, 1983.
22. De Rosa, G.P., and Kettelkamp, D.B.: Fracture of the Coracoid Process of the Scapula: A Case Report. J. Bone Joint. Surg., 59A: 696–697, 1977.
22a. Dumas, J.L., and Walker, N.: Bilateral Scapular Fractures Secondary to Electrical Shock. Arch. Orthop. Trauma Surg., 111:287–288, 1992.
23. Dzioba, R.B., and Quinlan, W.J.: Avascular Necrosis of Glenoid. J. Trauma, 24:448–451, 1984.
24. Ebraheim, N.A., An, S., Jackson, W.T., et al.: Scapulothoracic Dissociation. J. Bone Joint Surg., 70A:428–432, 1988.
25. Ebraheim, N.A., Pearlstein, S.R., Savolaine, E.R., et al.: Scapulothoracic Dissociation (Avulsion of the Scapula, Subclavian Artery, and Brachial Plexus): An Early Recognized Variant, A New Classification, and a Review of the Literature and Treatment Options. J. Orthop. Trauma, 1:18–23, 1987.
26. Edeland, H.G., and Zachrisson, H.E.: Fracture of the Scapular Notch Associated With Lesion of the Suprascapular Nerve. Orthop. Scand., 46:758–763, 1975.
27. Fery, A., and Sommelet, J.: Fractures de l'Apophyse Coide. Rev. Chir. Orthop., 65:403–407, 1979.
28. Findlay, R.T.: Fractures of the Scapula and Ribs. Am. J. Surg., 38:489–494, 1937.
29. Findlay, R.T.: Fractures of the Scapula. Ann. Surg., 1001–1008, 1931.
30. Fischer, R.P., Flynn, T.C., Miller, P.W., and Thompson, D.A.: Scapular Fractures and Associated Major Ipsilateral Upper-Torso Injuries. Curr. Concepts Trauma Care, 1:14–16, 1985.
31. Fischer, W.R.: Fracture of the Scapula Requiring Open Traction: Report of a Case. J. Bone Joint Surg., 21:459–461, 1939.
31a. Fleischmann, W., and Kinzl, L.: Philosophy of Osteosynthesis in Shoulder Fractures. Orthopaedics, 16:59–63, 1993.
31b. Folman, Y., El-Masri, W., Gepstein, R., and Messias, R.: Fractures of the Scapula Associated with Traumatic Paralysis: A Pathomechanical Indicator. Injury, 24:306–308, 1993.
32. Friedrich, B., and Winter, G.: Zur Operativen Therapie Frakturen der Scapula. Chirurg, 44:37–39, 1973.
33. Froimson, A.I.: Fracture of the Coracoid Process of the Scapula. J. Bone Joint Surg., 60A:710–711, 1978.
34. Gagney, O., Carey, J.P., and Mazas, F.: Les Fractures recentes de l'Omoplate à propos de 43 Cas. Rev. Chir. Orthop., 443–447, 1984.
35. Garcia-Elias, M., and Salo, J.M.: Nonunion of a Fractured Coracoid Process After Dislocation of the Shoulder. J. Bone Joint Surg., 67B:722–723, 1985.
35a. Gil, J.F., and Haydar, A.: Isolated Injury of the Coracoid Process: Case Report. J. Trauma, 31:1696–1697, 1991.
36. Gleich, J.J.: The Fractured Scapula, A Significance in Prognosis. Mo. Med., 77:24–26, 1980.
37. Goldberg, R.P., and Vicks, B.: Oblique Angle to View Coracoid Fractures. Skeletal Radiol., 9:195–197, 1983.
37a. Goss, T.P.: Fractures of the Glenoid Cavity: Operative Principles and Techniques. Tech. Orthop., 8:199–204, 1993.
37b. Goss, T.P.: Fractures of the Glenoid Cavity. J. Bone Joint Surg., 74A:299–305, 1992.
37c. Goss, T.P.: Double Disruptions of the Superior Shoulder Suspensory Complex. J. Orthop. Trauma, 7:99–106, 1993.
37d. Goss, T.P.: Fractures of the Glenoid Neck. J. Shoulder Elbow Surg., 3(Part I):42–52, 1994.
37e. Goss, T.P.: Scapular Fractures and Dislocations: Diagnosis and Treatment. Journal of American Academy of Orthopedic Surgeons, 3:22–33, 1995.
38. Halpern, A.A., Joseph, R., Page, J., and Nagel, D.A.: Subclavian Artery Injury and Fracture of the Scapula. J. Am. Coll. Physicians, 8:19–20, 1979.
39. Hardegger, F.H., Simpson, L.A., and Weber, B.G.: The Emergency Treatment of Scapular Fractures. J. Bone Joint Surg., 725–731, 1984.
40. Harmon, P.H., and Baker, D.R.: Fracture of the Scapula with Displacement. J. Bone Joint Surg., 25:834–838, 1943.
40a. Harris, R.D., and Harris, J.H.: The Prevalence and Significance of Missed Scapular Fractures in Blunt Chest Trauma. A.J.R., 151:747–750, 1988.
41. Hayes, J., and Zehr, D.: Traumatic Muscle Avulsion Causing Winging of the Scapula. J. Bone Joint Surg., 68A:495–1981.
42. Heatly, M.D., Breck, L.W., and Higinbotham, N.L.: Bilateral Fracture of the Scapula. Am. J. Surg., 71:256–259, 1946.
43. Henneking, K., Hofmann, D., and Kunze, K.: Skapula frakturen nach electrounfall. Unfallchirurgie, 10:149–151, 1984.
44. Heyse-Moore, G.H., and Stoker, D.J.: Avulsion Fractures of the Scapula. Skeletal Radiol., 9:27–32, 1982.
45. Hitzrot, T., and Bolling, R.W.: Fracture of the Neck of Scapula. Ann. Surg., 63:215–234, 1916.
45a. Ho, K.M.T., Schranz, P., and Wallace, W.A.: "Stress Fracture" of the Scapula. Injury, 24:498, 1993.
46. Hollinshead, R., and James, K.W.: Scapulothoracic Dislocation (Locked Scapula). J. Bone Joint Surg., 61A:1102–1103, 1979.
47. Ideberg, R.: Unusual Glenoid Fractures: A Report on 92 Cases. Acta Orthop. Scand., 58:191–192, 1987.
48. Ideberg, R.: Fractures of the Scapula Involving the Glenoid Fossa. *In* Bateman, J.E., and Welsh, R.P. (eds.): Surgery of the Shoulder, pp. 63–66. Toronto, B.C. Decker, 1984.
49. Imatani, R.J.: Fractures of the Scapula: A Review of 53 Fractures. J. Trauma, 15:473–478, 1975.
50. Ishizuki, M., Yamaura, I., Isobe, Y., Furuya, K., Tanabe, K., and Nagatsuka, Y.: Avulsion Fracture of the Superior Border of the Scapula: A Report of Five Cases. J. Bone Joint Surg., 63A:820–822, 1981.
50a. Kavanaugh, B.F., Bradway, J.K., and Cofield, R.H.: Open Reduction and Internal Fixation of Displaced Intraarticular Fractures of the Glenoid Fossa. J. Bone Joint Surg., 75A:479–484, 1993.
51. Kelbel, J.M., Hardon, O.M., and Huurman, W.W.: Scapulothoracic Dissociation: A Case Report. Clin. Orthop., 210–214, 1986.
52. Kelly, J.P.: Fractures Complicating Electroconvulsive Ther-

apy in Chronic Epilepsy. J. Bone Joint Surg., 36B:70–79, 1954.
53. Key, J.A., and Conwell, H.E.: The Management of Fractures, Dislocations and Sprains. St. Louis, C.V. Mosby, 1964.
54. Kohler, A., and Zimmer, E.A.: Borderlands of the Normal Early Pathologic Skeletal Roentgenogram. New York, Grune & Stratton, 1968.
55. Kopecky, K.K., Bies, J.R., and Ellis, J.H.: CT Diagnosis of Fracture of the Coracoid Process of the Scapula. Comput. Radiol., 8:325–327, 1984.
56. Kozlowski, K., Colavita, N., Morris, L., and Little, K.E.T.: Bilateral Glenoid Dysplasia (Report of Eight Cases). Aust. qyol. Radiol., 29:174–177, 1985.
56a. Kuhn, J.E., Blasier, R.B., and Carpenter, J.E.: Fractures of the Acromion Process: A Proposed Classification System. J. Orthop. Trauma, 8:6–13, 1994.
56b. Kumar, A.: Management of Coracoid Process Fracture with Acromioclavicular Joint Dislocation. Orthopaedics, 13:770–772, 1990.
57. Kummel, B.M.: Fractures of the Glenoid Causing Chronic Dislocation of the Shoulder. Clin. Orthop., 69:189–191, 1970.
58. Laing, R., and Dee, R.: Fracture Symposium. Orthop. Review, 13:717–720, 1984.
58a. Landi, A., Schoenhuber, R., Funicello, R., Rasio, G., and Esposito, M.: Compartment Syndrome of the Scapula., Ann. Hand Surg., 11:383–388, 1992.
58b. Lange, R.H., and Noel, S.H.: Traumatic Lateral Scapular Displacement: An Expanded Spectrum of Associated Neurovascular Injury. J. Orthop. Trauma, 7:361–366, 1993.
59. Lasda, N.A., and Murray, D.G.: Fracture Separation of Coracoid Process Associated With Acromioclavicular Dislocation. Clin. Orthop., 134:222–224, 1978.
60. Leffmann, R.: A Case of "Rattling Shoulder Blade." Med. Orientalia, 6:292–295, 1947.
60a. Leung, K.S., and Lam, T.P.: Open Reduction and Internal Fixation of Ipsilateral Fractures of the Scapular Neck and Clavicle. J. Bone Joint Surg., 75A:1015–1018, 1993.
61. Liberson, F.: Os Acromiale—A Contested Anomaly. J. Joint Surg., 19:683–689, 1937.
62. Lindblom, A., and Leven, H.: Prognosis in Fractures of Body and Neck of the Scapula. Acta Chir. Scand., 140:33–47, 1974.
63. Longabaugh, R.I.: Fracture Simple, Right Scapula. U.S. Naval Med. Bull., 27:341–343, 1924.
63a. Madhavan, P., Buckingham, R., and Stableforth, P.G.: Avulsion Injury of the Subscapularis Tendon Associated with Fracture of the Acromion. Injury, 25:271–272, 1994.
64. Mariani, P.P.: Isolated Fracture of the Coracoid Process in an Athlete. Am. J. Sports Med., 8:129–130, 1980.
64a. Marr, D.C., and Misamore, G.W.: Acromion Nonunion After Anterior Acromioplasty: A Case Report. J. Shoulder Elbow Surg., 1:317–320, 1992.
64b. Martin, S.D., and Weiland, A.J.: Missed Scapular Fracture After Trauma. Clin. Orthop. 299:259–262, 1994.
64c. Martin-Herrero, T., Rodriguez-Merchan, C., and Munuera-Martinez, L.: Fractures of the Coracoid Process: Presentation of Seven Cases and Review of the Literature. J. Trauma, 30(12):1597–1599, 1990.
65. Mathews, R.E., Cocke, T.B., and D'Ambrosia, R.D.: Scapular Fractures Secondary to Seizures in Patients Without Osteodystrophy. J. Bone Joint Surg., 65A:850–853, 1983.
66. McCally, W.C., and Kelly, D.A.: Treatment of Fractures of the Clavicle, Ribs and Scapula. Am. J. Surg., 50:558–562, 1940.
67. McClure, J.G., and Raney, R.B.: Anomalies of the Scapula. Clin. Orthop., 110:22–31, 1975.
68. McGahan, J.P., and Rab, G.T.: Fracture of the Acromion Associated With Axillary Nerve Deficit. Clin. Orthop., 147:216–1980.
69. McGahan, J.P., Rab, G.T., and Dublin, A.: Fractures of Scapula. J. Trauma, 20:880–883, 1980.
69a. McGinnis, M., and Denton, J.R.: Fractures of the Scapula: A Retrospective Study of 40 Fractured Scapulae. J. Trauma, 29(11):1488–1493, 1989.
70. McLaughlin, H.L.: Trauma, pp. 236–237. Philadelphia, W.B. Saunders, 1959.
71. McLennen, J.G., and Ungersma, J.: Pneumothorax Complicating Fractures of the Scapula. J. Bone Joint Surg., 64A:598–599, 1982.
72. McWilliams, C.A.: Subscapular Exostosis With Adventitious Bursa. J.A.M.A., 63:1473–1474, 1914.
72a. Meister K, Andrews JR: Classification and Treatment of Rotator Cuff Injuries in the Overhand Athelete. Journal of Orthopedic Sports Physical Therapy, 18:413–421, 1993.
73. Mencke, J.B.: The Frequency and Significance of Injuries to the Acromion Process. Ann. Surg., 59:233–238, 1914.
74. Michele, A.A., and Davies, J.J.: Scapulocostal Syndrome (Fatigue-Postural Paradox). N.Y. State J. Med., 50:1353–1356, 1950.
75. Mick, C.A., and Weiland, A.J.: Pseudo-arthrosis of a Fracture of the Acromion. J. Trauma, 23:248–249, 1983.
76. Milch, H.: Snapping Scapula. Clin. Orthop., 20:139–150 1961.
77. Milch, H.: Partial Scapulectomy for Snapping in the Scapula. J. Bone Joint Surg., 32A:561–566, 1950.
78. Milch, H., and Burman, M.S.: Snapping Scapula and Humerus Varus. Arch. Surg., 26:570–588, 1933.
78a. Miller, M.E., and Ada, J.R.: Injuries to the Shoulder Girdle. *In* Browner, B.D., Jupiter, J.B., Levine, A.M., and Trafton, P.G. (eds.): Skeletal Trauma, pp. 1291–1310. Philadelphia, W.B. Saunders, 1992.
79. Moneim, M.S., and Balduini, F.C.: Coracoid Fractures—A Complication of Surgical Treatment by Coraclavicular Tape Traction: A Case Report. Clin. Orthop., 168:133–135, 1982.
80. Montgomery, S.P., and Loyd, R.D.: Avulsion Fracture of Coracoid Epiphysis With Acromioclavicular Separation. J. Bone Joint Surg., 59:963–965, 1977.
81. Moseley, H.F.: Shoulder Lesions, 2nd ed., pp. 171–175. New York, Paul Hoeber, 1953.
82. Mudge, M.K., Wood, V.E., and Frykman, G.K.: Rotator Tears Associated With Os Acromiale. J. Bone Joint Surg., 66A:427–429, 1984.
83. Neer, C.S., II: Fractures About the Shoulder. *In* Wood, C.A., and Green, D.P. (eds.): Fractures, pp. 713–721. Philadelphia, J.B. Lippincott, 1984.
83a. Neer CS II: Fractures. *In* Shoulder Reconstruction, p. 412. Philadelphia, W.B. Saunders, 1990.
84. Nettrour, L.F., Krufty, L.E., Mueller, R.E., and Raycroft, J.F.: Locked Scapula: Intrathoracic Dislocation of the Inferior Angle. J. Bone Joint Surg., 54A:413–416, 1972.
85. Neviaser, J.: Traumatic Lesions: Injuries in and About Shoulder Joint. Instr. Course Lect., XIII:187–216, 1956.
86. Newell, E.D.: Review of Over 2,000 Fractures in the Seven Years. South. Med. J., 20:644–648, 1927.
86a. Niggebrugge, A.H., van Heusden, H.A., Bode, P.J., van Vugt, A.B.: Dislocated Intraarticular Fracture of Anterior Rim of Glenoid Treated by Open Reduction and Internal Fixation. Injury, 24(2):130–131, 1993.
87. Norris, T.: Fractures and Dislocations of the Glenohumeral Complex. *In* Chapman, M. (ed.): Operative Orthopedics, pp. 205–210. Philadelphia, J.B. Lippincott, 1984.
88. Norris, T.R.: Unfused Epiphysis Mistaken for Acromion Fracture. Orthop. Today, 3:12–13, 1983.
88a. Nordqvist, A., and Petersson, C. Fracture of the Body, Neck, or Spine of the Scapula. Clin. Orthop. Rel. Res., 283:139–144, 1992.
89. Nunley, R.L., and Bedini, S.J.: Paralysis of the Shoulder Subsequent to Comminuted Fracture of the Scapula: Rationale and Treatment Methods. Phys. Ther. Rev., 40:442–447, 1960.
90. Ogden, J.A., and Phillips, S.B.: Radiology of Postnatal Skeletal Development. Skeletal Radiol., 9:157–169, 1983.
90a. Oni, O.O.A., Hoskinson, J., and McPherson, S.: Closed Traumatic Scapulothoracic Dissociation. Injury, 23(2):138–139, 1992.
90b. Oni, O.O.A., and Hoskinson, J.: The 'Stove-in Shoulder:' Re-

sults of Treatment by Early Mobilization. Injury, 23:444–446, 1992.
91. Oreck, S.L., Burgess, A., and Levine, A.M.: Traumatic Lateral Displacement of the Scapula: A Radiologic Sign of Neurovascular Disruption. J. Bone Joint Surg., 66A:758–763.
92. Orthopedic Knowledge Update, 1985, Scapular Fractures.
93. Parsons, T.A.: The Snapping Scapula and Subscapularis Extosis. J. Bone Joint Surg., 55B:345–349, 1973.
94. Pate, D., Kursunoglu, S., Resnick, D., and Resnick, C.S.: Scapula Foramina. Skeletal Radiol., 14:270–275, 1985.
95. Pettersson, H.: Bilateral Dysplasia of the Neck of the Scapula and Associated Anomalies. Acta Radiol. [Diagn.] (Stockh.), 22:81–84, 1981.
96. Protiss, J.J., Stampfli, F.W., and Osmer, J.C.: Coracoid Process Fracture Diagnosis in Acromioclavicular Separation. Radiology, 116:61–64, 1975.
97. Ramin, J.E., and Veit, H.: Fracture of the Scapula During Electroshock Therapy. Am. J. Psychiatry, 110:153–154, 1953.
97a. Rao, J.P., and Femino, F.P.: Repair of a Glenoid Fracture Using a Powered Stapler. Orthop Rev., 21:1449–1452, 1992.
98. Rask, M.R., and Steinberg, L.H.: Fracture of the Acromion Caused by Muscle Forces. J. Bone Joint Surg., 60A:1146–1147, 1978.
99. Resnick, D., Walter, R.D., and Crudale, A.S.: Bilateral Dysplasia of the Scapular Neck. A.J.R., 139:387–390, 1982.
99a. Riggs, J.H., III, Schultz, G.D., and Hanes, S.A.: Radiation Induced Fracture of the Scapula. J. Manip. Physiol. Ther., 13:477–481, 1989.
99b. Robinson, C.M., and Court-Brown, C.M.: Nonunion of Scapula Spine Fracture Treated by Bone Graft and Plate Fixation. Injury, 24(6):428–429, 1993.
100. Rockwood, C.A.: Personal communication, 1989.
101. Rockwood, C.A.: Management of Fractures of the Scapula. Orthop. Trans., 10:219, 1986.
102. Rorabeck, C.H.: The Management of the Flail Upper Extremity in Brachial Plexus Injuries. J. Trauma, 20:491–493, 1980.
103. Rounds, R.C.: Isolated Fracture of the Coracoid Process. J. Bone Joint Surg., 31A:662–663, 1949.
104. Rowe, C.R.: Fractures of the Scapula. Surg. Clin. North 43:1565–1571, 1963.
105. Rowe, C.R.: The Bankart Procedure: A Study of Late Results (Proceedings). J. Bone Joint Surg., 59B:122, 1977.
106. Rowe, C.R.: The Shoulder, pp. 373–381. New York, Churchill Livingstone, 1987.
107. Rowe, C.R., Patel, D., and Southmayd, W.W.: The Bankart Procedure: A Long-Term End-Result Study. J. Bone Joint Surg., 60A:1–16, 1978.
108. Rubenstein, J.D., Abraheim, N.A., and Kellam, J.F.: Traumatic Scapulothoracic Dissociation. Radiology, 157:297–298, 1985.
109. Rush, L.V.: Fracture of the Coracoid Process of the Scapula. Ann. Surg., 90:1113–1114, 1929.
110. Ruther, H.: Therapy of Pseudoarthroses of the Scaphoid, Internal Malleollus, and Acromion. Z. Orthop., 79:485–499, 1950.
110a. Sampson, L.N., Britton, J.C., Eldrup-Jorgensen, J., Clark, D.E., Rosenburg, J.M., and Bredenberg, C.E.: The Neurovascular Outcome of Scapulothoracic Dissociation. J. Vasc. Surg., 17:1083–1088, 1993.
111. Sandrock, A.R.: Another Sports Fatigue Fracture: Stress Fracture of the Coracoid Process of the Scapula. Radiology, 117:274, 1975.
112. Scudder, C.L. (ed.): The Treatment of Fractures, 4th ed., pp. 201–212. Philadelphia, W.B. Saunders, 1904.
112a. Sinha, J., and Miller, A.J.: Fixation of Fractures of the Glenoid Rim. Injury, 23:418–419, 1992.
113. Smith, D.M.: Coracoid Fracture Associated With Sternioclavicular Dislocation: A Case Report. Clin. Orthop., 165–167, 1975.
114. Stein, R.E., Bono, J., Korn, J., and Wolff, W.I.: Axillary Artery Injury in Closed Fracture of the Neck of the Scapula: A Case Report. J. Trauma, 11:528–531, 1971.
115. Steindler, A.: Traumatic Deformities and Disabilities of the Upper Extremity, pp. 112–118. Springfield, Ill., Charles C Thomas, 1946.
116. Strizak, A.M., and Cowen, M.H.: The Snapping Scapula Syndrome. J. Bone Joint Surg., 64A:941–942, 1982.
117. Tachdjian, M.O.: Pediatric Orthopedics, pp. 1553–1555. Philadelphia, W.B. Saunders, 1972.
118. Tarquinio, T., Weinstein, M.E., and Virgilio, R.W.: Bilateral Scapular Fractures From Accidental Electric Shock. J. Trauma, 19:132–133, 1979.
119. Thompson, D.A., Flynn, T.C., Miller, P.W., and Fischer, R.P.: The Significance of Scapular Fractures. J. Trauma, 25:974–977, 1985.
119a. Van Wellen, P.A.J., Casteleyn, P.P., and Opdecam, P.: Traction-Suspension Therapy for Unstable Glenoid Neck Fracture. Injury, 23:57–58, 1992.
120. Varriale, P.L., and Adler, M.L.: Occult Fracture of the Glenoid Without Dislocation. J. Bone Joint Surg., 65A:688–689, 1983.
120a. Veluvolu, P., Kohn, H.S., Guten, G.N., et al.: Unusual Stress Fracture of the Scapula in a Jogger. Clin. Nucl. Med., 13:531–532, 1988.
120b. Wang, K.C., Hsu, K.Y., and Shih, C.H.: Coracoid Process Fracture Combined with Acromioclavicular Dislocation and Coracoclavicular Ligament Rupture. Clin. Orthop., 300:120–122, 1994.
120c. Ward, W.G., Bergfeld, J.A., and Carson, W.G.: Stress Fracture of the Base of the Acromial Process. Am. J. Sports Med., 22:146–147, 1994.
120d. Warner, J.J.P., and Port, J.: Stress Fracture of the Acromion. J. Shoulder Elbow Surg., 3:262–265, 1994.
121. Wilbur, M.C., and Evans, E.B.: Fractures of the Scapula: An Analysis of Forty Cases and Review of Literature. J. Bone Joint Surg., 59A:358–362, 1977.
121a. Wilkes, R.A., and Halawa, M.: Scapular and Clavicular Osteotomy for Malunion: Case Report. J. Trauma, 34:309, 1993.
121b. Williamson, D.M., and Wilson-MacDonald, J.: Bilateral Avulsion Fractures of the Cranial Margin of the Scapula. J. Trauma, 28:713–714, 1988.
121c. Wilson, K.M., and Colwill, J.C.: Combined Acromioclavicular Dislocation with Coracoclavicular Ligament Disruption and Coracoid Process Fracture. Am. J Sports Med., 17:697–698, 1989.
122. Wilson, P.D. (ed.): Experience in the Management of Fractures and Dislocations (Based on an Analysis of 4390 Cases) by Staff of the Fracture Service MGH, Boston. Philadelphia, J.B. Lippincott, 1938.
122a. Wirth, M.A., Lyons F.R, and Rockwood, C.A.: Hypoplasia of the Glenoid. J. Bone Joint Surg., 75A:1175–1183, 1993.
123. Wolfe, A.W., Shoji, H., and Chuinard, R.G.: Unusual Fracture of the Coracoid Process: Case Report and Review of the Literature. J. Bone Joint Surg., 58A:423–424, 1976.
123a. Wong-Chung, J., and Quinlan, W.: Fractured Coracoid Process Preventing Closed Reduction of Anterior Dislocation of the Shoulder. Injury, Case Report 296–297, September 1989.
124. Wong-Pack, W.K., Bobechko, P.E., and Becker, E.J.: Fractured Coracoid With Anterior Shoulder Dislocation. J. Can. Assoc. Radiol., 31:278–279, 1980.
125. Zdravkovic, D., and Damholt, V.V.: Comminuted and Severely Displaced Fractures of the Scapula. Acta Orthop. Scand., 45:60–65, 1974.
126. Zettas, J.P., and Muchnic, P.D.: Fracture of the Coracoid Process Base and Acute Acromioclavicular Separation. Comp. Rev., 5:77–79, 1976.
127. Zilberman, Z., and Rejovitzky, R.: Fracture of the Coracoid Process of the Scapula. Injury, 13:203–206, 1982.
128. Zuckerman, J.D., Koval, K.J., and Cuomo, F.: Fractures of the Scapula. Shoulder, 2:271–281, 1993.

INDEX

Page numbers followed by *f* indicate illustrations; page numbers followed by *t* indicate tabular material.

B

C

D

E

F

K

L

M

O

S

T

U

V

W

X

Y

Z